THE
5-MINUTE
VETERINARY
CONSULT
CANINE AND FELINE
SECOND EDITION

THE
5-MINUTE
VETERINARY
CONSULT

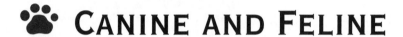

CANINE AND FELINE

SECOND EDITION

Larry Patrick Tilley, DVM
Diplomate, ACVIM (Internal Medicine)
President, Chief Medical Officer, VetMed Center
San Francisco, California
Director, Veterinary Specialty Referral Center
President, VET MED TELEMEDICINE Consultation Services
Santa Fe, New Mexico

Francis W. K. Smith, Jr., DVM
Diplomate, ACVIM (Internal Medicine & Cardiology)
Vice President, Editor-in-Chief, VetMedCenter
San Francisco, California
Clinical Assistant Professor, Department of Medicine
Tufts University, School of Veterinary Medicine
North Grafton, Massachusetts

LIPPINCOTT WILLIAMS & WILKINS
A **Wolters Kluwer** Company
Philadelphia • Baltimore • New York • London
Buenos Aires • Hong Kong • Sydney • Tokyo

Editor: Dan Limmer
Managing Editor: Matt Hauber
Marketing Manager: Anne Smith
Production Editor: Lisa JC Franko

Printed in the United States

First Edition, 1997

Library of Congress Cataloging-in-Publication Data

Tilley, Lawrence P.
  The 5-minute veterinary consult:canine and feline / Larry Patrick Tilley, Francis W.K. Smith.—2nd ed.
    p. cm.
  ISBN 0-683-30461-5
  1. Dogs—Diseases—Handbooks, manuals, etc. 2. Cats—Diseases—Handbooks, manuals, etc. I. Title: Five-minute veterinary consult. II. Smith, Francis W. K.
III. Title.
SF991 .T55 2000
636.7'0896—dc21   99-098181

The publishers have made every effort to trace the copyright holders for borrowed material. If they have inadvertently overlooked any, they will be pleased to make the necessary arrangements at the first opportunity.

To purchase additional copies of this book, call our customer service department at **(800) 638-3030** or fax orders to **(301) 824-7390.** For other book services, including chapter reprints and large quantity sales, ask for the Special Sales department.

For all other calls originating outside of the United States, please call **(301) 714-2324.**

Visit Lippincott Williams & Wilkins on the Internet: http://www.lww.com. Lippincott Williams & Wilkins customer service representatives are available from 8:30 am to 6:00 pm, EST, Monday through Friday, for telephone access.

00 01 02 03
1 2 3 4 5 6 7 8 9 10

To my ever-popular son, Ben, and his charming sister, Jade, thanks for the daily doses of joy. To my wife, May, thanks for your constant love and support.

Francis W. K. Smith, Jr.

To my wife Jeri and my son Kyle, in honor of that secret correspondence within our hearts; to family and animals, who represent the purity of life.

Larry Patrick Tilley

PREFACE

Keeping abreast of advances in veterinary internal medicine is extremely difficult, especially for the busy general practitioner. To keep current with all the veterinary journals while practicing medicine is impossible. The veterinarian in practice can be overwhelmed by all of the findings and conclusions of thousands of studies conducted by veterinary specialists. *The 5-Minute Veterinary Consult* is designed to provide the busy veterinary practitioner and student of veterinary medicine with concise practical reviews of almost all the diseases and clinical problems in dogs and cats. Our goal in creating this textbook was also to provide up-to-date information in an easy-to-use format. Emphasis is placed on diagnosis and treatment of problems and diseases likely to be seen by veterinarians.

Our fondest dream was realized when the first edition of this book was established as a comprehensive reference source for canine and feline medicine by veterinary students, practicing veterinarians, and boarded specialists. The format has proven easy to use and very popular with busy practitioners. We have made only minor changes in the format in the second edition. Some of the topic headings have been changed, and new ones have been added. The scope of the book and the number of consulting editors and authors have been expanded. We have also increased the number of authors from outside of North America, to provide the best advice in the world. The number of topics has been increased, and every topic has been updated to provide you with the most current information possible in a textbook. The Appendix has also been expanded to include more useful tables and the format of the Drug Formulary has been modified to make it even easier to use.

Several good veterinary internal medicine textbooks are available. The uniqueness and value of *The 5-Minute Veterinary Consult* as a quick reference is the consistency of presentation, the breadth of coverage, the contribution of large numbers of experts, and the timely preparation of the manuscript. The format of every clinical problem, laboratory abnormality, and disease is identical, making it easy to find information. An extensive list of topic headings ensures complete coverage of each topic.

The 5-Minute Veterinary Consult is divided into three basic sections: Presenting Problems and Physical Findings, Diagnostic Tests, and Diseases and Clinical Syndromes. These sections reflect the way one approaches a case. Veterinarians are first confronted with the chief complaints, signs, and abnormal physical findings. The first section deals with the diagnostic approach to these problems. Emphasis is placed on how to work up the case to determine the cause of the problem and how to provide symptomatic support while working toward a definitive diagnosis. After the veterinarian obtains the history and performs the physical examination, diagnostic tests are performed. The second section of the book is designed to assist the veterinarian in the diagnostic approach to laboratory test abnormalities and electrocardiograms. Diagnostic algorithms are used in these first two sections. The use of algorithms is not designed to encourage cookbook medicine, but rather to provide a logical framework for approaching a specific case. Once the database is complete, a definitive diagnosis is hopefully at hand. The final section covers the diseases likely to be encountered by veterinarians in practice. Common diseases are covered in a two-page, six-column format. Less common diseases are covered in a one-page, three-column format.

As the title implies, one objective of this book is to make information quickly available. To this end, we have organized topics alphabetically within sections. Most topics can be found without using the index. A table of contents broken out by section and by organ system and a detailed index are provided. Large volumes of useful information are summarized in charts in the Appendix. Included in the Appendix are an extensive and detailed Drug Formulary, toxicology tables, endocrine testing protocols, normal laboratory values, and conversion tables.

We are delighted and privileged to have had the assistance of numerous experts in veterinary internal medicine from around the world. For the second edition, we expanded the number of consulting editors and contributors. More than 300 veterinary specialists contributed to this text, allowing each chapter to be written by an expert on the subject. In addition to providing outstanding information, this large pool of experts allowed us to publish this major text in a timely manner.

Many large textbooks take several years to write, making some of the information outdated by the time the book is published. We are indebted to the many contributors and consulting editors, whose hard work allowed us to write, edit, and publish this work in 2 years, with most chapters completed within a year of publication. Our goal is to revise the text every 2 years, so that the contents will always be current.

We have also produced a CD-ROM disk to accompany this textbook. This medium combines text, sound, and graphics, in an interactive format. Now veterinarians can quickly access information about necessary clinical skills and new developments in diagnosis and treatment on their computer. Our *5-Minute Veterinary Consult* CD-ROM offers fast, affordable access to much of the accumulated wisdom in veterinary medicine by use of a simple search and retrieval process. This multimedia computer technology brings to the clinic examination room and doctor's office an-easy-to use "dynamic textbook" that will markedly improve the quality of continuing education and clinical practice.

The second edition of this textbook constitutes an important up-to-date medical reference source for your practice and clinical education. We strived to make it complete, yet practical and easy to use. Our dreams are realized if this text helps you to quickly locate and use the "momentarily important" information that is essential to the practice of high-quality veterinary medicine. We would appreciate your input, so that we can make future editions even more useful. If you would like to see any changes in content or format, additions, or deletions, please let us know. Send comments to the following:

Drs. Larry Tilley and Frank Smith
c/o Lippincott Williams & Wilkins
351 West Camden Street
Baltimore, MD 21201

ACKNOWLEDGMENTS

The completion of this textbook provides a welcome opportunity to recognize in writing the many individuals who have helped along the way. The Editors gratefully acknowledge the Consulting Editors and the contributors who, by their expertise, have so unmistakably enhanced the quality of this textbook.

Special gratitude goes to Christine MacMurray of VetMedCenter for her editorial supervision of the manuscript and her masterful precision and clarity. We would also like to acknowledge and thank our families for their support of this project and the sacrifices they made to allow us the time to complete this book.

In addition to thanking veterinarians who have referred patients to us, we would like to express our gratitude to each of the veterinary students, interns, and residents who we have had the privilege of teaching. Their curiosity and intellectual stimulation have enabled us to grow and have prompted us to undertake the task of writing this book.

Finally, a special thank you goes to all of the staff at Lippincott Williams & Wilkins and everyone in the Production and Editing departments. The Marketing and Sales departments must be acknowledged for generating such an interest in this book. They are all meticulous workers and kind people who have made the final stages of preparing this book both inspiring and fun. An important life goal of ours has been fulfilled: to provide expertise in small animal internal medicine worldwide and to teach the principles contained in this textbook to veterinarians and students everywhere.

CONSULTING EDITORS

LARRY G. ADAMS, DVM, PhD
Diplomate, ACVIM (Internal Medicine)
Purdue University School of Veterinary Medicine
West Lafayette, Indiana
Subject: Renal/Urologic

STEPHEN C. BARR, DVM
Diplomate, ACVIM (Internal Medicine)
Cornell University
New York State College of Veterinary Medicine
Ithaca, New York
Subject: Infectious Diseases

JAN BELLOWS, DVM
Diplomate, ABVP
Diplomate, AVDC
All Pets Dental Clinic
Weston, Florida
Subject: Dentistry

SHARON A. CENTER, DVM
Diplomate, ACVIM (Internal Medicine)
New York State College of Veterinary Medicine
Cornell University
Ithaca, New York
Subject: Hepatobiliary

SUSAN M. COTTER, DVM
Diplomate, ACVIM (Internal Medicine/Oncology)
Tufts University School of Veterinary Medicine
North Grafton, Massachusetts
Subject: Hematology/Immunology

MITCHELL A. CRYSTAL, DVM
Diplomate, ACVIM (Internal Medicine)
North Florida Veterinary Referral Center
Orange Park, Florida
Subject: Gastroenterology

BRETT M. FEDER, DVM
Diplomate, ACVIM (Internal Medicine)
Director, South Carolina Veterinary Internal Medicine
Columbia, South Carolina
Subject: Gastroenterology

DEBORAH S. GRECO, DVM
Diplomate, ACVIM (Internal Medicine)
Colorado State University
College of Veterinary Medicine
Veterinary Teaching Hospital
Fort Collins, Colorado
Subject: Endocrinology

ELEANOR C. HAWKINS, DVM
Diplomate, ACVIM (Internal Medicine)
North Carolina State University
College of Veterinary Medicine
Raleigh, North Carolina
Subject: Respiratory

SARA K. LYLE, DVM, MS
Diplomate, ACT
North Carolina State University
College of Veterinary Medicine
Raleigh, North Carolina
Subject: Theriogenology

PAUL E. MILLER, DVM
Diplomate, ACVO
School of Veterinary Medicine
University of Wisconsin-Madison
Madison, Wisconsin
Subject: Opthalmology

WALLACE B. MORRISON, DVM, MS
Diplomate, ACVIM (Internal Medicine)
Purdue University School of Veterinary Medicine
Veterinary Teaching Hospital
West Lafayette, Indiana
Subject: Oncology

CARL A. OSBORNE, DVM, PhD
Diplomate, ACVIM (Internal Medicine)
University of Minnesota
College of Veterinary Medicine
St. Paul, Minnesota
Subject: Renal/Urologic

GARY D. OSWEILER, DVM, PhD
Diplomate, ABVT
Director, Veterinary Diagnostic Laboratory
Iowa State University
College of Veterinary Medicine
Ames, Iowa
Subject: Toxicology

MARK PAPICH, DVM, MS
Diplomate, ACVCP
College of Veterinary Medicine
North Carolina State University
Raleigh, North Carolina
Subject: Drug Formulary

JOANE M. PARENT, DVM, MVSc
Diplomate, ACVIM (Neurology)
Ontario Veterinary College
Guelph, Ontario, Canada
Subject: Neurology

KAREN HELTON RHODES, DVM
Diplomate, ACVD
Dermatology Consultations
Goshen, New York
Subject: Dermatology

PETER D. SCHWARZ, DVM
Diplomate, ACVS
Veterinary Surgical Specialists of New Mexico, PC
Albuquerque, New Mexico
Subject: Musculoskeletal

FRANCIS W. K. SMITH, JR., DVM
Diplomate, ACVIM (Internal Medicine & Cardiology)
Vice President, Editor-in-Chief, VetMedCenter.com
San Francisco, California
Clinical Assistant Professor
Department of Medicine
Tufts University
School of Veterinary Medicine
North Grafton, Massachusetts

LARRY P. TILLEY, DVM
Diplomate, ACVIM (Internal Medicine)
President, Chief Medical Officer, VetMed Center
San Francisco, California
Director, Veterinary Specialty Referral Center
President, VET MED TELEMEDICINE Consultation Services,
Santa Fe, New Mexico

CONTRIBUTORS

JONATHAN A. ABBOTT, DVM
Diplomate, ACVIM (Cardiology)
Associate Professor
Department of Small Animal Clinical
Sciences
Virginia-Maryland Regional College of
Veterinary Medicine
Virginia Tech
Blacksburg, Virginia

LARRY G. ADAMS, DVM, PHD
Diplomate, ACVIM (Internal Medicine)
Associate Professor of Small Animal
Internal Medicine
Department of Veterinary Clinical
Sciences
Purdue University School of Veterinary
Medicine
West Lafayette, Indiana

ALBERT H. AHN, DVM
Clinician, Clinical Faculty, Tufts
University School of Veterinary Medicine
Manager, Veterinary Affairs
Hill's Pet Nutrition, Inc.
North Grafton, Massachusetts

RENEE AL-SARRAF, DVM
Diplomate, ACVIM (Oncology)
Veterinary Oncologist
Department of Oncology
Veterinary Referral Center
Little Falls, New Jersey

JAMES M. G. ANTHONY, BSc (AGR.), DVM,
MRCVS, FAVD
Diplomate, AVDC, EVDC
Private Dental Practice, Research
Pacific Dental Services for Animals
Vancouver, British Columbia, Canada

MAX J. G. APPEL, DVM, PHD
Professor Emeritus
Professor of Microbiology
Baker Institute
College of Veterinary Medicine
Cornell University
Ithaca, New York

LOUIS F. ARCHBALD, DVM, PhD
Diplomate, ACT
Professor
Department of Large Animal Clinical
Sciences
College of Veterinary Medicine
University of Florida
Gainesville, Florida

RODNEY S. BAGLEY, DVM
Diplomate, ACVIM (Neurology & Internal
Medicine)
Associate Professor
Department of Clinical Sciences
College of Veterinary Medicine
Washington State University
Pullman, Washington

E. MURL BAILEY, DVM, PhD
Diplomate, ABVT
Professor
Department of Veterinary Physiology and
Pharmacology
College of Veterinary Medicine
Texas A & M University
College Station, Texas

CLETA SUE BAILEY, DVM, PhD
Diplomate, ACVIM (Neurology)
Professor
Surgical and Radiological Sciences
University of California at Davis
School of Veterinary Medicine
Davis, California

LARRY BAKER, DVM, FAVD
Northgate Pet Clinic & Veterinary
Dentistry
Decatur, Illinois

STEPHEN C. BARR, BVSc, MVS, PhD
Diplomate, ACVIM (Internal Medicine)
Associate Professor of Medicine
Department of Clinical Sciences
College of Veterinary Medicine
Cornell University
Ithaca, New York

MARGARET C. BARR, DVM, PhD
Senior Scientist
Immune Complex Corporation
San Diego, California

JOSEPH W. BARTGES, DVM, PhD
Diplomate, ACVIM (Internal Medicine),
ACVN
Associate Professor, Internist, and
Nutritionist
Department of Small Animal Clinical
Sciences
College of Veterinary Medicine
University of Tennessee
Knoxville, Tennessee

BRIAN S. BEALE, DVM
Gulf Coast Veterinary Specialists, P.C.
Houston, Texas

KARIN M. BEALE, DVM
Diplomate, ACVD
Staff Dermatologist
Gulf Coast Veterinary Specialists
Houston, Texas

ANDREW W. BEARDOW, BVM&S, MRCVS
Diplomate, ACVIM (Cardiology)
Vice-President, Cardiopet, Inc.
President, Veterinary Referral Centre
Cardiopet, Inc.
Little Falls, New Jersey

ELLEN N. BEHREND, VMD, MS
Diplomate, ACVIM (Internal Medicine)
Assistant Professor
Department of SA Surgery and Medicine
Auburn University College of Veterinary
Medicine
Auburn, Alabama

JAMIE R. BELLAH, DVM
Diplomate, ACVS
Adjunct Professor, University of Florida
Staff Surgeon
Affiliated Veterinary Specialists—Orange
Park
Orange Park, Florida

JAN BELLOWS, DVM
Diplomate, ABVP, AVDC
Hometown Animal Hospital
Weston, Florida

MARC G. BERCOVITCH, DVM
Diplomate, ACVIM (Internal Medicine)
VCA—Veterinary Referral Associates
Gaithersburg, Maryland

CHRISTINE F. BERTHELIN-BAKER, DVM,
MRCVS
Diplomate, ACVIM (Neurology)
European College of Veterinary
Neurology,
Clinical Veterinary Neurologist
Neuropathology Unit
Veterinary Laboratories Agency
Weybridge, Addlestone, United Kingdom

NICHOLE BIRNBAUM, DVM
Diplomate, ACVIM (Internal Medicine)
Manassas, Virginia

JOHN D. BONAGURA, DVM, MS
Diplomate, ACVIM (Cardiology & Internal
Medicine)
Gilbreath-McLorn Professor of
Veterinary Cardiology
Department of Veterinary Medicine and
Surgery
College of Veterinary Medicine
University of Missouri
Columbia, Missouri

G. DANIEL BOON, DVM, MS
Diplomate, ACVP
Director of Laboratory Services
Virginia-Maryland Regional College of
Veterinary Medicine
Blacksburg, Virginia

MARIBETH J. BOSSBALY, VMD
Diplomate, ACVIM (Cardiology)
Cardiologist, Heartsound Consultants
Langhorn, Pennsylvania

RANDI BRANNAN, DVM
Fellow, Academy of Veterinary
Dentistry
Portland, Oregon

JANICE MCINTOSH BRIGHT, BSN, MS, DVM
Diplomate, ACVIM (Cardiology & Internal
Medicine)
CVMBS-VTH
Colorado State University
Fort Collins, Colorado

SCOTT A. BROWN, VMD, PhD
Diplomate, ACVIM (Internal Medicine)
Professor
Department of Small Animal Medicine
and Physiology
College of Veterinary Medicine
University of Georgia
Athens, Georgia

DONALD J. BROWN, BS, MSE, DVM, PhD
Diplomate, ACVIM (Cardiology)
Assistant Professor
Department of Clinical Sciences
School of Veterinary Medicine
Tufts University
North Grafton, Massachusetts

JÖRG BÜCHELER, DVM, PhD
Diplomate, ACVIM (Internal Medicine),
ECVIM-CA
Ross University School of Veterinary
Medicine
St. Kitts, West Indies

C. A. TONY BUFFINGTON, DVM, PhD
Diplomate, ACVN
Professor
Department of Clinical Sciences
College of Veterinary Medicine
Ohio State University
Columbus, Ohio

SUSAN E. BUNCH, DVM, PhD
Diplomate, ACVIM (Internal Medicine)
Professor of Medicine
Department of Clinical Sciences
North Carolina State University
College of Veterinary Medicine
Raleigh, North Carolina

COLIN F. BURROWS, BVetMed, PhD,
MRCVS
Diplomate, ACVIM (Internal Medicine)
Professor and Chair
Department of Small Animal Clinical
Sciences
College of Veterinary Medicine
University of Florida
Gainesville, Florida

NAOMI L. BURTNICK, MT (ASCP)
Chief Medical Officer
Southwest Veterinary Specialty Referral
Center
Ultrasound Consultant, VetMedCenter,
Telemedicine
Santa Fe, New Mexico

CATHRYN M. CALIA, DVM
Diplomate, ACVIM (Internal Medicine)
Staff Internist
Department of Internal Medicine
Veterinary Referral Centre
Little Falls, New Jersey

CLAY A. CALVERT, BS, DVM
Diplomate, ACVIM (Internal Medicine)
Professor
Department of Small Animal Medicine
and Surgery
College of Veterinary Medicine
University of Georgia
Athens, Georgia

KAREN CAMPBELL, DVM, MS
Diplomate, ACVIM (Internal Medicine),
Diplomate, ACVD
Department of Veterinary Clinical
Medicine
University of Illinois School of Veterinary
Medicine
Urbana, Illinois

LELAND CARMICHAEL, DVM, PHD
Diplomate, ACVM
John M. Olin Professor of Virology,
Emeritus
Department of Clinical Sciences
College of Veterinary Medicine
Cornell University
Ithaca, New York

LARRY CARPENTER, DVM, MS
Diplomate, ACVS
Surgeon
Department of Defense Military Working
Dog
Veterinary Services
Lackland Air Force Base
San Antonio, Texas

THOMAS L. CARSON, DVM, MS, PHD
Diplomate, ABVT
Toxicologist
Veterinary Diagnostic Laboratory
Iowa State University
College of Veterinary Medicine
Ames, Iowa

SHARON A. CENTER, DVM
Diplomate, ACVIM (Internal Medicine)
Professor of Medicine
Department of Veterinary Clinical
Sciences
College of Veterinary Medicine
Cornell University
Ithaca, New York

ERIN S. CHAMPAGNE, DVM
Diplomate, ACVO
Clinical Assistant Professor of
Ophthalmology
University of Missouri
Columbia, Missouri

DENNIS J. CHEW, DVM
Diplomate, ACVIM (Internal Medicine)
College of Veterinary Medicine
The Ohio State University
Columbus, Ohio

GEORGINA CHILD, BVSc
Diplomate, ACVIM (Neurology)
Neurology Specialty Practice
North Ryde, New South Wales, Australia

MARY M. CHRISTOPHER, DVM, PhD
Diplomate, ACVP (Clinical Pathology)
Department of Pathology, Microbiology,
and Immunology
University of California School of
Veterinary Medicine
Davis, California

RUTHANNE CHUN, DVM
Diplomate, ACVIM (Oncology)
Assistant Professor
Department of Clinical Sciences
School of Veterinary Medicine
Kansas State University
Manhattan, Kansas

SUSAN M. COCHRANE, DVM, DVSc
Diplomate, ACVIM (Neurology)
Specialty Practice
Morningside Animal Clinic
Scarborough, Ontario

ELLEN C. CODNER, BS, DVM, MS
Diplomate, ACVIM (Internal Medicine),
ACVD—Board Qualified
Animal Dermatology Clinic
Martinez, California

STEPHEN COLES, BVSc, MACVSC
Diplomate, AVDC
Melbourne, Victoria, Australia

B. KEITH COLLINS, DVM, MS
Diplomate, ACVO
Animal Eye Specialists
Waukesha, Wisconsin

JAMES L. COOK, DVM, PhD
Diplomate, ACVS
Assistant Professor, Small Animal
Orthopedics
Assistant Professor, Orthopedic Surgery
Director, Comparative Orthopedic
Laboratory
University of Missouri
Columbia, Missouri

ANGELYN M. CORNETTA, DVM
Diplomate, ACVIM (Internal Medicine)
Intern Director
VCA South Shore Animal Hospital
South Weymouth, Massachusetts

ROBERT M. CORWIN, DVM, PhD
Professor
Department of Veterinary Pathobiology
College of Veterinary Medicine
University of Missouri
Columbia, Missouri

SUSAN M. COTTER, DVM
Diplomate, ACVIM (Internal Medicine/Oncology)
Distinguished Professor of Medicine
Section Head of Small Animal Medicine
Department of Clinical Sciences
Tufts University School of Veterinary Medicine
North Grafton, Massachusetts

LAINE COWAN, DVM, MS
Diplomate, ACVIM (Internal Medicine)
Associate Professor
Department of Veterinary Clinical Sciences
College of Veterinary Medicine
Kansas State University
Manhattan, Kansas

LARRY D. COWGILL, DVM, PHD
Diplomate, ACVIM (Internal Medicine)
Professor, Department of Medicine and Epidemiology
Director, Companion Animal Hemodialysis Unit of the Veterinary Medical Teaching Hospital
School of Veterinary Medicine
University of California—Davis
Davis, California

MITCHELL A. CRYSTAL, DVM
Diplomate, ACVIM (Internal Medicine)
Chief of Medicine
North Florida Veterinary Specialists, P.A.
Orange Park, Florida

PAUL A. CUDDON, BVSc
Diplomate, ACVIM (Neurology)
Associate Professor
Department of Clinical Sciences
College of Veterinary Medicine
Colorado State University
Fort Collins, Colorado

ELIZABETH A. CURRY-GALVIN, DVM
Assistant Director, Scientific Activities
American Veterinary Medical Association
Schaumburg, Illinois

GEORGE H. D'ANDREA, BS, DVM, MS
Diplomate, ACVP
Diagnostic Specialist
Department of Pathology/Toxicology
CSR-Veterinary Diagnostic Laboratory
Auburn, Alabama

TANIA N. DAVEY, BSC, BVMS, MACVSC
Associate Clinician
West Chermside Veterinary Clinic and Specialist Referral Service
Brisbane, Australia

THOMAS KEVIN DAY, DVM, MS
Diplomate, ACVA, ACVECC
Emergency & Critical Care Veterinarian
Louisville Veterinary Specialty and Emergency Services
Louisville, Kentucky

HELIO AUTRAN DE MORAIS, DVM, MS, PhD
Diplomate, ACVIM (Internal Medicine & Cardiology)
Associate Professor, Departamento de Clinicas Veterinarias
Departmento de Clinicas Veterinarias
Universidade Estadual de Londrina
Londrina, Parana, Brazil

LINDA J. DEBOWES, DVM, MS
Diplomate, ACVIM (Internal Medicine), AVDC
Associate Professor
Department of Clinical Sciences
Veterinary Medical Teaching Hospital
Kansas State University
Manhattan, Kansas

TERESA C. DEFRANCESCO, DVM
Diplomate, ACVIM (Cardiology)
Clinical Assistant Professor
Department of Clinical Sciences
North Carolina State University College of Veterinary Medicine
Raleigh, North Carolina

ROBERT C. DENOVO, DVM, MS
Diplomate, ACVIM (Internal Medicine)
Associate Professor of Medicine
Department of Small Animal Clinical Science
College of Veterinary Medicine
University of Tennessee
Knoxville, Tennessee

NISHI DHUPA, BVM, MRCVS
Diplomate, ACVIM (Internal Medicine), ACVECC
Angell Memorial Animal Hospital
Boston, Massachusetts

SHARON M. DIAL, DVM, PhD
Director
Animal Diagnostic Laboratory
Tucson, Arizona

STEPHEN P. DIBARTOLA, DVM
Diplomate, ACVIM (Internal Medicine)
Professor
Veterinary Clinical Sciences
College of Veterinary Medicine
Ohio State University
Columbus, Ohio

KELLY J. DIEHL, DVM, MS
Diplomate, ACVIM (Internal Medicine)
Staff Veterinarian
Internal Medicine Section
Veterinary Referral Center of Colorado
Englewood, Colorado

BRADFORD C. DIXON, DVM, MS
Diplomate, ACVS
Staff Surgeon
Southwest Veterinary Surgical Service
Phoenix, Arizona

DAVID CHRISTOPHER DORMAN, DVM, PhD
Diplomate, ABVT
Chemical Industry Institute of Toxicology
Research Triangle Park, North Carolina

SUE DOWNING, DVM
Candidate, ACVIM (Internal Medicine)
Veterinary Cancer Referral Group
Los Angeles, California

DAVID DUCLOS, DVM
Diplomate, ACVD
Private Practitioner
Animal Skin and Allergy Clinic
Lynnwood, Washington

DEREK S. DUVAL, BA, VMD
Diplomate, ACVIM (Internal Medicine)
Associate Veterinarian
Veterinary Specialty Services
St. Louis, Missouri

DAVID F. EDWARDS, DVM
Diplomate, ACVIM (Internal Medicine), ACVP (Clinical Pathology)
Professor
Department of Pathology
University of Tennessee
Knoxville, Tennessee

ERICK EGGER
Diplomate, ACVS
Colorado State University
College of Veterinary Medicine
Fort Collins, Colorado

BRUCE E. EILTS, DVM, MS
Diplomate, ACT
Professor
Department of Veterinary Clinical Sciences
Louisana State University
School of Veterinary Medicine
Baton Rouge, Lousiana

MARC ELIE, BS, DVM
Diplomate, ACVIM (Internal Medicine)
Staff Internist
Department of Medicine
Veterinary Referral Centre
Little Falls, New Jersey

ROBYN ELMSLIE, DVM
Diplomate, ACVIM (Oncology)
Veterinary Cancer Specialists
Englewood, Colorado

RICHARD A. FAYRER-HOSKEN, BVSC, PHD, MRCVS
Diplomate, ACT
Professor
Department of Large Animal Medicine
University of Georgia
College of Veterinary Medicine
Athens, Georgia

BRETT M. FEDER, BS, DVM
Diplomate, ACVIM (Internal Medicine)
Director
South Carolina Veterinary Internal Medicine
Columbia, South Carolina

LINDA S. FINEMAN, DVM
Diplomate, ACVIM (Oncology)
Veterinary Tumor Institute
Santa Cruz, California

SCOTT D. FITZGERALD, DVM
Diplomate, ACVP
Associate Professor
Department of Pathology and Animal Health Diagnostic Lab
Michigan State University
Lansing, Michigan

SHANNON FLOOD, DVM
Diplomate, ACVIM (Internal Medicine)
Department of Clinical Sciences
School of Veterinary Medicine
Cornell University
Ithaca, New York

CAROL S. FOIL, DVM, MS
Diplomate, ACVD
Professor of Dermatology
Department of Veterinary Clinical
Sciences
Louisiana State University
School of Veterinary Medicine
Baton Rouge, Louisiana

SHARON K. FOOSHEE, MS, DVM
Diplomate, ACVIM (Internal Medicine),
ABVP
Lecturer, Academic Program
Mississippi State University
College of Veterinary Medicine
Mississippi State, Mississippi

S. DRU FORRESTER, DVM, MS
Diplomate, ACVIM (Internal Medicine)
Associate Professor
Department of Small Animal Clinical
Sciences
Virginia-Maryland Regional College of
Veterinary Medicine
Blacksburg, Virginia

THERESA W. FOSSUM, DVM, PhD
Diplomate, ACVS
Professor and Chief of Surgery
Department of Small Animal Medicine
and Surgery
Texas A & M University
College of Veterinary Medicine
College Station, Texas

GREGORY O. FREDEN, BS, DVM
Diplomate, ACVP
Director of Operations
Charles River Pharmaceutical Services
Southbridge, Massachusetts

JONI L. FRESHMAN, DVM, MS
Diplomate, ACVIM (Internal Medicine)
East Springs Animal Hospital
Colorado Springs, Colorado

VIRGINIA LUIS FUENTES, MA, VetMB, Cert
VR, DVC, MRCVS
RCVS Specialist in Veterinary Cardiology
Assistant Professor
Department of Veterinary Medicine and
Surgery
College of Veterinary Medicine
University of Missouri—Columbia
Columbia, Missouri

TOM GARLAND, DVM
Texas A & M University
College of Veterinary Medicine
College Station, Texas

BRIAN C. GILGER, DVM, MS
Diplomate, ACVO
Associate Professor
Department of Clinical Sciences
North Carolina State University College
of Veterinary Medicine
Raleigh, North Carolina

JOHN-KARL GOODWIN, DVM
Diplomate, ACVIM (Cardiology)
Director, Staff Cardiologist
Veterinary Heart Institute
Gainesville, Florida

JOHN G. GORDON, DVM
Diplomate, ACVD
Private Practice
MedVet Associates, Inc.
Columbus, Ohio

CECILIA GORREL, BSc, Vet MB, DDS, Hon
FAVD, MRCVS
Diplomate, EUCD
Dentist, Oral Pathologist & Veterinary
Surgeon
Pilley, Nr Lymington, Hants,
United Kingdom

JOANNE C. GRAHAM, DVM, MS
Diplomate, ACVIM (Internal Medicine)
Animal Medical Referral Center
Franklin Park Animal Hospital
Franklin Park, Illinois

W. DUNBAR GRAM, DVM
Diplomate, ACVD
Animal Allergy and Dermatology
Virginia Beach, Virginia

GREGORY F. GRAUER, DVM, MS
Diplomate, ACVIM (Internal Medicine)
Professor and Section Chief of Small
Animal Medicine
Department of Clinical Sciences
Colorado State University
College of Veterinary Medicine and
Biomedical Sciences
Fort Collins, Colorado

THOMAS K. GRAVES, DVM
Diplomate, ACVIM (Internal Medicine)
Department of Pharmacology and
Physiology
University of Rochester
School of Medicine and Dentistry
Rochester, New York

DEBORAH SUSAN GRECO, DVM, PhD
Diplomate, ACVIM (Internal Medicine)
Associate Professor
Department of Clinical Sciences
Colorado State University
College of Veterinary Medicine
Fort Collins, Colorado

JEAN SWINGLE GREEK, DVM
Diplomate, ACVD
Veterinary Specialists
Overland Park, Kansas

AMY M. GROOTERS, DVM
Diplomate, ACVIM (Internal Medicine)
Assistant Professor and Service Chief
Department of Companion Animal
Medicine
Louisana State University Veterinary
Clinical Sciences
Baton Rouge, Louisiana

NITA KAY GULBAS, DVM
Phoenix, Arizona

TIM HACKETT, DVM, MS
Diplomate, ACVECC
Assistant Professor, Emergency and
Critical Care Medicine
Department of Clinical Sciences
Colorado State University
College of Veterinary Medicine
Fort Collins, Colorado

DEBORAH J. HADLOCK, BS, VMD
Diplomate, ABVP
Staff Consultant
Department of Cardiology
Cardiopet, Inc
Bayville, New York

KEVIN A. HAHN, DVM, PhD
Gulf Coast Veterinary Oncology
Houston, Texas

JEFFERY O. HALL, DVM, PhD
Diplomate, ABVT
Assistant Professor, Diagnosic
Veterinary Toxicologist
Department of Animal, Dairy and
Veterinary Sciences
Utah State University
Logan, Utah

TERRANCE A. HAMILTON, DVM
Diplomate, ACVIM (Oncology)
Staff Oncologist
Veterinary Referral Clinic
Cleveland, Ohio

ROBERT L. HAMLIN, DVM, PhD
Diplomate, ACVIM (Cardiology, Internal
Medicine)
Professor
Department of Veterinary Biosciences,
Exercise Physiology and Biomedical
Engineering
The Ohio State University
College of Veterinary Medicine
Columbus, Ohio

STEVEN R. HANSEN, DVM, MS
Diplomate, ABVT
Vice President
ASPCA/National Animal Poison Control
Center
Urbana, Illinois

ROBERT HARDY, DVM, MS
Diplomate, ACVIM (Internal Medicine)
Professor
Department of Small Animal Clinical
Sciences
College of Veterinary Medicine
University of Minnesota
St. Paul, Minnesota

NEIL K. HARPSTER, DVM
Diplomate, ACVIM (Cardiology)
Department of Cardiology
Angell Memorial Hospital
Boston, Massachusetts

DANIEL P. HARRINGTON, DVM
Diplomate, ACVP
Veterinary Medical Referral Service
Riverwoods, Illinois

JOHN HART, JR., QDVM
Diplomate, ACVIM (Internal Medicine)
Staff Internist
Veterinary Specialty Hospital of San
Diego
Rancho Santa Fe, California

JOHN W. HARVEY, DVM, PhD
Diplomate, ACVP
Department of Physiological Sciences
University of Florida
College of Veterinary Medicine
Gainesville, Florida

ELEANOR C. HAWKINS, DVM
Diplomate, ACVIM (Internal Medicine)
Associate Professor of Internal Medicine
Department of Companion Animal &
Special Species Medicine
North Carolina State University
College of Veterinary Medicine
Raleigh, North Carolina

KAREN HELTON RHODES, DVM
Diplomate, ACVD
Dermatology Consultations
Dermatology Consultations
Goshen, New York

JOAN C. HENDRICKS, VMD, PhD
Diplomate, ACVIM (Internal Medicine)
Professor
Department of Clinical Sciences
University of Pennsylvania
School of Veterinary Medicine
Philadelphia, Pennsylvania

ROSEMARY A. HENIK, DVM, MS
Diplomate, ACVIM (Internal Medicine)
Clinical Associate Professor
Department of Medical Sciences
University of Wisconsin
School of Veterinary Medicine
Madison, Wisconsin

LORA STAHL HITCHCOCK, DVM
Diplomate, ACVIM (Cardiology)
Clinical Instructor, Cardiology
Department of Veterinary Medicine and
Surgery
University of Missouri
College of Veterinary Medicine
Columbia, Missouri

MARK E. HITT, DVM, MS
Diplomate, ACVIM (Internal Medicine)
Atlantic Veterinary Internal Medicine of
Annapolis and Greater Baltimore
Annapolis, Maryland

KEITH HNILICA, DVM
Diplomate, ACVD
Assistant Professor Veterinary
Dermatology
Department of Small Animal Medicine
College of Veterinary Medicine
University of Georgia
Athens, Georgia

WALTER E. HOFFMANN, DVM, PhD
Veterinary Pathobiology
University of Illinois
College of Veterinary Medicine
Urbana, Illinois

HARM HOGENESCH, DVM, PhD
Diplomate, ACVP
Associate Professor
Department of Veterinary Pathobiology
School of Veterinary Medicine
Purdue University
West Lafayette, Indiana

JUDY HOLDING, RN, DVM, BS
Veterinary Poison Information Specialist
ASPCA—National Animal Poison Control
Center
Urbana, Illinois

MOLLYANN HOLLAND, DVM
Diplomate, ACVIM (Internal Medicine)
Oklahoma City, Oklahoma

WILLIAM E. HORNBUCKLE, DVM
Diplomate, ACVIM (Internal Medicine)
Professor of Medicine
Department of Clinical Sciences
College of Veterinary Medicine
Cornell University
Ithaca, New York

JOHNNY D. HOSKINS, DVM, PHD
Diplomate, ACVIM (Internal Medicine)
Professor Emeritus
Department of Clinical Sciences
School of Veterinary Medicine
Louisiana State University
Baton Rouge, Louisiana

KATHERINE A. HOUPT, VMD, PhD
Diplomate, ACVB
Professor of Physiology
Department of Physiology
College of Veterinary Medicine
Cornell University
Ithaca, New York

KAREN DYER INZANA, DVM, PhD
Diplomate, ACVIM (Neurology)
Associate Professor
Department of Small Animal Clinical
Sciences
Virginia-Maryland Regional College of
Veterinary Medicine
Virginia Polytechnic Institute and State
University
Blacksburg, Virginia

FREDERIC JACOB, DVM
Resident in Nutrition and Internal
Medicine
Department of Small Animal Clinical
Sciences
University of Minnesota
College of Veterinary Medicine
St. Paul, Minnesota

CHRISTINE CAROLYN JENKINS, DVM
Diplomate, ACVIM (Internal Medicine)
Technical Services Veterinarian, CAD
Technical Services—Pfizer Adjunct
Associate Professor of Veterinary
Medicine, Department of Small
Animal Clinical Sciences
University of Tennessee
Companion Animal Division
Pfizer Animal Health
Exton, Pennsylvania

ALBERT E. JERGENS, DVM, MS
Diplomate, ACVIM (Internal Medicine)
Associate Professor
Department of Veterinary Clinical
Sciences
Iowa State University
College of Veterinary Medicine
Ames, Iowa

KENNETH A. JOHNSON, MVSc, PhD,
FACVSc
Diplomate, ACVS, ECVS
Professor of Orthopaedics
Department of Veterinary Clinical
Science
The Ohio State University
Columbus, Ohio

SUSAN E. JOHNSON, DVM, MS
Diplomate, ACVIM (Internal Medicine)
Associate Professor
Department of Veterinary Clinical
Sciences
The Ohio State University
Columbus, Ohio

LYNELLE R. JOHNSON, DVM, PhD
Diplomate, ACVIM (Internal Medicine)
Research Assistant Professor
Department of Veterinary Biomedical
Sciences
University of Missouri College of
Veterinary Medicine
Columbia, Missouri

SHIRLEY D. JOHNSTON, DVM, PhD
Diplomate, ACT
Dean, College of Veterinary Medicine
College of Veterinary Medicine, Western
University of Health Sciences
Pomona, California

RICHARD J. JOSEPH, DVM
Diplomate, ACVIM (Neurology)
Staff Neurologist/Acupuncturist
Department of Medicine
The Animal Medical Center
New York, New York

BRUCE W. KEENE, DVM, MS
Diplomate, ACVIM (Cardiology)
Associate Professor of Cardiology
College of Veterinary Medicine
North Carolina State University
Raleigh, North Carolina

ROBERT J. KEMPPAINEN, DVM, PhD
Professor
Department of Anatomy, Physiology and
Pharmacology
Auburn University
College of Veterinary Medicine
Auburn, Alabama

MARGARET R. KERN, DVM
Diplomate, ACVIM (Internal Medicine)
Associate Professor
Animal Health Center
College of Veterinary Medicine
Mississippi State University
Mississippi State, Mississippi

RICHARD D. KIENLE, DVM
Diplomate, ACVIM (Cardiology)
Mission Valley Veterinary Cardiology
Gilroy, California

LESLEY G. KING, MVB, MRCVS
Diplomate, ACVIM (Internal Medicine),
ACVECC
Associate Professor, Section of Critical
Care
Department of Clinical Studies
School of Veterinary Medicine
University of Pennsylvania
Philadelphia, Pennsylvania

PETER P. KINTZER, DVM
Diplomate, ACVIM (Internal Medicine)
Staff Internist
Boston Road Animal Hospital
Springfield, Massachusetts

Clinical Assistant Professor
Department of Medicine
Boston Road Animal Hospital
School of Veterinary Medicine
Tufts University
North Grafton, Massachusetts

REBECCA KIRBY, DVM
Diplomate, ACVIM (Internal Medicine),
ACVECC
Chief of Medicine
Animal Emergency Center
Glendale, Wisconsin

MARK D. KITTLESON, DVM, PhD
Diplomate, ACVIM (Cardiology)
Professor
Medicine and Epidemiology
University of California
Davis, California

JEFFREY S. KLAUSNER, DVM
Diplomate, ACVIM (Internal Medicine,
Oncology)
Small Animal Clinical Sciences
College of Veterinary Medicine
University of Minnesota
St. Paul, Minnesota

THOMAS KLEIN, DVM
Adjunct Professor of Dentistry
The Ohio State University
College of Veterinary Dentistry
Owner
East Hilliard Veterinary Services
Hilliard, Ohio

JOYCE S. KNOLL, VMD, PhD
Diplomate, ACVP
Associate Professor
Department of Biomedical Sciences
Tufts University
School of Veterinary Medicine
North Grafton, Massachusetts

GARY J. KOCIBA, DVM, PhD
Diplomate, ACVP
Professor
Department of Veterinary Biosciences
Ohio State University
College of Veterinary Medicine
Columbus, Ohio

JOHN M. KRUGER, DVM, PhD
Diplomate, ACVIM (Internal Medicine)
Associate Professor
Small Animal Clinical Sciences
Veterinary Clinical Center
Michigan State University
East Lansing, Michigan

NED F. KUEHN, DVM, MS
Diplomate, ACVIM (Internal Medicine)
Department of Internal Medicine
Michigan Veterinary Specialists
Southfield, Michigan

KAREN A. KUHL, DVM
Diplomate, ACVD
Veterinary Specialty Clinic
Midwest Veterinary Dermatology Center
Riverwoods, Illinois

MARY ANNA LABATO, DVM
Diplomate, ACVIM (Internal Medicine)
Staff Veterinarian, Clinical Associate
Professor
Department of Clinical Sciences
Tufts University
School of Veterinary Medicine
North Grafton, Massachusetts

MICHAEL S. LAGUTCHIK, DVM
Veterinary Teaching Hospital
College of Veterinary Medicine
Colorado State University
Fort Collins, Colorado

INDIA F. LANE, DVM, MS
Diplomate, ACVIM (Internal Medicine)
Assistant Professor, Internal Medicine
Department of Small Animal Clinical
Sciences
University of Tennessee
College of Veterinary Medicine
Knoxville, Tennessee

ROLF E. LARSEN, DVM, PhD
Diplomate, ACT
Associate Professor
Department of Large Animal Clinical
Sciences
College of Veterinary Medicine
University of Florida
Gainesville, Florida

KENNETH S. LATIMER, DVM, PhD
Diplomate, ACVP (Clinical Pathology)
Professor of Pathology
Veterinary Pathology
College of Veterinary Medicine University
of Georgia
Athens, Georgia

DENNIS F. LAWLER, DVM
Veterinary Services Manager
Ralston Purina Company
St. Louis, Missouri

SUZETTE LECLERC, DVM, MVSc
Diplomate, ACVP
Clinical Associate
Prairie Diagnostic Services
Saskatoon, Saskatchewan, Canada

GEORGE E. LEES, DVM, MS
Diplomate, ACVIM (Internal Medicine)
Professor
Small Animal Medicine and Surgery
College of Veterinary Medicine
Texas A&M University
College Station, Texas

ALFRED M. LEGENDRE, DVM, MS
Diplomate, ACVIM (Internal Medicine)
Professor of Medicine
Veterinary Teaching Hospital
University of Tennessee
College of Veterinary Medicine
Knoxville, Tennessee

LINDA LEHMKUHL, DVM
Diplomate, ACVIM (Cardiology)
Staff Cardiologist
Med Vet
Columbus, Ohio

MICHAEL B. LESSER, DVM
Diplomate, ACVIM (Cardiology)
Advanced Veterinary Care Center
Lawndale, California

STEVEN A. LEVY, VMD
Durham Veterinary Hospital, PC
Durham, Connecticut

DAVID C. LEWIS, BVSc, PhD
Diplomate, ACVIM (Internal Medicine)
Antech Diagnostics
Portland, Oregon

DENISE M. LINDLEY, DVM
Diplomate, ACVO
Department of Veterinary Clinical
Sciences
Animal Eye Consultants
Crestwood, Illinois

DAVID LIPSITZ, BS, DVM
Diplomate, ACVIM (Neurology)
Clinical Assistant Professor
Department of Medical Sciences
School of Veterinary Medicine
University of Wisconsin—Madison
Madison, Wisconsin

SUSAN E. LITTLE, DVM, PhD
Assistant Professor
Department of Parasitology
College of Veterinary Medicine University
of Georgia
Athens, Georgia

HEIDI B. LOBPRISE, DVM
Diplomate, AVDC
Associate Veterinarian
Dallas Dental Service Animal Clinic
Dallas, Texas

DAWN E. LOGAS, DVM
Diplomate, ACVD
Assistant Professor
Department of Small Animal Clinical
Sciences
University of Florida
Gainesville, Florida

RANDALL C. LONGSHORE, DVM
Diplomate, ACVIM (Neurology)
Staff Neurologist
Veterinary Neurological Center
Phoenix, Arizona

CARROLL LOYER, DVM
Diplomate, ACVIM (Cardiology)
Boulder, Colorado

JODY P. LULICH, DVM, PhD
Diplomate, ACVIM (Internal Medicine)
Department of Small Animal Clinical
Sciences
College of Veterinary Medicine
University of Minnesota
St. Paul, Minnesota

JOHN E. LUND, BS, MS, DVM, PhD
Diplomate, ACVP
Distinguished Research Veterinary
Pathologist Worldwide Toxicology
Pharmacia and Upjohn, Inc.
Kalamazoo, Michigan

PATRICIA J. LUTTGEN, DVM, MS
  Diplomate, ACVIM (Neurology)
  Specialty Practice
  Neurological Center for Animals
  Lakewood, Colorado

SARA K. LYLE, DVM, MS
  Diplomate, ACT
  North Carolina State University
  Raleigh, North Carolina

JOHN MACDONALD, DVM
  Diplomate, ACVD
  Associate Professor
  Department of Small Animal Medicine
  and Surgery
  Auburn University
  College of Veterinary Medicine
  Auburn, Alabama

PETER S. MACWILLIAMS, DVM, PhD
  Diplomate, ACVP
  Professor of Clinical Pathology
  Department of Pathobiological Sciences
  School of Veterinary Medicine
  University of Wisconsin—Madison
  Madison, Wisconsin

JILL MADDISON, BVSc, PhD, FACVSc
  Department of Pharmacology
  University of Sydney
  Sydney, New South Wales, Australia

ORLA M. MAHONY, MVB, MRCVS
  Diplomate, ACVIM (Internal Medicine)
  and ECVIM
  Clinical Assistant Professor
  Department of Small Animal Medicine
  Tufts University School of Veterinary
  Medicine
  North Grafton, Massachusetts

STANLEY L. MARKS, BVSc, PhD
  Diplomate, ACVIM (Internal Medicine,
  Oncology), ACVN
  Assistant Professor
  Medicine and Epidemiology
  School of Veterinary Medicine
  University of California, Davis
  Davis, California

STEVEN L. MARKS, BVSc, MS, MRCVS
  Diplomate, ACVIM (Internal Medicine)
  Assistant Professor
  Department of Veterinary Clinical
  Sciences
  Louisiana State University
  Baton Rouge, Lousisiana

ROBERT A. MASON, DVM, DVSc
  Diplomate, ABVP (Companion Animal),
  ACVIM (Internal Medicine)
  Oceanview Veterinary Specialists
  Poulsbo, Washington

KENNETH V. MASON, BVSc, MVSc,
FACVSc
  Animal Allergy and Dermatology Service
  Albert Animal Hospital
  Springwood, Australia

TERRI L. MCCALLA, DVM, MS
  Diplomate, ACVO
  Associate Veterinary Opthalmologist
  The Animal Eye Clinic
  Camarillo, California

PATRICK L. MCDONOUGH, MS, PhD
  Assistant Professor of Microbiology
  Assistant Director of Bacteriology—
  Mycology
  Department of Population Medicine and
  Diagnostic Sciences
  Diagnostic Laboratory
  College of Veterinary Medicine
  Cornell University
  Ithaca, New York

BRENDAN C. MCKIERNAN, DVM
  Diplomate, ACVIM (Internal Medicine)
  Denver Veterinary Specialists
  Wheat Ridge, Colorado

RONALD M. MCLAUGHLIN, JR., DVM
  Animal Health Center
  College of Veterinary Medicine
  Mississippi State University
  Mississippi State, Mississippi

CHRISTOPHER A. MCREYNOLDS, DVM, MS
  Diplomate, ACVIM (Internal Medicine)
  Pikes Peak Veterinary Specialists
  Colorado Springs, Colorado

LINDA MEDLEAU, DVM, MS
  Diplomate, ACVD
  Professor of Dermatology
  Department of Small Animal Medicine
  College of Veterinary Medicine
  University of Georgia
  Athens, Georgia

LYNDA D. MELENDEZ, DVM, MS
  Diplomate, ACVIM (Internal Medicine)
  Assistant Professor, Small Animal
  Medicine
  Department of Veterinary Clinical
  Sciences
  Oklahoma State University
  Stillwater, Oklahoma

TONATIUH MELGAREJO, DVM, MS, PhD
  Department of Clinical Studies
  Veterinary Hospital
  University of Pennsylvania
  Philadelphia, Pennsylvania

LINDA M. MESSINGER, DVM
  Diplomate, ACVD
  Veterinary Skin and Allergy Specialist PC
  Veterinary Referral Center of Colorado
  Englewood, Colorado

KATHRYN M. MEURS, DVM
  Diplomate, ACVIM (Cardiology)
  Veterinary Clinical Sciences, CVM
  The Ohio State University
  Columbus, Ohio

VICKI MEYERS-WALLEN, VMD, PhD
  Diplomate, ACT
  Associate Professor
  Department of Biomedical Sciences
  J.A. Baker Institute College of Veterinary
  Medicine
  Cornell University
  Ithaca, New York

ELLEN MILLER, DVM, MS
  Diplomate, ACVIM (Internal Medicine)
  Veterinary Specialists of Northern
  Colorado
  Loveland, Colorado

MATT W. MILLER, DVM, MS
  Diplomate, ACVIM (Cardiology)
  Associate Professor
  Department of Veterinary Small Animal
  Medicine and Surgery
  Texas A & M University
  College Station, TX

MICHAEL S. MILLER, MS, VMD
  Diplomate, ABVP (Canine and Feline)
  Director, Cardiology-Ultrasound Referral
  Service
  West Chester, Pennsylvania

PAUL E. MILLER, DVM
  Diplomate, ACVO
  Clinical Associate Professor of
  Opthalmology
  Department of Surgical Sciences
  School of Veterinary Medicine
  University of Wisconsin—Madison
  Madison, Wisconsin

LISA E. MOORE, DVM
  Diplomate, ACVIM (Internal Medicine)
  Assistant Professor
  College of Veterinary Medicine
  Kansas State University
  Manhattan, Kansas

DANIEL O. MORRIS, DVM
  Diplomate, ACVD
  Assistant Professor of Dermatology
  Veterinary Hospital
  University of Pennsylvania
  Philadelphia, Pennsylvania

WALLACE B. MORRISON, DVM, MS
  Diplomate, ACVIM (Internal Medicine)
  Professor
  Department of Veterinary Clinical
  Sciences
  Purdue University School of Veterinary
  Medicine
  West Lafayette, Indiana

BRADLEY L. MOSES, DVM
  Diplomate, ACVIM (Cardiology)
  Clinical Assistant Professor
  Department of Clinical Sciences
  Tufts University School of Veterinary
  Medicine
  Grafton, Massachusetts
  Roberts Animal Hospital
  Hanover, Massachusetts

JOCELYN MOTT, DVM
  Diplomate, ACVIM (Internal Medicine)
  North Florida Veterinary Specialists
  Jacksonville, Florida

MICHAEL J. MURPHY, DVM, PhD
  Diplomate, ABVT
  Toxicologist
  Department of Veterinary Diagnostic
  Medicine
  College of Veterinary Medicine
  University of Minnesota
  St. Paul, Minnesota

K. MARCIA MURPHY, DVM
  Dermatology Resident
  College of Veterinary Medicine,
  Veterinary Teaching Hospital
  North Carolina State University
  Raleigh, North Carolina

NATHANIEL C. MYERS III, DVM
Diplomate, ACVIM (Internal Medicine)
Pittsburgh Veterinary Internal Medicine
Pittsburgh, Pennsylvania

KRISTINA NARFSTRÖM, DVM, PhD
Diplomate, ECVO
Professor
Section for Opthalmology
Faculty of Veterinary Medicine
Swedish University of Agricultural
Sciences
Uppsala, Sweden

MARK P. NASISSE, DVM
Diplomate, ACVO
Carolina Veterinary Specialists
Greensboro, North Carolina

T. MARK NEER, DVM
Diplomate, ACVIM (Internal Medicine)
Professor of Internal Medicine
Department of Clinical Sciences
College of Veterinary Medicine
Louisiana State University
Baton Rouge, Louisiana

REGG D. NEIGER, DVM, PhD
Professor
Department of Veterinary Science
South Dakota State University
Brookings, South Dakota

RHETT NICHOLS, DVM
Diplomate, ACVIM (Internal Medicine)
Regional Director of Consulting Services
Antech Diagnostics
Farmingdale, New York

KATHLEEN E. NOONE, VMD
Diplomate, ACVIM (Internal Medicine)
Staff Internist
Department of Medicine
The Animal Medical Center
New York, New York

GARY D. NORSWORTHY, DVM
Diplomate, ABVP (Feline)
Practitioner
Alamo Feline Health Center
San Antonio, Texas

FREDERICK W. OEHME, DVM, PhD
Diplomate, ABVT, ABT, ATS
Professor of Toxicology, Pathobiology,
Medicine, and Physiology; Director,
Comparative Toxicology Laboratories
College of Veterinary Medicine
Kansas State University
Manhattan, Kansas

CARL A. OSBORNE, DVM, PhD
Diplomate, ACVIM (Internal Medicine)
Professor
Department of Small Animal Clinical
Sciences
College of Veterinary Medicine
University of Minnesota
St. Paul, Minnesota

GARY D. OSWEILER, DVM, PhD
Diplomate, ABVT
Director, Veterinary Diagnostic Lab
Veterinary Diagnostic Laboratory
College of Veterinary Medicine
Iowa State University
Ames, Iowa

KAREN L. OVERALL, MA, VMD, PhD
Diplomate, ACVB
Department of Clinical Studies
School of Veterinary Medicine
Veterinary Hospital
University of Pennsylvania
Philadelphia, Pennsylvania

DALE PACCAMONTI, DVM, MS
Diplomate, ACT
Department of Veterinary Clinical
Sciences
School of Veterinary Medicine
Louisiana State University
Baton Rouge, Louisiana

MARK G. PAPICH, DVM, MS
Diplomate, ACVCP
Associate Professor of Clinical
Pharmacology
Advisor of Clinical Pharmacology
Laboratory
Department of Anatomy, Physiological
Sciences & Radiology
College of Veterinary Medicine
North Caroline State University
Raleigh, North Carolina

JOANE M. PARENT, DVM, MVSc
Diplomate, ACVIM (Neurology)
Department of Veterinary Clinical Studies
Ontario Veterinary College
University of Guelph
Guelph, Ontario

NIKOLA A. PARKER, DVM, MS
Diplomate, ACT
Assistant Professor
Department of Large Animal Clinical
Sciences
Virginia-Maryland Regional College of
Veterinary Medicine
Virginia Polytechnic Institute and State
University
Blacksburg, Virginia

ALLAN J. PAUL, DVM, MS
Professor
Department of Veterinary Pathobiology
College of Veterinary Medicine
University of Illinois
Urbana, Illinois

MICHAEL E. PETERSON, DVM, MS
Reid Veterinary Hospital
Albany, Oregon

J. PHILLIP PICKETT, DVM
Diplomate, ACVO
Associate Professor of Ophthalmology
Department of Small Animal Clinical
Sciences
Virginia-Maryland Regional College of
Veterinary Medicine
Virginia Polytechnic Institute and State
University
Blacksburg, Virginia

JON D. PLANT, DVM
Diplomate, ACVD
President
Animal Dermatology Specialty Clinic
Marina del Ray, California

KONSTANZE H. PLUMLEE, DVM, MS
Diplomate, ABVT, ACVIM (Internal
Medicine)
Senior Toxicologist
ASPCA National Animal Poison Control
Center
Urbana, Illinois

DAVID J. POLZIN, DVM, PhD
Diplomate, ACVIM (Internal Medicine)
Professor
Department of Small Animal Clinical
Sciences
College of Veterinary Medicine
University of Minnesota
St. Paul, Minnesota

ROBERT H. POPPENGA, DVM, PhD
Diplomate, ABVT
Associate Professor of Veterinary
Toxicology
Director, Toxicology Laboratory at New
Bolton Center
Department of Pathobiology
University of Pennsylvania
Kennett Square, Pennsylvania

KLAAS POST, DVM, M Vet Sc
Professor, Department Chairman
Department of Veterinary Internal
Medicine
Western College of Veterinary Medicine
University of Saskatchewan
Saskatoon, Saskatchewan, Canada

JAMES C. PRUETER, DVM
Diplomate, ACVIM (Internal Medicine)
Director
Veterinary Referral Clinic of Cleveland
Cleveland, Ohio

BEVERLY J. PURSWELL, DVM, PhD
Diplomate, ACT
Associate Professor
Large Animal Clinical Sciences
College of Veterinary Medicine
Virginia Tech
Blacksburg, Virginia

ANDRÉE D. QUESNEL, DVM, DVSC
Diplomate, ACVIM (Neurology)
Assistant Professor
Departement des Sciences Cliniques
Faculte de Medecine Veterinaire
Universite de Montreal
St. Hyacinthe, Quebec

CYNTHIA C. RAMSEY, DVM, MS
Diplomate, ACVIM (Internal Medicine),
ACVECC
Assistant Professor
Department of Small Animal Clinical
Sciences
Veterinary Teaching Hospital
Michigan State University
East Lansing, Michigan

KENNETH M. RASSNICK, DVM
Diplomate, ACVIM (Oncology)
Clinical Assistant Professor
Harrington Oncology Program
Tufts University
School of Veterinary Medicine
North Grafton, Massachusetts

CLARENCE A. RAWLINGS, DVM, PhD
Diplomate, ACVS
Professor and Head
Department of Small Animal Medicine
University of Georgia
College of Veterinary Medicine
Athens, Georgia

WILLIAM J. REAGAN, DVM, PhD
Diplomate, ACVP
Director, Veterinary Diagnostic
Laboratories
Heska Corporation
Fort Collins, Colorado

ALAN H. REBAR, DVM, PhD
Diplomate, ACVP
Dean, School of Veterinary Medicine
Department of Veterinary Administration
Purdue University
School of Veterinary Medicine
West Lafayette, Indiana

LLOYD M. REEDY, DVM
Diplomate, ACVD
Animal Dermatology Clinic
Dallas, Texas

RALPH C. RICHARDSON, DVM
Diplomate, ACVIM (Oncology & Internal
Medicine)
Professor and Dean
College of Veterinary Medicine
Kansas State University
Manhattan, Kansas

KEITH P. RICHTER, DVM
Diplomate, ACVIM (Internal Medicine)
Internal Medicine Staff
Veterinary Specialty Hospital of San
Diego
Rancho Santa Fe, California

MICHAEL J. RINGLE, DVM
Diplomate, ACVO
Veterinary Opthalmologist
The Animal Eye Clinic of New Jersey
Red Bank, New Jersey

MARK RISHNIW, BVSC, MS
Diplomate, ACVIM (Cardiology & Internal
Medicine)
Lecturer Cardiology
Department of Cardiology
Cornell University New York State
College of Veterinary Medicine
Ithaca, New York

MARGARET V. ROOT KUSTRITZ, DVM, PhD
Diplomate, ACT
Assistant Clinical Specialist, Small
Animal Reproduction
Department of Small Animal Clinical
Sciences
College of Veterinary Medicine
University of Minnesota
St. Paul, Minnesota

WAYNE STEWART ROSENKRANTZ, DVM
Diplomate, ACVD
Owner
Animal Dermatology Clinics
Garden Grove, California

PHILIP ROUDEBUSH, DVM
Diplomate, ACVIM (Internal Medicine)
Veterinary Fellow
Hill's Science and Technology Center
Topeka, Kansas

ELIZABETH A. ROZANSKI, DVM
Diplomate, ACVECC, ACVIM (Internal
Medicine)
Assistant Professor
Department of Clinical Sciences
Tufts University School of Veterinary
Medicine
North Grafton, Massachusetts

JOHN E. RUSH, DVM, MS
Diplomate, ACVIM (Cardiology), ACVECC
Associate Professor and Associate
Department Chair
Clinical Sciences
School of Veterinary Medicine
Tufts University
North Grafton, Massachusetts

CARL D. SAMMARCO, BVSc, MRCVS
Diplomate, ACVIM (Cardiology)
Cardiopet, Veterinary Referral Centre
Little Falls, New Jersey

SHERRY L. SANDERSON, DVM, PhD
Diplomate, ACVIM (Internal Medicine)
Assistant Professor
Department of Small Animal Medicine
University of Georgia
College of Veterinary Medicine
Athens, Georgia

JUAN CARLOS SARDINAS, DVM
Diplomate, ACVS, ECVS
Palm Beach Veterinary Referral Services
Palm Beach, Florida

THOMAS SCHERMERHORN, VMD
Diplomate, ACVIM (Internal Medicine)
Department of Molecular Medicine
NYS College of Veterinary Medicine
Cornell University
Ithaca, New York

DONALD PAUL SCHROPE, DVM
Diplomate, ACVIM (Cardiology)
Staff Cardiologist
Department of Cardiology
Veterinary Referral Centre
Little Falls, New Jersey

PETER D. SCHWARZ, DVM
Diplomate, ACVS
Veterinary Surgical Specialists of New
Mexico, PC
Albuquerque, New Mexico

FRED W. SCOTT, DVM, PhD
Diplomate, ACVM, AFM
Professor Emeritus
Department of Microbiology and
Immunology
College of Veterinary Medicine
Cornell University
Ithaca, New York

J. CATHARINE R. SCOTT-MONCRIEFF, MA,
Vet MB, MS
Diplomate, ACVIM (Internal Medicine),
ECVIM
Diploma, Small Animal Medicine
Associate Professor
Department of Veterinary Clinical
Medicine
Purdue University School of Veterinary
Medicine
West Lafayette, Indiana

KEVIN SHANLEY, DVM
Diplomate, ACVD
Staff Dermatologist, Metropolitan
Veterinary Associates & Delaware
Veterinary Specialty Group
Dermatology Clinic for Animals
Valley Forge, Pennsylvania

DARCY SHAW, DVM, MVSc
Diplomate, ACVIM (Internal Medicine)
Associate Professor
Department of Companion Animals
Atlantic Veterinary College
University of Prince Edward Island
Charlottetown, Prince Edward Island,
Canada

LINDA G. SHELL, DVM
Diplomate, ACVIM (Neurology)
Professor
Small Animal Clinical Sciences
VA-MD Regional College of Veterinary
Medicine
Virginia Polytechnical Institute and State
University
Blacksburg, Virginia

G. DIANE SHELTON, DVM, PhD
Diplomate, ACVIM (Internal Medicine)
Associate Adjunct Professor
Department of Pathology, School of
Medicine
University of California, San Diego
LaJolla, California

KENNETH W. SIMPSON, BVM&S, PhD,
MRCVS
Diplomate, ACVIM (Internal Medicine),
ECVIM
Assistant Professor of Medicine
Department of Clinical Sciences
Cornell University College of Veterinary
Medicine
Ithaca, New York

BARBARA S. SIMPSON, DVM, PhD
Diplomate, ACVB
The Veterinary Behavior Clinic
Southern Pines, North Carolina
Adjunct Associate Professor
Department of Clinical Sciences
North Carolina State University
College of Veterinary Medicine
Raleigh, North Carolina

ALLEN FRANKLIN SISSON, DVM, MS
Diplomate, ACVIM (Neurology)
Staff Neurologist
Department of Medicine
Angell Memorial Animal Hospital
Boston, Massachusetts

STEPHANIE L. SMEDES, DVM
Diplomate, ACVO
Oceanview Veterinary Specialists, Inc., PS
Poulsbo, Washington

FRANCES O. SMITH, DVM, PhD
Diplomate, ACT
Smith Animal Hospital, Inc.
Burnsville, Minnesota

MARY O. SMITH, BVMS, PhD
Diplomate, ACVIM (Neurology)
Department of Clinical Sciences
College of Veterinary Medicine
Colorado State University
Fort Collins, Colorado

PATRICIA J. SMITH, DVM, MS, PhD
Diplomate, ACVO
Ophthalmologist
Animal Eye Care
Fremont, California

FRANCIS W. K. SMITH, JR., DVM
Diplomate, ACVIM (Internal Medicine and
Cardiology)
Vice President Editor-in-Chief,
VetMedCenter
San Francisco, California
Clinical Assistant Professor
Department of Medicine
Tufts University
School of Veterinary Medicine
North Grafton, Massachusetts

PAUL W. SNYDER, DVM, PhD
Diplomate, ACVP
Assistant Professor of Pathology
Department of Veterinary
Pathobiology
School of Veterinary Medicine
Purdue University
West Lafayette, Indiana

PATTI S. SNYDER, DVM, MS
Diplomate, ACVIM (Internal Medicine)
Assistant Professor
Small Animal Clinical Sciences
College of Veterinary Medicine
University of Florida
Gainesville, Florida

DON C. SORJONEN, DVM, MS
Diplomate, ACVIM (Neurology)
Professor of Neurology, Neurosurgery
Small Animal Surgery and Medicine
Auburn University
College of Veterinary Medicine
Auburn, Alabama

BARI L. SPIELMAN, DVM, BS
Diplomate, ACVIM (Internal Medicine)
Staff Internist
Department of Medicine
Angell Memorial Animal Hospital
Boston, Massachusetts

REBECCA L. STEPIEN, DVM
Diplomate, ACVIM (Cardiology)
Clinical Assistant Professor
Department of Medical Sciences
University of Wisconsin
School of Veterinary Medicine
Madison, Wisconsin

JERRY B. STEVENS, DVM, PhD
Professor, Clinical Pathology
College of Veterinary Medicine
North Carolina State University
Raleigh, North Carolina

ELIZABETH ARNOLD STONE, DVM
Diplomate, ACVS
Professor of Surgery
Department of Clinical Sciences
North Carolina State University
College of Veterinary Medicine
Raleigh, North Carolina

JUSTIN H. STRAUS, DVM
Diplomate, ACVIM (Internal Medicine)
Animal Emergency & Ref. Center
West Caldwell, NJ

MARGARET S. SWARTOUT, DVM, MS
Diplomate, ACVIM (Internal Medicine)
Owner
Veterinary Specialty Consultation
Service
Knoxville, Tennessee

CHERYL L. SWENSON, DVM, PhD
Diplomate, ACVP (Clinical Pathology)
Associate Professor
Department of Pathology
Veterinary Medical Center
Michigan State University
East Lansing, Michigan

HARRIET MERLIN SYME, BSc, BVetMed,
MRCVS
Diplomate, ACVIM (Internal Medicine)
Royal Veterinary College
London, England

JOSEPH TABOADA, DVM
Diplomate, ACVIM (Internal Medicine)
Professor and Director of Professional
Instruction
Department of Veterinary Clinical
Sciences
School of Veterinary Medicine
Louisiana State University
Baton Rouge, Louisiana

ROBERT A. TAYLOR, DVM
Diplomate, ACVS
Alameda East Veterinary Hospital
Denver, Colorado

WILLIAM B. THOMAS, DVM, MS
Diplomate, ACVIM (Neurology)
Associate Professor
Department of Small Animal Clinical
Sciences
College of Veterinary Medicine
University of Tennessee
Knoxville, Tennessee

JAMES P. THOMPSON, DVM, PhD
Diplomate, ACVIM (Internal Medicine and
Oncology), ACVM (Virology, Immunology,
Bacteriology, Mycology)
Professor
Small Animal Clinical Sciences
University of Florida
College of Veterinary Medicine
Gainesville, Florida

LELAND THOMPSON, DVM
Manager
Companion Animal Pharmaceuticals
Clinical Development
Pfizer, Inc. Animal Health Group
Lee's Summit, Missouri

JERRY A. THORNHILL, DVM
Diplomate, ACVIM (Internal Medicine)
Consultant, Veterinary Internal Medicine
and Nephrology
University of Missouri
Barrington, Illinois

MARY ANNA THRALL, BA, DVM, MS
Diplomate, ACVP
Professor
Department of Pathology
College of Veterinary Medicine &
Biomedical Sciences
Colorado State University
Fort Collins, Colorado

LARRY P. TILLEY, DVM
Diplomate, ACVIM (Internal Medicine)
President, Chief Medical Officer,
VetMedCenter
San Francisco, California
Director, Veterinary Specialty Referral
Center
President, VET MED TELEMEDICINE
Consultation Services
Sante Fe, New Mexico

ANDREA TIPOLD, PD Dr
Diplomate, ECVN
Associate Professor
Veterinary Virology and Veterinary
Neurology
Division Immunology
Bern, Switzerland

SHEILA M.F. TORRES, DVM, MS, PhD
Diplomate, ACVD
Assistant Professor
Small Animal Clinical Sciences
University of Minnesota College of
Veterinary Medicine
Minneapolis, Minnesota

DAVID C. TWEDT, DVM
Diplomate, ACVIM (Internal Medicine)
Professor
Clinical Sciences
Veterinary Teaching Hospital College of
Veterinary Medicine
Colorado State University
Fort Collins, Colorado

JOHN WILLIAM TYLER, DVM
Diplomate, ACVIM (Internal Medicine)
Assistant Professor
Small Animal Internal Medicine
Animal Health Center
Mississippi State University
College of Veterinary Medicine
Mississippi State, Mississippi

SHELLY L. VADEN, DVM, PhD
Diplomate, ACVIM (Internal Medicine)
Associate Professor
Internal Medicine
Department of Clinical Science
North Carolina State University
College of Veterinary Medicine
Raleigh, North Carolina

MARY ANN VONDERHAAR, DVM, MS
Visiting Assistant Professor
Small Animal Medicine
University of Illinois
College of Veterinary Medicine
Urbana, Illinois

MARK C. WALKER, BVSc, MACVSc
Diplomate, ACVIM (Internal Medicine)
North Florida Veterinary Specialists, P.A.
Jacksonville / Orange Park, Florida

MELISSA S. WALLACE, DVM
Diplomate, ACVIM (Internal Medicine)
Staff Internist
Department of Medicine
The Animal Medical Center
New York, New York

MICHELLE JOY WASCHAK, DVM, MS
Diplomate, ACVS
Associate Surgeon
South Carolina Surgical Referral
Service
Columbia, South Carolina

ROBERT J. WASHABAU, VMD, PhD
Diplomate, ACVIM (Internal Medicine)
Associate Professor and Section Chief of
Medicine
Department of Clinical Studies
School of Veterinary Medicine
University of Pennsylvania
Philadelphia, Pennsylvania

CYNTHIA R. WEBSTER, DVM
Diplomate, ACVIM (Internal Medicine)
Assistant Professor
Department of Clinical Sciences
School of Veterinary Medicine
Tufts University
North Grafton, Massachusetts

M. GLADE WEISER, DVM
Diplomate, ACVP (Clinical Pathology)
Vice President, Diagnostics
Heska Corporation
Fort Collins, Colorado

ALEXANDER H. WERNER, VMD
Diplomate, ACVD
Staff Dermatologist
Valley Veterinary Specialty Services
Studio City, California

MICHAEL D. WILLARD, DVM, MS
Diplomate, ACVIM (Internal Medicine)
Professor of Small Animal Medicine &
Surgery
Department of Small Animal Medicine &
Surgery
College of Veterinary Medicine
Texas A & M University
College Station, Texas

DAVID A. WILLIAMS, MA, Vet MB, PhD,
MRCVS
Diplomate, ACVIM (Internal Medicine),
ECVIM (Companion Animals)
Professor and Department Head
Department of Small Animal Medicine
and Surgery
College of Veterinary Medicine
Texas A&M University
College Station, Texas

JAMES E. WILLIAMS, JR., DVM, MS
Department of Veterinary Medicine &
Surgery
University of Missouri
Veterinary Teaching Hospital
Columbia, Missouri

RONALD B. WILSON, DVM
Diplomate, ACVP
Diagnostic Laboratory Director
Department of Agriculture
C.E. Kord Animal Disease
Laboratory
Nashville, Tennessee

J. PAUL WOODS, DVM, MS
Diplomate, ACVIM (Internal Medicine)
Certificate of Specialization in Small
Animal Internal Medicine
Canadian Veterinary Medical
Association
Associate Professor of Medicine
Department of Clinical Studies
Ontario Veterinary College
University of Guelph
Guelph, Ontario

KAREN M. YOUNG, VMD, PhD
Associate Professor
Department of Pathobiological
Sciences
School of Veterinary Medicine
University of Wisconsin—Madison
Madison, Wisconsin

CONTENTS *by section*

DIAGNOSTICS— LABORATORY TESTS

DIAGNOSTICS— ELECTROCARDIOGRAPHY

DISEASES AND CLINICAL SYNDROMES

TOPIC	

CONTENTS *by subject*

ENDOCRINOLOGY

GASTROENTEROLOGY

HEMATOLOGY/ IMMUNOLOGY

MUSCULOSKELETAL

Oncology

OPHTHALMOLOGY

RENAL/UROLOGIC

RESPIRATORY

THERIOGENOLOGY

TOXICOLOGY

PRESENTING PROBLEMS AND PHYSICAL FINDINGS

ABORTION, SPONTANEOUS (PREGNANCY LOSS)—CATS

BASICS

DEFINITION
• Abortion—expulsion of one or more live or dead fetuses that cannot sustain extrauterine life • Pregnancy loss—all pregnancy wastage, including embryonic death, reabsorption of early fetal losses, mummification, abortion, and dystocia

PATHOPHYSIOLOGY
• Primary causes—(lethal genetic defects, infections) kill the embryo or fetus directly • Secondary fetal wastage—death from defective or compromised placentation, inadequate uterine vascular or nutritional support, or failure of supportive endocrine development and function • Dam-related events (e.g., dystocia, trauma, extreme stress, and metabolic disease)—usually terminate fetal life indirectly • Possible outcomes (in descending order of frequency)—reabsorption during early gestation, abortion or mummification during later gestation, and stillbirth at term; reabsorption relatively difficult to document • Frequency of early embryonic death—unknown

SYSTEMS AFFECTED
• Reproductive • Other organs—if events leading to pregnancy wastage originate in another body system or externally; if pregnancy wastage leads to complications (e.g., toxemia or shock)

SIGNALMENT
• Nonspecific • More common at first parity and in queens > 6 years old, except with infectious cause

SIGNS

General Comments
• May be asymptomatic, especially early in gestation
• **NOTE:** not all signs are seen in every patient; any combination may occur.

Historical Findings
• Failure to litter on time • Decrease in abdominal size • Expulsion of recognizable fetuses or placental structures • Anorexia • Vomiting and diarrhea • Weight loss

Physical Examination Findings
• Bloody or purulent vulvar discharge—may not be observed in fastidious queens • Disappearance of vesicles or fetuses previously documented by palpation, ultrasound, or radiography • Abdominal straining and discomfort • Depression • Dehydration • Fever

CAUSES

Infectious
• Viruses—feline panleukopenia virus; feline rhinotracheitis virus; FeLV

• Bacteria—*Escherichia coli; Streptococcus* spp.; *Staphylococcus* spp.; *Salmonella* spp.; *Mycobacterium* spp.; *Mycoplasma* spp.
• Rickettsia—*Coxiella burnetii* (Q fever)
• Parasite—*Toxoplasma gondii*

Noninfectious—Reproductive
• Dystocia (fetal)—fetal malposition (relatively uncommon); fetal deformity; excessively large fetal size (e.g., small litter and prolonged gestation); multiple simultaneous fetal presentation; breed-based fetal–maternal disproportion (e.g., Persians and Himalayans) • Dystocia (maternal)—small pelvic diameter because of immaturity; previous injury; congenital abnormality; insufficient dilation of the soft tissue of the birth canal; fibrosis or malformation of the birth canal; uterine inertia (common); torsion of the uterine horn; prolapse; metabolic disease predisposing to episodic weakness, pain, and fatigue • Endocrinopathy—endometrial disease (e.g., cystic endometrial hyperplasia); hypoluteoidism (indirect evidence, but not documented conclusively) • Structural or functional placental inadequacy • Fetal defects—genetic or developmental (anatomic, metabolic, and chromosomal abnormalities); possibly gamete aging • Excessive or poorly planned inbreeding and poor choices of breeding stock—usually indirect evidence; difficult diagnosis without thorough family history and test matings • Abortifacient drugs—luteolytics (e.g., $PGF_{2\alpha}$); estrogens; prolactin inhibitors (cabergoline); glucocorticoids • Drugs reported in dogs—prolactin inhibitors (e.g., bromocriptine); antiestrogens (e.g., tamoxifen citrate); progesterone antagonists (e.g., mifepristone); progesterone synthesis inhibitors (e.g., espostane)

Noninfectious—Nonreproductive
• Nutrition—taurine < 200 ppm of diet
• Severe stress—environmental; physiologic; psychologic
• Trauma
• Some drugs
• Consequence of nonreproductive systemic disease

RISK FACTORS
• Previous history of pregnancy loss
• Concurrent acute or chronic disease
• Possibly excessive inbreeding
• First parity
• Age (> 6 years)

DIAGNOSIS

DIFFERENTIAL DIAGNOSIS

Vulvar Discharge

• Impending parturition
• Estrus—discharge usually not copious; behavioral signs of estrus noted; vaginal cytologic examination documents estrus (**NOTE:** sample collection may induce ovulation)
• Metritis
• Pyometra—neutrophilic leukocytosis, polydipsia and polyuria, and signs of systemic illness characteristic; large uterus noted on ultrasonography or radiography; inflammation confirmed on vaginal cytologic examination
• Severe vaginitis
• Uterine trauma or hemorrhage—history of recent injury and clinical signs (bloody discharge, weakness, shock, and pallor characteristic); acute blood loss noted from CBC; uterine fluid or blood clots seen on ultrasonography; bleeding without inflammation determined from vaginal cytologic examination
• Abnormal vaginal or rectovaginal anatomy—revealed on ultrasonography and contrast radiography; discharge of intestinal contents from vulva (fistula) characteristic
• Uterine or vaginal neoplasia
• Uterine stump infection
• Ovarian remnant syndrome—discharge usually not copious; history of ovariohysterectomy and behavioral signs of estrus characteristic; estrus documented on vaginal cytologic examination

Abdominal Signs
• Obstructive uropathy or nonobstructive lower urinary tract disease
• Severe renal disease—pyelonephritis
• Pancreatitis
• Liver disease
• Severe gastrointestinal disease
• Peritonitis
• Abdominal trauma

CBC/BIOCHEMISTRY/URINALYSIS
• Inflammatory or stress leukocyte response—except with panleukopenia
• Serum biochemistry profile and urinalysis—usually normal; may reveal systemic involvement if another disease led to secondary pregnancy wastage or if primary pregnancy wastage resulted in secondary systemic involvement
• Examination of discharge fluid—may reveal fetal or placental tissue

OTHER LABORATORY TESTS

Infectious Causes
• Feline panleukopenia—virus isolated from lungs, kidneys, urine, and feces; rising antibody titer from paired sera, 14–21-day interval; histologic changes in gastrointestinal tract; perform on patients early in course of disease
• Feline rhinotracheitis—immunofluorescent antibody test of conjunctival scrapings; rising

ABORTION, SPONTANEOUS (PREGNANCY LOSS)—CATS

antibody titer from paired sera, 14–21-day interval; frozen oropharyngeal, tonsillar, or nasal swabs for virus isolation (probably most practical in catteries, because virus is often endemic and serum antibody titers may be positive; contact regional diagnostic laboratory first for instructions or refer to specialized laboratory); perform on patients early in course of disease
• FeLV—immunofluorescent antibody and ELISA; perform on entire cattery or all cats in the household
• Mycoplasma—complement fixation, hemagglutination inhibition, culture (contact laboratory; special media required); perform on patients early in course of disease; test unaffected cats; isolation of organisms preferred.
• Coxiella—antibody titers from paired sera, 2–4-week intervals (contact regional diagnostic laboratory first for instructions or refer to specialized laboratory)

Noninfectious Causes
Hypoluteoidism—serial serum progesterone determinations; start before time of suspected fetal loss

IMAGING
• Radiography and palpation—establish existence of fetuses if performed at appropriate intervals of gestation
• Ultrasonography—essential for precise evaluation of fetal status
• Radiography and ultrasound—helpful to confirm several differential diagnoses

DIAGNOSTIC PROCEDURES
• Bacterial diseases—culture and sensitivity of the cervix, anterior vaginal canal, or uterus; obtain specimen by ultrasound guidance, laparoscopy, or laparotomy (contact laboratory before shipping samples for *Salmonella* or *Mycobacterium* culture); perform early in course of disease.
• Placental inadequacy—histologic and microbiologic evaluation of placenta

Fetal Defects
• Necropsy
• Karyotype—submit ear tip of necropsied patient; ship in heparinized dam's blood; contact karyotype laboratory at University of Minnesota; save gonad in Bouin solution for histopathologic examination
• Screen for inborn errors of metabolism—submit urine from necropsy or live patient; contact the Medical Genetics Section at the University of Pennsylvania
• Collect history of involved or related sires and dams

Poor Reproductive Planning
• Extensively review breeding records, including inbreeding coefficients, performance records, and records of related individuals

• History of high neonatal or pediatric mortality, poor growth of surviving subjects, and increased susceptibility to infectious diseases—often suggests excessive inbreeding or poor choice of breeding stock
• NOTE: the inbreeding coefficient is the probability that the two alleles from a randomly chosen autosomal locus are identical by descent; a measure of the effect of relatedness on an individual's genome

TREATMENT
• Inpatient—when aborting visible fetal and placental material; if patient is likely to abort; with clinical illness; patients with potential zoonoses, unless safe and effective outpatient management is ensured; obtain informed consent.
• Abortus or discharge—may be infectious; isolate patient with suspected infectious agent
• Practice strict sanitation for inpatient and outpatient treatment.
• Usually not possible to predict outcome of subsequent pregnancies without a complete diagnosis
• Ovariohysterectomy—considered for stable patients with no breeding value
• Prostaglandin or hysterotomy—considered to empty and clean uterus of breeding cats
• Normosol or lactated Ringer—management of dehydration; intravenous or subcutaneous, depending on severity of problem and cooperation of patient
• Potential contraindications for surgery—serious risk to patient; ability to resolve the problem by less invasive means
• For catteries, discuss history or possibility of multiple occurrences.
• Help client establish a monitoring system and encourage careful records of reproductive performance.

MEDICATIONS
DRUGS OF CHOICE
• Depend on underlying cause
• Amoxicillin—11–22 mg/kg PO q8–12h, pending results of bacterial culture
• $PGF_{2\alpha}$—no live fetuses but significant uterine contents noted on ultrasonography; 0.10–0.25 mg/kg SQ q24h for up to 5 days, if needed

CONTRAINDICATIONS
• Potential contraindications for prostaglandin—advanced age; live fetuses; mummified fetuses; closed cervix; sepsis; peritonitis; high risk of uterine rupture; other organ dysfunction
• Use caution if uterine rupture is possible.

PRECAUTIONS
$PGF_{2\alpha}$—intense grooming; salivation; defecation; vomiting; urination; tachycardia; vocalization; nervousness; panting; mydriasis; lordosis posture; tail flagging; (occasionally) hypotension

POSSIBLE INTERACTIONS
Check cautions when administering drugs to manage specific differential diagnoses.

ALTERNATIVE DRUGS
N/A

FOLLOW-UP
PATIENT MONITORING
• Physical examination—7–14 days after treatment • Repeat ultrasound—document complete evacuation of the uterus; establish continued existence of live fetuses

POSSIBLE COMPLICATIONS
• Depend on underlying cause • Sepsis • Shock • Uterine rupture • Peritonitis • Metritis • Pyometra • Subsequent infertility

MISCELLANEOUS
ASSOCIATED CONDITIONS
N/A

AGE-RELATED FACTORS
• Fertility declines naturally after 6 years of age. • Ovariohysterectomy—recommended in stable patients > 6 years old

ZOONOTIC POTENTIAL
• Bacterial causes • *Coxiella burnetii* • *Toxoplasma gondii*

PREGNANCY
N/A

ABBREVIATIONS
• FeLV = feline leukemia virus • ELISA = enzyme-linked immunoadsorbent assay

Suggested Reading
Feldman EC, Nelson RW. Canine and feline endocrinology and reproduction. Philadelphia: Saunders, 1987:525–548.
Papich MG. Effects of drugs on pregnancy. In: Kirk RW, Bonagura JD, eds. Current veterinary therapy X. Philadelphia: Saunders, 1989:1291–1299.
Troy GC, Herron MA. Infectious causes of infertility, abortion, and stillbirths in cats. In: Morrow DA, ed. Current therapy in theriogenology. Philadelphia: Saunders, 1986:834–837.

Author Dennis F. Lawler
Consulting Editor Sara K. Lyle

ABORTION, SPONTANEOUS (PREGNANCY LOSS)—DOGS

BASICS

DEFINITION
Loss of a fetus because of resorption in early stages or expulsion in later stages of pregnancy

PATHOPHYSIOLOGY
• Direct causes—congenital abnormality; infectious disease; trauma
• Indirect causes—infectious placentitis; abnormal ovarian or uterine maternal environment

SYSTEMS AFFECTED
• Reproductive
• Any dysfunction of a major body system can adversely affect pregnancy.

SIGNALMENT
Intact bitches

SIGNS
N/A

CAUSES

Infectious
• *Brucella canis*
• Canine herpesvirus
• Toxoplasma
• Mycoplasma and ureaplasma
• Miscellaneous bacteria—*E. coli; Streptococci; Campylobacter; Salmonella*
• Miscellaneous viruses—distemper virus, parvovirus

Uterine
• Cystic endometrial hyperplasia and pyometra
• Trauma—acute and chronic
• Neoplasia
• Embryotoxic drugs
• Chemotherapeutic agents
• Chloramphenicol—early gestation
• Estrogens
• Glucocorticoids—high dosage

• Prostaglandins—lysis of corpora lutea

Hormonal Dysfunction
• Hypothyroidism
• Hypoluteoidism

Fetal Defects
• Lethal chromosomal abnormality
• Lethal organ defects

RISK FACTORS
• Exposure of the brood bitch to carrier animals
• Old age
• Hereditary

DIAGNOSIS

DIFFERENTIAL DIAGNOSIS
• Differentiate infectious from noninfectious causes—*B. canis* of immediate concern
• Differentiate resorption from infertility—helped by early diagnosis of pregnancy
• History of drug use during pregnancy—particularly during the first trimester, or use of drugs known to cause fetal death
• Vulvar discharges during diestrus—may mimic abortion; evaluate discharge and origin to differentiate uterine from distal reproductive tract disease.
• Necropsy of aborted fetus, placenta, and stillborn puppies—enhances chances of definitive diagnosis
• History of systemic or endocrine disease—may indicate problems with the maternal environment

CBC/BIOCHEMISTRY/URINALYSIS
• Usually normal
• May reveal systemic disease—uterine infection; viral infection; endocrine abnormality

OTHER LABORATORY TESTS
• Serologic testing—for *B. canis,* canine herpesvirus, and toxoplasma; collect serum as soon as possible after abortion. Repeat testing for raising titers for canine herpesvirus and toxoplasma.

• Slide test for *B. canis*—very sensitive; negative results reliable; prevalence of false positives as high as 60%
• Tube agglutination test for *B. canis*—gives titers; < 1:200 considered insignificant
• Agar gel immunodiffusion test for *B. canis*—effectively differentiates between false and true positives
• Baseline T_4 serum concentration—when no infectious agents are identified; hypothyroidism is a common endocrine disease and has been suggested as causing fetal wastage.
• Progesterone serum concentration—when no infectious agents are identified; hypoluteoidism may cause fetal wastage; dogs depend on ovarian progesterone production throughout gestation (minimum of 2 ng/mL required to maintain pregnancy); determine as soon as possible after abortion; in subsequent pregnancies, we need to start monitoring @ week 3 which may be before we can document with ultrasound.
• Vaginal culture—*B. canis;* with positive serologic test

IMAGING
• Radiography—identify fetal structures after > 45 days of gestation; earlier, can determine uterine enlargement but cannot assess uterine contents
• Ultrasonography—identify uterine size and contents; assess fluid and its consistency; assess fetal remains or viability by noting heartbeats (normal, > 200 bpm; stress, < 200 bpm)

DIAGNOSTIC PROCEDURES
• Vaginoscopy—identify source of vulvar discharges and vaginal lesions; use a long enough scope to examine the entire length of the vagina (16–20 cm)
• Cytologic examination and bacterial culture—vagina; may reveal an inflammatory process (e.g., uterine infection); technique for culture: use a guarded swab culture instrument to ensure an anterior sample (distal reproductive tract is normally heavily contaminated with bacteria)

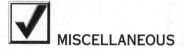

ABORTION, SPONTANEOUS (PREGNANCY LOSS)—DOGS

• Histopathologic examination and culture of fetal and placental tissue—may reveal infectious organisms; tissue culture, particularly of stomach contents, to identify infectious bacterial organisms

TREATMENT

• Most bitches should be confined and isolated pending diagnosis.
• *B. canis*—highly infective to dogs; shed in high numbers during abortion; if confirmed, euthanasia recommended owing to lack of successful treatment and to prevent spread of infection; may try ovariohysterectomy and long-term antibiotics
• Partial abortion—may attempt to salvage the live fetuses; administer antibiotics if a bacterial component is identified; institute cage rest; monitor pregnancy by ultrasonography to document continued fetal viability; monitor dam (temperature and CBC) for the remainder of the pregnancy.

MEDICATIONS

DRUGS OF CHOICE

• $PGF_{2\alpha}$—uterine evacuation after abortion; 0.1 mg/kg SC q8–24h; not approved for use in dogs, but adequate documentation legitimizes its use; do not substitute analogues (inadequate documentation of safe dosages); use only if all living fetuses have been expelled.
• Antibiotics—for bacterial disease; initially institute broad-spectrum agent; specific agent depends on culture and sensitivity testing of vaginal tissue and necropsy of fetus
• Progesterone (Regu-mate®) at 0.088 mg/kg (2 mL/110 lb) PO or progesterone in oil at 2 mg/kg IM—for documented hypoluteodism only.

CONTRAINDICATIONS

Progestogen supplementation is contraindicated except in those dogs with hypoluteodism.

PRECAUTIONS

$PGF_{2\alpha}$—metabolized in the lung; side effects: related to smooth muscle contraction, dose related, diminish with each injection; panting, salivation, vomition, and defecation common; dosing critical (LD_{50}, 5 mg/kg)

ALTERNATIVE DRUGS

Oxytocin—1 U/5 kg SC q6–24h; for uterine evacuation; most effective in the first 24–48 hr after abortion

FOLLOW-UP

PATIENT MONITORING

• Vulvar discharges—daily; for decreasing amount, odor, and inflammatory component; for consistency (increasing mucoid component)
• $PGF_{2\alpha}$—continued for 5 days or until most of the discharge ceases (3–15 days)
• *B. canis*—monitor after neutering and antibiotic therapy; yearly serologic testing to identify recrudescence
• Hypothyroidism—treat appropriately; neutering recommended (hereditary nature); see Hypothyroidism

POSSIBLE COMPLICATIONS

• Septicemia
• Toxemia
• Death owing to untreated pyometra
• Diskospondylitis
• Endophthalmitis
• Recurrent uveitis

✓ MISCELLANEOUS

ASSOCIATED CONDITIONS
N/A

AGE-RELATED FACTORS
N/A

ZOONOTIC POTENTIAL
B. canis—may be transmitted to humans, especially when handling the aborting bitch; massive number of organisms expelled during abortion

PREGNANCY
N/A

SEE ALSO
Infertility, Female

Suggested Reading

Carmichael LE, Greene CE. Canine brucellosis. In: Greene CE, ed. Infectious diseases of the dog and cat. Philadelphia: Saunders, 1990:573–584.

Evermann JF. Diagnosis of canine herpetic infections. In: Kirk RW, ed. Current veterinary therapy X. Philadelphia: Saunders, 1989:1313–1316.

Feldman EC, Nelson RW. Canine and feline endocrinology and reproduction. Philadelphia: Saunders, 1987:399–480.

Lein DH. Infertility and reproductive diseases in bitches and queens. In: Roberts SJ, ed.Veterinary obstetrics and genital diseases (theriogenology). Woodstock, VT: Roberts, 1986:728–734.

Roberts SJ. Diseases and accidents during the gestation period. In: Roberts SJ, ed. Veterinary obstetrics and genital diseases (theriogenology). Woodstock, VT: Roberts, 1986:206–210.

Authors Beverly J. Purswell and Nikola A. Parker
Consulting Editor Sara K. Lyle

ABORTION, TERMINATION OF PREGNANCY

 BASICS

DEFINITION
Induced termination of pregnancy; may accomplish by drugs that prevent fertilization, prevent implantation, or terminate an established pregnancy

PATHOPHYSIOLOGY
• Corpus luteum—must be functional throughout pregnancy in dogs and most likely in cats; suggested that pituitary rather than uterine or placental influences most important for maintenance
• LH and PRL—principal hormones involved in maintaining corpus luteum; reduced concentration may cause regression of corpus luteum and termination of pregnancy.
• Compounds that inhibit progesterone secretion or compete with progesterone receptors should lead to termination.

SYSTEMS AFFECTED
• Reproductive Gastrointestinal, Respiratory, Neurologic, and Cardiac—affected by drugs used in treatment

SIGNALMENT
Unwanted pregnancies

SIGNS
• Depend on stage of gestation
• May have no visible signs
• Vaginal discharge or expulsion of fetus(es)

CAUSES
• Withdrawing luteotrophic support
• Inhibiting progesterone synthesis
• Using a progesterone receptor antagonist

RISK FACTORS
Causal drugs—undesirable side effects; require a great deal of time and effort for administration and monitoring; many not approved for use in therapeutic abortions

 DIAGNOSIS

DIFFERENTIAL DIAGNOSIS
• Important to establish that a breeding has taken place
• Determine stage of estrous cycle—examine vaginal smears; measure plasma progesterone concentration (see Breeding, Timing)
• Look for sperm—examine vaginal smears; absence does not mean that breeding did not take place
• Patient in estrus with very high index of suspicion that she is pregnant—examine vaginal smears daily or every other day; determine day 1 of diestrus and start treatment on day 6
• Patient in very early diestrus—wait 5 days and start treatment
• Definitive diagnosis of pregnancy—ultrasound examination after day 20–30 of diestrus; radiographic examination after day 40 of diestrus
• Patient remains pregnant—treat again on day 31–35 of diestrus; usually will accomplish termination

CBC/BIOCHEMISTRY/URINALYSIS
• Before treatment as screening tests only for old patients
• Normal, unless concurrent underlying disease

OTHER LABORATORY TESTS
• Vaginal cytologic testing—determine stage of estrous cycle and presence of sperm
• Plasma progesterone concentration—determine stage of estrous cycle; monitor success of luteolysis

IMAGING
Ultrasound—4–5 weeks after breeding to determine pregnancy; diagnostic test of choice for documenting pregnancy and uterine evacuation

OTHER DIAGNOSTIC PROCEDURES
N/A

 TREATMENT

• Discuss patient's future; if breeding is not a consideration, ovariohysterectomy may be best alternative.
• Inform client of all options, and come to a mutually agreeable treatment regimen.
• Inpatient—use of off-label drugs; monitor for side effects; if owner insists on taking patient home, wait at least 1 hr after each treatment before discharging the patient.
• Many mismated (accidentally mated) bitches do not become pregnant; therefore, treatment may not be necessary.
• Pregnancy status in early diestrus is unknown, because ultrasound confirmation of pregnancy is not possible until 4–5 weeks after breeding.
• Treat on day 6–10 of diestrus—treatment in midgestation is more unpleasant (more discharge and fetuses may pass) and may have a psychologic effect on the patient
• $PGF_{2\alpha}$ (Lutalyse) and bromocriptine (Parlodel)—100% success in a small study ($n = 15$) in suppressing progesterone concentration below basal concentration

ABORTION, TERMINATION OF PREGNANCY

MEDICATIONS

DRUGS OF CHOICE
• PFF$_{2\alpha}$—luteolytic; causes cervical dilation and intense uterine contractions; initiate on day 6 of diestrus; (250 µg/kg SC q12h for 5 days); perform ultrasound examination at day 28–30 diestrus; if patient is pregnant, repeat regimen on day 31–35.
• Bromocriptine mesylate (Parlodel)—a prolactin inhibitor; administer on day 31–35 of diestrus; 30 µg/kg PO q12h or 100 µg/kg PO q24h for 5–6 days; induces abortion
• PGF$_{2\alpha}$ (250 µg/kg SC q12h) and bromocriptine (10 µg/kg PO q12h)—combination produces excellent results; administered on day 6–10 of diestrus; feed patient 2 hr after morning treatment to reduce side effects (vomiting).
• Miferprestone (progesterone and glucocorticoid receptor antagonist) and Epostane (an inhibitor of steroid synthesis)—potentially useful; not currently available to veterinarians in North America

CONTRAINDICATIONS
• PGF$_{2\alpha}$—may increase blood pressure and cause bronchoconstriction in some species; do not use in patients with high blood pressure or asthma; do not attempt treatment with synthetic analogues (safe dosages not determined).
• Bromocriptine—some patients are sensitive to ergot alkaloids.
• Estrogens—may cause cystic endometrial hyperplasia, pyometra, and bone marrow suppression leading to pancytopenia

PRECAUTIONS
• PGF$_{2\alpha}$—side effects are dose-dependent; hyperpnea, hypersalivation, vomition, and loose stools; may note mild locomotor incoordination and slight CNS depression with high dosage (440 µg/kg) LD$_{50}$ 5mg/kg)
• Bromocriptine—minimal side effects; some vomiting; evacuation of uterus takes longer than with PGF$_{2\alpha}$

POSSIBLE INTERACTIONS
Bromocryptine—concomitant use of erythromycin may increase plasma concentration of bromocriptine

ALTERNATIVE DRUGS
N/A

FOLLOW-UP

PATIENT MONITORING
Uterine ultrasonography—confirm evacuation of uterine contents

POSSIBLE COMPLICATIONS
• May shorten interestrous interval (interval to next estrous cycle)
• Treatment with estrogenic compounds contraindicated

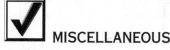

MISCELLANEOUS

ASSOCIATED CONDITIONS
N/A

AGE-RELATED FACTORS
N/A

ZOONOTIC POTENTIAL
N/A

PREGNANCY
N/A

SYNONYMS
Induced abortion

ABBREVIATIONS
• LH = luteinizing hormone
• PRL = prolactin
• PGF$_{2\alpha}$ = prostaglandin F$_{2\alpha}$

Suggested Reading

Braakman A, Okkens AC, van Haaften B. Medical methods to terminate pregnancy in the dog. Compend Contin Educ Pract Vet 1993;15:1505–1512.

Concannon PW, Verstegen J, Wanke P. Pregnancy termination in dogs and cats: use of prostaglandins, dopamine agonists, or Dexamethasone. Paper presented at the annual meeting of the Society of Theriogenology, 1997. Montreal, Canada, 240–244.

Olson PN, Johnston SD, Root MV, et al. Terminating pregnancy in dogs and cats. Annu Reprod Sci 1992;28:399–406.

Post K. Induced pregnancy termination in dogs. Paper presented at the annual meeting of the Society of Theriogenology, 1993. Jacksonville, Florida, pp. 215–221.

Author Klaas Post
Consulting Editor Sara K. Lyle

ACUTE ABDOMEN

 BASICS

DEFINITION
Characterized by historical and physical examination findings of a tense, painful abdomen; cardinal sign is acute abdominal pain; an acute abdominal presentation may be life-threatening and should be treated as an emergency.

PATHOPHYSIOLOGY
• A patient with an acute abdomen has pain associated with either distension of an organ, inflammation, traction on the mesentery or peritoneum, or ischemia. • The abdominal viscera are sparsely innervated, and diffuse involvement is often necessary to elicit pain; nerve endings also exist in the submucosa-muscularis of the bowel wall. • Any process that causes fluid or gaseous distension (i.e., intestinal obstruction, gastric dilatation-volvulus, ileus) may produce pain. • Inflammation produces abdominal pain by releasing vasoactive substances that directly stimulate nerve endings. • Many nerves exist in the peritoneum and are sensitive to a diffuse inflammatory response.

SYSTEMS AFFECTED
• Behavioral—trembling, inappetance, crying, lethargy or depression, and abnormal postural changes such as the praying position to achieve comfort • Cardiovascular—severe inflammation, ischemia, and sepsis may lead to acute circulatory collapse (shock). • Gastrointestinal—vomiting, diarrhea, inappetance, generalized functional ileus; pancreatic inflammation, necrosis, and abscesses may lead to cranial abdominal pain, vomiting, and ileus. • Hepatobiliary—jaundice associated with extrahepatic cholestasis from biliary obstructions (including pancreatitis) and bile peritonitis • Renal/Urologic—azotemia can be due to prerenal causes (dehydration, hypovolemia, and shock), renal causes (acute pyelonephritis and acute renal failure), and postrenal causes (urethral obstruction and uroperitoneum from bladder rupture). • Respiratory—increased respiratory rate due to pain or metabolic disturbances; possible aspiration pneumonia associated with vomiting

SIGNALMENT
• Dog and cat • Younger animals tend to have a higher incidence of trauma-related problems, intussusceptions, and acquired diet- and infection-related diseases; old animals have a greater frequency of malignancies. • Male cats and dogs are at higher risk for urethral obstruction. • Male dalmatians in particular have a higher risk of urethral obstruction because of the high incidence of urate urinary calculi. • German shepherds with pancreatic atrophy have a higher risk of mesenteric volvulus. • Patients treated with corticosteroids and nonsteroidal antiinflammatory drugs (NSAIDs) are at higher risk for gastrointestinal (GI) ulceration and perforation.

SIGNS

General Comments
Clinical signs vary greatly depending on the type and severity of the disease leading to an acute abdomen.

Historical Findings
• Trembling, reluctance to move, inappetance, vomiting, diarrhea, crying, and abnormal postures (tucked up or praying position)—signs that the owner may notice • Question owner carefully to ascertain what system is affected; for example, hematemesis with a history of NSAID treatment suggests GI ulceration.

Physical Examination Findings
• Abnormalities include abdominal pain, splinting of the abdominal musculature, gas- or fluid-filled abdominal organs, abdominal mass, ascites, pyrexia or hypothermia, tachycardia, and tachypnea. • Once abdominal pain is confirmed, attempt to localize the pain to cranial, middle, or caudal abdomen. • Perform a rectal examination to evaluate the colon, pelvic bones, urethra, and prostate, as well as the presence of melena. • Rule out extraabdominal causes of pain by careful palpation of the kidneys and thoracolumbar vertebrae. • Pain associated with intervertebral disk disease often causes referred abdominal splinting and is often mistaken for true abdominal pain.

CAUSES

Gastrointestinal
• Stomach—gastritis, ulcers, perforation, foreign bodies, gastric dilatation-volvulus • Intestine—obstruction (foreign bodies, intussusception, hernias), ulcers, perforations • Rupture after obstruction, ulceration, blunt or penetrating trauma or due to tumor growth • Vascular compromise from infarction, mesenteric volvulus, or torsion

Pancreas
• Pain associated with inflammation, abscess, ischemia, and tumors of the pancreas • Pancreatic masses or inflammation obstructing the biliary duct/papilla will cause jaundice.

Hepatic and Biliary System
• Rapid distension of the liver and its capsule can cause pain. • Gall bladder obstructions, ruptures, or necrosis may lead to bile leakage and peritonitis. • Hepatic abscess

Spleen
Splenic torsion, ruptured splenic masses, splenic abscess

Urinary Tract
• Distension is the main cause of pain in the urinary tract. • Lower urinary tract obstruction can be due to tumors of the trigone area of the bladder or urethra, urinary calculi, or granulomatous urethritis. • Traumatic ruptures of the ureters or bladder are associated with blunt trauma and increased intraabdominal pressure. • Urethral tears can be associated with pelvic fractures from acute trauma. • Free urine in the peritoneal cavity leads to a chemical peritonitis. • Acute pyelonephritis, acute renal failure, nephroliths, and ureteroliths are uncommon causes of acute abdomen.

Genital Tract
• Prostatitis and prostatic abscess, pyometra; a ruptured pyometra or prostatic abscess can cause endotoxemia, sepsis, and cardiovascular collapse. • Infrequent causes include ruptures of the gravid uterus after blunt abdominal trauma, uterine torsion, ovarian tumor or torsion, and intraabdominal testicular torsion (cryptorchid).

Abdominal Wall/Diaphragm
• Umbilical, inguinal, scrotal, abdominal, or peritoneal hernias with strangulated viscera • Trauma or congenital defects leading to organ displacement or entrapment in the hernia will lead to abdominal pain if the vascular supply of the organs involved becomes impaired or ischemic.

RISK FACTORS
• Exposure to NSAIDs or corticosteroid treatment—gastric, duodenal, or colonic ulcers • Garbage or inappropriate food ingestion—pancreatitis • Foreign body ingestion—intestinal obstructions • Abdominal trauma—hollow viscus rupture • Hernias—intestinal obstruction/strangulation

 DIAGNOSIS

DIFFERENTIAL DIAGNOSIS
• Renal associated pain, retroperitoneal pain, spinal or paraspinal pain, and disorders causing diffuse muscle pain may mimic abdominal pain; careful history and physical examination are essential in pursuing the appropriate problem. • Parvoviral enteritis can present similarly to intestinal obstructive disease; fecal parvoviral antigen assay and CBC (leukopenia) are helpful differentiating diagnostic tests.

CBC/BIOCHEMISTRY/URINALYSIS
• Inflammation or infection may be associated with leukocytosis or leukopenia. • Anemia may be seen with blood loss associated with GI ulceration. • Azotemia is associated with prerenal, renal, and postrenal causes. • Electrolyte abnormalities can help to evaluate GI disease (i.e., hypochloremic metabolic alkalosis with gastric outflow obstruction) and renal disease (i.e., hyperkalemia with acute renal failure or postrenal obstruction). • Hyperbilirubinemia and elevated hepatic enzymes help localize a problem to the liver or biliary tract. • Urine specific gravity (before fluid therapy) needed

to differentiate prerenal, renal, and postrenal problems. • Urine sediment may be helpful in acute renal failure, ethylene glycol intoxication, and pyelonephritis.

OTHER LABORATORY TESTS
Serum amylase, lipase, and trypsin-like immunoreactivity (TLI) can be useful in evaluating pancreatitis.

IMAGING

Abdominal Radiography
• May see abdominal masses or changes in shape or shifting of abdominal organs • Loss of abdominal detail with abdominal fluid accumulation is an indication for a peritoneal tap. • Free abdominal gas is consistent with a ruptured GI viscus or infection with gas-producing bacteria and is an indication for emergency surgery. • Use caution when evaluating postoperative radiographs; free gas is a normal finding for a few days postoperatively. • Ileus is a consistent sign with peritonitis. • Contrast in the area of the pancreas can be lost with pancreatic inflammation. • Foreign bodies may be radiopaque. • Characterize ileus as functional (due to metabolic or infectious causes) or mechanical (due to obstruction). • Upper GI barium contrast radiographs are useful in evaluating the GI tract, particularly for determination of GI obstruction. • Ingested radiopaque markers can also be useful for determination of obstruction.

Abdominal Ultrasound
• One of the most sensitive diagnostic tools available for the detection of abdominal masses, abdominal fluid, abscesses, cysts, lymphadenopathy, and biliary or urinary calculi • Like radiography, this can be extremely useful for differentiating medical and surgical acute abdomens.

DIAGNOSTIC PROCEDURES

Abdominocentesis/Abdominal Fluid Analysis
• Perform abdominocentesis on all patients presenting with acute abdomen. Fluid can often be obtained for diagnostic evaluation even when only a small amount of free abdominal fluid exists, well before detectable radiographic sensitivity. Although ultrasonography is much more sensitive than radiography for the detection of fluid, the lack of such detection does not preclude abdominocentesis. Abdominal fluid analysis with elevated WBC count, degenerate neutrophils, and intracellular bacteria is consistent with septic peritonitis and is an indication for emergency surgery. • Pancreatitis patients may have an abdominal effusion characterized as a nonseptic (sterile) peritonitis. Amylase and lipase determinations in abdominal fluid also help with this diagnosis and may avoid potentially unnecessary surgery. • Creatinine concentration higher in abdominal fluid than in serum indicates urinary tract leakage. • Similarly, higher bilirubin concentration in

abdominal fluid than in serum indicates bile peritonitis.

Sedation and Abdominal Palpation
Because of abdominal splinting associated with pain, a thorough abdominal palpation is often not possible without sedation; this is particularly useful for detecting intestinal foreign bodies that do not appear on survey radiographs.

Exploratory Laparotomy
Surgery may be useful diagnostically (as well as therapeutically) when ultrasonography is not available or when no definitive cause of the acute abdomen has been established with appropriate diagnostics.

 TREATMENT
Inpatient management with supportive care until decision about whether the problem is to be treated medically or surgically.

Supportive Care
• Keep patient NPO if vomiting, until a definitive cause is determined and addressed. • Intravenous fluid therapy is usually required because of the large fluid loss associated with an acute abdomen; the goal is to restore the normal circulating blood volume. • If severe circulatory compromise (shock) exists, supplement initially with isotonic crystalloid fluids (90 mL/kg, dogs; 70 mL/kg, cats) over 1–2 h; hypertonic fluids or colloids may also be beneficial. • Evaluate hydration and electrolytes (with appropriate treatment adjustments) frequently after commencement of treatment.

Surgical Considerations
• Many different causes of an acute abdomen (with both medical and surgical treatments) exist; make a definitive diagnosis whenever possible prior to surgical intervention. • This can prevent both potentially unnecessary and expensive surgical procedure and associated morbidity and mortality. • It will also allow the surgeon to prepare for the task and to educate the owner on the prognosis and costs involved.

 MEDICATIONS

DRUGS OF CHOICE

Corticosteroids (Soluble Glucocorticoids)
• When indicated for shock treatment; limit to single doses to avoid adverse effects on the GI tract • Dexamethasone sodium phosphate 2–4 mg/kg IV or prednisolone sodium succinate 15–30 mg/kg IV

Histamine H₂ Antagonists
• Reduce gastric acid production. • Cimetidine 5–10 mg/kg IV q8h or ranitidine 0.5–1 mg/kg IV q12h

Sucralfate
• Gastric mucosal protectant • 0.25–1 g PO q8h

Metoclopramide
Antiemetic as needed, 0.2–0.4 mg/kg IV q6–8h (or 24h continuous rate infusion)

Antibiotics
• Broad spectrum for gram-positive, gram-negative, and anaerobic bacteria • Gram stain and cultures prior to treatment if possible

CONTRAINDICATIONS
Do not use metoclopramide if GI obstruction is suspected.

PRECAUTIONS
Gentamicin and most NSAIDs can be nephrotoxic and should be used with caution in hypovolemic patients and those with renal impairment.

 FOLLOW-UP

PATIENT MONITORING
Patients usually require intensive medical care and frequent evaluation of physical examination and laboratory parameters.

 MISCELLANEOUS

SYNONYMS
Colic

SEE ALSO
• Gastric Dilatation • Volvulus Syndrome • Gastroduodenal Ulcer Disease • Gastrointestinal Obstruction • Intussusception • Pancreatitis • Prostatitis and Prostatic Abscess • Urinary Tract Obstruction

Suggested Reading
Bjorling DE. Acute abdomen syndrome. In: Morgan RV, ed. Handbook of small animal practice. New York: Churchill Livingstone, 1992:483–487.
Bjorling DE, Latimer KS, Rawlings CA, et al. Diagnostic peritoneal lavage before and after abdominal surgery in dogs. Am J Vet Res 1983;44:816–819.
Cowan LA. Abdominal pain. In: Lorenz MD, Cornelius LM, eds. Small animal medical diagnosis. Philadelphia: Lippincott, 1987: 291–298.
Crowe DT, Crane SW. Diagnostic abdominal paracentesis and lavage in the evaluation of abdominal injuries in dogs and cats: Clinical and experimental investigations. J Am Vet Med Assoc 1976;168:700–705.
Strombeck DR, Guilford WG. Small animal gastroenterology. 2nd ed. Davis, CA: Stonegate Publishing, 1990:81–86.
Author Juan Carlos Sardinas
Consulting Editors Brett M. Feder and Mitchell A. Crystal

AGGRESSION—CATS

 BASICS

DEFINITION
• Can be adaptive and appropriate if it helps the animal protect itself, its resources, or its present or future genetic contribution
• Behavioral medicine—concerned with recognizing when behavior is maladaptive or abnormal

Aggression Owing to Lack of Socialization
• No human contact before 3 months of age—cat misses sensitive period important for development of normal approach responses to people; if not handled until 14 weeks of age, it is fearful and aggressive to people; if handled for only 5 min/day until 7 weeks, it interacts with people, approaches inanimate objects, and plays with toys.
• Lack of social interaction with other cats—may result in lack of normal inquisitive response to other cats; negative response may be augmented by suboptimal nutritional conditions for the pregnant queen.
• These cats are never normal, cuddly pets; may eventually attach to one person or a small group of people; if forced into a situation involving restraint, confinement, or intimate contact, may become extremely aggressive

Play Aggression
• Weaned early and hand-raised by humans—cat may never learn to temper play responses; if not taught as a kitten to modulate responses, it may not learn to sheathe claws or inhibit bite; bottle-fed cats overrepresented
• Social play—peaks early; replaced by predatory activities by weeks 10–12 and social fighting by week 14

Fearful, Fear, or Fear-induced Aggression
• Fearful—cat may hiss, spit, arch the back, and piloerect if flight is not possible; combination of offensive and defensive postures and overt and covert aggressive behaviors are usually involved.
• Flight—virtually always a component of fearful aggression
• Pursued—if cornered, cat will stop, draw its head in, crouch, growl, roll on its back when approached (not submissive but overtly defensive), and paw at the approacher; if pursuit is continued, cat will strike then hold the approacher with its forepaws while kicking with the back feet and biting.
• If threatened, cat will defend itself; any cat can become fearfully aggressive.

Pain Aggression
Pain may cause aggression; with extended painful treatment, cat may exhibit fearful aggression.

Intercat Aggression
• Male–male aggression associated with mating or hierarchical status within the social group; mating may also involve social hierarchy issues.
• Maturity—in peaceful multicat households, problems may occur, regardless of sex composition, when a cat reaches social maturity (2–4 years of age).

Maternal Aggression
• May occur in the periparturient period
• Protection—queens may guard nesting areas and kittens by threatening with long approach distances, rather than attack; usually directed toward unfamiliar individuals; may inappropriately be directed toward known individuals; as kittens mature, aggression resolves.
• Unknown if kittens learn aggressive behavior from an aggressive mother

Predatory Aggression
• Occurs under different behavioral circumstances
• Normal predatory behavior—develops at 5–7 weeks of age; cat may be proficient hunter by 14 weeks; commonly displayed with field voles, house mice, and birds at feeders; more common in cats that have to fend for themselves; if well fed, cat may kill and only behead prey.
• Aggression—stealth, silence, heightened attentiveness, body posture associated with hunting (slinking, head lowering, tail twitching, and pounce postures), lunging or springing at prey, exhibiting sudden movement after a quiet period
• Free-ranging groups—when a new male enters, he may kill kittens to encourage queen to come into estrus.
• Inappropriate context distinctions about prey—potentially dangerous if "prey" is a foot, hand, or infant; cats exhibiting pre-pounce behaviors in these contexts are at risk.

Territorial Aggression
• May be exhibited toward other cats, dogs, or people; owing to transitive nature of social hierarchies, a cat aggressive to one housemate may not be to another.
• Turf may be delineated by patrol, chin rubbing, spraying, or nonspraying marking; threats and/or fight may occur if a perceived offender enters the area; if the struggle involves social hierarchy, the challenger may be sought out and attacked after the territory is invaded.
• May be difficult to treat, particularly if there is marking; marking problems suggest a possible underlying aggression.

Redirected Aggression
• Difficult to recognize and may be reported as incidental to another form of aggression
• Occurs when a motor pattern appropriate for a specific motivational state is redirected to an accessible target, because the primary target is unavailable (e.g., interruption of an aggressive event between two parties by a third party results in redirection of the aggressive behavior to the third party or to an uninvolved individual); cat may remain reactive for some time after being thwarted in an aggressive interaction.
• Often precipitated by another inappropriate behavior; important to treat that behavior as well

Assertion or Status-Related Aggression
• If unprovoked, most frequently occurs when being petted; a need to control when attention starts and ceases; cat may bite and leave or may take hand in teeth but not bite.
• May be accompanied by territorial aggression

Idiopathic Aggression
Rare; poorly understood and poorly defined; unprovoked, unpredictable, toggle-switch aggression

SYSTEMS AFFECTED
• Cardiovascular—signs consistent with sympathetic stimulation
• Endocrine/Metabolic—signs consistent with alterations in the HPA axis
• Hemic—stress leukogram
• Musculoskeletal—damage to teeth and gums, abscesses, abrasions, and lacerations common
• Nervous—increased motor activity, repetitive activity, trembling, and increased reactivity may accompany or follow outbursts of aggression
• Renal/Urologic—urine marking (spraying and nonspraying)
• Respiratory—tachypnea and the attendant metabolic changes possible in extreme situations
• Skin/Exocrine—skin lesions usually secondary and may result from injury; if consistently stressed by aggressive situations, may cease to groom

SIGNALMENT
• No breed differences, except for those resulting from a lack of socialization and play
• Appears at onset of social maturity (2–4 years)
• Males—may be more prone to intercat aggression

SIGNS

General Comments
Elimination behaviors—tightly coupled with aggression; take a thorough behavioral and medial history.

Historical Findings
Abuse—cat may learn aggression as a pre-emptive strategy.

Physical Examination Findings
• Usually nonremarkable except for injuries and a lack of condition associated with increased motor activity and withdrawal

• Continuous anxiety—decreased grooming

CAUSES
Part of the normal feline behavior; greatly influenced by the early socialization history, sex, social context, handling, and many other variables

RISK FACTORS
N/A

DIAGNOSIS

DIFFERENTIAL DIAGNOSIS
• Conditions that cause similar behavioral changes—seizures; brain disease; metabolic disease (thyroid or adrenal conditions)
• Hepatic encephalopathy
• Feline ischemic encephalopathy
• Lead poisoning
• Hyperthyroidism
• Epilepsy
• Rabies
• Behavioral aggression is usually directed; aggression from organic disease is unexpected, inappropriate, and more continuous.

CBC/BIOCHEMISTRY/URINALYSIS
• All should be performed.
• Urinalysis—relationship between aggression and elimination disorders

OTHER LABORATORY TESTS
• Hyperthyroidism—test, if indicated
• Urine culture and sensitivity—may be indicated when unexplained aggression correlates with urinary tract disease

IMAGING
CT and MRI—rule out structural brain disease.

DIAGNOSTIC PROCEDURES
• ECG—evaluate for arrhythmia or base line before treatment.
• CSF analysis—rule out inflammatory brain disease.

TREATMENT
• Avoid provocation.
• Teach client to observe signs (tail flicking, ears flat, pupils dilated, head hunched, claws possibly unsheathed, stillness or tenseness, low growl) and interrupt the behavior by letting the cat fall from his or her lap, abandoning it, and refusing to interact until appropriate behavior is displayed.
• Discourage direct physical correction; may intensify aggression
• Separate cats; keep the active aggressor in a less favored area to passively reinforce more desirable behavior.
• Desensitization, counterconditioning, flooding, and habituation—if subtleties of

social systems and communication are understood

MEDICATIONS

DRUGS OF CHOICE
• Antianxiety medications that increase CNS levels of serotonin—tricyclic antidepressants and selective serotonin reuptake inhibitors
• Amitriptyline—2.5–5.0 mg/cat (to start) PO q12h for 30 days
• Imipramine—2.5–5.0 mg/cat (to start) PO q12h for 30 days
• Buspirone—2.5–10 mg/cat/day; may make some cats more assertive; thus works well for anxiety-associated aggression
• Clomipramine—0.5 mg/kg PO q24h for 30 days
• Fluoxetine—0.5 mg/kg PO q24h for 30 days
• Buspirone, clomipramine, and fluoxetine—may take 3–5 weeks to be effective; best for active, overt aggressions
• Nortriptyline—active intermediate metabolite of amitriptyline; use instead of amitriptyline or imipramine, at the same dosage, if side effects appear.
• Anxious and fearful aggression with concomitant elimination disorders—diazepam (0.2–0.4 mg/kg PO as needed) or other benzodiazepine; use with caution because benzodiazepines facilitate and worsen inhibited aggressions.
• Some behaviors may be seizure activity and may respond to sedative or antiepileptic medications.

CONTRAINDICATIONS
• Cats experience more drug-related side effects than do dogs.
• Hepatic and renal compromise—some drugs contraindicated
• Cardiac conduction anomalies—give tricyclic antidepressants only with extreme caution and monitoring.
• Fat or pre-existing hepatic disease—may develop idiosyncratic, diazepam-induced hepatotoxicity

PRECAUTIONS
• Use of the listed medications is extra-label; Health and Human Services recommendations should be followed.
• Tricyclic antidepressants—overdoses can cause profound cardiac conduction disturbances; ECG evaluation before treatment is advised.

POSSIBLE INTERACTIONS
• Benzodiazepines—lipophilic; may be potentiated by other lipophilic drugs; if combination treatment is warranted, use lower dosages.
• Medications that impair the glucuronidation of active metabolites into

inactive compounds cause increases of the active metabolites.

FOLLOW-UP

PATIENT MONITORING
• CBC, serum biochemistry, and urinalysis—before treatment; semiannually in older patients; yearly in younger patients if treatment is continuous; adjust dosages accordingly.
• As warranted by clinical signs—vomiting; gastrointestinal distress; tachycardia, tachypnea

POSSIBLE COMPLICATIONS
• Early treatment using both behavioral modification and pharmacological intervention crucial
• Left untreated, these disorders always progress.

MISCELLANEOUS

ASSOCIATED CONDITIONS
Many occur with elimination disorders—substrate and location aversions and preferences; particularly, spraying and nonspraying marking

AGE-RELATED FACTORS
Social maturity—associated with development of intercat aggression, fear aggression, territorial aggression, redirected aggression, and status-related aggression

ZOONOTIC POTENTIAL
• Cat scratch disease (*Bartonella henselae* and *Afipia felis*)
• Rabies

PREGNANCY
Listed medications—avoid use of most in pregnant animals.

ABBREVIATIONS
CSF = cerebrospinal fluid
HPA = hypothalamic–pituitary–adrenal

Suggested Reading
Chapman BL. Feline aggression: classification, diagnosis, and treatment. Vet Clin North Am Small Anim Pract 1991;21:315–328.
Overall KL. Feline aggression. Part III: The role of social status in hierarchical systems. Feline Pract 1994;22:16–17.
Overall KL. Understanding the interactions between feline aggression and elimination disorders. Paper presented at the North American Veterinary Conference, 1994.
Author Karen L. Overall
Consulting Editor Joane M. Parent

AGGRESSION—DOGS

BASICS

DEFINITION
• Action by one dog directed against another organism with the result of harming, limiting, or depriving that organism; offensive, defensive, or predatory • Offensive—unprovoked attempt to gain some resource at the expense of another; includes dominance, intermale, and interfemale aggression • Defensive—by a victim toward another that is perceived as an instigator or threat; includes fear-induced, territorial defense, protective, irritable (pain-associated or frustration-related), and parental aggression

PATHOPHYSIOLOGY
• Not necessarily a pathologic condition • Rage—inappropriate offensive aggression; reported to be associated with biochemical abnormalities in the CSF • Some pathologic states are associated with an increase in aggression because of their effects on the CNS.

SYSTEMS AFFECTED
Nervous

SIGNALMENT
• Any age, sex, or breed • Cocker spaniels, springer spaniels, and German shepherds—most common; regional differences exist • Pit bulls, German shepherds, huskies, malamutes, Doberman pinschers, and rottweilers—associated with fatal dog bites • Dominance-related offensive aggression—escalates as dog approaches social maturity (1–2 years of age) • Males—intact or castrated; more common

SIGNS

General Comments
• Expressed by behavioral signs—staring; postures; growls; baring the teeth; snapping; frank attack • History—forms the basis for risk analysis and details of the treatment program; important questions: When were signs of aggression first noted? How often does the aggression occur? Against whom is the aggression directed? Under what circumstances does the aggression occur?

Historical Findings
Vary according to the situation and the functional type of aggression
Dominance-related Aggression
• Directed toward household members • Head up; tail up; staring; stiff gait • Resents—being reached out to, patted on head, and pushed off favored sleeping sites; having its food approached
Intermale and Interfemale Aggression
• Directed toward other dogs • Directed toward humans only when they interfere with fights • Head up; tail up; staring; stiff gait
Fear-Induced Aggression
• Directed to approaching or reaching humans

• Certain familiar people may be exempt • Head down; eyes wide; tail tucked
Territorial Aggression
• Directed toward strangers approaching house, yard, or car • May be exacerbated if restrained • Barking; agitation; rushing forward; baring teeth
Protective Aggression
• Directed toward stranger approaching owner • Escalates with decreasing distance
Irritable (Pain, Frustration) Aggression
• Restricted to specific context associated with pain (e.g., nail trim, injection) • Rule out dominance-related and fear-induced aggression.
Parental (Maternal) Aggression
• Directed toward individuals approaching the whelping area or puppies • Severity usually inversely related to age of puppies

Physical Examination Findings
• Usually unremarkable • Use extreme care when handling aggressive dogs; use muzzles and other restraints to prevent injury to the examiner. • Dominance-related, fear-related aggression, or irritable aggression—may be evident during the examination • Neurologic examination—abnormalities may suggest an organic disease process (e.g., rabies).

CAUSES
• Part of the normal range of behavior; strongly influenced by breed, sex, early socialization, handling, and other variables • Manifestation of an organic condition—possible but rare • In all cases, rule out medical causes of aggression.

RISK FACTORS
• Poor socialization to certain types of stimuli (e.g., children)—adult dog may display fear-related aggression • Predisposing environmental conditions—associating with other dogs in a pack; barrier frustration or tethering; cruel handling and abuse; and dog baiting and fighting

DIAGNOSIS

DIFFERENTIAL DIAGNOSIS
Pathologic conditions associated with aggression must be identified before a purely behavioral diagnosis can be made.

CBC/BIOCHEMISTRY/URINALYSIS
• Usually normal • Abnormalities—may suggest metabolic or endocrine causes

OTHER LABORATORY TESTS
As indicated (e.g., thyroid panel or ACTH-stimulation test)

IMAGING
• May be indicated to identify sources of pain

• MRI or CT—if cerebral neoplasia suspected

DIAGNOSTIC PROCEDURES
Postmortem fluorescent antibody test—any aggressive dog for which rabies is a differential diagnosis

RISK ASSESSMENT

General Comments
• Importance in cases of aggression cannot be overemphasized • Considered a separate procedure; perform before initiating treatment • Consists of historical questions, observation, and confirmation with supporting data (medical, legal, veterinary records)

Questions
• Has the dog ever broken the skin or otherwise injured a person? If yes, how many times in the past year? • Has anyone sought medical attention for injuries caused by this dog? If yes, describe the circumstances in detail. • Have the injuries by this dog been reported to authorities, resulting in quarantine or citation? If yes, describe. • Is the weight of this dog > 18.2 kg? • Are there children, elderly people, or others at high risk in this household? • Is there any doubt that this dog must be restrained behind a fence, on a leash, fitted with a muzzle, or in other ways effectively controlled by the owner to protect people from injury? • Does this dog ever run free, without being under the owner's strict control? • Does aggression appear to occur unpredictably? • If the owner responds yes to any of these questions, consider the personal and legal liability risks to the owner and the treating veterinarian.

TREATMENT
• The first tenet of management is to prevent human injury. • Euthanasia—appropriate solution in cases of vicious dogs; offer as the only safe solution. • Risk assessment may help the owner objectively evaluate the situation; all parties must understand that aggressive dogs are never cured, although sometimes the behavior can be managed • Recommend techniques to reduce human risk from the aggressive dog until the owner seeks treatment. • Management success—combination of multiple modalities: environmental control, behavior modification, and pharmacotherapy

Dominance-related Aggression
• Environmental—use barriers and restraint to prevent human injury.

- Devices—train the dog to a muzzle and head halter.
- Behavior modification, step 1—withdraw all attention from the dog for 2 weeks; list situations in which aggression occurs; devise a method of avoiding each situation; daily, list all aggressive incidents and circumstances to avoid in the future.
- Behavior modification, step 2—use nonconfrontational means to establish the owner's dominance; teach the dog to reliably sit/stay on command in gradually more challenging situations (dog must acquiesce to the owner to obtain attention and other benefits); no free benefits (dog must sit/stay before eating, being petted, going for walk, etc.; the owner initiates all interactions)
- Behavior modification, step 3—gain greater control; situations that previously elicited aggression are gradually introduced with the dog controlled in a sit/stay position (muzzle if necessary).
- Surgery—neuter

Intermale and Interfemale Aggression
- Environmental—use barriers to prevent contact between the dogs except when well supervised; note dominance order between dogs; if apparent, comply with dogs' rules (dominant dog is fed first, travels through doorways first, etc.).
- Devices—head halter, muzzle
- Behavior modification, step 1—owner must withdraw all attention to both dogs; teach sit/stay program (as for dominance-related aggression).
- Behavior modification, step 2—desensitize or countercondition by gradually decreasing distance between dogs while under leash control; reinforce acceptable behavior.
- Surgery—neuter males; OHE recommended only if aggression is associated with heat cycle (otherwise it will not improve behavior)

FEAR-INDUCED AGGRESSION
- Environmental—use barriers and restraint to prevent human injury.
- Devices—muzzle
- Behavior modification, step 1—list all situations in which the dog appears fearful or exhibits aggression; avoid those situations initially; teach dog basic obedience commands and reinforce under nonfearful conditions (generalize by training in many locations).
- Behavior modification, step 2—desensitize and countercondition; subject the dog to mildly fearful conditions with the stimulus (e.g., a stranger) far away; keep the dog attentive and performing obedience commands; gradually decrease the distance of the stranger; if the dog exhibits fear, the stranger should withdraw and work should continue at an easier level, then gradually progress.
- Surgery—castration or OHE probably will not improve the behavior.

Territorial Aggression
- Environmental—use barriers and restraint to prevent human injury; initially, when visitors come, isolate the dog to prevent it from exhibiting the behavior
- Devices—head halter, muzzle
- Behavior modification, step 1—teach the dog sit/stay, first at neutral locations, then near the door and at other sites of territorial aggression; later, control the dog while a familiar person approaches; reward the dog for calm, obedient behavior.
- Behavior modification, step 2—gradually introduce strangers (owner can dress in unfamiliar garb to represent a stranger); increase the difficulty until the dog is under control; move the exercises to the door; add entering the door, ringing the door bell, and other variables.
- Surgery—castration or OHE probably will not improve behavior.

MEDICATIONS

DRUGS OF CHOICE
- None approved by the FDA for the treatment of aggression
- Inform the client of the experimental nature of these treatments and the risk involved; document discussion in the medical record.
- Azaperone—buspirone hydrochloride at 2.5–10 mg/dog q8–12h; side effects: GI signs
- Tricyclic antidepressants—amitriptyline at 2.2–4.4 mg/kg q12–24h, side effects: sedation, anticholinergic effects; clomipramine at 1–3 mg/kg q12–24h, side effects: sedation, anticholinergic effects, cardiac conduction disturbances if predisposed; imipramine at 2.2–4.4 mg/kg q12–24h, side effects: sedation, anticholinergic effects
- Selective serotonin reuptake inhibitor—fluoxetine at 1 mg/kg q24h; side effects: inappetence, irritability

CONTRAINDICATIONS
Tricyclic antidepressants—contraindicated in patients with cardiac conduction disturbances, glaucoma, and fecal or urinary incontinence

PRECAUTIONS

Benzodiazepines (e.g., Diazepam)
- Use with caution for fear-induced aggression.
- These drugs can reduce fear but also may reduce fear-based inhibition.
- Dogs can become more aggressive when they lose their fear of the repercussions of biting.

POSSIBLE INTERACTIONS
Do not use listed drugs with monoamine oxidase inhibitors, including amitraz.

ALTERNATIVE DRUGS
Megestrol acetate—1 mg/kg PO q24h for 2 weeks; then taper to lowest effective dosage;

successful with dominance-related and intermale aggression; side effects: obesity, blood dyscrasias, pyometra, polyuria/polydipsia, diabetes mellitus, mammary hyperplasia, and carcinoma

FOLLOW-UP

PATIENT MONITORING
- Weekly to biweekly contact—recommended in the initial phases • Clients frequently need feedback and assistance with behavior modification plans and medication management.

PREVENTION/AVOIDANCE N/A

EXPECTED COURSE AND PROGNOSIS
Aggressive dogs are never cured, although sometimes the behavior can be managed.

POSSIBLE COMPLICATIONS
- Human injury • Dominance aggression—can be directed toward owners • Interdog aggression—humans often seriously injured when interfering with fighting dogs, either by accident or by redirected or irritable aggression; owners should not reach for fighting dogs; spray with water or push apart with a broom or a sturdy partition.

MISCELLANEOUS

ASSOCIATED CONDITIONS N/A

AGE-RELATED FACTORS
Adult-onset aggression—in the absence of any positive historical findings, suggests a medical cause; carefully evaluate sources of pain and sensory acuity.

ZOONOTIC POTENTIAL
Rabies is a potential cause of aggression.

PREGNANCY
Tricyclic antidepressants—contraindicated in pregnant animals

ABBREVIATIONS
- CSF = cerebrospinal fluid • OHE = ovariohysterectomy

Suggested Reading
Landsberg G, Hunthausen W, Ackerman L. Canine aggression. In: Handbook of behaviour problems of the dog and cat. Oxford, UK: Butterworth-Heinemann, 1997:129–150.
Simpson BS, Simpson DM. Behavioral pharmacotherapy. In: Borchelt P, Voith V, eds. Readings in companion animal behavior. Trenton, NJ: Veterinary Learning Systems, 1996:100–115.
Author Barbara S. Simpson
Consulting Editor Joane M. Parent

ALOPECIA—CATS

 BASICS

DEFINITION
• Common problem
• Pattern of hair loss—varied or symmetrical
• Causes—multifactorial

PATHOPHYSIOLOGY
Specific and unique for each cause

SYSTEMS AFFECTED
• Skin/Exocrine and associated adnexa
• Endocrine/Metabolic

SIGNALMENT
• No specific age, breed, or sex predilection
• Neoplastic and paraneoplastic associated alopecias—generally recognized in old cats

SIGNS
N/A

CAUSES
• Neurologic/behavioral—obsessive compulsive disorder
• Endocrine—sex hormone alopecia, hyper-thyroidism, hyperadrenocorticism, diabetes mellitus
• Immunologic—allergic dermatitis, alopecia areata
• Parasitic—demodicosis, dermatophytosis
• Physiologic—sebaceous adenitis
• Neoplastic—paraneoplastic dermatitis, squamous cell carcinoma in situ, epidermotropic lymphoma
• Idiopathic/inherited—alopecia universalis, hypotrichosis, spontaneous pinnal alopecia, anagen and telogen defluxion

RISK FACTORS
FeLV/FIV—for demodicosis

 DIAGNOSIS

DIFFERENTIAL DIAGNOSIS

Endocrine Alopecia/Sex Hormone
• Rarely a hormonal abnormality
• Rare hormonal cases—primarily castrated males; alopecia along the caudal aspect of the hindlimbs, which may extend along the perineum

Obsessive Compulsive Disorder
• Often misdiagnosed as endocrine
• The pattern of alopecia is frequently symmetrical with no associated inflammation.

Allergic Dermatitis
• Varies from mild partial alopecia with little inflammation to severe excoriation and ulceration
• Distribution—varied; often the head and neck region are most severely affected.
• Food allergy and inhalant/percutaneous causes

Hyperthyroidism
• Partial to complete alopecia from self-barbering
• Varied pattern
• Middle-aged to old cats
• Often mistaken for allergic dermatoses, obsessive compulsive disorder, or hormonal

Diabetes Mellitus
• Partial alopecia with an unkempt hair coat
• Poor wound healing
• Increased susceptibility to infections
• Cutaneous xanthomatosis secondary to hyperlipidemia (nodular to linear, yellow-pink alopecic plaques that tend to ulcerate)

Hyperadrenocorticism
• Rare; characterized by alopecia and extreme fragility of the skin
• Truncal alopecia, with or without a rattail and a curling of the pinnal tips
• Extreme skin fragility noted in approximately 70%
• Occurs secondary to pituitary or adrenal tumors
• Iatrogenic form less common in cats than in dogs

Paraneoplastic Alopecia
• Most cases associated with pancreatic exocrine adenocarcinomas
• Middle-aged to old cats (9–16 years)
• Acute onset
• Progresses rapidly
• Bilaterally symmetrical, ventrally distributed (also located along the bridge of the nose and periocular)
• Hair epilates in clumps
• Rare pruritus
• Erythema with dry fissuring footpads
• Glistening appearance to the alopecic skin
• Skin is thin and hypotonic.
• Rapid weight loss

Sebaceous Adenitis
• Slowly progressive partial alopecia associated with scaling along the dorsum of the body and the extremities

• Sebaceous glands are selectively destroyed by toxic intermediate metabolites or immunologic mechanisms.
• Possible dramatic pigment accumulation along the eyelid margins
• Questionable association with systemic disease (e.g., inflammatory bowel disease, lupus-like syndromes, upper respiratory tract infections)

Squamous Cell Carcinoma In Situ
• Multicentric premalignant dermatosis in old cats
• Slightly elevated, plaque-like or papillated lesions with scaling and partially alopecic surfaces
• Often misdiagnosed as seborrhea
• About 25% may convert to squamous cell carcinoma with in situ lesions along the borders (histologically).

Epidermotrophic Lymphoma
• Early stages—varying degrees of alopecia associated with scaling and erythema
• Later stages—plaques and nodules
• Old cats

Alopecia Areata
Rare, complete alopecia in a patchy distribution with no inflammation

Alopecia Universalis (Sphinx Cat)
• Hereditary
• Complete absence of primary hairs; decreased secondary hairs
• Thickened epidermis; normal dermis
• Sebaceous and apocrine ducts open directly onto the skin surface; oily feel to skin
• Wrinkled foreheads; gold eyes; no whiskers; downy fur on paws, tip of tail, and scrotum

Feline Hypotrichosis
• Siamese and Devon Rex cats (autosomal recessive alopecia)
• Poorly developed primary telogen hair follicles
• Born with a normal coat; thin and sparse by young adult

Spontaneous Pinnal Alopecia
• Siamese cats predisposed
• May represent form of alopecia areata or pattern baldness

Anagen and Telogen Defluxion
• Acute loss of hair owing to interference with the growth cycle
• Causes—stress, infection, endocrine disorder, metabolic disorder, fever, surgery, anesthesia, pregnancy, drug therapy

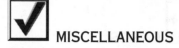

Demodicosis
• Rare; unlike dogs
• Partial to complete multifocal alopecia of the eyelids, periocular region, head, and neck
• Variable pruritus with erythema, scale, and crust, and ceruminous otitis externa
• *Demodex cati* (elongated shape) often associated with metabolic disease (e.g., FIV, systemic lupus erythematosus, diabetes mellitus)
• Unnamed short/blunted *Demodex* mite is rarely a marker for metabolic disease, this form may be transferable from cat to cat and has been associated with pruritus

Dermatophytosis
Numerous clinical manifestations; always associated with alopecia of some degree

CBC/BIOCHEMISTRY/URINALYSIS
Abnormalities may be noted with diabetes mellitus, hyperadrenocorticism, and hyperthyroidism.

OTHER LABORATORY TESTS
• FeLV and FIV—risk factors for demodicosis
• Thyroid hormones—document hyperthyroidism
• ANA titer—look for lupus-like syndromes
• ACTH-response test, LDDST, and HDDST—diagnose hyperadrenocorticism

IMAGING
• Abdominal ultrasound—assess adrenals in hyperadrenocorticism and look for cancer in animals with paraneoplastic syndrome
• CT scan—look for pituitary tumors in animals with hyperadrenocorticism

DIAGNOSTIC PROCEDURES
• Skin biopsy
• Skin scraping
• Fungal culture
• T-shirts to prove self-trauma
• Food elimination trials
• Intradermal skin testing

TREATMENT
• Therapy is limited for many of these disorders.
• Behavioral modification or application of a T-shirt may help prevent self-barbering.
• Removal of an offending dietary item may alleviate the symptoms of food allergy.
• If the pet is compliant, shampoo and topical therapy may help secondary problems, such as hyperkeratosis in sebaceous adenitis, crusting in demodicosis, secondary bacterial infections, and malodor for greasy conditions.

MEDICATIONS
DRUGS OF CHOICE
• Obsessive compulsive disorder—amitriptyline (10 mg/cat/day for a 21-day trial)
• Endocrine alopecia (males)—testosterone supplementation
• Allergic dermatitis—antihistamines, diet, corticosteroids, hyposensitization vaccine
• Hyperthyroidism—oral medications such as methimazole (tapazole) or radioactive iodine therapy
• Diabetes mellitus—regulation of glucose levels (insulin)
• Hyperadrenocorticism—surgery; no known effective medical therapy
• Paraneoplastic alopecia—no therapy; often fatal
• Epidermotropic lymphoma—retinoids (isotretinoin), corticosteroids, interferon
• Sebaceous adenitis—retinoids, corticosteroids
• Squamous cell carcinoma in situ—surgical excision, retinoids (topical and oral)
• Alopecia areata—no therapy; possibly counterirritants
• Demodicosis—lime sulfur dips at weekly intervals for 4–6 dips; Mitaban and ivermectin have been tried with variable success (dose and frequency of application are questionable)
• Dermatophytosis—griseofulvin (**CAUTION:** idiosyncratic toxicity), ketoconazole, itraconazole (best choice)

CONTRAINDICATIONS
N/A

PRECAUTIONS
Toxicity with griseofulvin (see Dermatophytosis)

POSSIBLE INTERACTIONS
N/A

ALTERNATIVE DRUGS
N/A

FOLLOW-UP
PATIENT MONITORING
Depends on specific diagnosis

PREVENTION/AVOIDANCE
Depends on specific diagnosis

POSSIBLE COMPLICATIONS
Depends on specific diagnosis

EXPECTED COURSE AND PROGNOSIS
Depends on specific diagnosis

MISCELLANEOUS
ASSOCIATED CONDITIONS
N/A

AGE-RELATED FACTORS
N/A

ZOONOTIC POTENTIAL
Dermatophytosis—can cause skin lesions in humans

PREGNANCY
Retinoids and griseofulvin should not be administered to pregnant animals

SYNONYMS
N/A

SEE ALSO
• Demodicosis
• Dermatophytosis
• Diabetes Mellitus, Uncomplicated
• Epidermotropic Lymphoma
• Feline Paraneoplastic Syndrome
• Hyperthyroidism
• Sebaceous Adenitis

ABBREVIATIONS
• ANA = antinuclear antibody
• FeLV = feline leukemia virus
• FIV = feline immunodeficiency virus
• HDDST = high-dose dexamethasone-suppression test
• LDDST = low-dose dexamethasone-suppression test

Suggested Reading
Baer KE, Helton KA. Multicentric squamous cell carcinoma in situ resembling Bowen's disease in cats. Vet Pathol 1993;30:535–543.

Helton Rhodes KA, Wallace M, Baer KE. Cutaneous manifestations of feline hyperadrenocorticism. In: Ihrke PJ, Mason IS, White SD. Advances in veterinary dermatology. New York: Perjamon, 1993.

Scott DW, Griffin CE, Miller BH. Acquired alopecia. In: Muller & Kirk's small animal dermatology. 5th ed. Philadelphia: Saunders, 1995:720–735.

Scott DW, Griffin CE, Miller BH. Congenital and hereditary defects. In: Muller & Kirk's small animal dermatology. 5th ed. Philadelphia: Saunders, 1995:736–805.

Scott DW, Griffin CE, Miller BH. Endocrine and metabolic diseases. In: Muller & Kirk's small animal dermatology. 5th ed. Philadelphia: Saunders, 1995:627–719.

Author Karen Helton Rhodes
Consulting Editor Karen Helton Rhodes

ALOPECIA—DOGS

 BASICS

DEFINITION
• Common disorder
• Characterized by a complete or partial lack of hair in areas where it is normally present
• May be associated with a multifactorial cause
• May be the primary problem or only a secondary phenomenon

PATHOPHYSIOLOGY
• Multifactorial causes
• All of the disorders represent a disruption in the growth of the hair follicle from infection, trauma, immunologic attack, mechanical "plugging," endocrine abnormalities, or blockage of the receptor sites for stimulation of the cycle.

SYSTEMS AFFECTED
• Skin/Exocrine
• Endocrine/Metabolic
• Hemic/Lymphatic/Immune

SIGNALMENT
No specific age, breed, or sex predilection

SIGNS
• May be acute in onset or slowly progressive.
• Multifocal patches of circular alopecia—most frequently associated with folliculitis from bacterial infection of demodicosis
• Large more diffuse areas of alopecia—may indicate a follicular dysplasia or metabolic component.
• The pattern and degree of hair loss are important for establishing a differential diagnosis.

CAUSES

Multifocal
• Localized demodicosis—partial to complete alopecia with erythema and mild scaling; lesions may become inflamed and crusted
• Dermatophytosis—partial to complete alopecia with scaling; with or without erythema; not always ring-like
• Staphylococcal folliculitis—circular patterns of alopecia with epidermal collarettes, erythema, crusting, and hyperpigmented macules*
• Injection reactions—inflammation with alopecia and/or cutaneous atrophy from scarring
• Rabies vaccine vasculitis—patch of alopecia observed 2–3 months postvaccination
• Localized scleroderma—well-demarcated, shiny, smooth, alopecic, thickened plaque
• Alopecia areata—noninflammatory areas of complete alopecia
• Sebaceous adenitis (short-coated breeds)—annular to polycyclic areas of alopecia and scaling

Symmetrical
• Hyperadrenocorticism—truncal alopecia associated with atrophic skin, comedones, and pyoderma
• Hypothyroidism—alopecia is an uncommon presentation
• Growth hormone–responsive dermatosis—symmetrical truncal alopecia associated with hyperpigmentation; alopecia often starts along the collar area of the neck
• Hyperestrogenism (females)—symmetrical alopecia of the flanks and perineal and inguinal regions with enlarged vulva and mammary glands
• Hypogonadism in intact females—perineal, flank, and truncal alopecia
• Testosterone-responsive dermatosis in castrated males—slowly progressive truncal alopecia
• Male feminization from Sertoli cell tumor—alopecia of the perineum and genital region with gynecomastia
• Castration-responsive dermatosis—hair loss in the collar area, rump, perineum, and flanks
• Estrogen-responsive dermatosis in spayed female dogs—alopecia of the perineum and genital regions
• Seasonal flank alopecia—serpiginous flank alopecia with hyperpigmentation

Patchy to Diffuse
• Demodicosis—often associated with erythema, folliculitis, and hyperpigmentation
• Bacterial folliculitis—multifocal area of circular alopecia to coalescing large areas of hair loss; epidermal collarettes
• Dermatophytosis—often accompanied by scale
• Sebaceous adenitis—alopecia with a thick adherent scale; predominantly on the dorsum of the body, including the head and extremities
• Color mutant alopecia—thinning of the hair coat with secondary folliculitis
• Follicular dysplasia—slowly progressive alopecia
• Anagen defluxion and telogen defluxion—acute onset of alopecia
• Hypothyroidism—diffuse thinning of the hair coat
• Hyperadrenocorticism—truncal alopecia with thin skin and formation of comedones
• Epidermotropic lymphoma—diffuse, generalized truncal alopecia with scaling and erythema, later nodule and plaque formation
• Pemphigus foliaceus—hair loss associated with scale and crust formation
• Keratinization disorders—alopecia associated with excessive scale and greasy surface texture

Specific Locations
• Pinnal alopecia—miniaturization of hairs and progressive alopecia
• Traction alopecia—hair loss on the top and lateral aspect of the cranium secondary to having barrettes or rubber bands applied to the hair

- Postclipping alopecia—failure to regrow after clipping
- Melanoderma (alopecia of Yorkshire terriers)—symmetrical alopecia of the pinnae, bridge of the nose, tail, and feet
- Seasonal flank alopecia—serpiginous flank alopecia that may connect over the dorsum
- Black hair follicular dysplasia—alopecia of the black-haired areas only
- Dermatomyositis—alopecia of the face, tip of ears, tail, and digits; associated with scale and crusting

RISK FACTORS
N/A

DIAGNOSIS

DIFFERENTIAL DIAGNOSIS
- Pattern and degree—important features for formulating a differential diagnosis
- Inflammation, scale, crust, and epidermal collarettes—important for determining diagnosis

CBC/BIOCHEMISTRY/URINALYSIS
Rule out metabolic causes such as hyperadrenocorticism

OTHER LABORATORY TESTS
- Thyroid testing—diagnose hypothyroidism
- ACTH-response test, LDDST, and HDDST—evaluate for hyperadrenocorticism
- Sex hormone profiles (questionable validity)

IMAGING
Ultrasonography—evaluate adrenal glands for evidence of hyperadrenocorticism

DIAGNOSTIC PROCEDURES
- Response to therapy as a trial
- Fungal culture
- Skin scraping
- Cytology
- Skin biopsy

TREATMENT

- Demodicosis—Mitaban, ivermectin, interceptor

- Dermatophytosis—griseofulvin, ketoconazole, itraconazole, lime sulfur dips
- Staphylococcal folliculitis—shampoo and antibiotic therapy
- Sebaceous adenitis—keratolytic shampoo, essential fatty acid supplementation, retinoids
- Keratinization disorders—shampoos, retinoids, vitamin D
- Endocrine—ovariohysterectomy, castration, Lysodren, adrenalectomy

MEDICATIONS

DRUGS OF CHOICE
Varies with specific cause; see Treatment

CONTRAINDICATIONS
N/A

PRECAUTIONS
Toxicity with griseofulvin, retinoids, and ivermectin

POSSIBLE INTERACTIONS
None

ALTERNATIVE DRUGS
None

FOLLOW-UP

PATIENT MONITORING
Varies with cause

POSSIBLE COMPLICATIONS
N/A

MISCELLANEOUS

ASSOCIATED CONDITIONS
N/A

AGE-RELATED FACTORS
N/A

ZOONOTIC POTENTIAL
Dermatophytosis can cause skin lesions in people

PREGNANCY
Avoid retinoids and griseofulvin in pregnant animals.

SYNONYMS
None

SEE ALSO
- Demodicosis
- Dermatomyositis
- Dermatophytosis
- Epidermotropic lymphoma
- Growth Hormone–Responsive Dermatoses
- Hyperadrenocorticism (Cushing Disease)
- Hypothyroidism
- Pemphigus
- Sebaceous Adenitis
- Sertoli Cell Tumor

ABBREVIATIONS
- HDDST = high-dose dexamethasone-suppression test
- LDDST = low-dose dexamethasone-suppression test

Suggested Reading
Helton-Rhodes KA. Cutaneous manifestations of canine and feline endocrinopathies. In: Nichols R, ed. Probl Vet Med 1990;12:617–627.

Schmeitzel LP. Growth hormone responsive alopecia and sex hormone associated dermatoses. In: Birchard SJ, Sherding RG, eds. Saunders manual of small animal practice. Philadelphia: Saunders, 1994:326–330.

Scott DW, Griffin CE, Miller BH. Acquired alopecia. In: Muller & Kirk's small animal dermatology. 5th ed. Philadelphia: Saunders, 1995:720–735.

Scott DW, Griffin CE, Miller BH. Endocrine and metabolic diseases. In: Muller & Kirk's small animal dermatology. 5th ed. Philadelphia: Saunders, 1995:627–719.

Scott DW, Griffin CE, Miller BH. Keratinization defects. In: Muller & Kirk's small animal dermatology. 5th ed. Philadelphia: Saunders, 1995:736–805.

Authors Karen Helton Rhodes and Karin M. Beale

Consulting Editor Karen Helton Rhodes

ANISOCORIA

BASICS

DEFINITION Inequality of pupil size

PATHOPHYSIOLOGY
• Interruption of sympathetic or parasympathetic innervation of the pupil—causes altered pupil size • Ocular disease

SYSTEMS AFFECTED
• Nervous • Ophthalmic

SIGNALMENT
Dogs and cats

SIGNS N/A

CAUSES
Neurologic
• See Table 1 • Disease affecting optic nerve, optic tract, oculomotor nerve, or cerebellum
Ocular
• See Table 2 • Anterior uveitis • Glaucoma • Iris atrophy or hypoplasia • Posterior synechia • Pharmacologic blockade • Neoplasia • Spastic pupil syndrome

RISK FACTORS N/A

DIAGNOSIS

DIFFERENTIAL DIAGNOSIS
• Must determine which pupil is abnormal—see Algorithm 1. • Distinguish between neurologic and ocular causes.

CBC/BIOCHEMISTRY/URINALYSIS N/A

OTHER LABORATORY TESTS N/A

IMAGING
• See Table 1 • Ultrasound—identifying ocular and retrobulbar lesions • CT and MRI—localizing and identifying CNS lesions

DIAGNOSTIC PROCEDURES
• See Table 1 • CSF tap—evaluate CNS disease. • ERG—evaluate retinal function • VEP—evaluate optic nerve function • Pharmacologic testing—see Algorithm 1; postganglionic lesions cause denervation supersensitivity; direct-acting (para)sympathomimetic drugs cause the pupil to constrict or dilate. • Preganglionic lesions—respond to indirect-acting (para)sympathomimetics

TREATMENT

Depends on underlying disease

MEDICATIONS

DRUGS OF CHOICE
Depend on underlying disease

CONTRAINDICATIONS N/A

PRECAUTIONS N/A

POSSIBLE INTERACTIONS N/A

ALTERNATIVE DRUGS N/A

FOLLOW-UP

PATIENT MONITORING N/A

POSSIBLE COMPLICATIONS
N/A

MISCELLANEOUS

ASSOCIATED CONDITIONS N/A

AGE-RELATED FACTORS N/A

ZOONOTIC POTENTIAL N/A

PREGNANCY N/A

SYNONYMS N/A

SEE ALSO
• Anterior Uveitis—Cats • Anterior Uveitis—Dogs • Glaucoma • Horner Syndrome • Iris atrophy • Optic Neuritis

ABBREVIATIONS
• CSF = cerebrospinal fluid • ERG = electroretinography • FeLV = feline leukemia virus • PLR = pupillary light reflex • VEP = visual-evoked potential

Suggested Reading
Neer TM, Carter JD. Anisocoria in dogs and cats. Ocular and neurologic causes. Compend Contin Educ Pract Vet 1987;9:817–824.
Scagliotti RH, Neuro-ophthalmology. In: Birchard SJ, Sherding RG, eds. Saunders manual of small animal practice. Philadelphia: Saunders, 1994:1242–1248.
Author David Lipsitz
Consulting Editor Paul E. Miller

Table 1.

Neurologic Lesions Causing Anisocoria

Lesion	Neurologic Signs	Differential Diagnosis	Diagnostic Plan
Optic nerve	Ipsilateral mydriasis	Optic neuritis	CT/MRI
	Ipsilateral monocular anopia	Neoplasm	CSF
	(total blindness in one eye)		electroretinogram (ERG)
	No direct PLR affected eye		
	Consensual PLR affected eye		
Optic tract	Contralateral blindness in	Neoplasm	CT/MRI
	Nasal/temporal visual fields	Infectious/inflammatory disease	CSF
	Ipsilateral pupil smaller in light	Trauma	
	Other neurologic deficits		
Oculomotor nerve	Ipsilateral dilated pupil	Neoplasm	CT/MRI
Parasympathetic nucleus CN III	Normal vision/no direct PLR	Infectious/inflammatory disease	CSF
	No consensual PLR from opposite eye	Trauma	ultrasound orbit
	Ptosis upper eyelid	Brain herniation	
	Ventrolateral strabismus	Retrobulbar mass	
Cerebellar disease	Contralateral mydriasis	Neoplasm	CT/MRI
	Normal PLR/normal vision	Infectious/inflammatory disease	CSF
	Ipsilateral lack of menace response	Trauma	
	Other cerebellar signs		

Table 2.

Ocular Diseases Causing Anisocoria

Lesion	Associated Signs	Causes
Anterior uveitis	Miosis, aqueous flare, Corneal edema Conjunctival hyperemia	infectious/inflammatory disease trauma
Glaucoma	Mydriasis Sluggish/absent PLR Increased intraocular pressure Corneal edema	primary glaucoma secondary glaucoma
Neoplasm	Miosis/mydriasis Change in iridial coloration	lymphoma melanoma
Posterior synechia	Variable pupil shape Sluggish/absent PLR Anterior uveitis	secondary to anterior uveitis
Iris atrophy Iris hypoplasia	Variable pupil shape, iridal thinning Sluggish/absent PLR Irregular pupil margin Other ocular abnormalities	old age change congenital
Pharmacological blockade	Mydriasis Absent direct/consensual PLR Normal vision	atropine
Spastic pupil syndrome	Miosis Normal vision	FeLV

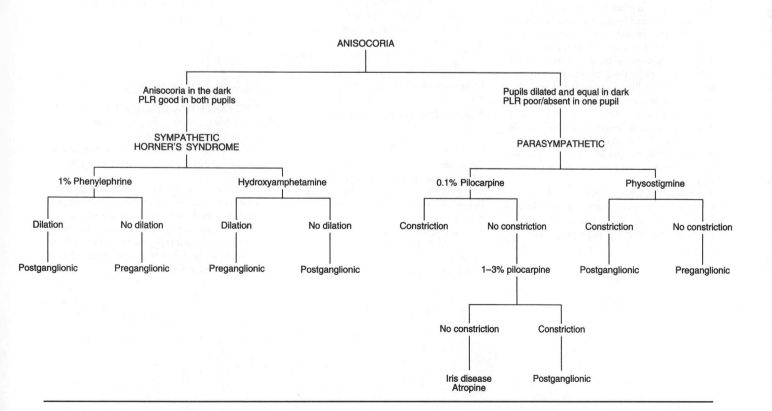

ANOREXIA

 BASICS

DEFINITION
The lack or loss of appetite for food; appetite is psychologic and depends on memory and associations, compared with hunger, which is physiologically aroused by the body's need for food; the existence of appetite in animals is assumed.

PATHOPHYSIOLOGY
• The control of appetite is a complex interaction between the CNS and the periphery.
• The CNS classically involves the hypothalamus, which includes the satiety center (ventromedial hypothalamus) and the feeding center (lateral hypothalamus); a number of other areas including the area postrema, paraventricular nucleus, ventral tegmental area, amygdala, and globis pallidus are involved in the central control of appetite.
• Recently, the concept of specific appetite centers in the hypothalamus has been challenged because satiety is also mediated by a serotonergic tract that passes near the ventromedial hypothalamus; the lateral hypothalamus is associated with dopaminergic tracts.
• Appetite regulation is more appropriately viewed as neuropharmacologic interactions mediated via neurotransmitters rather than as anatomic centers in the hypothalamus.
• The regulation of food intake also depends on the peripheral control of appetite.
• The gastric distension theory suggests that gastric distension promotes satiety, which is probably mediated by the hormone bombesin.
• Beyond the stomach, satiety can be induced by placing food in the small intestine.
• Cholecystokinin—a peripheral regulator of satiety; released by the gastrointestinal tract; its effect on food intake is mediated by the vagus nerve because abdominal vagotomy abolishes the satiation.
• Other postulated "satiety hormones" include somatostatin and pancreatic glucagon.
• A new system for appetite regulation involves leptin, a peptide hormone normally expressed by adipocytes.
• Genetically engineered mice, unable to produce leptin, were hyperphagic and obese; parenteral administration of recombinant leptin to mice decreased hyperphagia and obesity.

• Inflammatory, infectious, metabolic, or neoplastic diseases can cause inappetence, probably as a result of the release of a variety of chemical mediators such as cachectin and interleukin-1.

SYSTEMS AFFECTED
• Dog and cat
• All body systems are affected; breakdown of the intestinal mucosal barrier is particularly important in sick patients.

SIGNALMENT
Depends on the underlying cause

SIGNS
• Refusal to eat is a common complaint presented by pet owners, because a poor appetite is strongly associated with illness.
• Reluctance to eat may be the only abnormality identified after an evaluation of the patient history and physical examination; this is typical in psychologic causes of anorexia and food aversion.
• Patients with disorders causing dysfunction or pain of the face, neck, oropharynx, and esophagus may display an interest in food but be unable to complete prehension and swallowing.
• Pseudoanorectic patients commonly display weight loss, halitosis, excessive drooling, difficulty in prehension and mastication of food, dysphagia, and odynophagia (painful eating).
• Odynophagia is exhibited as repeated efforts at swallowing and vocalization when eating.
• Most underlying causes of pseudoanorexia can be identified by a thorough examination of the face, neck, oropharynx, and esophagus for traumatic lesions, masses, foreign bodies, dental disease, ulceration, and neuromuscular dysfunction.
• Clinical signs in true anorexia vary and are related to the underlying cause.

Historical Findings
N/A

Physical Examination Findings
N/A

CAUSES
Anorexia
• Almost any systemic disease process
• Psychologic—unpalatable diets, alterations in routine or environment, stress
• Acid–base disorders
• Cardiac failure
• Toxicosis and drugs
• Pain
• Endocrine and metabolic disease

• Neoplasia involving any site
• Infectious disease
• Immune-mediated disease
• Respiratory disease
• Gastrointestinal disease
• Musculoskeletal disorders
• Neurologic disease
• Miscellaneous—motion sickness, high environmental temperature, etc.

Pseudoanorexia
• Any disease process that interferes with the swallowing reflex
• Diseases causing painful prehension and mastication; stomatitis, glossitis, gingivitis (e.g., physical agents, caustics, bacterial infections, viral infections, Candida, foreign bodies, autoimmune diseases, immune-mediated disorders, uremia), oral or glossal neoplasia, neurologic disorders (rabies, tetanus, trigeminal paralysis, polyneuropathies, CNS lesions, neuropathies of cranial nerves VII, IX, X, XII), musculoskeletal disorders (masticatory myositis, temporomandibular joint arthropathy, mandible fracture or subluxation, craniomandibular osteopathy), dental disease, salivary gland disorders, and retrobulbar abscess
• Diseases causing oropharyngeal dysphagia; glossal disorders (neurologic, neoplastic), pharyngitis, tonsillitis, pharyngeal neoplasia, retropharyngeal disorders (lymphadenopathy, abscess, hematoma, sialocele), neuromuscular disorders (CNS lesions, cricopharyngeal achalasia, myasthenia gravis, botulism)
• Diseases of the esophagus—esophagitis, neoplasia, and neuromuscular disorders

RISK FACTORS
N/A

 DIAGNOSIS

DIFFERENTIAL DIAGNOSIS
• Systemic disease is the most common cause of anorexia in dogs and cats.
• Obtain a minimum database to help eliminate the possibility of underlying medical disorders.
• Questioning about the patient's interest in food and its ability to prehend, masticate, and swallow food, along with a thorough examination of the animal's oropharynx, face, and neck, will help identify pseudoanorexia; if the owners are poor historians the patient should be observed while eating.

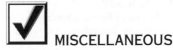
- A thorough history regarding the animals' environment, diet, other animals and people in the household, and any recent changes involving any of these helps identify psychologic anorexia.
- Any abnormalities detected in the physical examination or historical evidence of illness mandates a diagnostic workup for the identified problem.
- Only if the history, physical examination, and minimum database strongly suggest psychologic anorexia should further diagnostic workup be dropped; in such cases contact with the pet owner daily until the anorexia has resolved.

CBC/BIOCHEMISTRY/URINALYSIS
- Normal in patients with psychologic causes of anorexia
- Abnormalities vary with different underlying diseases and causes of pseudoanorexia and anorexia.

OTHER LABORATORY TESTS
Special tests may be necessary to rule out specific diseases suggested by the history, physical examination, or minimum database (See other topics on specific diseases).

IMAGING
- If underlying disease is suspected but no abnormalities are revealed by the physical examination or minimum database, consider thoracic and abdominal radiography and abdominal ultrasonography to identify hidden conditions.
- The need for further diagnostic imaging varies with the underlying condition suspected (see other topics on specific diseases).

DIAGNOSTIC PROCEDURES
Vary with underlying condition suspected (see other topics regarding specific diseases)

TREATMENT
- Treat underlying cause.
- Symptomatic therapy includes attention to fluid and electrolyte derangements, reduction in environmental stressors, and modification of the diet to improve palatability.
- Improve food palatability by adding flavored toppings such as chicken and beef broths, seasoning with condiments such as garlic powder, increasing the fat or protein content of the food, and heating the food to body temperature.

- As a general rule, dogs and cats with debilitating disease conditions should not go without food for longer than 3–5 days before enteral or parenteral feeding is used.
- Other factors to consider when deciding whether enteral or parenteral feeding is indicated include ≥10% body weight loss, hypoalbuminemia, lymphopenia, and/or a condition/disease likely to lead to prolonged anorexia.
- Techniques for providing enteral nutrition include force-feeding or placement of nasogastric, esophagostomy, gastrostomy, or jejunostomy tubes.

MEDICATIONS

DRUGS OF CHOICE
- Benzodiazepines given 10–20 min prior to feeding such as diazepam (0.1 mg/kg IV) and oxazepam (0.5 mg/kg PO) may increase appetite in some cats and rare dogs.
- Cyproheptadine, an antihistamine with antiserotonergic properties has been used as an appetite stimulant in dogs and cats (0.2–0.5 mg/kg PO 10–20 min prior to feeding), with mixed success.
- Analgesics may promote appetite in painful conditions.
- Metoclopramide (0.2–0.4 mg/kg SC or PO) and cisapride (0.5 mg/kg PO q8h) are useful if anorexia is associated with delayed gastric emptying or ileus.

CONTRAINDICATIONS
Avoid antiemetics if gastrointestinal obstruction is present/suspected.

PRECAUTIONS
N/A

POSSIBLE INTERACTIONS
N/A

ALTERNATIVE DRUGS
N/A

FOLLOW-UP

PATIENT MONITORING
Body weight and hydration to determine if management is effective

POSSIBLE COMPLICATIONS
- Dehydration, malnutrition, and cachexia are most likely; these exacerbate the underlying disease.
- Feline hepatic lipidosis is a possible complication of anorexia in obese cats.
- Breakdown of the intestinal mucosal barrier is a concern in debilitated patients.

☑ MISCELLANEOUS

ASSOCIATED CONDITIONS
Hypoglycemia may occur in anorectic puppies/kittens, toy breed dogs, and cachectic patients and in some medical conditions (e.g., advanced liver disease).

AGE-RELATED FACTORS
Nutritional support and/or glucose-containing fluids may be necessary to treat or prevent hypoglycemia in anorectic puppies and kittens.

ZOONOTIC POTENTIAL
N/A

PREGNANCY
N/A

SYNONYMS
Inappetance

SEE ALSO
Causes

ABBREVIATION
CNS = central nervous system

Suggested Reading

Guilford WG. Nutritional management of gastrointestinal diseases. In: Guilford WG, Center SA, Strombeck DR, et al., eds. Strombeck's small animal gastroenterology. 3rd ed. Philadelphia: Saunders, 1996:889–910.

Monroe WE. Anorexia and polyphagia. In: Ettinger SJ, ed. Veterinary internal medicine. 4th ed. Philadelphia: Saunders, 1995:18–21.

Phinney SD, Halstead CH. Obesity, anorexia nervosa, and bulimia. In: Feldman M, Scharschmidt BF, Sleisenger MH, eds. Gastrointestinal and liver disease. 6th ed. Philadelphia: Saunders, 1998:278–297.

Author Mark C. Walker

Consulting Editors Mitchell A. Crystal and Brett M. Feder

ASCITES

BASICS

DEFINITION
The escape of fluid, either transudate or exudate, into the abdominal cavity between the parietal and visceral peritoneum

PATHOPHYSIOLOGY
Ascites can be caused by the following:
• CHF and associated interference in venous return
• Depletion of plasma proteins associated with inappropriate loss of protein from renal or gastrointestinal disease—protein-losing nephropathy or enteropathy, respectively
• Obstruction of the vena cava or portal vein, or lymphatic drainage due to neoplastic occlusion
• Overt neoplastic effusion
• Peritonitis—infective or inflammatory
• Electrolyte imbalance, especially hypernatremia
• Liver cirrhosis

SYSTEMS AFFECTED
• Cardiovascular
• Gastrointestinal
• Renal/Urologic
• Hemic/Lymph/Immune

SIGNALMENT
• Dogs and cats
• No species or breed predisposition

SIGNS
• Episodic weakness
• Lethargy
• Abdominal fullness
• Abdominal discomfort when palpated
• Dyspnea from abdominal distension or associated pleural effusion
• Anorexia
• Vomiting
• Weight gain
• Scrotal or penile edema
• Groaning when lying down

CAUSES
• Nephrotic syndrome
• Cirrhosis of liver
• Right-sided CHF
• Hypoproteinemia
• Ruptured bladder
• Peritonitis
• Abdominal neoplasia
• Abdominal hemorrhage

RISK FACTORS
N/A

DIAGNOSIS

DIFFERENTIAL DIAGNOSIS

Differentiating Abdominal Distension Without Effusion
• Organomegaly—hepatomegaly, splenomegaly, renomegaly, and hydrometra
• Abdominal neoplasia
• Pregnancy
• Bladder distension
• Obesity
• Gastric dilatation

Differentiating Diseases
• Transudate—nephrotic syndrome, cirrhosis of liver, right-sided CHF, hypoproteinemia, and ruptured bladder
• Exudate—peritonitis, abdominal neoplasia, and hemorrhage

CBC/BIOCHEMISTRY/URINALYSIS
• Neutrophilic leukocytosis occurs in patients with systemic infection.
• Albumin is low in patients with impaired liver synthesis, gastrointestinal loss, or renal loss.
• Cholesterol is low in patients with impaired liver synthesis

Liver Enzymes
• Low to normal in patients with impaired liver synthesis
• High in patients with liver inflammation, hyperadrenocorticism, gallbladder obstruction, and chronic passive congestion

Total and Direct Bilirubin
• Low to normal in patients with impaired liver synthesis
• High in patients with biliary obstruction caused by tumor, gallbladder distension, or obstruction

BUN and Creatinine
• High in patients with renal failure
• BUN low in patients with impaired liver synthesis or hyperadrenocorticism

Glucose
Low in patients with impaired liver synthesis

OTHER LABORATORY TESTS
• To detect hypoproteinemia—protein electrophoresis and immune profile
• To detect proteinuria—urinary protein:creatinine ratio (normal < 0.5:1)

IMAGING
• Thoracic and abdominal radiography is sometimes helpful.
• Ultrasonography of the liver, spleen, pancreas, kidney, bladder, and abdomen can often determine cause.

DIAGNOSTIC PROCEDURES

Ascitic Fluid Evaluation
Exfoliative cytologic examination and bacterial culture and antibiotic sensitivity—remove approximately 3–5 mL of abdominal fluid via aseptic technique.

Transudate
• Clear and colorless
• Protein < 2.5 g/dL
• Specific gravity < 1.018
• Cells < 1000/mm³—neutrophils and mesothelial cells

Modified Transudate
• Red or pink; may be slightly cloudy
• Protein 2.5–5.0 g/dL
• Specific gravity > 1.018
• Cells < 5000 /mm³—neutrophils, mesothelial cells, erythrocytes, and lymphocytes

Exudate (Nonseptic)
• Pink or white; cloudy
• Protein 2.5–5.0 g/dL
• Specific gravity > 1.018
• Cells 5,000–50,000/mm³—neutrophils, mesothelial cells, macrophages, erythrocytes, and lymphocytes

Exudate (Septic)
• Red, white, or yellow; cloudy
• Protein > 4.0 g/dL
• Specific gravity > 1.018
• Cells 5,000–100,000/mm³—neutrophils, mesothelial cells, macrophages, erythrocytes, lymphocytes, and bacteria

Hemorrhage
• Red; spun supernatant clear and sediment red
• Protein > 5.5 g/dL
• Specific gravity 1.007–1.027
• Cells consistent with peripheral blood
• Does not clot

Chyle
• Pink, straw, or white
• Protein 2.5–7.0 g/dL
• Specific gravity 1.007–> 1.040

• Cells < 10,000/mm³—neutrophils, mesothelial cells, and large population of small lymphocytes
• Other—fluid in tube separates into cream-like layer when refrigerated; fat droplets stain with Sudan III.

Pseudochyle
• White
• Protein > 2.5 g/dL
• Specific gravity 1.007–1.040
• Cells < 10,000/mm³—neutrophils, mesothelial cells, and small lymphocytes
• Other—fluid in tube does not separate into creamlike layer when refrigerated; does not stain with Sudan III.

Urine
• Clear to pale yellow
• Protein > 2.5 g/dL
• Specific gravity 1.000–> 1.040
• Cells 5,000–50,000/mm³—neutrophils, erythrocytes, lymphocytes, and macrophages
• Other—if the urinary bladder ruptured < 12 h before, urinary glucose and protein could be negative; if bladder ruptured > 12 h before, urine becomes a dialysis medium with ultrafiltrate of plasma, and urine contains glucose and protein.

Bile
• Slightly cloudy and yellow
• Protein > 2.5 g/dL
• Specific gravity > 1.018
• Cells 5,000–750,000/mm³—neutrophils, erythrocytes, macrophages, and lymphocytes
• Other—bilirubin confirmed by urine dipstick; nonicteric patient may have gallbladder rupture, biliary tree leakage, or rupture in the proximal bowel.

TREATMENT
• Can design treatment on an outpatient basis, with follow-up or inpatient care, depending on physical condition and underlying cause
• If patients are markedly uncomfortable when lying down or become more dyspneic with stress, consider removing enough ascites to reverse these signs.
• Dietary salt restriction may help control transudate fluid accumulation due to CHF, cirrhosis, or hypoproteinemia.
• For exudate ascites control, address the

underlying cause; corrective surgery is often indicated, followed by specific therapeutic management (e.g., patient with splenic tumor: tumor removed, abdominal bleeding controlled, blood transfusion administered).
• Can recirculate nonseptic ascitic fluid in patients with liver insufficiency or nephrotic syndrome that has become refractory to conservative medical and dietary management; use the LeVeen peritoneovenous shunt concept—a unidirectional shunt conveys ascitic fluid to the jugular vein via a surgically placed one-way catheter from the midabdominal region; this autologous infusion has had limited success in dogs.

MEDICATIONS
DRUGS OF CHOICE
• Patients with liver insufficiency or CHF—restrict sodium and give a diuretic combination of hydrochlorothiazide (2–4 mg/kg ql2h PO) and spironolactone (1–2 mg/kg ql2h PO); if control is inadequate, furosemide (1–2 mg/kg q8h PO) can be substituted for the thiazide with spironolactone continued; must monitor serum potassium concentration to prevent potassium imbalances
• Patients with hypoproteinemia, nephrotic syndrome, and associated ascitic fluid accumulation—can treat as above with the addition of hetastarch (6% hetastarch in 0.9% NaCl); administer an IV bolus (dogs, 20 mL/kg; cats, 10–15 mL/kg) slowly over ~ 1 h; hetastarch increases plasma oncotic pressure and pulls fluid into the intravascular space for up to 24–48 h.
• Systemic antibiotic therapy is dictated by bacterial identification and sensitivity testing in patients with septic exudate ascites.

CONTRAINDICATIONS
N/A

PRECAUTIONS
N/A

POSSIBLE INTERACTIONS
N/A

ALTERNATIVE DRUGS
N/A

FOLLOW-UP
PATIENT MONITORING
• Varies with the underlying cause
• Check sodium, potassium, BUN, creatinine, and weight fluctuations periodically if the patient is maintained on a diuretic.

POSSIBLE COMPLICATIONS
Aggressive diuretic administration may cause hypokalemia, which could predispose to metabolic alkalosis and exacerbation of hepatic encephalopathy in patients with underlying liver disease; alkalosis causes a shift from NH_4 to NH_3.

MISCELLANEOUS
ASSOCIATED CONDITIONS
N/A

AGE-RELATED FACTORS
N/A

ZOONOTIC POTENTIAL
N/A

PREGNANCY
N/A

SYNONYMS
Abdominal effusion

SEE ALSO
• Nephrotic Syndrome
• Cirrhosis and Fibrosis of the Liver
• Congestive Heart Failure, Right-sided

ABBREVIATION
CHF = congestive heart failure

Suggested Reading
Lewis LD, Morris ML Jr, Hand MS. Small animal clinical nutrition. 3rd ed. Topeka, KS: Mark Morris Associates, 1987.
Porayko MK, Wiesner RH. Management of ascites in patients with cirrhosis. Postgrad Med 1992;2:155.
Author Jerry A. Thornhill
Consulting Editors Larry P. Tilley and Francis W. K. Smith, Jr.

ATAXIA

 BASICS

DEFINITION
• A sign of sensory dysfunction that produces incoordination of the limbs, head, and/or trunk
• Three clinical types—sensory (proprioceptive), vestibular, and cerebellar; all produce changes in limb coordination, but vestibular and cerebellar ataxia also produce changes in head and neck movement.

PATHOPHYSIOLOGY

Sensory
• Proprioceptive pathways in the spinal cord (i.e., fasciculus gracilis, fasciculus cuneatus, and spinocerebellar tracts) relay limb and trunk position to the brain.
• When the spinal cord is slowly compressed, proprioceptive deficits are usually the first signs observed, because these pathways are located more superficially in the white matter and their larger-sized axons are more susceptible to compression than are other tracts.
• Generally accompanied by weakness owing to early concomitant upper motor neuron involvement; weakness not always obvious early in the course of the disease

Vestibular
• Changes in head and neck position are relayed through the vestibulocochlear nerve to the brainstem.
• Diseases that affect the vestibular receptors, the nerve in the inner ear, or the nuclei in the brainstem cause various degrees of disequilibrium with ensuing vestibular ataxia.
• Affected animal leans, tips, falls, or even rolls toward the side of the lesion; accompanied by head tilt

Cerebellar
• The cerebellum regulates, coordinates, and smooths motor activity.
• Proprioception is normal, because the ascending proprioceptive pathways to the cortex are intact; weakness does not occur, because the upper motor neurons are intact.
• Inadequacy in the performance of motor activity; strength preservation; no proprioceptive deficits

SYSTEMS AFFECTED
Nervous—spinal cord (and brainstem); cerebellum; vestibular system

SIGNALMENT
Any age, breed, or sex

SIGNS
• Important to define the type of ataxia to localize the problem
• Only one limb involved—consider a lameness problem.
• Only hindlimbs affected—likely a spinal cord disorder
• All or both ipsilateral limbs affected—cerebellar
• Head tilt—vestibular

CAUSES

Neurologic
Cerebellar
• Degenerative—abiotrophy (Kerry blue terriers, Gordon setters, rough-coated collies, Australian kelpies, Airedales, Bernese mountain dogs, Finnish harriers, Brittany spaniels, border collies, beagles, Samoyeds, wire fox terriers, Labrador retrievers, great Danes, chow chows, Rhodesian ridgebacks, domestic shorthair cats); storage diseases often have cerebellomedullary involvement.
• Anomalous—hypoplasia secondary to perinatal infection with parvo virus (cats); malformed cerebellum owing to herpesvirus infection (newborn puppies)
• Neoplastic—any tumor of the CNS (primary or secondary) localized to the cerebellum
• Infectious—canine distemper virus; FIP; and any other CNS infection affecting the cerebellum
• Inflammatory, idiopathic, immune-mediated—granulomatous meningoencephalomyelitis
• Toxic—metronidazole
Vestibular—CNS
• Infectious—FIP; canine distemper virus; rickettsial diseases
• Inflammatory, idiopathic, immune-mediated—granulomatous meningoencephalomyelitis
• Toxic—metronidazole

Vestibular—PNS
• Infectious—otitis media interna
• Idiopathic—geriatric vestibular disease (dogs); idiopathic vestibular syndrome (cats); nasopharyngeal polyps (cats)
• Metabolic—hypothyroidism
• Neoplastic—squamous cell carcinoma, bone tumors
• Traumatic
Spinal Cord
• Degenerative—degenerative radiculomyelopathy (old German shepherds)
• Vascular—fibrocartilaginous embolic myelopathy
• Anomalous—hemivertebrae; other spinal cord and vertebral malformation
• Neoplastic—primary bone tumors; multiple myeloma and metastatic tumors that infiltrate the vertebral body
• Infectious—discospondylitis; myelitis
• Traumatic—intervertebral disc herniation; fracture or luxation; cervical vertebral instability; atlanto-axial subluxation-luxation

Metabolic
• Anemia
• Electrolyte disturbances—especially hypokalemia and hypoglycemia

Miscellaneous
• Drugs—acepromazine; antihistamines; antiepileptic
• Respiratory compromise
• Cardiac compromise

RISK FACTORS
• Intervertebral disk disease—dachshunds, poodles, cocker spaniels, and beagles
• Cervical cord compression—Doberman pinschers and Great Danes
• Fibrocartilaginous embolism—young, large-breed dogs and miniature schnauzers

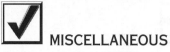
 DIAGNOSIS

DIFFERENTIAL DIAGNOSIS
- Differentiate the types of ataxia
- Differentiate from other disease processes that can affect gait—musculoskeletal; metabolic; cardiovascular; respiratory
- Musculoskeletal disorders—typically produce lameness and a reluctance to move
- Systemic illness and endocrine, cardiovascular, and metabolic disorders—can cause intermittent ataxia, especially of the pelvic limbs; with fever, weight loss, murmurs, arrhythmias, hair loss, or collapse with exercise suspect a non-neurologic cause; obtain minimum data from hemogram, biochemistry analysis, and urinalysis.
- Head tilt or nystagmus—likely vestibular
- Intention tremors of the head or hypermetria—likely cerebellar
- Only limbs affected—likely spinal cord dysfunction; all four limbs affected: lesion is in the cervical area or is multifocal to diffuse; only pelvic limbs affected: lesion is anywhere below the second thoracic vertebra

CBC/BIOCHEMISTRY/URINALYSIS
Normal unless metabolic cause (e.g., hypoglycemia, electrolyte imbalance, and anemia)

OTHER LABORATORY TESTS
- Hypoglycemia—determine serum insulin concentration on the same sample; calculate an amended insulin:glucose ratio (rule out insulinoma).
- Anemia—differentiate as nonregenerative or regenerative on the basis of the reticulocyte count.
- Electrolyte imbalance—correct the problem; see if ataxia resolves.
- Antiepileptic drugs—if being administered, evaluate serum concentration for toxicity.

IMAGING
- Spinal radiographs—if spinal cord dysfunction suspected
- Bullae radiographs—if peripheral vestibular disease suspected; CT or MRI scans superior but more expensive
- Thoracic radiographs—for old patients; identify neoplasia
- CT or MRI—if cerebellar disease suspected; evaluate potential brain disease
- Abdominal ultrasonography—if hepatic, renal, adrenal or pancreatic dysfunction suspected

DIAGNOSTIC PROCEDURES
- CSF—confirm nervous system causes
- Myelography—may establish evidence of spinal cord compression

 TREATMENT

- Usually outpatient, depending on the severity and acuteness of clinical signs
- Exercise—decrease or restrict if spinal cord disease suspected
- Client should monitor gait for increasing dysfunction or weakness; if paresis worsens or paralysis develops, other testing is warranted.
- Avoid drugs that could be contributing to the problem; may not be possible in patients on antiepileptic drugs for seizures

 MEDICATIONS

DRUG(S) OF CHOICE
Not recommended until the source or cause of the problem is identified.

CONTRAINDICATIONS
N/A

PRECAUTIONS
N/A

POSSIBLE INTERACTIONS
N/A

ALTERNATIVE DRUGS
N/A

 FOLLOW-UP

PATIENT MONITORING
Periodic neurologic examinations to assess condition

POSSIBLE COMPLICATIONS
- Spinal cord or neuromuscular disease—progression to weakness and possibly paralysis
- Hypoglycemia—seizures
- Cerebellar disease—head tremors and bobbing

✔ **MISCELLANEOUS**

ASSOCIATED CONDITIONS
N/A

AGE RELATED FACTORS
N/A

ZOONOTIC POTENTIAL
N/A

PREGNANCY
N/A

SYNONYMS
N/A

SEE ALSO
- See specific diseases
- Cerebellar Degeneration
- Head tilt (Vestibular Disease)
- Paralysis

ABBREVIATIONS
- CSF = cerebrospinal fluid
- CT = computed tomography
- FIP = feline infectious peritonitis
- MRI = magnetic resonance imaging
- PNS = peripheral nervous system

Suggested Reading

Chrisman CL. Vestibular diseases. Vet Clin North Am Small Anim Pract 1980;10:103–129.

Oliver JE, Lorenz MD, Kornegay JN. Handbook of veterinary neurology. 3rd ed. Philadelphia: Saunders, 1997:216–239.

Author Linda G. Shell

Consulting Editor Joane M. Parent

BLIND QUIET EYE

 BASICS

DEFINITION
Loss of vision in one or both eyes without ocular vascular injection or other externally apparent signs of ocular inflammation

PATHOPHYSIOLOGY
Results from abnormalities in focusing images on the retina, retinal image detection, optic nerve transmission, or CNS interpretation

SYSTEMS AFFECTED
• Ophthalmic
• Nervous

SIGNALMENT
• Dogs and cats
• Any age, breed, or sex
• Many causes (e.g., cataracts and progressive retinal atrophy) have a genetic basis and are often highly breed- and age-specific.
• SARDS—tends to occur in old dogs
• Optic nerve hypoplasia—congenital

SIGNS

Historical Findings
• Depend on underlying cause
• Bumping into objects
• Clumsy behavior
• Reluctance to move
• Impaired vision in dim light

Physical Examination Findings
• Depend on underlying cause
• Decreased or absent menace response
• Impaired visual placing responses

CAUSES
• Cataracts—generally, entire lens must become opaque to produce complete blindness; may note a reduction in visual performance during visually demanding tasks even with incomplete opacification
• Loss of focusing power of the lens—rarely completely blinding; substantial hyperopia (far-sightedness) occurs after lens extraction in which the optical power of the lens is not replaced and when the lens luxates posteriorly out of the pupillary plane and into the vitreous
• Retina—SARDS; PRA; retinal detachment; taurine deficiency (cats)
• Optic nerve—optic neuritis; neoplasia of the optic nerve or adjacent tissues; trauma; optic nerve hypoplasia; lead toxicity; excessive traction on the optic nerve during enucleation, resulting in trauma to the contralateral optic nerve or optic chiasm (especially cats and brachycephalic dogs)
• CNS (amaurosis)—lesions of the optic chiasm or tract; optic radiation; visual cortex

RISK FACTORS
• Poorly regulated diabetes mellitus—cataracts
• Related animals with genetic cataracts or

PRA
• Systemic hypertension—retinal detachment
• CNS hypoxia—blindness may become apparent after excessively deep anesthesia or revival from cardiac arrest.

 DIAGNOSIS

DIFFERENTIAL DIAGNOSIS

Signs
• Anterior segment inflammation and glaucoma—conjunctiva typically injected
• Young patients—may lack menace responses; usually successfully navigate a maze or visually track hand movements or cotton balls
• Postictal period—transient vision loss
• Abnormal mentation—may be difficult to determine whether an animal is visual; other neurologic abnormalities help localize the problem.

Causes
• Optic neuritis, retinal detachment, SARDS, or visual cortex hypoxia—sudden vision loss (over hours to weeks)
• SARDS—often proceeded by polyuria, polydipsia, or polyphagia and weight gain
• PRA—gradual vision loss, especially in dim light; apparently acute vision loss with sudden change in environment
• Cataract—history of either gradual or rapidly increasing opacification and vision loss in a quiet eye
• Optic nerve hypoplasia—congenital; may be unilateral or bilateral
• Optic neuropathy or CNS disease—signs of other neurologic abnormalities
• Pupillary light responses—usually normal with cataracts or visual cortex lesions; sluggish to absent with retinal or optic nerve diseases
• Ophthalmoscopy—normal with SARDS, retrobulbar optic neuritis, and higher visual pathway lesions; abnormal with retinal detachment and neuropathies of the optic nerve head

CBC/BIOCHEMISTRY/URINALYSIS
• Usually normal, unless underlying systemic disease
• Hyperglycemia or glucosuria—may note with diabetic cataracts
• Elevated ALP and changes consistent with hyperadrenocorticism (Cushing syndrome)—suggest SARDS
• Retinal detachment secondary to systemic hypertension (cats)—mildly high BUN or serum creatinine; changes consistent with hyperthyroidism

OTHER LABORATORY TESTS
• Blood lead and serology for deep fungal or viral infections—consider for suspected optic neuritis (see Optic Neuritis).
• LDDST—may help rule out Cushing syndrome with SARDS

IMAGING
• Ocular ultrasound—may demonstrate a retinal detachment (especially if the ocular media are opaque) or optic nerve mass lesion
• Plain skull radiographs—seldom informative
• CT or MRI—often helpful with orbital or CNS lesions

DIAGNOSTIC PROCEDURES
• Ophthalmic examination with a penlight—usually permits diagnosis of cataracts or retinal detachments severe enough to cause blindness
• Ophthalmoscopy—may reveal PRA or optic nerve disease; normal examination suggests SARDS, retrobulbar optic neuritis, or a CNS lesion.
• Systemic blood pressure—determine in retinal detachments
• Electroretinography—differentiates retinal from optic nerve or CNS disease when the diagnosis is in doubt
• CSF tap—may be of value with a neurogenic cause of vision loss

 TREATMENT

• Try to obtain a definitive diagnosis on an outpatient basis before initiating treatment.
• Consider referral before attempting empirical therapy.
• Most causes are not fatal, but must perform a workup to rule out potentially fatal diseases.
• Reassure client that most causes of a blind quiet eye are not painful and that blind animals can lead a relatively normal and functional life.
• Warn client that the environment should be examined for potential hazards to a blind animal.
• Advise client that patients with progressive retinal atrophy or genetic cataracts should not be bred and that related animals should be examined.
• Retinal detachment—recommend severely restricted exercise until the retina is firmly reattached.
• Calorie-restricted diet—to prevent obesity; owing to reduced activity level
• Cats with nutritionally induced retinopathy—ensure diet has adequate levels of taurine.
• SARDS, progressive retinal atrophy, optic nerve atrophy, and optic nerve hypoplasia—no effective treatment
• Cataracts, luxated lenses, and some forms of retinal detachment—best treated surgically

 MEDICATIONS

DRUGS OF CHOICE
• Depend on cause
• Workup is declined, infectious disease is unlikely, and the likely diagnosis is SARDS or

retrobulbar optic neuritis—consider systemic prednisolone (1–2 mg/kg/day for 7–14 days, then taper); may concurrently administer oral chloramphenicol or other systemic broad-spectrum antibiotic

CONTRAINDICATIONS
Do not use systemic corticosteroids and other immunosuppressive drugs with optic neuritis and retinal detachments that are infectious in origin.

PRECAUTIONS
Pretreatment with corticosteroids may mimic or mask liver enzyme changes in SARDS.

POSSIBLE INTERACTIONS
N/A

ALTERNATIVE DRUGS
• Flunixin meglumine (dogs)—may try a single dose (0.5 mg/kg IV) in place of corti-costeroids if infectious causes have not been ruled out
• Oral azathioprine—1–2 mg/kg/day for 3–7 days, then taper; may be used to treat immune-mediated retinal detachments if systemic corti-costeroids are not effective; perform a CBC, platelet count, and liver enzyme every 1–2 weeks for the first 8 weeks, then periodically.

FOLLOW-UP

PATIENT MONITORING
• Repeat ophthalmic examinations—as required to ensure that ocular inflammation is controlled, and, if possible, vision is maintained
• Recurrence of vision loss—common in optic neuritis; may occur weeks, months, or years after initial presentation

POSSIBLE COMPLICATIONS
• Death
• Permanent vision loss
• Loss of the eye
• Chronic ocular inflammation and pain
• Obesity from inactivity or as a sequela of SARDS

MISCELLANEOUS

ASSOCIATED CONDITIONS
• SARDS (dogs)—signs similar to those of hyperadrenocorticism
• Neurologic disease—may note seizures, behavior or personality changes, circling or other CNS signs
• Cardiomyopathy (cats)—taurine deficiency

AGE-RELATED FACTORS
• PRA and many cataracts—breed-specific ages of onset

• SARDS—tend to occur in old dogs
• Optic nerve hypoplasia—congenital

ZOONOTIC POTENTIAL
N/A

PREGNANCY
Corticosteroids and immunosuppressive drugs may complicate pregnancy.

SEE ALSO
See Causes

ABBREVIATIONS
ALP = alkaline phosphatase
CSF = cerebrospinal fluid
LDDST = low-dose dexamethasone-suppression test
PRA = progressive retinal atrophy
SARDS = sudden acquired retinal degeneration syndrome

Suggested Reading
Gelatt KN, ed. Veterinary ophthalmology. 3rd ed. Baltimore: Lippincott Williams & Wilkins 1999.
Millichamp NJ. Retinal degeneration in the dog and cat. Vet Clin North Am Sm Anim Pract 1990;20:799–835.
Rubin LF. Inherited eye disease in purebred dogs. Baltimore: Williams & Wilkins, 1989.
Slatter DS. Fundamentals of veterinary oph-thalmology. 2nd ed. Philadelphia: Saunders, 1990.
Author Paul E. Miller
Consulting Editor Paul E. Miller

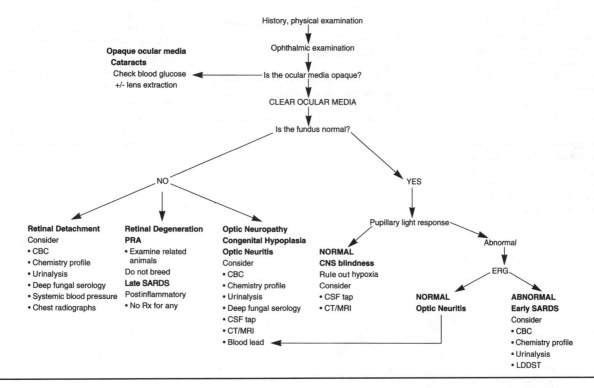

Blind Quiet Eye

History, physical examination

Ophthalmic examination

Is the ocular media opaque? → **Opaque ocular media / Cataracts** — Check blood glucose +/- lens extraction

CLEAR OCULAR MEDIA

Is the fundus normal?

NO

YES

Retinal Detachment
Consider
• CBC
• Chemistry profile
• Urinalysis
• Deep fungal serology
• Systemic blood pressure
• Chest radiographs

Retinal Degeneration / PRA
• Examine related animals
Do not breed
Late SARDS
Postinflammatory
• No Rx for any

Optic Neuropathy / Congenital Hypoplasia / Optic Neuritis
Consider
• CBC
• Chemistry profile
• Urinalysis
• Deep fungal serology
• CSF tap
• CT/MRI
• Blood lead

Pupillary light response

NORMAL / CNS blindness
Rule out hypoxia
Consider
• CSF tap
• CT/MRI

Abnormal

ERG

NORMAL / Optic Neuritis

ABNORMAL / Early SARDS
Consider
• CBC
• Chemistry profile
• Urinalysis
• LDDST

BREEDING, TIMING

BASICS

DEFINITION
Timing of inseminations during estrus to maximize fertility

PATHOPHYSIOLOGY
Dogs
• Multiple breedings—breed every other day during estrus to maximize fertility
• Fresh, cooled or frozen semen—usually limited to one or two inseminations; requires insemination to be timed with ovulation for maximum fertility
• Precise estimation of day of ovulation—variations in time of ovulation in relation to onset of behavioral or cytologic estrus; reduced longevity of semen; bitch that refuses to allow natural mating
• LH—controls ovulation; peaks on same day or up to 2 days after full cornification is observed; ovulation occurs approximately 2 days after the surge; 2–3 days more required for oocyte maturation; mature oocytes viable for another 2–3 days; thus fertile period is 4–8 days after the surge and fertility peaks 5–6 days after the surge; assay is a precise method for determining the day of the surge.
• Physical signs alone—may be unreliable for precise determination of fertile period
• Onset of estrus—usually associated with a change in the vaginal discharge from sanguinous to straw-colored and a reduction of vulvar swelling; sanguinous discharge may continue during estrus and cease only at the onset of diestrus (fertile period has passed; bitch no longer receptive).
• Receptivity—may be detected by stroking the near the tailhead; if receptive, female will flag by elevating the tail to one side
• Vaginal cytologic examination—good indicator of fertile period; cornification of vaginal epithelium controlled by estrogen; full cornification usually coincides with sexual receptivity; imprecise indicator of day of ovulation
• Serum progesterone—increase closely associated with the LH peak; useful for predicting the surge and thus the fertile period; concentration: < 1 ng/mL before the surge, 1.5–2.0 ng/mL on the day of the surge, and continues to rise during diestrus or pregnancy

Cats
• Ovulation—induced; timing of breeding is not as critical as with dogs; depends on adequate LH release, which is triggered by stimulation of the vagina and cervix
• Inadequate stimulation—characterized by lack of both a copulatory cry and a postcoital reaction; may fail to induce ovulation; frequency of coital stimuli important in determining adequacy of coital contact
• LH—peak concentration and duration of the elevation determine ovulation; higher plasma concentration with multiple copulations (more likely to result in ovulation than single matings); response to copulation depends on the day of estrus (greater release on estrus day 3 than on estrus day 1); release partially depends on duration of exposure to estrogen

SYSTEMS AFFECTED
• Renal
• Urogenital

SIGNALMENT
N/A

SIGNS
General Comments
Dogs
• Normal bitch—sanguinous discharge during proestrus becomes straw-colored during estrus; vulvar swelling of proestrus decreases slightly during estrus; receptive to male during estrus
• Limited number of available breedings—must know ovulation day
Cats
• LH response to a single mating—may vary substantially
• Neither single nor multiple copulations ensure ovulation.

Historical Findings
Dogs
• Refusal to accept male at the expected time
• Sanguinous vulvar discharge during estrus
Cats
• Return to estrus in < 30 days—indicates failure to ovulate

Physical Examination Findings
Dogs
• Fully cornified vaginal epithelium
• Interest shown by male
• Swollen vulva
• Vaginal discharge
• Flagging

CAUSES
Dogs
• Limited number of breedings
• Female unreceptive to male
Cats
• Coitus—too early or too late in estrus; too few times
• Breeding by artificial insemination (fresh, cooled or frozen semen)

RISK FACTORS
N/A

DIAGNOSIS

DIFFERENTIAL DIAGNOSIS
Vaginal discharge—proestrus or estrus; vaginitis; neoplasia

CBC/BIOCHEMISTRY/URINALYSIS
N/A

OTHER LABORATORY TESTS
Dogs
• In-house semiquantitative progesterone testing—as an adjunct to vaginal cytologic examination; to establish a baseline, begin when vaginal cytologic examination reveals 60%–75%; with no cytologic examination, begin early (day 3 or 4) in proestrus; perform every other day.
• In-house LH testing—must run samples daily to observe the LH peak

Cats
Submit samples for progesterone testing to verify ovulation.

IMAGING
Ultrasonographic imaging of the ovaries—may help determine ovulation; not reliable as the sole method of verifying ovulation

BREEDING, TIMING

DIAGNOSTIC PROCEDURES

Dogs

• Vaginal cytologic examination—at the onset of proestrus, most epithelial cells appear noncornified (nucleus appears stippled like a normal viable cell); percent cornified epithelial cells (cells with angular cytoplasm and pyknotic nuclei or nuclei that fail to take up stain) increases by approximately 10% per day during proestrus, reaching 90% or more by estrus. At the onset of diestrus, an abrupt decline in the percent cornified epithelin cells (usually 20–30%, often as great as 50%) occurs in a single day; the first day of noticeable decline in cornifaction is defined as Day 1 of diestrus (D1); normal to neutrophils on days 2–4 of diestrus
• Vaginoscopy—hyperplastic and wrinkled vaginal epithelium from proestrus to estrus

TREATMENT

DOGS

• Multiple breedings—inseminate every other day after the initial rise in progesterone is observed until D1.
• Two breedings—inseminate either on days 3 and 5 or on days 4 and 6 after the LH peak (day 0) or initial rise in progesterone (peak fertility); use fresh, chilled semen (viability reduced)
• Frozen semen—less viable than fresh chilled; thus timing is more critical; inseminate vaginally on days 4, 5, and 6 after the LH rise; a single surgical insemination more common; inseminate surgically on day 5 or 6 after the LH peak or initial rise in progesterone (day 0).
• May treat as outpatient—every-other-day visits for blood collection and vaginal cytologic examination
• Normal activity and diet
• Surgical artificial insemination requires routine postoperative care

CATS

• Increase the likelihood of ovulation by maximizing the number of matings; breed on successive days during estrus
• Breed four times a day spaced at least 2–3 hr apart on days 2 and 3 of estrus to maximize LH release
• May induce ovulation by administration of exogenous hormones—GnRH or hCG after mating

MEDICATIONS

DRUGS OF CHOICE
Cats—hCG (500 IU IM); GnRH (25–50 µg IM or IV)

CONTRAINDICATIONS
N/A

PRECAUTIONS
N/A

POSSIBLE INTERACTIONS
N/A

ALTERNATIVE DRUGS
N/A

FOLLOW-UP

PATIENT MONITORING
• Follow-up pregnancy examination
• Dogs—continue to obtain vaginal specimens after breeding throughout estrus to determine day 1 of diestrus; retrospective estimation of the day of ovulation is 6 days before D1; repeat semiquantitative progesterone test 3–4 days after the initial rise recommended to verify a continued rise
• Cats—progesterone assay to verify ovulation

POSSIBLE COMPLICATIONS

Dogs
• Vaginal cytologic examination—determine day 1; allows retrospective estimation of the day of ovulation (6 days before day 1); compare with the prospective estimation based on progesterone; if the estimates differ, pregnancy rates are reduced.
• Semiquantitative progesterone kits—must come to room temperature before use; false high values common when using a cold kit
• Serum progesterone—allow blood to clot at a cool temperature; separate cells from serum or plasma as soon as possible (within 20 min of collection); false low values when using serum mixed with RBCs (progesterone will be bound)
• A hemolyzed or lipemic specimen—may give a false low progesterone value
• Quantitative progesterone—performed by a commercial laboratory more accurate than semi-quantitative kits; perferable in cases of questionable fertility; turn around times make it difficult to use for prospective timing of breeding
• Serum LH—unidentified factors in the serum of some bitches interferes with the LH

kits causing the positive control line and test result to be obscured; must rely on serum progesterone.

MISCELLANEOUS

ASSOCIATED CONDITIONS
Vaginal stricture

AGE-RELATED FACTORS
Split heats in young bitches—typified by a period of proestrus, followed by cessation of signs, and subsequent resumption of the estrus cycle (1–3 wks later); no initial rise in progesterone of LH occurs with the first proestrus/estrus; subsequent estrus is usually normal with a LH peak and progesterone rise; fertility should be normal if breeding is based on LH peak or initial progesterone rise (most confirm continued rise 3–4 days later) rather than vaginal bleeding or cytology.

ZOONOTIC POTENTIAL
N/A

PREGNANCY
N/A

SEE ALSO
• Infertility, Female
• Vaginal Discharge

ABBREVIATIONS
• GnRH = gonadotropin-releasing hormone
• hCG = human chorionic gonadotropin
• LH = luteinizing hormone
• D1 = day 1 diestrus

Suggested Reading
Eilts BE, Paccamonti DL, Causey RC. Reproductive disorders. In: Norsworthy GD ed. Feline practice. Philadelphia: Lippincott, 1993:458–476

Holst PA. Vaginal cytology in the bitch. In: Morrow DA ed. Current therapy in theriogenology 2. Philadelphia: Saunders, 1986:457–462

Olson PN, Nett TM. Reproductive endocrinology and physiology of the bitch. In: Morrow DA, ed. Current therapy in theriogenology 2. Philadelphia: Saunders, 1986:453–457.

Author Dale Paccamonti
Consulting Editor Sara K. Lyle

CARDIOPULMONARY ARREST

BASICS

DEFINITION
- Cessation of effective perfusion and ventilation because of the loss of coordinated cardiac and respiratory function
- Cardiac arrest invariably follows respiratory arrest if not recognized and corrected.

PATHOPHYSIOLOGY
- Generalized or cellular hypoxemia may be the cause or effect of sudden death.
- After 1–4 min of airway obstruction, breathing efforts stop while circulation remains intact.
- If obstruction continues for 6–9 min, severe hypotension and bradycardia lead to dilated pupils, absence of heart sounds, and lack of palpable pulse.
- After 6–9 min, myocardial contractions cease even though the ECG may look normal—electrical mechanical dissociation
- Ventricular fibrillation, ventricular asystole, and electrical mechanical dissociation are rhythms indicating cessation of myocardial contractility.

SYSTEMS AFFECTED
- All systems are affected, but those requiring the greatest supply of oxygen and nutrients are affected first.
- Cardiovascular
- Renal/Urologic
- Neurologic

SIGNALMENT
- Dogs and cats
- Any age, breed, or sex

SIGNS
- Loss of consciousness
- Dilated pupils
- Cyanosis
- Agonal gasping or absence of ventilation
- Absence of peripheral pulses
- Hypothermia
- Absence of audible heart sounds
- Lack of response to stimulation

CAUSES
- Hypoxemia caused by ventilation perfusion mismatch, diffusion barrier impairment, hypoventilation, or shunting
- Poor oxygen delivery due to anemia or vasoconstriction
- Myocardial disease—infectious, inflammatory, infiltrative, traumatic, neoplastic, or embolic
- Acid–base abnormalities
- Electrolyte derangements—hyperkalemia, hypocalcemia, and hypomagnesemia

- Hypovolemia
- Shock
- Anesthetic agents
- Toxemia
- CNS trauma
- Electrical shock

RISK FACTORS
- Cardiovascular disease
- Respiratory
- Trauma
- Anesthesia
- Septicemia
- Endotoxemia
- Ventricular arrhythmias—ventricular flutter, R on T phenomenon, multiform
- Increased parasympathetic tone—gastrointestinal disease, respiratory disease, manipulation of eyes, larynx, or abdominal viscera
- Prolonged seizing
- Invasive cardiovascular manipulation—pericardiocentesis, surgery, angiography

DIAGNOSIS
- Sudden cardiovascular collapse associated with inadequate cardiac output can lead to severe consequences.
- Quick assessment and diagnosis is critical.
- Assess the ABCs—airway, breathing, circulation

DIFFERENTIAL DIAGNOSIS
- Severe hypovolemia and absence of palpable pulses
- Pericardial effusion, decreased cardiac output, and muffled heart sounds
- Pleural effusion with respiratory arrest
- Respiratory arrest can be confused with CPA
- Upper airway obstruction can rapidly progress to CPA

CBC/BIOCHEMISTRY/URINALYSIS
May help identify an underlying cause for CPA but should not be part of initial triage

OTHER LABORATORY TESTS
Blood gas evaluation may be useful during or after resuscitative procedures, but is not part of initial emergency management.

IMAGING
- Thoracic radiographs may help identify underlying disease processes but only consider after the patient has been stabilized.
- Echocardiography may confirm pericardial effusion or underlying myocardial disease but should not interfere with resuscitative procedures.

DIAGNOSTIC PROCEDURES
Once CPA has developed, continuous ECG monitoring, blood pressure monitoring, pulse oximetry, and capnography may be useful in monitoring effectiveness of resuscitative procedures.

TREATMENT
Institute cardiopulmonary resuscitation (CPR) immediately upon diagnosing CPA; can divide CPR into basic cardiac life support and advanced cardiac life support

BASIC CARDIAC LIFE SUPPORT

A—Airway
- Assessment—Visualize the airway by extending the patient's head and neck and pulling the tongue forward; clear any debris (e.g., secretions, blood, or vomitus), manually or with suction.
- Establish an airway by either oral endotracheal intubation or, if complete obstruction exists, emergency tracheostomy.

B—Breathing
- Assessment—make sure animal is not breathing.
- Institute artificial ventilation—administer two short breaths of ~2-sec duration each and reassess; if no spontaneous respiration occurs continue ventilations at a rate suitable for this animal (normal respiratory rate).
- Techniques for ventilation include mouth to mouth, mouth to nose, or mouth to endotracheal tube; these techniques provide ~16% oxygen; use of an Ambu bag and room air provides 21% oxygen.
- The preferred technique is endotracheal intubation and ventilation with 100% oxygen using an Ambu bag or an anesthesia machine.
- The suggested rate of oxygen administration is 150 mL/kg/min.

C—Circulation
- Assessment—palpate peripheral pulses and auscultate heart to confirm CPA.
- External cardiac massage provides at best ~30% of normal cardiac output; internal cardiac massage is two to three times more effective in improving cerebral and coronary perfusion.
- Hemodynamic studies in animal models suggest that several different mechanisms exist for generation of blood flow (artifical systole) during chest compressions; during external cardiac massage the cardiac pump theory takes advantage of direct compression of the heart in patients weighing <7 kg; in patients >7 kg the thoracic pump theory is used; this techniques uses increases in

CARDIOPULMONARY ARREST

intrathoracic pressures to increase cardiac output via the major arteries.

Compression/Ventilation Techniques
• Perform chest compressions rapidly, at a rate of between 80–100 compressions/min; the chest should be displaced ~30%.
• Use the cardiac pump in patients weighing <7 kg body weight; with the patient in right lateral recumbency, perform compressions directly over the heart (intercostal spaces 3–5); this can be done using one or two hands.
• Use the thoracic pump for patients weighing >7 kg body; with the patient in right lateral or dorsal recumbency, apply thoracic compressions at the widest portion of the thorax.
• If ventilation is provided without an endotracheal tube in place, one breath is given for every five compressions.
• If ventilation is provided via an endotracheal tube, one breath is given simultaneously with every compression or every other on compression.
• Interposing abdominal compressions between chest compressions enhances cerebral and coronary blood flow by increasing aortic diastolic pressure.

OPEN-CHEST CPR
• Indicated if closed-chest CPR is ineffective or preexisting conditions such as flail chest, obesity, diaphragmatic hernia, or pericardial effusion preclude closed-chest techniques
• Perform through a left thoracotomy at the fifth or sixth intercostal space.
• Perform a pericardectomy.
• The palmar surface of the fingers and thumb are used to push the ventricular blood toward the great vessel; digital compression of the descending aorta may help cranial perfusion.

ADVANCED CARDIAC LIFE SUPPORT
D—Drugs
• Base drug selection on the arrhythmia present.
• Atropine and epinephrine are most often correct selections.
E—ECG
• Accurate ECG interpretation is imperative.
• Check ECG leads.
F—Fibrillation Control and Fluids
• Defibrillation is time-dependent; perform immediately.
• Administer fluids cautiously.

MEDICATIONS

DRUGS OF CHOICE
• Base drug selection on the arrhythmia present.
• Administer drugs via central vein, intratracheal, intraosseous, or peripheral vein, in descending order of preference.
• Use intracardiac drug administration only as a last resort unless open-chest CPR is being performed.

CONTRAINDICATIONS
N/A

PRECAUTIONS
Only use high rates of fluid administration if there is a known history of hypovolemia; excessive fluid administration may lead to decreased coronary perfusion.

POSSIBLE INTERACTIONS
N/A

ALTERNATIVE DRUGS
N/A

FOLLOW-UP

PATIENT MONITORING
• Maintain normal heart rate and blood pressure with fluids and inotropic agents.
• Arterial blood pressure
• Central venous pressure
• Blood gas analysis
• Support respiration with artificial ventilation and supplemental oxygen.
• Neurological statis—if signs of increased intracranial pressure develop, consider mannitol, corticosteroids, and furosemide
• ECG—continuously
• Urine output
• Body temperature
• Radiograph thorax to assess resuscitative injury.
• Diagnose and correct factors that led to initial CPA.

PREVENTION/AVOIDANCE
Careful monitoring of all critically ill patients

POSSIBLE COMPLICATIONS
• Vomiting
• Aspiration pneumonia
• Fractured ribs or sternebrae
• Pulmonary contusions and edema
• Pneumothorax
• Acute renal failure
• Neurologic deficits

• Cardiac arrhythmias

EXPECTED COURSE AND PROGNOSIS
• Prognosis depends on underlying disease process.
• Rapid return to spontaneous cardiac and respiratory function improves the prognosis.
• Overall prognosis is poor; <10% of patients are discharged.

MISCELLANEOUS

ASSOCIATED CONDITIONS
N/A

AGE-RELATED FACTORS
N/A

ZOONOTIC POTENTIAL
N/A

PREGNANCY
N/A

SYNONYMS
• Cardiac arrest
• Heart attack

SEE ALSO
• Ventricular Fibrillation
• Ventricular Asystole

ABBREVIATIONS
CPA = cardiopulmonary arrest
CPR = cardiopulmonary resuscitation

Suggested Reading
American Heart Association. Guidelines for cardiopulmonary resuscitation and emergency cardiac care. JAMA 1992;268:16.
Beardow AW, Dhupa N. Cardiopulmonary arrest and resuscitation. In: Miller MS, Tilley LP, eds. Manual of canine and feline cardiology. 2nd ed. Philadelphia: Saunders, 1995:425.
Hackett TB, Van Pelt DR. Cardiopulmonary resuscitation. In: Bonagura JD, Kirk RW, eds. Kirks current veterinary therapy XII. Philadelphia: Saunders, 1995:167.
Kass PH, Haskins SC. Survival following cardiopulmonary resuscitation in dogs and cats. Vet Emerg Crit Care 1992;2:57.
Van Pelt DR, Wingfield WE. Controversial issues in drug treatment during cardiopulmonary resuscitation. J Am Vet Med Assoc 1992;200:1938.
Authors Andrew W. Beardow and Steven L. Marks
Consulting Editors Larry P. Tilley and Francis W. K. Smith, Jr.

CONSTIPATION AND OBSTIPATION

 BASICS

DEFINITION
• Constipation—infrequent, incomplete, or difficult defecation with passage of hard or dry feces
• Obstipation—intractable constipation caused by prolonged retention of hard, dry feces; defecation is impossible in the obstipated patient.

PATHOPHYSIOLOGY
• Constipation can develop with any disease that impairs the passage of feces through the colon.
• Delayed fecal transit allows removal of additional salt and water, producing drier feces.
• Peristaltic contractions may increase during constipation, but eventually motility diminishes because of smooth muscle degeneration secondary to chronic overdistention.

SYSTEMS AFFECTED
Gastrointestinal

SIGNALMENT
• Dogs and cats
• More common in cats

SIGNS

Historical Findings
• Straining to defecate with small or no fecal volume
• Hard, dry feces
• Infrequent defecation
• Small amount of liquid, mucoid stool—blood produced after prolonged tenesmus
• Occasional vomiting, inappetence, and/or depression

Physical Examination Findings
• Colon filled with hard feces
• Other findings depend on cause
• Rectal examination may reveal mass, stricture, perineal hernia, anal sac disease, foreign body or material, prostatic enlargement, or narrowed pelvic canal

CAUSES

Dietary
• Bones
• Hair

• Foreign material
• Excessive fiber

Environmental
• Lack of exercise
• Change of environment—hospitalization, dirty litter box
• Inability to ambulate

Drugs
• Anticholinergics
• Antihistamines
• Opioids
• Barium sulfate
• Sucralfate
• Antacids
• Kaopectolin
• Iron supplements
• Diuretics

Painful Defecation
• Anorectal disease—anal sacculitis, anal sac abscess, perianal fistula, anal stricture, anal spasm, rectal foreign body, rectal prolapse, pseudocoprostasis, proctitis
• Trauma—fractured pelvis, fractured limb, dislocated hip, perianal bite wound or laceration, perineal abscess

Mechanical Obstruction
• Extraluminal—healed pelvic fracture with narrowed pelvic canal, prostatic hypertrophy, prostatitis, prostatic neoplasia, intrapelvic neoplasia, pseudocoprostasis, sublumbar lymphadenopathy
• Intraluminal and intramural—colonic or rectal neoplasia or polyp, rectal stricture, rectal foreign body, rectal diverticulum, perineal hernia, rectal prolapse, and congenital defect (atresia ani)

Neuromuscular Disease
• Central nervous system—paraplegia, spinal cord disease, intervertebral disk disease, cerebral disease (lead toxicity, rabies)
• Peripheral nervous system—dysautonomia, sacral nerve disease, sacral nerve trauma (e.g., tail fracture/pull injury)
• Colonic smooth muscle dysfunction—idiopathic megacolon in cats

Metabolic and Endocrine Disease
• Impaired colonic smooth muscle function—hyperparathyroidism, hypothyroidism, hypokalemia (chronic renal failure)

• Debility—general muscle weakness, dehydration, neoplasia

RISK FACTORS
• Drug therapy—anticholinergics, narcotics, barium sulfate
• Metabolic disease causing dehydration
• Intact male—perineal hernia, prostatic disease
• Low tail carriage—perianal fistula
• Pica—foreign material
• Excessive grooming—hair
• Decreased grooming/inability to groom—long-haired cats, pseudocoprostasis
• Pelvic fracture

 DIAGNOSIS

DIFFERENTIAL DIAGNOSIS
• Dyschezia and tenesmus (e.g., caused by colitis)—unlike constipation, associated with increased frequency of attempts to defecate, and frequent production of small amounts of liquid feces containing blood and/or mucus; rectal examination reveals diarrhea and lack of hard stool.
• Stranguria (e.g., caused by cystitis)—unlike constipation, can be associated with hematuria and abnormal findings on urinalysis (pyuria, crystalluria, bacturia)

CBC/BIOCHEMISTRY/URINALYSIS
• Usually normal
• May detect hypokalemia, hypercalcemia
• High packed cell volume (PCV) and total protein in dehydrated patients
• High WBC in patients with abscess, perianal fistula, prostatic disease
• Pyuria and hematuria with prostatitis

OTHER LABORATORY TESTS
• If patient (dog) is hypercholesterolemic, consider T4 and TSH assay to rule out hypothyroidism.
• If patient is hypercalcemic, consider parathyroid hormone assay.

IMAGING
• Abdominal radiography may reveal colonic or rectal foreign body, colonic or rectal mass, prostatic enlargement, fractured pelvis, dislocated hip, or perineal hernias.

• Barium enema (after enemas to clean colon) may better define an intraluminal mass or stricture.
• Ultrasonography may help define extraluminal mass and prostatic disease.

DIAGNOSTIC PROCEDURES
Colonoscopy may be needed to identify a mass, stricture, other colonic or rectal lesion; biopsy specimens can also be obtained

TREATMENT
• Remove or ameliorate any underlying cause if possible.
• May need to treat as inpatient if obstipation and/or dehydration present
• Dehydrated patients should receive IV (preferably) or SC balanced electrolyte solution (with potassium supplementation if indicated).
• Dietary supplementation with a bulk-forming agent (bran, methylcellulose, canned pumpkin, psyllium) is often helpful, though they can sometimes worsen colonic fecal distension; in this case, feed a low-residue-producing diet.
• Manual removal of feces with the animal under general anesthesia (after rehydration) may be required if enemas and medications are unsuccessful.
• Subtotal colectomy may be required with recurring obstipation that responds poorly to assertive medical therapy.
• Discontinue any medications that may cause constipation.

MEDICATIONS

DRUGS OF CHOICE
• Emollient laxatives—docusate sodium or docusate calcium (dogs, 50–100 mg PO q12–24h; cats, 50 mg PO q12–24h)
• Lubricants—mineral oil and white petrolatum are not recommended because of danger of fatal lipoid aspiration pneumonia due to lack of taste.
• Stimulant laxative—bisocodyl (5 mg/animal PO q8–24h)

• Saline laxatives—isosmotic mixture of polyethylene glycol and poorly absorbed salts; usually used to prepare the colon for colonoscopy (GoLytely, 30–50 mL/ kg PO once to twice 6–12 h prior to procedure)
• Disaccharide laxative—lactulose (1 mL/4.5 kg PO q8–12h to effect)
• Warm water enemas may be needed; a small amount of mild soap or docusate sodium can be added but is usually not needed; sodium phosphate retention enemas (e.g. Fleet, C.B. Fleet Co., Inc.) are contraindicated because of their association with severe hypocalcemia.
• Suppositories can be used as a replacement for enemas; use glycerol, bisocodyl, or docusate sodium products.
• Motility modifiers can be tried—cisapride (dogs, 0.1–0.5 mg/kg PO q8–12h; cats, 2.5–10.0 mg/cat PO q8–12h) may stimulate motility; indicated with early megacolon

CONTRAINDICATIONS
• Fleet enemas
• Anticholinergics
• Diuretics

PRECAUTIONS
Metoclopramide, cisapride, and cholinergics—can be used with caution; contraindicated in obstructive processes

POSSIBLE INTERACTIONS
N/A

ALTERNATIVE DRUGS
Ranitidine causes contraction of colonic smooth muscle in vitro

FOLLOW-UP

PATIENT MONITORING
Monitor frequency of defecation and stool consistency at least twice a week initially, then weekly or biweekly.

POSSIBLE COMPLICATIONS
• Chronic constipation or recurrent obstipation can lead to acquired megacolon.
• Overuse of laxatives and enemas can cause diarrhea.

• Colonic mucosa can be damaged by improper enema technique, repeated rough mechanical breakdown of feces, or ischemic necrosis secondary to pressure of hard feces.
• Perineal irritation and ulceration can lead to fecal incontinence.

MISCELLANEOUS

ASSOCIATED CONDITIONS
Vomiting—with severe/prolonged obstipation

AGE-RELATED FACTORS
N/A

ZOONOTIC POTENTIAL
N/A

PREGNANCY
N/A

SYNONYMS
• Fecal impaction
• Colonic impaction

SEE ALSO
Megacolon

ABBREVIATIONS
TSH = thyroid-stimulating hormone

Suggested Reading

Bright RM. Management of constipation and megacolon in cats. In: Proceedings 17th Annual Waltham/OSU Symposium, 1993: 73–78.

Burrows CF. Medical diseases of the colon. In: Jones BD, ed. Canine and feline gastroenterology. Philadelphia: Saunders, 1986:221–256.

Burrows CF, Sherding RG. Constipation and dyschezia. In: Anderson NV, ed. Veterinary gastroenterology. Philadelphia: Lea & Febiger, 1992:484–503.

Hoskins JD. Management of fecal impaction. Compend Cont Ed Pract Vet, 1990;12: 1579–1585.

Authors Lisa E. Moore and Colin F. Burrows
Consulting Editors Mitchell A. Crystal and Brett M. Feder

COPROPHAGIA

 BASICS

DEFINITION
Ingestion of feces

PATHOPHYSIOLOGY
- Common in dogs; rare in cats
- Dogs are often attracted to herbivore, cat, and human (soiled diapers) feces.
- This phenomenon is so ubiquitous that it is considered normal canine behavior.
- Malnourished dogs may eat the feces from herbivores because they contain the products of intestinal (horses) and rumenal (cattle, sheep) fermentation.
- It is normal for bitches to ingest their puppies' feces for several weeks after they are born, presumably to keep the nest area clean until the puppies are strong enough to leave the nest to eliminate.
- Some dogs eat their own feces and those of other dogs; this is considered abnormal behavior.
- Hypothetical causes include nest cleaning, displacing behavior from unavailable herbivore feces to any feces, imitating the owners' behavior of removing feces, and responding to punishment for inappropriate soiling by removing the evidence.
- Dogs and cats with polyphagia secondary to drug administration, an underlying endocrinopathy, or a disease causing malassimilation of nutrients may exhibit coprophagia; the benefit of this behavior to dogs is unknown.

SYSTEMS AFFECTED
Gastrointestinal—potential for gastrointestinal parasites, gastroenteritis, and halitosis

SIGNALMENT
- Dogs and cats
- Nursing bitches frequently eat the feces of their pups
- Otherwise no age, sex, or breed predisposition

SIGNS
- Halitosis
- Vomiting
- Diarrhea
- Flatulence
- Borborygmus
- Weight loss—certain gastrointestinal or endocrine conditions

Historical Findings
N/A

Physical Examination Findings
N/A

CAUSES

Behavioral Causes
- Nest cleaning
- Displacement activity from unavailable herbivore feces
- Responding to punishment, by removing evidence of soiling
- Imitating owners' behavior—cleaning the nest

Medical Causes
- Exocrine pancreatic insufficiency
- Inflammatory bowel disease
- Small intestinal bacterial overgrowth
- Megaesophagus and/or esophageal stricture
- Intestinal parasitism
- Hyperthyroidism
- Diabetes mellitus
- Hyperadrenocorticism
- Dietary deficiencies—unproven
- Drug induced (e.g., glucocorticoids, progestins, phenobarbital)

RISK FACTORS
N/A

 DIAGNOSIS

DIFFERENTIAL DIAGNOSIS
- The diagnosis is based on the owners' history.
- Must distinguish medical and behavioral causes of coprophagia.
- A thorough evaluation of the animals diet, environment, appetite, and handling is essential.
- A complete physical examination is necessary to evaluate for underlying diseases.

CBC/BIOCHEMISTRY/URINALYSIS
- Iron-deficiency anemia uncommonly results from chronic gastrointestinal blood loss caused by parasites.
- Peripheral eosinophilia may occur with gastrointestinal parasitism or eosinophilic inflammatory bowel disease.
- Results may suggest diabetes mellitus, hyperthyroidism, hyperadrenocorticism, or drug-induced causes of polyphagia.

OTHER LABORATORY TESTS
- Multiple fecal flotations or a treatment trial with fenbendazole (dogs, 50 mg/kg PO q24h for 3 days; cats, 25 mg/kg PO q24h for 3 days), to evaluate for gastrointestinal parasitism
- Trypsin-like immunoreactivity (TLI) to evaluate for exocrine pancreatic insufficiency
- Cobalamin/folate to evaluate for small intestinal bacterial overgrowth and severe small intestinal mucosal disease
- ACTH stimulation test or low-dose dexamethasone suppression test to evaluate for hyperadrenocorticism
- Serum total T4 or T3 suppression test to evaluate for hyperthyroidism

COPROPHAGIA

IMAGING
• Thoracic radiographs to evaluate for mega-esophagus
• Swallowing studies (via contrast radiography or contrast fluoroscopy) to evaluate for mega-esophagus or esophageal stricture

DIAGNOSTIC PROCEDURES
• Esophagoscopy to evaluate for megaesophagus or esophageal stricture
• Small intestinal biopsy specimens obtained at surgery or via endoscopy to evaluate for infiltrative small bowel disease
• Quantitative cultures of the small intestine to evaluate for small intestinal bacterial overgrowth

TREATMENT
• Varies depending on whether the cause is medical or behavioral
• Treat any underlying endocrinopathies, gastrointestinal disease, or pancreatic disorders, and withdraw any drugs that could cause polyphagia.
• Correct any dietary deficiencies.
• Can treat behavioral coprophagia in a number of ways: can decrease access to feces by prompt disposal; walk dogs on a leash to facilitate removal from vicinity of feces.
• If unsuccessful, can use a muzzle or head halter on walks.
• Can give the dog a food reward when it defecates, thereby counterconditioning it to expect food rather than search for feces.
• Other recommendations, although unsupported by any published data, include feeding a highly digestible, predominantly meat diet; use of a meat tenderizer or pancreatic enzymes; and sprinkling noxious tasting/smelling substances on feces.

• Bitter and hot substances such as quinine, cayenne pepper, and commercial products (e.g., FOR-BID, Alpar Laboratories, Inc., La Grange, IL) have yielded variable results.
• Taste aversion learning is another potentially effective method—treat feces with an emetic agent that has a short duration of action; after a few experiences of coprophagy followed by nausea/malaise, the dog may learn to avoid feces.

MEDICATIONS

DRUGS OF CHOICE
Only use medications to treat coprophagia related to an underlying medical condition, and select them specifically to treat that condition.

CONTRAINDICATIONS
N/A

PRECAUTIONS
N/A

POSSIBLE INTERACTIONS
N/A

ALTERNATIVE DRUGS
N/A

FOLLOW-UP

PATIENT MONITORING
N/A

POSSIBLE COMPLICATIONS
• Intestinal parasitism
• Gastroenteritis
• Halitosis

✓ MISCELLANEOUS

ASSOCIATED CONDITIONS
See Complications

AGE-RELATED FACTORS
N/A

ZOONOTIC POTENTIAL
N/A

PREGNANCY
N/A

SYNONYMS
N/A

SEE ALSO
See Causes

ABBREVIATIONS
N/A

Suggested Reading
Houpt KA. Feeding and drinking behavior problems. Vet Clin North Am Small Anim Prac 1991;21:288–289.
Voith VL. Feeding behaviors. In Wills JM, Simpson KW, eds. The Waltham book of clinical nutrition. Oxford: Pergamon, 1994:121–129.
Author Mark C. Walker
Consulting Editors Mitchell A. Crystal and Brett M. Feder

CORNEAL AND SCLERAL LACERATIONS

BASICS

DEFINITION
• Penetrating—a wound or foreign body enters but does not pass completely through the cornea or sclera • Perforating—a wound or foreign body passes completely through the cornea or sclera; greater risk of vision loss than penetrating • Simple—involve only the cornea or sclera; may be penetrating or perforating; other ocular structures intact • Complicated—perforating; involve other structures besides the cornea or sclera; uveal, vitreal, or retinal incarceration or prolapse through the wound; traumatic cataract; hyphema; lid lacerations

PATHOPHYSIOLOGY
• Sharp trauma—wounds by an outside-in mechanism • Blunt trauma—wounds by an inside-out mechanism; eye undergoes sudden changes in its equatorial and axial dimensions and IOP; actual wound may be at a site other than the point of impact; more intraocular damage may result than from sharp trauma • All or a portion of the foreign object initiating the injury may be retained in the wound or eye.

SYSTEMS AFFECTED
• Ophthalmic • Musculoskeletal—surrounding skull or orbital tissue • Nervous—unconsciousness or brain injury

GENETICS
N/A

INCIDENCE/PREVALENCE
Common

GEOGRAPHIC DISTRIBUTION
N/A

SIGNALMENT

Species
Dogs and cats

Breed Predilections
None

Mean Age and Range
N/A

Predominant Sex
N/A

SIGNS

Historical Findings
• Usually acute onset • History of running through heavy vegetation, being hit by gunshot pellets or other projectiles, or being scratched by a cat common • Trauma may not be observed.

Physical Examination Findings
• Depend on tissues affected • Common—corneal, scleral, or eyelid deformity; edema; hemorrhage • May see a retained foreign body • Often rapidly seal; may appear only as a subconjunctival hematoma • May also see iris defects, pupil distortion, hyphema, cataract, vitreal hemorrhage, retinal detachment, and exophthalmia

CAUSES
Blunt or sharp trauma

RISK FACTORS
• Pre-existing visual impairment • Young, naive, or highly excitable animals • Hunting or running through heavy vegetation • Fighting

DIAGNOSIS

DIFFERENTIAL DIAGNOSIS
• History or a retained foreign body usually diagnostic • Traumatic event not observed and no foreign body found—consider non-traumatic corneal ulcer, hyphema, etc. • Traumatic Ulcerative keratitis—acute onset; linear, stellate or V-shaped; possibly multiple • Traumatic hyphema—almost invariably accompanied by corneal or scleral lesions and subconjunctival or periocular hemorrhage • Traumatic cataracts—disrupted lens capsule common • Traumatic retinal detachment—almost invariably accompanied by intraocular hemorrhage

CBC/BIOCHEMISTRY/URINALYSIS
• Usually noncontributory • Consider as a preanesthesia screen or when nontraumatic cause is possible.

OTHER LABORATORY TESTS
• Cytologic examination and aerobic culture and sensitivity testing of the wound and foreign body—recommended even if infection is not apparent; may need to collect specimen under general anesthesia at the time of surgery • Consider other tests (platelet count, coagulation profile, etc.) if nontraumatic causes are possible.

IMAGING
• Ocular ultrasonography—if the ocular media are opaque; may clarify the extent and nature of intraocular disease; may detect foreign body • Orbital radiographs or CT—may help determine projectile's course; may detect foreign body

DIAGNOSTIC PROCEDURES
• Determine the nature, force, and direction of impact of the object—help identify which tissues may be involved • Do not put pressure on the eye until rupture or laceration of the globe has been ruled out. • Assess vision—menace response; aversion to bright light • Periocular skin and orbit—examine for lacerations or deformities; suspect globe involvement if a lid laceration crosses the eyelid margin or penetrates the orbital septum; entry sites are often small and quickly seal. • Abnormal ocular motility—suggests extraocular muscle trauma, orbital hemorrhage or edema, retained foreign bodies or peripheral nerve or CNS damage • Scleral rupture—consider with subconjunc-

tival hemorrhage, especially if the anterior chamber is abnormally deep or shallow, there is vitreal hemorrhage, or the eye is abnormally soft. • Pupils—size; shape; symmetry; direct and consensual light reflexes • Detailed ophthalmoscopy—assess clarity of ocular media and fundus integrity; rule out intra-ocular foreign body • Seidel test—if any question of corneal or scleral leaking; use a dry to slightly moist fluorescein strip to paint a thin coat of fluorescein over the surface of the defect; leaking aqueous combines with the orange fluorescein, forming a bright green rivulet (seen best with cobalt illumination).

PATHOLOGIC FINDINGS
• Depend on wound and affected tissues • Usually correlate closely with clinical examination findings • Vitreal hemorrhage—may organize into a fibrous band, that applies traction to the retina, causing it to detach • Post-traumatic sarcoma (cats)—may occur months to years after severe ocular trauma

TREATMENT

APPROPRIATE HEALTH CARE
• Depends on severity • Outpatient—if integrity of the globe is ensured

NURSING CARE
• Sedation—considered for excited or fractious patients • When walking—apply an E-Collar and put ipsilateral foreleg through the leash to avoid increasing intraocular pressure in affected eye • Avoid third eyelid flaps in patients with perforations or deep or long penetrating wounds.

Injuries Considered for Medical Treatment
• Nonperforating wounds with no wound edge override or gape—apply an E-collar; give topical antibiotic or atropine ophthalmic solutions • Nonperforating wounds with mild wound gape or shelved edges—apply a therapeutic soft contact lens Bausch & Lomb (Plano T) and an E-collar; give topical antibiotic or atropine ophthalmic solutions • Simple full-thickness, pinpoint corneal perforation with a negative Seidel test that has a formed anterior chamber and no uveal prolapse—sedentary patients; use a therapeutic soft contact lens and an E-collar; give topical antibiotic or atropine ophthalmic solutions; re-examine a few hours after applying the lens and at 24 and 48 hr.

ACTIVITY
Usually confined indoors (cats) or limited to leash walks until healing is complete

DIET
N/A

CLIENT EDUCATION
Warn client that the full extent of the injury (cataracts, retinal detachment, infection) may

CORNEAL AND SCLERAL LACERATIONS

not be apparent until several days or weeks after the injury and that long-term follow-up is necessary.

SURGICAL CONSIDERATIONS

Injuries Requiring Surgical Exploration or Repair
• Full-thickness corneal lacerations with a positive Seidel test positive • Full-thickness wounds with iris incarceration or prolapse • Full-thickness scleral or corneoscleral lacerations • Suspected retained foreign body or a posterior scleral rupture • Simple nonperforating wound with edges that are moderately or overtly gaping and that are long or more than two-thirds the corneal thickness

Injuries Considered for Surgical Exploration or Repair
• Small full-thickness corneal lacerations with a negative Seidel test and no uveal incarceration or prolapse • Large conjunctival lacerations • Partial-thickness corneal or scleral lacerations in an active patient

MEDICATIONS

DRUGS OF CHOICE

Antibiotics
• Complicated wounds, those with retained plant material, and those caused by blunt trauma with tissue devitalization—infection common • Bacterial endophthalmitis—5%–7% of perforations; very rare in penetrating wounds • Penetrating—topical antibiotics alone (e.g., neomycin, polymyxin B, and bacitracin) or gentamicin solution q6– 8h; usually sufficient • Perforating wounds with negative Seidel test—systemic ciprofloxacin (dogs, 10–20 mg/kg PO SID); topical cefazolin (33 mg/mL by adding injectable cefazolin to artificial tears) and fortified gentamicin or tobramycin (add injectable aminoglycoside to the commercial ophthalmic solution to achieve a final concentration of 14 mg/mL) both drugs q4–6h • Perforating wounds with positive Seidel test positive—systemic ciprofloxacin (dogs, 10–20 mg/kg PO SID); topical cefazolin and fortified gentamicin or tobramycin as noted above, only when defect has been made watertight

Anti-Inflammatories
• Topical 1% prednisolone acetate or 0.1% dexamethasone solution—q6–12h; as soon as the wound is sutured or epithelized if there is no infection • Systemic prednisone—0.5–1.0 mg/kg SID to BID; for sutured or epithelialized wounds when inflammation is severe; when the lens or more posterior structures are involved; when the wound is infected or not epithelialized and control of inflammation is mandatory to preserve the eye • Topical NSAIDs—suprofen or flurbiprofen; may be used if topical corticosteroids are contraindi-

cated and control of inflammation is mandatory to preserve the eye

Mydriatics
1% atropine ophthalmic solution—q6–12h; when there is significant miosis or anterior chamber reaction

Analgesics
• Topical atropine or oral aspirin (dogs, 10–15 mg/kg PO BID to TID)—may provide sufficient pain relief • Butorphanol—dogs, 0.2–0.4mg/kg; cats, 0.1–0.2mg/kg IV, SC, or IM q2–4h or as needed; acute mild pain; sedation not required • Oxymorphone—dogs, 0.05–0.1 mg/kg; cats, 0.05 mg/kg IV, SC, or IM q4–6h or as needed; acute severe pain; sedation required • Naloxone—0.04 mg/kg IV, SC, or IM; to reverse narcotics

CONTRAINDICATIONS
• Topical ophthalmic preparations—avoid for perforations with positive Seidel test. • Ciprofloxacin—avoid in small and medium dog breeds aged 2–8 months; avoid in large dog breeds aged 2–12 months; avoid in giant dog breeds aged 2–18 months; potential for damaging rapidly growing articular cartilage

PRECAUTIONS
• Aminoglycosides—topical application may be irritating and may impede re-epithelization if used frequently or at high concentrations; possibility of toxicity when given to very small patients or when giving by more than one route • Topical solutions may be preferable to ointments if corneal perforation is possible. • Atropine—may exacerbate KCS and glaucoma • Topical or systemic NSAIDs—use cautiously with hyphema; safety of topical NSAIDs in cats unknown

POSSIBLE INTERACTIONS
Systemic NSAIDs—may potentiate the nephrotoxicity of aminoglycosides; ensure good hydration and adequate renal function, especially in small dogs.

ALTERNATIVE DRUGS
Topical ciprofloxacin ophthalmic solution—may be used instead of the combination of topical cefazolin and a fortified aminoglycoside; some streptococci are resistant.

FOLLOW-UP

PATIENT MONITORING
• Deep or long penetrating wounds that have not been sutured and perforating wounds—rechecked every 24–48 hr for the first several days to ensure integrity of the globe, to monitor for infection, and to check control of ocular inflammation. • Superficial penetrating wounds—usually may be rechecked at 3–5-day intervals until healed • Antibiotic therapy—altered according to culture and sensitivity results

PREVENTION/AVOIDANCE
• Take care when introducing new puppies to households with cats that have front claws. • Minimize running through dense vegetation or the owner should consider having a bottle of saline eyewash to irrigate foreign debris from the eye. • Minimize visually impaired or blind dogs' exposure to dense vegetation.

POSSIBLE COMPLICATIONS
• Loss of the eye or vision • Chronic ocular inflammation or pain • Post-traumatic sarcoma—may develop in blind cat eyes that have been severely traumatized; consider enucleation for all blind, traumatized feline eyes to prevent occurrence.

EXPECTED COURSE AND PROGNOSIS
• Most eyes with corneal lacerations or a retained corneal foreign body are salvageable. • The more posterior the injury, the poorer the prognosis for retention of vision. • Poor prognosis—scleral or uveal involvement; no light perception; perforating injuries involving the lens, cause significant vitreal hemorrhage, or retinal detachment • Penetrating injuries usually better prognosis than perforating injuries. • Blunt trauma carries a poorer prognosis than sharp trauma.

MISCELLANEOUS

ASSOCIATED CONDITIONS
Depends on nature and extent of injury

AGE-RELATED FACTORS
N/A

ZOONOTIC POTENTIAL
N/A

PREGNANCY
• Systemic corticosteroids—may complicate pregnancy • Systemic ciprofloxacin—probably should be avoided during pregnancy

SEE ALSO
• Cataracts • Hyphema • Keratitis, Ulcerative • Proptosis • Retinal Detachment

ABBREVIATIONS
• IOP = intraocular pressure • KCS = keratoconjunctivitis sicca

Suggested Reading
Kuhn F, Morris R, Witherspoon D, et al. A standardized classification of ocular trauma. Ophthalmology 1996;103:240–243.

Pieramici DJ, Sternberg P, Aaberg TM, et al. A system for classifying mechanical injuries of the eye (globe). Am J Ophthalmol 1997;123:820–831.

Gilger BC, Whitley RO. Surgery of the cornea and sclera. In: Gerlatt KN, ed. Veterinary ophthalmology 3rd ed. Baltimore: Lippincott Williams & Wilkins, 1999:675–700.

Author Paul E. Miller

Consulting Editor Paul E. Miller

COUGH

BASICS

DEFINITION
A sudden forceful expiration of air through the glottis, usually accompanied by an audible sound, which is preceded by an exaggerated inspiratory effort

PATHOPHYSIOLOGY
• One of the most powerful reflexes in the body
• Induced by stimulation of either afferent fibers of the pharyngeal distribution of the glossopharyngeal nerves or sensory endings of the vagus nerves located in the larynx, trachea, and larger bronchi
• Begins with an inspiratory phase followed in sequence by an inspiratory pause, glottis closure, increased intrathoracic pressure, and glottis opening
• Serves as an early warning system for the pharynx and respiratory system and as a protective mechanism

SYSTEMS AFFECTED
• Respiratory
• Musculoskeletal—because of the role played in the reflex by inspiratory and expiratory muscles of respiration
• Cardiovascular
• Nervous—result of cough syncope

SIGNALMENT
Dogs and cats of all ages and breeds

SIGNS
N/A

CAUSES
Upper Respiratory Tract Diseases
• Nasopharyngeal—rhinitis; sinusitis; nasopharyngeal foreign body or tumor; tonsillitis; tonsillar tumor
• Laryngeal—inflammation; foreign body; injuries; tumors
• Tracheal—inflammation (inhalation of irritating substances and heat); infections (viral and bacterial); foreign body; tracheal collapse; tumor

Lower Respiratory Tract Diseases
• Bronchial—inflammation; infection (viral, bacterial, and parasitic); allergy; foreign body; tumor
• Pulmonary—inflammation; infection (viral, bacterial, and fungal); aspiration pneumonia; pulmonary edema; tumor
• Pulmonary/vascular—heartworm disease; thrombosis or embolism; CHF; pulmonary hypertension; tumor

Other Diseases
• Esophageal—inflammation; foreign body; tumor
• Pleural—inflammation; infection (bacterial and fungal); hernia; tumor

RISK FACTORS
• Congenital and acquired esophageal, gastroesophageal, and upper gastrointestinal disorders—predispose the patient to aspiration pneumonia
• Hyperadrenocorticism and chronic administration of corticosteroids—may increase incidence of pulmonary thromboembolism
• Genetic predisposition to certain cardiac disorders—increases risk of pulmonary edema secondary to CHF
• Environmental factors—exposure to certain viral, bacterial, fungal, and parasitic diseases; exposure of dogs to mosquitoes without effective heartworm prophylaxis

DIAGNOSIS

DIFFERENTIAL DIAGNOSIS
Similar Signs
• Sneezing and coughing—expiratory events that may occur together in certain conditions (e.g., rhinitis, sinusitis, and regurgitation); may confuse both the owner and the history; forceful expiration of a sneeze: mouth usually closed; cough: mouth usually open
• Reverse sneeze—commonly misinterpreted as a cough by owners; associated with both an audible inspiratory and an expiratory component without the forceful expiratory event that characterizes both the sneeze and the cough; nasopharyngeal irritation usual cause; some of the same conditions that cause sneezing and coughing may be a cause.

Causes
• Patterns and characteristics—frequently suggest underlying cause
• Nocturnal—commonly associated with early stages of left-sided CHF and tracheal collapse
• Precipitated by exercise or excitement—frequently the result of inflammation or irritation involving the larynx, trachea, and bronchi
• Harsh and prolonged—suggests involvement of the major airways
• Soft and infrequent—likely the result of pulmonary alveolar disease or CHF
• Productive—suggests fluid or mucus in the expectorated material
• Dry—indicates lack of mucus or fluid production

CBC/BIOCHEMISTRY/URINALYSIS
• CBC—may suggest possible causes: neutrophilia with a left shift (e.g., infection and inflammation) or eosinophilia (e.g., allergic response)
• High liver enzymes with exaggerated SAP elevation—suggests hyperadrenocorticism
• Mild to moderate elevations in SAP—suggest liver congestion secondary to pulmonary disease or right heart failure
• Proteinuria—may be associated with pulmonary thromboembolism in patients with glomerulonephritis, amyloidosis, or hyperadrenocorticism

OTHER LABORATORY TESTS
• Filter test for microfilaria and/or filaria serologic test—evaluate for heartworm disease
• Low-dose dexamethasone suppression test or ACTH-response test—further evaluate elevations in liver enzymes
• Coagulation profile—for any patient that presents with a cough associated with either epistaxis or hemoptysis

IMAGING
• Radiographs—particularly useful for evaluating patients with nasal, sinus, tracheal, and lower respiratory tract disorders
• Thoracic ultrasound—useful for patients with primary cardiac disease, right heart disease secondary to a pulmonary condition, and pleural effusion

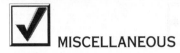

DIAGNOSTIC PROCEDURES
• Direct, flotation, Baermann, and sedimentation fecal tests—detect respiratory parasites and ova
• Transtracheal aspirate with cytologic examination and culture—evaluate lower respiratory tract disorders
• Laryngoscopy, tracheoscopy, and bronchoscopy—evaluate suspected foreign body, tumor, or other disorders in these regions; combine endoscopy with biopsy and bronchoalveolar lavage.
• Thoracocentesis—with pleural effusion
• Barium swallow—for suspected aspiration pneumonia
• CT scan—better evaluate nasal and sinus disorders

TREATMENT
• Outpatient—unless CHF is diagnosed or marked alteration in pulmonary function or hemoptysis noted
• Exercise restriction—best enforced until a cause is established and corrected, especially when activity aggravates the condition
• Inform client that a wide variety of conditions can be responsible for the cough, and a fairly extensive workup may be required to define and treat the underlying cause.
• Surgical intervention—may be indicated with tracheal collapse and for tumors involving the respiratory system

MEDICATIONS

DRUGS OF CHOICE
• Symptomatic treatment without other abnormalities—broad-spectrum antibiotics; bronchodilator-expectorant; appropriate follow-up evaluations
• Collect airway specimens for bacterial culture and sensitivity testing before administering antibiotics.
• Broad-spectrum antibiotics—for suspected infection when results of bacterial culture and sensitivity testing are pending
• Bronchodilator (e.g., theophylline and terbutaline) with or without the use of expectorants—may be beneficial for a variety of diseases affecting the trachea and lower respiratory airways

• Cough suppressants (e.g., hydrocodone and torbutrol)—avoid in patients with coughs secondary to bacterial respiratory infection and CHF; frequently beneficial for coughs of other origin
• Therapeutic thoracocentesis—perform for any patient with a marked pleural effusion.

CONTRAINDICATIONS
• Corticosteroids—do not use until a definitive allergy or inflammation is defined in the absence of infection, parasitic infestation, or cardiac disease; may potentiate the development of pulmonary thrombo-embolism; may reduce the efficacy of capar-solate in the treatment of heartworm disease
• Cough suppressants—do not use in any patient in which either a respiratory infection or clinically important heart disease is suspected.

PRECAUTIONS
• Cough suppressants—indiscriminate use may obscure the warning signs of serious cardiac and pulmonary disorders and pre-dispose the patient to serious complications or even death.
• Bronchodilator therapy—intravenous use of aminophylline may cause tachyarrhythmias.
• Diuretics—do not use in patients with primary airway disease; drying of secretions decreases clearance of mucus and exudate.

POSSIBLE INTERACTIONS
Theophylline bronchodilators—clearance may be inhibited by other drugs (e.g., enrofloxacin and chloramphenicol); signs of toxicity may develop with the addition of such drugs.

ALTERNATIVE DRUGS
N/A

FOLLOW-UP

PATIENT MONITORING
• Communicate with client concerning control of the cough.
• Follow-up thoracic radiographs—in 10–14 days with bronchopulmonary disease; in 3–4 weeks to monitor potential tumors

POSSIBLE COMPLICATIONS
• Complete control does not guarantee resolution of the inciting cause.
• Serious respiratory dysfunction and even death may be caused by underlying disease.

MISCELLANEOUS

ASSOCIATED CONDITIONS
• Heavy breathing
• Dyspnea

AGE-RELATED FACTORS
N/A

ZOONOTIC POTENTIAL
N/A

PREGNANCY
N/A

SEE ALSO
• Hypoxemia
• Nasal Discharge (Sneezing, Reverse Sneezing, Gagging)
• Respiratory parasites

ABBREVIATIONS
• CHF = congestive heart failure
• SAP = serum alkaline phosphatase

Suggested Reading
Ettinger SJ. Coughing. In: Ettinger SJ, ed. Textbook of veterinary internal medicine. 5th ed. Philadelphia: Saunders, 2000; 162–166
Kopos J, Tomori Z. Cough and other respiratory reflexes. Prog Respir Res 1979;12:15–188.
Langlands J. The dynamics of cough in health and in chronic bronchitis. Thorax 1967;22:88–96.
Yanagihara N, von Ledan H, Werner-Kukuk E. The physical parameters of cough: the larynx in a normal single cough. Acta Oto-laryngol (Stockh) 1965;61:495–510.
Author Neil K. Harpster
Consulting Editor Eleanor C. Hawkins

CYANOSIS

BASICS

DEFINITION
A bluish discoloration of the skin and mucous membranes owing to an increase in the amount of reduced, or deoxygenated, hemoglobin within the blood

PATHOPHYSIOLOGY
• Concentration of deoxygenated hemoglobin—must be > 5 g/dL to detect condition; thus anemia (PCV $< 15\%$) may obscure detection. • Central—associated with systemic arterial hypoxemia or hemoglobin abnormalities • Peripheral—limited to one or more extremities of the body; associated with diminished peripheral blood flow; arterial oxygen tension and saturation typically normal

Arterial Hypoxemia
• Decreased fraction of inspired oxygen—high altitude • Hypoventilation—upper airway obstructive disorders; restrictive or obstructive lung disease; pleural space disorders; neuromuscular failure • Ventilation–perfusion mismatching—pulmonary parenchymal or thromboembolic diseases • Diffusion impairment—thickening of the alveolar barrier through which oxygen must pass to reach the RBCs • Addition of venous blood to the arterial circulation—congenital right-to-left shunting cardiac defects (e.g., tetralogy of Fallot, transposition of the great vessels); reversed shunting cardiac defects caused by high pulmonary vascular resistance (e.g., right-to-left shunting PDA, ASD, VSD) • Anatomic shunts—distinguished from other causes of hypoxemia by the failure to respond to supplemental oxygen

Abnormal Hemoglobin
• Methemoglobin—most common abnormal heme pigment; unable to bind oxygen; normally formed at a low rate in erythrocytes • NADH-MR—intracellular reductive enzyme; maintains the methemoglobin:hemoglobin ratio at $< 2\%$; deficiency and/or exposure to oxidizing agents cause methemoglobinemia. • Hypoxia—when $> 20\%$–40% of hemoglobin has been oxidized to methemoglobin

Other
• Peripheral—results from increased oxygen extraction from the arterial supply to an area, e.g., a limb; caused by severe vasoconstriction, poor peripheral blood flow, obstruction to flow associated with arterial thromboembolism, or stagnation or obstruction of venous blood flow • Differential—with reverse shunting PDA, the head and neck receive oxygenated blood via the brachiocephalic trunk and left subclavian artery that arise from the aortic arch; the rest of the body receives desaturated

blood through the ductus located in the descending aorta.

SYSTEMS AFFECTED
• Central—all systems affected • Peripheral—may diminish or abolish the neuromuscular function of the affected limb(s)

SIGNALMENT
• Right-to-left cardiac shunts in association with high pulmonary vascular resistance and pulmonary hypertension (Eisenmenger physiology)—dogs: Keeshonds, English bulldogs, and beagles; some cats; generally young animals • Tracheal collapse—usually young or middle-aged small-breed dogs (e.g., Pomeranians, Yorkshire terriers, poodles) • Congenital laryngeal paralysis—young animals; reported in Dalmatians, Bouvier des Flandres, and Siberian huskies • Acquired laryngeal paralysis—most common in old large-breed dogs (e.g., Labrador retrievers, Afghans, setters, and greyhounds) • Hypoplastic trachea—identified in young English bull terriers; occasionally other breeds • Asthma (cats)—reported to have a higher incidence in Siamese

SIGNS

Historical Findings
• Central—stridor; dyspnea; cough; voice change; episodic weakness; syncope; exposure to oxidizing substances or drugs causing methemoglobinemia • Peripheral—limb paresis or paralysis

Physical Examination Findings
• Heart murmur or splitting of the second heart sound—with cardiac disease or pulmonary hypertension • Pulmonary crackles or wheezes—with pulmonary edema or respiratory disease • Muffled heart sounds—owing to pleural space or pericardial disease • Upper airway stridor with laryngeal paralysis • Honking cough—typical of tracheal collapse; may be induced by tracheal palpation • Dyspnea—may be inspiratory, expiratory or a combination (see Differential Diagnosis) • Limbs—may be cyanotic, cool, pale, painful, and edematous; may pulse in conditions causing peripheral cyanosis • Weakness—may be generalized and persistent with severe cardiac diseases; may be episodic and especially noticeable with exercise or excitement • Posterior paresis or paralysis—may be seen with distal aorta arterial thromboembolism; differentiated from primary neuromuscular disease by absence (or near absence) of pulses

CAUSES

Respiratory System
• Larynx—paralysis (acquired or congenital); collapse; spasm; edema; trauma; neoplasia; granulomatous disease • Trachea—collapse; neoplasia; foreign body; trauma; hypoplasia • Lower airway and parenchyma—pneu-

monia* (viral, bacterial, fungal, allergic, mycobacteria, aspiration); chronic bronchitis; hypersensitivity bronchial disease (allergic, asthma);* bronchiectasis; neoplasia; foreign body; parasites (filarioidea, *Paragonimus,* protozoa); pulmonary contusion or hemorrhage; noncardiogenic edema (inhalation, snake bite, electric shock); near drowning • Pleural space—pneumothorax; infectious (bacterial, fungal, FIP); chylothorax; hemothorax; neoplasia; trauma • Thoracic wall or diaphragm—congenital (pericardial, diaphragmatic hernia); trauma (diaphragmatic hernia, fractured ribs, flail chest); neuromuscular disease (tick paralysis, coonhound paralysis)

Cardiovascular System
• Congenital defects—Eisenmenger physiology (right-to-left shunting PDA, VSD, ASD); tetralogy of Fallot; truncus arteriosis; double outlet right ventricle; anomalous pulmonary venous return; atresia of aortic or tricuspid or pulmonary valves • Acquired disease—mitral valve disease; cardiomyopathy • Pericardial effusion—idiopathic disease; neoplasia • Pulmonary thromboembolic disease—hyperadrenocorticism; immune-mediated hemolytic anemia; protein-losing nephropathy; dirofilariasis • Pulmonary hypertension—idiopathic; right-to-left cardiac shunts • Peripheral vascular disease—arterial thromboembolism (feline cardiomyopathies); venous obstruction; reduced cardiac output; shock, arteriolar constriction

Neuromusculoskeletal System
• Brainstem dysfunction—encephalitis; trauma; hemorrhage; neoplasia; drug-induced depression of respiratory center (morphine, barbiturates) • Spinal cord dysfunction—edema; trauma; vertebral fractures; disk prolapse • Neuromuscular dysfunction—overdose of paralytic agents (succinylcholine, pancuronium); tick paralysis; botulism; acute polyradiculoneuritis (coonhound paralysis); dysautonomia; myasthenia gravis

Methemoglobinemia
• Congenital—NADH-MR deficiency (dogs) • Ingestion of oxidant chemicals—acetaminophen; nitrates; nitrites; phenacetin; sulfonamides; benzocaine; aniline dyes; dapsone

RISK FACTORS
N/A

DIAGNOSIS

DIFFERENTIAL DIAGNOSIS
• Generalized—systemic hypoxemia or heme abnormality • Peripheral only—reduced blood flow to extremities • Caudal body—right-to-left shunting PDA • Cardiac versus respiratory causes—differentiation may be difficult; cardiac murmur may suggest cardiac disease; murmurs may be heard in old patients with primary respiratory disease; thoracic radiography and echocardiography useful for differentiation
• Central or peripheral neurologic signs—should prompt concern of arterial hypoxemia owing to primary neuromuscular disease

Breathing Pattern
• May help define cause
• Inspiratory dyspnea—often associated with obstructive upper airway or pleural space disease; stridor frequently localizes problem to the larynx
• Expiratory dyspnea—generally seen with obstructive lower airway disease
• Rapid shallow (restrictive)—may be associated with pleural space disease or neuromuscular abnormalities of the thoracic wall

CBC/BIOCHEMISTRY/URINALYSIS
• Color of blood—often noticeably darkened with condition; chocolate brown with methemoglobinemia
• Polycythemia—often accompanies congenital heart disease; may occur with chronic hypoxemia owing to severe respiratory disease
• Proteinuria—accompanies protein-losing nephropathies, which may cause pulmonary thromboembolism

OTHER LABORATORY TESTS
• Methemoglobin concentrations—measure through a laboratory; alternatively, shake a blood sample in air 15 min: red, reduced hemoglobin with cardiac or respiratory disease; chocolate brown, methemoglobin
• Arterial blood gas analysis
• Urine protein:creatinine ratio—with suspected pulmonary thromboembolism secondary to a protein-losing nephropathy

IMAGING
• Radiography—essential for determining cause
• Echocardiography with Doppler—aids in diagnosis of congenital or acquired cardiac disease, pulmonary hypertension, and pulmonary thromboembolism

DIAGNOSTIC PROCEDURES
• Pulse oximetry—determine oxygen saturation
• Laryngoscopic examination—evaluate laryngeal structure and arytenoid function
• Bronchoscopy—may be used in the diagnosis of tracheal and pulmonary diseases
• Transtracheal wash, bronchoalveolar lavage, or fine-needle lung aspirate—may be required to characterize bronchopulmonary diseases
• Thoracocentesis—required for diagnosis and treatment of pleural space disorders
• Electrocardiography—may reveal heart enlargement changes; unreliable; echocardiography better

TREATMENT
• Inpatient—immediate diagnostic testing and treatment
• Stabilization therapy (e.g., oxygen, thoracocentesis, tracheostomy)—usually institute before aggressive diagnostics
• Specific therapy—depends on the ultimate diagnosis; usually exercise restriction and dietary modification required
• Surgical treatment—depends on primary disease process and the extent of cardiac or respiratory involvement
• Warn client when admitting the patient that diseases associated with cyanosis can have dire outcomes.

MEDICATIONS

DRUGS OF CHOICE
• Depends on final diagnosis
• Oxygen therapy—provide as soon as possible
• Diuretics (furosemide)—aggressive use indicated with suspected cardiogenic pulmonary edema
• Methemoglobinemia as a result of ingestion of oxidizing substances (acetaminophen)—give acetylcysteine (140 mg/kg PO, IV; then 70 mg/kg q4h for 3–5 treatments) as soon as possible; cimetidine (10 mg/kg PO; then 5 mg/kg PO q6h for 48 hr) useful adjunct to acetylcysteine; ascorbic acid (30 mg/kg PO q6h for 7 treatments) may be of some value but do not use as the sole agent.
• Plasminogen activators (alteplase, streptokinase)—may use for thrombolysis in cats with aortic thromboembolism; best administered by experienced clinicians

CONTRAINDICATIONS
Avoid using paralytic agents (succinylcholine, pancuronium) and agents that cause profound depression of the respiratory center (morphine, barbiturates).

PRECAUTIONS
N/A

POSSIBLE INTERACTIONS
N/A

ALTERNATIVE DRUGS
N/A

FOLLOW-UP

PATIENT MONITORING
• Patients in an oxygen cage should be disturbed as infrequently as possible for monitoring. • Assess efficacy of therapy—changes in depth and rate of respiration; color of mucous membranes (return to a normal pink color) if the cause is not an anatomic shunt and patient has adequate reserves; pulse oximetry or arterial blood analysis • Instruct client to monitor mucous membrane color and respiratory effort and advise immediate veterinary care if condition returns.

POSSIBLE COMPLICATIONS
Advanced pulmonary or airway disease and severe cardiac disease—poor long-term prognosis

MISCELLANEOUS

ASSOCIATED CONDITIONS
N/A

AGE-RELATED FACTORS
Congenital cardiac abnormalities—usually the cause in young patients

ZOONOTIC POTENTIAL
N/A

PREGNANCY
• Advanced pregnancy may exacerbate symptoms because of pressure on the diaphragm and reduced lung expansion. • Fetuses are likely to be harmed or aborted by the hypoxemia associated with cyanosis.

SEE ALSO
• Dyspnea, Tachypnea, and Panting • Stertor and Stridor • See also Causes

ABBREVIATIONS
• ASD = atrial septal defect • FIP = feline infectious peritonitis • MR = methemoglobin reductase • PCV = packed cell volume • PDA = patent ductus arteriosus • VSD = ventricular septal defect

Suggested Reading
Jacobs G. Cyanosis. In: Ettinger SJ, Feldman EC, eds. Textbook of veterinary internal medicine. 4th ed. Philadelphia: Saunders, 1995:192–196.
Krotje LJ. Cyanosis: physiology and pathogenesis. Compend Contin Educ Pract Vet 1987;9:271–278.
Author Ned F. Kuehn
Consulting Editor Eleanor C. Hawkins

DEAFNESS

 BASICS

DEFINITION
Lack or loss of sense of hearing, complete or partial

PATHOPHYSIOLOGY
• Either conduction deafness or nerve deafness
• Conduction—caused by diseases that obliterate the external ear canal, rupture the tympanum, or interfere with the function of the ear ossicles in the middle ear
• Nerve—acquired or congenital disease
• Acquired—caused by destruction of the normal inner ear structures; **NOTE:** for brainstem disease to cause deafness, extensive damage to auditory pathways is necessary, and such lesions would produce severe neurologic deficits from interference with the other systems adjacent to the auditory pathways.
• Congenital—caused by degeneration, hypoplasia, or aplasia of the spiral organ

SYSTEMS AFFECTED
Nervous—inner ear

SIGNALMENT
• Congenital—very young age; > 30 dog breeds known to be predisposed (Table 1); white cats with blue irises
• Acquired—any age; more common in geriatric dogs

SIGNS

General Comments
• Unilateral deafness difficult for most owners to ascertain; thus most animals brought to clinics have bilateral deafness.
• Conduction—usually relatively small hearing losses

Historical Findings
• Animal no longer responds to everyday sounds, does not respond to its name, or cannot be aroused from sleep by a loud noise.
• Puppy does not respond to the sounds of squeaky toys.

CAUSES

Conduction
• Otitis externa and other external ear canal disease (e.g., stenosis of canal, neoplasia, or ruptured tympanum)
• Otitis media

Nerve
• Degenerative changes in the cochlea of an old dog
• Anatomic—hypoplasia or aplasia of the spiral organ; hydrocephalus caused by damage to auditory cortex
• Neoplastic—acoustic neuroma; neurofibroma; neurofibrosarcoma
• Inflammatory and infectious—otitis interna;

canine distemper virus (may cause alterations in hearing, not complete deafness); nasopharyngeal polyps invading inner ear (cats)
• Trauma

Toxins and Drugs
• Antibiotics—aminoglycosides; polymixin B; erythromycin; vancomycin; chloramphenicol
• Antiseptics—ethanol; chlorhexidine; cetrimide
• Antineoplastics—cisplatin
• Diuretics—furosemide
• Heavy metals—arsenic; lead; mercury
• Miscellaneous—ceruminolytic agents; propylene glycol; salicylates

RISK FACTORS
• Chronic otitis externa, media, or interna
• Merle, piebald gene, or white coat color
• Use of certain drugs

 DIAGNOSIS

DIFFERENTIAL DIAGNOSIS
• Attempt to differentiate causes.
• Early age onset—usually suggests congenital causes in predisposed breeds
• History—use of ototoxic drugs; chronic ear disease
• Subtle behavioral changes—with slowly progressive disease of the cerebral cortex (e.g., senility, neoplasia), the brain may not be able to register what the ear can hear.
• Assess status of external ear canal and tympanum.
• Assess signs of hydrocephalus or canine distemper.

CBC/BIOCHEMISTRY/URINALYSIS
Usually normal

OTHER LABORATORY TESTS
Bacterial culture and sensitivity testing of ear canal—with otitis externa, media, or interna

IMAGING
• Tympanic bullae and skull radiographs—detect otitis media or otitis interna
• Ultrasound through open fontanelles—detect hydrocephalus

DIAGNOSTIC PROCEDURES
BAER—objectively assess hearing; essential for determining unilateral hearing loss and selecting breeding dogs

 TREATMENT

• Directed toward acquired causes; congenital deafness irreversible
• Otitis externa, media, or interna—medical or surgical approaches depend on culture and sensitivity test results and radiographic findings.

• Conduction—may improve as otitis externa or media resolves
• Hearing aids—have been used; apparatus must be modified for practical use.

 MEDICATIONS

DRUGS OF CHOICE
• None specific for deafness
• Used to treat otitis externa, media, and interna

CONTRAINDICATIONS
N/A

PRECAUTIONS
• Aminoglycosides or other ototoxic drugs—use with caution to prevent additional damage or damage to the normal side, if one exists.
• Topical treatment of external ear canal—avoid if tympanic membrane is ruptured.

POSSIBLE INTERACTIONS
N/A

ALTERNATIVE DRUGS
N/A

 FOLLOW-UP

PATIENT MONITORING
• Weekly to assess treatment of ear disease until resolved
• BAER—assess response to treatment of otitis interna

POSSIBLE COMPLICATIONS
Environment—may need to control for patient's protection

 MISCELLANEOUS

ASSOCIATED CONDITIONS
N/A

AGE-RELATED FACTORS
N/A

ZOONOTIC POTENTIAL
N/A

PREGNANCY
N/A

SYNONYMS
N/A

SEE ALSO
Otitis Media and Interna

ABBREVIATION
BAER = brainstem auditory-evoked response

Suggested Reading
Braund KG. Clinical syndromes in veterinary neurology. 2nd ed. St. Louis: Mosby, 1994.

Hayes HM, et al. Canine congenital deafness: epidemiologic study of 272 cases. J Am Anim Hosp Assoc 1981;17:473–476.

Mansfield PD. Ototoxicity in dogs and cats. Compend Contin Educ Pract Vet 1990;112:331–337.

Marshall AE. Hearing loss in aged dogs. Adv Small Anim Med Surg 1990;2:6–???.

Oliver JE, Lorenz MD. Handbook of veterinary neurology. 2nd ed. Philadelphia: Saunders, 1993.

Strain GM. Congenital deafness in dogs and cats. Compend Contin Educ Pract Vet 1991;13:245–254.

Strain GM, Kearney MT, Gignac IJ, et al. Brainstem auditory-evoked potential assessment of congenital deafness in Dalmatians: associations with phenotypic markers. J Vet Intern Med 1992;5:175–182.

Author T. Mark Neer
Consulting Editor Joane M. Parent

Table 1

Breeds with Reported Congenital Deafness	
Akita	Ibizan hound
American Staffordshire terrier	Jack Russell terrier
Australian heeler	Kuvasz
Australian shepherd	Maltese
Beagle	Miniature pinscher
Border collie	Miniature poodle
Boston terrier	Mongrel
Boxer	Norwegian dunkerhound
Bull terrier	Old English sheepdog
Catahoula leopard dog	Papillon
Cocker spaniel	Pointer
Collie	Rhodesian ridgeback
Dalmatian	Rottweiler
Dappled dachshund	St. Bernard
Doberman pinscher	Schnauzer
Dogo Argentino	Scottish terrier
English bulldog	Sealyham terriers
English setter	Shetland sheepdog
Fox terrier	Shropshire terrier
Foxhound	Siberian husky
German shepherd	Toy poodle
Great Dane	Walker American foxhound
Great Pyrenees	West Highland white terrier

BASICS

DEFINITION
Pathologic or cosmetic condition involving depigmentation of the skin and/or hair coat

SYSTEMS AFFECTED
Skin/Exocrine

SIGNALMENT
• SLE and DLE—collies, Shetland sheepdogs, German shepherds
• DLE—may occur more often in females
• Pemphigus foliaceus—chow chows, akitas
• Uveodermatologic syndrome—akitas, Samoyeds, Siberian huskies
• Vitiligo—Dobermans and Rottweilers, typically < 3 years old
• Seasonal nasal hypopigmentation—Siberian huskies, Alaskan malamutes, Labrador retrievers
• Cutaneous T cell lymphoma (mycosis fungoides)—typically dogs > 10 years old

SIGNS
• Leukotrichia
• Leukoderma
• Erythema
• Erosion and ulcerations

CAUSES
• Nasal solar dermatitis
• DLE
• SLE
• Pemphigus foliaceus
• Pemphigus erythematosus
• Uveodermatologic syndrome
• Contact hypersensitivity
• Vitiligo
• Seasonal nasal depigmentation
• Albinism
• Schnauzer gilding syndrome
• Drug reaction

RISK FACTORS
• Sun exposure—nasal solar dermatitis, DLE, SLE, pemphigus foliaceus, and pemphigus erythematosus
• Poorly pigmented nose—nasal solar dermatitis

DIAGNOSIS

DIFFERENTIAL DIAGNOSIS

Nasal Solar Dermatitis
• Lesions confined to nose and precipitated by heavy sunlight exposure
• Begins in poorly pigmented skin at the junction of the nasal planum and dorsal muzzle
• Negative for direct immunofluorescence

DLE
• Primarily affects nasal area
• Exacerbated by sunlight
• Positive direct immunofluorescence at basement membrane zone
• Biopsy—interface dermatitis

SLE
• Multisystemic disease
• Skin lesions—often involve nose, face, and mucocutaneous junctions; multifocal or generalized
• ANA—positive
• Positive direct immunofluorescence at basement membrane zone

Pemphigus Foliaceus
• Lesions—usually start on face and ears; commonly involve footpads; eventually generalized
• Biopsy—subcorneal pustules with acantholysis
• Positive direct immunofluorescence in intercellular spaces of epidermis

Pemphigus Erythematosus
• Lesions—primarily confined to face and ears
• Biopsy—intraepidermal pustules with acantholysis and interface dermatitis
• Positive direct immunofluorescence at basement membranes zone and intercellular spaces
• ANA—positive

Uveodermatologic Syndrome
• Typical breed
• Uveitis and cutaneous macular depigmentation with inflammation on nose, lips, and eyelids
• Biopsy of early lesions—interface dermatitis, pigmentary incontinence

Others
• Plastic or rubber dish dermatitis—depigmentation and erythema of the rostral nasal planum and lips; no ulceration and minimal crusting; history of exposure
• Vitiligo—cutaneous macular depigmentation without inflammation on nose, lips, eyelids, footpads, and nails; leukotrichia may be present with leukoderma.
• Seasonal nasal hypopigmentation—normal black coloration of nasal planum fades to light tan or pink; usually seasonal or slowly progressive with age
• Albinism—hereditary lack of pigment of the skin, hair coat, and irises
• Schnauzer gilding syndrome—young miniature schnauzers may develop idiopathic golden hair coat coloration, primarily of the trunk.
• Drug reaction—may resemble various cutaneous disorders such as DLE, SLE, pemphigus foliaceus, and pemphigus erythematosus; pruritus is variable; onset of signs is usually within 2 weeks of administration.

CBC/BIOCHEMISTRY/URINALYSIS
• Usually normal
• SLE—may see hemolytic anemia, thrombocytopenia, or evidence of glomerulonephritis

OTHER LABORATORY TESTS
N/A

IMAGING
N/A

DIAGNOSTIC PROCEDURES
• Cytology—acantholytic cells (pemphigus)
• Joint tap—evidence of polyarthritis in SLE
• ANA—positive in most cases of SLE
• Ocular examination—uveitis in uveodermatologic syndrome

DERMATOSES, DEPIGMENTING DISORDERS

• Direct immunofluorescence—deposition of immunoglobulin at the basement membrane zone with DLE, SLE, and pemphigus erythematosus, and in the intercellular spaces of the epidermis with pemphigus foliaceus and pemphigus erythematosus
• Skin biopsy

PATHOLOGIC FINDINGS

• Interface dermatitis—DLE, SLE, uveodermatologic syndrome
• Intraepidermal pustules with acantholysis—pemphigus foliaceus and pemphigus erythematosus
• Hypomelanosis—vitiligo, uveodermatologic syndrome, seasonal nasal hypopigmentation, and Schnauzer gilding syndrome
• Apoptosis—drug reaction (individual cell necrosis of keratinocytes)

TREATMENT

• Outpatient, except for SLE when severe multiorgan dysfunction is present
• Reduce exposure to sunlight—DLE, SLE, pemphigus erythematosus, and nasal solar dermatitis
• Avoid contact with topical drugs.
• Replace plastic or rubber dishes.
• Application of water-resistant ointments or gels with a SPF > 15 to depigmented areas

MEDICATIONS

DRUGS OF CHOICE

• Nasal solar dermatitis—topical corticosteroids; sunscreens (SPF > 15); tattoo hypopigmented skin
• SLE—immunosuppressive therapy with prednisolone, azathioprine (dogs), chlorambucil, or gold salts (cats)
• Vitiligo and nasal depigmentation—no treatment

CONTRAINDICATIONS

• Avoid chrysotherapy in patients with renal disease.
• Azathioprine therapy—not recommended in cats; may cause fatal leukopenia or thrombocytopenia

PRECAUTIONS

Ketoconazole—may cause anorexia, gastric irritation, hepatotoxicity, lightening of the hair coat or lethargy and inappetence owing to decreased glucocorticoid levels

POSSIBLE INTERACTIONS

N/A

ALTERNATIVE DRUGS

N/A

FOLLOW-UP

PATIENT MONITORING

Varies with specific disease and treatment prescribed

POSSIBLE COMPLICATIONS

SLE—associated scarring with ulcerative dermatitis

MISCELLANEOUS

ZOONOTIC POTENTIAL

None

SYNONYMS

None

SEE ALSO

• Cutaneous Drug Eruptions
• Lymphosarcoma, Epidermotropic
• Lupus Erythematosus, Cutaneous (Discoid)
• Lupus Erythematous, Systemic (SLE)
• Pemphigus
• Uveodermatologic syndrome (VKH)

ABBREVIATIONS

• ANA = antinuclear antibody
• DLE = discoid lupus erythematosus
• SLE = systemic lupus erythematous

Suggested Reading

Scott DW, Miller WH, Griffin CE. Muller & Kirk's small animal dermatology. 5th ed. Philadelphia: Saunders, 1995.

Author John G. Gordon

Consulting Editor Karen Helton Rhodes

DERMATOSES, EROSIVE OR ULCERATIVE

BASICS

DEFINITION
A heterogenous group of skin disorders characterized by disruption of the epidermis (erosions) or, if the basement membrane is compromised, the epidermis and dermis (ulcers).

PATHOPHYSIOLOGY
Varies widely, depending on the cause; may include congenital or developmental disorders that compromise tissue cohesion; cell-mediated (inflammatory or neoplastic) injury; anoxic injury; destruction by trauma, toxins, irritants, contactants, microbial organisms, or parasitic migration; and antigen-specific autoimmune disorders.

SYSTEMS AFFECTED
Skin/Exocrine

SIGNALMENT
Age, breed, and sex predispositions vary according to the disease in question.

SIGNS
N/A

CAUSES

Autoimmune
- Pemphigus foliaceus
- Pemphigus vulgaris
- Bullous pemphigoid
- Systemic or discoid lupus erythematosus
- Cold agglutinin disease

Immune-Mediated
- Erythema multiforme and toxic epidermal necrolysis (usually drug-induced or idiopathic)
- Vasculitis
  Canine eosinophilic furunculosis of the face (may be insect-related)
- Canine juvenile cellulitis (puppy strangles)
- Cutaneous histiocytosis
- Feline indolent ulcer (rodent ulcer)
- Feline hypereosinophilic syndrome

Infectious
- Superficial or deep staphylococcal pyoderma
- Deep fungal (e.g., sporotrichosis, coccidiodomycosis)
- Superficial fungal (malasseziasis, dermatophytosis)
- Atypical mycobacteriosis
- Actinomycetic bacteria (e.g., *Nocardia* spp., *Actinomyces* spp., *Streptomyces* spp.)
- Pythiosis
- Protothecosis
- Leishmaniasis
- Feline cow pox
- FIV/FeLV-related

Parasitic
- Demodicosis
- Sarcoptic/notoedric and demodectic acariases
- Flea bite allergy
- Feline mosquito bite hypersensitivity
- Pelodera and hookworm migration

Congenital/Hereditary
- Canine juvenile dermatomyositis
- Junctional epidermolysis bullosa
- Cutaneous asthenia (Ehlers-Danlos syndrome)
- Aplasia cutis (epitheliogenesis imperfecta)

Metabolic
- Diabetes mellitus
- Necrolytic migratory erythema (hepatocutaneous syndrome)
- Hyperadrenocorticism (especially when complicated by secondary infections or calcinosis cutis)
- Uremia (mucous membranes)

Neoplastic
- Squamous cell carcinoma
- Squamous cell carcinoma in situ (Bowen's disease)
- Mast cell tumors
- Cutaneous T cell lymphoma (mycosis fungoides)

Nutritional
- Zinc-responsive dermatosis
- Generic dog food dermatosis

Physical/Conformational Dermatoses
- Pressure point ulcers
- Intertrigo
- Self-trauma as a result of pruritic dermatoses

Idiopathic
- Ulcerative dermatosis of collies and shelties
- Feline ulcerative dermatosis with linear subepidermal fibrosis
- Lupoid dermatosis of German short-haired pointers
- Canine and feline acne
- Feline plasma cell pododermatitis

Miscellaneous
- Thermal, electrical, solar, or chemical burns
- Frost bite
- Chemical irritants
- Venomous snake and insect bites
- Thallium toxicosis

DIAGNOSIS

DIFFERENTIAL DIAGNOSIS
- History and physical examination—especially important owing to the extensive differential list (see Causes)
- Ascertain history of pruritus (self-induced ulcers or erosions), exposure to infectious organisms, travel history (for some fungal diseases), diet, and signs of systemic disease.
- Many of the causes have subtle differences in appearance and distribution of lesions.

CBC/BIOCHEMISTRY/URINALYSIS
Most helpful when metabolic disease is suspected or in any patient with signs of systemic disease

OTHER LABORATORY TESTS
Fungal serology and tests for immune-mediated diseases (e.g., ANA titer) may be indicated on a case-by-case basis.

DERMATOSES, EROSIVE OR ULCERATIVE

IMAGING
- Rarely indicated
- Thoracic radiographs—for deep/systemic fungal disease
- Thoracic or abdominal radiographs—identify calcinosis associated with hyperadrenocorticism

DIAGNOSTIC PROCEDURES
- Skin scrapings—suspected parasitism
- Direct impression cytology (Tzanck prep)—identify acantholytic cells if pemphigus is suspected
- Fine needle aspirate with cytology—indurated or nodular lesions
- Bacterial (aerobic and anaerobic), mycobacterial, and/or fungal cultures—suspected infectious disease (especially in cats with ulcers or draining tracts)
- Skin biopsy for histopathology—most informative test; for cavitary lesions, the leading edge should be harvested with a scalpel blade if the defect is too large to be excised in total; punch biopsy sufficient for diffuse erosive lesions

 TREATMENT
- Outpatient for most diseases
- Varies widely according to the cause
- Supportive therapy with fluid and nutritional supplementation is indicated in cases with severe fluid and protein loss through transepidermal exudation.

 MEDICATIONS

DRUGS OF CHOICE
Vary widely according to cause

CONTRAINDICATIONS
A definitive diagnosis can be imperative, because some immune-mediated cases that require immunosuppression may mimic infectious diseases that require specific antimicrobial chemotherapy (and for which immunosuppression could be fatal).

PRECAUTIONS
Side effects—associated with many antimicrobial, immunosuppressive, and antineoplastic drugs; consult a veterinary drug text.

POSSIBLE INTERACTIONS
Case-by-case basis

ALTERNATIVE DRUGS
N/A

 FOLLOW-UP

PATIENT MONITORING
Case-by-case basis, depending on the disease process, concurrent systemic disease(s), drugs used, and potential side effects expected

POSSIBLE COMPLICATIONS
- Depend on cause
- Some diseases are potentially life-threatening.
- Some diseases have zoonotic potential.
- Superinfections and drug side effects are possible in cases requiring immunosuppression.
- Some infectious diseases (nocardiosis, atypical mycobacteriosis) may be controlled but not cured.

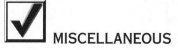 MISCELLANEOUS

ASSOCIATED CONDITIONS
N/A

AGE-RELATED FACTORS
N/A

ZOONOTIC POTENTIAL
- Sarcoptic acariasis
- Dermatophytosis
- Sporotrichosis
- Mycelial phase of some fungi (e.g., *Coccidioides immitis, Blastomyces dermatitidis*), when grown on culture media, can be infectious to humans through inhalation.
- In-clinic fungal culturing (other than for dermatophytes) is not advised.

PREGNANCY
N/A

SYNONYMS
N/A

SEE ALSO
Specific chapters devoted to diseases listed under Causes

ABBREVIATIONS
- ANA = antinuclear antibody
- FeLV = feline leukemia virus
- FIV = feline immunodeficiency virus

Suggested Reading
Angarano DW. Erosive and ulcerative skin disease. In: Kunkle GA, ed. Veterinary clinics of North America: small animal practice. Feline dermatology. Philadelphia: Saunders, 1995:871–885.

Beale KM. Nodules and draining tracts. In: Kunkle GA, ed. Veterinary clinics of North America: small animal practice. Feline dermatology. Philadelphia: Saunders, 1995:887–900.

Scott DW, Miller WH, Griffin CE, eds. Muller & Kirk's small animal dermatology. 5th ed. Philadelphia: Saunders, 1995.

Author Daniel O. Morris
Consulting Editor Karen Helton Rhodes

DERMATOSES, EXFOLIATIVE

BASICS

DEFINITION
Excessive or abnormal shedding of epidermal cells resulting in the clinical presentation of cutaneous scaling

PATHOPHYSIOLOGY
• An increase in the production, an increase in the desquamation, or a decrease in the cohesion of keratinocytes results in abnormal shedding of epidermal cells individually (fine scale) and in sheets (coarse scale).
• Primary exfoliative disorders—keratinization defects, in which the genetic control of epidermal cell proliferation and maturation is abnormal
• Secondary exfoliative disorders—from the affects of disease states on the normal maturation and proliferation of epidermal cells

SYSTEMS AFFECTED
• Skin/Exocrine—epidermal tissues, including nails

SIGNALMENT
• Primary—apparent by 2 years of age; characteristic in affected breeds (see Causes)
• Secondary—any age; any breed of dog or cat.

SIGNS

Historical Findings
• Excessive scaling
• Malodorous skin
• Pruritus

Physical Examination Findings
• Dry or greasy accumulations of fine scale or coarse rafts of epidermal cells located diffusely throughout the hair coat or focally in keratinaceous plaques
• "Rancid fat" odor common
• Comedones
• Follicular casts (accumulation of adherent debris around the hair shaft)
• Alopecia
• Pruritus
• Secondary pyoderma
• *Malassezia* overgrowth infrequent finding

CAUSES

Primary
• Primary idiopathic seborrhea (primary keratinization disorder)—primary cellular defect; accelerated epidermopoiesis and hyperproliferation of the seborrheic epidermis, follicular infundibulum, and sebaceous gland identified in some breeds; breeds at highest risk: cocker and springer spaniels, West Highland white terriers, basset hounds, Doberman pinschers, Irish setters, and Labrador retrievers; dry (sicca) and greasy (oleosa) forms exist, but determination of type has little prognostic value.

• Vitamin A–responsive dermatosis—nutritionally responsive; seen primarily in young cocker spaniels; clinical signs similar to severe idiopathic seborrhea; distinguished by the response to dietary vitamin A supplementation
• Zinc-responsive dermatosis—nutritionally responsive; results in alopecia, scaling, crusting, and erythema around the eyes, ears, feet, lips, and other external orifices; two syndromes: young adult dogs (especially Siberian huskies and Alaskan malamutes) and rapidly growing, large-breed puppies
• Ectodermal defects—follicular dysplasias; seen as color mutant or dilution alopecia; represent abnormalities in melanization of the hair shaft and structural hair growth; keratinization defects theorized as causative for several syndromes; breeds commonly affected: blue and fawn Doberman pinschers, Irish setters, dachshunds, chow chows, Yorkshire terriers, poodles, great Danes, whippets, salukis, and Italian greyhounds; signs include the failure to regrow blue or fawn hair with normal "point" hair growth, excessive scaliness, comedone formation, and secondary pyoderma.
• Idiopathic nasodigital hyperkeratosis—excessive accumulation of scale and crusts on the nasal planum and footpad margins; common in middle-aged spaniels; lesions generally asymptomatic, unless severe enough to result in cracking and secondary bacterial infection
• Sebaceous adenitis—inflammatory disease; breeds: middle-aged standard poodles, akitas, and Samoyeds; characteristic diffuse hair loss and excessive scaling; tightly adherent follicular casts; most dogs are generally healthy and asymptomatic; akitas: frequently develop severe and deep bacterial pyoderma; Vizslas: disease appears distinctly different and granulomatous
• Epidermal dysplasia and ichthyosis—rare and severe congenital disorder of keratinization; reported in West Highland white terriers; generalized accumulations of scale and crusts at an early age; secondary infections (bacterial and yeast) common; prognosis in severe cases is poor

Secondary
• Cutaneous hypersensitivity—atopy, flea allergic dermatitis, food allergy, and contact dermatitis; pruritus and resultant skin trauma and irritation
• Ectoparasitism—scabies, demodicosis, and cheyletiellosis; inflammation and exfoliation
• Pyoderma—skin infection; bacterial enzymatic dyshesion and increased exfoliation of keratinocytes in the attempt to shed pathogenic organisms
• Dermatophytosis—commonly exfoliative; increased shedding of affected keratinocytes is

a primary skin mechanism in resolving fungal infection.
• Endocrinopathy—hypothyroidism and hyperadrenocorticism commonly produce excessive scaling; hypothyroidism: abnormalities in keratinization, failure to regrow hair, and excessive sebum production; hyperadrenocorticism: abnormal keratinization and decreased follicular activity; secondary pyoderma common in both syndromes; other hormonal abnormalities (e.g., sex hormone abnormalities, hyperthyroidism, and diabetes mellitus) may also be associated with excessive scaling.
• Age—geriatric animals may have a dull, brittle, and scaly hair coat; changes may be caused by natural alterations in epidermal metabolism associated with age; no specific defect identified
• Nutritional disorders—malnutrition and generic dog food dermatosis; result in scaling from abnormalities in keratinization
• Autoimmune skin diseases—pemphigus complex: may appear exfoliative owing to rupturing of fragile vesicles and secondary pyoderma; cutaneous and systemic lupus erythematosus: cutaneous signs frequently appear as regions of alopecia and scaling.
• Neoplasia—primary epidermal neoplasia (epidermotropic lymphoma): may produce alopecia and scaling as epidermal structures are damaged; preneoplastic conditions (alopecia mucinosis, actinic keratosis): initially appear exfoliative
• Miscellaneous—any disease process may result in excessive scale formation owing to metabolic dyscrasia or cutaneous inflammation.

RISK FACTORS
N/A

DIAGNOSIS

DIFFERENTIAL DIAGNOSIS
• Signalment and history—paramount in distinguishing the possible causes of exfoliation
• Occurrence of pruritus—assists in determining the possibility of a cutaneous hypersensitivity; primary keratinization defects are often nonpruritic, unless secondary pyoderma develops.
• Concurrent signs (e.g., lethargy, weight gain, polyuria/polydipsia, reproductive failure, change in body conformation, and lack of hair regrowth), with or without inflammation, can assist in differentiation.

CBC/BIOCHEMISTRY/URINALYSIS
• Normal with primary keratinization disorders
• Mild, nonregenerative anemia and hypercholesteremia are consistent with hypothyroidism.
• Neutrophilia, monocytosis, eosinopenia, lymphopenia, elevated serum alkaline

phosphatase, hypercholesterolemia, and hyposthenuria suggest hyperadrenocorticism.

OTHER LABORATORY TESTS

Thyroid hormone levels and adrenal function tests if an endocrinopathy is suspected; see specific chapters for test recommendations.

IMAGING

N/A

DIAGNOSTIC PROCEDURES

• Skin scrapings—diagnose ectoparasitism
• Skin biopsy—rule out particular differential diagnoses; strongly recommended for most cases
• Intradermal skin testing—identify atopy
• Food-elimination trial—identify food allergy
• Epidermal exudate preparations—determine type of microflora on the skin

TREATMENT

• Frequent and appropriate topical therapy—cornerstone of proper treatment
• Underbathing, rather than overbathing, is a common error.
• Diagnose and control all treatable primary and secondary diseases.
• Recurrence of secondary pyoderma may require repeated therapy and further diagnostics.
• Maintaining control is often lifelong.

MEDICATIONS

DRUGS OF CHOICE

Shampoos

• Contact time—5–15 min required; > 15 min discouraged, because it results in epidermal maceration, loss of barrier function, and excessive epidermal drying.
• Hypoallergenic (soap free)—useful only in mild cases of dry scale and to maintain secondary exfoliation after the primary disease has been controlled
• Sulfur/salicylic acid—keratolytic, keratoplastic, and bacteriostatic; an excellent first choice for the moderately scaly patient; not overly drying
• Benzoyl peroxide—strongly keratolytic, antimicrobial, and follicle flushing; may cause irritation and severe dryness; benzoyl peroxide best for recurrent bacterial infection and/or extreme greasiness
• Ethyl lactate—less effective than benzoyl peroxide for follicular flushing and antimicrobial activity, but not as irritating or drying; most useful for moderate pyoderma and dry scale
• Tar—keratolytic, keratoplastic, and antipruritic; degreasing, but less so than

benzoyl peroxide; use for moderate scale associated with pruritus

Moisturizers

• Excellent for restoring skin hydration (frequent shampooing may result in excessive dryness and discomfort) and increasing effectiveness of subsequent shampoos
• Humectants—encourage hydration of the stratum corneum by attracting water from the dermis; at high concentrations may be keratolytic
• Microencapsulation—recent advances may improve the residual activity of moisturizers by permitting sustained release after bathing.
• Emollients—coat the skin; smooth the roughened surfaces produced by excessive scaling; usually combined with occlusives to encourage hydration of the epidermis

Systemic Therapy

• Specific causes require specific treatments (i.e., thyroxine replacement for hypothyroidism; zinc supplements for zinc-responsive dermatosis).
• Systemic antibiotics—always indicated for secondary pyoderma
• Retinoid drugs—varied success for idiopathic or primary seborrhea; reports of individual response to retinoids (especially cocker spaniels with a primary keratinization defect); generally, topical therapy provides more benefits for dogs than does retinoid administration; vitamin A analogs (etretinate, soriatane, and isotretinoin) used in limited studies; vitamin D analogs are currently being evaluated for use in keratinization defects

CONTRAINDICATIONS

N/A

PRECAUTIONS

• Corticosteroids—may be used judiciously to control the inflammation resulting from many exfoliative disorders; will mask signs of pyoderma and prevent accurate diagnosis of primary disease
• Vitamin A and D analogs—side effects can be severe, thus, patients should be referred to a dermatologist before being treated with these experimental drugs.

POSSIBLE INTERACTIONS

N/A

ALTERNATIVE DRUGS

N/A

FOLLOW-UP

PATIENT MONITORING

• Antibiotics and topical therapy—recheck every 3 weeks to monitor response; patients may respond differently to the various topical therapies.

• Seasonal changes, development of additional diseases (especially cutaneous hypersensitivity), and recurrence of pyoderma—may cause previously controlled patients to worsen; re-evaluation critical for determining if new factors are involved and if changes in therapy are necessary
• Endocrinopathies—after pill administration, routine 4–6-hr thyroid monitoring or ACTH-stimulation tests should be used for proper management
• Autoimmune disorders—re-evaluate frequently during the initial phase of induction; less often after remission; clinical evaluation and laboratory data required

POSSIBLE COMPLICATIONS

N/A

✓ MISCELLANEOUS

ASSOCIATED CONDITIONS

N/A

AGE-RELATED FACTORS

N/A

ZOONOTIC POTENTIAL

Dermatophytosis and several ectoparasites have either zoonotic potential or the ability to produce human lesions.

PREGNANCY

• Sulfonamide antibiotics and chloramphenicol—do not use in pregnant animals.
• Systemic retinoids and vitamin A in therapeutic dosages—do not use in intact females, because of severe and predictable teratogenicity and the extremely long withdrawal period

SYNONYMS

Keratinization disorders—seborrhea, idiopathic seborrhea, keratinization defect, dyskeratinization, and incorrect human terms (eczema and psoriasis); sebopsoriasis: correct term to describe the similarities between some human and canine keratinization defects

SEE ALSO

• Atopy
• Demodicosis
• Hyperadrenocorticism (Cushing Disease)
• Hypothyroidism
• *Malassezia* Dermatitis
• Pyoderma
• Sarcoptic Mange

Suggested Reading

Griffin CE, Kwochka KW, Macdonald JM. Current veterinary dermatology: the science and art of therapy. St. Louis: Mosby, 1993.
Author Alexander H. Werner
Consulting Editor Karen Helton Rhodes

DERMATOSES, PAPULONODULAR

  BASICS

DEFINITION
Diseases whose primary lesions may manifest as papules and nodules, which are solid, elevated lesions of the skin.

PATHOPHYSIOLOGY
• Papules—usually the result of tissue infiltration by inflammatory cells; accompanying intraepidermal edema or epidermal hyperplasia and dermal edema
• Nodules—larger than papules; usually the result of a massive infiltration of inflammatory cells into the dermis or subcutis

SYSTEMS AFFECTED
Skin/Exocrine

SIGNALMENT
Any age, breed, or sex

CAUSES
• Superficial and deep bacterial folliculitis
• Dermatophytosis
• Sebaceous adenitis
• Sterile eosinophilic pustulosis
• Canine and feline acne
• Kerions
• Demodicosis
• Rhabditic dermatitis
• Actinic conditions

RISK FACTORS
• Folliculitis, dermatophytosis, and demodicosis—any disease or medication that causes immune compromise predisposes animals
• Rhabditic dermatitis—may be associated with contact with decaying organic debris (straw or hay) containing *Pelodera strongyloides*
• Actinic conditions—seen more frequently in outdoor, short-haired dogs living in areas with ample sunlight

 DIAGNOSIS

DIFFERENTIAL DIAGNOSIS
• See Causes
• These diseases can be most easily differentiated by diagnostic tests (see below).

CBC/BIOCHEMISTRY/URINALYSIS
• Should be within normal range in most patients
• A circulating eosinophilia may be present with sterile eosinophilic pustulosis.

OTHER LABORATORY TESTS
N/A

IMAGING
N/A

DIAGNOSTIC PROCEDURES
• Skin scrapings—identify possible *Demodex* mites or rhabditiform larvae
• Dermatophyte cultures—identify possible dermatophytosis
• Tzanck preparations—determine if bacteria and degenerative neutrophils are present; compatible with bacterial folliculitis; eosinophils indicate eosinophilic pustulosis or furunculosis is more likely.
• Skin biopsy—if none of these tests has revealed a definitive diagnosis

 TREATMENT

• For nearly all causes, animal can be treated as an outpatient.
• Generalized demodicosis and secondary sepsis require hospitalized.
• Alteration of activity or diet should not be necessary.

MEDICATIONS

DRUGS OF CHOICE
Bacterial Folliculitis
• Superficial pyoderma—appropriate antibiotics based on bacterial culture and sensitivity should be given for 3–4 weeks
• Deep pyoderma—appropriate antibiotics based on bacterial culture and sensitivity should be given for 6–8 weeks or more

Sebaceous Adenitis
• A 50%–75% mixture of propylene glycol and water once daily as a spray to affected areas or bathing and soaking in baby oil weekly
• Essential fatty acid dietary supplements (PO q12h) in addition to evening primrose oil (500 mg PO q12h)
• Refractory cases—isotretinoin (1 mg/kg PO q12–24h); if response is seen, taper dosage (1 mg/kg q48h or 0.5 mg/kg q24h)
• Cyclosporine has also been used (5 mg/kg PO q12h).
• Most cases are refractory to corticosteroids.

Canine Acne
• May resolve without therapy in mild cases
• More severe cases—benzoyl peroxide shampoos and gels every 24 hr until lesions resolve; then as needed
• Mupirocin—topical antibiotic; apply every 24 hr or alternate with the benzoyl peroxide therapies
• Recurrent or very deep infection (furunculosis)—systemic antibiotics and warm water soaks
• Very refractory cases—topical tretinoin (every 12 hr) or isotretinoin (1–2 mg/kg PO q24h)
Feline Acne
• Underlying cause should be sought and treated accordingly
• No underlying cause found—Stri-Dex pads or benzoyl peroxide gels used daily or alternated daily

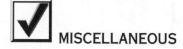

• Cats can be sensitive to the irritant effects of benzoyl peroxide.
• Refractory cases—try systemic antibiotics

Rhabditic Dermatitis
• Remove and destroy bedding.
• Wash kennels, beds, and cages and treat with a premise insecticide or flea spray.
• Bathe affected animal and remove crusts.
• Parasiticidal dip—at least 2 times at weekly intervals
• Severe infection—antibiotics may be necessary

Actinic Conditions
• Sunlight—avoid between 10 A.M. and 4 P.M; apply sunscreen with an SPF ≥ 15 every 12 hr
• Severe inflammation—topical or systemic corticosteroids may provide comfort; topical, 1%–2.5% hydrocortisone usually sufficient; systemic, prednisone (initially, 1 mg/kg PO for 3–5 days)
• Secondary infection—antibiotics may be necessary
• Squamous cell carcinoma—prognosis is guarded to poor, depending on the stage of the disease; therapy includes synthetic retinoids, hyperthermia, cryosurgery, photochemotherapy, radiation therapy, and surgical excision

Other
• Dermatophytosis—see specific chapter
• Sterile eosinophilic pustulosis—prednisolone/prednisone (2.2–4.4 mg/kg q24h; then taper to an alternate-day low dosage).
• Kerion—see Dermatophytosis
• Demodicosis—see specific chapter

CONTRAINDICATIONS
Corticosteroids and other immune suppressants should be avoided with folliculitis, dermatophytosis, kerions, and demodicosis.

PRECAUTIONS
• Fatty acids—use with caution in dogs with inflammatory bowel disease or recurrent bouts of pancreatitis

• Isotretinoin—may cause keratoconjunctivitis sicca, hyperactivity, ear pruritus, erythematous mucocutaneous junction, lethargy with vomiting, abdominal distension and erythema, anorexia with lethargy, collapse, and swollen tongue; CBC and chemistry screen abnormalities include high platelet count, hypertriglyceridemia, hypercholesterolemia, and high alanine transaminase.
• Cyclosporine—may cause vomiting and diarrhea, gingival hyperplasia, B lymphocyte hyperplasia, hirsutism, papillomatous skin lesions, and high incidence of infection; potential toxic reactions include nephrotoxicity and hepatotoxicity.

POSSIBLE INTERACTIONS
N/A

ALTERNATIVE DRUGS
N/A

 FOLLOW-UP

PATIENT MONITORING
• CBC, chemistry screen, and urinalysis—monitor monthly for 4–6 months in patients receiving cyclosporine and synthetic retinoid therapy
• Tear production—monitor monthly for 4–6 months, then every 6 months in patients receiving synthetic retinoid therapy
• Skin scrapings—monitor therapy in patients with demodicosis (see Demodicosis)
• Repeat fungal cultures—monitor therapy in patients with dermatophytosis (see Dermatophytosis)
• Resolution of lesions—monitor progress of sebaceous adenitis, and actinic conditions, and all other diseases

POSSIBLE COMPLICATIONS
Actinic conditions may progress to squamous cell carcinoma.

✓ MISCELLANEOUS

ASSOCIATED CONDITIONS
N/A

AGE-RELATED FACTORS
N/A

ZOONOTIC POTENTIAL
Dermatophytosis—contagious to humans in 30%–50% of cases of *Microsporum canis*.

PREGNANCY
• Synthetic retinoids—very teratogenic; do not use in pregnant animals, animals intended for reproduction, or intact animals; should not be used by women of childbearing age
• Corticosteroids—do not use in pregnant animals

SYNONYMS
N/A

SEE ALSO
• Demodicosis
• Dermatophytosis
• Pyoderma

Suggested Reading
Griffin CE, Kwochka KW, MacDonald JM, eds. Current veterinary dermatology. St. Louis: Mosby, 1993.
Gross TL, Ihrke PJ, Walder EJ. Veterinary dermatopathology. St. Louis: Mosby, 1992.
Muller GH, Kirk RW, Scott DW, eds. Small animal dermatology. 4th ed. Philadelphia: Saunders, 1989.
Authors Karen A. Kuhl and Jean Swingle Greek
Consulting Editor Karen Helton Rhodes

DERMATOSES, STERILE NODULAR/GRANULOMATOUS

BASICS

DEFINITION
Diseases whose primary lesions are nodules that are solid, elevated, and > 1 cm in diameter

PATHOPHYSIOLOGY
• Nodules—usually result from an infiltration of inflammatory cells into the dermis and subcutis; may be secondary to endogenous or exogenous stimuli
• Inflammation is typically, but not always, granulomatous to pyogranulomatous.

SYSTEMS AFFECTED
• Skin/Exocrine
• Several of these conditions may affect internal organs.

SIGNALMENT
• Nodular dermatofibrosis—German shepherds, 3–5 years old
• Calcinosis circumscripta—German shepherds, < 2 years old
• Malignant histiocytosis—Bernese mountain dogs
• May affect any age, breed, or sex, although Bernese mountain dogs are at higher risk for malignant histiocytosis and German shepherds are at higher risk for nodular dermatofibrosis

CAUSES
• Amyloidosis
• Foreign body reaction
• Sperulocytosis
• Idiopathic sterile granuloma and pyogranuloma
• Canine eosinophilic granuloma
• Calcinosis cutis
• Calcinosis circumscripta
• Malignant histiocytosis
• Cutaneous histiocytosis
• Sterile panniculitis
• Nodular dermatofibrosis
• Cutaneous xanthoma

RISK FACTORS
• Foreign body reaction—induced by exposure to any irritating material (e.g., concrete dust or fiberglass)
• Hair foreign bodies—increased risk for large dogs that rest on very hard surfaces
• Calcinosis cutis—increased risk with exposure to high doses of exogenous glucocorticoids
• Panniculitis—increased risk with vitamin E–deficient diet

DIAGNOSIS

DIFFERENTIAL DIAGNOSIS
• See Causes
• Sterile nodular dermatoses—must be differentiated from deep bacterial and fungal infections and dermal neoplasias
• All of these diseases can be diagnosed by histopathology and deep tissue cultures.

CBC/BIOCHEMISTRY/URINALYSIS
• Normal in most conditions causing sterile nodules.
• Amyloidosis—possible changes in biochemistry and/or urinalysis if internal organs are affected
• Malignant histiocytosis—pancytopenia
• Calcinosis cutis—changes characteristic of hyperglucocorticoidism (e.g., stress leukogram, high ALP, hyperglycemia, low urine specific gravity)
• Cutaneous xanthomas—may be glucosuria, hyperglycemia and/or lipid profile abnormalities

OTHER LABORATORY TESTS
Serum ferritin levels—may be high with malignant histiocytosis but not with cutaneous histiocytosis

IMAGING
• Radiology and ultrasonography—delineate involvement of internal organs in amyloidosis and histiocytosis
• Radiology—identify other areas of dystrophic calcification in dogs with calcinosis cutis
• Ultrasonography—identify cystadenocarcinomas in dogs with nodular dermatofibrosis

DIAGNOSTIC PROCEDURES
Skin biopsies for histopathology and cultures (fungal, aerobic, and mycobacterial) are essential for nodular dermatoses.

TREATMENT
• Most of these disorders can be treated on an outpatient basis.
• A few of these disorders (e.g., malignant histiocytosis, amyloidosis, and nodular dermatofibrosis) are almost always fatal.
• Dogs with calcinosis cutis may need to be hospitalized for sepsis and intense topical therapy.

MEDICATIONS

DRUGS
• Amyloidosis—no known therapy, unless the lesion is solitary and can be surgically removed.
• Sperulocytosis—only effective treatment is surgical removal.
• Idiopathic sterile granuloma and pyogranuloma—prednisone (2.2–4.4 mg/kg divided PO q12h) is the first line of therapy; continue steroids for 7–14 days after complete remission; then taper dose; for cases that are refractory to glucocorticoids, azathioprine (2.2 mg/kg PO q48h) in combination with prednisone or sodium iodide may be tried.

DERMATOSES, STERILE NODULAR/GRANULOMATOUS

• Foreign body reactions—best treated by removal of the offending substance if possible; for hair foreign bodies, the dog should be placed on softer bedding and topical therapy with keratolytic agents should be initiated; many dogs with hair foreign bodies also have secondary deep bacterial infections that need to be treated with both topical and systemic antibiotics.
• Canine eosinophilic granuloma—prednisone (1.1–2.2 mg/kg PO q24h) produces a good response
• Malignant histiocytosis—no effective therapy; it is rapidly fatal.
• Cutaneous histiocytosis—high-dose glucocorticoids and cytotoxic drugs results in remission; recurrences are common; L-asparginase has been helpful in some cases.
• Calcinosis cutis—underlying disease must be controlled if possible; most cases require antibiotics to control secondary bacterial infections; hydrotherapy and frequent bathing in antibacterial shampoos minimize secondary problems; topical DMSO is useful (applied to no more than one-third of the body once daily until lesions resolve); if lesions are extensive, serum calcium levels should be monitored closely.
• Calcinosis circumscripta—surgical excision is the therapy of choice in most cases.
• Sterile panniculitis—single lesions can be removed surgically; prednisone (2.2 mg/kg PO q24h or divided PO q12h) is the treatment of choice; administered until lesions regress; then tapered; some dogs remain in long-term remission, but others require prolonged alternate-day therapy; a few cases respond to oral vitamin E (400 IU q12h).

• Nodular dermatofibrosis—no therapy for most cases, because the cystadenocarcinomas are usually bilateral; for rare unilateral case of cystadenocarcinoma or a cystadenoma, removal of the single affected kidney may be helpful.
• Cutaneous xanthoma—correction of the underlying diabetes mellitus or hyperlipoproteinemia is usually curative.

CONTRAINDICATIONS
Corticosteroids and other immunosuppressive drugs should be avoided, if possible, in any animal with a secondary infection.

PRECAUTIONS
DMSO—handle with care; monitor serum calcium levels if used to treat calcinosis cutis.

POSSIBLE INTERACTIONS
N/A

ALTERNATIVE DRUGS
N/A

 FOLLOW-UP

PATIENT MONITORING
• Patients on long-term glucocorticoids should have a CBC, chemistry screen, urinalysis, and urine culture done every 6 months.
• Dogs being treated with DMSO for calcinosis cutis should have calcium levels checked every 7–14 days, starting at the beginning of therapy.

POSSIBLE COMPLICATIONS
Systemic amyloidosis, malignant histiocytosis, and nodular dermatofibrosis—invariably fatal

 MISCELLANEOUS

ASSOCIATED CONDITIONS
• Calcinosis cutis—hyperglucocorticoidism, chronic renal failure, and diabetes mellitus
• Calcinosis circumscripta—(occasionally) hypertrophic osteodystrophy and idiopathic polyarthritis
• Nodular dermatofibrosis—cystadenocarcinomas
• Cutaneous xanthoma—diabetes mellitus and hyperlipoproteinemia

SEE ALSO
• Adenocarcinoma, Renal
• Amyloidosis
• Hyperadrenocorticism (Cushing Disease)

ABBREVIATIONS
• ALP = alkaline phosphatase
• DMSO = dimethyl sulfoxide

Suggested Reading
Griffin CE, Kwochka KW, MacDonald JM, eds. Current veterinary dermatology. St Louis: Mosby, 1993.
Gross TL, lhrke PJ, Walder EJ. Veterinary dermatopathology. St Louis: Mosby, 1992.
Scott DW, Miller BH, Griffin CE, eds. Muller & Kirk's small animal dermatology. 5th ed. Philadelphia: Saunders, 1995.
Author Dawn E. Logas
Consulting Editor Karen Helton Rhodes

DERMATOSES, VESICULOPUSTULAR

 BASICS

DEFINITION
• Pustule—small, circumscribed elevation of the epidermis filled with pus
• Vesicle—small, circumscribed elevation of the epidermis filled with clear fluid

PATHOPHYSIOLOGY
Pustules and vesicles—produced by edema, acantholysis (pemphigus), ballooning degeneration (viral infections), proteolytic enzymes from neutrophils (pyoderma), degeneration of basal cells (lupus), or dermoepidermal separation (bullous pemphigoid)

SYSTEMS AFFECTED
• Multiple systems with SLE
• Skin/Exocrine—integument and muscle with dermatomyositis

SIGNALMENT
• Lupus—collies, shelties, and German shepherds may be predisposed
• Pemphigus erythematosus—collies and German shepherds may be predisposed
• Pemphigus foliaceus—akitas, chow chows, dachshunds, bearded collies, Newfoundlands, Doberman pinschers, and schipperkes may be predisposed
• Bullous pemphigoid—collies and Doberman pinschers may be predisposed
• Dermatomyositis—young collies and shelties
• Subcorneal pustular dermatosis—schnauzers affected most frequently
• Linear IgA dermatosis—dachshunds exclusively
• Dermatophytosis—young animals

SIGNS
N/A

CAUSES
Pustules
• Superficial pyoderma—impetigo, superficial spreading pyoderma, superficial bacterial folliculitis, acne
• Pemphigus complex—pemphigus foliaceus, pemphigus erythematosus, pemphigus vegetans
• Subcorneal pustular dermatosis
• Dermatophytosis
• Sterile eosinophilic pustulosis
• Linear IgA dermatosis

Vesicles
• SLE
• DLE
• Bullous pemphigoid
• Pemphigus vulgaris
• Dermatomyositis

RISK FACTORS
• Drug exposure—SLE and bullous pemphigoid
• Pyodermas are usually secondary to a predisposing factor (e.g., demodicosis, hypothyroidism, allergy, or steroid administration)
• Sunlight—pemphigus erythematosus, bullous pemphigoid, SLE, DLE, and dermatomyositis

 DIAGNOSIS

DIFFERENTIAL DIAGNOSIS
Pustular
Superficial Pyodermas
• Most common cause
• Readily respond to appropriate antibiotic therapy if the underlying cause is effectively managed
• Intact pustule—direct smear reveals neutrophils engulfing bacteria; culture usually yields *Staphylococcus intermedius;* biopsy shows intraepidermal neutrophilic pustules or folliculitis.
Pemphigus Complex
• A group of immune-mediated diseases characterized histologically by acantholytic cells
• Direct smears—many acantholytic cells, nondegenerate neutrophils, and no bacteria
• Culture of an intact pustule negative
• Direct immunofluorescence—deposits in the intercellular spaces of the epidermis in approximately 50% of the cases
• Tends to wax and wane irrespective of antibiotic therapy; responds to immunosuppressive therapy
Subcorneal Pustular Dermatosis
• A rare idiopathic pustular dermatosis of dogs
• Tends to wax and wane
• Intact pustules—direct smears reveal numerous neutrophils, no bacteria, and occasional acantholytic cells; cultures negative
• Direct immunofluorescence negative

• Poor response to glucocorticoids and antibiotics
Dermatophytosis
• Common disease of both dogs and cats
• Dermatophyte culture positive
• Secondary bacterial infection common
• Biopsy—folliculitis with fungal elements
Sterile Eosinophilic Pustulosis
• A rare idiopathic dermatosis of dogs
• Direct smears—numerous eosinophils, nondegenerate neutrophils, occasional acantholytic cells, and no bacteria
• Biopsy—eosinophilic intraepidermal pustules, folliculitis, and furunculosis
• Direct immunofluorescence negative
• Rapid response to glucocorticoids
Linear IgA Dermatosis
• A rare idiopathic dermatosis of dachshunds.
• Tends to wax and wane
• Pustules—sterile and subcorneal
• Direct immunofluorescence positive for IgA at the basement membrane zone

Vesicles/Ulceration
SLE
• A multisystemic disease with variable clinical signs and cutaneous manifestations, including mucocutaneous ulceration
• Direct immunofluorescence positive at the basement membrane zone
• ANA positive
DLE
• Affects only the skin; lesions usually confined to the face
• Depigmentation, erythema, and ulceration of the nasal planum common
• Biopsy—interface dermatitis
• Direct immunofluorescence positive at the basement membrane zone
• ANA negative
Bullous Pemphigoid
• Ulcerative disorder of the skin and/or mucous membranes
• Biopsy—subepidermal cleft formation
• Direct immunofluorescence positive at the basement membrane zone
• Acantholysis is not seen.
Pemphigus Vulgaris
• Most severe form of pemphigus
• Characterized by ulceration of the oral cavity, mucocutaneous junction, and skin
• Biopsy—suprabasal acantholysis and cleft formation

- Direct immunofluorescence positive at the intercellular spaces of the epidermis Dermatomyositis
- An idiopathic inflammatory disease of the skin and muscle of young collies and shelties
- Lesions affect the face, ear tips, tail tip, and pressure points of the extremities.
- Characterized by alopecia, crusting, pigmentation disturbances, erosions/ulceration, and scarring
- Biopsy—follicular atrophy, perifolliculitis, and hydropic degeneration of the basal cells
- Direct immunofluorescence negative
- Muscle biopsy and EMG—evidence of inflammation

CBC/BIOCHEMISTRY/URINALYSIS
- Results usually unremarkable
- SLE—anemia, thrombocytopenia or glomerulonephritis may develop
- Eosinophilic pustular dermatosis—most affected dogs have peripheral eosinophilia.

OTHER LABORATORY TESTS
N/A

IMAGING
N/A

DIAGNOSTIC PROCEDURES
- Direct smear from intact pustule
- Culture of intact pustule
- Biopsy for histopathology
- Direct immunofluorescence, including IgA
- ANA titer
- EMG
- Muscle biopsy

 TREATMENT
- Periodic bathing with an antimicrobial shampoo—helps remove surface debris and control secondary bacterial infections
- Usually treated as an outpatient
- SLE, pemphigus vulgaris, and bullous pemphigoid may be life-threatening and require inpatient intensive care.

 MEDICATIONS

DRUGS OF CHOICE

Subcorneal Pustular Dermatosis
- Dapsone—1 mg/kg PO q8h until remission (usually 1–4 weeks); then tapered to 1 mg/kg q24h or twice weekly
- Sulfasalazine (Azulfidine)—10–20 mg/kg PO q8h until remission; then as needed

Linear IgA Dermatosis
- Prednisolone—2.2–4.4 mg/kg PO q24h until remission; then taper to alternate-day therapy
- Dapsone—1 mg/kg PO q8h until remission; then taper and give as needed; individual patients may respond to one drug and not the other.

Sterile Eosinophilic Pustulosis
- Prednisolone: 2.2–4.4 mg/kg PO q24h until remission (usually 5–10 days); then as needed to prevent relapses (usually long-term, alternate-day therapy required)

See specific diseases

CONTRAINDICATIONS
N/A

PRECAUTIONS

Prednisolone
- Secondary infections
- Iatrogenic Cushing disease
- Muscle wasting
- Steroid hepatopathy
- Behavioral changes
- Polydipsia, polyuria
- Polyphagia

Dapsone
- Dogs—mild anemia, mild leukopenia, and mild elevation of ALT, which are not associated with clinical signs, are frequently noted; usually return to normal when dosage is reduced for maintenance
- Occasionally, fatal thrombocytopenia or severe leukopenia
- Occasional vomiting, diarrhea, or pruritic skin eruption
- Cats—more susceptible to dapsone toxicity; hemolytic anemia and neurotoxicity reported

Sulfasalazine
Keratoconjunctivitis sicca

POSSIBLE INTERACTIONS
N/A

ALTERNATIVE DRUGS
N/A

 FOLLOW-UP

PATIENT MONITORING
- Dapsone—monitor hemogram, platelet count, and ALT every 2 weeks initially and if any clinical side effects develop.
- Long-term sulfasalazine therapy—monitor tear production.
- Immunosuppressive therapy—monitor every 1–2 weeks initially; then every 3–4 months during maintenance therapy.

POSSIBLE COMPLICATIONS
N/A

 MISCELLANEOUS

ASSOCIATED CONDITIONS
N/A

AGE-RELATED FACTORS
N/A

ZOONOTIC POTENTIAL
Dermatophytosis

PREGNANCY
N/A

SYNONYMS
None

SEE ALSO
- Acne–Cats; Acne–Dogs
- Dermatomyositis
- Dermatophytosis
- Lupus Erythematosus, Cutaneus (Discoid)
- Lupus Erythematosus, Systemic (SLE)
- Pemphigoid, Bullous
- Pemphigus
- Pyoderma

ABBREVIATIONS
- ALT = alanine aminotransferase
- ANA = antinuclear antibody
- DLE = discoid lupus erythematosus
- EMG = electromyography
- SLE = systemic lupus erythematosus

Suggested Reading

Muller GH, Kirk RW, Scott DW. Small animal dermatology. 4th ed. Philadelphia: Saunders, 1989.

Authors Ellen C. Codner and Karen Helton Rhodes

Consulting Editor Karen Helton Rhodes

DIARRHEA, ACUTE

BASICS

DEFINITION
Abrupt or recent onset of abnormally frequent discharge and fluid content of fecal matter

PATHOPHYSIOLOGY
• Caused by imbalance in the absorptive, secretory, and motility actions of the intestines
• May or may not be associated with inflammation of the intestinal tract (enteritis) • Foodstuffs and products of digestion exert osmotic forces. • Ingestion of osmotically active foodstuffs that are poorly digestible, dietary malassimilation, malabsorption, or osmotically active medications (e.g., lactulose or magnesium sulfate) can increase intestinal lumen osmotic force, which holds and draws fluid into the gut lumen, producing osmotic diarrhea. • Fiber content contributes to the osmotic force exerted by a diet. • The clinical signs of osmotic diarrhea often abate or resolve with fasting.
• Normally, the intestinal epithelium secretes fluid and electrolytes to aid in the digestion, absorption, and propulsion of foodstuffs. • In disease states this secretion can overwhelm the absorptive activity and produce a secretory diarrhea. • Stimulation of the parasympathetic nervous system or exposure to a variety of secretogogues can increase intestinal secretion.
• Many of the infectious causes of diarrhea are related to increased secretion. • Forward intestinal motility propels intestinal chyme toward the colon and out of the body; segmental motility tends to slow forward progression and increase time for digestion and absorption of food; increased forward propulsion or decreased segmental contractions can produce diarrhea due to motility changes and secondary decreases in absorption. • Diarrhea can result from a combination of factors. • Inflammatory and infectious diarrhea—often produced by changes in secretion, motility, and absorptive ability; inflammation can also cause changes in intestinal wall permeability, causing loss of fluid and electrolytes and decreased absorptive ability.

SYSTEMS AFFECTED
• Endocrine/Metabolic • Gastrointestinal

SIGNALMENT
• Dogs and cats • Any animal can suffer from acute diarrhea; kittens and puppies are most frequently affected.

SIGNS

General Comments
• Diarrhea can occur with or without systemic illness. • Signs can vary from diarrhea in an apparently healthy patient to severe systemic signs. • The choice of diagnostic and therapeutic measures depends on the severity of illness. • Patients that are not systemically ill will have normal hydration and minimal systemic signs. • Signs of more severe illness (e.g., concurrent vomiting, abdominal pain, blood in the diarrhea or vomit, severe dehydration, and depression) should prompt more-aggressive diagnostic and therapeutic measures.

Historical Findings
• Increased fecal fluidity and frequency of short duration • Owner may report fecal accidents, vomiting, changes in fecal consistency and volume, blood or mucus in the feces, or straining to defecate. • A period of listlessness and anorexia may precede the onset of viral enteritis. • Owners may be able to report exposure to toxins, dietary changes, or dietary indiscretion.

Physical Examination Findings
• Vary with the severity of disease • Dehydration, depression, or lethargy often present to some degree. • Abdominal pain, abdominal discomfort, fever, signs of hypotension, nausea, and weakness may occur in more severely affected individuals.

CAUSES
• Can present acutely, but are generally dealt with under that heading • Systemic illness may also result in diarrhea as a secondary event.
• Dietary indiscretion—ingestion of garbage, nonfood material, or spoiled food • Dietary changes—abrupt changes in amount or type of foodstuffs • Dietary intolerance—maldigestion or malassimilation of foodstuffs, dietary hypersensitivity • Metabolic diseases—hypoadrenocorticism (Addison's disease), liver disease, renal diseases, and pancreatic disease can cause acute or chronic diarrhea. • Obstruction or foreign bodies—ingestion of foreign bodies, intussusception, or intestinal volvulus • Idiopathic—hemorrhagic gastroenteritis • Infectious
  Viral—parvovirus (CPV and feline panleukopenia), coronavirus, rotavirus, canine distemper virus
  Bacterial—*Salmonella, Campylobacter, Clostridium* spp., *Escherichia coli*, etc.
  Parasitic—verminous (hookworms, ascarids, whipworms, strongyles, and cestodes) or protozoal (*Giardia*, coccidia, and *Entamoeba*)
  Rickettsial—salmon poisoning (*Neorickettsia*)
• Drugs and toxins—heavy metals (i.e., lead), organophosphates, nonsteroidal antiinflammatories, steroids, antimicrobials, antihelminthic, antineoplastic agents, lawn and garden products, etc.

RISK FACTORS
Young dogs and cats present for diarrhea from dietary indiscretion, intussusception, foreign bodies, and infectious causes more often than older patients.

DIAGNOSIS

DIFFERENTIAL DIAGNOSIS
• Many cases of mild acute diarrhea resolve spontaneously or with minimal care. • Patients should have a complete physical examination, fecal examination, and a minimal database to assess their hydration status. • Further diagnostic tests depend on the extent of illness and other clinical signs.

CBC/BIOCHEMISTRY/URINALYSIS
• Generally normal; not necessary with mild illness • More-severe illness should prompt a more complete evaluation. • Can see leukopenia (especially neutropenia) with parvoviral enteritis • Electrolytes are commonly abnormal because of intestinal losses (hypokalemia, hypochloremia, hyponatremia). • Altered protein levels because of intestinal loss (decreased) or dehydration (increased)
• Altered renal values with dehydration or gastrointestinal hemorrhage (prerenal azotemia) or with renal disease • Liver and pancreatic enzymes can be elevated with disease in these organ systems.

OTHER LABORATORY TESTS
N/A

IMAGING
• Abdominal radiographs can help identify or rule out intestinal foreign bodies or obstruction.
• Ileus—commonly seen with acute diarrhea, regardless of cause
• Radiographs—generally not necessary in patients with mild illness
• More-severe signs (i.e., abdominal pain or persistent vomiting) may increase the likely diagnostic benefit of radiology.
• Contrast abdominal radiography and ultrasonography may be useful with some patients.

DIAGNOSTIC PROCEDURES
• Perform fecal analysis for parasites on all patients.
• Because helminth ova and *Giardia* oocytes can be shed in low numbers or intermittently, multiple fecal analyses are recommended, and empiric treatment may be advisable.
• Can perform fecal ELISA tests for parvovirus antigen in dogs
• Endoscopy and biopsy—useful in select cases; more commonly needed in chronic diarrhea

TREATMENT
• Depends largely on the severity of illness; patients with mild illness can most often be handled as outpatients with symptomatic

therapy; patients with more-severe illness or that fail to respond to therapy should be treated more aggressively.
• Fluid therapy and correction of electrolyte imbalances is the mainstay of treatment in most cases.
• Can give crystalloid fluid therapy orally, subcutaneously, or intravenously, as required; can give oral fluids (water or carbohydrate- and electrolyte-containing fluids) to patients that are not vomiting
• Aim to return the patient to proper hydration status (over 12–24 h) and replace any ongoing losses.
• Severe volume depletion can occur with acute diarrhea; aggressive shock fluid therapy may be necessary.
• Fluid choice for intravenous or subcutaneous use should take into consideration the electrolyte and hydration status.
• Use potassium supplementation (potassium chloride 20–40 mEq/L) in most patients, but not during shock fluid therapy.
• Patients with severe hypokalemia may require more-aggressive potassium supplementation.
• Patients with mild illness that are not vomiting—a period of fasting (12–24 h) is often followed by a bland diet such as boiled rice and chicken or a prepared diet.
• Limiting exposure to garbage, foods other than the patient's normal diet, and potential foreign bodies is also recommended.
• Patients with obstruction or foreign bodies may require endoscopy or surgery to evaluate the intestine and remove the foreign objects.

MEDICATIONS

DRUGS OF CHOICE
• Antidiarrheal drugs can be classified as motility-modifying drugs, antisecretory drugs, or intestinal protectants.
• Motility-modifying drugs generally operate by increasing segmental motility and thus increasing transit time (i.e., narcotic antidiarrheals such as loperamide; 0.1 mg/kg PO q8–12h in dogs; 0.08 mg/kg PO q12h in cats) or by decreasing forward motility (i.e., anticholinergics); these medications are not necessary in mild disease, which is generally self-limiting.
• In severe disease, give proper fluid therapy and seek underlying problems; do not use these medications longer than 1–2 days because of adverse effects.
• Acute diarrhea that does not resolve antidiarrheal drugs merits further investigation.
• Anticholinergics (i.e., atropine, propantheline) can produce a generalized ileus because they decrease segmental and peristaltic motion; this decrease in tone can

increase the severity of diarrhea in some patients.
• Antisecretory drugs are used to decrease the volume of fluid in the feces; opiates, anticholinergics, chlorpromazine, and salicylates may decrease secretion into the intestinal lumen.
• Intestinal protectants are generally not helpful in patents with acute diarrhea and have not been shown to change intestinal fluid or electrolyte loss.
• Bismuth subsalicylate may be of some benefit because of the antisecretory properties of salicylate.
• Anthelminthics (i.e., fenbendazole 50 mg/kg PO q24h for 3 days) and antiprotozoal drugs (i.e., metronidazole 30–60 mg/kg PO q24h for 5 days) are recommended as empiric treatment for patients with acute diarrhea or those with positive fecal analyses.
• Can use coccidiostatic (i.e., sulfadimethoxine) drugs if fecal analysis warrants
• Antibiotic therapy is probably unnecessary for most cases of mild illness and may cause diarrhea in its own right.
• Patients with bacterial enteritis, severe illness, concomitant leukopenia, or suspected breakdown of the gastrointestinal mucosal barrier (as evidenced by blood in the feces) should be treated with broad-spectrum antimicrobial agents.

CONTRAINDICATIONS
• Anticholinergics in patients with suspected intestinal obstruction, glaucoma, or intestinal ileus
• Narcotic analgesics—can cause CNS depression; undesirable in patients with more-severe illness that are already depressed or lethargic
• Narcotic analgesics in patients with liver disease and bacterial or toxic enteritis

PRECAUTIONS
• Most cases of acute mild diarrhea resolve with minimal treatment; be cautious of excessive diagnostics and overtreating these patients.
• Almost any drug can produce adverse effects (often including diarrhea and vomiting); these may be more severe than the initial problem.

POSSIBLE INTERACTIONS
N/A

ALTERNATIVE DRUGS
N/A

FOLLOW-UP

PATIENT MONITORING
• Most acute diarrhea resolves within a few days. • If clinical signs persist, additional diagnostics and treatments may be necessary.

• Upon completion of medication, recheck patients that exhibited parasites by fecal analysis.

POSSIBLE COMPLICATIONS
• Intussusception is thought to be associated with increased intestinal motility.
• Monitor for this complication in patients with acute diarrhea due to other causes, especially young dogs with parvoviral enteritis and parasitism.

MISCELLANEOUS

ASSOCIATED CONDITIONS
Acute vomiting commonly occurs concurrently with acute diarrhea.

AGE-RELATED FACTORS
• Young dogs and cats present for diarrhea from dietary indiscretion, intussusception, foreign bodies, and infectious causes more often than older patients. • Younger and smaller animals are also more prone to dehydration and may require more-aggressive fluid therapy.

ZOONOTIC POTENTIAL
• *Campylobacter* enteritis is contagious to people. • Some strains of *Giardia* may be contagious to people. • Parasitic larvae can cause visceral larval migrans (ascarids) and cutaneous larval migrans (hookworms) in people, particularly children.

PREGNANCY
N/A

SYNONYMS
N/A

SEE ALSO
See Causes.

ABBREVIATIONS
• CPV = canine parvovirus • ELISA = enzyme-linked immunosorbent assay

Suggested Reading

Burrows CF, Batt RM, Sherding RG. Disease of the small intestine. In: Ettinger SJ, Feldman EC, eds. Textbook of veterinary internal medicine. Philadelphia: Saunders, 1995:1169–1232.
Jergens AE. Acute diarrhea. In: Bonagura JD, ed. Kirk's current veterinary therapy XII. Philadelphia: Saunders, 1995:701–705.
Lewis LD, Morris ML, Hand MS. Gastrointestinal, pancreatic and hepatic diseases. In: Small animal clinical nutrition III. Topeka, KN: Mark Morris Associates, 1989.
Author Derek S. Duval
Consulting Editors Brett M. Feder and Mitchell A. Crystal

DIARRHEA, CHRONIC—CATS

BASICS

DEFINITION
• A change in the frequency, consistency, and volume of feces for more than 3 weeks or with a pattern of episodic recurrence
• Can be either small bowel or large bowel in origin

PATHOPHYSIOLOGY
• High solute and fluid secretion—secretory diarrhea
• Low solute and fluid absorption—osmotic diarrhea
• High intestinal permeability
• Abnormal GI motility

SYSTEMS AFFECTED
• GI
• Endocrine/metabolic/fluid, electrolyte, and acid–base
• Nutritional
• Lymphatic
• Exocrine

SIGNALMENT
Cats

SIGNS

General Comments:
Underlying disease process determines extent of clinical signs.

Historical Findings:
Small Bowel
• Larger volume of feces than normal
• Frequency of defecation is mild to moderately above normal (2–4 per day)
• Weight loss
• Polyphagia with malabsorption/maldigestion and hyperthyroidism
• May be melena; no hematochezia and mucus
• No tenesmus or dyschezia
• Vomiting is common.
Large Bowel
• Smaller volume of feces per defecation than normal
• Frequency of defecation significantly higher than normal (>4 times per day)
• No weight loss
• Melena absent; usually hematochezia and mucus
• Tenesmus and urgency; dyschezia with rectal or distal colonic disease
• Vomiting in some cats

Physical Examination Findings:
• Poor body condition associated with infiltrative bowel diseases, chronic obstruction, and metabolic disorders

• Diffuse intestinal thickening suggests infiltrative disease (lymphoma, IBD)
• Segmental thickening caused by neoplasia (especially lymphoma), foreign body, mesenteric lymphadenopathy, and eosinophilic or granulomatous enteritis (both rare)
• Aggregation of bowel loops may be palpated in a cat with a linear foreign body.
• A palpable thyroid nodule suggests hyperthyroidism.
• Small kidneys may indicate chronic renal disease.
• Hepatomegaly or icterus may indicate hepatic lipidosis, feline infectious peritonitis (FIP), hepatic neoplasia, or biliary disease.
• Rectal palpation may reveal abnormal rectal mucosa, intraluminal or extraluminal rectal mass, or rectal stricture; small or large bowel diarrhea
• Fundic examination may reveal lesions suggestive of toxoplasmosis, FIP, histoplasmosis, or feline leukemia virus (FeLV)

CAUSES
• IBD—lymphoplasmacytic enterocolitis, granulomatous enteritis, eosinophilic enteritis/hypereosinophilic syndrome, and idiopathic inflammatory colitis
• Neoplasia—lymphoma, adenocarcinoma, mast cell tumor, and polyps
• Obstruction—neoplasia, foreign body, IBD, intussusception, and stricture
• Parasitic—*Giardia, Toxoplasma gondii, Toxocara cati, Toxascaris leonina, Cryptosporidium* spp., *Cystoisospora* spp.
• Metabolic disorders—hyperthyroidism, renal disease, hepatobiliary disease, diabetes mellitus, toxins, and drug administration
• Bacterial—*Campylobacter jejuni, Salmonella* spp., *Yersinia pseudotuberculosis,* and *Clostridium perfringens*
• Viral—FeLV, FIV, and FIP
• Mycotic—histoplasmosis, mycobacteriosis, pythiosis, and aspergillosis
• Noninflammatory malabsorption—lymphangiectasia, small intestinal bacterial overgrowth, short bowel syndrome, villous atrophy, and duodenal ulcers
• Maldigestion—hepatobiliary disease and exocrine pancreatic insufficiency (uncommon in cats)
• Dietary—dietary sensitivity, dietary indiscretion, and diet changes
• Congenital anomalies—short colon, portosystemic shunt, and persistent pancreaticomesojejunal ligament

RISK FACTORS
Dietary changes and feeding poorly digestible or high-fat diet

DIAGNOSIS

DIFFERENTIAL DIAGNOSIS
First localize the origin of the diarrhea to the small or large bowel or both on the basis of historical signs.

CBC/BIOCHEMISTRY/URINALYSIS
• Eosinophilia in some cats with parasitism, eosinophilic enterocolitis/hypereosinophilic syndrome, or mast cell tumor
• Macrocytosis in some cats with hyperthyroidism or FeLV infection
• Anemia and microcytosis suggest chronic GI bleeding and iron deficiency
• Leukopenia in some cats with FeLV or FIV infection
• Biochemical and urinalysis abnormalities may suggest renal disease, hepatobiliary disease, or endocrinopathy
• Panhypoproteinemia caused by protein-losing enteropathy is uncommon in cats with intestinal disease

OTHER LABORATORY TESTS

Fecal and/or Rectal Scraping Examination
• Direct fecal examination, routine fecal flotation, and zinc sulfate centrifugation (for *Giardia*) may reveal GI parasites.
• Cytologic examination of rectal scrapings may reveal specific organisms (e.g., *Histoplasma* or *Prototheca*.
• Sudan stain for fecal fats may indicate steatorrhea, suggesting malabsorption or maldigestion.
• Culture feces if *Campylobacter, Salmonella,* or pythiosis are suspected—special media required; check with your laboratory prior to submission.

Thyroid Function Tests
• High serum total T_4 concentration indicates hyperthyroidism
• If hyperthyroidism is suspected but the total T_4 is normal, perform a T_3 suppression test, TRH response test, or technetium thyroid scan; free T_4 by dialysis can also be used but some false-positive results can occur.

Serologic Testing
Test for FeLV and FIV—especially if hematologic abnormalities are present

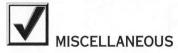

Test Exocrine Pancreatic Function
- Feline-specific TLI—fasted serum TLI < 8 μg/L is diagnostic of exocrine pancreatic insufficiency.
- Can measure fecal proteolytic activity in fecal samples from 3 consecutive days

IMAGING
- Survey abdominal radiography may indicate intestinal obstruction, mass, organomegaly, foreign body, small kidneys, hepatobiliary disease, or abdominal effusion.
- Contrast radiography (upper GI series or barium enema) may indicate bowel wall thickening, mucosal irregularity, mass, radiolucent foreign body, or stricture.
- Abdominal ultrasonography may demonstrate bowel wall thickening, abnormal bowel wall layering, GI or extra-GI masses, intussusception, foreign body, ileus, abdominal effusion, hepatobiliary disease, renal disease, or mesenteric lymphadenopathy.

DIAGNOSTIC PROCEDURES
If maldigestive (EPI), metabolic, parasitic, dietary, and infectious causes have been excluded, endoscopy and mucosal biopsy or GI ultrasound and fine-needle aspiration or microcore biopsy are indicated for definitive diagnosis and treatment.

Endoscopy
- Upper GI endoscopy allows examination and biopsy of the gastric and duodenal mucosa; always obtain multiple mucosal specimens from both duodenum and stomach.
- Flexible colonoscopy allows examination of the entire colon, cecum, and often the distal ileum; rigid colonoscopy limits examination to the descending colon and rectum; always obtain multiple mucosal specimens from all areas examined.

Ultrasound-guided GI Biopsy
Can use ultrasound-guided fine-needle aspiration on most GI lesions and guided microcore (true-cut) biopsy on noncystic lesions >2 cm in diameter

TREATMENT
- Often must be specific for the underlying cause to be successful
- When no definitive diagnosis is possible, empirical treatment with dietary management and metronidazole sometimes results in clinical improvement
- Surgery is needed to treat obstructive disease and GI mass

SURGICAL CONSIDERATIONS
Pursue exploratory laparotomy and surgical biopsy if there is evidence of obstruction, an intestinal mass, mid–small bowel disease unreachable via ultrasound-guided procedure, or if a diagnosis based on endoscopic biopsy or ultrasound-guided procedure is questioned because of poor response to therapy.

NURSING CARE
- Give fluid therapy with balanced electrolyte solution (e.g., normal saline or lactated Ringer's solution) for dehydration.
- Correct electrolyte and acid–base imbalances.

MEDICATIONS
DRUGS OF CHOICE
- A bland or hypoallergenic diet may be beneficial.
- A therapeutic trial with fenbendazole (25 mg/kg PO q24h for 3 days) or metronidazole (10–20 mg/kg PO q12h for 10–14 days) is often used to rule out occult *Giardia* infection. Fenbendazole has the additional benefit of anthelmintic therapy; metronidazole may have nonspecific antiinflammatory GI effects and is effective in treating small intestinal bacterial overgrowth.

CONTRAINDICATIONS
Anticholinergics exacerbate most types of chronic diarrhea and should not be used for empirical treatment.

PRECAUTIONS
Opiate antidiarrheals such as diphenoxylate and loperamide can cause hyperactivity and respiratory depression in cats and should not be used for more than 3 days.

POSSIBLE INTERACTIONS
N/A

ALTERNATIVE DRUGS
N/A

FOLLOW-UP
PATIENT MONITORING
- Fecal volume and character, frequency of defecation, and body weight
- Resolution usually occurs gradually with treatment; if diarrhea does not resolve, consider reevaluating the diagnosis.

POSSIBLE COMPLICATIONS
- Dehydration
- Abdominal effusion with intestinal adenocarcinoma

MISCELLANEOUS
ASSOCIATED CONDITIONS
N/A

AGE-RELATED FACTORS
N/A

ZOONOTIC POTENTIAL
- *Toxoplasma*
- *Giardia*
- *Cryptosporidium*
- *Salmonella, Campylobacter*

PREGNANCY
N/A

SYNONYMS
N/A

SEE ALSO
See Causes

ABBREVIATIONS:
FeLV = feline leukemia virus
FIP = feline infectious peritonitis
FIV = feline immunodeficiency virus
GI = gastrointestinal
IBD = inflammatory bowel disease
TLI = trypsin-like immunoreactivity

Suggested Reading
Crystal MA. Diarrhea. In: The feline patient. Essentials of diagnosis and treatment. Baltimore: Williams & Wilkins 1998:42–46.
Dennis JS, Kruger JM, Mullaney TP. Lymphocytic/plasmacytic colitis in cats: 14 cases (1985–1990). J Am Vet Med Assoc 1993;202:313–318.
Jergens AE. Feline idiopathic inflammatory bowel disease. Comp Contin Educ Pract Vet 1992;14:509–518.
Sherding RG. Diseases of the intestines. In: Sherding RG, ed. The cat: diseases and clinical management. New York: Churchill Livingstone, 1989:955–1006.
Steiner JM, Medinger TL, Williams DA. Feline trypsin-like immunoreactivity in feline exocrine pancreatic disease. Comp Contin Educ Pract Vet 1996;18:543–547.
Zajac AM. Giardiasis. Comp Contin Educ Pract Vet 1992;14:604–611.
Author Amy M. Grooters
Consulting Editor Mitchell A. Crystal and Brett M. Feder

BASICS

DEFINITION
• A change in the frequency, consistency, and volume of feces for more than 3 weeks or with a pattern of episodic recurrence • Can be either small bowel or large bowel in origin

PATHOPHYSIOLOGY
• High solute and fluid secretion—secretory diarrhea • Low solute and fluid absorption—osmotic diarrhea • High intestinal permeability • Abnormal GI motility

SYSTEMS AFFECTED
• GI • Endocrine/metabolic/fluid, electrolyte, and acid–base • Nutritional • Lymphatic • Exocrine

SIGNALMENT
Dogs

SIGNS
General Comments
Underlying disease process determines extent of clinical signs

Historical Findings
Small Bowel
• Larger volume of feces than normal • Frequency of defecation—mildly to moderately above normal (2–4 per day) • Weight loss • Polyphagia with malabsorption/maldigestion • May be melena; no hematochezia and mucus • No tenesmus or dyschezia • May be flatulence and borborygmus • Vomiting in some dogs
Large bowel
• Smaller volume of feces per defecation than normal • Frequency of defecation is significantly higher than normal (>4 times per day) • No weight loss • No melena; usually hematochezia and mucus • Tenesmus and urgency; dyschezia with rectal or distal colonic disease • Flatulence and borborygmus—variable • Vomiting—uncommon

Physical Examination Findings
Small Bowel
• Poor body condition associated with malabsorption, maldigestion, and PLE • May be dehydration • Abdominal palpation may reveal thickened small bowel loops associated with infiltrative small bowel disease, abdominal effusion as a result of hypoproteinemia from PLE, or an abdominal mass such as a foreign body, neoplastic mass, intussusception, or enlarged mesenteric lymph node. • Rectal palpation normal aside from small bowel diarrhea
Large bowel
• Body condition typically normal • Dehydration—uncommon • Abdominal palpation may reveal thickened large bowel loops or an abdominal mass such

as a foreign body, neoplastic mass, intussusception, or enlarged mesenteric lymph node. • Rectal palpation may reveal irregularity and thickening of the rectal mucosa, intraluminal or extraluminal rectal masses, rectal stricture, or sublumbar lymphadenopathy; large bowel diarrhea

CAUSES
Small Bowel
Primary small intestinal disease
• Inflammatory bowel disease (e.g., lymphoplasmacytic enteritis, eosinophilic enteritis, granulomatous enteritis, immunoproliferative enteropathy of basenjis and sprue)
• Lymphangiectasia
• Neoplasia (e.g., lymphoma and adenocarcinoma)
• Infection (e.g., histoplasmosis, *Salmonella* spp., *Clostridium perfringens,* and pythiosis)
• Parasites (e.g., *Giardia, Toxocara* spp., *Ancylostoma caninum,* and *A. strongyloides*)
• Partial obstruction (e.g., foreign body, intussusception, and neoplasia)
• Small intestinal bacterial overgrowth
• Short bowel syndrome
• Gastroduodenal ulcers
Maldigestion
• EPI (e.g., juvenile pancreatic acinar atrophy and chronic pancreatitis)
• Hepatobiliary disease
Dietary
• Dietary intolerance or allergy
• Gluten-sensitive enteropathy in Irish setters
Metabolic disorders
• Hepatobiliary disease, hypoadrenocorticism, uremia, toxins, and drug administration (e.g., anticholinergics and antibiotics)
• Apudoma (rare)

Large Bowel
Primary large intestinal disease
• Inflammatory bowel disease (e.g., lymphoplasmacytic colitis, eosinophilic colitis, histiocytic ulcerative colitis, and granulomatous colitis)
• Neoplasia (e.g., benign polyp, lymphoma, adenocarcinoma, leiomyoma, and leiomyosarcoma)
• Infection (e.g., histoplasmosis, *Clostridium perfringens, Salmonella* spp., *Campylobacter jejuni, Prototheca,* and pythiosis)
• Parasites (e.g., *Trichuris vulpis, Giardia, Ancylostoma caninum, Entamoeba histolytica,* and *Balantidium coli*)
• Noninflammatory causes (e.g., ileocolic intussusception and cecal inversion)
Dietary
• Diet—dietary indiscretion, diet changes, and foreign material (e.g., bones and hair)
• Fiber—responsive large bowel diarrhea
• Idiopathic—irritable bowel syndrome
• Metabolic disorders—uremia,

hypoadrenocorticism, toxins, drug administration

RISK FACTORS
Small Bowel
• Dietary changes and feeding poorly digestible or high-fat diets
• Large-breed dogs, especially German shepherds, have the highest incidence of EPI.
• Pythiosis occurs most often in young, large-breed dogs living in states bordering the Gulf of Mexico.

Large Bowel
• Dietary changes or indiscretion, stress, and psychologic factors may play a role.
• Histiocytic ulcerative colitis occurs most often in boxers < 3 years old.
• Pythiosis occurs most often in young, large-breed dogs living in states bordering the Gulf of Mexico.

 DIAGNOSIS

DIFFERENTIAL DIAGNOSIS
First localize the origin of the diarrhea to the small or large bowel or both on the basis of historical signs.

CBC/BIOCHEMISTRY/URINALYSIS
• Eosinophilia may be associated with parasitism, eosinophilic enterocolitis, or hypoadrenocorticism.
• Lymphopenia and hypocholesterolemia may be associated with lymphangiectasia.
• Anemia and microcytosis suggest chronic GI bleeding and iron deficiency.
• Panhypoproteinemia resulting from PLE is associated with infiltrative small bowel disorders and lymphangiectasia.
• Biochemical and urinalysis abnormalities may suggest renal disease, hepatobiliary disease, or endocrinopathy.

OTHER LABORATORY TESTS
Fecal and/or Rectal Scraping Examination
• Direct fecal examination, routine fecal flotation, and zinc sulfate centrifugation (for *Giardia*) may indicate GI parasites.
• Cytologic examination of rectal scrapings may reveal specific organisms, such as *Histoplasma* or *Prototheca.*
• Sudan stain for fecal fats may indicate steatorrhea, suggesting malabsorption or maldigestion.
• Culture feces if *Campylobacter, Salmonella,* or pythiosis are suspected—special media required; check with your laboratory prior to submission.

Tests of Exocrine Pancreatic Function
• TLI—test of choice for confirming EPI in dogs; fasted serum TLI < 2.5 μ g/L is diagnostic.

• Oral bentiromide (BT-PABA) test—a negligible rise in plasma PABA is consistent with a diagnosis of EPI.

Tests for Malabsorption
• Xylose absorption test—an insensitive and nonspecific test of intestinal malabsorption; peak plasma xylose concentration <45 mg/dL indicates malabsorption, but a normal value does not rule it out.
• Serum folate and B_{12} (cobalamin)—low serum B_{12} may be associated with EPI or distal small bowel malabsorption; low serum folate may be associated with proximal small bowel malabsorption; small intestinal bacterial overgrowth may increase serum folate and decrease serum B_{12}.

Tests for Metabolic Disease
• ACTH stimulation test—if hypoadrenocorticism is suspected; subnormal results indicate hypoadrenocorticism.
• Fasting and 2-h postprandial serum bile acids—test if hepatobiliary disease is suspected; significantly increased values suggest hepatic dysfunction, cholestasis, or portosystemic shunting.

IMAGING
• Survey abdominal radiography may indicate intestinal obstruction, organomegaly, mass, foreign body, hepatobiliary disease, renal disease, or abdominal effusion
• Contrast radiography (upper GI series or barium enema) may indicate bowel wall thickening, intestinal ulcers, mucosal irregularities, mass, radiolucent foreign body, or stricture.
• Abdominal ultrasonography may demonstrate bowel wall-thickening, abnormal bowel wall-layering, GI or extra-GI masses, intussusception, foreign body, ileus, abdominal effusion, hepatobiliary disease, renal disease, or mesenteric lymphadenopathy.

DIAGNOSTIC PROCEDURES
If maldigestive (EPI), metabolic, parasitic, dietary, and infectious causes have been excluded, perform endoscopy and mucosal biopsy or ultrasound and fine-needle aspiration or microcore biopsy for definitive diagnosis and treatment.

Endoscopy
• Upper GI endoscopy allows examination and biopsy of the gastric and duodenal mucosa; always obtain multiple mucosal specimens from both duodenum and stomach.
• Flexible colonoscopy allows examination of the entire colon, cecum, and often the distal ileum; rigid colonoscopy limits examination to the descending colon and rectum; always obtain multiple mucosal specimens from all areas examined.

Ultrasound-guided GI Biopsy
Can perform ultrasound-guided fine-needle aspiration on most GI lesions and guided microcore (true-cut) biopsy on noncystic lesions > 2 cm in diameter.

TREATMENT
• Treat the underlying cause—symptomatic or empirical therapy rarely resolves chronic diarrhea.
• Inform the owner that complete resolution of signs is not always possible despite a correct diagnosis and proper treatment; this is especially true for lymphangiectasia, intestinal neoplasia, pythiosis, and histoplasmosis.
• Fecal examinations are often negative in whipworm-infested dogs because of intermittent shedding of ova; because parasites are a common cause of diarrhea, perform therapeutic deworming with fenbendazole before pursuing additional diagnostic tests.
• Feeding a low-fat, highly digestible diet for 3–4 weeks may resolve diarrhea due to dietary intolerance or allergy.

SURGICAL CONSIDERATIONS
Pursue exploratory laparotomy and surgical biopsy if there is evidence of obstruction, an intestinal mass, or mid–small bowel disease unreachable via ultrasound-guided procedure or if a diagnosis based on endoscopic biopsy or ultrasound-guided procedure is questioned because of poor response to therapy.

NURSING CARE
• Give fluid therapy with balanced electrolyte solution such as normal saline or lactated Ringer solution if patient is dehydrated.
• Consider colloids for hypoproteinemic patients requiring fluid therapy.
• Correct electrolyte and acid–base imbalances.

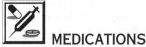

MEDICATIONS

DRUGS OF CHOICE
Perform therapeutic deworming with fenbendazole (50 mg/kg PO q24h for 3 days, repeat in 3 weeks and 3 months) before pursuing diagnostic testing.

CONTRAINDICATIONS
Anticholinergics exacerbate most types of chronic diarrhea; they are sometimes used to relieve cramping associated with irritable bowel syndrome; do not use them for empiric treatment of diarrhea.

PRECAUTIONS
N/A

POSSIBLE INTERACTIONS
N/A

ALTERNATIVE DRUGS
N/A

FOLLOW-UP

PATIENT MONITORING
• Fecal volume and character, frequency of defecation, and body weight • In dogs with PLE—serum proteins and clinical signs (ascites, subcutaneous edema, pleural effusion)
• Resolution of diarrhea is usually gradual after treatment; if it does not resolve with treatment, consider reevaluating the diagnosis. • Some dogs with inflammatory bowel disease or EPI have secondary small intestinal bacterial overgrowth, which must be treated along with the primary disorder.

POSSIBLE COMPLICATIONS
• Dehydration • Ascites, subcutaneous edema and/or pleural effusion with hypoalbuminemia from PLEs

MISCELLANEOUS

ASSOCIATED CONDITIONS
N/A

AGE-RELATED FACTORS
N/A

ZOONOTIC POTENTIAL
• *Giardia*
• *Salmonella, Campylobacter*

PREGNANCY
N/A

SYNONYMS
N/A

SEE ALSO
See Causes

ABBREVIATIONS
• B_{12} = vitamin B_{12}, cobalamin • EPI = exocrine pancreatic insufficiency • GI = gastrointestinal • PLE = protein-losing enteropathy • TLI = trypsin-like immunoreactivity

Suggested Reading
Leib MS, Codner EC, Monroe WE. A diagnostic approach to chronic large bowel diarrhea in dogs. Vet Med 1991;86:892–899.
Leib MS, Monroe WE, Codner EC. Management of chronic large bowel diarrhea in dogs. Vet Med 1991;86:922–929.
Strombeck DR, Guilford WG. Strombeck's small animal gastroenterology. 3rd ed. Philadelphia: Saunders, 1996.
Author Amy M. Grooters
Consulting Editors Mitchell A. Crystal and Brett M. Feder

DISCOLORED TOOTH/TEETH

BASICS

DEFINITION
• Any change from the norm—the normal color varies and depends on the shade, translucency, and thickness of enamel.
• Extrinsic—from surface accumulation of exogenous pigment
• Intrinsic—secondary to endogenous factors discoloring the underlying dentin

PATHOPHYSIOLOGY

Extrinsic Discoloration
• Bacterial stains—chromogenic bacteria give a green to black-brown to orange color.
• Plaque-related—a black-brown stain; usually secondary to the formation of ferric sulfide from the interaction of bacterial ferric sulfide and iron in the saliva
• Foods—charcoal biscuits and similar products penetrate the pits and fissures of the enamel; food that contains abundant chlorophyll can produce a green discoloration.
• Gingival hemorrhage—gives a green staining; results from the breakdown of hemoglobin into green biliverdin
• Dental restorative materials—amalgam gives a black-gray discoloration
• Medications—products containing iron or iodine give a black discoloration; those containing sulfides, silver nitrate, or manganese give a gray-to-yellow to brown-to-black discoloration; those containing copper or nickel give a green discoloration; products containing cadmium give a yellow-to-golden brown discoloration (e.g., 8% stannous fluoride combines with bacterial sulfides, giving a black stain; chlorhexidine gives a yellowish-brown discoloration)
• Metals—wear from chewing on cages or food dishes

Intrinsic Discoloration
• Hyperbilirubinemia—affects all teeth; occurs during the developmental stages of the dentition (during dentin formation); bilirubin accumulation in the dentin occurs from excess red blood cell breakdown; extent of tooth discoloration depends on the length of hyperbilirubinemia (one can see lines of resolution on the teeth once the condition has been resolved); gives a green discoloration

• Localized red blood cell destruction, usually one tooth—usually follows a traumatic injury to the tooth; discoloration comes from hemoglobin breakdown within the pulp from a pulpitis and secondary release into adjacent dentinal tubules; discoloration goes from pink (pulpitis) to gray (pulpal necrosis or resolution) to black (liquefactive necrosis); blood factors that cause tooth discoloration are hemoglobin, methemoglobin, hematoidin, hemosiderin, hematin, hemin, and sulfmethemoglobin.
• Amelogenesis imperfecta—developmental alteration in the structure of enamel affecting all teeth; teeth have a chalky appearance and a pinkish hue; can be a problem in the formation of the organic matrix, mineralization of the matrix, or the maturation of the matrix
• Dentinogenesis imperfecta—developmental alteration in the dentin formation; enamel separates easily from the dentin, resulting in grayish discoloration
• Infectious agents (systemic)—parvovirus, distemper virus, or any infectious agent that causes a sustained body temperature rise; affects the formation of enamel; a distinct line of resolution is visible on the teeth; affects all teeth; results in enamel hypoplasia where the pitted areas have black edges and the dentin is brownish
• Dental fluorosis—affects all teeth; excess fluoride consumption affects the maturation of enamel, resulting in pits (enamel hypoplasia) with black edges; the enamel is a lusterless, opaque white, with yellow brown zones of discoloration.

Internal/External Resorption
• Internal—follows pulpal injury (trauma) causing vascular changes with increased oxygen tension and a decreased pH, resulting in destruction (resorption) of the tooth from within the pulp from dentinoclasts; tooth has pinkish hue; usually one tooth affected
• External—many factors cause this, such as trauma, orthodontic treatment, excessive occlusal forces, periodontal disease, tumors, and periapical inflammation; reabsorption can occur anywhere along the periodontal ligament and can extend to the pulp; osteoclasts resorb the tooth structure.

Medications and Discoloration
• Tetracycline—binds to calcium, forming a calcium orthophosphate complex that is laid

down into the collagen matrix of enamel; occurs on all teeth; occurs only when the enamel is being formed; results in a yellow brown discoloration
• Amalgam (as with extrinsic stains)
• Iodine/essential oils
• From endodontically treated teeth with the mendicants penetrating the dentinal tubules

SYSTEMS AFFECTED
N/A

GENETICS
• Both amelogenesis imperfecta and dentinogenesis imperfecta in humans are inherited conditions that have many modes of inheritance: X-linked dominant, X-linked recessive, autosomal dominant, autosomal recessive.
• The mode of inheritance in animals has not been studied.

INCIDENCE/PREVALENCE
• Discoloration of the teeth or a tooth is extremely common in all animals.
• Extrinsic staining is very common, especially bacterial stains; others are less common.
• Intrinsic staining is likewise very common, especially internal and external resorption, followed by localized red blood cell destruction; the other causes are rare.

GEOGRAPHIC DISTRIBUTION
N/A

SIGNALMENT
• Dog and cat
• Affects all species, breeds
• No sex predilections
• The reported age range varies—when the condition affects the maturing enamel or dentin it can be first noted after 6 months.

SIGNS

Historical Findings
Owner reports a variation in color of a tooth or teeth

Physical Examination
• Abnormal coloration to tooth or teeth
• Pitted enamel with staining
• Fractured tooth
• Rings or lines of discoloration around tooth or teeth

CAUSES AND RISK FACTORS
• Extrinsic discoloration—bacterial stains from plaque and calculus; foods; gingival

DISCOLORED TOOTH/TEETH

hemorrhage; dental restorative materials, medications (chlorhexidine, 8% stannous fluoride), metal
• Intrinsic discoloration—internal (trauma); external (feline osteoblastic resorptive lesions) resorption; localized red blood cell destruction in the tooth (trauma); systemic infections; medications (tetracycline); fluorosis; hyperbilirubinemia; amelogenesis imperfecta; dentinogenesis imperfecta

DIAGNOSIS

DIFFERENTIAL DIAGNOSIS
• Calculus on the teeth
• Normal tooth aging—increased translucence

CBC/BIOCHEMISTRY/URINALYSIS
N/A

OTHER LABORATORY TESTS
N/A

IMAGING
Dental radiography is extremely useful in identifying internal or external resorption, restorative materials, or bacterial stain from coronal percolation.

DIAGNOSTIC PROCEDURES
If many teeth are affected, one tooth can be extracted and sent for histologic evaluation.

PATHOLOGIC FINDINGS
• Tooth or teeth are discolored; enamel and or dentin can be pitted or broken with staining.
• Extrinsic discoloration—all stain is in the enamel or exposed dentin, otherwise the tooth structure is normal.
• Intrinsic discoloration—hyperbilirubinemia; enamel hypoplasia; lines of resolution on the tooth; all teeth affected
• Localized red blood cell destruction—stain in dentinal tubules; pulpitis/liquefactive necrosis of the pulp
• Internal resorption—well-circumscribed enlargement of an area of the endodontic system with granulation tissue containing many odontoclasts
• External resorption—moth-eaten loss of tooth structure anywhere along the periodontal ligament; can extend into the endodontic system; areas of tooth resorption have granulation tissue with many osteoclasts
• Fluorosis—enamel hypoplasia; medications; systemic (e.g., tetracycline has irregular matrix formation to the enamel and dentin),

all teeth affected
• Amelogenesis imperfecta—irregular formation of the enamel matrix, mineralization, or maturation
• Dentinogenesis imperfecta—irregular formation of dentin; enamel may be separated from the dentin

TREATMENT

APPROPRIATE HEALTH CARE
• Nonemergency
• Extrinsic stain removal—mainly cosmetic
• Intrinsic stain treatment—functional and pain relieving

NURSING CARE
• Extrinsic stain—remove inciting cause.
• Intrinsic stain—soft food; remove chew toys.

ACTIVITY
N/A

DIET
Intrinsic stain—soften food.

CLIENT EDUCATION
• To prevent it in future animals or litters
• Intrinsic causes—if untreated the tooth or teeth are more likely to accumulate plaque and calculus, leading to subsequent periodontal disease; tooth fracture is more prevalent, which could result in tooth abscessation.

SURGICAL CONSIDERATIONS
• Extrinsic stain (cosmetic)—internal and/or external bleaching; veneers or crowns
• Intrinsic stain (functional and pain relief)—possible endodontic treatment (internal resorption and localized red blood cell destruction)
• Restorative procedures such as crowns or veneers to protect both tooth and pulp

MEDICATIONS

DRUGS OF CHOICE
N/A

CONTRAINDICATIONS
N/A

PRECAUTIONS
N/A

POSSIBLE INTERACTIONS
N/A

ALTERNATIVE DRUGS
N/A

FOLLOW-UP

PATIENT MONITORING
N/A

PREVENTION/AVOIDANCE
See Pathophysiology

POSSIBLE COMPLICATIONS
See Client Education

EXPECTED COURSE AND PROGNOSIS
N/A

MISCELLANEOUS

ASSOCIATED CONDITIONS
Juvenile purpura

AGE-RELATED FACTORS
Most common in young dogs and cats

ZOONOTIC POTENTIAL
N/A

PREGNANCY
N/A

SYNONYMS
• Intrinsic staining
• Tetracycline staining
• Extrinsic staining
• Chlorhexidine staining

SEE ALSO
N/A

ABBREVIATIONS
N/A

Suggested Reading

Harvey CE, Emily PP. Small animal dentistry. Philadelphia: Mosby, 1993.
Wiggs RB, Lobprise HB. Veterinary dentistry: principles and practice. Philadelphia: Lippincott-Raven, 1997.
Author James M. G. Anthony
Consulting Editor Jan Bellows

DYSCHEZIA AND HEMATOCHEZIA

BASICS

DEFINITION
• Dyschezia—painful or difficult defecation
• Hematochezia—bright red blood in the feces

PATHOPHYSIOLOGY
• Result from various causes of inflammation or irritation of the rectum or anus
• Hematochezia may also occur with diseases of the colon.

SYSTEMS AFFECTED
Gastrointestinal

SIGNALMENT
• Dogs and cats
• No breed or sex predilection

SIGNS

Historical Findings
• Crying and whimpering during defecation
• Tenesmus common
• Lack of defecation with obstipation may occur if pain is severe.
• Mucoid, bloody diarrhea in patients with colonic disease

Physical Examination
• Rectal examination may reveal hard feces (constipation or obstipation), diarrhea (colorectal disease), polyps, masses, rectoanal thickening, anal gland enlargement/pain, prostatomegaly, or perineal hernias.
• Fistulous tracts or wounds occur with perianal fistulas.
• Anal occlusion with matted hair and feces occurs with pseudocoprostasis.

CAUSES

Rectal/Anal Disease
• Stricture or spasm
• Anal sacculitis or abscess
• Perianal fistulas
• Rectal or anal foreign body
• Pseudocoprostasis
• Rectal prolapse
• Trauma—bite wounds, etc.
• Neoplasia—adenocarcinoma, lymphoma, and anal sac tumors
• Rectal polyps

Colonic Disease
• Neoplasia—adenocarcinoma, lymphoma
• Idiopathic megacolon—cats
• Inflammation—IBD, infectious or parasitic agents, allergic colitis (see Colitis and Proctitis)
• Constipation (see Constipation and Obstipation)

Extraintestinal Disease
• Fractured pelvis or hind limb
• Prostatic disease
• Perineal hernia
• Intrapelvic neoplasia

RISK FACTORS
• Ingestion of hair, bone, foreign material may contribute to constipation and subsequent dyschezia.
• Environmental factors such as a dirty litter pan and infrequent outside walks may contribute to constipation and subsequent dyschezia.

DIAGNOSIS

DIFFERENTIAL DIAGNOSIS
• Dysuria, stranguria, or hematuria—abnormal findings on urinalysis, such as pyuria, crystalluria, bacteriuria
• Dystocia—differentiate with history and imaging

CBC/BIOCHEMISTRY/URINALYSIS
• Usually normal
• Neutrophilia with infection or inflammation

OTHER LABORATORY TESTS
Fecal examination to rule out infectious/parasitic causes of colitis

IMAGING
• Pelvic radiographs may reveal intrapelvic disease, foreign body, or fracture.
• Ultrasonography may demonstrate prostatic disease or caudal abdominal masses.

DIAGNOSTIC PROCEDURES
Colonoscopy/proctoscopy to evaluate for inflammatory or neoplastic disease

TREATMENT
• Usually outpatient
• Consider laxatives to ease defecation if rectoanal disease.
• Balloon dilation of strictures
• Rectoanal diseases may need surgical correction—perianal fistulas, perineal hernias, rectoanal polyps

MEDICATIONS

DRUGS OF CHOICE
• Antibiotics—if bacterial infection (e.g., anal sac abscess); amoxicillin/clavulanic acid 15 mg/kg PO q12h
• Antiinflammatory drugs—sulfasalazine or prednisone if colitis is present (see Colitis)
• Laxatives—lactulose, 1 ml per 4.5 kg PO q8–12h to effect; docusate sodium or docusate calcium, dogs 50–100 mg PO q12–24h, cats 50 mg PO q12–24h

CONTRAINDICATIONS
Avoid agents that cause increased fecal bulk (fiber), unless specifically indicated (colitis).

PRECAUTIONS
N/A

POSSIBLE INTERACTIONS
N/A

ALTERNATIVE DRUGS
N/A

FOLLOW-UP

PATIENT MONITORING
Clinical signs every 2–3 weeks initially

POSSIBLE COMPLICATIONS
May see fecal incontinence if aggressive surgical therapy is needed—perianal fistulas

MISCELLANEOUS

ASSOCIATED CONDITIONS
N/A

AGE-RELATED FACTORS
N/A

ZOONOTIC POTENTIAL
N/A

PREGNANCY
Caution with corticosteroids, antibiotics

SYNONYMS
N/A

SEE ALSO
• Constipation and Obstipation
• Colitis and Proctitis

ABBREVIATION
IBD = inflammatory bowel disease

Suggested Reading
Burrows CF, Sherding RG. Constipation and dyschezia. In: Anderson NV, ed. Veterinary gastroenterology. Philadelphia: Lea & Febiger, 1992:484–503.
Authors Lisa E. Moore and Colin F. Burrows
Consulting Editors Mitchell A. Crystal and Brett M. Feder

DYSPHAGIA

 BASICS

DEFINITION
• Difficulty swallowing, resulting from the inability to prehend, form, and move a bolus of food through the oropharynx into the esophagus
• Esophageal dysphagia is discussed under the topics Megaesophagus and Regurgitation.

PATHOPHYSIOLOGY
• Swallowing difficulties can be caused by mechanical obstruction of the oral cavity or pharynx, neuromuscular dysfunction resulting in weak or uncoordinated swallowing movements, or pain associated with prehension, mastication, or swallowing.
• Oral dysphagia refers to difficulty with the voluntary components of swallowing—prehending and forming a bolus of food at the base of the tongue
• Pharyngeal dysphagia occurs when there is a malfunction of the involuntary movement of the food bolus through the oropharynx.
• Cricopharyngeal dysphagia refers to abnormal movement of the food bolus from the pharynx through the cricopharyngeus muscle, caused by either failure of the cricopharyngeus to relax (cricopharyngeal achalasia) or asynchrony between pharyngeal contractions and cricopharyngeus opening (cricopharyngeal asynchrony).
• Deglutition is coordinated by the swallowing center in the brainstem; sensory afferents are transmitted to the swallowing center by CNs V and IX.
• Motor efferents responsible for swallowing are carried by CN V, VII, XII (prehension and mastication) and IX and X (pharyngeal contraction); disorders in any of these areas may result in dysphagia.

SYSTEMS AFFECTED
• Neuromuscular
• Nervous
• Gastrointestinal
• Respiratory

SIGNALMENT
• Dogs and cats
• Congenital disorders that cause dysphagia (e.g., cricopharyngeal achalasia and cleft palate) are usually diagnosed in animals <1 year old.
• Acquired pharyngeal dysphagias are more common in older patients.

SIGNS

Historical Findings
• Drooling, gagging, weight loss, ravenous appetite, repeated attempts at swallowing, swallowing with the head in an abnormal position, coughing (due to aspiration), regurgitation, painful swallowing, and occasionally anorexia are all possible.
• Ascertain onset and progression.
• Foreign bodies cause acute dysphagia; pharyngeal dysphagia may be chronic and intermittent.

Physical Examination Findings
• A thorough oral examination, with the patient sedated or anesthetized, if necessary, is most important.
• Observe for asymmetry, anatomic defect, foreign body, inflammation, tumor, edema, abscessed teeth, and loose teeth.
• Must observe the patient eating; this may localize the abnormal phase of swallowing.
• Perform a complete neurologic examination, with emphasis on the cranial nerves.

Oral Dysphagia
• Modified eating behavior (e.g., eating with head tilted to one side and throwing head back while eating) may compensate for oral dysphagia.
• Mandibular paralysis, tongue paralysis, dental disease, masticatory muscle swelling or atrophy, inability to open the mouth, and food packed in the buccal folds without retention of saliva suggest oral dysphagia.

Pharyngeal Dysphagia
• Prehension of food is normal.
• Repeated attempts at swallowing while repeatedly flexing and extending the head and neck, excessive chewing, and gagging suggest pharyngeal dysphagia.
• Saliva-coated food retained in the buccal folds, a diminished gag reflex, and nasal discharge from aspiration may also exist.

Cricopharyngeal Dysphagia
• Patients make repeated, nonproductive efforts to swallow, gag, and cough, then forcibly regurgitate immediately after swallowing.
• Gag reflex and prehension are normal.
• Emaciation is more common with this form of dysphagia than others.

CAUSES
• Anatomic or mechanical lesions include pharyngeal inflammation (e.g., abscess, inflammatory polyps, and oral eosinophilic granuloma), retropharyngeal lymphadenomegaly, neoplasia, pharyngeal and retropharyngeal foreign body, sialocele, temporomandibular joint disorders (e.g., luxation, fracture, and craniomandibular osteopathy), mandibular fracture, cleft palate, lingual frenulum disorder, and pharyngeal trauma.
• Pain because of dental disease (e.g., tooth fractures and abscess), mandibular trauma, stomatitis, glossitis, and pharyngeal inflammation may also disrupt normal prehension, bolus formation, and swallowing.
• Neuromuscular disorders that impair prehension and bolus formation include cranial nerve deficits (e.g., idiopathic trigeminal neuropathy CN V, lingual paralysis CN XII) and masticatory muscle myositis.
• Pharyngeal weakness, paresis, or paralysis can be caused by infectious polymyositis (e.g., toxoplasmosis and neosporosis), immune-mediated polymyositis, muscular dystrophy, polyneuropathies, and myoneural junction disorders (e.g., myasthenia gravis, tick paralysis, and botulism).
• Rabies can cause dysphagia by affecting both the brainstem and peripheral nerves.
• Other CNS disorders, especially those involving the brainstem

RISK FACTORS
Many of the causative neuromuscular conditions have breed predispositions.

 DIAGNOSIS

DIFFERENTIAL DIAGNOSIS
• Must be differentiated from vomiting and regurgitation from esophageal disease
• Exaggerated or repeated efforts to swallow—characteristic of dysphagia; most useful means of distinguishing it from vomiting or regurgitation
• Vomiting is associated with abdominal contractions; dysphagia is not.

CBC/BIOCHEMISTRY/URINALYSIS
• Inflammatory conditions often cause a leukocytosis, sometimes with a left shift.
• High serum creatine phosphokinase activity is usually found in patients with muscular disorders resulting in dysphagia.
• May find evidence of renal disease (e.g., azotemia and low urine concentration) in patients with oral and lingual ulcers

OTHER LABORATORY TESTS

- Type 2M muscle antibody serology (masticatory muscle myositis)
- Acetylcholinesterase receptor antibody serology (acquired myasthenia gravis)
- Antinuclear antibody serology (immune-mediated diseases)
- Low-dose dexamethasone suppression test or ACTH stimulation test (hyperadrenocorticism—patients with chronic infections or myopathy)

IMAGING

- Obtain survey radiographs of the skull and neck, including the hyoid apparatus; give particular attention to the mandibles and temporomandibular joint, teeth, pharyngeal and retropharyngeal area, and position of the hyoid apparatus.
- Ultrasonography of the pharynx may be useful in patients with mass lesions and for obtaining ultrasound-guided biopsy specimens.
- Fluoroscopy, with or without positive contrast, is useful in evaluating pharyngeal movement in patients with suspected pharyngeal or cricopharyngeal dysphagia.
- Computed tomography (CT) and/or magnetic resonance imaging (MRI) for a suspected intracranial mass

DIAGNOSTIC PROCEDURES

- Excisional or incisional biopsies of a mass lesion
- Pharyngoscopy
- Electromyography of the pharyngeal musculature to confirm the presence of a neuromuscular disorder; also evaluate the patient for systemic neuromuscular disease.
- Repetitive nerve stimulation and edrophonium chloride (0.1–0.2 mg/kg IV) test for suspected myasthenia gravis
- Cerebrospinal fluid analysis in patients with a CNS disorder
- Cricopharyngeal manometry if cricopharyngeal achalasia is suspected.

TREATMENT

- Determine the underlying cause to develop a treatment plan and accurate prognosis.
- Direct primary treatment at the underlying cause.
- Nutritional support is important for all dysphagic patients.
- Patients with oral dysphagia may be able to swallow if a bolus of food is place in the caudal pharynx; other patients may find a gruel that can be lapped easier to swallow; take care to avoid aspiration when feeding orally.
- Elevating the head and neck may make swallowing easier for patients with pharyngeal or cricopharyngeal dysphagia and help prevent aspiration of food.
- If nutritional requirements cannot be met orally a gastrotomy may be necessary.
- Surgical excision of a mass lesion and foreign body may be curative or temporarily improve the signs of dysphagia.
- Cricopharyngeal myotomy may benefit patients with cricopharyngeal dysphagia; a correct diagnosis is essential before surgery, because cricopharyngeal myotomy will exacerbate dysphagia of patients with oropharyngeal dysphagia.

MEDICATIONS

DRUGS OF CHOICE

- Dysphagia is not immediately life-threatening; direct drug therapy at the underlying cause.
- Empirical treatment may consist of a broad-spectrum antibiotic (e.g., cephalexin 22 mg/kg PO q8h).

CONTRAINDICATIONS

NA

PRECAUTIONS

- Use barium sulfate with caution in patients with evidence of aspiration.
- Use corticosteroids with caution or not at all in patients with evidence of, or at risk for, aspiration.

POSSIBLE INTERACTIONS

N/A

ALTERNATIVE DRUGS

NA

FOLLOW-UP

PATIENT MONITORING

- Daily for signs of aspiration pneumonia (e.g., depression, fever, mucopurulent nasal discharge, coughing, and dyspnea)
- Body condition and hydration status daily; if oral nutrition does not meet requirements, use gastrostomy tube feeding.

POSSIBLE COMPLICATIONS

- Aspiration pneumonia is a common complication with swallowing disorders.
- Feeding multiple small meals with the patient in an upright position and maintaining this position for 10–15 min after feeding helps prevent aspiration of food.

MISCELLANEOUS

ASSOCIATED CONDITIONS

- Megaesophagus
- Aspiration pneumonia

AGE-RELATED FACTORS

- Young dogs are more likely to ingest foreign objects and suffer facial trauma.
- Young cats are more likely to form inflammatory polyps.

ZOONOTIC POTENTIAL

- Consider rabies in any patient with dysphagia, especially if the animal's rabies vaccination status is unknown or questionable or it has been exposed to a potentially rabid animal.
- If a dysphagic animal dies of rapidly progressive neurologic disease, submit the head to a qualified laboratory designated by the local or state health department for rabies examination.

PREGNANCY

N/A

SYNONYMS

N/A

SEE ALSO

- Megaesophagus
- Regurgitation
- Pneumonia, Bacterial

ABBREVIATION

CNs = cranial nerves

Suggested Reading

Watrous BJ. Clinical presentation and diagnosis of dysphagia. Vet Clin North Am 1983;13:437–459.

Willard MD. Dysphagia and swallowing disorders. In: Kirk's current veterinary therapy XI. Philadelphia: Saunders, 1992:572–577.

Author Randall C. Longshore

Consulting Editors Brett M. Feder and Mitchell A. Crystal

DYSPNEA, TACHYPNEA, AND PANTING

 BASICS

DEFINITION
• Dyspnea—distressful feeling associated with difficult or labored breathing; often applied to labored breathing that appears to be uncomfortable • Tachypnea—rapid breathing (not necessarily labored) • Hyperpnea—deep breathing • Hyperventilation—increased air entering the pulmonary alveoli; brought about by prolonged, rapid, and deep breathing • Panting—swift and shallow breathing with a fast respiratory frequency and a small tidal volume

PATHOPHYSIOLOGY
• Nonrespiratory causes of dyspnea—abnormalities in pulmonary vascular tone (e.g., CNS disease and shock), pulmonary circulation (e.g., CHF and pulmonary thromboembolism), oxygenation (e.g., methemoglobinemia and anemia), ventilation (e.g., obesity, ascites, and abdominal organomegaly) • Primary respiratory diseases—upper; lower (subdivided into obstructive or restrictive causes)

SYSTEMS AFFECTED
• Behavioral—panting or tachypnea from fear, nervousness, and response to pain • Cardiovascular • Endocrine/Metabolic—panting from endogenous or exogenous corticosteroid excess • Hemic/Lymphatic/ Immune—acid–base disturbances; secondary to hyperventilation or hypoventilation • Nervous—secondary to CNS hypoxia • Respiratory

SIGNALMENT
• Depends on underlying cause • Toy breeds and tracheal collapse • Old dogs and mitral valvular insufficiency • Male cats and pyothorax

SIGNS

Historical Findings
• Orthopnea (recumbent dyspnea), restlessness, and poor sleeping—may be noted with pleural space disease (e.g., diaphragmatic hernia, effusions, pneumothorax) or CHF • Coughing—may accompany dyspnea; character may relate to cause (e.g., soft and moist with CHF; dry and honking with tracheal collapse)

Physical Examination Findings
• Nasal obstruction—diminished or absent nasal airflow • Upper airway obstruction—tracheal collapse: stridor, stertor, tracheal sensitivity, honking cough; fixed obstruction: may affect inspiration and expiration (mass lesions); dynamic obstruction: affects mainly inspiration • Pneumonia—harsh inspiratory and expiratory wheezes and crackles • Bronchitis—harsh wheezes with or without crackles; prominent expiratory effort • Pneu-

mothorax—hyperresonant percussion of chest wall; diminished or absent lung sounds • Pleural effusion—dull percussion of chest wall; absent lung sounds ventrally; harsh bronchial sounds dorsally

CAUSES

Nonrespiratory
• Cardiac disease—CHF (e.g., mitral valvular insufficiency); low-output failure (e.g., cardiomyopathy and subaortic stenosis); cyanotic heart disease (e.g., right-to-left shunt in patients with reverse patent ductus arteriosus and tetralogy of Fallot); severe arrhythmia; cardiogenic shock • Neuromuscular disease—severe CNS disease (e.g., trauma, neoplasia, and inflammation); polyradiculoneuritis (e.g., coonhound paralysis); spinal disease (e.g., disk extrusion and trauma); myasthenia gravis (e.g., aspiration pneumonia, megaesophagus, and hypoventilation); polymyopathy • Metabolic disease—acidosis; diabetic ketoacidosis; uremia • Hematologic—methemoglobinemia (e.g., acetaminophen intoxication); anemia; hyperviscosity syndrome • Vascular—dirofilariasis; pulmonary thromboembolism (e.g., nephrotic syndrome and hyperadrenocorticism) • Endocrine disease—excessive panting with hyperadrenocorticism (e.g., Cushing disease) • Other—pain; fever; anxiety; heat stroke; obesity (e.g., Pickwickian syndrome or excessive fat in the chest wall, intrathoracic fat, and cranial displacement of the diaphragm owing to abdominal obesity); ascites; abdominal organomegaly

Respiratory
Upper Tract
• Brachycephalic syndrome—stenotic nares; elongated soft palate; laryngeal edema; everted laryngeal saccules • Nasal obstruction—granuloma; foreign body; neoplasia; cuterebriasis • Tonsillar enlargement—owing to hyperplasia or neoplasia • Laryngeal paralysis • Tracheal stenosis or hypoplasia • Cervical tracheal collapse • Laryngotracheal foreign body or neoplasia—adenocarcinoma in Siamese cats • Traumatic airway rupture and extraluminal compression—mediastinal mass; hilar lymphadenopathy
Lower Tract
Obstructive
• Intrathoracic tracheal disease—tracheal collapse; foreign body; neoplasia • Bronchial disease—bronchial collapse; compression by large left atrium in patients with mitral insufficiency; chronic bronchitis; feline asthma; bronchoconstriction; bronchogenic carcinoma • Pulmonary edema—cardiac; noncardiac • Pneumonitis—allergic; parasitic • Pneumonia—fungal; bacterial; viral • Neoplasia—primary; metastatic • Pulmonary contusion—trauma • Lung lobe torsion
Restrictive
• Interstitial fibrosis • Fibrosing pleuritis • Pyothorax • Pleural effusion—right heart failure;

pericardial disease • Hemothorax—coagulopathy; trauma • Chylothorax and nonseptic exudates—FIP; pancreatitis • Pneumothorax—open; closed; tension • Hernias—diaphragmatic; pericardioperitoneal • Mediastinal mass • Rib fracture • Flail chest

RISK FACTORS
• Poor ventilation or secondhand smoke—allergic or irritant bronchitis
• Blunt chest trauma
• Bite wounds—pyothorax; septic shock
• Ingestion of rodenticide—hemothorax

 DIAGNOSIS

DIFFERENTIAL DIAGNOSIS
• Tachypnea without dyspnea—may be physiologic response to fear, physical exertion, anxiety, fever, heat, pain, or acidosis
• Primary cardiac disease—may note a constellation of other signs (e.g., heart murmurs, gallop rhythms, tachycardia, distended jugular veins, pulse deficits, weak femoral pulses, and moist cough)
• Upper respiratory tract dyspnea—often more pronounced on inspiration; may be associated with stridor
• Voice changes—often accompany laryngeal paralysis
• Lower respiratory tract obstructions—more often associated with expiratory effort
• Fixed obstructions (e.g., intraluminal mass or foreign body)—may be accompanied by both inspiratory and expiratory dyspnea
• Pleural space disease—exaggerated chest excursions that generate only minimal airflow at the mouth or nares common

CBC/BIOCHEMISTRY/ URINALYSIS
• Anemia and polycythemia—cyanotic heart disease
• Inflammatory leukon—pneumonia; pyothorax
• Eosinophilia—allergic and parasitic pneumonitis
• Basophilia—heartworm disease
• Uremia—azotemia
• Acidosis—low P_{CO_2}
• Diabetes—hyperglycemia
• Hypothyroidism—high cholesterol; low T_4 and free T_4; high cTSH
• Renal azotemia—isosthenuria
• Proteinuria—predisposes patient to pulmonary thromboembolism
• Pyuria—pyelonephritis; sepsis

OTHER LABORATORY TESTS
• Heartworm test
• Arterial blood gas—assess oxygenation (PaO_2) and ventilation ($PaCO_2$); if unavailable in your clinic, make arrangements with a stat laboratory in a local human hospital and deliver the sample immediately.

• ACTH stimulation—rule out hyperadrenocorticism as a cause of pulmonary thromboembolism

IMAGING

Radiography

• Skull—nasal obstruction (e.g., fungal or neoplastic bony destruction)
• Cervical—tracheal collapse; may best be seen fluoroscopically
• Thoracic—tracheal collapse; pleural space disease (e.g., effusion, pneumothorax, and hernia); pulmonary disease (peribronchiolar: small airway disease; alveolar: pulmonary edema and pneumonia; interstitial: neoplastic or granulomatous disease, pulmonary contusions, and interstitial pneumonia); radiographs that show severe dyspnea with normal to hyperlucent lungs strongly suggest pulmonary thromboembolism or asthma
• Cardiac shadow—globose with pericardial effusion; generalized cardiomegaly with cardiomyopathy; valentine-shaped with hypertrophic cardiomyopathy (cats); left atrial enlargement with mitral regurgitation
• Size of heart and pulmonary veins with pulmonary edema—evidence of left atrial enlargement and pulmonary venous distension with cardiogenic; may be normal with noncardiogenic (e.g., electrocution)

Other

• Contrast arteriography—may demonstrate obstruction with pulmonary thromboembolism.
• Ventilation–perfusion scintigraphy—mismatch consistent with pulmonary thromboembolism
• Echocardiography—sensitive and noninvasive; evaluate pericardial effusion, cardiomyopathy, congenital defects, and valvular disease
• Thoracic ultrasound—may be beneficial with mediastinal mass lesions; beam is greatly attenuated by any air in surrounding lung lobes.

DIAGNOSTIC PROCEDURES

• Thoracentesis—fluid analysis and culture
• Laryngopharyngoscopy—evaluate laryngeal function; determine obstruction
• Tracheoscopy—assess and stage tracheal collapse
• Bronchoscopy—evaluate lower airways
• Lung wash—obtained by transtracheal wash or tracheobronchoscopy; cytologic examination and culture
• CSF—rule out CNS disease

TREATMENT

A: AIRWAY

Obstructed upper respiratory tract—may require intubation (if possible) or tracheostomy

B: BREATHING

• Oxygen enrichment—nasal, oxygen cage, or induction chamber
• Ventilate—only with bradypnea, pulmonary arrest, or hypoventilation owing to exhaustion; little benefit for hypoventilation owing to pleural space disease until the chest is evacuated

C: CHEST TAP

• May be both diagnostic and therapeutic for pleural space disease
• Perform before radiography in all acutely dyspneic patients, especially trauma patients
• Negative tap for air or fluid—suggests solid pleural space disease (e.g., mass or herniated viscus), primary pulmonary disease (e.g., contusion in the trauma patient), or cardiac disease
• Positive tap—**REMEMBER:** small animals may accommodate up to 50 mL/kg free fluid in the chest before becoming dyspneic.
• Remove as much fluid as possible; do not stop after obtaining a diagnostic sample.
• Dyspneic cats—especially fragile; even very stressed patients can be quickly clipped and prepped with minimal restraint
• Sedation—may be desirable, especially for a frantically air-starved cat; it may also be more prudent during sedation to perform for diagnostic procedures (e.g., thoracentesis, radiographs, and ultrasound); try low-dose morphine or butorphanol tartrate

MEDICATIONS

DRUGS OF CHOICE

• Oxygen—single most underused agent in the treatment of acute severe dyspnea.
• Fragile cats—if thoracentesis is not possible or the tap is dry, administer oxygen, furosemide (2–4 mg/kg IM PRN), nitroglycerin (2–4 mg q1h) topically, and glucocorticoids (dexamethasone at 0.1–0.25 mg/kg IM); status asthmaticus and acute heart failure may have very similar appearance; unlikely this shotgun approach will exacerbate either disease
• Cats with respiratory distress from asthma—terbutaline (0.01 mg/kg SC, repeat once in 5–10 min if needed) once cardiac disease has been ruled out; epinephrine reserved for life-threatening, nonresponsive condition
• See primary disorder for definitive treatment.

CONTRAINDICATIONS

• With CHF and blunt chest trauma—iatrogenic fluid overload may cause pulmonary edema; intravenous administration of crystalloids should be done judiciously.

• Carefully and frequently monitor respiratory rate and effort

PRECAUTIONS

• Epinephrine—may induce arrhythmias
• β-blockers—may potentiate bronchoconstriction in asthmatic patients

POSSIBLE INTERACTIONS

N/A

ALTERNATIVE DRUGS

N/A

FOLLOW-UP

PATIENT MONITORING

• Repeat abnormal tests. • CBC—with inflammatory, infectious, parasitic, anemic or polycythemic disease • Cardiac ultrasound—in 3–12 weeks, depending on the condition
• Radiographs—pulmonary edema should be visibly improved within 12 hr of treatment, if effective; monitor recurrence of pleural effusion

POSSIBLE COMPLICATIONS

• Relapse, progression, and death common
• Prognosis—depends on underlying disease

MISCELLANEOUS

ASSOCIATED CONDITIONS

N/A

ZOONOTIC POTENTIAL

N/A

PREGNANCY

N/A

SEE ALSO

• Congestive Heart Failure, Left-Sided • Congestive Heart Failure, Right-Sided • Hyperadrenocorticism (Cushing Disease) • Methemoglobinemia • Myasthenia Gravis • Pleural Effusion • Coonhound paralysis

ABBREVIATIONS

• CHF = congestive heart failure • CSF = cerebrospinal fluid • cTSH = canine thyroid-stimulating hormone • FIP = feline infectious peritonitis

Suggested Reading

Turnwald GH. Dyspnea and tachypnea. In: Ettinger SJ, Feldman EC, eds. Textbook of small animal internal medicine. 3rd ed. Philadelphia: Saunders, 1995:61–64.
Ware W. Dyspnea: diagnosis and management. In: August JR, ed. Consultations in feline medicine. Philadelphia: Saunders, 1991:147–169.
Author Robert A. Mason
Consulting Editor Eleanor C. Hawkins

DYSTOCIA

BASICS

DEFINITION
Difficult birth

PATHOPHYSIOLOGY
• Centers around a small or deformed birth canal, fetal oversize, or uterine weakness (e.g., insufficient uterine force to propel fetus through birth canal)
• Three stages of labor

Stage 1
• Begins with onset of uterine contractions; ends when cervix is fully dilated; averages 6–12 hr
• Bitches—may be restless, nervous, and anorectic; may shiver, pant, vomit, or pace; near end will usually seek a place to nest
• Queens—tend to vocalize initially; purr as delivery approaches

Stage 2
• Begins with full dilation of cervix, entry of the first fetus into the cervical canal, and rupture of the chorioallantois; ends with delivery of the last of the litter
• Bitch—obvious abdominal contractions in attempt to deliver
• From beginning of stage to delivery of first offspring usually < 4 hr; time between delivery of subsequent offspring usually 20–60 min (may be as long as 2–3 hr in bitches)

Stage 3
• Begins after delivery of the offspring; ends with passage of all placentae
• Bitch with multiple puppies—may alternate between stage 2 and 3

SYSTEMS AFFECTED
• Reproductive
• Cardiovascular

SIGNALMENT
• Dogs—common in brachycephalic, miniature, and small breeds; occasionally noted in large breeds with an extremely large litter
• Cats—frequently seen in Persians and Himalayans
• Prevalence increases with age.

SIGNS

Historical Findings
• Female undergoes 30 min of persistent, strong, abdominal contractions without expulsion of offspring
• More than 4 hr from the onset of stage 2 to delivery of first offspring
• More than 2 hr between delivery of offspring
• Failure to deliver 24 hr after rectal temperature falls < 37.2°C (99°F) or within 36 hr of serum progesterone < 2 ng/mL
• Female cries, displays signs of pain, and constantly licks the vulvar area when delivering
• Prolonged gestation—> 70 days from day of first mating; > 59 days from the first day of cytologic diestrus (dogs); > 66 days from LH peak (dogs)

CAUSES

Fetal
• Oversize—one-pup litter; monster, anasarcous fetus; and hydrocephalus
• Malposition in birth canal

Maternal
• Abnormal pelvic canal from previous pelvic fracture
• Congenitally small pelvis—Welsh corgis; brachycephalic breeds
• Pelvic immaturity
• Abnormality of the vaginal vault—stricture; septate; hyperplasia; intraluminal or extra luminal cyst; neoplasia
• Insufficient cervical dilation
• Lack of adequate lubrication
• Uterine torsion
• Poor uterine contractions—myometrial defect; biochemical imbalance; psychogenic disturbance; exhaustion (see Uterine Inertia)
• Ineffective abdominal press—pain; debility (exhaustion); diaphragmatic hernia; age

RISK FACTORS
• Age
• Brachycephalic and toy breeds
• Persian and Himalayan breeds
• Obesity
• Abrupt changes in environment peripartum
• Previous history of dystocia

DIAGNOSIS

DIFFERENTIAL DIAGNOSIS
• Uterine inertia—distinguished from obstructive dysecoia by previously diagnosed pelvic or vaginal anomaly and type of breed
• Complete physical examination—essential; determine concurrent or contributing problems (e.g., hypoglycemia, hypocalcemia, dehydration, and fever); careful abdominal palpation to confirm the existence of fetuses
• Detailed and meticulous digital vaginal examination—identify a fetus engaged in the vaginal canal; find abnormalities of the maternal pelvic canal or vaginal vault; determine the strength of abdominal press in response to stimulation of the roof of the vagina (feathering).
• Bitches that fail to produce abdominal contractions in response to feathering or oxytocin—more likely to have uterine inertia than obstructive dystocia, unless the obstruction is of several hours' duration

CBC/BIOCHEMISTRY/URINALYSIS
• Minimum database—PCV, total protein, BUN, and serum glucose and calcium concentrations
• Depend on duration of condition—may be normal; may note hypoglycemia, dehydration, and hypocalcemia
• Perform analyses although results might not be available until after resolution of the condition.

OTHER LABORATORY TESTS
N/A

IMAGING
• Radiography (abdomen and pelvic area)—paramount; determine state of pregnancy, pelvic structure, number and malposition of fetuses, fetal oversize, and fetal death
• Ultrasonography—recommended for monitoring fetal viability; detects fetal stress (e.g., fetal heart rate < 200 bpm)

DIAGNOSTIC PROCEDURES
N/A

TREATMENT

- Inpatient—until delivery of all offspring and mother has stabilized
- Fluid replacement—balanced electrolyte solutions; for clinical dehydration
- Uterine inertia—initiate treatment if no evidence of fetal stress; administer balanced electrolyte solution (adjusted to correct for any identified electrolyte imbalance).

Manual Delivery

- To deliver a fetus lodged in vaginal vault
- Apply lubrication liberally; place patient in a standing position.
- Use of fingers—safest and most reliable approach
- Instrument delivery (dogs)—vaginal vault too small for digital manipulations; use with adequate lubrication; always place a finger in the vaginal vault to direct the instrument; spay hook or nonratcheted forceps recommended; apply traction in a posterior and ventral direction.
- Use extreme caution; undesirable sequelae include mutilation of the fetus and laceration of the dam.
- Traction on a distal extremity—definitely contraindicated
- Cats—use of instruments not recommended because of the small size of the vaginal vault
- Failure to deliver within 25–30 min—cesarean section indicated
- Severely depressed queen—fluid and electrolyte balance must be restored before induction of anesthesia.

Surgical Delivery

- Indicated cesarean section—uterine inertia unresponsive to oxytocin; pelvic or vaginal obstruction; uncorrectable fetal malposition; fetal oversize; fetal stress; in utero fetal death
- Elective cesarean section—breeds highly prone to dystocia; bitches with a history of dystocia

MEDICATIONS

DRUG(S) OF CHOICE

Anesthesia

- Healthy or depressed bitch—premedication with diazepam (0.2–0.4 mg/kg IM) and butorphanol (0.2–0.4 mg/kg IM) with or without anticholinergics; isoflurane and mask for induction; intubate to maintain; provide intravenous fluids.
- Healthy queen—premedication with diazepam (0.4 mg/kg IV) and ketamine (6 mg/kg IV); administer intravenous fluids; 0.5% lidocaine spray for intubation; isoflurane preferred but may use halothane
- Severely depressed queen (exhausted from prolonged labor)—premedication with diazepam or midazolam (0.2–0.4 mg/kg IV, IM) with either butorphanol (0.4 mg/kg IV, IM) or oxymorphone (0.2 mg/kg IM); low-dose ketamine (1–2 mg/kg IV) for intubation; etomidate or propofol for induction
- After surgery all effects of drugs can be reversed.
- Oxytocin—for uterine inertia

CONTRAINDICATIONS

Oxytocin—contraindicated with obstructive dystocia of fetal or maternal cause, fetal stress, and longstanding in utero fetal death

PRECAUTIONS
N/A

POSSIBLE INTERACTIONS
N/A

ALTERNATIVE DRUGS
N/A

FOLLOW-UP

PATIENT MONITORING

Ultrasonography—recommended; monitor fetal heart rate during medical management of uterine inertia

POSSIBLE COMPLICATIONS

- Increased risk in future pregnancies
- Neonatal loss if treatment is not begun promptly

MISCELLANEOUS

ASSOCIATED CONDITIONS
N/A

AGE-RELATED FACTORS

Old, obese bitches—increased risk of uterine inertia

ZOONOTIC POTENTIAL
N/A

PREGNANCY
N/A

SEE ALSO
Uterine Inertia

ABBREVIATIONS

- PCV = packed cell volume
- LH = luteinizing hormone

Suggested Reading

Feldman EC, Nelson RW. Canine and feline endocrinology and reproduction. Philadelphia: Saunders, 1987:438–442, 536.

Paddleford RR. Anesthetic management of the cesarean section. In: Manual of small animal anesthesia. Churchill Livingstone, 1988:290–296.

Shille VM. Diagnosis and management of dystocia in the bitch and queen. In: Bojrab MJ, ed., Current techniques in small animal surgery. Philadelphia: Lea & Febiger, 1983;338–346.

Tranquilli WJ. Anesthesia for cesarean section in the cat. Vet Clin North Am Small Anim Pract 1992;22;484–486.

Author Louis F. Archbald
Consulting Editor Sara K. Lyle

DYSURIA AND POLLAKIURIA

BASICS

DEFINITION
• Dysuria—difficult or painful urination
• Pollakiuria—voiding small quantities of urine with increased frequency

PATHOPHYSIOLOGY
The urinary bladder and urethra normally serve as a reservoir for storage and periodic release of urine. Inflammatory and non-inflammatory disorders of the lower urinary tract may decrease bladder compliance and storage capacity by damaging structural components of the bladder wall or by stimulating sensory nerve endings located in the bladder or urethra. Sensations of bladder fullness, urgency, and pain stimulate premature micturition and reduce functional bladder capacity. Dysuria and pollakiuria are caused by lesions of the urinary bladder and/or urethra and provide unequivocal evidence of lower urinary tract disease; these clinical signs do not exclude concurrent involvement of the upper urinary tract or disorders of other body systems.

SYSTEMS AFFECTED
Renal/Urologic—bladder, urethra, and prostate gland

SIGNALMENT
N/A

SIGNS
N/A

CAUSES

Urinary Bladder
• Urinary tract infection—bacterial, viral, fungal, parasitic, or mycoplasmal
• Urocystolithiasis
• Neoplasia—e.g., transitional cell carcinoma
• Trauma
• Anatomic abnormalities—e.g., ureterocele, persistent uterus masculinus, perineal hernias containing the urinary bladder, and spay granulomas
• Detrusor atony—e.g., chronic partial obstruction and dysautonomia
• Chemicals/drugs—e.g., cyclophosphamide
• Iatrogenic—e.g., catheterization, palpation, reverse flushing, overdistension of the bladder during contrast radiography, urohydropropulsion, urethrocystoscopy, and surgery

• Idiopathic—e.g., idiopathic feline lower urinary tract disease

Urethra
• Urinary tract infection—see previous section
• Urethrolithiasis—see previous section
• Urethral plugs—e.g., matrix and matrix-crystalline
• Neoplasia—see previous section; local invasion by malignant neoplasms of adjacent structures
• Trauma
• Anatomic anomalies—e.g., congenital or acquired strictures, urethrorectal fistulas, and pseudohermaphrodites
• Urethral sphincter hypertonicity—e.g., upper motor neuron spinal cord lesions, reflex dyssynergia, and urethral spasm
• Iatrogenic—see previous section
• Idiopathic—see previous section

Prostate Gland
• Prostatitis or prostatic abscess
• Neoplasia—adenocarcinoma and transitional cell carcinoma
• Cystic hyperplasia
• Paraprostatic cysts

RISK FACTORS
• Diseases, diagnostic procedures, or treatments that (1) alter normal host urinary tract defenses and predispose to infection, (2) predispose to formation of uroliths, or (3) damage the urothelium or other tissues of the lower urinary tract
• Mural or extramural diseases that compress the bladder or urethral lumen

DIAGNOSIS

DIFFERENTIAL DIAGNOSIS

Differentiating from Other Abnormal Patterns of Micturition
• Rule out polyuria—increased frequency and volume of urine > 50 mL/kg/day
• Rule out urethral obstruction—stranguria, anuria, overdistended urinary bladder, signs of postrenal uremia
• Rule out urinary incontinence—involuntary urination, urine dribbling, enuresis, incomplete bladder emptying
• Rule out urine spraying or marking—voiding small amounts of urine on vertical surfaces or other socially significant places

Differentiate Causes of Dysuria and Pollakiuria

• Rule out urinary tract infection—hematuria; malodorous or cloudy urine; small, painful, thickened bladder
• Rule out urolithiasis—hematuria; palpable uroliths in urethra or bladder
• Rule out neoplasia—hematuria; palpable masses in urethra or bladder
• Rule out neurogenic disorders—flaccid bladder wall; residual urine in bladder lumen after micturition; other neurologic deficits to hind legs, tail, perineum, and anal sphincter
• Rule out prostatic diseases—urethral discharge, prostatomegaly, pyrexia, depression, tenesmus, caudal abdominal pain, stiff gait
• Rule out cyclophosphamide cystitis—history
• Rule out iatrogenic disorders—history of catheterization, reverse flushing, contrast radiography, urohydropropulsion, urethrocystoscopy, or surgery

CBC/BIOCHEMISTRY/URINALYSIS
• Results often normal. Lower urinary tract disease complicated by urethral obstruction may be associated with azotemia, hyperphosphatemia, acidosis, and hyperkalemia. Patients with concurrent pyelonephritis may have impaired urine-concentrating capacity, leukocytosis, and azotemia. Patients with acute prostatitis or prostatic abscesses may have leukocytosis. Dehydrated patients may have elevated total plasma protein.
• Disorders of the urinary bladder are best evaluated with a urine specimen collected by cystocentesis. Urethral disorders are best evaluated with a voided urine sample or by comparison of results of analysis of voided and cystocentesis samples (Caution: cystocentesis may induce hematuria).
• Pyuria, hematuria, and proteinuria indicate urinary tract inflammation, but these are nonspecific findings that may result from infectious and noninfectious causes of lower urinary tract disease.
• Identification of bacteria, fungi, or parasite ova in urine sediment suggests, but does not prove, that urinary tract infection is causing or complicating lower urinary tract disease. Consider contamination of urine during collection and storage when interpreting urinalysis results.
• Identification of neoplastic cells in urine sediment indicates urinary tract neoplasia. Use caution in establishing a diagnosis of neoplasia based on urine sediment examination. Urinary tract inflammation or extremes in urine pH or osmolality can cause epithelial cell atypia that is difficult to differentiate from neoplasia.

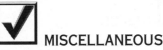

DYSURIA AND POLLAKIURIA

• Crystalluria occurs in normal patients, patients with urolithiasis, or patients with lower urinary tract disease unassociated with uroliths. Interpret the significance of crystalluria cautiously.

• Hematuria, proteinuria, and variable crystalluria occur in cats with nonobstructive idiopathic lower urinary tract disease. Significant pyuria is rare in these patients.

OTHER LABORATORY TESTS

• Quantitative urine culture—the most definitive means of identifying and characterizing bacterial urinary tract infection; negative urine culture results suggest a noninfectious cause (e.g., uroliths and neoplasia) or inflammation associated with urinary tract infection caused by fastidious organisms (e.g., mycoplasmas or viruses)

• Cytologic evaluation of urine sediment, prostatic fluid, urethral or vaginal discharges or biopsy specimens obtained by catheter or needle aspiration—may help in evaluating patients with localized urinary tract disease; may establish a definitive diagnosis of urinary tract neoplasia, but cannot rule it out

IMAGING

Survey abdominal radiography, contrast urethrocystography and cystography, urinary tract ultrasonography, and excretory urography are important means of identifying and localizing causes of dysuria and pollakiuria.

DIAGNOSTIC PROCEDURES

• Use urethrocystoscopy in patients with persistent lesions of the lower urinary tract for which no definitive diagnosis has been established by other, less-invasive, means.

• Use light microscopic evaluation of tissue biopsy specimens from patients with persistent lesions of the urinary tract for which no definitive diagnosis has been established by other, less-invasive, means. Tissue specimens may be obtained by catheter biopsy, urethrocystoscopy and pinch biopsy, or surgery.

TREATMENT

• Patients with nonobstructive lower urinary tract diseases are typically managed as outpatients; diagnostic evaluation may require brief hospitalization.

• Dysuria and pollakiuria associated with systemic signs of illness (e.g., pyrexia, depression, anorexia, vomiting, and dehydration) or laboratory findings of azotemia or leukocytosis warrant aggressive diagnostic evaluation and initiation of supportive and symptomatic treatment.

• Treatment depends on the underlying cause and specific sites involved. See specific chapters describing diseases listed in section on causes.

• Clinical signs of dysuria and pollakiuria often resolve rapidly following specific treatment of the underlying cause(s).

MEDICATIONS

DRUGS OF CHOICE

• Patients with urge incontinence, severe or persistent signs, or untreatable lower urinary tract disease may benefit from symptomatic therapy with propantheline or oxybutynin, anticholinergic agents that may reduce the force and frequency of uncontrolled detrusor contractions.

• Patients with transitional cell carcinoma of the urinary bladder or urethra may be symptomatically managed with the nonsteroidal antiinflammatory drug piroxicam, which reduces the severity of clinical signs, improves quality of life, and in some cases, induces tumor remission.

CONTRAINDICATIONS

• Glucocorticoids or other immunosuppressive agents in patients suspected of having urinary or genital tract infection.

• Potentially nephrotoxic drugs (e.g., gentamicin) in patients who are febrile, dehydrated, or azotemic or who are suspected of having pyelonephritis, septicemia, or preexisting renal disease.

PRECAUTIONS
N/A

POSSIBLE INTERACTIONS
N/A

ALTERNATIVE DRUGS
N/A

FOLLOW-UP

PATIENT MONITORING

• Response to treatment by clinical signs, serial physical examinations, laboratory testing, and radiographic and ultrasonic evaluations appropriate for each specific cause

• Refer to specific chapters describing diseases listed in section on causes.

POSSIBLE COMPLICATIONS

• Dysuria and pollakiuria may be associated with formation of macroscopic vesicourachal diverticula.

• Refer to specific chapters describing diseases

listed in section on causes.

✓ MISCELLANEOUS

ASSOCIATED CONDITIONS

• Hematuria, pyuria, and proteinuria
• Disorders predisposing to urinary tract infection
• Disorders predisposing to formation of uroliths
• Macroscopic vesicourachal diverticula

AGE-RELATED FACTORS
N/A

ZOONOTIC POTENTIAL
N/A

PREGNANCY
N/A

SYNONYMS
• Feline urological syndrome (FUS)
• Lower urinary tract disease

SEE ALSO
• Lower Urinary Tract Infection
• Urolithiasis
• Urinary Retention, Functional
• Urinary Tract Obstruction
• Feline Lower Urinary Tract Disease
• Vesicourachal Diverticula

ABBREVIATIONS
N/A

Suggested Reading

Hammer AS, LaRue S. Tumors of the urinary tract. In: Ettinger SJ, Feldman EC, eds. Textbook of veterinary internal medicine. 4th ed. Philadelphia: Saunders, 1995:1788–1796.

Lulich JP, Osborne CA. Bacterial infections of the urinary tract. In: Ettinger SJ, Feldman EC, eds. Textbook of veterinary internal medicine. 4th ed. Philadelphia: Saunders, 1995:1775–1788.

Lulich JP, Osborne CA, Bartges JW, et al. Feline lower urinary tract disease. In: Ettinger SJ, Feldman EC, eds. Textbook of veterinary internal medicine. 4th ed. Philadelphia: Saunders, 1995:1805–1832.

Authors John M. Kruger and Carl A. Osborne

Consulting Editors Larry G. Adams and Carl A. Osborne

EPIPHORA

BASICS

DEFINITION
Abnormal overflow of the aqueous portion of the precorneal tear film

PATHOPHYSIOLOGY
Caused by overproduction of the aqueous portion of tears (usually in response to ocular irritation), poor eyelid function secondary to malformation or deformity, or blockage of the nasolacrimal drainage system

SYSTEMS AFFECTED
Ophthalmic

SIGNALMENT
See Causes

SIGNS
N/A

CAUSES

Overproduction of Tears Secondary to Ocular Irritants
Congenital
• Distichiasis or trichiasis—young shelties; shih tzus; lhasa apsos; cocker spaniels; miniature poodles
• Entropion—shar peis; chow chows
• Eyelid agenesis—domestic shorthaired cats
Acquired
• Corneal or conjunctival foreign bodies—usually young, large-breed, active dogs
• Eyelid neoplasms—old dogs (all breeds)
• Blepharitis—infectious or immune-mediated
• Conjunctivitis—infectious or immune-mediated
• Ulcerative keratitis
• Anterior uveitis
• Glaucoma

Eyelid Abnormalities or Poor Eyelid Function
Tears never reach the nasolacrimal puncta but instead spill over the eyelid margin.
Congenital
• Macropalpebral fissures—brachiocephalic breeds
• Ectropion—Great Danes; bloodhounds; spaniels
• Entropion—especially of the medial lower lid
Acquired
• Post-traumatic eyelid scarring
• Facial nerve paralysis

Obstruction of the Nasolacrimal

Drainage System
Congenital
• Imperforate nasolacrimal puncta—cocker spaniels; bulldogs; poodles
• Ectopic nasolacrimal openings—extra openings along the side of the face ventral to the medial canthus
• Nasolacrimal atresia—lack of distal openings into the nose
Acquired
• Rhinitis or sinusitis—causes swelling adjacent to the nasolacrimal duct
• Trauma or fractures of the lacrimal or maxillary bones
• Foreign bodies—grass awns; seeds; sand; parasites
• Neoplasia—of the third eyelid, conjunctiva, medial eyelids, nasal cavity, maxillary bone, or periocular sinuses
• Dacryocystitis—inflammation of the canaliculi, lacrimal sac, or nasolacrimal ducts

RISK FACTORS
• Breeds prone to congenital eyelid abnormalities (see Causes)
• Active outdoor dogs—at risk for foreign bodies

DIAGNOSIS

DIFFERENTIAL DIAGNOSIS
• Other ocular discharges (e.g., mucus or purulent)—epiphora is a watery, serous discharge.
• Eye—usually red when caused by overproduction of tears; quiet when secondary to impaired outflow
• Irritative causes and some congenital causes of obstruction—thorough ocular examination
• Acute onset, unilateral condition with ocular pain (blepharospasm)—usually indicates a foreign body or corneal injury
• Chronic, bilateral condition—usually indicates a congenital problem
• Facial pain, swelling, nasal discharge, or sneezing—may indicate nasal or sinus infection; may indicate obstruction from neoplasm
• With mucus or purulent discharge at the medial canthus—may indicate dacryocystitis

CBC/BIOCHEMISTRY/URINALYSIS
N/A

OTHER LABORATORY TESTS
N/A

IMAGING

• Skull radiographs—may show a nasal, sinus, or maxillary bone lesion
• Dacryocystorhinography—radiopaque contrast material to help localize obstruction
• MRI or CT—may help localize obstruction and characterize associated lesions

DIAGNOSTIC PROCEDURES
• Bacterial culture and sensitivity testing and cytologic examination of the material—with purulent material at the medial canthus (e.g., dacryocystitis); performed before instilling any substance into the eye
• Topical fluorescein dye application to the eye—most physiologic test for nasolacrimal function; should be performed first; dye flows through the nasolacrimal system and reaches the external nares in approximately 10 sec in normal dogs.
• Rhinoscopy—with or without biopsy or bacterial culture; may be indicated if previous tests suggest a nasal or sinus lesion
• Surgical exploratory—may be the only way to obtain a definitive diagnosis
• Temporary tacking out of the lower medial eyelid with suture—may help determine whether repair of medial lower entropion or repositioning of the eyelid would reduce epiphora secondary to eyelid conformational abnormalities

Nasolacrimal flush
• Confirms obstruction
• May dislodge foreign material
• A nasolacrimal cannula is inserted into the upper nasolacrimal punctum
• Eyewash is flushed through the cannula—if fluid does not exit the lower nasolacrimal punctum, the obstruction is in the upper or lower canaliculi, the nasolacrimal sac, or the lower punctum (imperforate).
• Lower punctum is manually obstructed—if flushed fluid does not exit the external nares, the obstruction is in the nasolacrimal duct or at its distal opening (atresia or blockage from a nasal sinus lesion).

TREATMENT
• Remove cause of ocular irritation—removal of a conjunctival or corneal foreign body; treatment of the primary ocular disease (e.g., conjunctivitis, ulcerative keratitis, and uveitis); cryosurgery or electroepilation for distichiasis, entropion correction; medial or lateral canthoplasty (for medial trichiasis and

macropalpebral fissures); correction of cicatricial eyelid abnormalities
• Treat primary obstructing lesion (e.g., third eyelid mass, nasal or sinus mass, and infection)—do initially; successful management may allow normal nasolacrimal flow to resume.
• Warn client that patient is predisposed to nasolacrimal obstruction and that recurrence is common.
• Inform client that early detection and intervention provides a better long-term prognosis.

SURGICAL CONSIDERATIONS

Imperforate Puncta
• Surgical opening of the puncta is indicated.
• If one of the puncta is patent (usually the upper punctum), flushing eyewash through the upper opening will cause "tenting" of the conjunctiva at the site of the lower punctum.
• Place patient under topical or general anesthesia.
• Grasp conjunctiva overlying the lower canaliculi with forceps and cut with scissors to leave a patent punctum.
• Puncta closed by conjunctival scarring (symblepharon) caused by severe conjunctivitis (e.g., herpesvirus conjunctivitis in cats)—use same procedure.
• Recurrent disease—may be necessary to suture silastic tubing in place to prevent stricture formation.

Obstructed or Obliterated Distal Nasolacrimal Duct
• Dacryocystorhinotomy or conjunctivorhinostomy—create an opening to drain the tears into the nasal cavity
• See Suggested Reading for surgical technique.

MEDICATIONS

DRUGS OF CHOICE
• Topical broad-spectrum antibiotic ophthalmic solutions—while waiting for results of diagnostic tests (e.g., bacterial culture and sensitivity testing; diagnostic radiographs); q4–6h; may try neomycin, gramicidin, polymyxin B triple ophthalmic antibiotic solutions, or ophthalmic chloramphenicol solution
• Dacryocystitis—based on bacterial culture and sensitivity test results; continued for at least 21 days

CONTRAINDICATIONS
• Topical corticosteroids or antibiotic–corticosteroid combinations—avoid unless a definitive diagnosis has been made.
• Topical corticosteroids—never use if the cornea retains fluorescein stain.

PRECAUTIONS
N/A

POSSIBLE INTERACTIONS
N/A

ALTERNATIVE DRUGS
Tetracycline—5 mg/kg PO q24h; may help reduce idiopathic tear staining of the periocular facial hair; staining recurs when the drug is discontinued.

FOLLOW-UP

PATIENT MONITORING

Dacryocystitis
• Re-evaluate every 7 days until the condition is resolved.
• Continue treatment for at least 7 days after resolution of clinical signs to help prevent recurrence.
• Problem persists more than 7–10 days with treatment or recurs soon after cessation of treatment—indicates a foreign body or nidus of persistent infection; requires further diagnostics (e.g., dacryostorhinography) Nasolacrimal Catheter
• Commonly required for persistent dacryocystitis
• Maintains patency of the duct and prevents stricturing
• Catheter—silastic or polyethylene (PE90) tubing; left in place 2–4 weeks
• Procedure—pass 2–0 nylon via the upper punctum and thread it through the nasolacrimal duct to exit the external nares; pass tubing retrograde over the suture; suture the upper and lower portions of the tubing to the face.
• Most dogs tolerate the tubing well.
• Continue topical antibiotics as before.

Dacryocystorhinotomy/Conjunctivorhinostomy
• Tubing—reevaluate every 7 days to ensure it remains intact; may need to resuture if it becomes loosened or dislodged

• After tubing has been removed—reevaluate in 14 days; for this and future examinations, place fluorescein on the eye and check nasolacrimal patency by examining the external nares for fluorescein; may evaluate the nasolacrimal system further by cannulating and flushing with eyewash
• Dacryocystorhinography contrast study—repeated 3–4 months after surgery to evaluate size of the nasal opening; repeated for recurrence or with no nasolacrimal fluorescein drainage

POSSIBLE COMPLICATIONS
• Recurrence—most common complication; caused by recurrence of ocular irritation (e.g., corneal ulceration, distichiasis, entropion), recurrence of dacryocystitis, or closure of the dacryocystorhinotomy or conjunctivorhinostomy openings into the nasal cavity

MISCELLANEOUS

ASSOCIATED CONDITIONS
• Chronic conjunctivitis—Cats
• Chronic conjunctivitis—Dogs
• Recurrent eye "infections"
• Moist dermatitis (hot spots) ventral to the medial canthus
• Nasal discharge

AGE-RELATED FACTORS
N/A

ZOONOTIC POTENTIAL
N/A

PREGNANCY
N/A

SEE ALSO
• Conjunctivitis—Cats
• Conjunctivitis—Dogs
• Eyelash Disorders (Trichiasis/Distichiasis/Ectopic Cilia)
• Keratitis, Ulcerative
• Third Eyelid, Protrusion

Suggested Reading
Grahn BH. Diseases and surgery of the canine nasolacrimal system. In: Gelatt KN, ed. Veterinary ophthalmology. 3rd ed. Philadelphia: Williams & Wilkins 1999; 569–581.
Author Brian C. Gilger
Consulting Editor Paul E. Miller

EPISTAXIS

BASICS

DEFINITION
Bleeding from the nose

PATHOPHYSIOLOGY
Results from one of three abnormalities—coagulopathy; space-occupying lesion; vascular or systemic disease

SYSTEMS AFFECTED
• Respiratory—hemorrhage; sneezing
• Hemic/Lymphatic/Immune—anemia
• Gastrointestinal—melena

SIGNALMENT
Depends on underlying cause

SIGNS

Historical Findings
• Nasal hemorrhage
• Sneezing
• With coagulopathy—hematochezia, melena, hematuria, or hemorrhage from other areas of the body
• Melena

Physical Examination Findings
• Melena—may be from swallowing blood
• Nasal hemorrhage
• With coagulopathy—possibly petechia, ecchymosis, hematomas, hematochezia, melena, and hematuria.
• With coagulopathy or hypertension—possibly retinal hemorrhages

CAUSES

Coagulopathy
Thrombocytopenia
• Immune-mediated disease—idiopathic disease; SLE; drug reaction; MLV reaction
• Rickettsial disease—ehrlichiosis; Rocky Mounted spotted fever
• Bone marrow disease—neoplasia; aplastic anemia; infectious (fungal, rickettsial, or viral)
• DIC
Thrombopathia
• Congenital—Willebrand disease; thrombasthenia; thrombopathia
• Acquired—NSAIDs; hyperglobulinemia (*Ehrlichia*, multiple myeloma); uremia; DIC
• Coagulation factor defect—congenital: hemophilia A (factor VIIIc deficiency) and hemophilia B (factor IX deficiency); acquired: anticoagulant rodenticide (warfarin) intoxication, hepatobiliary disease, and DIC

Space-occupying Lesion
• Foreign body
• Trauma

• Infection—fungal (aspergillus, cryptococcus, and *Rhinosporidium*); viral or bacterial. Usually blood tinged mucopfrom exudate rather than frank hemorrhage
• Neoplasia—adenocarcinoma; carcinoma; chondrosarcoma; squamous cell carcinoma; fibrosarcoma; transmissible venereal tumor

Vascular or Systemic Disease
• Hypertension—renal disease; hyperthyroidism; hyperadrenocorticism; idiopathic disease
• Hyperviscosity—multiple myeloma; *Ehrlichia;* polycythemia
• Vasculitis—immune-mediated and rickettsial diseases

RISK FACTORS

Coagulopathy
• Immune-mediated disease—young to middle-aged, small to medium female dogs
• Rickettsial disease—dogs living or traveling to endemic areas
• Thrombasthenia—otter hounds
• Thrombopathia—basset hounds
• von Willebrand disease—Doberman pinschers, Airedales, German shepherds, Scottish terriers, Chesapeake Bay retrievers, and many other breeds; cats
• Hemophilia A—German shepherds and many other breeds; cats
• Hemophilia B—Cairn terriers, coonhounds, St. Bernards, and other breeds; cats

Space-occupying Lesions
• Aspergillosis—German shepherds
• Neoplasia—dolicephalic breeds

DIAGNOSIS

DIFFERENTIAL DIAGNOSIS
See Causes.

CBC/BIOCHEMISTRY/URINALYSIS
• Anemia—if enough hemorrhage has occurred
• Thrombocytopenia—possible (see Thrombocytopenia)
• Neutrophilia—infection; neoplasia
• Pancytopenia—bone marrow disease
• Hypoproteinemia—if enough hemorrhage has occurred
• High BUN with normal creatinine—possible, owing to gastrointestinal blood
• Hyperglobulinemia-ehrlichiosis, multiple myeloma
• Azotemia-renal failure–induced hypertension
• High ALT, AST, and total bilirubin-severe hepatic disease with coagulopathy possible
• Urinalysis usually normal

• Hematuria (coagulopathy), isosthenuria-renal failure–induced hypertension, and proteinuria (SLE)—possible

OTHER LABORATORY TESTS
• Coagulation profile—prolonged times with coagulation factor defects; normal with thrombocytopenia and thrombopathia
• Antinuclear antibody test—for suspected SLE
• Platelet function testing (e.g., bleeding time, von Willebrand factor analysis)—for suspected coagulopathy despite normal platelet count and coagulation profile
• *Ehrlichia* and Rocky Mountain spotted fever titers—with possible exposure
• Thyroid hormone assay—in old cats when coagulopathies and space-occupying lesions have been ruled out

IMAGING
• Thoracic radiograph—screen for metastasis with suspected neoplasia
• Nasal series—under anesthesia; including open mouth view and frontal sinus view; with suspected space-occupying lesions; osteolysis noted with neoplasia and fungal sinusitis; foreign bodies usually not seen
• CT scan—more sensitive than radiographs for some diseases

DIAGNOSTIC PROCEDURES
• Rhinoscopy, nasal lavage, nasal biopsy (blind or via rhinoscopy)—indicated for suspected space-occupying disease; aimed at removing foreign bodies and evaluating and sampling nasal tissue for a causal diagnosis (e.g., neoplasia and infection)
• Cytologic and histopathologic examination and bacterial and fungal culture and sensitivity testing—nasal tissue sample
• Bone marrow aspiration biopsy—with pancytopenia
• Blood pressure evaluation—when coagulopathies and space-occupying lesions have been ruled out and azotemia is noted

TREATMENT
• Coagulopathy—usually inpatient
• Space-occupying lesion or vascular or systemic disease—outpatients or inpatients, depending on the disease and its severity
• Minimize activity or stimuli that precipitate hemorrhage episodes.
• Inform client about the disease process.
• Teach client how to recognize a serious hemorrhage (e.g., weakness, collapse, pallor, and blood loss > 30 mL/kg of body weight).
• Whole blood or packed RBC transfusion—may be needed with severe anemia

Coagulopathy
- von Willebrands disease—plasma or cryoprecipitate for acute bleeding
- Hemophilia A—plasma or cryoprecipitate for acute bleeding; no long-term treatment
- Hemophilia B—plasma for acute bleeding; no long-term treatment
- Anticoagulant rodenticide intoxication—plasma for acute bleeding
- Liver disease and DIC—treat and support the underlying cause; plasma may be beneficial.
- Discontinue all NSAIDs
- Hyperglobulinemia plasmapheresis

Space-occupying lesion
- Topical soak * If desired!
- Radiotherapy—nasal tumors, various response rates, depending on tumor type
- Surgery—foreign body unremovable by rhinoscopy or blind attempt; fungal rhinitis (e.g., aspergillus and *Rhinosporidium*) can be treated via surgical exposure and delayed closure of the nasal cavity with daily application of povidone iodine solution.

 MEDICATIONS

DRUGS OF CHOICE

Coagulopathy
- Immune-mediated disease—prednisone (1.1 mg/kg q12h; taper over 4–6 months); other drugs may be used in addition to prednisone for refractive cases: (azathioprine, 2.2 mg/kg q24h for 14 days; then q48h, dogs only; danazol, 5 mg/kg q12h)
- Rickettsial disease—doxycycline (5 mg/kg q12h for 2–3 weeks)
- Bone marrow neoplasia—see Myelodysplasia Thrombopathia and thrombasthenia–no treatment
- Thyroid supplementation for chronic management of hypothyroidism
- DDAVP—1 μg/kg SC, IV diluted in 20 mL of 0.9% NaCl given over 10 min; may help control hemorrhage owing to von Willebrand's disease; intranasal formulation (less expensive) may be used if first passed through a bacteriostatic filter
- Anticoagulant rodenticide intoxication—plasma for acute bleeding; [vitamin K at 5.0 mg/kg loading dose followed by 1.25 mg/kg q12h for 1 (warfarin) to 4 (longer-acting formulations) weeks)]

Space-occupying Lesion
- Serious hemorrhage—control with cage rest and acepromazine (0.05–0.1 mg/kg SC, IV) to lower blood pressure and promote clotting if the patient is not hypovolemic; intranasal instillation of neosynephrine or dilute epinephrine may help (promotes vaso-constriction).
- Bacterial infection—antibiotics; based on culture and sensitivity testing
- Fungal infection—itraconazole (5 mg/kg PO q12h); topical treatment with 1-hr nonsurgical soaking throughout the nasal cavity and frontal sinuses with 1% clotrimazole effective; topical treatment with clotrimazole or enilconazole administered by surgically laced tubes (either q12h for 7–10 days or for 1-hr soaks) reported

Vascular or Systemic Disease
- Hyperviscosity—treat underlying disease (e.g., ehrlichiosis and multiple myeloma); plasmapheresis
- Vasculitis—doxycycline for rickettsial disease (5 mg/kg q12h for 2–3 weeks); prednisone for immune-mediated disease (1.1 mg/kg q12h; taper over 4–6 months) Hypertension
- Treat underlying disease—renal disease, hyperthyroidism, and hyperadrenocorticism
- Reduce weight
- Restrict sodium
- ACE inhibitors—benazepril (0.25–0.5 mg/kg q24h); enalapril (0.25–0.5 mg/kg q12–24h)
- β-blockers—propranolol (0.5–1.0 mg/kg q8h); atenolol (2.0 mg/kg q24h)
- Calcium channel blockers—diltiazem (0.5–1.5 mg/kg q8h, dogs; 1.75–2.5 mg/kg q8h, cats); amlodipine (0.625 mg/cat q24h) treatment of choice in cats
- Diuretics—hydrochlorothiazide (2–4 mg/kg q12h); furosemide (0.5–2.0 mg/kg q8–12h)

CONTRAINDICATIONS
- Avoid drugs that may predispose patient to hemorrhage—NSAIDs; heparin; phenothiazine tranquilizers
- Topical antifungals—do not use in dogs with disruption of the cribriform plate

PRECAUTIONS
- Chemotherapeutic drugs (e.g., azathioprine)—monitor neutrophil counts weekly until a pattern has been established that shows that the patient is tolerating the drug.
- Enalapril and/or diuretics—closely monitor patient with renal failure; avoid severe salt restriction when using enalapril.

POSSIBLE INTERACTIONS
N/A

ALTERNATIVE DRUGS
N/A

 FOLLOW-UP

PATIENT MONITORING
- Platelet count with thrombocytopenia
- Coagulation profile with coagulation factor defects
- Blood pressure with hypertension
- Monitor clinical signs

POSSIBLE COMPLICATIONS
Anemia and collapse rare

✓ MISCELLANEOUS

ASSOCIATED CONDITIONS
N/A

AGE-RELATED FACTORS
N/A

ZOONOTIC POTENTIAL
N/A

PREGNANCY
N/A

SEE ALSO
See Causes.

ABBREVIATIONS
ACE = angiotensin-converting enzyme
ALT = alanine transferase
AST = aspartate aminotransferase
DDAVP = 1 deamino-8-D-arginine vasopressin
DIC = disseminated intravascular coagulation
MLV = modified live virus
SLE = systemic lupus erythematosus

Suggested Reading

Cowgill LD, Kallet AJ. Systemic hypertension. In: Kirk RW, ed. Current veterinary therapy IX. Philadelphia: Saunders, 1986:360–364.

Dodds JW. Hemostasis. In: Kaneko JJ, ed. Clinical biochemistry of domestic animals. 4th ed. New York: Academic, 1989:274–315.

Feldman BF, ed. Hemostasis. Vet Clin North Am Small Anim Pract. 1988;18.

Pavletic MM, Clark GN. Open nasal cavity and frontal sinus treatment of chronic canine aspergillosis. Vet Surg 1991;20:43–48.

Snyder PS, Henik RA. Feline systemic hypertension. Paper presented at the 12th annual Veterinary Medicine Forum of the American College of Veterinary Internal Medicine, San Francisco,1994: 126–128.

Author Mitchell A. Crystal
Consulting Editor Eleanor C. Hawkins

FEARS AND PHOBIAS—DOGS

 BASICS

DEFINITION

Fear
• A feeling of apprehension associated with the presence or proximity of an object, individual, social situation, or class of these
• Part of normal behavior; can be an adaptive response
• Context determines whether response is abnormal or inappropriate.
• Normal and abnormal—usually manifests as graded responses; intensity of the response proportional to the perceived or actual proximity of the stimulus
• Reactions develop relatively gradually; within a bout of fearful behavior, animal may display some variation in response.
• Most reactions are learned and can be unlearned with gradual exposure.

Phobias
• Sudden, all-or-nothing, profound, abnormal responses that result in extremely fearful behaviors (catatonia, panic)
• Do not extinguish with gradual exposure to the object or with no exposure over time
• Immediate, excessive anxiety response is characteristic; little change among bouts
• It has been postulated that once a phobic event has been experienced, any event associated with it or the memory of it is sufficient to generate the response; without reinforcement, response can remain at or exceed its former high level for years.
• Origin—extremely scary and traumatic event; dog may have profound problems with internal fear (the fear itself acts as a reinforcer)
• Animal avoids trigger situation at all costs or, if unavoidable, endures it with intense anxiety or distress.
• Most common—associated with noises (e.g., thunderstorms or firecrackers)
• May co-occur or co-vary with separation anxiety; it is prudent to question the owner of a dog with separation anxiety about the animal's response to loud noises.

Anxiety
• Apprehensive anticipation of future danger or misfortune accompanied by a feeling of dysphoria (humans) and/or somatic signs of tension (vigilance and scanning, autonomic hyperactivity, increased motor activity, tension)
• Focus of the reaction can be internal or external.
• Separation anxiety—most common specific anxiety in companion dogs; when alone, the animal exhibits anxiety or excessive distress.

• Most common visible behaviors—elimination, destruction, and excessive vocalization; drooling, panting, and cognitive signs are not observed but probably occur.

PATHOPHYSIOLOGY
• Unclear
• Clinical signs—consistent with alterations in CNS transmitter levels and/or increases in ACTH levels (primary or secondary)
• Animal is usually brought to the clinic because the client becomes concerned about perceived changes in the animal's behavior or believes that the animal has never been normal.

SYSTEMS AFFECTED
• Cardiovascular—tachycardia
• Endocrine/Metabolic—alterations in the HPA axis
• Gastrointestinal—inappetence; aberrant appetite; gastrointestinal distress (salivation, vomiting, diarrhea, tenesmus, hematochezia)
• Hemic/Lymphatic/Immune—stress leukogram
• Musculoskeletal—poor condition attributable to increased motor activity and self-injury (weight loss, injured pads, damage to teeth and gums, and abrasions and lacerations)
• Nervous—increased motor activity; repetitive activity; trembling; self-injury
• Respiratory—tachypnea and the attendant metabolic changes
• Skin/Exocrine—lesions, usually secondary to self-injury (lick granulomas)

SIGNALMENT
• No age, breed, or sex is over-represented.
• Most develop at the onset of social maturity (18–36 months of age).
• Old-age onset idiopathic separation anxiety—may be a variant of cognitive dysfunction; reported in elderly dogs
• Profound form of idiopathic fear and withdrawal—occurs at 8–10 months of age; noted in Siberian huskies, German shorthaired pointers, Chesapeake Bay retrievers, Bernese mountain dogs, Great Pyrenees, border collies, and standard poodles; appears to be a strong familial component

SIGNS

General Comments
• Fears and anxieties—variable; diagnosis may be made only on the basis of nonspecific signs for which no discrete, identifiable stimulus is present.
• The extent to which the animal is experiencing the fear or phobia may affect the presentation.
• Mild fears—trembling, tail tucked, withdrawal, and hiding; reduced activity and passive escape behaviors

• Panic—active escape behavior; increased, out-of-context, and potentially injurious motor activity
• Classical signs of sympathetic autonomic nervous system activity

Historical Findings
• Fear—from a horrific experience; may have been forced into an unfamiliar experience
• Uncommon for a dog to be fearful, anxious, or phobic because of lack of exposure early in puppyhood (neophobia)
• Dogs that are absolutely deprived of variable social and environmental exposure until 14 weeks of age may become pathologically fearful; can be avoided with only little exposure
• Separation anxiety—history of abandonment, multiple owners, rehoming, or prior neglect common

Physical Examination Findings
• Usually nonremarkable, except for self-induced injuries and the lack of condition that may be associated with increased motor activity and withdrawal
• Anxieties—lesions such as lick granulomas may more common than has generally been appreciated.

CAUSES
• Any illness or painful physical condition can increase anxiety and contribute to the development of fears, phobias, and anxieties (rare).
• Degenerative (e.g., associated with age and concomitant neurologic changes), anatomic, infectious (primarily CNS viral conditions) and toxic (lead toxicosis) conditions—may lead to behavioral problems through primary or secondary aberrant neurochemical activity

 DIAGNOSIS

DIFFERENTIAL DIAGNOSIS
Rule out conditions that cause similar behavioral changes—seizures; brain disease; metabolic disease (e.g., thyroid or adrenal)

CBC/BIOCHEMISTRY/URINALYSIS
• Should be normal
• Perform before initiating drug treatment.

OTHER LABORATORY TESTS
Thyroid or adrenal tests—depending on clinical signs and serum biochemistry results

IMAGING
CT or MRI—rule out structural brain disease

DIAGNOSTIC PROCEDURES
• Biopsy of dermatologic lesions—determine if primary or secondary
• CSF analysis—rule out inflammatory CNS disease
• Endoscopy—evaluate primary bowel disease
• ECG—rule out cardiac disease that may produce physical signs mimicking anxiety

TREATMENT
- Usually outpatient
- Inpatient—patients with profound panic and separation anxiety who need to be protected until antianxiety medications reach effective plasma and CSF levels (days to weeks); patients who must be treated for or protected from physical injury (e.g., throwing itself from a window); constant daycare, dog-sitting, or inpatient monitoring and stimulation may be best
- Affected animals respond to some extent to a combination of behavior modification and pharmacologic treatment with antianxiety medication.
- Diagnose and control any atopic and painful condition because pruritus and pain are both neurochemically related to anxiety and its perception; may include dietary management
- Some profound, idiopathically fearful patients may need to live in a protected environment with as few social stressors as possible; these animals do not do well in dog shows.

Behavior Modification
- Gear toward teaching the dog to relax in a variety of environmental settings.
- Client may reassure the dog when it is experiencing fear or panic; inform client that the dog may interpret this as a reward for its behavior.
- Client must encourage calmness but not reinforce the fear reaction.
- Client must absolutely avoid punishment.
- Desensitization and counterconditioning—most effective if the fear, anxiety, or phobia is treated early; goal is to decrease the reaction to a specific stimulus (e.g., being left alone in the dark).
- Help client understand the subtlety of the signs involved and learn to recognize physical signs associated with the underlying physiologic state characterized by sympathetic stimulation.

MEDICATIONS
DRUGS OF CHOICE

Anxiety
- Antianxiety medications that increase CNS levels of serotonin—tricyclic antidepressants and selective serotonin reuptake inhibitors
- Amitriptyline—1–2 mg/kg PO q12h for 30 days to start
- Imipramine—1–2 mg/kg PO q12h for 30 days
- Buspirone—1 mg/kg PO q24h; takes 3–5 weeks to be effective

- Clomipramine—1 mg/kg PO q12h for 14 days; then 2 mg/kg PO q12h for 14 days; then 3 mg/kg PO q12h for 28 days (if successful, use as maintenance level); takes 3–5 weeks to be effective
- Fluoxetine—1 mg/kg PO q24h for 2 months; takes 3–5 weeks to be effective

Phobias and True Panic Disorders
- Respond to benzodiazepines; work best if administered before any signs of anxiety, fear, or panic; must be given 30–60 min before the anticipated provocative stimulus
- Diazepam—0.5–2.2 mg/kg PO as needed
- Chlorazepate—0.55–2.2 mg/kg PO q8–12h or as needed (phobias)
- Alprazolam—0.125–1.0 mg/kg as needed, not to exceed 4 mg/day
- Severe separation anxiety (e.g., dog breaks out of crates or throw itself from windows) and thunderstorm phobia that is accompanied by panic—alprazolam can be used concomitantly with other medications on an as-needed basis.

CONTRAINDICATIONS
- Hepatic and renal compromise—some listed drugs contraindicated because of their main route of metabolism
- Use caution when prescribing drugs to old patients that have generally diminished volume of distribution and decreased metabolism.
- Cardiac conduction anomalies—use extreme caution and monitoring when giving tricyclic antidepressants.

PRECAUTIONS
- All listed medications are extra-label—follow Health and Human Services recommendations.
- Overdose of tricyclic antidepressants—may cause profound cardiac conduction disturbances; perform a cardiac evaluation (preferably with ECG) before treatment.

POSSIBLE INTERACTIONS
- Benzodiazepines—lipophilic and may be potentiated by other lipophilic drugs; if combination treatment is warranted, use lower doses of either medication.
- Medication that impairs the glucuronidation of active metabolites into inactive compounds may cause increases of the active metabolites.

FOLLOW-UP
PATIENT MONITORING
- Chronic treatment—CBC, biochemistry, and urinalysis: as indicated by clinical signs, annually for young patients, and semiannually for old patients; adjust dosages accordingly.
- Advise clients to observe for vomiting, gastrointestinal distress, and tachypnea.

POSSIBLE COMPLICATIONS
Early treatment with both behavioral modification and pharmacologic intervention is key; if left untreated, these disorders always progress.

MISCELLANEOUS
ASSOCIATED CONDITIONS
Irritable bowel syndrome and lick granulomas—common; may indicate underlying anxiety-related conditions

AGE-RELATED FACTORS
Idiopathic separation anxiety in old dogs—frequently undiagnosed because it is insidious and not associated with social or environmental changes; changes appear to be in the dog's perception.

ZOONOTIC POTENTIAL
N/A

PREGNANCY
Most of the listed drugs are either not evaluated in or contraindicated in pregnant animals.

SYNONYMS
Generalized anxiety, neophobia, noise phobia, and thunderstorm phobia—not synonymous but are frequently discussed under the same heading.

ABBREVIATIONS
- CSF = cerebrospinal fluid
- HPA = hypothalamic–pituitary–adrenal

Suggested Reading
Chapman BL, Voith VL. Behavioral problems in old dogs. J Am Vet Med Assoc 1990;196:944–946.

McCrave EA. Diagnostic criteria for separation anxiety in the dog. Vet Clin North Am Small Anim Pract 1991; 21:247–256.

Overall KL. Clinical behavioral medicine for small animals. St. Louis: Mosby, 1997.

Tuber DS, Hothersall D, Peters MF. Treatment of fears and phobia in dogs. Vet Clin North Am Small Anim Pract 1982;12:607–623.

Young MS. Treatment of fear-induced aggression in dogs. Vet Clin North Am Small Anim Pract 1982;12:645–653.
Author Karen L. Overall
Consulting Editor Joane M. Parent

FEVER

BASICS

DEFINITION
Higher than normal body temperature because of a changed thermoregulatory set point in the hypothalamus; normal body temperature in dogs and cats is 100.2–102.8°F (37.8–39.3°C) Fever of unknown origin (FUO)—at least 103.5°F (39.7°C) on at least four occasions over a 14-day period and illness of 14 days' duration without an obvious cause

PATHOPHYSIOLOGY
Exogenous or endogenous pyrogens cause release of endogenous substances (e.g., interleukin-1 and prostaglandins) that reset the hypothalamic thermoregulatory center to a higher temperature, activating appropriate physiologic responses to raise the body temperature to this new set point. Physiologic consequences include increased metabolic demands, muscle catabolism, bone marrow suppression, heightened fluid and caloric requirements, and possibly disseminated intravascular coagulation (DIC) and shock.

SYSTEMS AFFECTED
• Cardiovascular—tachycardia • Nervous—cerebral edema • Hemic/Lymph/Immune—bone marrow depression and DIC

SIGNALMENT
• Dog and cat • Any age, breed, and sex

SIGNS

General Comments
• Prolonged fever > 105°F (> 40.5°C) leads to dehydration, anorexia, and depression.
• Fevers > 106°F (> 41.1°C) may lead to cerebral edema, bone marrow depression, and DIC.

Physical Examination Findings
• Hyperthermia • Lethargy • Inappetence
• Tachycardia • Hyperpnea • Dehydration
• Shock

CAUSES

Infectious Agents (Most Common)
• Viruses—feline leukemia (FeLV), feline immunodeficiency (FIV), parvovirus, distemper, herpes, and calicivirus
• Bacteria—gram-positive and gram-negative endotoxins
• Systemic fungi—*Histoplasma, Blastomyces, Coccidioidomyces,* and *Cryptococcus*
• Rickettsia—*Ehrlichia, Rickettsia rickettsii* (Rocky Mountain spotted fever), *Haemobartonella*
• Parasites and protozoa—*Babesia, Toxoplasma,* aberrant larva migrans, *Dirofilaria thromboemboli, Leishmania*
• *Borrelia burgdorferi* (Lyme disease)

Immune-mediated Processes
Systemic lupus erythematosus, immune-mediated hemolytic anemia, immune-mediated thrombocytopenia, pemphigus, polyarthritis, polymyositis, vasculitis, hypersensivity reactions, transfusion reaction, and infection secondary to inherited or acquired immune defects

Endocrine and Metabolic
Hyperthyroidism, hypoadrenocorticism (rare), pheochromocytoma, hyperlipidemia, and hypernatremia

Neoplasia
Lymphoma, myeloproliferative disease, plasma cell neoplasm, mast cell tumor, metastatic disease, and solid tumor, particularly in liver, kidney, bone, lungs, and lymph nodes

Other Inflammatory Conditions
Cholangiohepatitis, hepatic lipidosis, toxic hepatopathy, cirrhosis, inflammatory bowel disease, pancreatitis, peritonitis, pleuritis, granulomatous diseases, thrombophlebitis, infarctions, pansteatitis, panniculitis, hypertrophic osteodystrophy, blunt trauma, cyclic neutropenia, intracranial lesions (encephalitis, trauma), and pulmonary thromboembolism

Drugs and Toxins
Tetracycline, sulfonamide, penicillins, nitrofurantoin, amphotericin B, barbiturates, iodine, atropine, cimetidine, salicylates (high dosages), antihistamines, procainamide, and heavy metals

FUO—Dogs
• Recurrent bacteremia caused by endocarditis or localized abscess of organ or tissue—liver, pancreas, prostate, retroperitoneal and pleural space (pyothorax), lungs, kidneys and genitourinary system (chronic pyelonephritis and prostatitis), osteomyelitis, arthritis, discospondylitis, and meningitis
• Systemic infection—particularly early, chronic, or latent infection, including brucellosis, systemic mycoses, ehrlichiosis, Rocky Mountain spotted fever, toxoplasmosis
• Neoplasia—as above
• Immune disorders—as above
• Other causes—chronic hepatic diseases and chronic granulomatous disease

FUO—Cats
• Most are virally mediated (e.g., FeLV, FIV, FIP, less commonly parvovirus, herpes, and calicivirus)
• Persistent occult bacterial infection with atypical bacteria, sometimes secondary to bite wounds (e.g., *Yersinia, Mycobacteria, Nocardia, Actinomyces,* and *Brucella*)
• Pyothorax common
• Additional causes—pyelonephritis, blunt trauma, penetrating intestinal lesion, dental abscess, systemic mycoses (e.g., *Histoplasma,*

Blastomyces, Coccidioides), lymphoma, and solid tumors
• Immune disorders are rare, as are prostatitis, endometritis, discospondylitis, pneumonia, and endocarditis.

RISK FACTORS
• Recent travel
• Exposure to biologic agents
• Immunosuppression
• Very young or old animals

DIAGNOSIS

DIFFERENTIAL DIAGNOSIS
• Good clinical history (e.g., contact with infectious agents, recent vaccination, drug administration, insect bites, allergies) and thorough physical examination may help identify an underlying disease condition.
• Elucidation of patterns of fever (e.g., sustained, intermittent) is rarely helpful.
• True fever must be differentiated from hyperthermia. Stress and anxiety in the hospital may cause a mild temperature rise. Temperatures up to 103°F (39.4°C) may be caused by stress or illness. Temperatures > 104°F (> 40°C) are almost always important. Temperatures > 107°F (> 41.7°C) are usually not fever, more likely to be primary hyperthermia.

CBC/BIOCHEMISTRY/URINALYSIS
• CBC—leukopenia or leukocytosis, left shift, monocytosis, lymphocytosis, thrombo-cytopenia or thrombocytosis
• Biochemistry profile and urinalysis vary with the organ system involved

OTHER LABORATORY TESTS
• Additional laboratory testing depends on history, physical examination findings, and abnormalities in CBC, serum biochemistry profile, and urinalysis.
• If infectious disease is suspected, attempt to culture an organism—urine culture, blood cultures (i.e., three anaerobic and three aerobic cultures, taken during a rise in temperature or 30 min apart), fungal culture, and cultures of CSF, synovial fluid, and biopsy specimens, if clinically indicated
• FeLV and FIV test, serologic tests for *Toxoplasma,* Lyme disease, systemic mycoses, and rickettsial infection
• Fecal examination if gastrointestinal signs
• Tracheal wash or bronchoalveolar lavage, if respiratory involvement
• Occult heartworm test if pulmonary embolism suspected
• If immune disorders suspected—cytologic examination of synovial fluid; Coombs', antinuclear antibody, and rheumatoid factor tests; serum protein electrophoresis
• T4 to rule out hyperthyroidism

IMAGING

Radiography

- Abdominal radiographs to scan for tumors
- Thoracic radiographs to rule out pneumonia, neoplasia, and pyothorax
- Survey skeletal radiographs for bone tumors, multiple myeloma, osteomyelitis, discospondylitis, panosteitis, and hypertrophic osteodystrophy
- Dental and skull radiographs to look for tooth root abscess, sinus infections, and neoplasia
- Contrast radiography (e.g., gastrointestinal and excretory urography) to look for evidence of neoplasia or infection

Ultrasonography

- Abdominal (plus directed biopsy, if indicated) to look for abdominal neoplasia and abscess or other site of infection (e.g., pyelonephritis and pyometra)
- Echocardiography if endocarditis suspected

Nuclear Imaging

Radionuclide scanning procedures to evaluate for bone tumors, osteomyelitis, and pulmonary embolism

DIAGNOSTIC PROCEDURES

- Endoscopy and biopsy if gastrointestinal signs
- Bone marrow aspirate and biopsy if malignancy suspected
- Lymph node, skin, or muscle biopsy if clinically indicated
- Examination of fine-needle aspirate of any mass or large organ
- CSF tap if neurologic signs suggest brain tumor or meningitis
- Exploratory laparotomy—last resort if all other diagnostic tests fail to determine the cause and the patient is not improving

TREATMENT

- Restrict activity.
- Febrile patients are in a hypercatabolic state and require high caloric intake.
- Explain to the owner that the diagnostic workup of patients with fever of unknown origin is often extensive, expensive, and invasive and does not always provide a definitive diagnosis.
- Surgery may be necessary in some animals with underlying infectious (e.g., pyometra, peritonitis, pyothorax, and liver abscess) or localized neoplastic cause of fever.

MEDICATIONS

DRUGS OF CHOICE

- Goal of treatment—reset the thermoregulatory set point to a lower level.
- Selection depends on the diagnosis and specific cause.
- Do not use broad-spectrum (i.e., "shotgun") treatment in place of a thorough diagnostic workup unless the patient's status is critical and deteriorating rapidly.
- Fever may help the body fight the disease condition (e.g., by suppressing bacterial replication and facilitating host defenses). Only use antipyretic treatment when fever is prolonged and life-threatening (> 106°F, >41.1°C) and topical cooling is unsuccessful. Impaired patients (e.g., those with heart failure, seizures, or respiratory disease) require antipyretic treatment earlier. Antipyretic treatment may preclude elucidation of the cause, delay correct treatment, and complicate patient monitoring (e.g., reduction of fever is an important indication of response to treatment).
- Fluid administration often lowers body temperature.
- If the patient is dehydrated, initiate isotonic fluids (i.e., lactated Ringer's or 0.9% saline)

Antibiotics

- Based on results of bacterial culture
- In emergency situations, combination antibiotic therapy can be started after culture specimens have been obtained (e.g., cephalothin, 20 mg/kg IV q6–8h; gentamicin 2 mg/kg IV q8h).
- Do not give antibiotics longer than 1–2 weeks if the response is not favorable.

Antipyretics

- Salicylates—dogs, 10 mg/kg PO q12h; cats, 6 mg/kg PO q48h
- Flunixin meglumine—dogs, 0.5–1 mg/kg IV or IM once

Glucocorticoids

- Do not use unless infectious causes have been ruled out.
- May mask clinical signs, may lead to immunosuppression, and are not recommended for use as antipyretics; administration of corticosteroids to cats with intractable FUO after ruling out infectious diseases may promote a favorable response.
- Primarily indicated for fever associated with immune-mediated disease and certain steroid-responsive tumors (e.g., lymphoma)

CONTRAINDICATIONS

N/A

PRECAUTIONS

Side effects of antipyretics include emesis, diarrhea, gastrointestinal ulceration, renal damage, hemolysis, hepatotoxicity (acetaminophen, particularly dangerous in cats), and muscle stiffness (flunixin meglumine).

POSSIBLE INTERACTIONS

Combination of nonsteroidal antiinflamatory drugs (NSAIDS) and steroids raises the risk of gastrointestinal hemorrhage

ALTERNATIVE DRUGS

N/A

FOLLOW-UP

PATIENT MONITORING

- Patient's temperature at least q12h. • If the cause of the fever continues to elude the clinician, repeat the history and physical examination along with screening laboratory tests. • If fever develops or worsens during hospitalization, consider nosocomial infection or superinfection.

PREVENTION/AVOIDANCE

N/A

POSSIBLE COMPLICATIONS

Depend on cause

EXPECTED COURSE AND PROGNOSIS

Vary with cause; in some patients (more commonly in cats), an underlying cause cannot be determined.

MISCELLANEOUS

ASSOCIATED CONDITIONS

N/A

AGE-RELATED FACTORS

- Young animals—infectious disease more likely than other causes; prognosis better than in old animals • Old animals—common causes are neoplasia and intraabdominal infection; signs tend to be more nonspecific; prognosis often guarded

ZOONOTIC POTENTIAL

Depends on cause

PREGNANCY

N/A

SYNONYMS

Pyrexia

SEE ALSO

- Heatstroke and Hyperthermia

ABBREVIATIONS

N/A

Suggested Reading

Couto CG. Fever of undetermined origin. In: Nelson RW, Couto CG, eds. Essentials of small animal internal medicine. Philadelphia: Mosby Year Book, 1992:974–977.

Hardie EM. Sepsis versus septic shock. In: Murtaugh RJ, Kaplan PM, eds. Veterinary emergency and critical care medicine. Philadelphia: Mosby Year Book, 1992:176–193.

Author Jörg Bücheler
Consulting Editors Larry P. Tilley and Francis W. K. Smith, Jr.

FLATULENCE

BASICS

DEFINITION
Excessive formation of gases in the stomach or intestine, released through the anus

PATHOPHYSIOLOGY
• Occurs more commonly in dogs than cats
• Often results from dietary indiscretion, but may herald a more serious gastrointestinal disease
• The two main sources of intestinal gas are swallowed air and bacterial fermentation of nutrients.
• Intestinal gas—primarily composed of nitrogen, oxygen, hydrogen, methane, and carbon dioxide, all of which are odorless
• Malodorous gases (e.g., ammonia, hydrogen, sulfides, skatoles, indoles, mercaptans, volatile amines, and short-chain fatty acids)—compose less than 1% of intestinal gas
• Poorly digestible diets that escape intestinal assimilation and hence are available for colonic fermentation, and diets that liberate malodorous gases are associated with flatulence; these include diets with a high concentration of legumes (e.g., soy-bean meal), which contain indigestible oligosaccharides), spoiled diets, diets high in fat, and milk products.
• Dogs and cats are lactose intolerant; a dietary concentration of 1.5 g/kg/day (1 cup of milk contains 11 g of lactose/cup) may produce diarrhea and flatulence in dogs.
• A rapid change in diet or an increase in the concentration of a dietary component, especially carbohydrate or fiber, may cause flatulence during a period of intestinal adaptation.
• Aerophagia caused by gluttony or dyspnea can also cause intestinal gaseousness.
• Disease states causing malassimilation of nutrients, making them available for colonic fermentation, can cause flatulence.

SYSTEMS AFFECTED
Gastrointestinal

SIGNALMENT
• Dogs and cats
• No gender, age, or breed predisposition
• A 1998 study (Jones, et al.) reported that 43% of randomly chosen dog owners detected flatulence, most commonly in sedentary pets, with no association to an individual food or diet.

SIGNS
• Increased frequency and, possibly, volume of flatulence detected by the owner
• Mild abdominal discomfort caused by gastrointestinal distension
• Concurrent gastrointestinal signs—vomiting, borborygmus, diarrhea, and weight loss

Historical Findings
N/A

Physical Examination Findings
N/A

CAUSES

Increased Aerophagia
• Gluttony
• Respiratory disease

Diet-related
• Diets high in legumes—soybean meal
• Diets high in fermentable fiber—psyllium, lactulose, fibrim, oat bran
• Spoiled diets
• Milk products
• Abrupt dietary change

Disease Conditions
• Acute and chronic small bowel disease—inflammatory bowel disease, small intestinal bacterial overgrowth, neoplasia, irritable bowel syndrome, parasitism, bacterial enteritis, and viral enteritis
• Exocrine pancreatic insufficiency

RISK FACTORS
• Nervous or gluttonous eating, often caused by competition for food
• Inappropriate diets
• Abrupt dietary changes

DIAGNOSIS

DIFFERENTIAL DIAGNOSIS
• Distinguish dietary and behavioral causes of flatulence from gastrointestinal disease by thorough evaluation of the patient history; this allows the clinician to ascertain the type of diet, amount fed, frequency of feeding, frequency of changes or additions, and the environment in which the patient is fed.
• Observation of the patient eating may be required to identify gluttony.
• Perform a complete physical examination including careful abdominal palpation and rectal examination.
• Concurrent signs (e.g., vomiting, diarrhea, and weight loss) should prompt a search for underlying gastrointestinal disease.

CBC/BIOCHEMISTRY/URINALYSIS
Usually normal

OTHER LABORATORY TESTS
• Repeated fecal flotation tests and direct fecal smears or a treatment trial with fenbendazole (dogs, 50 mg/kg PO q24h for 3 days; cats, 25 mg/kg PO q24h for 3 days) to evaluate for small intestinal parasitism
• Serum trypsin-like immunoreactivity (TLI) to evaluate for exocrine pancreatic insufficiency
• Serum cobalamin/folate test to evaluate for small intestinal bacterial overgrowth or severe small intestinal mucosal disease
• Fecal cultures to evaluate for salmonellosis or campylobacteriosis
• Zinc sulfate flotation tests (×3) to evaluate for giardiasis

IMAGING
Abdominal ultrasound to diagnose gastro-intestinal masses or areas of mural thickening

DIAGNOSTIC PROCEDURES
• Small-intestinal biopsy specimens obtained at surgery or via endoscopy to evaluate for infiltrative small bowel disease
• Quantitative cultures taken from the small intestine to evaluate for small intestinal bacterial overgrowth

TREATMENT
• Treat any underlying gastrointestinal disease.
• If a dietary cause is suspected—change to a highly digestible, low-fiber/low-fat diet
• Suitable commercial diets are available (Eukanuba Low Residue Formula, Hill's i/d Diet, Innovative Veterinary Diet Select Care Neutral or Sensitive Formula, Purina EN Formula) or feed homemade diets containing boiled white rice (dogs) or rice baby cereal (cats) with skinned chicken or cottage cheese.
• Homemade diets must be fortified with vitamins and minerals if they are fed for prolonged periods.
• Discourage gluttony by providing smaller meals more frequently in a noncompetitive, quiet environment.
• Discourage dietary indiscretions (e.g., garbage ingestion or coprophagia).
• Encourage an active lifestyle so intestinal gas and feces can be expelled during exercise.
• If dietary and behavioral manipulations are unsuccessful, pharmacologic therapy may be necessary.

MEDICATIONS

DRUGS OF CHOICE
• Simethicone—an antifoaming agent that reduces the surface tension of intestinal mucus, allowing easier coalescence and release of intestinal gas; does not reduce gas production, but it helps prevent gas accumulation; can be used safely in dogs and cats (25–200 mg q6–8h); effectiveness as an antiflatulent in dogs and cats is unknown.
• Antiflatulent enzyme supplements—may reduce the severity of flatulence by helping to digest poorly digestible fermentable nutrients; anecdotal evidence suggests that these products may be effective.
• Bismuth subsalicylate—antibacterial and antiendotoxic properties that protect the gastrointestinal tract; may help decrease flatulence after dietary indiscretion (dogs, 1 mL/kg PO initially, then 0.25 mL q6h)
• Charcoal—questionable effectiveness and practicality

CONTRAINDICATIONS
Avoid bismuth subsalicylate in patients with gastroduodenal ulcer disease and those with preexisting bleeding disorders.

PRECAUTIONS
Use bismuth subsalicylate with caution in cats.

POSSIBLE INTERACTIONS
N/A

ALTERNATIVE DRUGS
N/A

FOLLOW-UP

PATIENT MONITORING
N/A

POSSIBLE COMPLICATIONS
N/A

MISCELLANEOUS

ASSOCIATED CONDITIONS
Gastrointestinal disease

AGE-RELATED FACTORS
N/A

ZOONOTIC POTENTIAL
N/A

PREGNANCY
N/A

SYNONYMS
N/A

SEE ALSO
• Exocrine Pancreatic Insufficiency
• Inflammatory Bowel Disease
• Small intestinal Bacterial Overgrowth
• Salmonellosis
• Campylobacteriosis
• Irritable Bowel Syndrome

ABBREVIATIONS
N/A

Suggested Reading

Guilford WG. New ideas for management of gastrointestinal tract disease. J Small Anim Pract 1994;35:620–624.
Guilford WG. Approach to problems in gastroenterology. In: Guilford WG, Center SA, Strombeck DR, et al., eds. Strombeck's small animal gastroenterology. 3rd ed. Philadelphia: Saunders, 1996:50–76.
Jones BR, Jones KS, Turner K, et al. Flatulence in pet dogs. NZ Vet J 1998;46:191–193.
Plumb DC. Bismuth subsalicylate. In: Plumb DC, ed. Veterinary drug handbook. 2nd ed. Ames: Iowa State Press, 1995:75–77.

Author Mark C. Walker
Consulting Editors Mitchell A. Crystal and Brett M. Feder

GINGIVITIS

 BASICS

DEFINITION
A reversible inflammatory response of the marginal gumline; the earliest phase of periodontal disease

PATHOPHYSIOLOGY
• The gingiva covers the alveolar processes of the mandible and maxilla and conforms closely to the neck of the tooth.
• The gingiva is divided into attached and free, or marginal, portions—the attached gingiva is tightly bound to the periosteum overlying the alveolar processes; the marginal gingiva extends above the crest of the alveolar bone and tapers to a knifelike edge that lies in contact with surface of the tooth.
• The gingival sulcus—the narrow cleft between the inner wall of the marginal gingiva and the tooth; in dogs, normally <3 mm but may be deeper around the canine teeth in large-breed dogs; in cats, normally =1 mm
• The junction between the gingiva and oral mucosa appears as a distinct line or furrow called the mucogingival line.
• The connective tissue of the gingiva (lamina propria) contains an extensive array of blood vessels, lymphatics, nerves, and collagen fibers; plasma cells, lymphocytes, and neutrophils are also abundant and are important in local defense mechanisms.
• Crevicular fluid—plasma-derived; passes from the gingival connective tissue through the crevicular epithelium to lavage the gingival sulcus; flow occurs in response to bacteria (plaque) in the gingival sulcus; contains immunoglobulins, other nonspecific antibacterial substances, and neutrophils as the predominant cells; important in controlling the bacterial population
• In healthy animals, gram-positive aerobic cocci and rods predominate in supragingival plaque; anaerobes are more abundant subgingivally, and spirochetes are found tightly packed in the apical region of the gingival sulcus.
• As gingivitis develops, anaerobes and spirochetes become increasingly more abundant in the subgingival sulcus.

• In dogs the bacteroides organisms (*Bacteroides, Prevotella, Porphyromonas* spp.) and *Fusobacterium* spp. appear to be important pathogens; *Porphyromonas* and *Peptostreptococcus* spp. are common in samples from cats with gingivitis.
• Gram-negative organisms—increase in number as gingivitis develops; invade tissues and elaborate endotoxins that can result in tissue destruction
• The fact that these bacteria are present in disease and health and that periodontal disease does not progress in linear fashion (i.e., periods of active disease are followed by quiescent periods) indicates that host–bacteria interaction is important in the pathogenesis of periodontal disease.
• Plaque—composed of bacteria, PMNs, and salivary glycoproteins; forms within 24 h on clean tooth surfaces; the gingiva's inflammatory response to plaque consists of vasculitis, edema, and collagen loss.
• Gingivitis of different severity can exist in one patient's mouth, based on the host's immunocompetency and local oral factors.
• Stage 1—early gingivitis; a small amount of plaque, mild gumline erythema, and smooth gingival surfaces
• Stage 2—advanced gingivitis; subgingival plaque and calculus, moderate-to-severe erythema, and irregular gingival surfaces

SYSTEMS AFFECTED
Oral cavity

SIGNALMENT
• Dogs and cats
• Over 80% of pets 3 years old and older have gingivitis.
• Higher prevalence earlier in life in toy breeds
• Cats generally are affected later in life than dogs.

SIGNS

Historical Findings
• Usually detected during routine wellness examinations
• Gingival swelling or bleeding
• Halitosis

Physical Examination Findings
• Halitosis
• Erythremic or edematous gingiva, especially buccal maxillary surfaces

• Variable degrees of plaque and calculus formation
• Gingival surfaces bleed easily on contact.

CAUSES
Plaque accumulation

RISK FACTORS
• Age
• Head shape and occlusive pattern; crowding of teeth reduces natural cleaning mechanisms (toy and brachycephalic breeds).
• Toy breeds affected earlier in life
• Soft foods
• Open-mouth breathing
• Chewing habits
• Lack of oral health care
• Metabolic diseases such as uremia and diabetes mellitus predispose to more pathogenic oral bacteria
• Autoimmune disease—pemphigus vulgaris, systemic lupus erythematosus

 DIAGNOSIS

DIFFERENTIAL DIAGNOSIS
• Periodontitis
• Stomatitis
• FeLV
• FIV

CBC/BIOCHEMISTRY/URINALYSIS
May help identify risk factors

OTHER LABORATORY TESTS
FeLV and FIV testing in cats

IMAGING
N/A

DIAGNOSTIC PROCEDURES
• Anesthetized oral examination allows more-thorough visual examination of all dental surfaces; use of a periodontal probe helps distinguish between gingivitis (normal sulcal depths of < 3 mm in dogs and < 1 mm in cats) and periodontitis.
• The use of plaque-disclosing agents helps identify plaque and bacterial accumulations on enamel surfaces.
• Biopsy and histopathology

TREATMENT

- Modify behavior to avoid chewing hard objects such as rocks and sticks and eliminate repetitive trauma, if possible.
- Stress the importance of home care and regular dental prophylaxis before lesions develop; daily or at least twice-weekly brushing is recommended, using an enzymatic toothpaste or zinc-ascorbic acid solution to remove and retard plaque accumulation; if the owner is unwilling to brush the teeth but the patient is manageable, the owner might possibly bring the pet to the clinic for brushing.
- Rawhide chew strips help to clean the teeth mechanically and exercise the attachment apparatus but should not be relied upon as the sole method of home care.
- Hard food leaves less substrate on the teeth than soft food; chewing also helps to clean teeth mechanically; Prescription Diet t/d (Hill's Pet Nutrition, Inc., Topeka, KS) is formulated to reduce plaque and tartar accumulation and reduce staining.
- Professional periodontal therapy followed by postoperative home care completely reverses gingivitis.
- Proper dental cleaning—complete oral examination; supragingival removal of plaque and calculus; subgingival scaling and root planing (if needed); polishing; subgingival irrigation; postcleaning examination; home care instructions; and follow-up examinations
- Eliminate predisposing factors such as retained deciduous teeth and crowded teeth.

MEDICATIONS

DRUGS OF CHOICE

- Lactoperoxidase- and chlorhexidine-containing dentifrices are effective in retarding plaque.
- Topically applied chlorhexidine, 0.4% stannous fluoride gel, and zinc ascorbate also reduce the inciting plaque formation.

- Antibiotics are generally not necessary at this stage.

CONTRAINDICATIONS
N/A

PRECAUTIONS
N/A

POSSIBLE INTERACTIONS
N/A

ALTERNATIVE DRUGS
N/A

FOLLOW-UP

PATIENT MONITORING

Regular oral reexaminations are necessary so the clinician can determine the proper interval between periodontal therapies and assess the effectiveness of oral home care; these steps can cure gingivitis and help to avoid the progression to periodontitis.

POSSIBLE COMPLICATIONS

- Gingivitis begins when bacteria invade the sulcular epithelium and connective tissue; the inflammatory response results in swelling and reddening of the marginal gingiva, which also becomes friable and bleeds easily; these lesions are reversible with dental prophylaxis and home care; if not controlled at this point, the attached gingiva and attachment apparatus (alveolar bone, periodontal ligament, and tooth root cementum) become involved, signifying the transition to periodontitis.
- Once periodontitis is established the lesions are generally considered controllable but not reversible.
- Uncontrolled periodontitis invariably leads to tooth loss.

MISCELLANEOUS

ASSOCIATED CONDITIONS

Always look for dental resorptive lesions (neck lesions) in cats, especially if gingivitis is focal or has the appearance of granulation tissue.

AGE-RELATED FACTORS

Transient gingivitis is a common, self-limiting problem in teething animals; if inflammation persists after adult tooth eruption, the cause should be determined.

ZOONOTIC POTENTIAL
None

PREGNANCY

Dental prophylaxis for simple gingivitis can be delayed until the puppies or kittens are weaned.

SYNONYMS
None

SEE ALSO
- Periodontal Disease
- Stomatitis

ABBREVIATIONS

FeLV = feline leukemia virus
FIV = feline immunodeficiency virus

Suggested Reading

Colmery B, Frost P. Periodontal disease: etiology and pathogenesis. Vet Clin North Am Small Anim Pract 1986;16:817–834.

Bojrab MJ, Tholen M, eds. Small animal medicine and oral surgery. Philadelphia: Lea & Febiger, 1990.

Harvey CE, Emily PP. Small animal dentistry. St. Louis, MO: Mosby, 1993.

West-Hyde L, Floyd M. Dentistry. In: Ettinger SJ; Feldman EC, eds. Textbook of veterinary internal medicine. 4th ed. Philadelphia: Saunders, 1995:1097–1121.

Wiggs RB, Lobprise HB. Veterinary dentistry: principles and practice. Philadelphia: Lippincott-Raven. 1997.

Author Thomas Klein
Consulting Editor Jan Bellows

HALITOSIS

BASICS

DEFINITION
An offensive odor emanating from the oral cavity; also called bad breath, foul breath, malodor, fetor ex ore, and fetor oris

PATHOPHYSIOLOGY
• The sour milk odor accompanying periodontal disease may result from bacterial populations associated with plaque, calculus, unhealthy tissues, decomposing food particles retained within the oral cavity, or from the rotten meat odor from tissue necrosis.
• Contrary to common belief, neither normal lung air or stomach aroma contribute.
• The most common cause is periodontal disease caused by plaque—bacteria are attracted to an acellular film formed from the precipitation of salivary glycoproteins (the pellicle).
• This biofilm forms over a freshly cleaned and polished tooth as soon as the patient starts to salivate; bacteria attach to the pellicle within 6–8 h; within days, the plaque becomes mineralized, producing calculus; as plaque ages and gingivitis develops into periodontitis (bone loss), the bacterial flora changes from a predominantly nonmotile gram-positive aerobic coccoid flora to a more motile, gram-negative anaerobic population including *Bacteroides, Fusobacterium,* and *Actinomyces* spp.
• The rough surface of calculus attracts more bacteria while irritating the free gingiva; as the inflammation continues, the gingival sulcus is pathologically transformed into a periodontal pocket; the pocket accumulates putrefied food debris, bacterial breakdown products, and resorbing bone, leading to halitosis.
• The primary cause of malodor is gram-negative anaerobic bacterial putrefaction that generates volatile sulfur compounds, such as hydrogen sulfide, methyl mercaptan, dimethyl sulfide, and volatile fatty acids.
• Volatile sulfur compounds may also play a role in periodontal disease affecting the integrity of the tissue barrier, allowing endo-toxins to produce periodontal destruction, endotoxemia, and bacteremia.

SYSTEMS AFFECTED
N/A

SIGNALMENT
• Dog and cat
• Small breeds and brachycephalic breeds are more prone to oral disease because the teeth are closer together, smaller animals live longer, and their owners tend to feed softer food.
• Older animals are predisposed.

SIGNS
• If due to oral disease, ptyalism, pawing at mouth, anorexia, may occur.
• In most cases, no clinical signs other than the odor

CAUSES
• Multiple causes
• Eating malodorous food
• Metabolic—diabetes, uremia
• Respiratory—rhinitis, sinusitis, neoplasia
• Gastrointestinal—megaesophagus, neoplasia, foreign body
• Dermatologic—lip-fold pyoderma
• Dietary—fetid foodstuffs, coprophagy
• Oral disease—periodontal disease and ulceration, orthodontic, pharyngitis, tonsillitis, neoplasia, foreign bodies
• Trauma—electric cord injury, open fractures, caustic agents
• Infectious—bacterial, fungal, viral
• Autoimmune diseases
• Eosinophilic granuloma complex

RISK FACTORS
N/A

DIAGNOSIS

CBC/BIOCHEMISTRY/URINALYSIS
N/A

OTHER LABORATORY TESTS
N/A

IMAGING
N/A

DIAGNOSTIC PROCEDURES
• Hydrogen sulfide, mercaptans, and volatile fatty acids are the primary components of halitosis; an industrial sulfide monitor can be used to measure sulfide concentration in peak parts per billion.
• Other diagnostic procedures to evaluate periodontal disease include intraoral radiography, probing pocket depths, attachment levels, and tooth mobility.

TREATMENT

• Once the specific cause of halitosis is known, direct therapy at correcting existing pathology.
• Topical treatment with zinc ascorbate cysteine gel usually reduces halitosis within 30 min because of cysteine's effect on sulfur compounds in the mouth.
• Clean the teeth when physical examination reveals gingivitis and/or when calculus exists on the maxillary fourth premolar; cleaning removes plaque and calculus above and below the gumline (with the help of hand instruments or scaler tips designed to be used subgingivally), irrigates debris from the mouth, and polishes the teeth.

MEDICATIONS

DRUGS OF CHOICE

• Clindamycin—destroys most periodontal pathogens; can be used as pulse therapy, administering the label dose the first 5 days of each month.
• Controlling periodontal pathogens helps control dental infections and accompanying malodor.
• The use of oral care products that contain metal ions, especially zinc, inhibits odor formation because of the affinity of the metal ion to sulfur; zinc complexes with hydrogen sulfide to form insoluble zinc sulfide; zinc interferes with microbial proliferation and calcification of microbial deposits (by interfering with the crystal development of calculus).
• Chlorhexidine used as a rinse or paste also helps control plaque, decreasing eventual odor; supplied as CHX Guard, CHX Guard LA, CET Oral Hygiene Spray (VRx Products, Harbor City, CA); DentiVet toothpaste and Hexarinse (Virbac, Fort Worth, TX); zinc ascorbate plus amino acid (Maxi/Guard Oral Cleansing Gel-Addison Biologicals)
• DentTreats (VRx Products)—a breath tablet for dogs; contains zinc citrate, sodium copper chlorophyllin, and essential oils (parsley seed, mint, and rosemary); does not treat a specific disease but neutralizes odor.

CONTRAINDICATIONS
N/A

PRECAUTIONS
N/A

POSSIBLE INTERACTIONS
N/A

ALTERNATIVE DRUGS
N/A

FOLLOW-UP

PATIENT MONITORING
Daily brushing to remove plaque and control dental disease and odor; periodic examinations to monitor care

POSSIBLE COMPLICATIONS
N/A

MISCELLANEOUS

ASSOCIATED CONDITIONS
N/A

AGE-RELATED FACTORS
N/A

ZOONOTIC POTENTIAL
N/A

PREGNANCY
N/A

SEE ALSO
N/A

ABBREVIATIONS
N/A

Suggested Reading

Harvey CE, Emily PP. Small animal dentistry. Philadelphia: Mosby, 1993.
Wiggs RB, Lobprise HB. Veterinary dentistry: Principles and practice. Philadelphia: Lippincott-Raven, 1997.
Author Jan Bellows
Consulting Editor Jan Bellows

HEAD TILT (VESTIBULAR DISEASE)

 BASICS

DEFINITION
Tilting of the head away from its normal orientation with the trunk and limbs; associated with disorders of the vestibular system

PATHOPHYSIOLOGY
• Vestibular system—coordinates position and movement of the head with that of the eyes, trunk, and limbs by detecting linear acceleration and rotational movements of the head; includes vestibular nuclei in the rostral medulla of the brainstem, vestibular portion of the vestibulocochlear nerve (cranial nerve VIII), and receptors in the semicircular canals of the inner ear • Head tilt—most consistent sign of diseases affecting the vestibular system and its projections to the cerebellum, spinal cord, cerebral cortex, reticular formation, and extraocular eye muscles via the medial longitudinal fasciculus; usually directed toward the same side as the lesion

SYSTEMS AFFECTED
Nervous—peripheral or CNS

SIGNALMENT N/A

SIGNS
Be sure that abnormal head posture is not head turning (turning the head and neck to the side as if to turn in a circle), which is of thalamocortical origin and is not associated with other vestibular signs (e.g., abnormal nystagmus).

CAUSES

Peripheral Disease
• Anatomic—congenital head tilt • Metabolic—hypothyroidism; pituitary chromophobe adenoma; paraneoplastic disease; cranial nerve polyneuropathy • Neoplastic—nerve sheath tumor of cranial nerve VIII; neoplasia of the bone and surrounding tissue (e.g., osteosarcoma, fibrosarcoma, chondrosarcoma, and squamous cell carcinoma) • Inflammatory—otitis media and interna;* primarily bacterial but also related to parasitic (e.g., *Otodectes*), mycotic, and fungal origins; foreign body; nasopharyngeal polyps • Idiopathic—canine geriatric vestibular disease;* feline idiopathic vestibular disease* • Immune mediated—polyneuropathy • Toxic—aminoglycosides; lead; hexachlorophene • Traumatic—tympanic bulla or petrosal bone fracture; ear flush

Central Disease
• Degenerative—storage disease; demyelinating disease; vascular event • Anatomic—hydrocephalus • Neo-plastic—glioma; choroid plexus papilloma; meningioma; lymphosarcoma; nerve sheath tumor; medulloblastoma; skull tumor (e.g.,

osteosarcoma); metastasis (e.g., hemangiosarcoma and melanoma) • Nutritional—thiamine deficiency • Inflammatory, infectious—viral (e.g., FIP, canine distemper virus); protozoal (e.g., toxoplasmosis); fungal (e.g., cryptococcosis, blastomycosis, histoplasmosis, coccidioidomycosis, and nocardiosis); bacterial (e.g., central erosion caused by otitis media and interna); parasitic (e.g., *Cuterebra* larvae); rickettsial (e.g., ehrlichiosis); algae (prototethcosis) • Inflammatory, noninfectious—granulomatous meningoencephalomyelitis • Trauma—petrosal bone fracture with brainstem injury • Toxic—metronidazole

RISK FACTORS
• Hypothyroidism • Administration of ototoxic drugs • Thiamine-deficient diet (e.g., exclusively fish diet) • Otitis externa, media, and interna

 DIAGNOSIS

DIFFERENTIAL DIAGNOSIS

Vestibular Disease
• Unilateral disease—head tilt usually directed toward the side of the lesion; may be accompanied by other vestibular signs; abnormal nystagmus (resting, positional) with fast phase usually in the direction opposite the tilt; mild ventral deviation of the eye (vestibular strabismus) ipsilateral to the tilt that is exacerbated by elevation of the head; ataxia and disequilibrium with a tendency to fall, lean, or circle toward the side of the tilt • Bilateral disease—head tilt may be absent or mild in the direction of the more severely affected side; abnormal nystagmus may be seen; physiologic nystagmus (e.g., normal vestibular nystagmus or conjugate eye movements) may be depressed or absent with wide side-to-side swaying movements of the head (especially evident in cats); may note a wide-based stance, especially in the thoracic limbs, or a crouched posture with reluctance to move • Head tilt—must be localized in the peripheral (e.g., vestibular portion of cranial nerve VIII or receptors in the inner ear) or central (e.g., vestibular nuclei and their neuronal pathways) nervous system • Peripheral deficits—horizontal or rotatory nystagmus with fast phase always in the direction opposite the head tilt; patient may have concomitant ipsilateral facial nerve paresis or paralysis or Horner syndrome, because of the close association of cranial nerves VIII and VII in the petrosal bone and the sympathetic nervous system in the tympanic bulla. • Central deficits—vertical, horizontal, or rotatory nystagmus that can change with the position of the head; altered mentation; ipsilateral paresis or proprioceptive

deficits; other signs related to the cerebellum, rostral medulla, and caudal pons; in some patients, multiple cranial nerve involvement other than cranial nerve VII. • Paradoxical vestibular syndrome—caused by lesions in the cerebellar peduncles, cerebellar medulla, or flocculonodular lobes of the cerebellum; vestibular signs (e.g., head tilt and nystagmus) are opposite the side of the lesion, whereas the cerebellar signs and the proprioceptive deficits are ipsilateral to the lesion.

Nonvestibular Head Tilt and Head Posture
• Uncommon • Must be differentiated from vestibular head tilt • Unilateral lesions of the midbrain—cause severe rotation of the head (rare) of > 90° toward the side opposite the lesion; no other vestibular signs; tilt corrects when the patient is blindfolded. • Circling of adversive syndrome (secondary to rostral thalamic lesions)—the head turn, lean, or neck curvature can be misinterpreted as a vestibular tilt; no vestibular signs; contralateral postural, menace, or sensory deficits reflect a thalamic lesion; compulsive turning, usually in large circles and without the disequilibrium of vestibular circling

CBC/BIOCHEMISTRY/URINALYSIS
• Usually normal
• Mild anemia—hypothyroidism
• Leucocytosis with neutrophilia—otitis media or interna
• Thrombocytopenia—ehrlichiosis
• Hypercholesterolemia—hypothyroidism
• High serum globulin concentration—FIP

OTHER LABORATORY TESTS
• TSH response test and T_4, free T_4, and endogenous TSH levels—when hypothyroidism is suspected on the basis of physical examination findings and unilateral or bilateral involvement of cranial nerve VIII and possibly VII
• Bacterial culture and sensitivity testing—sample from myringotomy or surgical drainage of tympanic bulla if otitis media or interna is suspected
• Microscopic examination of ear swab—parasites (e.g., ear mites)
• Serologic testing—infectious causes (e.g., canine distemper; FIP; and protozoal, fungal, and rickettsial diseases)

IMAGING
• Tympanic bullae and skull radiography—normal radiographs do not rule out bulla disease.
• CT and MRI—valuable for confirming bulla lesions and CNS extension from peripheral document or localized tumor, granuloma, and extent of inflammation

DIAGNOSTIC PROCEDURES
• CSF analysis—sample from the cerebellomedullary cistern; valuable for evaluating central vestibular disease; detect

HEAD TILT (VESTIBULAR DISEASE)

inflammatory process; protein electrophoresis and titers to match with serologic testing may be indicated; sample collection may put the patient at risk for herniation if there is a mass or high intracranial pressure.
• BAER—assess cochlear portion of cranial nerve VIII and brainstem auditory pathways; particularly valuable for evaluating peripheral vestibular disease, because some diseases may cause ipsilateral deafness (e.g., otitis media and interna), whereas other diseases (e.g., canine geriatric vestibular disease and hypothyroidism) affect only the vestibular portion of cranial nerve VIII
• Biopsy—bone: when a tumor or osteomyelitis is suspected; brainstem masses (e.g., cerebellomedullary angle): difficult to approach and to remove surgically

TREATMENT

• Inpatient vs. outpatient—depends on severity of the signs (especially vestibular ataxia), size, and age of the patient, and need for supportive care
• Supportive fluids—replacement or maintenance fluids (depend on clinical state); may be required in the acute phase when disorientation, nausea, and vomiting preclude oral intake; especially important in geriatric patients
• Activity—restrict (e.g., avoid stairs and slippery surfaces) according to the degree of disequilibrium
• Diet—usually no need for modification unless the cause is thiamine deficiency (e.g., exclusively fish diet without vitamin supplementation); oral intake may need to be restricted with nausea and vomiting;
CAUTION: be aware of aspiration secondary to abnormal body posture in patients with severe head tilt and vestibular disequilibrium or brainstem dysfunction.
• Advise client that the prognosis for central vestibular disorders is usually poorer than that for peripheral disorders.
• Inform client of the risks associated with biopsy, surgery, and radiation of a brainstem mass.
• Surgical treatment—may be required to drain bulla with otitis media or interna, to remove nasopharyngeal polyps in cats, and to resect tumor, if accessible

MEDICATIONS

DRUGS OF CHOICE

• Otitis media or interna—broad-spectrum antibiotic (parenteral or oral) that penetrates bone while awaiting culture results; trimethoprim-sulfa (15 mg/kg PO q12h or 30 mg/kg PO q12–24h); first-generation cephalosporins, such as cephalexin (10–30 mg/kg PO q6–8h) and amoxicillin/clavulanic acid (12.2–25 mg/kg PO q12h for dogs or 62.5 mg/cat PO q12h); treatment often required for 4–6 weeks
• Hypothyroidism—T$_4$ replacement (dogs, levothyroxine 22 μg/kg PO q12h) should be introduced gradually in geriatric patients, especially with cardiac disease; response varies, partly depending on the duration of signs (e.g., in some patients, neuropathy is not reversible)
• Drug affecting vestibular function—discontinue offending agent; signs are usually, but not always, reversible.
• Infectious—specific treatment, if indicated; for bacterial diseases, antibiotic that penetrates the blood–brain barrier (e.g., trimethoprim-sulfa, 15 mg/kg PO q12h); for protozoal diseases, sulfa or clindamycin (12.5–25 mg/kg PO q12h); for fungal diseases, itraconazole (dogs, 2.5 mg/kg PO q12h or 5 mg/kg PO q24h; cats, 5 mg/kg PO q12h); prognosis usually grave for protozoal, fungal, and viral diseases (e.g., canine distemper and FIP)
• Granulomatous meningoencephalo-myelitis—usually initially treated with steroids: dexamethasone (dogs, 0.25 mg/kg PO, IM q12h for 3 days; then 0.25 mg/kg PO q24h for 3 days), followed by prednisone (1 mg/kg PO q24h for 1–2 weeks; then decrease slowly); depending on progress, may need stronger immunosuppression—azathioprine (dogs, 2 mg/kg PO q24h initially; then 0.5–1 mg/kg PO q48h)—or radiation
• Trauma—supportive care (e.g., anti-inflammatory drugs, antibiotics, intravenous fluid administration); specific fracture repair or hematoma removal is difficult, considering the location.
• Canine geriatric and feline idiopathic vestibular disease—supportive care only
• Cranial polyneuropathy—response to prednisone usually good if the patient has a primary immune disorder
• Thiamine deficiency—diet modification and thiamine replacement

CONTRAINDICATIONS

Drugs potentially toxic to the vestibular system—aminoglycoside antibiotics; prolonged high-dose metronidazole

PRECAUTIONS

• Long-term trimethoprim sulfa administration—keratoconjunctivitis sicca (dry eye)
• Avoid topical drugs (especially oil based) if the tympanic membrane is ruptured.

POSSIBLE INTERACTIONS N/A

ALTERNATIVE DRUGS N/A

FOLLOW-UP

PATIENT MONITORING

• Encourage client to keep a progress report.
• Repeat the neurologic examination at a frequency dictated by the underlying cause
• Head tilt may persist. • Hypothyroidism—measure T$_4$ concentration 6 hr after treatment at 4–6 weeks after initiation of hormone replacement therapy to evaluate dosage
• Repeat CSF and brain imaging—with some central vestibular disorders • Monitor tear production (Schirmer tear test) with long-term trimethoprim sulfa administration.

POSSIBLE COMPLICATIONS

• Progression of disease with deterioration of mental status • Brain herniation

MISCELLANEOUS

ASSOCIATED CONDITIONS

• Facial nerve (cranial nerve VII) paresis or paralysis • Horner syndrome

AGE-RELATED FACTORS

Canine geriatric vestibular syndrome affects only old dogs.

ZOONOTIC POTENTIAL N/A

PREGNANCY N/A

SYNONYMS N/A

SEE ALSO

• Encephalitis
• Meningoencephalomyelitis, Granulomatous
• Nasal and Nasopharyngeal Polyps • Otitis Media and Interna • Vestibular Disease, Geriatric—Dogs • Vestibular Disease, Idiopathic—Cats

ABBREVIATIONS

• BAER = brainstem auditory-evoked response • CSF = cerebrospinal fluid
• FIP = feline infectious peritonitis • TSH = thyroid-stimulating hormone

Suggested Reading
de Lahunta A. Veterinary neuroanatomy and clinical neurology. 2nd ed. Philadelphia: Saunders, 1983.
Oliver JE, Lorenz MD. Handbook of veterinary neurologic diagnosis. 2nd ed. Philadelphia: Saunders, 1993.
Parent JM, Cochrane SM. Head tilt. In: Allen DG, ed. Small animal medicine. Philadelphia: Lippincott, 1991:753–759.
Author Susan M. Cochrane
Consulting Editor Joane M. Parent

HEMATEMESIS

BASICS

DEFINITION
Vomiting of blood

PATHOPHYSIOLOGY
Vomiting in association with
• Esophageal, gastric, or upper small intestinal mucosal barrier disruption
• Coagulopathy
• Swallowing blood from an extragastrointestinal source (oral, respiratory, dermatologic, etc.)

SYSTEMS AFFECTED
• Gastrointestinal (GI)—inflammation, ulceration and/or neoplasia in the oral cavity, esophagus, stomach, and/or duodenum
• Cardiovascular—tachycardia, systolic heart murmur and/or hypotension may occur with acute/severe hemorrhage
• Respiratory—respiratory hemorrhage with ingestion can lead to hematemesis; tachypnea may occur with severe anemia; rarely, aspiration pneumonia may occur with severe vomiting.
• Hematologic—coagulopathy with GI hemorrhage can lead to hematemesis.

SIGNALMENT
• Dogs and cats
• No age, breed, or sex predilection

SIGNS

Historical Findings
• Vomiting with blood—blood in the vomitus may appear as fresh flecks of blood, blood clots, or digested blood that looks like "coffee grounds"
• Melena
• Anorexia
• Abdominal pain
• Hematochezia, melena, petechiation, ecchymosis, epistaxis, and/or hematuria—if coagulopathy
• Dyspnea, epistaxis, hemoptysis, and/or coughing—if respiratory disease
• Pallor, weakness, and/or collapse—if the patient is anemic

Physical Examination Findings
• Abdominal pain • Melena • Hematochezia, melena, petechiation, ecchymosis, epistaxis, and/or retinal hemorrhage—if coagulopathy
• Dyspnea, epistaxis, hemoptysis, and/or coughing—if respiratory disease is present
• Pallor, weakness, and/or collapse—if the patient is anemic

CAUSES

Coagulopathies
• Thrombocytopenia
• Thrombocytopathia—Von Willebrand's disease, NSAIDs, hyperglobulinemia
• Disseminated intravascular coagulation

• Anticoagulant rodenticide toxicity
• Coagulation factor deficiency

Drugs
• NSAIDs
• Glucocorticoids

Gastrointestinal Diseases
• Gastroduodenal ulcers
• Esophagitis
• Parasitism
• Oral, esophageal, gastric, or duodenal neoplasia
• Oral, esophageal, gastric, or duodenal foreign body
• Hemorrhagic gastroenteritis
• Inflammatory bowel disease

Heavy Metal Poisoning
Arsenic, zinc, or lead

Infectious Diseases
• *Helicobacter* spp.
• Viral and bacterial gastroenteritis
• Pythiosis

Metabolic Diseases
• Renal failure
• Liver disease
• Hypoadrenocorticism
• Pancreatitis

Neoplasia
• Oral, nasal, respiratory, or GI tumors
• Mastocytosis
• Gastrinoma

Neurologic Diseases
• Head trauma
• Spinal cord disease

Respiratory Disease
• Nasal disease—neoplasia, fungal infection
• Pulmonary and airway disease—neoplasia, severe pneumonia, fungal infection, foreign body, heartworm disease

Stress/Major Medical Illness
• Septic or hypovolemic shock
• Severe illness
• Major surgery
• Heat stroke
• Trauma
• Burns

RISK FACTORS
• Administration of ulcerogenic drugs—NSAIDs
• Critically ill patients
• Hypovolemic or septic shock
• Thrombocytopenia
• Gastric, duodenal, and/or esophageal disease

DIAGNOSIS

DIFFERENTIAL DIAGNOSIS

Differentiating Similar Signs
• Hemoptysis—physical examination findings may differentiate; thoracic radiographs may reveal presence of airway or pulmonary disease
• Regurgitation or vomiting of swallowed blood from extragastrointestinal diseases (e.g., oropharyngeal, nasopharyngeal, cutaneous, urogenital tract, and anal sac disease)—physical examination findings may differentiate; may need observation of patient for ingestion of blood and thorough examination ± imaging under sedation or anesthesia
• Ingestion and vomiting of foreign materials or foods that look like fresh or digested blood

CBC/BIOCHEMISTRY/URINALYSIS
• If acute (3–5 days) blood loss, nonregenerative anemia (normocytic, normochromic, minimal reticulocytosis)
• If blood loss >5 days duration—regenerative anemia (macrocytic, hyperchromic, reticulocytosis)
• If chronic blood loss—iron deficiency anemia (microcytic, hypochromic, poor reticulocytosis, ± thrombocytosis)
• May be thrombocytopenia if underlying cause
• May be panhypoproteinemia due to alimentary hemorrhage
• May see mature neutrophilia or left-shift neutrophilia with sepsis and gastroduodenal ulcer perforation
• Blood urea nitrogen (BUN):creatinine ratio may be elevated with GI hemorrhage
• May be elevated BUN and creatinine, hyperphosphatemia, and isosthenuria if renal disease– induced ulcers
• May be elevated liver enzymes, hyperbilirubinemia, and/or hypoalbuminemia if hematemesis is due to liver disease–induced ulcers
• May be hyperkalemia, hyponatremia, and azotemia if due to hypoadrenocorticism-induced ulcers—atypical hypoadrenocorticism will not have electrolyte abnormalities
• May be elevated lipase and amylase if due to pancreatitis-induced ulcers

OTHER LABORATORY TESTS
• Fecal occult blood test may be positive—test is accurate if dog is eating dry food.
• Fecal floatation—to screen for GI parasitism
• Coagulation profile—if bleeding disorder suspected
• Bile acids—if suspect disease
• ACTH stimulation—if suspect hypoadrenocorticism
• Buffy coat—if suspect systemic mast cell disease
• Gastrin levels—if more-common causes excluded

IMAGING
• Abdominal radiography may identify changes consistent with kidney or liver disease if these are a cause of ulcer-induced hematemesis; gastric or duodenal foreign body or masses occasionally identified
• A positive- or double-contrast GI study may identify foreign objects and irregularities in the esophageal, gastric, and/or duodenal mucosa.
• Thoracic radiographs may reveal an esophageal foreign body or mass or pulmonary metastasis
• Abdominal ultrasonography may identify a gastric or duodenal mass, gastric or duodenal wall-thickening, and/or abdominal lymphadenopathy.
• Abdominal ultrasound can also screen for abnormalities in the pancreas, liver, kidneys, and other abdominal organs as a source of hematemesis.

DIAGNOSTIC PROCEDURES
• Endoscopy to evaluate esophagus, stomach, and upper small intestinal tract if extragastrointestinal causes are ruled out; biopsy the esophageal, gastric, and/or duodenal lesions for histopathology to determine the nature of the underlying GI disease.
• If an infectious etiology is suspected, submit biopsy specimens for culture.
• If abdominal ultrasound shows a gastric or duodenal mass or gastroduodenal wall-thickening, an abdominal ultrasound-guided biopsy can be performed; occasionally the ultrasound-guided gastroduodenal biopsy is diagnostic and the endoscopic biopsies are not.
• Urease testing of gastric biopsy specimens may reveal *Helicobacter* organisms.
• Pythiosis-induced ulceration/hematemesis requires deep biopsies (ultrasound guided or surgical); samples should be submitted unrefrigerated in saline for culture and in formalin for histopathology with special staining.
• May use abdominocentesis to identify septic gastroduodenal ulcer perforation/peritonitis
• Obtain fine-needle aspirates or biopsy specimens of cutaneous or intraabdominal masses to identify mast cell tumor-induced ulcer disease/hematemesis.

 TREATMENT
• Generally hospitalization and inpatient treatment required
• Treat underlying disease.
• Supportive care may involve intravenous fluids to correct hydration status and acid–base and electrolyte abnormalities.
• Severe hematemesis may need aggressive intravenous fluid treatment for shock—crystalloids and/or colloids.

• Anemic patients may require whole blood, packed red blood cells, or oxygen-carrying hemoglobin solution (Oxyglobin).
• Patients with an underlying coagulopathy as the cause of hematemesis may need whole blood, fresh plasma, or fresh frozen plasma to replace clotting factor deficiencies.
• Discontinue oral intake until vomiting ceases; when feeding is resumed, feed small amounts in multiple feedings.
• Recommended diet depends on the underlying cause.
• Severe hematemesis may require surgical treatment.

 MEDICATIONS

DRUGS OF CHOICE

For Primary GI Disease
• Histamine H$_2$-receptor antagonists competitively inhibit gastric acid secretion—famotidine 0.5 mg/kg PO, IV q12–24h; ranitidine 1–4 mg/kg SC, PO, IV q8–12h; cimetidine 5–10 mg/kg PO, SC, IV q8h
• Sucralfate suspension (0.5–1 g PO q8h) protects ulcerated tissue (cytoprotection) by binding to ulcer sites
• Parenteral administration of antibiotics
• Antiemetics (chlorpromazine 0.5–4 mg/kg SC, IM, IV q6–8h; prochlorperazine 0.1–0.5 mg/kg PO, SC, IM, IV q6–8h) are administered if vomiting occurs frequently or results in significant fluid losses.
• See Gastroduodenal Ulcer Disease and/or Gastritis, Acute and Chronic, for specific drug therapy.

For Extragastrointestinal Disease
See specific chapters on causes of hematemesis for appropriate drug therapy; treat for gastroduodenal ulcer disease until this diagnosis is excluded.

CONTRAINDICATIONS
Avoid drugs that might damage the gastroduodenal mucosal barrier (e.g., NSAIDs and corticosteroids).

PRECAUTIONS
N/A

POSSIBLE INTERACTIONS
• Cimetidine binds to hepatic cytochrome P450 enzyme and may interfere with metabolism of other drugs.
• Sucralfate may alter absorption of other drugs.

ALTERNATIVE DRUGS
Omeprazole (0.7 mg/kg PO q24h) is a potent inhibitor of gastric acid secretion.

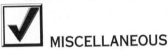 FOLLOW-UP

PATIENT MONITORING
• May assess improvement by resolution of clinical signs; can use the PCV, TP, and BUN to detect continued blood loss.
• Depending on the underlying cause, specific laboratory or imaging tests may be necessary to follow response to therapy.

POSSIBLE COMPLICATIONS
• Severe blood loss requiring transfusion
• Sepsis
• Ulcer perforation
• Death—secondary to ulcer perforation, sepsis, hemorrhage
• Aspiration pneumonia—rare

 MISCELLANEOUS

ASSOCIATED CONDITIONS
• Anemia
• Hypovolemic shock
• Melena

AGE-RELATED FACTORS
• Neoplasia in middle-aged to old animals
• Ingestion of foreign materials by young animals

ZOONOTIC POTENTIAL
Zoonosis of *Helicobacter* spp. is controversial.

SEE ALSO
• Gastroduodenal Ulcer Disease
• Melena
• Hemoptysis
• Chapters on specific causes

ABBREVIATIONS
N/A

Suggested Reading
Davenport D. Hematemesis: diagnosis and treatment. In: Kirk RW, Bonagura J, eds. Current veterinary therapy XI. Philadelphia: Saunders, 1992:132–137.
Guilford WG, Strombeck DR. Strombeck's small animal gastroenterology. 3rd ed. Philadelphia: Saunders, 1996.
Willard M. Diseases of the stomach. In: Ettinger SJ, Feldman EC, eds., Textbook of veterinary internal medicine. Philadelphia: Saunders, 1994:1143–1168.
Author Jocelyn Mott
Consulting Editors Mitchell A. Crystal and Brett M. Feder

HEMATURIA

BASICS

DEFINITION
The presence of blood in the urine

Pathophysiology
Secondary to loss of endothelial integrity in urinary tract, clotting factor deficiency, or thrombocytopenia

Systems Affected
• Renal/Urologic
• Reproductive

SIGNALMENT
• Dogs and cats
• Familial hematuria in young animals, neoplasia in older animals
• Females at greater risk for urinary tract infection

SIGNS

Historical Findings
Red-tinged urine with or without pollakiuria

Physical Examination Findings
• Palpable mass in patients with neoplasia
• Abdominal pain in some patients
• Painful prostate gland in males
• Petechia or ecchymoses in patients with coagulopathy

CAUSES

Systemic
• Coagulopathy
• Thrombocytopenia
• Vasculitis

Upper Urinary Tract
• Anatomic—e.g., cystic kidney disease and familial
• Metabolic—e.g., nephrolithiasis
• Neoplastic—e.g., renal lymphoma, adenocarcinoma, and hemangiosarcoma
• Infectious—e.g., leptospirosis, feline infectious peritonitis (FIP), and bacteria
• Inflammatory—e.g., glomerulonephritis
• Idiopathic
• Trauma

Lower Urinary Tract
• Anatomic—e.g., bladder malformations
• Metabolic—e.g., uroliths
• Neoplasia—e.g., transitional cell carcinoma, and lymphosarcoma
• Infectious—e.g., bacterial, fungal, and viral disease
• Idiopathic—cats
• Trauma
• Cyclophosphamide-induced hemorrhagic cystitis

Genitalia
• Metabolic—e.g., estrous
• Neoplastic—e.g., transmissible venereal tumor, leiomyoma, and prostatic adenocarcinoma
• Infectious—e.g., bacterial and fungal disease
• Inflammatory—e.g., benign prostatic hyperplasia
• Trauma

RISK FACTORS
Breed predisposed to urolithiasis and coagulopathy

DIAGNOSIS

DIFFERENTIAL DIAGNOSIS
• Other causes of discolored urine (e.g., myoglobinuria, hemoglobinuria, and bilirubinuria)

LABORATORY FINDINGS

Drugs That May Alter Laboratory Results
Substantial doses of vitamin C (ascorbic aid) may cause false-negative reagent test strip results; newer generations of reagent strips are more resistant to interference by reducing substances such as ascorbic acid.

Disorders That May Alter Laboratory Results
• Common urine reagent strip tests for blood are designed to detect red blood cells, hemoglobin, or myoglobin.
• Low specific urine gravity (polyuric syndromes) lyses RBCs.
• Bacteriuria (bacterial peroxidase) causes false-positive reagent test strip results
• Formalin preservative causes false-negative reagent test strip results.

Valid If Run in a Human Laboratory?
Yes

CBC/BIOCHEMISTRY/URINALYSIS
• Thrombocytopenia and severe anemia in some patients
• Azotemia in some patients with bilateral renal disease
• RBCs and possibly infectious agents may be seen in urine sediment.
• Crystalluria in some patients with urolithiasis

OTHER LABORATORY TESTS
• Activated clotting time (ACT) or clotting profile to rule out coagulopathy
• Bacterial culture of urine to identify urinary tract infection
• Examination of an ejaculate to identify prostatic disease

IMAGING
Ultrasonography, radiography, and possibly contrast radiography may be useful in obtaining a diagnosis.

DIAGNOSTIC PROCEDURES
• Biopsy of mass lesion
• Vaginoscopy or cystoscopy in females

TREATMENT
• Hematuria may indicate a serious disease process.
• Urolithiasis and renal failure may require diet modification.
• Urinary tract infection may be caused by another disease, local (e.g., neoplasia and urolithiasis) or systemic (e.g., hyperadreno-corticism and diabetes mellitus) that also requires treatment.

MEDICATIONS

DRUGS OF CHOICE
• Blood transfusion may be necessary if patient is severely anemic.
• Crystalloids to treat dehydration
• Antibiotics to treat urinary tract infection and septicemia
• Heparin for disseminated intravascular coagulation (DIC)

CONTRAINDICATIONS
Immunosuppressive drugs, except to treat immune-mediated disease

PRECAUTIONS
N/A

POSSIBLE INTERACTIONS
Intravenous contrast media can cause acute renal failure.

ALTERNATIVE DRUGS
N/A

FOLLOW-UP

PATIENT MONITORING
Depends on primary or associated diseases

POSSIBLE COMPLICATIONS
• Anemia
• Hypovolemia if severe hemorrhage
• Ureteral or urethral obstruction due to blood clots

MISCELLANEOUS

ASSOCIATED CONDITIONS
N/A

AGE-RELATED FACTORS
• Neoplasia tends to occur in older animals.
• Immune-mediated diseases tend to occur in young adult animals.

ZOONOTIC POTENTIAL
Leptospirosis

PREGNANCY
N/A

SYNONYMS
N/A

SEE ALSO
• Coagulopathies
• Crystalluria

• Cylindruria
• Dysuria and Pollakiuria
• Feline Idiopathic Lower Urinary Tract Disease
• Glomerulonephritis
• Hemoglobinuria and Myoglobinuria
• Lower Urinary Tract Infection
• Nephrolithiasis
• Prostatitis
• Prostatomegaly
• Proteinuria
• Pyelonephritis
• Thrombocytopenia
• Urolithiasis

ABBREVIATIONS
• ACT = activated clotting time
• DIC = disseminated intravascular coagulation
• FIP = feline infectious peritonitis

Suggested Reading
Lage AL. Diagnostic approach to canine and feline hematuria. In: Kirk RW, ed. Current veterinary therapy X. Philadelphia: Saunders, 1989:1117–1123.
McCall Kaufman G. Hematuria-dysuria. In: Ettinger SJ, ed. Textbook of veterinary internal medicine. 3rd ed. Philadelphia: Saunders, 1989:160–164.
Author Joseph W. Bartges
Consulting Editors Larry G. Adams and Carl A. Osborne

HEPATOMEGALY

 BASICS

DEFINITION
Large liver, detected on physical examination, abdominal radiography, ultrasonography, or direct visualization; liver normally 1.3%–6.0% of body weight

PATHOPHYSIOLOGY
Normal size—determined by hepatatrophic factors (produced in the gut and pancreas and delivered in portal blood); sinusoidal capacitance; and parenchymal or sinusoidal accumulation of cells, substrates, or storage products
Diffuse or Generalized
• Inflammatory—immune-mediated or infectious hepatitis; classified according to cell type • Lymphoreticular hyperplasia—response to antigens or accelerated erythrocyte destruction • Congestion—impaired venous drainage • Infiltration—cellular (usually neoplastic) invasion or accumulation of abnormal substances (glycogen, amyloid, storage disease) • Cystic lesions • Cholestasis—EHBDO; intrahepatic cholestasis • Extramedullary hematopoiesis
Nodular, Focal, or Asymmetric
• Neoplasia • Hemorrhage • Infection or inflammation • Nodular hyperplasia • Anteriovenous fistula—involved lobe larger than other lobes • Asymmetric regeneration after large-volume hepatic resection • Cystic lesions

SYSTEMS AFFECTED
• Gastrointestinal—gastric compression or displacement with severe condition • Pulmonary—compromised ventilatory space

SIGNALMENT
• Dogs and cats • Old animals more commonly affected • Puppies and kittens have a larger liver:body mass ratio than do adults.

SIGNS

Historical Findings
• Abdominal distention or palpable mass
• Depend on underlying cause

Physical Examination Findings
• Dogs—liver palpable beyond costal margin (normal or small liver no palpable) • Cats—liver palpable 1.5 cm beyond costal margin (normal liver palpable) • May remain undetected in markedly obese patients

CAUSES

Inflammation
• Infectious hepatitis—chronic active hepatitis (early) • Acute hepatic necrosis—toxins; drugs; ischemia; other • Feline cholangiohepatitis complex • Biliary cirrhosis • Lymphoreticular hyperplasia—immune-mediated disease (rickettsial, hemolytic anemia, systemic lupus erythematosus, idiopathic)

Venous Outflow Occlusion
• High central venous pressure—right-sided congestive heart failure secondary to tricuspid valve disease; cardiomyopathy; congenital anomaly (cor triatriatum dexter); neoplasia; pericardial disease; heartworm disease; pulmonary hypertension; severe arrhythmia
• High vena caval or hepatic venous resistance—vena caval occlusion secondary to thrombosis; tumor invasion or extramural occlusion; heartworm vena cava syndrome; vena caval stenosis; congenital kink in the vena cava; diaphragmatic hernia; hepatic vein occlusion secondary to Budd-Chiari syndrome (thrombosis, other occlusion); extramural tumor invasion or stricture; liver lobe torsion; veno-occlusive disease

Infiltration
• Neoplasia • Metabolic abnormalities—amyloid; glycogen (vacuolar or glucocorticoid hepatopathy in dogs); lipid (hepatic lipidosis: especially cats, also neonatal cats and dogs and dogs with diabetes mellitus); metabolic products of storage disease

Neoplasia
• Infiltrative, diffuse, or large focal tumors
• Primary hepatic—lymphoma; hepatocellular adenoma; hepatocellular carcinoma; cholangiocarcinoma (bile duct carcinoma) • Hemangioma or hemangiosarcoma • Fibroma or fibrosarcoma • Leiomyoma or leiomyosarcoma • Osteosarcoma • Various metastatic tumors

Biliary Obstruction
• Pancreatitis; pancreatic neoplasia; other neoplasms arising near the common bile duct or involving the bile duct (bile duct carcinoma); granuloma of the common bile duct • Inspissated bile • Cholelithiasis • Abscess • Proximal duodenitis; duodenal foreign body • Fluke migration (cats)

Cystic Lesions
• Hepatic or biliary cysts • Cystadenoma • Polycystic disease—may be associated with renal cysts • Acquired cysts—tumors • Hepatic abscesses. • Extramedullary hematopoiesis • Regenerative anemias—hemolytic (immune mediated, congenital or metabolic); chronic oxidant injury; erythroparasitemia; idiopathic

Other
• Drugs—phenobarbital • Nodular hyperplasia

RISK FACTORS
• Cardiac disease • Heartworm disease • Neoplasia • Primary hepatic disease—inflammatory, neoplastic, or cystic • Corticosteroids—treatment or endogenous • Phenobarbital • Poorly controlled diabetes mellitus • Obesity complicated by anorexia (cats)—hepatic lipidosis • EHBDO • Certain anemias

 DIAGNOSIS

DIFFERENTIAL DIAGNOSIS
• Similar Signs
Distinguished from gastric, splenic, or other cranial abdominal masses or effusions via radiographic and ultrasonographic imaging

Causes
• History or physical examination findings—cardiac disorders (e.g., heart murmur, weak femoral pulses, hepatojugular reflex, jugular distention and pulses, muffled heart sounds); significant anemia (pallor with or without jaundice); tachycardia; tachypnea; exercise intolerance; bounding pulses • Parenchymal liver disease—characterized by lethargy, anorexia, vomiting, diarrhea, weight loss, jaundice, bleeding tendency, hepatic encephalopathy, polydipsia and polyuria, and ascites
• Ultrasonography—mass lesions; EHBDO; cystic lesions; pancreatic disease • Signs of hyperadrenocorticism—common in dogs with glucocorticoid-induced vacuolar hepatopathy
• Hepatic lipidosis—suggested by poorly controlled diabetes mellitus (dogs or cats) or jaundice (obese anorectic cats)

CBC/BIOCHEMISTRY/URINALYSIS

CBC
• Identify anemia and cause; spherocytes (immune-mediated hemolytic anemia); schistocytes (vascular shearing, vena cava syndrome, hemangiosarcoma, DIC, *Haemobartonella, Babesia*) • Circulating blast cells—myeloproliferative or lymphoproliferative disease • Nucleated red cells—extramedullary hematopoiesis • Macrocytosis and nonregenerative anemia—feline retroviral infection • Leukogram—underlying conditions • Thrombocytopenia—increased consumption; increased destruction; reduced production

Biochemistry
• Inflammatory disorders—usually associated with high liver enzymes; hyperglobulinemia; variable bilirubin and albumin concentrations • Lymphoreticular hyperplasia—mild to moderately high liver enzymes; abnormalities consistent with disease in other organs • Venous outflow obstruction—mild to moderately high liver enzymes • Primary hepatic neoplasia—markedly high liver enzymes (ALP) • Metastatic neoplasia—normal to moderately high liver enzymes; may see hypercalcemia or hyperglobulinemia • Infiltrative disorders—minor liver enzyme abnormalities; hyperbilirubinemia • Vacuolar hepatopathy (dogs)—markedly high ALP with few other abnormalities; high cholesterol with glucocorticoids • Hepatic lipidosis (cats)—markedly high ALP, AST, and ALT; minor increases in GGT • Storage disorders—few abnormalities • EHBDO— markedly high ALP; moderately high AST, ALT, and GGT; severe hyperbilirubinemia and hypercholesterolemia • Cystic lesions—normal, except with hepatic abscess (markedly high ALT and AST) • Phenobarbital associated—high liver enzymes (especially ALP) • Nodular hyperplasia—normal or moderately high ALP

OTHER LABORATORY TESTS
• FeLV and immunodeficiency virus testing • Buffy coat smears—circulating blast cells (neoplasia) • Coagulation panel—DIC

common with hepatic hemangiosarcoma or diffuse lymphoma; prolonged coagulation times (especially PIVKA) commonly seen with EHBDO • TSBA—high with diffuse disorders; redundant if hemolysis ruled out as a cause of jaundice • Pituitary–adrenal axis (dogs)—evaluated with vacuolar hepatopathy • Heartworm testing—in endemic area • Fungal serology—in endemic area

IMAGING

Abdominal Radiography
• Hepatomegaly—extension of a rounded liver margin caudal to the costal arch; caudal-dorsal displacement of stomach; caudal displacement of cranial duodenal flexure, right kidney, and transverse colon • May suggest cause

Thoracic Radiography
• Right and left lateral views—screen for metastasis and underlying disorders • Cardiac, pulmonary, pericardial, vena caval disorders • Sternal lymphadenopathy—reflects abdominal inflammation or neoplasia • Puppies, kittens, and deep inspirations—spurious hepatomegaly

Abdominal Ultrasonography
• Liver size and contour • Abdominal effusions—distribution and echogenic patterns • Diffuse enlargement with normal echogenicity—congestion; cellular infiltration; inflammation; extramedullary hematopoiesis, reticuloendothelial hyperplasia • Diffuse enlargement with hypoechoic parenchyma—normal variation; diffuse sarcoma; amyloidosis • Diffuse enlargement with hyperechoic parenchyma (minor nodularity)—lipidosis; glycogen accumulation; inflammation; diffuse early fibrosis • Distinguish intrahepatic from posthepatic cholestasis—EHBDO • Identify concurrent abdominal disease—liver; kidneys; intestines; lymph nodes • Cannot differentiate benign from malignant disease

Thoracic Ultrasonography
• Right atrium—with evidence of hemangiosarcoma • Pericardium—pericardial tamponade • Mediastinum—masses or lymphadenopathy • Cardiac—functional abnormalities; masses (right heart, pulmonary trunk, vena cava) • Caudal vena cava at the diaphragm and hepatic venules—distention; oscillatory flow; mass lesions

OTHER DIAGNOSTIC PROCEDURES
• Fine-needle aspiration—23- or 25-gauge 2.5–3.75-cm (1–1.5-in) needle; diffusely enlarged liver aspirated without ultrasonography; nodules (> 0.5 cm) aspirated with ultrasound guidance • Cytology—may reveal infectious agents (especially in macrophages), neoplasia, inflammation, or extramedullary hematopoiesis • Hepatic biopsy—if findings suggest primary hepatic disease and imaging rules out EHBDO and other obvious diagnoses; via percutaneous blind or ultrasound-guided needle, laparos-

copy, or laparotomy • Microbial culture—aerobic and anaerobic bacterial; fungal • Staining—trichrome; copper; PAS (glycogen); acid fast (mycobacterial); Congo red (amyloid) • Coagulation—before liver biopsy; PT, APTT, ACT, fibrinogen, PIVKA, and mucosal bleeding time • Abdominal effusion paracentesis—cytology; protein content; cultures

TREATMENT

APPROPRIATE HEALTH CARE
• Outpatient—except with cardiac or hepatic failure • General supportive goals—eliminate inciting cause; optimize conditions for hepatic regeneration; prevent complications; reverse derangements associated with hepatic failure (see Hepatic Failure, Acute; Hepatitis, Chronic Active; Hepatic Encephalopathy) • Important derangements—dehydration and hypovolemia; hepatic encephalopathy; hypoglycemia; acid–base and electrolyte abnormalities; coagulopathies; gastrointestinal ulcerations; sepsis; endotoxemia

NURSING CARE
• Heart failure or ascites—avoid sodium-rich fluids. • Supplement potassium chloride in maintenance fluids—20 mEq/L fluid

ACTIVITY
Restricted, cage rest while undergoing primary therapy

DIET
• Restrict dietary protein—only with hepatic encephalopathy • Well-balanced with adequate energy; positive nitrogen balance; adequate vitamins and micronutrients • Restrict sodium—with cardiac failure or liver disease that causes ascites

CLIENT EDUCATION
• Inform client that treatment depends on underlying cause. • Warn client that many causes are life-threatening, although others are less serious and amenable to treatment. • Inform client that a thorough workup is essential for attaining a definitive diagnosis.

SURGICAL CONSIDERATIONS
Indicated for EHBDO; resection of primary or focal hepatic mass lesions (neoplasia, abscess) and large cystic lesions; pericardectomy if effusion recurs after initial pericardiocentesis

MEDICATIONS

DRUGS OF CHOICE
• Cardiac causes—diuretics (e.g., furosemide) and an angiotensin-converting enzyme inhibitor (enalapril) often warranted • Infectious (e.g., bacterial) diseases—appropriate antimi-

crobial agents • Metabolic disorders—depend on underlying cause; see Hyperadrenocorticism (Cushing Disease); Hepatic Lipidosis; Storage Disorders, Glycogen; Diabetes Mellitus, Uncomplicated

CONTRAINDICATIONS
• Avoid hepatotoxic medications. • Vacuolar hepatopathy (dogs)—avoid glucocorticoids. • Hepatic lipidosis (cats)—avoid catabolism or drugs that invoke a catabolic response.

POSSIBLE INTERACTIONS N/A

ALTERNATIVE DRUGS N/A

FOLLOW-UP

PATIENT MONITORING
• Physical assessment and hepatic imaging—reassess liver size • CBC, biochemistry, TSBA—assess progression of hepatic dysfunction • Thoracic radiographs, ECG, and echocardiography—assess previous abnormalities • Pituitary–adrenal axis—with hyperadrenocorticism • Glucose profile—with diabetes • Adjust drug dosages according to status of liver function. • Reticulocyte count and CBC—with anemia

POSSIBLE COMPLICATIONS
Many causes are life-threatening.

MISCELLANEOUS

ASSOCIATED CONDITIONS N/A

AGE-RELATED FACTORS N/A

ZOONOTIC POTENTIAL N/A

PREGNANCY N/A

ABBREVIATIONS
• ALP = alkaline phosphatase • ALT = alanine aminotransferase • APTT = activated partial thromboplastin time • AST = aspartate aminotransferase • DIC = disseminated intravascular coagulation • EHBDO = extrahepatic bile duct obstruction • FeLV = feline leukemia virus • GGT = γ-glutamyltransferase • PIVKA = proteins invoked by vitamin K absence or antagonism • PT = prothrombin time • TSBA = total serum bile acids

Suggested Reading
Guilford WG, Center SA, Strombeck DR, et al. eds., Strombeck's small animal gastroenterology. 3rd ed. Philadelphia: Saunders, 1996.

Author Keith P. Richter
Consulting Editor Sharon A. Center

HOUSESOILING IN CATS, URINE

BASICS

DEFINITION
Includes inappropriate urination, characterized by simple (squat) urination on horizontal surfaces outside the litter box, and urine spraying on vertical surfaces outside the litter box

PATHOPHYSIOLOGY
• Inappropriate urination—behavior may be a normal response to dissatisfaction with litter box environment or may reflect an underlying pathophysiologic state such as a negative (pain) association with the litter box • Urine spraying—a normal marking behavior observed in feral and domestic cats; behavior may have a heritable component

SYSTEMS AFFECTED
• Behavior • Renal/urologic

SIGNALMENT
• Inappropriate urination can occur in any age, breed, or sex. • Urine spraying is more common in intact and neutered males than in females.

SIGNS

Inappropriate urination
• Acute or chronic problem • History of lower urinary disease or systemic illness may suggest an underlying medical problem. • History may suggest dissatisfaction with features of the litter box or change in environment. • Presence of abnormal physical findings depends on whether problem is pathophysiologic or behavioral.

Urine spraying
• The cat orients caudally to a vertical surface, stiffens its posture, raises and quivers its tail, and directs a small burst of urine caudally.
• The owner may detect urine marks at prominent vertical sites such as around doorways or windows or selectively sprayed on new objects brought into the house. • Spraying around doors or windows suggests a marking response to the presence of an outdoor cat. More-generalized spraying may be a response to another cat in the home. Spraying on grocery bags or new furniture suggests olfactory marking associated with arousal in response to new stimuli. Urine marking on clothing or bedding associated with specific humans or visitors may occur.

CAUSES

Medical Abnormalities Associated with Inappropriate Urination
• Diabetes mellitus • Urolithiasis • Hyperthyroidism • Iatrogenic—administration of fluids, corticosteroids, diuretics • FeLV • FIV • FIP
• Lower urinary tract disease including interstitial cystitis • Intracranial *Cuterebra* migration • Dysautonomia • Seizures

Environmental Factors Contributing to Inappropriate Urination
Litter Box Characteristics
• Soiled box; inadequate number of boxes (one box per cat is recommended) • Box located in remote or unpleasant surrounding
• Inappropriate type of box—a covered litter box may maintain odors at an offensive level or may be too small to allow large cats to move around comfortably; a covered litter box allows other cats, pet dogs, and young children to target the cat as it exits • Time factors—daily or weekly temporal patterns of inappropriate urination suggests an environmental cause; acute onset in a cat that has previously used the litter box reliably suggests a medical problem; long-term (months to years) problems have a guarded prognosis for complete resolution.
• Substrate—wrong litter type; preference tests indicate that more cats prefer unscented, fine-grained (clumping) litter; coincident change in litter box habits with new litter type suggests an association; a sudden shift from one substrate (e.g., litter) to an unusual substrate (e.g., a porcelain sink) suggests a lower urinary tract disorder • Location—urination outside the litter box may suggest a location preference or influential social factors • Social dynamics—consider any concomitant changes in the social world of the cat at the time the problem started (e.g., addition of a new cat)

Environmental Factors Contributing to Urine Spraying
• Probability of urine spraying is directly proportional to the number of cats in the household. • The presence of outdoor cats may elicit spraying around doorways and windows.

RISK FACTORS

Inappropriate Urination
• Infrequently changed litter box (or boxes)
• Frequent travel by owner

Urine Spraying
• History of urine spraying by a parent
• Multiple-cat households

DIAGNOSIS

DIFFERENTIAL DIAGNOSIS
• *Must* differentiate inappropriate urination from urine spraying • Inappropriate urination—most common behavioral cause is dissatisfaction with the litter box • Urine spraying—most common cause is urine marking in response to the presence of other cats

CBC/BIOCHEMISTRY/URINALYSIS
Usually normal when urine spraying and inappropriate urination are strictly behavioral problems; urinalysis is the minimum database in any cat examined because of inappropriate urination; collect serial samples from cats whose behavioral signs wax and wane

OTHER LABORATORY TESTS
Cats with refractory inappropriate urination or progressive signs should be tested for hyperthyroidism, FeLV, and FIV.

IMAGING
Abdominal radiographs to rule out urolithiasis as an underlying cause for inappropriate urination

DIAGNOSTIC PROCEDURES
In multicat households it may be difficult to determine which cat is responsible for inappropriate elimination. Identify the offending cat in one of two ways:
1. Isolate each cat, one at a time, in a small room to identify the culprit by process of elimination; however, this protocol may alter the social milieu enough to stop inappropriate elimination during the serial confinement.
2. Administer the dye fluorescein (fluorescein test strips or solution in a gel capsule PO) sequentially to each cat. Urine outside the litter box fluoresces under a Wood's light for approximately 24 h; if negative after 36 h, the test can be repeated on another cat. Negative results are common in households in which the frequency of spraying is low.

TREATMENT
• Treat any underlying medical condition.
• Use environmental and behavioral therapies before or with pharmacologic treatment.
• If the owner requires immediate cessation of the problem to keep the cat, it is helpful to confine it to one room in the owner's absence. Provide a litter box, water, food, and resting sites. The cat can be let out of the room when the owner returns and is available for strict supervision of the cat. Initiate other, more permanent treatments.

Inappropriate Urination
Environmental Management Techniques
• Scoop out the litter box daily and clean thoroughly weekly. • Avoid deodorizers or other strong odors in the vicinity of the litter box. • Provide at least one litter box per cat, distributed in more than one location, and avoid high traffic or noisy areas. • Move food bowls away from the litter box. • If the litter box is covered, provide an additional large, plain, uncovered litter box filled with unscented, fine-grained, clumping litter, with no liner. • If one site in the home is preferred for inappropriate urination, place another litter box over this site. After it is in regular use, move it several inches a day to a site more acceptable to the owner. • If numerous sites outside the litter box are used, use tactile (e.g., aluminum foil, plastic drop clothes) or olfactory (e.g., citrus odor eliminator or mothballs) deterrents at those sites.

Behavior Modification

• Some owners have sufficient patience to monitor the cat and take it to the litter box at an appropriate time (e.g., first thing in the morning). The cat is then rewarded with a favored treat for using the litter box. • Punishment (e.g., a water pistol or sound alarm) is only effective if initiated at the start of the behavior sequence. Punishment associated with sounds or movements by the owner will condition the cat to avoid the owner. • Feeding or playing with the cat at inappropriate elimination sites may countercondition the unacceptable behavior.

Urine Spraying

• Neuter intact animals—this curbs spraying behavior in up to 90% of males and 95% of females • If there are signs that the cat is spraying in response to cats outside, prevent visual or olfactory access to those cats. A new environmental product (Feliway, Abbott Labs), a concentrate of synthesized feline facial pheromone, is now commercially available as a treatment for urine marking. The product is sprayed regularly in the environment at sites of urine spraying and other prominent locations in the environment. Although data from blinded clinical trials are not yet available, the product shows promise in decreasing arousal and the incidence of urine spraying in some cases. • To focus the affected cat's attention away from other cats, the owner should spend time interacting with the cat daily. • Pharmacotherapy plays an important role in the control of urine spraying.

MEDICATIONS

DRUGS OF CHOICE

Inappropriate Urination

Usually are not indicated, except in cases of generalized anxiety

Urine Spraying

Drugs from a number of drug classes may be used. All have the general effect of decreasing arousal and anxiety. Side Effects can be sedation and/or altered social behavior. (See Appendix VIII-Formulary). Options are listed in Table 1.

Table 1

CONTRAINDICATIONS

• Benzodiazepines in cats with hepatic disease, because of the potential for fatal idiopathic hepatic necrosis • Tricyclic antidepressants in cats with a history of cardiac conduction disturbances, megacolon, lower urinary tract blockages, and glaucoma

PRECAUTIONS

• All drugs listed are used in an extra-label fashion. Explain to the client the experimental nature of these treatments and common side effects; document the discussion by a notation in the medical record or use a release form. Start using psychotropic drugs when the owner is present to monitor the patient. • Some psychotropic drugs have human abuse potential. Dispense not more than a 4-week supply, with refills available. • Benzodiazepines rarely cause idiopathic hepatic necrosis in apparently healthy cats. Use tricyclic antidepressants with caution in patients with urinary or fecal retention.

POSSIBLE INTERACTIONS

• Benzodiazepine drugs can interact with cimetidine. • Do not use monoamine oxidase inhibitors (including amitraz) concurrently with tricyclic antidepressants or selective serotonin reuptake inhibitors.

ALTERNATIVE DRUGS

Synthetic progestins—the risk of serious side effects, including blood dyscrasias, pyometra, mammary hyperplasia, mammary carcinoma, diabetes mellitus, and obesity, has diminished their once-common use; dosage: 5 mg q24h 1–2 weeks, then taper gradually to 2.5 mg 2×/week.

FOLLOW-UP

PATIENT MONITORING

The owner should keep a daily log of elimination pattern so that treatment success can be evaluated and appropriate adjustments in therapy can be made.

POSSIBLE COMPLICATIONS

Client expectations must be realistic. Immediate control of a longstanding problem

of housesoiling is unlikely; the goal is gradual improvement over time. Treatment failure may result in the cat being euthanized, dropped at an animal shelter, or released outside.

MISCELLANEOUS

ASSOCIATED CONDITIONS

N/A

AGE-RELATED FACTORS

N/A

ZOONOTIC POTENTIAL

Pregnant women should not clean up cat urine because of the risk of toxoplasmosis.

PREGNANCY

Tricyclic antidepressants are contraindicated in pregnant animals.

SYNONYMS

Feline inappropriate elimination (FIE), feline housesoiling, squat urination, urination outside the litter box, urine marking, urine spraying

SEE ALSO

N/A

ABBREVIATIONS

• FeLV = feline leukemia virus • FIE = feline inappropriate elimination • FIP = feline infectious peritonitis • FIV = feline immunodeficiency virus

Suggested Reading

Cooper LL. Feline inappropriate elimination. Vet Clin North Am (Small Anim Pract) 1997;27(3):569–600.
Overall KL. Treating feline elimination disorders. Vet Med 1998;93:367–382.
Simpson BS, Simpson DM. Behavioral pharmacotherapy. In: Voith VL, Borchelt PL, eds. Readings in companion animal behavior. Trenton, NJ: Veterinary Learning Systems, 1996:100–115.
Author Barbara S. Simpson
Consulting Editor Larry G. Adams and Carl A. Osborne

Drugs and Dosages Used to Manage Feline Urine Housesoiling				
Drug Class	Drug	Dosage in Cats (mg/cat; PO)	Frequency	Latency to Effect
Benzodiazepine	Diazepam	1–2	q12h	Immediate
Benzodiazepine	Alprazolam	0.125–0.25	q12h	Immediate
Azaperone	Buspirone	5–7.5	q12h	3 weeks
Tricyclic antidepressant	Amitriptyline	2.5–7.5	q12–24h	3–4 weeks
Tricyclic antidepressant	Clomipramine	1–2.5	q12–24h	3–4 weeks
Selective serotonin reuptake inhibitor	Fluoxetine	1–5	q24h	3–4 weeks

HYPOTHERMIA

 BASICS

DEFINITION
• Body temperature below normal in a homothermic organism
• Mild hypothermia—90–99°F (32–35°C)
• Moderate hypothermia—82–90°F (28–32°C)
• Severe hypothermia—any temperature < 82°F (28°C)

PATHOPHYSIOLOGY
• The hypothalamus regulates body temperature in response to changes in blood and skin temperature. Animals conserve heat by behavioral responses and physiologic responses (e.g., peripheral vasoconstriction to reduce heat loss to the environment, and piloerection to trap a layer of air next to the skin to provide thermal insulation. Active heat production—increased cardiac output, metabolic rate, and muscle activity (i.e., shivering).
• Thermoregulatory responses may be inadequate in neonates, geriatric animals, and hypothyroid or anesthetized animals. During prolonged exposure to cold, thermal homeostasis may fail, even in healthy animals.
• Hypothermia causes CNS depression. Peripheral vasoconstriction and fluid shifts increase blood viscosity and reduce cardiac output. Severe hypothermia is associated with hypotension. Reduced respiratory rate and depth leads to hypercapnia and respiratory acidosis. Fluid shifts into the alveoli affect alveolar gas exchange, resulting in hypoxemia. Increased hemoglobin affinity for oxygen causes reduced oxyhemoglobin unloading at the tissue level. Reduction of cellular metabolism may have a protective effect in animals with severe hypothermia.

SYSTEMS AFFECTED
• Nervous—impaired consciousness ranging from obtundation to coma
• Cardiovascular—arrhythmias, conduction disturbances, changes in vasomotor tone, hypotension, and low cardiac output
• Respiratory—respiratory depression, respiratory acidosis, and hypoxemia
• Hemic/Lymph/Immune—reversible platelet and coagulation factor dysfunction and disseminated intravascular coagulation (DIC)

SIGNALMENT
• Any animal exposed to severe cold
• Most common—small animals with a predisposition to surface heat loss, neonates, and geriatric, cachectic, and hypothyroid animals with impaired response mechanisms, low body fat and glycogen stores or reduced metabolic rates

SIGNS

Historical Findings
• Known prolonged exposure to cold ambient temperatures
• Possibly, disappearance from home or a history of trauma
• Cold, unresponsive animal

Physical Examination Findings
Mild hypothermia (90–99°F)
• Mental depression
• Lethargy
• Weakness
• Shivering
Moderate hypothermia (82–90°F)
• Muscle stiffness
• Bradycardia
• Hypotension
• Reduced respiratory rate and depth
• Stupor/obtundation
Severe hypothermia (< 82°F)
• Inaudible heart sounds
• Difficulty breathing
• Coma
• Fixed and dilated pupils

CAUSES
• Cold ambient temperature
• Impaired thermoregulation (e.g., neonates, geriatrics, animals with hypothyroidism or hypothalamic disease)
• Impaired behavioral responses—as seen in neonates, sick, debilitated, or injured animals)
• Predisposition to surface heat loss—as in neonates and small animals
• Inadequate heat generation—as in neonates and cachectic and hypothyroid animals

RISK FACTORS
• Hypothyroidism
• Hypothalamic disease
• Very young or old age

 DIAGNOSIS

DIFFERENTIAL DIAGNOSIS

Differentiating Similar Signs
Must differentiate from death in animals with severe hypothermia

Differentiating Causes
• Must differentiate from other causes of CNS depression, including primary CNS disease, metabolic disorders, such as hypoglycemia and hepatic encephalopathy, electrolyte disturbances, systemic infection, and neoplasia
• Must differentiate from other causes of bradycardia and cardiac arrhythmias, such as primary cardiac disease, hyperthyroidism in cats, and anesthetic or sedative agents

CBC/BIOCHEMISTRY/URINALYSIS
• Usually normal
• Mild hemoconcentration and hyperglycemia in some animals

OTHER LABORATORY TESTS
• Platelet count and coagulation panel may reveal thrombocytopenia and prolongation of activated partial thromboplastin and prothrombin times.
• Thyroid hormone evaluation may confirm underlying hypothyroidism.

IMAGING
N/A

DIAGNOSTIC PROCEDURES
Rectal or esophageal probes or low recording thermometers may be useful for monitoring body temperatures below 93°F in patients with severe hypothermia.

Electrocardiography
• Sinus bradycardia with lengthening of PR, QRS, and QT intervals
• Atrial arrhythmias initially in some patients
• Ventricular arrhythmias (e.g., ventricular premature complex and ventricular tachycardia) occur as body temperature decreases further.
• Ventricular fibrillation likely at body temperatures < 82°F.

 ## TREATMENT
• Treat most as inpatients until normothermia is reached.
• Minimize movement to prevent lethal cardiac arrhythmias, especially in patients with severe hypothermia.
• Anticipate further decline in body temperature during initial rewarming, because of contact of warmer "core" blood with the colder surface of the body.
• Aim to support vital organ systems, rewarm the patient, and prevent further heat loss.
• Airway management and oxygen supplementation are essential; ventilatory support may be required in animals with severe hypothermia.
• Mild hypothermia—use passive rewarming techniques, including thermal insulation with blankets.
• Mild hypothermia—use active external rewarming with heat sources such as heating pads and radiant heat; apply heat to the trunk to rewarm the body's "core" without causing peripheral vasodilation in the limbs; provide a protective layer between the heat source and the patient's skin.

• Severe hypothermia—use core rewarming techniques, including warm water gastric and peritoneal lavage, warm water enemas, warm IV fluid administration, and airway rewarming (using warmed air).

 ## MEDICATIONS

DRUGS OF CHOICE
• Oxygen supplementation may be provided via a face mask or endotracheal tube.
• Blood volume support—essential; most isotonic, balanced electrolyte solutions can be used.
• Fluid solutions should be warm to prevent additional heat loss.
• Fluid supplementation with dextrose may be helpful.

CONTRAINDICATIONS
• Severe hypothermia—avoid lactated Ringer's solution because of impaired hepatic metabolism of lactate.
• At temperatures < 82°F the heart is refractory to atropine and antiarrhythmic agents.

PRECAUTIONS
N/A

POSSIBLE INTERACTIONS
N/A

ALTERNATIVE DRUGS
N/A

 ## FOLLOW-UP

PATIENT MONITORING
• Core body temperature during rewarming
• ECG and blood pressure to assess cardiovascular status during rewarming

POSSIBLE COMPLICATIONS
• Peripheral vasodilation during rewarming may further drop body temperature.
• Return of cool peripheral blood to the heart may precipitate cardiac arrhythmias.
• Severe hypothermia may cause cardiac arrest.

✓ MISCELLANEOUS

ASSOCIATED CONDITIONS
N/A

AGE-RELATED FACTORS
Sick or hypoglycemic neonates can become markedly hypothermic in normal environments; treatment may extend to long-term management of ambient temperature of environment.

ZOONOTIC POTENTIAL
N/A

PREGNANCY
N/A

SYNONYMS
None

SEE ALSO
Shock, Cardiogenic

ABBREVIATIONS
DIC = disseminated intravascular coagulation

Suggested Reading
Dhupa N. Hypothermia in dogs and cats. Compend Contin Educ Pract Vet 1995;17:61–69.
Murtaugh RJ, Kaplan PM. Hypothermia. In: Veterinary and emergency critical care medicine. Philadelphia: Mosby Year Book, 1992:199–200.

Author Nishi Dhupa
Consulting Editors Larry P. Tilley and Francis W. K. Smith, Jr.

INCONTINENCE, FECAL

BASICS

DEFINITION
Inability to retain feces, resulting in involuntary passage of fecal material

PATHOPHYSIOLOGY
• Reservoir fecal incontinence develops when disease processes reduce the capacity or compliance of the rectum.
• Sphincter incontinence develops when the external anal sphincter is anatomically disrupted (i.e. nonneurogenic sphincter incontinence) or denervated (i.e. neurogenic sphincter incontinence).
• Neurogenic sphincter incontinence can be caused by pudendal nerve damage, sacral spinal cord disease, autonomic dysfunction, and generalized peripheral neuropathy or myopathy.
• Damage to, or degeneration of, the levator ani and coccygeus muscles may also contribute.

SYSTEMS AFFECTED
• Nervous
• Gastrointestinal

SIGNALMENT
• Dogs and cats
• Although any age animal may be affected, incidence increases in older patients.

SIGNS

Historical Findings
• Reservoir incontinence—promotes an urge to defecate; signs include frequent, conscious defecation without dribbling of feces; defecation may be associated with tenesmus, dyschezia, or hematochezia.
• Sphincter incontinence—associated with involuntary expulsion or dribbling of fecal material, especially during excitement or barking and coughing
• Question clients about previous neurologic disease, anorectal surgery and/or trauma, house training, deworming, and whether the pet seems to defecate voluntarily or involuntarily; also obtain information regarding the pet's diet, current medications, and concurrent systemic clinical signs, especially neurologic signs.
• Concurrent urinary incontinence suggests neurogenic sphincter incontinence.

Physical Examination Findings
• Reservoir incontinence—may include anorectal sensitivity or pain on digital palpation, a rectal mass or thickening of the rectal mucosa; external anal sphincter tone and nonneurogenic sphincter incontinence anal reflex are normal.
• Nonneurogenic sphincter incontinence—may include evidence of perineal trauma or perianal fistulas; the anal reflex is present, but the external anal sphincter may not completely close if the sphincter has been anatomically disrupted.
• Neurogenic sphincter incontinence—may include loss of tone to the external anal sphincter, but anal tone is a poor indicator of anal sphincter function; the anal reflex is absent or diminished.
• Do a complete neurologic examination on all animals with sphincter incontinence; additional findings suggesting lumbosacral spinal cord disease include loss of voluntary movement and tone to the tail, lumbosacral pain, flaccid posterior paresis or paralysis, and hyporeflexic myotatic reflexes to the pelvic limbs.
• Diffuse lower motor neuron signs suggest generalized peripheral neuropathy or myopathy; upper motor neuron signs to the pelvic limbs suggest CNS disease cranial to the lumbosacral plexus.

CAUSES

Reservoir Incontinence
• Colorectal disease—colitis and neoplasia
• Diarrhea—large volumes of feces from any cause can overwhelm the absorptive and storage capacity of the colon.

Nonneurogenic Sphincter Incontinence
• Traumatic anal injuries—bite wounds, laceration, or gunshot
• Iatrogenic—the external anal sphincter and levator ani muscles can be anatomically disrupted during anorectal surgery.
• Perianal fistulas

Neurogenic Sphincter Incontinence
• CNS—degenerative myelopathy, spinal dysraphism, spina bifida, trauma, intervertebral disk extrusion, neoplasia, meningomyelitis (various causes), fibrocartilaginous embolism, other vascular compromises
• Cauda equina syndrome—L6-L7 or L7-S1 intervertebral disk extrusion, spondylosis deformans, congenital spinal canal stenosis, lumbosacral instability, diskospondylitis, and neoplasia
• Peripheral neuropathy—infectious, immune-mediated, drug-induced (e.g., vincristine sulfate), dysautonomia, and idiopathic
• Myopathy/neuromuscular disorder
• Degeneration (aging)—multiple factors are likely involved, including atrophy of the muscles involved in fecal continence, weakness, degenerative neuropathy, and senility.

RISK FACTORS
• Anorectal disease and surgery
• CNS disease and peripheral neuropathy

DIAGNOSIS

DIFFERENTIAL DIAGNOSIS
• Gastrointestinal disease from any cause can increase the urge to defecate without directly altering the reservoir capacity of the colon.
• Unlike sphincter incontinence, gastrointestinal disease is often associated with weight loss, vomiting, tenesmus, dyschezia, and hematochezia.
• Behavior disorders (e.g., separation anxiety), unlike fecal incontinence, are often associated with destructive activities or excessive vocalization.
• Inadequate house training usually occurs in young dogs or dogs recently introduced to an indoor environment.

CBC/BIOCHEMISTRY/URINALYSIS
• Results usually normal
• Urinalysis may show evidence of lower urinary tract infection (e.g., pyuria, hematuria), especially with concurrent urinary incontinence.

OTHER LABORATORY TESTS
Perform fecal flotation to help rule out parasitism as a cause of diarrhea.

IMAGING
• Lateral and ventrodorsal survey radiography of the lumbosacral spine may show evidence of intervertebral disk extrusion, diskospondylitis, vertebral neoplasia, spina bifida, lumbosacral trauma, or vertebral malformation.
• Myelography and epidurography are also useful in demonstrating compressive lesions within the spinal canal.
• CT and MRI may be necessary to demonstrate some compressive lesions and intraparenchymal spinal cord lesions.

INCONTINENCE, FECAL

OTHER DIAGNOSTIC PROCEDURES

• Electromyography (EMG) to evaluate external anal sphincter, levator ani, and coccygeus muscles for evidence of denervation or myopathy
• Evaluation of other muscles recommended to help localize the neurologic lesion—diffuse denervation versus focal spinal cord lesion
• Can evaluate the pudendal-anal reflex electrophysiologically
• Muscle and nerve biopsy for myopathy and peripheral neuropathy
• Analysis of cerebrospinal fluid (CSF) collected by lumbar puncture may reveal evidence of a CNS infectious or inflammatory process, neoplasia, or trauma.
• Perform colonoscopy and colorectal mucosal biopsy if reservoir incontinence is suspected.

TREATMENT

• If possible, identify the underlying cause; fecal incontinence may resolve if the underlying cause is successfully treated (e.g., spinal cord decompression).
• Dietary—fecal volume can be reduced by feeding low-residue diets such as cottage cheese and rice and/or tofu.
• Frequent warm water enemas will diminish the volume of feces in the colon and thus decrease the incidence of inappropriate defecation.
• Environmental changes (e.g., making the pet an outside pet) may increase client satisfaction and thus avoid euthanasia of an otherwise healthy animal.
• Reflex defecation can sometimes be induced in animals with posterior paralysis (e.g., a mild pinch of the toe on a pelvic limb or tail); similarly, applying a warm washcloth to the anus or perineum may stimulate defecation.
• Surgical reconstruction of anorectal lesions may markedly improve fecal continence in patients with nonneurogenic sphincter incontinence.
• Fascial slings and silicone elastomer slings have met with variable success in treating neurogenic sphincter incontinence in dogs.
• Prognosis is poor if the underlying cause cannot be identified and successfully corrected; discuss the prognosis with the client early in the evaluation, to avoid unrealistic expectations.

MEDICATIONS

DRUGS OF CHOICE

• Opiate motility-modifying drugs (e.g., diphenoxylate hydrochloride and loperamide hydrochloride) increase segmental contraction of the bowel and slow passage of fecal material, thus increasing the amount of water absorbed from the feces.
• Anti-inflammatory agents, such as glucocorticoids and sulfasalazine, may benefit patients with suspected reservoir incontinence due to inflammatory bowel disease.

CONTRAINDICATIONS

• Do not use motility-modifying drugs in patients with diarrhea if an infectious or toxic cause is suspected.
• Do not use opiate motility-modifiers in patients with respiratory disease; use cautiously in patients with liver disease.
• Use of opiates in cats is generally not recommended.

PRECAUTIONS

• Motility-modifying drugs may cause constipation and bloat.
• Opiate motility-modifying drugs may cause sedation.

POSSIBLE INTERACTIONS

Increased sedation and respiratory depression are possible when opiates are used concurrently with other CNS depressants (e.g., barbiturates, general anesthetics, and tranquilizers).

ALTERNATIVE DRUGS

N/A

FOLLOW-UP

PATIENT MONITORING

• If fecal incontinence is due to an underlying neurologic cause, use serial neurologic examinations to monitor patient progress.
• Radiographic procedures, EMG, CSF analysis, and electrodiagnostic studies can also be used to follow progress.
• Check fecal consistency and volume.
• Adjust diet and motility-modifying drug dosages to find the appropriate therapy for each individual patient.

POSSIBLE COMPLICATIONS

• Neurogenic sphincter incontinence is often unresponsive despite appropriate dietary, medical, and surgical treatment.
• Fifty percent of pets with fecal incontinence were euthanatized in one recent study.

MISCELLANEOUS

ASSOCIATED CONDITIONS

N/A

AGE-RELATED FACTORS

N/A

ZOONOTIC POTENTIAL

• Exposure to animal feces increases the risk of exposure to zoonotic parasites.
• Advise clients about zoonotic diseases (e.g., cutaneous and visceral larval migrans and toxoplasmosis).

PREGNANCY

N/A

SYNONYMS

N/A

SEE ALSO

• Incontinence, Urinary
• Intervertebral Disk Disease

ABBREVIATIONS

CSF = cerebrospinal fluid
CT = computed tomography
EMG = electromyography
MRI = magnetic resonance imaging

Suggested Reading

Guilford WG. Fecal incontinence in dogs and cats. Compend Contin Educ Pract Vet 1990;12:313–326.
Richter KP. Diseases of the rectum and anus. In: Kirk's current veterinary therapy XI. Philadelphia: Saunders, 1992:615–616.
Washabau RJ, Brockman DJ. Recto-anal disease. In: Ettinger SJ, Feldman EC, eds., Textbook of veterinary internal medicine. 4th ed. Philadelphia: Saunders, 1995:1408–1409.

Author Randall C. Longshore
Consulting Editors Brett M. Feder and Mitchell A. Crystal

INCONTINENCE, URINARY

 BASICS

DEFINITION
Loss of voluntary control of micturition, usually observed as involuntary urine leakage

PATHOPHYSIOLOGY
Usually a disorder of the storage phase of micturition. Urine storage failure is caused by failure of urinary bladder accommodation, failure of urethral continence mechanisms, or anatomic bypass of urinary storage structures. Partial outlet obstruction and other causes of urinary bladder overdistension may result in paradoxical, or overflow, urinary incontinence.

SYSTEMS AFFECTED
• Renal/Urologic
• Nervous
• Skin/Exocrine—urine scald and perineal and ventral dermatitis

SIGNALMENT
• Dogs and cats
• Most common in middle-aged to old, neutered female dogs; also observed in juvenile females and (rarely) neutered males
• Medium to large-breed dogs most often affected

SIGNS
N/A

CAUSES

Neurologic
• Disruption of local neuroreceptors, peripheral nerves, spinal pathways, or higher centers involved in the control of micturition can disrupt urine storage.
• Lesions of the sacral spinal cord, such as a congenital malformation, cauda equina compression, lumbosacral disk disease, or traumatic fractures or dislocation can result in a flaccid, overdistended urinary bladder with weak outlet resistance. Urine retention and overflow incontinence develop.
• Lesions of the cerebellum or cerebral micturition center affect inhibition and voluntary control of voiding, usually resulting in frequent, involuntary urination or leakage of small volumes of urine.

Urinary Bladder Storage Dysfunction
• Poor accommodation of urine during storage or urinary bladder hypercontractility leads to frequent leakage of small amounts of urine.
• Urinary tract infection, chronic inflammatory disorder, infiltrative neoplastic lesion, external compression, and chronic partial outlet obstruction

• Congenital urinary bladder hypoplasia may accompany ectopic ureters or other developmental disorders of the urogenital tract.
• Idiopathic detrusor instability has been associated with FeLV infection in cats and unknown causes in dogs.

Urethral Disorders
• If urethral closure provided by urethral smooth muscle, striated muscle, and connective tissue does not prevent leakage of urine during storage, intermittent urinary incontinence is observed.
• Examples—congenital urethral hypoplasia or incompetence, acquired urethral incompetence (i.e., reproductive hormone-responsive urinary incontinence), urinary tract infection or inflammation, prostatic disease or prostatic surgery (males), and vestibulovaginal anomaly (females)

Anatomic
• Developmental or acquired anatomic abnormalities that divert urine from normal storage mechanisms or interfere with urinary bladder or urethral function
• Ectopic ureters can terminate in the distal urethra, uterus, or vagina.
• Patent urachal remnants divert urine outflow to the umbilicus.
• Vestibulovaginal anomalies, congenital urocystic hypoplasia, or urethral hypoplasia

Urine Retention
Observed when intravesicular pressure exceeds outlet resistance

Mixed Urinary Incontinence
Mixed or multiple causes are observed in humans and probably occur in dogs and cats. Combinations of urethral and bladder storage dysfunction and combinations of anatomic and functional disorders are most likely.

RISK FACTORS
• Neutering increases the risk of development of urethral incompetence.
• Conformational characteristics such as bladder neck position, urethral length, and concurrent vaginal anomalies may increase the risk of urinary incontinence in female dogs.
• Obesity may increase the risk of urinary incontinence in neutered female dogs.

 DIAGNOSIS

DIFFERENTIAL DIAGNOSIS

Differentiating Similar Signs
• Voluntary but inappropriate urination

• Urethral discharges, often associated with prostatic disease in male dogs and vaginal disorders in female dogs
• Urine spraying in cats can be confused with urinary incontinence or inappropriate urination; spraying is more likely to be done by cats in an upright position, with urine soiling found on vertical surfaces of furniture, walls, and drapes.

Differentiating Causes
• Polyuria—may precipitate or exacerbate urinary incontinence or lead to nocturia and inappropriate urination; measure urine specific gravity in a random urine sample to rule in or out clinically important polyuria.
• Neurogenic causes of urinary incontinence—usually cause a large, distended urinary bladder and other neurologic deficits such as weak anal or tail tone, depressed perineal sensation, and proprioceptive deficits
• Dogs with urethral incompetence typically exhibit intermittent occurrences of urinary incontinence, observed most often at night or while the animal is sleeping. Physical examination reveals a small urinary bladder and no other defects.
• Historical and physical findings in patients with urinary bladder storage dysfunction resemble those observed in patients with urethral incompetence, although increased frequency of urination may be an additional clinical sign.
• Anisocoria is found frequently in cats with urinary incontinence associated with FeLV infection.
• Historical signs in male dogs with prostatic disease include tenesmus, hind limb weakness, dysuria, and pollakiuria. Physical findings include prostatomegaly, lumbosacral pain, pain on prostatic palpation, and hind limb trembling or weakness.

CBC/BIOCHEMISTRY/URINALYSIS
• Hematologic and biochemical analyses may be indicated in patients with polyuric disorders (see Polyuria and Polydipsia).
• Urinalysis may reveal evidence of urinary tract infection (e.g., pyuria, hematuria, and bacteria) or polyuria (e.g. low urine specific gravity).

OTHER LABORATORY TESTS
Test cats for FeLV infection.

IMAGING

Radiographic Findings
• Contrast radiography indicated in juvenile animals and animals exhibiting urinary incontinence shortly after surgical procedures or traumatic incidents

• Excretory urography allows visualization of the kidneys, ureteral terminations, and urinary bladder.

• Retrograde vaginourethrography allows visualization of the vaginal vault, urethra, and urinary bladder. Ectopic ureters usually fill with contrast media in these retrograde studies as well.

• Double-contrast cystography may be required for full visualization of urinary bladder structure and identification of urinary bladder lesions.

Ultrasonographic Findings

Can use evaluation of the kidneys and urinary bladder to identify uroliths, masses, hydronephrosis or hydroureter, or evidence of pyelonephritis

DIAGNOSTIC PROCEDURES

• Neurologic examination—examination of anal tone, tail tone, perineal sensation, and bulbospongiosus reflexes provides a brief assessment of caudal spinal and peripheral nerve function

• Urethral catheterization—may be required to assess patency of the urethra if urine retention is observed

• Urodynamic procedures—consider cystometrography, urethral pressure profilometry, and electromyography to evaluate urinary bladder, urethral, and neurologic function more objectively.

TREATMENT

• Usually as outpatient

• Address partial obstructive disorders and primary neurologic disorders specifically if possible.

• Identify urinary tract infection and treat appropriately.

• Ectopic ureters and congenital urethral hypoplasia can be surgically corrected; functional abnormalities of urethral competence or urinary bladder storage function may accompany the anatomic disorder and require ancillary medical treatment.

• Surgical procedures such as colposuspension, cystourethropexy, Teflon or collagen implants, and prosthetic sphincter implantation have been described for the treatment of refractory incontinence.

MEDICATIONS

DRUGS OF CHOICE

Urethral Incompetence

• Manage with reproductive hormones (e.g., stilbestrol, diethylstilbestrol, conjugated estrogens, estriol, and testosterone) or α-adrenergic agonists (e.g., phenylpropanolamine, phenylephrine, pseudoephedrine).

• α-Adrenergic agents and reproductive hormones can be administered in combination for a synergistic therapeutic effect.

• Imipramine, a tricyclic antidepressant with anticholinergic and α-agonist actions, provides an alternative method of treatment.

Detrusor Instability

Manage with anticholinergic or antispasmodic agents (e.g., oxybutynin, propantheline, imipramine, flavoxate, and dicyclomine).

Prostatic Disease

See Prostatomegaly, Prostatitis, and Prostatic Abscesses.

CONTRAINDICATIONS

• Adrenergic agonists in patients with cardiac disease, renal disease, and hypertensive disorders

• Anticholinergic agents in patients with glaucoma or cardiac disease

PRECAUTIONS

• Estrogen compounds (rarely) cause signs of estrus, bone marrow suppression, and exacerbate immune-mediated disease.

• Testosterone administration can cause signs of aggression or libido, exacerbate prostatic disease, and contribute to the development of perineal hernia or perianal adenoma.

• Adrenergic agonists can cause restlessness, tachycardia, and hypertension.

• Anticholinergic agents can cause nausea, vomiting, and constipation.

POSSIBLE INTERACTIONS
N/A

ALTERNATIVE DRUGS
N/A

FOLLOW-UP

PATIENT MONITORING

• Patients receiving α-adrenergic agents—observe during the initial treatment period for adverse effects of the drug including tachycardia, anxiety, and hypertension.

• Patients receiving estrogen—periodic hemogram

• Periodic urinalysis

• Expect excellent response to medical treatment in 60–90% of treated patients.

• Once a therapeutic effect has been observed, slowly reduce the dosage and frequency of administration of pharmacologic agents to the minimum required.

POSSIBLE COMPLICATIONS

• Recurrent and ascending urinary tract infection

• Urine scald and perineal and ventral dermatitis

• Refractory and unmanageable incontinence

MISCELLANEOUS

ASSOCIATED CONDITIONS
Urinary tract infection

AGE-RELATED FACTORS
See Signalment.

ZOONOTIC POTENTIAL
N/A

PREGNANCY
Although urinary incontinence is rare in pregnant animals, the use of estrogens or anticholinergic agents is not advised.

SYNONYMS
Enuresis

SEE ALSO
• Polyuria and Polydipsia
• Prostatitis and prostatic abscess
• Urinary Tract Obstruction
• Urine Retention, Functional

ABBREVIATION
FeLV = feline leukemia virus

Suggested Reading

Arnold S. Relationship of incontinence to neutering. In: Kirk RW, Bonagura J, eds., Current veterinary therapy XI. Philadelphia: Saunders, 1992:875–877.

Holt PE. Pathophysiology and treatment of urethral sphincter mechanism incompetence in the incontinent bitch. Vet Int 1992;3:15.

Lane IF, Barsanti JA. Urinary incontinence. In: August J. ed., Consultations in feline internal medicine. 2nd ed., Philadelphia: Saunders, 1994:373–382.

Moreau PM, Lappin MR. Pharmacologic manipulation of micturition. In: Kirk RW, ed., Current veterinary therapy X. Philadelphia: Saunders, 1989:1214–1222.

Richter K. Use of urodynamics in micturition disorders in dogs and cats. In: Kirk RW, ed., Current veterinary therapy X. Philadelphia, Saunders, 1989:1145–1150.

Author India F. Lane

Consulting Editors Larry G. Adams and Carl A. Osborne.

INFERTILITY, FEMALE

BASICS

DEFINITION
Historical complaint that occurs in bitches showing abnormal cycling, copulation failure, conception failure, or pregnancy loss

PATHOPHYSIOLOGY
• Normal fertility—requires normal estrus cycling with ovulation of normal ova into a patent, healthy reproductive tract; fertilization by normal spermatozoa; implantation of the conceptus into the endometrium; formation of the normal zonary placenta; and maintenance of pregnancy in the presence of high progesterone concentration throughout the approximately 2-month gestation
• Breakdown in any of the processes causes infertility.

SYSTEMS AFFECTED
Reproductive

SIGNALMENT
• Animals of all ages; may be more common in old animals
• Dogs > 6 years old—more likely to have underlying cystic endometrial hyperplasia; may be predisposed to uterine infection and failure of conception or implantation
• Dog breeds predisposed to thyroid insufficiency—may have a higher prevalence; golden retrievers, Doberman pinschers, dachshunds, Irish setters, miniature schnauzers, Great Danes, poodles, and boxers

SIGNS

Historical Findings
• Failure to cycle
• Failure to copulate
• Normal copulation with no subsequent pregnancy or parturition

Physical Examination Findings
Positive pregnancy with no subsequent parturition

CAUSES
Animals acquired when already mature—possibility of previous ovariohysterectomy

Dogs
• Insemination at the improper time in the estrous cycle—most common
• Subclinical uterine infection
• Male infertility factors
• Thyroid insufficiency

• Hypercortisolism
• Anatomic abnormality
• Chromosomal abnormality
• Abnormal ovarian function
• *Brucella canis*—always a possibility

Cats
• Similar to those of dogs
• Lack of sufficient copulatory stimulus to induce ovulation
• Systemic viral or protozoal infection

RISK FACTORS
• *B. canis* (dogs)
• Thyroid insufficiency (dogs)
• Hypercortisolism (dogs and cats)—endogenous or exogenous
• Systemic viral infection (dogs and cats)—canine herpesvirus; FeLV; FIV
• Systemic protozoal infection (dogs and cats)—toxoplasmosis
• Any chronic, debilitating disease condition (dogs and cats)
• Congenital vaginal anomaly (dogs and cats)

DIAGNOSIS

DIFFERENTIAL DIAGNOSIS

Historical Information
• Extremely useful in distinguishing causes
• Is the patient cycling?
• Has the patient conceived or given birth in the past? If so, how recently? What was the litter size? What percentage of the litter was weaned?
• Is the patient free of systemic viral or protozoal infection?
• Is the patient capable of normal copulation?
• Was the patient bred to a male of proven fertility at the proper time of the estrous cycle?
• Did the patient ovulate during the estrous cycle and maintain progesterone concentration consistent with pregnancy during the entire gestation?
• Is the bitch euthyroid?

CBC/BIOCHEMISTRY/URINALYSIS
Usually normal

OTHER LABORATORY TESTS

Serologic Test for B. canis (Dogs)
• Rapid slide agglutination test—used as a screen
• Sensitive but not specific
• Positive results—recommend recheck by an agar gel immunodiffusion test (Cornell University Diagnostic Laboratory, 607-253-3900) or bacterial culture of whole blood or lymph node aspirate

Serum Progesterone Measurement
• Should remain high throughout gestation
• May measure at the time of examination
• Concentration < 2 ng/mL in midgestation and pregnancy loss occurs, insufficient luteal function indicated (Hypoluteodism). (See Abortion—Dogs)
• Concentration > 2 ng/mL—may indicate silent heat; estrus with no overt behavioral or physical changes; or pathologic production of progesterone from a luteal ovarian structure, functional ovarian neoplasm, or the adrenal gland
Dogs
• May be measured during proestrus and estrus to predict ovulation time and optimize breeding management
• Concentration and ovulation—1.0–1.9 ng/mL, ovulation in 3 days; 2.0–2.9 ng/mL, ovulation in 2 days; 3.0–3.9 ng/mL, ovulation in 1 day; 4.0–10.0 ng/mL, ovulation that day
• Optimal breeding day for maximum litter size—2 days after ovulation
• Day of ovulation—extremely variable; not well correlated with standing behavior (see Breeding, Timing)
Cats
• May be measured after breeding to assess induction of ovulation
• Concentration > 2 ng/mL—indicates functional luteal tissue

Other
• Bacterial culture for uterine organisms (dogs and cats)—vaginal discharge originating in the uterus during proestrus or estrus collected directly by hysterotomy or indirectly from the anterior vagina by a guarded swab
• Thyroid hormone testing (dogs)—may measure resting serum concentration of T_3 or T_4; may measure T_4 after challenge with TSH to assess insufficiency
• Serologic testing—canine herpesvirus and toxoplasmosis (see Abortion, Spontaneous [Pregnancy Loss]—Dogs); FeLV, FIV, and toxoplasmosis (see Abortion, Spontaneous [Pregnancy Loss]—Cats)
• Karyotype (dogs and cats)—performed on heparinized blood samples of patients with primary or persistent anestrus; look for chromosomal abnormalities that can cause abnormal sexual differentiation (University of Minnesota Cytogenetics Laboratory, 612-624-3067; see Sexual Development Disorders)
• Serum cortisol assay (dogs and cats)—if the resting serum concentration is high, investigate the underlying cause.

• Semen evaluation (dogs and cats)—direct evaluation to rule out oligospermia or azoospermia recommmended; alternatively, may test-breed the male to another female to prove fertility; rule out azoospermia in tom cat by finding spermatozoa in a vaginal flush or swab specimens from the queen or in urine collected by cystocentesis from the tom (See Infertility, male—Dogs).

IMAGING

• Radiography and ultrasonography—normal ovaries and a nongravid uterus not visible; large ovaries may indicate cystic ovarian disease or neoplasia; visible uterus may indicate cystic endometrial hyperplasia.
• Positive-contrast procedures—vaginography in dogs; hysterography in dogs and cats; performed prepuberally or when the patient is in estrus; may reveal anatomic abnormality (e.g., abnormal structure and impatency)
• Ultrasound—may diagnose pregnancy as early as 20–24 days after ovulation; useful for documenting pregnancy loss

DIAGNOSTIC PROCEDURES

• Laparotomy (dogs and cats)—assess anatomy of the tubular tract and gonads
• Hysterotomy—to obtain a direct uterine culture specimen; biopsy of the uterus or ovaries

TREATMENT

• Cats—seasonal breeders; depend on photoperiod; cycle when exposed to long day length, normally from late January to mid-October; induce year-round cycling by a daily light exposure of ≥ 12 hr; for a noncycling cat during the physiologic breeding season, ask client about the queen's housing and exposure to light.
• Heritable cause (e.g., thyroid insuffi-ciency)—counsel owner regarding the advisability of retaining the patient in the breeding program.
• Surgical resection of vaginal anomalies (dogs)—may ease natural service and vaginal delivery
• Surgical repair of impatent tubular tract (dogs and cats)—difficult procedure; prognosis for future fertility guarded
• Surgical drainage of ovarian cysts (dogs and cats)—efficacy unknown
• Unilateral ovariectomy of neoplastic ovary (dogs and cats)—future fertility depends on resumption of normal function of the remaining ovary and lack of metastasis.
• Prognosis for future fertility—initially good, because the most common cause is improper breeding management; worsens for other causes

MEDICATIONS

DRUGS OF CHOICE

• Antibiotics (dogs and cats—for uterine infection; choice depends on bacterial culture and sensitivity test of the uterus or of vaginal discharge during proestrus or estrus.
• L-Thyroxine—for thyroid insufficiency; dogs: 0.01 mg/kg PO q12h; prognosis for future fertility with return to euthyroid state guarded

Gonadotropin Therapy

• For induction of ovulation
• GnRH, which causes release of endogenous LH from the pituitary, or hCG, which has LH-like activity
• Cats not adequately stimulated to ovulate at the time of copulation—GnRH (25 µg/cat IM or hCG 250 IU/cat IM) at time of breeding
• Ovarian cystic disease—cats: GnRH (25 µg/cat IM) or hCG (250 IU/cat IM); dogs: GnRH (50 µg/dog IM) or hCG (1000 IU/dog half IV, half IM); causes ovulation or luteinization of cystic ovarian tissue

CONTRAINDICATIONS
N/A

PRECAUTIONS
N/A

POSSIBLE INTERACTIONS
N/A

ALTERNATIVE DRUGS
N/A

FOLLOW-UP

PATIENT MONITORING

• L-Thyroxine (dogs)—blood concentrations of T_3 and T_4 rechecked after 1 month of supplementation to ensure adequate absorption of medication and resumption of a euthyroid state
• Ultrasonography (dogs and cats)—definitively diagnose pregnancy; monitor gestation.
• Progesterone assay (dogs and cats)

POSSIBLE COMPLICATIONS
N/A

MISCELLANEOUS

ASSOCIATED CONDITIONS

• Infertility caused by endocrinopathy—dermatologic abnormality (e.g., alopecia with thyroid insufficiency or hypercortisolism); systemic signs of disease (e.g., polydipsia and polyuria with hypercortisolism)
• Bitches with a vaginal anatomic abnormality—persistent or recurrent urinary tract disease or vaginitis

AGE-RELATED FACTORS
N/A

ZOONOTIC POTENTIAL

B. canis infection—organism is less readily shed if affected animals are gonadectomized; stress good hygiene.

PREGNANCY
N/A

SEE ALSO
• See Causes

ABBREVIATIONS

FeLV = feline leukemia virus
FIV = feline immunodeficiency virus
GnRH = gonadotropin-releasing hormone
hCG = human chorionic gonadotropin
LH = luteinizing hormone
T_3 = triiodothyronine
T_4 = thyroxine
TSH = thyroid-stimulating hormone

Suggested Reading

Freshman JL. Clinical approach to infertility in the cycling bitch. Vet Clin North Am Small Anim Pract 1991;21:427–436.
Johnston SD, Olson PNS, Root MV. Clinical approach to infertility in the bitch. Semin Vet Med Surg Small Anim 1994;9:2–6.
Authors Margaret V. Root and Shirley D. Johnston
Consulting Editor Sara K. Lyle

INFERTILITY, MALE—DOGS

BASICS

DEFINITION
• Diminished or absent fertility; does not imply sterility
• Results from a wide range of problems that prevent the delivery of sufficient numbers of spermatozoa to fertilize ovulated, mature oocytes in the bitch

PATHOPHYSIOLOGY
• Spermatogenesis—encompasses the formation and development of spermatozoa from primordial germ cells; a coordinated, hormonally controlled, cyclic process; approximately 60 days required for a complete phase (46 days for the testicular phase; remainder for the epididymal phase); thus testicular problems require at least 60 days, and epididymal problems, 2 weeks.
• Azoospermia—ejaculate completely devoid of spermatozoa
• Oligozoospermia—ejaculate with low numbers of spermatozoa
• Primary causes—impaired or arrested spermatogenesis; blockage of the excurrent ducts; genitourinary inflammation; testicular neoplasia; environmental stress; congenital abnormality; endocrine abnormality

SYSTEMS AFFECTED
• Reproductive
• Endocrine/Metabolic
• Musculoskeletal
• Nervous

SIGNALMENT
• Prevalence increases with age.
• Relatively higher prevalence of specific problems seen in certain breeds.

SIGNS

General Comments
General complaint—no puppies produced; owner suspects male dog infertility

Historical Findings
• Age of testicular decent
• Age at first attempted mating
• Libido and breeding behavior
• Frequency and number of matings
• Method used to time breedings
• Litter size(s)
• Familial history of infertility
• Degree of inbreeding
• Fertility status of bitches bred
• *Brucella canis* status of all breeding partners
• Current and previous drug and dietary therapies
• Previous medical or surgical illnesses

Physical Examination Findings
• Sheath and penis—palpated to identify masses or adhesions
• Nonerect penis—exteriorized to determine if the superficial mucosa contains any clinically important lesions and if the os penis is undamaged
• Testes and epididymis—palpated and examined, size and symmetry of the epididymis relative to the testes noted
• Internal urethra and prostate—digital rectal palpation to determine location, size, and symmetry

CAUSES
Incorrect timing of breeding—most common cause

Congenital
• Chromosomal abnormalities (XXY syndrome) and XX sex reversal (XX "males")—phenotypic males with hypoplastic testes and no spermatogenesis
• Biopsy—reveals some have Sertoli cells (see Sexual Development Disorders)
• Unilateral or bilateral segmental aplasia of the epididymis or vas deferens—causes either oligospermia or azoospermia

Acquired
• Incomplete ejaculation—unfamiliar surroundings; slippery flooring; no estrous bitch; dominant owner or bitch present
• Obstruction of the efferent ductules, epididymides, or ductus deferens—leads to azoospermia; sperm granuloma, spermatocele, acute inflammation, chronic inflammatory stenosis, segmental aplasia, neoplasia, previous vasectomy, and attempts to tack testes into a scrotal location
• Inflammation or infection of the testes—especially *B. canis* and *Escherichia coli*; requires prompt and aggressive treatment to prevent infertility
• Hypothyroidism—role unclear; evaluate thyroid function with poor semen quality; may be associated with decreased libido
• Hyperadrenocorticism—causes testicular atrophy; probably reversible
• Drugs—parasiticides, corticosteroids, anabolic steroids, chemotherapeutic agents, and some antifungal agents may interfere with or interrupt spermatogenesis; assess all topical and systemic therapies.
• Environmental toxins—effect unknown
• Trauma, environmental damage, testicular neoplasia, systemic disease, ischemia, and heat stress—may cause transient infertility or sterility
• Prostatic disease—appears to markedly reduce semen quality

• Inbreeding—initially reduces fertility; eventually a rebound effect and fertility starts to return to near normal if the breeder selects for fertile individuals.
• Lymphocytic orchitis—familial in some breeds (e.g., beagles and Borzois); affected animals may be fertile when young; fertility declines at an accelerated rate with age.
• Retrograde ejaculation—some retrograde flow into the bladder normal; complete retrograde ejaculation (aspermia) rare; diagnosis aided by urinalysis after ejaculation

RISK FACTORS
• Congenital disorders affecting reproductive function—not uncommon; tend to occur in selected breeds
• Test bitches and stud dogs not tested for infectious disease (e.g., *B. canis* and bacterial culture of genital tract) before breeding.

DIAGNOSIS

DIFFERENTIAL DIAGNOSIS
Before extensive diagnostic work on the male, determine that the bitches are fertile (previous litters) and that the breedings were optimally timed (see Infertility, Female; and Breeding, Timing)

CBC/BIOCHEMISTRY/URINALYSIS
• Usually normal
• Brucellosis or prostatitis—variable changes in the leukogram (normal or leukocytosis) and urinalysis (high numbers of leukocytes); depends on the time-course of the infection
• Systemic illness—may impair reproductive function, but infertility is usually not the primary complaint on examination

OTHER LABORATORY TESTS

Endocrine Profile
• Resting testosterone—normal, intact dogs, 0.4–10 ng/mL; most common range, 1–4 ng/mL
• Androgenic tissue—confirmed if serum concentration of testosterone increases 100% over the resting value 2–3 hr after injection with either 1–2 μg/kg GnRH or 40 IU/kg hCG; useful to detect bilaterally cryptorchid condition
• Serum FSH concentration—rises with marked reduction in spermatogenesis because of loss of inhibin secretion (Cornell Laboratories)
• Serum LH concentration—difficult to interpret because of its episodic secretion
• Thyroid function—evaluated by baseline T_3 and T_4 values and TSH test

IMAGING
Ultrasonography—helps identify lesions that alter the testicular and epididymal architecture (e.g., neoplasia and spermatocele); evaluates the prostate gland for hyperplasia, chronic prostatitis, cyst, abscess, or neoplasia (see Benign Prostatic Hyperplasia; Prostatic Cysts; Prostatitis and Prostatitis Abscess)

DIAGNOSTIC PROCEDURES

Breeding Soundness Examination
• Pivotal to ensure that all appropriate information is collected
• Sperm-rich and prostatic portions of the ejaculate—collected as separate fractions by use of a sterile artificial vagina and sterile, graduated, nontoxic plastic tubes in the presence of an estrous bitch; use 4 × 4 gauze pads or swabs containing estrual vaginal discharge (can be frozen and stored) if estrous bitch unavailable
• Semen volume, concentration and motility of sperm cells, morphologic and cytologic characteristics of sperm cells, and qualitative and quantitative cultures—sperm-rich fraction
• Cytologic examination and qualitative and quantitative cultures—prostatic fraction and urine (collected by cystocentesis)
• Culture results—must be correlated with clinical and cytologic evidence of an active infection; evidence of inflammation if greater than 1 WBC/hpf observed (especially sperm rich fraction)
• Prostatic fraction that indicates a clinically important infection—re-evaluate by other sampling techniques that avoid contamination from the penile mucosa and prepuce.
• Azoospermic or oligospermic ejaculate—recollect 1 hr later and again on several occasions before confirming infertility.

Epididymal Markers
ALP concentration in seminal fluid—normal, 8,000–40,000 U/mL; of epididymal origin; may indicate obstruction if < 5,000 U/mL and a complete ejaculate was obtained

Testicular Biopsy
• Determines the degree of spermatogenesis and the integrity of the blood–testis barrier
• Differentiates obstruction of efferent ducts from testicular hypoplasia and degeneration
• Allows an informed prognosis
• Incisional biopsy—superior to aspiration or needle biopsy for obtaining a diagnostic sample; Bouin's fixative required for processing the tissue

TREATMENT
• Supportive regimens—reducing environmental heat or other stress; ensuring adequate diet and mineral supplementation
• Specific medications—must be administered long enough and at a dosage that will ensure tissue penetration
• Inform client that the testis will require at least 60 days to return to function.
• Stress patience while the patient is regularly checked to ensure there is no worsening of the condition.
• Reanastomosis of blocked excurrent ducts—being attempted; little data available on success rates

MEDICATIONS

DRUGS OF CHOICE
• Antibiotics (for penetration and spectrum)—chloramphenicol, trimethoprim-sulfa, erythromycin, and enrofloxacin; usually recommended for a minimum of 3–4 weeks to allow adequate and sustained levels within the reproductive tract
• Pseudoephedrine—used with limited success in humans with retrograde ejaculation

CONTRAINDICATIONS
• Trimethoprim-sulfas—contraindicated if predisposed to keratitis sicca
• Chloramphenicol and trimethoprim-sulfas—reportedly induce blood dyscrasias

PRECAUTIONS
N/A

POSSIBLE INTERACTIONS
N/A

ALTERNATIVE DRUGS
N/A

FOLLOW-UP

PATIENT MONITORING
Recheck at intervals that take into account the length of the spermatogenic cycle (60 days) but are frequent enough to allow detection of deteriorating condition.

POSSIBLE COMPLICATIONS
N/A

MISCELLANEOUS

ASSOCIATED CONDITIONS
• Brucellosis infection—diskospondylitis, polyarthritis, posterior paresis, fever, and uveitis
• Prostatic disease—obstipation, locomotor difficulties, fever, hematuria, pollakiuria, and dysuria
• Lymphocytic orchitis—lymphocytic thyroiditis

AGE-RELATED FACTORS
• Reduction in daily sperm output and morphologically normal sperm cells—with age
• Difficult to assess the effect of age alone on fertility
• Most old, infertile dogs have concurrent diseases (e.g., systemic or prostatic disease and testicular neoplasia) that have documented effects on fertility.

ZOONOTIC POTENTIAL
N/A

PREGNANCY
N/A

SEE ALSO
See Causes

ABBREVIATIONS
ALP = alkaline phosphatase
FSH = follicle-stimulating hormone
GnRH = gonadotropin-releasing hormone
hCG = human chorionic gonadotropin
LH = luteinizing hormone
TSH = thyroid-stimulating hormone

Suggested Reading
Fayrer-Hosken RA, Caudle AB. Canine semen examination, with special reference to proximal cytoplasmic droplets and their relation to fertility. Georgia Vet 1990;42:11–13.
Kennelly JJ. Coyote reproduction. The duration of the spermatogenic cycle and sperm transport. J Reprod Fertil 1972;31:163–170.
Meyers-Wallen, VN. Clinical approach to infertile dogs with sperm in the ejaculate. Vet Clin North Am Small Anim Pract 1991;21:609–633.
Olson PN. Clinical approach for evaluating dogs with azoospermia. Society For Theriogenology, San Diego, CA 1991:202–207.
Wallace MS. Infertility in the male dog. Probl Vet Med 1992;4:531–544.
Authors Richard A. Fayrer-Hosken and Frances O. Smith
Consulting Editor Sara K. Lyle

LAMENESS

BASICS

DEFINITION
A disturbance in gait and locomotion in response to pain or injury

PATHOPHYSIOLOGY
• Severe, sharp pain—when moving, patient carries or puts no weight on the affected limb.
• Milder, dull, or aching pain—when moving, patient limps or bears little weight on the affected limb; at rest, the patient bears less weight on the affected limb.
• Pain produced only during certain phases of movement—patient adjusts its motion and gait to minimize discomfort.

SYSTEMS AFFECTED
• Musculoskeletal
• Nervous

SIGNALMENT
• Any age or breed of dog
• Age, breed, and sex predilection—depend on specific disease

SIGNS

General Comments
• Unilateral forelimb—compensated for by moving the head and neck upward as the affected limb is placed on the ground and dropping the head and neck when the sound limb bears the weight
• Bilateral hindlimb—head and neck movement less pronounced; more weight shifted to the forelimbs by dropping the forequarters
• Unilateral hindlimb—may drop lower on the sound limb when it strikes the ground; elevated hindquarters when the affected limb is on the ground

• Always assess the patient's neurologic status, especially with a suspected proximal lesion.

Historical Findings
• Complete history—mandatory; signalment; identification of affected limb(s); known trauma; changes with weather, exercise, or rest; responsiveness to previous treatments
• Determine onset of lameness—acute or chronic
• Determine progression—static; slow; rapid
• Is the patient demonstrably painful?

Physical Examination Findings
• Perform a complete routine examination.
• Observe gait—walking; trotting; climbing stairs; doing figure-eights
• Palpate—asymmetry of muscle mass; bony prominences
• Manipulate bones and joints, beginning distally and working proximally.
• Assess—instability; incongruency; luxation or subluxation; pain; abnormal range of motion; abnormal sounds
• Examine suspected area of involvement last—by starting with normal limbs, patient may relax, allowing assessment of normal reaction to maneuvers.

CAUSES

Forelimb
Growing Dog (< 12 Months of Age)
• Osteochondrosis of the shoulder
• Shoulder luxation or subluxation—congenital
• Osteochondrosis of the elbow
• Un-united anconeal process
• Fragmented medial coronoid process
• Elbow incongruity
• Avulsion or calcification of the flexor muscles—elbow
• Asymmetric growth of the radius and ulna
• Panosteitis

• Hypertrophic osteodystrophy
• Trauma—soft tissue; bone; joint
• Infection—local; systemic
• Nutritional imbalances
• Congenital anomalies
Mature Dog (> 12 Months of Age)
• Degenerative joint disease
• Bicipital tenosynovitis
• Calcification or mineralization of supraspinatus or infraspinatus tendon
• Contracture of supraspinatus or infraspinatus muscle
• Soft tissue or bone neoplasia—primary; metastatic
• Trauma—soft tissue; bone; joint
• Panosteitis
• Polyarthropathies
• Polymyositis
• Polyneuritis

Hindlimb
Growing Dog (< 12 Months of Age)
• Hip dysplasia
• Avascular necrosis of femoral head—Legg-Calvé-Perthes disease
• Osteochondrosis of stifle
• Patella luxation—medial or lateral condyle
• Osteochondrosis of hock
• Panosteitis
• Hypertrophic osteodystrophy
• Trauma—soft tissue; bone; joint
• Infection—local; systemic
• Nutritional imbalances
• Congenital anomalies

Mature dog (> 12 Months of age)
• Degenerative joint disease
• Cruciate ligament disease
• Avulsion of long digital extensor tendon—stifle
• Soft tissue or bone neoplasia—primary; metastatic
• Trauma—soft tissue; bone; joint

- Panosteitis
- Polyarthropathies
- Polymyositis
- Polyneuritis

RISK FACTORS
N/A

 DIAGNOSIS

DIFFERENTIAL DIAGNOSIS
Must differentiate musculoskeletal from neurogenic causes

CBC/BIOCHEMISTRY/URINALYSIS
Usually normal

OTHER LABORATORY TESTS
Depend on suspected cause

IMAGING
- Radiographs—recommended for all suspected musculoskeletal causes
- CT, MRI, and bone scans with radio-isotopes—help identify and delineate causative lesions

DIAGNOSTIC PROCEDURES
- Cytologic examination of joint fluid—identify and differentiate intra-articular disease
- EMG—differentiate neuromuscular from musculoskeletal disease
- Muscle and/or nerve biopsy—reveal and identify neuromuscular disease

 TREATMENT
Depends on underlying cause

 MEDICATIONS

DRUGS OF CHOICE
- Analgesics and NSAIDs—often indicated for symptomatic treatment; try buffered or enteric-coated aspirin (10–25 mg/kg PO q8h or q12h), caroprofen (2.2 mg/kg PO q12h), etodolac (10–15 mg/kg PO q24h), phenyl-butazone (3–7 mg/kg PO q8h, total dose < 800 mg/day), meclofenemic acid (0.5 mg/kg PO q12h), or piroxicam (0.3 mg/kg PO q24h for 3 days, then q48h)
- Corticosteroids—use judiciously, unless specifically indicated (potential side effects; articular cartilage damage associated with long-term use).

CONTRAINDICATIONS
N/A

PRECAUTIONS
NSAIDs—gastrointestinal irritation may preclude use in some patients.

POSSIBLE INTERACTIONS
N/A

ALTERNATIVE DRUGS
- Chondroprotective drugs (e.g., polysulfated glycosaminoglycans, glucosamine, and chondroitin sulfate)—for degenerative joint disease; may be of benefit in limiting cartilage damage and degeneration; may help alleviate pain and inflammation

 FOLLOW-UP

PATIENT MONITORING
Depends on underlying cause

POSSIBLE COMPLICATIONS
N/A

 MISCELLANEOUS

ASSOCIATED CONDITIONS
N/A

AGE-RELATED FACTORS
N/A

ZOONOTIC POTENTIAL
N/A

PREGNANCY
N/A

SEE ALSO
Chapters covering musculoskeletal and neuromuscular disorders

Suggested Reading

Brinker WO, Piermattei DL, Flo GL. Physical examination for lameness. In: Handbook of small animal orthopedics and fracture repair. 3rd ed. Philadelphia: Saunders, 1997:228–230.
Brinker WO, Piermattei DL, Flo GL. In: Handbook of small animal orthopedics and fracture repair. 3rd ed. Philadelphia: Saunders, 1997:393–394.

Author Peter D. Schwarz
Consulting Editor Peter D. Schwarz

LYMPHADENOPATHY (LYMPHADENOMEGALY)

BASICS

DEFINITION
Abnormally large lymph nodes, generalized or localized to a single node or group of regional nodes

PATHOPHYSIOLOGY
• Can result from hyperplasia of lymphoid elements, inflammatory infiltration, or neoplastic proliferation within the lymph node.
• Because of their filtration function, lymph nodes often act as sentinels of disease in the tissues they drain; inflammation of any tissue is often accompanied by enlargement of the draining nodes, which most likely results from reactive lymphoid hyperplasia but may also be caused by extension of the inflammatory process into the nodes (lymphadenitis).
• Reactive hyperplasia involves proliferation of lymphocytes and plasma cells in response to antigenic stimulation.
• Lymphadenitis—implies active migration of neutrophils, activated macrophages, or eosinophils into the lymph node.
• Infectious agents may be involved.
• Neoplastic proliferation may be either primary (malignant lymphoma) or metastatic.

SYSTEMS AFFECTED
Hemic/Lymph/Immune

SIGNALMENT
• Dogs and cats
• No breed, sex, or age predilection

SIGNS
• Typically does not cause clinical signs
• Severe—may cause mechanical obstruction and interference with the function of adjacent organs, signs of which depend on the affected lymph node and may include dysphagia, regurgitation, respiratory distress, dyschezia, and limb swelling.
• Dogs and cats may be systemically ill from the underlying disease process.

CAUSES

Lymphoid Hyperplasia
• Localized or systemic infection caused by infectious agents of all categories (i.e., bacteria, viruses, fungi, protozoa, and algae) when infection does not directly involve the node
• Some infectious agents may produce lymphadenitis of certain lymph nodes with concurrent hyperplasia of other nodes that are not directly infected.

• Other infectious agents (e.g., rickettsia and *Brucella canis*)—hyperplasia without overt lymphadenitis
• FIV and FeLV infection—generalized hyperplasia, although lymphoid depletion may occur late in the course of the disease; lymphadenitis can develop with a secondary infection.
• Antigenic stimulation by factors other than infectious agents (e.g., allergens)
• May develop in animals with immune-mediated disease (e.g, SLE and rheumatoid arthritis)

Lymphadenitis
• Bacteria—capable of causing purulent lymphadenitis, which may progress to abscessation; a few (e.g., *Mycobacterium* spp.) induce granulomatous lymphadenitis; other agents include aerobic and anaerobic organisms, *Pasteurella*, *Bacteriodes*, fusobacterium, *Yersinia pestis*, and *Francisella tularensis*.
• Fungi—systemic infections from histoplasmosis, blastomycosis, cryptococcosis, and sporotrichosis
• Uncommon—protozoa, algae, and metazoan parasites
• Several involved lymph nodes—frequently a manifestation of systemic infection, such as histoplasmosis or blastomycosis
• Although primary infection of the lymph nodes does occur, lymphadenitis is usually accompanied by (and often results from) infection of other tissues being drained by the affected node.
• Eosinophilic—may be associated with allergic inflammation of the organ being drained by the affected lymph node (e.g., skin affected with flea allergy dermatitis); may be encountered in a patient with multisystemic idiopathic eosinophilic disease, such as feline hypereosinophilic syndrome, or in a lymph node draining a mast cell tumor.

Neoplasia
• Cats—neoplastic transformation of lymphocytes by FeLV
• Dogs—lymphoma, cause unknown
• Most tumors that metastasize to the lymph nodes—unknown

RISK FACTORS
• Impaired immune function predisposes to infection and, therefore, to lymphadenitis.
• Animals with allergic diseases are likely to develop lymph node hyperplasia or eosinophilic lymphadenitis.
• Malignant lymphoma (cats)—infection with the FeLV
• Lymphadenomegaly caused by metastatic neoplasms—vary with the type of primary neoplasm

DIAGNOSIS

DIFFERENTIAL DIAGNOSIS
• A mass in a location characteristic of a lymph node usually can be assumed to be one; cytologic evaluation of a fine-needle aspirate usually resolves any doubt.
• Palpable lymph nodes in normal dogs—mandibular, prescapular, axillary, superficial inguinal, and popliteal nodes; facial, retropharyngeal, and iliac nodes are palpable when larger than normal.
• Severe lymph node enlargement (> 5 times normal size)—most likely to develop in patients with abscessation (lymphadenitis) and lymphoma
• Lesser degrees of enlargement—attributable to reactive hyperplasia, lymphadenitis, or neoplasia
• Extent of enlargement in patients with metastatic disease varies widely.
• Multiple lymph nodes affected throughout the body—likely the result of lymphoma or systemic infection that causes either lymphadenitis or lymphoid hyperplasia
• Abscessation and metastatic neoplasms usually affect a single lymph node.

CBC/BIOCHEMISTRY/URINALYSIS
• Cytopenias—seen with lymphoma, anemia of chronic disease, stress, splenic disease, or neoplastic infiltration of the bone marrow; also seen with rickettsial or viral disease.
• Lymphocytosis—suggests rickettsial disease (dogs) and lymphoid neoplasia (dogs and cats); atypical lymphocytes in the blood help establish a diagnosis of lymphoid neoplasia.
• Eosinophilia—may occur in animals with lymphadenopathy owing to allergic or parasitic skin disease
• Neutrophilia, with or without a left shift—may develop in patients with lymphadenitis, lymphoid hyperplasia, or neoplasia
• Hypercalcemia—relatively common in dogs and rare in cats with lymphoma
• Hyperglobulinemia—may develop in patients with chronic inflammatory disease or lymphoid neoplasia

OTHER LABORATORY TESTS
• Cats—test for FeLV antigen and FIV in animals with large lymph nodes; infected animals may have lymphoma, lymphoid hyperplasia, or even lymphadenitis caused by immunosuppression.
• Serologic tests for antibodies against systemic fungal agents such as *Blastomyces* and *Cryptococcus* may help establish those diagnoses.

LYMPHADENOPATHY (LYMPHADENOMEGALY)

IMAGING
• Radiography and ultrasonography—involvement of lymph nodes within the body cavity
• Lesions associated with lymph node enlargement may be detected in other organs, e.g., diffuse pneumonia in dogs with blastomycosis, and primary tumor in animals with lymphadenomegaly caused by metastatic neoplasia.

DIAGNOSTIC PROCEDURES

Cytologic Examination
• Aspirates from affected lymph nodes help determine the major category of lymphadenomegaly (i.e., hyperplasia, inflammation, or neoplasia) and may provide a specific diagnosis in patients with certain infectious diseases or neoplasms; a differential stain (e.g., Diff-Quik) is suitable in most cases.
• Gram staining can be performed in animals suspected of bacterial lymphadenitis.
• Aspirates from hyperplastic lymph nodes contain a mixed cell population in which small lymphocytes predominate along with large lymphocytes, plasma cells, occasional neutrophils and (perhaps) a few eosinophils and mast cells.
• Hyperplastic and normal lymph nodes are cytologically indistinguishable.
• Aspirates from lymph nodes affected by lymphadenitis contain high proportions of neutrophils, macrophages, and/or eosinophils, depending on the cause of the inflammation; specific infectious agents, such as bacteria and systemic fungi, may be evident.
• Frequently the means of diagnosis in animals with systemic fungal infection, such as blastomycosis and cryptococcosis.
• Aspirates from lymph nodes affected by lymphoma typically contain a high proportion of (usually > 50%) large lymphocytes.
• Aspirates from lymph nodes containing metastatic neoplasia contain populations of cells that are not seen in normal nodes; the appearance of such cells varies widely, depending on the type of neoplasm.

Other
• In cats, severe lymphoid hyperplasia has been misdiagnosed as lymphoma; thus a biopsy is essential for animals with lymphadenomegaly.
• When a diagnosis cannot be made by cytologic examination, a surgical biopsy may be needed; excisional biopsy is preferable to needle biopsy.

• The cytologic diagnosis of lymphoma should be confirmed by histopathologic examination of an excised lymph node for accurate grading and to obtain potential prognostic information.

TREATMENT
• Because of the many disease processes and specific agents that can cause lymphadenomegaly, treatment depends on establishing the underlying cause
• In animals suspected of lymphoma, corticosteroids should not be administered before completing staging tests if chemotherapy may be instituted.

MEDICATIONS

DRUGS OF CHOICE
Appropriate medications vary with the cause of lymph node enlargement.

CONTRAINDICATIONS
N/A

PRECAUTIONS
N/A

POSSIBLE INTERACTIONS
N/A

ALTERNATIVE DRUGS
N/A

FOLLOW-UP

PATIENT MONITORING
Lymph node size to assess efficacy of treatment

POSSIBLE COMPLICATIONS
N/A

MISCELLANEOUS

ASSOCIATED CONDITIONS
• Lymph node hyperplasia and lymphadenitis are often components or manifestations of systemic disease
• Lymphoma may involve other organs (e.g., liver, spleen, intestines, kidneys, and meninges) with a variety of clinical consequences.

• Clinical disease in animals with metastatic neoplasms in the lymph nodes is usually attributable to the primary tumor rather than to the metastasis; however, exceptions are dogs with tonsillar carcinoma, who may have massively large mandibular lymph nodes, and dogs with adenocarcinoma of the anal sac, who often have dramatically large sublumbar lymph nodes.

AGE-RELATED FACTORS
None

ZOONOTIC POTENTIAL
• Direct transmission of diseases that cause lymphadenitis to humans is unlikely, with the exception of systemic mycotic disease, sporotrichosis, tularemia, and plague.
• Caution should be exercised when performing fine-needle aspiration in animals that may have systemic fungal disease.

PREGNANCY
N/A

SEE ALSO
• Lymphadenitis
• Lymphosarcoma (lymphoma)—Cats
• Lymphosarcoma (lymphoma)—Dogs

ABBREVIATIONS
FeLV = feline leukemia virus
FIV = feline immunodeficiency virus
SLE = systemic lupus erythematosus

Suggested Reading
Day MJ, Whitbread TJ. Pathological diagnoses in dogs with lymph node enlargement. Vet Rec 1988;136:72–73.
Duncan JR. The lymph nodes. In: Cowell RL, Tyler RD, eds. Diagnostic cytology of the dog and cat. Goleta, CA: American Veterinary, 1989:93–98.
Rogers KS, Barton CL, Landis M. Canine and feline lymph nodes. II. Diagnostic evaluation of lymphadenopathy. Compend Contin Ed Pract Vet 1993;15:1493–1503.
Author Kenneth M. Rassnick
Consulting Editor Susan M. Cotter

MELENA

BASICS

DEFINITION
Presence of digested blood in the feces, which gives a black, tarry appearance

PATHOPHYSIOLOGY
Usually results from upper GI bleeding, but can be associated with ingested blood from the oral cavity or respiratory tract

SYSTEMS AFFECTED
• Gastrointestinal
• Respiratory
• Coagulation

SIGNALMENT
• More common in dogs than cats
• No breed or sex predilection

SIGNS

Historical Findings
• Patients with upper GI tract hemorrhage may demonstrate vomiting, inappetance, weight loss, weakness, and/or mucous membrane pallor.
• Patients with respiratory tract hemorrhage may demonstrate epistaxis, sneezing, hemoptysis, mucous membrane pallor, weakness, and/or dyspnea.
• Patients with abnormal coagulation may demonstrate petechia, ecchymosis, mucous membrane pallor, epistaxis, hematuria, hyphema, and/or weakness.

Physical Examination Findings
Depends on the underlying cause

CAUSES

Primary GI Ulceration/Erosion
• Neoplasia—lymphoma, adenocarcinoma
• Infectious—pythiosis, fungal, parasitic

Helicobacter
• Mechanical—foreign body
• Inflammatory—acute gastritis; hemorrhagic gastroenteritis, lymphoplasmacytic, eosinophilic, granulomatous, and/or histiocytic enteritis
• Drugs—corticosteroids, NSAIDs

Metabolic/Other Diseases That Cause GI Ulceration
• Renal failure
• Hepatic disease
• Pancreatitis
• Hypoadrenocorticism
• Neoplasia—gastrinoma, mast cell tumor
• Shock, poor perfusion

Ingestion of Blood
• Diet
• Esophageal lesion—neoplasia, esophagitis
• Oral or pharyngeal lesion—neoplasia, abscess
• Nasal lesion—neoplasia, fungal rhinitis
• Respiratory lesion—lung lobe torsion, neoplasia, pneumonia, trauma

Coagulopathy
• Thrombocytopenia
• Platelet dysfunction—von Willebrand's disease, thrombasthenia, thrombopathia, NSAIDs
• Clotting factor abnormalities—anticoagulant rodenticide ingestion, clotting factor deficiency
• DIC

RISK FACTORS
Arthritis or other conditions requiring use of NSAIDs or corticosteroids

DIAGNOSIS

DIFFERENTIAL DIAGNOSIS
• Medications that cause dark stool—bismuth subsalicylate, oral iron therapy
• Must distinguish intestinal and extra-intestinal disease

CBC/BIOCHEMISTRY/URINALYSIS
• Microcytic, hypochromic, poorly regenerative anemia if chronic blood loss
• Regenerative anemia in early blood loss—may be poorly regenerative if <3 days
• Panhypoproteinemia if significant blood loss
• Thrombocytopenia, neutrophilia in some patients; pancytopenia in some
• Biochemistry analysis may reveal extra-intestinal cause of melena—renal failure, hepatic disease, hypoadrenocorticism
• Urinalysis may demonstrate hematuria in patients with coagulation defects.

OTHER LABORATORY TESTS
• Coagulation profile may reveal clotting abnormality.
• Bleeding time may be prolonged.
• Fecal examination may reveal infectious cause—parasites
• ACTH stimulation test abnormally low with hypoadrenocorticism
• Urease testing for *Helicobacter* spp.

IMAGING
• Abdominal radiography may reveal a mass, foreign body, or abnormalities in renal or hepatic size/shape.
• Thoracic radiographs may identify intrathoracic lesions.
• Nasal radiographs may indicate intranasal lesions.

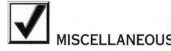
- Ultrasonography may reveal a mass, hepatic disease, pancreatitis, or renal disease.
- Upper GI barium series may delineate gastric or upper small intestinal mass, ulceration, or filling defect.

DIAGNOSTIC PROCEDURES

- Endoscopy allows visualization of masses and/or ulcers (esophageal, gastric, and/or duodenal), retrieval of GI foreign bodies, and biopsy.
- Rhinoscopy occasionally allows visualization of nasal lesions (endoscope or bronchoscope retroflexion and choanal evaluation is often helpful).
- Bronchoscopy allows visualization of airway lesions.
- Bone marrow aspiration and cytology indicated if pancytopenia is present

TREATMENT

- Inpatient—exception may be animal with intestinal parasites
- Treat underlying disease—renal failure, hepatic disease, hypoadrenocorticism, respiratory disease, etc.
- Fluid replacement with balanced electrolyte solutions and potassium supplementation
- Whole blood or packed red cell transfusions if anemia is severe
- Whole blood or plasma transfusion if the patient has a coagulopathy
- Temporarily discontinue oral intake if vomiting
- Surgery may be required for severe gastroduodenal ulceration or neoplasia

MEDICATIONS

DRUGS OF CHOICE

- Mucosal protectants for gastroduodenal ulceration/erosion— H_2-receptor antagonists (e.g., ranitidine 2 mg/kg IV or PO q12h or famotidine 0.5 mg/kg IV or PO q12–24h); sucralfate 0.5–1g PO q6–8h)
- Triple therapy if *Helicobacter* suspected or confirmed (see *Helicobacter*)

CONTRAINDICATIONS

Avoid corticosteroids and NSAIDs in patients with gastroduodenal ulceration/erosion

PRECAUTIONS

N/A

POSSIBLE INTERACTIONS

N/A

ALTERNATIVE DRUGS

Na/K-ATPase pump blocker (omeprazole 0.7 mg/kg PO q24h) can be used if H_2-receptor antagonists are unsuccessful or initially in severe gastroduodenal ulcer disease.

FOLLOW-UP

PATIENT MONITORING

- PCV daily until anemia stabilized, then weekly
- Hydration daily if patient vomiting
- Daily for respiratory distress if respiratory tract involved

POSSIBLE COMPLICATIONS

- Gastric or duodenal perforation and peritonitis
- Hypovolemic shock and death if severe, acute blood loss

MISCELLANEOUS

ASSOCIATED CONDITIONS

N/A

AGE-RELATED FACTORS

N/A

ZOONOTIC POTENTIAL

Helicobacter spp. may have zoonotic potential.

PREGNANCY

N/A

SYNONYMS

N/A

SEE ALSO

Individual causative diseases—
Hypoadrenocorticism, *Helicobacter,* etc.

ABBREVIATIONS

DIC = disseminated intravascular coagulation
GI = gastrointestinal
NSAIDs = nonsteroidal antiinflammatory drugs

Suggested Reading

Willard MD. Diseases of the stomach. In: Ettinger SJ, Feldman EC, eds. Textbook of veterinary internal medicine. Philadelphia: Saunders, 1995:1143–1168.

Authors Lisa E. Moore and Colin F. Burrows
Consulting Editors Mitchell A. Crystal and Brett M. Feder

MURMURS, HEART

BASICS

DEFINITION
Vibrations caused by disturbed blood flow

Timing of Murmurs
• Systolic murmurs occur between S1 and S2 (systole).
• Diastolic murmurs occur between S2 and S1 (diastole).
• Continuous and to-and-fro murmurs occur throughout all or most of the cardiac cycle.
• Continuous murmurs are usually accentuated near S2 and to-and-fro murmurs are usually absent near S2.

Grading Scale for Murmurs
• Grade I—barely audible
• Grade II—soft, but easily auscultated
• Grade III—intermediate loudness; most hemodynamically important murmurs are at least grade III.
• Grade IV—loud with palpable thrill
• Grade V—very loud, audible with stethoscope barely touching the chest; palpable thrill
• Grade VI—very loud, audible without the stethoscope touching the chest; palpable thrill

Configuration
• Plateau murmurs have uniform loudness and are typical of regurgitant murmurs such as mitral and tricuspid insufficiency and ventricular septal defect.
• Crescendo-decrescendo murmurs get louder and then softer and are typical of ejection murmurs such as pulmonic and aortic stenosis and atrial septal defect.
• Decrescendo murmurs start loud and then get softer and are typical of diastolic murmurs such as aortic or pulmonic insufficiency and mitral or tricuspid stenosis.

Location
Dogs
• Mitral area—left fifth intercostal space at costochondral junction
• Aortic area—left fourth intercostal space above costochondral junction
• Pulmonic area—left second to fourth intercostal space at sternal border
• Tricuspid area—right third to fifth intercostal space near costochondral junction

Cats
• Mitral area—left fifth to sixth intercostal space 1/4 ventrodorsal distance from sternum
• Aortic area—left second to third intercostal space just above the pulmonic area
• Pulmonic area—left second to third intercostal space 1/3–1/2 ventrodorsal distance from sternum
• Tricuspid area—right fourth to fifth intercostal space 1/4 ventrodorsal distance from sternum

PATHOPHYSIOLOGY
• Disturbed blood flow associated with high flow through normal or abnormal valves or with structures vibrating in the blood flow
• Flow disturbances associated with outflow obstruction or forward flow through stenosed valves or into a dilated great vessel
• Flow disturbances associated with regurgitant flow through an incompetent valve, septal defect, or patent ductus arteriosus

SYSTEMS AFFECTED
Cardiovascular

SIGNALMENT
Dogs and cats

SIGNS
Relate to cause of the murmur

CAUSES
Systolic Murmurs
• Mitral and tricuspid valve endocardiosis
• Cardiomyopathy
• Physiologic flow murmurs
• Anemia
• Mitral and tricuspid valve dysplasia
• Atrial septal defect
• Ventricular septal defect
• Pulmonic stenosis
• Aortic stenosis
• Tetralogy of Fallot
• Mitral and tricuspid valve endocarditis
• Hyperthyroidism
• Heartworm disease
• Continuous or to-and-fro murmurs
• Patent ductus arteriosus
• Ventricular septal defect with aortic regurgitation
• Aortic stenosis with aortic regurgitation

Diastolic Murmurs
• Mitral and tricuspid valve stenosis
• Aortic and pulmonic valve endocarditis

RISK FACTORS
Cardiac disease

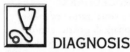

DIAGNOSIS

DIFFERENTIAL DIAGNOSIS
Differential Signs
• Must differentiate from other abnormal heart sounds—split sounds, ejection sounds, gallop rhythms, and clicks
• Must differentiate from abnormal lung sounds and pleural rubs; listen to see if timing of abnormal sound is correlated with respiration or heart beat.

Differential Causes
• Pale mucous membranes support anemic murmur.
• Location and radiation of murmur and timing during cardiac cycle can help determine cause; see algorithm.

CBC/BIOCHEMISTRY/URINALYSIS
• Anemia in animals with anemic murmurs
• Polycythemia in animals with right-to-left shunting congenital defects
• Leukocytosis with left shift in animals with endocarditis

OTHER LABORATORY TESTS
N/A

IMAGING
• Thoracic radiography—useful for evaluating heart size and pulmonary vasculature in hopes of determining cause and significance of murmur
• Echocardiography—recommended when a cardiac cause is suspected and the nature of the defect is unknown

Diagnostic Procedures
Electrocardiography may be useful in assessing heart enlargement patterns in animals with murmurs.

TREATMENT
• Outpatient unless heart failure is evident
• Base decisions on the cause of the murmur and associated clinical signs.
• None indicated for murmur alone

MURMURS, HEART

MEDICATIONS

DRUGS OF CHOICE
N/A

CONTRAINDICATIONS
N/A

PRECAUTIONS
N/A

POSSIBLE INTERACTIONS
N/A

ALTERNATIVE DRUGS
N/A

FOLLOW-UP

PATIENT MONITORING
Low-grade systolic ejection murmurs in puppies may be physiologic; most resolve by 6 months of age. If murmur still present after 6 months, include diagnostic imaging.

POSSIBLE COMPLICATIONS
If murmur is associated with structural heart disease, may see signs of congestive heart failure (e.g., coughing, dyspnea, and ascites) or exercise intolerance)

MISCELLANEOUS

ASSOCIATED CONDITIONS
N/A

AGE-RELATED FACTORS
• Murmurs present since birth generally associated with a congenital defect or physiologic flow murmur
• Acquired murmurs in geriatric, small-breed dogs usually associated with degenerative valve disease
• Acquired murmurs in large-breed dogs usually associated with dilated cardiomyopathy
• Acquired murmurs in geriatric cats usually associated with cardiomyopathy or hyperthyroidism

ZOONOTIC POTENTIAL
N/A

PREGNANCY
N/A

SYNONYMS
N/A

SEE ALSO
See Causes

ABBREVIATIONS
S1—first heart sound
S2—second heart sound

Suggested Reading
Smith FWK Jr., Tilley LP. Rapid interpretation of heart sounds, murmurs, and arrhythmias. Philadelphia: Lea & Febiger, 1992.
Authors Francis W. K. Smith, Jr., and Robert L. Hamlin
Consulting Editors Larry P. Tilley and Francis W. K. Smith, Jr.

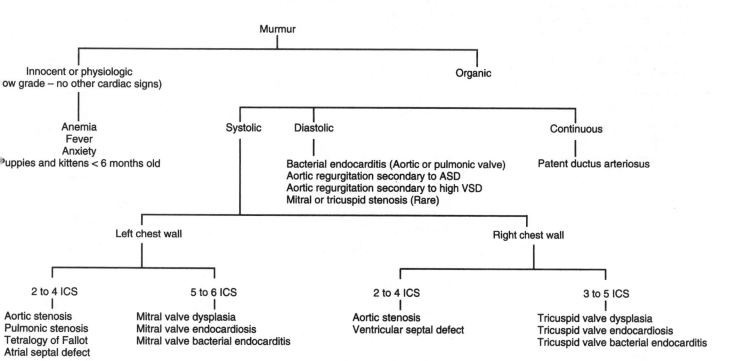

Figure 1

Differential diagnosis of cardiac disease based on the timing and location of murmurs. Adapted from Allen DG. Murmurs and abnormal heart sounds. By permission of Mosby-Year Book, Inc. In: Allen DG, Kruth SA, eds. Small animal cardiopulmonary medicine. Philadelphia: BC Decker, 1988:13.

MYOCLONUS

BASICS

OVERVIEW
• A coarse, repetitive, involuntary, and rhythmic contraction of a portion of a muscle, entire muscle, or group of muscles
• May affect one or several muscle groups
• May occur synchronously or asynchronously in several areas
• A CNS dysfunction involving the lower motor neurons and interneurons at the segmental level of the spinal cord or the brainstem
• A clinical sign; although reported most commonly with canine distemper virus infection, may be caused by other encephalitides and degenerative processes

SIGNALMENT
Acquired
• Dogs and rarely cats
• No breed, sex, or age predispositions

Congenital
• Dogs
• Reflex myoclonus—Labrador retrievers and Dalmatians; develops in the first few weeks of life
• Neonatal myoclonus of the paravertebral muscles—silky terriers; caused by spongy degeneration

SIGNS
Historical Findings
• With distemper—observed after a bout of gastrointestinal signs, cough, and/or ocular or nasal purulent discharge; persists at rest and even during sleep or light anesthesia; consistent frequency within a given patient; distemper diagnosis may precede the myoclonus by months to years; occurs more frequently in chronic phase of distemper
• With familial reflex—observed when the patient starts to walk; intermittent muscle contractions induced by auditory or tactile stimulus and by exercise; involves all limbs, neck, and head (e.g., the facial and masticatory muscles); patient unable to rise without assistance

Physical Examination Findings
• Masticatory and appendicular muscles—most frequently affected with distemper-induced disease; may be paresis of the affected limb
• May see other signs suggesting distemper (e.g., hard pads, ocular and nasal purulent discharge, and chorioretinitis)
• Neurologic deficits suggesting multifocal lesions in some patients
• The patient may be otherwise healthy.

CAUSES & RISK FACTORS
Congenital
• Familial in Labrador retrievers
• Spongy degeneration in silky terriers
• Other congenital anomalies of unknown cause

Acquired
• Canine distemper virus—most frequent cause; the only CNS disease repeatedly associated with myoclonus in dogs; unvaccinated dogs are at risk.
• Encephalitis of any cause—dogs and cats
• Degenerative disease—especially spongy degeneration
• Described in a dog with lead poisoning

DIAGNOSIS

DIFFERENTIAL DIAGNOSIS
• Canine distemper virus—systemic signs (e.g., gastroenteritis, pneumonia, and ocular or nasal purulent discharge)
• Other disorders that are limited to parts of the body—differentiate from acquired form

MYOCLONUS

• Partial seizures—Dobermans, Labrador retrievers, and English bulldogs; occasional head nods in a yes or no direction; occur infrequently and intermittently; limited to the head; last from few seconds to minutes; affected dog continues its activity and is otherwise normal.
• Dancing Doberman disease—differentiated on the basis of breed and the movements observed (e.g., the dog holds one pelvic limb flexed while standing; both limbs usually become affected, giving a dancing aspect to the standing position)

CBC/BIOCHEMISTRY/URINALYSIS
• Congenital or secondary to a past canine distemper virus infection—normal
• Other acquired forms—may suggest a specific cause if the patient has infectious encephalomyelitis; otherwise, normal

OTHER LABORATORY TESTS
N/A

IMAGING
N/A

DIAGNOSTIC PROCEDURES
Acute development—CSF analysis, serologic testing, and brain imaging (CT and MRI) may help determine the diagnosis.

TREATMENT
• Active encephalomyelitis—inpatient; establish a diagnosis and initiate treatment.
• Exercise—as tolerated
• Diet—ensure proper nutrition with active CNS disease; modify, if necessary, with vomiting or diarrhea
• Usually persists for years but spontaneous remission can occur
• Familial—clinical signs in Labrador retrievers and Dalmatians are severe and usually not compatible with quality of life.

MEDICATIONS

DRUGS
• With chronic, inactive canine distemper—treatment often unnecessary; alleviation may be obtained with procainamide (125–250 mg/dog PO q6–12h).
• Chlorazepate or acetylpromazine—reflex disease; may see improvement
• Active encephalomyelitis—treat accordingly

CONTRAINDICATIONS/POSSIBLE INTERACTIONS
N/A

FOLLOW-UP
• Monitor CNS disease.
• Usually persists indefinitely; remission occasionally seen
• Active distemper virus infection—poor to grave prognosis

✓ MISCELLANEOUS

SYNONYMS
• Flexor spasm
• Canine chorea

ABBREVIATION
CSF = cerebrospinal fluid

Suggested Reading
Oliver JE, Lorenz MD, Kornegay JN. Handbook of veterinary neurology. 3rd ed. Philadelphia: Saunders, 1997.
Author Joane M. Parent
Consulting Editor Joane M. Parent

NAIL AND NAILBED DISORDERS

 BASICS

DEFINITION
• Paronychia—inflammation of soft tissue around the nail
• Onychomycosis—fungal infection of the nail
• Onychorrhexis—brittle nails that tend to split or break
• Onychomadesis—sloughing of the nail
• Nail dystrophy—deformity caused by abnormal growth

PATHOPHYSIOLOGY
• Nails and nailfolds—subject to trauma, infection, vascular insufficiency, immune-mediated disease, neoplasia, defects in keratinization, and congenital abnormalities.
• A particular nail deformity may be caused by a variety of diseases.
• A single disease can present with various nail lesions.
• Sometimes, the cause is unknown and there is no response to treatment.

SYSTEMS AFFECTED
Skin/Exocrine

SIGNALMENT
• Dogs and cats
• Dachshund—predisposed to onychorrhexis

SIGNS
• Licking
• Lameness
• Pain
• Swelling, erythema, and exudate of nailfold
• Deformity or sloughing of nail

CAUSES

Paronychia
• Infection—bacteria, dermatophyte, yeast (*Candida*), demodicosis, leishmaniasis
• Immune-mediated—pemphigus, bullous pemphigoid, SLE, drug eruption, lupoid onychodystrophy
• Neoplasia—squamous cell carcinoma, melanoma, eccrine carcinoma, osteosarcoma, subungual keratoacanthoma, inverted squamous papilloma
• Arteriovenous fistula

Onychomycosis
• Dogs—*Trichophyton mentagrophytes*—usually generalized
• Cats—*Microsporum canis*

Onychorrhexis
• Idiopathic—especially in dachshunds; multiple nails
• Trauma
• Infection—dermatophytosis, leishmaniasis

Onychomadesis
• Trauma
• Infection
• Immune-mediated—pemphigus, bullous pemphigoid, SLE, drug eruption, lupoid onychodystrophy
• Vascular insufficiency—vasculitis, cold agglutinin disease
• Neoplasia—see above
• Idiopathic

Nail Dystrophy
• Acromegaly
• Feline hyperthyroidism
• Zinc-responsive dermatosis
• Congenital malformations

RISK FACTORS
• Paronychia (infectious)—immunosuppression (endogenous or exogenous), FeLV infection, trauma, and diabetes mellitus
• Bacterial onychomadesis—excessively short nail trimming (into the quick) postulated to predispose animal

 DIAGNOSIS

DIFFERENTIAL DIAGNOSIS
• Trauma or neoplasia often affects a single nail.
• Involvement of multiple nails suggests a systemic disease.
• Immune-mediated diseases (except lupoid onychodystrophy) usually have other skin lesions in addition to nail/nailfold lesions.

CBC/BIOCHEMISTRY/URINALYSIS
May show evidence of SLE, diabetes mellitus, hyperthyroidism or other systemic illness

OTHER LABORATORY TESTS
• FeLV
• T_4
• ANA titer

IMAGING
Radiographs—osteomyelitis of third phalanx

OTHER DIAGNOSTIC PROCEDURES
• Biopsy—histopathology and direct immunofluorescence; often involves a third phalanx amputation
• Cytology of exudate
• Skin scraping
• Bacterial and fungal culture

 TREATMENT

PARONYCHIA
• Surgical removal of nail plate (shell)—provide adequate drainage; grasp nail firmly with hemostat and strip it from its attachments with one swift downward motion; bandage foot following procedure.
• Antimicrobial soaks
• Identify underlying condition and treat specifically.

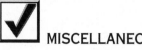

NAIL AND NAILBED DISORDERS

ONYCHOMYCOSIS
• Antifungal soaks—chlorhexidine, povidone iodine, lime sulfur
• Surgical removal of nail plate—may improve response to systemic medication
• Amputation of third phalanx

ONYCHORRHEXIS
• Repair with fingernail glue (type used to attach false nails in humans).
• Remove splintered pieces.
• Amputation of third phalanx
• Treat underlying cause.

ONYCHOMADESIS
• Antimicrobial soaks
• Treat underlying cause

NEOPLASIA
• Depends on biologic behavior of specific tumor
• Surgical excision
• Amputation of digit
• Amputation of leg
• Chemotherapy
• Radiation therapy

NAIL DYSTROPHY
Treat underlying cause

MEDICATIONS

DRUGS OF CHOICE
• Bacterial paronychia—systemic antibiotics based on culture and sensitivity; cephalosporins pending culture result
• *Candida paronychia*—ketoconazole (10 mg/kg PO q12h); topical nystatin or miconazole
• Onychomycosis—griseofulvin (50–150 mg/kg PO per day) or ketoconazole (10 mg/kg PO q12h) for 6–12 months until negative cultures; itraconazole (10 mg/kg PO daily) for 3 weeks and then pulse therapy twice a week until resolved
• Onychomadesis—depends on cause; immunosuppressive therapy for immune-mediated diseases.

CONTRAINDICATIONS
Griseofulvin—do not use in pregnant animals.

PRECAUTIONS
• Griseofulvin—may cause bone marrow suppression, anorexia, vomiting, and diarrhea; absorption enhanced if given with a high-fat meal
• Ketoconazole—may cause anorexia, gastric irritation, hepatic toxicity, and lightening of the hair coat

POSSIBLE INTERACTIONS
N/A

ALTERNATIVE DRUGS
N/A

FOLLOW-UP

PATIENT MONITORING
Depends on underlying cause

POSSIBLE COMPLICATIONS
N/A

EXPECTED COURSE AND PROGNOSIS
• Bacterial or fungal paronychia and onycho-mycosis—treatment may be prolonged and response may be influenced by underlying immunosuppressive factors.
• Onychomycosis and onychorrhexis—may require amputation of the third phalanx for resolution
• Nail dystrophy—prognosis is good when underlying cause can be effectively treated (e.g., hyperthyroidism, zinc-responsive dermatosis).
• Onychomadesis—prognosis depends on underlying cause; immune-mediated diseases and vascular problems carry a more guarded prognosis than do trauma or infectious causes.
• Neoplasia—some can be totally excised or removed by amputation of the digit; others are highly malignant and may have already spread by the time of diagnosis.

✓ MISCELLANEOUS

ASSOCIATED CONDITIONS
N/A

AGE-RELATED FACTORS
N/A

ZOONOTIC POTENTIAL
Dermatophyte infections

PREGNANCY
N/A

SYNONYMS
Nailfold = nail bed

SEE ALSO
• Demodicosis
• Dermatophytosis
• Pemphigoid, Bullous
• Pemphigus
• Pododermatitis
• Pyoderma
• Vasculitis, Cutaneous

ABBREVIATIONS
• ANA = antinuclear antibody
• FeLV = feline leukemia virus
• SLE = systemic lupus erythematosus

Suggested Reading
Muller GH, Kirk RW, Scott DW. Small animal dermatology. 4th ed. Philadelphia: Saunders, 1989.
Authors Ellen C. Codner and Karen Helton Rhodes
Consulting Editor Karen Helton Rhodes

NASAL DERMATOSES

 BASICS

DEFINITION
Pathologic condition of the nasal skin involving either the haired portion (bridge of the nose) or nonhaired portion (nasal planum)

PATHOPHYSIOLOGY
N/A

SYSTEMS AFFECTED
- Skin/exocrine
- Multisystemic—SLE

SIGNALMENT
- Dermatophytosis, zinc-responsive dermatosis, dermatomyositis, and demodicosis—more likely in dogs < 1 year of age
- Zinc-responsive dermatosis—Siberian huskies, Alaskan malamutes
- Dermatomyositis—collies, Shetland sheepdogs
- Uveodermatologic syndrome—akitas, Samoyeds, Siberian huskies
- SLE and DLE—collies, Shetland sheepdogs, German shepherds; DLE may occur more often in females
- Epidermotropic lymphoma—old dogs

SIGNS
- Depigmentation
- Hyperpigmentation
- Erythema
- Erosion/ulceration
- Vesicles/pustules
- Crusts
- Scarring
- Alopecia
- Nodules/plaques

CAUSES
- Nasal pyoderma
- Demodicosis
- Dermatophytosis
- Other fungal infections—cryptococcosis, sporotrichosis, aspergillosis
- DLE and SLE
- Pemphigus foliaceus
- Pemphigus erythematosus
- Nasal solar dermatitis
- Dermatomyositis
- Zinc-responsive dermatosis
- Uveodermatologic syndrome
- Vitiligo
- Nasal depigmentation
- Contact hypersensitivity—plastic dish dermatitis, topical drug hypersensitivity (neomycin)
- Tumors—squamous cell carcinoma, basal cell carcinoma, mycosis fungoides, fibrosarcoma
- Trauma
- Idiopathic sterile granuloma
- Idiopathic nasal hyperkeratosis

RISK FACTORS
- Adult cats—may be inapparent carriers of dermatophytes
- Rooting behavior—pyoderma, dermatophytosis
- Sun exposure—nasal solar dermatitis, DLE, SLE, pemphigus erythematosus
- Poorly pigmented nose—nasal solar dermatitis, squamous cell carcinoma
- Large, rapidly growing breeds oversupplemented with calcium or fed high-cereal diet—zinc-responsive dermatosis
- Immunosuppression—demodicosis, pyoderma, dermatophytosis

 DIAGNOSIS

DIFFERENTIAL DIAGNOSIS

Nasal Solar Dermatitis
- Lesions—confined to nose; precipitated by heavy sunlight exposure
- Begins in poorly pigmented skin at junction of nasal planum and bridge of nose
- Negative DIF

DLE
- Primarily affects nasal area
- Exacerbated by sunlight
- Positive DIF at basement membrane zone
- Biopsy—interface dermatitis

SLE
- Multisystemic disease
- Skin lesions—often involve nose, face, mucocutaneous junctions; multifocal or generalized
- ANA positive
- Positive DIF at basement membrane zone

Pemphigus Foliaceus
- Lesions—usually start on face and ears; commonly involve footpads; eventually generalize
- Biopsy—subcorneal pustules with acantholysis
- Positive DIF in intercellular spaces of epidermis

Pemphigus Erythematosus
- Lesions—primarily confined to face and ears
- Biopsy—intraepidermal pustules with acantholysis
- Positive DIF at basement membrane zone and intercellular spaces

Demodicosis
- Often starts on face or forelimbs
- May generalize
- Diagnose with skin scrapings

Plastic (or Rubber) Dish Dermatitis
- Depigmentation and erythema of anterior nasal planum and anterior lips
- No ulceration or crusting
- History of exposure

Dermatomyositis
- Typical breed
- Nasal, facial, and extremity lesions—characterized by erosion, alopecia, scarring, and hyperpigmentation
- Polymyositis or megaesophagus may be seen.
- Biopsy—interface dermatitis with follicular atrophy
- Negative DIF

Uveodermatologic Syndrome
- Typical breed
- Uveitis and cutaneous macular depigmentation without inflammation—nose, lips, and eyelids
- Biopsy of early lesions—interface dermatitis, pigmentary incontinence

Zinc-responsive Dermatosis
- Typical signalment or diet (i.e., high-fiber or calcium supplementation)
- Crusted lesions—face, mucocutaneous junctions, pressure points, footpads
- Biopsy—parakeratotic hyperkeratosis

Other
- Nasal pyoderma—acute onset of folliculitis on haired portion of nose
- Dermatophytosis—haired portion of the nose; diagnose with culture or biopsy
- Vitiligo—cutaneous macular depigmentation without inflammation on nose, lips, eyelids, footpads, and nails; leukotrichia with leukoderma may be seen.
- Nasal hypopigmentation—normal black coloration of nasal planum fades to light brown or whitish color; may be seasonal or wax and wane

NASAL DERMATOSES

• Idiopathic nasal hyperkeratosis—dry, horny growths of keratin localized to nasal planum
• Other diseases—differentiate with history or biopsy

CBC/BIOCHEMISTRY/URINALYSIS

• Usually normal
• SLE —may see hemolytic anemia, thrombocytopenia, or evidence of glomerulonephritis (high BUN, proteinuria)

OTHER LABORATORY TESTS

N/A

IMAGING

N/A

DIAGNOSTIC PROCEDURES

• Skin scrapings—*Demodex*
• Cytology—fungal organisms, bacteria, or acantholytic cells (pemphigus)
• Dermatophyte test medium—dermatophytosis
• Culture on Sabouraud agar—other fungal infections
• Bacterial culture and sensitivity or cytologic evaluation—pyoderma
• Joint tap—evidence of polyarthritis in SLE
• ANA—positive in most cases of SLE
• Ocular examination—uveitis in uveodermatologic syndrome
• ECG—evidence of myocarditis in SLE
• EMG—evidence of polymyositis in SLE and dermatomyositis
• DIF—deposition of immunoglobulin at the basement membrane zone in DLE, SLE and pemphigus erythematosus and intercellular spaces of epidermis in pemphigus foliaceus and pemphigus erythematosus
• Skin biopsy

IMAGING

N/A

PATHOLOGIC FINDINGS

• Folliculitis/furunculosis (± mites, bacteria, or fungal elements)—demodicosis, dermatophytosis, nasal pyoderma
• Follicular atrophy and perifollicular fibrosis—dermatomyositis
• Interface dermatitis—DLE, SLE, dermatomyositis, uveodermatologic syndrome
• Intraepidermal pustules with acantholysis—pemphigus foliaceus and pemphigus erythematosus
• Parakeratotic hyperkeratosis—zinc-responsive dermatosis
• Hypomelanosis—vitiligo, uveodermatologic syndrome
• Granulomatous/pyogranulomatous dermatitis—pyoderma, fungal, foreign body, idiopathic sterile granuloma

TREATMENT

• Outpatient, except SLE with severe multiorgan dysfunction or tumors requiring surgical excision or radiation therapy
• Reduce exposure to sunlight—DLE, SLE, pemphigus erythematosus, nasal solar dermatitis, squamous cell carcinoma
• Discourage rooting behavior—pyoderma, dermatophytosis
• Warm soaks—aid removal of exudate and crusts
• Replace plastic or rubber dish and avoid contact with topical drug or other agent causing hypersensitivity reaction.

MEDICATIONS

DRUGS

• Fungal infections—systemic antifungals: griseofulvin, ketoconazole, itraconazole (drug of choice in the cat); topical enilconazole for aspergillosis; surgical excision of early discrete lesions
• Nasal solar dermatitis—topical corticosteroids; antibiotics for secondary infection; sunscreens; tattoo hypopigmented skin (not currently used)
• Idiopathic sterile granuloma—surgical excision when feasible; immunosuppressive therapy with glucocorticoids ± azathioprine
• SLE—immunosuppressive therapy with prednisolone ± azathioprine (dogs), chlorambucil, or gold salts (cats)
• Vitiligo/nasal depigmentation—no treatment
• Tumors—surgical excision; chemotherapy; radiation therapy
• Idiopathic nasal hyperkeratosis—antibiotic-corticosteroid cream for fissures
• Other diseases—see specific disease

CONTRAINDICATIONS

• Avoid chrysotherapy in patients with renal disease.
• Azathioprine—use cautiously in cats; may cause fatal leukopenia or thrombocytopenia

PRECAUTIONS

• Griseofulvin—can cause anorexia, vomiting, diarrhea, and bone marrow suppression; feed with high-fat diet
• Ketoconazole—may cause anorexia, gastric irritation, hepatotoxicity, and lightening of hair coat

POSSIBLE INTERACTIONS

N/A

ALTERNATIVE DRUGS

N/A

FOLLOW-UP

PATIENT MONITORING

Varies with specific disease and treatment prescribed

POSSIBLE COMPLICATIONS

Scarring with deep infections or overly vigorous cleaning

MISCELLANEOUS

ASSOCIATED CONDITIONS

N/A

AGE-RELATED FACTORS

N/A

ZOONOTIC POTENTIAL

Dermatophytosis

PREGNANCY

Griseofulvin is teratogenic.

SYNONYMS

Uveodermatologic = Vogt-Koyanagi-Harada syndrome

ABBREVIATIONS

• ANA = antinuclear antibody
• DIF = direct immunofluorescence
• DLE = discoid lupus erythematosus
• EMG = electromyography
• SLE = systemic lupus erythematosus

Suggested Reading

Muller GH, Kirk RW, Scott DW. Small animal dermatology. 4th ed. Philadelphia: Saunders, 1989.

Authors Ellen C. Codner and Karen Helton Rhodes

Consulting Editor Karen Helton Rhodes

NASAL DISCHARGE (SNEEZING, REVERSE SNEEZING, GAGGING)

BASICS

DEFINITION
• May be serous, mucoid, mucopurulent, purulent, blood tinged, frank blood (epistaxis), or contain food debris • Sneezing—reflexive expulsion of air through the nasal cavity; commonly associated with nasal discharge • Reverse sneezing—repetitive, forceful inspiratory efforts elicited after irritation of the caudal-dorsal nasopharynx • Gagging and retching—involuntary, reflexive attempts to clear secretions from the pharynx, upper respiratory, or gastrointestinal tract

PATHOPHYSIOLOGY
• Secretions—produced by mucous cells of the epithelium and submucosal glands; increased production owing to irritation of the nasal mucosa by mechanical, chemical, or inflammatory stimuli • Mucosal irritation and accumulated secretions—potent stimulus of the sneeze reflex, which may be first sign of nasal discharge • Sneezing—frequency often diminishes with chronic disease • Reverse sneezing—caused by irritation of the mucosa of the caudo-dorsal nasopharynx • Gagging—protective reflex elicited by oropharyngeal stimulation; usually functions to clear material from the oropharynx; often follows a coughing episode as secretions are brought through the larynx into the oropharynx

SYSTEMS AFFECTED
• Respiratory—mucosa of the upper tract, including the nasal cavities, sinuses, and nasopharynx; lower tract disease may produce secretions that affect the upper airways. • Cardiovascular—systemic hypertension • Gastrointestinal—signs may be observed with extranasal diseases (e.g., swallowing disorders and esophageal or gastrointestinal diseases) • Hemic/Lymphatic/Immune—blood-tinged discharge or epistaxis owing to platelets or primary defects of hemostasis

SIGNALMENT
• Dogs and cats • Young animals—cleft palate; ciliary dyskinesia; immunoglobulin deficiency; nasal polyps • Old animals—nasal tumors; primary dental disease • Hunting dogs—foreign body • Dolichocephalic dogs—aspergillosis • Irish wolfhounds—hyperplastic rhinitis • Nasal aspergillosis and rhinosporidiosis—not reported in cats. • Male dogs may have a higher incidence of nasal fungal infection than do females.

SIGNS

Historical Findings
• Sneezing—commonly reported as a concurrent problem • Important to collect information concerning both the initial and current character of the discharge and whether it was originally unilateral or bilateral • Response to previous antibiotic therapy—may help determine secondary bacterial involvement; foreign body and dental-related disease usually respond initially to antibiotic treatment but commonly relapse days to weeks after treatment; nasal tumors and fungal rhinitis typically show little response.

Physical Examination Findings
• Secretions or dried discharge on the hair of the muzzle or forelimbs • May note reduction in nasal air flow • Concurrent dental disease • Bony involvement—with a tumor or fourth premolar abscess; may be detected as facial or hard palate swelling or as pain secondary to osteomyelitis owing to fungal or bacterial infection or tumor invasion • Mucosal depigmentation of the nasal cartilages—often observed with chronic nasal discharge, especially dogs with nasal aspergillosis • Mandibular lymphadenomegaly—neoplasia, fungal infection, dental disease • Polyp—may be visible on otoscopic exam • Chorioretinitis—may be seen with distemper or cryptococcosis

CAUSES
• Unilateral—often associated with non-systemic processes; foreign body; dental-related disease (e.g., abscess and oronasal fistula); fungal infections (e.g., aspergillosis, penicilliosis, cryptococcosis, and *Sporothrix*); nasal tumor (e.g., adenocarcinoma, squamous cell carcinoma, and fibrosarcoma) • Bilateral—infectious agent (e.g., feline viral rhinotracheitis, feline calci virus, canine distemper, and secondary bacterial infection); airborne irritant; allergy; ciliary dyskinesia; IgA deficiency; lymphoplasmacytic or hyperplastic rhinitis • Unilateral progressing to bilateral—*Aspergillus;* nasal tumor • Either unilateral or bilateral—epistaxis (e.g., coagulopathy and systemic hypertension); foreign body; nasal parasites (dogs, *Pneumonyssoides;* dogs and cats, *Cuterebra* and *Capillaria;* cats, *Linguatula*) • Extranasal diseases—pneumonia, megaesophagus, chronic vomiting, cricopharyngeal achalasia; secretions may be forced into the nasopharynx, resulting in discharge

RISK FACTORS
• Exposure to other animals • Dental disease • Foreign bodies—more common in outdoor animals • Infectious—poorly vaccinated animal; kennel situations • Nasal aspergillosis—dogs bedded on straw • Nasal mites—kennel-raised dogs • Immunosuppression, chronic corticosteroid use, and FeLV or FIV infection • Chronic pneumonia • Chronic vomiting

DIAGNOSIS

DIFFERENTIAL DIAGNOSIS

Similar Signs
Differentiate reverse sneezing (occurs on inspiration) from regular sneezing (occurs on expiration)—localize the site of irritation to the caudal-dorsal nasopharynx

Causes
• Serous—mild irritation; viral and parasitic (e.g., nasal mites) disorders • Mucoid—allergy; early neoplastic condition • Purulent (or mucopurulent)—secondary bacterial or fungal infection • Serosanguinous to epistaxis—destructive process (e.g., primary nasal tumor and aspergillosis in dogs); after violent or paroxysmal sneezing episodes (e.g., traumatic capillary rupture); associated with selected systemic disease (e.g., coagulopathy, platelet disorder, and systemic hypertension)

CBC/BIOCHEMISTRY/URINALYSIS
• Results not specific for any particular cause • Valuable—detect concurrent problems; part of a thorough evaluation before general anesthesia for diagnostic procedures

OTHER LABORATORY TESTS
• Serologic tests—diagnose fungal (e.g., aspergillosis and cryptococcosis) and rickettsial (e.g., ehrlichiosis and Rocky Mountain spotted fever) diseases • Coagulation studies—determine platelet numbers and function • Immunoglobulin quantification—diagnose IgA deficiency

IMAGINING

Skull Radiography
• Anesthetize and carefully position patient • Perform before rhinoscopy and periodontal probing, which may cause nasal bleeding and alter the radiographic density observed in the nasal cavity. • Lateral view—detect any periosteal reaction over the nasal bone; note gross changes in the maxillary teeth, nasal cavity, and frontal sinuses (without identifying which side is involved); evaluate air column outlining the nasopharynx • Open-mouth ventrodorsal and the intraoral views (using mammography sheet film)—excellent for evaluating nasal cavities and turbinates • Rostrocaudal view—evaluate each frontal sinus (periosteal reaction and filling) • CT scans—help detect the extent of bony changes associated with nasal tumors and fungal rhinitis

Dental Radiography
• Lateral oblique views (use high-speed screen film)—best for detecting maxillary tooth abnormalities • Ultraspeed, nonscreen,

NASAL DISCHARGE (SNEEZING, REVERSE SNEEZING, GAGGING)

intraoral dental film—provides excellent detail of nasal and dental disorders in cats

Thoracic Radiography
May reveal areas of alveolar infiltrates—coughed-up secretions in a patient with chronic pneumonia may cause nasopharyngeal irritation and nasal discharge.

DIAGNOSTIC PROCEDURES
• Rhinoscopy—indicated with chronic or recurrent nasal discharge; may be indicated with reverse sneezing and acute epistaxis; both anterior and posterior procedures; may be contraindicated with bleeding disorders • Nasal cytologic examination—nonspecific inflammation (nondegenerative polymorphonuclear cells) most commonly found; large numbers of eosinophils suggest hypersensitivity or allergic rhinitis; hyphae or microconidia diagnostic for *Aspergillus;* yeast bodies diagnostic for *Cryptococcus;* may note neoplastic cells • Fungal culture—difficult to interpret; up to 40% of normal dogs may have positive fungal cultures; heavy bacterial growth of a single organism may be important; deep culture specimens obtained by rhinotomy or deep rhinoscopy more reliable • Biopsy of the nasal cavity—indicated with chronic nasal discharge and with suspected tissue growth (tumor or granuloma); various techniques may be used (direct endoscopic biopsy, rigid catheter or the blind coring technique, and rhinotomy); multiple samples required to ensure adequate representation because necrosis of the leading edge is common; perform electron microscopy with suspected ciliary dyskinesia. • Bronchoscopy—indicated when rhinoscopy reveals only minimal changes; exudate often observed in the middle lung lobes of dogs that do not show typical lower respiratory signs and serves as an extranasal source of discharge • Periodontal probing of all upper teeth—part of every evaluation of sneezing and nasal discharge; perform after rhinoscopy; the normal gingival sulcus: dogs, < 4.0 mm; cats, < 1.0 mm • Blood pressure—with epistaxis and a normal coagulation profile

TREATMENT
• Outpatient—acceptable except when surgery is required
• Surgery—for exploratory rhinotomy; to treat *Rhinosporidium* or foreign body; to place tubes to deliver antifungal medications
• Adequate hydration, nutrition, warmth and hygiene (keeping nares clean)—important with chronic sneezing and nasal discharge

MEDICATIONS

DRUGS OF CHOICE
• Secondary bacterial infection—antibiotics; choose a good gram-positive spectrum of activity (e.g., amoxicillin, clavamox, clindamycin, and one of the cephalosporins); tetracyclines are actively secreted into the gingival sulcus and may be used with chronic rhinitis secondary to dental disease.
• Attempt to dry up nasal secretions—decongestants (ephedrine at 10–50 mg total PO q8–12h, to a maximum of 4 mg/kg, dogs; 2–4 mg/kg q8–12h, cats); topical vasoconstrictors (neosynephrine at 0.25%–0.5% q8–24h or oxymetazoline at 0.25% q24h)
• Dental-associated rhinitis—antibiotics; dental work (e.g., extractions, gingivectomy, and flap closure to treat fistula)
• Foreign body removal—antibiotics
• Nasal parasites—ivermectin (200–300 μg/kg PO weekly for 2–3 weeks) to treat *Pneumonyssoides;* fenbendazole (50 mg/kg q6h for 10 days) to treat *Capillaria*
• Allergy—prednisolone (1–2 mg/kg PO q12–24h)
• Fungal rhinitis—topical treatment with an antifungal agent delivered through surgically or endoscopically placed frontal sinus tubes (e.g., enilconazole or clotrimazole, or systemic treatment with itraconazole at 5–10 mg/kg PO q12–24h); surgical curettage in selected cases
• Neoplasia—radiotherapy and chemotherapy

CONTRAINDICATIONS
• Ephedrine—in cardiac patients
• Ivermectin—in collies

PRECAUTIONS
• Itraconazole—anorexia, nausea, vomiting, and high liver enzymes (e.g., ALT) reverse when the drug is discontinued
• Rebound phenomenon—reported with overuse of topical nasal vasoconstrictors

POSSIBLE INTERACTIONS
N/A

ALTERNATIVE DRUGS
• *Cryptococcus* or *Sporothrix* (cats)—itraconazole and fluconazole

FOLLOW-UP

PATIENT MONITORING
• Nasal discharge and sneezing—note changes in frequency, volume, and character. • Surgically placed nasal tubes—inpatient monitoring; watch for subcutaneous emphysema and local cellulitis. • Repeat rhinoscopy—indicated to ensure adequate response to treatment for fungal rhinitis • Recheck thoracic radiographs or bronchoscopy—monitor response to treatment for chronic pneumonia

POSSIBLE COMPLICATIONS
• Loss of appetite—especially in cats • Extension of primary disease (e.g., fungal infection and tumor) into the mouth, eye, or brain
• Dyspnea—caused by nasal obstruction
• Involvement of the cribriform plate in dogs with aspergillosis—may cause CNS damage during topical drug therapy and tube placement

MISCELLANEOUS

ASSOCIATED CONDITIONS
• Sinusitis • Dental disease • Secondary causes—coagulopathy, pneumonia, cricopharyngeal disease, megaesophagus • Cats—immunosuppression caused by FeLV or FIV; fungal disease (e.g., cryptococcosis and *Sporothrix*); upper respiratory viral infection

AGE-RELATED FACTORS
Middle-aged to old patients—often associated with dental or neoplastic conditions

ZOONOTIC POTENTIAL
Sporothrix infection may represent a zoonotic health concern.

PREGNANCY
The safety of most recommended drugs has not been established in pregnant animals.

SEE ALSO
• Aspergillosis • Ciliary Dyskinesia, Primary • Cryptococcosis • Epistaxis • Nasal and Nasopharyngeal Polyps • Nasopharyngeal Stenosis • Rhinitis and Sinusitis

ABBREVIATIONS
• ALT = alanine aminotransferase • FeLV = feline leukemia virus • FIV = feline immunodeficiency virus

Suggested Reading

McKiernan BC. Sneezing and nasal discharge. In: Ettinger SJ, Feldman EC, eds. Textbook of veterinary internal medicine. 4th ed. Philadelphia: Saunders, 1994:79–85.

Ogilvie GK, LaRue SM. Canine and feline nasal and paranasal sinus tumors. Vet Clin North Am 1992;22:1133–1144.

Van Pelt DR, Lappin MR. Pathogenesis and treatment of feline rhinitis. Vet Clin North Am 1994;24:807–823.

Van Pelt DR, McKiernan BC. Pathogenesis and treatment of canine rhinitis. Vet Clin North Am Small Anim Pract 1994;24:789–806.

Author Brendan C. McKiernan
Consulting Editor Eleanor C. Hawkins

NECK AND BACK PAIN

 BASICS

DEFINITION
Discomfort along the spinal column

PATHOPHYSIOLOGY
Pain may originate in the epaxial muscle, vertebrae and associated structures, spinal nerves, nerve roots or dorsal root ganglia, and meninges.

SYSTEMS AFFECTED
- Nervous
- Musculoskeletal

SIGNALMENT
- Dogs and cats
- Disk disease—dogs: usually develops at 3–8 years old, occasionally outside this range; rare in cats
- Wobbler syndrome—large-breed dogs; more often in middle-aged to old Doberman pinschers and young Great Danes
- Atlantoaxial luxation and subluxation—occurs in young to middle-aged miniature breeds

SIGNS

Historical Findings
Complaints—relate to perceived discomfort; reluctance in going up or down stairs most common

Physical Examination Findings
- Head down posture—neck
- Arched back—neck or back
- Pain on epaxial palpation
- Guarded posture
- Reluctance to walk
- Epaxial muscle rigidity
- Palpable heat in the epaxial musculature
- Low grade fever—primarily in patients with meningeal involvement

CAUSES

Epaxial Muscle
- Traumatic myositis
- Exertional rhabdomyolysis
- Muscle neoplasia—rhabdomyosarcoma
- Inflammatory myositis—parasitic, bacterial, protozoal, or immune mediated
- Foreign body myositis—grass awn migration

Vertebrae and Associated Structures
- Disk disease
- Diskospondylitis
- Osteoarthritis of facets
- Unstable vertebral anomalies—hemivertebrae and atlantoaxial luxation or subluxation
- Vertebral neoplasia—osteosarcoma, chondrosarcoma, multiple myeloma, and metastatic tumors
- Vertebral osteomyelitis
- Fracture
- Luxation and subluxation
- Malformation and malarticulation

Spinal Nerves
- Entrapment by disk herniation
- Neoplasia—neurofibroma and neurofibrosarcoma
- Traumatic entrapment, tearing, or laceration
- Neuritis—viral, bacterial, and parasitic
- Compression or inflammation of dorsal root ganglion
- Meninges
- Meningioma and metastatic neoplasia
- Meningitis—bacterial, viral, parasitic, protozoal, rickettsial, immune mediated, or idiopathic

RISK FACTORS
- Trauma
- Very active animal
- Previous diagnosis of cancer

 DIAGNOSIS

DIFFERENTIAL DIAGNOSIS
- Diseases involving thoracic structures—pleura, cardiovascular system, and lungs
- Diseases involving abdominal structures—kidneys, prostate gland, pancreas, and intestines
- Rule out limb musculoskeletal pain.
- Degenerative radiculomyelopathy and fibrocartilaginous myelopathy—nonpainful diseases of the spinal cord
- Often associated with neoplasia in cats

CBC/BIOCHEMISTRY/URINALYSIS

Epaxial Muscle
- Creatine kinase—can be high with any diseases affecting the muscle
- High WBC count—may indicate an abscess
- Myoglobinuria—may reflect the extent of damage

Vertebrae and Associated Structures
- Usually normal with degenerative, anomalous, and neoplastic disease
- Hemogram—may be abnormal with inflammatory diseases (e.g., acute diskospondylitis and multisystemic involvement)

Spinal Nerves
Usually normal

Meninges
- Usually normal, even with severe meningitis
- Leucocytosis—some patients with aseptic meningitis

OTHER LABORATORY TESTS

Vertebrae and Associated Structures
Multiple myeloma—may note Bence Jones protein in the urine; bone marrow examination may reveal neoplastic cells.

Meninges
- Specific serologic tests—depend on suspected cause; canine distemper, ehrlichiosis, Rocky Mountain spotted fever, neosporosis, toxoplasmosis
- Serum IgA—often high with aseptic meningitis

IMAGING

Epaxial Muscle
- Applicable only in patients with suspected neoplasia or foreign body
- Thoracic radiography—detect metastasis

Vertebrae and Associated Structures
- Survey radiography—thoracic: detect metastasis; spinal: detect obvious bony abnormalities (e.g., fracture or luxation, diskospondylitis, neoplasia, osteoarthritis, and extruded calcified disk)
- Myelography—delineate extradural (e.g., disk herniation), intradural-extramedullary (e.g., meningioma), and intramedullary (e.g., spinal neoplasia) lesions
- Discography—best used at the lumbosacral junction; identify stenosis and disk herniation
- CT—cross-sectional and other special views; more clearly defines bony lesions
- MRI—cross-sectional and other special views; more clearly defines soft tissue lesions

Spinal Nerves
- Survey radiograph—seldom of benefit
- Myelography—seldom of benefit unless the lesion is pressing or invading the meninges
- MRI—most rewarding imaging technique for identifying the location and extent of the lesion

Meninges
- Myelography—can identify neoplastic involvement (e.g., meningioma)
- MRI—more clearly defines soft tissue lesions

NECK AND BACK PAIN

DIAGNOSTIC PROCEDURES

Epaxial Muscle
• Muscle biopsy—may reveal neoplastic or inflammatory cells
• EMG—may identify an irritating or denervating process affecting the muscles

Vertebrae and Associated Structures
• Bone biopsy—helps confirm vertebral neoplasia and infection
• Cytology and culture (diskospondylitis)—obtain aspirate from the affected intervertebral space; may help identify cause

Spinal Nerves
• Electrodiagnostic testing—EMG, nerve conduction velocity, and F waves; helps differentiate and confirm muscle versus nerve disease and location of the lesion

Meninges
CSF analysis—diagnostic test of choice; include measurement of immunoglobulins, serologic testing, and bacterial culture.

TREATMENT
• Varies widely according to the nature and extent of the tissues involved
• **CAUTION:** symptomatic treatment without first establishing a diagnosis can be dangerous.
• Inpatient vs. outpatient—depends on severity of disease
• Surgical intervention—inpatient; indicated for disk herniation, trauma, congenital anomalies, and neoplasia; foreign body may require removal or drainage to treat an associated abscess.

MEDICATIONS

DRUGS OF CHOICE

Epaxial Muscle
• Antimicrobial therapy—for infection; depends on the causative agent
• Glucocorticosteroids—may be required; depends on the diagnosis
• Chemotherapy or radiotherapy—for neoplasia; depends on tumor type

Vertebrae and Associated Structures
• Glucocorticosteroids—indicated in some patients and contraindicated in others; establish a diagnosis, if at all possible, before initiating
• Antimicrobials—indicated when a specific organism can be identified or is suspected (e.g., with diskospondylitis)
• Chemotherapy and radiotherapy—depends on tumor type

Spinal Nerves
Corticosteroids—useful for trauma, inflammation, and nerve compression; may help some patients with neoplasia

Meninges
• Antimicrobials that cross the blood–brain barrier—when delivery to the CNS is desired
• Corticosteroids—may be indicated; establish a diagnosis, if at all possible, before initiating.

CONTRAINDICATIONS
Glucocorticosteroids—may be detrimental for patients with infectious conditions and with gastroenteritis or cystitis

PRECAUTIONS
• Glucocorticosteroids—watch for signs of gastroenteritis or cystitis before initiating and while administering.
• With instability or possible disk disease—cage rest indicated for patients using drugs with analgesic effects to prevent exacerbation of the primary problem and further neurologic damage.
• Steroids and NSAIDs—do not use in combination; life-threatening gastroenteritis may result.

POSSIBLE INTERACTIONS
N/A

ALTERNATIVE DRUGS
• NSAIDs
• Polysulfated glycosaminoglycan
• Methocarbamol—muscle relaxation
• Benzodiazepines (e.g., diazepam)—muscle relaxation and antianxiety effects
• Phenylbutazone—may alleviate musculoskeletal pain; ineffective against neurologic pain

FOLLOW-UP

PATIENT MONITORING
• Monitor response to treatment closely and make adjustments as necessary.
• Instruct client to watch for signs of gastroenteritis and cystitis.

POSSIBLE COMPLICATIONS

Epaxial Muscle
• Abscess
• Chronic pain
• Fibrous replacement of muscle fibers, causing chronic pain and immobility

Vertebrae and Associated Structures
• Frequent recurrence in patients with disk disease that receive medical management only
• Permanent paralysis or dysfunction
• Urinary and fecal incontinence
• Chronic pain
• Spread to adjacent tissues

Spinal Nerves
• Permanent paralysis or dysfunction
• Chronic pain

Meninges
• Death
• Involvement of surrounding spinal cord and brain tissue

MISCELLANEOUS

ASSOCIATED CONDITIONS
• Cardiac muscle disease in patients with myositis
• Sites of infection in other tissues as a source of CNS or vertebral involvement (e.g., bacterial endocarditis or cystitis as a cause of diskospondylitis)
• Metastatic disease from a primary tumor in another organ system
• Immunologic incompetence

AGE-RELATED FACTORS
• Anomalous conditions—usually seen in younger animals
• Disk disease—most frequently seen in active, middle-aged dogs
• Neoplastic conditions—more often seen in middle-aged to old animals

ZOONOTIC POTENTIAL
N/A

PREGNANCY
Use of glucocorticosteroids is contraindicated.

SEE ALSO
See causes

ABBREVIATION
EMG = electromyelography
NSAIDS = nonsteroidal antiinflammatory drugs

Suggested Reading
Aron DM. Pain. In: Lorenz MD, Cornelius LM, eds. Small animal medical diagnosis. Philadelphia: Lippincott, 1987:411–424.
Oliver JE, Lorenz MD, Kornegay JN. Pain. In: Handbook of veterinary neurology. Philadelphia: Saunders, 1997:333–340.
Author Patricia J. Luttgen
Consulting Editor Joane M. Parent

NEONATAL MORTALITY (FADING SYNDROME)

BASICS

DEFINITION
Death occuring from birth to 2 weeks of age

PATHOPHYSIOLOGY
• Inadequate thermoregulatory activity, immunologic responses, and glucose control allows greater susceptibility to a number of insults, usually combination of environmental, infectious, nutritional, and metabolic factors
• Hypothermia, hypoglycemia, dehydration, and hypoxia—common preludes

SYSTEMS AFFECTED
• Respiratory
• Endocrine/Metabolic
• Cardiovascular
• Nervous
• Hepatobiliary
• Renal/Urologic

SIGNALMENT
• Dogs and cats
• Pedigree puppies and kittens—more prone to congenital (and hereditary) defects

SIGNS

General Comments
• Preweaning losses—typically 10%–30%; about 65% occur during the first week; greater losses in a cattery or kennel should be considered abnormal.
• Historical and physical examination findings rarely narrow the differential diagnosis, because of the limited number of ways neonates can respond to illness.

Historical Findings
• Low birth weight, loss of weight, and/or failure to gain weight
• Decreased activity and appetite
• Weakness
• Constantly vocal or restless early, quiet and inactive later
• Tendency to remain separate from the dam and the rest of the litter

Physical Examination Findings
• Nonspecific
• Weakness, hypothermia (newborn temperature is about 35.5°C [96°F], rising to 37–37.8°C [99°–100°F] during the fourth week of life), hypoglycemia, dehydration—common and inter-related
• Respiratory distress, diarrhea, or hemoglobinuria—may be seen
• Gross anatomic defects—may be detectable

CAUSES

Noninfectious
• Dam-related—dystocia or prolonged labor; cannibalism; lactation failure; trauma; inattention or overattention; inadequate nutrition, including taurine deficiency in kittens
• Environmental—any factor that discourages nursing and allows hypothermia, including temperature extremes, humidity extremes, inadequate sanitation, overcrowding, and stress
• Nutritional—inadequate or ineffective nursing; hypoglycemia; hypothermia-induced digestive malfunction
• Neonatal isoerythrolysis—queen with blood type B; kitten with blood type A
Birth Defects
• Gross anatomic defects—more frequently in kittens (about 10% of nonsurviving neonates) than in puppies
• Gastrointestinal abnormalities—cleft palate; segmental intestinal agenesis or atresia
• Craniofacial abnormalities—failure of midline closure, causing herniation
• Cardiac defects—valvular dysplasia; VSD; atrioventricular fistula
• Respiratory defects—thoracic wall abnormalities; pectus excavatum; primary ciliary dyskinesia; surfactant deficiency
• Inborn errors of metabolism—usually autosomal recessive traits

Infectious
• Viral (kittens)—feline calicivirus; FeLV; FIV; feline herpesvirus type 1, feline panleukopenia virus
• Viral (puppies)—canine adenovirus type 1; canine distemper virus; canine herpesvirus; canine parvovirus type 1
• Bacterial—acquired mainly across the placenta, in the birch canal, via the umbilicus, gastrointestinal tract, respiratory tract, urinary tract, or skin wounds
• Neonatal sepsis—primarily from *E. coli*, β-hemolytic streptococcus, coagulase-positive staphylococcus, and gram-negative enteric organisms
• Respiratory—*Bordetella bronchiseptica; Pasteurella multocida*
• Enteric—*E. coli; Salmonella* spp.; *Campylobacter* spp.
• *Brucella canis*—puppies
• Parasitic—heavy infection with helminths *Toxocara canis, Toxocara cati, Toxascaris leonina, Ancylostoma caninum,* or *Ancylostoma tubaeforme;* coccidian parasites such as *Toxoplasma, Neospora, Isospora, Cryptosporidium,* or *Giardia*

RISK FACTORS
• Subnormal birth weight or failure to grow normally—kittens: minimum daily gain of 7–10 g; puppies: should double in weight by 10–12 days; both: 5%–10% gain per day generally acceptable
• Dystocia or prolonged labor
• Inbreeding—higher incidence of homozygous recessive genotype
• Sire with blood type A and queen with blood type B

DIAGNOSIS

DIFFERENTIAL DIAGNOSIS
Excessive losses often owing to a combination of environmental, immunologic, nutritional, infectious, and metabolic factors; detection and correction of problems in each area necessary to prevent ongoing losses

CBC/BIOCHEMISTRY/URINALYSIS
Premortem blood samples from affected individuals usually not obtainable and not pathognomonic

CBC
• Hydration status and age influence results.
• Mild normocytic, normochromic anemia
• White cell counts variable; may note thrombocytopenia and mild to moderate neutrophilia (with left shift) if septic

Biochemistry
• Hypoglycemia
• Other changes depend on organ system involved.

Urinalysis
• Hemoglobinuria—with neonatal isoerythrolysis
• Bacteria—with infection
• Urine specific gravity—> 1.017 suggests inadequate hydration

OTHER LABORATORY TESTS
• FeLV antigen test
• FIV antibody test
• Serology—*Brucella canis;* canine herpesvirus; *Toxoplasma; Neospora*

IMAGING
N/A

NEONATAL MORTALITY (FADING SYNDROME)

DIAGNOSTIC PROCEDURES
- Histopathologic—examination of multiple tissues collected at necropsy
- Metabolic screening of urine sample—rule out inborn errors of metabolism.
- Virus isolation
- Bacterial culture
- Blood typing in pedigree cats
- Fecal examination—parasites

PATHOLOGIC FINDINGS
- Postmortem—extremely important; examine as soon after death as possible advisable to minimize autolysis; give special notice to the following items.
- Stomach—devoid of contents: lack of nursing; consider dam-related causes (e.g., inappropriate behavior or lactation) or neonatal problems (e.g., weakness, trauma, or physiologic abnormality); filled with milk: suggests sudden death (e.g., trauma, peracute illness) or gastrointestinal dysfunction (body temperature <35°C [95°F])
- Thymus subnormal size—not pathognomonic; can be a result of multiple causes (e.g., viral infection, nutrition, and defective immune system)
- Petechiation—common; accompanied by hemorrhage in other organ systems suggests coagulopathy or septicemia
- Urine in the urinary bladder—implies a degree of renal dysfunction or inadequate care by the dam
- Lungs—should appear the same as an adult's; homogeneous dark red color typical of a stillborn animal that has not taken a breath; hemorrhage, edema, congestion, and mottled color abnormal but nonspecific
- Note malformations.
- Multiple tissue samples—submit to a diagnostic laboratory; virus isolation, bacterial culture and sensitivity, and histopathology; check with laboratory for proper submission

 TREATMENT
- Correct any underlying deficiencies in husbandry or breeding selection.
- Warmth—slowly warm neonate to 36–36.7°C (97°–98°F) over several hours, if necessary; provide ambient temperature of 29–35°C (85°– 95°F) and relative humidity of 55%–65%.
- Oxygen—supplement at 30%–40%, if necessary

- Intravenous fluids—consider administration of warmed D_5W solution if hypoglycemic; administer warm lactated Ringer's solution or half-strength lactated Ringer's and $D_{2.5}W$ (intravenously, intraosseously, or subcutaneously) at 1.0 mL/30 g body weight
- Do not attempt to feed if body temperature < 35°C (95°F) and no sucking reflex; once warmed, encourage nursing.
- Neonatal isoerythrolysis—disallow nursing for first 24 hr after birth.

 MEDICATIONS

DRUGS OF CHOICE
- Antibiotics—commonly used are penicillins (penicillin G, ampicillin, amoxicillin, amoxicillin with clavulanic acid) and first-generation cephalosporins; reduce adult dose by one-half and use same dosage interval.
- Supplement—milk replacer formula
- Vitamin K_1—0.01–0.1 mg SC or IM once

CONTRAINDICATIONS
Aminoglycosides, tetracyclines, fluoroquinolones, trimethoprim/sulfonamide, and chloramphenicol—avoid during the neonatal period

PRECAUTIONS
Drug absorption, distribution, metabolism, and excretion for dogs and cats differ significantly during the first 5 weeks of life from that of adults

POSSIBLE INTERACTIONS
N/A

ALTERNATIVE DRUGS
N/A

 FOLLOW-UP

PATIENT MONITORING
- Hydration status—check daily; dryness of mouth and yellow golden urine indicate dehydration.
- Body weight—monitor daily or every other day in growing neonates.
- Dam—check that nursing and care is adequate; supplement with milk replacer formula, if necessary.

POSSIBLE COMPLICATION
N/A

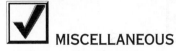 MISCELLANEOUS

ASSOCIATED CONDITIONS
N/A

AGE-RELATED FACTORS
N/A

ZOONOTIC POTENTIAL
N/A

PREGNANCY
N/A

SYNONYMS
- Wasting syndrome
- Fading puppy or kitten syndrome

SEE ALSO
See Causes

ABBREVIATIONS
- FeLV = feline leukemia virus
- FIV = feline immunodeficiency virus
- VSD = ventricular septal defect

Suggested Reading
Hoskins JD. Clinical evaluation of the kitten: from birth to eight weeks of age. Compend Contin Educ Pract Vet 1990;12:1215–1225.
Hoskins JD. Fading puppy and kitten syndromes. Feline Pract 1993;21:19–22.
Jones RL. Special considerations for appropriate antimicrobial therapy in neonates. Vet Clin North Am Small Anim Pract 1987;17:577–602.
Lawler DF. Care and diseases of neonatal puppies and kittens. In: Kirk RW, Bonagura JD, eds. Current veterinary therapy X. Philadelphia: Saunders, 1989:1325–1333.
Lawler DF. Investigating kitten deaths in catteries. In: August JR, ed., Consultations in feline internal medicine. Philadelphia: Saunders, 1991:47–54.
Author Johnny D. Hoskins
Consulting Editor Stephen C. Barr

NEPHROTIC SYNDROME

 BASICS

DEFINITION
The combination of significant proteinuria, hypoalbuminemia, ascites or edema, and hypercholesterolemia; in addition, systemic hypertension and hypercoagulability are commonly associated; usually occurs secondary to either glomerulonephritis or renal amyloidosis

PATHOPHYSIOLOGY
• Persistent protein loss exceeding 3.5 g/day often leads to clinical signs; consequences of severe proteinuria include sodium retention and edema, hypercholesterolemia, hypertension, hypercoagulability, muscle wasting and weight loss. • A combination of low plasma oncotic pressure and hyperaldosteronism causing sodium retention often causes the ascites and edema, but it has been hypothesized that intrarenal mechanisms, independent of aldosterone, may also contribute to sodium retention. The hypercholesterolemia probably results from a combination of decreased catabolism and increased hepatic synthesis of proteins and lipoproteins, which results in accumulation of large-molecular-weight, cholesterol-rich lipoproteins that are not lost through the damaged capillary wall as are the smaller-molecular-weight proteins such as albumin.
• Systemic hypertension is a frequent complication in dogs. It probably results from a combination of sodium retention, glomerular capillary and arteriolar scarring, decreased renal production of vasodilators, increased responsiveness to normal pressor mechanisms, and activation of the renin-angiotensin system. In one study, 84% of dogs with glomerular disease (e.g., glomerulonephritis, glomerulosclerosis, and amyloidosis) had systemic hypertension.
• Hypercoagulability and thromboembolism occur secondary to several abnormalities in the clotting system. In addition to a mild thrombocytosis, hypoalbuminemia-related platelet hypersensitivity increases platelet adhesion and aggregation in proportion to the magnitude of hypoalbuminemia. Loss of antithrombin III in urine also contributes to hypercoagulability. Antithrombin III works in concert with heparin to inhibit serine proteases (clotting factors II, IX, X, XI, and XII) and normally plays a vital role in modulating thrombin and fibrin production. • Finally, altered fibrinolysis and an increased concentration of large-molecular-weight clotting factors (fibrinogen, and clotting factors V, VII, VIII, and X) may lead to a relative increase in clotting factors compared with regulatory proteins.

SYSTEMS AFFECTED
• Renal/Urologic—proteinuria initially; often the underlying disease is progressive, resulting in irreversible glomerular damage, loss of nephrons, azotemia, and chronic renal failure • Cardiovascular—edema, ascites, hypercholesterolemia/hyperlipidemia, hypertension hypercoagulability, and thromboembolic disease

GENETICS
• Familial glomerulonephritis has been reported in Bernese mountain dogs, samoyeds, dobermans, English cocker spaniels, rottweilers, greyhounds, and soft-coated wheaten terriers, as well as cats. • Familial amyloidosis has been reported in Abyssinian, Oriental shorthair, and Siamese cats and Chinese shar pei dogs.

INCIDENCE/PREVALENCE
More common in dogs than in cats

GEOGRAPHIC DISTRIBUTION
N/A

SIGNALMENT

Species
Dogs and cats

Breed Predilection
In some glomerulonephritis studies, golden retrievers, miniature schnauzers, and long-haired dachshunds appear to be overrepresented. Beagles, collies, and Walker hounds are reportedly at increased risk for renal amyloidosis.

Mean Age and Range
• Mean age of dogs with glomerulonephritis—6.5–7.0 years; range, 0.8-17 years • Cats with glomerulonephritis—mean age at presentation is 4.0 years • Most dogs and cats with renal amyloidosis are over 5 years of age.

Predominant Sex
None

SIGNS

Historical Findings
• Edema and/or ascites are the most common presenting complaint. • Occasionally, signs associated with an underlying infectious, inflammatory, or neoplastic disease may be why owners seek veterinary care. • Rarely, dogs may exhibit acute dyspnea or severe panting due to a pulmonary thromboembolism or acute blindness due to retinal hemorrhage or detachment.

Physical Examination Findings
• Edema and ascites • Retinal hemorrhage, detachment, and papilledema can indicate systemic hypertension. • Arrhythmias and/or murmurs secondary to left ventricular hypertrophy caused by systemic hypertension • Dyspnea and cyanosis in dogs with pulmonary thromboembolism

CAUSES
Glomerulonephritis and amyloidosis occur secondary to chronic inflammatory conditions (e.g., infection, neoplasia, and immune-mediated disease).

RISK FACTORS
See Causes above.

 DIAGNOSIS

DIFFERENTIAL DIAGNOSIS

Proteinuria
• Most common cause is inflammatory urinary tract disease (e.g., bacterial cystitis/pyelonephritis, urolithiasis, and neoplasia); inflammation of the urinary tract is usually associated with active urine sediment—increased numbers of RBCs, WBCs, epithelial cells, and bacteria observed in the urine sediment • Glomerulonephritis and renal amyloidosis often cause severe proteinuria with inactive urine sediment (hyaline casts may be present); renal biopsy is the only accurate way to distinguish amyloidosis from glomerulonephritis.

Hypoalbuminemia
Can be associated with decreased albumin production (severe liver disease) and increased albumin loss (protein-losing enteropathies and protein-losing nephropathies)

CBC/BIOCHEMISTRY/URINALYSIS
• Persistent, significant proteinuria with inactive urine sediment (hyaline casts may be observed) is the hallmark laboratory abnormality associated with protein-losing nephropathies. • Hypoalbuminemia and hypercholesterolemia are common.

OTHER LABORATORY TESTS

Urine Protein:Creatinine Ratio
Used to confirm and quantify abnormal proteinuria; the magnitude of proteinuria roughly correlates with the severity of glomerular lesions, making this ratio a useful parameter for assessing response to therapy or progression of disease.

Protein Electrophoresis
• Of urine and serum—may help identify the source of the proteinuria and establish a prognosis • Proteinuria associated with hemorrhage into the urinary tract may have an electrophoretic pattern similar to that of the serum.
• Early glomerular damage usually results principally in albuminuria; with progression of the glomerular disease, an increasing amount of globulin may be lost as well. • Marked decreases in serum albumin and increased concentrations of larger-molecular-weight proteins, such as IgM, in the serum suggest severe proteinuria and the nephrotic syndrome. As the glomerular disease progresses and causes loss of at least three-quarters of the nephrons, the resultant decreased glomerular filtration usually results in decreased proteinuria.

IMAGING
Protein-losing nephropathies do not cause specific changes on abdominal radiographs or renal ultrasound (with severe renal cortical amyloidosis there may increased renal cortical echogenicity and the cortex may be thickened);

NEPHROTIC SYNDROME

however, these tests are useful in ruling out other concurrent conditions. Ultrasound can be used to guide percutaneous renal biopsies.

DIAGNOSTIC PROCEDURES

Do a renal biopsy if significant and persistent proteinuria with inactive urine sediment exists. Histopathologic evaluation of renal tissue will establish a diagnosis (e.g., glomerulonephritis vs. amyloidosis) and help in formulating a prognosis. Consider renal biopsy only after less-invasive tests (CBC, serum biochemistry profile, urinalysis, quantitation of proteinuria) are completed and blood clotting ability has been assessed.

TREATMENT

APPROPRIATE HEALTH CARE
Most nephrotic syndrome patients can be treated as outpatients; exceptions include severely azotemic and/or hypertensive patients and patients with thromboembolic disease.

NURSING CARE
Paracentesis—reserved for patients with respiratory distress and abdominal discomfort caused by ascites

ACTIVITY
Restrict activity because of the possibility of thromboembolic disease.

DIET
Sodium-reduced, high quality, low quantity protein diets

CLIENT EDUCATION
• If the underlying cause cannot be identified and corrected, glomerulonephritis and amyloidosis are usually progressive, resulting in chronic renal failure. • Biopsy required to differentiate between glomerulonephritis and amyloidosis

SURGICAL CONSIDERATIONS
N/A

MEDICATIONS

DRUGS OF CHOICE

Systemic Hypertension
• If hypertension is not controlled with dietary sodium restriction, consider vasodilator therapy. • Angiotensin-converting enzyme (ACE) inhibitors such as enalapril (0.5 mg/kg PO q24h) have decreased glomerular capillary pressure, proteinuria, and incidence of glomerulosclerosis in some studies with rats. Results of clinical trials in dogs with glomerulonephritis are lacking, but the effects of enalapril on renal function in dogs with congestive heart failure have been described. • Individual responses to ACE

inhibitors vary, and acute renal decompensation associated with hypotension is a potential adverse side effect.

Edema and Ascites
• Cage rest and dietary sodium restriction
• Reserve paracentesis and diuretics for patients with respiratory distress and abdominal discomfort. Overzealous use of diuretics may cause dehydration and acute renal decompensation. • Plasma transfusions provide only temporary benefit. • Dietary protein supplementation was formerly recommended to offset the effects of proteinuria; however, normal or high dietary protein may contribute to the progression of renal disease by causing glomerular hyperfiltration, increased proteinuria, and, subsequently, glomerulosclerosis. Thus dietary therapy should include a reduced (not restricted) amount of high-quality protein such as Hill's prescription diets canine and feline k/d. • Dietary protein modulates the renin-angiotensin-aldosterone axis, and angiotensin II may be responsible for the increased glomerular permselectivity mediated by dietary protein. Enalapril and low dietary protein have an additive antiproteinuric effect in rats, and enalapril attenuates hypercholesterolemia and glomerular injury in hyperlipidemic rats. Thus, besides decreasing glomerular capillary hydraulic pressure, ACE inhibitors may attenuate proteinuria by another mechanism.

Antithrombotic
• Prophylactic anticoagulant treatment may benefit patients with significant proteinuria and measurement of antithrombin III and fibrinogen concentrations may help identify patients at greatest risk of thromboembolism. Dogs with antithrombin III concentrations below 70% of normal and fibrinogen concentrations above 300 mg/dL have increased risk for thrombus formation and are candidates for anticoagulant treatment. • Warfarin is highly protein-bound. Individualize its dosage for each patient. An initial dosage of 0.22 mg/kg PO q24h is recommended for dogs. Monitor prothrombin time (with the goal of increasing the baseline prothrombin time by 150%). If new drugs (especially highly protein-bound drugs like aspirin, which may displace warfarin from protein-binding sites) are added to the treatment regimen or if marked changes occur in serum albumin concentrations, reevaluate the patient's prothrombin time. • Low-dose aspirin (5–10 mg/kg PO q12–24h) is easily administered on an outpatient basis and does not require the extensive monitoring of warfarin treatment.

CONTRAINDICATIONS
Do not use corticosteroids in azotemic patients.

PRECAUTIONS
• Dosages of highly protein-bound drugs (e.g., aspirin) may need adjustment; serum albumin concentrations change with treatment or progression of disease. • Use enalapril with

caution in azotemic patients.

POSSIBLE INTERACTIONS
See Precautions

ALTERNATIVE DRUGS
N/A

FOLLOW-UP

PATIENT MONITORING
Urinary protein:creatinine ratio, serum urea nitrogen, creatinine, albumin, and electrolyte concentrations, blood pressure, and body weight; ideally, recheck examinations should occur 1, 3, 6, 9, and 12 months after initiation of treatment.

POSSIBLE COMPLICATIONS
Chronic renal insufficiency or failure

MISCELLANEOUS

ASSOCIATED CONDITIONS
• Hypertension • Hypercoagulability

AGE-RELATED FACTORS
N/A

ZOONOTIC POTENTIAL
N/A

PREGNANCY
High risk in those patients with severe hypoalbuminemia and/or hypertension

SYNONYMS
• Glomerulopathy • Protein-losing nephropathy

SEE ALSO
• Glomerulonephritis • Amyloidosis • Proteinuria

ABBREVIATIONS
ACE = angiotensin-converting enzyme

Suggested Reading

Center SA, Smith CA, Wilkinson E, et al. Clinicopathologic, renal immunofluorescent, and light microscopic features of glomerulonephritis in the dog: 41 cases (1975–1985). J Am Vet Med Assoc 1987;190:81–90.

Cook AK, Cowgill LD. Clinical and pathologic features of protein-losing glomerular disease in the dog. A review of 137 cases (1985–1992). J Am Anim Hosp Assoc 1996;32:313–322.

DiBartola SP, Benson MD. Review: the pathogenesis of reactive systemic amyloidosis. J Vet Int Med 1989;3:31–41.

Grauer GF. Glomerulonephritis. Semin Vet Med Surg (Small Anim) 1992;7:187–197.

Author Gregory F. Grauer

Consulting Editors Larry G. Adams and Carl A. Osborne

OBESITY

BASICS

DEFINITION
The presence of body fat in sufficient excess to compromise normal physiologic function or predispose to metabolic, surgical, and/or mechanical problems

PATHOPHYSIOLOGY
• Animal factors—although breed predispositions have been reported, any animal may become obese; inactivity is an important risk factor in both dogs and cats, as are increasing age and neutering.
• Dietary factors—no specific diet other than a surfeit of "table scraps" and "treats" has been shown to increase risk in dogs; in cats, consumption of "high-fat" diets reportedly increases risk.
• Feeding management—many animals are overfed; reasons for excessive food consumption include ignorance of proper feeding practices, inappropriately generous feeding recommendations by manufacturers, emphasis on food palatability both by owners and manufacturers, and inadequate explanation by veterinarians of appropriate body condition for the pet and how to maintain it.
• Owner factors—many owners of overweight pets are overweight themselves and engage in feeding as a social activity; clients also may consider their pet to be "one of the family" and be unwilling to deprive a loved one of food; these factors may undermine simple-minded "eat less and exercise more!" approaches to management of obesity; they must be identified and acknowledged by both client and therapist for long-term resolution of obesity.

SYSTEMS AFFECTED
• Patients more than 40% above "optimum" (moderate) body weight are at increased risk.

Dogs
• Cardiovascular
• Musculoskeletal—articular and locomotor problems, including developmental orthopedic disease in growing dogs

Cats
• Endocrine/Metabolic—diabetes mellitus
• Musculoskeletal—lameness
• Dermatologic—nonallergic skin problems
• Hepatobiliary—hepatic lipidosis may occur if food intake ceases.

SIGNALMENT
• Dogs and cats
• Breeds predisposed include the Labrador retriever, Cairn terrier, cocker spaniel, dachshund, sheltie, basset hound, beagle, King Charles spaniel, collie, and, in our practice, Norwegian elkhounds
• Female dogs are at increased risk.
• In cats, apartment dwelling, inactive, middle-aged neutered males of mixed-breed ancestry are at increased risk.

SIGNS
• Excess amounts of body fat for body size, often measured as body condition score of ≥4 on a 1–5 scale in which 1 = cachectic (>20% underweight), 2 = lean (10–20% underweight), 3 = moderate, 4 = stout (20–40% overweight), 5 = obese (>40% overweight)
• Sites of adipose tissue to evaluate during physical examination include the ribcage and abdomen; one should be able to feel the ribs easily and see an abdominal "waist" when viewing the animal either from above or from the side.
• Cats often exhibit excessive inguinal fat.

CAUSES
• Most commonly, excessive access to highly palatable food, often combined with insufficient activity; clinically, at least two types of owners may be distinguished: "mindless," for whom feeding the animal is an automatic chore, and "timeless," for whom feeding is a significant social, time-filling activity.
• Hypothyroidism
• Hyperadrenocorticism
• Insulinoma

RISK FACTORS
• Owner lifestyle
• Diet palatability and energy density
• Breed
• Activity level

DIAGNOSIS

DIFFERENTIAL DIAGNOSIS
Differentiating Similar Signs
• Pregnancy
• Increased muscle mass
• Hypothyroidism
• Cushing's disease
• Insulinoma
• Intraabdominal neoplasia or organomegaly

Differentiating Causes
• Similar problems/diseases should be differentiated via history, physical examination, laboratory evaluation, and imaging.
• Document body condition score ≥4

CBC/BIOCHEMISTRY/URINALYSIS
Normal

OTHER LABORATORY TESTS
Normal

IMAGING
Demonstrates excess body fat

DIAGNOSTIC PROCEDURES
N/A

TREATMENT

Success is lifelong amelioration of the problem.

DIET

• Any of the many reduced-calorie diets currently available may be dispensed or prescribed.

• Changing the diet may help to reeducate the client about feeding, but diet per se does not cause obesity and is ancillary to its long-term treatment.

CLIENT EDUCATION

• Most important part of obesity therapy; must be tailored to each particular circumstance

• Mindless—demonstrate appropriate body condition score, explain that the pet should be fed the amount of food necessary to achieve this condition in this particular animal; reducing food availability to achieve the desired body condition often suffices.

• Timeless—much more careful investigation of the circumstances and consideration of the necessity for maintaining a lower weight are necessary for this group; clients must come to want the animal to maintain a lower weight for demonstrable reasons and need the means and support to achieve this, while retaining the desired relationship with the pet. Therapeutic suggestions include reasonable, functional weight loss goals, rather than recommending achieving a poorly defined "optimal adult weight" for aesthetic reasons (e.g., sufficient weight loss to enhance glycemic control of a non–insulin-dependent diabetic or ability to walk for 20 min without exhaustion or lameness). Keeping a food record that identifies all food sources may help some clients appreciate how many the pet consumes. Suggest that "snacks" *replace* regular food rather than *supplement* it and that the snacks consist of a portion of the regularly allotted food.

 ## MEDICATIONS

DRUGS OF CHOICE
N/A

CONTRAINDICATIONS
N/A

PRECAUTIONS
N/A

POSSIBLE INTERACTIONS
N/A

ALTERNATIVE DRUGS
N/A

 ## FOLLOW-UP

PATIENT MONITORING

• As with any other chronic metabolic problem, lifelong follow-up, coaching, and support are essential to maintain the reduced weight.

• At the initial visit instruct clients to recognize moderate body condition score and to feed the quantity of food necessary to maintain this condition during the changing physiologic and environmental conditions of the pet's life; remind them at checkups.

• When clients express concern about how little food is needed to maintain moderate body condition, recommend increased activity and/or a reduced-calorie diet *before* the animal becomes obese.

POSSIBLE COMPLICATIONS
N/A

 ## MISCELLANEOUS

ASSOCIATED CONDITIONS
• Orthopedic problems
• Skin problems
• Respiratory problems
• Increased anesthetic risk
• Cardiovascular problems—dogs
• Diabetes mellitus—cats
• Hepatic lipidosis—cats

AGE-RELATED FACTOR
N/A

ZOONOTIC POTENTIAL
N/A

PREGNANCY
Obesity may increase risk of dystocia; but because of potential risk to the fetus, do not treat pregnant animals.

SYNONYMS
N/A

SEE ALSO
• Hyperadrenocorticism
• Hypothyroidism
• Insulinoma

ABBREVIATIONS
N/A

Suggested Reading

Obesity in cats and dogs. Int J Obesity 1994;18(Suppl 1).

Scarlett JM, Donoghue S. Associations between body condition and disease in cats. JAVMA 1998;212(11):1725–1731.

Ohio State University Weight Loss Plan on the world wide web at http://www.nss.vet.ohio-state.edu

Author C. A. Tony Buffington

Consulting Editors Mitchell A. Crystal and Brett M. Feder

ODONTOCLASTIC RESORPTIVE LESIONS—CATS

BASICS

DEFINITION
Dental resorptions of unknown etiology affecting cats

PATHOPHYSIOLOGY
• Unlike cavities in humans, which result from bacterial enzymes and acids digesting the tooth substance, the cause of feline odontoclastic resorptive lesions (FORLs) is presently unknown; cells called odontoclasts, found in the defects, cause tooth structure to dissolve; odontoclasts originate from monocytes.
• In the acute phase, odontoclasts attach to the lacunar surface of intact dental tissue; resorption progresses and reparative bonelike or cementum-like tissue covers the excavated dentin; granulomatous tissue often occupies the excavated sites.
• Resorption also occurs in the periodontal ligament and alveolar bone; both external and internal resorption may take place; in time, remodeling replaces dentinal tissue with bonelike or cementum-like tissues, radio-graphically appearing as ankylosis.

SYSTEMS AFFECTED
Oral cavity

GENETICS
N/A

INCIDENCE/PREVALENCE
• A relatively newly recognized syndrome
• A large percentage of cats older than 1 year have at least one FORL.
• Most feline patients presented for diagnosis or treatment of oral or dental disease have their teeth affected with FORLs; presence consistently increases with age.

GEOGRAPHIC DISTRIBUTION
N/A

SIGNALMENT

Species
Cat

Breed Predilections
Asian short-haired, Siamese, Persian, and Abyssinian cats may show a breed predisposition.

Mean Age and Range
N/A

Predominant Sex
N/A

SIGNS

Historical Findings
• Most affected cats show no clinical signs; some show hypersalivation; others, oral bleeding or difficulty chewing; some cats pick up and drop food (especially hard food) when eating; others hiss while chewing.
• Some cats have behavior changes—reclusive or aggressive

Physical Examination Findings
• A cotton-tipped applicator applied to the suspected FORL (classes 2–4) usually cause pain evidenced by jaw spasms.
• FORLs can occur above or below the free gingival margin; most occur at the labial or buccal surface near the cementoenamel junction where the free gingiva meets the tooth surface; calculus and hyperplastic gingival tissue may obscure the lesion.
• FORLs can be found on any tooth; most commonly affected are the mandibular third premolar and molar, followed by the maxillary third and fourth premolars.
• Under general anesthesia, the lesions are examined with an explorer; a fine Shepherd's hook type is preferred; the explorer helps identify subgingival lesions coronal to the alveolar bone; the furcation area is a frequent site, and the examiner must distinguish a resorptive lesion from disease limited to alveolar bone loss.
• Class I FORL—enamel defect less than 0.5 mm deep; minimally sensitive because it has not entered the dentin
• Class 2 FORL—penetrates the enamel and dentin, but does not enter the endodontic system; these teeth may be treated with glass ionomer restoratives, which release fluoride ions to desensitize the exposed dentin,

strengthen the enamel, and chemically bind to tooth surfaces; only 20% success rate, longterm (> 2 yr).
• Class 3 FORL—penetrates into the endodontic system; radiographs are needed to determine the full extent of penetration.
• Class 4 FORL—the crown has been eroded or fractured; gingiva growing over the root fragments leave a painful bleeding lesion upon probing
• Class 5 FORL—the tooth crown is gone; gingival swelling covers the retained root.

CAUSES
• The etiology is unknown; likely a multitude of initiating factors exist.
• Affected cats may have calcium regulation problems; an improper ratio of dietary calcium, magnesium, and phosphorus; or parathyroid gland malfunction producing calcium imbalance.
• Hyperreactivity to inflammatory cells; dental plaque, and/or calculus, endotoxins; prostaglandins, cytokines, and proteinases, are also under investigation.

RISK FACTORS
N/A

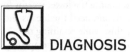

DIAGNOSIS

DIFFERENTIAL DIAGNOSIS
Lymphocytic plasmacytic stomatitis syndrome

CBC/BIOCHEMISTRY/URINALYSIS
N/A

IMAGING
• Intraoral radiology is helpful in making definitive diagnosis and planning treatment.
• Radiographic appearance varies from minute radiolucent defects of the tooth primarily at the cementoenamel junction to internal resorption and ankylosis of the apex to the supporting bone.

PATHOLOGIC FINDINGS
• Odontoclasts are arranged regularly along the edge of resorptive lesions.

ODONTOCLASTIC RESORPTIVE LESIONS—CATS

• No decalcification in the dentin, suggesting that the resorptive lesions are not derived from dental caries.
• Resorptive lesions appear to be induced by granulation tissue.

 TREATMENT

APPROPRIATE HEALTH CARE
N/A

NURSING CARE
• Controversial; FORLs are considered to be progressive; treatment may be attempted if the lesion is shallow and does not involve the pulp chamber.
• Class 1—an enamel defect is noted; the lesion is minimally sensitive because it has not entered dentin; therapy includes thorough cleaning and polishing; gingivectomy and odontoplasty have been adjunctive; pulse antibiotics (given the first 5 days of each month) may help control plaque accumulation in all stages; application of fluoride varnish and dental sealers has been advocated but not evaluated to determine effectiveness in halting or slowing lesion progression.
• Class 2 lesions—penetrate the enamel and dentin; are painful and must be treated by extraction or glass ionomer restoration, which provides short-term results in most cases.
• Glass ionomer restoratives release fluoride ions to desensitize the exposed dentin, strengthen enamel, and chemically bind to tooth surfaces; application does not automatically stop disease progression.
• Class 2 FORL treatment procedure with self-cured glass ionomer—(1) clean the area to be treated, with a curette or scaler; use flower pumice and water as a polish (not prophy paste); (2) isolate the gingiva by packing with gingival retraction cord or perform a gingivectomy; (3) irrigate and dry the area (but not bone dry); (4) once mixed, glass ionomer cement is placed on top of the lesion; when set, a varnish or nonfilled, light-cured resin is place over the restoration; and (5) finish and shape the restoration with a

finishing bur; place a second coat of varnish or resin over the restoration to maintain proper moisture levels while curing.
• Class 3 lesions—enter the endodontic system; require either endodontics to seal the canal from oral bacteria or extraction; restoration with glass ionomer restoratives as the sole treatment is not an option.

ACTIVITY
N/A

DIET
Prewet diet to soften

CLIENT EDUCATION
Daily home brushing may help control plaque.

SURGICAL CONSIDERATIONS
• Class 4 FORLs—the crown is eroded or fractured with part of the crown remaining; gingiva grows over the root fragments, yielding a sensitive bleeding lesion upon probing; treatment of choice is flap surgery and extraction of the root fragments.
• Class 5 FORLs—the crown is gone and roots remain; the decision to perform surgery to find and extract the retained root(s) is based on inflammation and/or pain; if the cat feels discomfort when the lesion is probed, then the root(s) is extracted via flap exposure.

 MEDICATIONS

DRUGS OF CHOICE
N/A

CONTRAINDICATIONS
N/A

PRECAUTIONS
N/A

POSSIBLE INTERACTIONS
N/A

 FOLLOW-UP

PATIENT MONITORING
N/A

PREVENTION/AVOIDANCE
N/A

POSSIBLE COMPLICATIONS
N/A

EXPECTED COURSE AND PROGNOSIS
N/A

 MISCELLANEOUS

ASSOCIATED CONDITIONS
N/A

AGE-RELATED FACTORS
N/A

ZOONOTIC POTENTIAL
N/A

PREGNANCY
N/A

SYNONYMS
• External osteodontoclastic resorptive lesions
• Neck lesions
• Idiopathic buccocervical erosion
• Chronic subgingival tooth erosion
• Cervical line erosion
• Subgingival resorptive lesions

SEE ALSO
See Causes

ABBREVIATIONS
FORL = feline odontoclastic resorptive lesions

Suggested Reading
Harvey CE, Emily PP. Small animal dentistry. Philadelphia: Mosby, 1993.
Wiggs RB, Lobprise HB. Veterinary dentistry: principles and practice. Philadelphia: Lippincott-Raven, 1997.
Author Jan Bellows
Consulting Editor Jan Bellows

OLIGURIA AND ANURIA

BASICS

DEFINITION
• Oliguria—the production of an abnormally small amount of urine (urine production rate < 0.25 mL/kg/h)
• Anuria—formation of essentially no urine (urine production rate < 0.08 mL/kg/h)

PATHOPHYSIOLOGY
• Physiologic oliguria occurs when the kidneys limit renal water loss during episodes of low renal perfusion to preserve body fluid and electrolyte balance. High plasma osmolality or low effective circulating fluid volume stimulate ADH synthesis and release. ADH acts on the kidneys to induce formation of small quantities of concentrated urine (the hallmark of physiologic oliguria).
• Pathologic oliguria results from severe renal parenchymal impairment. Factors include (1) high resistance in afferent glomerular vessels, (2) low glomerular permeability, (3) increased leakage ("back leak") of filtrate from damaged renal tubules, (4) renal intratubular obstruction, and (5) extensive loss of nephrons resulting in marked reduction in the quantity of glomerular filtrate produced.
• Anuria may be of renal or postrenal origin. Severe renal disease occasionally causes anuria. Mechanisms are the same as for pathologic oliguria (e.g., obstruction of urinary flow or rupture of the excretory pathway).

SYSTEMS AFFECTED
Renal/Urologic

SIGNALMENT
Dogs and cats

SIGNS
N/A

CAUSES
• Physiologic oliguria—renal hypoperfusion (caused by low blood volume or hypotension) or hypertonicity (usually caused by hypernatremia)
• Pathologic oliguria—acute oliguric renal failure or end-stage chronic renal failure
• Anuria—complete urinary tract obstruction, rupture of the urinary excretory pathway, or very severe, primary renal failure

RISK FACTORS
• Physiologic oliguria—dehydration, low cardiac output, hypotension
• Pathologic oliguria and anuria caused by primary renal failure (risk factors for acute renal failure)—preexisting renal disease,* exposure to nephrotoxins,* dehydration,* low cardiac output, hypotension,* electrolyte imbalance, acidosis, advanced age,* fever, sepsis, liver disease, multiple organ failure,

trauma, diabetes mellitus, hypoalbuminemia, hyperviscosity syndrome
• Anuria—urolithiasis, urinary tract neoplasia, idiopathic feline lower urinary tract disease (obstruction), micturition disorder, trauma

DIAGNOSIS

DIFFERENTIAL DIAGNOSIS
• Physiologic oliguria is suggested by physical signs of poor tissue perfusion (e.g., dehydration, prolonged capillary refill time, pale mucous membranes, weak pulse, rapid or irregular pulse, cool extremities); patient may have a history of recent fluid loss (vomiting, diarrhea, polyuria, hemorrhage); signs of uremia are typically absent and oliguria resolves rapidly when renal hypoperfusion is corrected
• Suspect pathologic oliguria and renal anuria with any of the risk factors given; the more risk factors, the more likely the patient has or will develop acute renal failure. Patients with pathologic oliguria caused by chronic renal failure typically have a history of progressive renal disease (including longstanding polyuria, polydipsia, poor appetite, and weight loss). Patients with chronic renal failure are at risk of developing acute renal failure. Signs of uremia are commonly observed, and fluid therapy and other measures designed to restore adequate renal perfusion often fail to increase urinary flow.
• Suspect anuria due to urinary obstruction or rupture of the excretory pathway in patients that repeatedly strain to void but cannot produce urinary flow. They may have a previous history of pollakiuria, dysuria, stranguria, hematuria, urolithiasis, trauma, or instrumentation of the urinary tract. In patients with urinary obstruction, physical examination may reveal an enlarged urinary bladder, painful posterior abdomen, and masses or uroliths in the urethra or bladder. Physical examination of patients with rupture of the urinary tract may reveal ascites, fluid infiltration in tissues around the urinary tract, painful caudal abdomen, masses or uroliths in the bladder or urethra, or evidence of trauma (e.g., pelvic fracture). Urinary obstruction caused by disorder of micturition may be suspected in patients with enlargement of the urinary bladder, increased resistance to manual expression of the bladder, and neurologic signs affecting the hind limbs and/or tail. Signs of uremia may develop. Restoration of urinary flow or correcting rents in the excretory pathway rapidly restores adequate urinary flow.

CBC/BIOCHEMISTRY/URINALYSIS
• Serum urea nitrogen and creatinine concentrations are typically high unless the onset of oliguria or anuria is very recent.
• Hyperkalemia is common with pathologic

oliguria and anuria, less common and less severe in animals with physiologic oliguria (except in those with hypoadrenocorticism).
• Physiologic oliguria is characterized by urinary specific gravity values above 1.030 in dogs and 1.035 in cats. Oliguria associated with lower urinary specific gravity values suggests primary renal failure. Patients with urine-concentrating defects from other diseases or drugs are the exception to this rule.
• Renal anuria is often characterized by urinary specific gravity values above 1.030 (dogs) or 1.035 (cats). Urinary specific gravity in patients with postrenal anuria varies. Adequate urine-concentrating ability is often lost after urinary obstruction but may persist with rupture of the excretory pathway.

OTHER LABORATORY TESTS
N/A

IMAGING
• Abdominal radiographs and ultrasound are useful to rule out urinary obstruction and rupture of the excretory pathway. Distension of any portion of the excretory pathway or observation of uroliths within the ureters, bladder neck, or urethra suggests urinary obstruction.
• Detection of fluid within the peritoneal cavity or adjacent to the urinary tract supports a diagnosis of rupture of the excretory pathway.
• Excretory urography, retrograde urethrocystography, or vaginourethrocystography may provide definitive proof of urinary obstruction or rupture of the excretory pathway.

DIAGNOSTIC PROCEDURES
• Electrocardiography may quickly establish whether the patient has clinically important hyperkalemia. Hyperkalemic cardiotoxicity is characterized (in order of progressing hyperkalemia) by tall, peaked T waves with a narrow base; prolongation of the P-R interval and QRS complex; decreased amplitude and increased width of P waves; bradycardia; atrial standstill; QRS-T fusion causing a widecomplex, idioventricular rhythm; ventricular fibrillation or asystole.
• Urethrocystoscopy may provide evidence for obstruction or rupture of the urinary tract.
• Placing a urinary catheter may provide information about the integrity of the lower urinary tract, but this approach is not recommended as a diagnostic procedure because it may be misleading, it may cause additional trauma to the urinary tract, and it may introduce bacteria.

TREATMENT
• Oliguria and anuria are medical emergencies; left untreated, they may lead to death within hours to days. Death typically

results from uremia, hyperkalemia, or sepsis (in patients with urinary tract infection).
• Correct persistent renal hypoperfusion rapidly; it may lead to acute ischemic renal injury.
• Correct renal hypoperfusion by intravenous administration of normal saline or lactated Ringer solution. In selected animals, other fluids may be more appropriate (e.g., blood to correct hypoperfusion resulting from hemorrhage).
• Therapy for primary renal oliguria and anuria is usually limited to symptomatic and supportive care designed to allow the patient to survive long enough for some spontaneous recovery of renal function to occur. Elimination of causative factor may slow or stop further renal injury (e.g., terminating aminoglycoside administration, correcting hypercalcemia, or restoring adequate renal perfusion); however, once oliguria or anuria has developed, few if any renal diseases will be amenable to specific treatment.
• Postrenal causes for anuria may be corrected by nonsurgical or surgical methods. Nonsurgical methods include hydropropulsion of uroliths or urethral plugs or placement of urinary catheters to restore low-pressure urinary flow. Surgical methods may include removal of uroliths, polyps, or neoplastic tissue or surgical correction of rents, strictures, or malposition of the excretory pathway.

MEDICATIONS

DRUGS OF CHOICE
• In patients with renal oliguria, diuretics are usually indicated after correcting renal hypoperfusion. Diuretic-induced increased urinary flow rate does not necessarily indicate improved renal function, but converting oliguria to nonoliguria facilitates managing the patient by fluid and electrolyte administration. Increased urinary flow after diuretic administration suggests a more favorable prognosis.
• Furosemide (2 mg/kg/IV q8h) is often used initially in patients with oliguric renal failure. Urinary flow should increase within 1 h. If diuresis does not ensue within an hour, dosage may be increased to 4–6 mg/kg IV.
• Dopamine (1–5 μg/kg/min) is generally administered concurrently with furosemide. Diuresis should ensue within 1–2 h. If urinary flow does not increase within 2 h, discontinue dopamine. In one study in dogs, infusion of dopamine with furosemide was more effective than furosemide alone. However, most recent data suggest that dopamine is usually ineffective in reversing established oliguria.
• Mannitol (0.5–1.0 g/kg IV) can be given as a

10 or 20% solution over 15–20 min. Urinary flow should increase within 1 h. Do not repeat administration of mannitol if diuresis does not ensue; it may cause excessive volume expansion.
• A safer but possibly less effective alternative to mannitol is infusion of 10–20% dextrose solution (25–50 mL/kg/IV q8–12h) over 1–2 h. Because dextrose is metabolized, the potential for volume expansion is minimized.

CONTRAINDICATIONS
Nephrotoxic drugs

PRECAUTIONS
• Administer fluids judiciously to patients that are persistently oliguric or anuric to avoid overhydration. In patients with unresponsive renal oliguria, peritoneal dialysis may be the only means of correcting severe fluid-induced volume overexpansion.
• Correct fluid deficits before initiating diuretic administration. Otherwise renal hypoperfusion and ischemic renal injury may be exacerbated.
• Use drugs requiring renal excretion with caution. If resolution of oliguria or anuria can reasonably be expected within minutes to a few hours (e.g., physiologic oliguria and anuria due to urinary obstruction), normal dosages of drugs requiring renal excretion may be used.
• Avoid electrolyte solutions containing more than 4 mEq of potassium per liter in most animals.
• Dopamine can cause cardiac arrhythmias, particularly in animals with hyperkalemia.
• ECG monitoring is recommended when high dosages are used and in animals with hyperkalemia.

POSSIBLE INTERACTIONS
Furosemide may promote the nephrotoxicity associated with aminoglycoside antibiotics.

ALTERNATIVE DRUGS
Mannitol may be used in preference to furosemide in patients with aminoglycoside-induced oliguric acute renal failure.

FOLLOW-UP

PATIENT MONITORING
• Urinary flow rate—urinary catheterization may be necessary for accurate determination of urine volume, but it can induce bacterial urinary tract infection, an important cause of morbidity and mortality in patients with acute renal failure. Catheters must be placed using aseptic technique. Intermittent catheterization is less likely to cause urinary tract infection than an indwelling catheter. The shorter the time that a catheter is indwelling, the lower the risk of urinary tract infection. Attach indwell-

ing catheters to a closed, sterile, urinary drainage system.
• Creatinine, serum urea nitrogen and potassium concentrations after 12–24 h; patients with severe hyperkalemia may need more frequent monitoring of serum potassium concentrations.
• ECG to assess cardiac effects of dopamine, hyperkalemia, and response to therapy

POSSIBLE COMPLICATIONS
• Hyperkalemia and associated cardiotoxicity
• Uremia leading to death
• Dehydration caused by vomiting, diarrhea, respiratory losses
• Overhydration caused by excessive fluid intake or administration leading to pulmonary edema
• Bacterial urinary tract infection

MISCELLANEOUS

ASSOCIATED CONDITIONS
N/A

AGE-RELATED FACTORS
N/A

ZOONOTIC POTENTIAL
N/A

PREGNANCY
N/A

SYNONYMS
N/A

SEE ALSO
• Creatinine and Blood Urea Nitrogen (BUN)—Azotemia and Uremia
• Hyperkalemia
• Nephrotoxicity, Drug-induced
• Renal Failure, Acute and Chronic
• Urinary Tract Obstruction

ABBREVIATION
ADH = antidiuretic hormone

Suggested Reading
Cowgill LD, Langston CE. Role of hemodialysis in the management of dogs and cats with renal failure. Vet Clin North Am Small Anim Pract 1996;26(6):1347–1348.
Grauer GF, Lane IF. Acute renal failure. In: Ettinger SJ, Feldman EC, eds. Textbook of veterinary internal medicine. Philadelphia: Saunders, 1995:1720–1733.
Lane IF, Grauer GF, Fettman MJ. Acute renal failure. Part II. Diagnosis, management, and prognosis. Compend Cont Educ 1994;16:625–645.
Author David J. Polzin
Consulting Editors Larry G. Adams and Carl A. Osborne

ORAL ULCERATION

BASICS

DEFINITION
Destruction of the oral epithelium, exposing underlying connective tissue

PATHOPHYSIOLOGY
• Cell–cell and cell–matrix adhesion proteins are responsible for maintaining the integrity of the mucosal lining of the oral cavity.
• Disease processes that destroy keratinocytes or adversely affect their adhesion to one another or to the subjacent basement membrane result in erosions, ulcerations, and desquamation.
• Immunologic processes that have a deleterious effect on the integrity of the epithelial–basement membrane submucosa complex may be involved in causing ulcers to form.

SYSTEMS AFFECTED
Oral cavity—hard palate, attached and unattached gingiva, and tongue

SIGNALMENT
• Dog and cat
• Ulcerative eosinophilic stomatitis in Cavalier King Charles spaniels—lesions are similar in gross appearance to palatine eosinophilic granulomas, but histologically lack granuloma formation.
• Maltese are prone to oral ulceration caused by periodontal disease.

SIGNS
• Ptyalism
• Anorexia
• Painful chewing

CAUSES
See Differential Diagnosis

RISK FACTORS
N/A

DIAGNOSIS

DIFFERENTIAL DIAGNOSIS
• Periodontal disease
• Uremia—tongue and buccal mucosa ulcers
• Lymphocytic plasmacytic stomatitis—feline
• Viral diseases in the cat—calicivirus, herpesvirus
• Autoimmune disease—pemphigus vulgaris, bullous disease; erythema multiforme; systemic lupus erythematosus
• Gum chewers disease—chronic chewing of the cheeks
• Malignancy
• Trauma
• Chemical injury
• Eosinophilic ulceration
• Infection—bacterial, viral, and fungal

CBC/BIOCHEMISTRY/URINALYSIS
N/A

OTHER LABORATORY TESTS
N/A

IMAGING
Use intraoral radiographs to evaluate periodontal disease–caused ulcers.

DIAGNOSTIC PROCEDURES
• Exfoliative cytology—place an applicator stick on the lesion, then on a stained microscopic slide for examination; helps differentiate infection from autoimmune or neoplastic disease
• Toluidine blue stain outlines ulcers—if presence questionable
• Oral examination for adjacent teeth in various stages of periodontal disease

TREATMENT
• Uremic ulcers—Pepcid, clindamycin, Carafate; suspend 1/4- to 1/2-g tablet in water and give once or twice a day; promotes oral epithelialization and binds phosphorus
• If secondary to periodontal disease, treat periodontal disease and advise home care. If oral ulceration continues, extract tooth rubbing on ulcer.

MEDICATIONS

DRUGS OF CHOICE
- Topical antimicrobial and antifungal agents
- Topical and systemic corticosteroids
- Carboxymethylcellulose preparations (Orabase)
- Zinc—membrane-stabilizing and anti-oxidant effects; zinc-containing oral rinses and gels (Maxi-Guard- Addison Biologicals) are helpful because zinc is required for wound healing

CONTRAINDICATIONS
N/A

PRECAUTIONS
N/A

POSSIBLE INTERACTIONS
N/A

ALTERNATIVE DRUGS
N/A

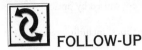 FOLLOW-UP

PATIENT MONITORING
Weekly then monthly

 MISCELLANEOUS

N/A

ASSOCIATED CONDITIONS
N/A

AGE-RELATED FACTORS
N/A

ZOONOTIC POTENTIAL
N/A

PREGNANCY
N/A

SYNONYMS
N/A

SEE ALSO
N/A

ABBREVIATIONS
N/A

Suggested Reading

Harvey CE, Emily PP. Small animal dentistry. Philadelphia: Mosby, 1993.
Wiggs RB, Lobrise HB. Veterinary dentistry: principles and practice. Philadelphia: Lippincott-Raven, 1997.

Author Jan Bellows
Consulting Editor Jan Bellows

ORBITAL DISEASES (EXOPHTHALMUS, ENOPHTHALMUS, STRABISMUS)

BASICS

DEFINITION
• Abnormal position of the eye
• Exophthalmus—anterior displacement of the globe
• Enophthalmus—posterior displacement of the globe
• Strabismus—deviation of the globe from the correct position of fixation, which the patient cannot correct

PATHOPHYSIOLOGY
• Orbit cannot be examined directly; orbital disease manifested only by signs that alter the position, appearance, or function of the globe and adnexa
• Malpositioned eye—caused by changes in volume (loss or gain) of the orbital contents or abnormal extraocular muscle function
• Exophthalmus—caused by space-occupying lesions posterior to the equator of the globe
• Enophthalmus—caused by loss of orbital volume or space-occupying lesions anterior to the equator of the globe
• Strabismus—usually caused by an imbalance of extraocular muscle tone or lesions that restrict extraocular muscle mobility

SYSTEMS AFFECTED
• Ophthalmic
• Respiratory—because of the close proximity, the nasal cavity and frontal and maxillary sinuses are often involved.

SIGNALMENT
• Dogs/Cats
• Orbital abscess or cellulitis and myositis—more common in young adult dogs
• Myositis—predisposed breeds: German shepherds, golden retrievers, Weimaraners, and English springer spaniels
• Orbital neoplasia—more common in middle-aged to old dogs

SIGNS

Exophthalmus
• Secondary signs of space-occupying orbital disease
• Difficulty in retropulsing the globe
• Serous to mucopurulent ocular discharge
• Chemosis
• Eyelid swelling
• Lagophthalmos—inability to close the eyelids over the cornea adequately during blinking
• Exposure keratitis—with or without ulceration
• Pain on opening the mouth
• Third eyelid protrusion

• Visual impairment caused by optic neuropathy
• Fundic abnormalities, including retinal detachment
• Retinal vascular congestion
• Focal inward deviation of the posterior globe
• Optic disk swelling
• Neurotropic keratitis after damage to the ophthalmic branch of cranial nerve V
• Fever and malaise—with orbital abscess or cellulitis
• IOP—rarely high

Enophthalmus
• Ptosis
• Third eyelid protrusion
• Extraocular muscle atrophy
• Entropion—with severe disease

Strabismus
• Deviation of one or both eyes from the normal position
• May note exophthalmous or enophthalmus

CAUSES

Exophthalmus
• Neoplasm—primary or secondary
• Abscess or cellulitis—bacterial or fungal; fungal more likely in cats; look for foreign bodies.
• Zygomatic mucocele—not described in cats
• Myositis—muscles of mastication or extra-ocular muscles
• Orbital hemorrhage secondary to trauma
• Arteriovenous fistula—rare

Enophthalmus
• Ocular pain
• Microphthalmia
• Phthisis bulbi
• Collapsed globe
• Horner syndrome
• Dehydration
• Loss of orbital fat or muscle
• Conformational enophthalmus in dolicho-cephalic breeds

Strabimus
• Abnormal innervation of extraocular muscle
• Restriction of extraocular muscle motility by scar tissue from previous trauma or inflammation
• Destruction of extraocular muscle attachments after proptosis
• Convergent strabismus—congenital; results from abnormal crossing of visual fibers in the CNS (Siamese cats)

RISK FACTORS
Proptosis—more readily occurs in brachycephalic dogs with shallow orbits

DIAGNOSIS

DIFFERENTIAL DIAGNOSIS

Similar Signs
• Buphthalmic globe—may simulate a space-occupying mass and cause the eye to be displaced anteriorly owing to its size in relationship to the orbital volume; IOP usually high; corneal diameter is greater than normal.
• Episcleritis—may cause severe diffuse or focal thickening of the fibrous tunic, often imitating a buphthalmic globe; corneal edema; low IOP; aqueous flare

Causes
• Acute onset of exophthalmus—often caused by inflammatory orbital disease; pain, especially on opening the mouth, is more likely the result of an inflammatory orbital disease than orbital neoplasia, which generally is less painful and has a slower onset and progression.
• Mucoceles—more variable in speed of onset and degree of patient discomfort
• Myositis—may be unilateral but is often bilateral

CBC/BIOCHEMISTRY/URINALYSIS
• Usually normal
• Leukogram—may show inflammation with abscess or cellulitis or myositis
• Peripheral eosinophilia—occasionally seen in dogs with masticatory muscle myositis

OTHER LABORATORY TESTS
N/A

IMAGING
• Skull radiographs (especially of the frontal sinuses and nasal cavity), orbital ultrasonography, and CT—are extremely helpful in defining the extent of the lesion
• Thoracic radiographs—may help identify metastatic disease

DIAGNOSTIC PROCEDURES
• Lack of globe retropulsion—confirms a space-occupying mass
• Oral examination, skull radiographs, and fine-needle aspiration of the orbit—may be completed after anesthetizing the patient
• Fine-needle aspiration (18–20-gauge)—submit samples for aerobic, anaerobic, and fungal cultures; gram staining; and cytologic examination
• Cytology—often diagnostic for abscess or cellulitis, zygomatic salivary gland mucocele, and neoplasia
• Biopsy—probably indicated if needle aspiration is undiagnostic; histopathologic examination of masseter, temporal, or extraocular muscle to determine myositis

ORBITAL DISEASES (EXOPHTHALMUS, ENOPHTHALMUS, STRABISMUS)

• Forced duction of the globe (strabismus)—grasp the conjunctiva with a fine pair of forceps with the patient under topical anesthesia; differentiation of neurologic disease (in which the globe moves freely) from restrictive condition (in which the globe cannot be moved manually)

TREATMENT

PROPTOSIS
• See Proptosis.

ORBITAL ABSCESS OR CELLULITIS
• Inpatient—intravenous fluids to maintain hydration and replace fluid deficits until patient is able to eat
• Establish ventral orbital drainage while the patient is anesthetized.
• Incise the surgically prepared mucosa for approximately 1 cm behind the last molar.
• Push a blunt-tipped forceps (e.g., Kelly or Carmalt) into the orbital space and open; in general, advance the forceps to the level of the box lock, or if movement of the eye occurs with forceps opening.
• Apparent drainage is seen in less than half of patients.
• Take care to minimize retrobulbar trauma and optic nerve damage; use only blunt dissection; never crush tissue or use scissors to cut.
• Samples for bacterial culture and cytologic examination may be obtained through this port.
• Hot packing—q6h; helps lessen swelling and cleans discharges

ORBITAL NEOPLASMS
• Usually primary and malignant
• Early exenteration or orbital exploratory surgery and debulking of the mass via a lateral approach to the orbit to save the globe—rational therapeutic choices
• Chemotherapy or radiotherapy—may be employed as adjuncts, depending on neoplasm type and extent of the lesion
• Without adjunct therapy—survival is weeks to months when the malignancy is diagnosed because the patient is usually examined late in the course of disease.
• Consultation with an oncologist is recommended once the diagnosis is made.

ZYGOMATIC MUCOCELE
May resolve with antibiotic and corticosteroid administration; if not, surgical excision is usually curative.

STRABISMUS
• Neurologic—best treated by identifying the underlying cause and addressing that, if possible
• Restrictive or posttraumatic—may be treated surgically; repositioning the attachments of the extraocular muscles; relieving excessive tension on those muscles; usually a very difficult procedure

MEDICATIONS

DRUGS OF CHOICE
• Exophthalmus (all patients)—lubricate cornea (e.g., artificial tear ointment q6h) to prevent desiccation and ulceration.
• Ulceration—topical antibiotic (e.g., bacitracin-neomycin-polymyxin, q8h) and cycloplegic (e.g., 1% atropine q12–24h), to prevent infection and reduce ciliary spasm

Orbital Abscess or Cellulitis
• Intravenous antibiotics—sodium ampicillin (20 mg/kg q6–8h) or chloramphenicol (25 mg/kg q8h); while awaiting results of bacterial culture and cytologic examination; if owners decline diagnostic testing
• Bacterial orbital infections—may be mixed; *Pasteurella multocida* and *Enterobacteriaceae* common
• Oral antibiotics—after patient begins to eat; based on culture and sensitivity
• Most patients recover within approximately 2 weeks of treatment.
• Itraconazole—2.5 mg/kg q12h; may be considered for orbital aspergillosis
• Prednisolone acetate—1 mg/kg SC or IM q24h, once or twice; minimize optic neuritis and reduce orbital swelling and globe exposure

Acute Myositis
• Difficult prehension—systemic corticosteroids (prednisolone acetate, 2 mg/kg SC or IM); then oral corticosteroids for the following 4–6 weeks (prednisone, 2 mg/kg q24h) until the swelling subsides; then taper
• Azathioprine—1–2mg/kg PO q24h for 3–7 days; then q48h and taper; with or without corticosteroids, may be used chronically to manage recurrent disease

CONTRAINDICATIONS
N/A

PRECAUTIONS
• Systemic corticosteroids—use with extreme caution with deep fungal orbital disease.
• Azathioprine—may be hepatotoxic and cause myelosuppression

• Follow CBC platlet count and liver enzymes every 1–2 weeks for 8 weeks, then periodically thereafter.

POSSIBLE INTERACTIONS
N/A

ALTERNATIVE DRUGS
N/A

FOLLOW-UP

PATIENT MONITORING
• Inflammatory orbital disease—examine at least weekly until clinical signs abate.
• Advise client to watch for recurrence of signs, especially if an orbital foreign body is likely.
• Treat fungal infections with itraconazole for 60 days after signs cease.

POSSIBLE COMPLICATIONS
• Vision loss
• Loss of the eye
• Permanent malposition of the globe
• Death

MISCELLANEOUS

ASSOCIATED CONDITIONS
N/A

AGE-RELATED FACTORS
N\A

ZOONOTIC POTENTIAL
N/A

PREGNANCY
Avoid systemic corticosteroids, antifungal medications, and azathioprine in pregnant animals.

SEE ALSO
• Proptosis
• Red Eye

Suggested Reading
Lindley DM. Disorders of the orbit. In: Kirk RW, Bonagura, JD., eds., Current veterinary therapy XI. Phildadelphia: Saunders, 1992:1081–1085.
Speiss BM, Wallin-Hakenson N. Diseases of the canine orbit. In: Gelatt KN, ed. Veterinary Ophthalmology, 3rd ed. Philadelphia: Lippincott Williams & Wilkins, 1999:511–533.
Author Denise M. Lindley
Consulting Editor Paul E. Miller

PARALYSIS

BASICS

DEFINITION
• Paresis—weakness of voluntary movement
• Paralysis—lack of voluntary movement
• Quadriparesis (tetraparesis)—weakness of voluntary movements in all limbs
• Quadriplegia (tetraplegia)—absence of all voluntary limb movement
• Paraparesis—weakness of voluntary movements in pelvic limbs
• Paraplegia—absence of all voluntary pelvic limb movement

PATHOPHYSIOLOGY
• Weakness—may be caused by lesions in the upper or lower motor neuron system
• Cell bodies or nuclei for the upper motor neuron system—located within the brain; responsible for initiating voluntary movement
• Axons from these cell bodies—form tracts (rubrospinal, corticospinal, vestibulospinal, reticulospinal) that descend from the brain to synapse on interneurons in the spinal cord
• Interneuronal axons—then synapse on large (α) motor neurons in the ventral gray matter of the spinal cord
• Large motor neurons—cell bodies of origin for the lower motor neuron system, which is responsible for spinal reflexes
• Collections of lower motor neurons in the cervical and lumbar intumescences—give rise to axons that form the ventral nerve roots, the spinal nerves, and (ultimately) the peripheral nerves that innervate limb muscles
• Evaluation of limb reflexes—determine which system (upper or lower motor neuron) is involved
• Upper motor neurons and their axons—inhibitory influence on the large motor neurons of the lower motor neuron system; maintain normal muscle tone and normal spinal reflexes; if injured, spinal reflexes are no longer inhibited or controlled and reflexes become exaggerated or hyperreflexic.
• Large α motor neurons or their processes (peripheral nerves)—if injured, spinal reflexes cannot be elicited (areflexic) or are reduced (hyporeflexic).

SYSTEMS AFFECTED
Nervous

SIGNALMENT
Any species

SIGNS

General Comments
Limb weakness—acute or gradual onset

Historical Findings
• Owner may describe the patient as being unable to move, walk, or get up
• Many focal compressive spinal cord diseases begin with ataxia and progress to weakness and finally to paralysis.

Physical Examination Findings
• Usually normal, unless the disease process is systemic
• Patient usually alert
• If in pain, patient may resent handling and manipulation during the examination.
• Aortic emboli—patient may be paraplegic on examination; femoral pulses absent; limbs should be cold; nail beds often blue

Neurologic Examination Findings
• Confirm that the problem is weakness or paralysis.
• Localize problem to either lower or upper motor neuron system.
• Paraplegia—likely bladder is also paralyzed, negating voluntary urination

CAUSES

Generalized Quadriplegia
• Lower motor neuron—acute onset: coonhound paralysis; botulism; tick paralysis; fulminating form of myasthenia gravis; protozoal myoneurosis; more gradual onset: polyneuropathies; polymyopathies
• Upper motor neuron—cervical spinal cord or multifocal cord diseases: disk herniation; diskospondylitis; fibrocartilaginous embolism; trauma; neoplasia; myelitis of many causes; malformations

Paraplegia
• Upper motor neuron—disk herniation; diskospondylitis; fibrocartilaginous embolism; neoplasia; trauma
• Lower motor neuron—fibrocartilaginous embolism; disk herniation; lumbosacral instability; diskospondylitis; trauma; neoplasia; spina bifida

Generalized Quadriplegia with Cranial Nerve Deficits, Seizures, or Stupor
Upper motor neuron—diseases of the brain: encephalitis; neoplasia; trauma; vascular accidents; congenital or inherited disorders

RISK FACTORS
• Breeds at risk for degenerative disk disease—dachshunds, poodles, cocker spaniels, and beagles
• Hunting dogs—at risk for coonhound paralysis
• Roaming animals—at risk for spinal cord trauma

DIAGNOSIS

DIFFERENTIAL DIAGNOSIS
• Weak or paralyzed pelvic limbs—make sure femoral pulses are present and normal; aortic or femoral artery emboli may lead to lower motor neuron paraparesis or paraplegia.
• Spinal reflexes—localize weakness to the cervical, thoracolumbar, or lower lumbar cord segments.
• Acute onset—be careful when moving the patient because of the possibility of trauma.

CBC/BIOCHEMISTRY/URINALYSIS
Usually normal, unless inflammatory diseases involved

OTHER LABORATORY TESTS
• Urinary tract inflammation—bacterial culture of urine
• Diskospondylitis—diagnose by spinal radiographs; perform a Brucella titer; consider blood and urine bacterial cultures.
• Exercise-induced weakness—determine acetylcholine receptor antibody titers (test for myasthenia gravis); check serum creatine kinase concentration (polymyositis).
• Lower motor neuron weakness or muscle pain, muscle atrophy, or hypertrophy—determine creatine kinase concentration to help diagnose polymyositis.
• Suspected myelitis or meningitis—perform titers for *Neospora caninum, Ehrlichia canis,* and canine distemper virus.

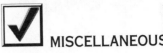

IMAGING

- Spinal radiographs—lesion localized to the spinal cord; may reveal disk herniation, diskospondylitis, bony tumor, congenital vertebral malformation, and fracture or luxation
- Myelography—required if survey radiography is not diagnostic and when considering surgery
- CT or MRI—if lesion can be precisely localized or if more information is required after myelography localizes the lesion; will likely replace myelography for imaging the spine once the technology becomes more accessible
- Diskospondylitis—may collect aspirate of the intervertebral space using fluoroscopy; perform cytology and culture to isolate the infectious agent.

DIAGNOSTIC PROCEDURES

- CSF analysis—do before myelography to detect myelitis and meningitis; if high protein or cell numbers are found, a culture is warranted.
- Needle electromyography and motor nerve conduction velocity—generalized lower motor neuron signs; better characterize the lesion and help determine the prognosis
- Muscle and nerve biopsy—generalized lower motor neuron weakness

 TREATMENT

- Inpatient—with severe weakness or paralysis until bladder function can be ascertained
- Hand feeding—with diffuse lower motor neuron signs, swallowing can be affected; until it is certain that the patient can swallow properly
- Feeding from an elevated platform—recommended for animals with megaesophagus
- Activity—restrict until spinal trauma and disk herniation can be ruled out
- Physical therapy—important for paralyzed patients; tone muscles and keep joints flexible
- Bedding—move paralyzed patients away from soiled bedding, check and clean frequently to prevent urine scalding and superficial pyoderma; use padded bedding or a waterbed to help prevent decubital ulcer formation.
- Turning—turn quadriplegic patients from side to side four to eight times daily; prevent hypostatic lung congestion and decubital ulcer formation
- Surgery—for disk herniation, fracture, and some neoplasias and congenital conditions; often the quickest and most effective method of improving the neurologic status

 MEDICATIONS

DRUGS OF CHOICE

- Methylprednisolone sodium succinate—30 mg/kg IV followed by 15 mg/kg 2 and 6 hr later; may be beneficial for suspected trauma, disk herniation, or fibrocartilaginous embolism; acute upper motor neuron signs
- Pyridostigmine bromide—0.5–3.0 mg/kg PO q8–12h; for suspected myasthenia gravis; administer while waiting for titer results.
- Acute generalized lower motor neuron signs—check for ticks; dip with appropriate insecticides, if necessary.

CONTRAINDICATIONS

Corticosteroids—do not use with diskospondylitis; do not use with myasthenia gravis associated with aspiration pneumonia.

PRECAUTIONS

Corticosteroids—associated with gastrointestinal ulceration and hemorrhage, delayed wound healing, and heightened susceptibility to infection

POSSIBLE INTERACTIONS

N/A

ALTERNATIVE DRUGS

- Dexamethasone—0.5–1 mg/kg q24–48h
- Prednisolone—1–2 mg/kg q12–24h

 FOLLOW-UP

PATIENT MONITORING

- Neurologic examinations—daily to monitor status
- Bladder—evacuate (via manual expression or catheterization) three to four times a day to prevent overdistension and subsequent bladder atony; once bladder function has returned, patient can be managed at home.

POSSIBLE COMPLICATIONS

- Urinary tract infection, bladder atony, urine scalding and pyoderma, constipation, decubital ulcer formation
- Aspiration pneumonia—with generalized lower motor neuron disease
- Myelomalacia—with severe spinal cord trauma or disk herniations
- Respiratory compromise or paralysis—with myelomalacia or generalized lower motor neuron disease

✓ MISCELLANEOUS

ASSOCIATED CONDITIONS

N/A

AGE-RELATED FACTORS

N/A

ZOONOTIC POTENTIAL

N/A

PREGNANCY

Contraindicated in paralyzed patients

ABBREVIATION

CSF = cerebrospinal fluid

Suggested Reading

Chrisman CL. Paraplegia, paraparesis, and ataxia of the pelvic limbs. In: Problems in small animal neurology. Philadelphia: Lea & Febiger, 1991:397–431.

de Lahunta A. Veterinary neuroanatomy and clinical neurology. 2nd ed. Philadelphia: Saunders, 1983.

Oliver JE, Lorenz MD, Kornegay JN. Tetra-paresis, hemiparesis, and ataxia. In: Hand-book of veterinary neurology. 3rd ed. Philadelphia: Saunders. 1997:173–215.

Withrow SJ. Localization and diagnosis of spinal cord lesions in small animals. Part 1. Compend Contin Educ Pract Vet 1980;2:464–474.

Author Linda G. Shell
Consulting Editor Joane M. Parent

PERIODONTAL DISEASE

 BASICS

DEFINITION
Inflammation of some or all of the tooth's support structures (gingiva, cementum, periodontal ligament, and alveolar bone); compared with gingivitis (inflammation of the marginal gingiva), periodontitis indicates bone loss.

PATHOPHYSIOLOGY
• An intact epithelial barrier and high rate of epithelial turnover and surface desquamation prevent bacteria from gaining direct access to tissue.
• Some bacterial products may diffuse through the junctional epithelium to reach the underlying gingival connective tissue; normal host defense mechanisms limit the penetration of these products and their damaging effects.
• Fluctuations in the host–parasite equilibrium may result in cycles of either diminished or increased intensity of the inflammatory response; it may be possible to think of periodontitis as the outcome of an imperfectly balanced host–parasite interaction.
• Caused by bacteria located in the gingival crevice; initially a pellicle forms on the enamel surface of a clean tooth; the pellicle is composed of proteins and glycoproteins deposited from saliva and gingival crevicular fluid; the pellicle attracts aerobic Gram-positive bacteria (mostly actinomyces and streptococci); more bacteria soon adhere, forming plaque; within days the plaque thickens, becomes mineralized and transforms into calculus, which is rough and irritating to the gingiva; the underlying bacteria run out of oxygen and anaerobic motile rods and spirochetes begin to populate the subgingival area; more plaque builds on top of the calculus; endotoxins released by anaerobic bacteria cause tissue destruction and bone-loss periodontitis.

SYSTEMS AFFECTED
Microscopic hepatic, renal, and CNS lesions are found in some animals.

SIGNALMENT
Dogs and cats 6 months and older may be affected.

SIGNS
Physical Examination Findings
• Grade 1 inflammation—confined to tissues of the marginal gingiva
• Grade 2 inflammation—edema; gingival bleeding on probing
• Grade 3—as above; pustular discharge; slight-to-moderate bone loss (25–50% attachment loss)
• Grade 4—as above; mobility; severe bone loss (>50% attachment loss)

CAUSES
• Gingivitis—dogs; *Streptococcus* and *Actinomyces* spp.
• Periodontitis—dogs; pigmented and nonpigmented bacteroides (*Porphyromonas gingivalis, Prevotella* spp., *Bacteroides* spp.), *Fusobacterium* spp.
• Cats—*Peptostreptococcus, Actinomyces,* and *Porphyromonas* spp.
• Soft diet promotes periodontal disease through accumulation of plaque.

RISK FACTORS
• Toy breeds with crowded teeth
• Dogs that groom themselves—causes hair to be imbedded in the gingival sulcus
• Other debilitating illnesses
• Poor nutritional state

 DIAGNOSIS

DIFFERENTIAL DIAGNOSIS
• Pemphigus
• Lupus
• Oral neoplasia
• Stomatitis

CBC/BIOCHEMISTRY/URINALYSIS
N/A

OTHER LABORATORY TESTS

IMAGING
• Radiography—important diagnostic tool; as much as 60% of disease is hidden below the gum line.

• No radiographic changes in grades 1 and 2 disease (gingivitis).
• Early radiographic signs of grade 3 disease include loss of density and sharpness of the crestal bone; as periodontal disease progresses, loss of lamina dura mineralization apically and furcation involvement in multirooted teeth.
• Severe periodontal disease radiographically appears as loss of bone support around one or more roots; bone loss may be horizontal (a decrease in bone height around one or more teeth), vertical (infrabony defect), or oblique (a combination of both).

DIAGNOSTIC PROCEDURES
• Periodontal probing—"probing depth": distance between free gingival margin and apical extent of pocket; probing depths >2 mm in the dog and 1 mm in the cat are abnormal.
• "Attachment loss" measures between CEJ and apical extent of pocket; normally the gingival sulcus is located at the CEJ junction; any attachment loss is abnormal.

 TREATMENT

• The ultimate goal of periodontal therapy is to control plaque; a willing patient and a client who can provide home care are important considerations in creating a therapy plan.
• Grade 1 or 2—professional cleaning, hand scaling, polishing, irrigation, application of fluoride
• Grade 3—pocket depths: 3–6 mm in dogs, 2–4 mm in cats; above plus closed-root planing and subgingival curettage
• Grade 4—pocket depth >6 mm in dogs, 4 mm in cat; surgery needed to either expose the root for treatment (open-flap curettage) or extract
• If 2–3 mm of healthy, attached gingiva is present—apically reposition flap to decrease pocket depth in areas of alveolar bone loss; if not enough healthy gingiva remains to apically reposition flap; rotated flap (from adjacent gingiva), free gingival flap, or extraction

• Bone replacement procedures—with two-, three-, four-walled infrabony pockets
• Guided tissue regeneration—use tissue barriers to separate gingival tissue and root surface.
• Periodontal splinting—can be used especially in the incisor areas to help stabilize mobile teeth; criteria for splinting include normal periodontal support on both sides of the tooth (teeth) to be stabilized, strict home care, and a cooperative patient who will not chew on hard objects and destroy the splint.

MEDICATIONS

DRUGS OF CHOICE
Clindamycin is approved for dental infections; may be used for a week before periodontal treatment, 20 min before anesthesia, postoperatively for 7–10 days, and/or, in a pulse therapy fashion, given the first 5 days of each month.

Home Care
• Fluoride—stannous fluoride preparations (Omni Gel and Gel Kam) help control periodontal disease by reducing plaque deposition on the surface of enamel and also decrease dental pain; use 0.4% strength in patients with stage 3 and 4 periodontal disease, especially those with exposed root surfaces.
• Chlorhexidine—the most effective product to inhibit plaque formation in humans; bacteriostatic and bactericidal against bacteria, fungi, and some viruses; once absorbed it continues to be effective for up to 24 h; in humans, to be maximally effective, it is swished in the mouth for 1 min twice daily; the contact time of application is important for binding to the tooth and gingival sulcus; 1-min oral rinsing is difficult to accomplish in animals; chlorhexidine can be applied with a gauze sponge or cotton-tipped applicators, as a spray, or with finger brushes.
• CHX Guard solution (VRx Products, Harbor City, CA) contains chlorhexidine gluconate 0.12% plus zinc gluconate, which

promotes healing of ulcerated tissue; CHX gel chlorhexidine gluconate 0.12%; the gel allows greater binding time and has a pleasant taste.
• DentiVet toothpaste (Virbac, Fort Worth, TX) contains chlorhexidine gluconate, zinc, and sodium hexamethylphosphate; Hexarinse contains 0.12% chlorhexidine, cetylpyridinium, chloride, and zinc.
• Novaldent—chlorhexidine acetate 0.1%
• Lactoperoxidase system enhanced enzyme products—have antibacterial properties that decrease plaque (CET, CET Forte toothpastes, CET Chews, CET Spray-VRx Product).
• Diet-hard biscuit foods are preferable to soft sticky foods.
• T/D tartar control diet (Hills)—specifically indicated to control tartar in dogs and cats
• Amount and type of home care products dispensed depends on dental periodontal pathology.
Stage 1 and 2—daily brushing with dentifrice
Stage 3, established periodontal disease—daily brushing with fluoride-containing toothpaste plus twice-weekly application of stannous fluoride gel and pulse therapy antibiotics
Stage 4, advanced periodontal disease—zinc ascorbate gel (Maxi-Guard-Addison Biologics Inc) 3–4 times daily to help regenerate cellular collagen, plus 0.2% chlorhexidine spray twice daily; or CHX-Guard (VRx Products), a combination of chlorhexidine gluconate and zinc, and pulse therapy antibiotics; after 2 weeks, can substitute stannous fluoride gel twice weekly for the chlorhexidine spray

CONTRAINDICATIONS
N/A

PRECAUTIONS
N/A

POSSIBLE INTERACTIONS
Do not use chlorhexidine and fluoride products concurrently; binding both products may inactivate them; better to wait 30 min to 1 h between use of a dentifrice containing fluoride and a chlorhexidine rinse or gel

ALTERNATIVE DRUGS
• Tetracycline
• Clavamox
• Flagyl

FOLLOW-UP

PATIENT MONITORING
The degree of periodontal pathology dictates recall interval; some patients are checked weekly, while others can be evaluated every 3–6 months.

POSSIBLE COMPLICATIONS
N/A

MISCELLANEOUS

ASSOCIATED CONDITIONS
N/A

AGE-RELATED FACTORS
N/A

ZOONOTIC POTENTIAL
N/A

PREGNANCY
N/A

SYNONYMS
N/A

SEE ALSO
N/A

ABBREVIATIONS
CEJ = cementoenamel junction

Suggested Reading
Harvey CE. Periodontal disease in dogs. Vet Clin North Am 1998;28:1111–1128.
Wiggs RB, Lobprise HB. Veterinary dentistry: principles and practice. Philadelphia: Lippincott-Raven, 1997.
Author Jan Bellows
Consulting Editor Jan Bellows

PETECHIA/ECCHYMOSIS/BRUISING

 BASICS

DEFINITION
Disorders of primary hemostasis (platelet- or vessel-wall-mediated) that result in bleeding into the skin or mucous membranes to a degree out of proportion to the trauma

PATHOPHYSIOLOGY
• Thrombocytopenia and, less commonly, defective platelet function cause impaired primary hemostasis (i.e., failure of platelet plug formation).
• Thrombocytopenia—caused by shortened platelet life span, impaired thrombopoiesis, or platelet sequestration
• Acquired platelet function deficits—most often associated with uremic inhibition of cyclooxygenase; occasionally associated with drugs (e.g., aspirin), dysproteinemia, and myeloproliferative disease
• Congenital platelet function defects—varied and, other than von Willebrand disease, rare; sequestration of platelets in a large spleen or liver occurs rarely.
• Vascular hemostatic defects—generally caused by one of three mechanisms: (1) heightened permeability, as in patients with hyperadrenocorticism; (2) reduced vessel strength, as in patients with Ehlers-Danlos syndrome or scurvy (seen only in guinea pigs and primates); and (3) lack of contraction

SYSTEMS AFFECTED
• Hemic/Lymph/Immune
• Skin/Exocrine—petechia/ecchymosis/bruising
• Respiratory—epistaxis
• Renal/urologic—hematuria
• Gastrointestinal—melena

SIGNALMENT
• Most causes of thrombocytopenia and platelet function defects are not associated with a breed, age, or sex predisposition.
• All are more common in dogs than in cats.

SIGNS
N/A

CAUSES
Thrombocytopenia
• Increase in platelet use or destruction—immune-mediated disease, consumptive coagulopathy, or infectious disease such as ehrlichiosis
• Immune-mediated disease—primary autoimmune; isoimmune in the newborn; or secondary to viruses, bacteria, *Ehrlichia, Rickettsia* (e.g., Rocky Mountain spotted fever), or protozoa
• Some infectious diseases cause thrombocytopenia by immune-mediated mechanisms.
• Low platelet production—myelophthisis, aplastic anemia, and drug reactions (e.g., estrogen toxicity)
• Sequestration of platelets in a large spleen, liver, or other sizable mass of microvasculature usually does not lead to bleeding.

Thrombocytopathy
• Congenital platelet function disorders—von Willebrand disease, Glanzmann thrombasthenia (rare), and thrombopathia of basset hounds (rare).
• Acquired platelet function disorders—uremia, DIC, liver disease, myeloproliferative and lymphoproliferative disease, paraproteinemia, congenital heart disease, and treatment with NSAIDs

Vascular Disease
Secondary purpura can be seen in patients with Cushing disease, uremia, dysproteinemia, drug reaction, and some infectious diseases (e.g., Rocky Mountain spotted fever).

Coagulation Factors
Deficiencies do not result in this type of bleeding disorder; rather they are more commonly associated with hematomas and hemarthroses.

RISK FACTORS
• The occurrence of any of the diseases mentioned.
• Previous administration of aspirin or other NSAID is particularly important to know if bleeding time is to be measured (see Diagnosis).

 DIAGNOSIS

DIFFERENTIAL DIAGNOSIS
• Usually are not mistaken for anything else; however, injuries causing an expected amount of bleeding or bruising must be ruled out by history and physical examination.
• Evidence of any of the diseases mentioned (see Causes) should raise suspicion that it may be the underlying cause of petechiae or bruising.
• Many breeds are predisposed to von Willebrand disease, including Doberman pinschers, standard and toy Manchester terriers, Pembroke Welsh corgis, miniature schnauzers, Scottish terriers, golden retrievers, Shetland sheepdogs, and standard poodles.

CBC/BIOCHEMISTRY/URINALYSIS
• Platelets are low either by estimation on a well-made blood smear or by a direct count in patients with thrombocytopenia; if the platelet count is > 100,000/μL, consider other causes of defective primary hemostasis.
• RBC fragmentation suggests DIC or other vascular disease.
• Patients with myeloproliferative and lymphoproliferative diseases may be leukemic or cytopenic.
• Biochemical analysis—rule out hepatic, renal, and hormonal (e.g., Cushing disease) causes; hyperproteinemia may be the first indication of paraproteinemia.

OTHER LABORATORY TESTS
• Coagulation studies (APTT, PT, FDP, thrombin time)—help rule out DIC
• Von Willebrand factor assay—necessary to confirm von Willebrand disease
• Platelet function tests—may be necessary to rule out platelet function disorders
• Serum protein electrophoresis and examination of the urine for light chains (e.g., Bence-Jones protein)—indicated if the patient has hyperproteinemia
• Dexamethasone suppression or ACTH stimulation test—may be indicated if Cushing disease is suspected.

IMAGING
Abdominal radiography or ultrasonography may help identify splenomegaly or hepatomegaly associated with hypersplenism or Cushing disease, respectively.

DIAGNOSTIC PROCEDURES
• The buccal mucosa simplate bleeding time—long in patients with most of the thrombopathies in addition to thrombocytopenia; normal range 1.7–4.2 min; most useful in patients with platelet concentrations > 100,000/uL.
• Most invasive procedures are contraindicated in patients with bleeding disorders.
• Bone marrow examination—indicated if cytopenia or hyperproteinemia is detected

 TREATMENT
• Usually as inpatient until a definitive diagnosis is made
• Minimize activity to reduce the risk of even minor trauma.
• Discontinue any medications that may alter platelet function (e.g., aspirin and other NSAIDs).
• Maintenance of fluid volume by administration of balanced electrolyte solutions is recommended for all conditions.
• Blood or platelet transfusion may be necessary to survival before a definitive diagnosis is made; obtain serum, whole blood, and any other samples necessary before initiating such treatment.
• No specific treatment available for the congenital thrombocytopathies; in patients with acquired thrombocytopathy, the underlying disease must be treated; see specific diseases for details.

 MEDICATIONS

DRUGS OF CHOICE
Vary with the cause of the bruising

CONTRAINDICATIONS
N/A

PRECAUTIONS
Aspirin and other NSAIDs should be avoided unless patient has DIC or other cause of platelet activation.

POSSIBLE INTERACTIONS
N/A

ALTERNATIVE DRUGS
N/A

 FOLLOW-UP

PATIENT MONITORING
In patients with thrombocytopenia, conduct a daily platelet count daily until a response is noted; see specific diseases for details.

POSSIBLE COMPLICATIONS
• Death or morbidity caused by hemorrhage into the brain or other vital organs
• Shock caused by hemorrhagic hypovolemia

 MISCELLANEOUS

ASSOCIATED CONDITIONS
N/A

AGE-RELATED FACTORS
None

ZOONOTIC POTENTIAL
None

PREGNANCY
N/A

SYNONYMS
• Hemorrhagic diatheses
• Bleeding

SEE ALSO
• Disseminated Intravascular Coagulation (DIC)
• Hyperadrenocorticism (Cushing Disease)
• Myeloproliferative Disorders
• von Willebrand Disease

ABBREVIATIONS
• APTT = activated partial thromboplastin time
• DIC = disseminated intravascular coagulation
• FDP = fibrin degradation product
• PT = prothrombin time

Suggested Reading

Boon GD, Rebar AH. The clinical approach to disorders of hemostasis. In: Ettinger SJ, ed. Textbook of veterinary internal medicine. Philadelphia: Saunders, 1989:105–107.

Forbes CD, Printice CRM. Vascular and non-thrombocytopenic purpura. In: Bloom AL, Thomas DP, eds. Haemostasis and thrombosis. Edinburgh: Churchill Livingstone, 1987:321–332.

Green RA. Hemostatic disorders: coagulopathies and thrombotic disorders. In: Ettinger SJ, ed. Textbook of veterinary internal medicine. Philadelphia: Saunders, 1989:2246–2264.

Jergens AE, Turrentine MA, Kraus KH, Johnson GS. Buccal mucosa bleeding times of healthy dogs and of dogs in various pathologic states, including thrombocytopenia, uremia, and von Willebrand's disease. Am J Vet Res 1987;48:1337–1342.

Author G. Daniel Boon
Consulting Editor Susan M. Cotter

PODODERMATITIS

 BASICS

DEFINITION
An inflammatory, multifaceted complex of diseases that involves the feet of dogs and, less commonly, cats

PATHOPHYSIOLOGY
• Depends on the underlying cause
• Causes include infectious, allergic, autoimmune, endocrine/metabolic, neoplastic, and environmental diseases
• Psychogenic dermatoses rarely involved

SYSTEMS AFFECTED
Skin/Exocrine—primary or secondary infection (bacterial, fungal, or parasitic); neoplasia; target organ for underlying autoimmune, endocrine, or other systemic disease; paronychia (ungual folds, claw folds)

GENETICS
N/A

INCIDENCE/PREVALENCE
• Dogs—common
• Cats—uncommon

GEOGRAPHIC DISTRIBUTION
N/A

SIGNALMENT

Species
Dogs and cats

Breed Predilections
• Short-coated breeds (dogs)—most commonly affected; English bulldogs, great Danes, basset hounds, mastiffs, bull terriers, boxers, dachshunds, Dalmatians, German short-haired pointers, and weimaraners
• Long-coated breeds (dogs)—German shepherds, Labrador retrievers, golden retrievers, Irish setters, and Pekingese
• Cats—none

Mean Age and Range
Any age

Predominant Sex
• Dogs—male
• Cats—none

SIGNS

General Comments
The history and physical findings vary considerably depending on the underlying cause.

Historical Findings
• History—extremely important; determine environment and general husbandry (e.g., indoor vs. outdoor, working dog vs. pet, unsanitary conditions, other pets affected, trauma, contact irritants, hookworms)
• Seasonality—suggests atopic dermatitis, allergic contact dermatitis, or irritant contact dermatitis
• Lesions elsewhere on the body—may aid in diagnosis of cause

• Response to previous therapy—antibiotics, antifungals, and corticosteroids
• Diet, travel history, and other medical problems—important in investigation

Physical Examination Findings
Infectious (Dogs)
• Tissues—may be erythematous and edematous, nodules, inflammatory plaques (fungal "kerions"), ulcers, fistulae, hemorrhagic bullae, or serosanguineous or seropurulent discharge
• Feet—may be grossly swollen, may have pitting edema of the metacarpal and metatarsal areas
• Skin—may be alopecic and moist owing to constant licking; patient may have some degree of pain, pruritus, and paronychia
• Regional lymph nodes may be enlarged.
Infectious (Cats)
• Painful paronychia, involving one or more claws
• Higher incidence of nodular, often ulcerated lesions, compared to dog
• Footpads and periungual areas—commonly involved
• Interdigital spaces—seldom affected
• Scaly and crusted lesions—occasionally seen
Allergic (Dogs)
• Feet—erythematous and alopecic, secondary to pruritus; dorsal surface usually more severely affected
• Salivary staining may be evident.
• Allergic contact dermatitis—uncommon cause; dermatitis of the ventral interdigital surfaces is usually worse, although the whole paw may be involved.
Allergic (Cats)
Single or multiple, exudative or ulcerated, eosinophilic, pruritic plaques of the digits, periungual, and interdigital spaces.
Immune-Mediated (Dogs)
• Crusts and ulcerations—most common lesions; occasionally vesicles or bullae are seen.
• All four feet may be affected, especially the nailbeds and footpads.
• Hyperkeratotic and erosive dermatitis of the footpads—common finding in pemphigus foliaceus
Immune-Mediated (Cats)
• Lesions—generally involve the footpad, including hyperkeratosis and ulceration
• Lameness and paronychia—may occur
Endocrine/Metabolic (Dogs)
• Lesions—usually consistent with secondary infectious pododermatitis.
• Hepatocutaneous syndrome—rare condition; signs of skin disease precedes the onset of signs of internal disease; lesions include hyperkeratosis and ulceration of the footpads.
Endocrine/Metabolic (Cats)
Whitish nodules resembling candle wax; may be caused by cutaneous xanthomatosis; seen with diabetes mellitus.

Neoplastic
• Dogs—lesions usually nodules, possible ulceration or pruritus; usually only one foot is involved; multiple foot involvement with nailbed squamous cell carcinoma reported
• Cats—tumors appear as nodules; variably ulcerated and painful; localized destruction variable, depends on the tumor type
Environmental (Dogs and Cats)
• Depends on underlying cause
• Lesions—involve one digit or foot (foreign body, trauma) or multiple digits (irritant contact dermatitis, thallium toxicity, housed on rough surface or in moist environment)
• Chronic interdigital inflammation, ulceration, pyogranulomatous abscesses, draining tracts, or swelling, with or without pruritus
Miscellaneous
• Hyperkeratosis of the footpads (dogs)—associated with several diseases (e.g., zinc-responsive dermatosis, generic dog food dermatosis, and idiopathic digital hyperkeratosis)
• Nodules without draining tracts (dogs)—associated with sterile pyogranulomas in several breeds and nodular dermatofibrosis of the German shepherds and golden retrievers
• Hypomelanosis of the footpads (cats)—associated with vitiligo
• Hypermelanosis of the footpads (cats)—associated with lentigo simplex
• Polydactylism and syndactylism (cats)—common in certain families

CAUSES

Infectious (Dogs)
• Bacterial—*Staphylococcus intermedius*, *Pseudomonas* spp., *Proteus* spp., *Mycobacterium* spp., *Nocardia* spp., or *Actinomyces* spp.
• Fungal—dermatophytes, intermediate mycoses (sporotrichosis, mycetoma), or deep mycoses (blastomycosis, cryptococcosis)
• Parasitic—*Demodex canis, Pelodera strongyloides,* and hookworms)
• Protozoal—leishmaniasis

Infectious (Cats)
• Bacterial—same as dog, plus *Pasteurella* spp.
• Fungal—same as dog, excluding blastomycosis
• Parasitic—*Neotrombicula autumnalis, Notoedres cati,* or *Demodex* spp.
• Protozoal—*Anatrichosoma cutaneum*

Allergic
• Dogs—atopy; food hypersensitivity; allergic contact dermatitis
• Cats—atopy; rare for flea allergy dermatitis, adverse food reaction (food hypersensitivity), or contact dermatitis to involve paws

Immune-Mediated
• Dogs—pemphigus foliaceus; systemic lupus erythematosus; erythema multiforme; toxic epidermal necrolysis; vasculitis; cold agglutinin disease; pemphigus vulgaris; bullous pemphigoid; epidermolysis bullosa acquisita
• Cats—pemphigus foliaceus; systemic lupus

erythematosus; erythema multiforme; toxic epidermal necrolysis; vasculitis; cold agglutinin disease; plasma cell pododermatitis

Endocrine/Metabolic
• Dogs—hypothyroidism; hyperadrenocorticism; hepatocutaneous syndrome (necro-lytic migratory erythema)
• Cats—hypothyroidism; hyperadrenocorticism; cutaneous xanthomatosis (secondary to diabetes mellitus); endocrine pododermatitis rare

Neoplastic
• Higher incidence in cats than in dogs
• Dogs—squamous cell carcinomas; melanomas; mast cell tumors; keratoacanthomas; inverted papillomas, eccrine adenocarcinomas
• Cats—papillomas; spinocellular epithelioma; trichoepithelioma; fibrosarcoma; malignant fibrous histiocytoma; metastatic primary adenocarcinoma of the lung; other metastatic carcinomas

Environmental
• Dogs—irritant contact dermatitis; trauma; concrete and gravel dog runs; excessive exercise; clipper burn; foreign bodies (grass awns, bristle-like hairs of short-coated dogs); thallium toxicity
• Cats—irritant contact dermatitis; foreign bodies; thallium toxicity

Miscellaneous
• Dogs—sterile interdigital granulomas; see Physical Examination Findings
• Cats—see Physical Examination Findings

RISK FACTORS
• Lifestyle and general husbandry conditions—influence development
• Excess exercise, abrasive or moist housing, poor grooming, and/or lack of preventative medical practice may predispose an animal or exacerbate condition

DIAGNOSIS

DIFFERENTIAL DIAGNOSIS
See Signs and Causes

CBC/BIOCHEMISTRY/URINALYSIS
• Depend on the underlying cause
• Rarely used in the initial workup

OTHER LABORATORY TESTS
Endocrine tests, serology, or immune studies—rarely used in the initial workup; indications depend on results of initial workup.

IMAGING
• Radiographs and ultrasound—rarely used in the initial workup
• Neoplastic—depending on the underlying cause, may be necessary to confirm system disease or stage tumors

DIAGNOSTIC PROCEDURES
• Skin scrapings, fungal culture, and a stained

smear of any exudate or pustule contents
• Biopsy—histopathology, bacterial and fungal culture, and potentially for immunopathology
• Food elimination diet
• Intradermal skin testing
• Endocrine tests
• Dogs—biopsies indicated if skin scrapings are negative and lesions (nodules, draining tracts) are seen
• Cats—biopsies may be indicated in all cases, because pedal dermatosis is relatively rare.

PATHOLOGIC FINDINGS
Vary depending on the underlying cause

TREATMENT

APPROPRIATE HEALTH CARE
Outpaient, unless surgery is indicated

NURSING CARE
Foot soaks, hot packing, and/ or bandaging may be necessary, depending on cause.

ACTIVITY
Depends on severity of the lesions and the underlying cause

DIET
Hypoallergenic diet—determine food hypersensitivity

CLIENT EDUCATION
• Depends on underlying cause and severity of condition
• Discuss husbandry, lifestyle, and preventative medical practices.
• For allergic, immune-mediated, or endocrine causes, client must understand that condition will be managed, not cured.

SURGICAL CONSIDERATIONS
• Melanomas and squamous cell carcinomas—very poor prognosis; early diagnosis necessitates removal of the digit, digits, or paw.
• Infectious—may benefit from surgical débridement of devitalized tissue before medical therapy

MEDICATIONS

DRUGS OF CHOICE
• Long-term antibiotics, antifungals, anti-inflammatory or immunosuppressive levels of corticosteroids, chemotherapeutic agents, hormone-replacement therapy, or zinc supplementation
• Depend on the underlying cause and secondary infections

CONTRAINDICATIONS
N/A

PRECAUTIONS
Depend on the treatment protocol selected for the underlying cause; see specific drugs and their precautions

POSSIBLE INTERACTIONS
Depend on the underlying cause and treatment protocol selected

ALTERNATIVE DRUGS
N/A

FOLLOW-UP

PATIENT MONITORING
Depends on the underlying cause and treatment protocol selected

PREVENTION/AVOIDANCE
• Environmental cause—good husbandry and preventative medical practices should avoid recurrence.
• Allergic cause—important to avoid the allergen (inhalant or food), if possible

POSSIBLE COMPLICATIONS
Depend on the underlying cause and treatment protocol selected

EXPECTED COURSE AND PROGNOSIS
• Success of therapy depends on finding the underlying cause; often the cause is unknown; even when the cause is known, management can be frustrating owing to relapses or lack of affordable therapeutics.
• Often the disease can only be managed and not cured.
• Surgical intervention is sometimes the only option.

MISCELLANEOUS

ASSOCIATED CONDITIONS
N/A

AGE-RELATED FACTORS
Depend on the underlying cause

ZOONOTIC POTENTIAL
Not usually; depends on the underlying cause

PREGNANCY
Avoid systemically administered corticosteroids, antifungals, chemotherapeutic agents, azathioprine, and certain antimicrobials (e.g., enrofloxacin) in pregnant animals.

SYNONYMS
N/A

SEE ALSO
See Causes

Suggested Reading
Foil CS. Disorders of the feet and claws. Paper presented at the 11th Kal Kan Symposium.
Guaguere E, Hubert B, Delabre C. Feline pyodermatoses. Vet Dermatol 1992;3:1–12.
White SD. Pododermatitis. Vet Dermatol 1989;1:1–18.
Author K. Marcia Murphy
Consulting Editor Karen Helton Rhodes

POISONING (INTOXICATION)

BASICS

DEFINITION
- Acutely ill patients are often diagnosed as poisoned when no other diagnosis is obvious.
- Direct efforts toward stabilizing the patient.
- Make the diagnosis after determining pre-existing conditions and initially controlling clinical signs.
- Goals of treatment—providing emergency intervention; preventing further exposure; preventing further absorption; applying specific antidotes; hastening elimination; providing supportive measures; offering client education
- Suspected intoxication—suspected toxic materials and specimens may be valuable from a medicolegal aspect; maintain a proper chain of physical evidence; keep good medical records.
- Valuable time can be saved by applying the appropriate treatment for a suspected or known intoxicant.

Initial Instructions to Client
- May be beneficial to subsequent treatment
- Transport patient to a veterinarian as soon as possible.
- Delayed transport—keep patient warm; avoid any other stress.
- Warn onlookers about the condition of the patient.
- May need to muzzle the patient.
- Transport uncontaminated vomitus and suspected toxic materials and their containers to the hospital.
- Use clean plastic containers or glass jars for the specimens.

DIAGNOSIS

DIFFERENTIAL DIAGNOSIS
- Definitive diagnosis—difficult; animals come in contact with a vast array of toxicants; see Appendix IV: Clinical Toxicosis—Systems Affected and Clinical Effects
- Resources for emergencies—National Poison Control Center; state diagnostic laboratories; local poison control centers; great value for cases of suspected intoxication, especially when labels or containers are available
- When suspected compound and clinical signs do not concur—treat the signs; disregard the label
- Confirmation of diagnosis—by chemical analysis (may occur after the fact); accurate diagnosis and detailed records may help with future patients affected by the same intoxicant and are invaluable in medicolegal proceedings.

TREATMENT

SUPPORTIVE
- Control of body temperature
- Maintenance of respiratory and cardiovascular function
- Control of acid–base balance
- Alleviation of pain
- Control of CNS disorders—see specific topics

EMERGENCY
- Establishment of a patent airway
- Artificial respiration
- Cardiac massage—external or internal
- Application of defibrillation techniques
- After stabilization—may proceed with more specific therapeutic measures

PREVENT ABSORPTION
- Major treatment factor
- First remove patient from the affected environment.
- Available measures—washing; judicious use of emetics; gastric lavage techniques; use of adsorbents and cathartics

Washing Skin
- External toxicants
- Wash patient's skin to remove the noxious agent.
- **CAUTION:** avoid contamination of the people handling the patient.

Emetics
- Of little value beyond 4 hr after ingestion; most material will have passed to the duodenum.
- Do not induce in unconscious or severely depressed patients or after ingestion of strong acids, alkalis, petroleum distillates, tranquilizers, or other antiemetics.
- Apomorphine—most effective and most reliable for use in dogs and cats; availability at any given time unknown; small animals, 0.04 mg/kg IV or 0.08 mg/kg IM, SC; control adverse clinical signs caused by apomorphine with an appropriate intravenous narcotic antagonist (e.g., naloxone at 0.04 mg/kg).
- Ipecac—little efficacy; never use when activated charcoal is part of the therapeutic regimen.
- Xylazine—intravenous administration; used with some success in dogs and cats

Activated Charcoal
- Does not detoxify but prevents absorption if properly used
- Highly absorptive of many toxicants—organophosphate insecticides; other insecticides; rodenticides; mercuric chloride; strychnine; other alkaloids (e.g., morphine and atropine); barbiturates; ethylene glycol
- Ineffective against cyanide

POISONING (INTOXICATION)

• Administered in combination with emetics—increases efficacy of toxicant elimination by emesis

• Use a bathtub or some other easily cleansed area when administering activated charcoal to small animals.

• Dosage—1–5 g/kg body weight in a concentration of 1 g charcoal/5–10 mL water three to four times a day for 2–3 days

• Some charcoal should remain in the stomach and be followed by a cathartic to prevent desorption of the toxicant.

• Cathartic—sodium sulfate; administered 30 min after administration of the charcoal

Gastric Lavage

• An effective means of emptying the stomach

• Stomach tube size—use the largest possible; a good rule: use the same size as the cuffed endotracheal tube (1 mm = 3 Fr).

• Volume of water or lavage solution for each washing—5–10 mL/kg body weight

• Infusion and aspiration cycle—repeated 10–15 times

• Activated charcoal in the solution enhances the effectiveness.

• Precautions—(1) use low pressure to prevent forcing the toxicant into the duodenum; (2) reduce the infused volume in obviously weakened stomachs (e.g., in a patient that has ingested a caustic or corrosive toxicant); (3) do not force the stomach tube through either the esophagus or the stomach wall.

Oils

• Mineral or vegetable oil—of value for lipid-soluble toxicants

• Mineral oil (liquid petrolatum)—inert; less likely to be absorbed

• Use with a cathartic.

• Sodium sulfate—1 g/kg PO; more efficient agent for evacuation of the bowel than is magnesium sulfate; preferred with activated charcoal and mineral oil

Enemas

• Colonic lavage or high enema—may hasten the elimination of toxicants from the gastrointestinal tract

• Warm water with Castile soap—excellent solution

• Commercially available preparations are available that act as osmotic agents.

• Take care to avoid the induction of dehydration and electrolyte imbalances with overzealous treatment.

• Avoid hexachlorophene soaps in cats.

ENHANCE ELIMINATION

• Absorbed toxicants—generally excreted by the kidneys; may be excreted by other routes (e.g., bile, feces, lungs, and other body secretions)

• Renal excretion—may be manipulated in many animals

• Urinary excretion—may be enhanced by the use of diuretics or by altering the pH of the urine

Diuretics

• To enhance urinary excretion of toxicants—requires maintenance of adequate renal function

• Minimum urine flow cannot be established—must use peritoneal dialysis

• Agents of choice—mannitol (1.0–2.0 g/kg IV q6h) and furosemide (5 mg/kg q6–8h)

Manipulating Urine pH

• Classic pharmacologic technique

• Acidic compounds remain ionized in alkaline urine; alkaline compounds remain ionized in acidic urine

• Long-term urinary acidification—ammonium chloride (200 mg/kg PO daily in divided doses) and ethylenediamine dihydrochloride (1–2 tablets q8h for the average-sized dog)

• Physiologic saline—good, rapid, urinary acidifying agent

• Sodium bicarbonate—5 mEq/kg/hr; may be used as an alkalinizing agent

Peritoneal Dialysis

• Indicated for oliguria or anuria

• Indicated for simple removal of absorbed toxicants in patient with normal renal function

• pH of the solution—may be altered to maintain the ionized state of the offending compound

MEDICATIONS

Specific antidotes or procedures are available for the more common toxicants; see specific topic

FOLLOW-UP

Specific monitoring depends on the toxicant and the patient's signs and laboratory abnormalities.

MISCELLANEOUS

Suggested Reading

Bailey EM, Garland T. Toxicologic emergencies. In: Murtaugh RJ, Kaplan PM, eds., Veterinary emergency and critical care medicine. St. Louis: Mosby Year Book, 1992:427–452.

Authors E. Murl Bailey and Tom Garland
Consulting Editor Gary D. Osweiler

POLYURIA AND POLYDIPSIA

BASICS

DEFINITION
• Polyuria—greater than normal urine production (dogs, >45 mL/kg/day; cats, > 40 mL/kg/day) • Polydipsia—greater than normal water consumption (dogs, >90 mL/kg/day; cats, >45 mL/kg/day)

PATHOPHYSIOLOGY
• Urine production and water consumption (thirst) are controlled by interactions between the kidneys, pituitary gland, and hypothalamus. Volume receptors within the cardiac atria and aortic arch also influence thirst and urine production. Polyuria may occur when the quantity of functional antidiuretic hormone (ADH) synthesized in the hypothalamus or released from the posterior pituitary is limited or when the kidneys fail to respond normally to ADH. Polydipsia occurs when the thirst center in the anterior hypothalamus is stimulated. • In most patients, polydipsia occurs as a compensatory response to polyuria to maintain hydration. The patient's plasma becomes relatively hypertonic and activates thirst mechanisms. Occasionally, polydipsia is the primary process and polyuria is the compensatory response. Then, the patient's plasma becomes relatively hypotonic because of excessive water intake, and ADH secretion is reduced, resulting in polyuria.

SYSTEMS AFFECTED
• Renal/urologic—kidneys • Endocrine-metabolic—pituitary gland and hypothalamus • Cardiovascular—alterations in "effective" circulating volume

SIGNALMENT
• Dogs and cats • Congenital (e.g., central diabetes insipidus, nephrogenic diabetes insipidus, portal-vascular anomalies, and certain renal diseases), hypoadrenocorticism, and some causes of primary polydipsia predominantly affect young dogs. • Renal failure, hyperadrenocorticism, hyperthyroidism, and neoplastic disorders affecting the pituitary and hypothalamus predominantly affect middle-aged and older dogs and cats.

SIGNS
N/A

CAUSES
• Primary polyuria due to impaired renal response to ADH—renal failure, hyperadrenocorticism (dogs), hyperthyroidism (cats), pyelonephritis, hypoadrenocorticism, pyometra, hepatic failure, hypercalcemia, hypokalemia, renal medullary solute washout, dietary protein restriction, drugs, congenital nephrogenic diabetes insipidus • Primary polyuria caused by osmotic diuresis—diabetes mellitus, primary renal glucosuria, post-obstructive diuresis, some diuretics (e.g., mannitol and furosemide), ingestion or administration of large quantities of solute (e.g., sodium chloride or glucose), and hypersomatotropism • Primary polyuria due to ADH deficiency—idiopathic, traumatic, neoplastic, or congenital-origin central diabetes insipidus; some drugs (e.g., alcohol and phenytoin) • Primary polydipsia—behavioral problem, pyrexia, pain, or organic disease of the anterior hypothalamic thirst center of neoplastic, traumatic, or inflammatory origin

RISK FACTORS
• Renal disease or liver disease • Selected endocrine and electrolyte disorders • Administration of diuretics, corticosteroids, and anticonvulsants • Low-protein diets designed for dissolution of struvite uroliths in dogs • Young, hyperactive, large-breed dogs appear to be at higher than normal risk for primary polydipsia.

DIAGNOSIS

DIFFERENTIAL DIAGNOSIS

Differentiating Similar Signs
• Differentiate polyuria from an abnormal increase in the frequency of urination (pollakiuria). Pollakiuria is often associated with dysuria, stranguria, or hematuria. Patients with polyuria void large quantities of urine; patients with pollakiuria typically void small quantities of urine. Confirm polyuria/polydipsia by measuring 24-h water intake or urine output (a 3- to 5-day collection period is used to increase reliability). • Alternatively, measuring urinary specific gravity may provide evidence of adequate urine-concentrating ability (dogs, 1.030; cats, 1.035), which rules out polyuria/polydipsia.

Differentiating Causes
• Renal failure, hyperadrenocorticism, and diabetes mellitus are common causes of polyuria/polydipsia in dogs. Renal failure, hyperthyroidism, and diabetes mellitus are common causes of polyuria/polydipsia in cats. Rule out these conditions before seeking less common disorders. • If associated with progressive weight loss—consider renal failure, diabetes mellitus, hyperthyroidism, hepatic failure, pyometra, pyelonephritis, and malignancy-induced hypercalcemia • If associated with polyphagia—consider diabetes mellitus, hyperthyroidism, and hyperadrenocorticism • If associated with bilateral alopecia and other cutaneous problems—consider hyperadrenocorticism and other endocrinologic disorders • If associated with uremic breath and uremic stomatitis—consider renal failure • If associated with vomiting—consider renal failure, hypoadrenocorticism, pyelonephritis, hepatic failure, hypercalcemia, hypokalemia, and diabetes mellitus; occasionally, vomiting occurs after rapid consumption of a large quantity of water • If associated with recent estrus (within the previous 2 months) in a middle aged intact female—consider pyometra • If associated with abdominal distention—consider hepatic failure, hyperadrenocorticism, pyometra, and nephrotic syndrome • If associated with lymphadenopathy or anal sac mass—consider hypercalcemia of malignancy • If associated with palpable thyroid nodule—consider hyperthyroidism • If associated with hypertensive retinopathy—consider renal failure, hyperthyroidism, and hyperadrenocorticism • If associated with behavioral or neurologic disorder—consider hepatic failure, primary polydipsia, or central diabetes insipidus • If associated with marked polydipsia, in which patients almost continuously seek and consume water from any source—consider primary polydipsia, central diabetes insipidus, and congenital nephrogenic diabetes insipidus

CBC/BIOCHEMISTRY/URINALYSIS
• Serum sodium concentration may help differentiate primary polyuria from primary polydipsia. Measuring serum osmolality is preferred; calculated serum osmolality is not an acceptable substitute. • Relative hypernatremia or high serum osmolarity suggests primary polyuria (values typically trend to or exceed the high end of the normal range). • Hyponatremia or low serum osmolarity suggests primary polydipsia (values typically trend to or decline below the normal range), except in animals with hypoadrenocorticism, which have hyponatremia and primary polyuria. • Azotemia is consistent with renal causes for polyuria/polydipsia but may also indicate dehydration resulting from inadequate compensatory polydipsia. • Unexpectedly low BUN concentrations suggest hepatic failure. • High hepatic enzyme activities are consistent with hyperadrenocorticism (especially when the value for ALP exceeds that for ALT), hyperthyroidism, hepatic failure, pyometra, and diabetes mellitus. Administration of some drugs that promote polyuria/polydipsia (e.g., anticonvulsants and corticosteroids) elevates hepatic enzyme activities. • Persistent hyperglycemia is consistent with diabetes mellitus. • Hyperkalemia, particularly if associated with hyponatremia, suggests possible hypoadrenocorticism or therapy with potassium-sparing diuretics. • Hypercalcemia and hypokalemia can cause, or occur in association with, other diseases that cause polyuria/polydipsia (e.g., chronic renal failure may be associated with both; hypoadrenocorticism may be associated with hypercalcemia). • Hypercalcemia induces polyuria only when it results from increased ionized calcium concentration. • Hypoalbuminemia supports renal or hepatic causes or polyuria/polydipsia. • Neutrophilia is consistent with pyelonephritis, pyometra, hyperadrenocorticism, and cortico-

steroid administration. • Urinary specific gravity values between 1.001 and 1.005 particularly suggest primary polydipsia, central diabetes insipidus, or congenital nephrogenic diabetes insipidus. • Glucosuria supports a diagnosis of diabetes mellitus or renal glucosuria; pyuria, white blood cell casts, and/or bacteriuria should prompt consideration of pyelonephritis.

OTHER LABORATORY TESTS
• ACTH stimulation or dexamethasone suppression tests to rule out hyperadrenocorticism in middle-aged to older dogs in which initial findings do not explain polyuria/polydipsia.
• Serum thyroxine concentration to rule out hyperthyroidism in middle-aged and old cats
• Urine culture—chronic pyelonephritis cannot be conclusively ruled out by absence of pyuria or bacteriuria.
• Cytologic examination of lymph node aspirate may provide evidence of lymphosarcoma, which induces polyuria by hypercalcemic nephrotoxicity or direct infiltration of renal tissues.

IMAGING
Abdominal survey radiography and ultrasonography may provide additional evidence of renal (e.g., primary renal diseases and urinary obstruction), hepatic (e.g., microhepatica, portal vascular anomalies, and hepatic infiltrate), adrenal (e.g., adrenal mass and bilateral adrenal hypertrophy suggesting hyperadrenocorticism), or uterine (e.g., pyometra) disorders that can contribute to polyuria/polydipsia.

DIAGNOSTIC PROCEDURES
Modified Water Deprivation with ADH Response Testing (see Appendix):
• Differentiates central diabetes insipidus from primary polydipsia and nephrogenic diabetes insipidus. Rule out other causes for polyuria/polydipsia before performing this test.
• Most useful for patients with marked polyuria/polydipsia and hyposthenuria.
• Water deprivation testing is contraindicated in dehydrated and azotemic patients, but ADH response testing may be performed safely in these patients.
• Patients that concentrate urine adequately in response to water deprivation are presumed to have primary polydipsia.
• Patients that fail to concentrate urine adequately in response to properly designed water deprivation tests but further concentrate their urine in response to administration of exogenous ADH have central diabetes insipidus.
• Patients that fail to concentrate urine adequately in response to water deprivation and also fail to further concentrate urine in response to administration of exogenous ADH have nephrogenic diabetes insipidus.

TREATMENT
• Serious medical consequence for the patient is rare if patient has free access to water and is willing and able to drink. Until the mechanism of polyuria is understood, discourage owners from limiting access to water. Direct treatment at the underlying cause.
• Provide polyuric patients with free access to water unless they are vomiting. If polyuric patients are vomiting, give replacement maintenance fluids parenterally. Also provide fluids parenterally when other conditions limit oral intake or dehydration persists despite polydipsia.
• Base fluid selection on knowledge of the underlying cause for fluid loss. In most patients, lactated Ringer's solution is an acceptable replacement fluid.
• When dehydration has resulted from withholding water, or when urine is hyposthenuric, providing oral water or parenteral administration of dextrose 5% in water may be preferred to lactated Ringer's solution.
• Primary polydipsia—treat by limiting water intake to a normal daily volume. It may be necessary to reduce water intake over days to weeks to avoid such undesirable behavior as increased barking, urine consumption, or other patterns of bizarre behavior. Monitor the patient closely to avoid iatrogenic dehydration. Salt (1 g/30 kg q12 h) or sodium bicarbonate (0.6 g/30 kg q12 h) may be given orally to help reestablish the renal medullary solute gradient. Consider behavior modification if water restriction alone is unsuccessful.

MEDICATIONS
DRUGS OF CHOICE
Vary with underlying cause

CONTRAINDICATIONS
Do not administer ADH (or any of its synthetic analogs, such as DDAVP) to patients with primary polydipsia because of the risk of inducing water intoxication.

PRECAUTIONS
Until renal and hepatic failure have been excluded as potential causes for polyuria/polydipsia, use caution in administering any drug eliminated via these pathways.

POSSIBLE INTERACTIONS
N/A

ALTERNATIVE DRUGS
N/A

FOLLOW-UP
PATIENT MONITORING
• Hydration status by clinical assessment of hydration and serial evaluation of body weight
• Fluid intake and urine output—provide a useful baseline for assessing adequacy of hydration therapy

POSSIBLE COMPLICATIONS
Dehydration

MISCELLANEOUS
ASSOCIATED CONDITIONS
• Bacterial urinary tract infection—patients appear to be at particular risk of developing urinary tract infection as a consequence of urinary catheterization • Urinary incontinence may develop in dogs with concurrent urethral sphincter dysfunction, presumably because of increased bladder-filling associated with polyuria.

AGE-RELATED FACTORS
N/A

ZOONOTIC POTENTIAL
N/A

PREGNANCY
N/A

SYNONYMS
N/A

SEE ALSO
• Calcium, Hypercalcemia • Congenital/Developmental Renal Disorders • Diabetes Insipidus • Diabetes Mellitus • Fanconi's Syndrome • Hepatic Failure, Acute • Hyperadrenocorticism • Hyperthyroidism • Hypoadrenocorticism • Portovascular Anomalies • Potassium, Hypokalemia • Pyelonephritis • Pyometra • Renal Failure, Acute and Chronic • Urinary Tract Obstruction

ABBREVIATIONS
ADH = antidiuretic hormone

Suggested Reading
Feldman EC, Nelson RW. Canine and feline endocrinology and reproduction. Philadelphia: Saunders, 1996:2–37.
Meric SM. Polyuria and polydipsia. In: Ettinger SJ, Feldman EC, eds. Textbook of veterinary internal medicine. Philadelphia: Saunders, 1995:159–163.
Author David J. Polzin
Consulting Editors Larry G. Adams and Carl A. Osborne

PROSTATOMEGALY

BASICS

DEFINITION
Abnormally large prostate gland determined by rectal or abdominal palpation or by abdominal radiography or prostatic ultrasonography; enlargement can be symmetrical or asymmetrical, painful or nonpainful. Normal prostate size varies with age, body size, castration status, and breed, so determination of enlargement is subjective.

PATHOPHYSIOLOGY
Enlargement can result from epithelial cell hyperplasia or hypertrophy (e.g., benign prostatic hyperplasia), neoplasia of prostatic epithelium or stroma, cystic change within the prostatic parenchyma, or inflammatory cell infiltration (e.g., acute and chronic bacterial prostatitis and prostatic abscess).

SYSTEMS AFFECTED
• Renal/Urologic
• Reproductive

SIGNALMENT
• Dogs
• Typically noted in middle-aged to older males

SIGNS
• Maybe none
• Straining to defecate
• Ribbonlike stools
• Dysuria
• Urethral outflow obstruction

CAUSES
• Benign prostatic hyperplasia
• Squamous metaplasia
• Adenocarcinoma
• Transitional cell carcinoma
• Sarcoma
• Metastatic neoplasia
• Acute bacterial prostatitis
• Prostatic abscess
• Chronic bacterial prostatitis
• Prostatic cyst

RISK FACTORS
• Castration lowers the risk of benign prostatic hyperplasia and bacterial prostatitis.
• Risk of adenocarcinoma may be increased in neutered dog.

DIAGNOSIS

DIFFERENTIAL DIAGNOSIS
• Benign prostatic hyperplasia—typically causes nonpainful symmetrical enlargement of the prostate gland; not found in neutered dogs
• Primary or metastatic neoplasia—typically causes painful, nonsymmetrical enlargement of the prostate gland; weight loss, impaired appetite, rear limb weakness observed in some patients; suspect neoplasia in neutered dogs.
• Acute bacterial prostatitis—typically results in slight-to-moderate symmetric or nonsymmetrical enlargement of the prostate gland with prostatic pain; fever, impaired appetite, rear limb weakness, and painful abdomen observed in some patients.
• Chronic bacterial prostatitis—signs similar to those seen in animals with acute prostatitis or those related to recurrent lower urinary tract infection (e.g., dysuria and hematuria); bacterial prostatitis uncommon in neutered dogs
• Prostatic abscess—may result in signs similar to those in patients with acute or chronic prostatitis; abscess rupture causes fever and caudal abdominal pain.
• Prostatic cysts—may cause a palpable caudal abdominal mass, straining to urinate, or straining to defecate; patient may also be asymptomatic.

CBC/BIOCHEMISTRY/URINALYSIS
• CBC normal in patients with benign prostatic hyperplasia
• Leukocytosis in patients with acute and chronic (occasionally) bacterial prostatitis, prostatic abscess, and prostatic neoplasia (occasionally)
• High bilirubin and alkaline phosphatase (ALP) in some patients with prostatic abscess
• Urinalysis—normal or hematuria in patients with benign prostatic hyperplasia
• Pyuria, hematuria, proteinuria, bacteriuria in patients with bacterial prostatitis
• Pyuria, hematuria, proteinuria, and, occasionally, neoplastic cells in dogs with prostatic neoplasia

OTHER LABORATORY TESTS
Serum prostatic esterase concentration is high in dogs with benign prostatic hyperplasia.

IMAGING

Radiographic Findings
• Prostatomegaly
• Prostatic mineralization more likely in dogs with prostatic neoplasia

Ultrasonographic Findings
• Abscess or cyst—hypoechoic or anechoic lesions with distal enhancement
• Acute bacterial prostatitis—uniform prostatic echogenicity
• Benign prostatic hyperplasia—uniform prostatic echogenicity; small fluid-filled cysts in some patients
• Chronic bacterial prostatitis—focal or diffuse hyperechogenicity
• Prostatic neoplasia—focal to multifocal areas of coalescing echogenicity and acoustic shadowing (if mineralization)

DIAGNOSTIC PROCEDURES
• Examination of prostatic fluid obtained by ejaculation or prostatic massage may reveal

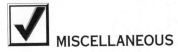
changes similar to those seen on urinalysis.
• Bacterial culture of prostatic fluid typically reveals >10,000 bacteria/mL in dogs with bacterial prostatitis.
• Transrectal aspiration biopsy (specimen obtained by a Franzen needle guide) or urethral catheter biopsy reveals neoplastic cells in some dogs with prostatic carcinoma.
• Needle biopsy with ultrasound guidance provides visualization of the area to be sampled and increases the likelihood of obtaining a diagnostic sample; take care to avoid rupturing a prostatic abscess.

TREATMENT

• Varies with the cause of prostatomegaly
• Surgical castration—indicated in symptomatic dogs with benign prostatic hyperplasia and after acute infection resolves in dogs with bacterial prostatitis
• Surgical drainage—indicated in dogs with prostatic abscess or large prostatic cysts
• External beam radiotherapy may provide palliation in patients with prostatic carcinoma.

MEDICATIONS

DRUGS OF CHOICE

Benign Prostatic Hyperplasia
If castration is not acceptable, the following drugs may produce a temporary response:
• Finasteride (0.5 mg/day)
• Megestrol acetate (0.11 mg/kg PO daily for 3 weeks)
• Medroxyprogesterone (3 mg/kg SC)

Bacterial Prostatitis
Chose antibiotics on the basis of antibacterial sensitivity testing of the isolated organism and ability of the antibiotic to diffuse into prostatic fluid in therapeutic concentrations; good choices for latter include trimethoprim/sulfa, chloramphenicol, and enrofloxacin.

Prostatic Carcinoma
Chemotherapy has not been proved beneficial; can consider combination therapy with cyclophosphamide and doxorubicin

CONTRAINDICATIONS
N/A

PRECAUTIONS
Long-term administration of megestrol acetate or medroxyprogesterone can cause diabetes mellitus.

POSSIBLE INTERACTIONS
N/A

ALTERNATIVE DRUGS
N/A

FOLLOW-UP

PATIENT MONITORING
• Abdominal radiographs or prostatic ultrasonography to assess efficacy of treatment in benign prostatic hyperplasia, prostatic carcinoma, or bacterial prostatitis
• Urine and prostatic fluid culture to access efficacy of treatment in patients with bacterial prostatitis

POSSIBLE COMPLICATIONS
• Urethral obstruction
• Rectal obstruction

MISCELLANEOUS

ASSOCIATED CONDITIONS
N/A

AGE-RELATED FACTORS
Prostatic carcinoma typically diagnosed in 8- to 10-year-old dogs

ZOONOTIC POTENTIAL
N/A

PREGNANCY
N/A

SYNONYMS
N/A

SEE ALSO
• Adenocarcinoma, Prostate
• Benign Prostatic Hyperplasia
• Prostatic Cysts
• Prostatitis/Prostatic Abscess

ABBREVIATIONS
ALP = alkaline phosphatase

Suggested Reading
Barsanti JA, Finco DR. Canine prostatic diseases. In: Ettinger SJ, ed. Textbook of veterinary internal medicine. Philadelphia: Saunders, 1989:1662–1685.
Kay ND. Diseases of the prostate gland. In: Birchard SJ, Sherding, RD, eds. Saunders manual of small animal practice. Philadelphia: Saunders, 1994:865–871.
Author Jeffrey S. Klausner
Consulting Editors Larry G. Adams and Carl A. Osborne

PRURITUS

BASICS

DEFINITION
The sensation that provokes the desire to scratch, rub, chew, or lick; an indicator of inflamed skin

PATHOPHYSIOLOGY
• A specific end organ has not been found.
• The sensation of itch is conducted by A δ fibers and C fibers of the peripheral nervous system to the dorsal root of the spinal cord.
• The axons, some of which cross over, ascend via the lateral spinothalamic tract and synapse in the caudal thalamus and then to the sensory cortex.
• Other factors can modify the perception of pruritus at this level.

SYSTEMS AFFECTED
Skin/Exocrine—in severe cases, the mental state of the animal may also be affected.

SIGNALMENT
Highly variable; depends on the underlying cause

SIGNS
• The act of scratching, licking, biting, or chewing
• For some animals, evidence of self-trauma and cutaneous inflammation is necessary to make the diagnosis if the history is incomplete.
• Cats—can be secretive lickers; alopecia without inflammation may be the only sign

CAUSES
• Parasitic—fleas, scabies, *Demodex, Otodectes, Notoedres, Cheyletiella,* trombicula, lice, *Pelodera,* endoparasite migration
• Allergic—parasite, atopy, food, contact, drug, bacterial hypersensitivity
• Bacterial/fungal—pachydermatis
• Miscellaneous—primary and secondary seborrhea, calcinosis cutis, cutaneous neoplasia, immune-mediated dermatosis; psychogenic diseases and endocrine dermatosis variable

RISK FACTORS
N/A

DIAGNOSIS

DIFFERENTIAL DIAGNOSIS
• Alopecia—in most cases, a clear history of pruritus is noted; without pruritus, may accompany endocrine diseases; some animals may excessively lick themselves without the owners knowledge; demodicosis, dermatophytosis, bacterial pyoderma, seborrhea, some cutaneous neoplasms, and unusual diseases (e.g., leishmaniasis) may cause alopecia with varying degrees of inflammation and pruritus.
• History—often the most important guide to necessary tests; severe condition, which constantly keeps the patient and owner awake, suggests scabies, flea allergy/infestation, food allergy, or cutaneous yeast infection; all but the latter typically have an acute onset.
• Uncomplicated atopy—initially very steroid responsive; originally seasonal; often progresses to nonseasonal, pruritic disease with a predilection for the face, feet, ears, forelimbs, axilla, and rump; flea- and food-allergic animals are predisposed to atopy and may show similar signs.

CBC/BIOCHEMISTRY/URINALYSIS
N/A

OTHER LABORATORY TESTS
N/A

IMAGING
N/A

DIAGNOSTIC PROCEDURES
• Skin scrapes, epidermal cytology and dermatophyte cultures (with microscopic identification)—identify primary or co-existing diseases caused by parasites or other microorganisms
• Wood's lamp—do not use as the sole means of diagnosing or excluding dermatophytosis, owing to false negatives and misinterpretations of florescence.

Allergy Testing
• Two methods—skin testing (intradermal skin testing) and blood testing; skin testing is the historical standard and the preferred method; some veterinary dermatologists use both tests.

• Skin testing—identify individual allergens; takes into account the important allergy-associated immunoglobulins (IgGd and systemic as well as localized IgE)
• Blood testing—commercial tests for allergies measure only serum IgE, not IgGd; disadvantage, some tests determine groups or mixes of allergens
• Allergy extract—correlate positive reactions with the history; then formulate the immunotherapy solution; contains a mixture of specific allergens, based on the history, test results, and the veterinarian's (or the laboratory's) clinical experience; concentration may vary with the type of test done and may affect the success rate

Skin Biopsy
• Useful when associated lesions are unusual and an immune-mediated disease is expected or the history and physical findings do not correlate
• Results should be interpreted by a trained veterinary dermatopathologist.

Trial Courses
Canine Scabies
• Can be difficult to diagnose
• Skin scrapes often negative
• Trial course (lime sulfur, ivermectin) often necessary to rule out
• Ivermectin—use caution; associated with idiosyncratic reactions and death
Food Allergy
• Blood and skin tests—not recommended for diagnosis
• Hypoallergenic dietary trial most appropriate test
• Trial—must include only novel food; use a diet that has been confirmed as hypoallergenic through clinical trials; avoid meat-flavored treats and medicines (heartworm preventatives); continue trial until patient improves or for 8–10 weeks; if improvement is noted, reintroduce original diet and monitor for itching for 7–14 days; return of itching may occur within hours; reintroduction of original diet confirms food allergy

TREATMENT
• More than one disease may be contributing to the itching; if treatment for an identified condition does not result in improvement, consider other causes.
• Use of a mechanical restraint (e.g., Elizabethan collar) can help but is seldom feasible in the long term.

MEDICATIONS

DRUGS OF CHOICE

Topical Therapy
- Helpful for mild cases
- Localized—sprays, lotions, and creams
- Generalized—shampoos
- Colloidal oatmeal—available in all forms; may be very beneficial; duration of effect usually < 2 days
- Antihistamines—beneficial effect not demonstrated
- Anesthetics—very short duration of effect
- Antibacterial shampoo—controls bacterial infections; some (e.g., benzoyl peroxide or iodine) may exacerbate the condition
- Lime sulfur—may be antipruritic; has anti-parasitic, antibacterial, and antifungal properties; disadvantages are bad odor and staining
- Steroids—most useful topical medication; excessive use causes localized and systemic side effects; hydrocortisone mildest and most common; stronger drugs (e.g., betamethasone) more effective, more expensive, and cause more side effects; some contain ingredients (e.g., alcohol) that increase irritation.
- Sometimes the application of any substance, including water (especially warm water), can worsen itching sensation; cool water is often soothing.

Systemic Therapy
- Three pathways lead to inflammation and itching.
- Steroids—block all three pathways; undesirable side effects; consider drugs that block individual pathways
- Antihistamines—hydroxyzine, diphenhydramine, and chlorpheniramine; block only one pathway
- ω-3 and ω-6 fatty acids—available as powder, liquid, and capsules; help block individual pathways that lead to inflammation; 6–8 weeks until maximum effect is observed; prevent rather than stop inflammation; help control dry or flaky skin
- Psychogenics—can help control itching; amitriptyline (Elavil; a human antidepressant) has rather potent antihistaminic actions in dogs, with side effects similar to antihistamines; doxepin is similar; fluoxetine (Prozac) used with variable success in treating canine lick granuloma (acral lick dermatitis); diazepam (Valium) has been beneficial; reports of acute hepatotoxicity in cats

- The use of nonsteroid drugs is less convenient but diminishes the potential for serious side effects; if not totally effective in controlling clinical signs, they often help reduce the amount of steroids necessary to decrease itching.

CONTRAINDICATIONS
- Sometimes the application of anything topically, including water and products containing alcohol, iodine, and benzoyl peroxide, can exacerbate itching; cool water may be soothing.
- Steroids—avoid with infectious causes

PRECAUTIONS

Steroids
- Most well-known drug used to control itching
- Significant long-term and not always obvious side effects
- Used wisely, usually safe
- Avoid long-term daily administration of oral corticosteroids (including prednisone or methylprednisolone).
- Avoid long-term daily or alternate-day administration of triamcinolone (Vetalog).
- Short-term use seldom causes serious problems.
- Avoid with a history of pancreatitis, diabetes mellitus, calcinosis cutis, demodicosis, dermatophytosis, and other infectious diseases.

POSSIBLE INTERACTIONS
N/A

ALTERNATIVE DRUGS
Immunosuppressive drugs (e.g., azathioprine)—use in extremely rare cases; because of potential profound side effects, reserve for cases in which euthanasia is being considered or when all other treatments have failed.

FOLLOW-UP

PATIENT MONITORING
- Multiple causes (e.g., flea allergy, inhalant allergy, and pyoderma) common; eradication or control of one cause may not be enough to reduce the condition.
- Food- and airborne/inhalant-allergic animals may do well during winter on a hypoallergenic diet; clinical signs may return in the warmer months in association with inhalant allergies.
- Monitor patients receiving chronic steroids every 3–6 months for signs of iatrogenic Cushing disease.

POSSIBLE COMPLICATIONS
- Client frustration owing to the chronic nature of pruritus
- Skin scrapes and other tests may be initially negative or normal but may later become diagnostic.
- Complications common with chronic steroid use

MISCELLANEOUS

ASSOCIATED CONDITIONS
N/A

AGE-RELATED FACTORS
N/A

ZOONOTIC POTENTIAL
Some causes (e.g., sarcoptic mange)

PREGNANCY
N/A

SEE ALSO
See Causes

Suggested Reading
Bevier DE. Long-term management of atopic disease in the dog. In: DeBoer DJ, ed. Vet Clin North Am Small Anim Pract 1995;25:1487–1505.

Author W. Dunbar Gram

Consulting Editor Karen Helton Rhodes

PTYALISM

 BASICS

DEFINITION
• Excessive production of saliva
• Pseudoptyalism is the excessive release of saliva that has accumulated in the oral cavity.

PATHOPHYSIOLOGY
• Saliva is constantly produced and secreted into the oral cavity from the salivary glands (parotid, sublingual, mandibular, zygomatic, buccal).
• Normal saliva production may appear excessive in patients with an anatomic abnormality that allows saliva to dribble out of the mouth or a condition that affects swallowing.
• Salivation increases because of excitation of the salivary nuclei in the brainstem.
• Stimuli that lead to this are taste and tactile sensations involving the mouth and tongue.
• Higher centers in the CNS can also excite or inhibit the salivary nuclei.
• Lesions involving either the CNS or the oral cavity can cause excessive salivation.
• Diseases that affect the pharynx, esophagus, and stomach can also stimulate excessive production of saliva.

SYSTEMS AFFECTED
N/A

SIGNALMENT
• Dogs and cats
• Young animals are more likely to have ptyalism caused by a congenital problem such as portosystemic shunt and from ingestion of a toxin, caustic agent, or foreign body.
• Yorkshire terrier, Maltese terrier, Australian cattle dog, miniature schnauzer, and Irish wolfhound breeds have a relatively higher incidence of congenital portosystemic shunt.
• Megaesophagus is hereditary in wire-haired fox terriers and miniature schnauzers; familial predispositions have been reported in the German shepherd, Newfoundland, Great Dane, Irish setter, Chinese shar-pei, greyhound, and retriever breeds, as well as in Siamese cats.
• Congenital hiatal hernia has been recognized in the Chinese shar-pei.
• Giant breeds, such as St. Bernard and mastiff, are known for excessive drooling.

SIGNS

Historical Findings
• Anorexia—seen most often in patients with oral lesions, gastrointestinal disease, and systemic disease
• Eating behavior changes—patients with oral disease or cranial nerve dysfunction may refuse to eat hard food, not chew with the affected side (patients with unilateral lesions), hold the head in an unusual position while eating, or drop prehended food.
• Other behavioral changes—irritability, aggressiveness, and reclusiveness are common, especially in patients with a painful condition.
• Dysphagia—may be seen if inability to swallow
• Regurgitation—in patients with esophageal disease
• Vomiting—secondary to gastrointestinal or systemic disease
• Pawing at the face or muzzle—patients with oral discomfort or pain
• Neurologic signs—patients that have been exposed to causative drugs or toxins and those with hepatic encephalopathy

Physical Examination Findings
• Periodontal disease—inflammation may cause ptyalism
• Stomatitis—ulceration and inflammation of many different causes is associated with ptyalism
• Mass in the oral cavity
• Lesions of the tongue—inflammation, ulceration, mass, and foreign body
• Lesions of the oropharynx—inflammation, ulceration, and mass, especially involving the soft palate and glossopalatine arch
• Blood in the saliva—suggests bleeding from the oral cavity, pharynx, or esophagus
• Halitosis—usually caused by oral cavity disease, but also by esophageal and gastric disease
• Facial pain—caused by oral cavity or pharyngeal disease
• Dysphagia—caused by oral cavity, pharyngeal, or neuromuscular disease or abnormally large retropharyngeal lymph nodes
• Cranial nerve deficits—trigeminal nerve (CN V) lesions can cause drooling due to inability to close the mouth; facial nerve palsy (CN VII) can cause drooling from the affected side; glossopharyngeal (CN IX), vagus (CN X), and hypoglossal (CN XII) nerve lesions can cause a loss of the gag reflex or inability to swallow.
• Salivary gland problem—inflamed, necrotic, or painful salivary glands can cause ptyalism (rare).
• Cheilitis or acne—persistent drooling can lead to dermatologic lesions.

CAUSES

Conformational Disorder of the Lips
Particularly in giant-breed dogs

Oral and Pharyngeal Diseases
• Foreign body
• Neoplasm
• Gingivitis or stomatitis—secondary to periodontal disease, FeLV infection in cats, viral upper respiratory infection, immune-mediated disease (e.g., lymphoplasmacytic stomatitis, pemphigus vulgaris), uremia, ingestion of a caustic agent, poisonous plant, or burns (e.g., those from biting on an electrical cord)
• Neurologic or functional disorder of the pharynx

Salivary Gland Diseases
• Foreign body
• Neoplasm
• Sialoadenitis
• Hyperplasia
• Infarction
• Sialocele (ranula)

Esophageal or Gastrointestinal Disorders
• Esophageal foreign body
• Esophageal neoplasm
• Esophagitis—secondary to ingestion of a caustic agent or poisonous plant
• Gastroesophageal reflux
• Hiatal hernia
• Megaesophagus
• Gastric distension/volvulus
• Gastric ulcer

Metabolic Disorders
• Hepatoencephalopathy (especially in cats)—caused by congenital or acquired portosystemic shunt or hepatic failure
• Hyperthermia
• Uremia

Neurologic Disorders
• Rabies
• Pseudorabies in dogs
• Botulism
• Tetanus
• Disorders that cause dysphagia
• Disorders that cause facial nerve palsy or a dropped jaw
• Disorders that cause seizures—during a seizure, ptyalism may occur because of autonomic discharge or reduced swallowing of saliva and may be exacerbated by chomping of the jaws
• Nausea associated with vestibular disease

Drugs and Toxins
• Those that are caustic (e.g., household cleaning products and some common house plants)
• Those with a disagreeable taste (especially in cats)—many antibiotics and anthelminthics
• Those that induce hypersalivation, including organophosphate compounds, cholinergic drugs, insecticides containing boric acid, pyrethrin and pyrethroid insecticides, iver

mectin (dogs), fluids containing benzoic acid derivatives (cats), caffeine, and illicit drugs such as amphetamines, cocaine, and opiates
• Animal venom (e.g., black widow spiders, Gila monsters, and North American scorpions)
• Toad and newt secretions

RISK FACTORS
N/A

DIAGNOSIS

DIFFERENTIAL DIAGNOSIS
• Differentiating causes of ptyalism and pseudoptyalism requires a thorough history, including vaccination status, current medications, and possible toxin exposure.
• May be able to distinguish salivation associated with nausea (signs of depression, lip smacking, and retching) from dysphagia by observing the patient
• Complete physical examination (with special attention to the oral cavity and neck) and neurologic examination are critical; wear examination gloves when rabies exposure is possible.

CBC/BIOCHEMISTRY/URINALYSIS
• CBC—often normal; leukocytosis in patients with immune-mediated or infectious disease
• Stress leukogram—common in animals that have ingested a caustic agent or organophosphate
• FeLV-infected cats may have leukopenia and nonregenerative anemia.
• Possible microcytosis with portosystemic shunts
• Biochemical analysis—usually normal except in patients with renal disease (azotemia, hyperphosphatemia, decreased urine specific gravity) and hepatoencephalopathy (possibly elevated hepatic enzyme activities, decreased BUN, and decreased albumin)
• Marked ptyalism can result in hypokalemia and acidosis from the loss of potassium and bicarbonate-rich saliva.

OTHER LABORATORY TESTS
• Serologic FeLV and FIV testing in cats with oral lesions
• Fasting and postprandial bile acids when hepatoencephalopathy is suspected
• Serum cholinesterase concentration to detect organophosphate toxicosis
• Postmortem fluorescent antibody testing of the brain if rabies is suspected

IMAGING
• Survey radiography of the oral cavity, neck, and thorax when foreign body or neoplasm is suspected
• Ultrasonographic evaluation, portal venography, or portal scintigraphy may help diagnose a portosystemic shunt.
• Fluoroscopic evaluation of swallowing may be useful in dysphagic patients.

DIAGNOSTIC PROCEDURES
• Biopsy and histopathology of mucocutaneous lesions—possibly including immunofluorescence testing when immune-mediated disease (e.g., pemphigus vulgaris) is suspected
• Cytologic examination of oral lesions or fine-needle aspiration of oral mass
• Biopsy and histopathology of oral lesion, salivary gland, or mass
• Consider esophagoscopy or gastroscopy if lesions distal to the oral cavity are suspected.

TREATMENT
• Treat the underlying cause (refer to sections pertaining to specific conditions)
• Symptomatic treatment to reduce the flow of saliva—generally unnecessary, may be of little value to the patient, and may mask other signs of the underlying cause and so delay diagnosis; only recommended when hypersalivation is prolonged and severe and, if possible, after the underlying condition has been diagnosed

MEDICATIONS

DRUGS OF CHOICE
• Atropine (0.05 mg/kg SC q8h)—can give symptomatically to reduce the flow of saliva
• Petroleum jelly—can apply to areas of the face constantly wet from saliva, to help prevent moist dermatitis
• Astringent solutions applied for 10 min q8–12h—can be used to treat areas of moist dermatitis
• Crystalloid fluids—give IV or SC to treat dehydration caused by prolonged or severe ptyalism

CONTRAINDICATIONS
N/A

PRECAUTIONS
N/A

POSSIBLE INTERACTIONS
N/A

ALTERNATIVE DRUGS
N/A

FOLLOW-UP

PATIENT MONITORING
• Depends on the underlying cause (see Causes)
• Continually monitor hydration, serum electrolytes, and nutritional status, especially in dysphagic or anorexic animals.

POSSIBLE COMPLICATIONS
• Dehydration
• Hypokalemia
• Acidosis
• Moist dermatitis

MISCELLANEOUS

ASSOCIATED CONDITIONS
N/A

AGE-RELATED FACTORS
N/A

ZOONOTIC POTENTIAL
Rabies

PREGNANCY
N/A

SYNONYMS
• Hypersalivation
• Drooling
• Sialorrhea

SEE ALSO
• Gingivitis
• Stomatitis
• Hepatic Encephalopathy
• Megaesophagus
• Gastroesophageal Reflux

ABBREVIATIONS
CN = cranial nerve
FeLV = feline leukemia virus
FIV = feline immunodeficiency virus

Suggested Reading
DeBowes LJ. Ptyalism. In: Ettinger SJ, ed., Veterinary internal medicine. 4th ed. Philadelphia: Saunders, 1995:125–128.
Spangler WL, Cubertson MR. Salivary gland disease in dogs and cats: 245 cases (1985–1988). J Am Vet Med Assoc 1991;198:465–469.
Authors Daniel P. Harrington and Nathaniel C. Myers III
Consulting Editors Brett M. Feder and Mitchell A. Crystal

RED EYE

BASICS

DEFINITION
Hyperemia of the eyelids, ocular vasculature or hemorrhage within the eye

PATHOPHYSIOLOGY
• Active dilation of ocular vessels—in response to extraocular or intraocular inflammation or passive congestion
• Hemorrhage from existing or newly formed blood vessels

SYSTEMS AFFECTED
Ophthalmic—eye and/or ocular adnexa

SIGNALMENT
Dogs and cats

SIGNS

Historical Findings
Depend on cause

Physical Examination Findings
• Depend on cause
• May affect one or both eyes
• Result of systemic disease—abnormalities in other organ systems common

CAUSES
• Virtually every case fits into one or more of the following categories.
• Blepharitis
• Conjunctivitis
• Keratitis
• Episcleritis or scleritis
• Anterior uveitis
• Glaucoma
• Hyphema
• Orbital disease—usually the orbital abnormality is more prominent.

RISK FACTORS
• Systemic infectious or inflammatory diseases
• Immunocompromise
• Coagulopathies
• Systemic hypertension
• Topical ophthalmic medications—aminoglycosides; pilocarpine; epinephrine
• Neoplasia
• Trauma

DIAGNOSIS

DIFFERENTIAL DIAGNOSIS
More than one cause may occur simultaneously.

Similar Signs
• Rule out normal variations.
• Palpebral conjunctiva—normally redder than bulbar conjunctiva
• One or two large episcleral vessels—may be normal if the eye is otherwise quiet

• Transient mild hyperemia—with excitement, exercise, and straining
• Horner's syndrome—may cause mild conjunctival vascular dilation; differentiated by other signs and pharmacologic testing

Causes
• Superficial (conjunctival) vessels—originate near the fornix; move with the conjunctiva; branch repeatedly; blanch quickly with topical 2.5% phenylephrine or 1:100,000 epinephrine; suggest ocular surface disorders (e.g., conjunctivitis, superficial keratitis, blepharitis)
• Deep (episcleral) vessels—originate near the limbus; branch infrequently; do not move with the conjunctiva; blanch slowly or incompletely with topical sympathomimetics; suggest episcleritis or intraocular disease (e.g., anterior uveitis or glaucoma)
• Discharge—mucopurulent to purulent: typical of ocular surface disorders and blepharitis; serous or none: typical of intraocular disorders
• Swollen or inflamed eyelids—indicate blepharitis
• Corneal opacification, neovascularization, or fluorescein stain retention—suggests keratitis
• Aqueous flare or cell (increased protein or cells in the anterior chamber)—confirms diagnosis of anterior uveitis
• Pupil—miotic: common with anterior uveitis; dilated: common with glaucoma; normal: with blepharitis and conjunctivitis
• Abnormally shaped or colored irides—suggests anterior uveitis
• Luxated or cataractous lenses—suggests glaucoma or anterior uveitis
• IOP—high: diagnostic for glaucoma; low: suggests anterior uveitis
• Loss of vision—suggests glaucoma, anterior uveitis, or severe keratitis
• Glaucoma and anterior uveitis—may complicate hyphema

CBC/BIOCHEMISTRY/URINALYSIS
• Typically normal, except with anterior uveitis, glaucoma, or hyphema secondary to systemic disease
• See Anterior Uveitis—Dogs; Anterior Uveitis—Cats; Hyphema

OTHER LABORATORY TESTS
Depend on cause

IMAGING
• Chest radiographs—consider with anterior uveitis or for which intraocular neoplasia is a possibility.
• Abdominal radiography or ultrasonography—may help rule out infectious or neoplastic causes
• Ocular ultrasonography—if the ocular media are opaque; may define the extent and nature of intraocular disease or identify an intraocular tumor

DIAGNOSTIC PROCEDURES
Tonometry—must perform in every patient with an unexplained red eye

Ocular Surface Disorders
• Aerobic bacterial culture and sensitivity profile—with a purulent discharge, chronic disease, or if the response to treatment is poor
• Schirmer tear test
• Cytologic examination of affected tissue—lid; conjunctiva; cornea
• Cats—consider PCR or IFA test on corneal or conjunctival scrapings for feline herpesvirus and *Chlamydia;* collect sample before fluorescein staining to avoid false-positive results on IFA
• Fluorescein stain
• Conjunctival biopsies—with chronic conjunctivitis or with a mass lesion
• See specific disease—conjunctivitis; blepharitis; keratitis

Intraocular Disorders
• Fluorescein stain
• See specific disease—uveitis; hyphema; glaucoma

TREATMENT
• Usually outpatient
• Elizabethan collar—considered to prevent self-trauma
• Avoid dirty environments or those that may lead to ocular trauma, especially if topical corticosteroids are used.
• Because there is a narrow margin for error, consider referral if you cannot attribute the condition to one of the listed causes, if you cannot rule out glaucoma on the initial visit, or if the diagnosis is so uncertain that administration of a topical antibiotic alone or a topical corticosteroid alone would be questionable.
• Few causes are fatal; however, a workup may be indicated (especially with anterior uveitis and hyphema) to rule out potentially fatal systemic diseases.
• Deep corneal ulcers and glaucoma—may be best treated surgically

MEDICATIONS

DRUGS OF CHOICE
• Depends on specific cause
• Generally, control ocular pain, inflammation, and infection and IOP
• Aspirin—10–15 mg/kg PO q8–12h; may control mild ocular inflammation and pain pending test results
• Flunixin meglumine—0.5 mg/kg IV one time; may be used in dogs with severe ocular inflammation pending test results

RED EYE

CONTRAINDICATIONS
• Topical corticosteroids—contraindicated if the cornea retains fluorescein stain
• Systemic corticosteroids—avoid until infectious systemic causes have been ruled out.

PRECAUTIONS
• Topical aminoglycosides—may be irritating; may impede reepithelization if used frequently or at high concentrations
• Topical solutions—may be preferable to ointments if corneal perforation is possible
• Atropine—may exacerbate KCS and glaucoma
• NSAIDs—use with caution in hyphema

POSSIBLE INTERACTIONS
N/A

ALTERNATIVE DRUGS
N/A

FOLLOW-UP

PATIENT MONITORING
• Depends on cause
• Repeat ophthalmic examinations—as required to ensure that IOP, ocular pain, and inflammation are well controlled

• The greater the risk of loss of vision, the more closely the patient needs to be followed; may require daily or more frequent examination

POSSIBLE COMPLICATIONS
• Death
• Loss of the eye or permanent vision loss
• Chronic ocular inflammation and pain

MISCELLANEOUS

ASSOCIATED CONDITIONS
Numerous systemic diseases

AGE-RELATED FACTORS
N/A

ZOONOTIC POTENTIAL
See Anterior Uveitis—Dogs; Anterior Uveitis—Cats

PREGNANCY
Systemic corticosteroids may complicate pregnancy.

SEE ALSO
See Causes.

ABBREVIATIONS
IFA = immunofluorescent antibody
IOP = intraocular pressure
KCS = keratoconjunctivitis sicca
PCR = polymerase chain reaction

Suggested Reading
Gelatt KN, ed. Veterinary ophthalmology. 3rd ed. Philadelphia: Lippincott Williams & Wilkins, 1999.
Glaze MB. Ocular manifestations of systemic disease. In: Kirk RW, Bonagura JD, eds. Current veterinary therapy XI. Philadelphia: Saunders, 1992:1061–1070.
Slatter DS. Fundamentals of veterinary ophthalmology. 2nd ed. Philadelphia: Saunders, 1990.
Walde I, Schäffer EH, Köstlin RG. Atlas of ophthalmology in dogs and cats. Philadelphia: Decker, 1990.
Author Paul E. Miller
Consulting Editor Paul E. Miller

RED EYE

History, physical examination

Ophthalmic examination

Determine:

CONJUNCTIVITIS		superficial	← • Nature of injection	→ deep/hyphema			ANTERIOR UVEITIS
	Suggests Ocular Surface Disorder Perform	across/mucoid/ mucopurulent	← • Nature of discharge	→ none/serous			
		reddened/ swollen	← • Appearance of eyelids	→ normal	Suggests Intraocular Disorder		
KERATITIS	• Culture/sensitivity • Schirmer tear test	opacified	← • Corneal opacity	→ normal/edema	Perform		
	• Cytology	thickened/ normal	← • Scleral thickening	→ thickened/none	• Tonometry		GLAUCOMA
BLEPHARITIS	• Fluorescein stain • Tonometry	none	← • Aqueous flare or cell	→ present/none	• Fluorescein stain		
	• Biopsy	normal	← • Pupil size	→ miotic/mydriatic/ normal			HYPHEMA
EPISCLERITIS		normal	← • Iris color/shape	→ altered/normal			
		normal	← • Lens clarity/position	→ altered/normal			
		normal	← • Fundus	→ altered/normal			
		normal/ decreased	← • Vision	→ decreased/ normal			

REGURGITATION

BASICS

DEFINITION
Passive retrograde flow of ingesta to a level proximal to the upper esophageal sphincter

PATHOPHYSIOLOGY
• The esophagus acts via a series of coordinated peristaltic contractions moving ingesta from the oral cavity to the stomach.
• Usually results from abnormal peristalsis altering the motility of ingesta, allowing it to accumulate in the esophagus and ultimately be expelled through the oral cavity

SYSTEMS AFFECTED
• Respiratory—aspiration pneumonia
• Musculoskeletal—weight loss; cachexia (if chronic)

SIGNALMENT
• More common in dogs than cats
• Megaesophagus is hereditary in wire-haired fox terriers and miniature schnauzers.
• Familial predisposition—German shepherd, Newfoundland, Great Dane, Irish setter, sharpei, and Siamese-related breeds of cats
• Congenital causes of megaesophagus tend to present after weaning.
• Acquired forms—reported most often in young to middle-aged adult animals

SIGNS

Historical Findings
• Chief complaint often vomiting
• Take a thorough history to differentiate vomiting (forceful abdominal contractions) from regurgitation (passive).
• The character of the expelled ingesta and the time interval from ingestion to expulsion may also help differentiate vomiting and regurgitation.

• Often there is a ravenous appetite, sometimes accompanied by profound weight loss.
• Ptyalism is common.
• Dysphagia, or distress shortly after eating, may be noted.
• Coughing and/or dyspnea may be the complaint when aspiration pneumonia is present.

Physical Examination Findings
• May vary considerably; often animals appear normal on examination.
• Some may be emaciated and weak.
• The cervical esophagus may bulge on expiration or with compression of the thorax.
• Fever and abnormal lung sounds on auscultation may be present in those with aspiration pneumonia.
• Ptyalism may be present.

CAUSES

Congenital
• Congenital megaesophagus
• Vascular ring anomaly
• Esophageal stenosis

Acquired
• Idiopathic megaesophagus
• Megaesophagus—secondary to systemic illness
• Esophagitis
• Esophageal foreign body
• Esophageal stricture

Congenital/Acquired
• Hiatal hernia
• Esophageal diverticulum
• Diaphragmatic hernia
• Gastroesophageal intussusception

RISK FACTORS
N/A

DIAGNOSIS

DIFFERENTIAL DIAGNOSIS
• Must distinguish from vomiting
• Forceful retching and involuntary abdominal contractions associated with the expulsion of digested and bile-stained ingesta or liquid support vomiting
• Effortless expulsion of foam, liquid, or partially digested or undigested food supports regurgitation.

CBC/BIOCHEMISTRY/URINALYSIS
• Most often normal
• Leukocytosis may be seen in patients with a secondary aspiration pneumonia.
• Useful for evaluation of systemic disease associated with secondary megaesophagus (e.g., electrolyte imbalance with hypoadrenocorticism or hypercholesterolemia with hypothyroidism)

OTHER LABORATORY TESTS
Evaluation for secondary causes of mega-esophagus—can include thyroid function tests (TSH/free T_4), blood lead and cholinesterase levels, serum creatine phosphokinase (for polymyositis), ACTH stimulation test (adrenal function), antinuclear antibody test (for immune-mediated disease), and acetylcholine receptor antibody serology (for acquired myasthenia gravis)

IMAGING
• Survey thoracic radiographs—may reveal an esophagus dilated with gas, fluid, or ingesta (in patients with megaesophagus) or may be within normal limits; may also reveal pulmonary infiltrates consistent with aspiration pneumonia
• Contrast esophagram (with liquid barium and/or barium-coated food) may confirm

obstructive disorders (vascular ring anomalies, foreign bodies, strictures, neoplasia, or granulomas).
• Fluoroscopy can detect pharyngeal dysfunction and esophageal motility disorders.

DIAGNOSTIC PROCEDURES
Esophagoscopy—can be useful with obstructive disorders of the esophagus; usually unrewarding with megaesophagus

TREATMENT
• Generally outpatients; managed medically unless there is aspiration pneumonia or severe debilitation
• For other causes than primary idiopathic megaesophagus, aim treatment at the primary cause.
• If the patient is dehydrated, a balanced electrolyte solution may be indicated.
• If no known underlying cause, treatment goals include minimizing risk of aspiration pneumonia and providing and maintaining adequate nutrition.
• Feeding and watering in an upright position and maintaining that position for 10–15 min has been recommended.
• Individualize the consistency of the diet for each patient—gruel vs. solid food.
• Liquid gruel may have less potential for regurgitation but may increase the risk of aspiration.
• Limit activity to leash walks immediately after eating.
• Occasionally, bypassing the esophagus via a gastrostomy tube is necessary.

MEDICATIONS
DRUGS OF CHOICE
• Broad-spectrum antibiotics are necessary for patients with aspiration pneumonia.
• Specific medications are recommended if regurgitation is secondary to identifiable, treatable disorders.
• Metoclopramide (0.2–0.4 mg/kg PO, SC q8–12h)—increases gastric emptying and may increase esophageal motility; occasionally, affected individuals respond favorably.
• Cisapride (0.5 mg/kg PO q8–12h)—a gastrointestinal prokinetic drug; increases lower esophageal pressure and esophageal peristalsis; the author has found it to be less effective than metoclopramide.

CONTRAINDICATIONS
N/A

PRECAUTIONS
N/A

POSSIBLE INTERACTIONS
N/A

ALTERNATIVE DRUGS
N/A

FOLLOW-UP
PATIENT MONITORING
• Check clinical signs in patients treated symptomatically.
• Obtain thoracic radiographs if aspiration pneumonia is suspected—fever, cough, nasal discharge

POSSIBLE COMPLICATIONS
Aspiration pneumonia

MISCELLANEOUS
ASSOCIATED CONDITIONS
Aspiration pneumonia

AGE-RELATED FACTORS
N/A

ZOONOTIC POTENTIAL
N/A

PREGNANCY
N/A

SYNONYMS
N/A

SEE ALSO
• Megaesophagus
• Myasthenia Gravis
• Esophageal Foreign Bodies
• Esophageal Diverticula
• Pneumonia, Bacterial
• Dysphagia

ABBREVIATIONS
N/A

Suggested Reading
Tams TR. Vomiting, regurgitation, and dysphagia. In: Ettinger SJ, Feldman EC, eds. Textbook of veterinary internal medicine. 4th ed. Philadelphia: Saunders, 1995: 103–111.
Author Bari L. Spielman
Consulting Editors Brett M. Feder and Mitchell A. Crystal

RENOMEGALY

 BASICS

DEFINITION
One or both kidneys are abnormally large as detected by abdominal palpation or radiography.

PATHOPHYSIOLOGY
The kidneys may become abnormally large because of abnormal cellular infiltration (e.g., inflammation, infection, and neoplasia), urinary tract obstruction, acute tubular necrosis, or development of renal cysts or pseudocysts.

SYSTEMS AFFECTED
- Renal/Urologic
- Gastrointestinal—inappetence, vomiting, diarrhea, or melena due to gastrointestinal irritation or ulceration in patients with uremia
- Endocrine/Metabolic—metabolic acidosis due to decreased elimination of acid by kidneys and inability to reclaim bicarbonate
- Hemic/Lymph/Immune—anemia due to blood loss or decreased red blood cell survival in patients with uremia; increased susceptibility to infections due to immune dysfunction in patients with uremia
- Nervous—depression, lethargy associated with effect of uremic toxins on central nervous system
- Respiratory—tachypnea or dyspnea due to uremic pneumonitis or compensatory response for metabolic acidosis

SIGNALMENT
Dogs and cats

SIGNS
Historical Findings
- Lethargy
- Loss of appetite
- Weight loss
- Vomiting
- Diarrhea
- Polyuria and polydipsia
- Discolored urine
- Lameness (rarely) because of hypertrophic osteopathy associated with renal neoplasia

Physical Examination Findings
- Abnormally large abdomen
- Abdominal mass
- One or both kidneys palpably large
- Dehydration
- Pale mucous membranes
- Oral ulcers
- Foul-smelling breath

CAUSES
Neoplasia
- Lymphoma—most often occurs in cats and causes bilateral renomegaly; some patients have unilateral renomegaly.
- Renal carcinoma—most common renal tumor of dogs; often causes unilateral renomegaly; very malignant and rapidly metastatic to distant sites such as lungs
- Nephroblastoma—also called Wilms' tumor; a congenital renal tumor that affects young dogs, although it may not be diagnosed until the patient is much older; biologic behavior varies, usually unilateral
- Sarcomas—usually cause unilateral renomegaly and behave malignantly
- Cystadenocarcinoma—bilateral renal tumor that occurs in German shepherd dogs; often associated with skin lesions (i.e., nodular dermatofibrosis)

Inflammation/Infection
- Leptospirosis—may cause bilateral renomegaly and acute renal failure in dogs
- Feline infectious peritonitis—causes bilateral renomegaly in cats; some cats have unilateral renomegaly
- Renal abscess—localized abscess within renal parenchyma usually causes unilateral renomegaly in dogs and cats.

Developmental/Acquired Disorders
- Hydronephrosis—can cause unilateral or bilateral renomegaly in dogs and cats; develops secondarily to ureteral obstruction (e.g., urolithiasis, ureteral strictures, and neoplasia at trigone of urinary bladder) and ectopic ureters

- Polycystic kidney disease—causes bilateral renomegaly in cats and often leads to chronic renal failure; may be more common in Persians and domestic longhair cats
- Hematoma—occurs secondarily to trauma; infrequent cause of renomegaly in dogs and cats
- Compensatory hypertrophy—causes unilateral renomegaly and occurs secondarily to abnormality of the other kidney (e.g., renal hypoplasia, renal dysplasia, or nephrectomy)
- Ethylene glycol toxicosis—can cause bilateral renomegaly secondary to renal tubular swelling and renal infiltration by calcium oxalate crystals

RISK FACTORS
- Feline leukemia virus infection predisposes cats to development of renal lymphoma.
- Exposure to infectious diseases such as leptospirosis and feline infectious peritonitis increases risk of developing renomegaly associated with these disorders.

 DIAGNOSIS

DIFFERENTIAL DIAGNOSIS
- Must distinguish from other abdominal masses
- Confirmation may require diagnostic imaging procedures or exploratory celiotomy.

CBC/BIOCHEMISTRY/URINALYSIS
- Leukocytosis in patients with infectious, inflammatory, and neoplastic causes of renomegaly
- Nonregenerative anemia secondary to chronic renal failure or inflammatory disorders in some
- Polycythemia and extreme leukocytosis accompany some renal neoplasms (rare).
- Hyperglobulinemia in some patients with infectious or inflammatory disorders (e.g., feline infectious peritonitis)
- Azotemia, hyperphosphatemia, and low urine specific gravity (dogs, <1.030; cats, <1.035) in patients with renal failure

• Hematuria and proteinuria in some patients with renal neoplasia
• Neoplastic cells rarely observed in urine of patients with renal neoplasia

OTHER LABORATORY TESTS
• Test cats for feline leukemia virus infection.
• Do serum protein electrophoresis to distinguish between polyclonal and monoclonal hyperglobulinemia in patients with hyperglobulinemia.
• Do paired titers for *Leptospira* spp. 3–4 weeks apart in dogs with suspected leptospirosis.

IMAGING
Radiographic Findings
• Survey indicated abdominal radiographs to confirm
• Kidneys on the ventrodorsal view are >3 or 3.5 times the length of the second lumbar vertebra in cats or dogs, respectively.
• Can use excretory urography to confirm presence of renomegaly, hydronephrosis, and space-occupying masses of the kidneys
• Thoracic radiography indicated to detect metastases in patients with renal neoplasia.

Ultrasonographic Findings
Helpful to confirm diagnosis and identify potential causes such as polycystic kidney disease, perirenal pseudocysts, hydronephrosis, neoplastic mass, abscess, and subcapsular hematoma

DIAGNOSTIC PROCEDURES
• Examination of fine-needle aspirate can confirm presence of renal cyst, abscess, and neoplasia (especially lymphoma).
• If no definitive diagnosis is made by cytologic evaluation of renal aspirates, renal biopsy may be indicated.

 TREATMENT
• Diagnose and treat underlying cause if possible.
• Usually treat as an outpatient unless patient is dehydrated or has decompensated renal failure.
• If the patient is healthy otherwise, feed normal diet and allow normal exercise.

• If the patient cannot maintain hydration, administer lactated Ringer's solution or a maintenance fluid either intravenously or subcutaneously.
• If the patient has dehydration or continuing fluid losses such as vomiting or diarrhea, administer fluids intravenously to correct hydration deficits, maintain daily fluid requirements, and replace ongoing losses.

 MEDICATIONS

DRUGS OF CHOICE
Vary with the cause

CONTRAINDICATIONS
Avoid nephrotoxic drugs.

PRECAUTIONS
N/A

POSSIBLE INTERACTIONS
N/A

ALTERNATIVE DRUGS
N/A

 FOLLOW-UP

PATIENT MONITORING
Perform physical examination and weigh patient to assess hydration status.

POSSIBLE COMPLICATIONS
• Renal failure, depending on underlying cause of renomegaly
• Paraneoplastic syndromes caused by production of hormone-like substances by renal neoplasms

 MISCELLANEOUS

ASSOCIATED CONDITIONS
N/A

AGE-RELATED FACTORS
N/A

ZOONOTIC POTENTIAL
Leptospirosis can be spread by contact with infected urine.

PREGNANCY
N/A

SYNONYMS
None

SEE ALSO
• Ethylene Glycol Toxicosis
• Feline Infectious Peritonitis
• Hydronephrosis
• Leptospirosis
• Lymphosarcoma—Feline
• Polycystic Kidneys
• Renal Carcinoma

ABBREVIATIONS
None

Suggested Reading

Cuypers MD, Grooters AM, Williams J, et al. Renomegaly in dogs and cats. Part I. Differential diagnosis. Compend Contin Educ Pract Vet 1997;19:1019–1033.

Klein MK, Cockerell GL, Harris CK, et al. Canine primary renal neoplasms: A retrospective review of 54 cases. J Am Anim Hosp Assoc 1988;24:443–452.

Lulich JP, Osborne CA, Walter PA, et al. Feline idiopathic polycystic kidney disease. Compend Contin Educ Pract Vet 1988;10:1030–1041.

Mooney SC, Hayes AA, Matus RE, et al. Renal lymphoma in cats: 28 cases (1977–1984). J Am Vet Med Assoc 1987;191:1473–1477.

Osborne C, Stevens J, Perman V. Kidney biopsy. Vet Clin North Am (Small Anim Pract) 1974;4:351–365.

Author S. Dru Forrester
Consulting Editors Larry G. Adams and Carl A. Osborne

RETINAL DEGENERATION

BASICS

DEFINITION
• Degeneration of the retina from any cause, inherited or acquired • Inherited—generalized PRA; a group of progressive retinal diseases; may subdivided into photoreceptor degenerations (begin after the retina matures) and photoreceptor dysplasias (begin before the retina fully develops, < 12 weeks)

PATHOPHYSIOLOGY
• PRA—a variety of inherited defects (e.g., reduced rod outer segment production, abnormal cyclic nucleotide metabolism) have been found. • Secondary to retinal pigment epithelial or choroidal disease (central PRA, ornithine deficiency, and the mucopolysaccharidoses)—metabolic defects have been described. • May be idiopathic or secondary to diffuse or focal inflammation and scarring (e.g., chorioretinitis), nutritional deficiency, or previous retinal detachment

SYSTEMS AFFECTED
Ophthalmic

GENETICS
Dogs
• PRA—autosomal recessive in most breeds, especially collies, Irish setters, miniature poodles, cocker spaniels, and Labrador retrievers • Central PRA—autosomal dominant with incomplete penetrance in Labrador retrievers • Inheritance in many breeds not determined • Neuronal ceroid lipofuscinosis—autosomal recessive (proven or presumed) in most breeds studied • Hemeralopia—autosomal recessive cone dysplasia in Alaskan malamutes; undetermined inheritance in miniature poodles

Cats
• Rod–cone dysplasia (Abyssinians)—autosomal dominant: clinical signs at 4 months; autosomal recessive: clinical signs at 2 years • Isolated reports of both dominant and recessive inheritance in young Persians and domestic shorthair cats • Gyrate atrophy—autosomal recessive; ornithine aminotransferase deficiency

INCIDENCE/PREVALENCE
• Hereditary—prevalence greater in dogs than in cats • Taurine deficiency—uncommon in cats because cat foods are now appropriately supplemented

GEOGRAPHIC DISTRIBUTION
Central PRA—more common in dogs from Europe than from the United States

SIGNALMENT
Species
Dogs and cats

Breed Predilections
Hereditary—Dogs
• Early-onset PRA—Irish setters; collies; Norwegian elkhounds; miniature schnauzers; Belgian shepherds • Late-onset PRA—miniature and toy poodles; American and English cocker spaniels; Labrador retrievers; Tibetan terriers; miniature longhair dachshunds; akitas; Samoyeds • Central PRA—Labradors; golden retrievers; border collies; collies; Shetland sheepdogs; Briards; others • Neuronal ceroid lipofuscinosis—English setters; Dalmatians; Tibetan terriers; collies • SARD—Brittany spaniels; miniature schnauzer; dachshunds
Hereditary—Cats
• Abyssinians • Siamese • Persians • Domestic shorthairs

Mean Age and Range
• Early PRA and dystrophies—3–4 months to 2 years • Late PRA—clinical signs > 4–6 years • SARD—middle-aged to old

Predominant Sex
• PRA—none, except possibly X-linked recessive condition in Siberian huskies • SARD—70% of affected animals are female

SIGNS
Historical Findings
• PRA (dog)—a gradually progressing nyctalopia (night blindness) that ultimately affects vision in bright light; may note dilated pupils or brighter tapetal reflex at night; may appear to become acutely blind (when patient finally becomes totally blind or is moved to unfamiliar surroundings) • Hemeralopia—rare; cones degenerate; day vision lost • Central PRA (dogs)—rare in the US; central vision lost; may never become completely blind; may have difficulty locating stationary objects in bright light (especially hunting breeds) • SARD—vision lost in 1–4 weeks; polyuria, polydipsia, and polyphagia common

Physical Examination Findings
• Severe—direct and contralateral consensual pupillary light reflexes impaired or nearly abolished • Manifests as tapetal hyperreflectivity and nontapetal depigmentation or hyperpigmentation; eventually, retinal blood vessel attenuation and optic nerve atrophy • PRA (dogs)—cataracts common • SARD (dogs)—obesity; hepatomegaly; may note slow or absent pupillary light reflexes • Taurine-deficient retinopathy (cats)—begins as a spot in area centralis; then horizontal band forms superior to the optic nerve; finally, diffuse degeneration and hyperreflectivity • Post-inflammatory retinal scars—focal or multifocal lesions manifest as areas of tapetal hyperreflectivity or altered pigmentation.

CAUSES
Degenerative
• PRA—genetic; affects both eyes symmetrically • Chronic or uncontrolled glaucoma—retinal and optic nerve atrophy • May occur secondary to scarring from previous multifocal or diffuse retinal detachment or inflammation

Anomalous
• Rod–cone photoreceptor dysplasias—genetically inherited; affect both eyes • Other dysplasias—may be multifocal and nonblinding (e.g., in English springer spaniels and Labrador retrievers)

Metabolic
• Mucopolysaccharidosis—mixed-breed dogs; Siamese and domestic shorthair cats • Ornithine aminotransferase deficiency—a mitochondrial enzyme; progressive and total gyrate atrophy of the choroid and retina

Neoplastic
Scars from previous retinal detachment or neoplastic cell infiltrate

Nutritional
• Severe deficiency of vitamin E or A (dogs and cats)—experimentally may cause partial or complete degeneration • Taurine deficiency (cats)—causes retinal degeneration and dilated cardiomyopathy

Infectious/Immune
See Retinal Detachment; Chorioretinitis

Idiopathic
• SARD—dogs; one possible case reported in a cat. • See Retinal Detachment; Chorioretinitis

Toxic
• Idiosyncratic reaction to griseofulvin (cats)—induces diffuse retinal inflammation and subsequent atrophy • Concurrent administration of ketamine hydrochloride and methylnitrosourea (cats)—induces diffuse degeneration

RISK FACTORS
• Ocular disease—cataracts; posterior segment inflammation; chorioretinitis; retinal detachment; glaucoma • Taurine-deficient diet—dog food fed to cats • Heredity

DIAGNOSIS

DIFFERENTIAL DIAGNOSIS
• See Blind Quiet Eye
• Acute vision loss—pupillary light reflex slow or absent: SARD, optic neuritis, retinal detachment, unrecognized PRA, or glaucoma; pupillary light reflex normal: rapidly developing diabetic cataracts or visual cortex disease • Slowly progressive visual loss—PRA; cataracts; severe corneal disease (e.g., pigmentation, scarring, or edema); chronic retinitis; chorioretinitis; vitreal inflammation (e.g., posterior uveitis); differentiated by ophthalmic examination

CBC/BIOCHEMISTRY/URINALYSIS
• Usually normal, unless secondary to a systemic disease

• SARD (dogs)—results may be consistent with hyperadrenocorticism, which patient may have

OTHER LABORATORY TESTS
• ACTH-stimulation and dexamethasone-suppression tests—with SARD; confirm and help localize central versus adrenal hyperadrenocorticism
• Taurine concentration (cats)—diffuse degeneration, especially with dilated cardiomyopathy
• Serum and urinary (may collect on dry filter paper) ornithine concentrations (cats)—elevated with ornithine aminotransferase deficiency

IMAGING
• Thoracic radiographs and cardiac ultrasound (cats)—may be indicated with suspected taurine-deficient condition
• Abdominal radiographs and ultrasound (dogs)—may be indicated with SARD
• CT or MRI—may help localize and identify causes of central blindness (e.g., optic nerve damage, cortical blindness, and SARD with pituitary adenoma)

DIAGNOSTIC PROCEDURES
• Complete ophthalmic examination
• Electroretinography—confirms blindness not apparent on ophthalmoscopy; minimal or no response with severe condition (SARD, late PRA); normal with optic neuritis and CNS blindness

PATHOLOGIC FINDINGS
• Thin retina
• Edges of focal retinal scars—sharply delineated; course of blood vessels not altered
• Hyperpigmented areas—associated with postinflammatory scars or central PRA
• Histologic characteristics of end-stage degenerations—marked photoreceptor atrophy; generalized reduction in retinal cell destiny
• Lipopigment accumulated in the neuroepithelium—central PRA

TREATMENT

APPROPRIATE HEALTH CARE
Outpatient

NURSING CARE
N/A

ACTIVITY
See Client Education

DIET
Cats—food should contain 500–750 ppm taurine.

CLIENT EDUCATION
• Patient visually impaired—inform client that the condition is irreversible but nonpainful.

• Advise client that blind dogs should be watched or kept on a leash if they are outside, not in fenced yards, or in an area with a pool.
• Suggest playing with toys that make sounds.
• Inform client that dogs can memorize their environment and that unless the family moves or rearranges the furniture, most blind animals function well.
• Suggest applying perfume to legs of furniture to help the patient memorize the environment and identify the location of objects
• Warn client that some old blind animals with other problems such as hearing loss or senility may not adapt well to blindness.
• Warn client that some blind animals experience behavioral changes such as increased aggression or reduced activity.
• Assure clients that animals with only one blind eye can function normally.
• Blind cats may adapt better than dogs but should probably be kept indoors.

SURGICAL CONSIDERATIONS
Not indicated in patients with blind, nonpainful eyes

MEDICATIONS

DRUG(S) OF CHOICE
• None currently effective
• Pyridoxine supplementation (cats)—for ornithine aminotransferase deficiency; may increase activity of the enzyme; has not clinically arrested or reversed degeneration
• Adequate dietary taurine—may halt the progression of the taurine-deficient retinopathy

CONTRAINDICATIONS
N/A

PRECAUTIONS
Cataract surgery—do not perform in patients with retinal degeneration; electroretinography is useful for avoiding unnecessary surgery.

POSSIBLE INTERACTIONS
N/A

ALTERNATIVE DRUGS
N/A

FOLLOW-UP

PATIENT MONITORING
• Serial fundic examinations—at 3–6-month intervals; confirm progressive degeneration if the diagnosis is in doubt; will note obvious signs of degeneration over weeks in the retinas of dogs with SARD • Developing and progressing cataracts—with PRA; watch for painful complications (e.g., glaucoma and uveitis).

PREVENTION/AVOIDANCE
• Do not breed animals suspected of having inherited PRA. • Do not breed known carriers (e.g., offspring of an affected animal).

POSSIBLE COMPLICATIONS
• Cataracts • Glaucoma • Uveitis • Ocular trauma as a result of visual impairment—corneal trauma with ulceration or perforation
• Obesity—secondary to reduced activity

EXPECTED COURSE AND PROGNOSIS
• Inherited PRA—progresses to complete blindness; progression often slow enough for patient to adapt to visual loss; nonpainful
• Degeneration from previous inflammation or trauma—usually does not progress unless a systemic disease causes persistent (e.g., uveodermatologic syndrome) or recurrent ocular inflammation (e.g., blastomycosis and toxoplasmosis) • SARD—irreversible blindness • Transient taurine deficiency (cats)—degeneration may halt at any stage (e.g., a horizontal hyperreflective band over the optic nerve).

MISCELLANEOUS

ASSOCIATED CONDITIONS
SARD—adrenal or pituitary hyperadrenocorticism

AGE-RELATED FACTORS
N/A

ZOONOTIC POTENTIAL
N/A

PREGNANCY
N/A

SYNONYMS
• PRA—progressive rod–cone degeneration; retinal atrophy; retinal dystrophy; dysplasia
• Taurine-deficient retinopathy—previously called feline central retinal degeneration

SEE ALSO
• Blind Quiet Eye • Chorioretinitis • Retinal Detachment

ABBREVIATIONS
• PRA = progressive retinal atrophy • SARD = sudden acquired retinal degeneration

Suggested Reading
Narfström K, Ekesten B. Diseases of the canine ocular fundus. In: Gelatt KN ed., Veterinary Ophthalmology 3rd ed. Philadelphia: Lippincott Williams & Wilkins 1999;869– 933.
Author Patricia J. Smith
Consulting Editor Paul E. Miller

RETINAL HEMORRHAGE

BASICS

DEFINITION
• Focal or generalized areas of bleeding into part or all layers of the retina
• May be acute or chronic

PATHOPHYSIOLOGY
• Depends on cause
• May result from a variety of causes
• Trauma-induced retinal detachments—may tear retinal blood vessels
• Often involved in congenital malformations, concurrent vascular abnormalities, and neo-vascularization syndromes
• May note a retinopathy in conjunction with diabetes mellitus—includes the formation of vascular microaneurysms with accompanying hemorrhage or exudation
• Intoxications, systemic clotting, neoplastic disorders, systemic fungal disease—may cause focal or more widespread hemorrhage
• Systemic hypertension and immune-mediated diseases (e.g., those causing anemia)—may cause local hemorrhage in conjunction with vascular abnormalities and/or complete or partial retinal detachments

SYSTEMS AFFECTED
Ophthalmic

SIGNALMENT
• Any breed, age, or sex
• Cause may have a genetic basis and be highly breed and age specific—young collies with collie eye anomaly; Labrador retrievers with congenital vitreoretinal dysplasia
• Hereditary breed-specific congenital defects that might cause detachment or severe retinal dysplasia—collies and shelties with collie eye anomaly; Labradors, Sealyhams, Bedlington terriers, and springer spaniels with retinal dysplasia

SIGNS

Historical findings
• Often none
• Vision loss
• Bumping into objects

Physical Examination Findings
• Depend on underlying cause
• Evidence of bleeding elsewhere—petechia; ecchymoses; melena; hematuria
• Leukocoria (whitish appearing pupil) with or without reddish coloration behind the lens
• Absent of menace response
• Abnormal pupillary responses

CAUSES

Congenital
• Retinal detachment secondary to congenital malformation
• Vitreoretinal dysplasia

Acquired
• Trauma
• Systemic hypertension (especially old cats)—renal disease; cardiac disease; hyper-thyroidism; hyperadrenocorticism; idiopathic
• Intoxication—dicumarol; paracetamol; sulfonamide; Estradurin
• Systemic mycosis—cryptococcosis
• Neoplasia—lymphosarcoma
• Plasma cell myeloma
• Hematologic disorders—blood-clotting disorder (von Willebrand disease); severe anemia; thrombocytopenia; monoclonal gammopathy and hyperviscosity syndrome
• Diabetic retinopathy
• Retinal detachment

RISK FACTORS
• Systemic hypertension
• Hematologic

DIAGNOSIS

DIFFERENTIAL DIAGNOSIS

Signs
• Reddish coloration of the pupil—may indicate vitreal hemorrhage; impossible to rule out concurrent retinal hemorrhage
• Generalized or local blurring or lack of fundus detail—usually no reddish coloration without vitreal or retinal hemorrhage

Causes (Vitreal Hemorrhage)
• Young dogs—may be associated with abnormal persistence of the hyaloid vascular system (e.g., hereditary PHTVL/PHPV and some forms of multiple developmental ocular anomalies)
• Neoplasia
• Lens luxation
• Uveitis
• Glaucoma
• Severe inflammatory changes in the vitreous—associated with ocular infections owing to penetrating injuries, foreign bodies, and spread from local or systemic diseases (e.g., systemic mycosis)

CBC/BIOCHEMISTRY/URINALYSIS
• Usually normal unless secondary to a systemic disease
• Hyperglycemia and/or glucosuria—may note with diabetic retinopathy
• High BUN or serum creatinine and proteinuria—common in cats with retinal detachment and hemorrhage secondary to systemic hypertension

OTHER LABORATORY TESTS
Complete workup—suspected systemic disease; includes thyroid and adrenal endocrine tests, serologic tests for infectious agents, and immune studies

IMAGING
Ocular ultrasound—may demonstrate retinal detachment

DIAGNOSTIC PROCEDURES
• Ophthalmic examination with a penlight—usually permits diagnosis of complete retinal detachment with partial retinal hemorrhage; detached neuroretina may often be visualized through the pupil as a whitish veil of tissue.
• Indirect ophthalmoscopy—diagnosis of funduscopic and vitreal changes; may evaluate depth of the hemorrhage by its shape and color; preretinal (between the external limiting membrane and the vitreous body): often shaped as a boat keel and light red; intraretinal: more rounded and darker
• Vitreous paracentesis and cytologic examination—aid in the diagnosis for suspected neoplasia
• Blood pressure measurement—indicated in all patients with severe retinal and vitreal hemorrhage

TREATMENT
• Usually initially treated as inpatients—sometimes in intensive care for maximal follow-up
• Intoxications—often require specific

RETINAL HEMORRHAGE

treatment
• Consider referral for a more detailed ophthalmic examination, including ultrasound, before attempting empirical therapy.
• Retinal detachment—cage rest until the retina is reattached
• Discuss euthanasia for severe bilateral hemorrhage in young pups with congenital abnormalities (of the breeds listed under Signalment)
• Advise client that unilaterally affected dogs can function as pets but should not be used for breeding, a fact not always obvious to the owner.
• Surgery—for some forms of retinal detachment; refer patient to an ophthalmologist.

MEDICATIONS

DRUGS OF CHOICE
• Depend on underlying cause
• Systemic corticosteroids—workup is declined and infectious disease is unlikely; prednisolone (1–2 mg/kg/day for 7–14 days, then taper; long-term treatment up to 4–6 weeks); especially for retinal detachment as a sequela to trauma
• Chloramphenicol or other systemic broad-spectrum antibiotic—suspected infectious disease; may be administered concurrently with corticosteroids
• Primary systemic hypertension—treat as required; often combined with corticosteroid treatment (as above) and diuretics (e.g., furosemide, 3–4 mg/kg/day for 5–7 days)
• Oral azathioprine—1–2 mg/kg/day up to a week, then taper; for immune-mediated retinal detachments; combine with systemic corticosteroids; perform a CBC, platelet count, and liver enzyme analysis every 2 weeks for the first 2 months, then periodically.
• Itraconazole—for cryptococcosis or other deep fungal infection; see Cryptococcosis or appropriate systemic mycosis

CONTRAINDICATIONS
• Systemic corticosteroids and other immunosuppressive drugs—do not use in manifest infectious processes in the posterior segment of the eye
• Systemic NSAIDs—contraindicated with bleeding disorders, impaired renal function, or pre-existing hypersensitivities; predispose patient to gastrointestinal ulceration

PRECAUTIONS
NSAIDs—flunixin meglumine and aspirin commonly used but may exacerbate bleeding; either may be administered to control intraocular inflammation in dogs. Use with caution in cats. (see Contraindications).

POSSIBLE INTERACTIONS
N/A

ALTERNATIVE DRUGS
• Flunixin meglumine—0.5 mg/kg UV; single dose; may be used in dogs if infectious causes have not been ruled out
• Oral azathioprine—may be used in immune-mediated fundus disease; see Drugs of Choice

FOLLOW-UP

PATIENT MONITORING
• Repeated monitoring—required to ensure that condition subsides and retinal morphology normalizes
• Preretinal hemorrhages—usually absorbed within a few weeks to several months if localized
• Larger or repeated hemorrhages—may be followed by fibroblastic processes; may lead to the formation of fibrous preretinal membranes and vitreoretinal adhesions, which may cause vitreoretinal traction and retinal detachment
• Intraretinal hemorrhage—resorbed within several weeks to months; may produce retinal scarring

POSSIBLE COMPLICATIONS
• Blindness
• Impaired vision
• Chronic uveitis
• Glaucoma

MISCELLANEOUS

ASSOCIATED CONDITIONS
• Trauma—may often note concurrent lesions in other parts of the eye or body
• Hypertension cardiac, renal disease, hyperthyroidism, or hyperadrenocorticism—common; may cause systemic medical problems that must be monitored
• Intoxication—often a generalized bleeding disorder affecting other organs

• *Cryptococcus* infection—often causes concurrent leptomeningitis and pneumonitis
• Lymphosarcoma—may affect several parts of the body; fatal disease
• Hematologic disorders—cause systemic disease; symptoms depend on pathophysiology; anemia and recurrent bleeding common
• Secondary cataracts—may develop within weeks after the onset of diabetes mellitus in dogs

AGE-RELATED FACTORS
• May occur at any age
• May be a sequela to congenital diseases (usually have a hereditary background) or to developmental disease processes (see Causes)

ZOONOTIC POTENTIAL
N/A

PREGNANCY
Corticosteroids and immunosuppressive drugs may cause complications.

SEE ALSO
• Chorioretinitis
• Hypertension, Systemic
• Hyphema
• Retinal Detachment

ABBREVIATIONS
PHPV = persistent hyperplastic primary vitreous
PHTVL = persistent hyperplastic tunica vasculosa lentis

Suggested Reading
Narfström K, Eksten B. Diseases of the canine ocular fundus. In: Gelatt KN ed., Veterinary Ophthalmology 3rd ed. Philadelphia: Lippincott Williams & Wilkins: 1999; 869–933.
Peiffer RL, Petersen-Jones SM. Small animal ophthalmology. A problem-oriented approach. London: Saunders, 1997.
Petersen-Jones SM, Crispin SM. Manual of small animal ophthalmology. Gloucestershire, UK: British Small Animal Veterinary Association, 1993.
Slatter D. Fundamentals of veterinary ophthalmology. Philadelphia: Saunders, 1990.
Author Kristina Narfström
Consulting Editor Paul E. Miller

SEIZURES (CONVULSIONS, STATUS EPILEPTICUS)—CATS

BASICS

DEFINITION
- Clinical manifestation of excessive discharges of hyperexcitable cerebrocortical neurons
- Clinical signs vary depending on the area of the brain involved.

PATHOPHYSIOLOGY
- Intracranial and extracranial—result in focal or diffuse hyperexcitability of cerebrocortical neurons
- High-frequency and sustained activity may recruit other parts of the brain into the epileptic discharge and cause neuronal damage, leading to more frequent and refractory seizures (in both acute and chronic disorders).

SYSTEMS AFFECTED
Nervous

SIGNALMENT
Cats of any age, breed, and sex

SIGNS

General Comments
- Sudden onset; short duration (usually < 2 min); abrupt termination; often followed by postictal disturbances (e.g., mental confusion, apparent blindness)
- May occur as isolated events, cluster seizures (more than two within 24 hr), or status epilepticus (one sustained or serial seizures lasting > 30 min)
- Generalized—diffuse onset within both cerebral hemispheres; manifest with unconsciousness and bilateral, symmetrical motor signs involving the whole body (e.g., tonic–clonic or convulsive, and atonic seizures)
- Partial—focal onset in one cerebral hemisphere; limited spreading within one or both cerebral hemispheres; indicated by aura and localized postictal motor deficits, even if seizure appears to be generalized from the onset
- Simple partial—no consciousness alterations; unilateral, often localized motor signs (e.g., facial twitching); contralateral to the seizure focus
- Complex partial—most common; consciousness alterations; unilateral or bilateral (symmetrical or asymmetrical) motor signs; bizarre behavior common
- Aura—behavior changes within the few seconds or minutes of the ictus onset

Historical Findings
- Seizure history (e.g., age at first seizure; type; initial and subsequent frequency)—may reveal important clues about the underlying cause (e.g., partial seizures are always caused by structural brain lesions)

Physical Examination Findings
- Physical or fundic abnormalities—may be related to the seizures, indicating multisystemic disease (e.g., infectious, metabolic)
- Unilateral or bilateral but asymmetrical deficits in the menace response, nasal septum sensation, hopping, and proprioceptive positioning—structural brain lesion in the contralateral forebrain; common but often subtle and must be looked for carefully
- Bilateral symmetrical deficits—may be caused by diffuse brain dysfunction owing to intracranial or extracranial diseases or to postictal disturbances
- Multifocal neurologic deficits—multifocal CNS involvement; usually caused by infectious or noninfectious encephalomyelitides

CAUSES

Extracranial Causes
- Metabolic—severe hypoglycemia and hypocalcemia; advanced hepatic encephalopathy
- Toxicities—many intoxications in their advanced stages
- Hypoxic—polycythemia; cardiovascular diseases

Intracranial causes
- Functional (idiopathic and genetic) epilepsy—poorly documented
- Structural brain lesions—most common; active: meningoencephalitis of unknown but suspected viral or perhaps immune-mediated origin, feline ischemic encephalopathy (seizures may be the only sign in the atypic form), and brain tumors (e.g., meningiomas) common; infectious encephalitides (FIP, toxoplasmosis, bacterial and fungal infections, and cuterebral myiasis) less frequent; inactive: postencephalitic, postanoxic and ischemic (e.g., birth-related, polycythemia-related cerebrovascular accidents, feline ischemic encephalopathy), and post-traumatic epilepsy

RISK FACTORS
Any brain lesion involving the forebrain

DIAGNOSIS

DIFFERENTIAL DIAGNOSIS

Similar Signs
- Syncope—sudden loss of consciousness and muscle tone resulting in flaccid recumbency and followed by complete recovery within seconds; differentiated by history and physical examination (e.g., episodes induced by stress or exercise, cardiovascular abnormalities such as heart murmur and arrhythmias)

- Sleep disorders—violent movements occurring exclusively during sleep; patient can be aroused by external stimulations and exhibits a normal waking behavior (no postictal disturbances).

Causes
- Extracranial—rare; cause an acute onset of multiple or continuous generalized convulsive seizures and no focal neurologic deficits
- Metabolic and hypoxic disorders—other historical, clinical, and laboratory signs
- Toxins—a progression from shaking to trembling and finally to sustained status epilepticus until treatment or death
- Structural brain lesions—look for carefully; acute onset of high-frequency seizures (status epilepticus, cluster seizures or more than one seizure within the first 4–6 weeks) with no sign of extracranial causes; partial seizures, including auras or localized postictal deficits; neurologic deficits of forebrain origin
- FeLV and FIV—rare causes of primary clinical CNS disease

CBC/BIOCHEMISTRY/URINALYSIS
- Usually normal unless multisystemic disease (e.g., fungal, bacterial, and protozoal encephalitides) exists
- Polycythemia—PCV usually > 60%.

OTHER LABORATORY TESTS
- Serologic testing—FeLV, FIV, FIP, and *Toxoplasma gondii;* usually noncontributory without concurrent systemic signs; FIP and *Toxoplasma* tests do not reliably identify active infection.
- Bile acid testing—indicated only with classical signs of hepatic encephalopathy (e.g., episodic depression, dementia, and salivation that develop and resolve over hours)

IMAGING
- Skull radiography—usually unrewarding; may reveal calcified meningiomas or associated calvarial hyperostosis
- CT or MRI (brain)—most useful to identify and define structural brain lesions

DIAGNOSTIC PROCEDURES
CSF analysis—detect active brain diseases; findings often nonspecific

TREATMENT
- Known cause—treat, if possible
- Prompt and aggressive antiepileptic drug therapy—> 1 single seizure every 6–8 weeks; cluster seizures (more than one seizure per 24 hr); status epilepticus (convulsive or nonconvulsive)
- Goal—< 1 single seizure every 6–8 weeks.

SEIZURES (CONVULSIONS, STATUS EPILEPTICUS)—CATS

• Inpatient—severe cluster seizures or status epilepticus; treat aggressively with parenteral antiepileptic drugs.

CLIENT EDUCATION
• Emphasize the importance of the diagnostic workup.
• Discuss the treatment goals, potential drug side effects and toxicity, and the need for follow-up examinations.
• Instruct the client to keep a seizure calendar.
• Discuss the importance of consulting the clinic before modifying treatment and the risks of abrupt medication withdrawal.
• Outline an emergency plan.

MEDICATIONS

DRUGS OF CHOICE

Chronically Recurrent Seizures
• Phenobarbital—first choice; 1–2.5 mg/kg PO q12h
• Diazepam—second choice; 0.5–1.0 mg/kg divided q8–12h

Severe Cluster Seizures and Status Epilepticus
• Diazepam—0.5–1.0 mg/kg IV bolus; may repeat if gross seizure activity has not stopped within 5 min; immediately start a 0.25–0.5 mg/kg/hr infusion in maintenance fluids in an in-line burette; prepare only 1–2 h of infusion at a time to avoid adsorption into the plastic
• Persistent seizures—increase diazepam dosage and/or add phenobarbital (2–5 mg/kg IV bolus and raise the diazepam infusion to 0.5–1.0 mg/kg/hr, diluting the phenobarbital solution for dosage accuracy)
• When seizures have been controlled for at least 6 hr, slowly decrease the infusion rate by 25% every 4–6 hr.
• Phenobarbital—initiate orally as soon as possible.
• Dexamethasone—0.25 mg/kg; may give for extremely severe seizures (prolonged or frequent, convulsive or nonconvulsive); may be contraindicated in patients with infectious diseases; interferes with CSF analysis

CONTRAINDICATIONS
• Thiamine, glucose, and calcium—do not administer unless a deficiency is documented.
• Acepromazine, ketamine, xylazine, tricyclic antidepressor (e.g., amitriptyline), bronchodilators (e.g., aminophylline, terbutaline, theophylline), and estrogens—do not administer to any patient with documented or potential seizures; lower seizure threshold

PRECAUTIONS
• Intensive parenteral antiepileptic drug therapy—requires constant monitoring and care; hypothermia common; persistent subtle seizure activity difficult to recognize; potential cardiovascular and respiratory depression with overdosage
• Never leave a patient with historical, actual, or potential seizures hospitalized without constant supervision; if monitoring cannot be provided on a 24-hr basis, send the patient home or refer to an emergency clinic.

POSSIBLE INTERACTIONS
• Cimetidine, ranitidine, and chloramphenicol—decrease the metabolism of phenobarbital
• Glucocorticosteroids—increase the metabolism of phenobarbital (dose related)

ALTERNATIVE DRUGS
Potassium bromide—10–20 mg/kg/day in 1 or 2 daily doses; may be used as a third-line drug

FOLLOW-UP

PATIENT MONITORING
• Rational and aggressive diagnostic and therapeutic procedures lead to a good outcome in most patients (well-controlled epileptic episodes or seizures stop), including many with severe and initially refractory seizures
• CBC, biochemistry, and urinalysis—evaluate before initiation of maintenance oral antiepileptic drug therapy; then monitor along with drug concentration every 6–12 months.
• Measure serum drug concentration 10–14 days (phenobarbital) or 5–7 days (diazepam) after treatment initiation and after any dosage modification; adjust dosage as needed to reach the optimal concentration: 100–130 μmol/L (23–30 μg/L) for phenobarbital or 200–500 ng/L for diazepam.
• Benzodiazepine assays—not readily available; therapeutic serum concentrations are not well defined
• If the patient remains seizure free for > 6–12 months, attempt to wean from antiepileptic drug over a few months; if seizures recur more often than one single seizure every 6–8 weeks, resume treatment.
• Adequate seizure control not obtained despite optimal serum concentration of phenobarbital or diazepam—add diazepam to phenobarbital or vice versa; if seizures are still not well controlled, add potassium bromide: measure serum bromide concentration every 8 weeks; adjust dosage to reach an optimal concentration of 15–20 mmol/L; feed a regular diet to ensure stable chloride intake (increases bromide elimination); consult a veterinary neurologist for fourth-line drugs.

POSSIBLE COMPLICATIONS
• Hypersensitivity to phenobarbital—thrombocytopenia, neutropenia, pruritus, and swelling of the feet (noted in a few patients); repeat the CBC within a few weeks of treatment initiation; may need to discontinue (substitute diazepam)
• Diazepam—acute hepatic necrosis: monitor liver enzyme 5–7 days after treatment initiation; discontinue drug if elevated (substitute potassium bromide)

MISCELLANEOUS

ASSOCIATED CONDITIONS
N/A

AGE-RELATED FACTORS
• Kittens may have a higher metabolic rate than adults and may require a higher phenobarbital dosage to reach an optimal serum concentration; may need to decrease dosage when maturity is reached (measure serum concentration at 12–14 months of age and adjust dosage, if necessary)

ZOONOTIC POTENTIAL
N/A

PREGNANCY
N/A

ABBREVIATIONS
CSF = cerebrospinal fluid
FeLV = feline leukemia virus
FIP = feline infectious peritonitis
FIV = feline immunodeficiency virus
PCV = packed cell volume

Suggested Reading
Parent JM, Quesnel AD. Seizures in cats. Vet Clin North Am Small Anim Pract 1996;26:811–825.
Quesnel AD, Parent JM. Diagnostic approach and medical treatment of seizure disorders. In: August T, ed. Consultations in feline internal medicine 3. Philadelphia, Saunders, 1997:389–402.
Quesnel AD, Parent JM, McDonell W. Clinical management and outcome of cats with seizure disorders: 30 cases (1991–1993). J Am Vet Med Assoc 1997;210:72–77.
Quesnel AD, Parent JM, McDonell W, et al. Diagnostic evaluation of cats with seizure disorders: 30 cases (1990–1993). J Am Vet Med Assoc 1997;210:65–71.
Author Andrée D. Quesnel
Consulting Editor Joane M. Parent

SEIZURES (CONVULSIONS, STATUS EPILEPTICUS)—DOGS

BASICS

DEFINITION
• The manifestation of abnormal neuronal hyperactivity involving the cerebral cortical neurons • Clinical appearance depends on the extent and location of the neuronal hyperactivity; frequently convulsive • Status epilepticus—results from continuous seizure activity lasting at least 30 min or from seizures repeated at brief intervals for 30 min or more, without complete recovery between seizures; may be convulsive, which is a life-threatening medical emergency • Epilepsy—recurrence of seizures from primary brain origin; primary: no gross or microscopic structural abnormalities; secondary: seizures are the result of a structural cerebral disease; cryptogenic: seizure pattern strongly suggests a secondary cause (e.g., partial seizure) but the diagnostic work up fails to reveal a cause

PATHOPHYSIOLOGY
• Originate from the thalamocortex; result in a paroxysmal disorganization of one or several brain functions; part or entire brain may be involved. • Type largely determined by extent of brain involvement • Basic disorder—most commonly localized in the brain, but metabolic abnormalities may lead to encephalopathies and seizure activity. • As more seizures occur, the tendency for neuronal damage and the propensity for developing more seizures or status epilepticus increase.

SYSTEMS AFFECTED
Nervous

SIGNALMENT
Dogs of any breed, age, or sex

SIGNS

General Comments
• Generalized or partial • Generalized—patient is unconscious; convulsions (tonic–clonic motor seizures) predominate; nonconvulsive (absence seizures) rare • Partial—patient is conscious; localized onset; indicate focal cerebral disease; may generalize; complex: alteration of consciousness; simple: normal mental status • Partial complex—often symmetrical; motor activity, if it occurs, often predominates on one side (the side opposite to the cerebral lesion).

Historical Findings
• Obtain a description of the entire event. • Determine if the patient knows a seizure is coming (aura). • Aura—beginning of a seizure; indicates a partial onset even if the seizure rapidly generalizes

Physical Examination Findings
N/A

CAUSES

Extracranial
• Metabolic—hypoglycemia; hypocalcemia; acute renal failure; hepatic encephalopathy • Toxins (e.g., metaldehyde in slug bait)—in advanced stages of poisoning

Intracranial
• Degenerative—storage diseases; anoxia; vascular accident; senile changes • Anomalous—hydrocephalus; other congenital malformations • Neoplasia—primary (gliomas, meningioma); secondary (metastatic) • Inflammatory or infectious—viral (e.g., canine distemper); fungal; protozoal (*Neospora*, *Toxoplasma*); rickettsial (ehrlichiosis, Rocky Mountain spotted fever); bacterial • Idiopathic or immune-mediated—granulomatous meningoencephalomyelitis; eosinophilic meningoencephalomyelitis; pug encephalitis; necrotizing meningoencephalitis of Maltese dogs; necrotizing encephalitis of Yorkshire terriers • Traumatic—acute • Epilepsy—primary (idiopathic or genetic); secondary (postencephalitic or post-traumatic glial scar)

RISK FACTORS
• Any disease that affects the thalamocortex can cause seizure activity during the acute phase of the disease or, later, as a result of a glial scar formation. • In-breeding

DIAGNOSIS

DIFFERENTIAL DIAGNOSIS

Similar Signs
• Seizures—transient altered mentation, salivation, urination, and defecation during the ictal phase; aimless pacing, blindness, polydipsia, or polyphagia during the postictal phase; recumbency usually the result of involuntary tonic–clonic muscle activity; aura may precede ictus; period of disorientation, confusion, and apparent blindness follows; most occur while patient is resting • Syncope—sudden loss of consciousness and muscle tone; results in recumbency and flaccidity; may be difficult to differentiate from absence seizure (nonconvulsive generalized seizure) without EEG and ECG recordings; sudden onset; rapid and complete recovery • Narcolepsy—excessive daytime sleepiness; periods of unconsciousness are frequent daily; elicited by excitement such as eating and playing • Obsessive–compulsive behaviors or stereotypies—complex and goal-directed behaviors; abnormal behavior can be stopped early in the course of the disorder.

Causes
• Extracranial—generalized seizures; no lateralizing neurologic deficits; no aura at the onset • Seizurogenic toxins—progression

from shaking to trembling to status epilepticus; seizures continue until treatment or death. • Active brain diseases—likely with an acute onset of multiple seizures in the absence of extracranial causes (more than two seizures within the first week), occurrence of partial seizures, and/or presence of neurologic deficits interictally • Idiopathic or primary epilepsy—differentiated by age and breed; progressive onset of generalized seizures; and a normal CBC, biochemical profile, and urinalysis

CBC/BIOCHEMISTRY/URINALYSIS
• Usually identify extracranial cause when combined with the history, signalment, seizure pattern, and physical examination • Infectious CNS diseases—blood test results may reflect multisystemic involvement. • Metabolic acidosis—common • Hyperglycemia—in the early stages • Hypoglycemia—in the advanced stages (especially in the small breeds) • Creatine kinase—mild to markedly high; with or without myoglobinuria; result of muscle necrosis

OTHER LABORATORY TESTS
• Suspected hepatic encephalopathy—bile acid testing; seizures are rare; accompanied interictally by abnormal behavior such as unawareness, dementia, and aimless pacing • Hypoglycemia—fasting blood glucose and an amended insulin:glucose ratio; dogs > 5 years old with an onset of occasional seizures • Viral, fungal, rickettsial, and protozoal diseases—serology indicated if systemic signs are noted and laboratory abnormalities suggest such a disease.

IMAGING
• Skull radiographs—usually unrewarding • MRI scan (brain)—most useful imaging modality; define location, extent, and nature of structural abnormalities

DIAGNOSTIC PROCEDURES
• CSF analysis—indicated whenever an intracranial structural cause is suspected; titers may be useful for diagnosing some infectious diseases when combined with serum titers. • Surface EEG—usually unrewarding for detecting epileptic waves; may be of some help for assessing background cortical activity

TREATMENT
• Outpatient—isolated seizures • Inpatient—cluster seizures (> 3 seizures/24 hr); status epilepticus; treat rapidly and aggressively. • Treat early: the more seizures occur, the more drugs required for control and the more time needed for recovery.

SEIZURES (CONVULSIONS, STATUS EPILEPTICUS)—DOGS

NURSING AND SUPPORTIVE CARE

Constantly supervise the hospitalized patient.

DIET

Withhold food until the patient can swallow.

CLIENT EDUCATION

• Emphasize the importance of a diagnostic workup if a metabolic or intracranial structural cerebral disease is suspected.
• Inform client that antiepileptic treatment in such cases is only symptomatic and may not help until the primary cause is addressed.

MEDICATIONS

DRUGS OF CHOICE

Convulsive Cluster Seizures or Status Epilepticus

Diazepam
• Administer as a 0.5–1.0 mg/kg IV bolus; repeat 5 min later if gross motor activity has not subsided; follow immediately with 0.5–1.0 mg/kg/hr as a constant-rate infusion added to the maintenance fluids in an in-line burette (prepare only 1–2 hr of infusion at a time to avoid adsorption to the plastic).
• Rectal—should not replace intravenous administration in an emergency situation; use only in the rare instance when an IV access cannot be obtained; may diminish or stop the gross motor seizure activity to allow IV catheter placement

Phenobarbital
• Add if seizures persist; administer at a constant rate of infusion if the patient is already being treated with the drug or as a loading dose if the patient is new to the drug
• Loading dose (total mg) = (desired serum level µg/mL) × (body weight kg) × (0.8 L/kg); optimal therapeutic range = 100–120 µmol/L (23–28 µg/mL)
• Administer one-quarter of the loading dose every 15 min until the desired effect is reached. • If the patient is already on the drug, obtain a serum level before administering the IV bolus.
• Administer as a 2–5 mg/kg IV bolus; follow with 2–6 mg/dog/hr as a constant-rate infusion added to the diazepam infusion; once seizures have been controlled for 4–6 hr, gradually wean the patient off the infusion over as many hours.
• Start or resume oral maintenance antiepileptic treatment using phenobarbital and/or potassium bromide as soon as the patient can swallow.

Other
• Potassium bromide—no place in the treatment of convulsive status epilepticus; takes too long to reach therapeutic serum levels
• Dexamethasone—0.25 mg/kg 1–3 times a

day for 1–3 days; reduce cerebral edema
• Corticosteroids—use for acute treatment of cerebral edema secondary to severe inflammatory CNS disease, even if infectious

Partial Complex Status

• Frequently difficult to control; unknown if recurrence worsens the underlying epilepsy; thus usually not treated aggressively
• If treatment is applied, treat as for convulsive cluster seizures or status epilepticus.
• Diazepam and phenobarbital—both have been proven effective experimentally
• Potassium bromide—in humans, more effective against generalized seizures

CONTRAINDICATIONS

• Acepromazine, ketamine, aminophylline, and xylazine—do not use in patients with historical, ongoing, or potential seizure disorders; lower seizure threshold
• Steroids—avoid if considering a CSF analysis; alter CSF parameters

PRECAUTIONS

• Phenobarbital—highly protein bound and metabolized by the liver; with hypoalbuminemia or liver disease, lower dose and monitor levels closely; do not abruptly discontinue (may precipitate seizure activity); for status epilepticus, add cautiously to diazepam because the drugs potentiate each other, and cardiac and respiratory depression may ensue.
• Steroids—contraindicated in infectious diseases, but one dose of dexamethasone (0.25 mg/kg) may help decrease brain edema when impending brain herniation or life-threatening brain edema is suspected.

POSSIBLE INTERACTIONS

• Cimetidine and chloramphenicol—interfere with the metabolism of phenobarbital
• Each time a drug is added to phenobarbital or to other chronic antiepileptic treatment, refer to pharmacology texts for possible interactions.

ALTERNATIVE DRUGS

Propofol or pentobarbital—anaesthetize patients in status epilepticus that fail to respond to intravenous diazepam and phenobarbital; antiepileptic activity of propofol is superior to pentobarbital; if possible, monitor anesthetized patient with surface EEG to evaluate treatment response.

FOLLOW-UP

PATIENT MONITORING

• Inpatients should be under constant supervision and monitored for seizure activity. • Note that eyelid or lip twitching in a heavily sedated patient is a sign of ongoing seizure activity. • Patient may need 7–10 days before returning to normal after status epilepticus; vision returns last. • Epilepsy

secondary to treated primary disease (e.g., *Ehrlichia canis*)—slowly and gradually (over months) wean patient off the antiepileptic drug after 6 months without seizures; if seizures recur, reinstate the drug.

POSSIBLE COMPLICATIONS

• Phenobarbital—hepatotoxicity after chronic treatment with serum drug levels in the middle to upper therapeutic range; acute neutropenia (rare) in the first few weeks of use requires permanent withdrawal from the drug. • Seizures may continue despite adequate antiepileptic drug serum levels; refractoriness to diazepam may develop rapidly. • Status epilepticus, leading to death. • Permanent neurologic deficits (e.g., blindness, abnormal behavior, cerebellar signs) may follow severe status epilepticus regardless of the cause.

MISCELLANEOUS

ASSOCIATED CONDITIONS

Status Epilepticus

• Hyperthermia • Acid–base and electrolyte imbalances • Anoxia • Pulmonary edema • Arrhythmias • Aspiration pneumonia • Cardiovascular collapse • Death

AGE-RELATED FACTORS

• Primary and idiopathic epilepsy—6 months to 5 years of age; more severe and often refractory when onset is at < 2 years of age
• Phenobarbital—higher dose needed in puppies (< 5 months) to reach the therapeutic range; minimum initial dose of 5 mg/kg q12h is advised; measure serum levels every 5 days until optimal levels are reached.

ZOONOTIC POTENTIAL

N/A

PREGNANCY

N/A

SYNONYMS

N/A

SEE ALSO

• Epilepsy, Idiopathic, Genetic, Primary • Narcolepsy and Cataplexy • Stupor and Coma • Syncope

ABBREVIATION

CSF = cerebrospinal fluid

Suggested Reading
Indrieri RJ. Status epilepticus. Prob Vet Med 1989;1:606–618.
Podell M. Canine epilepsy. In: Standards of care: emergency and critical care medicine. Vol. 1.1999:1–8.

Author Joane M. Parent
Consulting Editor Joane M. Parent

SEPSIS AND BACTEREMIA

BASICS

DEFINITION
• Bacteremia—defined as the presence of bacterial organisms in the bloodstream
• Sepsis—systemic response to bacterial infection (e.g., fever, hypotension)
• Terms are not synonymous, although often used interchangeably

PATHOPHYSIOLOGY
• Shedding of bacterial organisms into the bloodstream—may occur transiently, intermittently, or continually
• The most critical host response for elimination of bacteremia—provided by mononuclear phagocyte system of the spleen and liver; activation leads to release of numerous cellular mediators (cytokines), some of which are beneficial and others detrimental; may lead to death of the host
• Neutrophils—relatively more important for defense against extravascular infection
• Bacteremia—transient, subclinical event or may escalate to overt sepsis when the immune system is overwhelmed; generally of more pathologic significance when the bloodstream is invaded from venous or lymphatic drainage sites

SYSTEMS AFFECTED

Cardiovascular
• With peracute development of septicemia—increased or decreased cardiac output, decreased systemic vascular resistance, and increased vascular permeability; ultimately, refractory hypotension develops, leading to multiorgan failure and death.
• Endocarditis—may develop; presence of bacteremia alone is not sufficient for induction; multiple factors involving both the host and the bacterial organism must be favorable for bacterial adherence to heart valves.

Hemic/Lymphatic/Immune
• Coagulation disorders and thromboembolism
• Kidney and myocardium especially prone to septic embolization
• With chronic bacteremia—antigenic stimulation of the immune system may lead to immune-complex deposition.

Other
• Respiratory
• Gastrointestinal
• Hepatobiliary

SIGNALMENT
• Dogs and cats
• No age, sex, or breed predispositions reported.
• Large-breed male dogs—predisposed to bacterial endocarditis and discospondylitis

SIGNS

General Comments
• Development may be acute or may occur in a vague or episodic fashion.
• Variable and may involve multiple organ systems
• May be confused with those of immune-mediated disease
• Clinical—more severe when gram-negative organisms are involved
• Dogs that develop overt sepsis—the earliest signs are usually referable to the gastrointestinal tract
• Cats—respiratory system more commonly involved

Physical Examination Findings
• Intermittent or persistent fever
• Lameness
• Depression
• Tachycardia
• Heart murmur
• Weakness

CAUSES
• Dogs—gram-negative organisms (especially *E. coli*) most common; gram-positive cocci and obligate anaerobes also important; polymicrobial infection reported in about 20% of dogs with positive blood cultures
• Cats—bloodstream pathogens usually gram-negative bacteria from the Enterobacteriaceae family or obligate anaerobes; *Salmonella* most common gram-negative organism cultured
• *Pseudomonas aeruginosa*—uncommon isolate from animal blood cultures

RISK FACTORS
• Peracute—pyometra and disruption of the gastrointestinal tract most often associated
• More protracted onset—infections of the skin, upper urinary tract, oral cavity, and prostate
• Hyperadrenocorticism, diabetes mellitus, liver or renal failure, splenectomy, malignancy, and burns—predisposing factors
• Immunodeficient state—chemotherapy, FIV, splenectomy; particular risk
• Glucocorticoids—considered an important risk factor for bacteremia; allows greater multiplication of bacteria in extravascular tissues
• Intravenous catheter—provides rapid venous access for bacteria
• Indwelling urinary catheters—may be a predisposing factor

DIAGNOSIS

DIFFERENTIAL DIAGNOSIS
• Consider other causes of fever, heart murmur, joint or back pain, or hypotension.

• Clinical signs of more chronic bacteremia may be confused with immune-mediated disease.

CBC/BIOCHEMISTRY/URINALYSIS
• Neutrophilic leukocytosis with a left shift and an associated monocytosis—most common hematologic abnormalities
• Neutropenia—may develop
• Hypoalbuminemia and a high ALP (up to two times upper limit of normal)—up to 50% of affected dogs
• Hypoglycemia—about 25% of affected dogs

OTHER LABORATORY TESTS
• With suspected catheter-induced sepsis—submit catheter tip for culture.
• Urine culture—may be useful; positive culture does not determine if urinary tract is primary or secondary source of infection.

IMAGING
May identify source of bacteremia (e.g., pyometra) or secondarily infected organs (e.g., discospondylitis)

DIAGNOSTIC PROCEDURES

Blood Culture
• Indications—any patient that develops fever (or hypothermia), leukocytosis (especially with a left shift), neutropenia, shifting leg lameness, recent onset or changing heart murmur, or any sign of sepsis that cannot be explained
• Essential for confirming suspected bacteremia and for optimizing management of the patient; one study of critically ill animals reported approximately 75% of cats and 50% of dogs had positive blood cultures.
• Clinical findings—not reliable for discriminating between particular types of bacteria Guidelines
• Current antimicrobial therapy—does not preclude collection of blood cultures; advise laboratory that patient is receiving antibiotics; steps can be taken to inactivate certain medications.
• Anaerobic cultures—special bottles may not be necessary.
• Sets (pairs) of samples—inform laboratory that for each submitted pair of bottles, one is for aerobic culture and the other for anaerobic.
• Collect at least two (and preferably three) sets of samples—improves chance of obtaining a positive culture and facilitates interpretation of results

SEPSIS AND BACTEREMIA

• Volume—the greater the volume of collected blood, the better the chances of obtaining positive cultures; often only a few organisms present per milliliter of blood; 10 mL of blood per culture recommended; may not be possible for cats and small dogs; have an assortment of culture bottles available (including 25, 50, and 100 mL); small bottles useful for small patients for maintaining appropriate blood-to-culture broth ratio
• Timing—for most patients, sufficient to take three cultures over a 24-hr period; for critically ill patients, take three cultures over a 2-hr period.
Collection
• Bottles—warm to room temperature; apply alcohol or iodine to the rubber stopper.
• Patient—clip hair; thoroughly disinfect skin before venipuncture, to avoid contamination; wipe with 70% alcohol, then apply an iodine-based disinfectant; allow a minimum of 1 min of contact time with the skin.
• Withdrawing blood—wearing a sterile glove, palpate the vein; draw blood into a sterile syringe; evacuate all air from the syringe; attach a new needle before inoculating blood into the bottles.
• Samples—maintain culture bottles at room temperature for transport to the laboratory.
Media
• Commercial multipurpose nutrient broth media—recommended
• A medium that supports growth of both aerobes and anaerobes—ideal
• Often the laboratory that processes the culture will supply culture bottles.
Interpretation of Results
• Single positive culture—not possible to distinguish true bacteremia from sample contamination
• Two or more positive cultures identified as the same organism desired
• Coagulase-negative staphylococci, α-hemolytic streptococci, and *Acinetobacter*—probably contamination
• *Enterobacteriaceae, Bacteroidaceae, Pseudomonas aeruginosa, Staphylococcus aureus, Staphylococcus intermedius,* β-hemolytic streptococci, and yeasts—nearly always clinically significant bacteremia
• Negative results from two or three successive cultures—generally eliminates bacteremia owing to common pathogens; some less common bacteria may take several weeks to grow.

TREATMENT

• Success—requires early identification of the problem and aggressive intervention; careful monitoring essential, because the status of patient may change rapidly

• Hypotension—intravenous fluids; isotonic fluids (e.g., lactated Ringer) at a rate up to 90 mL/kg/hr in dogs and 55 mL/kg/hr in cats; use caution when hypoalbuminemia or increased vascular permeability is a concern
• Volume expanders (e.g., hydroxyethyl starch)—may help maintain oncotic pressure
• With hypoglycemia—may add dextrose to intravenous fluids
• Electrolytes and acid–base balance—correct abnormalities.
• Abscesses—locate and drain
• External sources of infection—give appropriate attention to wound care and bandage changes.
• Internal sources of infection (e.g., pyometra or disruption of the bowel)—surgical intervention essential
• Nutritional support—provide by assisted feeding or placement of a feeding tube.

MEDICATIONS

DRUGS OF CHOICE
• Antibiotics—usually selected before culture and sensitivity results available; empiric therapy acceptable while waiting for results; do not delay treatment.
• Antimicrobials—give intravenously; direct therapy to cover all possible bacterial organisms (gram-positive and negative; aerobic and anaerobic)
• If patient not in shock—a good choice is a first-generation cephalosporin; dogs and cats: administer cefazolin at 40 mg/kg IV as a loading dose; then 20–30 mg/kg IV q6–8h (dogs and cats).
• Aminoglycosides—add to protocol if more aggressive therapy is warranted; administer gentamicin at 2–4 mg/kg IV q8h (dogs and cats).

CONTRAINDICATIONS
Glucocorticoids and NSAIDs—value in treating septic shock; do not improve survival unless given within the first few hours of the onset; may complicate the clinical picture in potentially ischemic organs (e.g., gastro-intestinal tract and kidneys)

PRECAUTIONS
• Aminoglycosides—use with caution with renal impairment.

POSSIBLE INTERACTIONS
None

ALTERNATIVE DRUGS
None

FOLLOW-UP

PATIENT MONITORING
• Aminoglycoside therapy—monitor renal function.
• Blood pressure and ECG—monitor, if indicated.

POSSIBLE COMPLICATIONS
Gram-negative septicemia—high rate of mortality; death owing to hypotension, electrolyte and acid–base disturbances, and endotoxemic shock

MISCELLANEOUS

ASSOCIATED CONDITIONS
• Suspected discospondylitis (dogs)—may need to screen for *Brucella canis*
• See Risk Factors for possible underlying diseases

AGE-RELATED FACTORS
N/A

ZOONOTIC POTENTIAL
N/A

PREGNANCY
N/A

SYNONYMS
• Septic shock
• Septicemia

SEE ALSO
• Abscessation
• Anaerobic Infection
• Endocarditis, Bacterial
• Shock, Septic

ABBREVIATIONS
• ALP = alkaline phosphatase
• FIV = feline immunodeficiency virus

Suggested Reading
Dow SW, Jones RL. Bacteremia: pathogenesis and diagnosis. Compend Contin Educ Pract Vet 1989;11:432–444.
Purvis D, Kirby R. Systemic inflammatory response syndrome: septic shock. Vet Clin North Am Small Anim Pract 1994;24:1225–1247.
Author Sharon K. Fooshee
Consulting Editor Stephen C. Barr

SHOCK, CARDIOGENIC

 BASICS

DEFINITION
Results from profound impairment of cardiac function leading to a decrease in stroke volume and cardiac output, venous congestion, and peripheral vasoconstriction.
• Cardiac dysfunction may be caused by hypertrophic or dilated cardiomyopathies, pericardial tamponade, outflow obstructions, thrombosis, severe endocardiosis, heartworm disease, or severe arrhythmias.
• Cardiac "pump" failure may also be secondary to systemic diseases causing myocardial dysfunction such as sepsis.
• Results in hypotension and compromised tissue perfusion, with reduced tissue oxygen delivery

PATHOPHYSIOLOGY
• Most causative conditions are associated with markedly depressed left or right ventricular function, but conditions that cause cardiac compression, leading to inadequate ventricular filling, such as pericardial effusion, or conditions causing severe ventricular inflow or outflow obstruction, may also play a role.
• Associated with greatly diminished stroke volume and cardiac output.
• Severe hypotension causes tissue hypoperfusion.
• Compensatory neuroendocrine responses cause peripheral vasoconstriction, which further impairs tissue perfusion. Tissue hypoperfusion causes organ ischemia and energy depletion, leading to abnormal organ function, which exacerbates the shock state. Secondary organs affected include the brain, heart, lung, liver, and kidneys.
• Patients display signs of low output failure. As shock progresses, CHF may develop.
• Rises in left atrial pressure and pulmonary venous pressure may lead to pulmonary edema.

SYSTEMS AFFECTED
• Cardiovascular—primary cardiac dysfunction is causative; cardiac dysfunction (i.e., reduced myocardial contractility) may occur secondary to sepsis; low cardiac output affects coronary blood flow, resulting in myocardial hypoperfusion that exacerbates myocardial dysfunction; cardiac arrhythmias may develop, further compromising myocardial function.
• Respiratory—as cardiac dysfunction progresses, increases in left atrial pressure result in pulmonary venous congestion and development of pulmonary edema; pulmonary gas exchange is affected and hypoxemia results.
• Renal/urologic—systemic hypotension and renal hypoperfusion may result in oliguria, ischemic tubular damage, and development of acute renal failure.
• Hepatobiliary—hepatic congestion may result from right-sided CHF (R-CHF) in cases of right ventricular dysfunction. Hepatic hypoperfusion may lead to increased hepatocellular enzyme concentration.
• Musculoskeletal—low cardiac output and muscle hypoperfusion lead to skeletal muscle weakness.
• Nervous—central nervous system depression occurs in response to organ hypoperfusion.

SIGNALMENT
• Dogs and cats
• Any breed, age, or sex

SIGNS

Historical Findings
• Cardiac decompensation may be associated with a history of previously compensated heart disease and cardiac drug administration.
• A suspicion of previously undiagnosed cardiac disease may result from a history of coughing, exercise intolerance, weakness or syncope.

Physical Examination Findings
• Pale mucous membranes
• Prolonged capillary refill time
• Weak femoral pulse
• Muscle weakness
• Mental dullness
• Possible cardiac arrhythmias
• Cool extremities and hypothermia
• Variable heart rate and respiratory rate
• Harsh lung sounds and crackles
• Cough

CAUSES

Primary Cardiac Disease
• Dilated cardiomyopathy—large-breed dogs, or cats with taurine deficiency
• Hypertrophic or intermediate cardiomyopathy in young male cats
• Severe mitral insufficiency or other end-stage valvular disease in dogs
• Tachy- or bradyarrhythmias
• Pericardial tamponade or constriction

Secondary Cardiac Dysfunction
• Sepsis may result in reduced cardiac contractility.
• Hyperkalemia
• Pulmonary thromboembolism
• Tension pneumothorax

RISK FACTORS
Concurrent illness causing hypoxemia, acidosis, electrolyte imbalances, or the release of cytokines that may affect myocardial function

 DIAGNOSIS

DIFFERENTIAL DIAGNOSIS

Differentiating Similar Signs
Differentiate cardiogenic shock associated with circulatory collapse from compensated cardiac failure; cardiogenic shock is associated with significant reduction in cardiac output, hypotension, tissue hypoperfusion, and evidence of multiorgan dysfunction as evidenced by oliguria, muscle weakness, and mental depression.

Differentiating Causes
• Severe mitral insufficiency—detect by auscultation of a left-sided systolic murmur and the presence of bounding femoral pulses.
• Pericardial effusion—muffled heart sounds, tachycardia, and weak femoral pulses (possibly pulsus paradoxus)
• Dilated cardiomyopathy—weak apex beat and weak femoral pulses
• Cardiac arrhythmias—auscultation and asynchrony of femoral pulses

CBC/BIOCHEMISTRY/URINALYSIS
Usually normal; hyponatremia, high hepatocellular enzyme concentrations, and mild hypoalbuminemia in some patients

OTHER LABORATORY TESTS
Blood gas analysis or pulse oximetry may reveal hypoxemia or metabolic acidosis.

SHOCK, CARDIOGENIC

IMAGING

Radiographic Findings

Thoracic radiography may reveal cardiomegaly (cardiomyopathy, pericardial effusion) or evidence of pulmonary edema (CHF).

Echocardiography

May document cardiomyopathy, valvular disease, depressed myocardial contractility, or pericardial tamponade

DIAGNOSTIC PROCEDURES

• Blood pressure measurement may document hypotension.
• Electrocardiography may aid in the detection of arrhythmias.

TREATMENT

• Treat as inpatient; the degree of cardiac dysfunction necessitates intensive medical treatment.
• Pericardiocentesis is essential for patients displaying pericardial tamponade.
• Provide minimal fluid therapy until cardiac function is improved, with the use of positive inotropes or vasodilators or by decompression of a pericardial effusion, as CHF may be exacerbated.
• Oxygen supplementation is important; it can be administered by oxygen cage, mask, or nasal cannula.
• Inform owner of the danger of imminent cardiac arrest in all patients.

MEDICATIONS

DRUGS OF CHOICE

• Provide positive inotropic cardiac support to patients with reduced myocardial contractility—digoxin (0.005 mg/kg hourly for up to 4 doses) or dobutamine (5–20 µg/kg/min), given intravenously (dogs)
• Cats with hypertrophic cardiomyopathy may benefit from the use of a calcium channel blocker or a β-blocker.
• Dogs with ventricular arrhythmias may require antiarrhythmic therapy with lidocaine hydrochloride (2 mg/kg loading dose followed by 50 µg/kg/min), given intravenously. Ventricular tachycardia is rare in cats; if lidocaine is needed in a cat, use 1/10 the dose recommended for dogs and administer it slowly while monitoring for signs of neurotoxicity.
• Diuretic therapy may be required for patients in CHF.
• Vasodilator therapy (enalapril 0.25–0.5 mg/kg PO or sodium nitroprusside 5–10 µg/kg/min IV) may improve cardiac output by reducing afterload; monitor blood pressure closely.

CONTRAINDICATIONS

• Avoid diuretic therapy in patients with pericardial effusion.
• Avoid calcium channel and β-blockers in patients with reduced myocardial contractility.

PRECAUTIONS

• Vasodilator therapy without positive inotropic support may further compromise tissue perfusion in patients with myocardial dysfunction.
• Monitoring blood pressure and indicators of perfusion (mental status, urine production, body temperature, muscle strength, capillary refill time) may be helpful.
• Use infusion pumps for constant rate infusions of sodium nitroprusside or dobutamine.

POSSIBLE INTERACTIONS
N/A

ALTERNATIVE DRUGS

Dopamine may be used as an alternative to dobutamine at a dose of 5–10 µg/kg/min (dogs).

FOLLOW-UP

PATIENT MONITORING

• Heart rate, pulse intensity, mucous membrane color, respiratory rate, lung sounds, urine output, mentation, and rectal temperature during treatment with inotropic drugs or fluids; cardiovascular monitoring by ECG, measurement of central venous pressure, and blood pressure is useful; must monitor blood pressure if sodium nitroprusside therapy is used.

• Blood gas analysis and pulse oximetry to follow tissue oxygenation and acid-base balance
• PCV, serum total protein, serum electrolytes, hepatocellular enzymes, blood urea nitrogen, and serum creatinine

POSSIBLE COMPLICATIONS

• Cardiac arrhythmias
• Acid-base disturbances
• Pulmonary edema
• Renal dysfunction
• Syncope
• Hepatic dysfunction
• Cardiac arrest

MISCELLANEOUS

ASSOCIATED CONDITIONS
N/A

AGE-RELATED FACTORS
N/A

ZOONOTIC POTENTIAL
N/A

PREGNANCY
N/A

SYNONYMS
N/A

SEE ALSO

• Atrioventricular Valve Endocardiosis
• Congestive Heart Failure, Left-Sided
• Congestive Heart Failure, Right-Sided
• Dilated Cardiomyopathy—Dogs
• Hypertrophic Cardiomyopathy—Cats
• Pericardial Effusion

ABBREVIATIONS

CHF = congestive heart failure

Suggested Reading

Shoemaker WC. Diagnosis and treatment of shock syndromes. In: WC Shoemaker, et al., eds. Textbook of critical care. Philadelphia: Saunders, 1995:85–101.
Author Nishi Dhupa
Consulting Editors Larry P. Tilley and Francis W. K. Smith, Jr.

SHOCK, HYPOVOLEMIC

 BASICS

DEFINITION
Hypovolemia occurs when blood volume is diminished by whole blood loss or extracellular fluid losses. If initial blood loss is severe or compensatory mechanisms fail, adequate coronary and cerebral perfusion cannot be achieved, and hypovolemic shock exists.

PATHOPHYSIOLOGY
Caused by significant whole blood loss or extracellular fluid losses (third-space accumulations, vomiting, diarrhea, burns) lead to hypovolemic shock; normal compensatory mechanisms include splenic and venous constriction to shunt blood from venous capacitance vessels to the central arterial circulation, peripheral arteriolar vasoconstriction to help maintain diastolic blood pressure, and increased heart rate to increase cardiac output. The aim is to support coronary and cerebral perfusion, which occurs at the expense of visceral and other peripheral organ perfusion; the resultant compromise of oxygen and nutrient delivery to the tissues is characteristic. Therapeutic steps that restore blood volume via exogenous administration of fluids can reestablish visceral organ perfusion. If excessive hypoperfusion and hypotension persist, peripheral tissue ischemia leads to multiorgan failure. In the presence of hypoxia and accumulation of noxious metabolic products, peripheral arterioles lose their ability to remain constricted; as they dilate, blood begins to pool in tissue capillary beds. At this stage the animal has moved from early, compensatory, vasoconstrictive shock to the decompensatory, vasodilative, irreversible stage of hypovolemic shock. Essential blood volume becomes sequestered, venous return and cardiac output are compromised, and organs fail.

SYSTEMS AFFECTED
• Cardiovascular—compensatory responses to all forms of early shock involve increased heart rate, contractility, and peripheral vasoconstriction, effects that result from sympathetic activation and serve to maintain blood pressure. Sympathetic activation of the heart increases oxygen demands in the face of reduced oxygen delivery. Arrhythmias may result and can intensify shock by further decreasing cardiac output. Prolonged shock decreases cardiac function because of poor coronary perfusion and hypoxia.
• Respiratory—hyperventilation may occur in an attempt to compensate for the progressive metabolic acidosis that develops; as shock progresses, respiratory failure may result from respiratory muscle fatigue secondary to ischemia.
• Renal/Urologic—renal function is compromised because of splanchnic vasoconstriction and reduced renal blood flow and glomerular filtration. Progressive renal ischemia leads to oliguria, azotemia, and acute renal failure.
• Gastrointestinal—compromise of gastrointestinal mucosal blood flow during compensation for hypovolemia leads to ischemic mucosal necrosis, hemorrhage, mucosal sloughing, and potential for bacterial translocation; intense pancreatic vasoconstriction may cause release of vasoactive and cardiodepressant polypeptides.
• Hepatobiliary—hepatic ischemia results in release of hepatocellular enzymes; hepatic reticuloendothelial system dysfunction leads to reduced bacterial clearance and predisposes to bacteremia and endotoxemia.

SIGNALMENT
N/A

SIGNS

Historical Findings
May be associated with a history of trauma and blood loss, burn injury, severe vomiting and diarrhea, or bleeding associated with surgery

Physical Examination Findings
Early or compensatory shock
• Tachycardia
• Normal or high arterial blood pressure
• Bounding peripheral pulses
• Hyperemic mucous membranes
• Rapid capillary refill time
• Tachypnea
• Pale mucous membranes, if associated with blood loss; evidence of bleeding or traumatic injuries, if trauma related
Late or decompensatory shock
• Tachycardia or bradycardia
• Poor peripheral pulses
• Pale mucous membranes
• Prolonged capillary refill time
• Cool extremities
• Hypothermia
• Mental depression or stupor
• Oliguria
• Tachypnea
• Extreme weakness

CAUSES
• Traumatic blood loss into body cavities or lungs, into fracture sites, or from wounds
• Severe gastrointestinal bleeding associated with corticosteroids or nonsteroidal antiinflammatory drug therapy, neoplasia, or thrombocytopenia
• Severe epistaxis secondary to intranasal infection, neoplasia, or thrombocytopenia
• Intrathoracic or intraabdominal hemorrhage secondary to coagulation disorders or anticoagulant rodenticide toxicity
• Fluid loss from extensive burn injury, severe vomiting, or diarrhea

RISK FACTORS
• Exposure to possible trauma or burn injury
• Exposure to anticoagulant rodenticides
• Concurrent illness causing thrombocytopenia or coagulopathy
• Exposure to potentially hazardous situations such as roadways

 DIAGNOSIS

DIFFERENTIAL DIAGNOSIS
Must differentiate hypovolemic shock associated with circulatory collapse from compensated hypovolemia or dehydration. Circulatory collapse is associated with tachycardia or

bradycardia, reduced cardiac output, hypotension, reduced tissue perfusion and evidence of multiorgan dysfunction such as skeletal muscle weakness, mental depression and oliguria.

CBC/BIOCHEMISTRY/URINALYSIS
• Anemia and hypoproteinemia in animals with blood loss
• Hemoconcentration and electrolyte disturbances in patients with fluid loss caused by gastrointestinal disease or burns
• Hypoproteinemia associated with protein loss in gastrointestinal disease or burns
• Urinalysis may support a diagnosis of hypovolemia and a renal water conservation response (high urine specific gravity).
• If renal ischemia progresses, may be evidence of renal failure (casts in urine)

OTHER LABORATORY TESTS
Blood gas analysis may reveal hypoxemia and acid–base disturbances.

IMAGING
Thoracic radiography may reveal microcardia and pulmonary vascular underperfusion associated with severe hypovolemia.

DIAGNOSTIC PROCEDURES
• Blood pressure measurement may document hypotension.
• Electrocardiography may reveal cardiac arrhythmias.
• Central venous pressure monitoring allows objective monitoring of hypovolemia and guides fluid therapy.
• Coagulation profile may document coagulopathy or thrombocytopenia with body cavity or mucosal blood loss.
• Endoscopy or abdominal ultrasonography may help locate a source of blood loss in the gastrointestinal tract.

TREATMENT
• Inpatient because of circulatory collapse
• Vigorous fluid therapy to increase effective circulatory volume
• Use balanced electrolyte solutions at initial rate of up to 90 mL/kg for dogs and 40

mL/kg for cats. May use colloidal solutions such as whole blood, hydroxyethyl starch (Hetastarch), or dextrans in combination with crystalloid solutions to retain fluid within the vascular space. Colloids—20 mL/kg will allow concurrent reduction of crystalloid fluid dosage to 1/4–1/2 the usual shock dosage; indicated for severe hypovolemia; also use in severe protein loss (e.g., burn patients). A 7.5% solution of hypertonic saline may also be used (5 mL/kg IV bolus) for rapid volume resuscitation.
• Refractory hypovolemic shock—may use positive inotropic therapy (dobutamine 5–10 μg/kg/min) or vasopressor therapy (dopamine 5–20 μg/kg/min) to raise systemic blood pressure
• Oxygen supplementation—essential; can be administered by oxygen cage, mask, or nasal cannula

MEDICATIONS
CONTRAINDICATIONS
N/A
PRECAUTIONS
N/A
POSSIBLE INTERACTIONS
N/A
ALTERNATIVE DRUGS
May use vasopressor agents (e.g., phenylephrine or norepinephrine) instead of dopamine

FOLLOW-UP
PATIENT MONITORING
• The aim of aggressive therapy is to obtain a positive trend and reverse the hypovolemic shock state.
• Physical parameters such as heart rate, pulse intensity, mucous membrane color, respiratory rate, urine output, mentation, and rectal temperature

• Cardiovascular—ECG, central venous pressure, and blood pressure recommended; can use blood gas analysis and pulse oximetry to follow tissue oxygenation and acid–base balance
• Should measure PCV, serum total protein, serum electrolytes, hepatocellular enzymes, blood urea nitrogen, and serum creatinine

POSSIBLE COMPLICATIONS
• Electrolyte and acid–base disturbances
• Severe anemia and hypoproteinemia
• Cardiac arrhythmias
• Renal dysfunction
• Hepatic dysfunction
• Gastrointestinal ischemia and hemorrhage and bacterial translocation
• Cardiac arrest

MISCELLANEOUS
ASSOCIATED CONDITIONS
N/A
AGE-RELATED FACTORS
N/A
ZOONOTIC POTENTIAL
N/A
PREGNANCY
N/A
SYNONYMS
N/A
SEE ALSO
• Hypoxemia
• Anemia, Regenerative
• Albumin, Hypoalbuminemia
ABBREVIATIONS
N/A

Suggested Reading
Shoemaker WC. Diagnosis and treatment of shock syndromes. In: WC Shoemaker, et al., eds. Textbook of critical care. Philadelphia: Saunders, 1995:85–101.
Author: Nishi Dhupa
Consulting Editors: Larry P. Tilley and Francis W. K. Smith, Jr.

SHOCK, SEPTIC

BASICS

DEFINITION
Develops as a complication of overwhelming systemic infection. Sepsis is defined as a systemic inflammatory response to infection. Occurs in severe sepsis and is associated with hypoperfusion or hypotension that may or may not respond to fluids or pharmacologic cardiovascular support to maintain arterial pressure.

PATHOPHYSIOLOGY
Results from cardiovascular and/or vasomotor failure caused by circulating endotoxin and inflammatory mediator release. Gram-positive or Gram-negative, aerobic or anaerobic, systemic bacterial infection is the most common underlying cause. The primary event is hypovolemia caused by pyrexia, dehydration, and vascular fluid leakage (because of increased microvascular permeability). Differential vasoconstriction and vasodilation of microvascular beds causes pooling of blood and differential tissue perfusion. Vasculitis and thromboembolic events further compromise tissue perfusion. The ultimate result is tissue hypoxemia and metabolic acidosis, leading to multiple organ failure. In Gram-negative bacterial sepsis, endotoxin (a lipopolysaccharide component of the outer bacterial membrane) plays a key role in the activation of the complement and fibrinolytic pathways. Endotoxin also stimulates macrophages to release cytokines, including tumor necrosis factor and interleukin-1, which in turn amplify the systemic response to endotoxin by stimulating neutrophils, endothelial cells, and platelets, and the release of other cellular mediators that are ultimately responsible for the cardiorespiratory and systemic manifestations of septic shock. Gram-positive bacteria produce other bacterial products capable of activating the same mediator responses.

SYSTEMS AFFECTED
• Cardiovascular—cardiac dysfunction (i.e., reduced myocardial contractility) may occur secondary to sepsis due to ischemia and circulating myocardial depressant factors. Differential vasoconstriction and vasodilation occur in capillary beds because of a loss of local vascular autoregulation, in response to ischemia and locally vasoactive metabolites and inflammatory mediators. Vascular endothelial damage results in permeability changes, fluid leakage, and DIC. Increased blood

viscosity impairs microcirculatory flow and leads to aggregation of red blood cells and platelets in low-flow vessels. Peripheral circulatory failure is typical of septic shock and leads to tissue hypoxemia.
• Respiratory—pulmonary edema and pulmonary thromboembolism may be associated with sepsis. Pulmonary edema may be caused by myocardial failure or may be noncardiogenic in origin (i.e., related to vascular leakage of fluids). Noncardiogenic edema may progress to ARDS following development of widespread lung injury. Pulmonary changes may cause potentially severe hypoxemia.
• Renal/Urologic—the kidney initially compensates for reduced blood flow by increasing efferent arteriolar tone, which helps maintain glomerular filtration rate. As circulatory compromise progresses, the protective mechanisms fail, causing a diminished glomerular filtration rate and abnormalities of intrarenal blood flow. Renal ischemia lead to oliguria and acute renal failure.
• Gastrointestinal—severe vasoconstriction and ischemia can lead to necrosis of gastric and intestinal mucosa, in turn leading to erosions, mucosal sloughing, and hemorrhage. Bowel injury results in absorption of bacteria and toxins, which predisposes to bacteremia and endotoxemia.
• Hepatobiliary—hepatic ischemia causes high hepatocellular enzyme concentrations, hyperbilirubinemia, and possible coagulation factor deficiency. Reticuloendothelial system dysfunction reduces bacterial clearance.

SIGNALMENT
Dogs and cats of any breed, age, and sex

SIGNS

Historical Findings
• Possible history of known infection such as urinary tract infection or prostatitis
• Previous surgery possible
• Immunosuppressive conditions, such as diabetes mellitus, hyperadrenocorticism, or chemotherapy regimens, possible

Physical Examination Findings
Early or compensatory shock
• Tachycardia
• Normal or high arterial blood pressure
• Bounding peripheral pulses
• Hyperemic mucous membranes
• Rapid capillary refill time
• Pyrexia
• Tachypnea
Late or decompensatory shock
• Tachycardia or bradycardia
• Poor peripheral pulses
• Pale mucous membranes
• Prolonged capillary refill time

• Cool extremities
• Hypothermia
• Mental depression or stupor
• Oliguria
• Dyspnea
• Petechiation
• Peripheral edema
• Dyspnea and tachypnea
• Gastrointestinal bleeding
• Extreme weakness

CAUSES
• Gastrointestinal mucosal compromise from hypovolemia or ischemia resulting in bacterial translocation and endotoxemia
• Urinary tract infection (e.g., pyelonephritis)
• Prostatitis and prostatic abscessation
• Gastrointestinal rupture
• Septic peritonitis
• Pneumonia
• Bacterial endocarditis
• Bite wounds

RISK FACTORS
• Concurrent condition causing immunocompromise and predisposing to sepsis; examples include diabetes mellitus, hyperadrenocorticism, high-dosage steroids, or chemotherapy
• Old or young age

DIAGNOSIS

DIFFERENTIAL DIAGNOSIS
Clinical features include fever, inflammatory response, and circulatory collapse. Septic shock associated with circulatory collapse must be differentiated from systemic infection with adequate compensatory cardiovascular response. Circulatory collapse is associated with tachycardia or bradycardia, reduced cardiac output, hypotension, reduced tissue perfusion, and evidence of multiorgan dysfunction such as mental depression, oliguria, and DIC.

CBC/BIOCHEMISTRY/URINALYSIS
• Leukocytosis with a left shift and possible toxic changes in cells; overwhelming septic shock may be associated with marked leukopenia.
• Hemoconcentration, or anemia and hypoproteinemia in patients with blood loss.
• Hypoalbuminemia secondary to vascular permeability changes and fluid leakage
• High hepatocellular enzyme concentrations and bilirubinemia
• Azotemia (e.g., high BUN, high creatinine)
• Thrombocytopenia
• Urinalysis may show evidence of urinary

tract infection (bacteria, whole cells, blood) or acute renal failure (casts).

OTHER LABORATORY TESTS

• Coagulation profile may show prolongation of the activated partial thromboplastin and prothrombin times, increased fibrin degradation products and thrombocytopenia; all consistent with DIC
• Blood gas analysis may reveal hypoxemia and acid–base disturbances.

IMAGING

• Thoracic radiography may reveal evidence of pneumonia, pyothorax, pulmonary edema, or pulmonary thromboembolism.
• Echocardiography may document depressed myocardial contractility, vegetative valvular lesions secondary to bacterial endocarditis, or right ventricular overload secondary to pulmonary hypertension (due to ARDS or pulmonary thromboembolism).
• Abdominal ultrasonography may help detect underlying abdominal disease such as pyelonephritis, abscessation, and peritonitis.

DIAGNOSTIC PROCEDURES

• Electrocardiography may document arrhythmias associated with myocardial depression, ischemia, and acidosis.
• Blood pressure measurement may document hypotension.
• Aerobic and anaerobic blood cultures may identify an infectious source of sepsis.

 TREATMENT

• Inpatient because of circulatory collapse
• Surgically excise any source of sepsis (e.g., an abscess); aggressive treatment and life support may be required. Vigorous fluid therapy is needed to increase effective circulating volume. Use balanced electrolyte solutions at initial rate of up to 90 mL/kg/h for dogs and 40 mL/kg/h for cats. Colloidal solutions such as hydroxyethyl starch (Hetastarch) or dextrans may be used in combination with crystalloid solutions to retain fluid within the vascular space. Synthetic colloids (20 mL/kg) allow reducing the concurrent crystalloid fluid dosage to 1/4–1/2 the usual dosage for shock. A 7.5% solution of hypertonic saline may be used (5 mL/kg IV bolus) for rapid volume resuscitation.
• Oxygen supplementation—as important as fluid replacement; administer by oxygen cage, mask, or nasal cannula.

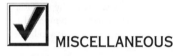 MEDICATIONS

DRUGS OF CHOICE

• Refractory septic shock—systemic blood pressure may be raised through the use of positive inotropic agents or vasopressors. Dobutamine (5–20 µg/kg/min) can be used as a positive inotrope in myocardial depression. Dopamine (5–20 µg/kg/min) can be used for vasopressor support. Supply both drugs as constant-rate infusions.
• Broad-spectrum antibiotics administered intravenously are essential; while awaiting results of blood, urine, or tissue cultures, initiate treatment with one of the following combinations: ampicillin or cephalexin and gentamicin or enrofloxacin; metronidazole can be used with either of these combinations.
• Sodium bicarbonate may be given intravenously to a patient with severe metabolic acidosis. Calculate the bicarbonate dose with the equation 0.3 mEq × body weight (kg) × base deficit. Give 1/2 the dose slowly IV over a 20-min period and the rest in crystalloid fluids over 4 h. If unable to calculate the plasma bicarbonate, administer 0.5–1 mEq/kg as directed above.

CONTRAINDICATIONS
N/A

PRECAUTIONS
When using dopamine or dobutamine, watch for development of tachyarrhythmias; high doses of dopamine may also cause excessive peripheral vasoconstriction.

POSSIBLE INTERACTIONS
Sodium bicarbonate and dopamine or dobutamine cannot be administered in the same intravenous line.

ALTERNATIVE DRUGS
Vasopressor agents (e.g., phenylephrine or norepinephrine) may be used instead of dopamine.

 FOLLOW-UP

PATIENT MONITORING
• Heart rate, pulse intensity, mucous membrane color, respiratory rate, lung sounds, urine output, mentation; and rectal temperature during aggressive treatment with fluids or inotropic drugs

• ECG and measurement of central venous pressure and blood pressure are useful; use blood gas analysis and pulse oximetry to follow tissue oxygenation and acid–base balance.
• PCV, serum total protein, serum electrolytes, hepatocellular enzymes, blood urea nitrogen, and serum creatinine

POSSIBLE COMPLICATIONS

• Electrolyte and acid–base disturbances
• Cardiac arrhythmias
• Pulmonary edema or ARDS
• Pulmonary thromboembolism
• DIC
• Renal dysfunction
• Hepatic dysfunction
• Gastrointestinal ischemia and bacterial translocation
• Cerebral edema and seizures
• Pancreatitis
• Vasculitis and peripheral edema
• Cardiac arrest

 MISCELLANEOUS

ASSOCIATED CONDITIONS
N/A

AGE-RELATED FACTORS
N/A

ZOONOTIC POTENTIAL
N/A

PREGNANCY
N/A

SYNONYMS
N/A

SEE ALSO
• Disseminated Intravascular Coagulation
• Hypoxemia
• Bacteremia and Septicemia

ABBREVIATIONS
ARDS = acute respiratory distress syndrome
DIC = disseminated intravascular coagulation

Suggested Reading
Shoemaker WC. Diagnosis and treatment of shock syndromes. In: WC Shoemaker, ed. Textbook of critical care. Philadelphia: Saunders, 1995:85–101.
Author Nishi Dhupa
Consulting Editors Larry P. Tilley and Francis W. K. Smith, Jr.

SPLENOMEGALY

BASICS

DEFINITION
Enlargement of the spleen; characterized as either diffuse or nodular

PATHOPHYSIOLOGY
• Spleen—removal of senescent and abnormal erythrocytes; filtration and phagocytosis of antigenic particles; production of lymphocytes and plasma cells; reservoir for erythrocytes and platelets; hematopoiesis, as required
• Many disorders are related to and reflect splenic functions.

Diffuse
• Four general pathologic mechanisms
• Inflammatory (splenitis)—associated with infectious agents; classified according to cell type (e.g., suppurative, necrotizing, eosinophilic, lymphoplasmacytic, and granulomatous-pyogranulomatous)
• Lymphoreticular hyperplasia—hyperplasia of mononuclear phagocytes and lymphoid elements (in response to antigens); accelerated erythrocyte destruction
• Congestion—associated with impaired venous drainage
• Infiltration—involves cellular invasion of the spleen or deposition of abnormal substances

Nodular
Associated with neoplastic (tumor) or nonneoplastic disorders (hemorrhage, infection, or inflammation)

SYSTEMS AFFECTED
N/A

SIGNALMENT
• Splenic torsion—overrepresented in large deep-chested dog breeds (German shepherds and Great Danes)
• Hemangiosarcoma—predilection in German shepherds, golden retrievers, Labrador retrievers, and standard poodles
• Prominent spleen—may be normal in certain breeds (German shepherds, Scottish terriers)

SIGNS

General Comments
• May reflect the underlying disease rather than splenic enlargement
• Often nonspecific

Historical Findings
• Hemoabdomen secondary to splenic hematoma or hemangiosarcoma (dogs)—weakness; collapse
• Lymphosarcoma, mast cell tumor, FIP, and lymphoplasmacytic enteritis (cats)—diarrhea; vomiting; anorexia

Physical Examination Findings
• Enlarged spleen on abdominal palpation; nonpalpable spleen does not preclude enlargement.
• Dogs—smooth or irregular surface
• Cats—usually diffuse; uniform enlargement
• Splenic hemorrhage—may note pallor and tachycardia
• Massive enlargement and/or splenic rupture—may note abdominal distension
• Coagulopathy owing to primary splenic or underlying disease—may result in petechiae and ecchymoses
• Infiltrative or inflammatory disease—implied by hepatomegaly, thickened intestines, and/or enlarged mesenteric lymph nodes
• Lymphosarcoma—suggested by concurrent peripheral lymphadenopathy

CAUSES

Nodular
Dogs
• Nonneoplastic—nodular hyperplasia; hematoma; abscess
• Neoplastic—malignant: hemangiosarcoma, lymphosarcoma, fibrosarcoma, leiomyosarcoma; benign: hemangioma, lipoma, myelolipoma, leiomyoma
Cats
• Nonneoplastic—extramedullary hematopoiesis; hematoma; abscess
• Neoplastic—lymphosarcoma; hemangiosarcoma; metastatic carcinoma

Diffuse
Dogs
Inflammation (Splenitis)
• Suppurative—penetrating abdominal wound; migrating foreign body; endocarditis; sepsis; infection secondary to splenic torsion
• Necrotizing—anaerobes; *Salmonella* (usually secondary to torsion or neoplasia)
• Eosinophilic—eosinophilic gastroenteritis
• Lymphoplasmacytic—subacute or chronic infectious disorder; infectious canine hepatitis; ehrlichiosis; pyometra; brucellosis
• Granulomatous—histoplasmosis; mycobacteriosis
• Pyogranulomatous—blastomycosis; mycobacteriosis
Hyperplasia
• Infection—bacterial endocarditis; diskospondylitis; brucellosis
• Immune-mediated disease—SLE; hemolytic disease
• Congestion—tranquilizers; barbiturates; portal hypertension; right-sided heart failure; splenic torsion
Infiltration
• Neoplasia—lymphosarcoma; acute and chronic leukemia; malignant histiocytosis; multiple myeloma; systemic mastocytosis

• Extramedullary hematopoiesis—immune-mediated hemolytic anemia or thrombocytopenia; chronic anemia; infectious disease; malignancy; SLE
• Amyloidosis
Cats
Inflammation
• Lymphoplasmacytic—lymphoplasmacytic enteritis; *Haemobartonella*
• Pyogranulomatous—FIP
• Eosinophilic—hypereosinophilic syndrome
• Granulomatous—histoplasmosis; mycobacteriosis
• Suppurative—penetrating wound or abscess; septicemia; salmonellosis; toxoplasmosis
Hyperplasia
• Haemobartonellosis
• Chronic hemolysis
• Congestion
• Portal hypertension
• Congestive heart failure
Infiltration
• Neoplastic—mast cell tumor (most common); lymphosarcoma; myeloproliferative disease; lymphoproliferative disease
• Nonneoplastic—amyloidosis, extramedullary hematopoiesis

RISK FACTORS
N/A

DIAGNOSIS

DIFFERENTIAL DIAGNOSIS
Other cranial organomegaly or masses

CBC/BIOCHEMISTRY/URINALYSIS

Dogs
• Schistocytes or acanthocytes—may indicate splenic neoplasia
• Spherocytes—hemolysis
• Leukocytosis with a left shift—may indicate infectious and inflammatory conditions or extramedullary hematopoiesis
• Thrombocytopenia—from increased consumption (DIC) secondary to hemangiosarcoma, increased destruction, sequestration, or decreased production
• Hypercalcemia and hyperglobulinemia—may be associated with neoplasia
• Hemoglobinemia and hyperbilirubinemia—may be seen with splenic torsion

Cats
• Direct examination for hemoparasites
• Regenerative anemia and splenomegaly—may indicate haemobartonellosis
• Macrocytosis and nonregenerative anemia—suggest retroviral infection
• Eosinophilia—suggests hypereosinophilic syndrome or systemic mastocytosis

• Circulating blast cells—indicate myeloproliferative or lymphoproliferative disorder
• Nucleated RBCs—may accompany extramedullary hematopoiesis
• Severe thrombocytopenia—reflects myeloproliferative disease
• Hyperglobulinemia—from FIP, chronic inflammation, or myeloma

OTHER LABORATORY TESTS
• FeLV and FIV testing
• Buffy coat smears—circulating mast cells
• Coagulation panel—DIC commonly seen with hemangiosarcoma (includes prolonged clotting times, hypofibrinogenemia, and increased fibrin degeneration products)

IMAGING
Abdominal Radiography
• Confirm or detect splenomegaly
• May provide evidence for the underlying cause—concurrent hepatomegaly may indicate infiltrative disease or right-sided heart disease; splenic torsion may occur secondary to gastric dilatation or volvulus
• Effusion—may indicate hemorrhage from splenic rupture (hemangiosarcoma, hematoma)

Thoracic Radiography
• Right and left lateral views—screen for metastasis and underlying disease
• Sternal lymphadenopathy—may reflect abdominal inflammation or neoplasia

Abdominal Ultrasonography
• Distinguishes between diffuse and nodular
• Diffuse enlargement with normal parenchyma—may be noted with congestion or cellular infiltration
• Reduced echogenicity—may be seen with splenic torsion, splenic vein thrombosis, lymphosarcoma, and leukemia
• Nodular abnormalities easily identified
• Complex, mixed echogenic pattern—hemangiosarcoma
• Hematomas—variable echogenicity; may have internal septation and encapsulation
• Can identify concurrent abdominal diseases affecting liver, kidneys, intestines, and lymph nodes
• Cannot differentiate between benign and malignant disease

Echocardiography
Evaluation of the right atrium—indicated with evidence for hemangiosarcoma (based on ultrasonographic appearance and hematologic findings); mass supports diagnosis of hemangiosarcoma

DIAGNOSTIC PROCEDURES
Fine-Needle Aspiration
• Procedure—place patient in right lateral or dorsal recumbency; use a 23- or 25-gauge, 2.5–3.75-cm (1–1.5-in) needle; diffuse: may aspirate without ultrasonography; nodular: requires ultrasound guidance
• Specimens—evaluate cytologically for infectious agents (most commonly found in macrophages); identify the predominant inflammatory cell type.
• Neoplastic infiltrates—classified as hematopoietic, lymphatic, carcinoma, or sarcoma.

Bone marrow aspiration
• Indicated with cytopenias before splenectomy (spleen may be the main source of circulating blood cells)
• May yield a diagnosis of infectious disease (e.g., ehrlichiosis or mycosis) or hematopoietic neoplasia

 TREATMENT
• Depends on underlying cause; supportive nursing care as needed
• Important to determine if the spleen is the cause of disease and if a splenectomy is appropriate
• Treatment and prognosis after splenectomy—based on histopathologic results

SURGICAL CONSIDERATIONS
Splenectomy
• With anemia or leukopenia—rule out bone marrow aplasia; spleen may be providing hematopoietic activity
• Indicated for splenic torsion, splenic rupture, splenic masses, and mast cell infiltration (cats)
• Exploratory celiotomy—permits direct evaluation of all abdominal organs

 MEDICATIONS
DRUG(S) OF CHOICE
Depend on underlying disease

CONTRAINDICATIONS
N/A

PRECAUTIONS
N/A

POSSIBLE INTERACTIONS
N/A

ALTERNATIVE DRUGS
N/A

 FOLLOW-UP
PATIENT MONITORING
Ventricular arrhythmias (dogs)—associated with splenic mass lesions; may occur before, during, and up to 3 days after surgery; evaluate (auscultation and electrocardiogram) surgical candidates before anesthesia; continuous cardiac monitoring during surgery and the postoperative period recommended

POSSIBLE COMPLICATIONS
• Postoperative sepsis—uncommon complication after surgery
• Antibiotics—indicated in patients that are receiving immunosuppressive therapy

 MISCELLANEOUS
ASSOCIATED CONDITIONS
N/A

AGE-RELATED FACTORS
N/A

ZOONOTIC POTENTIAL
N/A

PREGNANCY
N/A

SEE ALSO
See Causes

ABBREVIATIONS
DIC = disseminated intravascular coagulation
FeLV = feline leukemia virus
FIP = feline infectious peritonitis
FIV = feline immunodeficiency virus
SLE = systemic lupus erythematosus

Suggested Reading
Hammer AS, Couto CG. Disorders of the lymph nodes and spleen. In: Scherding RG, ed. The cat: diseases and clinical management. 2nd ed. New York: Churchill Livingstone, 1994:671–689.
Neer MT. Clinical approach to splenomegaly in dogs and cats. Compendium 1996;18:35–48.
Spangler WL, Culbertson MR. Prevalence and type of splenic diseases in cats: 455 cases (1985–1991). J Am Vet Med Assoc 1992;201:773–776.
Spangler WL, Kass PH. Pathologic factors affecting postsplenectomy survival in dogs. J Vet Intern Med 1997;11:166–171.
Author Angelyn M. Cornetta
Consulting Editor Sharon A. Center

STEREOTYPIES—CATS

BASICS

DEFINITION
• Repetitive, relatively invariant behavior patterns without apparent function
• Controversial in their classification and interpretation; behaviors such as psychogenic alopecia, compulsive pacing, repetitive vocalizing, and fabric sucking/chewing may be included under this heading when other causes cannot be identified.

PATHOPHYSIOLOGY
• Diagnosis of exclusion; must rule out pathophysiologic causes before the diagnosis may be made
• May be a behavioral response to undefined environmental conditions (e.g., stress or boredom); over time, may become fixed and independent of the environment
• Species, breed, and family lines may be predisposed.
• Behaviors may be self-reinforcing, possibly caused by the release of endogenous opioids in the CNS; may allow some animals to cope with conditions that do not meet their species-specific needs

SYSTEMS AFFECTED
• Skin/Exocrine—psychogenic alopecia
• Musculoskeletal—repetitive vocalization, compulsive pacing
• Gastrointestinal—fabric sucking/chewing

SIGNALMENT
• Any age, sex, or breed
• Siamese and other Asian breeds and crosses—may be overrepresented for repetitive vocalization and fabric sucking/chewing

SIGNS

General Comments
• These behaviors, once started, may quickly increase in frequency if they are reinforced in some way by the owner.
• Client's response to the behavior is an important part of the history.

Historical Findings
• Psychogenic alopecia—excessive grooming to the exclusion of other activities; behavior may occur secretly; duration of the problem variable; onset may be coincident with an environmental change (e.g., move or new household member)
• Compulsive pacing—behavior may begin intermittently and increase in frequency; initiation may occur at a time of confinement (e.g., restricted from going outdoors)

• Repetitive vocalization
• Fabric sucking/chewing—often spontaneously appears; suggested that patients may have been weaned early; some patients show preference for a specific fabric type (wool); may suck in a manner reminiscent of suckling; may chew and ingest fabric; patient may become adept at detecting opportunities for engaging in the behavior.

Physical Examination Findings
• Psychogenic alopecia—focal, partial, and bilateral; most commonly in the groin, ventrum, and medial thigh regions; appearance of skin variable (normal or abnormal; erythematous to abraded)
• Compulsive pacing—typically within normal limits; rule out neurologic abnormalities.
• Repetitive vocalization—typically within normal limits
• Fabric sucking/chewing—typically within normal limits; secondary gastrointestinal inflammation or obstruction may occur.

CAUSES
• Unidentified
• Rule out organic causes before a psychogenic basis is presumed.

RISK FACTORS
• Changes in surroundings predispose cat.
• More commonly reported in indoor cats; may be an artifact of the higher level of attention such pets receive or may be related to the stress of confinement or social isolation, as the pacing and other forms of barrier frustration seen in felids in zoologic parks

DIAGNOSIS

DIFFERENTIAL DIAGNOSIS
Rule out medical differentials before a behavioral diagnosis is made.

Psychogenic Alopecia
• Skin conditions—especially those associated with pruritus
• External parasites
• Fungal dermatitis
• Bacterial dermatitis
• Allergic dermatitis—including food allergy
• Cutaneous neoplasia
• Eosinophilic granuloma complex
• Nervous system disorders
• Disk rupture and associated neuritis
• Feline hyperesthesia syndrome
• Pain

Compulsive Pacing
• Normal sexual behavior
• Nervous system disorders
• Chronic pain

• Focal brain lesions—tumor; vascular accident
• Postictal seizure disorder
• Metabolic and endocrine disorders
• Biotin deficiency
• Hepatic encephalopathy
• Hyperthyroidism
• Lead intoxication
• Renal failure
• Thiamin deficiency

Repetitive Vocalization
• Normal sexual behavior
• Deafness
• Hyperthyroidism
• Lead intoxication

Fabric Sucking/Chewing
• Lead intoxication
• Hyperthyroidism
• Thiamin deficiency

CBC/BIOCHEMISTRY/URINALYSIS
Rule out metabolic abnormalities.

OTHER LABORATORY TESTS

Psychogenic Alopecia
• Microscopic examination of hairs—typically shafts are cleanly broken off at variable length as a result of trauma from the tongue.
• Skin scraping, fungal culture, bacterial culture, skin biopsy, and intradermal allergy testing—rule out dermatologic condition.

Compulsive Pacing
• CSF analysis—if indicated by abnormal neurologic examination
• Serum T_4 and T_3

Repetitive Vocalization
• CSF analysis—if indicated by abnormal neurologic examination
• Serum T_4 and T_3

Fabric Sucking/Chewing
• Serum lead level—if indicated for pica
• Serum T_4 and T_3

IMAGING
• CT or MRI—if indicated by abnormalities on the neurologic examination
• Thyroid imaging—if indicated by questionable serum thyroid levels

DIAGNOSTIC PROCEDURES
Psychogenic alopecia—examine for fleas and their products; may attempt an elimination diet

TREATMENT

ENVIRONMENTAL AND SURGICAL CONTROL

• Reduce environmental stress—increase the predictability of household events (feeding, play, exercise, and social time with the client); eliminate unpredictable events as much as possible; confinement contraindicated
• Psychogenic alopecia—topical agents as deterrents usually ineffective
• Compulsive pacing—allowing the patient to go outside after the start of this behavior may reinforce it; if possible, let the patient out before the behavior begins.
• Repetitive vocalizations—breed or spay an intact female; castrate an intact male.
• Fabric chewing/sucking—keep fabrics of interest out of the patient's reach; increase dietary roughage.

BEHAVIOR MODIFICATION

• Do not reward the behavior.
• Instruct client to ignore the behavior as much as possible.
• Advise client to note details of the time, place, and social milieu so that an alternative behavior (play or feeding) may be scheduled then.
• Inform client that punishment associated with his or her voice, movement, and touch increase the unpredictability of the patient's environment, may increase the patient's fear or aggressive behavior, and may disrupt the human/animal bond.

MEDICATIONS

DRUGS OF CHOICE

• Environmental control—preferred method of management; psychoactive drugs may be needed concurrently.
• Goal—use the drugs until control is achieved for 2 months; then attempt gradual withdrawal.
• Drugs are listed with dosage used to manage behavior, the latency, and common side effects.
• Benzodiazepine (diazepam)—1–2 mg/cat q12h; immediate; sedation, idiopathic hepatic necrosis
• Phenothiazine (acepromazine)—0.125–0.25 mg/cat PO q12h; immediate; sedation, paradoxical excitation
• Azaperone (buspirone)—5–7.5 mg/cat PO q12h; 3–4 weeks; gastrointestinal signs, alterations in behavior
• Tricyclic antidepressant—amitriptyline: 2.5–7.5 mg/cat PO q12–24h; 3–4 weeks; sedation, anticholinergic effects; or clomipramine: 1–2.5 mg/cat PO q12–24h;

3–4 weeks; sedation, anticholinergic effects, cardiac conduction disturbances
• Selective serotonin re-uptake inhibitor (fluoxetine)—1–5 mg/cat PO q24h; 3–4 weeks; inappetence, irritability
• Narcotic antagonist (naltrexone)—25–50 mg/cat PO q24h; immediate

CONTRAINDICATIONS

• Diazepam—idiopathic hepatic necrosis (a rare but potentially fatal condition) may develop spontaneously after short-term use.
• Tricyclic antidepressants—potent antihistamine and anticholinergic (atropine-like) side effects; contraindicated with cardiovascular abnormalities (cardiac conduction disturbances, glaucoma, and urinary and fecal retention)

PRECAUTIONS

• Drug abuse—psychotropic drugs have human abuse potential; take sensible precautions to ensure that prescriptions for pets are not abused by humans
• Tricyclic antidepressants—overdose (e.g., ingesting a bottle of pills) by pets or humans can cause fatal cardiac disturbances; no antidote; dispense in small quantities (not more than a 4-week supply) with refills to decrease the risk of fatalities; generally well tolerated but numerous potential side effects, including anticholinergic (atropine-like) and antihistaminic effects; use with caution in patients with urinary or fecal retention.
• Extralabel drug use—no drugs are approved by the FDA for the treatment of these disorders in cats; inform client of the experimental nature of these treatments and the risks involved; document the discussion in the medical record or with a dedicated release form.
• Side effects—provide written instructions along with common side effects (e.g., benzodiazepines and tricyclic antidepressants may cause sedation until drug tolerance develops); initiate psychotropic drugs and monitor the patient in the presence of the owner.
• Phenothiazines—may cause akathisia, expressed as motor restlessness and paradoxical excitation; extrapyramidal side effects include ataxia and tremors.
• Diazepam—rarely, idiopathic hepatic necrosis may occur in apparently healthy patients given therapeutic doses of either generic or proprietary (Valium) formulations

POSSIBLE INTERACTIONS

Benzodiazepines—can interact with cimetidine

ALTERNATIVE DRUGS

N/A

FOLLOW-UP

PATIENT MONITORING

• Successful treatment requires a schedule of follow-up examinations.
• Environmental modification program and/or psychoactive medications must be adjusted according to patient response.
• If a medication is not effective after dosage adjustment, select an agent from another drug class.

POSSIBLE COMPLICATIONS

• Realistic expectations must be made; immediate control of a long-standing problem is unlikely.
• Before initiating treatment, record the frequency of stereotypic bouts that occur each week so that progress can be monitored.

MISCELLANEOUS

ASSOCIATED CONDITIONS

Avoidance behavior or aggression toward the owner—if the owner punishes the patient when it exhibits a stereotypic behavior.

ZOONOTIC POTENTIAL

N/A

PREGNANCY

Tricyclic antidepressants—contraindicated in pregnant animals

SYNONYMS

• Compulsive behavior
• Obsessive–compulsive behavior
• Psychogenic alopecia
• Neurodermatitis
• Psychic eczema
• Pacing
• Repetitive vocalizations
• Crying
• Vocalizing
• Fabric chewing/sucking
• Wool chewing/sucking

ABBREVIATION

CSF = cerebrospinal fluid

Suggested Reading

Landsberg G, Hunthausen W, Ackerman L. Stereotypic and compulsive disorders. In: Handbook of behaviour problems of the dog and cat. Oxford, UK: Butterworth-Heinemann, 1997:169–184.
Simpson BS, Simpson DM. Behavioral pharmacotherapy. In: Borchelt P, Voith V, eds., Readings in companion animal behavior. Trenton, NJ: Veterinary Learning Systems, 1996:100–115.

Author Barbara S. Simpson
Consulting Editor Joane M. Parent

STEREOTYPIES—DOGS

 BASICS

DEFINITION
• A repetitious, relatively unvaried sequence of movements that has no obvious purpose or function, usually derived from contextually normal maintenance behaviors (e.g., grooming, eating, walking); inherent is that the behavior interferes with normal behavioral functioning.
• Also called OCD
• An American Psychiatric Association classification of abnormal behavior characterized by recurrent, frequent thoughts or actions that are out of context to the situations in which they occur; may involve cognitive or physical rituals and are deemed excessive (given the context) in duration, frequency, and intensity
• One hallmark distinguishing it from motor tics (humans)—behaviors follow a set of rules created by the patient.
• Condition in domestic animals—probably similar and analogous through descent; probably includes stereotypies, self-directed behaviors, etc.; behavior must be sufficiently pronounced to interfere with normal functioning.
• Most common—spinning; tail chasing; self-mutilation; hallucinating ("fly biting"); circling; fence running; hair/air biting; pica; pacing; staring and vocalizing; self-directed vocalization; potentially some aggression

PATHOPHYSIOLOGY
• Unclear; clinical signs consistent with alterations in CNS transmitter function
• Main neurotransmitters implicated in stereotypic behavior—dopamine; serotonin; endorphins, for conditions involving mutilation
• Humans—basal nuclei, particularly the putamen and the caudate nuclei, are the regions most commonly implicated in aberrant neurochemistry.
• Pet brought to the clinic because the client perceives changes in the patient's behavior or because the client believes patient has never been normal

SYSTEMS AFFECTED
• Cardiovascular—tachycardia
• Endocrine/Metabolic—signs caused by alterations in the HPA axis
• Gastrointestinal—inappetence; aberrant appetite (including pica and coprophagia); gastrointestinal distress (salivation, vomiting, diarrhea, tenesmus, hematochezia)
• Hemic/Lymphatic/Immune—stress leukogram common
• Musculoskeletal—poor condition attributable to increased motor activity and

self-injury; weight loss, injured pads, damage to teeth and gums, and abrasions and lacerations common
• Nervous—increased motor activity, repetitive activity, trembling, and self-injury common
• Respiratory—tachypnea and the attendant metabolic changes possible in extreme situations

Skin/Exocrine
• Skin lesions—usually secondary; may be a result of self-injury, overgrooming, barbering, sucking, or abrasion from repetitive activity
• Lick granulomas—not uncommon; may be a dermatologic manifestation; mild type usually not the only sign; type associated with deep tissue damage may occur

SIGNALMENT
• No age, breed, or sex over-represented
• Begin to develop at onset of social maturity (18–36 months), like other anxiety disorders
• Bull terriers—tail chasing not uncommon and seems to run in families
• German shepherds—reported to be over-represented for spinning
• Great Danes and German short-haired pointers—some lines display self-mutilation, stereotypic motor behavior (fence running), or hallucinations; prevalence only recently appreciated, so likely more widespread than now thought; may be more familial than breed-associated
• Breed vs. familial association—confounded in dogs; not all family members show the same manifestation (e.g., spinning, grooming, or hallucinating) and, in fact, the opposite may be true; humans: occurrence of any one characteristic behavior is associated with an increased risk of another manifestation in first-degree relatives.

SIGNS
General Comments
• May be nonspecific
• One hallmark—immutable rule structure that specifies how and when the patient is to perform the activity
• The behavior may be a manifestation of an OCD if the client cannot interrupt it and if it intensifies over time, increases in frequency or duration, and interferes with normal functioning.

Historical Findings
• Patient may have begun to chase its tail as part of play but now the tip is missing and even physical restraint does not stop the behavior.
• May be seen in young dogs, but its onset is more common during social maturity; play decreases with age, OCD increases.
• A solitary focus may have seemed to spur the behavior (e.g., chasing a mouse that the patient could not catch), but usually no provocative stimulus is noted.

• One hallmark—behavior worsens with time.

Physical Examination Findings
• Usually unremarkable
• May see self-induced injuries and the lack of condition that may be associated with increased motor activity and the repetitive behaviors; may note self-mutilation with a focus on the tail, forelimbs, and distal extremities

CAUSES
• Illness or painful physical condition—may increase an animal's anxieties and contribute to these problems; few of these conditions actually cause OCD
• Kenneling and incarceration—may be associated with spinning
• Degenerative (e.g., aging and concomitant neurologic changes), anatomic, infectious (primarily CNS viral conditions), and toxic (lead toxicosis) causes—may be causal, but abnormal behavior likely rooted in primary or secondary aberrant neurochemical activity

 DIAGNOSIS

DIFFERENTIAL DIAGNOSIS
• Conditions that cause similar behavioral changes—seizures; brain disease; metabolic disease (e.g., thyroid or pancreatic conditions)
• Some behavioral conditions (play and attention seeking) may look like the early stages of OCD.

CBC/BIOCHEMISTRY/URINALYSIS
Perform; results within the laboratory's reference range

OTHER LABORATORY TESTS
Thyroid or liver profile—rule out hypo-thyroidism and hepatic encephalopathy if there is any doubt that the signs are behavioral

IMAGING
CT and MRI—rule out structural brain disease

DIAGNOSTIC PROCEDURES
• Biopsies of skin lesions—confirm if they are primary or secondary
• CSF analysis—rule out inflammatory CNS disease
• Endoscopy—evaluate primary bowel disease
• ECG—diagnostic; premedication precaution; cardiac disease may produce physical signs of anxiety.
• Aberrant endorphin metabolism—evaluate by administrating naloxone (11–22 μg/kg IV); if behavior does not decrease dramatically in intensity or frequency within 15–20 min, endorphin metabolism unlikely to be the main driving mechanism

TREATMENT

• Most patients respond to a combination of behavior modification and pharmacologic treatment with antianxiety medication.
• Pharmacologic intervention—implement early; may be a prerequisite to effecting any behavioral therapy
• Usually outpatient
• Inpatient—patients with severe self-mutilation and self-induced injury; patients that must be protected from the environment until the antianxiety medications reach effective plasma and CSF levels (days to weeks); constant monitoring, stimulation, and care
• Sedation—profound cases; only a stop-gap measure
• Behavior modification—geared toward teaching the patient to relax in a variety of environmental settings and to substitute a calm, competitive behavior for the stereotypic one
• Discourage the client from reassuring the patient that it does not have to spin, chew, etc.; this inadvertently rewards the repetitive behavior.
• Desensitization and counterconditioning—most effective if instituted early; may be coupled to a verbal cue that signals the patient to execute a behavior that is competitive with the abnormal one (e.g., instead of circling, the patient is taught to relax and lie down with its head and neck stretched prone on the floor when the client says "Head down")
• Help client understand the subtlety of the signs and learn to recognize the outward physical signs associated with the underlying physiologic state characterized by sympathetic stimulation.
• Punishment—contraindicated; may make the behavior worse and render the patient more secretive
• Atopic and painful conditions—diagnose and control (including the use of dietary management); pruritus and pain neurochemically related to anxiety and its perception
• Amputation—avoid; eliminates the outward signs but does nothing to alleviate the condition

MEDICATIONS

DRUGS OF CHOICE
• TCAs and selective serotonin reuptake inhibitors—increase CNS levels of serotonin
• Mild—amitriptyline (1–2 mg/kg PO q12h for 30 days, to start); imipramine (1–2 mg/kg PO q12h for 30 days)

• Long-standing—clomipramine (1 mg/kg PO q12h for 14 days; then 2 mg/kg PO q12h for 14 days; then 3 mg/kg PO q12h for 28 days; if successful, this will be the maintenance dosage); fluoxetine (1 mg/kg PO q24h for 2 months); some combination of the above; these drugs may take 3–5 weeks to be effective.
• Self-mutilation—narcotic antagonists (naltrexone 2.2 mg/kg PO q8–12–24h) may be useful.
• Unlikely to work if the behavior was not first blocked by intravenous administration.
• Thioridazine—occasionally used as an adjuvant treatment; newer more specific treatments appear more effective.
• Treatment is lifelong; any attempt to withdraw medication should be gradual; recurrence is common.

CONTRAINDICATIONS
• Hepatic and renal compromise—medications for which these are the main routes of metabolism
• Cardiac conduction anomalies—give TCA with extreme caution; monitor closely.

PRECAUTIONS
• All listed medications are extralabel; recommendations from Health and Human Services should be followed.
• TCA overdose (human and animal)—profound cardiac conduction disturbances; perform a cardiac evaluation with an ECG before treatment.

POSSIBLE INTERACTIONS
• Medications that impair the glucuronidation of active metabolites into inactive compounds—may increase the active metabolites
• TCA and selective serotonin reuptake inhibitors—most have active intermediate metabolites; pharmacokinetics may differ from that of the parent compound
• Combination therapy with two antianxiety agents—may potentiate either or both medications; lower the dosages.

FOLLOW-UP

PATIENT MONITORING
• CBC, biochemistry and urinalysis—semiannually or yearly if the patient is on chronic treatment; adjust dosages accordingly.
• Advise client to observe for vomiting, gastrointestinal distress, and tachypnea.

POSSIBLE COMPLICATIONS
Early intervention, using both behavioral modification and pharmacologic intervention, is crucial; if left untreated, these conditions always progress.

MISCELLANEOUS

ASSOCIATED CONDITIONS
• Irritable bowel syndrome
• Lick granulomas

AGE-RELATED FACTORS
• Appears most frequently at social maturity
• Little is known about contributory and developmental factors, but any condition that contributes to the patient's underlying anxiety or to its perception of it can worsen the condition.

ZOONOTIC POTENTIAL
N/A

PREGNANCY
• Most of the drugs used to treat these conditions either are not evaluated in or are contraindicated in pregnant animals; their use should be avoided.

SYNONYMS
Obsessive–compulsive disorder

ABBREVIATIONS
CSF = cerebrospinal fluid
HPA = hypothalamic–pituitary–adrenal
OCD = obsessive–compulsive disorder
TCA = tricyclic antidepressant

Suggested Reading
Brown SA, Crowell-Davis S, Malcom T, Edwards P. Naloxone-responsive compulsive tail chasing in a dog. J Am Vet Med Assoc 1987;190:884–886.
Dodman NH, Shuster L, White SD, et al. Use of narcotic antagonists to modify stereotypic self-licking, self-chewing, and scratching behavior in dogs. J Am Vet Med Assoc 1988;193:815–819.
Luescher UA, McKeown DB, Halip J. Stereotypic or obsessive-compulsive disorders in dogs and cats. Vet Clin North Am Small Anim Pract 1991;21:401–414.
Overall KL. Recognition, diagnosis, and management of obsessive-compulsive disorders. Part I. Canine Pract 1992;17:40–44.
Overall KL. Use of clomipramine to treat ritualistic stereotypic motor behavior in three dogs. J Am Vet Med Assoc 1994;205:1733–1741.
Author Karen L. Overall
Consulting Editor Joane M. Parent

STERTOR AND STRIDOR

BASICS

DEFINITION
• Abnormally loud sounds that result from air passing through an abnormally narrowed pharynx or larynx and meeting resistance because of partial obstruction of these regions
• Stertor—low-pitched snoring sound that usually arises from the vibration of flaccid tissue or fluid; usually arises from pharyngeal airway obstruction
• Stridor—higher-pitched sounds that result when relatively rigid tissues are vibrated by the passage of air; result of nasal or laryngeal obstruction

PATHOPHYSIOLOGY
• Airway obstruction causes turbulence as air passes through a narrowed passage; with worsening obstruction or increasing air velocity, the amplitude of the sound increases as the tissue, secretion, or foreign body composing the obstruction is vibrated.
• Obstruction sufficient enough to increase the work of breathing—respiratory muscles increase their effort and the turbulence is exacerbated; inflammation and edema of the tissues in the region of the obstruction may develop, further reducing the airway lumen and further increasing the work of breathing, creating a vicious circle.

SYSTEMS AFFECTED
Respiratory

SIGNALMENT
• Dogs and cats
• Common in brachycephalic breeds
• Inherited laryngeal paralysis—identified in Bouvier des Flandres, Siberian husky crosses, and Dalmatians
• Acquired laryngeal paralysis—over-represented by certain giant breeds (e.g., St. Bernards and Newfoundlands) and large breeds (e.g., Irish setters, Labradors, and golden retrievers)
• Affected brachycephalic dogs—typically younger than 1 year of age when owners detect a problem
• Cats—diagnosed less commonly than are dogs; no obvious age pattern
• Tumor—usually old animal
• No sex predilection for any cause, except inherited laryngeal paralysis, which has a 3:1 male predominance

SIGNS
• Partial obstruction—produces an increase in airway sounds before producing an obvious change in respiratory pattern and long before producing a change in the respiratory function of gas exchange; increased sound may precede any obvious change in behavior.
• Owners may indicate that the sound has existed for as long as several years.
• Breath sounds audible from a distance without a stethoscope—suspect narrowing of the upper airway
• Nature of the sound—ranges from abnormally loud to obvious fluttering to high-pitched squeaking, depending on the degree of airway narrowing
• May note increased respiratory effort and paradoxical respiratory movements (chest wall collapses inward during inspiration and springs outward during expiration) when the effort is extreme; are often accompanied by obvious postural changes (e.g., abducted forelimbs, extended head and neck, and open-mouth breathing)

CAUSES
• Brachycephalic airway syndrome
• Laryngeal paralysis—inherited or acquired
• Airway tumors and middle ear polyps
• Acromegaly
• Neuromuscular dysfunction—myasthenia gravis; brainstem disease; polyneuropathy; polymyopathy; hypothyroidism
• Anesthesia or sedation—only if predisposing anatomy exists
• Edema or inflammation of the palate, pharynx, and larynx (including everted mucosal lining of the laryngeal ventricles)—secondary to coughing, vomiting or regurgitation, turbulent airflow, upper respiratory infection, and hemorrhage
• Secretions (e.g., pus, mucus, and blood) in the airway lumen—acutely after surgery; a normal conscious animal would cough these out or swallow them
• Foreign bodies in the airway lumen

RISK FACTORS
• High ambient temperature
• Fever
• High metabolic rate—as occurs with hyperthyroidism or sepsis
• Exercise
• Anxiety
• Any respiratory or cardiovascular disease that increases ventilation
• Turbulence caused by the increased airflow may lead to swelling and worsen the airway obstruction.

DIAGNOSIS

DIFFERENTIAL DIAGNOSIS
• Must differentiate sounds from pharyngeal and laryngeal narrowing from sounds arising elsewhere in the respiratory system
• Nasal and tracheal narrowing and severe or extensive narrowing of the bronchi—may cause increased respiratory sounds
• If the sound persists when the patient opens its mouth, a nasal cause can virtually be ruled out.
• If the sound occurs only during expiration, it is likely that intrathoracic narrowing is the cause.
• If the owner describes a change in voice, the larynx is the likely abnormal site.
• Without helpful indicators, systematically auscultate over the nose, pharynx, larynx, and trachea to identify the point of maximal intensity of any abnormal sound and to identify the phase of respiration when it is most obvious.
• Important to identify the anatomic location from which the abnormal sound arises and to seek exacerbating causes (see Risk Factors; e.g., a chronic airway obstruction may become manifest when the patient is exposed to extremely high ambient temperatures)

CBC/BIOCHEMISTRY/URINALYSIS
N/A

OTHER LABORATORY TESTS
N/A

IMAGING
• Lateral radiographs of the head and neck—may help identify abnormal soft tissues of the airway (e.g., elongated soft palate or a nasal polyp); limited use for identifying laryngeal disease, although experienced radiographers can identify abnormally dilated or swollen laryngeal saccules; may allow further evaluation of external masses compressing the upper airway
• Radiography and fluoroscopy—important for assessing the cardiorespiratory system; rule out other or additional causes of respiratory difficulty; such conditions may add to an underlying upper airway obstruction, causing a subclinical condition to become symptomatic.

DIAGNOSTIC PROCEDURES

Pharyngoscopy and Laryngoscopy

• Definitive diagnostic tests for direct visualization of pharyngeal or laryngeal changes

• Require general anesthesia; must consider risk to patient

• Remember that the patient's ability to use muscles to open the airway is compromised by anesthesia; veterinarian and clients must determine if they are prepared to carry out surgical remedies if indicated.

• Remediable condition not identified and corrected—patient's recovery from anesthesia may be complicated by severe airway obstruction; must be prepared to perform a tracheostomy if airway is obstructed and a definitive surgical remedy cannot be pursued immediately

• Assess timing and degree of movement of the vocal folds during light anesthesia—evaluate laryngeal paralysis

• Normal palate—thin; just barely overlaps the tip of the epiglottis; easily displaced dorsally using the blade of the laryngoscope

• Overlong soft palate—thick; usually inflamed; may lie as much as 1 cm or more past the tip of the epiglottis

• Patient should be as stable as possible before undergoing general anesthesia, but do not unduly delay procedure; appropriate surgical treatment is usually the only means of reducing the airway obstruction.

TREATMENT

• Hypoxia and hypoventilation—occur only after prolonged severe obstruction; supplemental oxygen not always critical for sustaining with partial airway collapse

• Keep patient cool, quiet, and calm—anxiety, exertion, and pain lead to increased ventilation, potentially worsening the obstruction

• All sedatives—may relax the upper airway muscles and worsen the obstruction; closely monitor effects of sedatives; be prepared with emergency means for securing the airway if complete obstruction occurs.

• Extreme airway obstruction—attempt an emergency intubation; if obstruction prevents intubation, emergency tracheostomy or passage of a tracheal catheter to administer oxygen may be the only available means for sustaining life; a tracheal catheter can only briefly sustain oxygenation while a more permanent solution is sought.

MEDICATIONS

DRUGS

• Medical approaches—appropriate only if the underlying cause is infection, edema, inflammation, or hemorrhage; anatomic or neurologic causes are not amenable to symptomatic medical treatment.

• Steroids—may be indicated if edema or inflammation is thought to be an important contributor; effect with intravenous administration should be apparent in approximately 1 hr.

• Diuretics—may be administered; efficacy doubtful

CONTRAINDICATIONS

N/A

PRECAUTIONS

• Atropine—reduces fluid secretions, makes mucus more tenacious; not advisable other than as an adjunct to emergency resuscitative procedures

• Sedatives and anesthetics

POSSIBLE INTERACTIONS

N/A

ALTERNATIVE DRUGS

N/A

FOLLOW-UP

PATIENT MONITORING

• When owner elects to try medical treatment—recommend telephone follow-up; the excitement of an office visit may precipitate a crisis.

• Even after surgical treatment, some degree of obstruction may remain; advise client to avoid exercise, high ambient temperatures, and extreme excitement.

POSSIBLE COMPLICATIONS

• Serious complications—may occur and persist despite efforts to relieve the obstruction; include airway edema, pulmonary edema (may progress to life-threatening acute lung injury), and hypoventilation; may require tracheostomy and/or artificial ventilation

• Take particular care when inducing general anesthesia or when using sedatives in any patient with upper airway obstruction.

• Inform client that the patient can make the transition from being a noisy breather to having an obstructed emergency in a few minutes or even seconds.

• When owner chooses to take an apparently stable patient home, or if continual observation is not feasible, inform client that complete obstruction could occur.

MISCELLANEOUS

ASSOCIATED CONDITIONS

N/A

AGE-RELATED FACTORS

N/A

ZOONOTIC POTENTIAL

N/A

PREGNANCY

N/A

SYNONYM

Snoring

SEE ALSO

• Acromegaly—Cats
• Brachycephalic Airway Syndrome
• Hypothyroidism
• Laryngeal Disease
• Myasthenia Gravis
• Nasal and Nasopharyngeal Polyps

Suggested Reading

Hendricks JC. Brachycephalic airway syndrome. Update on respiratory disease. Vet Clin North Am Small Anim Pract 1992; 22:1145–1153.

Hendricks JC. Respiratory condition in critical patients. Critical care. Vet Clin North Am Small Anim Pract 1989;19:1167–1188.

Nelson AW. Upper respiratory system. In: Slatter D, ed. Textbook of small animal surgery. 2nd ed. Philadelphia: Saunders, 1993:733–776.

Author Joan C. Hendricks
Consulting Editor Eleanor C. Hawkins

STOMATITIS

BASICS

DEFINITION
An inflammation of the soft tissues of the oral cavity, which may be caused by many different stimuli of local or systemic origin.

PATHOPHYSIOLOGY
Inflammation and other changes may develop in the normal oral mucosa because of the tremendous amount of vasculature in the area and its proximity to the external environment.

SYSTEMS AFFECTED
• Gastrointestinal—prehension and mastication
• May be affected because of pain
• Behavioral—varying degrees of interest in food may result; patients may approach food and attempt to masticate with varying degrees of difficulty.
• Ophthalmic—periorbital swelling, exophthalmos, protrusion of nictitating membrane, resistance to retropulsion of the globe, orbital cellulitis, conjunctivitis, and other ophthalmic manifestations of posterior maxillary disease because of its proximity to the orbital structures
• Skin/Exocrine—may be inflammation of the skin around the lips because of ptyalism; other conditions may affect the skin around the oral cavity because of its proximity to lesions affecting the cheek or lips

SIGNALMENT
• Dog and cat
• Ulcerative stomatitis in Maltese—higher incidence in males
• Juvenile-onset periodontitis in young cats
• Oral eosinophilic granuloma—most commonly in Siberian husky (may be

hereditary)
• Gingival hyperplasia in large breeds
• Rapidly progressive periodontitis seen mostly in young adult animals such as the greyhound and the shih tzu
• Lymphocytic plasmocytic stomatitis in cats
• Localized juvenile periodontitis in the maxillary or mandibular incisor region—especially common in miniature schnauzer

SIGNS
• Halitosis
• Pain
• Ulcerated lesions
• Ptyalism
• Edema
• Extensive plaque and calculus

CAUSES

Anatomic
• Periodontal disease due to overcrowding of teeth
• Lip frenulum attachment
• Tight-lip syndrome in shar-pei

Metabolic
• Uremia and high ammonia levels in saliva
• Vasculitis and xerostomia seen with diabetes mellitus
• Macroglossia and puffy lips as seen with hypoparathyroidism

Immune-Mediated
• Pemphigus foliaceous
• Pemphigus vulgaris
• Bullous pemphigoid
• Systemic lupus erythematosus and discoid lupus erythematosus in the dog
• Acute hypersensitivity to drugs

Infectious
• Opportunistic oral flora secondary to oral lesions
• Mycotic stomatitis
• Systemic infections

• Leptospirosis—*Mycobacterium lepraemurium* in cats
• Calicivirus or herpesvirus infections—cat
• Canine distemper
• Viral papillomatosis—dogs

Trauma
• Irritation from calculus
• Foreign objects—gum-chewers syndrome
• Electrical cord shock
• Chemical burns
• Lacerations
• Snake bite
• Blows
• Trauma of the palate from base-narrow mandibular canine teeth

Toxic
• Certain plants
• Chemotherapy
• Radiotherapy
• Chemical irritants

RISK FACTORS
N/A

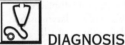

DIAGNOSIS

DIFFERENTIAL DIAGNOSIS
N/A

CBC/BIOCHEMISTRY/URINALYSIS
Useful to detect systemic disease

OTHER LABORATORY TESTS
• Immunologic testing
• Mycotic cultures
• Virus isolation
• Toxicologic studies
• Serum protein electrophoresis
• Endocrine tests

IMAGING
Radiography to identify osseous or dental abnormalities

DIAGNOSTIC PROCEDURES
Biopsy

TREATMENT

• Correct nutritional or hydration deficiencies as needed, on an inpatient or outpatient basis
• Can place feeding tube if necessary
• Dental disease or periodontal disease present should be treated
• Sometimes most or all teeth must be extracted to resolve stomatitis.

MEDICATIONS

DRUGS OF CHOICE

Antimicrobials
• Broad-spectrum antibiotics
• Amoxicillin-clavulanate
• Clindamycin
• Metronidazole—10 mg/kg ql2h PO or 40–50 mg/kg as a loading dose on the first day, followed by 20–25 mg/kg q8h for 7 days or less
• Doxycycline—5 mg/kg PO loading dose, 2.5 mg/kg PO 12 h later, and 2.5 mg/kg PO once daily thereafter
• Chlorhexidine solution or gel (CHX, VRx Products, Harbor City, CA)-plaque retardant
• Maxi-Guard (Addison Biological Laboratory, Fayette, MO) zinc-organic acid solutions and gels to promote tissue healing and retard plaque accumulation

Antiinflammatory Drugs
• Prednisolone or prednisone
• For eosinophilic ulcer: 2–4.4 mg/kg PO once a day; for chronic cases use 0.5–1.0 mg/kg PO every other day.
• For adjunctive therapy of feline plasma cell gingivitis–pharyngitis; may improve inflammation and appetite

CONTRAINDICATIONS
• Hypersensitivity to medication
• Glucocorticoid use with systemic mycotic infections

PRECAUTIONS
N/A

POSSIBLE INTERACTIONS
N/A

ALTERNATIVE DRUGS
N/A

FOLLOW-UP

PATIENT MONITORING
• Laboratory tests when systemic disease is involved
• Oral rinses and brushing the teeth with oral medications may be helpful, especially with periodontal disease.

POSSIBLE COMPLICATIONS
Bacteremia from periodontal disease can cause renal, cardiac, hepatic, and pulmonary disease.

MISCELLANEOUS

ASSOCIATED CONDITIONS
Periodontal disease is probably the leading cause of other oral disorders.

AGE-RELATED FACTORS
Periodontal disease associated with calculus is seen most often in old dogs and cats and in susceptible breeds.

ZOONOTIC POTENTIAL
• Dental prophylaxis procedures have caused human infections
• Safety glasses and a mask are recommended when performing such procedures.

PREGNANCY

SYNONYMS
• Trench mouth
• St. Vincent's stomatitis, an ulceromembranous stomatitis due to *Fusobacterium* spp. and spirochetes

SEE ALSO
N/A

ABBREVIATIONS
N/A

Suggested Reading
Harvey CE, Emily PP. Oral lesions of soft tissues and bone: differential diagnosis. In: Harvey CE, Emily PP, eds. Small animal dentistry. St. Louis: CV Mosby, 1993:42–88.
Wiggs RB, Lobprise HB. Veterinary dentistry. Philadelphia: Lippincott-Raven. 1997:104–139.
Author Larry Baker
Consulting Editor Jan Bellows

STUPOR AND COMA

BASICS

DEFINITION
• Stupor—unconscious but arousable with noxious stimuli • Coma—unconscious and not arousable with noxious stimuli

PATHOPHYSIOLOGY
ARAS—network of neurons situated in the core of the brainstem; functions as the arousal system for the cerebral cortex; any severe pathologic change (either anatomic or metabolic) that causes interruption can lead to depression, stupor, or coma.

SYSTEMS AFFECTED
• Nervous • Cardiovascular • Respiratory • Ophthalmic

SIGNALMENT
• Dogs and cats • No breed, age, or sex predilection

SIGNS

Historical Findings
• The possibility of trauma or unsupervised roaming • Past medical problems of significance—diabetes mellitus and insulin therapy; hypoglycemia; cardiovascular problems; hypoxic episodes; renal failure; liver failure; neoplasia • Record a description of the patient's environment—possible heatstroke; hypothermia; drowning; exposure to drugs, narcotics, and toxins (e.g., ethylene glycol, lead, anticoagulants), including owner's medications • Onset may be acute or slowly progressive, depending on underlying cause.

Physical Examination Findings
• Look for evidence of external or internal trauma. • Examine for severe hypothermia or hyperthermia. • Evidence of hypoxia or cyanosis, ecchymosis or petechiation, or cardiac or respiratory insufficiency—warrants investigation for metabolic causes • Carefully palpate for evidence of neoplasia. • Retinal hemorrhages or distended vessels—hypertension • Papilledema—cerebral edema • Retinal detachment—infectious, neoplastic, or hypertensive causes • Chorioretinitis—infectious causes (distemper, FeLV-related diseases, toxoplasmosis, cryptococcosis, or FIP) • Sustained bradycardia (with normal serum potassium)—midbrain, pontine, or medullary lesion

Neurologic Examination Findings
• Determine level of consciousness and whether patient is arousable.
• Pupillary light reflexes—small responsive pupils: cerebral or diencephalic lesion; dilated unresponsive pupils (unilateral or bilateral) or fixed in midposition: midbrain or severe medullary lesions
• Oculocephalic reflex (when cervical manipulation is possible)—loss of physiologic vestibular nystagmus: brainstem involvement.
• Respiratory patterns—Cheyne-Stokes respiration: severe, diffuse cerebral or diencephalic lesion; hyperventilation: midbrain lesion; ataxic or apneustic breathing: pons or medulla lesion
• Cranial nerves—no deficits with lesion of cerebrum-diencephalon; deficits of cranial nerve III: midbrain lesion; deficits of cranial nerves V–XII: pons and medulla lesions
• Postural changes—decerebrate rigidity: midbrain lesion

CAUSES
• Drugs—narcotics; depressants; ivermectin
• Anatomic—hydrocephalus
• Metabolic—severe hypoglycemia; hyperglycemia; hyperosmolar syndromes; hypernatremia; hyponatremia; hepatic encephalopathy; hypoxemia; hypercarbia; hypothermia; hyperthermia; hypotension; coagulopathies; renal failure; lysosomal storage disease
• Nutritional—hypoglycemia; thiamine deficiency
• Neoplastic (primary)—meningioma; astrocytoma; gliomas; choroid plexus papilloma; pituitary adenoma; others
• Metastatic—hemangiosarcoma; lymphosarcoma; mammary carcinoma; others
• Inflammatory noninfectious—granulomatous meningoencephalomyelitis
• Infectious—bacterial; viral (distemper, FIP); parasitic (aberrant larva migrans); protozoal (neosporosis, toxoplasmosis); fungal (cryptococcosis, blastomycosis, histoplasmosis, coccidioidomycosis, actinomycosis); rickettsial
• Idiopathic—epilepsy (poststatus epilepticus)
• Immune-mediated—vasculitis and thrombocytopenia leading to hemorrhage
• Traumatic
• Toxins—ethylene glycol; lead; rodenticide anticoagulants; others
• Vascular—hemorrhage (bleeding disorders, hypertension); infarction (feline ischemic encephalopathy, microfilaria, or migrating adult heartworm)

RISK FACTORS
• Diabetes mellitus—insulin therapy
• Insulinomas
• Severe heat or cold exposure without protection
• Free-roaming animals—trauma
• Young and unvaccinated animals

DIAGNOSIS

DIFFERENTIAL DIAGNOSIS

Similar Signs
• Other altered states of consciousness—narcolepsy (intermittent episodes of deep sleep with spontaneous recovery); syncope (temporary loss of consciousness with spontaneous recovery); collapse and severe depression (patient is conscious with depressed mentation and motor activity)

Causes
• Acute onset—most commonly caused by toxins, drugs, trauma, or vascular accidents
• Slow progression of neurologic signs without systemic abnormalities—suggests primary neurologic disorders of inflammatory, neoplastic, or anatomic causes
• Bilateral diffuse cortical signs—metabolic diseases, toxins, systemic infection, drugs, and nutritional causes
• Brainstem signs—trauma, inflammation, neoplasia, vascular accidents or commonly from progression of cerebral disease causing tentorial herniation

CBC/BIOCHEMISTRY/URINALYSIS

CBC
• Lead toxicity—may show nucleated red blood cells or basophilic stippling
• Severe infection—inflammatory hemogram
• Severe anemia—suggests hypoxemia

Biochemistry
May see hypoglycemia, hyperglycemia, hypernatremia, azofemia, hyperosmolarity, and other metabolic derangements

Urinalysis
• Diabetes mellitus—glycosuria
• End-stage renal disease—isosthenuria
• Immune-mediated disease or severe infection—proteinuria
• Hepatic encephalopathy—ammonium biurate crystals
• Ethylene glycol toxicity—calcium oxalate or hippurate crystals

OTHER LABORATORY TESTS
• Serum ethylene glycol test and measure osmolar gap—acute onset
• Serum ammonia concentrations and preprandial and postprandial bile acids—high levels indicate hepatic encephalopathy.
• Serum and CSF titers—suspected infectious disease (e.g. distemper, FIP, rickettsial diseases, cryptococcosis, blastomycosis, histoplasmosis, Neospora caninum, toxoplasmosis)
• Arterial blood gases—evidence of hypoxemia; severe pH changes; hypercarbia
• Coagulogram—including PT, PTT, fibrinogen, FDP, platelet count, antithrombin III, and buccal bleeding time; suspected intracranial bleeding or thrombosis
• Serologic testing—FeLV, FIV, and heartworm disease

IMAGING
• Survey radiographs (chest and abdomen)—evidence of organ compromise, infiltration, or neoplasia
• Skull radiographs—fractures in trauma cases

• MRI—best modality for detecting acute hemorrhage within the cranial vault or brain
• CT (skull)—method of choice for detecting depressed fractures or penetrating foreign bodies

DIAGNOSTIC PROCEDURES

• CSF analysis—include immunoglobulin concentrations and titers for infectious diseases; perform when there is no evidence of trauma, increased ICP, coagulopathies, or metabolic disease.
• BAER—determine brainstem function
• ECG—determine cardiac dysfunction; abnormalities may contribute to stupor or coma or may be caused by brain disease.

 TREATMENT

• Hydration—maintained with a balanced electrolyte crystalloid solution
• The head should be level with the body or elevated to a 20° angle; the head should never be lower than the body to avoid increase in ICP.
• Avoid triggering a cough or sneeze reflex during intubation or oxygen supplementation by nasal cannula; may severely elevate ICP; lidocaine (dogs: 0.75 mg/kg IV) given before intubation can blunt the gag and cough reflex.
• PaO_2—maintain between 35 and 45 mm Hg; hyperventilating may reduce cerebral blood flow and ICP; must be above 50 mm Hg to maintain cerebral blood flow autoregulation; use peripheral veins, leaving the jugular vein blood flow unobstructed; shifting blood volume into the jugular veins is an important compensatory mechanism during high ICP.
• Prevent thrashing, seizures, or any other form of uncontrolled motor activity; may elevate ICP; diazepam infusion (0.5–1 mg/kg/hr) may be required for seizures.
• Meticulous nursing care to prevent secondary complications of recumbency—eye lubrication; aseptic technique with catheters; turning to avoid hypostatic lung congestion; hygiene
• Surgical decompression and exploration—seriously consider if neurologic signs worsen, including cerebral dysfunction that is progressing to midbrain signs with a history of trauma or bleeding (tentorial herniation), high ICP not responsive to medical therapy (if monitoring instrumentation available), depressed skull fracture fragments, and penetrating foreign body.
• Nutrition—maintain during the unconscious period; adjust nutritional requirements to compensate for metabolic demands.

 MEDICATIONS

DRUGS OF CHOICE

Poor Perfusion

• Use a minimal amount of crystalloids, because they contribute to brain edema; a combination of large molecular weight colloids (e.g., hetastarch) with crystalloids allows small fluid volume resuscitation.
• Do not use colloids if there is intracranial hemorrhage.
• Maintain systolic arterial blood pressure > 90 mm Hg with crystalloids and/or colloids; avoid hypertension.

High ICP

• Hyperventilation or diuretic therapy
• Furosemide—0.75 mg/kg IV; lowers CSF production and ICP
• Mannitol—0.1–0.5 g/kg IV bolus q2h for 3–4 doses in dogs and 2–3 doses in cats); improves brain blood flow and lowers ICP; given after furosemide

Underlying Disease

• Glucocorticosteroids—inflammatory and space-occupying intracranial abnormalities
• Lactulose enemas and fluid support—hepatic encephalopathy
• Fluid diuresis—renal failure
• Rehydration and insulin—diabetes mellitus with hyperosmolality; lower glucose slowly.
• Glucose supplementation—hypoglycemia
• Support the intravascular volume; cool—Hyperthermia.
• Support the intravascular volume; warm—Hypothermia.
• Gastric lavage and instillation of activated charcoal with a cathartic—suspected toxic ingestion
• Specific toxins may require specific therapeutics (e.g., ethylene glycol treated with ethanol and peritoneal dialysis).
• Antibiotics—use agents that cross the blood–brain barrier for suspected bacterial infections (e.g., trimethoprim-sulfa, chloramphenicol, and metronidazole) use broad-spectrum agents if the blood–brain barrier is interrupted (e.g., first-generation cephalosporins).

CONTRAINDICATIONS

• Do not allow the head to lie below plane of body.
• Colloids—do not use when there is intracranial hemorrhage.

PRECAUTIONS

• Avoid hypertension.
• Avoid intravascular volume overload.
• Mannitol and hypertonic saline—may worsen neurologic status when there is intracranial hemorrhage

• Hyperventilating—maintain $PaCO_2$ > 25 mm Hg; do not perform for extended time periods (> 48 hr).

POSSIBLE INTERACTIONS

N/A

ALTERNATIVE DRUGS

N/A

 FOLLOW-UP

PATIENT MONITORING

• Repeat neurologic examinations—detect deterioration of function that warrants aggressive therapeutic intervention • Blood pressure—keep fluid therapy adequate for perfusion while avoiding hypertension • Blood gases—assess need for oxygen supplementation or ventilation; monitor PCO_2 when hyperventilating • Blood glucose—ensure an adequate blood level to maintain brain functions while avoiding hyperosmolality
• ECG—detect arrhythmias that may affect perfusion, oxygenation, and cerebral blood flow • ICP—detect marked elevations; track success of therapeutics

POSSIBLE COMPLICATIONS

N/A

 MISCELLANEOUS

SEE ALSO

Brain Injury (Head Trauma and Hypoxia)

ABBREVIATIONS

• ARAS = ascending reticular activating system • BAER = brainstem auditory-evoked response • CSF = cerebrospinal fluid • FDP = fibrin degradation product • FeLV = feline leukemia virus • FIP = feline infectious peritonitis • FIV = feline immunodeficiency virus • ICP = intracranial pressure • PT = prothrombin time • PTT = partial thromboplastin time

Suggested Reading

Chrisman CL. Coma and altered states of consciousness. In: Problems in small animal neurology. Philadelphia: Lea & Febiger, 1991:219–233.
Author Rebecca Kirby
Consulting Editor Joane M. Parent

SYNCOPE

 ## BASICS

DEFINITION
Temporary loss of consciousness and vascular tone associated with loss of postural tone, with spontaneous recovery

PATHOPHYSIOLOGY
Inadequate cerebral perfusion and delivery of oxygen and metabolic substrates leads to loss of consciousness and motor tone; impaired cerebral perfusion can result from changes in vasomotor tone, cerebral disease, and low cardiac output caused by structural heart disease or arrhythmias.

SYSTEMS AFFECTED
• Nervous
• Cardiovascular

SIGNALMENT
More common in old animals

SIGNS
N/A

CAUSES

Cardiac Causes
• Bradyarrhythmias—sinus bradycardia, sinus arrest, second-degree atrioventricular (AV) block, complete AV block, atrial standstill
• Tachyarrhythmias—ventricular tachycardia, supraventricular tachycardia, atrial fibrillation
• Low cardiac output (nonarrhythmic)—cardiomyopathy, AV valve endocardiosis, subaortic stenosis, pulmonic stenosis, heartworm disease, pulmonary embolism, cardiac tumor, cardiac tamponade

Neurologic and Vasomotor Instability
• Vasovagal syncope—emotional stress and excitement may cause heightened sympathetic stimulation leading to transient tachycardia and hypertension, which is followed by a compensatory rise in vagal tone, leading to excessive vasodilation without a compensatory rise in heart rate and cardiac output; bradycardia often occurs.
• Situational syncope refers to syncope associated with coughing, defecation, urination, and swallowing.
• Carotid sinus hyperactivity may cause hypotension and bradycardia—often the cause of syncope when one pulls on a dog's collar

Miscellaneous Causes
• Drugs that affect blood pressure and regulation of autonomic tone
• Hypoglycemia, hypocalcemia, and hyponatremia (rare)
• Hyperviscosity syndromes (e.g., polycythemia and paraproteinemia) cause sludging of blood and impaired cerebral perfusion (rare).

RISK FACTORS
• Heart disease
• Sick sinus syndrome—breeds at risk include cocker spaniel, miniature schnauzer, pug, and dachshund; most common in old females
• Drug therapy—vasodilators (e.g., calcium channel blockers, ACE inhibitors, hydralazine, and nitrates), phenothiazines (e.g., acepromazine), antiarrhythmics, and diuretics

 ## DIAGNOSIS

DIFFERENTIAL DIAGNOSIS

Differential Signs
• Must differentiate from other altered states of consciousness, including seizures and narcolepsy (a sleep disorder)
• Seizures are often associated with a prodromal and postictal period; syncope occurs without warning, and animal usually has rapid, spontaneous recovery. Unlike syncope, seizure activity is usually associated with tonic clonic muscle activity rather than flaccidity.
• Like syncope, narcolepsy occurs suddenly, results in muscle flaccidity, and resolves spontaneously. Unlike syncope, narcolepsy can last for minutes and can be terminated by loud noises or harsh external stimuli.
• Must differentiate from other causes of collapse such as musculoskeletal disease and neuromuscular disease (e.g., myasthenia gravis), which are not associated with loss of consciousness

Differential Causes
• Syncope with excitement or stress suggests vasovagal syncope.
• Syncope with coughing, urination, or defecation suggests situational syncope.
• Syncope with exercise suggests low output states associated with arrhythmias or structural heart disease.
• A murmur supports heart disease but does not confirm cardiac cause for syncope.

CBC/BIOCHEMISTRY/URINALYSIS
• Usually normal
• Hypoglycemia or electrolyte disturbance in some animals

OTHER LABORATORY TESTS
• If animal is hypoglycemic, measure insulin concentration on same sample. Calculate an amended insulin:glucose ratio to rule out insulinoma.
• If animal is hyponatremic or hyperkalemic, consider an ACTH stimulation test.
• If low cardiac output is suspected, rule out occult heartworm disease.

IMAGING

Echocardiography
May detect structural heart disease that could lower cardiac output

DIAGNOSTIC PROCEDURES
• Have owner monitor heart rate during any syncopal episode.
• Electroencephalogram, computed tomography of the head, cerebrospinal fluid (CSF) tap if CNS origin suspected

Electrocardiographic Findings
• Postexercise ECG may reveal intermittent arrhythmia.
• Holter monitoring (24-h ECG recording) or use of an ECG event (loop) recorder—useful for evaluating arrhythmic causes
• Carotid sinus massage with ECG and blood pressure monitoring useful in evaluating carotid sensitivity

 ## TREATMENT

• Treat as outpatient unless important heart disease evident
• Minimize stimuli that precipitate episodes:
• Low cardiac output—minimize activity.
• Vasovagal—minimize excitement and stress.
• Cough—remove collar.
• Assure owner that most noncardiac causes are not life threatening; cardiac causes may be treated, but syncope in patients with cardiac disease may suggest higher mortality risk.
• Avoid or discontinue medications likely to precipitate syncope.

MEDICATIONS

DRUGS OF CHOICE

Bradyarrhythmias
• Correct metabolic causes.
• Anticholinergics (e.g., atropine, propantheline bromide)
• Sympathomimetics (e.g., isoproterenol, bronchodilators)
• Pacemaker implantation in some patients

Tachyarrhythmias
• Atrial arrhythmias—administer digoxin, β-blocker, or diltiazem.
• Ventricular arrhythmias—administer lidocaine, procainamide, quinidine, mexiletine, sotalol, or β-blockers.

Low Cardiac Output
Institute treatment to improve cardiac output, which varies according to specific cardiac disease.

Vasovagal
• β-Blockers (e.g., atenolol, propranolol, and metoprolol) may indirectly prevent vagal stimulation by blocking the initial sympathetic response.
• Theophylline or aminophylline—sometimes helpful; mechanism of action in this setting is unclear
• Anticholinergics (e.g., propantheline bromide and scopolamine) may blunt the vagal response.

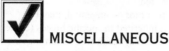

CONTRAINDICATIONS
N/A

PRECAUTIONS
Drugs that lower blood pressure

POSSIBLE INTERACTIONS
N/A

ALTERNATIVE DRUGS
N/A

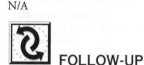 **FOLLOW-UP**

PATIENT MONITORING
ECG or Holter monitoring to assess efficacy of antiarrhythmic therapy

POSSIBLE COMPLICATIONS
• Death
• Trauma when collapse occurs

✓ **MISCELLANEOUS**

ASSOCIATED CONDITIONS
N/A

AGE-RELATED FACTORS
N/A

ZOONOTIC POTENTIAL
N/A

PREGNANCY
N/A

SYNONYMS
Fainting

SEE ALSO
• Seizures
• Narcolepsy and Cataplexy
• Myasthenia Gravis

ABBREVIATIONS
N/A

Suggested Reading
Kapoor WN. Syncope and hypotension. In: Braunwald E, ed. Heart disease: a textbook of cardiovascular medicine. 5th ed. Philadelphia: Saunders, 1997;863–876.
Rush JE. Syncope and episodic weakness. In: Fox PR, Sisson D, Moise NS eds. Textbook of canine and feline cardiology. Philadelphia: Saunders, 1999:446–455.
Author Francis W. K. Smith, Jr.
Consulting Editors Larry P. Tilley and Francis W. K. Smith, Jr.

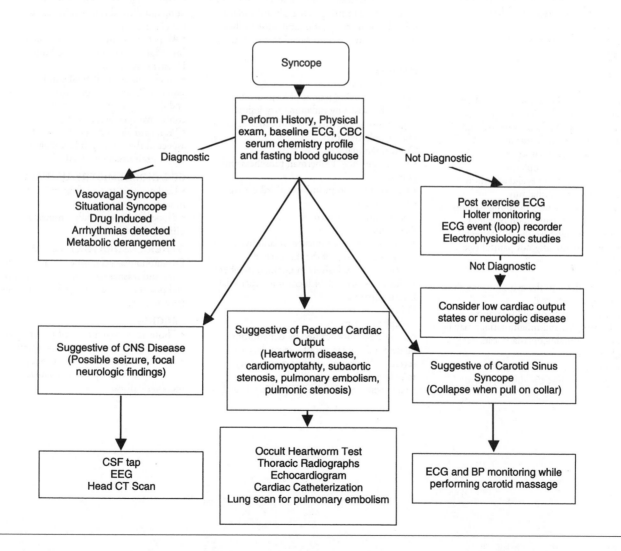

THIRD EYELID PROTRUSION

 BASICS

DEFINITION
Abnormal protrusion (elevation) of the third eyelid

PATHOPHYSIOLOGY
• Dogs—movement of the third eyelid is passive.
• Cats—partial sympathetic nervous control of the third eyelid
• Results from a space-occupying mass in the orbit pushing the third eyelid forward, enophthalmia, sympathetic denervation of the eye, or a painful eye

SYSTEMS AFFECTED
• Ophthalmic—third eyelid(s); orbit; eyeball
• Nervous—autonomic nervous system

SIGNALMENT
See Causes.

SIGNS
• May have none
• May be associated with primary condition—exophthalmus; enophthalmus; blepharospasm; Horner syndrome
• Unilateral or bilateral—depending on cause

CAUSES
Unilateral
Blepharospasm
• Painful ocular condition—corneal ulcer; glaucoma; uveitis; or ocular foreign body
• May cause the globe to be retracted and secondary third eyelid elevation
Space-Occupying Orbital Mass
• Often an abscess or neoplasm
• May displace the third eyelid anteriorly
• Usually causes exophthalmus
• Abscess—generally seen in young patients; usually acute onset; painful on palpation
• Neoplasm—usually seen in old patients; gradual onset; frequently not painful (see Orbital Diseases)
Enophthalmus
• Globe—recedes into the orbit, causing third eyelid to appear elevated
• Unilateral—may be caused by trauma, orbital fat atrophy, and inflammation; may be secondary to orbital neoplasia in cats (see Orbital Diseases)
Microphthalmos or Phthisis Bulbi
• Small globes—cause the third eyelid to

appear elevated
• Microphthalmos—congenital; may be idiopathic; inherited in specific breeds (collie eye anomaly); may result from toxin ingestion (griseofulvin in pregnant cats)
• Phthisis bulbi—occurs with severe damage to the globe (severe uveitis, glaucoma, or trauma); ciliary body fails to produce aqueous humor; diminished; small, fibrotic globe from chronic inflammation
Other
• Horner's Syndrome—clinical signs develop after sympathetic denervation; elevated third eyelid; enophthalmus; ptosis (drooping upper eyelid); miosis (see Horner's Syndrome)
• Neoplasia of the third eyelid—adenocarcinoma of the gland of the third eyelid and squamous cell carcinoma of eyelid most common
• Cherry eye—see Prolapsed Gland of the Third Eyelid (Cherry Eye)
• Everted or scrolled cartilage of the third eyelid—seen in Wiemaraners, Great Danes, German short-haired pointers, and other breeds; the T-shaped cartilage of the third eyelid is rolled away from the surface of the eye instead of conforming to the corneal surface.
• Symblepharon—postinflammatory adhesions between the third eyelid and cornea or conjunctiva

Bilateral
Exophthalmus
• Space-occupying lesions of both orbits
• Usually caused by inflammatory lesions (e.g., eosinophilic myositis and extraocular muscle polymyositis)
Conformational
• Breed-specific—Doberman pinschers and pointers
• Deep orbits and prominent third eyelids
• Not pathologic
• No treatment needed
Plasmoma
• Immune-mediated thickening and hyperemia of the leading edge of the third eyelid
• Seen almost exclusively in German shepherds
• May be associated with chronic superficial keratitis (pannus)
Other
• Blepharospasm
• Enophthalmus—caused by dehydration, bilateral orbital fat atrophy secondary to severe cachexia, and chronic masticatory muscle myositis
• Haw syndrome (cats)—idiopathic bilateral

elevation of the third eyelids; all other aspects of the ophthalmic examination are normal; usually resolves in 3–4 weeks without treatment
• Dysautonomia (Key-Gaskell syndrome)—bilateral elevated third eyelids; dilated nonresponsive pupils; KCS; dry mucosal surfaces; anorexia; lethargy; regurgitation; megaesophagus; bradycardia; megacolon; distended bladder (see Dysautonomia)
• Tranquilizers—many (e.g., acepromazine) cause bilateral third eyelid elevation
• Fatigue—may cause transient third eyelid elevation, especially in dogs prone to ectropion

RISK FACTORS
Depend on cause

 DIAGNOSIS

DIFFERENTIAL DIAGNOSIS
• Most common causes of acute onset of unilateral condition—ocular pain (e.g., corneal ulcer and uveitis); orbital inflammation (e.g., orbital abscess and cellulitis)
• Middle-aged or old patient with unilateral, nonpainful condition—third eyelid or orbital neoplasm likely
• All patients—must rule out a small eye (microphthalmos or phthisis bulbi) and Horner's syndrome
• Likely causes of bilateral condition—systemic illness (e.g., dehydration, cachexia, and dysautonomia); associated with conformational abnormalities
• Prolapsed gland of the third eyelid—medial aspect of the third eyelid swollen; the third eyelid itself usually normal

CBC/BIOCHEMISTRY/URINALYSIS
• Leukocytosis and a left shift—with orbital inflammatory processes
• Blood work—generally unrewarding in differentiating causes

OTHER LABORATORY TESTS
Dysautonomia—confirmed by measuring urine and plasma catecholamine concentrations and pharmacologic testing of the autonomic nervous system

IMAGING
• Thoracic radiography—all patients with Horner's syndrome to rule out intrathoracic cause of sympathetic denervation; patients with suspected neoplasia to evaluate for metastatic disease

• Orbital ultrasound—recommended to help localize suspected orbital mass and define its nature (e.g., solid or cystic)
• CT or MRI—further define suspected or known orbital mass
• Skull radiographs—rarely show signs of orbital disease unless the lesion is very large and destructive

DIAGNOSTIC PROCEDURES
• Thorough ophthalmic examination
• Slit-lamp biomicroscope or some other source of magnification—recommended to help localize any potential ocular abnormality
• All patients with unilateral condition—examine both surfaces of the third eyelid and the conjunctival cul-de-sac carefully for a foreign body or symblepharon.
• Pharmacologic testing—localize lesion(s) with Horner syndrome (see Horner Syndrome)
• Exploratory surgery and biopsy—may be only means to make a definitive diagnosis for a suspected orbital or third eyelid mass

Cytology
• For suspected mass lesions—orbital mass or mass of the third eyelid; fine-needle aspirate; may help make the diagnosis
• Unguided fine-needle aspiration—attempt only if the mass is anterior to the equator of the eye.
• Ultrasonography guided fine-needle aspiration—for masses posterior to the eye; help avoid delicate retrobulbar structures
• Third eyelid scrapings (German shepherds with suspected plasmoma)—reveal plasma cells and lymphocytes

TREATMENT
• Depends on cause
• Painful condition—remove the cause of the irritation (e.g., foreign body); treat the primary ocular condition
• Orbital cellulitis and abscess—generally respond well to systemically administered antibiotics
• Orbital neoplasms—usually require wide surgical excision via an orbital exenteration; may require adjunct therapeutic modalities (e.g., radiotherapy or chemotherapy) if excision is incomplete
• Microphthalmic eyes—usually none required; remove the globes if painful or subject to recurrent conjunctivitis.

• Pathologic globes—enucleate to prevent formation of intraocular sarcomas (cats).
• Horner syndrome—treat cause, if known (~ 50% of dogs and cats); otherwise will usually resolve without treatment in 4–12 weeks
• Surgical removal of the entire third eyelid—indicated for third eyelid neoplasia; may require adjunct therapeutic modalities (e.g., radiotherapy or chemotherapy) if the surgical margins are not free of neoplasm
• Radiotherapy around the eye—may result in severe keratitis, dry eye, and cataracts; discuss enucleation with the client before initiating treatment.
• Orbital exenteration—may be warranted if the mass extends into the orbit
• Plasmomas—usually controlled with topically applied medications; not cured; inform client that some form of treatment will likely be needed for the life of the patient; topical corticosteroids (0.1% dexamethasone or 1% prednisolone acetate; q6h initially, reduced to q24h when the lesion appears resolved); topical 1% cyclosporine (q12h) also effective
• Haw syndrome—usually resolves in 3–4 weeks without treatment
• Dysautonomia—see Dysautonomia.

MEDICATIONS

DRUGS OF CHOICE
See Treatment.

CONTRAINDICATIONS
Topical corticosteroids—never use with a corneal ulcer.

PRECAUTIONS
N/A

POSSIBLE INTERACTIONS
N/A

ALTERNATIVE DRUGS
N/A

FOLLOW-UP

PATIENT MONITORING
Malignant neoplasm—take thoracic radiographs every 3–6 months to monitor for metastatic disease.

POSSIBLE COMPLICATIONS
Neoplasm—extension to or infection of adjacent orbital structures (e.g., eye, orbit,

orbital sinuses, and cranial cavity) possible; metastasis to distant sites (usually thorax or liver) possible (approximately 90% are malignant)
• Vision loss—from the lesion itself; from the elevation; from treatment (e.g., radiotherapy and exenteration)

MISCELLANEOUS

ASSOCIATED CONDITIONS
N/A

AGE-RELATED FACTORS
• Middle-aged to old patients—at risk for neoplastic diseases of the third eyelid and orbit
• Young patients—at risk for congenital abnormalities; affected by inflammatory conditions of the third eyelid more frequently than are old animals

ZOONOTIC POTENTIAL
N/A

PREGNANCY
N/A

SYNONYMS
• Elevated third eyelid
• Haw syndrome (cats)

SEE ALSO
• Ectropion
• Entropion
• Horner's Syndrome
• Orbital Diseases (Exophthalmus, Enophthalmus, Strabismus)
• Prolapsed Gland of the Third Eyelid (Cherry Eye)

ABBREVIATIONS
KCS = keratoconjunctivitis sicca

Suggested Reading
Sharp NH, Nash AS, Griffiths IR. Feline dysautonomia (the Key-Gaskell syndrome): a clinical and pathological study of forty cases. J Small Anim Pract 1985;25:599–615.
Ward DA. Diseases and surgery of the canine nictitating membrane. In: Gelatt KN, ed. Veterinary Ophthalmology, 3rd ed. Philadelphia: Lippincott Williams & Wilkins, 1999; 609–618.
Author Brian C. Gilger
Consulting Editor Paul E. Miller

TREMORS

BASICS

DEFINITION
Rhythmic, oscillatory, involuntary movement of all or part of the body

PATHOPHYSIOLOGY
• Abnormal movement caused by the alternate or synchronous contraction of reciprocally innervated, antagonistic muscles
• Synchronous contraction—force or duration of contraction is slightly different in the opposing muscles, resulting in biphasic, to-and-fro, movement.

SYSTEMS AFFECTED
• Nervous
• Musculoskeletal—muscle weakness or pain

SIGNALMENT
• Dogs and cats
• Age depends on cause.

Dogs
• Generalized tremor syndrome—usually young to middle-aged
• Variety of hair coat colors, including white
• Hypomyelination—6–8 weeks old; chow chows, springer spaniels, Samoyeds, Weimaraners, and Dalmatians
• Idiopathic head tremor—Doberman pinschers and Labrador retrievers

SIGNS
• Localized or generalized
• Localized—most often involves the head or the pelvic limbs

CAUSES

Head
• Cerebellar abnormalities—degenerative; congenital; inflammatory; immune-mediated; toxic causes
• Idiopathic—Doberman pinschers and English bulldogs overrepresented
• Genetic
• Inflammatory—encephalitides
• Trauma
• Drug administration—doxorubicin; diphenhydramine; metoclopramide
• Abnormalities of the central or peripheral vestibular system

Pelvic Limb Tremor
• May be a sign of weakness or pain in the lumbosacral area
• Metabolic—renal failure; hypoparathyroidism; hypoglycemia
• Compressive lesions of the spine or nerve roots—lumbosacral stenosis; cauda equina syndrome; spinal cord tumor; diskospondylitis
• Peripheral neuropathy; neuromuscular junction abnormality; myopathy
• Poor perfusion to pelvic muscles—right-to-left shunting patent ductus arteriosus; other cardiopulmonary diseases
• Unknown—pelvic limbs in older dogs (senile tremor)

Generalized Tremor
• Hypomyelination
• Intoxications—organophosphates; hexachlorophene; bromethalin
• Degenerative neurologic disease—storage disease; spongiform encephalopathy
• Idiopathic generalized tremor syndrome—white shaker dog syndrome

RISK FACTORS
• Any encephalitis or degenerative neurologic disease—storage disease and spongiform encephalopathy
• Treatment with doxorubicin, diphenhydramine, or metoclopramide
• White hair coat—may predispose for generalized tremor syndrome

DIAGNOSIS

DIFFERENTIAL DIAGNOSIS

Similar Signs
• Shaking, shuddering, myotonia, and myoclonus—tremor usually more consistent, rhythmic, to-and-fro movements of similar amplitude that persist throughout the waking state and stops during sleep
• Weakness—tremor associated with weakness usually occurs when the muscles are forced to work (e.g., during standing, walking, and running).

• Tetany—usually a more consistent extension of the limbs and facial muscles without an extension–flexion cycle of movement
• Seizures—short duration; may be associated with autonomic disturbances (e.g., urination, defecation, and salivation) and alterations of consciousness
• Reflex myoclonus—Labrador retrievers and Dalmatians; characterized by prolonged episodes of extensor rigidity with tactile or auditory stimulus and voluntary exercise

CAUSES
• May be localized or generalized
• Localized to the pelvic limbs—diseases of the lumbosacral spinal cord and associated peripheral nerves

Localized to the Head
• Assess for additional neurologic deficits suggesting cerebellar disease; often a clinical sign of cerebellar disease; intention tremor that worsens when the patient attempts to move the head in a goal-oriented manner; may also involve the whole body; ataxia and dysmetria help determine the neuroanatomic diagnosis.
• Idiopathic condition—breed-specific (e.g., Doberman pinschers); patient usually young at onset; sporadic; occurs at a frequency of 2–4 Hz; up-and-down (yes) or side-to-side (no) direction; anatomic origin unknown; may be a partial seizure

Generalized
• Young dog (6–8 weeks)—congenital myelination abnormality; check breed incidences
• Young adult dog—assess history for toxin exposure; consider generalized tremor syndrome, especially with a white hair coat.

CBC/BIOCHEMISTRY/URINALYSIS
• Usually normal with an associated primary brain disease
• Localized to the head or pelvic limbs—assess for occult metabolic disease; may find hypoglycemia, hypocalcemia, and abnormal renal function
• Some myopathies are characterized by high creatine kinase.

OTHER LABORATORY TESTS
N/A

IMAGING
• Localized to the pelvic limbs—radiography, myelography, epidurography, CT, and MRI; reveal lumbosacral, spinal, or vertebral abnormalities
• Generalized or localized to the head—CT and MRI of the brain and radiography of the spine usually normal
• Maltese dogs with generalized tremor syndrome—CT; reveals hydrocephalus; importance of this finding uncertain
• Hypomyelination—MRI; may reveal evidence of lack of myelin

DIAGNOSTIC PROCEDURES
• CSF analysis—usually helpful in establishing diagnosis of generalized tremor syndrome and other causes of encephalitis
• Suspected lumbosacral syndrome—survey radiography; CSF analysis; electromyography of limb muscles; myelography; epidurography with or without discography; CT; and MRI; look for evidence of a lumbar spinal compressive lesion.
• Suspected primary brain disease—CSF analysis (assess underlying brain inflammation); CT or MRI (assess intracranial structures); BAER (assess central auditory pathways and overall brainstem function)

 TREATMENT
• Treat the underlying primary disease.
• Outpatient, unless surgical treatment is indicated (lumbosacral disease that requires decompression and stabilization)
• Avoid excitement and exercise—may worsen many tremors
• Generalized tremor of primary brain origin—patient may lose weight; monitor weight and modify oral intake accordingly.
• Most of the causes in adult dogs are treatable.
• Degenerative neurologic diseases (e.g., storage disease and spongiform encephalopathy)—no treatment available

• Hypomyelination—generally not treatable; some breeds improve with maturity (e.g., chow chows)
• Idiopathic head tremor—no effective treatment available; benign tremor that occurs sporadically; has few health consequences
• Drug-induced—consider an alternate drug.
• Suspected intoxication—remove patient from further exposure; consult with a poison control center for possible antidote.

 MEDICATIONS

DRUGS OF CHOICE
• Usually do not respond to muscle relaxants or anticonvulsants (e.g., phenobarbital or diazepam)
• Corticosteroids—immunosuppression; for generalized tremor syndrome
• Antibiotics—for diskospondylitis; choose on the basis of culture and sensitivity of the lesion, blood, or urine.
• Cerebellar diseases—depends on the diagnosis

CONTRAINDICATIONS
Sympathomimetic drugs—may worsen condition

PRECAUTIONS
N/A

POSSIBLE INTERACTIONS
N/A

ALTERNATIVE DRUGS
N/A

 FOLLOW-UP

PATIENT MONITORING
• Monitor the primary disease.
• Corticosteroids for generalized tremor syndrome—monitor weekly initially to assess response to treatment.

POSSIBLE COMPLICATIONS
N/A

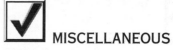 **MISCELLANEOUS**

ASSOCIATED CONDITIONS
N/A

AGE-RELATED FACTORS
N/A

ZOONOTIC POTENTIAL
N/A

PREGNANCY
N/A

SYNONYMS
• Shaking
• Shuddering

SEE ALSO
• Cerebellar Degeneration
• Hypomyelination, Central and Peripheral Nervous System
• See also Causes

ABBREVIATIONS
• BAER = brainstem auditory-evoked response
• CSF = cerebrospinal fluid

Suggesting Reading

Bagley RS. Tremor syndromes in dogs: diagnosis and treatment. J Small Anim Pract 1992;33:485–490.

Cuddon PA. Tremor syndromes. Prog Vet Neurol 1990;1:285–299.

De Lahunta A. Veterinary neuroanatomy and clinical neurology. 2nd ed. Philadelphia: Saunders, 1983.

Farrow BH. Generalized tremor syndrome. In: Kirk RW, ed. Current veterinary therapy IX. Philadelphia: Saunders, 1986:880–881.

Kornegay JN, Thomson CE. Trembling and shaking. In: Ettinger SJ, ed. Textbook of veterinary internal medicine: diseases of the dog and cat. 3rd ed. Philadelphia: Saunders, 1989:54–56.

Wagner SO, Podell M, Fenner WR. Generalized tremors in dogs: 24 cases (1984–1995). J Vet Med Assoc 1997;211:731–735.

Author Rodney S. Bagley
Consulting Editor Joane M. Parent

URINE RETENTION, FUNCTIONAL

 BASICS

DEFINITION
Incomplete voiding not associated with urinary obstruction

PATHOPHYSIOLOGY
Usually a disorder of the voiding phase of micturition; incomplete voiding results from hypocontractility of the urinary bladder (detrusor atony) or from inappropriately excessive outlet resistance (functional urinary obstruction).

SYSTEMS AFFECTED
• Renal/Urologic
• Endocrine/Metabolic
• Nervous

SIGNALMENT
More common in male than female dogs and cats; see Causes.

SIGNS
• Palpably distended resting urinary bladder; after attempts by the animal to void, palpable distension may persist or inappropriate residual urine can be measured (normal < 0.5 mL/kg).
• Affected animals may demonstrate ineffective, frequent, or no attempts to void.
• Urine stream may be weak, attenuated, or interrupted.
• Abdominal distension, abdominal pain, or signs of postrenal azotemia may predominate in rare cases or with urinary tract rupture.
• May be an occult finding in patients with recurrent urinary tract infection
• May be overflow urinary incontinence

CAUSES

Hypocontractility of the Urinary Bladder Detrusor Muscle (Detrusor Atony)
• Most commonly develops as a sequel to acute or chronic urinary bladder overdistension; many patients have a history of neurologic dysfunction or previous urinary obstruction.
• Neurogenic causes include lesions of the pelvic nerves, sacral spinal cord, and suprasacral spinal cord.
• Lesions of the sacral spinal cord (e.g., congenital malformations, cauda equina compression, lumbosacral disk disease, and vertebral fractures/dislocations) can result in a flaccid, overdistended urinary bladder with weak outlet resistance. Urine retention and overflow (paradoxical) urinary incontinence are observed.
• Lesions of the suprasacral spinal cord (e.g., intervertebral disk protrusion, spinal fractures, and compressive neoplasms) can result in a distended, firm urinary bladder

that is difficult to express.
• Electrolyte disturbances, including hyperkalemia, hypokalemia, hypocalcemia, and hypercalcemia, and other metabolic disturbances associated with generalized muscle weakness can also affect detrusor muscle contractility.
• Detrusor atony with urine retention may be a feature of dysautonomia, a disturbance of autonomic ganglia primarily encountered in cats in Great Britain; the disorder has also been described in dogs in certain geographic regions of the United States.

Functional Urinary Obstruction
• Occurs when excessive or inappropriate outlet resistance prevents complete voiding during urinary bladder contraction
• In patients with suprasacral spinal lesions or midbrain disorders, urethral outlet resistance becomes uninhibited and remains inappropriately excessive or fails to coordinate with voiding contractions (detrusor-urethral dyssynergia). The condition has been associated with sacral lesions, local neuropathy, and idiopathic causes.
• Excessive urethral resistance, usually attributed to smooth or striated muscular components of the urethra (urethrospasm), may be seen after urethral obstruction or urethral or pelvic surgery, urethral inflammation, or prostatic disease.

RISK FACTORS
• Feline lower urinary tract disease
• Urethral obstruction
• Pelvic or urethral surgery
• Anticholinergic medications

DIAGNOSIS

DIFFERENTIAL DIAGNOSIS
• When no voiding is observed, must be differentiated from oliguria, anuria, and urinary tract rupture
• Must be differentiated from physical and mechanical obstruction; clinical signs of urinary obstruction include pollakiuria, stranguria, and hematuria; patients with mechanical obstruction may void a few drops of urine after long periods of straining.
• Neurologic findings in dogs with supraspinal lesions affecting micturition include paralysis or paresis of pelvic ± thoracic limbs, hyper-reflexia of affected limbs, and cervical, thoracolumbar, and lumbar pain. The urinary bladder is usually distended, firm, and difficult to express. In patients with chronic or partial lesions, reflexive voiding may return, characterized by incomplete, involuntary

detrusor contractions with outlet spasticity.
• Neurologic findings in dogs with sacral lesions affecting micturition include pelvic limb paresis with hyporeflexia, depressed anal and tail tone, perineal sensory loss, and depressed bulbospongiosus reflexes. The urinary bladder is typically distended, flaccid, and fairly easy to express.
• A urine stream that can be initiated but is abruptly tapered or halted is typical of idiopathic detrusor-urethral dyssynergia. Manual palpation may confirm detrusor contractions, which persist after flow terminates, and may suggest a high residual volume of urine.
• In patients recovering from urinary obstruction, inability to void may result from reobstruction, excessive (functional) urethral resistance, or detrusor atony caused by over-distension. If the urinary bladder can be expressed with gentle manual compression of the urinary bladder, detrusor atony is likely. If resistance to manual expression is encountered and urethral obstruction can be ruled out by examination or catheterization, functional obstruction is likely.
• Clinical signs accompanying urine retention in patients with dysautonomia include mydriasis, prolapsed third eyelids, regurgitation or vomiting, and diarrhea or constipation.

CBC/BIOCHEMISTRY/URINALYSIS
• Results of hemogram and serum biochemical profile may rule in or rule out metabolic causes of muscle weakness; also used to detect severity of postrenal azotemia
• Urinalysis and urine sediment examination may reveal evidence of urinary tract infection or inflammation.

OTHER LABORATORY TESTS
N/A

IMAGING
• Contrast cystourethrography or vagino-urethrography—use to rule out obstructive lesions
• Myelography or epidurography—use to localize neurologic lesions

DIAGNOSTIC PROCEDURES
• Neurologic examination—a brief assessment of caudal spinal and peripheral nerve function is provided by examination of anal tone, tail tone, perineal sensation, and bulbospongiosus reflexes.
• Urethral catheterization—may be required to rule out urethral obstruction; catheters should pass easily in animals with no mechanical obstruction and in those with extramural urethral compression (e.g., that caused by a smooth bladder neck mass, a large

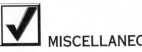

URINE RETENTION, FUNCTIONAL

prostate gland, or a caudal abdominal mass).
• Testing for dysautonomia includes a number of tests of autonomic responses.
• Urodynamic procedures—may use to confirm detrusor atony or functional urethral obstruction or to document detrusor-urethral dyssynergia; detrusor areflexia may be documented by cystometrographic studies; inappropriate urethral resistance or urethral spasm occasionally is documented by resting urethral profilometry; combined cystometry and urethral pressure measurements, or uroflow studies, are necessary to document dyssynergia.

TREATMENT

• Usually managed as inpatients until adequate voiding function returns
• Address primary disorders such as electrolyte disturbances and neurologic lesions and correct if possible.
• Manage azotemia, electrolyte imbalances, and acid–base disturbances associated with acute urine retention appropriately.
• Identify urinary tract infection and treat appropriately.
• May consider surgical options for salvaging urethral patency in some patients; perineal urethrostomy may be required in male cats with unmanageable distal urethral resistance
• Keep the urinary bladder small by intermittent or indwelling catheterization or frequent manual compression; intermittent or indwelling urinary catheterization may be required temporarily to ensure urine flow.

MEDICATIONS

DRUGS OF CHOICE

Detrusor Atony
• Bethanechol—a cholinergic, parasympathomimetic agent; may increase detrusor contractile input in partially denervated or acutely overdistended urinary bladders
• Metoclopramide—a dopamine antagonist with prokinetic activity in the gastrointestinal tract; may stimulate detrusor contraction as well
• Cisapride—a smooth muscle prokinetic agent; thought to enhance acetylcholine release; may promote bladder emptying

Functional Urethral Obstruction
• Phenoxybenzamine—an α-adrenergic antagonist; reduces smooth muscle contraction in the urethra; more effective in dogs than in cats; prazosin is an alternative, potent α-antagonist.

• Diazepam—a short-acting, central skeletal muscle relaxant; relaxes striated muscle of the external urethral sphincter
• Acepromazine—a phenothiazine tranquilizer; has general muscle relaxant and α-blocking effects on urethral tone; may be effective in cats with excessive urethral resistance
• Dantrolene—another striated muscle relaxant; acts via calcium antagonist properties; appears to be effective in reducing distal urethral resistance in cats
• Baclofen—a spinal reflex inhibitor; acts as a skeletal muscle relaxant; clinical use in small animals has been limited.

CONTRAINDICATIONS
• Baclofen in cats
• Acepromazine, phenoxybenzamine, and prazosin have vasodilatory effects—avoid volume-depleted or azotemic patients as well as those with cardiac disease.
• Acepromazine and diazepam—can cause sedation; avoid in lethargic patients

PRECAUTIONS
• Ensure an adequate outlet for urine flow before administering bethanechol. Phenoxybenzamine or prazosin is frequently administered concurrently, since bethanechol can increase muscular contraction of the urinary bladder neck and proximal urethra.
• Acute hepatopathy—described as a rare complication of prolonged oral administration of diazepam in cats

POSSIBLE INTERACTIONS
N/A

ALTERNATIVE DRUGS
N/A

FOLLOW-UP

PATIENT MONITORING
• As treatment progresses, assess residual urine volume by urinary bladder palpation or by periodic urinary catheterization.
• In most patients, can slowly withdraw medications after primary causes are corrected and adequate voiding function has been sustained for several days
• Perform periodic urinalysis in patients with chronic urine retention to detect urinary tract infection.
• Advise clients that complete voiding function may not return and that pets should be monitored for signs of complete obstruction or uremia.

POSSIBLE COMPLICATIONS
• Lower urinary tract and ascending infection
• Permanent detrusor muscle injury and atony; urinary bladder or urethral rupture
• Postrenal azotemia

☑ MISCELLANEOUS

ASSOCIATED CONDITIONS
• Urinary tract infection
• Azotemia

AGE-RELATED FACTORS
N/A

ZOONOTIC POTENTIAL
N/A

PREGNANCY
Bethanechol is contraindicated.

SYNONYMS
• Dysfunctional voiding
• Neuropathic bladder
• Reflex dyssynergia, detrusor-urethral dyssynergia
• Urethrospasm

SEE ALSO
• Urinary Tract Obstruction
• Intervertebral Disk Disease, Thoracolumbar
• Lumbosacral Stenosis
• Prostatitis and Prostatic Abscess
• Feline Idiopathic Lower Urinary Tract Disease
• Dysuria and Pollakiuria
• Creatinine and Blood Urea Nitrogen (BUN)—Azotemia and Uremia

ABBREVIATIONS
N/A

Suggested Reading

Barsanti JA. Urinary incontinence. In: Lorenz MD, Cornelius LM, eds. Small animal medical diagnosis. 2nd ed. Philadelphia: Lippincott, 1993:345–356.

Lees GE. Management of voiding disability following relief of urethral obstruction. In: August J, ed. Consultations in feline internal medicine. 2nd ed. Philadelphia: Saunders, 1994:365–372.

Moreau PM, Lappin MR. Pharmacologic manipulation of micturition. In: Kirk RW, ed. Current veterinary therapy X. Small animal practice. Philadelphia: Saunders, 1989: 1214–1222.

Moreau PM, Lees GE. Urinary obstruction and atony. In: Ettinger SJ, ed. Textbook of veterinary internal medicine. 3rd ed. Philadelphia: Saunders, 1989:155–159.

Author India F. Lane
Consulting Editors Larry G. Adams and Carl A. Osborne

URINARY TRACT OBSTRUCTION

BASICS

DEFINITION
Restricted flow of urine from the kidneys through the urinary tract to the external urethral orifice

PATHOPHYSIOLOGY
• Excess resistance to urine flow through the urinary tract develops because of lesions affecting the excretory pathway, which cause increased pressure in the urinary space proximal to the obstruction and may cause abnormal distension of this space with urine. Ensuing pathophysiologic consequences depend on the site, degree, and duration of obstruction. Complete obstruction produces a pathophysiologic state equivalent to oliguric acute renal failure.
• Perforation of the excretory pathway with extravasation of urine is functionally equivalent.

SYSTEMS AFFECTED
• Renal/Urologic
• Gastrointestinal, Cardiovascular, Nervous, and Respiratory systems as uremia develops

SIGNALMENT
More common in males than females

SIGNS

Historical Findings
• Pollakiuria (common)
• Stranguria
• Reduced velocity or caliber of the urine stream or no urine flow during voiding
• Gross hematuria
• Signs of uremia that develop when urinary tract obstruction is complete (or nearly complete): lethargy, dull attitude, reduced appetite, and vomiting

Physical Examination Findings
• Excessive (i.e., overly large or turgid) or inappropriate (i.e., remains after voiding efforts), palpable distension of the urinary bladder
• Uroliths are often palpable in the urethras of obstructed male dogs.
• Occasionally, palpable renomegaly is discovered in an animal with chronic partial ureteral obstruction, especially when the lesion is unilateral.
• Signs of severe uremia—dehydration, weakness, hypothermia, bradycardia with moderate hyperkalemia, high rate of shallow respirations, stupor or coma, seizures occurring terminally, tachycardia resulting from ventricular dysrhythmias induced by severe hyperkalemia
• Signs of perforation of the excretory pathway—leakage of urine into the peritoneal cavity causes abdominal pain and distension; leakage of urine into periurethral spaces causes pain and swelling in intrapelvic or

perineal tissues, depending on the site of the urethral injury; fever

CAUSES

Intraluminal Causes
• Solid or semisolid structures including uroliths, urethral plugs in cats, blood clots, and sloughed tissue fragments
• Most common site—the urethra
• Urolithiasis—most common cause in male dogs*
• Urethral plugs—most common cause in male cats*

Intramural Causes
• Neoplasia of the bladder neck or urethra—common cause in dogs
• Pyogranulomatous inflammatory lesions in the urethra—seen occasionally in dogs
• Fibrosis at a site of prior injury or inflammation can cause stricture or stenosis, which may impede urine flow or may be a site where intraluminal debris becomes lodged.
• Prostatic disorders in male dogs
• Edema, hemorrhage, or spasm of muscular components can occur at sites of intraluminal (e.g., urethral) obstruction and contribute to persistent or recurrent obstruction to urinary flow after removal of the intraluminal material. Tissue changes might develop because of injury inflicted by the obstructing material, by the manipulations used to remove the obstructing material, or both.
• Ruptures, lacerations, and punctures—usually caused by traumatic incidents

Miscellaneous Causes
• Displacement of the urinary bladder into a perineal hernia
• Neurogenic (see Urinary Retention, Functional)

RISK FACTORS
• Urolithiasis, particularly in males
• Feline lower urinary tract disease, particularly in males
• Prostatic disease in male dogs

DIAGNOSIS

DIFFERENTIAL DIAGNOSIS
• Repeated unproductive squatting in the litter box by a cat that has a urethral obstruction can be misinterpreted as constipation.
• Animals whose efforts to urinate are not observed by their owners can be examined because of signs referable to uremia without a history of possible obstruction.
• Evaluation of any patient with azotemia should include consideration of possible postrenal causes (e.g., urinary obstruction). See Creatinine and Blood Urea Nitrogen (BUN)—Azotemia and Uremia, for differential diagnosis of this problem.

• Patients with a ruptured urinary bladder can exhibit clinical signs (e.g., anorexia, vomiting, diarrhea, depression, lethargy, weakness, and collapse) and laboratory test results (azotemia, hyperkalemia and hyponatremia) similar to those commonly seen in patients with hypoadrenocorticism (Addison's disease).
• Once existence of urinary obstruction is recognized, diagnostic efforts focus on detecting the presence and evaluating the magnitude of abnormalities secondary to obstruction, and identifying the location, cause, and completeness of the impediment(s) to urine flow.

CBC/BIOCHEMISTRY/URINALYSIS
• Results of a hemogram are usually normal, but a stress leukogram may be seen.
• Biochemistry analysis reveals azotemia, hyperphosphatemia, metabolic acidosis, and hyperkalemia proportional to the duration of complete obstruction.
• Hematuria and proteinuria are common; crystalluria supports a diagnosis of urolithiasis, and atypical epithelial cells may be seen in patients with neoplasia.

OTHER LABORATORY TESTS
Uroliths passed or retrieved should be sent for crystallographic analysis to determine their composition.

IMAGING

Abdominal Radiography
• Uroliths—often demonstrated by survey radiography; some are difficult or impossible to see because of their size, composition, or location.
• Positive-contrast urethrography is the most sensitive method of detecting intraluminal and intramural lesions of the urethra; double-contrast cystography is the most sensitive method of detecting lesions of the bladder lumen and wall.
• Upper urinary tract (i.e., ureter or renal pelvis) obstruction can be detected by excretory urography if enough renal function is preserved on the affected side(s) so that radiographic contrast media is excreted and sufficiently concentrated to be seen proximal to the obstruction.

Abdominal Ultrasonography
Ultrasonography is highly sensitive for detecting lesions of the bladder and proximal urethra (including the prostate gland in male dogs) and upper urinary tract (i.e., ureter or renal pelvis) obstruction.

DIAGNOSTIC PROCEDURES
• Electrocardiography may detect abnormalities secondary to hyperkalemia, including tall T waves, prolonged PR interval, bradycardia, and atrial standstill.
• Urinary catheterization has diagnostic and therapeutic value. As the catheter is inserted, the location and nature of obstructing material

may be determined. Some or all of the obstructing material (e.g., small uroliths and feline urethral plugs) may be induced to pass out of the urethra distally for identification and analysis. Retrograde irrigation of the urethral lumen may propel intraluminal debris toward the bladder. Although intramural lesions sometimes are detected during catheterization, catheter insertion can be normal. Animals that cannot urinate despite generating adequate intravesicular pressure (i.e., excessive outlet resistance) and have urethras that can be readily catheterized and irrigated either have intramural lesions or functional urinary retention.

• Cytologic evaluation of specimens obtained from the urinary tract with the assistance of catheters may be diagnostic, particularly for carcinoma of the urethra or bladder and some prostatic diseases. Prostatic massage or physical manipulation of the catheter tip positioned near the suspected lesion is used to produce cell-rich specimens that are retrieved through the catheter by aspiration or washing with saline in an attached syringe.

• Cystoscopy can be helpful, particularly in female dogs with intramural lesions of the bladder neck or urethra.

TREATMENT

APPROPRIATE HEALTH CARE
• Complete obstruction is a medical emergency that can be life-threatening; treatment should usually be started immediately.
• Partial obstruction—not necessarily an emergency, but these patients may be at risk for developing complete obstruction; may cause irreversible urinary tract damage if not treated promptly
• Treat as an inpatient until the patient's ability to urinate has been restored.
• Surgery is sometimes required.
• Long-term management and prognosis depend on the cause of the obstruction.
• Treatment has three major components: combating the metabolic derangements associated with postrenal uremia (e.g., dehydration, hypothermia, acidosis, hyperkalemia, and azotemia); restoring and maintaining a patent pathway for urine outflow; and implementing specific treatment for the underlying cause of urine retention.

NURSING CARE
Give fluid therapy to patients with dehydration or azotemia. Give fluids intravenously if systemic derangements are moderately severe or worse. Lactated Ringer's solution is the fluid of choice, except for patients with severe hyperkalemia (i.e., >8.0 mEq/L and/or ECG changes), in which the fluid of choice is 0.45% saline and 2.5% dextrose solution

with addition of sodium bicarbonate (1–2 mEq/kg slow bolus). Normal saline with added dextrose (2.5% IV) is an alternative fluid choice for patients with dehydration and hyperkalemia. Combat cardiotoxic effects of hyperkalemia that are immediately life-threatening by giving calcium gluconate (2–10 mL 10% solution IV slowly to effect). As soon as hyperkalemia and its effects have abated, use lactated Ringer's solution.

MEDICATIONS

DRUGS OF CHOICE
Procedures for relief of obstruction often require, or are facilitated by, giving sedatives or anesthetics. When substantial systemic derangements exist, start fluid administration and other supportive measures first. Careful decompression of the bladder by cystocentesis may be performed before anesthesia and catheterization. Calculate the dosage of sedative or anesthetic drug using the low end of the recommended range or give only to effect. Isoflurane is the anesthetic of choice; however, certainly a variety of other anesthetics or sedatives can give satisfactory results.

CONTRAINDICATIONS
Avoid intramuscular ketamine in patients with complete obstruction, because it is excreted through the kidneys. If the obstruction cannot be eliminated, prolonged sedation may result.

PRECAUTIONS
Avoid drugs that reduce blood pressure or induce cardiac dysrhythmia until dehydration and hyperkalemia are resolved.

POSSIBLE INTERACTIONS
None

ALTERNATIVE DRUGS
N/A

FOLLOW-UP

PATIENT MONITORING
• Assess urine production and hydration status frequently, and adjust fluid administration rate accordingly.
• Verify ability to urinate adequately or use urinary catheterization to combat urine retention.
• Indwelling catheterization with closed drainage is appropriate if catheter insertion requires chemical restraint or is unduly traumatic, but frequent brief catheterization is a better choice if catheter can readily be inserted repeatedly (i.e., as in some male dogs).
• When the ECG indicates life-threatening changes, use continuous monitoring initially to guide treatment and evaluate response.

POSSIBLE COMPLICATIONS
• Death
• Injury to the excretory pathway while trying to relieve obstruction
• Hypokalemia during postobstruction diuresis
• Recurrence of obstruction

MISCELLANEOUS

ASSOCIATED CONDITIONS
• Bradycardia secondary to hyperkalemia
• Azotemia, hyperphosphatemia, and metabolic acidosis

AGE-RELATED FACTORS
In old dogs, the underlying cause of obstruction (e.g., tumor and prostate disease) often is difficult to treat effectively.

ZOONOTIC POTENTIAL
N/A

PREGNANCY
N/A

SYNONYMS
Urethral obstruction

SEE ALSO
• Creatinine and Blood Urea Nitrogen (BUN)—Azotemia and Uremia
• Feline Idiopathic Lower Urinary Tract Disease
• Hydronephrosis
• Potassium, Hyperkalemia
• Urinary Retention, Functional

ABBREVIATIONS
None

Suggested Reading

Barsanti JA, Finco DR, Brown SA. Feline urethral obstruction: medical management. In: Kirk RW, Bonagura JD, eds. Current veterinary therapy, XI, 9th ed. Philadelphia: Saunders, 1992:883–885.

Labato MA. Urologic emergencies. In: Murtaugh RJ, Kaplan PM, eds. Veterinary emergency and critical care medicine. St. Louis: Mosby-Year Book, 1992:295–320.

Littman MP. Urinary obstruction and atony. In: Ettinger SJ, Feldman EC, eds. Textbook of veterinary internal medicine. 4th ed. Philadelphia: Saunders, 1995:169–172.

Stone EA, Barsanti JA. Urologic surgery of the dog and cat. Philadelphia: Lea & Febiger, 1992.

Author George E. Lees
Consulting Editors Larry G. Adams and Carl A. Osborne

VAGINAL DISCHARGE

BASICS

DEFINITION
Any substance emanating from the vulvar labia

PATHOPHYSIOLOGY
May originate from several distinct sources, depending in part on the age and reproductive status of the patient; from urinary tract, uterus, vagina, vestibule, clitoris, or perivulvar skin; may be normal or abnormal

SYSTEMS AFFECTED
• Reproductive
• Renal/Urologic
• Skin/Exocrine

SIGNALMENT
• Prepubertal bitches—anomalies and prepubertal vaginitis more common
• Estrual and postpartum bitches—normal discharges common
• Postestrual, pregnant, and postpartum bitches—may be more serious

SIGNS

Historical Findings
• Discharge from the vulva
• Spotting
• Scooting
• Attracting males
• Parturition—with postpartum discharge
• Estrus during the preceding 2 months—with pyometra

PHYSICAL EXAMINATION FINDINGS
• Blood
• Lochia
• Pus
• Urine
• Feces

CAUSES

Serosanguinous
• Normal during proestrus and sometimes into estrus
• Urinary tract infection
• Foreign body
• Vaginal neoplasia—transmissible venereal tumor; leiomyoma
• Vaginal trauma
• Fetal death
• Vaginal hematoma
• Ovarian neoplasia

Lochia and Postpartum
• Normal postpartum discharge—for 6–8 weeks
• Subinvolution of placental sites—discharge lasting longer than 8 weeks
• Retained placentas
• Metritis

Purulent Exudate
• Normal in early diestrus (slight)
• Prepubertal vaginitis
• Primary vaginitis
• Secondary vaginitis—from anomaly, foreign body, urinary tract infection, clitoral hypertrophy, vaginal neoplasia, and fetal death
• Pyometra
• Embryonic and fetal death
• Postpartum metritis
• Perivulvar dermatitis
• Zinc toxicity—reported

Other
• Urine or feces—with congenital anomaly
• Acquired perivulvar dermatitis can also be mistaken for vaginal discharge
• Urine from ectopic ureters or incontinence from hypoestrogenism
• Normal mucus discharge during pregnancy

RISK FACTORS
• Exogenous androgens—may cause clitoral hypertrophy
• Prophylactic antibiotics—may alter the normal vaginal flora
• Exogenous estrogens given during late estrus and diestrus—predispose patient to pyometra

DIAGNOSIS

DIFFERENTIAL DIAGNOSES
• History and signalment—establish risk of anomaly and hormonal influences (e.g., estrus, diestrus, pregnancy, and parturition)
• Source and type of the discharge—must be identified by appropriate diagnostics

CBC/BIOCHEMISTRY/URINALYSIS
• Leukocytosis with a left shift—with pyometra or metritis
• High BUN and creatinine—with pyometra
• Isosthenuria—with polyuria and polydipsia associated with pyometra
• Urinary tract infection—may be noted
• Otherwise, unremarkable

OTHER LABORATORY TESTS
• Serum progesterone concentration—determine if the bitch is in diestrus and more likely to have pyometra
• Rapid slide agglutination test—helps rule out *Brucella canis*

IMAGING
• Radiography—detect a large uterus in patients with metritis or pyometra and later stages of fetal death; cannot differentiate early pregnancy from pyometra
• Contrast radiography of the vagina—helps rule out vaginal neoplasia, urethrovaginal stricture, and rectovaginal stricture
• Ultrasonography—determine pregnancy as early as the 14th day of diestrus; heartbeats seen as early as the 20th day of diestrus; fetal heartbeats and movement rule out fetal death; fetal distress considered if fetal heart rate < 200 bpm

VAGINAL DISCHARGE

DIAGNOSTIC PROCEDURES

- Vaginal bacterial culture—via guarded Culturette (AccuCulShure); perform before doing any other vaginal procedure.
- Vaginal cytologic examination—determine if the discharge is purulent, blood, or feces; extent of cornification determines the estrogen influence and helps establish whether the bitch is in proestrus or estrus.
- Vaginoscopy—reveal anomalies and bands; may need an endoscope to see the anterior vagina; cervix not usually seen by endoscopy (except possibly in large dogs); differentiates fluid emanating from the uterus from vaginal and vestibular discharges
- Digital examination of the vagina—help identify vaginal anomalies (e.g., bands, strictures, and persistent hymen) and tumors
- Cystocentesis and bacterial culture—help rule out urinary tract infection
- Biopsy of vaginal mass—rule out neoplasia

TREATMENT

- Outpatient, unless metritis or pyometra noted (ovariohysterectomy may be indicated)
- Medical treatment for pyometra—performed in a hospital and with great care
- Remove or treat any inciting cause—foreign body; neoplasia; anomaly; urinary tract infection; exogenous androgens or estrogens
- Prepubertal vaginitis—usually resolves spontaneously after the first estrus
- Supportive fluids—for pyometra if the patient is not extremely ill; for metritis if the patient is ill
- Subinvolution of placental sites

MEDICATIONS

DRUGS OF CHOICE

- Pyometra—prostaglandin and systemic antibiotics if the patient is not extremely ill (see Pyometra and Cystic Endometrial Hyperplasia)
- Prepubertal vaginitis—diethylstilbestrol to induce estrus may help; long-term effects not documented; 5 mg PO q24h for up to 7 days; day 1 of bleeding is day 1 of the induced cycle; continue treatment for an additional 2 days.
- Primary vaginitis—systemic antibiotics; vaginal douches
- Metritis—systemic antibiotics if the patient is ill
- Transmissible venereal tumor—vincristine

CONTRAINDICATIONS

Many antibiotics are contraindicated during pregnancy.

PRECAUTIONS

- Estrogens—increase the risk of pyometra if given during diestrus
- Prostaglandins—cause transient vomiting, diarrhea, and possibly hypotension

POSSIBLE INTERACTIONS

Estrogen during diestrus—associated with increased risk of pyometra

ALTERNATIVE DRUGS

N/A

FOLLOW-UP

PATIENT MONITORING

Ultrasonography or radiography—determine uterine size and contents with pyometra or metritis

POSSIBLE COMPLICATIONS

Toxic shock—with severe pyometra or metritis

MISCELLANEOUS

ASSOCIATED CONDITIONS

N/A

AGE-RELATED FACTORS

- Puppies—prepubertal vaginitis; anomalies; ectopic ureters
- Old—pyometra

ZOONOTIC POTENTIAL

B. canis—common with postpartum lochia caused by abortion or stillbirth; rare with vaginitis

PREGNANCY

Many antibiotics are contraindicated during pregnancy.

SEE ALSO

See Causes

Suggested Reading

Bouchard G. Estrus induction in the bitch using DES. Proceedings of the Annual Meeting of the Society of Theriogenology, 1994:176–184.

Johnson CA. Diagnosis and treatment of chronic vaginitis in the bitch. Vet Clin North Am Small Anim Pract 1991;21:523–531.

Memon MA, Mickelson WD. Clinical management of bitches with vaginal discharge during pregnancy. Semin Vet Med Surg Small Anim 1994;9:38–40.

Reberg SR, Peter AT, Blevins WE. Subinvolution of placental sites in dogs. Compend Contin Educ Pract Vet 1992;14:789–793.

Romagnoli SE, Johnston SD. Vulvar discharge. In: Allen DG, ed., Small animal medicine. Philadelphia: Lippincott, 1991:763–779.

Wykes PM, Soderberg SF. Disorders of the canine vagina. In: Morgan RV, ed. Handbook of small animal practice. 2nd ed. New York: Churchill Livingstone, 1992:661–666.

Author Bruce E. Eilts

Consulting Editor Sara K. Lyle

VOMITING, ACUTE

BASICS

DEFINITION
• Forceful, reflex expulsion of gastric contents from the oral cavity
• Acute vomiting is defined as vomiting of short duration (<7 days) and variable frequency.

PATHOPHYSIOLOGY
• A complex set of reflex activities under central neurologic control involving the coordination of GI, abdominal, and respiratory musculature
• Often preceded by prodromal signs of nausea that can include depression, shivering, hiding or seeking comfort, hypersalivation, lip licking, frequent swallowing, and retching
• Occurs when the VC in the medulla is stimulated by afferent activity from several sources
• Stimulation can occur from stretch receptors, chemoreceptors, and osmoreceptors located throughout the GI tract, hepatobiliary system, genitourinary system, peritoneum, and pancreas.
• The CTZ, when stimulated by a variety of drugs and toxins, can also stimulate the VC.
• Higher centers can lead to psychogenic vomiting and input from the vestibular apparatus (e.g., motion sickness, vestibular disease) can stimulate the VC.

SYSTEMS AFFECTED
• Cardiovascular—hypovolemia, causing tachycardia, pale mucous membranes, and weak pulses; hypokalemia can cause arrhythmias.
• GI—reflux esophagitis
• Metabolic—electrolyte and acid–base abnormalities (e.g., hypokalemia, hyponatremia, hypochloremia, metabolic alkalosis), prerenal azotemia, and dehydration
• Respiratory—aspiration pneumonia, rhinitis from ingesta refluxed into the nasopharynx
• Nervous—depression

SIGNALMENT
No age, breed, or sex predisposition

SIGNS

Historical Findings
• Variable vomiting of food, fluid (either clear or bile or blood-stained), or both
• Ingestion of foreign material
• Variable lethargy and appetite; may be diarrhea, and melena

Physical Examination Findings
• May include dehydration, (e.g., dry mucous membranes, reduced skin turgor, pale mucous membranes, tachycardia, weak pulses), fluid-filled bowel loops, excessive gut sounds, abdominal pain (localized [e.g., foreign body, pancreatitis, pyelonephritis, hepatic disease] vs. diffuse [e.g., peritonitis, severe enteritis]), or abdominal mass (e.g., foreign body, intussusceptum, torsed viscus)
• May note diarrhea or melena on rectal examination
• May see fever with infectious and inflammatory causes

CAUSES
• Adverse food reactions—indiscretions (eating rapidly, ingestion of foreign material); intolerances (e.g., sudden diet change, allergies)
• Drugs—antibiotics, antiinflammatories (corticosteroid and NSAIDs), chemotherapeutics, digitalis, narcotics, xylazine, thiacetarsamide
• Gastrointestinal inflammation—infectious enteritis: viruses (parvo, distemper, corona), bacteria (salmonella, Campylobacter); hemorrhagic gastroenteritis
• Gastroduodenal ulcers
• Gastrointestinal obstruction—foreign bodies, intussusception, neoplasia, volvulus, ileus, constipation
• Systemic disease—uremia, hepatic failure, sepsis, acidosis, electrolyte imbalance (hypokalemia, hypocalcemia, hypercalcemia)
• Abdominal disorders—pancreatitis, peritonitis, pyometra
• Endocrine disease—hypoadrenocorticism, diabetic ketoacidosis
• Neurologic disease—vestibular disturbances, meningitis, encephalitis, CNS trauma
• Parasitism—*Tricuspis* (dogs), ascarids, *Giardia, Physaloptera* (dogs), *Ollulanus tricuspis* (cats), salmon poisoning (dogs)
• Toxins—lead, ethylene glycol, zinc, mycotoxins, household plants
• Miscellaneous—anaphylaxis, heat stroke, motion sickness, pain, fear

RISK FACTORS
N/A

DIAGNOSIS

DIFFERENTIAL DIAGNOSIS

Differentiating Similar Signs
• Vomiting usually includes hypersalivation, retching, and forceful contractions of the abdominal muscles and diaphragm.
• Must always be differentiated from regurgitation, which is the effortless expulsion of fluid or food from the esophagus or pharyngeal cavity, and dysphagia (difficulty in swallowing), which is observed during eating or drinking
• Animals that are vomiting may have disorders that additionally cause regurgitation, and frequent vomiting can lead to reflux esophagitis and regurgitation.

Differentiating Causes
• Classify patients as serious or nonserious cases.
• If no signs of serious vomiting (e.g., dehydration, lethargy, fever, anorexia, or abdominal pain), can assess with a thorough history and physical examination alone.
• When indications of serious vomiting exist, when frequency intensifies, or signs do not resolve over 2–3 days, obtain a minimum database (including CBC, biochemical analysis, urinalysis, and survey abdominal radiographs) in an attempt to find the primary cause.

CBC/BIOCHEMISTRY/URINALYSIS
• In nonsevere vomiting the hemogram, biochemical profile, and urinalysis are typically normal.
• Dehydration—may see hemoconcentration (high PCV and total protein)
• May see a stress leukogram
• Infectious or inflammatory causes—may see an inflammatory leukogram
• Differentiate prerenal azotemia from renal causes by urine specific gravity.
• Acute hepatopathies—may see elevated liver enzymes and serum bilirubin or hypoglycemia
• Pancreatitis—may see elevated lipase, amylase, and liver enzymes and hypocalcemia
• Hyponatremia, hyperkalemia, and azotemia suggest hypoadrenocorticism.
• Hyperglycemia with glucosuria and ketonuria indicates ketoacidotic diabetic mellitus.

VOMITING, ACUTE

OTHER LABORATORY TESTS

Additional blood tests for specific diseases when indicated (e.g., blood lead level, ethylene glycol assay, ACTH stimulation for hypoadrenocorticism)

IMAGING

• Survey abdominal radiographs are often normal, but radiodense foreign bodies, segmental ileus, or gastric distension indicating volvulus or outflow obstruction may be observed; serosal detail may be lost ("ground glass" appearance) with pancreatitis or peritonitis; a mass effect or haziness in the right cranial quadrant or persistent gas in the descending duodenum may indicate pancreatitis.
• Can use contrast radiography to evaluate for radiolucent foreign bodies, obstruction, intussusception, or volvulus.
• Can use abdominal ultrasonography to visualize a focally dilated bowel loop indicating an obstruction or a multilamellar abdominal mass indicating an intussusception or to confirm an enlarged hypoechoic pancreas typical of pancreatitis

DIAGNOSTIC PROCEDURES

Endoscopy may be useful to assess for gastroduodenal ulceration and gastric and proximal duodenal foreign bodies.

TREATMENT

• The most frequent cause of acute vomiting is dietary indiscretion.
• Patients with nonserious vomiting are treated on an outpatient basis, resting the GI tract by keeping the animal NPO for 12–24 h.
• If vomiting resolves, initially offer small amounts of water and/or ice cubes, followed by an easily digestible, low-fat, single-carbohydrate, and single-protein source diet, such as non-fat cottage cheese and rice.
• Recovery from nonserious vomiting is usually rapid and spontaneous.
• If vomiting does not recur, wean the patient back onto the normal diet over 4–5 days.
• Patients with serious vomiting should be hospitalized and treated initially NPO with intravenous crystalloid fluids while further diagnostics are performed.

MEDICATIONS

• NPO followed by a bland diet usually will control nonserious vomiting.
• Antiemetics can be used for frequent vomiting.

DRUGS OF CHOICE

• May use antiemetics in patients with severe vomiting causing electrolyte and/or acid–base disturbances or reflux esophagitis
• Several antiemetics are available for both dogs and cats—phenothiazine derivatives that act at the CTZ and VC include chlorpromazine (0.5–4 mg/kg SC q8h) and metoclopramide, a dopamine antagonist and motility modifier that acts at the CTZ and on local receptors in the gut (0.2–0.5 mg/kg PO or SC q6–8h , or 1–2 mg/kg/day as a CRI); H_1-receptor antagonists acting on the CTZ can be used in motion sickness (e.g., diphenhydramine 2–4 mg/kg PO, IM q6–8h)
• Patients with ulceration—can use H_2-receptor antagonists such as ranitidine (1–2 mg/kg PO, SC, IV q12h) and/or the gastric mucosal protectant, sucralfate (250 mg/cat PO q8–12h, 250–1000 mg/dog PO q8–12 h)
• Fever or mucosal injury (hematemesis, melena)—antibiotics may be indicated (e.g.. ampicillin, cephalothin).

CONTRAINDICATIONS

• Use phenothiazines with caution in dehydrated patients because of possible hypotension from their α-receptor antagonist effect; they also lower the seizure threshold and should be avoided in epileptics.
• Do not use anticholinergics; they can cause gastric atony and intestinal ileus, which could exacerbate vomiting.
• Do not use metoclopramide in patients with GI obstruction, because of its prokinetic effect.

PRECAUTIONS

Use antiemetics carefully; they may suppress vomiting and mask progressive disease or hamper an important means of monitoring response to primary therapy.

POSSIBLE INTERACTIONS

Anticholinergics negate the effect of metoclopramide.

ALTERNATIVE DRUGS

N/A

FOLLOW-UP

PATIENT MONITORING

• If frequency of vomiting increases or serious problems occur, hospitalize animals for treatment and obtain appropriate data.
• If vomiting persists beyond 7 days despite conservative therapy, pursue appropriate testing for chronic vomiting.

POSSIBLE COMPLICATIONS

N/A

MISCELLANEOUS

ASSOCIATED CONDITIONS

See Systems Affected

AGE-RELATED FACTORS

Young animals are more likely to ingest foreign objects and acquire viral, bacterial, and parasitic disease.

ZOONOTIC POTENTIAL

N/A

PREGNANCY

Misoprostol, a synthetic prostaglandin used most often in treatment or prevention of gastric ulceration, is contraindicated in pregnant animals.

SYNONYMS

N/A

SEE ALSO

• Gastroduodenal Ulcer Disease
• Diarrhea, Acute

ABBREVIATIONS

CRI = continuous-rate infusion
CTZ = chemoreceptor trigger zone
GI = gastrointestinal
PCV = packed cell volume
VC = vomiting center

Suggested Reading

Guilford WG, Strombeck DR. Acute gastritis. In: Guilford WG, et al., eds., Small animal gastroenterology. Philadelphia: Saunders, 1996:261–274.

Willard MD. Diseases of the stomach. In: Ettinger SJ, Feldman EC, eds., Textbook of veterinary internal medicine. Philadelphia: Saunders, 1995:1143–1168.

Author John Hart Jr.

Consulting Editors Brett M. Feder and Mitchell A. Crystal

VOMITING, CHRONIC

BASICS

DEFINITION
• Chronic vomiting is defined as either intermittent episodes of vomiting that have not responded to symptomatic treatment or persistent vomiting of long duration with variable frequency.

PATHOPHYSIOLOGY
• Vomiting occurs when the vomiting center, located within the medulla oblongata, is activated by humoral or neural stimulation of various peripheral receptors sensitive to chemicals, inflammation, and changes in osmolality.

SYSTEMS AFFECTED
• Endocrine/Metabolic—dehydration, electrolyte and acid–base imbalances, prerenal azotemia • Cardiovascular—hypovolemia or electrolyte and acid–base imbalances can cause arrhythmias • Gastrointestinal—gastroesophageal reflux, esophagitis and subsequent esophageal stricture • Respiratory system—aspiration pneumonia • Neurologic system—altered mentation

SIGNALMENT
• Dogs and cats • Young animals are more likely to ingest foreign bodies; linear foreign bodies are more common in cats. • Confirmed or suspected breed predispositions—Lhasa apso, shih tzu, and other brachycephalic breeds are prone to pyloric stenosis; basenjis, German shepherds and shar-peis are prone to inflammatory bowel diseases; rottweilers are prone to gastric eosinophilic granuloma; airdale terriers are prone to pancreatic carcinoma; beagles, Bedlington terriers, cocker spaniels, Doberman pinschers, Labrador retrievers, Skye terriers, and standard poodles are prone to chronic hepatitis.

SIGNS

Historical Findings
• Vomiting, regurgitation, or both, of food, clear or bile-stained fluid, hematemesis, decreased appetite or anorexia, pica, melena, polydipsia, and abdominal distension are typical of gastric disease. • Diarrhea and weight loss are more characteristic of intestinal disease. • Signs such as weakness, polyuria, or jaundice relate to other underlying metabolic diseases.

Physical Examination Findings
• May see poor haircoat, weight loss, abdominal distension, abdominal pain, palpably thickened bowel loops, or abdominal masses may be observed • Dry, pale, mucous membranes occur if the patient is dehydrated or anemic. • Increased gut sounds occasionally auscultated • Rectal examination may detect diarrhea, hematochezia, or melena.

CAUSES

Esophageal Disease
• Hiatal hernia • Gastroesophageal reflux • Distal esophagitis

Infectious Disease
• *Helicobacter*-related gastritis • Histoplasmosis • Pythiosis • Small intestinal bacterial overgrowth (SIBO) • Disseminated aspergillosis • Gastric parasites—*Physaloptera* spp. • Intestinal parasitism

Metabolic Diseases
• Renal disease • Hepatic disease • Biliary disease • Hypoadrenocorticism • Chronic pancreatitis • Ketoacidotic diabetes mellitus • Metabolic acidosis • Electrolyte abnormalities—hypokalemia, hyperkalemia, hyponatremia, hypercalcemia can alter motility

Inflammatory Bowel Disease (IBD)
• Lymphocytic, plasmacytic, eosinophilic, or granulomatous • Gastritis, enteritis, or colitis

Obstructive GI Disease
• Foreign body • Congenital pyloric stenosis • Chronic pyloric hypertrophic gastropathy • Intussusception

Neoplastic Disease
• Gastric polyps • GI lymphosarcoma, adenocarcinoma, fibrosarcoma • Pancreatic adenocarcinoma • Pancreatic gastrin-secreting tumor (gastrinoma) • Systemic mastocytosis

Neurologic
• Cerebral edema • CNS tumors • Encephalitis/meningoencephalitis • Vestibulitis

Motility Disorders
• Chronic enterogastric reflux • Diabetic gastroparesis • Postgastric dilatation • Postsurgical—gastric, pyloric, duodenal • Electrolyte imbalances

Miscellaneous
• Drug-induced (e.g., NSAIDs, glucocorticoids, antibiotics, antifungals) • Food intolerance/allergy • Toxicity

Additional Causes in Cats
• Parasitic—dirofilariasis, *Ollulanus tricuspis,* giardiasis • Inflammatory—cholecystitis, cholangiohepatitis • Metabolic—hyperthyroidism • Functional—obstipation

RISK FACTORS
Breed-associated disease (see Signalment).

DIAGNOSIS

DIFFERENTIAL DIAGNOSIS
• Initially, vomiting must be differentiated from dysphagia and regurgitation. • Dysphagia—characterized by difficulty with prehension and initiation of swallowing; indicates abnormality in the oral cavity, pharynx, or proximal esophagus • Regurgitation is a passive retrograde movement into the oronasal cavity of fluid and undigested food that has not yet reached the stomach. • Regurgitation—occurs without retching (forceful abdominal contractions); localizes disease to the esophagus • Vomiting is often preceded by restlessness, nausea, salivation, and repeated swallowing. • Retching and expulsion of partially digested food and clear or bile-stained liquid, sometimes with digested blood that resembles coffee-grounds—typical observations of vomiting patients • Vomiting patients may also regurgitate because of secondary esophagitis. • Vomiting—the hallmark of gastric disease; however, many intestinal and nongastrointestinal diseases cause vomiting. • Diarrhea, abnormal stool, or significant weight loss is more suggestive of intestinal disease. • Changes in activity or mentation, or signs, such as polyuria, weakness, or jaundice, indicate that vomiting is secondary to metabolic abnormalities caused by renal, adrenal, or hepatic disease. • If vomiting persists for 5–7 days or if vomiting occurs intermittently several days per week, it is classified as chronic vomiting. • A thorough diagnostic workup is indicated.

CBC/BIOCHEMISTRY/URINALYSIS
• CBCs are usually normal with primary gastric disease. • Chronic GI bleeding can cause a nonregenerative anemia, often with characteristics of iron deficiency (microcytosis, hypochromasia, thrombocytosis). • Acute GI bleeding can cause either regenerative or nonregenerative anemia, depending on severity and duration. • Nonregenerative anemia occurs secondary to chronic metabolic or chronic inflammatory diseases. • Inflammatory bowel diseases, chronic pancreatitis, cholangiohepatitis, and cholecystitis may cause neutrophilic leukocytosis and monocytosis. • Eosinophilia can occur from eosinophilic gastroenteritis, adrenocortical insufficiency, and GI nematodes. • Dehydration increases the packed cell volume and total protein. • Biochemistry—diagnostic and therapeutic information; normal results rule out metabolic disease as a cause of chronic vomiting. • Electrolyte and acid–base imbalances usually do not indicate the cause of vomiting but do reflect severity of losses and can help to localize disease. • Include total CO_2 in the biochemical assessment of any chronically vomiting patient. • Hypochloremic metabolic alkalosis, often with hypokalemia, indicates substantial loss of gastric content, most consistent with gastric outflow obstruction; vomiting from acute pancreatitis or renal failure can cause similar changes. • Hyperkalemia in the vomiting patient indicates hypoadrenocorticism or oliguric or anuric renal failure; occasionally, enteritis caused by trichuriasis or bacterial infection (salmonellosis) mimics hypoadrenocorticism. • Metabolic acidosis is common in dehydrated patients and those with renal failure, diabetic ketoacidosis, and severe gastroenteritis with diarrhea. • Increased liver enzyme activity, hypoalbuminemia, hyperbilirubinemia, hypoglycemia, or low urea nitrogen concentration indicates liver disease. • Increased blood and urine glucose concentration, with or without ketonemia or ketonuria, is diagnostic for diabetes mellitus. • Hyperglobulinemia may indicate chronic inflammation or infection. • Hypoalbuminemia and lymphopenia occur secondary to a protein-losing enteropathy caused by infiltrative intestinal diseases such as lymphocytic plasmacytic gastroenteritis,

neoplasia, histoplasmosis, or primary intestinal lymphangiectasia. • Hypocholesterolemia may also be seen with lymphangiectasia. • Urinalysis is used to rule out such nongastrointestinal causes of chronic vomiting as renal failure or diabetic ketoacidosis. • Acid urine in the hypokalemic, hypochloremic, alkalotic patient indicates substantial loss of gastric content as would occur with gastric outflow obstruction.

OTHER LABORATORY TESTS
• ACTH stimulation test is used to confirm hypoadrenocorticism. • Amylase, lipase, and trypsin-like immunoreactivity help confirm pancreatitis. • Bile acid concentration is used to help confirm hepatobiliary disease.

IMAGING
• Survey radiographs of the abdomen help identify foreign bodies, GI distension with fluid or gas, and displacement, malposition, and shape or size changes of abdominal organs. • Survey thoracic radiographs are used to evaluate for pulmonary metastatic or infectious disease. • Abdominal contrast radiographs help identify foreign bodies, GI wall masses or infiltrative disease, mucosal ulceration, delayed gastric emptying, and motility disorders. • Abdominal ultrasonography is done to seek parenchymal abnormalities of the liver, kidneys, pancreas, and GI tract to identify an underlying cause of chronic vomiting. • CT and MRI further evaluate for parenchymal abnormalities of abdominal organs.

DIAGNOSTIC PROCEDURES
• Gastroduodenoscopy—allows direct inspection of the gastric and intestinal lumen to identify gross mucosal lesions and foreign bodies and provides a method of biopsy to evaluate for microscopic disease • Laparoscopy or exploratory laparotomy is used for more extensive diagnostic and therapeutic procedures.

TREATMENT
• Specific treatment, elimination of underlying causes, and supportive therapy • If vomiting persists, stop oral intake of food and water for several days. • Use fluid therapy to replace deficits and to provide for maintenance and ongoing losses. • If acid–base status is unknown or if hypochloremic metabolic alkalosis is present, use 0.9% normal saline. • If metabolic acidosis is present, use lactated Ringer's solution. • Supplement potassium if hypokalemia is present; 20 mEq of KCl/L of fluid can be safely added for replacement and maintenance. • Debilitated patients and those in poor nutritional condition may need parenteral or enteral nutrition. • Dietary therapy for patients with suspected food allergy or with IBD should use a diet containing a single-source protein novel to the patient, given for a minimum of 4–6 weeks. • Give blood transfusion to severely anemic patients with evidence of active GI

bleeding. • Use surgical treatment if uncontrolled hemorrhage, obstruction, or perforation are seen.

MEDICATIONS
DRUGS OF CHOICE
• Use anti-ulcer medications for patients with evidence of upper GI bleeding (e.g., hematemesis or melena). • Antisecretory drugs such as H_2-receptor blockers (e.g., cimetidine, ranitidine, famotidine, nizatidine) or proton-pump inhibitors such as omeprazole (more potent than H_2-receptor blockers and permits once-daily dosing)—ranitidine 2 mg/kg PO, IV q12h; Omeprazole 0.7 mg/kg PO q24h • Protectants such as sucralfate (0.5–1 g/dog PO q8–12h; 0.25 g/cat PO q 8–12h) to accelerate gastric mucosal healing • Antibiotics—indicated for treatment of *Helicobacter*-associated gastritis, as an adjunct to corticosteroids in the treatment of IBD, and to treat SIBO syndrome • Suggested treatment of *Helicobacter*-associated gastritis—amoxicillin 22 mg/kg PO q8h plus omeprazole 0.7 mg/kg PO qd; metronidazole 10 mg/kg PO q8h can be added if response is inadequate; azithromycin 5 mg/kg PO q12h is an effective alternative to amoxicillin • Metronidazole—effective in some cases of mild IBD and is used in combination with corticosteroids to treat IBD • SIBO syndrome—tetracycline, metronidazole, amoxicillin, and tylosin in addition to correcting the underlying cause • Use corticosteroids in conjunction with dietary changes and sometimes antibiotics to treat biopsy-confirmed IBD (e.g., lymphocytic-plasmacytic, eosinophilic, granulomatous) • Azathioprine or cyclophosphamide—can use as alternatives in patients that do not respond to corticosteroids or in conjunction with corticosteroids to decrease the dosage of corticosteroids required to control symptoms • Can use the prokinetic drugs metoclopramide, cisapride, or erythromycin to treat delayed gastric emptying not associated with obstructive disease • Pyrantel pamoate is effective for *Physaloptera*; fenbendazole is effective for *Ollulanus*. • Animals with chronic GI bleeding, that develop microcytic hypochromic anemia, may require iron supplementation. • Treatment for neoplasia depends on tumor type and location; most require surgical resection, some with adjunctive chemotherapy. • GI lymphosarcoma is usually treated with chemotherapy. • Paraneoplastic hypersecretion of gastric acid, as occurs with mastocytosis and gastrin-secreting pancreatic tumors, is best treated with potent antisecretory drugs such as omeprazole to diminish gastritis, gastric ulcer, and chronic vomiting. • Reserve antiemetics for patients with persistent vomiting unresponsive to treatment of the underlying disease. • Phenothiazines (e.g., chlorpromazine, phenylethylpirazine) block at both the CTZ and vomiting

center; limit use to 48–72 h—chlorpromazine 0.5 mg/kg SC, IM q6–8h • Prokinetic drugs (e.g., metoclopramide or cisapride)—metoclopramide also blocks the CTZ; can use both indefinitely to treat motility disorders; metoclopramide 0.2–0.5 mg/kg IV, IM, PO q6–8h • Vomiting caused by chemotherapy is best treated with ondansetron 0.5–1 mg/kg IV, PO given 30 min before chemotherapy.

CONTRAINDICATIONS
Do not give α-adrenergic blockers such as chlorpromazine to dehydrated patients; they can cause hypotension.

PRECAUTIONS
• Use antiemetics with caution; they can mask an underlying problem. • Metoclopramide can cause depression, restlessness, agitation, and other behavioral changes, particularly in cats. • Corticosteroids are immunosuppressive and are a risk factor for development of GI ulceration; use caution when treating IBD with corticosteroids at high dosages or for long periods. • Azathioprine is myelotoxic; do a CBC for neutropenia and thrombocytopenia every 2 weeks for the first 2 months of treatment and monthly thereafter. • Do not use anticholinergics as antiemetics; they can cause gastric atony and gastric retention, which can exacerbate vomiting. • Metoclopramide and cisapride are contraindicated in patients with GI obstruction.

POSSIBLE INTERACTIONS
Cimetidine and ranitidine interfere with hepatic metabolism of theophylline, phenytoin, and warfarin, and should not be used concurrently with these drugs.

MISCELLANEOUS
ZOONOTIC POTENTIAL
• *Helicobacter heilmanii* and *H. felis* may have zoonotic potential; they have been isolated from humans with chronic gastritis, most of whom have had close contact with dogs or cats. • Insufficient information exists to conclude that these or other *Helicobacter* species are zoonotic.

Suggested Reading
Fox JG. Gastric helicobacters. In: Greene CE, ed. Infectious diseases of the dog and cat. 2nd ed. Philadelphia: Saunders, 1998:229–235.
Strombeck DR, Guilford WG. Small animal gastroenterology. 2nd ed. Davis, CA: Stonegate Publishing 1990:186–207.
Willard M. Diseases of the stomach. In: Ettinger SJ, Feldman ED, eds. Textbook of veterinary internal medicine. 4th ed. Philadelphia: Saunders, 1995:1143–1167.
Authors Robert C. DeNovo and Christine C. Jenkins
Consulting Editors Brett M. Feder and Mitchell A. Crystal

WEIGHT LOSS AND CACHEXIA

BASICS

DEFINITION
• Weight loss is considered clinically important when it exceeds 10% of the normal body weight and is not associated with fluid loss.
• Cachexia is defined as the state of extreme poor health and is associated with anorexia, weight loss, weakness, and mental depression.

PATHOPHYSIOLOGY
• Weight loss can result from many different pathophysiologic mechanisms that share a common feature—insufficient caloric intake or availability to meet metabolic needs.
• Insufficient caloric intake can be caused by (1) a high energy demand (e.g., that characteristic of a hypermetabolic state); (2) inadequate energy intake, including insufficient quantity or quality of food, or inadequate nutrient assimilation (e.g., with anorexia, dysphagia, regurgitation, or malabsorption—maldigestion disorders); (3) excessive loss of nutrients or fluid, which can occur in patients with gastrointestinal losses, glucosuria, proteinuria, or extensive skin lesions (burns, excoriations, etc.)

SYSTEMS AFFECTED
Any can be affected by weight loss, especially if severe or the result of systemic disease.

SIGNALMENT
Dogs and cats

SIGNS

Historical Findings
• Clinical signs of particular diagnostic value in patients with weight loss are whether the appetite is normal, increased, decreased, or absent, and the presence or absence of fever.
• Historical information is very important, especially regarding type of diet, duration of storage of diet, the patient's daily activity or use, environment, pregnancy, appetite, signs of gastrointestinal disease, including dysphagia, regurgitation, vomiting, diarrhea, or signs of any specific disease.

Physical Examination Findings
Seek signs of systemic disease, gastrointestinal disease, neoplasia, cardiac disease, and neuromuscular disorders.

CAUSES

Dietary Causes
• Insufficient quantity
• Poor quality
• Inedible food—decreased palatability
• Spoiled diets
• Diets that have lost nutrients because of prolonged storage

Anorexia

Pseudoanorexia
• Inability to smell, prehend, or chew food
• Dysphagia
• Regurgitation
• Vomiting

Malabsorptive Disorders
• Infiltrative and inflammatory bowel disease
• Lymphangiectasia
• Severe intestinal parasitism

Maldigestive Disorders
• Exocrine pancreatic insufficiency

Metabolic Disorders
• Organ failure—cardiac failure, hepatic failure, and renal failure
• Hypoadrenocorticism
• Hyperthyroidism (especially cats)
• Cancer cachexia

Excessive Nutrient Loss
• Protein-losing enteropathy
• Protein-losing nephropathy
• Diabetes mellitus
• Extensive skin lesions

Neuromuscular Disease
• Lower motor neuron disease
• CNS disease—usually associated with anorexia or pseudoanorexia

Excessive Use of Calories
• Increased physical activity
• Prolonged or extreme cold environment
• Hyperthyroidism
• Pregnancy or lactation
• Increased catabolism—fever, inflammation, cancer

RISK FACTORS
See Causes above.

DIAGNOSIS

• First confirm weight loss by comparing the current weight to previous weights.
• If previous weights are not available, subjectively assess the patient for cachexia, emaciation, dehydration, or other clues that would confirm the owner's complaint of weight loss.
• After weight loss is confirmed, seek the underlying cause.

DIFFERENTIAL DIAGNOSIS
• First categorize the weight loss as occurring with a normal, increased, or decreased appetite.
• The list of likely differential diagnoses for a patient with weight loss despite a normal or increased appetite is much different and much shorter than that for patients with decreased appetite or anorexia.
• Determine what the patient's appetite was at the onset of weight loss; any condition can lead to anorexia if it persists long enough for the patient to become debilitated.
• The patient's age may provide a clue as to the underlying cause (e.g., portosystemic shunt in a young dog and hyperthyroidism in an older cat).
• Also seek causes of pseudoanorexia (e.g., loss of sense of smell, dysphagia, and disorders of the oral cavity, head and neck).
• Fever suggests that the underlying cause may be infectious or inflammatory (e.g., immune-mediated disease, pancreatitis, or neoplasia).
• Absence of fever is more consistent with metabolic causes of weight loss such as cardiac, renal, or hepatic failure.

CBC/BIOCHEMISTRY/URINALYSIS
• Help identify infectious, inflammatory, and metabolic diseases including organ failure
• Especially helpful when the history and physical examination do not provide much useful information

OTHER LABORATORY TESTS
• Determined by the clinician's list of most likely differential diagnoses on the basis of the specific findings of the history and physical examination
• Perform serologic feline leukemia virus (FeLV) and feline immunodeficiency virus

(FIV) tests in any cat with weight loss of unknown cause.
• Measure serum T4 concentration in any cat >5 years old with weight loss of unknown cause, especially (but not restricted to) cats with a normal or increased appetite.
• Examine a fecal flotation and direct smear to exclude intestinal parasitism.
• Specific organ function tests are necessary if indicated by historical, physical examination, and initial database findings.
• Examples include a serum TLI for exocrine pancreatic insufficiency, an ACTH stimulation test for hypoadrenocorticism, pre- and postprandial serum bile acids for hepatobiliary disease, and a urine protein:creatinine ratio if protein-losing nephropathy is suspected.
• Fecal digestive studies and assays of fecal α_1-protease inhibitor activity may help identify protein-losing enteropathies.

IMAGING
• The most useful diagnostic imaging techniques vary, depending on other clinical findings and suspected underlying causes.
• Thoracic radiography may be particularly helpful in diagnosing thoracic disease, including cardiac failure and metastatic neoplasia.
• Abdominal radiography or ultrasonography may be useful.

DIAGNOSTIC PROCEDURES
• Vary depending on initial diagnostic findings and the suspected underlying cause of weight loss
• If gastrointestinal disease is probable but unconfirmed, examine multiple biopsy specimens taken from the indicated portions of the gastrointestinal tract by endoscopy or exploratory laparotomy.
• Many indications for exploratory laparotomy exist—obtain multiple biopsy specimens from the suspected organ or organs as well as from other routinely biopsied abdominal organs such as liver, multiple sites along the gastrointestinal tract, ± pancreas, ± mesenteric lymph nodes.

TREATMENT
• The most important treatment principle is to treat the underlying cause of the weight loss.

• Must provide sufficient caloric nutrition in the form of adequate amounts of an appropriate, high-quality diet fed in the form or manner that best allows patient utilization; this requires calculating the patient's caloric needs and may require assisted enteral feeding with nasogastric, pharyngostomy, esophagostomy, or gastrostomy tubes.
• If enteral feeding is considered inappropriate, parenteral feeding may become necessary.
• Determine caloric requirements from formulas for basal (resting) energy requirement (BER) multiplied by an illness/infection/injury factor to yield a maintenance energy requirement (MER]):

$$BER = 70 \times (\text{patient's weight in kg})^{0.75}$$

or approximately 30 (patient's weight in kg) + 70 for animals weighing over 2 kg and less than 45 kg. Illness factors tend to range from 1.0 to 1.5, depending on the severity and nature of the underlying disorder. Recently proposed alternative formulas for MER include 1500 × (body surface area in square meters) for dogs, and 500 × (square root of body surface area in square meters) in cats.

MEDICATIONS

DRUGS OF CHOICE
• Depend on the underlying cause of the weight loss; see specific topic for each condition, including anorexia.
• See other sections regarding specific disorders or problems.

CONTRAINDICATIONS
N/A

PRECAUTIONS
N/A

POSSIBLE INTERACTIONS
N/A

ALTERNATIVE DRUGS
N/A

FOLLOW-UP

PATIENT MONITORING
The necessity for frequent patient monitoring and the methods required depends on the

underlying cause of the weight loss; however, the patient should be weighed regularly and often.

POSSIBLE COMPLICATIONS
See Causes.

MISCELLANEOUS

ASSOCIATED CONDITIONS
See Causes.

AGE-RELATED FACTORS
N/A

ZOONOTIC POTENTIAL
N/A

PREGNANCY
Pregnancy and lactation can be associated with weight loss due to increased calorie expenditure.

SYNONYMS
N/A

SEE ALSO
See Causes (refer to specific sections).

ABBREVIATIONS
BER = basal (resting) energy requirement
MER = maintenance energy requirement
TLI = trypsin-like immunoreactivity

Suggested Reading
Carnevale JM, et al. Nutritional assessment: guidelines to selecting patients for nutritional support. Comp Cont Ed 1991;13:255–261.
Greco DS. Changes in body weight. In: Ettinger SJ, ed. Veterinary internal medicine. 4th ed. Philadelphia: WB Saunders, 1995:2–5.
Hill RC. A rapid method of estimating maintenance energy requirement from body surface area in inactive dogs and in cats. J Am Vet Med Assoc 1993;202:1814–1816.
Willard M: Clinical manifestations of gastrointestinal disorders. In: Nelson RW, Couto CG, eds. Essentials of small animal internal medicine. St. Louis: Mosby Year Book, 1992:274–275.
Authors Daniel P. Harrington and Nathaniel C. Myers III
Consulting Editors Brett M. Feder and Mitchell A. Crystal

DIAGNOSTICS— LABORATORY TESTS

ACIDOSIS, METABOLIC

BASICS

DEFINITION
Primary decrease in plasma bicarbonate concentration ($[HCO_3^-]$; dogs, <18 mEq/L; cats, <16 mEq/L) with high hydrogen ion concentration ($[H^+]$), low pH, and a compensatory decrease in carbon dioxide tension (PCO_2)

PATHOPHYSIOLOGY
Acidosis results from loss of HCO_3^+-rich fluid, addition of acid, acid production by metabolism, or diminished renal excretion of acid. Loss of HCO_3^--rich fluids (which have low chloride concentration) is associated with retention of chloride, which causes hyperchloremic metabolic acidosis. Addition of acids containing chloride (e.g., NH_4Cl, cationic amino acids) and chloride retention by the kidneys (e.g., renal tubular acidosis and administration of carbonic anhydrase inhibitors) also cause hyperchloremic metabolic acidosis. Addition (e.g., ethylene glycol toxicity), excessive production (e.g., lactate produced by prolonged anaerobic metabolism), or renal retention (e.g., renal failure) of anions other than chloride causes metabolic acidosis without increasing chloride concentration (so-called normochloremic or high anion gap metabolic acidosis).

SYSTEMS AFFECTED
• Respiratory—increased $[H^+]$ stimulates peripheral and central chemoreceptors to increase alveolar ventilation; hyperventilation decreases PCO_2, which counters the effects of low plasma $[HCO_3]$ on pH. In dogs, a decrease of approximately 0.7 mm Hg in PCO_2 is expected for each 1 mEq/L decrease in plasma $[HCO_3^-]$. Little is known about compensation in cats, but it is less effective than in dogs.
• Renal/Urologic—the kidneys increase net acid excretion, primarily by increasing excretion of NH_4^+.
• Cardiovascular—myocardial contractility is diminished and acidosis may predispose the heart to ventricular arrhythmias and ventricular fibrillation when the pH falls below 7.1.

SIGNALMENT
Any breed, age, or sex of dog and cat

SIGNS

Historical Findings
Chronic disease processes that lead to metabolic acidosis (e.g., renal failure, diabetes mellitus, and hypoadrenocorticism), exposure to toxins (e.g., ethylene glycol, salicylate, and paraldehyde), diarrhea, administration of carbonic anhydrase inhibitors (e.g., acetazolamide and dichlorphenamide)

Physical Examination Findings
• Generally relate to the underlying disease
• Depression in severely acidotic patients
• Tachypnea in some patients results from compensatory increase in ventilation.
• Kussmaul's respiration, typically seen in human beings with metabolic acidosis, is not observed in dogs and cats.

CAUSES

Associated with Hyperchloremia (Hyperchloremic Metabolic Acidosis)
• Diarrhea
• Renal tubular acidosis
• Administration of carbonic anhydrase inhibitors, amiloride, spironolactone, potassium chloride, or NH_4Cl
• Total parenteral nutrition with fluids containing cationic amino acids, lysine, arginine, and histidine
• Rapid correction of hypocapnia (chronic respiratory alkalosis)

Associated with Normochloremia (High Anion-Gap Metabolic Acidosis)
• Uremic acidosis
• Diabetic ketoacidosis
• Lactic acidosis
• Ethylene glycol, salicylate, paraldehyde, and methanol intoxication
• Hyperphosphatemia

RISK FACTORS
• Patients with chronic renal failure, diabetes mellitus, and hypoadrenocorticism are at high risk of developing metabolic acidosis as a complication of the chronic disease process.
• Patients with poor tissue perfusion or hypoxia are at risk of developing lactic acidosis.

DIAGNOSIS

DIFFERENTIAL DIAGNOSIS
Low plasma $[HCO_3^-]$ may also be compensatory in animals with chronic respiratory alkalosis, in which PCO_2 is low and pH is low or near normal, despite decreased $[HCO_3^-]$.

Blood gas determination is required to differentiate.

LABORATORY FINDINGS

Drugs That May Alter Laboratory Results
Potassium bromide is measured as chloride in most analyzers, so potassium bromide administration artificially decreases the anion gap.

Disorders That May Alter Laboratory Results
• Too much heparin (>10% of the sample) decreases $[HCO_3^-]$
• Samples stored at room temperature for more than 20 min have low pH because of increased PCO_2.
• Some blood gas analyzers only report pH and PCO_2; $[HCO_3^-]$ must be calculated, which is a potential source of error.

Valid If Run in Human Laboratory?
Yes

CBC/BIOCHEMISTRY/URINALYSIS
• Low total CO_2 (total CO_2 in serum samples handled aerobically) closely approximates the $[HCO_3^-]$ concentration; unfortunately, patients with chronic respiratory alkalosis also have low total CO_2, and the distinction cannot be made without blood gas analysis.
• Metabolic acidoses are traditionally divided into hyperchloremic and high anion gap by means of the anion gap. Anion gap, the difference between the measured cations and the measured anions, is calculated as $AG = [Na^+] - ([HCO3^-] + [Cl^-])$ or $AG = ([Na^+] + [K^+]) - ([HCO_3^-] + [Cl^-])$, depending on the preference of the clinician or laboratory. Normal values with potassium included in the calculation are usually 12–24 mEq/L in dogs and 13–27 mEq/L in cats. The negative charges of albumin are the major contributors to the normal anion gap; thus estimation of anion gap is not reliable in patients with hypoalbuminemia.
• Normal anion gap (i.e., hyperchloremic metabolic acidosis)—most common cause is diarrhea; also, hypoadrenocorticism
• High anion gap (i.e., normochloremic metabolic acidosis)—most common causes are renal failure, diabetes mellitus, lactic acidosis (caused by tissue hypoperfusion), and hypoadrenocorticism (caused by lactic acidosis)
• Hyperglycemia—consider diabetes mellitus.
• Azotemia—consider renal failure.
• Hyperphosphatemia—consider renal failure, hypertonic sodium phosphate enema toxicity, and toxicity due to urinary acidifiers containing phosphate.

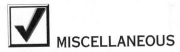
• High lactate concentration—consider lactic acidosis due to poor tissue perfusion or poor metabolism of lactate (e.g., liver disease and lymphoma).
• Hyperkalemia—the only form of metabolic acidosis that can be causative is acute hyperchloremic acidosis; otherwise, it results from the disease process causing the metabolic acidosis (e.g., renal failure and diabetes mellitus), not from the acidosis itself.

OTHER LABORATORY TESTS
Blood gas analysis reveals low $[HCO_3^-]$, low PCO_2, and low pH.

IMAGING
N/A

DIAGNOSTIC PROCEDURES
N/A

TREATMENT
• Acid–base disturbances—secondary phenomena; successful resolution depends on diagnosis and treatment of the underlying disease process.
• Treat patients with blood pH < 7.1 aggressively while pursuing the definitive diagnosis.
• Discontinue drugs that may cause metabolic acidosis.
• Nursing care—lactated Ringer's solution is the fluid of choice for patients with mild metabolic acidosis and normal liver function.

MEDICATIONS

DRUGS OF CHOICE
• Patients with metabolic acidosis and pH < 7.2 should receive $NaHCO_3$. Patients with high anion gap metabolic acidosis should receive enough $NaHCO_3$ to bring the pH to 7.2. These patients metabolize organic anions to HCO_3^-, and administration of HCO_3^- may predispose them to metabolic alkalosis. Patients with hyperchloremic acidosis are less likely to develop overshoot metabolic alkalosis.
• Estimation of HCO_3^- dose—dogs, $0.3 \times$ body weight (kg) $\times$ (21—patient $[HCO_3^-]$); cats, $0.3 \times$ body weight (kg) $\times$ (19—patient $[HCO_3^-]$). Give half of this dose slowly IV and reevaluate blood gases before deciding on the need for additional administration. An empirical dose of 2 mEq/kg followed by reevaluation of blood gas status is safe in most patients.

• Potential complications of $NaHCO_3$ administration—volume overload resulting from administered sodium, tetany from low ionized calcium concentration, increased affinity of hemoglobin for oxygen, paradoxical CNS acidosis, overshoot metabolic alkalosis, and hypokalemia

CONTRAINDICATIONS
• Avoid $NaHCO_3$ in patients with respiratory acidosis because it generates CO_2.
• Patients with respiratory acidosis cannot adequately excrete CO_2, and increased PCO_2 will further decrease the pH.
• Avoid diuretics that act in the distal nephron (e.g., spironolactone, triamterene, and amiloride).
• Avoid carbonic anhydrase inhibitors (e.g., acetazolamide, dichlorphenamide).

PRECAUTIONS
Use $NaHCO_3$ cautiously in patients with congestive heart failure because the sodium load may cause decompensation of the heart failure.

POSSIBLE INTERACTIONS
N/A

ALTERNATIVE DRUGS
• Carbicarb—an equimolar mixture of Na_2CO_3 and $NaHCO_3$; can use as alternative to bicarbonate; does not generate CO_2 and is especially useful in patients with concurrent respiratory acidosis; appears to be more effective than $NaHCO_3$ in the treatment of hypoxic lactic acidosis
• Dichloroacetate—activates pyruvate dehydrogenase complex; reduces blood lactate levels; can use as alternative to $NaHCO_3$ in patients with lactic acidosis

FOLLOW-UP

PATIENT MONITORING
Recheck acid–base status; frequency dictated by the underlying disease and patient response to treatment

POSSIBLE COMPLICATIONS
• Hyperkalemia
• Myocardial depression and ventricular arrhythmias

✓ MISCELLANEOUS

ASSOCIATED CONDITIONS
• Hyperkalemia
• Hyperchloremia

AGE-RELATED FACTORS
N/A

ZOONOTIC POTENTIAL
N/A

PREGNANCY
N/A

SYNONYMS
• Nonrespiratory acidosis
• Hyperchloremic acidosis—normal anion gap acidosis
• Normochloremic acidosis—high anion gap acidosis
• Hyperphosphatemic acidosis—metabolic acidosis resulting from high phosphate concentration
• Organic acidosis—metabolic acidosis resulting from accumulation of organic anions (e.g., ketoacidosis, uremic acidosis, and lactic acidosis)
• Dilutional acidosis—metabolic acidosis resulting from increased free water in plasma

SEE ALSO
• Diabetes mellitus, Ketoacidosis
• Potassium, Hyperkalemia
• Chloride, Hyperchloremia

ABBREVIATIONS
• AG = anion gap
• HCO_3^+ = bicarbonate
• $NaHCO_3$ = sodium bicarbonate
• PCO_2 = carbon dioxide tension
• H^+ = hydrogen ion
• O_2 = oxygen

Suggested Reading
de Morais HSA, Muir WW. Strong ions and acid-base disorders. In: Bonagura JD, Kirk RW, eds. Kirk's current veterinary therapy XII. Philadelphia: Saunders, 1995:121–127.
DiBartola SP. Metabolic acidosis. In: DiBartola, SP, ed. Fluid therapy in small animal practice. Philadelphia: Saunders, 1992:216–243.
Muir WW, de Morais HSA. Acid-base balance: traditional and modified approaches. In: Thurmon JC, Tranquilli WJ, Benson GJ, eds. Lumb & Jones' veterinary anesthesia. 3rd ed. Baltimore: Williams & Wilkins, 1996:558–571.
Author Helio Autran de Morais
Consulting Editors Larry G. Adams and Carl A. Osborne

ACTH RESPONSE TEST

BASICS

DEFINITION
- ACTH gel or synthetic ACTH is used
- Dogs—if ACTH gel (Acthar, Rhone-Poulenc Rorer Pharmaceuticals) is used, collect a pre-ACTH blood sample and then give 2.2 U/kg IM; one post-ACTH sample is collected 2 h later
- Cats—use the same dose of ACTH, but take blood samples before and 1 and 2 h after injection
- If using synthetic ACTH (Cosyntropin, Organon Inc.), give the drug intravenously; use 5 μg/kg for dogs, with a maximum of 250 μg/dog, or 0.125 mg (125 μg)/cat; in both species, draw blood samples before and 1 h after injection.
- Baseline, resting or pre-ACTH cortisol concentration in dogs is 10– 160 nmol/L (0.4–6.0 μg/dL) and in cats, 10– 110 nmol/L (0.4–4.0 μg/dL).
- Normal dogs and cats have a post-ACTH plasma cortisol concentration of 220–560 nmol/L (8–20 μg/ dL) and 220–330 nmol/L (8–12 μg/dL), respectively; normal values vary slightly between laboratories.

PATHOPHYSIOLOGY
- The dose of ACTH maximally stimulates cortisol secretion
- The test can be used to screen for hyperadrenocorticism (Cushing's syndrome), hypoadrenocorticism (Addison's disease), and adrenal reserve in dogs or cats receiving exogenous glucocorticoids or mitotane (Lysodren) or cats receiving progestins.
- An above-normal response is consistent with a diagnosis of Cushing's syndrome but could may also be a nonspecific finding in dogs with non-adrenal illness; a below-normal response is consistent with hypoadrenocorticism, previous glucocorticoid administration, Lysodren therapy in dogs or cats, or progestin treatment in cats.
- Cushing's syndrome can be caused by either an ACTH-secreting pituitary tumor (i.e., pituitary-dependent hyperadrenocorticism, PDH) or a cortisol-secreting AT; with PDH, constant overstimulation of the adrenal cortex by excess ACTH leads to bilateral adrenal hyperplasia and increased secretory ability; the adrenal tumor mass can similarly increase the ability to release cortisol; thus, ACTH usually elicits an above-normal cortisol response.
- An increased response to ACTH in dogs may also be due to nonadrenal illness and associated nonspecific activation of the hypothalamic-pituitary-adrenal axis and adrenal cortical hyperplasia; the effect of nonadrenal illness on ACTH response in cats is unknown.
- A false-negative response is seen in ~15% of patients with canine or feline Cushing's syndrome; in PDH, this may be attributable to early hyperadrenocorticism in which adrenal cortical hyperplasia is minimal; in AT, the tumor tissue may not have receptors for ACTH and so does not respond to an injection of ACTH.
- A below-normal response can be seen with destruction or atrophy of the adrenal cortex; destruction can be due to spontaneous primary Addison's disease or mitotane therapy; during long-term glucocorticoid therapy, a patient's ACTH secretion may be suppressed by negative feedback by the exogenous steroids on the pituitary; lack of ACTH in turn leads to atrophy of the adrenocortical zonae reticularis and fasciculata; thus, when therapy is discontinued, the adrenals secrete subnormal amounts of glucocorticoids; long-term glucocorticoid therapy results in adrenal atrophy and severely reduced or no response to ACTH; short-term glucocorticoid therapy can reduce the ACTH response moderately.
- Progestin therapy in cats also suppresses ACTH release; similarly, secondary Addison's disease, loss of ability to secrete ACTH, causes adrenal atrophy and a subnormal ACTH response.
- Because of the ability to detect hyper- and hypoadrenocorticism, this test is preferred if an animal has a definitive or questionable history of receiving exogenous glucocorticoids and signs compatible with Cushing's syndrome; the response to ACTH will differentiate spontaneous hyperadrenocorticism (an above-normal response in association with the clinical signs) from iatrogenic Cushing's syndrome (a below-normal response in association with the clinical signs).

SYSTEMS AFFECTED
- None are affected by an abnormal ACTH response per se; they are affected by the excess cortisol secreted in Cushing's syndrome or lack of cortisol in Addison's disease.
- See Hyperadrenocorticism or Hypoadrenocorticism.

SIGNALMENT
N/A

SIGNS

General Comments
No historical or physical examination findings are specifically due to an abnormal ACTH response; they are due to the underlying disease process.

Historical Findings
N/A

Physical Examination Findings
N/A

CAUSES

Above-normal Response
• Cushing's syndrome—dogs and cats
• Nonadrenal illness—dogs, cats unknown

Below-normal Response
• Primary or secondary hypoadrenocorticism—dogs and cats
• Glucocorticoid therapy—dogs and cats
• Mitotane therapy—dogs and cats
• Progestin therapy—cats

RISK FACTORS
See Causes

 DIAGNOSIS

DIFFERENTIAL DIAGNOSIS

Above-normal Response
• Historical findings of hyperadrenocorticism include polyuria/polydipsia, alopecia or failure to regrow hair, abdominal enlargement, polyphagia, obesity, panting, lethargy, muscle weakness, anestrus, and heat intolerance.
• Physical examination findings of hyperadrenocorticism include thin skin, abdominal enlargement, bilaterally symmetrical alopecia, abdominal enlargement, hepatomegaly, pyoderma, seborrhea, cutaneous hyperpigmentation, muscle wasting of extremities, calcinosis cutis, bruising, and testicular atrophy.
• Findings vary depending on which nonadrenal illness is present.

Below-normal Response
• Findings of glucocorticoid or mineralocorticoid deficiency are the same regardless of the cause. (See Hypoadrenocorticism.)

• A history of glucocorticoid, mitotane, or progestin administration helps to define the cause.

LABORATORY FINDINGS

Drugs That May Alter Laboratory Results
• Prednisone, prednisolone, and hydrocortisone cross-react in many cortisol radioimmunoassays and cause an artifactually high measured cortisol concentration.
• A subnormal cortisol concentration may be obscured, and a patient with subnormal or normal plasma cortisol concentrations may appear to have an above-normal ACTH response.

Disorders That May Alter Laboratory Results
• Delayed separation of plasma from blood cells may falsely lower measured cortisol concentration.
• Use plasma, preferably collected with EDTA as the anticoagulant; cortisol is stable stored at ≤ 25°C for 5 days; storage at higher temperatures or use of serum may lead to decay of cortisol and a spurious decrease in apparent cortisol concentration.

Valid If Run in Human Laboratory?
Yes, if assay is validated for dogs and cats

CBC/BIOCHEMISTRY/URINALYSIS

Above-normal Response
• CBC with hyperadrenocorticism—a mature leukocytosis, neutrophilia, lymphopenia, eosinopenia, or mild polycythemia
• Biochemistry—increased ALP, (elevation may be extreme), alanine aminotransferase (ALT), cholesterol, fasting blood glucose and lipase can be seen with hyperadrenocorticism; may see lipemia and decreased BUN
• Urinalysis—dilute urine (e.g., specific gravity < 1.015) and bacteriuria with or without

pyuria have been associated with Cushing's syndrome

Below-normal Response
CBC, biochemistry and urinalysis will be the same regardless of the underlying cause of hormone deficiency; hyperkalemia and hyponatremia are seen with loss of mineralocorticoids but not if only glucocorticoids were lacking.

OTHER LABORATORY TESTS

Above-normal Response
• Other tests used to screen for Cushing's syndrome include urinary cortisol:creatinine ratio (UCCR) and a low-dose dexamethasone suppression test (LDDST).
• If an ACTH stimulation test indicates Cushing's syndrome but the diagnosis is questionable (e.g., nonadrenal illness or results borderline), the diagnosis is best confirmed with the LDDST, which is more sensitive than the ACTH response; if the LDDST is normal, consider another diagnosis.
• If the ACTH response is normal but suspicion of Cushing's syndrome remains high, an LDDST can be performed; a positive LDDST but normal ACTH response may represent a false-negative ACTH response with a true-positive LDDST result.
• If the ACTH response is above normal and a diagnosis of Cushing's syndrome is likely on the basis of historical and clinical findings, perform a high-dose dexamethasone suppression test or measure endogenous ACTH concentrations to differentiate between PDH and AT.

Below-normal Response
• Measuring endogenous ACTH concentration and/or serum aldosterone concentrations pre- and post-ACTH injection can differentiate spontaneous primary and secondary Addison's disease.

ACTH RESPONSE TEST

• Measuring serum aldosterone concentrations can assess mineralocorticoid secretory ability after mitotane therapy.

IMAGING

Above-normal Response

• Abdominal radiography and ultrasonography can be used to differentiate PDH from AT.

• Computed tomography (CT) and magnetic resonance imaging (MRI) can reveal a pituitary tumor.

Below-normal Response

CT and MRI can reveal a pituitary abnormality (e.g., space-occupying lesion destroying the pituitary) in spontaneous secondary Addison's disease.

DIAGNOSTIC PROCEDURES

Above-normal Response

• With hyperadrenocorticism, urinary protein: creatinine ratio and systemic blood pressure may be mildly elevated, but neither are specific.

• A skin biopsy can confirm the diagnosis of calcinosis cutis, a pathognomonic finding for hyperadrenocorticism; other skin changes may suggest an endocrinopathy but are not specific.

• A liver biopsy can show changes consistent with steroid hepatopathy, a sensitive but nonspecific marker of Cushing's syndrome.

Below-normal Response

N/A

TREATMENT

Above-normal Response

• Lack of suppression does not need to be treated.

• If the test result is due to nonadrenal illness, direct therapy toward resolution of that disease.

• If Cushing's syndrome is believed present, direct therapy toward managing hyperadrenocorticism; unless a complication of Cushing's syndrome requires hospitalization (e.g., pulmonary thromboembolism), treat as outpatients.

Below-normal Response

• An acute addisonian crisis is a medical emergency requiring hospitalization and intensive fluid therapy (see Hypoadrenocorticism).

• Patients with chronic hypoadrenocorticism can be hospitalized or not, depending on the severity of clinical signs.

• Feeding must be altered if vomiting is present.

• Limit activity and avoid stress until the patient is stable and glucocorticoid replacement therapy has begun.

MEDICATIONS

DRUGS OF CHOICE

Above-normal Response

None needed while completing all tests for the diagnosis.

Below-normal Response

• Acute addisonian crisis requires glucocorticoids and fluid therapy.

• See Hypoadrenocorticism.

• Chronic glucocorticoid deficiency—may give physiologic doses of prednisone (0.2 mg/kg/day) as needed, depending on the severity of the deficiency.

• If cortisol lack is due to long-term steroid administration, taper the steroid dose slowly if possible to physiologic doses of prednisone, and then discontinue as adrenal function recovers; if the patient is receiving a synthetic glucocorticoid other than prednisone, taper medication slowly and then replace with prednisone; if a cat is receiving progestins, stop this medication and give physiologic doses of prednisone

• A repeat test can indicate when the adrenal reserve has returned to normal.

CONTRAINDICATIONS

Above-normal Response

Glucocorticoids

Below-normal Response

N/A

PRECAUTIONS

Above-normal Response

N/A

Below-Normal Response

Any medication that can lower blood pressure (e.g., calcium-channel blockers, phenothiazine tranquilizers, α_2-agonists); if administered, observe the patient for weakness or syncope and monitor mucous membrane color and heart rate; pale or cyanotic mucous membranes or tachycardia are consistent with severe hypotension.

POSSIBLE INTERACTIONS

N/A

ALTERNATIVE DRUGS

N/A

FOLLOW-UP

PATIENT MONITORING

Above-normal Response

• If hyperadrenocorticism, follow-up depends on the type of therapy chosen (see Hyperadrenocorticism)

• If nonadrenal illness is present and considered a possible cause of the abnormal response, treat the illness; once the animal is stable, repeat the ACTH response test after 4–8 weeks.

ACTH RESPONSE TEST

Below-normal Response
• If spontaneous Addison's disease, monitoring depends on the type of therapy chosen (see Hypoadrenocorticism).
• If subnormal response is due to glucocorticoid, mitotane, or progestin administration, use sequential ACTH response tests to assess recovery of glucocorticoid secretory ability; test every 7–14 days at first; subsequent frequency depends on how quickly the secretory ability is returning
• Rate of recovery after glucocorticoid or progestin administration depends on the form, route, and length of administration.
• After mitotane therapy, if only glucocorticoids are deficient, secretory ability usually returns within 2 months but can take up to 18; if mineralocorticoids are deficient as well, loss of both hormones is likely to be permanent.

POSSIBLE COMPLICATIONS
Above-normal Response
Untreated hyperadrenocorticism can lead to development of all classical signs if not already present (e.g., polyuria, polydipsia, panting, polyphagia) as well as such life-threatening complications as pulmonary thromboembolism or diabetes mellitus.

Below-normal Response
Untreated glucocorticoid deficiency can be fatal; if mineralocorticoids are deficient as well, clinical deterioration and death may occur rapidly.

MISCELLANEOUS
ASSOCIATED CONDITIONS
None related to abnormal ACTH response per se

AGE-RELATED FACTORS
Above-normal Response
• Nonadrenal illness can occur in an animal of any age.
• Hyperadrenocorticism is typically a disease of middle-aged to old cats and dogs but has been reported in dogs 1 year old.

Below-normal Response
• Spontaneous hypoadrenocorticism is seen in dogs <1–12 years, with a median of 4 years, and mainly in middle-aged cats, but the reported range is 1–9 years.
• Glucocorticoids can suppress the adrenal cortex in dogs or cats of any age.
• Similarly, progestin therapy can cause adrenal atrophy in cats of any age.
• Mitotane suppression of the adrenal cortex can be seen any time during the course of therapy; since this drug is used to treat dogs with Cushing's syndrome, it is mainly administered to middle-aged and older dogs.

ZOONOTIC POTENTIAL
N/A

PREGNANCY
N/A

SYNONYMS
N/A

SEE ALSO
• Hyperadrenocorticism
• Hypoadrenocorticism
• Low-Dose Dexamethasone Suppression Test
• Urine Cortisol:Creatinine Ratio

ABBREVIATIONS
• ACTH = adrenocorticotropic hormone
• ALP = alkaline phosphatase
• AT = adrenal tumor
• LDDST = low-dose dexamethasone suppression test
• MRI = magnetic resonance imaging
• PDH = pituitary-dependent hyperadrenocorticism
• UCCR = urinary cortisol:creatinine ratio

Suggested Reading
Feldman EC, Nelson RW. Hyperadrenocorticism (Cushing's syndrome). In: Canine and feline endocrinology and reproduction. 2nd ed. Philadelphia: Saunders, 1996:187–265.

Guptill L, Scott-Moncrieff JC, Widmer W. Diagnosis of canine hyperadrenocorticism. Vet Clin North Am Small Anim Pract 1997;27:215–235.

Kaplan AJ, Peterson ME, Kemppainen RJ. Effects of disease on the results of diagnostic tests for use in detecting hyperadrenocorticism in dogs. J Am Vet Med Assoc 1995;207:445–451.

Kintzer PP, Peterson ME. Primary and secondary canine hypoadrenocorticism. Vet Clin North Am (Small Anim Pract) 1997;27:349–358.

Van Liew CH, Greco DS, Salman MD. Comparison of results on adrenocorticotropic hormone stimulation and low-dose dexamethasone suppression tests with necropsy findings in dogs: 81 cases (1985–1995). J Am Vet Med Assoc 1997;211:322–325.

Authors Ellen N. Behrend and Robert Kemppainen
Consulting Editor Deborah S. Greco

ALANINE AMINOTRANSFERASE (ALT)/ASPARTATE AMINOTRANSFERASE

 BASICS

DEFINITION
• Major causes of high serum activity—hepatocellular injury; enzyme induction; myonecrosis
• Increased activity—may reflect both primary and secondary hepatocellular changes; magnitude may reflect activity of underlying disease but cannot discern severity, prognosis, or tissue of origin
• Sequential measurements—may infer continuation and relative severity of ongoing tissue damage or enzyme induction

PATHOPHYSIOLOGY
• Metabolic role—amino acid metabolism
• Both located in the cytosol; rapidly dispersed upon cell membrane alteration; present in large quantities in liver and striated muscle
• AST—cytosolic and mitochondrial enzyme; disproportionate increase relative to ALT suggests release of the mitochondrial isoenzyme; isoenzyme utility has not been demonstrated in companion animals.
• Values must be interpreted with knowledge of serum creatinine kinase activity to deduce myonecrosis.
• Plasma half-life—ALT: dogs, 4–72 hr; cats, 4–6 hr; AST: dogs, approximately 5 hr; cats, 1.3 hr
• Cleared from plasma by enzyme degradation in the monocyte–macrophage system

SYSTEMS AFFECTED
N/A

SIGNALMENT
• No breed or sex differences in expression reported
• Neonatal enzyme activity—onefold to twofold higher than the reference range for adults

SIGNS
• Depend on underlying causes, increased activity
• Serum enzyme activity does not contribute directly to clinical signs.
• Fulminant hepatic failure owing to diffuse hepatic necrosis—lethargy; jaundice; dehydration; hypoglycemia; hypokalemia; hypocholesterolemia; collapse
• Unifocal hepatic necrosis—may find none discernible
• Hyperthyroidism (cats)—specific induced enzymes and clinical signs

CAUSES
• Hepatocellular necrosis—initially associated with only marked transaminase activity; may occur with the following disorders
• Idiosyncratic drug toxicity—tetracycline (cats); anticonvulsants (e.g., primidone, phenytoin, phenobarbital; dogs); benzimida

zole anthelmintics (e.g., oxibendizole, mebendazole; dogs); halothane; diazepam (cats); carparsolate; carprofen (dogs)
• Toxin ingestion—mushroom alkaloids (e.g., amatoxin, phylladin); carbon tetrachloride; acetaminophen
• Severe acute hypoxia—severe anemia; DIC; cardiac failure; hypovolemia
• Endocrinopathies—mild to moderate transaminase activity in dogs and cats (diabetes mellitus, hyperthyroidism, hyperadrenocorticism, hypothyroidism); high ALP activity; normal total bilirubin
• Cholestatic disease—high transaminases; high ALP and GGT activity; hyperbilirubinemia
• Vacuolar hepatopathy (dogs)—high ALP and GGT activity; moderate increase in transaminase activity
• Hepatic lipidosis (cats)—high ALP; normal to slightly high GGT activity; hyperbilirubinemia
• Cholangiohepatitis (cats)—high ALP and GGT activity; variable hyperbilirubinemia; high transaminases
• Cirrhosis (dogs)—may develop high transaminase activity with end-stage disease
• Chronic active hepatitis (dogs)—mild to moderate transaminase activity; greater increase in serum ALP activity; variable hyperbilirubinemia
• Neoplasia (primary or metastatic)—high transaminase activity may be the only clinicopathologic indicator.
• Immunologic or infectious (bacterial, viral, parasitic, protozoal, fungal)—variable changes in transaminase activity, depending on extent of hepatocellular insult
• Myonecrosis—severely high serum creatinine kinase activity

RISK FACTORS
• Depend on cause
• Conditions that alter membrane permeability in certain tissues (reversible or irreversible)—may increase activity

 DIAGNOSIS

DIFFERENTIAL DIAGNOSIS
Generally, no specific aspects of the history or physical examination consistently help differentiate causes of high ALT or AST activity. If either is high, the clinician should first attempt to establish the presence of liver disease, whether it is primary or secondary, and the underlying cause.

LABORATORY FINDINGS
Drugs That May Alter Laboratory Results
• Many drugs and chemicals may cause hepatic transaminase liberation, as a result of either hepatocellular damage or induced enzyme synthesis (dogs).
• No known drugs interfere with the biochemical analysis.

Disorders That May Alter Laboratory Results
Hemolysis—false-high activity in species other than dogs and cats

Valid If Run in Human Laboratory?
Yes, if the animal reference range is determined

CBC/BIOCHEMISTRY/URINALYSIS
Adjunctive interpretation of routine screening tests—necessary to deduce liver disease or myonecrosis, to determine the importance of primary or secondary conditions, and to assess the patient's clinical status

CBC
• Poikilocytes (cats)—highly associated with liver disease
• Abnormal platelet function and thrombocytopenia—occur with some liver diseases

Serum Biochemistry Profile
• Albumin—low with hepatic failure; high with dehydration
• Globulins—high with stimulated acute-phase proteins or reduced hepatic monocyte–macrophage function; high fibrinogen indicates high acute-phase protein production.
• ALP—dogs: increased with many disorders as a result of the induction of the glucocorticoid isoenzyme; high with cholestasis and necroinflammatory disorders
• BUN—low with compromised urea cycle function, polyuria or polydipsia, induced high glomerular filtration rate, low protein intake, or protein malnutrition
• Glucose—low with portosystemic shunting, starvation, fulminant hepatic failure, and sepsis; high with diabetes mellitus, hepaticocutaneous syndrome, stress (cats), and treatment with glucocorticoids (cats)
• Cholesterol—low with portosystemic shunting, gut malabsorption, or pancreatic exocrine insufficiency; high with diabetes mellitus, hepaticocutaneous syndrome, nephrotic syndrome, major bile duct occlusion, pancreatitis, hypothyroidism, and impaired glomerular filtration rate owing to chronic interstitial nephritis (cats)
• Creatinine kinase—very high values with transaminase activities derived from myonecrosis
• Potassium—low concentrations in cats may induce myonecrosis, causing significant enzyme release.
• Hyperbilirubinemia—cholestatic disease; severe hemolysis, producing hypoxic liver damage and high transaminase activity

Urinalysis
• Bilirubinuria—cats: always abnormal, indicating hyperbilirubinemia; dogs: may conjugate in renal tubules
• Ammonium urate crystalluria—indicates hyperammonemia with fulminant hepatic

ALANINE AMINOTRANSFERASE (ALT)/ASPARTATE AMINOTRANSFERASE

failure or portosystemic shunting
• Hyposthenuria—indicates impaired urine concentration (medullary washout, primary polydipsia with hepatic encephalopathy)

OTHER LABORATORY TESTS
• Bile acids—12-hr fasting and 2-hr postprandial values; sensitive assessment of hepatic function, perfusion, and enterohepatic circulation
• Indocyanine green or sulfobromophthalein—cholephilic organic anion water-soluble dyes; assess hepatobiliary function and perfusion.
• Ammonia-tolerance testing—appraises hepatic function and hepatoportal perfusion; demonstrates hyperammonemia; utility impaired in routine practice owing to difficulties (lability, spurious values derived from frozen samples, analytic inaccuracies).
• Evaluations targeted at underlying disease conditions—pancreatitis (trypsin-like immunoactive, amylase, and lipase); endocrinopathies (thyroid profiles, adrenal function testing, insulin determinations); serologic tests for infectious disorders (FIP, leptospirosis, brucellosis, tick-borne disorders, fungal disease)
• Coagulation assessments—PT, APTT, or ACT; PIVKA; fibrinogen concentration; platelet count; mucosal bleeding time; evaluated in patients scheduled for liver aspirate or biopsy

IMAGING
• Radiography—evaluate liver size, position, shape, and margins; determine parenchymal density (mineralization, gas); evaluate other abdominal viscera (position, mass lesions); detect abdominal effusion
• Ultrasonography—evaluate echogenic patterns with hepatic parenchyma, biliary tree (wall thickness, luminal dilation, contents), vascular components (flow, thrombi, relative size of vessels), porta hepatis structures, perihepatic and peripancreatic lymph nodes, pancreatic tissue, and peripancreatic fat; appraise intestinal wall motility

DIAGNOSTIC PROCEDURES

Liver Biopsy
• Core—via ultrasound guidance, laparoscopy, or abdominal exploration; requires a minimum of 15 portal triads, necessitating four to six samples
• Wedge (laparotomy) or pinch (laparoscopy)—affords larger diagnostic samples; collected from visibly involved lobes

TREATMENT
• None specific is advised, unless the underlying cause of high activity is inferred from the history or deduced from the liver biopsy.
• Removal of the inciting cause (e.g., infectious disease, drugs)—most important

Fluids
• If indicated, balanced polyionic solutions are usually safe.
• Reduced lactate metabolism—may occur with fulminant hepatic failure or in cats with hepatic lipidosis; do not use lactated Ringer solution
• Ascites—reduced-sodium fluids recommended
• Hypoglycemia—supplement with dextrose, to effect
• Hypokalemia—correct by judicious administration of supplemental potassium chloride; especially important with hepatic encephalopathy and for cats with hepatic lipidosis
• Rate—based on patient hydration status and condition

Nutritional Support
• Essential—especially with hepatic encephalopathy
• After a necrotizing insult—positive nitrogen balance; adequate ingestion of vitamins and essential trace minerals
• Protein restriction—contraindicated with hepatic necrosis that is not symptomatic for hepatic encephalopathy

MEDICATIONS

DRUGS OF CHOICE
• Suspected free radical–induced damage—antioxidants; vitamin E (α-tocopherol; 10–40 IU/kg PO per day); possibly acetylcysteine (as for acetaminophen toxicity) or S-adenosylmethionine (20 mg/kg PO per day) as sources of glutathione
• Suspected fulminant hepatic necrosis—broad-spectrum bactericidal antibiotics effective against enteric gram-negative and anaerobic bacteria
• Control of emesis—metoclopramide
• Gastrointestinal ulceration (hematemesis, melena)—omeprazole or the H_2-blocker famotidine combined with sucralfate (0.25 g/5 kg PO q8–12h) to control gastric acidity
• Fulminant hepatic failure or evidence of bleeding tendencies—vitamin K_1 (0.5–1.5 mg/kg IM initially); may require transfusion of whole blood or fresh-frozen plasma; DDAVP (1–5 μg/kg) may control critical hemorrhage on a one-time basis (continued administration ineffectual; mechanism in liver patients unknown).

CONTRAINDICATIONS
N/A

PRECAUTIONS
N/A

POSSIBLE INTERACTIONS
N/A

ALTERNATIVE DRUGS
N/A

FOLLOW-UP

PATIENT MONITORING
• Depends on the underlying cause; consult specific disorders; treatment targeted at an underlying condition may require periodic enzyme assessment.
• High activities associated with mild disorders—some patients remain stable; may not require treatment; treatment may consist of outpatient supportive care.

POSSIBLE COMPLICATIONS
High activity—may indicate severe hepatobiliary disease, which may lead to severe debilitation or death; may be the only (early) indication of chronic hepatitis

MISCELLANEOUS

ASSOCIATED CONDITIONS
N/A

AGE-RELATED FACTORS
Neonatal activities—normally onefold to twofold greater than that for normal adults

ZOONOTIC POTENTIAL
A variety of infectious diseases may involve the liver—leptospirosis; brucellosis; systemic fungal infections; toxoplasmosis; campylobacteriosis

PREGNANCY
N/A

SYNONYMS
• Serum glutamic pyruvic transaminase (ALT)
• Serum glutamic oxaloacetate transaminase (AST)

SEE ALSO
Causes of liver disease

ABBREVIATIONS
• ACT = activated clotting time
• ALP = alkaline phosphatase
• APTT = activated partial thromboplastin time
• DDAVP = 1 deamino-8-D-arginine vasopressin
• DIC = disseminated intravascular coagulation
• FIP = feline infectious peritonitis
• GGT = gamma-glutamyltransferase
• PIVKA = proteins invoked by vitamin K absence or antagonism
• PT = prothrombin time

Suggested Reading
Center SA. Diagnostic procedures for evaluation of hepatic disease. In: Guilford WG, Center SA, Strombeck DR, et al., eds. Strombeck's small animal gastroenterology. Philadelphia: Saunders, 1996:130–188.
Author Sharon A. Center
Consulting Editor Sharon A. Center

ALBUMIN, HYPOALBUMINEMIA

BASICS

DEFINITION
• Low serum albumin concentration; varies with method of determination • Low serum albumin—for most assays, < 2.0 g/dL

PATHOPHYSIOLOGY
• Albumin—produced exclusively in the liver; provides 75%–80% of plasma colloid oncotic pressure; important in retaining fluid within the vascular compartment • Associated low oncotic pressure—permits loss of fluid into the interstitial space and potential third space compartments, causing edema and body cavity effusions • Serum albumin < 1.5 g/dL—edema and effusions • Serum albumin 1.5–2.5 g/dL—no edema or effusion unless other factors provoke fluid extravasation; increased hydrostatic pressure (venous occlusion, vascular bed hypertension), renal sodium retention, fluid overload, or increased vascular permeability • Symptomatic condition—develops as a result of chronic liver disease; extracorporeal loss in the gut (PLE), loss through the glomeruli (PLN), or cutaneous loss (severe exudative dermatitis, third-degree burns); malnutrition or starvation • Albumin:globulin concentration—may help differentiate cause; equivalent losses occur in PLE and nonselective proteinuria.

SYSTEMS AFFECTED
• Cardiovascular and Respiratory—transudative body cavity effusions (e.g., pleural effusion and ascites); peripheral edema; pulmonary edema • Renal/Urologic—prerenal azotemia, resulting from low plasma volume and impaired renal perfusion • Endocrine/Metabolic—altered protein binding, permitting increased unbound-free drug and adverse drug effects • Musculoskeletal—delayed wound healing (controversial)

SIGNALMENT
Dogs and cats

SIGNS

Historical Findings
• Abdominal distention with ascites • Dyspnea—owing to pulmonary edema or pleural effusion • Swollen limbs—with edema

Physical Examination Findings
• Ascites • Muffled heart sounds—with pleural effusion • Pulmonary crackles—with edema • Peripheral edema • Dyspnea

CAUSES

Decreased Albumin Production
• Chronic liver disease—chronic hepatitis; cirrhosis; idiopathic hepatic fibrosis • Inadequate intake—malnutrition; PLE

Extracorporeal Albumin Loss
• PLN—amyloidosis; glomerulonephritis

• PLE—lymphangiectasia; lymphoma; severe inflammatory bowel disease; histoplasmosis • Exudative cutaneous lesions • Chronic severe blood loss • Repeated large volume paracentesis of abdominal or pleural effusions

Sequestration in Body Cavities or Tissues
• Inflammatory effusions—pancreatitis; peritonitis; chylous effusions • Neoplasia—carcinomatosis • Vasculopathy—vasculitis (immune mediated); infectious (*Ehrlichia*, Rocky Mountain spotted fever)

Miscellaneous
• Hyperglobulinemia • Negative acute phase response • Catabolism • Dilution—iatrogenic vascular expansion; syndrome of inappropriate • ADH Hypoadrenocorticism

RISK FACTORS
• Diseases of the liver, kidney, intestines, blood vessels • Negative nitrogen balance

DIAGNOSIS

DIFFERENTIAL DIAGNOSIS
• Severe liver disease—patient may be anicteric or jaundiced; may note hepatic encephalopathy or polyuria/polydipsia; patient predisposed to ascites • PLE—diarrhea common; usually see thickened bowel segments • Cutaneous lesions—must be severe and exudative • External blood loss—associated with pallor; vital signs indicate anemia; extracorporeal evidence of blood loss • Malnutrition—mild hypoalbuminemia • Aggressive fluid therapy—may exacerbate condition or create spurious findings

LABORATORY FINDINGS

Drugs That May Alter Laboratory Results
Ampicillin—may cause falsely high values

Disorders That May Alter Laboratory Results
Extreme lipemia or excessive hemolysis—artificially high values with the bromcresol green method

Valid If Run in Human Laboratory?
Yes

CBC/BIOCHEMISTRY/URINALYSIS

CBC
• Depends on underlying cause • Severe liver disease—RBC microcytosis common • Severe blood loss—regenerative anemia • PLE—lymphopenia in lymphangiectasia

Biochemistry
• Fractionation of total protein may indicate underlying disorder. • Chronic liver disease—low albumin, normal-high globulin • PLE—low albumin, low globulins • PLN—low albumin, variable globulins • Exudative losses—low albumin, variable globulins • Malnutrition—low albumin, normal globulins • Severe blood loss—low albumin, low to normal globulins • Patterns—influenced by acute-phase response, which increases globulins and provides a negative feedback on albumin synthesis • Cholesterol—low with chronic liver disease, severe PLE, Addison disease, severe malnutrition; high with PLN • Liver enzymes—may be increased with chronic active liver disease, inflammatory bowel disease causing PLE, and with a general systemic response to inflammation • Total bilirubin—may be high with chronic liver disease • BUN—may be very low with chronic liver disease or when undergoing diuresis; high with substantially reduced renal function • Hyperkalemia and hyponatremia—indicate hypoadrenocorticism or gut-associated pseudohypoadrenocorticism • Spurious hypocalcemia—calculate predicted calcium: corrected calcium = measured calcium − measured albumin + midrange calcium for current laboratory

Urinalysis
• Complete urine examination—essential; rule out PLN • Proteinuria—if detected by dipstick method, substantiate by chemical determination • Urine protein:creatinine—essential; > 3.0 compatible with nephrotic syndrome; must interpret along with urine sediment; spurious positive values with active sediment composed of large positive blood (grossly visible) or severe pyuria

OTHER LABORATORY TESTS
• TSBA—high with severe liver disease; may note spurious low values with PLE (fat malabsorption) • Physicochemical examination of cavity effusions—transudates (pure or modified)

IMAGING
• Thoracic radiographs—may demonstrate pleural effusion and pulmonary edema • Barium contrast studies—limited utility for differential diagnosis • Abdominal radiographs—demonstrate ascites; may suggest alterations in liver size, mass lesions, or quadrant signs of pancreatic disease

• Abdominal ultrasonography—helps differentiate visceral abnormalities (e.g., small liver, thickened gut wall), mass lesions, fluid pockets, changes in portal blood flow, or mesenteric lymphadenopathy

DIAGNOSTIC PROCEDURES
• Antithrombin III—similar molecular weight to albumin; may not be detected with PLE, PLN, and other conditions associated with albumin loss; low with hepatic synthetic failure
• Liver biopsy—after evaluating coagulation (mucosal bleeding time, PIVKA, PT, APTT)
• Renal biopsy—differentiates amyloidosis from glomerulonephritis; limited use owing to few treatment options for these diseases
• Endoscopy—pinch biopsy or full-thickness bowl biopsy

TREATMENT

APPROPRIATE HEALTH CARE
• Depends on definitive cause
• Pleural effusion restricting ventilation—perform thoracentesis and place chest tube.
• Inpatient—during diagnostic procedures

NURSING CARE
Provide physical therapy and walk patient to improve drainage of peripheral edema fluid.

Fluid Therapy
• Avoid excessive sodium loading.
• Colloids—use to reduce the quantity of crystalloids required for volume expansion; anticipate continued intravenous administration; not retained by patients with extracorporeal losses (PLE, PLN, surface exudation), so administer during crisis situations only
• Plasma—best colloid; use for longer-term effect than that provided by synthetic colloid
• Antithrombin III—provided in plasma; lost extracorporeally along with albumin; reduced synthesis associated with reduced albumin synthesis owing to liver disease
• Dextran 70—polysaccharide; molecular weight = 70,000; alternative colloid; 6% solution in 0.9% NaCl (1 mL/kg/hr); may exacerbate or create bleeding tendencies; does not negate the loss in protein binding; avoid use with liver patients
• Hetastarch—synthetic polymer; increases oncotic pressure; 6% solution in 0.9% NaCl (10–20 mL/kg IV over 6–8 hr or dripped slowly for 24 hr); multiple doses usually given; may exacerbate or create bleeding tendencies; does not negate the loss in protein binding

DIET
• Achieve positive energy and nitrogen balance.
• Hepatic encephalopathy—restrict protein intake.

• PLE associated with lymphangiectasia—medium-chain triglycerides (dogs only) combined with a fat-restricted diet

CLIENT EDUCATION
Depends on definitive diagnosis

SURGICAL CONSIDERATIONS
Delayed wound healing (controversial)

MEDICATIONS

DRUGS OF CHOICE
• Glucocorticoids—use for some active nonsuppurative hepatopathies and inflammatory bowel disease; select agent with minimal mineralocorticoid effects (e.g., dexamethasone) to avoid sodium and water retention.
• Diuretics—assist in mobilization and excretion of excess body water and sodium; furosemide (1–4 mg/kg IV, IM, PO q4–12h), used judiciously to avoid intravascular volume contraction, in combination with spironolactone (1–4 mg/kg PO q12h) with liver disease
• Antithrombotic treatment—aspirin (0.5 mg/kg PO or rectally q12h) with low antithrombin III, especially with PLN

CONTRAINDICATIONS
Synthetic colloids—avoid with anuria, renal failure, congestive heart failure, severe coagulopathy, or von Willebrand disease

PRECAUTIONS
• Fluid therapy—large doses of synthetic colloids may cause volume overload and coagulopathies (dextrans); do not overload with crystalloid fluids (e.g., lactated Ringer, plasmalyte), which are rapidly distributed into the interstitial space (70% volume within 1 hr), worsening pulmonary edema, limb edema, and body cavity effusions.
• Plasma transfusion—may be complicated by transfusion reactions
• Diuretic therapy—may result in volume contraction, predisposing patients to azotemia and hypotension
• Unanticipated drug side effects—owing to reduced albumin concentration for drug binding

POSSIBLE INTERACTIONS
N/A

ALTERNATIVE DRUGS
N/A

FOLLOW-UP

PATIENT MONITORING
• Body weight—especially during fluid therapy; monitor fluid retention • Vital signs, thoracic auscultation for crackles—monitor

pulmonary edema • Serum albumin concentration • Blood pressure—monitor vascular expansion • Abdominal girth—monitor severity of ascites • Pulse oximetry—detect hypoxemia secondary to pulmonary edema

PREVENTION/AVOIDANCE
N/A

POSSIBLE COMPLICATIONS
• PLN—may be complicated by thromboembolism; minimize intravenous catheterization and iatrogenic trauma. • Hypovolemia—owing to translocation of fluid to interstitial and third spaces; predisposes patient to acute renal failure and DIC

EXPECTED COURSE AND PROGNOSIS
Depend on underlying cause

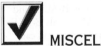

MISCELLANEOUS

ASSOCIATED CONDITIONS
N/A

AGE-RELATED FACTORS
N/A

PREGNANCY
Condition complicates pregnancy.

SEE ALSO
• Amyloidosis • Cirrhosis/Fibrosis of the Liver • Glomerulonephritis • Protein-losing enteropathy

ABBREVIATIONS
• ADH = antidiuretic hormone • APTT = activated partial thromboplastin time • DIC = disseminated intravascular coagulation
• PIVKA = proteins invoked by vitamin K absence or antagonism • PLE = protein-losing enteropathy • PLN = protein-losing nephropathy
• PT = prothrombin time
• TSBA = total serum bile acids

Suggested Reading
Center SA. Disorders of fluid accumulation. In: Willard MD, Tvedten H, Turnwald GH, eds. Small animal clinical diagnosis by laboratory methods. Philadelphia: Saunders, 1998.
Smiley LE, Garvey MS. The uses of hetastarch as adjunct therapy in 26 dogs with hypoalbuminemia: a phase two clinical trial. J Vet Intern Med 1994;8:195–202.
Turnwald GH, Barta O. Immunologic and plasma protein disorders. In: Willard MD, Tvedten H, Turnwald GH, eds. Small animal clinical diagnosis by laboratory methods. Philadelphia: Saunders, 1989:229–242.
Author Susan E. Johnson
Consulting Editor Sharon A. Center

ALKALINE PHOSPHATASE (ALP)/γ-GLUTAMYL TRANSFERASE (GGT)

BASICS

DEFINITION
• Serum enzymes useful for diagnosing liver disease
• ALP—useful for detecting other conditions; serum activity generally 30–150 U/L in healthy dogs and 30–100 U/L in healthy cats
• GGT—serum activity usually 1–7 U/L in healthy dogs and < 2 IU/L in healthy cats

PATHOPHYSIOLOGY
ALP
• Found in most organs; in greatest concentration in kidney, intestine, liver, and bone
• Isoenzymes contribute to serum enzyme activity—liver (L-ALP), bone (B-ALP), and corticosteroi-induced (C-ALP); only B-ALP and L-ALP found in healthy dogs and cats
• L-ALP—primarily found attached to the outer canalicular and sinusoidal surfaces of hepatocytes upon induction; released from sinusoidal surfaces with cholestasis, in which bile acids serve as potent enzyme inducers and facilitate membrane release; released in noncholestatic disorders after enzyme induction; release from sinusoidal membrane facilitated by normal bile acid flux
• B-ALP—found on osteoblasts and matrix vesicles; increases with increased osteogenesis (young animals) and owing to osteomyelitis and osteosarcoma
• C-ALP—produced in dog liver (not cat liver); released under the influence of glucocorticoids and other inducers
• Serum activity—lower in cats than in dogs owing to shorter plasma half-life (6 hr vs. 72 hr) and smaller magnitude of enzyme induction in cat liver
• Cats—mild increases in serum activity indicate disease (e.g., cholestasis, hyperthyroidism, hepatic lipidosis).
• Dogs—twofold to fourfold increases in serum activity often nonspecifically develop with illness.

GGT
• Membrane-bound enzyme found primarily on bile ductular epithelial cells
• Liver and serum—normally lower in dogs and cats than in other species (horses and humans)

• Release mechanism with cholestasis requires bile acids.
• Cats—activity primarily indicates cholestasis; more sensitive than ALP
• Dogs—activity reflects cholestasis and induction (e.g., glucocorticoids)

SYSTEMS AFFECTED
• High activity causes no injury.
• High enzymes—disease; cell proliferation; enzyme induction

SIGNALMENT
• Newborns—high GGT develops after colostrum ingestion
• Juveniles—high ALT common with bone growth and remodeling
• Adult dogs—modest to marked increase in ALT with diseases unrelated to the liver; may be associated with increased cortisol release, or from treatment with glucocorticoids (any route of application)

SIGNS
• None
• Clinical signs compatible with hepatic disease—determine ALP and GGT activities as indicators of cholestasis.
• Clinical signs compatible with hyperadrenocorticism (dogs)—determine ALP activity.

CAUSES
General
GGT—even minimal increases suggest hepatic disease; higher diagnostic specificity than ALP (less false-positives); marked and disproportionate increases (> 100 U/L) often associated with biliary hyperplasia or hepatic cancer (e.g., hepatocellular carcinoma, biliary adenocarcinoma)
Dogs
• Both enzymes—usually increase with cholestasis and vacuolar hepatopathy; induced by some drugs (e.g., anticonvulsants: phenobarbital, primidone, and phenytoin), especially ALP
• ALP—rarely increases with osteogenic activity; minor to modest increases common with a variety of diseases and usually reflect C-ALP derived from chronic stress and release of endogenous cortisol secondary to the primary disease process

Cats
• ALP—no drug or glucocorticoid induction (glucocorticoids lead to hepatic lipid vacuolation); mild to marked activity associated with hyperthyroidism
• GGT—more sensitive to hepatic disorders, except hepatic lipidosis (see below)

Associated Liver Disorders
• High ALP activity—cholestasis; cholangiohepatitis (cats); chronic active hepatitis (dogs); vacuolar hepatopathy (dogs); hepatic lipidosis (cats); primary hepatic neoplasia
• High GGT activity—cholestasis; chronic active hepatitis (dogs); vacuolar hepatopathy (dogs); primary hepatic neoplasia
• Hepatic lipidosis (cats)—uniquely associated with cholestasis that causes minor or no increase in serum GGT
• Minor increases in ALP—metastatic neoplasia (variable); portosystemic vascular anomaly; cirrhosis
• Acute disruption of hepatocellular membrane integrity (hepatic necrosis, liver trauma)—because of its relatively low liver concentration, ALP displays only minor acute increases compared to ALT and AST.

Glucocorticoid Hepatopathy (Dogs)
• ALP—minor to marked increases after treatment; initially owing to L-ALP and later to C-ALP; magnitude depends on drug dose, route of administration (increase greater with injectable than with oral), duration of treatment, pharmacologic preparation, and biological variation; increase also noted with ophthalmic and topically administered preparations.
• Hyperadrenocorticism—associated with increased C-ALP activity in > 83% of dogs, of which approximately 50% have some increase in GGT activity

Serum B-ALP
• Highest activity in the newborn; decreases continually until adulthood
• Diseases involving bone (e.g., bone fractures, fungal infections, metabolic disorders, primary or metastatic neoplasia) and chronic renal failure (secondary hyperparathyroidism)—may note high activity
• Osteosarcoma—may note normal to high activity (up to 2000 U/L)

RISK FACTORS
N/A

ALKALINE PHOSPHATASE (ALP)/γ-GLUTAMYL TRANSFERASE (GGT)

DIAGNOSIS

DIFFERENTIAL DIAGNOSIS
• ALP—may be associated with both hepatic and nonhepatic diseases; must interpret activity along with other liver function tests (e.g., TSBA, bilirubin, ALT, AST); mild to moderate increases consistently observed in young animals
• Chronic renal disease (renal azotemia; dogs)—mild to moderate increase in ALP common
• Significant hepatobiliary disease—high ALP and GGT in conjunction with and high TSBA and/or bilirubin
• Vacuolar hepatopathy owing to hyper-adrenocorticism or glucocorticoid administration or in a response to other primary disease processes (anicteric dogs)—high ALP with or without high GGT, with normal or mildly abnormal TSBA, and with minor increases or normal ALT and AST
• Hepatic lipidosis or hyperthyroidism (cats)—marked increase in ALP without comparable GGT activity

LABORATORY FINDINGS

Drugs That May Alter Laboratory Results
ALP (dogs)—numerous drugs and chemicals can induce activity.

Disorders That May Alter Laboratory Results
ALP and GGT—marked hemolysis may lower activity, depending on methods.

Valid If Run in Human Laboratory?
Yes

CBC/BIOCHEMISTRY/URINALYSIS
• CBC—not likely to assist in confirming hepatic disease; useful for identifying a primary disease
• ALP and GGT activity—lack specificity and/or sensitivity for hepatic disease; interpret in conjunction with urinalysis and other tests of hepatic disease
• ALT—often secondarily increased in cholestasis; primarily indicates liver necrosis or trauma

OTHER LABORATORY TESTS
• TSBA and bilirubin—identify hepatobiliary disorders

• High ALP activity in dogs with no evidence of cholestasis—rule out hyperadrenocorticism via history, clinical signs, and appropriate adrenal–pituitary axis evaluations (e.g., ACTH-response test, low-dose dexamethasone suppression test); measure C-ALP (high sensitivity, but low specificity)
• High ALP (cats)—evaluate hepatic lipidosis with abdominal ultrasonography and fine-needle hepatic aspirate; measure serum thyroxin to rule out hyperthyroidism.

IMAGING

Abdominal Radiography
• Microhepatia—with cirrhosis or PSVA; may see normal or mildly high ALP and GGT activity, unless an active acquired lesion is noted
• Hepatomegaly—vacuolar hepatopathy, hepatic neoplasia, hepatic lipidosis, or congestion; high ALP with or without high GGT likely

Abdominal Ultrasonography
• Rule out extrahepatic bile duct occlusion, pancreatitis, and focal hepatic mass lesions
• May increase suspicion for a diffuse hepatopathy

DIAGNOSTIC PROCEDURES
• Hepatic biopsy—when laboratory findings suggest hepatobiliary disease and ultrasonography rules out extrahepatic bile duct occlusion
• Fine-needle aspirates—initial evaluation of suspected hepatic lipidosis (cats), vacuolar hepatopathy (dogs), and neoplasia

TREATMENT
Based on underlying disease

MEDICATIONS

DRUG(S) OF CHOICE
Depend on underlying disease

CONTRAINDICATIONS
Depend on underlying disease

PRECAUTIONS
Depend on underlying disease

ALTERNATIVE DRUGS
Depend on underlying disease

FOLLOW-UP

PATIENT MONITORING
• Successful treatment of underlying disease—activity generally decreases within a few days to few weeks.
• Marked biliary hyperplasia—high GGT may persist.
• Hyperadrenocorticism or termination of very-long-term corticosteroid therapy—ALP may normalize after weeks to months.

POSSIBLE COMPLICATIONS
N/A

MISCELLANEOUS

ASSOCIATED CONDITIONS
N/A

AGE-RELATED FACTORS
ALP—mildly to moderately high activity is normal in growing puppies and kittens.

ZOONOTIC POTENTIAL
N/A

PREGNANCY
ALP—high activity may develop in pregnancy.

SEE ALSO
Cirrhosis/Fibrosis of the Liver
Hepatic Lipidosis
Hepatitis, Chronic Active
Hepatocellular Adenoma
Hepatocellular Carcinoma (HCCA)
Hepatotoxins
Steroid Hepatopathy

ABBREVIATIONS
• ALT = alanine aminotransferase
• AST = aspartate aminotransferase
• PSVA = portosystemic vascular anomaly
• TSBA = total serum bile acids

Suggested Reading
Center SA. Diagnostic procedures for evaluation of hepatic disease. In: Guilford WG, Center SA, Strombeck DR, et al., eds. Strombeck's small animal gastroenterology. Philadelphia: Saunders, 1996:130–188.
Kramer JW, Hoffmann WE. Clinical enzymology. In: Kaneko JJ, Harvey JW, Bruss ML, eds. Clinical biochemistry of domestic animals. 5th ed. San Diego: Academic Press, 1997:303–326.
Author Walter E. Hoffmann
Contributing Editor Sharon A. Center

DIAGNOSTICS—LAB

ALKALOSIS, METABOLIC

 BASICS

DEFINITION

Primary increase in plasma bicarbonate concentration ($[HCO_3^-]$) (dogs, >24 mEq/L; cats, >22 mEq/L) with low hydrogen ion concentration ($[H^+]$), high pH, and a compensatory increase in carbon dioxide tension (PCO_2)

PATHOPHYSIOLOGY

Loss of chloride and hydrogen ion-rich fluid via the alimentary tract or kidneys is usually accompanied by volume depletion. Loss of H^+ is associated with an increase in plasma HCO_3^- concentration. With chloride loss and volume depletion, the kidneys reabsorb sodium and HCO_3^- instead of chloride, perpetuating the metabolic alkalosis. Chronic administration of alkali also may result in transient metabolic alkalosis. Renal excretion of exogenously administered alkali is effective, and it is difficult to create metabolic alkalosis by increasing HCO_3^- intake, unless the patient has renal dysfunction.

SYSTEMS AFFECTED

• Respiratory—low $[H^+]$ reduces alveolar ventilation. Hypoventilation increases PCO_2 and helps offset the effects of high plasma $[HCO_3^-]$ on pH. In dogs, an increase of approximately 0.7 mm Hg in PCO_2 can be expected for each 1 mEq/L increase in plasma $[HCO_3^-]$.
• Renal/Urologic—the kidneys rapidly and effectively excrete excessive alkali. In patients with chloride deficiency (and less importantly, volume depletion), the kidneys cannot excrete the excessive alkali and metabolic alkalosis is maintained.
• Nervous—muscle twitching and seizures occur rarely in dogs.

SIGNALMENT

Any breed, age, or sex of dog and cat

SIGNS

Historical Findings
• Administration of loop diuretics (e.g., furosemide) or thiazides
• Vomiting

Physical Examination Findings
• Signs related to the underlying disease or accompanying potassium depletion (e.g., weakness, cardiac arrhythmias, and ileus)
• Muscle twitching caused by low ionized calcium concentration
• Dehydration in volume-depleted patients
• Muscle twitching and seizures in patients with neurologic involvement (rare)

CAUSES
• Chloride-responsive—diuretic administration, vomiting of stomach contents, and rapid correction of hypercapnia (respiratory acidosis)
• Chloride-resistant—hyperadrenocorticism and primary hyperaldosteronism
• Oral administration of alkali—administration of sodium bicarbonate or other organic anions with sodium (e.g., lactate, acetate, gluconate); administration of cation-exchange resin with nonabsorbable alkali (e.g., phosphorus binders)
• Miscellaneous—hypoalbuminemia, administration of large doses of sodium penicillin or carbenicillin

RISK FACTORS
• Administration of loop or thiazide diuretics
• Vomiting

 DIAGNOSIS

DIFFERENTIAL DIAGNOSIS

High plasma $[HCO_3^-]$ in animals can also be compensating for chronic respiratory acidosis, in which PCO_2 is high and pH is low despite high $[HCO_3^-]$; blood gas determination required to differentiate.

LABORATORY FINDINGS

Drugs That May Alter Laboratory Results
N/A

Disorders That May Alter Laboratory Results
• Too much heparin (>10% of the sample) decreases $[HCO_3^-]$
• Samples stored at room temperature for more than 20 min have low pH because of increased PCO_2.
• Some blood gas analyzers only report pH and PCO_2; bicarbonate must be calculated, a potential source for error.

Valid If Run in Human Laboratory?
Yes

CBC/BIOCHEMISTRY/URINALYSIS
• High total CO_2 (total CO_2 in samples handled aerobically closely approximates $[HCO_3^-]$)
• Low ionized calcium concentration
• Electrolyte abnormalities vary with underlying cause.
• Hypochloremia—consider hypochloremic metabolic alkalosis, the most common reason for metabolic alkalosis in dogs and cats, which usually results from diuretic administration or vomiting of stomach contents.
• High sodium but normal chloride concentration—consider chloride-resistant metabolic alkalosis (e.g., hyperadrenocorticism or primary hyperaldosteronism) or administration of alkali.
• Hypoalbuminemia—consider hypoalbuminemic metabolic alkalosis; albumin is a weak acid. In human beings, a decrease of 1 g/dL in albumin is associated with a 3.7 mEq/L increase in $[HCO_3^-]$.
• Hypokalemia—hypokalemia likely results from the metabolic alkalosis or the underlying problem (e.g., vomiting of stomach contents or loop diuretic administration); hypokalemia-induced metabolic alkalosis does not occur in dogs and cats.

OTHER LABORATORY TESTS

Blood gas analysis reveals high $[HCO_3^-]$, high PCO_2, and high pH.

IMAGING
N/A

DIAGNOSTIC PROCEDURES
N/A

TREATMENT

• Acid–base disturbances are secondary phenomena. Diagnosis and treatment of the underlying disease process is integral to the successful resolution of acid–base disorders.
• Discontinue drugs that may cause metabolic alkalosis.

NURSING CARE
The fluids of choice contain chloride; give patients with volume depletion an intravenous infusion of 0.9% NaCl supplemented with KCl; patients with hypokalemia may require large doses of KCl (see potassium, hypokalemia).

MEDICATIONS

DRUGS OF CHOICE
• If the underlying cause cannot be corrected (e.g., chronic heart failure patients receiving diuretics), oral compounds containing chloride without sodium (e.g., KCl, NH_4Cl) can be tried; also consider simultaneous use of distal tubule blocking agents (e.g., spironolactone, triamterene, and amiloride).
• Chloride-resistant metabolic alkalosis can only be corrected by resolution of the underlying disease; metabolic alkalosis is usually mild in these patients.

CONTRAINDICATIONS
• Avoid chloride-free fluids—they may correct volume depletion but will not correct metabolic alkalosis.
• Avoid drugs containing sodium without chloride (e.g., sodium penicillin, sodium bicarbonate)—they may worsen metabolic alkalosis.

• Avoid using salts of potassium without chloride (e.g., potassium phosphate)—potassium will be excreted in the urine and will correct neither the alkalosis nor the potassium deficit.

PRECAUTIONS
Do not use distal blocking agents (e.g., spironolactone, triamterene, and amiloride) in volume-depleted patients.

POSSIBLE INTERACTIONS
N/A

ALTERNATIVE DRUGS
N/A

FOLLOW-UP

PATIENT MONITORING
Acid–base status—frequency dictated by the underlying disease and patient response to treatment

POSSIBLE COMPLICATIONS
• Hypokalemia
• Neurologic signs

MISCELLANEOUS

ASSOCIATED CONDITIONS
• Hypokalemia
• Hypochloremia

AGE-RELATED FACTORS
N/A

ZOONOTIC POTENTIAL
N/A

PREGNANCY
N/A

SYNONYMS
• Nonrespiratory alkalosis
• Chloride-responsive metabolic alkalosis—metabolic alkalosis that responds to chloride administration

• Chloride-resistant metabolic alkalosis—metabolic alkalosis that does not respond to chloride administration
• Hypochloremic metabolic alkalosis—metabolic alkalosis caused by low chloride concentration
• Hypoalbuminemic alkalosis—metabolic alkalosis caused by low albumin concentration
• Concentration alkalosis—metabolic alkalosis caused by high sodium concentration
• Contraction alkalosis—metabolic alkalosis formerly attributed to volume-contraction, but now known to be caused by chloride depletion

SEE ALSO
• Potassium, Hypokalemia
• Chloride, Hypochloremia

ABBREVIATIONS
HCO_3^- = bicarbonate
PCO_2 = carbon dioxide tension
H^+ = hydrogen ion

Suggested Reading
de Morais HSA. Chloride ion in small animal practice: the forgotten ion. J Vet Emerg Crit Care 1992;2:11–24
DiBartola SP. Metabolic alkalosis. In: DiBartola SP, ed. Fluid therapy in small animal practice. Philadelphia: Saunders, 1992:244–257.
DiBartola SP, Green RA, de Morais HSA. Electrolytes and acid base disorders. In: Willard MD, Tvedten H, Turnwald GH, eds. Small animal clinical diagnosis by laboratory methods. 2nd ed. Philadelphia: Saunders, 1994:97–113.
Robinson EP, Hardy RM. Clinical signs, diagnosis, and treatment of alkalemia in dogs: 20 cases (1982–1984). J Am Vet Med Assoc 1988;192:943–949.
Authors Helio Autran de Morais and Stephen P. DiBartola
Consulting Editors Larry G. Adams and Carl A. Osborne

α_1-PROTEASE INHIBITOR (α_1-PI) FECAL

BASICS

DEFINITION
Fecal α_1-PI > 6.0 μg/g feces

PATHOPHYSIOLOGY
- α_1-PI is not normally present in the lumen of the gastrointestinal (GI) tract above trace background concentrations unless there is abnormal transmucosal loss of plasma, lymph, or intercellular fluid as a result of GI disease.
- In some disease states, excessive quantities of plasma proteins including α_1-PI are lost into the intestinal lumen.
- Most plasma proteins are rapidly degraded by digestive proteases, and constituent amino acids are reabsorbed. α_1-PI is resistant to such degradation by virtue of its inhibitory activity; it is excreted in feces with minimal loss of its immunoreactivity and can be detected by specific immunoassays.
- In hypoalbuminemic patients the GI tract is usually implicated as the site of protein loss by excluding significant proteinuria and hepatic disease.
- PLE occurs in association with mucosal disease processes (inflammation, ulceration) or by obstruction of lymphatic flow from the intestines.
- When plasma proteins are lost into the intestinal lumen, all (including albumin, α_1-PI, and globulins) are lost at an equal rate.
- If the enteric protein loss is great, the resultant panhypoproteinemia (hypoalbuminemia and hypoglobulinemia) is characteristic of PLEs.
- No such decreased protein concentration is observed if the protein loss is not severe enough to overcome compensatory mechanisms such as increased hepatic albumin synthesis.
- Fecal α_1-PI can reach abnormal concentrations before protein loss is severe enough to cause hypoalbuminemia.

SYSTEMS AFFECTED
- Gastrointestinal—protein-losing GI diseases can lead to this abnormality.
- Cardiovascular—right-sided congestive heart failure can rarely lead to this abnormality.

SIGNALMENT

Species
Dogs; immunoassay for α_1-PI is species-specific.

Breed Predilection
- Breeds with reported familial predisposition to intestinal protein loss include Norwegian lundehunds, soft-coated wheaten terriers, and basenjis.
- Other breeds including Yorkshire terrier, shar pei, and rottweiler may have an increased prevalence for intestinal protein loss.

Predominant Sex
N/A

Mean Age and Range
N/A

SIGNS

Historical Findings
- Weight loss
- Vomiting
- Anorexia
- Diarrhea
- All signs of GI disease, including diarrhea, may be absent.

Physical Examination Findings
- May be normal
- Poor body condition and dull hair coat are common.
- Lethargy and or thickened bowel loops may be present.
- Ascites and edema may be observed with severe or chronic hypoproteinemia.
- Dyspnea may be seen in cases of pulmonary thromboembolism.

CAUSES

Ulceration of the Mucosal Lining and Mucosal Inflammatory Disorders (Increased Mucosal Permeability)
- IBD—lymphocytic plasmacytic, eosinophilic, or granulomatous gastroenteritis
- GI neoplasia
- Foreign body, intussusception
- Intestinal parasitism
- Small intestinal bacterial overgrowth (SIBO)
- Fungal infection (e.g., histoplasmosis, pythiosis)
- Acute viral and bacterial enteritis
- Food allergies (e.g., gluten-sensitive enteropathy in the Irish setter)

Lymphatic Disorders
- Primary—congenital lymphangiectasia (ludehunds)
- Secondary—acquired lymphangiectasia, usually associated with lymphatic obstructive lesions; neoplasia (lymphosarcoma); lipogranulomatous lesions within and around the lymphatics; congestive heart failure

RISK FACTORS
- GI disease
- Compromised lymphatic system
- Right-sided heart failure

DIAGNOSIS

DIFFERENTIAL DIAGNOSIS
α_1-PI concentrations above 6 μg/g of feces indicate excessive loss of protein into the GI tract; the clinician should differentiate the various causes for PLE from other causes of hypoalbuminemia:
- Hepatic disease—decreased synthesis of albumin
- Renal disease—proteinuria due to amyloidosis or glomerulonephritis
- Blood loss—acute or chronic
- Vasculitis
- Hypoproteinemia from renal and hepatic disorders is characterized by low serum albumin concentrations and normal serum globulin concentrations; hypoalbuminemia from blood loss and vasculitis may be characterized by either panhypoproteinemia or hypoalbuminemia.

LABORATORY FINDINGS

Drugs That May Alter Laboratory Results
N/A

Disorders That May Alter Laboratory Results
- Fecal α_1-PI is labile, and concentrations decline when fecal specimens are kept at ambient temperatures for more than 36 h.
- Fecal samples can be stored at 4°C for up to 7 days with negligible loss of immunoreactivity.
- Freezing the specimens is advisable if samples will be stored for more than 7 days.

Valid If Run in Human Laboratory?
- No—immunoassay for human α_1-PI is species-specific; does not crossreact with canine α_1-PI
- ELISA for canine α_1-PI—can only be performed in a laboratory that has purified canine α_1-PI for use as a standard, and specific antibodies against canine α_1-PI.

CBC/BIOCHEMISTRY/URINALYSIS
- Findings vary, depending on the intestinal disease.
- Lymphopenia may be observed in lymphangiectasia.
- Regenerative anemia occurs with acute blood loss; nonregenerative anemia may occur with chronic blood loss.
- Nonregenerative anemia may occur with chronic diseases.
- Total serum calcium concentration may decrease because of lower serum albumin concentration.
- Hypocholesterolemia may occur in lymphangiectasia due to fat malabsorption.
- If hypoalbuminemia is associated with hypoglobulinemia (panhypoproteinemia), this pattern is characteristic of PLE.
- Proteinuria is absent unless there is concurrent protein-losing nephropathy or cystitis.

OTHER LABORATORY TESTS
- Measure pre- and postprandial bile acids to rule out hypoalbuminemia due to hepatic disease.
- Determine urinary protein:creatinine ratio to rule out significant proteinuria due to protein-losing nephropathy.
- Perform serial fecal examinations to rule out intestinal parasitism.
- Measure serum concentrations of cobalamin and folate to detect intestinal malabsorptive disorders or SIBO.

α₁-PROTEASE INHIBITOR (α₁-PI) FECAL

• Hydrogen breath testing may reveal concurrent carbohydrate malabsorption.
• Cytologic examination of fecal specimens or colonic and rectal mucosal swabs may disclose intestinal histoplasmosis.

IMAGING
• Thoracic and abdominal radiographs are useful to document some causes of PLE (e.g., intestinal obstruction, GI neoplasia, cardiac disease, and fungal enteropathies).
• Abdominal ultrasound may reveal hepatic, renal, or intestinal disorders; biopsy specimens can be collected in some cases.
• Contrast studies of the GI tract may help visualize thickened bowel loops in dogs with infiltrative disorders.

DIAGNOSTIC PROCEDURES
• Perform endoscopy to obtain duodenal/jejunal mucosal biopsy specimens, collect intestinal juice for bacterial culture, and directly visualize the mucosa of the stomach and proximal small intestine. Full-thickness biopsy specimens are required to document submucosal lymphatic obstruction in patients with primary or secondary lymphangiectasia.
• Surgical exploration and biopsy are indicated if endoscopic and/or ultrasound-guided biopsies are nondiagnostic or if the lesion cannot be assessed and/or biopsied by these procedures.

TREATMENT
• Usually outpatient medical management
• Nursing or supportive care depends on the underlying cause.
• Activity need not be restricted (unless severe anemia due to intestinal blood loss).
• Feed a low-fat high-protein diet if lymphangiectasia is confirmed; vitamin supplementation may benefit if documented cobalamin, folate, or other vitamin deficiencies
• Disorders associated with enteric protein loss are usually chronic, and owners must be prepared for long-term therapy.
• Some animals with PLE are severely hypoalbuminemic (i.e., <1.5 mg/dL) and thus may have delayed wound healing after surgery. With appropriate care these patients can be safely biopsied. Exercise special care when suturing enterotomies and closing the abdominal wall; use strong monofilament suture for intestinal and abdominal wall closure.

MEDICATIONS

DRUGS OF CHOICE
• Numerous disorders can cause PLEs in the dog; the specific therapy depends on the underlying disease.

• Plasma transfusions or colloids—no long-term value, but can be given as a palliative measure prior to anesthesia or when the hypoproteinemia is severe enough to cause edema or effusion
• If lymphangiectasia is documented, feed a low-fat, high-quality protein diet supplemented with medium-chain triglyceride oil (Mead Johnson; Evansville, IN, 1–2 mL/kg daily in food), to decrease distension of intestinal lymphatic vessels.
• Can give glucocorticoid therapy (to inhibit inflammation, exert an immunosuppressive effect, and to promote enterocyte function) if no underlying cause for intestinal lymphangiectasia can be found
• Immunosuppressive agents such as azathioprine may benefit patients with IBD and a poor response to corticosteroids.
• If SIBO can be documented, therapy with oxytetracycline or metronidazole may be effective.
• In patients with dietary sensitivity, direct treatment to feeding the patient with an appropriate antigen-restricted diet (e.g., a gluten-free diet). A diet with a single source of carbohydrate and a single source of protein (e.g., rice and low-fat cottage cheese–based diet) may prove helpful.

CONTRAINDICATIONS
N/A

PRECAUTIONS
Decrease dosage of protein-bound drugs in patients that are hypoproteinemic.

POSSIBLE INTERACTIONS
N/A

ALTERNATIVE DRUGS
Although controversial, some human patients with PLE have responded to antifibrinolytic therapy with *trans*-4-aminomethyl cyclohexane carboxylic acid (tranexamic acid) or aminocaproic acid. There are no reports of this therapeutic approach in canine patients with PLE.

FOLLOW-UP

PATIENT MONITORING
Recheck fecal α₁-PI concentration every 14–28 days to evaluate response to treatment. In human patients, fecal α₁-PI concentration has been used to evaluate response to chemotherapy for intestinal lymphosarcoma.

POSSIBLE COMPLICATIONS
• Pulmonary thromboembolism due to hypoproteinemia (loss of antithrombin III) may cause acute respiratory complications (rare).
• Respiratory distress from pleural effusion
• Postoperative complications due to slow wound healing
• Continued clinical problems from poor response to therapy

MISCELLANEOUS

ASSOCIATED CONDITIONS
Concurrent protein-losing gastroenteropathy and protein-losing nephropathy have been documented in soft-coated wheaten terriers.

AGE-RELATED FACTORS
N/A

ZOONOTIC POTENTIAL
Intestinal infectious diseases that cause PLE, such as histoplasmosis and hematophagus parasites (*Ancylostoma caninum*), are potentially zoonotic to human beings.

PREGNANCY
N/A

SYNONYMS
Fecal α₁-antitrypsin (α₁-AT)

SEE ALSO
• Diarrhea, Chronic—Dogs
• Dietary Intolerance
• Lymphangiectasia
• Inflammatory Bowel Disease
• Protein-losing Enteropathy
• Small Intestinal Bacterial Overgrowth

ABBREVIATIONS
• α₁-PI = α₁-protease inhibitor
• GI = gastrointestinal
• IBD = inflammatory bowel disease
• PLE = protein-losing enteropathy
• SIBO = small intestinal bacterial overgrowth

Suggested Reading

Fossum TW. Protein-losing enteropathy. Semin Vet Med Surg Small Anim 1989;190:60–64.
Melgarejo T, Tamayo A, Williams DA. Fecal alpha₁-protease inhibitor (α₁-PI) for the diagnosis of canine protein-losing enteropathy. J Vet Int Med 1997;11:115 (Abstract).
Melgarejo T, Williams DA, Asem E. Enzyme-linked immunosorbant assay for canine of α₁-protease inhibitor (α₁-PI). Am J Vet Res, in press, 1997.
Williams DA. Malabsorption, small intestinal bacterial overgrowth and protein-losing enteropathy. In: Guilford WG, Center SA, Strombeck DR, et al., eds. Small animal gastroenterology. 3rd ed. Philadelphia: Saunders, 1996:367–380.

Author Tonatiuh Melgarejo
Consulting Editors Mitchell A. Crystal and Brett M. Feder

AMMONIA

BASICS

DEFINITION
• A nonprotein nitrogenous compound that is normally detoxified in the hepatic urea cycle to water-soluble urea; to a lesser extent, also detoxified by temporary conversion to glutamine and predominantly stored in muscle
• Maintained as the relatively nondiffusible ammonium ion (NH_4^+)
• Maximum normal plasma values—approximately 165 μg/dL (μmol/L) in dogs and 130 μg/dL (μmol/L) in cats

PATHOPHYSIOLOGY
• Liver—primary site of urea synthesis (Krebs-Henseleit cycle); receives enterically produced ammonia via the portal vein
• Systemic—derived from endogenous catabolism of nitrogenous compounds from skeletal muscle; enteric microbial digestion of urea, exfoliated cellular debris, and dietary protein; and pathologic bleeding in the alimentary canal
• Impaired detoxification—reduced hepatic mass; impaired liver function; portosystemic shunting; inherited defects of the urea cycle

SYSTEMS AFFECTED
Nervous—cerebral dysfunction most common; hyperammonemia: abnormal function of the blood–brain barrier, impaired cerebral blood flow, abnormal neuronal excitability, deranged neurotransmitter metabolism, balance, interactions with neuroreceptors, degenerative neuronal changes (if chronic)

SIGNALMENT
• Dogs and cats
• Depends on underlying disorder
• Hyperammonemia in young animals—commonly congenital PSVA; rarely inborn errors of urea cycle enzymes

SIGNS

General Comments
• Primarily related to hepatic encephalopathy, which may occur sporadically and have a progressive course
• May worsen after feeding a high-protein (e.g., meat, fish, egg) meal

Historical Findings
• Ptyalism—especially cats
• Neurobehavioral abnormalities
• Visual deficits
• Circling
• Pacing
• Anxiety
• Head pressing
• Stupor
• Coma

Physical Examination Findings
PSVA
• Stunted growth
• Loss of body condition
• Cryptorchidism—males
• Copper-colored eyes in non-Persian and non-blue-eyed cats
• Mentation changes and aberrant behavior
Acquired Liver Disorders
• Depend on specific disease; may note icterus
• Chronically hepatic encephalopathy—neuronal degeneration; may become nonresolvable
• Hyperammonemia—urolithiasis owing to ammonium biurate crystalluria

CAUSES
• Reduced hepatic mass
• Impaired liver function
• Portosystemic shunting
• Inherited defects of the urea cycle—enzyme deficiencies
• Urease-producing organisms—combination of uro-obstruction and urinary tract infection
• Cats—obligate need for dietary arginine (part of the urea cycle); experimental arginine-deficient, high-protein diet may produce symptomatic hyperammonemia.

RISK FACTORS
• Reduced ammonia tolerance—high-risk patient; risk of hyperammonemia increases with the following factors.
• Transfusion—improperly stored or out-of-date RBC products that contain high levels of ammonia
• Gastrointestinal hemorrhage—causes an endogenous ammonia challenge (blood digested to its nitrogenous waste products)
• Large-volume hematoma formation or body cavity hemorrhagic effusions—heme protein overload
• Constipation—raises ammonia concentrations by increasing time for microbial production and colonic absorption
• Oral or rectal ammonium chloride administration when completing a tolerance test
• Loss of muscle mass—reduced ammonia storage as muscle glutamine
• Catabolic medication administration—cortisol, tetracycline
• Systemic infection
• Azotemia—25% of systemic urea diffuses into the gut, where it is transformed by ureases.
• Alkalemia—favors ammonia diffusion across cell membranes and the blood–brain barrier
• Hypokalemia—increases renal ammonia-genesis

DIAGNOSIS

DIFFERENTIAL DIAGNOSIS
• Must differentiate from primary neurologic disease and behavior problems.
• History; signalment; results of hemogram, serum biochemistry, and urinalysis (ammonium urate crystalluria); TSBA values; and results of hepatic biopsy and imaging (ultrasonography, contrast portography, or colorectal scintigraphy)—may be required for definitive diagnosis
• Hepatic encephalopathy—many associated toxins; do not rely on only high ammonia concentration to confirm diagnosis.

LABORATORY FINDINGS

Drugs That May Alter Laboratory Results
• The following alter ammonia concentration but not the validity of test results.
• Antibiotics—reduce bacterial intestinal flora; may lower plasma concentration
• Lactulose (orally or rectal)—may reduce systemic concentration by increasing nitrogen incorporation in enteric bacteria; produces an acidic enteric pH, which traps ammonia and NH_4^+; provides a cathartic effect (mechanical removal of ammonia and substrates)
• Cleansing or retention enemas (lactulose, lactose, neomycin, metronidazole, dilute vinegar solution)—facilitate removal of ammonia and ammoniagenic substrates; reduce enteric bacteria associated with ammonia formation; produces an acidic enteric pH, which traps NH_4^+
• Blood transfusion or administration of parenteral amino acids, narcotics, or diuretics—high concentrations may develop

Disorders That May Alter Laboratory Results
Venous occlusion during sampling—may cause high values, especially with muscle exertion during restraint

Valid If Run in Human Laboratory?
• Yes
• Keep samples in an ice bath and analyze within 30 min
• In-house dry chemistry analysis—has increased popularity of test; requires adequate controls, paired samples, and proper sample handling; spurious high values common

CBC/BIOCHEMISTRY/URINALYSIS
• Depend on associated liver disease
• CBC—erythrocyte microcytosis associated with portosystemic shunting
• Standard serum biochemistry—may be normal with PSVA; may note high liver enzymes and bilirubin, hypoglycemia, hypercholesterolemia or hypocholesterolemia, hypoalbuminemia, and low BUN with acquired liver disease

• Urinalysis—ammonia biurate crystals and low urine specific gravity owing to underlying liver disease

OTHER LABORATORY TESTS
TSBA—advised for nonicteric patients; confirms hepatic insufficiency; equivalent to ammonia for portosystemic shunting and liver dysfunction; more sensitive than ammonia for cholestasis; reliably tests enterohepatic circulation function with few confounding variables

IMAGING
• Abdominal radiography—assess hepatic size
• Ultrasonography—helpful; sensitivity and specificity depend on operator and patient
• Isotope studies—intravenous and colorectal radioisotope (technetium) perfusion techniques; require gamma-camera imaging; may assess portal blood flow; may be limited to referral centers

DIAGNOSTIC PROCEDURES
• Hepatic biopsy—usually necessary for definitive diagnosis
• ATT—may increase suspicion of hepatic insufficiency or portosystemic shunting; may precipitate hepatic encephalopathy; collect heparinized blood before and 30 min after administration of NH_4Cl (0.1 g/kg not to exceed 3 g) by enema (high rectal placement) or PO gelatin capsules; 3–10-fold increase above baseline indicates ammonia intolerance.

TREATMENT

APPROPRIATE HEALTH CARE
Inpatient intensive care—required with severe encephalopathy; see Hepatic Encephalopathy

NURSING CARE
• Fluids—correct dehydration, azotemia, hypoglycemia, and hypokalemia; see Hepatic Encephalopathy
• Lactate—use is of minimal concern, unless fulminant hepatic failure noted
• Chronic liver disease and acquired portosystemic shunting—water and sodium retention are concerns; avoid overhydration and high-sodium-containing fluids (e.g., 0.9% sodium chloride).
• Do not use jugular catheters with hyperammonemia, which often occurs with other disorders derived from hepatic insufficiency; bleeding tendencies may occur

ACTIVITY
Encephalopathy—keep patient quiet, warm, and adequately hydrated.

DIET
• Adequate calories—avoid catabolism
• Obtund—put patient on an initial fast.

• Dietary protein restriction—cornerstone of medical management for chronic hepatic encephalopathy and hyperammonemia; only as needed to ameliorate signs; dairy and vegetable proteins are best tolerated.
• Good-quality vitamin supplement (without methionine)—vitamin metabolism is often perturbed, with liver dysfunction.
• Ensure thiamine repletion—avoid Wernicke encephalopathy

MEDICATIONS

DRUGS OF CHOICE
• Medications that increase dietary protein tolerance—alter gastroenteric flora or enteric conditions; reduce production or availability of substances that precipitate hepatic encephalopathy
• Antibiotics—broad spectrum against aerobic and anaerobic intestinal flora; neomycin, nonabsorbable (10–20 mg/kg PO q8–12h) and metronidazole, local and systemic (7.5–10 mg/kg q12h); used in combination with lactulose
• Fermented carbohydrate, nonabsorbable
• Lactulose, lactitol, or lactose (if lactase deficient)—decrease production and absorption of ammonia; increase rate of stool transit; goal is passage of two to three soft stools per day; lactulose most commonly used (precise dose undetermined; start at 0.5–1 mL/kg PO q8–12h); may be administered as an enema with acute hepatic coma

Enemas
• Cleansing—10–15 mL/kg; warmed polyionic fluids; mechanically cleans the colon
• Retention—directly delivers fermentable substrates or alters colonic pH; dilute solutions containing lactulose, lactitol, or lactose 1:2 in water; neomycin in water (do not exceed oral dose); diluted Betadine (1:10, rinse well after 15 min); diluted vinegar (1:10 in water)

CONTRAINDICATIONS
Use caution with drugs that affect the CNS, because of common association of hyperammonemia with hepatic encephalopathy (depressed or altered mentation) and possibly impaired hepatic metabolism; barbiturates and benzodiazepam-like drugs are of particular concern.

PRECAUTIONS
N/A

POSSIBLE INTERACTIONS
• Carefully consider drugs that inhibit hepatic biotransformation or elimination pathways (e.g., cimetidine, ketoconazole, fluorinated quinolones) because of impaired hepatic metabolism

• Pathologic hypoalbuminemia permits increased free-drug concentrations of highly protein bound medications.

ALTERNATIVE DRUGS
N/A

FOLLOW-UP

PATIENT MONITORING
• Repeated assessments of plasma concentrations—may help assess severe hepatic encephalopathy when corrective therapy has been given
• Monitor ammonium urate crystalluria—assess success of medical management
• Monitor serum potassium and glucose—advised in critical patients; depletion of either augments encephalopathic signs caused by high concentrations.

POSSIBLE COMPLICATIONS
Test inaccuracy—biggest problem; ammonia labile in blood samples; delay in processing causes falsely high values; storage and temperature changes of samples may result in falsely high or low values.

MISCELLANEOUS

ASSOCIATED CONDITIONS
N/A

AGE-RELATED FACTORS
N/A

ZOONOTIC POTENTIAL
N/A

PREGNANCY
N/A

SEE ALSO
Hepatic Encephalopathy

ABBREVIATIONS
• ATT = ammonia-tolerance test
• PSVA = portosystemic vascular anomaly
• TSBA = total serum bile acids

Suggested Reading

Dimski DS. Ammonia metabolism and the urea cycle: function and clinical implications. J Vet Intern Med 1994;8:73–78.
Hitt ME, Jones BD. Effects of storage temperature and time on canine plasma ammonia concentrations. Am J Vet Res 1986;47:363–364.
Willard MD, Tvedten H, Turnwald GH. Small animal clinical diagnosis by laboratory methods. Philadelphia: Saunders, 1989.

Author Mark E. Hitt
Consulting Editor Sharon A. Center

AMYLASE AND LIPASE

BASICS

DEFINITION
Elevation in serum amylase and lipase concentrations above laboratory reference ranges

PATHOPHYSIOLOGY
• Only α-amylase is present in animals; the pancreas, liver, and small intestine serve as sources of serum amylase. • Serum amylase activity in health is derived primarily from extrapancreatic sources. • Considerable serum amylase activity (up to 1000 IU/L) is found in normal animals. • Hyperamylasemia may occur with pancreatitis, GI inflammation, and renal disease. • Serum lipase is derived from the pancreas and gastric mucosa; its activity is optimal at alkaline pH.
• Both amylase and lipase are inactivated by the kidney and eliminated in urine. • Hyperlipasemia may occur with pancreatitis, renal disease, hepatic disease, and neoplasia, and following the administration of dexamethasone.

SYSTEMS AFFECTED
N/A

SIGNALMENT
At-risk breeds for acute pancreatitis:
• Dogs—middle-aged and old miniature schnauzers, miniature poodles, cocker spaniels • Cats—middle-aged Siamese cats

SIGNS AND SYMPTOMS

General Comments
Clinical signs vary, depending upon the organ system or etiology involved.

Historical Findings
• Pancreatitis—lethargy, depression, anorexia, vomiting, diarrhea • Hepatic disease—anorexia, altered mentation, icterus, weight loss, vomiting, diarrhea, PU/PD, abdominal distention • Renal disease—PU/PD, lethargy, anorexia, weight loss, vomiting, diarrhea • GI disease—vomiting, diarrhea, anorexia, weight loss
• Exogenous glucocorticoids—PU/PD, polyphagia, weight gain

Physical Examination Findings
• Pancreatitis—lethargy, dehydration, abdominal pain, fever, icterus (more common in cats)
• Hepatic disease—icterus, hepatomegaly, depression, abdominal pain, weight loss, peritoneal effusion • Renal disease—weight loss, mucous membrane pallor, dehydration, altered renal size or contour • Gastrointestinal disease—weight loss, dehydration, palpable mass lesions or foreign bodies, variable fecal consistency

CAUSES

Pancreatitis and Hyperamylasemia
• Serum amylase activity increases in most dogs with pancreatitis, activity over 5000 IU/L strongly suggests acute pancreatitis. • Increased amylase concentration is a sensitive indicator of pancreatic inflammation, but it may also be increased by nonpancreatic diseases (poor specificity). • Serum amylase is best interpreted in light of serum lipase concentration. Amylase activities in dogs with pancreatitis do not correlate with lipase activity until serum lipase values exceed 800 IU/L. • Serum amylase activity decreases in cats with acute pancreatitis; determination of amylase values in cats is not recommended.

Pancreatitis and Hyperlipasemia
• Serum lipase consistently increases several-fold in dogs with pancreatitis. Using serum lipase concentrations of 500 IU/L, the sensitivity of the assay is 98%. • Lipase activities are also affected by a variety of nonpancreatic disorders (specificity of 78% using values of 500 IU/L as a cutoff). • Serum lipase values in cats with pancreatitis will be normal to high.
• Normal serum lipase activity does not rule out pancreatic disease. Up to 15–20% of patients with acute pancreatitis have normal lipase and/or amylase activity. • In general, lipase activity is a more reliable marker for pancreatitis in dogs and cats.

Renal Disease
• Renal failure is associated with hyperamylasemia and hyperlipasemia. • Increased serum concentrations may result from impaired renal degradation and/or inadequate clearance due to reduced glomerular filtration.

Hepatic Disease
The source for increased lipase activity in patients with liver disease is not known.

Gastrointestinal Disease
Increased serum amylase activity may occur in dogs as a consequence of enteritis, small intestinal obstruction, and GI perforation.

Miscellaneous
• A 3-fold or more increase is serum lipase activity may occur after routine laparotomy in dogs without clinical signs or gross evidence of pancreatitis. • Hyperlipasemia and decreased serum amylase activity have been reported in dogs following the administration of corticosteroids.

RISK FACTORS
• Obesity and the ingestion of high-fat diets for pancreatitis • Presence of underlying renal disease • Presence of underlying hepatic disease • Nonspecific GI inflammation
• Previous administration of dexamethasone
• Postoperative period

DIAGNOSIS

DIFFERENTIAL DIAGNOSIS
• Vomiting, depression, fever, and abdominal pain suggest pancreatitis. • PU/PD, anorexia, weight loss, vomiting, anemia, and altered renal size suggest renal disease. • Icterus, hepatomegaly, vomiting, PU/PD, and altered mentation suggest hepatic disease. • Vomiting, diarrhea, anorexia, and palpable abnormalities in intestinal loops suggest GI disease.

LABORATORY FINDINGS

Drugs That May Alter Laboratory Results
Corticosteroids increase serum lipase activity and decrease serum amylase activity.

Disorders That May Alter Laboratory Results
• Measure serum amylase activity with an amyloclastic method that measures the disappearance of starch from the assay. • Maltase activity in the plasma of dogs is high, and use of a saccharogenic method (measuring the appearance of glucose in the assay) will indicate a falsely high amylase activity, since maltase contributes to glucose formed in the assay.
• Measurement of serum lipase activity requires more time, is technically more cumbersome to perform, and yields results with more arbitrary interpretation. • Hemolysis inhibits lipase enzyme activity. • Lipemia falsely decreases serum lipase activity as measured by kinetic assays.
• Specific immunoassays are generally only useful for the species in which they were developed.

Valid If Run in Human Laboratory?
Yes

CBC/BIOCHEMISTRY/URINALYSIS
• Pancreatitis—leukocytosis with left shift, anemia in cats, hyperlipidemia, increased ALT, ALP, and total bilirubin, prerenal azotemia
• Renal disease—anemia (nonregenerative), renal azotemia, hyperphosphatemia, hypokalemia (cats), impaired urinary concentrating ability • Hepatic disease—increased ALT, ALP, and total bilirubin; hypoproteinemia; hypoalbuminemia; low BUN; impaired urinary concentrating ability • GI disease—variable, depends on cause

OTHER LABORATORY TESTS
• Serum TLI (dogs and cats) —increased in pancreatitis • TAP by ELISA (dogs)—increased with pancreatitis • Abdominocentesis or diagnostic peritoneal lavage and cytology—may reveal nonseptic suppurative peritonitis often seen with pancreatitis • Bile acid assay—increased hepatobiliary dysfunction and cholestasis • Tests to assess GI inflammation including serology for infectious agents, fecal cultures, etc.

IMAGING

• Pancreatitis—abdominal radiographs may demonstrate peritoneal effusion, focal soft tissue opacity in right cranial abdominal compartment, gas retention in proximal duodenum; thoracic radiographs may demonstrate mild pleural effusion; abdominal ultrasound may demonstrate peritoneal effusion and occasionally demonstrates a pancreatic mass or altered echogenicity in the area of the pancreas. • Renal disease—abdominal radiographs demonstrate normal or altered renal size, irregularity to renal cortical margins, skeletal osteodystrophy; abdominal ultrasound may demonstrate altered renal size and architecture and irregular renal margins. • Hepatic disease—abdominal radiographs demonstrate peritoneal effusion, hepatomegaly; abdominal ultrasound demonstrates hepatomegaly and alterations in hepatic parenchymal echogenicity. • GI disease—abdominal radiographs demonstrate radiopaque foreign bodies, obstructive lesions, increased bowel-loop diameter, mucosal irregularities (contrast), ulcers (contrast); abdominal ultrasound is variable but demonstrates foreign bodies, obstructive lesions, intramural infiltrative lesions, and masses.

DIAGNOSTIC PROCEDURES

• Renal biopsy (via laparotomy, laparoscopy, or ultrasound-guidance) to confirm diagnosis of renal disease • Hepatic biopsy (via laparotomy, laparoscopy, or ultrasound-guidance) to confirm diagnosis of hepatic disease • GI biopsy (via endoscopy, laporotomy or ultrasound guidance) to confirm GI disease • Foreign body removal (via endoscopy or laporotomy) for treatment of GI foreign body • Pancreatic abscesses—resection and/or open peritoneal drainage via laparotomy may be needed for pancreatic abscessation.

TREATMENT

GENERAL COMMENTS

• Treatment varies depending on the underlying cause for increased serum amylase and/or lipase activities, but most disease processes require inpatient medical management; surgery is occasionally necessary (see above). • Restricted activity is required for most patients. • Patients that are vomiting should be kept NPO until vomiting has ceased for more than 24–48 h. • Intravenous fluid therapy via a balanced electrolyte solution (such as lactated Ringer's solution) is typically necessary to restore hydration, provide maintenance (if NPO or adipsic/anorectic), and promote diuresis (renal disease). • Electrolyte assessment and management (especially potassium) is indicated; potassium supplementation should be based on measured serum levels but is usually

required (use 20 mEq of KCl/L of IV fluid if serum potassium levels are not available; do not exceed a potassium administration rate of 0.5 mEq/kg/h).

MEDICATIONS

DRUGS OF CHOICE

• Pancreatitis—use parenteral antibiotics (ampicillin 20 mg/kg IV q8h; penicillin 20,000 units/kg IV q6h; cefazolin 20 mg/kg IV q8h slowly) if sepsis; use antiemetics (chlorpromazine 0.5 mg/kg IM or SC q6–8h) if intractable vomiting occurs; use corticosteroids (prednisolone sodium succinate 20 mg/kg IV once or dexamethasone sodium phosphate 2–4 mg/kg IV once) if patient is in shock. • Renal disease—treat signs of uremia with antiemetics (metoclopramide 0.2–0.5 mg/kg IV, IM, or PO q6–8h) and H$_2$-receptor antagonists (famotidine 0.5 mg/kg IV or PO q24h, ranitidine 1–2 mg/kg IV or PO q12h, cimetidine 5 mg/kg IV or PO q8h); transfusion (packed red cells or whole blood) may be required in animals with severe anemia. • Hepatic disease—lactulose (1 mL/4.5 kg PO q8–12h) and metronidazole (10–15 mg/kg IV or PO q12h) can be used to reduce signs of hepatic encephalopathy. • GI disease—avoid antibiotics unless hemorrhagic diarrhea exists; avoid anticholinergic drugs that can cause ileus; avoid antiemetics unless profuse vomiting exists.

CONTRAINDICATIONS

• Avoid using azathioprine, chlorothiazide, estrogens, furosemide, tetracycline, and sulfamethazole in patients with pancreatitis. • Avoid aminoglycosides in patients with renal disease. • Adjust the dosage or dosing interval appropriately for all other drugs that are eliminated by the kidneys. • Adjust the dosage of drugs that require hepatic biotransformation or hepatic degradation in animals with liver disease. • Avoid metoclopramide or other promotility drugs in animals with GI obstruction.

PRECAUTIONS

Since pancreatitis is the most common cause for significant elevations in both serum amylase and lipase activities, use the following drugs cautiously:
• Corticosteroids—may aggravate lesions of pancreatitis • Phenothiazine antiemetics—have hypotensive properties and may exacerbate pancreatic ischemia • Dextrans—high dosages may promote bleeding in patients with hemorrhagic pancreatitis.

POSSIBLE INTERACTIONS

N/A

ALTERNATIVE DRUGS

N/A

FOLLOW-UP

PATIENT MONITORING

Pancreatitis

• Evaluate patient hydration status closely first 48 h (body weight, skin turgor, membrane moistness, etc.) • Repeat biochemistries and lipase as needed. • Gradually reintroduce oral alimentation.

Other Conditions

• Extremely variable; depends on the organ system involved and extent of disease

POSSIBLE COMPLICATIONS

• Severe episodes of pancreatitis can cause death. • Diabetes mellitus and exocrine pancreatic insufficiency may occur secondary to pancreatitis.

MISCELLANEOUS

ASSOCIATED CONDITIONS
N/A

AGE-RELATED FACTORS
N/A

ZOONOTIC POTENTIAL
N/A

PREGNANCY
N/A

SYNONYMS
N/A

SEE ALSO

• Pancreatitis • Renal Failure, Acute • Renal Failure, Chronic • Trypsin-Like Immunoreactivity

ABBREVIATIONS

• ALP = alkaline phosphatase • ALT = alanine aminotransferase • GI = gastrointestinal • NPO = nothing per os • PU/PD = polyuria/polydipsia • TLI = trypsin-like immunoreactivity

Suggested Reading

Murtaugh RJ. Acute pancreatitis: diagnostic dilemmas. Semin Vet Med Surg (Small Anim) 1987;2:282–295.

Polzin DJ, Osborne CA, Stevens JB, et al. Serum amylase and lipase activities in dogs with chronic primary renal failure. Am J Vet Res 1983;44:404–410.

Williams DA. The pancreas. In: Guilford WG, Center SA, Strombeck DR, et al., eds. Strombeck's small animal gastroenterology. 3rd ed. Philadelphia: Saunders, 1996:

Author Albert E. Jergens
Consulting Editors Mitchell A. Crystal and Brett M. Feder

ANEMIA, NONREGENERATIVE

BASICS

DEFINITION
Low RBC mass without evidence of a regenerative response (increased polychromasia or reticulocytosis) in the peripheral blood

PATHOPHYSIOLOGY
• Key feature is low or inadequate erythroid production or release • Onset of anemia and its related signs insidious unless RBC survival is concurrently shortened (e.g., hemorrhage and hemolysis) • May be caused by selective alteration in erythropoiesis or generalized bone marrow injury affecting leukocytes and platelets as well • Mechanisms for selectively altered erythropoiesis include deficient hormonal stimulation, deficient or defective nurture, and disturbed metabolism in or destruction of precursors; generalized bone marrow injury usually caused by a toxin, infection, or infiltrative process • These distinctions are not absolute; a cat with FeLV infection can have nonregenerative anemia alone, pancytopenia, or leukemia/erythroleukemia.

SYSTEMS AFFECTED
• Cardiovascular—heart murmur associated with low blood viscosity • Hepatobiliary—centrilobular degeneration associated with hypoxic injury

SIGNALMENT
• Varies with primary cause • Giant schnauzer—congenital cobalamin malabsorption

SIGNS

General Comments
• Usually a secondary condition • Signs associated with the primary disease often precede signs directly attributable to the anemia.

Historical Findings
• Lack of energy, exercise intolerance, inappetence, and cold intolerance • Other findings reflect the primary condition, such as polyuria and polydipsia (e.g., chronic renal failure), exposure to paint from remodeling old houses (e.g., lead poisoning), living in multicat households (e.g., FeLV), and treating female dogs for mismating or urinary incontinence and feminization in male dogs (e.g., hyperestrogenism).

Physical Examination Findings
• Pallor, heart murmur (relatively severe anemia), and possibly tachycardia or polypnea • Signs reflecting the primary condition include uremic breath and oral ulcerations (e.g., chronic renal failure), cachexia (e.g., cancer), lymphadenopathy (e.g., lymphoma), gastrointestinal or CNS signs (e.g., lead poisoning), symmetrical alopecia (e.g., hypothyroidism and hyperestrogenism).

CAUSES

Nonregenerative Anemia without Other Cytopenias
• Chronic disease—the most common cause; associated with chronic infection (e.g., gingivitis and abscess), chronic noninfectious inflammation (e.g., dermatologic disease), and certain malignancies; anemia typically mild; sequestration of iron within bone marrow macrophages, low serum iron and transferrin, and high concentration of serum ferritin causes impaired marrow response to anemia; RBC survival shortened • Chronic renal failure—kidneys fail to produce adequate amount of erythropoietin; uremic toxins shorten RBC lifespan and impair the response to erythropoietin. • Chronic liver disease—RBC morphologic changes (target cells and acanthocytes) and shortened RBC survival caused by changes in RBC membrane phospholipid and cholesterol content; mobilization of hepatic iron may be impaired. • Endocrine disease—thyroid hormones and cortisol stimulate erythropoiesis and facilitate the effect of erythropoietin; mild anemia is commonly associated with hypothyroidism and can occasionally be seen in patients with hypoadrenocorticism and hypopituitarism.

Nutritional or Mineral Deficiency
• Iron deficiency—usually caused by chronic blood loss; initially regenerative, but as severity increases, hemoglobin concentration cannot be maintained and anemia becomes nonregenerative. • Cobalamin (vitamin B_{12}) and/or folate deficiency—rare in dogs and cats but can be caused by dietary insufficiency, malabsorption, or chronic drug administration (e.g., methotrexate, sulfas, and anticonvulsants) that inhibits folate; congenital defect in cobalamin absorption reported in giant schnauzers • Disruption of precursor metabolism—chronic lead toxicity and possibly high concentrations of aluminum and cadmium inhibit heme synthesis; cadmium also reported to cause renal toxicity and impaired erythropoietin production • Immune-mediated destruction of precursors • Infectious destruction of precursors (although usually > 1 cell line is involved; e.g., FeLV and ehrlichiosis)

Nonregenerative Anemia with Other Cytopenias
• Toxicities—drugs or chemicals (e.g., cancer chemotherapeutics, chloramphenicol, phenylbutazone, trimethoprim-sulfadiazine, and benzene), hormones (e.g., estrogen toxicity secondary to abortifacient therapy and Sertoli cell tumor) • Infections—FeLV, ehrlichiosis, Rocky Mountain spotted fever, and parvoviral infection (although recovery usually precedes development of anemia) • Infiltrative processes—myelodysplasia, myeloproliferative disease, lymphoproliferative disease, metastatic neoplasia, myelofibrosis, and osteosclerosis

RISK FACTORS
• Renal failure • Inflammatory disease • Liver failure • Sertoli cell tumor • Chronic disease process • Cancer • Chronic blood loss • Cats from multicat households (FeLV) • Lead exposure

DIAGNOSIS

DIFFERENTIAL DIAGNOSIS
Sudden onset of signs more consistent with regenerative than nonregenerative anemia; however, the latter may appear to have an acute onset if associated with a sudden exacerbation of a chronic primary condition.

LABORATORY FINDINGS

Drugs That May Alter Laboratory Results
None

Disorders That May Alter Laboratory Results
Factors causing turbidity (lipemia) can falsely elevate hemoglobin and MCHC values.

Valid If Run in Human Laboratory?
• Yes; however, electronic counters used for human RBCs may underestimate counts of small RBCs in most domestic animals other than dogs, which produces a falsely low RBC count and PCV. • A centrifuge is preferable for measuring PCV.

CBC/BIOCHEMISTRY/URINALYSIS

CBC and Blood Smear
• PCV, RBC count, and hemoglobin low • Anemia usually normocytic, normochromic, with normal MCV and MCHC • Macrocytosis (high MCV)—without polychromasia suggests a nuclear maturation defect (cells skip a division); seen in cats with FeLV; caused by vitamin B_{12} or folate deficiency; uncommon in domestic animals • Microcytosis (low MCV)—suggests a cytoplasmic maturation defect (cells undergo an extra division); iron deficiency the most common cause; in late stages, concurrent hypochromasia (low MCHC) common in dogs but not in cats; also seen in approximately one-third of patients with hepatic insufficiency or vascular shunting • Schistocytes commonly associated with iron deficiency • Acanthocytes associated with cholestatic liver disease • Target cells associated with iron deficiency, liver disase, and hypothyroidism • An inflammatory leukogram supports anemia associated with inflammatory disease. • Thrombocytosis often accompanies iron deficiency. • A high number of nucleated RBCs without polychromasia or disproportionate to the degree of anemia and polychromasia seen in animals with lead toxicity; extramedullary hematopoiesis and injury to bone marrow stroma by endotoxemia or hypoxia are other sources of circulating nucleated RBCs. • RBC or WBC precursors in the peripheral blood without orderly progression to more mature forms suggests myelodysplasia or myeloproliferative disease (leukemia). • Concurrent cytopenia in other cell lines without evidence of marrow responsiveness (e.g., band

neutrophils and macroplatelets) suggests generalized bone marrow injury.

Serum Biochemistry and Urinalysis
• High BUN and creatinine with inadequate urine concentration (dogs, < 1.030; cats, < 1.035) support anemia of renal failure. • High ALT, bilirubinemia, and bilirubinuria suggest liver disease. • High serum cholesterol (> 500 mg/dL) strongly suggests hypothyroidism. • Hyponatremia with concurrent hyperkalemia, lymphopenia, and eosinopenia in ill dogs suggests hypoadrenocorticism.

OTHER LABORATORY TESTS
• Reticulocyte count—value of < 60,000/μL in dogs or < 50,000/μL in cats accompanied by a low PCV confirms nonregenerative anemia. • Because it takes the bone marrow 3–5 days to increase erythropoiesis in response to an acute demand, patients in the early stage of acute hemorrhage or hemolysis may appear to be affected with the disease. • Direct antiglobulin test (Coombs')—immune-mediated destruction of erythroid precursors can lead to anemia without reticulocytosis; spherocytosis or autoagglutination may suggest immune-mediated hemolytic anemia; positive Coombs' test with species-specific reagents provides support for immune-mediated anemia. • Serum iron profile—indicated for patients with microcytic anemia; in dogs, evaluation of iron stores in a bone marrow aspirate should precede iron assay; in patients with iron deficiency, serum iron is low, total iron-binding capacity varies, and serum ferritin is low; in patients with anemia associated with inflammatory disease, serum iron is low but serum ferritin is high (MCV and MCHC usually normal). • Bile acids measurement—may be indicated for evaluation of microcytic anemia and confirmation of hepatic insufficiency or vascular shunting • Serum lead measurement—indicated when nucleated red cells are present, especially when the patient has concurrent gastrointestinal or CNS signs; a value > 30 μL/dL (0.3 ppm) strongly supports lead intoxication. • Serologic testing—FeLV test in any cat with nonregenerative anemia; *Ehrlichia canis* and Rocky Mountain spotted fever titers indicated in dogs with unexplained anemia, especially when concurrent with other cytopenias or hyperglobulinemia • Endocrine testing—indicated when clinical signs and laboratory tests suggest a possible endocrine disorder; thyroid: T_4, free T_4, and TSH concentrations and adrenal: low-dose dexamethasone suppression test, and ACTH-stimulation test

IMAGING
N/A

DIAGNOSTIC PROCEDURES

Cytologic Examination of Bone Marrow and Core Biopsy
• Cytologic examination of an aspirate indicated in all patients, unless the primary cause is readily apparent (e.g., anemia of inflammatory

disease and chronic renal failure) • Erythroid hypoplasia or aplasia confirms the disease. • Myeloid hyperplasia and high iron stores support anemia associated with inflammatory disease. • Absence of bone marrow iron stores, which occurs before microcytosis, supports iron deficiency; classically, iron deficiency associated with an expanded erythron and high numbers of metarubricytes • Increased erythrophagocytosis suggests injury to cells (e.g., immune-mediated and toxic disease). • An incomplete maturation sequence suggests injury to a specific maturation stage (e.g., immune-mediated and toxic causes) or possibly incomplete recovery from a previous injury (recheck in 3–5 days). • A disorderly maturation sequence and atypical cellular morphology suggest myelodysplastic syndrome. • High number of blast cells (> 30% of nucleated cells) indicates hematopoietic neoplasia; morphologic examination of cells and cytochemical stains used to identify the affected cell line(s); circulating neoplastic cells may or may not be seen. • Nonmarrow cells indicate metastatic neoplasia. • If specimens are hypocellular, core biopsy should be done to evaluate bone marrow cellularity and to look for conditions such as myelofibrosis.

TREATMENT
• Nonregenerative anemia usually resolves with resolution of the underlying disease. • Conditions associated with severe anemia or pancytopenia often carry a guarded-to-poor prognosis and may involve long-term treatment without complete resolution. • Metabolic compensation occurs with slowly developing nonregenerative anemia; thus mild to moderately severe anemia (PCV > 15%) generally requires no supportive intervention; for patients with severe anemia (PCV < 10– 15%), the degree of hypoxia will probably require restricted exercise, transfusions, or both. • If blood volume and tissue perfusion are compromised by concurrent blood loss or shock, administer lactated Ringer's solution or colloids

MEDICATIONS

DRUGS OF CHOICE
• Erythropoietin in patients with anemia of chronic renal failure (see Anemia of Chronic Renal Disease) • Iron supplementation in patients with iron deficiency anemia (see Anemia, Iron-Deficiency) • May supplement with folic acid at a rate of 4–10 mg/kg/day. • May supplement with cobalamin (vitamin B_{12}) at a rate of 100–200 mg/day PO (dogs) or 50–100 mg/day PO (cats); parenteral administration (0.5–1 mg IM weekly to once

every few months) needed in giant schnauzers with inherited cobalamin malabsorption

CONTRAINDICATIONS
None

PRECAUTIONS
Monitor for transfusion reactions in patients receiving multiple transfusions.

POSSIBLE INTERACTIONS
None

ALTERNATIVE DRUGS
None

FOLLOW-UP

PATIENT MONITORING
• In patients with severe anemia, PCV and blood smear examination every 1–2 days • In stabilized animals with chronic or slowly improving disease course, re-evaluation every 1–2 weeks

POSSIBLE COMPLICATIONS
N/A

MISCELLANEOUS

ASSOCIATED CONDITIONS
N/A

AGE-RELATED FACTORS
N/A

ZOONOTIC POTENTIAL
N/A

PREGNANCY
A mildly low PCV caused by dilution of RBC mass by a high blood volume may be seen in some pregnant animals.

SYNONYMS
Nonresponsive anemia

SEE ALSO
See Causes

ABBREVIATIONS
• ALT = alanine aminotransferase • FeLV = feline leukemia virus • MCHC = mean corpuscular hemoglobin concentration • MCV = mean cell volume • PCV = packed cell volume • TSH = thyroid-stimulating hormone

Suggested Reading
Kristensen AT, Feldman BF. Blood banking and transfusion medicine. In: Ettinger SJ, Feldman EC, eds. Textbook of veterinary internal medicine: diseases of the dog and cat. Vol. 1. 4th ed. Philadelphia: Saunders, 1995:347–360.

Rogers K. Anemia. In: Ettinger SJ, Feldman EC, eds. Textbook of veterinary internal medicine: diseases of the dog and cat. Vol. 1. 4th ed. Philadelphia: Saunders, 1995:187–191.

Author Joyce S. Knoll
Consulting Editor Susan M. Cotter

ANEMIA, REGENERATIVE

 BASICS

DEFINITION
• Characterized by a low circulating RBC mass (as indicated by low PCV, hemoglobin, and total RBC count) accompanied by appropriate, compensatory increase in RBC production by the bone marrow (e.g., reticulocytosis in the peripheral blood and RBC hyperplasia in the bone marrow) • Regenerative response may not be evident until several days after the onset of anemia.

PATHOPHYSIOLOGY
• Regenerative anemia caused by blood loss or hemolysis • In patients with blood loss anemia, circulating RBC lifespan is normal and RBCs are lost from the body as a result of vascular injury; in patients with hemolytic anemia, vessels are intact but there is excessive intravascular or extravascular destruction of RBCs with shortened circulating RBC life span. • Hemolysis—caused by erythrocyte membrane abnormalities, physical damage, oxidative injury, release of hemolysins, osmotic changes, immune-mediated RBC destruction, and congenital RBC abnormalities • Intravascular hemolysis may lead to DIC and subsequent hemoglobinuria. • Hemolytic anemia usually more regenerative than blood loss anemia; blood loss depletes body of both cells and iron; hemolysis conserves iron, which is readily available for reuse in RBC production; availability of iron that makes hemolytic anemia generally more responsive.

SYSTEMS AFFECTED
• Hemic/lymph/immune—marked RBC hyperplasia in the bone marrow; splenomegaly also can be a feature of extravascular hemolytic anemia. • Cardiovascular—murmurs with marked anemia; tachycardia with severe rapid-onset anemia • Hepatic—anoxia causes centrilobular degeneration of the liver; hemolysis may cause icterus.

SIGNALMENT
• No breed, age, or sex predilections for the broad category of regenerative anemia • Congenital pyruvate kinase deficiency—basenjis, beagles, West Highland white terriers, Cairn terriers, and Abyssinian cats • Phosphofructokinase deficiency—English springer spaniels and American cocker spaniels • Hereditary nonspherocytic hemolytic anemia in some poodles and beagles • Feline congenital porphyria—Siamese and domestic shorthair cats • Some breeds of dogs have a genetic predisposition for certain heritable coagulopathies such as factor VIII deficiency and von Willebrand disease. • Middle-aged female dogs have a predisposition to immune-mediated syndromes, such as immune-mediated hemolytic anemia and SLE.

SIGNS
• Pallor • Weakness • Exercise intolerance • Anorexia • Possible heart murmur, tachycardia, and jaundice • Clinical signs depend on the degree of anemia and rapidity of onset • Rapid loss of 50–60% of the blood volume or acute hemolysis results in shock and possible death in patients with chronic anemia • Compensatory increases in heart rate, and eventually heart size, lessens the RBC circulation time; hemoglobin can drop to as low as 50% of the minimum normal value without overt signs of hypoxia.

CAUSES

Immune Mediated
• Antibodies and/or complement on the RBC surface shorten RBC lifespan. • Antibodies may target RBC membrane antigens or antibodies may be directed against tumor antigens, infectious agents, or drugs (e.g., trimethoprim-sulfadiazine, penicillins, and methimazole) adherent to RBC surface. • Hemolysis—depending on the antibody type, may be either intravascular or extravascular; may be caused by vaccination or transfusion of incompatible blood. • Neonatal isoerythrolysis seen in kittens born to a blood type B queen mated to a blood type A tom.

Oxidant Injury
• Exposure to oxidants can cause Heinz body formation (aggregates of oxidized hemoglobin), eccentrocytes (oxidative injury to RBC membranes), and methemoglobinemia. • Changes in RBC morphology results in premature removal of these cells from the circulation (extravascular hemolysis). • Oxidants include onions (especially in dogs), acetaminophen (especially in cats), zinc toxicity (from pennies minted after 1982, zinc oxide ointment, and zinc bolts), benzocaine, vitamin K_3 (dogs), DL-methionine (cats), phenolic compounds (moth balls), and phenazopyridine (cats) • In cats, some systemic diseases (e.g, diabetes mellitus, hyperthyroidism, and lymphoma) enhance Heinz body formation.

Erythrocyte Parasites
• *Haemobartonella felis* (cats); *H. canis* (rare cause of anemia in dogs) • *Babesia canis* and *B. gibsoni* (dogs) • *Cytauxzoon felis* (cats)

Mechanical RBC Fragmentation
• DIC • Heartworm disease • Cardiac disease • Liver disease • Vasculitis • Neoplasia (e.g. hemangiosarcoma) • Splenic torsion • Hemolytic-uremic syndrome.

Inherited RBC Abnormalities
• Pyruvate kinase deficiency—causes impaired erythrocyte glucose use and ATP formation, leading to premature destruction of RBCs.

• Phosphofructokinase deficiency—causes marked alkaline fragility caused by impaired synthesis of 2,3-diphosphoglycerate; hemolytic episodes triggered by hyperventilation-induced alkalemia such as occurs after vigorous exercise • Hereditary nonspherocytic hemolytic anemia—resembles pyruvate kinase deficiency, but the RBCs have normal glycolytic enzyme activities and the basic defect is undetermined; in poodles, an autosomal dominant mode of inheritance has been described. • Feline congential porphyria—deficiency in uroporphyrinogen III cosynthetase causes an inability to produce normal amounts of hemoglobin; coproporphyrin and uroporphyrin accumulate, causing brown-red discoloration of teeth and bones; autosomal dominant trait.

Blood Loss
• Trauma • Bleeding neoplasms (e.g., hemangiosarcoma and intestinal adenocarcinoma or leiomyoma) • Coagulopathies (e.g., warfarin poisoning, hemophilia, and thrombocytopenia) • Blood sucking parasites (e.g., fleas, ticks, and *Ancylostoma*) • Gastrointestinal ulcers

RISK FACTORS
N/A

 DIAGNOSIS

DIFFERENTIAL DIAGNOSIS
Differentiated from nonregenerative anemia by high reticulocyte count

LABORATORY FINDINGS

Drugs That May Alter Laboratory Results
None

Disorders That May Alter Laboratory Results
Lipemia in the sample can cause in vitro hemolysis, resulting in a falsely low PCV and total RBC count and falsely high MCHC.

Valid If Run in Human Laboratory?
• Dogs, yes • Cats, yes if lab's hematology instrument uses species-specific parameters • Automated instruments designed strictly for analysis of human specimens may fail to accurately count the small RBCs in cats; thus reticulocyte counts should be performed manually • Human labs may be unfamiliar with the punctuate reticulocytes found in cats and may include them in the reticulocyte count, thereby overestimating the regenerative response • Human labs may be unfamiliar with important RBC parasites such as *Haemobartonella*.

CBC/BIOCHEMISTRY/URINALYSIS
• PCV, RBC count, and hemoglobin low

ANEMIA, REGENERATIVE

• RBC indices vary depending on the cause of anemia and degree of regenerative response: MCV, normal to high; MCHC normal to low in most patients

• In patients with intravascular hemolytic anemia with hemoglobinemia, MCHC artifactually may be high.

• Dogs with iron deficiency owing to chronic blood loss may have a low MCV, MCH, and MCHC.

• Cats with iron deficiency often have a low MCV but normal MCH and MCHC.

• Anisocytosis and expanded RBC distribution width associated with increased polychromasia

• In patients with hemolytic anemia, specific morphologic RBC changes suggest cause: marked spherocytosis suggests immune-mediated disease; Heinz bodies suggest oxidant injury; and numerous schistocytes suggest microangiopathy

• Spherocytes cannot be readily detected in cats because of smallness and lack of central pallor of RBCs.

• Agglutinated RBCs indicate anemia is immune-mediated; autoagglutination must be distinguished from rouleaux by sample dilution with saline.

• Hemolysis may cause neutrophilia with a left shift and monocytosis. Blood loss may be accompanied by either thrombocytopenia or rebound thrombocytosis; iron deficiency often accompanied by thrombocytosis

• Total protein normal in patients with hemolytic anemia; may be low in those with blood loss anemia

• Hyperbilirubinemia and bilirubinuria accompany marked hemolysis; hemoglobinemia and hemoglobinuria seen if hemolysis is intravascular

OTHER LABORATORY TESTS

• In an anemic animal, an absolute reticulocyte count (RBC count × reticulocyte %) > 50,000/μL (cats) or > 60,000/μL (dogs) suggests regenerative anemia

• Formula for calculating a corrected reticulocyte count—reticulocyte % × (PCV/normal PCV) (normal PCV: 45, dog; 37, cat); corrected reticulocyte count > 1% suggests a regenerative response.

• If reticulocyte count is low in a patient with suspected regenerative anemia, it may mean that the anemia is in the early stages of response; it takes 3–5 days for the bone marrow to mount a peak regenerative response to anemia.

• Direct antiglobulin test (e.g., DAT and Coombs test) indicated when immune-mediated hemolytic anemia suspected; a positive test with species-specific reagents and evidence of spherocytosis and polychromasia in the peripheral blood is confirmatory; both false-negatives and false-positives are possible, so the test must be used judiciously and interpreted cautiously.

IMAGING
N/A

DIAGNOSTIC PROCEDURES

• Bone marrow aspirate—cytologic examination of bone marrow reveals RBC hyperplasia; needed only when there is no evidence of RBC responsiveness in the peripheral blood (i.e., no polychromasia and no reticulocytosis); absence of RBC hyperplasia means that the anemia is nonregenerative.

• Bone marrow biopsy—useful in evaluation of bone marrow architecture and overall cellularity; important for confirmation of a nonregenerative process.

TREATMENT

• Emergency if anemia is severe and develops rapidly

• Massive hemorrhage leads to hypovolemic shock and anoxia; acute hemolysis leads to anoxia and systemic toxemia

• Cage rest and careful observation indicated, depending on severity of clinical signs

Blood Loss Anemias

• Fluids to correct hypovolemia may be indicated in animals with acute traumatic blood loss anemia.

• If signs of hypoxia severe (i.e., extremely pale mucous membranes, weakness, tachycardia, and tachypnea), RBC replacement (volume depends on PCV of donor and patient) or oxyhemoglobin (30 mL/kg at rate of 10 mL/kg/hr) indicated

Hemolytic Anemias

• Blood transfusion, packed RBCs, or oxyhemoglobin may be indicated; in patients with an immune-mediated process, RBCs probably survive similarly to the patient's own RBCs, so transfusion should not be withheld if marked signs of anemia are present.

MEDICATIONS

DRUGS OF CHOICE

• Blood-loss anemias—administration of iron may be of benefit in animals with chronic blood-loss anemia (see Anemia, Iron-Deficiency)

• Hemolytic anemias—varies with cause of hemolysis

CONTRAINDICATIONS
N/A

PRECAUTIONS
N/A

POSSIBLE INTERACTIONS
N/A

ALTERNATIVE DRUGS
N/A

FOLLOW-UP

PATIENT MONITORING

• Measurements of RBC mass (e.g., PCV, RBC count, and hemoglobin) and morphologic evaluation of peripheral blood film to monitor effectiveness of treatment and bone marrow responsiveness • Initially, patients should be checked every 24 hr; as regeneration becomes apparent (indicated by rising RBC values and polychromasia), patients should be checked every 3–5 days; return to normal values should occur about 14 days after acute hemorrhage but may take longer with an immune-mediated process.

POSSIBLE COMPLICATIONS
None

MISCELLANEOUS

ASSOCIATED CONDITIONS
N/A

AGE-RELATED FACTORS
N/A

ZOONOTIC POTENTIAL
N/A

PREGNANCY
N/A

SYNONYMS
Responsive anemias

SEE ALSO

• Acetaminophen Toxicity • Anemia, Heinz Body • Anemia, Immune-Mediated • Anemia, Iron-Deficiency • Rodenticide Anticoagulant Toxicity • Babesiosis • Cytauxzoonosis • Disseminated Intravascular Coagulation (DIC) • Hemobartonellosis • Zinc Toxicity

ABBREVIATIONS

• DAT = direct antiglobulin (Coombs') test
• DIC = disseminated intravascular coagulation • MCHC = mean corpuscular hemoglobin concentration • MCV = mean cell volume • PCV = packed cell volume • SLE = systemic lupus erythematosus

Suggested Reading

Jain, NC. Essentials of veterinary hematology. Philadelphia: Lea & Febiger, 1993.

Weiser MG. Erythrocyte responses and disorders. In: Ettinger SJ, Feldman EC, eds. Textbook of veterinary internal medicine. Diseases of the dog and cat. 4th ed. Philadelphia: Saunders, 1995:1876–1886.

Author Joyce S. Knoll

Consulting Editor Susan M. Cotter

ANION GAP

 BASICS

DEFINITION

• The AG is a calculation used to help differentiate causes of metabolic (non-respiratory) acidosis and mixed acid–base disorders; it may be normal, increased, or decreased, depending on the underlying metabolic disorder.
• The AG is calculated by subtracting the summed values for the measured major anions in serum (Cl^- and HCO_3^-) from the summed values of the measured major cations (Na^+ and K^+); the formula is $(Na^+ + K^+) - (Cl^- + HCO_3^-)$.
• The normal anion gap in dogs is 12–24 mEq/L; the normal anion gap for cats is 13–27 mEq/L.

PATHOPHYSIOLOGY

• In addition to commonly measured electrolytes, serum also contains minor cations and anions that are not typically measured, but are important in regulating electroneutrality; these are called unmeasured cations (UC^+) and anions (UA^-).
• In reality, no true "gap" exists; electrolytes, unmeasured cations, and unmeasured anions in serum preserve electroneutrality: $(Na^+ + K^+ + UC^+) = (Cl^- + HCO_3^- + UA^-)$; this formula reduces to $AG = UA^- - UC^+$ to denote that any numerical gap calculated is a result of changes in either UA^- or UC^+.
• In metabolic acidosis, every time HCO_3^- decreases, Cl^- or UA^- must increase to maintain electroneutrality. A normal AG metabolic acidosis (hyperchloremic) develops when HCO_3^- is replaced with Cl^-; the resultant difference in $(UA^- - UC^+)$ is unchanged. An increased AG metabolic acidosis (normochloremic) develops when HCO_3^- is replaced by UA^-; the difference in $(UA^- - UC^+)$ increases, but the Cl^- concentration is unchanged.
• UCs include calcium and magnesium; UAs include albumin, phosphates, sulfates, and organic acids (e.g., lactate, ketones, ethylene glycol metabolites); clinically, an increased AG metabolic acidosis usually implies accumulation of organic acids.
• Because the measurement of total CO_2 content of blood (TCO_2) mostly represents the HCO_3^- concentration in the blood,

TCO_2 can be used in place of measured HCO_3^- in the formulas above.

SYSTEMS AFFECTED

• Acidosis affects many body organs, especially cardiovascular function and electrolyte distribution.
• Clinical signs usually relate more to the disease causing the acidosis than to direct effects of the acidosis itself.
• Cardiovascular effects include decreased myocardial contractility, ventricular dysrhythmias, shifts in the oxyhemoglobin dissociation curve, arterial vasodilating effects, and venous vasoconstrictive effects.
• Electrolyte changes include variable increases in serum potassium levels, an increase in ionized calcium levels, and natriuresis.

SIGNALMENT

Dog and cat

SIGNS

General Comments

Signs of acidosis usually relate more to the underlying disorder causing the acidosis than to direct effects of the acidosis itself.

Historical Findings

Disorders causing metabolic acidosis are common, and the history may prompt suspicion of an underlying acidosis.

Physical Examination Findings

• Tachypnea usually occurs in patients with metabolic acidosis as the patient attempts respiratory compensation.
• Most patients with metabolic acidosis are hypovolemic and thus demonstrate evidence of poor tissue perfusion or dehydration (dark mucous membranes, prolonged capillary refill time, increased skin turgor).
• Severely acidotic patients may have cardiac dysrhythmias and poor contractility.

CAUSES

• Metabolic acidosis with a normal AG (hyperchloremic metabolic acidosis)—disorders characterized by gastrointestinal loss of bicarbonate (e.g., diarrhea, metabolism of cationic amino acids in parenteral nutrition supplements, and hypoadrenocorticism), renal wasting of bicarbonate (e.g., renal tubular acidosis, use of carbonic anhydrase inhibitors, and use of ammonium chloride), and several miscellaneous causes (e.g., posthypocapnic metabolic acidosis, dilutional acidosis from rapid administration of 0.9% saline)

• Metabolic acidosis with an increased AG (normochloremic metabolic acidosis)—most commonly disorders characterized by increased levels of organic acids (e.g., diabetic ketoacidosis, lactic acidosis, ethylene glycol intoxication, aspirin intoxication, and uremic acidosis)
• Some causes of metabolic acidosis exhibit variations from typical AG findings—for example, patients with early hypoadrenocorticism typically have hyperchloremic metabolic acidosis (normal AG), yet when presented for emergency care have hypochloremia and an increased AG acidosis caused by advanced lactic acidosis due to water loss, decreased renal function, and decreased tissue perfusion.
• A decreased AG is uncommon; it usually is caused by hypoalbuminemia (true decrease or dilutional decrease due to crystalloid fluid administration) due to a decrease in the net negative charge provided by albumin; other potential causes include hypercalcemia, hypermagnesemia, and bromide toxicity, conditions characterized by an increased UC concentration.

RISK FACTORS

• Those for development of AG changes relate directly to risk factors for the specific disorders causing the underlying metabolic acid–base disorder.
• In general, young animals are more at risk for developing severe gastrointestinal disorders with vomiting and diarrhea (parvoviral enteritis, foreign body ingestion with obstruction) and are more likely to ingest toxicants (ethylene glycol, aspirin) that lead to changes in the AG.
• Older animals are more likely to develop metabolic disorders that lead to changes in the AG (renal failure, hypoadrenocorticism, diabetic ketoacidosis); consult Risk Factors for these specific disorders.

 DIAGNOSIS

DIFFERENTIAL DIAGNOSIS

• Those disorders described under Causes
• Any severely ill patient animal is suspect for an underlying metabolic acidosis; AG evaluation can aid in diagnosis.

LABORATORY FINDINGS

Drugs That May Alter Laboratory Results

• Using several drugs during initial treatment of underlying disorders that lead to an increased AG may blunt its increase, making the gap and the medical condition seem less severe; examples include crystalloid fluids, diuretics, and sodium bicarbonate.
• Calculation of the anion gap is best done using blood samples drawn before any therapeutic interventions.

Disorders That May Alter Laboratory Results

• Hypoalbuminemia may reduce and mask the severity of an increased AG for reasons explained above; alkalosis and dehydration also artificially increase the AG, as does long-term (>2 h) exposure of serum to room air.
• Recent reports demonstrate that the AG may be normal in critically ill patients with conditions that are typically associated with an increased AG acidosis; many of these patients have concurrent hypoalbuminemia, hyperchloremia, or mixed acid–base disorders that blunt the AG increase and confound interpretation.
• A normal AG does not rule out metabolic acidosis due to increased organic acids.

Valid If Run in Human Laboratory?

Yes, as long as the electrolyte testing required for the calculation is reliable for the species involved.

CBC/BIOCHEMISTRY/URINALYSIS

• Minimum requirements for determining the AG are serum electrolytes, including the TCO_2 or HCO_3^- concentration.
• Few specific CBC findings suggest etiologies for changes in the AG.
• Biochemical and urinalysis findings help determine the underlying cause for AG changes—examples include renal azotemia and markedly increased serum osmolality seen with ethylene glycol intoxication; renal azotemia, hyperkalemia, and tubular casts seen with acute renal failure; and increased lactate concentration, increased total protein, and increased hematocrit with dehydration and poor tissue perfusion.

OTHER LABORATORY TESTS

• Arterial blood gas analysis is useful in detecting and determining the extent of a concurrent respiratory disorder or mixed acid–base disorder.

• Additional tests (e.g., ethylene glycol, serum and urine glucose, serum and urine ketones) may be helpful, depending on the suspected cause.

IMAGING

• Ethylene glycol intoxication has characteristic ultrasonographic findings that may support this diagnosis.
• No specific imaging procedures diagnose changes in AG.

DIAGNOSTIC PROCEDURES

N/A

 TREATMENT

N/A

 MEDICATIONS

DRUGS OF CHOICE

• Specific drug and fluid use depends on the underlying cause.
• Many causes of metabolic acidosis are characterized by fluid volume deficits; aggressive fluid therapy is traditionally an initial step in treating conditions with AG changes.
• Prompt identification and treatment of the underlying disorder is critical.

CONTRAINDICATIONS

N/A

PRECAUTIONS

N/A

POSSIBLE INTERACTIONS

N/A

ALTERNATIVE DRUGS

N/A

 FOLLOW-UP

PATIENT MONITORING

Depends on the type and severity of the underlying disease process.

POSSIBLE COMPLICATIONS

N/A

✓ MISCELLANEOUS

ASSOCIATED CONDITIONS

• Metabolic acidosis may be associated with a normal or increased AG, depending on the cause.
• Hypoalbuminemia and hypercalcemia may be associated with a decreased AG.

AGE-RELATED FACTORS

N/A

ZOONOTIC POTENTIAL

N/A

PREGNANCY

N/A

SYNONYMS

N/A

SEE ALSO

• Metabolic Acidosis
• See Causes

ABBREVIATIONS

• AG = anion gap
• TCO_2 = total CO_2 content
• UA = unmeasured anions
• UC = unmeasured cations

Suggested Reading

DeMorais HSA, DiBartola SP. Mixed acid-base disorders. Part I. Clinical approach. Compend Cont Educ Pract Vet 1993;15:1619–1626.
DiBartola SP. Metabolic acidosis. In: Dibartola SP, ed. Fluid therapy in small animal practice. Philadelphia: Saunders, 1992:216–243.
Kellum JA, Kramer DJ, Pinsky MR. Strong ion gap: a methodology for exploring unexplained anions. J Crit Care 1995;10:51–55.
Rose BD. Metabolic acidosis. In: Rose BD, ed., Clinical physiology of acid-base and electrolyte disorders. 4th ed. New York: McGraw-Hill, 1994:545–551.
Salem MM, Mujais SK. Gaps in the anion gap. Arch Intern Med 1992;152:1625–1629.
Author Michael S. Lagutchik
Consulting Editor Deborah S. Greco

ANTINUCLEAR ANTIBODY (ANA) TITER/ LUPUS ERYTHEMATOSUS (LE) CELL TEST

BASICS

DEFINITION
Indicated in animals suspected of having SLE

Positive ANA Test
• Indicates development of autoantibodies directed against a wide variety of normal cellular components, which may be associated with several immune-mediated diseases, most notably SLE
• In dogs, primarily IgG directed against individual histones
• A more sensitive test for SLE than the LE cell test, but a positive result may be seen in animals with other diseases

Positive LE Cell Test
• Indicates neutrophils are phagocytizing nuclear material that has been depolymerized and opsonized by ANA
• Typically, these neutrophils contain a large pink-purple cytoplasmic inclusion (LE body) that causes peripheral displacement of the nucleus; the LE body is void of any nuclear chromatin material
• Neutrophils containing LE bodies are referred to as LE cells; their presence establishes a positive test result
• Can be performed in the clinic.
• Less sensitive than the ANA test but more specific for SLE; does not require species-specific reagents

PATHOPHYSIOLOGY
• In animals with SLE, autoantibody formation to cell tissue–nonspecific autoantigens is responsible for multisystemic lesions, which are generally characterized by a type III hypersensitivity reaction.
• In animals with SLE, autoantibody formation to cell tissue–specific autoantigens (involving antigens found on platelets and erythrocytes) results in fairly well defined or specific lesions, typical of a type II hypersensitivity response.
• LE cells develop in vitro when fresh clotted blood from a patient with ANAs is incubated.

SYSTEMS AFFECTED
• Musculoskeletal—symmetric nonerosive polyarthritis with shifting leg lameness; painful and swollen joints (especially the carpi, tarsi, metatarsi, stifle, and elbows); up to 75% of patients have symmetric polyarthritis during the course of disease.
• Renal/Urologic—glomerulonephritis (with deposition of immune complexes) in up to 50% of patients; urinalysis reveals proteinuria.
• Skin/Exocrine—dermatologic disease (bullous dermatitis) in up to 50% of patients.
• Hemic/Lymph/Immune—peripheral lymphadenopathy in up to 30% of patients; hemolytic anemia in 25% of dogs with SLG; thrombocytopenia in 20% of dogs with SLG
• Nervous—depression and seizures may be seen in dogs.

SIGNALMENT

Species
• Dogs and cats
• Healthy animals frequently have low positive ANA titer.

Breed Predilection
Shetland sheepdogs, poodles, Irish setters, Old English sheepdogs, German shepherds, beagles, collies

Mean Age and Range
• Middle-aged dogs (mean, 5.8 years)
• Reported in 2–12-year-old dogs

Predominant Sex
None

SIGNS

General Comments
• Severity of clinical signs does not parallel the magnitude of the titer.
• Vary with cause of positive test results

Historical Findings
• Lethargy
• Shifting leg lameness
• Dermatologic lesions
• Signs may modulate and change over time.

Physical Examination Findings
• Fever
• Lymphadenomegaly
• Swollen and painful joints
• Dermatologic lesions (e.g., scaling, ulceration, alopecia, and erythema), symmetrical or focal
• Lesions involving the mouth and other mucocutaneous junctions commonly observed

CAUSES
Unless causes of positive ANA titer noted, patient likely to have an ANA titer < 1:40.

Skin Disorders
• SLE—ANA titer (1:80–>1:160) most consistently high
• Pemphigus erythematosus (seldom pemphigus vulgaris)
• Discoid lupus
• Generalized demodicosis
• Flea bite hypersensitivity
• Plasma cell pododermatitis

Hematologic Disorders
• Immune-mediated hemolytic anemia
• Immune-mediated thrombocytopenia

Cardiopulmonary Disorders
• Bacterial endocarditis
• Heartworm disease

Drugs
• Griseofulvin
• Hydralazine
• Procainamide
• Sulfonamides
• Tetracyclines

Other Disorders
• Cholangiohepatitis
• FeLV
• FIP
• Rheumatoid arthritis
• Lymphocytic thyroiditis
• Various neoplasms
• Ulcerative autoimmune stomatitis—ANA titer 1:80–1:160

RISK FACTORS
Exposure to drugs known to induce ANA

DIAGNOSIS

DIFFERENTIAL DIAGNOSIS
• Polyarthritis/myositis, proteinuria, bullous dermatitis/vasculitis, hemolytic anemia, and thrombocytopenia—consider SLE; positive ANA test and/or a LE cell test in conjunction with appropriate clinical signs establishes diagnosis; ANA titer is preferred by most veterinary labs; however, no single test is diagnostic.

ANTINUCLEAR ANTIBODY (ANA) TITER/ LUPUS ERYTHEMATOSUS (LE) CELL TEST

- Fever, murmur, shifting leg lameness—consider bacterial endocarditis
- Chronic cough, dyspnea, ascites—consider heartworm disease
- Exposure to causative drugs—consider drug-induced positive test result
- Icteric cat—consider cholangiohepatitis and FIP
- Dermatologic condition with low-moderate ANA titer—consider pemphigus erythematosus and pemphigus vulgaris
- Evidence of mass or tumor—consider neoplasia

LABORATORY FINDINGS

Drugs That May Alter Laboratory Results
- Cytotoxic drugs and chronic or high-dose corticosteroids lower ANA concentration.
- LE test more sensitive than ANA test to effects of corticosteroids

Disorders That May Alter Laboratory Results
LE cell test—low levels of complement or excessive amounts of heparin can cause false-negative test results

Valid If Run in Human Laboratory?
- ANA requires species-specific reagent.
- LE test valid

CBC/BIOCHEMISTRY/URINALYSIS
- Regenerative anemia and thrombocytopenia—consider SLE
- Eosinophilia—consider heartworm disease
- Leukocytosis—consider heartworm disease
- Proteinuria—consider glomerulonephritis secondary to SLE, endocarditis, and heartworm disease

OTHER LABORATORY TESTS
Serologic tests for FeLV and heartworm disease

IMAGING
- Radiographs of affected joints—nonerosive arthritis characteristic of SLE
- Thoracic radiographs—rule out neoplasia and heartworm disease
- Echocardiography—rule out bacterial endocarditis in dogs with heart murmur
- Abdominal ultrasound—rule out neoplastic disease and cholangiohepatitis, if indicated

DIAGNOSTIC PROCEDURES
- Arthrocentesis of affected joints for fluid analysis—generally with SLE, fluid is characterized by a high neutrophil count and bacterial culture is negative

- Patients with skin lesions—biopsy for immunofluorescent and histopathologic testing
- Urine protein:creatinine ratio and possibly renal biopsy—might be indicated in dogs with marked proteinuria

TREATMENT
- No specific treatment done solely because of positive ANA titer or LE cell test.
- Discontinue medication if contributing to positive test result.
- Other treatment depends on the cause of the positive test result and clinical signs.

MEDICATIONS

DRUGS OF CHOICE
Depends on cause of disease and systems affected; see Lupus Erythematosus, Systemic (SLE) for specific treatment.

CONTRAINDICATIONS
Avoid aspirin administration in patients with thrombocytopenia.

PRECAUTIONS
N/A

POSSIBLE INTERACTIONS
N/A

ALTERNATIVE DRUGS
N/A

FOLLOW-UP

PATIENT MONITORING
- See Lupus Erythematosus, Systemic (SLE)
- Generally, monitoring of ANA or LE tests not useful in long-term care.

POSSIBLE COMPLICATIONS
Systemic infection secondary to immunosuppression; requires close monitoring and client education

MISCELLANEOUS

ASSOCIATED CONDITIONS
None

AGE-RELATED FACTORS
None

ZOONOTIC POTENTIAL
None

PREGNANCY
Use of prednisone and other immunosuppressive drugs in pregnant animals not advisable unless no other treatment options exist.

SYNONYMS
None

SEE ALSO
- Anemia, Immune-mediated
- Glomerulonephritis
- Lupus Erythematosus, Systemic (SLE)
- Polyarthritis, Nonerosive, Immune-mediated

ABBREVIATIONS
- FeLV = feline leukemia virus
- FIP = feline infectious peritonitis
- SLE = systemic lupus erythematosus

Suggested Reading
Lewis RM, Picut CA. Veterinary clinical immunology: classroom to clinic. Philadelphia: Lea & Febiger, 1989.
Meyer DJ, Harvey JW. Veterinary laboratory medicine: interpretation and diagnosis. 2nd ed. Philadelphia: Saunders, 1998.
Willard MD, Tvedten H, Turnwald GH. Small animal clinical diagnosis by laboratory methods. Philadelphia: Saunders, 1989.
Author Albert H. Ahn and Francis W. K. Smith, Jr.
Consulting Editor Susan M. Cotter

BILE ACIDS

BASICS

DEFINITION
• Detergent amphipathic organic anions synthesized in the liver
• Essential for facilitation of fat digestion
• Best application—adjunctive use of other routine diagnostic tests (hematologic, clinical chemistry, urinalysis, hepatic and pancreatic ultrasonography)
• Determine both fasting and postprandial values—2-hr postprandial values usually higher, reflecting the postprandial bile acid challenge; higher fasting values seen in approximately 20% of dogs and 5% of cats owing to delayed gastric emptying and slow enteric transit
• Indications for test—suspected hepatobiliary disease from routine evaluation; detected occult hepatic disease with normal enzymes (PSVA, cirrhosis, metastatic neoplasia); detected portosystemic shunting; to monitor hepatobiliary function (e.g., disease regression, recrudescence, or adverse or iatrogenic drug hepatotoxicity)

PATHOPHYSIOLOGY
• Synthesized in the liver from cholesterol
• Primary (cholic acid, chenodeoxycholic acid) transformed to secondary (deoxycholic acid, lithocholic acid, respectively) via dehydroxylation by enteric bacteria
• After synthesis—secreted in bile; stored in gallbladder; expelled into alimentary canal when animal eats under the influence of cholecystokinin
• In the intestines—facilitate fat digestion through formation of micelles and activation of pancreatic lipase; passive (upper small bowel) and, more important, active (ileum) absorption restricts fecal loss to < 5%.

• After enteric absorption—normal hepatoportal circulation and hepatic uptake maintain a highly efficient enterohepatic circulation (> 90% efficiency)
• Impaired hepatic function, cholestasis, or deviated or impaired portal circulation—produces high serum concentrations; cannot use serum values to differentiate among specific disorders (wide overlap of values), although particular patterns have been associated with general disease categories

SYSTEMS AFFECTED
• Hepatobiliary—hepatotoxic when retained, especially lithocholate and chenodeoxycholate
• Gastrointestinal—increased concentrations in the colon as a consequence of impaired ileal uptake may induce a secretory diarrhea; gastric reflux of bile may induce ulcer formation; ileal malabsorption results in very low serum concentrations.

SIGNALMENT
• Inherited defects in synthesis or hepatocellular uptake—not characterized in dogs or cats
• Congenital PSVA and microvascular dysplasia—more common in some purebred dogs; often first recognized via high serum bile acid values

SIGNS
• High serum concentration—may contribute to underlying hepatocellular damage and altered permeability of the blood–brain barrier, which may facilitate hepatic encephalopathy development; reflect deranged hepatic function and perfusion; expected with signs of hepatic encephalopathy
• Diarrhea—may occur with malabsorption

CAUSES
• Common liver disorders associated with high serum bile acid concentrations—chronic hepatitis; hepatic necrosis; hepatic lipidosis; vacuolar hepatopathy; infectious hepatitis; diffuse hepatic neoplasia; cirrhosis; toxic hepatopathy; feline cholangiohepatitis syndrome; hepatic infection with FIP; fulminant hepatic failure; portosystemic shunting of any cause

RISK FACTORS
• Hepatobiliary disorders and portosystemic shunting
• Pancreatitis—may increase concentration owing to induced hepatic inflammation and extrahepatic bile duct occlusion

DIAGNOSIS

DIFFERENTIAL DIAGNOSIS
• Hepatobiliary disease—may be initially suspected on physical examination from alterations in liver size or contour, jaundice, ascites, or neurobehavioral evidence of hepatic encephalopathy; may be suspected from results of laboratory tests: increased ALT, AST, ALP, or GGT; reduced serum albumin, BUN, cholesterol, or glucose; increased cholesterol with jaundice (e.g., extrahepatic bile duct occlusion or ammonium biurate crystalluria)
• PSVA—suspect in young patients with high concentrations and signs of hepatic encephalopathy or ammonium urate crystalluria or calculi with relatively few laboratory abnormalities
• Microvascular dysplasia—suspect solely on the basis of increased values
• Jaundice—hepatobiliary uptake and transport, storage, and biliary excretion are not competitive with bilirubin; test not clinically useful when hemolysis has been discounted as the underlying cause; test redundant because abnormal bile acid metabolism precedes abnormal bilirubin metabolism
• Impaired liver function—high sensitivity; may discover early dysfunction before histologic lesions are obvious; must couple test with routine clinical evaluation to avoid inappropriate liver biopsy (no discernible lesions when values are only mildly high)

LABORATORY FINDINGS

Drugs That May Alter Laboratory Results
Ursodeoxycholic acid—does not accumulate to abnormal values in healthy animals; accumulates in the serum of patients with liver disease associated with reduced hepatic function and/or cholestasis; measured by the total serum bile acid test; thus cannot use sequential serum bile acid values to monitor disease status

Disorders That May Alter Laboratory Results
• Inadequate meal consumption, delayed gastric emptying or intestinal transit, and a low-fat diet—may impair development of high postprandial values
• Ileum disease and large-volume diarrhea—impair enteric absorption, resulting in spurious low values
• Failure to clear lipemic samples—produces spuriously results (low or high); a serious problem in many diagnostic laboratories
• Hemolysis—complicates test end point determination, resulting in spurious values (low or high); avoid by using heparinized blood and gentle collection into appropriate Vacutainers.

• Handle postprandial samples gently, because RBCs tend to lyse in lipemic plasma; carefully preprocess lipemic plasma.

Valid If Run in Human Laboratory?
Yes, if done by a direct enzymatic procedure that detects all 3α-hydroxylated bile acids; values not valid for the radioimmunoassay method, which has not been as rigorously evaluated

CBC/BIOCHEMISTRY/URINALYSIS
• Serum bile acid values—major use is to evaluate anicteric liver disease; interpretation of routine screening tests helps verify hepatobiliary disease
• High bile acid values coupled with normal bilirubin and hepatic enzymes—suggest PSVA or acquired portosystemic shunting with quiet cirrhosis
• Normal to moderately high bile acid values coupled with high ALP and normal total bilirubin—suggest canine vacuolar hepatopathy (steroid hepatopathy)
• Markedly high bile acid values coupled with markedly high liver enzymes (especially ALP) and hyperbilirubinemia—common with cholestatic disorders
• High bile acid values coupled with normal, mild, or markedly increased serum enzymes and total bilirubin—cirrhosis
• Normal bile acid values—common with metastatic or primary hepatic neoplasia, unless disease is diffusely disseminated within the liver or has caused biliary tree occlusion

OTHER LABORATORY TESTS
Plasma ammonia concentration and indocyanine green clearances—usually parallel abnormal serum bile acid concentrations in disorders causing reduced hepatic mass or altered hepatic perfusion

IMAGING
Abdominal Radiography
• Microhepatia—associated with cirrhosis (dogs), PSVA, and fulminant hepatic necrosis; spurious condition may be recognized in deep-chested dogs, during maximal expiration, and with diaphragmatic hernia of the liver lobes.
• Hepatomegaly—seen with primary or metastatic neoplasia; parenchymal infiltration with lipid, glycogen, amyloid, or storage disease products; congestion; diffuse inflammation; hepatic or biliary cystic malformations; extramedullary hematopoiesis; reticuloendothelial hyperplasia; spurious condition may be recognized in puppies and

kittens and in adults during deep inspiration or when positioning with left side down enhances silhouetting of the caudate lobe.

Abdominal Ultrasonography
• May disclose hepatic surface contour changes; disorders involving the hepatic parenchyma, biliary tree, portal circulation, porta hepatis, perihepatic lymph nodes, and pancreas; and abdominal effusion
• Changes in parenchymal echogenicity—may reflect diffuse infiltration or multifocal distribution; diffuse hyperechogenicity seen with fatty infiltration, vacuolar hepatopathy, fibrosis, and hepatic cirrhosis
• Most reliable noninvasive means of distinguishing intrahepatic from extrahepatic bile duct occlusion

Nuclear Scintigraphy
Colorectal scintigraphy after rectal instillation of ^{99m}Tc—sensitive for detection of macroscopic portosystemic shunting

DIAGNOSTIC PROCEDURES
• Hepatic biopsy—necessary for definitive diagnosis when laboratory findings and hepatic imaging suggest hepatic disease without evidence of PSVA or extrahepatic bile duct obstruction; use blind percutaneous, ultrasound-guided, laparoscopy, or laparotomy technique.
• Exploratory laparotomy—indicated with suspected extrahepatic bile duct obstruction

TREATMENT
• Depends on underlying disease
• Surgery—necessary for extrahepatic bile duct obstruction and PSVA
• Chronic medical therapy—warranted for acquired intrahepatic disease; see specific disorder

MEDICATIONS
DRUGS OF CHOICE
Depend on underlying disease and extent of hepatobiliary dysfunction

CONTRAINDICATIONS
Depend on underlying disease and extent of hepatobiliary dysfunction

PRECAUTIONS
Depend on underlying disease and extent of hepatobiliary dysfunction

POSSIBLE INTERACTIONS
Depend on underlying disease and extent of hepatobiliary dysfunction

ALTERNATIVE DRUGS
N/A

FOLLOW-UP
PATIENT MONITORING
Re-evaluate serum chemistry profile, bile acid concentration, and hepatic imaging—frequency dictated by underlying disorder

POSSIBLE COMPLICATIONS
Many causes of high bile acid values are life-threatening.

MISCELLANEOUS
ASSOCIATED CONDITIONS
N/A

AGE-RELATED FACTORS
Puppies and kittens (> 6 weeks age)—serum values should be within the adult reference range; high values suggest PSVA.

ZOONOTIC POTENTIAL
N/A

PREGNANCY
N/A

SEE ALSO
See Causes

ABBREVIATIONS
• ALP = alkaline phosphatase
• ALT = alanine aminotransferase
• AST = aspartate aminotransferase
• FIP = feline infectious peritonitis
• GGT = gamma-glutamyltransferase
• PSVA = portosystemic vascular anomaly

Suggested Reading
Center SA. Diagnostic procedures for evaluation of hepatic disease. In: Guilford WG, Center SA, Strombeck DR, et al., eds., Strombeck's small animal gastroenterology. Philadelphia: Saunders, 1996:130–188.
Center SA. Pathophysiology of liver disease: normal and abnormal function. In: Guilford WG, Center SA, Strombeck DR, et al., eds. Strombeck's small animal gastroenterology. Philadelphia: Saunders, 1996:553–632.
Authors Sharon A. Center and Keith P. Richter
Consulting Editor Sharon A. Center

BILIRUBIN, HIGH

BASICS

DEFINITION
Serum concentration higher than reference range

PATHOPHYSIOLOGY
• Bilirubin—originates from degradation of heme-containing proteins; most (80%) comes from senescent erythrocytes; remainder from heme-containing proteins • Unconjugated—transported in plasma bound to albumin; after hepatocellular uptake, conjugated with glucuronic acid • Conjugated—transported (with other components of bile) into the biliary system; expelled into the intestines, where most is converted to urobilinogen, which can undergo an enterohepatic circulation • Hyperbilirubinemia—caused by increased production (RBC destruction; hemolysis) in excess of the liver's ability to take up and process it or by impaired clearance (disturbed handling by hepatocytes or interference with discharge into the intestines) • Nonhemolytic jaundice (dogs and cats)—caused by hepatobiliary disease

SYSTEMS AFFECTED
• Skin/Exocrine—discoloration of the skin (jaundice) when serum level > 2.5 mg/dL • Hepatobiliary—retained bile acids and possibly bilirubin lead to cholestasis and may contribute to hepatocellular injury. • Renal/Urologic—high concentration may cause renal tubular injury. • Nervous—very high unconjugated concentration may cause degenerative lesions in the brain.

SIGNALMENT
• All ages and breeds of dogs and cats affected • Most causes—diseases of adult animals • Familial hepatic diseases—described (e.g., Doberman pinschers, Bedlington terriers) • Young, unvaccinated dogs—at risk for infectious canine hepatitis

SIGNS

Historical Findings
Increased Formation—Hemolysis
• Lethargy • Anorexia • Weakness • Jaundice • Recent blood transfusion • Severe trauma or hematoma formation
Decreased Elimination— Cholestasis
• Lethargy • Anorexia • Jaundice • Pigmenturia • Abdominal enlargement • Altered mentation • Vomiting • Diarrhea • Polyuria or polydipsia

Physical Examination Findings
Increased Formation—Hemolysis
• Pallor • Jaundice • Hepatomegaly • Splenomegaly • Bleeding tendencies—thrombocytopenia • Orange feces • Lymphadenopathy • Fever

Decreased Elimination—Cholestasis
• Weight loss • Jaundice • Hepatomegaly • Splenomegaly • Abdominal effusion • Abdominal pain • Cranial abdominal mass • Melena • Fever • Acholic feces

CAUSES

Prehepatic Jaundice
• Hemolytic disorders causing destruction of RBCs • Immune-mediated hemolysis—certain drugs; SLE • Infectious—FeLV; *Haemobartonella* spp.; heartworms; *Babesia; Ehrlichia; Cytauxzoon* spp. • Oxidative injury—onions; phenolic compounds; zinc • Resorption of blood—large hematoma

Hepatic Jaundice
• Chronic idiopathic or familial hepatitis • Adverse drug reactions—anticonvulsants; acetaminophen; trimethoprim-sulfa; thiacetarsamide • Cholangitis or cholangiohepatitis • Infiltrative neoplasia—lymphoma • Cirrhosis—dogs • Hepatic lipidosis—cats • Massive hepatic necrosis • Systemic illnesses with a hepatic component—certain serovars of leptospirosis (dogs); histoplasmosis; FIP; hyperthyroidism (cats) • Bacterial sepsis—anywhere in the body; may elaborate bacterial products, impairing hepatic bilirubin processing

Posthepatic Jaundice
• Transient or persistent mechanical interference with the excretion of bilirubin and other bile elements • Pancreatitis • Neoplasia—bile duct; pancreatic; duodenal • Intraluminal duct occlusion—cholelithiasis; sludged bile; liver flukes (cats) • Sclerosing cholangitis—cats • Ruptured gallbladder or bile duct

RISK FACTORS
• Young dogs—infectious disease • Breed predisposition for familial hepatic disease—Dobermans, Bedlington terriers • Middle-aged obese dogs—pancreatitis • Anorectic obese cats—hepatic lipidosis • Hepatotoxic drugs • Blunt abdominal trauma or chronic biliary tract disease—bile peritonitis • Hemolytic anemia

DIAGNOSIS

DIFFERENTIAL DIAGNOSIS
• Prehepatic jaundice—usually abrupt onset; mucous membrane pallor; mild to moderate jaundice; weakness; tachypnea; cardiac murmur with severe anemia • Hepatic jaundice—breed risk for familial hepatic disease; variable jaundice, otherwise normal mucous membranes; alteration in liver size (large or very small); abdominal effusion or ascites (pure or modified transudate); polyuria or polydipsia; behavioral abnormalities; bleeding • Posthepatic jaundice—chronic and/or recurrent bouts of apparent gastroenteritis or pancreatitis; moderate or marked jaundice, otherwise normal mucous membranes; diffuse abdominal pain; cranial abdominal pain or mass; abdominal effusion (septic or nonseptic exudate); bleeding

LABORATORY FINDINGS

Drugs That May Alter Laboratory Results
N/A

Disorders That May Alter Laboratory Results
• Bilirubin assay—based on the diazo reaction; assesses quantity of direct-reacting and total serum bilirubins; most yield reasonable total bilirubin results; values for direct bilirubin vary. • Sample management—important, total bilirubin may decrease by 50%/hr with direct exposure to sunlight or artificial lighting • Hemolysis—variable effects on total bilirubin measured by spectrophotometry • Lipemia—falsely increases total bilirubin values measured by end-point assays • Fractionation into conjugated and unconjugated—unable to define causes of jaundice

Valid If Run in Human Laboratory?
Yes

CBC/BIOCHEMISTRY/URINALYSIS

Prehepatic Jaundice
• CBC—severe anemia (usually regenerative); RBC morphology may reveal spherocytes, Heinz bodies, and parasites; hemoglobinemia with severe hemolysis • Biochemistry—normal to high ALT, ALP, and BUN; normal albumin, glucose, and cholesterol

Hepatic Jaundice
• CBC—mild nonregenerative anemia • Biochemistry—mildly to markedly high ALT and ALP; normal to low albumin, BUN, glucose, and cholesterol • Urinalysis—normal to dilute urine; bilirubinuria precedes hyperbilirubinemia

Posthepatic Jaundice
• CBC—mild nonregenerative anemia • Biochemistry—mildly high ALT; moderate to markedly high ALP; usually normal albumin, BUN, and glucose; normal to high cholesterol

OTHER LABORATORY TESTS
• Saline-dispersion slide test—with suspected

RBC agglutination; very large MCV
• Direct Coombs test—with nonagglutination and spherocytes
• Osmotic fragility test
• Blood smears—for hemoparasites
• ANA—with hemolytic anemia
• Serum bile acids—no need if prehepatic causes for jaundice have been eliminated
• Serology—for infectious diseases (e.g., FeLV, leptospirosis, and mycoses) with signs of multisystemic illness and hepatic jaundice
• Abdominal effusion—characterize
• Coagulation tests—prolonged values, especially PIVKA and PT with bile duct occlusion
• Microbial culture and sensitivity—blood and/or other specimens; with an inflammatory leukon and potential focus of bacterial infection (e.g., urinary tract)

IMAGING
• Abdominal radiography—details obscured with moderate to marked abdominal effusion; may reveal hepatomegaly, a mass effect, or mineral or gas interfaces in liver; splenomegaly with hemolytic anemia, portal hypertension, or abdominal neoplasia; metallic foreign body with zinc-associated hemolysis
• Thoracic radiography—may reveal neoplastic nodules; sternal lymphadenopathy reflects abdominal (hepatobiliary or other visceral) inflammation or neoplasia
• Abdominal ultrasonography—may distinguish primary hepatobiliary disease from extrahepatic biliary obstruction; characterizes hepatic parenchymal lesions; may determine origin of abdominal effusion; to direct biopsy sampling

DIAGNOSTIC PROCEDURES
• Liver biopsy—bacterial culture of liver tissue and bile; specimens obtained via celiotomy, blind percutaneous, keyhole, laparoscopic, or ultrasound-guided technique
• Celiotomy and surgical intervention—required to confirm and correct most causes of posthepatic jaundice

TREATMENT
• Depends on underlying cause
• Inpatient—initial medical care
• Cage rest—facilitate liver regeneration
• Restricted activity—required with jaundice
• Diet—important for hepatic and posthepatic jaundice; nutritionally balanced with maximum protein tolerated by patient; carbohydrate based (dogs) with moderately restricted protein for hepatic encephalopathy; restricted sodium for ascites
• Vitamin supplementation—water-soluble vitamins in all patients; vitamin K_1 for bile duct obstruction or severe cholestasis

MEDICATIONS

DRUGS OF CHOICE
• Prehepatic jaundice—eliminate inciting cause; see Anemia, Immune-mediated; whole blood transfusion for life-threatening anemia
• Hepatic and posthepatic jaundice—treat medical causes as determined by results of liver biopsy and cultures.

CONTRAINDICATIONS
• Avoid known hepatotoxic drugs.
• Avoid tetracyclines—suppress hepatic protein synthesis
• Avoid analgesics, anesthetics, and barbiturates—with hepatic failure

PRECAUTIONS
• Most commonly used drugs are well tolerated by jaundiced patients with hepatobiliary disease.
• Antibiotics—use cautiously; for specific therapy only
• Sedatives—avoid; may precipitate hepatic encephalopathy
• Corticosteroids—use carefully for nonseptic inflammatory hepatobiliary disease; may increase the chance of intercurrent infections; may aggravate ascites by promoting water and sodium retention

POSSIBLE INTERACTIONS
• Use all drugs cautiously—the liver is the most important organ involved with drug metabolism; duration and intensity of action of many drugs requiring hepatic biotransformation may be increased; others may not be transformed to their effective form.

ALTERNATIVE DRUGS
N/A

FOLLOW-UP

PATIENT MONITORING
• Prehepatic jaundice—recheck PCV as needed; may require repeat transfusions; may be required; gradually taper off immunosuppressive drugs. • Hepatic and posthepatic jaundice—recheck serum biochemical profile as dictated by underlying disease; continue symptomatic and specific treatment

POSSIBLE COMPLICATIONS
Diseases causing jaundice may cause death.

MISCELLANEOUS

ASSOCIATED CONDITIONS
• Patients with immune-mediated hemolysis that are treated with immunosuppressive doses of corticosteroids are predisposed to thromboembolism, possible gastrointestinal ulceration, and infections. • Patients with hepatic failure are susceptible to infection and gastrointestinal bleeding. • Patients that have had reconstructive biliary surgery are at risk for recurrent ascending bacterial cholangitis.

AGE-RELATED FACTORS
N/A

ZOONOTIC POTENTIAL
Certain serovars of leptospirosis

PREGNANCY
N/A

SYNONYMS
• Icterus • Jaundice

SEE ALSO
• Anemia, Heinz Body • Anemia, Immune-mediated • Anemia, Regenerative • Antinuclear Antibody Titer and Lupus Erythematosus (LE) Cell Test • Babesiosis • Blood Transfusion Reactions • Cholangitis/Cholangiohepatitis • Cholelithiasis • Cirrhosis/Fibrosis of the Liver • Coombs Test • Copper Hepatopathy • Flukes, Liver and Hepatic • Haemobartonellosis • Hepatic Failure, Acute • Hepatic Lipidosis • Hepatitis, Chronic Active • Hepatitis, Infectious Canine • Hepatitis, Leptospirosis • Hepatitis, Suppurative and Hepatic Abscess • Hepatotoxins • Lupus Erythematosus, Systemic (SLE) • Pancreatitis • Zinc Toxicity

ABBREVIATIONS
• ALP = alkaline phosphatase • ALT = alanine aminotransferase • FeLV = feline leukemia virus • FIP = feline infectious peritonitis • MCV = mean cell volume • PCV = packed cell volume • PIVKA = proteins invoked by vitamin K absence or antagonism • PT = prothrombin time • SLE = systemic lupus erythematosus

Suggested Reading
Center SA. Pathophysiology of liver disease: normal and abnormal function. In: Guilford WG, Center SA, Strombeck DR, et al., eds. Strombeck's small animal gastroenterology. 3rd ed. Philadelphia: Saunders, 1996:553–632.

Duncan JR, Prasse KW, Mahaffey EA. Liver. In: Duncan RJ, Prasse KW, Mahaffey EA, eds. Veterinary laboratory medicine. 3rd ed. Ames: Iowa State University Press, 1994.

Johnson SE. Diseases of the liver. In: Ettinger SJ, Feldman ED, eds. Textbook of veterinary internal medicine. 4th ed. Philadelphia: Saunders, 1995:1313–1357.

Author Susan E. Bunch
Consulting Editor Sharon A. Center

CALCIUM, HYPERCALCEMIA

BASICS

DEFINITION
- Serum total calcium > 11.5 mg/dL (dogs)
- Serum total calcium > 10.5 mg/dL (cats)

PATHOPHYSIOLOGY
- Control of calcium is complex and is influenced by the actions of parathyroid hormone (PTH) and vitamin D and the interaction of these hormones with the gut, bone, kidneys, and parathyroid glands.
- Derangement in the function of these can lead to hypercalcemia.
- Secretory productions of some neoplastic cells can also disturb calcium homeostasis.

SYSTEMS AFFECTED
- Renal/Urologic—high levels of calcium are toxic to the renal tubules and can cause polyuria and polydipsia (PU/PD) and renal failure; can also lead to urolithiasis and associated lower urinary tract disease
- Gastrointestinal—reduces excitability of smooth muscle and can alter gastrointestinal function
- Neuromuscular—depressed skeletal muscle contractility causes weakness.
- Cardiovascular—hypertension and altered cardiac contractility

SIGNALMENT
- Dog and cat
- Primary hyperparathyroidism in the keeshond and Siamese cat

SIGNS

General Comments
- Depend on the cause of hypercalcemia
- Patients with underlying neoplasia, renal failure, or hypoadrenocorticism generally appear ill.
- Patients with primary hyperparathyroidism show mild clinical signs, if any, due solely to the effects of hypercalcemia.
- Signs become apparent when hypercalcemia is severe and chronic.

Historical Findings
- PU/PD—most common in dogs
- Anorexia
- Lethargy—most common in cats
- Vomiting
- Constipation
- Weakness
- Stupor and coma—severe cases

Physical Examination Findings
- Lymphadenopathy or abdominal organomegaly in patients with lymphosarcoma
- Usually unremarkable in dogs with primary hyperparathyroidism
- Parathyroid gland adenoma—not palpable in dogs; often palpable in cats with primary hyperparathyroidism

CAUSES
- Neoplasia—lymphosarcoma (most common in dogs, less common in cats), anal sac apocrine gland adenocarcinoma (dogs), multiple myeloma, lymphocytic leukemia, metastatic bone tumor, fibrosarcoma (cats), various types of carcinoma
- Primary hyperparathyroidism
- Renal failure—acute or chronic
- Blastomycosis
- Hypoadrenocorticism
- Vitamin D rodenticide intoxication—no longer marketed in the United States

RISK FACTORS
- Keeshond breed—hyperparathyroidism
- Renal failure
- Neoplasia
- Use of calcium supplements or calcium-containing intestinal phosphate binders
- Use of calcitriol or other vitamin D preparations

DIAGNOSIS

DIFFERENTIAL DIAGNOSIS
- History should include exposure to rat poison and any previous response to steroids.
- History of waxing/waning illness suggests hypoadrenocorticism.
- Complete lymph node, rectal, and abdominal palpation may raise index of suspicion for lymphosarcoma and other neoplasia.
- Assessment of hydration status, renal palpation, and urinary history points toward lower urinary tract disease or renal failure.

LABORATORY FINDINGS

Drugs That May Alter Laboratory Results
- Oxalate, citrate, and EDTA anticoagulants bind calcium and falsely lower calcium measurement.
- Vitamin D preparations and thiazide diuretics can raise serum calcium concentrations.

Disorders That May Alter Laboratory Results
- Hemolysis and lipemia can falsely raise calcium concentrations.
- Hypoalbuminemia can falsely lower total calcium concentration.

Valid If Run in Human Laboratory?
Yes

CBC/BIOCHEMISTRY/URINALYSIS
- Serum calcium—total calcium concentration depends on binding proteins; adjusted (corrected) calcium can be estimated by the following formulas:

$$\text{Corrected Ca} = \text{Ca (mg/dL)} - \text{albumin (g/dL)} + 3.5$$

or

$$\text{Corrected Ca} = \text{Ca (mg/dL)} - [0.4 \times \text{total protein (g/dL)}] + 3.3$$

- Azotemia and isosthenuria help define degree of renal impairment.
- Serum phosphorus is usually low or low-normal in patients with primary hyperparathyroidism or hypercalcemia associated with malignancy.
- Hyperphosphatemia in the absence of azotemia suggests a nonparathyroid cause of hypercalcemia.
- Combination of hyperphosphatemia and azotemia is difficult to interpret, since renal failure can be the cause or effect of hypercalcemia.
- Hyperkalemia and hyponatremia suggest hypoadrenocorticism.
- Hyperglobulinemia is associated with multiple myeloma.
- Cytopenias are seen in patients with myelophthisic disease.

OTHER LABORATORY TESTS
• Serum ionized calcium is high in patients with primary hyperparathyroidism or hypercalcemia associated with malignancy; usually normal or low in patients with hypercalcemia associated with renal failure
• Serum PTH measurement—intact molecule and two-site assay methods have the greatest specificity; high-normal or high concentration suggests primary hyperparathyroidism; low concentration suggests neoplasia.
• Serum PTH-rp measurement is often high in patients with hypercalcemia associated with malignancy.
• Vitamin D assays are not readily available.

IMAGING
• Radiography is useful for assessing renal size and shape, urolithiasis, bone lysis, and occult neoplasia.
• Ultrasonography valuable for assessing renal architecture, abdominal lymphadenopathy, and urolithiasis

DIAGNOSTIC PROCEDURES
• Cytologic examination of fine-needle aspirate of lymph nodes to confirm lymphosarcoma
• Examination of bone marrow aspirate to confirm occult hematopoietic neoplasia
• ACTH stimulation testing to confirm hypoadrenocorticism

TREATMENT
• Inpatient care because of the deleterious effects of hypercalcemia and the need for fluid therapy
• Consider severe hypercalcemia a medical emergency.

MEDICATIONS

DRUGS OF CHOICE
• Normal saline—fluid of choice
• Avoid calcium-containing fluids.
• Diuretics (furosemide) and corticosteroids can be useful.

CONTRAINDICATIONS
• Do not use glucocorticoids until the diagnosis of lymphoma is excluded; they can obfuscate the diagnosis; if hypoadrenocorticism is suspected, do not give glucocorticoids until after ACTH stimulation testing.
• Thiazide diuretics can cause calcium retention.

PRECAUTIONS
N/A

POSSIBLE INTERACTIONS
Avoid the use of calcium- or phosphorus-containing compounds; they can cause soft tissue mineralization in severely hypercalcemic and hyperphosphatemic patients.

ALTERNATIVE DRUGS
• Sodium bicarbonate (1–4 mEq/kg) may be useful in combination with other treatments.
• Mithramycin has been used in severe hypercalcemic crises; avoid its use if possible, because of associated nephrotoxicity and hepatotoxicity.
• Calcitonin may be useful in the treatment of hypervitaminosis D.

FOLLOW-UP

PATIENT MONITORING
• Serum calcium every 12 h
• Renal function tests—the first sign of tubular damage may be casts in the urine sediment.
• Must monitor urine output, particularly if oliguric renal failure is suspected, in which case urine output should be measured carefully; oliguria cannot be determined unless the patient is fully hydrated.
• Hydration status must be monitored; indicators of overhydration include increased body weight, increased central venous pressure, and edema (pulmonary or subcutaneous).

POSSIBLE COMPLICATIONS
• Irreversible renal failure
• Soft tissue mineralization

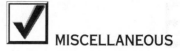

MISCELLANEOUS

ASSOCIATED CONDITIONS
Calcium-containing urolithiasis

AGE-RELATED FACTORS
• Mild elevations in calcium and phosphorus may be normal in growing animals.
• Middle-aged and older dogs and cats are at increased risk for cancer.

ZOONOTIC POTENTIAL
N/A

PREGNANCY
A fetus is at the same risk as the dam; do not alter treatment because of pregnancy.

SYNONYMS
N/A

SEE ALSO
• Hyperparathyroidism
• Renal Failure (Chronic or Acute)

ABBREVIATIONS
• Ca = calcium
• PTH = parathyroid hormone
• PTH-rp = parathyroid hormone–related peptide

Suggested Reading
Chew DJ, Nagode LA, Carothers M. Disorders of calcium: hypercalcemia and hypocalcemia. In: DiBartola SP, ed. Fluid therapy in small animal practice. Philadelphia: Saunders 1992;116–176.
Feldman EC. Disorders of the parathyroid glands, In: Ettinger SJ, Feldman EC, eds. Textbook of veterinary internal medicine. 4th ed. Philadelphia: Saunders, 1994;1437–1464.
Author Thomas K. Graves
Consulting Editor Deborah S. Greco

CALCIUM, HYPOCALCEMIA

 BASICS

DEFINITION
Low total serum calcium concentration

PATHOPHYSIOLOGY
Of the total circulating serum calcium, 50% is protein bound, 40% is ionized, and 10% is complexed with other substances. Protein-bound calcium cannot diffuse through membranes and thus is unusable by the tissues. Complexed calcium can diffuse through membranes but is unavailable for use by tissues. Only the ionized form is available to tissues, so only changes in this fraction of total serum calcium are responsible for clinical problems (hypo- and hypercalcemia). Measurement of ionized calcium is difficult for routine performance, and biochemical profiles record only total serum calcium. Mechanisms involved in hypocalcemia include
- Low concentrations of binding proteins—hypoalbuminemia
- Reduced intestinal absorption—deficient vitamin D (renal disease, severe intestinal disease)
- Reduced renal and bone resorption—hypoparathyroidism
- Inadequate dietary intake
- Excessive loss—lactation
- Sequestration—saponification (acute pancreatitis)
- Binding/complexing with administered or ingested chemicals—phosphate-containing enemas, citrate toxicity, ethylene glycol toxicity, low calcium/high phosphorus diet (nutritional secondary hyperparathyroidism)
- Impaired synthesis or refractoriness to PTH—hypomagnesemia

SYSTEMS AFFECTED
- Nervous/Neuromuscular—seizures, tetany, ataxia, and weakness
- Cardiovascular—ECG changes and bradycardia
- Gastrointestinal—anorexia and vomiting (especially cats)
- Ophthalmic—posterior lenticular cataracts
- Respiratory—panting

SIGNALMENT
- Dog and cat
- Varies depending on the underlying cause

SIGNS

General Comments
Signs of the underlying disease may be seen without clinical signs of hypocalcemia,
because the latter do not occur until total serum calcium falls below 6.7 mg/dL.

Historical Findings
- Seizures
- Muscle trembling, twitching, or fasciculations
- Ataxia or stiff gait
- Weakness
- Panting
- Facial rubbing
- Vomiting
- Anorexia

Physical Examination Findings
- Fever
- Posterior lenticular cataracts in patients with primary hypoparathyroidism

CAUSES

Nonpathologic Hypocalcemia
- Laboratory error—occurs up to 13% of the time; repeat serum calcium determination recommended to confirm true hypocalcemia, especially if results indicate significant hypocalcemia despite absence of clinical signs.
- Hypoalbuminemia—most common cause; accounts for over 50% of patients; leads to reduction of protein-bound calcium without affecting ionized calcium; not associated with clinical signs
- Correct for hypoalbuminemia by use of one of the following formulas:

$$\text{Corrected Ca} = \text{Ca (mg/dL)} - \text{albumin (g/dL)} + 3.5$$

or

$$\text{Corrected Ca} = \text{Ca (mg/dL)} - [0.4 \ 3 \ \text{total protein (g/dL)}] + 3.3$$

Note: In cats, hypoalbuminemia causes a drop in the calcium concentration; these formulas were developed in dogs and cannot be applied to cats.
- Alkalosis—causes a shift from protein-bound calcium to ionized calcium as well as a reduction in measured calcium. Not associated with clinical signs

Pathologic Hypocalcemia
- Primary hypoparathyroidism
- Hypoparathyroidism secondary to thyroidectomy and parathyroid damage
- Renal failure—acute or chronic
- Ethylene glycol toxicity
- Acute pancreatitis
- Puerperal tetany—eclampsia
- Phosphate-containing enemas
- Nutritional secondary hyperparathyroidism
- Hypomagnesemia
- Intestinal malabsorption
- Citrate toxicity—multiple blood transfusions or improper citrate–blood ratio

RISK FACTORS
Puerperal tetany (eclampsia)—usually seen in small-breed bitches during the first 21 days of nursing a litter

 DIAGNOSIS

DIFFERENTIAL DIAGNOSIS
- Clinical signs of hypocalcemia—rule out primary hypoparathyroidism, hypoparathyroidism secondary to thyroidectomy and parathyroid damage, and puerperal tetany (eclampsia); other causes rarely lower the serum calcium enough to cause clinical signs.
- Polyuria and polydipsia—rule out renal failure.
- Neurologic signs—rule out ethylene glycol toxicity.
- Vomiting and diarrhea—rule out acute pancreatitis, intestinal malabsorption, renal failure, and ethylene glycol toxicity.
- Bone pain or fractures—rule out nutritional secondary hyperparathyroidism.

LABORATORY FINDINGS

Drugs That May Alter Laboratory Results
- Sodium bicarbonate may cause alkalosis and lower the serum calcium concentration.
- Samples collected in EDTA tubes may have a falsely low serum calcium concentration because of calcium chelation.

Disorders That May Alter Laboratory Results
- Lipemia can raise the serum calcium significantly.
- Any cause of hypoalbumenia can falsely lower the serum calcium (see causes of nonpathogenic hypocalcemia).

Valid If Run in Human Laboratory?
Yes

CBC/BIOCHEMISTRY/URINALYSIS
- Low calcium
- Mild-to-moderate anemia possible in patients with chronic renal failure, nutritional secondary hyperparathyroidism, and intestinal malabsorption
- Leukocytosis possible in patients with acute pancreatitis
- Hypoalbuminemia in patients with hypoproteinemia-induced hypocalcemia—intestinal malabsorption, protein-losing nephropathy, other
- High total CO_2 in patients with alkalosis-induced hypocalcemia

• High BUN and creatinine in patients with acute and chronic renal failure and ethylene glycol toxicity
• High phosphorus in patients with acute and chronic renal failure, ethylene glycol toxicity, primary hypoparathyroidism, hypoparathyroidism secondary to thyroidectomy and parathyroid damage, and those receiving phosphate-containing enemas
• High amylase and lipase in many, but not all, patients with acute pancreatitis
• Isosthenuria in patients with chronic renal failure, moderate-to-advanced acute renal failure, and ethylene glycol toxicity
• Glucosuria in patients with acute renal failure and ethylene glycol toxicity

OTHER LABORATORY TESTS
• Ethylene glycol test—indicated in patients suspected of ingesting ethylene glycol within the previous 12–16 h
• PTH assay—indicated when primary hypoparathyroidism is suspected
• Serum magnesium concentration—hypomagnesemia is a rare cause of hypocalcemia; indicated when all other causes of hypocalcemia have been ruled out

IMAGING
• Radiography usually normal
• Possibly, small kidneys in patients with chronic renal failure and large kidneys in patients with acute renal failure and ethylene glycol toxicity
• Possibly, decreased bone density in patients with nutritional secondary hyperparathyroidism
• Possibly, mild pleural effusion and decreased abdominal detail from effusion with pancreatitis

DIAGNOSTIC PROCEDURES
ECG changes include prolongation of the ST and Q-T segments; sinus bradycardia and wide T waves or T wave alternans in some patients

TREATMENT
• Treat patients with clinical hypocalcemia whose underlying disease requires support as inpatients.
• Emergency treatment is usually only needed for patients with primary hypoparathyroidism, hypoparathyroidism secondary to thyroidectomy and parathyroid damage, puerperal tetany (eclampsia), recent phosphate-containing enema administration, and citrate toxicity (rare).

• Short-term and long-term treatment is usually only needed to treat primary hypoparathyroidism and puerperal tetany (eclampsia).
• Diet change recommended in patients with nutritional secondary hyperparathyroidism (to a balanced diet) and renal failure (see Renal Failure, Chronic).

MEDICATIONS

DRUGS AND FLUIDS
Emergency Treatment
• Calcium gluconate 10% solution—5–15 mg/kg (0.5–1.5 mL/kg) slowly to effect over a 10-min period; monitor heart rate and stop administration temporarily if bradycardia occurs; if ECG monitoring is possible, Q-T interval shortening is an indication to temporarily stop administration.
• Calcium chloride 10% solution—also effective; extremely caustic if administered extravascularly and three times more potent than calcium gluconate; the mg/kg dosage is the same, but one third the volume is needed (0.15–0.5 mL/kg).
• If the patient has puerperal tetany (eclampsia), remove the puppies from the mother and hand-nurse until weaned.

Short-term Treatment Immediately After Correction of Tetany
Calcium gluconate 10% solution—relapse of clinical signs after emergency treatment can be prevented by use of one of the following:
• Constant-rate IV infusion of 60–90 mg/kg/day (6.5–9.75 mL/kg/day) added to the fluids
• Subcutaneous administration 3–4 times daily of the dosage determined necessary for initial control of tetany; dilute this dose in an equal volume of saline.

Long-term Treatment
See Hypoparathyroidism.

CONTRAINDICATIONS
N/A

PRECAUTIONS
See Hypoparathyroidism.

POSSIBLE INTERACTIONS
See Hypoparathyroidism.

ALTERNATIVE DRUGS
N/A

FOLLOW-UP

PATIENT MONITORING
• Serum calcium concentration monthly for the first 6 months then every 2–4 months
• Goal is to maintain serum calcium concentration between 8 and 10 mg/dL.

POSSIBLE COMPLICATIONS
Hypocalcemia and hypercalcemia (which can lead to renal failure) are both concerns in patients on long-term therapy.

MISCELLANEOUS

ASSOCIATED CONDITIONS
N/A

AGE-RELATED FACTORS
N/A

ZOONOTIC POTENTIAL
N/A

PREGNANCY
• Hypocalcemia can lead to weakness and dystocia.
• Clinical hypocalcemia caused by puerperal tetany (eclampsia) usually is seen in small-breed bitches during the first 21 days of nursing a litter.

SYNONYMS
N/A

SEE ALSO
• See specific causes.
• Hypoparathyroidism

ABBREVIATIONS
• Ca = calcium
• PTH = parathyroid hormone

Suggested Reading
Feldman EC, Nelson RW. Hypocalcemia and primary hypoparathyroidism. In: Feldman EC, Nelson RW, eds., Canine and feline endocrinology and reproduction. Philadelphia: Saunders, 1996:497–516.
Meuten DJ, Armstrong PJ. Parathyroid disease and calcium metabolism. In: Ettinger SJ, ed., Textbook of veterinary internal medicine. Philadelphia: Saunders, 1989:1610–1631.
Waters CB, Scott-Moncrieff JCR. Hypocalcemia in cats. Compend Contin Educ Pract Vet 1992;14:497–507.
Author Mitchell A. Crystal
Consulting Editor Deborah Greco

CHLORIDE, HYPERCHLOREMIA

BASICS

DEFINITION
Serum chloride concentration >122 mEq/L in dogs and >129 mEq/L in cats

PATHOPHYSIOLOGY
• Chloride is the most abundant anion in the extracellular fluid.
• Hyperchloremia is associated with similar conditions to those that cause hypernatremia—water loss in excess of sodium and chloride or excessive NaCl intake
• Chloride concentration varies inversely to bicarbonate concentration; high bicarbonate loss (i.e., GI or renal wasting), followed by low renal chloride resorption in excess of bicarbonate, can cause hyperchloremia.

SYSTEMS AFFECTED
Relates to underlying cause

GENETICS
N/A

INCIDENCE
N/A

GEOGRAPHIC DISTRIBUTION
N/A

SIGNALMENT

Species
Dogs and cats

Breed Predilection
None

Predominant Sex
None

Mean Age and Range
N/A

SIGNS

General Comments
• Related to concurrent hypernatremia or the underlying disorder or both
• Severity of neurologic signs is related to the degree of hypernatremia and the rate at which it develops.

History and Physical Examination Findings
• Polydipsia
• Disorientation
• Coma
• Seizures

CAUSES

High Total Body Chloride
• Oral ingestion—rare
• NaCl administered IV during cardiovascular resuscitation

Normal Total Body Chloride with Water Deficit
• Low intake (e.g., no access to water)
• High urinary water loss (e.g., diabetes insipidus)
• High insensible water loss (e.g., panting)

Low Total Body Chloride with Hypotonic Fluid Loss
Urinary loss—diabetes mellitus, osmotic diuresis, and diuresis after urinary obstruction

Hyperchloremic Metabolic Acidosis
• Renal tubular acidosis—renal tubular disorders that cause renal wasting of bicarbonate or low hydrogen ion secretion
• Diarrhea associated with gastrointestinal loss of bicarbonate and renal resorption of chloride

RISK FACTORS
N/A

DIAGNOSIS

DIFFERENTIAL DIAGNOSIS
• Normal anion gap metabolic acidosis (e.g., renal tubular acidosis and gastrointestinal bicarbonate loss)
• Diabetes insipidus
• Hypertonic dehydration
• Severe forms of diabetes mellitus (e.g., diabetic ketoacidosis and hyperosmolar nonketotic syndrome)
• Salt ingestion—rare

LABORATORY FINDINGS

Drugs That May Alter Laboratory Results
• A wide variety of drugs can interfere with renal capacity to concentrate urine, leading to water loss in excess of sodium, and high sodium and chloride concentrations; these drugs include lithium, demeclocycline, and amphotericin.
• Other drugs that may increase chloride concentration include acetazolamide, ammonium chloride, androgens, and cholestyramine.
• A falsely high chloride concentration can occur with a high serum concentration of iodide or bromide—most commonly seen in patients with epilepsy treated with potassium bromide

Disorders That May Alter Laboratory Results
Hemoglobin and bilirubin cause falsely high chloride readings if colorimetric tests are used.

Valid If Run in Human Laboratory?
Yes

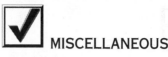

CHLORIDE, HYPERCHLOREMIA

CBC/BIOCHEMISTRY/URINALYSIS
- High chloride, often coupled with high sodium
- Diabetes insipidus—low urinary specific gravity, polyuria, and low urinary sodium
- Diabetic ketoacidosis and hyperosmolar nonketotic syndrome—high blood glucose
- Hypertonic dehydration—low urinary sodium and high urinary specific gravity (usually >1.030)
- Renal tubular acidosis—hyperchloremic acidosis, urine pH > 5.3, serum potassium often low, and other causes of metabolic acidosis have been ruled out

OTHER LABORATORY TESTS
Renal tubular acidosis—response to $NaHCO_3$ or NH_4CL.

IMAGING
CT scan or MRI in patients with diabetes insipidus to rule out pituitary tumor

OTHER DIAGNOSTIC PROCEDURES
N/A

TREATMENT
Hyperchloremia with hypernatremia—hypotonic fluids (5% dextrose in water); decrease sodium by 0.5 mEq/h or by no more than 20 mEq/L/day.

MEDICATIONS

DRUGS OF CHOICE
- Hypovolemia—isotonic saline (normal saline or lactated Ringer's solution) or isotonic fluid (5% dextrose with half-normal saline)
- Central diabetes insipidus—DDAVP (1–2 drops in the conjunctival sac q12–24h)
- Nephrogenic diabetes insipidus—chlorothiazide 10–40 mg/kg PO q12h
- Hyperchloremic metabolic acidosis—treat underlying cause; consider bicarbonate and potassium replacement if needed.

CONTRAINDICATIONS
N/A

PRECAUTIONS
- Rapid correction of hyperchloremia with hypernatremia can cause pulmonary edema.
- Hypocalcemia may develop during correction of hyperchloremia.

POSSIBLE INTERACTIONS
N/A

ALTERNATIVE DRUGS
N/A

FOLLOW-UP

PATIENT MONITORING
Electrolytes, body weight, and hydration status

POSSIBLE COMPLICATIONS
- Related to associated hypernatremia or the underlying disorder
- Neurologic complications include CNS thrombosis or hemorrhage; seizures; and hyperactivity

MISCELLANEOUS

ASSOCIATED CONDITIONS
N/A

AGE-RELATED FACTORS
N/A

ZOONOTIC POTENTIAL
N/A

PREGNANCY
N/A

SYNONYMS
N/A

SEE ALSO
Sodium, Hypernatremia

ABBREVIATIONS
- DDAVP = brand name for desmopressin, a synthetic antidiuretic hormone preparation
- GI = gastro intestinal

Suggested Reading
DiBartola SP. Fluid therapy in small animal practice. Philadelphia: Saunders, 1992.
Ross DB. Clinical physiology of acid-base and electrolyte disorders. 3rd ed. New York: McGraw-Hill, 1989.
Author Rhett Nichols
Editor Deborah S. Greco

DIAGNOSTICS—LAB

CHLORIDE, HYPOCHLOREMIA

 ## BASICS

DEFINITION
Serum chloride concentration below the lower limit of normal—dogs, <105 mEq/L; cats, <117 mEq/L

PATHOPHYSIOLOGY
• Chloride is the most abundant anion in the extracellular fluid.
• Chloride concentration is controlled by electrochemical gradients resulting from the active transport of sodium.
• In general, chloride concentration varies directly with sodium concentration and inversely with bicarbonate concentration.

SYSTEMS AFFECTED
Depend on underlying disorder

SIGNALMENT
Dog and cat

CAUSES
• Gastric vomiting
• Hypoadrenocorticism
• Metabolic alkalosis
• Salt-losing nephropathy
• Diuretic therapy

RISK FACTORS
N/A

 ## DIAGNOSIS

DIFFERENTIAL DIAGNOSIS
If the degree of hypochloremia exceeds that of hyponatremia, it suggests selective chloride loss as seen in patients with gastric vomiting.

LABORATORY FINDINGS

Drugs That May Alter Laboratory Results
Furosemide, thiazides, bicarbonate, and laxatives lower the serum concentration.

Disorders That May Alter Laboratory Results
Lipemia and hyperproteinemia can falsely lower chloride concentration if ion-specific electrodes are not used.

Valid If Run in Human Laboratory?
Valid

CBC/BIOCHEMISTRY/URINALYSIS
• Low chloride
• Other abnormalities depend on underlying disorder; possibly, hyponatremia, hyperkalemia, and high bicarbonate concentration

OTHER LABORATORY TESTS
• Measurement of urine fractional excretion of chloride may demonstrate high excretion.
• Blood gas measurement may reveal metabolic alkalosis.

IMAGING
N/A

DIAGNOSTIC PROCEDURES
N/A

 ## TREATMENT
• Depends on underlying disorder
• Use 0.9% NaCl if fluid administration is indicated.

DIET
No need to alter

CLIENT EDUCATION
Depends on underlying disorder

SURGICAL CONSIDERATIONS
N/A

MEDICATIONS

DRUGS OF CHOICE
Other fluid therapy and medication as dictated by underlying cause.

CONTRAINDICATIONS
N/A

PRECAUTIONS
N/A

POSSIBLE INTERACTIONS
N/A

ALTERNATIVE DRUGS
N/A

 FOLLOW-UP

PATIENT MONITORING
Serum electrolyte concentrations as needed to ensure appropriate response

POSSIBLE COMPLICATIONS
Depend on underlying disorder

PREVENTION/AVOIDANCE
Depends on underlying disorder

EXPECTED COURSE/PROGNOSIS
Depends on underlying cause

✓ MISCELLANEOUS

ASSOCIATED CONDITIONS
Often accompanied by hyponatremia

AGE-RELATED FACTORS
N/A

ZOONOTIC POTENTIAL
N/A

PREGNANCY
N/A

SYNONYMS
N/A

SEE ALSO
N/A

ABBREVIATIONS
N/A

Suggested Reading
DiBartola SP. Fluid therapy in small animal practice. Philadelphia: Saunders, 1992.
Rose DB. Clinical physiology of acid-base and electrolyte disorders. 3rd ed. New York: McGraw-Hill, 1989.
Author Peter P. Kintzer
Consulting Editor Deborah S. Greco

DIAGNOSTICS—LAB

CLOTTING FACTOR DEFICIENCIES

BASICS

DEFINITION
Hemostatic defects characterized by deficient activity of one or more coagulation factors

PATHOPHYSIOLOGY
• Coagulation mechanism involves a series of sequential enzyme activations leading to the generation of thrombin, which converts fibrinogen to fibrin monomers, and subsequent polymerization of the monomers into fibrin strands, which stabilize the platelet plugs at sites of vessel injury
• Severe deficiency or defective function of coagulation factors causes defective hemostasis.

SYSTEMS AFFECTED
• Coagulation defects can cause hemorrhage in any tissue or organ and anemia.
• Hemorrhage—most commonly in and around the joints and major muscle masses (causing large swellings) and into the body cavities; region of the larynx or pleural cavity of special concern because of the risk of asphyxia; brain or spinal cord of major concern because the rigid bony case limits expansion, and the risk for permanent damage is high

SIGNALMENT
• Factor VIII and factor IX deficiencies—severe defects usually recognized as spontaneous hemorrhages before 10 weeks of age; X-linked defects; males are clinically affected, whereas females are carriers and usually clinically normal. Females, of course, can have these deficiencies though relatively rarely.
• Von Willebrand disease—autosomal defect; both males and females are affected clinically; the most common inherited coagulation defect with high prevalence in many breeds.
• Factor X deficiency—detected in American cocker spaniels and Jack Russell terriers; manifests as stillborn puppies or neonatal deaths related to internal hemorrhage; autosomal trait: homozygotes severely affected; heterozygotes may be clinically normal or have only a mild bleeding tendency.
• Factor XI deficiency—rare defect described in the English springer spaniels, great Pyrenees, and Kerry blue terriers; mild autosomal defect with bleeding after surgery or injury.
• Factor XII deficiency—fairly common in cats but rarely detected because no bleeding tendency is associated with the defect

SIGNS
• Inactivity
• Swollen joints
• Subcutaneous swellings
• Abnormal bleeding from cuts or mucous membranes
• Hemorrhages in deeper tissues or body cavities

CAUSES
• True deficiency of clotting factors (e.g., genetic defect, liver disease, rodenticide anticoagulant toxicity, and vitamin K deficiency)
• Synthesis of defective factors
• Exposure to inhibitors (e.g., heparin)

RISK FACTORS
• Aspirin or NSAIDs can potentiate a bleeding defect.
• Environmental exposure to rodenticide anticoagulants
• Liver disease

DIAGNOSIS

DIFFERENTIAL DIAGNOSIS
• Factor VIII or factor IX deficiency—spontaneous bleeding noticed in young males but not female litter mates
• Von Willebrand disease or factor XI deficiency—usually detected as abnormal bleeding after injury or surgery in males or females
• Factor XII deficiency—no clinical bleeding defect
• DIC is secondary to severe systemic disease and may be associated with thrombocytopenia or platelet function defects causing petechiae.
• Rodenticide anticoagulants often cause major bleeding into body cavities.

LABORATORY FINDINGS

Drugs That May Alter Laboratory Results
Heparin and other anticoagulants used in treatment or from samples collected through heparinized catheters cause abnormal coagulation test results.

Disorders That May Alter Laboratory Results
• Shortening or prolonging of coagulation test results can be caused by contamination of blood with tissue fluid during problems with venipuncture; evidence of hemolysis should raise concern about possible tissue fluid contamination or prolonged time before testing.
• Extreme lipemia may interfere with clot detection by some automated coagulation analyzers.
• Because of the lability of some coagulation factors, especially factor VIII, plasma should be separated from the rest of the sample and sent on ice or frozen to the laboratory.

Valid If Run in Human Laboratory?
• Coagulation assays vary in sensitivity but generally should yield valid data; important to interpret results in relation to concurrent data from samples of normal plasma from the same species
• Some of the activators used in the APTT are not as effective on domestic animal samples as they are on human samples.
• Some tests for fibrin degradation products are species-specific.

CBC/BIOCHEMISTRY/URINALYSIS
• Regenerative anemia proportional to the blood loss caused by bleeding episodes
• Platelet count normal unless the patient has DIC or massive bleeding
• Resorption of blood from large hematoma may cause high bilirubin.

OTHER LABORATORY TESTS
• Measurement of PT the test of choice for screening for extrinsic mechanism defects
• Measurement of APTT the test of choice for screening for intrinsic mechanism defects; although not as sensitive or precise, ACT is a practical substitute for the APTT test.
• Specific assays for coagulation factors required for diagnosis of most inherited defects; these assays can be run with human deficient plasma as substrate, but the assays must be performed with dilutions of species-specific normal plasma for the activity curves.

IMAGING
N/A

DIAGNOSTIC PROCEDURES
• Bleeding time with a gauze tourniquet on the folded lip over the maxilla prolonged in patients with von Willebrand disease
• Bleeding time normal in patients with most other coagulation defects, except DIC

TREATMENT

• Most bleeding episodes in animals with inherited coagulation defects can be effectively treated by transfusion of fresh blood, fresh plasma, cryoprecipitate, or fresh frozen plasma.
• Because repeated transfusions may be required in the future, cryoprecipitate or plasma recommended unless the need for RBC replacement is severe.
• In patients with factor VIII deficiency, the short half-life of this factor (10–12 hr) may necessitate repeat transfusions at 12–24-hr intervals.

MEDICATIONS

DRUG OF CHOICE
Vitamin K₁ an effective treatment for patients with anticoagulant rodenticide poisoning or vitamin K deficiency; if PT is normal, no rationale for vitamin K₁ administration.

CONTRAINDICATIONS
Aspirin and NSAIDs should be avoided because of adverse effects on platelet function.

PRECAUTIONS
• Intramuscular injections should be avoided because of the risk of inducing additional bleeding.
• Intravenous administration of vitamin K not recommended because of the risk of anaphylaxis

POSSIBLE INTERACTIONS
None

ALTERNATIVE DRUGS
Desmopressin acetate (1 μg/kg SC) just before surgery may increase the concentration of von Willebrand factor and shorten the bleeding time in dogs with von Willebrand disease; results, however, are inconsistent.

 FOLLOW-UP

PATIENT MONITORING
• PT can be used to monitor effectiveness of vitamin K administration in animals with anticoagulant toxicity; with appropriate treatment, prolonged PT should be corrected within 24 hr; persistence after this time suggests incorrect diagnosis or undertreatment of poisoning.
• ACT a less-sensitive but reasonable substitute for monitoring response to vitamin K
• Most inherited defects can be monitored by clinical arrest of bleeding and improvement in results of coagulation screening tests.

POSSIBLE COMPLICATIONS
Animals with inherited defects at continual risk for repeated hemorrhagic episodes

 MISCELLANEOUS

ASSOCIATED CONDITIONS
None

AGE-RELATED FACTORS
None

ZOONOTIC POTENTIAL
None

PREGNANCY
May cause fluctuations in clotting factor activity, which generally do not lead to bleeding episodes

SYNONYMS
• Coagulation defects
• Coagulopathies

SEE ALSO
• Von Willebrand Disease
• Disseminated Intravascular Coagulation (DIC)

ABBREVIATIONS
• ACT = activated clotting time
• APTT = activated partial thromboplastin time
• DIC = disseminated intravascular coagulation
• PT = prothrombin time

Suggested Reading
Dodds WJ. Hemostasis. In: Kaneko JJ, Harvey JW, Bruss ML, eds. Clinical biochemistry of domestic animals. New York: Academic Press, 1997:241–283.
Fogh JM, Fogh IT. Inherited coagulation disorders. Vet Clin North Am Small Anim 1988;18:231–243.
Jain NC. Coagulation and its disorders. In: Jain NC, ed. Essentials of veterinary hematology. Philadelphia: Lea & Febiger, 1993:82–104.
Parry BW. Laboratory evaluation of hemorrhagic coagulopathies in small animal practice. Vet Clin North Am Small Anim 1989;19:729–742.
Author Gary J. Kociba
Consulting Editor Susan M. Cotter

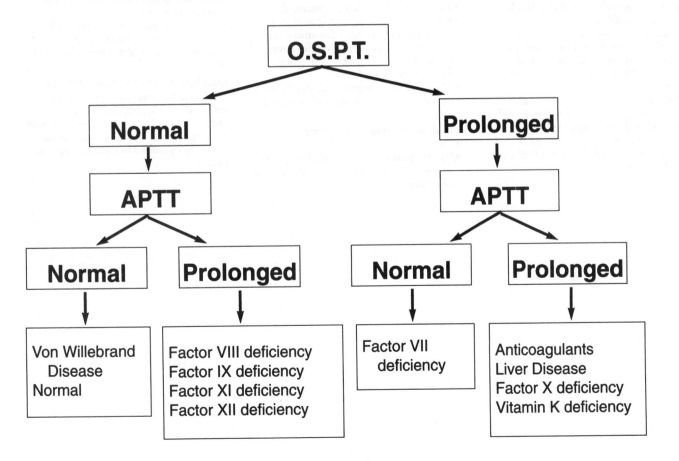

COBALAMIN AND FOLATE, SERUM

BASICS

DEFINITION
Subnormal serum cobalamin or folate concentrations or above-normal serum folate concentration, either alone or in combination, reflect consequences of chronic small intestinal disease or exocrine pancreatic insufficiency; this information may have diagnostic and therapeutic importance.

PATHOPHYSIOLOGY
• Folate is absorbed by carrier-mediated diffusion in the upper small intestine of the dog (and, it is assumed, of the cat).
• Chronic malabsorption of folate secondary to chronic small intestinal disease of sufficient severity and duration leads to depletion of body folate stores and subnormal serum folate concentration.
• Canine enteropathies associated with overgrowth of folate-synthesizing bacteria in the upper small intestine may lead to enhanced folate absorption and thus increased serum folate concentration. Increased serum folate is rarely observed in cats.
• Cobalamin is absorbed by specific receptors in the distal small intestine of dogs and cats only after it has been bound by intrinsic factor secreted exclusively (cat) or largely (dog) in pancreatic juice.
• Chronic malabsorption of cobalamin secondary to chronic small intestinal disease of sufficient severity and duration leads to depletion of body stores and subnormal serum cobalamin concentrations.
• Canine enteropathies associated with overgrowth of cobalamin-binding bacteria (especially obligate anaerobes) in the upper small intestine may impair cobalamin absorption, thus leading to subnormal serum cobalamin concentration.

• Available evidence suggests that abnormal proliferation of cobalamin-binding bacteria in the upper small intestine of cats is rare, if it occurs at all; this is presently not considered a cause of cobalamin malabsorption in cats.

SYSTEMS AFFECTED
• Gastrointestinal—anorexia, lethargy, failure to gain weight, weight loss
• Hemic/Lymphatic/Immune—mild nonregenerative anemia, neutropenia, hypersegmented neutrophils

SIGNALMENT
• Dogs and cats
• Inherited selective cobalamin malabsorption is reported in giant schnauzers and border collies; affected dogs present at less than 6 months of age.
• Dogs and cats with acquired causes of cobalamin malabsorption can present at any age, and, while some enteropathies are characteristically observed in some breeds (German shepherd dogs, basenjis, Norwegian lundehunds), any breed of dog may be affected.

SIGNS

Historical Findings
• Chronic diarrhea, weight loss, polyphagia, anorexia, vomiting, lethargy, borborygmus, coprophagia
• Low-folate diet (extremely rare)
• Folate supplementation (uncommon)
• Cats with exocrine pancreatic insufficiency consistently have severely subnormal serum cobalamin concentrations and often have moderately to severely subnormal serum folate concentrations.
• Dogs with exocrine pancreatic insufficiency often have increased serum folate concentrations.

Physical Examination Findings
• Often normal
• Possible findings include weight loss, poor haircoat, abdominal discomfort, and thickened bowel loops.

CAUSES
• Small intestinal diseases
• Exocrine pancreatic insufficiency
• Vitamin supplementation
• Coprophagia?
• Vitamin-deficient diets

RISK FACTORS
Unknown (except for inherited selective cobalamin malabsorption and causes of exocrine pancreatic insufficiency)

DIAGNOSIS

DIFFERENTIAL DIAGNOSIS
• Changes in serum cobalamin and folate concentrations are very specific for disorders of the exocrine pancreas and small intestine.
• If exocrine pancreatic function is normal (normal serum TLI), then abnormalities reflect changes in the small intestine with a high degree of specificity.

LABORATORY FINDINGS
• Lipemia, hemolysis, hyperbilirubinemia, and delayed separation of serum do not affect assay of serum cobalamin and folate.
• Serum folate concentration is increased by hemolysis, since red cell folate concentration is markedly greater than serum or plasma concentration.
• Serum cobalamin and folate are relatively stable at room temperature, but avoid prolonged exposure of samples to light and heat.

CBC/BIOCHEMISTRY/URINALYSIS
Abnormalities other than mild nonregenerative anemia, neutropenia, or hypersegmented neutrophils in patients with markedly subnormal serum vitamin concentrations should be considered to indicate coexistent disease.

COBALAMIN AND FOLATE, SERUM

OTHER LABORATORY TESTS
Serum cobalamin and folate concentrations cannot be used to diagnose small intestinal disease unless exocrine pancreatic function is known to be normal (normal serum TLI).

IMAGING
• Abdominal ultrasonography is generally not useful in the diagnosis of small intestinal disease, although lymphadenopathy and thickened intestinal loops can be identified in some cases.
• Needle aspiration of abnormal tissue may reveal neoplastic cells or infectious agents (*Histoplasma* spp.).

DIAGNOSTIC PROCEDURES
Additional testing of intestinal function and histologic examination of biopsy specimens from small intestine obtained at endoscopy or exploratory laparotomy may be required to define and characterize the underlying pathology fully.

 TREATMENT
When indicated, outpatient medical therapy is instituted.

 MEDICATIONS

DRUGS OF CHOICE
• Patients with severe cobalamin deficiency require parenteral supplementation (cyanocobalamin 250–500 μg SC or IM q7d for 4–6 weeks).
• Severe folate deficiency can usually be rectified by high doses of oral folate (0.5–2.0 mg PO q24h for 1 month.

CONTRAINDICATIONS
N/A

PRECAUTIONS
• Oral cobalamin is ineffective at normalizing subnormal serum cobalamin concentrations—parenteral administration is required.
• Oral multivitamin preparations often do not contain sufficient folate to normalize subnormal serum folate concentrations—selective high-dose oral supplementation is required.

POSSIBLE INTERACTIONS
N/A

ALTERNATIVE DRUGS
N/A

 FOLLOW-UP

PATIENT MONITORING
• Recheck serum cobalamin and folate concentrations after 1 month or so to verify that they have normalized.
• Retest patients with subnormal serum vitamin concentrations every 6–12 months to ensure that deficiency does not recur.
• Every 12 months or so test patients at risk of developing deficiency.

POSSIBLE COMPLICATIONS
• Cobalamin or folate deficiency (or other vitamin deficiencies, e.g., tocopherol) may develop over months to years in patients with malabsorption, despite apparent resolution of weight loss and diarrhea.
• Consider these acquired problems when patients develop unexplained anorexia, neuromuscular or retinal disease, or bleeding disorders.

 MISCELLANEOUS

ASSOCIATED CONDITIONS
Canine and feline patients with exocrine pancreatic insufficiency often have abnormal serum cobalamin and/or folate concentrations, either at the time of diagnosis or during subsequent treatment.

AGE-RELATED FACTORS
N/A

ZOONOTIC POTENTIAL
None

PREGNANCY
N/A

SYNONYMS
N/A

SEE ALSO
• Serum Trypsin-like Immunoreactivity
• Cobalamin Malabsorption in Giant
• Schnauzers and Border Collies

ABBREVIATION
TLI = trypsin like immunoreactivity

Suggested Reading
Williams DA. Malabsorption, small intestinal bacterial overgrowth, and protein-losing enteropathy. In: Strombeck DR, Guilford WG, Center SA, Meyer DJ, eds. Small animal gastroenterology. 3rd ed. Philadelphia: Saunders, 1996:367–380.

Williams DA, Guilford WG. Procedures for the evaluation of pancreatic and gastrointestinal tract diseases. In: Strombeck DR, Guilford WG, Center SA, Meyer DJ, eds. Small animal gastroenterology. 3rd ed. Philadelphia: Saunders, 1996:77–113.

Author David A. Williams

Consulting Editors Brett M. Feder and Mitchell A. Crystal

COOMBS' TEST

 BASICS

DEFINITION
- Positive results indicate the presence of RBCs that have been coated with antierythrocyte autoantibody as a result of primary AIHA or secondary IMHA.
- Test indicated in patients with anemia, especially regenerative anemia

PATHOPHYSIOLOGY
- Intravascular or extravascular hemolysis resulting in anemia can occur as a sequela to certain bacterial and parasitic infections, chemical and plant exposures, immune-mediated diseases, erythrocyte defects, fragmentation processes, and electrolyte abnormalities.
- Immune-mediated disease—antierythrocyte autoantibody production; RBCs bearing these immunoglobulins on their surface are phagocytized and cleared by the liver, spleen, lymph nodes, and macrophages.
- Affected animals may be severely anemic.
- Animals with intravascular hemolysis exhibit the classic signs of icterus, dark red (wine-colored) urine, and pallor; occasionally, they develop thromboembolic disorders and even DIC.

SYSTEMS AFFECTED
If Accompanied by Anemia
- Hemic/Lymph/Immune—hemolysis can result in marked reduction of PCV.
- Hepatobiliary—hemolysis can lead to hyperbilirubinemia with development of icterus.
- Respiratory—response to hypoxia in severely anemic patients includes compensatory mechanisms that lead to tachypnea.
- Cardiovascular—response to hypoxia results in a compensatory increase in heart rate.
- Renal/urologic—reduced perfusion and hypoxia can cause tubular necrosis.

SIGNALMENT

Primary AIHA
- Dogs and rarely cats
- Any age
- Predilection for females
- Cocker spaniels, poodles, Old English sheepdogs, Irish setters, English springer spaniels, and collies

SIGNS

Historical Findings
- No signs, associated with the positive test result
- Signs, if any, relate to associated anemia and its cause (e.g., weakness, exercise intolerance, lethargy, syncope, tachypnea, and dyspnea).

Physical Examination Findings
Findings associated with IMHA
- Hepatomegaly
- Splenomegaly
- Icterus
- Pale mucous membranes
- Tachypnea
- Tachycardia

CAUSES

Primary or True AIHA
Unknown, possible genetic predisposition

Secondary IMHA
- Infectious agents—viruses or modified live virus vaccines, *Hemobartonella, Babesia, Leptospira, Dirofilaria, Ehrlichia,* feline leukemia virus
- Microangiopathic processes
- Drugs—cephalosporins, heparin, quinidine, methimazole, propylthiouracil, sulfa compounds
- Neoplasia—especially lymphoma, malignant histiocytosis, and hemangiosarcoma

RISK FACTORS
N/A

 DIAGNOSIS

DIFFERENTIAL DIAGNOSIS
- Secondary problems must be ruled out.
- Some dogs with AIHA have nonregenerative anemia with or without a positive test.
- Between 25 and 30% of dogs with AIHA have a negative test.

Positive Test (Dogs)
- In animal with signs of hemolytic anemia confirms an immune-mediated cause
- Rare in normal dogs

Other Causes of Hemolysis
- Dogs—onion and zinc ingestion, splenic torsion, and pyruvate kinase deficiency
- Cats—oxidant toxicity (e.g., acetaminophen, propylene glycol, and methylene blue) and anemia secondary to retrovirus infection

LABORATORY FINDINGS

Drugs That May Affect Laboratory Results
- Cephalosporins rarely reported to cause positive test
- Antibodies to transfused RBCs (alloantibodies) may be present in dogs.
- Previous treatment with steroids not likely to interfere if hemolysis is ongoing

Disorders That May Alter Laboratory Results
None

Valid If Run in Human Laboratory?
Species-specific reagent must be used.

CBC/BIOCHEMISTRY/URINALYSIS

In Patients with Concurrent Anemia
- CBC—anisocytosis, polychromasia, presence of spherocytes and nucleated RBCs, neutrophilic leukocytosis with left shift, hemoglobinemia, and elevation of MCV
- Biochemistry—high concentration of ALT and hyperbilirubinemia
- Urinalysis—bilirubinuria and hemoglobinuria

OTHER LABORATORY TESTS
• Serologic tests for appropriate infectious agents
• Coagulation profile to diagnose DIC
• Platelet count to diagnose Evan's syndrome or early DIC
• Reticulocyte count to determine if anemia is regenerative

IMAGING
Radiography
• Splenomegaly
• Hepatomegaly

Ultrasonography
• Hepatomegaly–with hyperchoic or hypoechoic parenchymal changes
• Splenomegaly
• Hyperdynamic cardiac changes consistent with anemic state

DIAGNOSTIC PROCEDURES
Bone marrow aspiration typically reveals erythroid hyperplasia, although some animals with nonregenerative anemia may have low numbers of erythroid precursors.

TREATMENT
• See Anemia, Immune-Mediated
• Patients in hemolytic crisis should be hospitalized until their condition has been stabilized (hemolysis and anemia), after which they can be treated as outpatients.
• Transfusion with RBCs should be given if clinically indicated; transfusions do not exacerbate hemolytic processes.
• Strict cage rest required if anemia is severe

MEDICATIONS

DRUGS OF CHOICE
• Vary with the cause of the positive test result
• See Anemia, Immune-Mediated

CONTRAINDICATIONS
N/A

PRECAUTIONS
N/A

POSSIBLE INTERACTIONS
N/A

ALTERNATIVE DRUGS
N/A

FOLLOW-UP

PATIENT MONITORING
Monitor PCV and CBC in anemic patients to assess response to treatment.

PREVENTION/AVOIDANCE
N/A

POSSIBLE COMPLICATIONS
Vary with the cause of the positive test result

EXPECTED COURSE AND PROGNOSIS
Vary with the cause of the positive test result

MISCELLANEOUS

ASSOCIATED CONDITIONS
Other immune-mediated diseases such as SLE

AGE-RELATED FACTORS
N/A

ZOONOTIC POTENTIAL
None

PREGNANCY
The use of prednisone and other immunosuppressive drugs during pregnancy not advisable unless no alternative treatment options exist

SYNONYMS
Direct antiglobulin test

SEE ALSO
Anemia, Immune-mediated

ABBREVIATIONS
• AIHA = autoimmune hemolytic anemia
• ALT = alanine aminotransferase
• DIC = disseminated intravascular coagulation
• IMHA = immune-mediated hemolytic anemia
• MCV = mean cell volume
• PVC = packed cell volume
• SLE = systemic lupus erythematosus

Suggested Reading
Duncan JR, Prasse KW, Mahaffey EA. Veterinary laboratory medicine. Clinical pathology. 3rd ed. Ames: Iowa State University Press, 1994.
Lewis RM, Picut CA. Veterinary clinical immunology. Philadelphia: Lea & Febiger, 1989.
Meyer DJ, Coles EH, Rich LJ. Veterinary laboratory medicine. Interpretation and diagnosis. Philadelphia: Saunders, 1992.
Author Albert Ahn
Consulting Editor Susan M. Cotter

CREATINE KINASE

BASICS

DEFINITION
Serum concentrations above the reference range for the laboratory in use

PATHOPHYSIOLOGY
• Creatine kinase—three clinically important isoenzymes (two in skeletal and cardiac muscle; one in brain tissue); leakage enzyme
• Increased serum concentration—indicates reversible or irreversible injury to muscle cells; occurs within a few hours of the muscle injury; peaks by 12 hr; returns to normal within 24–48 hr unless damage is ongoing (remains persistently increased); does not usually reflect the brain isoenzyme unless the blood–brain barrier is broken
• Increase associated with CNS disease—often secondary to muscle trauma and degeneration

SYSTEMS AFFECTED
• Musculoskeletal
• Endocrine/Metabolic

SIGNALMENT
• Dogs and cats of any age, breed, or sex, depending on underlying cause
• Some breeds may be predisposed to hereditary myopathies (see Risk Factors).

SIGNS

Historical Findings
• Trauma
• Vigorous exercise
• Recent intramuscular injection
• Paralysis or persistent recumbency
• Exercise intolerance
• Dysphagia
• Dysphonia
• Dyspnea
• Regurgitation
• Discolored urine
• Weight loss
• Anorexia (cats)

Physical Examination Findings
• Bruising
• Muscle pain
• Paralysis or persistent recumbency
• Gait abnormality—stiff gait; hopping

• Ventriflexion of the neck (cats)
• Muscle atrophy or hypertrophy
• Pain on opening the mouth
• Fever
• Primary myopathies—conscious proprioception and spinal reflexes usually normal
• Neuropathies—more commonly associated with spinal reflex abnormalities, hyperesthesias or paresthesias, and decreased conscious proprioception

CAUSES
• Degenerative—inherited (muscular dystrophy, Labrador myopathy, Irish terrier myopathy, chow chow myotonia); acquired (atrophy, myotonia associated with hyperadrenocorticism)
• Immune-mediated—idiopathic; SLE; masticatory muscle myositis; dermatomyositis
• Metabolic/endocrine—hyperadrenocorticism; hypothyroidism; hyperthermia (malignant or exercise-induced)
• Neoplastic—paraneoplastic myopathy
• Nutritional—hypokalemia (cats); anorexia (cats); vitamin E and/or selenium deficiency
• Infectious—toxoplasmosis; clostridial myositis; neosporosis
• Trauma—most common cause; associated with vigorous exercise or exertional rhabdomyolysis, blunt trauma, intramuscular injections, hypothermia, hyperthermia (exercise induced, malignant, or environmental), persistent recumbency, electric shock, seizures, and lacerations

RISK FACTORS
• Breeds predisposed to inherited myopathies—Labradors; Irish terriers; golden retrievers; chow chows
• Breeds predisposed to immune-mediated myopathies—collies (ermatomyositis)
• Hypokalemia (cats)
• Endocrinopathies—hyperadrenocorticism; hypothyroidism
• Neurologic disease resulting in prolonged recumbency
• Muscle trauma
• Intramuscular injections
• Vigorous exercise
• Seizures
• Hyperthermia or hypothermia

DIAGNOSIS

DIFFERENTIAL DIAGNOSIS
• Signalment—may suggest inherited myopathy or immune-mediated myositide
• Pain opening the mouth or involvement of muscles of the head—suggests masticatory muscle myositis
• Systemic signs (polyuria or polydipsia and alopecia)—may suggest hyperadrenocorticism
• Obesity, lethargy, and cold intolerance—suggest hypothyroidism
• Old cats with polyuria or polydipsia and evidence of primary renal failure—consider hypokalemic polymyopathy
• Anorexia in cats—associated with significantly increased serum concentrations
• History of trauma, injections, electric shock, seizures, or vigorous exercise—may suggest the cause

LABORATORY FINDINGS

Drugs That May Alter Laboratory Results
Clofibrate, succinylcholine, any drug given by intramuscular injection, penicillin, D-penicillamine, sulfonamides, and phenytoin—may cause an immune-mediated polymyositis and increased serum concentrations

Disorders That May Alter Laboratory Results
• Hemolysis—falsely increases concentrations; controversial; only if severe
• Lipemia—no affect
• EDTA, citrate, fluoride, exposure to sunlight, and delayed analysis—falsely decrease concentrations
• Icterus—falsely increases concentrations
• Electromyography—increases concentrations

CBC/BIOCHEMISTRY/URINALYSIS
• CBC—may be inflammatory with infectious or immune-mediated myositis
• Stress leukogram—consistent with hyperadrenocorticism
• Eosinophilia—may be associated with masticatory muscle myositis
• Increased AST without evidence of liver disease—supports diagnosis of muscle disease

• Increased ALP without significant evidence of liver disease—consider hyperadrenocorticism
• Hypokalemia and azotemia (cats)—may result in polymyositis
• Hypercholesterolemia—may suggest hyperadrenocorticism or hypothyroidism
• Myoglobinuria—may be seen with exertional rhabdomyolysis

OTHER LABORATORY TESTS
• Positive ANA test—supports diagnosis of SLE if multisystemic disorder is identified
• Positive type II muscle fiber antibody test—helps confirm masticatory muscle myositis
• TSH-stimulation test—definitively diagnoses hypothyroidism; see Hypothyroidism
• ACTH-stimulation test or low-dose dexamethasone suppression test—reveals hyperadrenocorticism; see Hyperadrenocorticism (Cushing Disease)
• Serology for *Toxoplasma gondii*—may support toxoplasmal myositis
• Pre-exercise and postexercise plasma lactate concentrations—may identify metabolic myopathy associated with mitochondrial enzyme deficiencies

IMAGING
Chest and abdomen radiography—may help identify underlying neoplasia, assess kidney size (hypokalemic nephropathy in cats), confirm traumatic injuries (fractures), and support endocrinopathies (hepatomegaly or adrenomegaly with hyperadrenocorticism)

DIAGNOSTIC PROCEDURES
Muscle biopsy and electromyography—pursued when trauma, exercise, hyperthermia, hypothermia, seizures, injections, and drugs have been ruled out; performed with persistent and unexplained increased serum concentrations

Muscle Biopsy
• Helps definitively diagnose primary underlying cause (e.g., toxoplasmosis, neosporosis, and immune-mediated myositis), unless long-standing disease has resulted in fibrosis and atrophy
• Muscle specimens—formalin preserved for routine histopathology; cryopreserved for histochemical staining; glutaraldehyde preserved for electron microscopy

• Culture—muscle tissue, for suspected bacterial myositis

Electromyography
• May support the diagnosis of a primary muscle versus primary neurologic disorder; overlap may exist, depending on duration of the illness
• Spontaneous discharges—associated with primary myopathies
• Prolonged insertional activity, positive sharp waves, and fibrillation potentials—more common with primary neuropathies
• Pseudomyotonic discharges—common with endocrine disorders

TREATMENT
• Depends on underlying cause (see specific disease)
• Supportive care for recumbent patient—prevent pressure sores and minimize atrophy; soft bedding; turning; passive range of motion exercises
• Traumatized patient—may need emergency care for shock and/or wound and fracture management

MEDICATIONS
None specific for lowering serum concentration; condition not dangerous to the patient

FOLLOW-UP

PATIENT MONITORING
• Serum levels—assess response to treatment or recovery from a traumatic incident
• Clinical response to therapy—better indicator of the efficacy of treatment

POSSIBLE COMPLICATIONS
N/A

MISCELLANEOUS

ASSOCIATED CONDITIONS
Hypokalemia in cats with renal disease—associated with polymyositis and increased serum creatine kinase

AGE-RELATED FACTORS
None known

ZOONOTIC POTENTIAL
Toxoplasmosis—may have some potential, depending on species of patient and phase of disease

PREGNANCY
N/A

SYNONYMS
• Creatine phosphokinase (CPK)
• ATP–creatine transphosphorylase

SEE ALSO
See Causes

ABBREVIATIONS
• ALP = alkaline phosphatase
• ANA = antinuclear antibody
• AST = aspartate transaminase
• SLE = systemic lupus erythematosus
• TSH = thyroid-stimulating hormone

Suggested Reading
DiBartola SP, Tasker JB. Elevated serum creatine phosphokinase: a study of 53 cases and a review of its diagnostic significance in clinical veterinary medicine. J Am Anim Hosp Assoc 1977;13:744–753.
Fascetti AJ, Mauldin GE, Mauldin GN. Correction between serum creatine kinase activities and anorexia in cats. J Vet Intern Med 1997;11:9–13.
Kornegay JN, Gorgacz EJ, Dawe DL, et al. Polymyositis in dogs. J Am Vet Med Assoc 1980;176:431–438.
Scott-Moncrieff JC, Hawkings EC, Cook JR. Canine muscle disorders. Compend Contin Educ Pract Vet 1990;12:31–38.
Wilson JW. Serum creatine phosphokinase in the canine. J Am Anim Hosp Assoc 1976;12:522–524.
Author Ellen Miller
Consulting Editor Peter D. Schwarz

DIAGNOSTICS—LAB

BASICS

DEFINITION
Azotemia is an excess of urea, creatinine, or other nonprotein nitrogenous substances in blood, plasma, or serum. Uremia is the polysystemic toxic syndrome that results from abnormal renal function in animals with azotemia. Uremia occurs simultaneously in animals with increased quantities of urine constituents in blood.

PATHOPHYSIOLOGY
• Azotemia can be caused by 1) high production of nonprotein nitrogenous substances, 2) low glomerular filtration rate, or 3) reabsorption of urine that has escaped from the urinary tract into the bloodstream. High production of nonprotein nitrogenous waste substances may result from high intake of protein (diet or gastrointestinal bleeding) or accelerated catabolism of endogenous proteins. Glomerular filtration rate may decline because of reduced renal perfusion (prerenal azotemia), renal insufficiency or failure due to primary renal disease (renal azotemia), or urinary obstruction (postrenal azotemia). Reabsorption of urine into the systemic circulation may result from leakage of urine from the excretory pathways (also termed postrenal azotemia). • Pathophysiology of uremia—incompletely understood; may be related to 1) metabolic and toxic systemic effects of waste products retained because of renal excretory failure, 2) deranged renal regulation of fluids, electrolytes, and acid–base balance, and 3) impaired renal production and degradation of hormones and other substances (e.g., erythropoietin and 1,25-dihydroxycholecalciferol)

SYSTEMS AFFECTED
• Gastrointestinal—anorexia, nausea, vomiting, diarrhea, uremic stomatitis, xerostomia, uremic breath, constipation • Neuromuscular—dullness, drowsiness, lethargy, fatigue, irritability, tremors, gait imbalance, flaccid muscle weakness, myoclonus, behavioral changes, dementia, isolated cranial nerve deficits, seizures, stupor, coma • Endocrine/Metabolic—renal secondary hyperparathyroidism, inadequate production of 1,25-dihydroxycholecalciferol and erythropoietin, hypergastrinemia, weight loss • Cardiovascular—arterial hypertension, left ventricular hypertrophy, heart murmur, cardiomegaly, cardiac rhythm disturbances • Hemic/Lymph/Immune—nonregenerative anemia (normocytic, normochromic) and immunodeficiency
• Ophthalmic—scleral and conjunctival injection, retinopathy, acute-onset blindness • Respiratory—dyspnea • Skin/Exocrine—pallor, bruising, increased shedding, unkempt appearance, loss of normal sheen to coat

SIGNALMENT
Dogs and cats

SIGNS

General Comments
Azotemia may or may not be associated with historical or physical abnormalities. Unless patient has uremia, clinical findings are limited to the disease responsible for azotemia. Findings described here are those of uremia.

Historical Findings
• Weight loss • Declining appetite or anorexia • Reduced activity • Depression • Fatigue • Weakness • Vomiting • Diarrhea • Halitosis • Constipation • Poor haircoat or unkempt appearance

Physical Examination Findings
• Cachexia • Depression • Dehydration • Weakness • Pallor • Petechia and ecchymoses • Dull and unkempt haircoat • Uremic breath • Uremic stomatitis • Scleral and conjunctival injection

CAUSES

Prerenal Azotemia
• Reduced renal perfusion due to low blood volume or low blood pressure • Accelerated production of nitrogenous waste products because of enhanced catabolism of tissues in association with infection, fever, trauma, corticosteroid excess, or burns • Increased gastrointestinal digestion and absorption of protein sources (diet or gastrointestinal hemorrhage)

Renal Azotemia
Acute or chronic renal failure (primary renal disease affecting glomeruli, renal tubules, renal interstitium, or renal vasculature) that impairs at least 75% of renal function.

Postrenal Azotemia
Urinary obstruction; rupture of the excretory pathway

RISK FACTORS
• Medical conditions—renal disease, hypoadrenocorticism, low cardiac output, hypotension, fever, sepsis, polyuria, liver disease, pyometra, hypoalbuminemia, dehydration, acidosis, exposure to nephrotoxic chemicals, gastrointestinal hemorrhage, urolithiasis, urethral plugs in cats, urethral trauma and neoplasia • Advanced age may be a risk factor. • Drugs—potentially nephrotoxic drugs, nonsteroidal antiinflammatory drugs, diuretics, antihypertensive medications

DIAGNOSIS

DIFFERENTIAL DIAGNOSIS
• Dehydration, poor peripheral perfusion, low cardiac output, history of recent fluid loss, high protein diet, or black, tarry stools—rule out prerenal azotemia. • Recent onset of altered urine output (high or low), clinical signs consistent with uremia, exposure to possible nephrotoxicants or ischemic renal injury, or kidney size normal or enlarged—rule out acute renal failure. • Progressive weight loss, polyuria, polydipsia, small kidneys, pallor, and signs of uremia that have developed over several weeks to months—rule out chronic renal failure. • Abrupt decline in urine output and onset of signs of uremia; occasionally dysuria, stranguria, and hematuria; large urinary bladder or fluid-filled abdomen—rule out postrenal azotemia.

LABORATORY FINDINGS

Drugs That May Alter Laboratory Results
N/A

Disorders That May Alter Laboratory Results
N/A

Valid If Run in Human Laboratory?
Yes

CBC/BIOCHEMISTRY/URINALYSIS

CBC
• Nonregenerative anemia—often present with chronic renal failure • Hemoconcentration—often present with prerenal azotemia; can also be seen with acute renal failure and postrenal azotemia

Biochemistry
• Serial determinations of serum urea nitrogen and creatinine concentrations may help differentiate the cause of azotemia. Appropriate therapy to restore renal perfusion typically yields a dramatic reduction in azotemia in patients with prerenal azotemia (typically within 24–48 h). Correcting obstruction to urine flow or a rent in the excretory pathway typically gives a rapid reduction in the magnitude of azotemia in patients with postrenal azotemia. • Concurrent hyperkalemia may be consistent with postrenal azotemia, primary renal azotemia due to oliguric renal failure, or prerenal azotemia associated with hypoadrenocorticism.

Urinalysis
• A urine specific gravity value ≥ 1.030 in dogs and ≥ 1.035 in cats supports a diagnosis of prerenal azotemia. Administration of fluid therapy before urine collection may interfere with interpretation of low specific gravity values. • Azotemia patients that have not been treated with fluids and have urine specific gravity < 1.030 in dogs and < 1.035 in cats typically have primary renal azotemia. A notable exception to this rule is dogs and cats with glomerular disease. Glomerulopathy is sometimes characterized by glomerulotubular imbalance in which urine-concentrating ability may persist despite sufficient renal glomerular damage to cause primary renal azotemia; these patients are recognized by

CREATININE AND BLOOD UREA NITROGEN (BUN)—AZOTEMIA AND UREMIA

moderate to marked proteinuria in the absence of hematuria and pyuria. Urine specific gravity does not help differentiate postrenal azotemia from prerenal or primary renal azotemia.

OTHER LABORATORY TESTS

Endogenous or exogenous creatinine clearance tests or other specific tests of glomerular filtration rate may be used to confirm that azotemia is caused by reduced glomerular filtration rate.

IMAGING

• Abdominal radiographs—used to determine kidney size (small kidneys consistent with chronic renal failure; mild-to-moderate enlargement of kidneys may be consistent with acute renal failure or urinary obstruction) and to rule out urinary obstruction (marked dilation of the urinary bladder or mineral densities within the excretory pathway) • Ultrasonography—may detect changes in echogenicity of the renal parenchyma and size and shape of kidneys that support a diagnosis of primary renal azotemia; useful to rule out postrenal azotemia characterized by distension of the excretory pathway and uroliths or masses within or impinging on the excretory pathway and intraabdominal fluid accumulation (with rupture of the excretory pathway) • Excretory urography or cystourethrography—may help establish the diagnosis of postrenal azotemia due to urinary obstruction or rupture of the excretory pathway

DIAGNOSTIC PROCEDURES

Renal biopsy can be used to confirm the diagnosis of primary renal failure, to differentiate acute from chronic renal failure, and to attempt to establish the underlying disease process responsible for primary renal failure.

TREATMENT

• Prerenal azotemia caused by impaired renal perfusion—direct at correcting the underlying cause of renal hypoperfusion; aggressiveness of treatment depends on the severity of the underlying condition and the probability that persistent renal hypo–perfusion will lead to primary renal injury or failure.
• Primary renal azotemia and associated uremia—1) specific therapy directed at halting or reversing the primary disease process affecting the kidneys, and 2) symptomatic, supportive, and palliative therapies that ameliorate clinical signs of uremia; minimize the clinical impact of deficits and excesses in fluid, electrolyte, acid–base balances; minimize the effects of inadequate renal biosynthesis of hormones and other substances, and maintain adequate nutrition.

• Postrenal azotemia—direct at eliminating urinary obstruction or repairing rents in the excretory pathway; supplemental fluid administration is often required to prevent dehydration that may develop during the solute diuresis that follows correction of postrenal azotemia.
• Fluid therapy—indicated for most azotemic patients; preferred fluid selections include 0.9% saline or lactated Ringer's solution. Estimate the quantity of fluid to be administered on the basis of severity of dehydration or volume depletion. If no clinical dehydration is evident, cautiously assume that the patient is less than 5% dehydrated and administer a corresponding volume of fluid. Generally provide the bulk of volume replacement over 2–6 h, except in patients with overt or suspected cardiac failure.
• Treat patients in shock appropriately.

MEDICATIONS

DRUGS OF CHOICE
N/A

CONTRAINDICATIONS
Administration of nephrotoxic drugs

PRECAUTIONS
• Use caution when administering drugs requiring renal excretion. Consult appropriate references concerning dose-reduction schedules or adjustments of maintenance intervals.
• Use caution in administering fluids to patients that are oliguric or anuric. Monitor urine production rates and body weight during fluid therapy to minimize the likelihood of inducing overhydration.
• Use caution in administering drugs that may promote hypovolemia or hypotension (e.g., diuretics); carefully monitor the response to such drugs by assessing hydration status, peripheral perfusion, and blood pressure, with serial evaluation of renal function tests.
• Corticosteroids may worsen azotemia by increasing catabolism of endogenous proteins.

POSSIBLE INTERACTIONS
N/A

ALTERNATIVE DRUGS
N/A

FOLLOW-UP

PATIENT MONITORING
Serum urea nitrogen and creatinine concentrations 24 h after initiating fluid administration; also urine production, body weight, and hydration status

POSSIBLE COMPLICATIONS
• Failure to correct prerenal azotemia caused by renal hypoperfusion rapidly could result in ischemic primary renal failure. • Primary renal azotemia can progress to uremia. • Failure to restore normal urine flow in patients with postrenal azotemia can result in progressive renal damage or death due to hyperkalemia and uremia.

MISCELLANEOUS

ASSOCIATED CONDITIONS
An association may exist between hypokalemia and azotemia in cats. Preliminary findings suggest that hypokalemia may be associated with functional or structural renal changes leading to azotemia.

AGE-RELATED FACTORS
Primary renal failure may occur in animals of any age, but geriatric dogs and cats appear to be at substantially higher risk for both acute and chronic renal failure. However, do not assume that azotemia in geriatric dogs and cats indicates primary renal failure, because these patients are also at higher risk for prerenal and postrenal causes for azotemia.

ZOONOTIC POTENTIAL
Leptospirosis

PREGNANCY
• Data on azotemia and pregnancy in dogs and cats are very limited. Humans may tolerate minimal renal disease well during pregnancy; however, ability to sustain a viable pregnancy declines as renal function declines.
• Pregnant azotemic animals—pharmacologic agents excreted by nonrenal pathways are preferred.

SYNONYMS
N/A

SEE ALSO
• Renal Failure, Acute • Renal Failure, Chronic • Urinary Tract Obstruction

ABBREVIATIONS
N/A

Suggested Reading

Osborne CA, Polzin DJ. Azotemia: a review of what's old and what's new. Part I. Definition of terms and concepts. Compend Cont Educ 1983;5:497–508.

Osborne CA, Polzin DJ. Azotemia: a review of what's old and what's new. Part II. Localization. Compend Cont Educ 1983;5:561–574.

Author David J. Polzin

Consulting Editors Larry G. Adams and Carl A. Osborne

CRYSTALLURIA

 BASICS

DEFINITION
Appearance of crystals in urine

PATHOPHYSIOLOGY
• Crystals form only in urine that is, or recently has been, supersaturated with crystallogenic substances; thus crystalluria represents a risk factor for urolithiasis. However, detection of urine crystals is not synonymous with uroliths and clinical signs associated with them. Nor are urine crystals irrefutable evidence of a stone-forming tendency.
• Certain types indicate an underlying disease. Proper identification and interpretation of urine crystals is also important in formulation of medical protocols to dissolve uroliths. Evaluation of urine crystals may aid in 1) detection of disorders predisposing animals to urolith formation, 2) estimation of the mineral composition of uroliths, and 3) evaluation of the effectiveness of medical protocols initiated to dissolve or prevent urolithiasis.
• Crystalluria in individuals with anatomically and functionally normal urinary tracts is usually harmless because the crystals are eliminated before they grow large enough to interfere with normal urinary function. However, they represent a risk factor for urolithiasis.
• Crystals that form following elimination or removal of urine from the patient often are of little clinical importance. Identification of crystals that have formed in vitro does not justify therapy.
• Detection of some types of crystals (e.g., cystine and ammonium urate) in clinically asymptomatic patients, frequent detection of large aggregates of crystals (e.g., calcium oxalate or magnesium ammonium phosphate) in apparently normal individuals, or detection of any form of crystals in fresh urine collected from patients with confirmed urolithiasis may have diagnostic, prognostic, or therapeutic importance.

SYSTEMS AFFECTED
Renal/Urologic

SIGNALMENT
• Calcium oxalate in miniature schnauzer, Yorkshire terrier, Lhasa apso, and miniature poodle dogs and Burmese, Himalayan, and Persian cats
• Cystine in dachshund, English bulldog, and Newfoundland
• Ammonium urate in dalmatian and English bulldogs
• Xanthine uroliths in Cavalier King Charles spaniels

SIGNS
None or those caused by concomitant urolithiasis

CAUSES

In vivo variables
• Concentration of crystallogenic substances in urine (which in turn is influenced by their rate of excretion and urine concentration of water)
• Urine pH (struvite and calcium phosphate are most common in neutral-to-alkaline urine; ammonium urate, sodium urate, calcium oxalate, cystine, and xanthine crystals are most common in acid-to-neutral urine)
• Solubility of crystallogenic substances in urine
• Excretion of diagnostic agents (e.g., radiopaque contrast agents) and medications (e.g., sulfonamides)
• Dietary influence—hospital diet may differ from home diet; timing of collection (fasting vs. postprandial) may influence crystalluria.

In vitro variables
• Temperature
• Evaporation
• pH changes following sample collection
• Technique of specimen preparation—centrifugation vs. noncentrifugation, volume of urine examined
• Important in vitro changes that occur following urine collection may enhance formation or dissolution of crystals. When knowledge of in vivo urine crystal type and quantity is especially important, examine fresh specimens, ideally at body temperature. If this is not possible, they should be at room temperature, not refrigeration temperature.

RISK FACTORS
See discussion about in vivo and in vitro crystalluria

 DIAGNOSIS

DIFFERENTIAL DIAGNOSIS

Ammonium Urate, Sodium Urate, and Amorphous Urate Crystalluria
• Uncommonly observed in apparently healthy dogs and cats
• Frequently observed in dogs and occasionally observed in cats with portal vascular anomalies, with or without concomitant ammonium urate uroliths
• Observed in some dogs and cats with urate uroliths caused by disorders other than portal vascular anomalies

Bilirubin Crystalluria
• Observed in highly concentrated urine from some healthy dogs
• Large numbers in serial samples should arouse suspicion of an abnormality in bilirubin metabolism.
• Usually associated with underlying diseases in cats

Calcium Oxalate Monohydrate and Calcium Oxalate Dihydrate Crystalluria
• May be observed in apparently healthy dogs and cats and in dogs and cats with uroliths primarily composed of calcium oxalate
• Calcium oxalate dihydrate observed in some cats and dogs intoxicated with ethylene glycol, but calcium oxalate monohydrate crystals more common (ethylene glycol toxicity may also occur without crystalluria)

Calcium Phosphate Crystalluria
• Large numbers of crystals presumed to be composed of calcium phosphate have been observed in apparently healthy dogs, dogs with persistently alkaline urine, dogs with calcium phosphate uroliths, and dogs with uroliths composed of a mixture of calcium phosphate and calcium oxalate.
• Small numbers of calcium phosphate crystals may occur in association with infection-induced struvite crystalluria.

Struvite Crystalluria
• Observed in dogs and cats that are apparently healthy
• Observed in dogs and cats with infection-induced struvite uroliths, sterile struvite uroliths, nonstruvite uroliths, and uroliths of mixed composition (e.g., a nucleus composed of calcium oxalate and a shell composed of struvite)
• Observed in dogs and cats with urinary tract disease without uroliths

Uric Acid Crystalluria
• Uncommon in dogs and cats
• Importance as described for ammonium and amorphous urates

Xanthine Crystalluria
• Suggests administration of excessive dosages of allopurinol in conjunction with consumption of relatively high amounts of dietary purine precursors
• Primary xanthinuria has been observed in Cavalier King Charles spaniels.
• Primary xanthinuria and xanthine uroliths occur in cats.

Miscellaneous Crystalluria
• Cholesterol crystals—observed in humans with excessive tissue destruction, nephrotic syndrome, and chyluria; observed in apparently healthy dogs

- Cystine uroliths—develop in some dogs and cats with cystinuria
- Hippuric acid crystals—apparently rare in dogs and cats; importance unknown
- Leucine crystals in dogs—importance not determined; may occur in association with cystinuria
- Tyrosine crystals—occur in association with severe liver disease in humans; uncommonly observed in dogs and cats with liver disorders

Drug-induced Crystalluria
- May be observed following administration of radiopaque contrast agents
- May be observed following treatment with sulfadiazine, fluoroquinolones, primidone, and tetracycline

LABORATORY FINDINGS
Drugs That May Alter Laboratory Results
- Urinary acidifiers (e.g., *d,l*-methionine and ammonium chloride)
- Urinary alkalinizers (e.g., sodium bicarbonate and potassium citrate)

Disorders That May Alter Laboratory Results
N/A

Valid If Run in Human Laboratory?
Yes

CBC/BIOCHEMISTRY/URINALYSIS
- Bilirubin crystals may be associated with bilirubinemia and other laboratory abnormalities of hepatic disorders.
- Most dogs and cats with calcium oxalate and calcium phosphate crystalluria are normocalcemic; some are hypercalcemic.
- Some dogs and cats with calcium oxalate crystalluria may be acidemic.
- Serially examine fresh specimens when knowledge of in vivo urine crystal type is especially important; evaluate the number, size, and structure of crystals and their tendency to aggregate.
- Microscopic evaluation of the appearance of urine crystals gives only a tentative indication of their composition; variable conditions associated with their formation, growth, and dissolution may alter their appearance. Definitive identification of crystal composition depends on optical crystallography, infrared spectrophotometry, thermal analysis, x-ray diffraction, electron microprobe analysis, or a combination of these.
- To confirm the composition of microscopic crystalluria, prepare a large pellet of crystals by centrifuging an appropriate volume of urine in a cone-tipped centrifuge tube. Evaluate the pellet by methods designed for quantitative urolith analysis. The type of crystals identified by this method may only reflect the outer portions of uroliths.

OTHER LABORATORY TESTS
- Cystine crystalluria is usually associated with a positive urine cyanide-nitroprusside reaction.
- Sulfonamide crystalluria may be associated with a positive lignin test.
- Ammonium urate and amorphous urate crystals are insoluble in acetic acid; addition of 10% acetic acid to urine sediment containing these crystals often yields uric acid and sometimes sodium urate crystals.
- Most dogs and a few cats with struvite crystalluria have urinary tract infections caused by urease-producing bacteria (especially staphylococci and sometimes *Proteus* spp.).
- Dogs and cats with ammonium urate crystalluria and portosystemic shunts often have high serum bile acid levels and hyperammonemia.
- Dogs and cats with calcium oxalate crystalluria secondary to ethylene glycol poisoning have detectable levels of ethylene glycol in serum and urine up to 48 h after ingestion.

IMAGING
May be radiographically or ultrasonographically detectable uroliths

DIAGNOSTIC PROCEDURES
Voiding urohydropropulsion or aspiration through a transurethral catheter to retrieve small urocystoliths

TREATMENT
- Manage clinically important in vivo crystalluria by eliminating or controlling the underlying cause(s) or associated risk factors.
- Minimize clinically important crystalluria by increasing urine volume, by encouraging complete and frequent voiding, by dietary modification, in some instances by appropriate drug therapy, and, in some instances, by modifying pH.

MEDICATIONS
DRUGS OF CHOICE
N/A

CONTRAINDICATIONS
N/A

PRECAUTIONS
N/A

POSSIBLE INTERACTIONS
N/A

ALTERNATIVE DRUGS
N/A

FOLLOW-UP
PATIENT MONITORING
- Recheck urinalysis to determine if crystalluria is present.
- See chapters on specific urolith types for monitoring urolithiasis.

POSSIBLE COMPLICATIONS
- Persistent crystalluria may contribute to formation and growth of uroliths.
- Crystalluria may solidify crystalline-matrix plugs, resulting in urethral obstruction.

MISCELLANEOUS
ASSOCIATED CONDITIONS
N/A

AGE-RELATED FACTORS
N/A

ZOONOTIC POTENTIAL
N/A

PREGNANCY
N/A

SYNONYMS
N/A

SEE ALSO
- Nephrolithiasis
- Urolithiasis, Calcium Phosphate
- Urolithiasis, Cystine
- Urolithiasis, Struvite—Dogs
- Urolithiasis, Struvite—Cats
- Urolithiasis, Urate
- Urolithiasis, Xanthine

ABBREVIATIONS
N/A

Suggested Reading
Osborne CA, Davis LS, Sanna J, et al. Identification and interpretation of crystalluria in domestic animals. A light and scanning electron microscopic study. Vet Med 1990;85:18–37.
Osborne CA, Lulich JP, Bartges JW, et al. Drug-induced urolithiasis. Vet Clin North Am 1999;29:251–266.
Osborne CA, Lulich JP, Ulrich LK, et al. Feline crystalluria. Detection and interpretation. Vet Clin North Am 1996;26:369–391.
Authors Carl A. Osborne and Lisa K. Ulrich
Consulting Editors Larry G. Adams and Carl A. Osborne

CYLINDRURIA

BASICS

DEFINITION
Abnormally high number of casts (>2 casts/lpf) in urine sediment

PATHOPHYSIOLOGY
• May develop in animals with primary renal disease or systemic disorder that secondarily affects the kidneys
• High number of casts indicates accelerated renal cellular degeneration, glomerular leakage of protein, hemorrhage, or exudation into renal tubular lumens.

SYSTEMS AFFECTED
Renal/Urologic

SIGNALMENT
Dogs and cats

SIGNS
None

CAUSES

Nephrotoxicosis
• Toxin (e.g., ethylene glycol)*
• Nephrotoxic drug (e.g., aminoglycoside,* intravenously administered tetracycline, amphotericin B, cisplatin, thiacetarsamide, nonsteroidal antiinflammatory drug, angiotensin-converting enzyme inhibitor)
• Diagnostic agent (e.g., intravenously administered radiocontrast agent)

Renal Ischemia
• Dehydration
• Hypovolemia
• Low cardiac output (e.g., congestive heart failure, cardiac arrhythmia, or pericardial disease)
• Renal vessel thrombosis (e.g., emboli from bacterial endocarditis or DIC*)
• Hemoglobinuria (e.g., intravascular hemolysis)
• Myoglobulinuria (e.g., rhabdomyolysis)

Renal Inflammation
Infectious diseases (e.g., pyelonephritis, leptospirosis, feline infectious peritonitis, Rocky Mountain spotted fever, or ehrlichiosis)

Glomerular Disease
• Glomerulonephritis
• Amyloidosis

RISK FACTORS
• Any disorder that impairs renal perfusion
• Exposure to nephrotoxins

DIAGNOSIS

DIFFERENTIAL DIAGNOSIS
• History of potential exposure to toxins or nephrotoxic drugs—rule out acute tubular necrosis.
• Recent onset of vomiting or diarrhea—rule out renal ischemia caused by dehydration.
• Recent inhalation anesthesia—rule out tubular necrosis caused by ischemia.
• Potential for exposure to infectious diseases—rule out nephritis.
• Fever—rule out infectious, inflammatory, and neoplastic disease.
• Cardiac murmur, especially if diastolic and of recent onset—rule out bacterial endocarditis.
• Petechiae and ecchymoses—rule out systemic thrombosis.

LABORATORY FINDINGS

Drugs That May Alter Laboratory Results
N/A

Disorders That May Alter Laboratory Results
• Waiting longer than 2 h to perform urinalysis may result in disappearance of casts.
• Alkaline urine causes dissolution of casts.
• Dilute urine (specific gravity < 1.003) causes dissolution of casts; interpret numbers of casts in light of urine specific gravity.

Valid If Run in Human Laboratory?
Yes

CBC/BIOCHEMISTRY/URINALYSIS
• Anemia, hemoconcentration, leukocytosis, or thrombocytopenia in some patients
• High serum concentrations of urea nitrogen, creatinine, and phosphorus in patients with dehydration or renal failure
• Epithelial, granular, or waxy casts indicate diseases that cause degeneration and necrosis of renal tubular epithelial cells.
• RBC casts indicate severe glomerular disease or hemorrhage into renal tubules.
• WBC casts indicate renal inflammation, most often caused by pyelonephritis; most patients with pyelonephritis do not have WBC casts.
• Hyaline casts—commonly associated with disorders that cause proteinuria; also may be observed during diuresis and after dehydration

Laboratory Test Patterns
• Cylindruria plus azotemia and adequately concentrated urine (specific gravity 1.030 in dogs and 1.040 in cats) —consider prerenal disorders such as dehydration.

• Cylindruria plus azotemia and inadequately concentrated urine (specific gravity < 1.030 in dogs and < 1.035 in cats)—consider renal failure.
• Cylindruria plus leukocytosis—consider infectious and inflammatory disorders.
• Cylindruria plus thrombocytopenia—consider DIC.
• Cylindruria plus glucosuria and proteinuria—consider renal tubular necrosis.

OTHER LABORATORY TESTS
• If the patient has thrombocytopenia or RBC casts, perform coagulation studies (e.g., PTT, PT, and FDP) to rule out consumptive coagulopathy such as DIC.
• If the patient has proteinuria, determine urine protein:creatinine ratio to evaluate the magnitude of proteinuria.
• If the patient has pyuria or WBC casts, perform urine culture to rule out urinary tract infection.
• If systemic infectious diseases are suspected, submit serum for appropriate titers.

IMAGING
N/A

DIAGNOSTIC PROCEDURES
Consider renal biopsy if renal disease persists and progresses and the cause cannot be determined from routine and special laboratory tests.

TREATMENT

• Treat as outpatient unless the patient is dehydrated or has decompensated renal failure.
• If the patient is healthy otherwise, feed normal diet and allow normal exercise.

• If the patient cannot maintain hydration, administer lactated Ringer's solution or a maintenance fluid either intravenously or subcutaneously.
• If the patient has dehydration or continuing fluid losses such as vomiting or diarrhea, administer fluids intravenously to correct hydration deficits, maintain daily fluid requirements, and replace ongoing losses.

MEDICATIONS

DRUGS OF CHOICE
None

CONTRAINDICATIONS
Avoid nephrotoxic drugs.

PRECAUTIONS
N/A

POSSIBLE INTERACTIONS
N/A

ALTERNATIVE DRUGS
N/A

FOLLOW-UP

PATIENT MONITORING
Physical examination including patient's weight to assess hydration status

POSSIBLE COMPLICATIONS
Renal failure depending on underlying cause of cylindruria

MISCELLANEOUS

ASSOCIATED CONDITIONS
N/A

AGE-RELATED FACTORS
N/A

ZOONOTIC POTENTIAL
N/A

PREGNANCY
N/A

SYNONYMS
N/A

SEE ALSO
N/A

ABBREVIATIONS
• DIC = disseminated introvascular coagulation
• FDP = fibrin degradation products
• PT = prothrombin time
• PTT = partial thromboplastin time

Suggested Reading
Chew DJ, DiBartola, SP. Diagnosis and pathophysiology of renal disease. In: Ettinger SJ, ed. Textbook of veterinary internal medicine. Philadelphia: Saunders, 1994:1893–1961.

Lees GE, Willard MD, Green RA. Urinary disorders. In: Willard MD, Tvedten H, Turnwald GH, eds. Small animal clinical diagnosis by laboratory methods. Philadelphia: Saunders, 1994:15–146.

Osborne CA, Stevens JB. Handbook of canine and feline urinalysis. St. Louis: Ralston Purina Company, 1981:91–118.

Author S. Dru Forrester
Consulting Editors Larry G. Adams and Carl A. Osborne

EOSINOPHILIA AND BASOPHILIA

 BASICS

DEFINITION
• Peripheral blood eosinophil count > 750–1000/μL (reference range may vary regionally) • Peripheral blood basophil count > 200/μL or a minimum of 3–6% of the differential count

PATHOPHYSIOLOGY

Eosinophilia
• Develops in response to a primary disease process; highest counts seen in patients with hypereosinophilic syndrome, disseminated mast cell tumor, flea allergy, asthma, and some parasitic diseases • The level does not predict the degree of eosinophilic infiltration of tissues, which can be marked even in the absence of eosinophilia. • Results from heightened bone marrow production in response to specific stimuli (e.g., allergens, parasitic antigens, and products of tumor cells); repeated exposure to an antigen produces more rapid and dramatic eosinophilia. • Eosinophils can kill parasites and may contribute to host defense against tumors, but eosinophil-derived products can also cause destruction of host tissue. • Whether eosinophilic inflammation is beneficial or harmful varies according to the situation.

Basophilia
• Basophils play a role in immune-mediated inflammation, especially anaphylaxis and cutaneous hypersensitivity, but specific stimuli are not well characterized. • Basophils may participate in host rejection of parasites (especially ticks) and may play a role in tumor cytotoxicity. • Often accompanies eosinophilia, especially in patients with ectoparasites (mites) and dirofilariasis. • Basophil numbers may increase in the face of sustained lipemia or altered lipid metabolism.

SYSTEMS AFFECTED
• Skin • Respiratory • Gastrointestinal • Reproductive—during estrus • Patients with hypereosinophilic syndrome or eosinophilic leukemia—gastrointestinal tract, liver, spleen, and lymph nodes, especially mesenteric lymph nodes

SIGNALMENT
N/A

SIGNS

General Comments
Signs usually relate to underlying disease process

Historical Findings
• Skin—pruritus, flea infestation, alopecia, and crusty lesions • Respiratory tract—coughing and dyspnea • Gastrointestinal tract—vomiting, diarrhea, anorexia, and weight loss • Lethargy and depression

PHYSICAL EXAMINATION FINDINGS
• Skin—pruritus, alopecia, miliary dermatitis, oral lesions, other cutaneous lesions, regional lymphadenopathy, plaques, granulomas, and indolent ulcers • Respiratory—abnormal lung sounds, coughing, tachypnea, dyspnea, and pleural effusion • Gastrointestinal—thickened intestines, mesenteric lymphadenopathy, and abdominal effusion • Reproductive—estrus or vaginal discharge • Neoplasia—mass lesions and lymphadenopathy

CAUSES

Eosinophilia
• Causes are associated with tissue infiltrates of eosinophils with or without accompanying basophilic infiltration.
• Circulating eosinophilia is a variable finding.

Parasitism
• Especially parasites that invade tissues • Migrating helminthic parasites—particularly *Toxocara* spp., *Strongyloides stercoralis*, and *Ancylostoma* spp. • *Dirofilaria immitis* and *Dipetalonema reconditum* • Respiratory helminths—*Capillaria aerophila*, *Paragonimus kellicotti* (dogs and cats); *Aelurostrongylus abstrusus* (cats); *Oslerus osleri*, *Filaroides hirthi*, *Crenosoma vulpis*, and *Andersonstrongylus milksi* (dogs) • Ectoparasites—mites and fleas • Protozoa—*Giardia*, *Coccidia*, *Toxoplasma*, and *Neospora* • *Trichinella spiralis* • *Cuterebra*

Hypersensitivity Reactions and Other Inflammatory Conditions
• Skin—hypersensitivity to fleas and mites, reaction to insect bites (e.g., *Hymenoptera*), food allergy, inhalant allergic dermatitis (e.g., atopy), eosinophilic granuloma complex (e.g., indolent ulcer, plaque, and granuloma) in cats, eosinophilic granuloma in dogs, sterile eosinophilic folliculitis in cats, sterile eosinophilic pustulosis in dogs, chronic inflammation of skin
• Respiratory—chronic upper respiratory infection and rhinitis or sinusitis in cats, allergic bronchopulmonary disease (e.g., asthma, bronchitis, pneumonitis) in cats, less commonly seen in dogs as part of chronic obstructive pulmonary disease, parasitic pneumonia, granulomatous disease in dogs (mostly dirofilariasis), pulmonary infiltrates with eosinophilia (PIE—nonspecific term that includes pulmonary eosinophilic granulomatosis; eosinophilic pneumonia; bronchitis; bronchiolitis; and alveolitis caused by parasitism, allergic disease, dirofilariasis, drug reactions, bacterial and fungal infection, neoplasia, and idiopathic disease), focal pneumonia, interstitial pneumonia, pneumothorax, foreign body, chronic inflammation of the lung, and lymphomatoid granulomatosis
• Gastrointestinal—endoparasitism, oral or gastrointestinal eosinophilic granuloma, eosinophilic gastroenterocolitis (caused by dietary, bacterial, toxic, parasitic, and altered mucosal antigens) in dogs may be isolated to one segment of the GI tract; eosinophilic gastroenteritis in cats may be part of the hypereosinophilic syndrome and bacterial infection (including *Helicobacter*)
• Urogenital tract—estrus (occasionally in dogs), chronic inflammation of the reproductive tract, and urologic syndrome in cats
• Musculoskeletal (dogs)—eosinophilic myositis, panosteitis, immune-mediated polyarthritis, idiopathic eosinophilic polyarthritis, diskospondylitis (Airedales)
• Other inflammatory conditions—chronic fungal (e.g., gastric phycomycosis, disseminated coccidioidomycosis, and cryptococcosis of the CNS) and protozoal (e.g., hepatozoonosis and granulomatous meningoencephalitis)
• Tumor-associated eosinophilia (paraneoplastic syndrome)—most commonly observed in patients with mast cell tumor (visceral or disseminated) and lymphoma and occasionally other neoplasms (e.g., carcinoma and sarcoma)
• Myeloproliferative disease (dogs and cats)—hypereosinophilic syndrome (including gastroenteritis in cats), FeLV-associated eosinophilia (Rickard strain), and eosinophilic leukemia (rare)
• Miscellaneous—hypoadrenocorticism, eosinophilic meningoencephalitis (e.g., idiopathic steroid-responsive, protozoal, and migrating helminths), immune-mediated disease (e.g., SLE and AIHA), vaccine reaction (e.g., SQ rabies inoculation with granulomatous response), drug reaction (e.g., cyclophosphamide and phenol), administration of IL-2 or GM-CSF
• Miscellaneous (cats)—eosinophilic keratitis and conjunctivitis, hyperthyroidism, panleukopenia, infectious peritonitis, chronic gingivitis, infections with *Staphylococcus* and *Streptococcus* spp., and cardiac disease
• Most common diseases (cats)—flea allergy dermatitis, eosinophilic granuloma complex, allergic bronchitis, chronic upper respiratory infection, chronic rhinitis and sinusitis, and gastrointestinal disease with endoparasitism

Basophilia
• Parasitism—dirofilariasis (especially occult), tick infestation, other ectoparasites, and tracheal parasites
• Often accompanies eosinophilia (e.g., caused by chronic inflammation of mucosal and skin surfaces, disseminated mast cell tumor, and PIE)
• Lymphomatoid granulomatosis
• Basophilic leukemia

EOSINOPHILIA AND BASOPHILIA

• Possibly in animals with altered lipid metabolism that have sustained lipemia (e.g., chronic liver disease; nephrotic syndrome; genetic hyperlipoproteinemia; and endocrinopathy such as hyperadrenocorticism, diabetes mellitus, and hypothyroidism)

RISK FACTORS
• Parasitism
• Hypersensitivity disorder
• Inflammation
• Neoplasia

DIAGNOSIS

DIFFERENTIAL DIAGNOSIS
• Pruritus, alopecia, dermatitis, ulcer/plaque/granuloma, flea infestation—rule out atopy, flea or food allergy, eosinophilic granuloma complex, other disorders of hypersensitivity, and other inflammatory disorders of the skin.
• Coughing, dyspnea, tachypnea—rule out allergic diseases of respiratory tract (e.g., bronchitis and asthma), parasitic diseases (e.g., dirofilariasis and lungworm), PIE, and chronic inflammation.
• Nodular lung lesions with eosinophilia—rule out mycotic infection, idiopathic eosinophilic granuloma, primary or metastatic neoplasia, and lymphomatoid granulomatosis.
• Vomiting, diarrhea, weight loss—rule out eosinophilic gastroenterocolitis, parasitism, and hypereosinophilic syndrome.
• Lymphadenopathy or mass lesion—rule out mast cell tumor, lymphoma, other neoplasms, and hypereosinophilic syndrome.

LABORATORY FINDINGS

Drugs That May Alter Laboratory Results
Corticosteroid-induced eosinopenia can mask eosinophilia.

Disorders That May Alter Laboratory Results
None

Valid If Run in Human Laboratory?
Yes; laboratory should be informed that basophils in cats have beige-gray or mauve, round granules.

CBC/BIOCHEMISTRY/URINALYSIS
• Eosinophilia and basophilia
• Biochemical analysis may detect organ dysfunction.

OTHER LABORATORY TESTS
• Fecal flotation test to identify parasitic ova
• Baermann fecal sedimentation test to identify parasite larvae, especially nematode lungworms
• Heartworm test
• Cytologic examination of tracheobronchial fluid to identify eosinophilic inflammation, ova, and larvae
• Cytologic examination of skin, mucosal

(e.g., oral and rectal), and corneal or conjunctival scrapings for eosinophilic infiltrates and possible cause of eosinophilia
• Examination of buffy coat for mast cells, presence of which may indicate disseminated mast cell tumor
• Examination of bone marrow to rule out neoplasia

IMAGING
• Survey radiography of thorax to detect thoracic disease (e.g., diffuse, peribronchial, interstitial, or alveolar lung patterns, pleural fluid, and pneumothorax) and of abdomen to detect mass lesions or abdominal fluid
• Contrast studies of gastrointestinal tract to identify mucosal irregularities and wall thickenings
• Ultrasonography of thoracic or abdominal mass

DIAGNOSTIC PROCEDURES
• Intradermal skin testing (atopy)
• Transtracheal wash or bronchoalveolar lavage (respiratory disease)
• Thoracocentesis or abdominocentesis
• Examination of fine-needle aspirate or biopsy of mass lesion, skin, gastrointestinal tract, lung, lymph nodes, or bone marrow to rule out neoplasia
• Endoscopy (gastrointestinal disease)
• Laparotomy
• Exclusion diet
• Medical trial of corticosteroids or other medications

TREATMENT

• Treatment varies with the primary cause.
• Because eosinophils can cause damage to host cells, treatment aimed at decreasing or eliminating eosinophilic infiltrates may be required.

MEDICATIONS

DRUGS OF CHOICE
• Specific medications for the primary disease
• Corticosteroids are the most effective anti-inflammatory drug for treating eosinophil-related disorders (e.g., prednisolone, 1 mg/kg q12h, then taper by giving q24h, then alternate days to lowest dose that is still effective).
• For some conditions, cytotoxic drugs such as hydroxyurea may be required.
• Cyclosporin A may prove useful in controlling eosinophilic infiltrates induced by activated T cells.

CONTRAINDICATIONS
Corticosteroids are generally contraindicated in patients with sepsis.

PRECAUTIONS
• Corticosteroids are associated with hepatopathy and pancreatitis and affect the pituitary-adrenal axis.
• Chemotherapeutic and immunosuppressive agents have toxic effects (e.g., myelosuppression).

POSSIBLE INTERACTIONS
None

ALTERNATIVE DRUGS
None

FOLLOW-UP

PATIENT MONITORING
• Monitor primary disease as indicated.
• Recheck eosinophil and basophil counts.

POSSIBLE COMPLICATIONS
Eosinophilic infiltrates can cause severe tissue damage.

MISCELLANEOUS

ASSOCIATED CONDITIONS
Basophilia is often associated with eosinophilia.

AGE-RELATED FACTORS
None

ZOONOTIC POTENTIAL
Some parasitic diseases

PREGNANCY
Corticosteroids and chemotherapeutic agents may be contraindicated in pregnant animals.

SYNONYMS
None

SEE ALSO
Hypereosinophilic syndrome

ABBREVIATIONS
• AIHA = autoimmune hemolytic anemia
• FeLV = feline leukemia virus
• GM-CSF = granulocyte-macrophage colony-stimulating factor
• IL-2 = interleukin 2
• PIE = pulmonary infiltrates with eosinophilia
• SLE = systemic lupus erythematosus

Suggested Reading
Center SA, Randolph JF. Eosinophilia. In: August JR, ed. Consultations in feline internal medicine. Philadelphia: Saunders, 1991.
Tvedten H. Leukocyte disorders. In: Willard MD, Tvedten H, Turnwald GH, eds. Small animal clinical diagnosis by laboratory methods. Philadelphia: Saunders, 1994:63–66.
Author Karen M. Young
Consulting Editor Susan M. Cotter

FRUCTOSAMINE AND GLYCOSYLATED HEMOGLOBIN

BASICS

DEFINITION
Fructosamine and glycosylated hemoglobin (GHb) are blood proteins that can be used as adjunctive tests for diagnosing diabetes mellitus and monitoring glycemic control in the diabetic.

PATHOPHYSIOLOGY
• In the past metabolic control in diabetic patients was assessed primarily by evaluation of blood glucose measurements; unfortunately, these measurements indicate glycemic status only at one moment in time and are routinely affected by stress, diurnal variations, and medications.
• Chronic hyperglycemia results in increased glycosylation of serum proteins.
• Techniques for measuring fructosamine and GHb provide an objective means of evaluating average blood glucose concentration over several weeks.
• GHb is normally formed in a small percentage of red blood cells.
• Prolonged hyperglycemia increases the glycosylation of hemoglobin; prolonged hypoglycemia has the opposite effect.
• GHb accumulates over the life of a red blood cell and correlates with the average blood glucose concentration over the last 60–90 days in dogs, whose erythrocyte lifespan is 120 days.
• Cat's red blood cells have a shorter lifespan (~ 68 days), and thus GHb concentration reflects glycemic control over the preceding 30–45 days.
• Fructosamine is a serum protein that forms when glucose binds to a lysine residue on a protein, forming a ketoamine; the serum fructosamine concentration is a measure of glycosylation of all serum proteins; because serum proteins have a much shorter half-life than hemoglobin, fructosamine concentration reflects the glycemic status over the last 2–3 weeks.

SYSTEMS AFFECTED
• Endocrine/metabolic—weight loss secondary to impaired carbohydrate metabolism
• Hemic/lymphatic/immune—diabetic cats and dogs are significantly more prone to develop infections, because of impaired host defense mechanisms
• Neuromuscular—diabetic neuropathy can develop, most commonly in cats, which develop posterior weakness and plantigrade stance
• Ophthalmic—persistent hyperglycemia in a unregulated diabetic can result in cataract formation secondary to sorbitol accumulation within the lens
• Renal/urologic—osmotic diuresis caused by serum glucose exceeding the renal threshold results in polyuria and secondary polydipsia

SIGNALMENT
• Most dogs and cats affected with diabetes mellitus are >6 years of age.
• Female dogs are affected twice as frequently as males.
• Appears to be no breed predilection in cats; the following dog breeds are frequently affected with diabetes: cairn terriers, dachshunds, keeshonden, miniature schnauzers, and poodles

SIGNS

Historical Findings
• Most clients present their pets for one or a combination of the following complaints: polydipsia, polyuria, weight loss, and polyphagia; in a few instances clients may ignore these classic signs of diabetes mellitus.
• Dogs may then present for evaluation of suspected blindness caused by cataract formation or the cat for rear limb weakness secondary to diabetic neuropathy.

Physical Examination Findings
• The nonketotic diabetic has no classic examination findings.
• Some animals, in particular cats, may be obese.
• Bilateral cataracts can be seen in the canine diabetic.
• Diabetic cats may develop a plantigrade stance as a result of diabetic neuropathy.
• The diabetic patient with ketoacidosis can show varying degrees of dehydration, depression, tachypnea, and vomiting; the ketoacidotic patient may have a strong acetone odor to the breath.

CAUSES
• Elevated fructosamine and GHb concentrations only occur with persistently high blood glucose concentration as seen most commonly with diabetes mellitus.
• Other causes of hyperglycemia, including hyperadrenocorticism, progesterone or glucocorticoid administration, pancreatitis, feline acromegaly, diestrus in the bitch, renal insufficiency, pheochromocytoma, glucagonoma, and exocrine pancreatic neoplasia, can mildly increase fructosamine and GHb concentrations.
• Recent research indicates that GHb concentrations do not differ significantly in dogs with confirmed hyperadrenocorticism and normal dogs.
• Transient hyperglycemia from a stressful incident (e.g., a visit to the veterinarian) will not increase either fructosamine or glycosylated hemoglobin concentration.

RISK FACTORS
Hyperadrenocorticism, feline acromegaly, pancreatitis, diestrus in the bitch, chronic progesterone or glucocorticoid administration all cause insulin resistance that may result in carbohydrate intolerance and eventually overt diabetes

DIAGNOSIS

DIFFERENTIAL DIAGNOSIS
• Always evaluate fructosamine and GHb along with anamnesis, physical examination, and laboratory abnormalities; other causes of persistent hyperglycemia listed above must be ruled out.
• All other causes of hyperglycemia should increase fructosamine and GHb only mildly.

LABORATORY FINDINGS

Drugs That May Alter Laboratory Results
• Glucocorticoids and progestins (i.e., megestrol acetate [Ovaban])—the two most common drugs; long-term use could cause hyperglycemia and subsequent elevations in fructosamine and GHb.
• Thiazide diuretics, growth hormone, dextrose-containing fluids, and morphine can also induce hyperglycemia and if given longer than 5–7 days can induce mild fructosamine and GHb elevations.

Disorders That May Alter Laboratory Results
• Changes in the serum protein concentration and or composition may affect the serum fructosamine concentration; this appears to have little clinical importance.
• The concentration of GHb is affected by the lifespan of the erythrocyte and the glucose concentration during that period; thus the concentration of GHb can be decreased in conditions that decrease the lifespan of circulating erythrocytes or in conditions of persistent hypoglycemia.
• Similarly, polycythemia may cause elevations in the GHb concentration; always interpret GHb results in the context of the hematocrit.

Valid If Run in Human Laboratory?
Run in veterinary diagnostic laboratory in which the normal ranges for canine and feline patients have been determined

CBC/BIOCHEMISTRY/URINALYSIS
• Persistent hyperglycemia and glycosuria with elevated fructosamine or GHb concentration strongly suggests diabetes mellitus.
• Evaluating other laboratory test result helps to identify other diseases that may be causing or contributing to the carbohydrate intolerance.

CBC
• Hemogram is commonly normal in an uncomplicated diabetic.
• Can see inflammatory leukogram with concurrent infection or pancreatitis

Biochemistry
• Elevated liver enzymes are common in diabetic dogs and cats because of concurrent hepatic lipidosis or pancreatitis.

FRUCTOSAMINE AND GLYCOSYLATED HEMOGLOBIN

• Elevated BUN and creatinine may suggest concurrent renal insufficiency or prerenal azotemia secondary to dehydration.
• Hypercholesterolemia is seen in most diabetics.

Urinalysis
• Persistent glycosuria—all diabetics
• Bacteruria with or without pyuria, hematuria, and proteinuria suggests concurrent urinary tract infection.
• Trace ketones may be seen in healthy diabetics; large amounts of ketones along with systemic signs support a diagnosis of diabetic ketoacidosis.

OTHER LABORATORY TESTS
• Amylase/lipase/ and trypsin-like immuno-reactivity—run on all diabetics with history of anorexia, vomiting, and/or abdominal pain, to rule in concurrent pancreatitis
• If inappropriate response to insulin therapy—ACTH stimulation test or low-dose dexamethasone suppression test to rule in hyperadrenocorticism; serum thyroxine levels to evaluate for hyperthyroidism or hypothyroidism; insulin-like growth factor I (IGF-1) levels to rule in acromegaly; and urinary catecholamine levels to rule out pheochromocytoma

IMAGING
Abdominal radiography and ultrasonography may provide important information about such concurrent disorders as pancreatitis, hyperadrenocorticism, pheochromocytoma, and neoplasia.

DIAGNOSTIC PROCEDURES
N/A

TREATMENT
• Primary goal is elimination of owner-observed signs of diabetes mellitus (polyuria, polydipsia, polyphagia, weight loss) by attempting to normalize blood glucose concentrations without inducing hypoglycemia.
• Address other disorders that may have caused or contributed to carbohydrate intolerance.

DIET
A high-fiber diet will help minimize postprandial glucose fluctuations; avoid soft, moist foods because of high level of simple carbohydrates in them; controlled weight reduction in obese animals will reduce obesity-induced insulin resistance

EXERCISE
Daily routine should include period of moderate exercise; physical activity has a glucose-lowering effect; excessive physical activity can induce hypoglycemia and should be avoided or decrease the insulin dose on days of strenuous exercise

CLIENT EDUCATION
Owners are a crucial link in establishing glycemic control; explain the basics of the disease, appropriate insulin administration techniques, recognition and treatment of hypoglycemic signs that may result from therapy, and chronic complications.

MEDICATIONS
DRUGS OF CHOICE

Dogs
Healthy, nonketotic—initial insulin of choice is NPH or lente, initially at 0.5/kg BID

Cats
• Not all cats are insulin-dependent diabetics; can try treating healthy, nonketotic cats with oral hypoglycemic agents; 30% of cats have a complete or partial response to glipizide
• Insulin-dependent cats—can try long-acting ultralente 1–3 units SID initially, but it is poorly absorbed in 25% of cats
• Lente insulin at an initial dose of 2 units BID is the choice of this author
• PZI, the initial insulin of choice of cats, has recently come back on the market
• DKA (diabetic ketoacidosis) Fluid support and short-acting regular insulin

CONTRAINDICATIONS
Avoid diabetogenic drugs such as glucocorticoids and progestogens.

PRECAUTIONS
• The major complication in treating diabetic animals is the development of hypoglycemia.
• Instruct owners to watch for signs of ataxia, lethargy, dullness, weakness, and seizures that may indicate insulin overdose.
• Owners should attempt to feed their animal if they note any of the above signs and contact the veterinarian immediately.

POSSIBLE INTERACTIONS
N/A

ALTERNATIVE DRUGS
Consider oral hypoglycemic drugs, particularly the sulfonylurea glipizide, for healthy, nonketotic cats whose owners are adverse to administering insulin injections or those that have recurring bouts of hypoglycemia on insulin therapy (see Drugs of Choice).

FOLLOW-UP
PATIENT MONITORING
• Reevaluate patient 5–7 days after initiating insulin therapy; the author commonly performs a serial blood glucose curve at this time, primarily to ensure against hypoglycemia; later

changes in insulin dosage are determined by assessing historical decrease in polyuria/polydipsia, changes in body weight, physical examination findings, and decreases in fructosamine or GHb concentrations.
• Evaluation of fructosamine and GHb concentrations—does not eliminate the need for serial blood glucose curves; detects inadequate glycemic control and shows when a blood glucose curve is necessary.

POSSIBLE COMPLICATIONS
• Impaired host defense mechanisms render diabetic animals significantly more prone to developing infections.
• Instruct owners to watch closely for signs of urinary infections or recurrence of polyuria/polydipsia; in a well-regulated diabetic these could suggest insulin resistance secondary to a occult infection.
• Good glycemic control helps slow the progression of cataracts in the canine but is unlikely to prevent their formation.

MISCELLANEOUS
ASSOCIATED CONDITIONS
Pancreatitis, bacterial infections, and less commonly hyperadrenocorticism, diestrus in the bitch, and feline acromegaly may be seen concurrently in animals with diabetes mellitus.

AGE-RELATED FACTORS
N/A

ZOONOTIC POTENTIAL
N/A

PREGNANCY
Because of the insulin-antagonist effects of progesterone, intact female canine diabetics should be spayed.

ABBREVIATIONS
• GHb = glycosylated hemoglobin
• IGF1 = insulin-like growth factor 1
• NPH = isophane
• PZI = protomine zinc insulin

Suggested Reading
Feldman EC, Nelson RW. Glycosylated hemoglobin and fructosamine. In: Feldman EC, Nelson RW, eds. Canine and feline endocrinology and reproduction. Philadelphia: WB Saunders, 1996:
Jensen AL. Glycated blood proteins in canine diabetes mellitus. Vet Rec 1995;137:401–405.
Thoresen SI, Bredal WP. Clinical usefulness of fructosamine in diagnosing and monitoring feline diabetes mellitus. J Small Anim Pract 1996;37:64–68.
Author Christopher A. McReynolds
Consulting Editor Deborah S. Greco

GLOBULIN

BASICS

DEFINITION
• Heterogenous group of proteins; includes immunoglobulins, clotting factors, acute-phase proteins, and complement proteins
• Hyperglobulinemia—high serum globulin concentration
• Hypoglobulinemia—low serum globulin concentration
• Gammopathy—any abnormality in the concentration of immunoglobulins

PATHOPHYSIOLOGY
• Hyperglobulinemia—from increased production of immunoglobulins and hepatic synthesis of acute-phase proteins; falsely increased by dehydration; classified as either polyclonal or monoclonal; may result in hyperviscosity syndrome and impaired immune function
• Polyclonal gammopathies—from production of immunoglobulins by several different cell lines; usually in response to persistent antigenic stimulation
• Monoclonal gammopathies—from synthesis of one type of immunoglobulin by a single clone of cells; proliferation may be associated with lymphoid hyperplasia or neoplasia.
• Hypoglobulinemia—from either impaired synthesis or extracorporeal globulin loss
• Impaired synthesis—results in immunodeficiency syndromes; characterized by chronic infection and unthrifty appearance
• Extracorporeal loss—commonly from gastrointestinal disease; also secondary to blood loss; rarely from hepatic insufficiency and renal losses

SYSTEMS AFFECTED
Hyperglobulinemia
• Hemic/Lymphatic/Immune—monoclonal gammopathies: diminished synthesis of normal immunoglobulins (immune deficiency and chronic infections); cause decreased platelet adhesion (bleeding tendencies)
• Cardiovascular—production of para-proteins: hyperviscosity syndrome; increased cardiac work load; myocardial hypoxia (may result in cardiac failure); hypertension
• Nervous—poor perfusion of the CNS owing to hyperviscosity (severe depression, seizures, ataxia, and nystagmus)

• Ophthalmic—high serum viscosity: retinal hemorrhage; retinal detachment; blindness

Hypoglobulinemia
Hemic/Lymphatic/Immune—impaired immunoglobulin synthesis: impaired immune function; chronic or recurrent infections of the gastrointestinal tract, skin, and respiratory system

SIGNALMENT
Hyperglobulinemia
• No age, breed, or sex predilection
• Monoclonal gammopathies—commonly associated with neoplasia; thus more common in old animals

Hypoglobulinemia
• Mild—normal finding in young animals
• Immunodeficiency syndromes—most common in neonates and adolescents; shar peis, German shepherds, Doberman pinchers, beagles, basset hounds, Weimaraners, and Samoyeds

SIGNS
Hyperglobulinemia
• Relate to the underlying cause
• Bone pain and lameness—bony lesions of multiple myeloma
• Secondary to high serum viscosity—neuro-logic abnormalities, bleeding disorders, and cardiovascular impairment common

Hypoglobulinemia
• Relate to immunodeficiency
• Recurrent infections—pneumonia; gastro-enteritis; dermatitis; upper respiratory infections
• With PLE—vomiting; diarrhea; weight loss

CAUSES
Hyperglobulinemia
Polyclonal Gammopathy
• Chronic infection or inflammation—bacterial (pyoderma, pyometra, brucellosis, pneumonia); fungal (blastomycosis, histo-plasmosis, coccidioidomycosis, crypto-coccosis); protozoal or rickettsial (ehrlichiosis, babesiosis, leishmaniasis, trypanosomiasis, heamobartonellosis); viral (FIP, FeLV, FIV); parasitic (dirofilariasis, demodicosis, scabies)
• Immune-mediated disorders—SLE; hemo-lytic anemia; thrombocytopenia; pemphigus complex; bullous pemphigoid; rheumatoid arthritis; chronic polyarthritis; neoplasia
Monoclonal Gammopathy
• Neoplasia—multiple myeloma; lympho-sarcoma; chronic lymphocytic leukemia

• Infection or inflammation—*Ehrlichia canis;* FIP; leishmaniasis
• Idiopathic—macroglobulinemia; benign monoclonal gammopathy

Hypoglobulinemia
• Neonates—normal
• Increased loss—blood; gastrointestinal (lymphangiectasia, inflammatory bowel disease, intestinal neoplasia, other severe PLN); renal (PLN, rare)
• Humoral immunodeficiency—IgM; IgA; transient hypogammaglobulinemia

RISK FACTORS
• Chronic inflammation or immune stimulation or neoplasia—may predispose patient to develop hyperglobulinemia
• Inbreeding—may predispose animal to humoral immunodeficiency and subsequent hypoglobulinemia

DIAGNOSIS

DIFFERENTIAL DIAGNOSIS
Hyperglobulinemia
• Chronic infection or inflammation—upper respiratory infections; dermatitis
• Neoplasia—weight loss; severe bone pain; bleeding disorders; neurologic signs

Hypoglobulinemia
• Immune deficiency—unthriftiness and chronic infection in a young patient
• Gastrointestinal loss—chronic diarrhea

LABORATORY FINDINGS
Drugs That May Alter Laboratory Results
N/A

Disorders That May Alter Laboratory Results
Hyperglobulinemia—dehydration; hemolysis; lipemia

Valid If Run in Human Laboratory?
Yes

CBC/BIOCHEMISTRY/URINALYSIS
CBC—Hyperglobulinemia
• Anemia, leukopenia, and thrombo-cytopenia—may indicate bone marrow neoplasia, *E. canis* infection, or immune-mediated disorder
• Marked lymphocytosis—may indicate leukemia
• Rouleaux—common, owing to paraproteins and reduction of normal repulsion forces between erythrocytes

Biochemistry—Hypoglobulinemia
Concurrent hypoalbuminemia—indicates blood loss or severe PLE

Urinalysis
• Hyperglobulinemia—proteinuria may be associated with neoplasia (e.g., multiple myeloma) or immune-mediated glomerulonephritis.
• Hypoglobulinemia—nonselective severe proteinuria; rare
• Urinary tract infections—common with hyperglobulinemia and hypoglobulinemia owing to immunosuppression

OTHER LABORATORY TESTS
• Serum protein electrophoresis—quantitative means of determining cause of hyperglobulinemia not associated with dehydration; differentiates between polyclonal and monoclonal gammopathy
• Immunoelectrophoresis—qualitative measure of immunoglobulins; may identify specific immunoglobulins making up a monoclonal gammopathy; may identify deficient immunoglobulin concentrations
• Infectious disease titers and immunologic testing (e.g., ANA, Coombs test)—important for clarifying cause of hyperglobulinemia
• Serum viscosity—estimate with suspected hyperviscosity syndrome; usually associated with a monoclonal gammopathy; IgM and IgA dimers greatest causal potential, owing to their size
• Cryoprecipitation—with suspected cryoglobulins secondary to multiple myeloma or macroglobulinemia

IMAGING
• Thoracic radiographs—identify neoplastic or infectious diseases
• Skeletal radiographs—suspected multiple myeloma; search for typical punched-out osteolytic bone lesions
• Abdominal ultrasound—reveal neoplasia (hyperglobulinemia) or thickened gastrointestinal wall associated with PLE (hypoglobulinemia)

DIAGNOSTIC PROCEDURES
• Bone marrow aspirations—suspected multiple myeloma or leukemia (hyperglobulinemia)
• Bone biopsy—osteolytic lesions; may be needed to diagnose multiple myeloma
• Intestinal biopsy—suspected PLE (hypoglobulinemia)

TREATMENT

APPROPRIATE HEALTH CARE
Inpatient—depends on treatment (e.g., hyperviscosity syndrome)

NURSING CARE

Hyperglobulinemia
• Hemoconcentration—treated with judicious crystalloid fluid therapy
• Polyclonal or monoclonal gammopathy—initial supportive care; long-term therapy directed at the underlying cause (e.g., chemotherapy, antimicrobial therapy, immunosuppressive therapy)
• Hyperviscosity syndrome—plasmapheresis; if unavailable, try phlebotomy with crystalloid fluid replacement

Hypoglobulinemia
Humoral immunodeficiency—treat for opportunistic infections, as appropriate.

MEDICATIONS

DRUGS OF CHOICE
• Depend on the underlying cause
• See Treatment

CONTRAINDICATIONS
N/A

PRECAUTIONS
N/A

POSSIBLE INTERACTIONS
N/A

ALTERNATIVE DRUGS
N/A

FOLLOW-UP

PATIENT MONITORING
• Dictated by underlying cause
• Hyperviscosity—monitor frequently (hourly) until signs abate

POSSIBLE COMPLICATIONS
• Associated humoral immunodeficiency—susceptible to recurrent infection by opportunistic pathogens
• Hyperviscosity syndrome—may result in bleeding tendencies, neurologic abnormalities, or cardiac failure

MISCELLANEOUS

ASSOCIATED CONDITIONS
• PLE—commonly associated with hypoalbuminemia and hypocholesterolemia
• Panhypoproteinemia associated with PLN—usually accompanied by a marked hypercholesterolemia

AGE-RELATED FACTORS
• Low serum globulin concentration—normal in neonates
• Neoplasia—frequent cause of hyperglobulinemia in old patients
• Hypoglobulinemia associated with humoral immunodeficiency—more common in young patients

ZOONOTIC POTENTIAL
N/A

PREGNANCY
N/A

SYNONYMS
• Gammopathy
• Hypergammaglobulinemia
• Hypogammaglobulinemia

SEE ALSO
See Causes.

ABBREVIATIONS
• ANA = antinuclear antibody
• FeLV = feline leukemia virus
• FIP = feline infectious peritonitis
• PLE = protein-losing enteropathy
• PLN = protein-losing nephropathy
• SLE = systemic lupus erythematosus

Suggested Reading
Dorfman M, Diminski DS. Paraproteinemias in small animal medicine. Compend Contin Educ Pract Vet 1992;14:1259–1262.
Guilford WG. Primary immunodeficiency diseases in dogs and cats. Compend Contin Educ Pract Vet 1987;9:641–650.
Matus RE, Leifer CE. Immunoglobulin-producing tumors. Vet Clin North Am Small Anim Pract 1985;15:741–753.
Williams DA. Gammopathies. Compend Contin Educ Pract Vet 1981;3:815–822.
Author Shannon M. Flood
Consulting Editor Sharon A. Center

GLUCOSE, HYPERGLYCEMIA

BASICS

DEFINITION
High concentration of glucose in whole blood, plasma, or serum

PATHOPHYSIOLOGY
• May result from absolute or relative insulin deficiency, reduced use of glucose in peripheral tissue, increased gluconeogenesis in the liver, and increased glycogenolysis
• Insulin antagonists or counterregulatory hormones (e.g., cortisol, adrenocorticotropic hormone [ACTH], growth hormone, epinephrine, and glucagon) also contribute to hyperglycemia.

SYSTEMS AFFECTED
• Endocrine/Metabolic—primarily because of regulating carbohydrate metabolism
• Renal/Urologic—osmotic diuresis caused by hyperglycemia causes polyuria with secondary polydipsia.
• Nervous—severe hyperglycemia may cause CNS dysfunction by increasing serum osmolality.
• Ophthalmic—persistent hyperglycemia (e.g., diabetes mellitus) can cause cataracts in dogs.

SIGNALMENT
Dog and cat

SIGNS

General Comments
• Clinical signs vary and often reflect underlying disease.
• Some patients are asymptomatic, especially those with transient, stress-induced, and postprandial hyperglycemia.

Historical Findings
• Variable
• Polydipsia, polyuria, depression, weight loss, obesity, polyphagia
• CNS depression—severe hyperglycemia

Physical Examination Findings
Often normal, but can include nonhealing wounds, abscesses, obesity, cataracts, and hepatomegaly

CAUSES
• Low glucose use—diabetes mellitus, acute pancreatitis, acromegaly (increased growth hormone) in cats, high progesterone during diestrus (dogs), renal insufficiency, and pancreatectomy to treat insulinoma
• High glucose production—hyperadrenocorticism, pheochromocytoma, glucagonoma, exocrine pancreatic neoplasia
• Physiologic—postprandial fluctuation, exertion or excitement, and stress (epinephrine induced), especially in cats
• Drugs—thiazide diuretics, morphine, dextrose-containing fluids, progestins (e.g., megestrol acetate [Ovaban]), growth hormone, glucocorticoids, and ACTH
• Insulin administration problems in confirmed diabetics—Somogyi phenomenon, antiinsulin antibodies, and poor insulin absorption
• Parenteral administration of nutritional solutions
• Laboratory error

RISK FACTORS
• Concurrent disease—hyperadrenocorticism, acromegaly, and acute pancreatitis
• Diabetogenic drugs
• Dextrose-containing fluids

DIAGNOSIS

DIFFERENTIAL DIAGNOSIS
• Mild, transiently high blood glucose can be associated with stress and epinephrine-induced excitement or normal postprandial fluctuation.
• In patients with mild hyperglycemia and no history of polydipsia/polyuria, repeat blood glucose determination after 12-h fast and eliminate or minimize stress (i.e., allow time for acclimation to hospital environment).

LABORATORY FINDINGS

Drugs That May Alter Laboratory Results
• High blood glucose concentration—glucocorticoids, ACTH, dextrose-containing fluids, epinephrine, asparaginase, β-adrenergic agonists, and diazoxide
• Low blood glucose concentration determined enzymatically—aspirin, ascorbic acid, and acetaminophen

Disorders That May Alter Laboratory Results
• Lipemia, hemolysis, and icterus may interfere with spectrophotometric assays.
• Delayed serum separation artificially lowers glucose concentration; must separate serum within 1 h of collection to prevent cellular glucose use
• Refrigerate or freeze serum sample not analyzed within 12 h.
• Blood glucose reagent strips require whole blood.
• Measure glucose concentration in whole blood within 30 min of collection.
• Sodium fluoride collection tubes allow more-stable readings and can prevent artificially low readings by spectrophotometry; do not use for enzymatic assays.

Valid If Run in Human Laboratory?
Yes

CBC/BIOCHEMISTRY/URINALYSIS
• Hyperglycemia may be the only abnormal finding.
• CBC—may be normal; possible inflammatory leukogram in patients with infection
• Urinalysis—may be normal; possible abnormalities include glucosuria, pyuria, bacteruria, and ketonuria.
• Fasting hyperglycemia plus glucosuria suggests diabetes mellitus, although mild hyperglycemia and glucosuria can be physiologic in cats.
• Lipemia is associated with low lipoprotein lipase, hyperadrenocorticism, acute pancreatitis, and postprandial blood sampling.

- High amylase and lipase activity suggests acute pancreatitis, especially in nonazotemic patients.
- High liver enzyme activity may accompany fatty infiltration.

OTHER LABORATORY TESTS
- ACTH stimulation or low-dose dexamethasone suppression test to rule out hyperadrenocorticism
- Serum insulin concentration—hyperglycemia is usually accompanied by hyperinsulinemia.
- Hyperglycemia with low serum insulin suggests diabetes mellitus.
- Although rarely indicated, IV glucose and a glucagon tolerance test may help demonstrate carbohydrate intolerance; blood glucose should return to normal within 60 min and serum insulin should increase after IV glucose or glucagon administration.
- Determine serum osmolarity in patients with moderate-to-severe hyperglycemia.

IMAGING
Abdominal radiography and ultrasonography may provide valuable information regarding underlying causes.

DIAGNOSTIC PROCEDURES
N/A

TREATMENT
- Minimize or eliminate stress.
- Avoid abrupt decreases in blood glucose.
- Discontinue diabetogenic drugs or adjust their dosage to normalize blood glucose while maintaining therapeutic concentration.
- Dextrose-free fluids
- Avoid semimoist commercial foods because of the higher content of simple sugars.
- Offer a high-protein, low-carbohydrate, low-fat, high-fiber diet.

MEDICATIONS

DRUGS OF CHOICE
Insulin—regular (crystalline) insulin has a more rapid onset of effect but a shorter duration of action than other types of insulin.

CONTRAINDICATIONS
- Diabetogenic drugs (e.g., glucocorticoids)
- Dextrose-containing fluids

PRECAUTIONS
Avoid lowering blood glucose abruptly and causing hypoglycemia.

POSSIBLE INTERACTIONS
N/A

ALTERNATIVE DRUGS
Oral administration of hypoglycemic agents—sulfonylureas (e.g., glipizide [Glucotrol]) and biguanides are most useful in cats with type II (non-insulin-dependent) diabetes mellitus.

FOLLOW-UP

PATIENT MONITORING
- Blood glucose after initiating treatment and discontinuing diabetogenic drugs
- Glucose curves by measuring blood glucose hourly or every 2 h for 12–24 h after insulin administration
- Glycosylated hemoglobin and fructosamine on an outpatient basis to monitor long-term glucose control
- Insulin concentrations after treatment
- For return of clinical signs such as polyuria, polydipsia, and polyphagia

POSSIBLE COMPLICATIONS
- High incidence of sepsis (and infection)
- Severe hyperglycemia may be associated with CNS depression and coma because of hyperosmolarity

MISCELLANEOUS

ASSOCIATED CONDITIONS
- Severe hyperglycemia associated with hyperosmolarity
- Uremia may be associated with hyperglycemia.
- Hyperglycemia associated with acidosis, hyponatremia, hypokalemia, and hypophosphatemia; although total body concentrations of these electrolytes are low, serum chemistry measurements may be normal, high, or low.

AGE-RELATED FACTORS
N/A

ZOONOTIC POTENTIAL
N/A

PREGNANCY
Pregnancy-induced diabetes mellitus caused by high progesterone concentration is reported in humans.

SYNONYMS
"High blood sugar"

SEE ALSO
- Diabetes Mellitus
- Hyperosmolarity

ABBREVIATIONS
ACTH = adrenocorticotropic hormone

Suggested Reading
Kaneko JJ, ed. Carbohydrate metabolism and its diseases. In: Kaneko JJ, ed. Clinical biochemistry of domestic animals. 4th ed. San Diego: Academic Press, 1989:44–85.
Rich LJ, Coles EH. Tables of abnormal blood values as a guide to disease syndromes. In: Ettinger SJ, Feldman EC, eds. Textbook of veterinary internal medicine. 4th ed. Philadelphia: Saunders, 1995:11–17.
Willard MD, Tvedten H, Turnwald GH. Small animal clinical diagnosis by laboratory methods. 2nd ed. Philadelphia: Saunders, 1994:154–160.

Author Margaret R. Kern
Consulting Editor Deborah S. Greco

GLUCOSE, HYPOGLYCEMIA

BASICS

DEFINITION
Abnormally low blood glucose concentration

PATHOPHYSIOLOGY
Mechanisms responsible for hypoglycemia
• Excess insulin or insulin-like factors (e.g., insulinoma, extrapancreatic paraneoplasia, and iatrogenic insulin overdose)
• Reduction of hormones needed to maintain normal serum glucose (e.g., hypoadrenocorticism)
• Reduced hepatic gluconeogenesis (e.g., hepatic disease, glycogen storage diseases, and sepsis)
• Excessive use (e.g., hunting dogs, pregnancy, neoplasia, polycythemia, and sepsis)
• Reduced intake or underproduction (e.g., puppies and kittens, toy breeds, and severe malnutrition or starvation)

SYSTEMS AFFECTED
• Nervous
• Musculoskeletal

SIGNALMENT
• Dog and cat
• Variable, depending on the underlying cause

SIGNS
• Seizures
• Posterior paresis
• Weakness
• Collapse
• Muscle fasciculations
• Abnormal behavior
• Lethargy and depression
• Ataxia
• Polyphagia
• Weight gain
• PU/PD
• Exercise intolerance
• Some animals appear normal aside from findings associated with underlying disease.
• Many animals have episodic signs.

CAUSES
Endocrine
• Insulinoma
• Extrapancreatic paraneoplasia
• Iatrogenic insulin overdose
• Hypoadrenocorticism

Hepatic Disease
• Portosystemic shunt
• Cirrhosis
• Severe hepatitis (e.g., toxic and inflammatory)
• Glycogen storage diseases

Overuse
• Hunting dog hypoglycemia
• Pregnancy
• Polycythemia
• Neoplasia
• Sepsis

Reduced Intake/Underproduction
• Young puppies and kittens
• Toy-breed dogs
• Severe malnutrition or starvation

RISK FACTORS
• Low energy intake predisposes hypoglycemia in patients with conditions causing overuse and underproduction.
• Fasting, excitement, exercise, and eating may or may not increase the risk of hypoglycemic episodes in patients with insulinoma.

DIAGNOSIS

DIFFERENTIAL DIAGNOSIS
• Patients with hyperinsulinism—signs of hypoglycemia or a normal physical examination
• Patients with hypoadrenocorticism—waxing, waning, nonspecific signs (e.g., vomiting, diarrhea, melena, and weakness); addisonian patients that present in a crisis usually display hypovolemia and hyperkalemia rather than hypoglycemia (e.g., shock, bradycardia, and dehydration).
• Patients with portosystemic shunts—usually young to middle-aged; often thin or appear to have stunted growth; rarely, they have ascites or edema
• Patients with cirrhosis and severe hepatitis—usually have other signs of their disease (e.g., gastrointestinal signs, icterus, and ascites or edema).
• Patients with sepsis—critical; usually in shock; pyrexia or hypothermia revealed by examination; may have gastrointestinal signs
• Glycogen storage diseases—rare; usually seen in animals <1 year old

• Extrapancreatic paraneoplasia and large neoplastic processes that cause hypoglycemia can often be detected by physical examination.

LABORATORY FINDINGS
Drugs That May Alter Laboratory Results
N/A

Disorders That May Alter Laboratory Results
Delayed separation of serum causes falsely low serum glucose values; if blood cannot be centrifuged and the serum separated within 30 min of collection, it should be collected in a sodium fluoride tube.

Valid If Run in Human Laboratory?
Valid

CBC/BIOCHEMISTRY/URINALYSIS
• Patients with hyperinsulinism may have normal results.
• Patients with hypoadrenocorticism may have lymphocytosis, eosinophilia, hyperkalemia, hyponatremia, azotemia, or hypercalcemia.
• Patients with portosystemic shunts may have microcytosis, hypoalbuminemia, low BUN, mildly high liver enzyme activities, urate crystals, and low urinary specific gravity.
• Patients with cirrhosis, severe hepatitis, and hepatic neoplasia may have anemia associated with chronic disease, high liver enzyme activities, hyperbilirubinemia, hypoalbuminemia, bilirubinuria, and low urinary specific gravity.
• Patients with polycythemia have a PCV >65.

OTHER LABORATORY TESTS
• Simultaneous fasting glucose/insulin determination—indicated when insulinoma is suspected; high plasma insulin in the face of hypoglycemia suggests insulinoma
• AIGR—indicated when insulinoma is suspected;

$$AIGR = \frac{(\text{plasma insulin } [\mu U/mL] \times 100)}{(\text{plasma glucose } [mg/dL] - 30)}$$

as denominator if glucose is <30; AIGR > 30 suggests an insulinoma; AIGR = 19–30 is a gray zone, repeat test; AIGR < 19 indicates insulinoma is unlikely. (**Note:** False-positive results are possible, especially when the blood glucose concentration is <40 mg/dL.)
• ACTH stimulation test—indicated when hypoadrenocorticism is suspected

• Fasting and postprandial serum bile acids—indicated when a portosystemic shunt or functional hepatic disease is suspected
• Bacterial culture of blood—indicated when sepsis is suspected

IMAGING
• Abdominal radiography and ultrasonography—useful in patients with extrapancreatic paraneoplasia and large neoplastic processes (may see organomegaly or masses), as well as portosystemic shunt (microhepatica), cirrhosis (microhepatica, hyperechogenicity), and severe hepatitis (hepatomegaly)
• Thoracic radiography—to detect metastasis if neoplasia is suspected
• Technetium-99m per rectal quantitative hepatic scintigraphy—useful to detect portosystemic shunt
• Mesenteric portography—useful to detect portosystemic shunt (requires surgery)

DIAGNOSTIC PROCEDURES
• ECG—useful to evaluate bradycardia in patients with hypoadrenocorticism
• Ultrasound-guided or surgical biopsy—useful to evaluate for cirrhosis, hepatitis, and glycogen storage diseases

TREATMENT
• Treat animals with clinical hypoglycemia whose underlying disease needs support as inpatients.
• If able to eat (i.e., responsive, no vomiting), feeding should be part or all initial treatment.
• If unable to eat, start continuous fluid therapy with 2.5% dextrose; if clinical signs persist, use a 5% dextrose solution.
• Surgery is indicated if a portosystemic shunt or insulinoma is the cause of hypoglycemia.

MEDICATIONS

DRUGS OF CHOICE

Emergency/Acute Treatment
• In hospital—administer 50% dextrose, 1 mL/kg IV slow bolus (1–3 min).
• At home—do not attempt to have the owner administer medication orally during a seizure; hypoglycemic seizures usually abate within 1–2 min; if a seizure is prolonged, recommend transportation to hospital; if a

short seizure has ended or other signs of a hypoglycemic crisis exist, recommend rubbing corn syrup or 50% dextrose on the buccal mucosa, followed by 2 mL/kg of the same solution orally once the patient can swallow; then, seek immediate attention.
• Initiate frequent feeding of a diet low in simple sugars or, if unable to eat, continuous fluid therapy with 2.5% dextrose.

Long-term Treatment
• See Insulinoma for treatment of insulinoma and extrapancreatic paraneoplasia.
• Hunting dog hypoglycemia—feed moderate meal of fat, protein, and complex carbohydrates a few hours before hunting; can feed snacks (e.g., dog biscuits) every 3–5 h during the hunt
• Toy-breed hypoglycemia—increase the frequency of feeding.
• Puppy and kitten hypoglycemia—increase the frequency of feeding (nursing or hand feeding).
• Other causes of hypoglycemia require treating the underlying disease and do not usually need long-term treatment.

CONTRAINDICATIONS
• Insulin
• Barbiturates and diazepam in patients with hypoglycemic seizures—they do not treat the cause of the seizure and they may worsen hepatoencephalopathy in patients with portosystemic shunt and cirrhosis.

PRECAUTIONS
• 50% dextrose causes tissue necrosis and sloughing if given extravascularly; never give dextrose in concentrations over 5% without confirmed vascular access.
• Administering a dextrose bolus without following with frequent feedings or continuous IV fluids with dextrose can predispose to subsequent hypoglycemic episodes.

POSSIBLE INTERACTIONS
N/A

ALTERNATIVE DRUGS
N/A

FOLLOW-UP

PATIENT MONITORING
• At home—for return or progression of clinical signs of hypoglycemia; assess serum glucose if signs recur.

• Single, intermittent serum glucose determinations may not truly reflect the glycemic status of the patient because of normal production of counterregulatory hormones.
• Other monitoring is based on the underlying disease.

POSSIBLE COMPLICATIONS
Recurrent, progressive episodes of hypoglycemia

MISCELLANEOUS

ASSOCIATED CONDITIONS
Prolonged hypoglycemia can cause transient (hours to days) to permanent blindness from laminar necrosis of the occipital cerebral cortex.

AGE-RELATED FACTORS
Neonatal animals have poor glycogen storage capacity and a reduced ability to perform gluconeogenesis; thus, short periods of fasting (6–12 h) can cause hypoglycemia.

ZOONOTIC POTENTIAL
N/A

PREGNANCY
• Hypoglycemia can lead to weakness and dystocia.
• Pregnancy coupled with fasting causes hypoglycemia in rare instances.

SYNONYMS
N/A

SEE ALSO
• See specific causes.
• Insulinoma

ABBREVIATIONS
• AIGR = amended insulin:glucose ratio
• PU/PD = polyuria and polydipsia

Suggested Reading
Leifer CE. Hypoglycemia. In: Kirk RW, ed. Current veterinary therapy IX. Philadelphia: Saunders, 1986:982–987.
Nelson RW. Disorders of the endocrine pancreas. In: Ettinger SJ, ed. Textbook of veterinary internal medicine. Philadelphia: Saunders, 1989:1676–1720.
Author Mitchell A. Crystal
Consulting Editor Deborah S. Greco

GLUCOSURIA

 BASICS

DEFINITION
Urinary glucose concentration detectable by routine laboratory tests. The small quantity of glucose normally present in urine is not detected by routine laboratory tests; persistent glucosuria is abnormal.

PATHOPHYSIOLOGY
• Should be categorized as hyperglycemic or normoglycemic, and subcategorized as transient or persistent. • Glucose passes readily through glomerular capillary walls and has the same concentration in glomerular filtrate and blood. It is reabsorbed at the luminal membrane of proximal renal tubular cells by secondary active transport coupled with sodium reabsorption. In this way, glucose attains a high intracellular concentration. It is then transported into renal interstitium through basolateral membranes by a sodium-independent mechanism and returned to the peripheral circulation via renal peritubular capillaries.

Hyperglycemic Glucosuria
Occurs when the concentration of glucose in glomerular filtrate exceeds the transport maximum of tubular epithelial cells; the renal tubular threshold for glucose in dogs is 170–220 mg/dL; for cats, 260–310 mg/dL as measured in venous blood. When hyperglycemia is observed, the next step is to determine whether it is transient or persistent.

Transient Glucosuria
• Physiologic glucosuria—typically transient; associated with increases of "stress" hormones (glucagon, catecholamines, glucocorticoids), particularly in cats • Pharmacologic (iatrogenic) glucosuria—transient; results from administration of parenteral solutions (e.g., dextrose, total parenteral nutrition solutions) that contain sufficient glucose; parenteral administration of glucocorticoids is an uncommonly recognized cause of glucosuria in dogs and cats. • Adrenocorticotropic hormone, glucagon, epinephrine, morphine, and phenothiazines also have the potential to cause transient glucosuria.

Persistent (or Pathologic) Glucosuria
• Patient may be normoglycemic or hyperglycemic. • Normoglycemic glucosuria—includes renal tubular dysfunction associated with generalized and specific reabsorptive defects of proximal nephrons; can be further subdivided into congenital or acquired proximal renal tubular defects • Primary renal glucosuria—a congenital disorder in Scottish terriers and mixed-breed dogs; associated with specific reabsorptive defects for glucose in proximal renal tubular cells • Fanconi's syndrome (aminodiabetes)—characterized by generalized proximal renal tubular defects associated with glucosuria, phosphaturia, and aminoaciduria; dogs may also have varying degrees of hypercalciuria, hyperbicarbonaturia, hypernatriuria, hyperkaliuria, and hyperuricuria. See section entitled "Fanconi's syndrome." • A congenital (juvenile) renal disease associated with renal tubular transport dysfunction has been reported in Norwegian elkhounds. • Congenital glomerular diseases reported in Doberman pinschers, cocker spaniels, and Samoyed dogs are typically not associated with proximal renal tubular defects and glucosuria. • Acquired normoglycemic glucosuria may also be associated with some forms of acute renal failure; not commonly observed in association with chronic renal failure. • Etiologic agents include heavy metal poisons (e.g., lead, mercury), drugs (e.g., gentamicin, cisplatin), and chemicals (e.g., Lysol, maleic acid). In humans, multiple myeloma may lead to development of acquired Fanconi's syndrome.

SYSTEMS AFFECTED
• Renal/Urologic—in normoglycemia glucosuria, renal tubular cells function is abnormal. Dogs with Fanconi's syndrome commonly develop CRF and secondary multisystem involvement. Glucosuria may also predispose to a bacterial urinary tract infection and associated manifestations. • Endocrine—diabetes mellitus and hyperadrenocorticism cause hyperglycemic glucosuria.

SIGNALMENT
• Persistent hyperglycemic glucosuria is usually caused by adult-onset diabetes mellitus. • Onset of clinical disease in dogs with Fanconi's syndrome typically occurs after they reach maturity. Defective reabsorption of glucose and amino acids is recognized at 4–5 years of age. There is no sex predilection for the disease. • Primary renal glucosuria is an incidental finding that can be recognized at an early age. • Familial tubular disorders have been reported in Basenjis, border terriers, and Scottish terriers, and in Norwegian elkhounds with generalized familial (juvenile) nephropathies.

SIGNS

General Comments
Clinical signs—vary; depend on the primary cause

Historical Findings
• If glucosuria is of sufficient magnitude, polyuria secondary to osmotic diuresis and compensatory polydipsia develop. • The frequency of occurrence of polyuria and polydipsia with primary renal glucosuria is unknown; there have been too few documented cases to formulate generalities. However, dogs with primary renal glucosuria may form less concentrated urine. • Urinary tract infections that develop secondary to disease associated with glucosuria, show signs typical of lower and/or upper urinary tract disease. • Breed and drug history are important.

Physical Examination Findings
• Hyperglycemic glucosuria may be associated with systemic signs. • Body systems are often normal in patients with normoglycemic glucosuria. • Dogs with Fanconi's syndrome may develop signs of renal failure.

CAUSES

Hyperglycemic Glucosuria
• Transient physiologic—stress hyperglycemia is common in cats. • Transient pharmacologic—parenteral solutions (e.g., dextrose, total parenteral nutrition solutions), xylazine in cats, glucocorticoids, ACTH, glucagon, epinephrine, morphine, phenothiazine, diazoxide, l-asparaginase • Persistent hyperglycemic glucosuria—diabetes mellitus (100%), hyperadrenocorticism (5–10%), acute pancreatitis, CNS lesions, pheochromocytoma, progesterone-associated hyperglycemia, acromegaly, sepsis, glucagonoma, chronic liver failure (failure to clear glucagon)

Normoglycemic Glucosuria
• Congenital normoglycemic glucosuria—primary renal glucosuria (Scottish terriers and mixed-breed dogs); congenital Fanconi's syndrome (basenjis, Norwegian elkhound, Shetland sheepdog, miniature schnauzer); congenital diseases associated with renal dysfunction (Norwegian elkhound) • Acquired normoglycemic glucosuria—acute renal failure associated with significant proximal tubular lesions; CRF (rare); acquired Fanconi's syndrome due to heavy metal poisoning (lead, mercury, cadmium, uranium), drugs (gentamicin, cephalosporins, outdated tetracycline, cisplatin, streptozotocin, amoxicillin) and chemicals (Lysol, maleic acid)

RISK FACTORS
Vary with causes

 DIAGNOSIS

DIFFERENTIAL DIAGNOSIS
• Fasted, persistent, hyperglycemic glucosuria is most often associated with endocrinopathies (e.g., diabetes mellitus, hyperadrenocorticism). • Normoglycemic glucosuria is associated with renal tubular reabsorptive dysfunctions. • Further diagnostic procedures are required to find the cause of glucosuria. • Expect mild transient hyperglycemia in stressed animals.

LABORATORY FINDINGS

Screening Tests
• Normally too little glucose is present in urine to be detected by routine laboratory tests. • Dipsticks and reagent tapes impregnated with glucose oxidase, peroxidase, and other reagents that result in color changes when glucose is present involve interrelated sequential bienzymatic reactions. Glucose oxidase reacts specifically with glucose; the enzyme will not

react with nonglucose-reducing substances. Drugs containing azo dyes, nitrofurantoin, and riboflavin, or other causes of severe pigmenturia (hemoglobinuria, bilirubinuria) may affect the readability of the reagent pad and lead to mis-interpretation. • False-positive results—contamination of the sample or test system with small quantities of hydrogen peroxide (0.006%), hydrochlorite, chlorine, or other strong oxidizing agents • False-negative results—(1) Ascorbic acid concentration as low as 50 mg/dL can prevent detection of low concentrations (50 or 100 mg/dL) of urine glucose by the glucose oxidase test. Ascorbic acid concentrations as high as 90 mg/dL have been detected in urine samples collected from dogs; as high as 50 mg/dL in cats with diabetes mellitus. Consumption of large amounts of ascorbic acid or salicylates (e.g., vitamin C supplements, tetracycline drugs because of ascorbic acid in formulation) may yield false-negative results. (2) Moderately high ketonuria (40 mg/dL) may cause false-negative results for specimens containing small amounts of glucose (75–125 mg/dl). (3) Refrigerated urine may reduce the rate of enzymatic activity in glucose oxidase/peroxidase tests. (4) Reactivity of the glucose test area for Multistix reagents may decrease with increasing specific gravity. (5) Outdated reagents or reagents exposed to sunlight may also give erratic results. • Colori-metric copper reduction methods are based on the change from cupric acid (blue) to cuprous oxide (orange-red). The color change (blue to green to orange) depends on the concentration of reducing compounds (including glucose) in urine. Copper reduction methods are not specific for glucose and are less sensitive than glucose oxidase methods. • False-positive results may be caused by (1) sufficient concentrations of nonglucose-reducing substances, including fructose, lactose, galactose, pentose, and maltose; (2) sufficient quantities of glucuronic acids (e.g., conjugated bilirubin); penicillin, salicylates, and chloral hydrate act as reducing substances; and (3) formaldehyde; (4) no ascorbic acid concentrations high enough to cause false-positive results with copper reduction techniques have been observed at the University of Minnesota.

Confirmation Testing
When unsuspected results or unusual test pad colors from highly pigmented urine occur, results can be confirmed by measuring glucose in the urine. Hexokinase- or glucose dehydrogenase–based techniques are recommended for quantitation of urinary glucose.

Drugs That May Alter Laboratory Results
See Laboratory Findings—Screening Tests.

Disorders That May Alter Laboratory Results
See Laboratory Findings—Screening Tests.

Valid If Run in Human Laboratory?
Yes

CBC/BIOCHEMISTRY/URINALYSIS
Hyperglycemic Glucosuria
• Detection of ketonuria, hyperglycemia, and glucosuria indicates diabetic ketoacidosis.
• Mild hyperglycemia with concomitant transient glucosuria is physiologic in stressed animals. • Inflammatory leukogram, high serum lipase, and amylase activity in gluco-suric dogs with adequate renal function supports a diagnosis of acute pancreatitis.
• High serum ALP activity in dogs with hyperglycemic glucosuria should prompt consideration of hyperadrenocorticism.

Normoglycemic Glucosuria
• Glucosuria is typically the only abnormal finding in dogs with normoglycemic primary renal glucosuria. • In other conditions associated with normoglycemic glucosuria, high serum urea nitrogen, creatinine, and phosphorus with impaired urine-concentrating ability suggests renal tubular dysfunction. Hyperchloremic metabolic acidosis may occur secondary to decreased bicarbonate resorption by proximal renal epithelial cells (renal tubular acidosis type 2). If progressive renal failure develops, characteristic clinical and laboratory findings will result.

OTHER LABORATORY TESTS
• Normoglycemic glucosuria—measurement of phosphorus, glucose, and amino acid concentrations in timed urine collections permits differentiation of Fanconi's syndrome and renal primary glucosuria. • Hyperglycemic glucosuria—ACTH response test or low-dose dexamethasone suppression test if suspect hyperadrenocorticism; see chapters related to specific cause.

IMAGING
Ultrasonography may be helpful in diagnosis of hyperadrenocorticism.

DIAGNOSTIC PROCEDURES
N/A

TREATMENT
• Discontinue any drugs associated with acquired tubular transport defects. • Treatment varies with cause; see relevant chapters.

MEDICATIONS
DRUGS OF CHOICE
• No specific drugs for glucose transport defects • Treat underlying disease when possible.

CONTRAINDICATIONS
Diabetogenic drugs (e.g., corticosteroids) or dextrose-containing fluids

PRECAUTIONS
N/A

POSSIBLE INTERACTIONS
N/A

ALTERNATIVE DRUGS
N/A

FOLLOW-UP
PATIENT MONITORING
Varies with cause

POSSIBLE COMPLICATIONS
• Persistent glucosuria is predisposing for development of cystitis, ascending pyelonephritis, and sepsis. • Osmotic diuresis with obligatory polyuria and secondary polydipsia

MISCELLANEOUS
ASSOCIATED CONDITIONS
Urinary tract infections

AGE-RELATED FACTORS
N/A

ZOONOTIC POTENTIAL
N/A

PREGNANCY
Diestrus in bitches may induce diabetes mellitus (noninsulin-dependent) caused by high progesterone concentration.

SYNONYMS
N/A

SEE ALSO
• Diabetes Mellitus, Uncomplicated • Fanconi's Syndrome • Hyperadrenocorticism • Renal Disease, Congenital and Developmental

ABBREVIATIONS
CRF = chronic renal failure

Suggested Reading
Brown SA. Fanconi's syndrome; inherited and acquired. In: Kirk RW, Current veterinary therapy X. Philadelphia: Saunders, 1989:1163–1165.
Finco DR. Congenital, inherited, and familial renal diseases. In: Osborne CA, Finco DR, eds. Canine and feline nephrology and urology. Baltimore: Williams & Wilkins, 1995: 1471–1483.
Meyers DJ, Harvey JW. Veterinary laboratory medicine interpretation and diagnosis. 2nd ed. Philadelphia: Saunders, 1998:221–237.
Authors Frédéric Jacob and Carl A. Osborne
Consulting Editors Larry G. Adams and Carl A. Osborne

DIAGNOSTICS—LAB

HEMOGLOBINURIA AND MYOGLOBINURIA

 BASICS

DEFINITION

Loss of sufficient hemoglobin or myoglobin through the glomeruli to cause a positive reaction to a test for blood in the urine when tested by the pseudophosphatase-orthotoluidine method

PATHOPHYSIOLOGY

• Intravascular hemolysis causes release of free hemoglobin into plasma. Hemoglobin forms a complex with hepatoglobin. Once heptoglobin is saturated, free hemoglobin appears in the blood, divides into subunits, and is cleared from the blood by the kidneys. Some unbound plasma hemoglobin releases ferriheme, which binds reversibly to either albumin (methemalbumin) or a plasma protein called hemopexin. Free hemoglobin, hemoglobin–heptoglobin complex, hemoglobin subunits, methemalbumin, ferriheme–hemopexin complex, and bilirubin all contribute to the color of plasma. Hemoglobin complexes in concentrations over about 50 mg/dL of plasma are detectable as pink plasma.
• Myoglobin released from damaged muscle is not associated with pink plasma because it does not bind to serum proteins and so is rapidly cleared by the liver and kidneys.
• Both hemoglobin and myoglobin are reabsorbed and metabolized by proximal renal tubule cells; these proteins only appear in urine after the renal tubular uptake mechanism is saturated.

SYSTEMS AFFECTED

• Renal/Urologic—hemoglobin and myoglobin can be nephrotoxic, particularly when renal perfusion is compromised.
• Hemic/Lymph/Immune—intravascular hemolysis, extensive muscle damage, and hypoxia can precipitate disseminated intravascular coagulopathy (DIC).
• Low oxygen-carrying capacity (acute) can lead to secondary central lobular liver cell damage, lactic acid acidosis, and shock, which in turn exacerbates hypoxia.

SIGNALMENT

• Copper-associated liver disease in the Bedlington and West Highland white terriers
• Exertional lactic acidosis in the Old English sheepdog—hemoglobinuria
• Exertional myopathy in the racing greyhound; hematuria should clear within 6–12 h; if not, suspect myoglobinuria from muscle damage
• Neonatal isoerythrolysis (blood type A queen with type B kitten) in the British shorthair, Doven rex, Abyssinian, Birman, Himalayan, Persian, Scottish fold, and Somali breeds; neonates die within 2 days of birth.
• Phosphofructokinase deficiency in the English springer spaniel male
• Pyruvate kinase deficiency in the basenji and beagle; affected dogs <3 years old

SIGNS

General Comments

A wide variety of clinical signs are associated with specific causes; see Causes.

Historical Findings

Breed and drug treatment history are particularly important. See Signalment.

Physical Examination Findings

• Signs associated with anemia, such as tachycardia, lethargy, pale mucous membranes, fever, and icterus, are not seen in patients with muscle damage or hematuria.
• Fever may be associated with intravascular hemolysis.
• DIC secondary to intravascular hemolysis or muscle trauma may induce hematuria.
• Patients with muscle damage have muscle tenderness or bruising.

CAUSES

Hemoglobinuria

• Genetic associated—pyruvate kinase deficiency, phosphofructokinase deficiency, exertional lactic acidosis in the Old English sheepdog, copper-associated liver disease
• Toxins and drugs—chlorates, benzocaine, copper, DMSO, menadione (vitamin K_3), mercury, methylene blue, nitrates, methionine, phenazopyridine, paracetamol (acetaminophen), phenylhydrazine, propylene glycol, propylthiouracil, snake venom (Elapidae), zinc
• Plants—Onions
• Physical agents—burns (severe), crush injury, electric shock, extreme exercise, heatstroke, hypoosmotic solution, microangiopathy (e.g., caval syndrome and DIC)
• Infectious agents—Babesiasis (i.e., *B. canis* but usually not *B. gibsoni* or *B. vogeli*), feline hemobartonellosis (rarely causes intravascular hemolysis), leptospirosis (i.e., *L. icterohemorhagica*)
• Immune-mediated—idiopathic immune-mediated hemolytic anemia, incompatible blood transfusion, isoerythrolysis–blood type A queen with type B kittens, systemic lupus erythematosus
• Deficiencies—hypophosphatemia (induced by hyperalimentation or diabetes mellitus)

Myoglobinuria

• Acute myositis (e.g., toxoplasmosis)
• Compartment syndrome
• Crush injury
• Extreme exercise
• Tourniquet syndrome
• Prolonged seizures

RISK FACTORS

• Genetic predisposition (see Signalment)
• Exposure to selected drugs and toxins (e.g., zinc cage bolts and copper and zinc coins)
• Extreme physical exertion

 DIAGNOSIS

DIFFERENTIAL DIAGNOSIS

• Common urine reagent strip tests for blood are designed to detect RBCs, hemoglobin, or myoglobin that is not visible to the human eye.
• RBCs or ghost cells in the sediment suggest hematuria.
• Clear plasma suggests myoglobinuria or hematuria.
• Pink plasma with urine positive for occult blood suggests intravascular hemolysis.
• Chocolate-colored whole blood and urine positive for occult blood suggests hemolyzing, methemoglobin-producing toxins (oxidants).
• Hemoglobinuria without icterus suggests acute hemolytic anemia; both findings suggest chronic hemolytic anemia.

HEMOGLOBINURIA AND MYOGLOBINURIA

- Icterus without hemoglobinuria suggests extravascular hemolysis or liver disease.
- False-positive results (see below)

LABORATORY FINDINGS

Drugs That May Alter Laboratory Results

- Administration of substantial doses of vitamin C (ascorbic aid) may cause false-negative results with reagent test strips; newer generations of reagent strips are more resistant to interference by reducing substances such as ascorbic acid.
- Resuscitation fluids containing polymerized hemoglobin may give false-positive results.

Disorders That May Alter Laboratory Results

- Low urinary specific gravity (polyuric syndromes) lyses RBCs.
- Bacteriuria (bacterial peroxidase) causes false-positive test results.
- Formalin preservative causes false-negative results.

Valid If Run in Human Laboratory?
Yes

CBC/BIOCHEMISTRY/URINALYSIS

- Intravascular hemolysis
- Low and falling PCV, often accompanied by leukocytosis
- Blood smear evaluation—possibly spherocytes, parasites, and Heinz bodies
- Bilirubinemia and high alanine ALT activity
- Bilirubinuria
- Rhabdomyolysis
- High creatine kinase activity
- High aspartate transaminase (AST) activity

OTHER LABORATORY TESTS

- Ammonium sulfate precipitation test—mix 5 mL of urine well with 2.8 mg of ammonium sulfate and centrifuge. Hemoglobin precipitates, myoglobin does not. If the supernatant remains dark after centrifugation, suspect myoglobinuria.
- New methylene blue–stained blood film to detect Heinz bodies
- Methemoglobin in RBCs helps identify toxin as an oxidant.
- Haptoglobin concentration is low if the patient has acute or chronic progressive intravascular hemolysis.
- Serum copper and zinc concentrations

IMAGING

- Abdominal radiography or ultrasonography may reveal coins or cage bolts or nuts in the gastrointestinal tract.
- Abnormal liver size and conformation in patients with copper-associated liver disease

DIAGNOSTIC PROCEDURES

- Forced exercise (Old English sheepdog)
- Liver biopsy for copper concentration (copper-associated liver disease)
- Bone marrow biopsy (pyruvate kinase and phosphofructokinase deficiencies)

TREATMENT

- Copious amounts of fluids to maintain renal function, especially in the face of shock; lactated Ringer's solution or isotonic saline if the patient is dehydrated; maintenance fluids if not
- Exercise-induced hematuria has a benign, self-limiting course.
- Avoid stress and excitement if the patient has anemia or copper-associated liver disease.
- Avoid hyperventilation if the patient has phosphofructokinase deficiency.
- See suspected causes for specific treatment.

MEDICATIONS

DRUGS OF CHOICE
Vary with underlying cause

CONTRAINDICATIONS
See list of causes for contraindicated drugs.

PRECAUTIONS
N/A

POSSIBLE INTERACTIONS
N/A

ALTERNATIVE DRUGS
N/A

FOLLOW-UP

PATIENT MONITORING
PCV, pO_2, urinalysis, serum creatinine, and ALT (copper-associated liver disease)

POSSIBLE COMPLICATIONS
Renal damage (failure) can develop, especially in association with shock.

MISCELLANEOUS

ASSOCIATED CONDITIONS
N/A

AGE-RELATED FACTORS
Neonatal isoerythrolysis

ZOONOTIC POTENTIAL
- Leptospirosis
- Toxoplasmosis

PREGNANCY
N/A

SYNONYMS
- Hemosiderinuria
- Pigmenturia

SEE ALSO
See Causes.

ABBREVIATIONS
- ALT = alanine aminotransferase
- AST = aspartate aminotransferase
- DIC = disseminated intravascular coagulopathy
- DMSO = dimethyl sulfoxide
- PCV = packed cell volume

Suggested Reading

Ettinger S, ed. Textbook of veterinary internal medicine: disease of the dog and cat. 4th ed. Philadelphia: Saunders, 1995.

Jain NC, ed. Schalm's veterinary hematology. 4th ed. Philadelphia: Lea & Febiger, 1986.

Kaneko JJ, ed. Clinical biochemistry of domestic animals. 4th ed. San Diego: Academic Press, 1989.

Osborne CO, Stevens JB. Handbook of canine & feline urinalysis. St. Louis: Ralston Purina, 1981.

Sherding RG, ed. The cat: diseases and clinical management. 2nd ed. New York: Churchill Livingstone, 1994.

Authors Jerry B. Stevens and Carl A. Osborne

Consulting Editors Carl A. Osborne and Larry G. Adams

DIAGNOSTICS—LAB

HIGH-DOSE DEXAMETHASONE SUPPRESSION TEST AND PLASMA ACTH LEVELS

BASICS

DEFINITION
Tests used to differentiate PDH from hyper-adrenocorticism due to cortisol-secreting AT; not used to diagnose HAC

PATHOPHYSIOLOGY
• A high dose of dexamethasone (0.1 or 1.0 mg/kg administered IV or IM, depending on the laboratory used) will, through negative feedback, shut off ACTH production in most (75–80%) animals with PDH, with a subsequent decrease in serum cortisol concentration.
• Cortisol secretion by ATs is autonomous; cortisol levels are not suppressed following administration of high doses of dexamethasone.
• Plasma ACTH levels are high normal-to-increased in PDH and undetectable-to-low in AT, although in rare cases overlap can be seen unless multiple samples are evaluated.

SYSTEMS AFFECTED
Typical of HAC

SIGNALMENT
Species
Can be used in both dogs and cats

SIGNS
Typical of HAC

General Comments
• Follow your laboratory's protocol for performance and interpretation of these tests.
• Adding aprotonin before collecting samples for ACTH greatly simplifies handling the samples.

Historical Findings
Typical of HAC

Physical Examination Findings
Typical of HAC

CAUSES
• PDH
• Cortisol-secreting AT

RISK FACTORS
N/A

DIAGNOSIS

DIFFERENTIAL DIAGNOSIS
• PDH
• Cortisol-secreting AT

LABORATORY FINDINGS
• High-dose dexamethasone suppression test—suppression of serum cortisol levels below 1.5 μg/dL at 8 h excludes an adrenal tumor; failure to suppress means an approximately 50/50 chance of the patient having an adrenal tumor versus nonsuppressible PDH; use of an absolute cutoff value of 8 h is recommended; use of percentage suppression does not appear to be as accurate.
• ACTH levels—normal-to-elevated levels are consistent with PDH; undetectable-to-low levels are consistent with AT.

CBC/BIOCHEMISTRY/URINALYSIS
N/A

OTHER LABORATORY TESTS
N/A

Drugs That May Alter Laboratory Results
N/A

Disorders That May Alter Laboratory Results
N/A

Valid If Run in Human Laboratory?
N/A

IMAGING
• Recommended to back up results; necessary if test is inconclusive
• Use of ultrasound, CT, or MRI preferred

DIAGNOSTIC PROCEDURES
N/A

TREATMENT

Usually outpatient unless serious complications of HAC present

HIGH-DOSE DEXAMETHASONE SUPPRESSION TEST AND PLASMA ACTH LEVELS

MEDICATIONS

DRUGS OF CHOICE
- Lysodren, ketoconazole, or *l*-deprenyl for PDH
- Surgery, Lysodren, or ketoconazole for AT (see section on HAC)

CONTRAINDICATIONS
N/A

PRECAUTIONS
Rare adverse reaction to high doses of dexamethasone

POSSIBLE INTERACTIONS
N/A

ALTERNATE DRUGS
N/A

FOLLOW-UP

PATIENT MONITORING
See section on HAC.

POSSIBLE COMPLICATIONS
Depend on underlying disorder

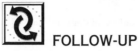

MISCELLANEOUS

ASSOCIATED CONDITIONS
See section on HAC.

AGE-RELATED FACTORS
N/A

ZOONOTIC POTENTIAL
N/A

PREGNANCY
N/A

SYNONYMS
N/A

SEE ALSO
N/A

ABBREVIATIONS
- AT = adrenocortical tumors
- HAC = hyperadrenocorticism
- PDH = pituitary-dependent hyperadrenocorticism

Suggested Reading
Guptill L, Scott-Moncrieff JC, Widmer WR. Diagnosis of canine hyperadrenocorticism. Vet Clin North Am 1997;27(2):215–236.

Kintzer PP, Peterson ME. Diagnosis and management of canine cortisol-secreting adrenal tumors. Vet Clin North Am. 1997.

Peterson ME. Hyperadrenocorticism. In: Kirk RW, ed. Current veterinary therapy IX. Philadelphia: Saunders, 1986.

Author Peter P. Kintzer

Consulting Editor Deborah S. Greco

DIAGNOSTICS—LAB

HYPERCAPNIA

 BASICS

DEFINITION
• An increase in the partial pressure of carbon dioxide in the arterial blood
• Normal $PaCO_2$ values—35–45 mm Hg

PATHOPHYSIOLOGY
• CO_2—end product of aerobic cellular metabolism; considered the primary drive to ventilation by stimulation of central chemoreceptors in the medulla oblongata; carried in the blood in three forms: bicarbonate (65%), bound to hemoglobin (30%), and dissolved in plasma (5%; the source of $PaCO_2$ values); constantly being added to alveolar gas from the pulmonary circulation and removed by alveolar ventilation
• Uncommon in nonanesthetized, clinically normal patient; result of alveolar hypoventilation

SYSTEMS AFFECTED
• Nervous—the brain is primary affected organ; cerebral blood flow related to $PaCO_2$ in a linear fashion; results in increased cerebral blood flow and intracranial pressure; $PaCO_2$ > 90 mm Hg may lead to CO_2 narcosis and unconsciousness.
• Hemic/Lymphatic/Immune—may alter acid–base balance; acute increase results in production of excess hydrogen ions and a decrease in pH (respiratory acidosis)
• Cardiovascular—may result in endogenous catecholamine release, which may induce cardiac arrhythmias

SIGNALMENT
Any breed, age, and sex of dogs and cats

SIGNS

Historical Findings
• Abnormal breathing pattern
• Weakness—secondary to concurrent hypoxemia or primary neuromuscular disease

Physical Examination Findings
• Anesthetized patients—usually no obvious signs; severe condition may lead to tachypnea
• Hypoventilation owing to muscle weakness or neuropathy—weak respiratory efforts; decreased thoracic excursion; possibly generalized weakness
• Upper airway obstruction—marked, prolonged inspiratory efforts with variable expirations, depending on whether the obstruction is fixed (e.g., mass) or nonfixed (e.g., laryngeal paralysis); stertor or stridor common
• Pleural effusion—may have shallow rapid respirations; may note a marked abdominal component; lung sounds normal to decreased

CAUSES
• Hypoventilation—an increase in $PaCO_2$ that results from a decrease in alveolar ventilation; owing to anesthesia, muscular paralysis, upper airway obstruction, air or fluid in the pleural space, restriction in movement of the thoracic cage, diaphragmatic hernia, pulmonary parenchymal disease, and CNS disease
• Spontaneously breathing patients during inhalation anesthesia (isoflurane or halothane)
• Increased inspired CO_2—rebreathing of expired gases because of exhausted CO_2 absorbent in an anesthesia machine most common cause; also inadequate fresh gas flow in a nonrebreathing anesthesia circuit (e.g., Bain and Ayres T-piece)
• Exogenous administration of sodium bicarbonate, which dissociates into CO_2, with inadequate ventilation

RISK FACTORS
• Deep planes of inhalation anesthesia
• Inadequate fresh gas flow of oxygen with nonrebreathing anesthesia circuits
• Bronchial or alveolar disease
• Upper airway obstruction
• Pleural disease
• Inadequate ventilation during administration of sodium bicarbonate

 DIAGNOSIS

DIFFERENTIAL DIAGNOSIS
• Conscious patient with tachypnea—excitement or anxiety; hyperthermia; hypoxemia; head trauma; pain
• Anesthetized patient with tachypnea—light plane of anesthesia; hypoxemia

LABORATORY FINDINGS

Drugs That May Alter Laboratory Results
N/A

Disorders That May Alter Laboratory Results
Air bubbles in the arterial blood sample and/or improper packaging of the arterial blood sample—falsely low $PaCO_2$ values after approximately 30 min

Valid If Run in Human Laboratory?
Yes

CBC/BIOCHEMISTRY/URINALYSIS
N/A

OTHER LABORATORY TESTS
• Arterial blood gas analysis—diagnosis determined from a blood sample collected in an anaerobic manner
• Use enough heparin to coat the needle and the inside of the syringe; place a rubber stopper on the needle or cover the hub of the syringe to prevent room air from entering the sample.
• Analyze sample within 15 min if left at room temperature; place sample on ice to extend time for safe and accurate analysis to 2–4 hr.

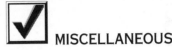

- Bedside or portable blood gas analyzers—several models available; make analysis more convenient

IMAGING
Thoracic radiography—may reveal bronchial, alveolar, or pleural space disease

OTHER DIAGNOSTIC PROCEDURES
- Alternative method of analysis—capnometer
- End tidal gas is almost entirely alveolar gas and provides nearly the same value as $PaCO_2$, which closely approximates the mean value of perfused alveoli
- Exception—during conditions of pulmonary thromboembolism, $PaCO_2$ much higher than $PETCO_2$
- Advantage of capnometry—may monitor $PaCO_2$ on a breath-by-breath basis, whereas a blood gas sample is a finite value at a finite time.

TREATMENT
- Provide adequate alveolar ventilation—most important
- Anesthesia—ventilation accomplished manually or mechanically
- Nonanesthetized patient with severe pulmonary or CNS disease—mechanical ventilation requires heavy sedation, muscle relaxants, or general anesthesia
- Supplemental oxygen—need determined by primary disease
- Definitive treatment—treat primary cause (e.g., discontinuing inhalation anesthesia is the definitive treatment for anesthesia-induced hypoventilation)

MEDICATIONS

DRUGS
- Respiratory stimulants (e.g., doxapram)—may administer; rarely indicated
- Doxapram—nonspecific stimulant of the respiratory center; does not provide definitive treatment; administer only as an infusion (just 1 bolus will increase ventilation and lower $PaCO_2$, decreasing the drive of ventilation and causing apnea).

CONTRAINDICATIONS
Anesthetic drugs or other respiratory depressants—contraindicated with CNS disease if adequate ventilatory support cannot be provided; increased $PaCO_2$ may result in dangerous elevations of intracranial pressure and predispose patient to herniation of the brainstem.

PRECAUTIONS
N/A

POSSIBLE INTERACTIONS
N/A

ALTERNATIVE DRUGS
N/A

FOLLOW-UP

PATIENT MONITORING
- Assess effectiveness of supportive (ventilation) and definitive treatment—decrease in respiratory effort
- Re-evaluate the arterial blood gas or capnometry—determine improvement; assess adequacy of ventilation

POSSIBLE COMPLICATIONS
- Concurrent CNS disease—may cause high intracranial pressure and predispose the patient to herniation of the brainstem and death.

MISCELLANEOUS

ASSOCIATED CONDITIONS
N/A

AGE-RELATED FACTORS
N/A

ZOONOTIC POTENTIAL
N/A

PREGNANCY
N/A

SYNONYMS
Hypercarbia

SEE ALSO
Dyspnea, Tachypnea, and Panting

ABBREVIATION
- $ETCO_2$ = end tidal carbon dioxide

Suggested Reading

Benumof JL. Respiratory physiology and respiratory function during anesthesia. In: Miller RD, ed. Anesthesia. 3rd ed. New York: Churchill Livingstone, 1990:529–532.
Nunn JE. Applied respiratory physiology. 3rd ed. London: Butterworths, 1987:207–226.
Author Thomas Kevin Day
Consulting Editor Eleanor C. Hawkins

HYPOSTHENURIA

BASICS

DEFINITION
Urinary specific gravity between 1.000 and 1.006

PATHOPHYSIOLOGY
The ability to concentrate urine normally (dogs, >1.030; cats, >1.035) depends on a complex interaction between ADH, the protein receptor for ADH on the renal tubule, and a hypertonic renal medullary interstitium; interference with the synthesis, release, or actions of ADH, damage to the renal tubule, and altered tonicity of the medullary interstitium (medullary washout) can cause hyposthenuria.

SYSTEMS AFFECTED
Depends on the underlying disorder

GENETICS
N/A

INCIDENCE
N/A

GEOGRAPHIC DISTRIBUTION
N/A

SIGNALMENT
Dogs and cats

Breed Predilection
None

Predominant Sex
None

Mean Age and Range
None

SIGNS
• Polyuria and polydipsia
• Urinary incontinence—occasional
• Other signs depend on the underlying disorder.

CAUSES
Any disorder or drug that interferes with the release or action of ADH, damages the renal tubule, causes medullary washout, or causes a primary thirst disorder (see Differential Diagnosis)

RISK FACTORS
N/A

DIAGNOSIS

DIFFERENTIAL DIAGNOSIS
• Pyometra
• Cushing's disease
• Diabetes insipidus
• Pyelonephritis
• Hypercalcemia
• Early renal failure
• Primary liver disease
• Hypokalemia
• Hypoadrenocorticism
• Primary polydipsia—compulsive water drinking

LABORATORY FINDINGS

Drugs That May Alter Laboratory Results
Cortisone, lithium, demeclocycline, methoxyflurane, thiazide diuretics, and intravenous administration of fluids can all lower urine specific gravity into the hyposthenuric range.

Disorders That May Alter Laboratory Results
N/A

Valid If Run in a Human Laboratory?
Yes

CBC/BIOCHEMISTRY/URINALYSIS
• Low urinary specific gravity (1.000 to 1.006), other abnormalities may point to the underlying cause.
• High serum ALP activity suggests hyperadrenocorticism or primary liver disease.
• High cholesterol common in patients with hyperadrenocorticism
• Leukocytosis with a left shift in some patients with pyometra or pyelonephritis
• Hyperkalemia and hyponatremia suggest hypoadrenocorticism.
• Low serum potassium confirms hypokalemia.
• Inflammatory sediment or bacteriuria consistent with pyelonephritis
• Proteinuria common in patients with pyelonephritis, pyometra, and hyperadreno-corticism

OTHER LABORATORY TESTS
ACTH levels to determine the cause of hyperadrenocorticism (i.e., pituitary dependent versus adrenal tumor)

IMAGING
• Radiography to assess renal size and shape and to detect calcified adrenal tumor or large uterus
• Intravenous pyelogram to help diagnose pyelonephritis

• Ultrasonography to assess adrenal size, renal and hepatic size and architecture, and uterine size
• MRI or CT scan to assess a pituitary or hypothalamic mass that may be the cause of central diabetes insipidus or hyperadrenocorticism

DIAGNOSTIC PROCEDURES

• ACTH stimulation test to screen for hyperadrenocorticism and hypoadrenocorticism
• Low-dose dexamethasone suppression test and urine/cortisol creatinine test to screen for hyperadrenocorticism
• Serum bile acids to evaluate liver function
• **Note:** dogs with hyperadrenocorticism often have mildly high bile acids.
• Modified water deprivation test to differentiate diabetes insipidus from psychogenic polydipsia; see Appendix for test protocol.

PATHOLOGIC FINDINGS
N/A

TREATMENT

• Depends on the underlying disorder
• Do not restrict patient's water intake unless appropriate to the definitive diagnosis.
• Depends on the underlying disorder

MEDICATIONS

DRUGS OF CHOICE
Depends on the underlying disorder

CONTRAINDICATIONS
N/A

PRECAUTIONS
N/A

POSSIBLE INTERACTIONS
N/A

ALTERNATE DRUGS
N/A

FOLLOW-UP

PATIENT MONITORING
Urine specific gravity, hydration status, renal function, and electrolytes

POSSIBLE COMPLICATIONS
Dehydration

MISCELLANEOUS

ASSOCIATED CONDITIONS
See Differential Diagnosis

AGE-RELATED FACTORS
N/A

ZOONOTIC POTENTIAL
N/A

PREGNANCY
N/A

SYNONYMS
N/A

SEE ALSO
• Hyperadrenocorticism
• Diabetes Insipidus

ABBREVIATIONS
• ACTH = adrenocorticotrophic hormone
• ADH = antidiuretic hormone
• ALP = alkaline phosphatase
• CT = computed tomography
• MRI = magnetic resonance imaging

Suggested Reading
DiBartola SP. Fluid therapy in small animal practice. Philadelphia: Saunders, 1992.
Rose DB. Clinical physiology of acid-base and electrolyte disorders. 3rd ed. New York: McGraw-Hill, 1989.
Author Rhett Nichols
Consulting Editor Deborah S. Greco

HYPOXEMIA

 BASICS

DEFINITION
• A decrease in PaO_2, resulting in marked desaturation of hemoglobin
• Clinically significant desaturation of hemoglobin begins at a $PaO_2 < 60$ mm Hg.

PATHOPHYSIOLOGY
Six physiologic causes—(1) low FIO_2; (2) hypoventilation (increase in $PaCO_2$); (3) mismatching of alveolar ventilation and perfusion so that areas of the lung that are not ventilated properly are still perfused adequately; (4) alveolar–capillary membrane diffusion defect; (5) right-to-left cardiac or pulmonary shunting; (6) low cardiac output

SYSTEMS AFFECTED
• All organs—oxygen essential for normal cellular function; individual tissue oxygen requirements vary by organ.
• Nervous—brain and CNS most important; may result in irreversible brain damage
• Cardiovascular—may result in focal or global ischemia; if prolonged, may develop arrhythmias and cardiac failure

SIGNALMENT
Any breed, age, and sex of dogs and cats

SIGNS

Historical Findings
• Episodes of coughing
• Breathing problems—especially open-mouth breathing
• Trauma
• Gagging
• Exercise intolerance
• Cyanosis
• Collapse

Physical Examination Findings
• Tachypnea
• Dyspnea
• Orthopnea
• Pale mucous membranes
• Cyanosis
• Coughing
• Open-mouth breathing
• Tachycardia
• Poor peripheral pulse
• Abnormal thoracic auscultation

CAUSES
• Low FIO_2—high altitude (the higher the elevation, the lower the FIO_2); suffocation; enclosure in small areas with improper ventilation
• Hypoventilation—result of inadequate alveolar ventilation; muscular paralysis; upper airway obstruction; air or fluid in the pleural space; restriction of the thoracic cage, diaphragmatic hernia; pulmonary parenchymal disease; CNS disease
• Mismatching of alveolar ventilation and perfusion—usually during anesthesia or prolonged recumbency in which a large area of lung becomes atelectatic; pulmonary edema; pulmonary thromboembolism; pulmonary parenchymal disease (infectious or neoplastic); lower airway disease; pneumonia; pulmonary contusions
• Alveolar–capillary membrane diffusion defect—rarely clinically important
• Right-to-left cardiac or pulmonary shunting—tetralogy of Fallot; ventricular septal defect; reversed patent ductus arteriosus; intrapulmonary arteriovenous shunt
• Low cardiac output—cardiac failure from any cause; shock from any cause

RISK FACTORS
• Sudden move to higher elevations
• Bronchial disease—chronic obstructive pulmonary disease; feline asthma
• Trauma
• Bronchopneumonia
• Pleural disease
• Anesthesia
• Cardiac disease
• Geriatric pulmonary or cardiac changes

DIAGNOSIS

DIFFERENTIAL DIAGNOSIS
• Signs of tachypnea and/or dyspnea
• Excitement or anxiety
• Hyperthermia
• Pyrexia
• Head trauma
• Pain

LABORATORY FINDINGS

Drugs That May Alter Laboratory Results
N/A

Disorders That May Alter Laboratory Results
• Air bubbles in the arterial blood sample—falsely high PaO_2 values

• Improper packaging of the arterial blood sample—falsely high PaO_2 values after approximately 30 min at room temperature

Valid If Run in Human Laboratory?
Yes

CBC/BIOCHEMISTRY/URINALYSIS
PCV—may be high with chronic condition; may be low if inflammatory cause

OTHER LABORATORY TESTS

Arterial Blood Gases
• Collect arterial blood sample in an anaerobic manner.
• Use enough heparin to coat the needle and the inside of the syringe.
• Place a rubber stopper on the needle or covering the hub of the syringe to prevent room air from entering the sample.
• Analyze sample within 15 min if left at room temperature; place sample on ice to extend safe time for analysis to 24 hr
• Bedside or portable blood gas analyzers—several models available; make analysis more convenient

IMAGING
Thoracic radiographs and echocardiography—evaluate intrathoracic disease; differentiate pulmonary and cardiac disease.

DIAGNOSTIC PROCEDURES

Pulse Oximetry
• Indirectly determines SaO_2; relation between PaO_2 and SaO_2 based on the oxyhemoglobin dissociation curve: $SaO_2 > 90\%$ when $PaO_2 > 60$ mm Hg
• $SaO_2 < 85\%$–90%—considered abnormal
• Best results when probe used on the tongue of animals; thus may be limited to anesthetized, heavily sedated, or seriously ill patients with a low level of consciousness; keep tongue moistened for most accurate readings
• Other successful probe sites—ear; vulva (female) and prepuce (male); skin between toes; thin skin in the flank area
• Poor results—least accurate in low-flow states such as hypotension (global low flow) or hypothermia (low flow to skin); falsely low values (usually $< 85\%$) during carboxyhemoglobinemia (smoke inhalation)
• Rectal probes—should become available; will allow readings in awake patients

TREATMENT

• Must identify and correct the primary cause

Oxygen Therapy

• Most common supportive treatment
• Corrects low-inspired oxygen, hypoventilation, and alveolar–capillary membrane diffusion defects; may not always correct mismatching of ventilation and perfusion; often does not correct right-to-left cardiac or pulmonary shunts and low cardiac output
• May not be completely beneficial until adequate blood volume is established
• Delivery—directly from an oxygen source from the anesthetic machine via a face mask placed securely around the muzzle; from an E-tank fitted with an oxygen regulator through a face mask, intranasal catheter, or oxygen cage
• Increase in FIO_2—determined by the oxygen flow rate and the amount of oxygen mixed with room air
• PPV—may be needed for ARDS or severe hypoventilation

Fluid Therapy

• Low cardiac output—fluid administration and inotropic support (e.g., dobutamine or dopamine) important
• Cardiac failure—requires aggressive medical treatment; diuretics; afterload and preload reduction; inotropic support; oxygen administration; fluids indicated after institution of primary treatment; use caution with type and rate of fluids after initial stabilization
• Hypovolemic, hemorrhagic, traumatic, or septic shock—requires aggressive fluid administration; crystalloids (90 mL/kg as fast as possible), hypertonic solutions (7% NaCl, 4 mL/kg), colloids (hetastarch, 20 mL/kg), or combination
• Severe pulmonary contusion—hypertonic fluids, colloids, or combination preferred

 MEDICATIONS

DRUGS

Bronchospasm—bronchodilators; aminophylline (dogs, 10 mg/kg PO, slow IV q8h; cats, 6.6 mg/kg PO, slow IV q12h); terbutaline (dogs, 0.02 mg/kg SC q8h; cats 0.1 mg/cat SC q12h)

CONTRAINDICATIONS

• Aggressive fluid administration—not indicated for cardiac failure and pulmonary edema
• Diuretics—not indicated for shock, low FIO_2, alveolar–capillary membrane diffusion defects, mismatching of alveolar ventilation and perfusion, and right-to-left shunts

PRECAUTIONS

• Inotropic drugs—arrhythmias may develop.
• Oxygen toxicity—from prolonged (> 12 hr) exposure to high-concentration (> 70%) oxygen; pulmonary edema, seizures, and death

POSSIBLE INTERACTIONS

N/A

ALTERNATIVE DRUGS

N/A

 FOLLOW-UP

PATIENT MONITORING

• Decrease in respiratory effort and a decrease in cyanosis (if initially noted)—efficacy of treatment and support
• Arterial blood gas—determine resolution
• Pulse oximetry—alternative; interpret results cautiously with hypotension, hypothermia, smoke inhalation, and nontongue probe site.

POSSIBLE COMPLICATIONS

• Brain damage—depends on severity and duration; partial or complete loss of neuronal function; dementia; seizures; loss of consciousness
• Arrhythmias—may develop secondary to myocardial hypoxia; may be very difficult to treat effectively

 MISCELLANEOUS

ASSOCIATED CONDITIONS
N/A

AGE-RELATED FACTORS
N/A

ZOONOTIC POTENTIAL
N/A

PREGNANCY
May adversely affect fetuses, especially during the first trimester of pregnancy

SEE ALSO
• Cyanosis
• Dyspnea, Tachypnea, and Panting
• See also Causes

ABBREVIATIONS
• ARDS = acute respiratory distress syndrome
• PCV = packed cell volume
• PPV = positive pressure ventilation

Suggested Reading

Benumof JL. Respiratory physiology and respiratory function during anesthesia. In: Miller RD, ed. Anesthesia. 3rd ed. New York: Churchill Livingstone, 1990:529–532.
Nunn JE. Applied respiratory physiology. 3rd ed. London: Butterworths, 1987.
Taylor AE, Rehder K, Hyatt RE, Parker JC. Clinical respiratory physiology. Philadelphia: Saunders, 1989:157–158.
Author Thomas Kevin Day
Consulting Editor Eleanor C. Hawkins

LACTIC ACIDOSIS (HYPERLACTATEMIA)

BASICS

DEFINITION
• Hyperlactatemia—serum lactate concentration > 1.5 mmol/L for dogs; no reported lactate kinetics for cats
• Lactic acidosis—hyperlactatemia with an arterial pH below the normal range

PATHOPHYSIOLOGY
• Lactic acid is the end product of both aerobic and anaerobic glucose metabolism; at physiological pH, lactic acid immediately dissociates to lactate and hydrogen ion; small amounts of lactate are formed daily in healthy individuals, but clinically significant lactate accumulation is from anaerobic glycolysis. Lactic acid is produced during normal physiologic processes (e.g., exercise) and during pathologic processes (e.g., shock).
• Cori cycle—the preferred route of lactate use by the liver and kidneys; helps maintain the balance between lactate production and clearance, while providing a consistent source of glucose to critical tissues such as the brain and red blood cells, which preferentially use glucose; important in maintaining acid–base balance because the hydrogen ion produced during lactic acid dissociation is used during gluconeogenesis
• In most critically ill patients, hyperlactatemia and lactic acidosis are due to conditions that induce tissue hypoxia, with the shift to anaerobic glycolysis.
• Inadequate perfusion, severe hypoxemia, increased oxygen demands, decreased hemoglobin concentration, or combinations of these factors cause tissue hypoxia.
• Depending on the duration and severity of hypoxia, hyperlactatemia and possibly lactic acidosis may develop.
• Hyperlactatemia generally develops when tissue perfusion is adequate and acid–base buffering systems are intact.
• Clinically evident tissue hypoperfusion does not usually occur in patients with hyperlactatemia alone, but "occult" hypoperfusion may be present that is not detectable by routine monitoring and may represent a precursor phase to overt hypoperfusion.
• Lactic acidosis is usually present in association with abnormal metabolic regulation secondary to marked tissue hypoxia and hypoperfusion, certain drugs or toxins, or congenital defects in carbohydrate metabolism; buffering systems usually cannot cope with the developing acidosis.
• The severity of hyperlactatemia and acidosis that develops in critically ill patients with inadequate tissue perfusion and oxygen delivery or inadequate oxygen uptake reflects the severity of tissue hypoxia; thus evaluation of lactate levels in these patients helps in assessing the degree of tissue hypoperfusion and hypoxia.
• Studies in human trauma and shock patients demonstrate that lactate predicts outcome and that mortality is correlated with the severity of the lactic acidosis: the higher the lactate level, the greater the mortality.
• Lactate measurement allows reliable assessment of the response by critically ill or injured people to initial and continuing resuscitative therapy.
• Lactate concentrations are increased in critically ill and injured dogs; and an apparent association exists between severity of increased lactate concentrations and outcome and differences in lactate concentrations between varying disease states and injury types (seizures, ethylene glycol and aspirin intoxication, and major trauma).
• Numerous clinical and experimental studies in critically ill human patients and recent results in critically ill and injured dogs clearly show blood lactate measurement to be a useful tool for assessing the severity of tissue hypoxia and the response to therapy and a prognostic tool for outcome.

SYSTEMS AFFECTED
• Persistent lactic acidosis directly affects myocardial function, reduces cardiac output, and increases organ hypoperfusion; these effects lead to deeper levels of tissue hypoxia.
• Hypoxia and acidosis eventually lead to such deleterious effects on cellular function, especially myocardial function, that multiple organ system failure ensues.

SIGNALMENT
Dog and cat

SIGNS

General Comments
Usually relate more to the underlying disorder causing the acidosis than to direct effects of the acidosis itself

Historical Findings
Disorders causing lactic acidosis are fairly common, and historical facts may prompt the clinician to suspect an underlying acidosis.

Physical Examination Findings
• Tachypnea is usually present in these patients as they attempt respiratory compensation.
• Most patients with acidosis are hypovolemic and thus demonstrate evidence of poor tissue perfusion or dehydration—dark mucous membranes, prolonged capillary refill time, and increased skin turgor.
• Severely acidotic patients may have cardiac dysrhythmias and poor contractility.

CAUSES
• Two types, A and B, based on the clinical presence or absence of hypoperfusion or tissue hypoxia
• Type A lactic acidosis—more common; due to decreased or inadequate oxygen delivery and oxygen consumption (i.e., poor tissue perfusion and tissue hypoxia)
• Causes of type A include shock, regional hypoperfusion, arterial obstruction, severe hypoxemia, severe anemia, carbon monoxide poisoning, severe asthma, and severe motor seizures.
• Type B lactic acidosis—includes all other causes of lactic acidosis; is subdivided into three subsets (B_1, B_2, B_3); is characterized by the absence of hypoxemia or poor tissue perfusion
• Many causes of type B lactic acidosis have recently been shown to be "occult" hypoperfusion not detectable by routine monitoring parameters or possibly combinations of types A and B lactic acidosis.
• The most common causes of type B lactic acidosis in veterinary medicine include neoplasia, alkalosis, sepsis, renal failure, liver disease, catecholamine use (norepinephrine, epinephrine), and intoxications (strychnine, cyanide, ethylene glycol, salicylates, acetaminophen, propylene glycol).

RISK FACTORS
• Risk factors for development of hyperlactatemia and lactic acidosis relate directly to risk factors for the specific disorders causing the underlying tissue hypoxia.
• In general, young animals are more at risk for traumatic shock and intoxications.
• Older animals are more likely to develop neoplasia, renal failure, heart failure, liver disease, severe anemias, and vascular disorders; consult Risk Factors for these specific disorders.

DIAGNOSIS

DIFFERENTIAL DIAGNOSIS
• Differential diagnoses for hyperlactatemia and lactic acidosis include those disorders described under Causes.
• Any severely ill animal is suspect for an underlying acidosis, and evaluating the lactate concentration can aid in diagnosis.

LABORATORY FINDINGS

Drugs That May Alter Laboratory Results
• Catecholamines, salicylates, acetaminophen, terbutaline, nitroprusside, halothane, bicarbonate, and propylene glycol all can cause mild-to-moderate increases in lactate concentrations in the absence of true tissue hypoperfusion and hypoxia.

LACTIC ACIDOSIS (HYPERLACTATEMIA)

• Lower lactate concentrations are found in samples with sodium citrate anticoagulant than in those with heparin and EDTA.

• Even small amounts of lactate-containing intravenous fluids (e.g., lactated Ringer's solution) may cause false increases in circulating lactate concentration in a blood sample if not properly cleared from the catheter or tubing through which the intravenous fluid was being given.

Disorders That May Alter Laboratory Results

• Several types of neoplasia increase lactate concentrations because the tumor cells preferentially use anaerobic glucose metabolism as part of the cancer cachexia syndrome.

• Alkalosis, sepsis, liver disease, and renal failure also can increase lactate concentrations by mechanisms other than poor tissue perfusion and hypoxia.

• Failure to detect elevated lactate concentrations does not ensure adequate perfusion to all organs; significant organ hypoperfusion may exist that may ultimately lead to multiple organ failure.

• Regional hypoperfusion, especially splanchnic, occurs in the absence of, or before, increases in systemic lactate and metabolic acidosis and often despite therapy that successfully maintains blood pressure, cardiac output, heart rate, DO_2, VO_2, and respiratory parameters.

Valid If Run in Human Laboratory?

• Yes; semiautomated and automated techniques are available for rapid measurement of lactate concentration in microliter samples of whole blood, serum, and plasma.

• Lactate concentration is ideally measured on an arterial sample; however, central venous and pulmonary artery samples are acceptable.

• Peripheral venous blood samples are not ideal, especially if the measurement will be used to assess global tissue perfusion.

CBC/BIOCHEMISTRY/URINALYSIS

• Few specific CBC findings would suggest causes for hyperlactatemia and lactic acidosis.

• Biochemical and urinalysis findings help determine the underlying cause; examples include renal azotemia and markedly increased serum osmolality seen with ethylene glycol intoxication; renal azotemia, hyperkalemia, and tubular casts seen with acute renal failure; and increased lactate concentration, increased total protein, and increased hematocrit with dehydration and poor tissue perfusion in a shock patient.

OTHER LABORATORY TESTS

• Arterial blood gas analysis may help define the extent of a concurrent respiratory disorder and a mixed acid–base disorder.

• Additional tests (e.g., ethylene glycol, serum and urine glucose, serum and urine ketones) may be helpful, depending on the suspected cause.

IMAGING
N/A

DIAGNOSTIC PROCEDURES
N/A

TREATMENT

• Hyperlactatemia alone is seldom significant enough to prompt specific therapy and is more important as a marker of possible severe or developing systemic problems.

• Lactic acidosis is often severe, and aggressive therapy to correct the underlying cause(s) and specifically treat the acidosis is usually indicated.

• Detection of hyperlactatemia, with or without acidosis, should drive the clinician to seek causes of hypoperfusion and should dictate early therapeutic interventions to improve tissue oxygen delivery to halt organ ischemia and avert progression to circulatory shock.

MEDICATIONS

DRUGS OF CHOICE

• Specific drug and fluid use depends on the underlying cause.

• Many causes of hyperlactatemia and lactic acidosis are characterized by fluid volume deficits; thus, aggressive fluid therapy is traditionally a hallmark initial step in treatment.

CONTRAINDICATIONS
N/A

PRECAUTIONS
N/A

POSSIBLE INTERACTIONS
N/A

ALTERNATIVE DRUGS
N/A

FOLLOW-UP

PATIENT MONITORING

• Serial lactate determinations are more valuable than single (admission, peak) lactate levels; monitor lactate over time in critical patients.

• The ability of a patient to clear lactate predicts response to therapy, and survival.

• Continue checking other parameters that help gauge the response to therapy for the underlying cause.

POSSIBLE COMPLICATIONS

• Persons with lactic acidosis are at greater risk of developing multiple organ failure and have a higher mortality rate than patients without lactic acidosis.

• Dogs and horses with elevated lactate concentrations and lactic acidosis have poorer outcomes as well.

MISCELLANEOUS

ASSOCIATED CONDITIONS
N/A

AGE-RELATED FACTORS
N/A

ZOONOTIC POTENTIAL
N/A

PREGNANCY
N/A

SYNONYMS
N/A

SEE ALSO
Metabolic Acidosis; see Causes

ABBREVIATIONS
N/A

Suggested Reading

Kruse JA. Lactic acidosis. In: Carlson RW, Geheb MA, eds. Principles and practice of medical intensive care. Philadelphia, Saunders, 1995:1231–1245.

Lagutchik MS, Ogilivie GK, Wingfield WE, Hackett TB. Lactate kinetics in veterinary critical care: a review. J Vet Emerg Crit Care 1996;6:81–95.

Mizock BA, Falk JL. Lactic acidosis in critical illness. Crit Care Med 1992;20:80–93.

Vail DM, Ogilive GK, Wheeler SL, et al. Alterations in carbohydrate metabolism in canine lymphoma. J Vet Intern Med 1990;4:8–11.

Author Michael S. Lagutchik
Consulting Editor Deborah S. Greco

LIPIDS, HYPERLIPIDEMIA

 BASICS

DEFINITIONS
- Concentration of lipid in the blood of a fasted (>12 h) patient that exceeds the upper range of normal for that species; includes both hypercholesterolemia and hypertriglyceridemia
- Lipemic—serum or plasma separated from blood that contains an excess concentration of triglycerides (>200 mg/dL)
- Lactescence—opaque, milklike appearance of serum or plasma that contains an even higher concentration of triglycerides (>1000 mg/dL) than lipemic serum

PATHOPHYSIOLOGY

Primary Hyperlipidemia
- Idiopathic hyperchylomicronemia—defect in lipid metabolism causing hypertriglyceridemia and hyperchylomicronemia; possibly caused by a defect in lipoprotein lipase activity or the absence of the surface apoprotein CII; familial disorder in the miniature schnauzer
- Hyperchylomicronemia in cats—familial, autosomal recessive defect in lipoprotein lipase activity
- Idiopathic hypercholesterolemia—occurs in some families of Doberman pinschers and rottweilers; LDL cholesterol is high.

Secondary Hyperlipidemia
- Postprandial—absorption of chylomicrons from the gastrointestinal tract occurs 30–60 min after ingestion of a meal containing fat; may increase serum triglycerides for 3–10 h
- Diabetes mellitus—low lipoprotein lipase (LPL) activity; high synthesis of very-low-density lipoprotein (VLDL) by the liver
- Hypothyroidism—low LPL activity and lipolytic activity by other hormones (e.g., catecholamines); reduced hepatic degradation of cholesterol to bile acids
- Hyperadrenocorticism—increased synthesis of VLDL by the liver and low LPL activity causes both hypercholesterolemia and hypertriglyceridemia.
- Liver disease—hypercholesterolemia caused by reduced excretion of cholesterol in the bile
- Nephrotic syndrome—common synthetic pathway for albumin and cholesterol and possibly low oncotic pressure leads to increased cholesterol synthesis.
- Obesity— excessive hepatic synthesis of VLDL

SYSTEMS AFFECTED
- Ophthalmic
- Nervous
- Endocrine/Metabolism
- Gastrointestinal
- Hepatobiliary

SIGNALMENT
- Dog and cat
- Variable, depending on the cause
- Hereditary hyperlipidemias—age of onset 8 months in cats and >4 years in predisposed breeds of dog such as the miniature schnauzer

SIGNS

Historical Findings
- Recent ingestion of a meal
- Seizures
- Abdominal pain and distress
- Neuropathies

Physical Examination Findings
- Lipemia retinalis
- Lipemic aqueous
- Neuropathy
- Cutaneous xanthomata
- Lipid granulomas in abdominal organs

CAUSES

Increased Absorption of Triglycerides or Cholesterol
Postprandial

Increased Production of Triglycerides or Cholesterol
- Nephrotic syndrome
- Pregnancy
- Defects in lipid clearance enzymes or lipid carrier proteins
- Idiopathic hyperchylomicronemia
- Hyperchylomicronemia in cats
- Idiopathic hypercholesterolemia

Decreased Clearance of Triglycerides or Cholesterol
- Hypothyroidism
- Hyperadrenocorticism
- Diabetes mellitus
- Pancreatitis
- Cholestasis

RISK FACTORS
- Obesity
- High dietary intake of fats
- Genetic predisposition in miniature schnauzer and Himalayan cat
- Idiopathic hypercholesterolemia observed in families of Doberman pinschers and rottweilers

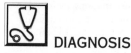 DIAGNOSIS

DIFFERENTIAL DIAGNOSIS

Fasting Hyperlipidemia
Rule out postprandial lipemia with a 12-h fast.

Primary Hyperlipoproteinemia
- Idiopathic hyperchylomicronemia is observed most commonly in the miniature schnauzer breed.
- Hyperchylomicronemia in cats often manifests as polyneuropathies and lipogranulomas.
- Idiopathic hypercholesterolemia is observed most frequently in the Doberman pinscher and rottweiler breeds; animals are often asymptomatic.

Secondary Hyperlipidemia
- Diabetes mellitus—signs include polyphagia, weight loss, polydipsia, and polyuria; glycosuria and fasting hyperglycemia confirm the diagnosis.
- Hypothyroidism—signs include lethargy, hypothermia, heat seeking, and dermatologic changes (e.g., alopecia and hyperpigmentation).
- Pancreatitis—signs include abdominal pain, vomiting, diarrhea, and anorexia; often hyperlipidemia is accompanied by high liver enzyme activities and high lipase and amylase.
- Hyperadrenocorticism—signs include polydipsia, polyuria, polyphagia, dermatologic changes (e.g., alopecia and thin skin), and hepatomegaly; hypercholesterolemia often is attended by high ALP isoenzyme.
- Hepatic disease and cholestatic disorders—signs include anorexia, weight loss, and icterus.
- Nephrotic syndrome—signs include ascites and peripheral edema; hypercholesterolemia is observed in conjunction with hypoproteinemia and proteinuria.

LABORATORY FINDINGS

Sample Handling
- Submit serum.
- Lipemia causes hemolysis if serum remains on RBC for a long time; inquire about the laboratory method of clearing lipemic samples before submission.
- Two samples may be submitted: one for biochemical analysis, which may be cleared, and one for triglycerides and cholesterol concentrations.

LIPIDS, HYPERLIPIDEMIA

Drugs That May Alter Laboratory Results
• Corticosteroids
• Phenytoin
• Prochlorperazine
• Thiazides
• Phenothiazines

Disorders That May Alter Laboratory Results
• Falsely high cholesterol
• Nonfasted samples (<12 h)
• Icterus—spectrophotometric techniques
• Fluoride and oxalate anticoagulants—enzymatic techniques
• Lipemia

Valid If Run in Human Laboratory?
Yes

CBC/BIOCHEMISTRY/URINALYSIS
• Results of hemogram usually normal
• Hyperadrenocorticism—polycythemia and nucleated RBC
• Hypothyroidism—mild normocytic, normochromic anemia
• High triglycerides—dogs, >150 mg/dL; cats, >100 mg/dL
• High cholesterol—dogs, >300 mg/dL; cats, >200 mg/dL
• Nephrotic syndrome—low albumin
• Diabetes mellitus—high serum glucose
• Hyperadrenocorticism— high ALP activity
• Pancreatitis—high serum lipase
• Results of urinalysis often normal
• Nephrotic syndrome—proteinuria

OTHER LABORATORY TESTS
• HDL and LDL determinations—used in human medicine; values reported for HDL and LDL in dogs and cats cannot be assumed to be reliable.
• Chylomicron test—obtain serum sample after a 12-h fast and refrigerate for 12–14 h; do not freeze; chylomicrons rise to the surface and form a creamy layer.
• Lipoprotein electrophoresis—separates LDL, VLDL, HDL1, and HDL2
• LPL activity—collect serum for triglycerides and cholesterol concentrations and lipoprotein electrophoresis before and 15 min after IV administration of heparin (90 IU/kg); if there is no change in values before and after heparin administration, a defective LPL enzyme system should be suspected.
• T_4 and T_3 determinations indicated if hypothyroidism is suspected
• Adrenocorticotropic hormone (ACTH) stimulation test indicated if hyperadrenocorticism is suspected

IMAGING
N/A

DIAGNOSTIC PROCEDURES
N/A

TREATMENT
Diet should contain <10% fat (e.g., Hill's r/d, Iams restricted calorie).

MEDICATIONS

DRUGS OF CHOICE
• Initial management is dietary.
• See Alternative Drugs if diet fails to control hyperlipidemia.

CONTRAINDICATIONS
N/A

PRECAUTIONS
N/A

POSSIBLE INTERACTIONS
N/A

ALTERNATIVE DRUGS
• Gemfibrozil—7.5 mg/kg PO q12h
• Fish oils—linolenic acid (omega-3 polyunsaturated fat)
• Clofibrate and niacin—not currently recommended in cats or dogs

FOLLOW-UP

PATIENT MONITORING
• Keep triglyceride concentrations < 500 mg/dL to avoid possibly fatal episodes of acute pancreatitis.
• Checking cholesterol often is not necessary because hypercholesterolemia is not associated with clinical signs.

POSSIBLE COMPLICATIONS
• Pancreatitis and seizures are common complications of hyperlipidemia in the miniature schnauzer.
• In cats with hereditary chylomicronemia, xanthoma formation, lipemia retinalis, and neuropathies have been reported; peripheral neuropathies usually resolve 2–3 months after institution of a low-fat diet.

MISCELLANEOUS

ASSOCIATED CONDITIONS
• Pancreatitis
• Seizures
• Neuropathies

AGE-RELATED FACTORS
N/A

ZOONOTIC POTENTIAL
N/A

PREGNANCY
Potential cause of high cholesterol

SYNONYMS
• Lipemia
• Hyperlipoproteinemia

SEE ALSO
See Causes.

ABBREVIATIONS
• HDL = high-density lipoproteins
• LDL = low-density lipoproteins
• LPL = lipoprotein lipase
• VLDL = very-low-density lipoproteins
• T_4 = thyroxine
• T_3 = triiodothyronine

Suggested Reading
Armstrong PJ, Ford RB. Hyperlipidemia. In: Kirk RW, ed. Current veterinary therapy X. Philadelphia: Saunders, 1989:1046–1050.
Ford R. Canine hyperlipidemias. In: Ettinger ST, Feldman EC, eds. Textbook of veterinary internal medicine. 4th ed. Philadelphia: Saunders 1994:1414–1418.
Jones B. Feline hyperlipidemias. In: Ettinger ST, Feldman EC, eds. Textbook of veterinary internal medicine. 4th ed. Philadelphia: Saunders, 1994:1410–1413.
Author Deborah S. Greco
Consulting Editor Deborah S. Greco

DIAGNOSTICS—LAB

LOW-DOSE DEXAMETHASONE SUPPRESSION TEST

BASICS

DEFINITION
• To perform a LDDST, administer dexamethasone (0.01–0.015 mg/kg IV for dogs and 0.1 mg/kg for cats).
• Can use dexamethasone or dexamethasone sodium phosphate as long as calculations are based on the concentration of the active ingredient
• Draw blood before and 4 and 8 h after injection.
• At baseline (i.e., predexamethasone), normal plasma cortisol concentrations in dogs are 10–160 nmol/L (~0.4–6.0 µg/dL) and in cats, 10–110 nmol/L (~0.4–4.0 µg/dL).
• A normal animal has a cortisol concentration below ~30 nmol/L (1.0 µg/dL) at both 4 and 8 h postdexamethasone. (**Note:** normal values vary slightly between laboratories.)
• Dexamethasone should be diluted in sterile saline if necessary for cats and small dogs, so that the patient is dosed accurately.
• If part or all of the dexamethasone is given out of the vein, the test should be stopped and attempted again after at least 48 h.

PATHOPHYSIOLOGY
• Used to screen for hyperadrenocorticism (Cushing's syndrome); lack of suppression in response to a low dose of dexamethasone is consistent with a diagnosis of hyperadrenocorticism but can be a nonspecific finding in dogs with nonadrenal illness.
• Cushing's syndrome can be caused either by an ACTH-secreting pituitary tumor (i.e. pituitary-dependent hyperadrenocorticism, PDH) or by a cortisol-secreting AT.
• Normally, dexamethasone feeds back onto the pituitary and turns off ACTH secretion; when systemic ACTH concentration falls, the secretory stimulus to the adrenal cortex diminishes, and cortisol release decreases; thus 4 and 8 h after dexamethasone, plasma cortisol concentration is low (<30 nmol/L).
• With PDH, the pituitary tumor is relatively resistant to feedback, and secretion of ACTH and in turn cortisol continues.
• Because of the continued autonomous secretion of cortisol from an AT, endogenous ACTH is already suppressed, administration of an exogenous glucocorticoid has no further effect on the pituitary, and autonomous cortisol secretion continues despite dexamethasone administration.

• A diagnosis of either PDH or AT is supported by a 4- and/or 8-h postdexamethasone plasma cortisol concentration > 30 nmol/L; in addition, if the 4-h postdexamethasone concentration is < 30 nmol/L but the 8-h sample is > 30 nmol/L or if one or both are less than 50% of baseline, PDH is likely; however, if both postdexamethasone concentrations are > 30 nmol/L and neither of these values is less than 50% of baseline, either PDH or AT is possible.
• A lack of suppression in dogs during an LDDST can also be due to nonadrenal illness and associated nonspecific activation of the hypothalamic-pituitary-adrenal axis; the effect of nonadrenal illness on the LDDST in cats is unknown.
• A false-negative test result is seen in ~5% of patients with Cushing's syndrome; this may be due to early PDH in which the tumor still responds to glucocorticoid feedback.

SYSTEMS AFFECTED
• Organ systems are not affected by an abnormal LDDST per se; they are affected by the excess cortisol secreted in Cushing's syndrome.
• See Hyperadrenocorticism.

SIGNALMENT
Dog and cat

SIGNS

General Comments
• No historical or physical examination findings are specifically due to abnormal suppression; they are due to Cushing's syndrome.
• See Hyperadrenocorticism.

Historical Findings
N/A

Physical Examination Findings
N/A

CAUSES
• Cushing's syndrome—dogs and cats
• Nonadrenal illness—dogs; cats unknown

RISK FACTORS
• See Causes
• Phenobarbital administration may cause lack of suppression.

DIAGNOSIS

DIFFERENTIAL DIAGNOSIS
• Historical findings of hyperadrenocorticism include polyuria/polydipsia, bilaterally symmetrical alopecia or failure to regrow hair, abdominal enlargement, polyphagia, obesity, panting, lethargy, muscle weakness, anestrus, heat intolerance.
• Physical examination findings of hyperadrenocorticism include thin skin, abdominal

enlargement, bilaterally symmetrical alopecia, hepatomegaly, pyoderma, seborrhea, cutaneous hyperpigmentation, muscle wasting of extremities, calcinosis cutis, bruising, testicular atrophy.
• Historical and physical examination findings vary, depending on the nonadrenal illness present.

LABORATORY FINDINGS

Drugs That May Alter Laboratory Results
• Phenobarbital administration may cause lack of suppression.
• Prednisone, prednisolone, and hydrocortisone cross-react in many cortisol radioimmunoassays and cause an artifactual increase in measured cortisol concentration; suppression in response to dexamethasone may be obscured.
• Prolonged glucocorticoid therapy may affect the pituitary-adrenal axis by continuously activating normal negative feedback mechanisms.
• The LDDST is unreliable in these patients because it may not cause adequate suppression, leading to a false-positive test result.

Disorders That May Alter Laboratory Results
• Delayed separation of plasma from blood cells may falsely lower measured cortisol concentration.
• Use plasma collected with EDTA as an anticoagulant because cortisol will be stable if stored at ≤25°C for 5 days; storage at higher temperatures or use of serum may lead to decay of cortisol and a spurious decrease in apparent cortisol concentration.

Valid If Run in Human Laboratory?
Yes, if assay is validated for dogs and cats.

CBC/BIOCHEMISTRY/URINALYSIS
• CBC—with hyperadrenocorticism, a mature leukocytosis, neutrophilia, lymphopenia, eosinopenia, or mild polycythemia
• Biochemistry—increased alkaline phosphatase (ALP; elevation may be extreme), alanine aminotransferase (ALT), cholesterol, fasting blood glucose, and lipase can be seen with hyperadrenocorticism; lipemia and decreased BUN may also be noted.
• Urinalysis—dilute urine (e.g., specific gravity < 1.015) and bacteriuria with or without pyuria have been associated with Cushing's syndrome.

OTHER LABORATORY TESTS
• Other tests used to screen for Cushing's syndrome include a urinary cortisol:creatinine ratio (UCCR), an ACTH response test, and a combined high-dose dexamethasone suppression/ACTH response.

LOW-DOSE DEXAMETHASONE SUPPRESSION TEST

• An elevated UCCR is a highly sensitive but nonspecific finding for Cushing's syndrome; a normal ratio signifies the patient has <10% chance of having hyperadrenocorticism.

• An ACTH response and the combined high-dose dexamethasone suppression/ACTH response are both less sensitive but more specific for Cushing's syndrome than the LDDST; if a patient does not suppress in response to dexamethasone but has a normal ACTH response or combination test, consider whether a nonadrenal illness is causing a false-positive LDDST result.

• If the results of the LDDST are abnormal but borderline (e.g., 4- and 8-h postdexamethasone cortisol concentrations are slightly above 30 nmol/L), retest the patient or, ideally, perform an ACTH response test to confirm the diagnosis of Cushing's syndrome.

• If nonadrenal illness is present and possible cause of abnormal LDDST results, treat the illness; when the patient is stable, perform an ACTH response test after 4–8 weeks.

• If there is no suppression on the LDDST, no nonadrenal illness known to be present, and the diagnosis of hyperadrenocorticism is likely on the basis of historical and clinical findings but the test did not determine if the cause was PDH, a high-dose dexamethasone suppression test can be performed or endogenous ACTH concentration measured for differentiation.

IMAGING

• Abdominal radiography and ultrasonography can be used to differentiate PDH from AT.

• CT and magnetic resonance imaging (MRI) can reveal a pituitary tumor.

DIAGNOSTIC PROCEDURES

• With hyperadrenocorticism, urinary protein:creatinine ratio and systemic blood pressure may be mildly elevated, but neither is specific.

• A skin biopsy can confirm the diagnosis of calcinosis cutis, a pathognomonic finding for hyperadrenocorticism; other skin biopsy changes may suggest an endocrinopathy but are not specific.

• A liver biopsy can show changes consistent with steroid hepatopathy, a sensitive but nonspecific marker of Cushing's syndrome.

 TREATMENT

• Lack of suppression per se does not need to be treated.

• If the test result is due to nonadrenal illness, direct therapy toward resolution of that disease.

• If Cushing's syndrome is believed to be present, direct therapy toward managing hyperadrenocorticism; unless a complication of Cushing's syndrome requires hospitalization (e.g. pulmonary thromboembolism), patients can be treated as outpatients.

 MEDICATIONS

DRUGS OF CHOICE
Lack of suppression does not need to be treated while completing all tests for the diagnosis.

CONTRAINDICATIONS
Glucocorticoids

PRECAUTIONS
N/A

POSSIBLE INTERACTIONS
N/A

ALTERNATIVE DRUGS
N/A

 FOLLOW-UP

PATIENT MONITORING
• If hyperadrenocorticism is present, follow-up depends on the type of therapy chosen (see Hyperadrenocorticism).

• If nonadrenal illness is present and believed possibly to be the cause of abnormal LDDST results, treat the illness; when the patient is stable, perform an ACTH response test after 4–8 weeks.

POSSIBLE COMPLICATIONS
Untreated hyperadrenocorticism can lead to development of all classical signs not already present (e.g., polyuria, polydipsia, panting, polyphagia), as well as such life-threatening complications as pulmonary thromboembolism or diabetes mellitus.

 MISCELLANEOUS

ASSOCIATED CONDITIONS
None related to lack of suppression per se

AGE-RELATED FACTORS
• Nonadrenal illness can occur in an animal of any age.

• Hyperadrenocorticism is typically a disease of middle-aged to old cats and dogs, although it has been reported in dogs 1 year old.

ZOONOTIC POTENTIAL
N/A

PREGNANCY
N/A

SYNONYMS
N/A

SEE ALSO
• Hyperadrenocorticism
• ACTH Response Test
• Urine Cortisol:Creatinine Ratio

ABBREVIATIONS
• ACTH = adrenocorticotropic hormone
• ALP = alkaline phosphatase
• AT = adrenal tumor
• CT = computed tomography
• LDDST = low-dose dexamethasone suppression test
• MRI = magnetic resonance imaging
• PDH = pituitary-dependent hyperadrenocorticism
• UCCR = urine cortisol:creatinine ratio

Suggested Reading

Feldman EC, Nelson RW, Feldman MS. Use of low- and high-dose dexamethasone tests for distinguishing pituitary-dependent from adrenal tumor hyperadrenocorticism in dogs. J Am Vet Med Assoc 1996;209:772–775.

Feldman EC, Nelson RW. Hyperadrenocorticism (Cushing's syndrome). In: Feldman EC, Nelson RW, eds. Canine and feline endocrinology and reproduction. 2nd ed. Philadelphia: Saunders, 1996.

Guptill L, Scott-Moncrieff JC, Widmer W. Diagnosis of canine hyperadrenocorticism. Vet Clin North Am: Small Anim Pract 1997;27:215–235.

Kaplan AJ, Peterson ME, Kemppainen RJ. Effects of disease on the results of diagnostic tests for use in detecting hyperadrenocorticism in dogs. J Am Vet Med Assoc 1995; 207:445–451.

Van Liew CH, Greco DS, Salman MD. Comparison of results on adrenocorticotropic hormone stimulation and low-dose dexamethasone suppression tests with necropsy findings in dogs: 81 cases (1985–1995). J Am Vet Med Assoc 1997;211:322–325.

Authors Ellen N. Behrend and Robert J. Kemppainen

Consulting Editor Deborah S. Greco

LYMPHOCYTOSIS

 BASICS

DEFINITION
• Absolute number of circulating lymphocytes greater than the reference range: dogs, $> 5 \times 10^9/L$ or $> 5000/\mu L$ or mm^3; cats, $> 7 \times 10^9/L$ or $> 7000/\mu L$ or mm^3
• Absolute lymphocyte counts are greater in juveniles than in adults.

PATHOPHYSIOLOGY
• Lymphocytes are imperative for humoral- (B lymphocytes) and cell-mediated immunity (T lymphocytes).
• B lymphocytes—derived from lymphoid stem cells in the bone marrow; responsible for the production of antibodies; differentiation of pre-B cells in the bone marrow is antibody independent; undergo transformation into antibody-producing plasma cells.
• T lymphocytes—derived from lymphoid stem cells in the bone marrow; differentiation in the thymus is influenced by interleukins and other substances produced by macrophages and cells in the thymic medulla and is antibody independent; responsible for cytotoxicity (a delayed-type hypersensitivity reaction), graft rejection, and regulation of the immune system through production of lymphokines.
• Lymphoid cells produced in the bone marrow and thymus migrate to secondary lymphoid organs (e.g., lymph nodes, spleen, and gut-associated lymphoid tissue) where they give rise to immunocompetent cells in response to antigenic stimulation.
• Under the proper stimulus, lymphocytes transform into lymphoblasts and then proliferate to make a clonal population of cells; the process is promoted by γ-interferon; some of the progeny become memory cells, but most express the appropriate immune response (humoral or cellular).
• Lymphocyte generation time is 6–8 hr; stimulated by antigens; suppressed by corticosteroids, sex hormones, and malnutrition.
• Most B lymphocytes are short lived, with a survival time of several hours to about 5 days; most T lymphocytes and memory B lymphocytes are long lived, with an average lifespan of about 4 years; some memory cells can persist for decades.
• B and T lymphocytes are responsible for approximately 95% of all lymphocytes; the remainder are "null" lymphocytes (i.e., large, granular lymphocytes), which serve as natural killer cells and other diverse functions.
• Generally, the different types of lymphocytes cannot be identified on a blood film; occasionally, activated B lymphocytes (reactive lymphocytes) can be recognized by their large size, deep blue cytoplasm, and perinuclear clear zone; large, granular lymphocytes can be recognized by the presence of small, red cytoplasmic granules.
• Reactive cells that have undergone blast transformation are known as immunoblasts.
• Cytokines secreted at sites of inflammation increase the expression of homing molecules that mediate lymphocyte adhesion to endothelial cells and migration into tissues. Recirculation
• Unlike granulocytes, about 70% of the lymphocytes that enter tissues return to the vasculature and recirculate.
• Most recirculating lymphocytes are T cells along with small numbers of B memory cells.
• Important for immune surveillance and provides a mechanism for distribution of lymphocytes during a systemic immune response
• Circulation through the bone marrow, spleen, and thymus is hematogenous.
• Re-entry to lymph nodes is through the lymph.

SYSTEMS AFFECTED
• Hemic/Lymph/Immune—spleen, liver, and bone marrow owing to hyperplasia or neoplasia
• Lymphoma can involve all systems and produce specific problems, including ocular, CNS, gastrointestinal, and renal.

SIGNALMENT
Dogs and cats

SIGNS
• Physiologic lymphocytosis—excited, vicious, or scared cat
• Lymphoma—large lymph nodes and, possibly, splenomegaly and hepatomegaly

CAUSES
Physiologic
• Epinephrine surge, especially common in excited cats
• The change occurs in minutes and lasts about 30 min.
• Can be produced by exogenous epinephrine injection, excitement, and fear; usually seen in young, healthy animals.
• Can be induced by difficulty collecting a blood sample.
• The change is much less common in cats that are sick.
• The absolute lymphocyte count can occasionally rise to $> 20,000/\mu L$ and is much greater than the relatively mild increase in mature neutrophils that accompanies this type of lymphocytosis.

Antigenic Stimulation
• Chronic inflammation, often with a suppurative component, such as pyometra and pyoderma
• Immune-mediated diseases, acquired and autoimmune
• Canine ehrlichiosis
• Vaccination
• The increase in lymphocyte numbers associated with these problems is relatively mild and can range from the higher end of the reference range to approximately $10,000/\mu L$.
• Lymphocytosis in the face of an obvious clinical disease is particularly important because lymphopenia is a common response to the stress of disease.
• Immunocytes and immunoblasts (activated B lymphocytes) in the circulation generally indicate antigenic stimulation; however, morphologically, reactive lymphocytes cannot be readily distinguished from neoplastic lymphocytes.

Lymphoma
• Peripheral blood lymphocyte count can range from lymphopenia to counts $> 100,000/\mu L$.
• Found in approximately 20% of dogs with lymphoma; usually mild to moderate (i.e., 5,000–15,000/μL); markedly high counts (i.e., $> 30,000/\mu L$) are uncommon.
• Lymphopenia occurs in $> 50\%$ of dogs with lymphoma and is more common than lymphocytosis in dogs with lymphoma because of the release of endogenous corticosteroids caused by the stress of the disease.
• Immature and atypical-appearing lymphocytes should be searched for in a blood film; careful examination of the feathered edge or lateral margins of the blood smear is a good place to search for these cells.

Acute Lymphoblastic Leukemia
• Lymphoid neoplasia arises from and primarily involves the bone marrow and is unassociated with solid tumor masses.
• Counts of $> 20,000/\mu L$ are usually seen owing to circulating lymphoblasts (usually T cells in cats and B cells in dogs).
• Occasionally, leukemia involves large granular lymphocytes characterized by large, pink, cytoplasmic granules.
• Some animals are "aleukemic" (neoplastic cells absent from the circulation).
• Pancytopenia may result from myelophthises, with lymphoblasts composing $> 30\%$ of the nucleated cells in the bone marrow.

Chronic Lymphocytic Leukemia
• Lymphoid neoplasm characterized by excessive numbers of small mature lymphocytes in the blood and bone marrow.
• Lymphocytes appear normal or may have slightly more cytoplasm than normal.
• Although the bone marrow usually contains high numbers of small lymphocytes, the level of infiltration is less than in patients with acute lymphoblastic leukemia.
• Pancytopenia is uncommon.

Hypoadrenocorticism
• Occurs in 25–33% of dogs with hypoadrenocorticism owing to the absence of glucocorticoids.
• Classically, accompanied by mild

eosinophilia and the absence of neutrophilia or monocytosis in a sick and stressed animal
• A normal lymphocyte count in a sick and stressed animal suggests low glucocorticoids and, therefore, the possibility of hypoadrenocorticism.

Hyperthyroidism
• Approximately 10% of cats with hyperthyroidism have lymphocytosis.
• Germ-free cats
• Lymphocyte count 4,000–14,000/µL.
• FeLV
• Although listed as a cause of lymphocytosis, FIV causes lymphopenia owing to selective loss of $CD4^+$ helper T cells and relative lymphocytosis of $CD8^+$ suppressor T cells; an inverted $CD4^+$:$CD8^+$ ratio is seen.

Drugs
• Methimazole associated with lymphocytosis in 7% of cats treated for hyperthyroidism
• Epinephrine and other β-adrenergic agonists can cause marked, transient lymphocytosis owing to recruitment from a noncirculating pool of lymphocytes.

RISK FACTORS
• FeLV infection—about 74% of feline lymphoma are positive for either FeLV antigen or DNA; insertion of viral DNA is thought to alter normal gene function and play a role in development of feline lymphoma.
• FIV infection—lymphoma reported in a small percentage of affected cats, although the role of this virus in tumorigenesis appears to be indirect; recurrent infections and subsequent polyclonal B cell activation may set up the potential for malignant transformation.

DIAGNOSIS

DIFFERENTIAL DIAGNOSIS
• Ill, lethargic dog—consider hypoadrenocorticism, lymphoma, and acute lymphoblastic leukemia
• Lymphadenopathy—consider lymphoma or ehrlichiosis
• Thin, hyperactive, polyphagic cat—consider hyperthyroidism
• Thin, lethargic cat—consider lymphoma

LABORATORY FINDINGS

Drugs That May Alter Laboratory Results
Corticosteroids cause lymphopenia.

Disorders That May Alter Laboratory Results
Incorrect identification of nucleated RBCs or monocytes as lymphocytes

Valid If Run in Human Laboratory?
Yes

CBC/BIOCHEMISTRY/URINALYSIS
• Severe lymphocytosis (> 15,000/µL)—consider acute lymphoblastic or chronic lymphocytic leukemia
• Immature, bizarre, and abnormal lymphocytes in circulation—consider lymphoma or acute lymphoblastic leukemia
• Mature neutrophilia—consider physiologic epinephrine response and chronic inflammation
• Nonregenerative anemia, leukopenia, and/or thrombocytopenia—consider intramarrow disease, such as lymphoma and lymphocytic leukemia
• Eosinophilia—consider hypoadrenocorticism
• Polycythemia—consider hyperthyroidism
• Hypercalcemia—consider lymphoma

OTHER LABORATORY TESTS
• Serum protein electrophoresis monoclonal gammopathy suggests lymphoma and ehrlichiosis.
• Thyroid testing—high resting T_3, T_4 diagnoses hyperthyroidism

IMAGING
Hepatosplenomegaly—consider lymphoma

DIAGNOSTIC PROCEDURES
• Biopsy helps confirm lymphoma.
• Examination of bone marrow aspirate used to diagnose acute lymphoblastic leukemia or stage lymphoma

TREATMENT
Treatment must be directed at the primary disease.

MEDICATIONS

DRUGS OF CHOICE
Lymphoma—chemotherapy (see appropriate topics)

CONTRAINDICATIONS
N/A

PRECAUTIONS
N/A

POSSIBLE INTERACTIONS
Complex interactions between levamisole, an immunomodulator that restores depressed immune function, and B and T lymphocytes affect their function.

ALTERNATIVE DRUGS
N/A

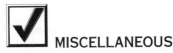

FOLLOW-UP

PATIENT MONITORING
N/A

POSSIBLE COMPLICATIONS
N/A

MISCELLANEOUS

ASSOCIATED CONDITIONS
None

AGE-RELATED FACTORS
• Young puppies—lymphocyte count increases from birth to a maximum of 6,000/µL at approximately 6 weeks of age; value is within adult reference range for adults by 8 weeks of age.
• Young kittens—absolute lymphocyte count increases from birth to a maximum of 10,500/µL at 12–14 weeks of age; value is within reference range for adults by 16–20 weeks of age.

ZOONOTIC POTENTIAL
None

PREGANCY
N/A

SYNONYMS
None

SEE ALSO
• Ehrlichiosis
• Hypoadrenocorticism (Addison's Disease)
• Leukemia, Acute Lymphoblastic
• Leukemia, Chronic Lymphocytic
• Lymphoma—Cats
• Lymphoma—Dogs

ABBREVIATIONS
• FeLV = feline leukemia virus
• FIV = feline immunodeficiency virus

Suggested Reading
Breitschwerdt EB, Woody BJ, Zerbe CA, et al. Monoclonal gammopathy associated with naturally occurring canine ehrlichiosis. J Vet Intern Med 1987;1:2–9.
Jain NC. Schalms' veterinary hematology. 4th ed. Philadelphia: Lea & Febiger, 1986.
Tompkins M, Nelson PD, English RV, et al. Novotney C. Early events in the immunopathogenesis of feline retrovirus infections. J Am Vet Med Assoc 1991;199:1311–1316.
Wellman ML, Couto CG, Starkey RJ, Rajok JL. Lymphocytosis of large granular lymphocytes in three dogs. Vet Pathol 1989; 26:158–163.
Author Joyce S. Knoll
Consulting Editor Susan M. Cotter

DIAGNOSTICS—LAB

LYMPHOPENIA

 BASICS

DEFINITION
Absolute number of circulating lymphocytes less than reference range: dogs, $< 1 \times 10^9/L$ or $< 1000/\mu L$ or mm^3; cats, $< 1.5 \times 10^9/L$ or $< 1,500/\mu L$ or mm^3

PATHOPHYSIOLOGY
• B lymphocytes—derived from lymphoid stem cells in the bone marrow; responsible for the production of antibodies (humoral immunity)
• T lymphocytes—derived from lymphoid stem cells in the bone marrow; undergo further differentiation in the thymus; responsible for cytotoxicity (a delayed-type hypersensitivity reaction), graft rejection, and regulation of the immune system through production of lymphokines.
• Lymphoid cells produced in the bone marrow and thymus migrate to secondary lymphoid organs (e.g., lymph nodes, spleen, and gut-associated lymphoid tissue) where they give rise to immunocompetent cells in response to antigenic stimulation.
• Most antibody production takes place in the lymph nodes and involves participation of macrophages, B lymphocytes, and T lymphocytes; the interaction of these cells stimulates a clonal expansion of B and T cells; some of the progeny become memory cells, but most express the appropriate immune response (humoral or cellular).
• Cytokines secreted at sites of inflammation increase the expression of these homing molecules and facilitate lymphocyte adhesion to endothelial cells and migration into tissues.
• The number of lymphocytes in the blood depends on rates of production, recirculation, use, and destruction and does not necessarily reflect the level of lymphopoiesis.
• B and T lymphocytes are responsible for approximately 95% of all lymphocytes; the remainder are "null" lymphocytes (i.e., large, granular lymphocytes), which serve as natural killer cells and other diverse functions.
• Generally, the different types of lymphocytes cannot be identified on a blood film.

Recirculation
• Unlike granulocytes, about 70% of the lymphocytes that enter tissues return to the vasculature and recirculate.
• Most recirculating lymphocytes are T cells along with small numbers of B memory cells.
• Important for immune surveillance and provides a mechanism for distribution of lymphocytes during a systemic immune response
• Circulation through the bone marrow, spleen, and thymus is hematogenous.
• Re-entry to lymph nodes is through the lymph.
• Mechanisms responsible for regulation are not entirely understood, but surface adhesion molecules on both lymphocytes and endothelial cells play a role.

SYSTEMS AFFECTED
Hemic/Lymph/Immune—atrophy of lymph nodes and lymphoid tissue in spleen can be caused by some infectious agents.

SIGNALMENT
Dogs and cats

SIGNS
Relate to primary cause

CAUSES
Corticosteroid-Induced
• Stress of systemic illness
• Hyperadrenocorticism—lymphopenia occurs in approximately 88% of affected dogs because of excess glucocorticoids
• Corticosteroid administration
• Corticosteroid-induced lympholysis and an increased shift of lymphocytes into tissue compartments
• Glucocorticoids inhibit interleukin synthesis by activated T lymphocytes and macrophages, resulting in immunosuppression.
• Classically accompanied by neutrophilia, monocytosis, and eosinopenia, but these are not consistent findings.

Acute Viral Infection
• FeLV—loss of both CD4+ helper T lymphocytes and CD8+ suppressor T lymphocytes; the CD4+:CD8+ ratio remains normal.

• FIV—selective loss of CD4+ helper T cells and a relative lymphocytosis of CD8+ suppressor T cells; an inverted CD4+:CD8+ ratio is seen.
• Canine distemper virus—widespread atrophy and necrosis of lymphoid tissue results in depletion of both B and T lymphocytes; viral inclusions are occasionally seen in leukocytes (especially lymphocytes) or erythrocytes during the early stage of disease.
• Inclusions are large (up to 3 μm), homogeneous structures that stain from pale blue to reddish purple with Romanowsky stains.
• Canine and feline parvovirus (feline panleukopenia virus)—destruction of rapidly dividing cells in both lymph nodes and bone marrow causes lymphopenia and neutropenia
• Infectious canine hepatitis

Loss of Lymphocytes
Loss of lymphocyte-rich lymph in patients with chylothorax, intestinal lymphangiectasia, or other protein-losing enteropathy.

RISK FACTORS
None

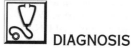 **DIAGNOSIS**

DIFFERENTIAL DIAGNOSIS
• Acute diarrhea—consider parvovirus or distemper infection
• Chronic diarrhea—consider protein-losing enteropathy
• Ill, lethargic cat—consider FeLV or FIV infection
• Cat with recurrent infection—consider FIV infection
• Thin-skinned, polyphagic, polyuric dog—consider hyperadrenocorticism
• Dyspnea—consider chylothorax
• Nasal discharge, cough—consider canine distemper infection
• Seizures—consider canine distemper infection

LABORATORY FINDINGS

Drugs That May Alter Laboratory Results
None

Disorders That May Alter Laboratory Results
Incorrect identification of nucleated RBCs or monocytes as lymphocytes

Valid If Run in Human Laboratory?
Yes

CBC/BIOCHEMISTRY/URINALYSIS
• Severe neutropenia—consider parvovirus
• Mature neutrophilia, monocytosis, and eosinopenia—consider glucocorticoid response to stress, exogenous glucocorticoid administration, and hyperadrenocorticism
• Marked elevation in alkaline phosphatase—consider canine hyperadrenocorticism
• Hyperglycemia, low serum total protein—consider protein-losing enteropathy and lymphangiectasia
• Nonregenerative anemia—consider FeLV
• Unresponsive to insulin administration—consider hyperadrenocorticism

OTHER LABORATORY TESTS
• Serology—detect FeLV antigen in serum, canine parvovirus antigen in feces, and serum antibody titers to FIV and canine distemper
• Adrenal function testing—ACTH stimulation and low-dose dexamethasone suppression tests to diagnose hyperadrenocorticism; urine cortisol:creatinine ratio is a quick screen to rule out hyperadrenocorticism.

IMAGING
Large adrenal gland(s)—consider hyperadrenocorticism

DIAGNOSTIC PROCEDURES
Intestinal biopsy if lymphangiectasia suspected

TREATMENT
Must be directed at the primary disease

MEDICATIONS

DRUGS OF CHOICE
Hyperadrenocorticism—Lysodren (see appropriate topics)

CONTRAINDICATIONS
None

PRECAUTIONS
None

POSSIBLE INTERACTIONS
Levamisole—an immunomodulator that restores depressed immune function; complex interactions with B and T lymphocytes affect their function.

ALTERNATIVE DRUGS
None

FOLLOW-UP

PATIENT MONITORING
N/A

POSSIBLE COMPLICATIONS
N/A

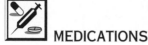

MISCELLANEOUS

ASSOCIATED CONDITIONS
None

AGE-RELATED FACTORS
• Young puppies—lymphocyte count increases from birth to a maximum of 6000/μL at approximately 6 weeks of age; value is within adult reference range for adults by 8 weeks of age
• Young kittens—absolute lymphocyte count increases from birth to a maximum of 10,500/μL at 12–14 weeks of age; value is within reference range for adults by 16–20 weeks of age

ZOONOTIC POTENTIAL
None

PREGANCY
N/A

SYNONYMS
None

SEE ALSO
• Distemper—Dogs
• Feline Immunodeficiency Virus
• Feline Panleukopenia
• Hyperadrenocorticism (Cushing disease)
• Protein-Losing Enteropathy

ABBREVIATIONS
• FeLV = feline leukemia virus
• FIV = feline immunodeficiency virus

Suggested Reading
Grindem CB. Blood cell markers. Vet Clin North Am Small Anim Pract 1996;26:1043–1064.
Jain NC. Schalm's veterinary hematology. 4th ed. Philadelphia: Lea & Febiger, 1986.
Tompkins M, Nelson PD, English RV, Novotney C, et al. Early events in the immunopathogenesis of feline retrovirus infections. J Am Vet Med Assoc 1991;199:1311–1316.
Author Joyce S. Knoll
Consulting Editor Susan M. Cotter

DIAGNOSTICS—LAB

MAGNESIUM, HYPERMAGNESEMIA

 BASICS

DEFINITION

- Dogs—serum magnesium >2.51 mg/dL
- Cats—serum magnesium >2.3 mg/dL

PATHOPHYSIOLOGY

- Magnesium—second only to potassium as the most abundant intracellular cation; most is found in bone and muscle; required for many metabolic functions
- Magnesium is an important cofactor in the sodium-potassium ATPase pump that maintains an electrical gradient across membranes and thus plays an important role in the activity of electrically excitable tissues.
- Interference with the electrical gradient can change resting membrane potentials; repolarization disturbances result in neuromuscular and cardiac abnormalities.
- Magnesium homeostasis is largely controlled by renal elimination; any condition that severely lowers the glomerular filtration rate can elicit hypermagnesemia.
- High magnesium concentration impairs transmission of nerve impulses and decreases the postsynaptic response at the neuromuscular junction.
- Magnesium has been called nature's calcium blocker; the most serious complications of hypermagnesemia result from calcium antagonism in the cardiac conduction system.

SYSTEMS AFFECTED

- Cardiovascular
- Musculoskeletal
- Nervous

SIGNALMENT

Dog and cat

SIGNS

General Comments

- Usually caused by renal failure; clinical signs may be referable to azotemia and renal insufficiency.
- Characterized by progressive loss of neuromuscular, respiratory, and cardiovascular function

Historical and Physical Examination Findings

- Earliest symptoms—nausea, vomiting, weakness, and hyporeflexia
- Hypotension and ECG changes, including delayed intraventricular conduction and prolonged QT interval, are noted as serum magnesium levels climb.
- Atrioventricular block, respiratory depression, coma, and cardiac arrest have been seen in people with serum magnesium concentrations >16 mg/dL.

CAUSES

- Renal failure
- Intestinal hypomotility disorders and constipation
- Endocrine disorders including hypoadrenocorticism, hypothyroidism, and hyperparathyroidism
- Excessive magnesium administration from magnesium-containing cathartic solutions given in conjunction with activated charcoal, magnesium-containing laxatives, and excess magnesium in peritoneal dialysis solutions

RISK FACTORS

- Renal disease
- Massive hemolysis
- Hypoadrenocorticism

- Hyperparathyroidism
- Excessive use of magnesium-containing cathartic solutions, especially in patients with renal insufficiency
- Intestinal hypomotility

 DIAGNOSIS

DIFFERENTIAL DIAGNOSIS

- Signs are most similar to those of hypocalcemia, which often occurs simultaneously.
- Bradycardia can be caused by neurologic disease, hyperkalemia, hypertension, hypothyroidism, sick sinus syndrome, and various drugs.

Laboratory Findings

Note: 12 mg of magnesium = 1 mEq of magnesium; to convert from mg/dL to mEq/L, divide by 1.2

Drugs That May Alter Laboratory Results

- Serum is favored over plasma because the anticoagulant used for plasma samples can contain citrate or other ions that may bind magnesium.
- EDTA, sodium fluoride-oxalate, sodium citrate, and intravenous calcium gluconate can cause falsely low serum magnesium values.

Disorders That May Alter Laboratory Results

- Hemolysis may cause false increases in serum magnesium; the magnesium concentration in erythrocytes is approximately three times that in serum.
- Holding serum or urine in metal containers can falsely elevate magnesium values.
- Hyperbilirubinemia can cause false decreases in serum magnesium.

MAGNESIUM, HYPERMAGNESEMIA

Valid If Run in Human Laboratory?
Yes

CBC/BIOCHEMISTRY/URINALYSIS
• Serum magnesium—dogs, >2.51 mg/dL; cats, >2.3 mg/dL
 • Hypocalcemia is common.
• Azotemia in some patients

OTHER LABORATORY TESTS
N/A

IMAGING
N/A

DIAGNOSTIC PROCEDURES
Electrodiagnostics (e.g. electromyelography and ECG) reveal effects of hypermagnesemia but do not help differentiate the cause.

TREATMENT
• Management involves enhancing elimination from the body and symptomatic therapy.
 • Discontinue all magnesium-containing medications and nutritional supplements.
• Saline diuresis enhances renal clearance of magnesium and provides fluid volume.
 • Patients with oliguria may require peritoneal dialysis to treat severe hypermagnesemia.
• Parenteral calcium directly antagonizes the effect of magnesium, reversing respiratory depression, cardiac arrhythmias, and hypotension; calcium also enhances magnesium excretion.
• Fluid therapy with 0.9% NaCl provides fluid volume to address hypotension and azotemia.

MEDICATIONS

DRUGS OF CHOICE
• Furosemide promotes renal excretion of magnesium by decreasing absorption of magnesium in the loop of Henle.
• Enteral and parenteral calcium administration helps reverse clinical manifestations of hypermagnesemia and correct concurrent hypocalcemia; oral supplementation with any preparation can be given at a dosage of 25–50 mg/kg/day; severe hypermagnesemia can be treated with 10% calcium gluconate: 1–2 mL/kg (diluted 1:1 with saline) IV or SC q8h, administered very slowly.

CONTRAINDICATIONS
Magnesium-containing compounds

PRECAUTIONS
Monitor ECG during calcium infusions.

POSSIBLE INTERACTIONS
N/A

ALTERNATIVE DRUGS
N/A

FOLLOW-UP

PATIENT MONITORING
• Serum magnesium and calcium concentrations
• Renal function—azotemia and urine output
• Continuous electrocardiogram if possible

POSSIBLE COMPLICATIONS
• Severe hypermagnesemia and hypocalcemia can be fatal.
• Hypermagnesemic dogs were 2.6 times more likely not to survive their illness than patients with normal serum Mg levels.

✓ MISCELLANEOUS

ASSOCIATED CONDITIONS
• Hypocalcemia
• Hyperphosphatemia
• Azotemia

AGE-RELATED FACTORS
N/A

ZOONOTIC POTENTIAL
N/A

PREGNANCY
Effects on the fetus identical to the effects on the dam

SYNONYMS
None

SEE ALSO
Calcium, Hypocalcemia

ABBREVIATIONS
N/A

Suggested Reading

Macintire DK. Disorders of potassium, phosphorus, and magnesium in critical illness. Compend Cont Educ 1997;19:41–48.
Marino PL. Magnesium. In: Marino PL, ed. The ICU book. Baltimore: Williams & Wilkins, 1998:660–672.
McClean RM. Magnesium and its therapeutic uses: a review. Am J Med 1994;96:63–76.
Van Hook JW. Hypermagnesemia. Crit Care Clin 1991;7:215–223.

Author Tim Hackett
Consulting Editor Deborah S. Greco

MAGNESIUM, HYPOMAGNESEMIA

 BASICS

DEFINITION
- Dogs—serum magnesium <1.89 mg/dL
- Cats—serum magnesium <1.8 mg/dL

PATHOPHYSIOLOGY
- Magnesium—second only to potassium as the most abundant intracellular cation; most is found in bone (60%) and soft tissue (38%); most of the soft tissue magnesium resides in skeletal muscle and liver; required for many metabolic functions; an activator or catalyst for over 300 enzyme systems including phosphatases and enzymes that involve ATP.
- Because only 1–2% of total magnesium resides in the extracellular compartment, serum magnesium concentration does not always reflect the whole-body magnesium status.
- Hypomagnesemia—many causes; incidence rates >50% have been reported in critically ill human patients, but it has often been ignored in veterinary practice.
- Magnesium is an important cofactor in the sodium–potassium ATPase pump that maintains an electrical gradient across membranes; as a result, it plays an important role in the activity of electrically excitable tissues.
- Magnesium is also important in the production and elimination of acetylcholine; a low concentration of magnesium in the extracellular fluid can increase concentrations of acetylcholine at motor endplates and cause tetany.
- Interference with the electrical gradient can change resting membrane potentials and repolarization disturbances resulting in neuromuscular and cardiac abnormalities.
- Magnesium regulates calcium movement into smooth muscle cells important to contractile strength and peripheral vascular tone.
- Hypomagnesemia can alter the functions of the skeletal muscles, resulting in tetany and a variety of myopathies seen in patients receiving cisplatin and other nephrotoxic drugs.
- Magnesium depletion can affect the membrane pump on cardiac cell membranes, resulting in the depolarization of cardiac cells and tachyarrhythmias; cardiac arrhythmias associated with hypomagnesemia include ventricular arrhythmias, torsades de pointes, QT prolongation, ST segment shortening, and widening of T waves; hypomagnesemia increases the risk of digoxin toxicity because both inhibit the membrane pump.
- Hypomagnesemia causes resistance to the effects of PTH and can increase the uptake of calcium into bone.

SYSTEMS AFFECTED
- Multiple organ systems
- Gastrointestinal
- Renal
- Endocrine

SIGNALMENT
Dog and cat

SIGNS
- Hypomagnesemia occurs with a variety of diseases with diverse signs:
- Weakness
- Muscle fibrillation
- Ataxia and depression
- Hyperreflexia
- Tetany
- Behavior changes
- Arrhythmias

CAUSES
- Four general categories—gastrointestinal, renal, endocrine, and miscellaneous
- Severe malnutrition or significant malabsorptive intestinal diseases can lead to hypomagnesemia; hypomagnesemia can occur after excessive loss of body fluids (e.g., severe, prolonged diarrhea); magnesium is found in high concentration in the lower gastrointestinal tract, so secretory diarrhea in humans has been associated with profound hypomagnesemia; this is not well documented in veterinary patients.
- Magnesium homeostasis is regulated by the kidney; renal control of tubular reabsorption takes place primarily in the ascending limb of the loop of Henle; renal magnesium loss can be due to nephrotoxic drugs, including cisplatin, aminoglycosides, and amphotericin B; magnesium reabsorption can also be impaired with osmotic diuresis (diabetes mellitus), loop diuretics, hypercalciuria, and tubular acidosis.
- Hypomagnesemia associated with diuretic administration is a significant problem in human heart failure patients but has not been noted in animals.
- Endocrine problems associated with hypomagnesemia include hypercalcemia, hyperthyroidism, and hyperparathyroidism.
- Magnesium can be redistributed by refeeding after starvation, insulin therapy in diabetic ketoacidotic patients, parathyroidectomy, use of a total parenteral nutrition formulation with inadequate magnesium content, and in patients with acute pancreatitis.
- Causes of hypomagnesemia in the critically ill include decreased intake, lack of magnesium in parenteral fluids in patients receiving long-term fluid therapy or dialysis, excessive gastrointestinal loss, redistribution, and sequestration.

- Hypomagnesemia is associated with diabetes mellitus, especially following aggressive insulin therapy for diabetic ketoacidosis; nearly 25% of human diabetic outpatients were found to have low serum magnesium.

RISK FACTORS
- Total parenteral nutrition
- Diuretic administration
- Peritoneal dialysis
- Intestinal lymphangiectasia
- Diabetes mellitus

 DIAGNOSIS

DIFFERENTIAL DIAGNOSIS
- Signs of hypomagnesemia are vague and multisystemic, and other causes of neuromuscular abnormalities, especially other electrolyte abnormalities, must be investigated.
- Consider cardiac abnormalities, intoxications, and renal diseases.

LABORATORY FINDINGS
Note: 12 mg of magnesium = 1 mEq of magnesium; to convert from mg/dL to mEq/L, divide by 1.2.

Drugs That May Alter Laboratory Results
- Serum is favored over plasma because the anticoagulant used for plasma samples can contain citrate or other ions that bind magnesium.
- EDTA, sodium fluoride-oxalate, sodium citrate, and intravenous calcium gluconate can cause falsely decreased serum magnesium values.

Disorders That May Alter Laboratory Results
- Hemolysis can falsely elevate serum magnesium.
- Hypercalcemia (> 16 mg/dL) and hyperproteinemia (> 10.0 g/dL) can also falsely elevate serum magnesium.
- Hyperbilirubinemia and lipemia can cause false decreases in serum magnesium.

Valid If Run in Human Laboratory?
Yes

CBC/BIOCHEMISTRY/URINALYSIS
- Serum magnesium < 1.89 mg/dL
- If patient is azotemic, consider renal causes.
- Tubular casts in urinary sediment may indicate nephrotoxicity.
- Hypokalemia, hyponatremia, and hypocalcemia are common findings, regardless of the cause of hypomagnesemia; because serum magnesium is not routinely measured, hypokalemia or hyponatremia should alert the clinician to the possibility of hypomagnesemia.

OTHER LABORATORY TESTS

• The diagnosis of magnesium depletion can be difficult since <1% of total body magnesium is located in serum; only 55% of the magnesium in plasma is in the active (ionized) form; 33% is bound to plasma proteins and 12% is chelated with divalent anions such as phosphate and sulfate; magnesium assays (spectrophotometry) measure all three fractions.

• Ionized magnesium can be measured with an ion-specific electrode or by ultrafiltration of plasma; alternative methods of evaluating magnesium status include mononuclear blood cell magnesium levels or quantifying retention from a loading dose.

• Urinary magnesium determination may help differentiate conditions associated with high urinary magnesium loss from conditions of low intake or absorption.

• Human studies suggest that retention of >40–50% of an administered magnesium load indicates magnesium depletion, while retention of <20% indicates adequate magnesium stores.

IMAGING

N/A

DIAGNOSTIC PROCEDURES

Electrodiagnostics (e.g., electromyelography and ECG) may reveal effects of hypomagnesemia but will not help differentiate the cause.

TREATMENT

• Treatment depends on the underlying cause of the abnormality and the severity of hypomagnesemia.

• Since experience in treating veterinary patients with hypomagnesemia is extremely limited, recommendations are difficult.

• Mild hypomagnesemia may resolve with treatment of the underlying disorder; however, if hypomagnesemia is severe, intensive care is needed.

MEDICATIONS

DRUGS OF CHOICE

Can dilute magnesium sulfate in 5% dextrose in water and administer 0.75–1 mEq/kg/day as a constant-rate intravenous infusion; the solution of magnesium sulfate should be less than 20%; the magnesium infusion should use a separate intravenous line to minimize interactions with other minerals.

CONTRAINDICATIONS

• Do not use aminoglycosides; hypomagnesemia potentiates their nephrotoxicity.

• Do not use cisplatin chemotherapy.

PRECAUTIONS

• Discontinue digoxin if possible.

• Use diuretics with caution.

• Hypermagnesemia is possible with overzealous treatment.

• Azotemic patients requiring magnesium therapy should receive a lower dose and more frequent monitoring than patients with normal kidney function, to prevent iatrogenic hypermagnesemia.

POSSIBLE INTERACTIONS

• Magnesium sulfate is incompatible with sodium bicarbonate, hydrocortisone, and dobutamine HCl; avoid mixing other drugs with magnesium sulfate solution.

• Avoid calcium-containing compounds; they lower the serum magnesium concentration.

• Additive CNS depression can occur when parenteral magnesium sulfate is used with CNS depressant sedatives, neuromuscular blocking agents, and anesthetics.

• Parenteral magnesium sulfate used with nondepolarizing neuromuscular blocking agents has caused excessive neuromuscular blockade.

• Use magnesium supplementation cautiously with digitalis compounds to avoid serious conduction disturbances.

• Calcium supplements may negate the effects of parenteral magnesium.

ALTERNATIVE DRUGS

N/A

FOLLOW-UP

PATIENT MONITORING

• Serum magnesium and calcium concentrations daily

• ECG continuously, especially during magnesium infusion

POSSIBLE COMPLICATIONS

Severe hypomagnesemia can be fatal.

MISCELLANEOUS

ASSOCIATED CONDITIONS

• Hypokalemia
• Hyponatremia
• Hypocalcemia
• Hypophosphatemia

AGE-RELATED FACTORS

N/A

ZOONOTIC POTENTIAL

N/A

PREGNANCY

Effects on the fetus are identical to the effects on the dam

SYNONYMS

None
See Causes.

ABBREVIATIONS

• ATP = adenosine triphosphate
• CNS = central nervous system
• ECG = electrocardiogram
• PTH = parathyroid hormone

Suggested Reading

Dhupa N. Magnesium therapy. In: Bonagura JD, ed. Kirk's current veterinary therapy XII. Philadelphia: Saunders, 1995:132–133.

Flanders JA, Neth S, Erb HN, et al. Functional analysis of ectopic parathyroid activity in cats. Am J Vet Res 1991;52:1336–1340.

Hebert P, Mehta N, Wang J, et al. Functional magnesium deficiency in critically ill patients identified using a magnesium-loading test. Crit Care Med 1997;25:749–755.

Macintire DK. Disorders of potassium, phosphorus, and magnesium in critical illness. Compend Cont Educ 1997; 19:41–48.

Marino PL. Magnesium. In: Marino PL, ed. The ICU book. Baltimore: Williams & Wilkins, 1998:660–672.

Martin LG, Wingfield WE, Van Pelt DR, et. al. Magnesium in the 1990's: Implications for veterinary critical care. J Vet Emerg Crit Care 1993;3:105–114.

Martin LG, Matteson VL, Wingfield WE, et al. Abnormalities of serum magnesium in critically ill dogs: incidence and implications. J Vet Emerg Crit Care 1994;4:15–20.

Rosol TJ, Capen CC. Calcium-regulating hormones and diseases of abnormal mineral metabolism. In: Kaneko JJ, Harvey JW, Bruss MJ, eds. Clinical biochemistry of domestic animals. 5th ed. San Diego: Academic Press, 1997:674–687.

Author Tim Hackett
Consulting Editor Deborah S. Greco

DIAGNOSTICS–LAB

METHEMOGLOBINEMIA

BASICS

DEFINITION
• Methemoglobin content in blood > 1.5% of total hemoglobin.
• Methemoglobin differs from hemoglobin in that the iron moiety of heme groups has been oxidized from the ferrous (+2) to the ferric (+3) state

PATHOPHYSIOLOGY
• About 3% of hemoglobin is oxidized to methemoglobin each day in normal animals as a result of autoxidation of hemoglobin or secondary to oxidants produced in normal metabolic reactions.
• Methemoglobin usually accounts for < 1% of total hemoglobin, because it is constantly reduced back to hemoglobin by a NADH-dependent methemoglobin reductase (cytochrome b_5 reductase) enzyme reaction within RBCs.
• Caused by either increased production of methemoglobin by oxidants or decreased level of methemoglobin associated with a deficiency of the RBC methemoglobin reductase enzyme.

SYSTEMS AFFECTED
• Hemic/Lymph/Immune—reduced oxygen-carrying capacity of blood, because methemoglobin cannot bind oxygen; if methemoglobin content reaches high values (e.g., > 50% of total hemoglobin), various organs may suffer hypoxic injury.
• Hepatobiliary—in addition to hypoxic injury, the liver may be damaged directly by oxidant drugs that it metabolizes.
• Renal/Urologic—in addition to hypoxic injury, the kidneys may be damaged if intravascular hemolysis occurs.

SIGNALMENT
• Dogs and cats
• Deficiency in RBC methemoglobin reductase has been recognized in Chihuahuas, borzois, English setters, terrier mixes, cockapoos, poodles, corgis, Pomeranians, and toy Eskimo dogs and in domestic short-haired cats.

SIGNS

Caused Directly
• Possibly none in animals with mild to moderate methemoglobinemia.
• Cyanotic-appearing mucous membranes—may be difficult to recognize in heavily pigmented animals.
• Lethargy, tachycardia, tachypnea, ataxia, and stupor caused by hypoxia when methemoglobin content reaches 50%.
• Coma-like state and death when methemoglobin content reaches 80%.

Caused by Associated Diseases
• Vomiting, anorexia, and diarrhea possible in patients with drug toxicity.
• Hemoglobinuria secondary to severe intravascular hemolysis in some patients with concomitant Heinz body hemolytic anemia
• Subcutaneous edema, especially involving the face, and salivation in cats with acetaminophen toxicity.

CAUSES
• Toxicity—acetaminophen,* benzocaine, and phenazopyridine in cats and dogs; these drugs can also cause Heinz body hemolytic anemia.
• Deficiency in RBC methemoglobin reductase.

RISK FACTORS
• Application of benzocaine to traumatized skin or mucous membranes increases the likelihood of systemic absorption and methemoglobinemia.
• Cats are much more likely to develop clinically significant methemoglobinemia than are dogs after acetaminophen administration; this drug is not recommended for use in cats.
• Methemoglobinemia secondary to methemoglobin reductase deficiency is presumed to be an inherited disorder.

DIAGNOSIS

DIFFERENTIAL DIAGNOSIS
• Both low blood oxygen tension and methemoglobinemia can cause cyanotic-appearing mucous membranes and dark-colored blood samples.
• Hypoxemia is documented by measuring low PO_2 in an arterial blood sample.
• Methemoglobinemia is suspected when arterial blood with normal or high PO_2 is dark colored.

LABORATORY FINDINGS

Drugs That Alter Laboratory Results
None

Disorders That May Alter Laboratory Results
Hemolysis in the sample may raise the methemoglobin value, especially if the methemoglobin assay is not conducted soon after sample collection.

Valid If Run in Human Laboratory?
• Valid, as long as the method to lyse RBCs does not cause methemoglobin formation in the animal being tested
• Saponin should not be used to lyse RBCs, because it raises the methemoglobin value in some species.

CBC/BIOCHEMISTRY/URINALYSIS
• Chronic methemoglobinemia secondary to methemoglobin reductase deficiency can result in a slightly high PCV; in contrast, anemia may accompany methemoglobinemia caused by oxidant drugs.
• If severe or induced by oxidant drugs, evidence of injury to various organs (e.g., high BUN and ALT) may be seen.

OTHER LABORATORY TESTS

• Spot test—determine if the patient's methemoglobin content is clinically important: one drop of blood from the patient is placed on a piece of absorbent white paper and a drop of normal control blood is placed next to it. If the methemoglobin content is ≥ 10%, the patient's blood will be noticeably browner than the bright red of the control blood.

• Accurate determination of methemoglobin content requires that blood be rapidly submitted to a laboratory.

• Methemoglobin content in dogs with methemoglobin reductase deficiency varies from 13 to 41%; the methemoglobin content in two deficient cats was 45% and 50%.

• A definitive diagnosis of methemoglobin reductase deficiency is made by measuring enzyme activity in RBCs; this assay is done in a few research laboratories and requires that arrangements be made before blood samples are submitted.

IMAGING
N/A

DIAGNOSTIC PROCEDURES

• Blood should be stained for Heinz bodies if evidence of toxicity is present.

• The presence of Heinz bodies indicates exposure to an oxidant drug that may also cause hemolytic anemia.

 TREATMENT

• Mild to moderate—does not require specific treatment to reduce the methemoglobin content.

• Drug-induced—the use of the drug should be discontinued; RBCs can convert much of the methemoglobin back to hemoglobin within 24 hr after elimination of drug exposure.

• Inherited methemoglobin reductase deficiency—animals have normal life expectancy and generally do not require treatment, although veterinarians may wish to give a single IV injection of methylene blue (see below) 1 hr before a deficient animal is anesthetized for surgery to maximize the amount of hemoglobin that is capable of binding oxygen.

• Whole blood transfusions should be given to patients with severe anemia and those with rapidly decreasing PCV and clinical signs suggesting a deteriorating condition.

• Severe intravascular hemolysis—IV fluid administration recommended

• Treatment of electrolyte or acid–base imbalances may also be indicated in patients with severe vomiting or diarrhea, concomitant renal injury, or impending shock.

• Administration of oxygen is of limited value because methemoglobin cannot bind oxygen, and an increase in dissolved oxygen results in only a small increase in blood oxygen content.

 MEDICATIONS

DRUGS OF CHOICE

• Methylene blue—given slowly over several minutes as a 1% solution (1 mg/kg IV), may be administered in patients with severe methemoglobinemia; a dramatic response should occur during the first 30 min of treatment; **CAUTION:** although this dose can be repeated if necessary, methylene blue can cause Heinz body hemolytic anemia in cats and dogs.

• *N*-acetylcysteine is efficacious in the treatment of acetaminophen toxicity in cats if given within a few hours after exposure; recommended dosage is 140 mg/kg PO followed by 70 mg/kg q6h for 7 treatments.

CONTRAINDICATIONS
None

PRECAUTIONS

In patients that have been given drugs that cause substantial Heinz body formation and methemoglobinemia, methylene blue treatment can potentiate the formation of Heinz bodies and anemia; consequently, it is prudent to measure the PCV for 3 days after methylene blue treatment to ensure that clinically important anemia does not develop.

POSSIBLE INTERACTIONS
None

ALTERNATIVE DRUGS
None

 FOLLOW-UP

PATIENT MONITORING

• The cyanotic appearance of skin and mucous membranes should disappear after reduction of methemoglobin to an amount that does not produce clinical signs.

• Blood on the spot test should appear bright red after reduction of methemoglobin to values < 10% of total hemoglobin.

• If methylene blue treatment is given or Heinz bodies are present within RBCs, the PCV should be monitored closely, because it usually does not reach its lowest point until approximately 3 days after initial oxidant exposure.

POSSIBLE COMPLICATIONS

Coma and death can occur if methemoglobin content reaches 80% of total hemoglobin.

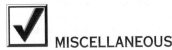 **MISCELLANEOUS**

ASSOCIATED CONDITIONS
Heinz body anemia

AGE-RELATED FACTORS
None

ZOONOTIC POTENTIAL
None

PREGNANCY
N/A

SYNONYMS
None

SEE ALSO
• Acetaminophen Toxicity
• Anemia, Heinz Body

ABBREVIATIONS
• ALT = alanine aminotransferase
• PCV = packed cell volume

Suggested Reading

Cullison RF. Acetaminophen toxicosis in small animals: clinical signs, mode of action, and treatment. Comp Cont Ed Pract Vet 1984;6:315–321.

Harvey JW. Methemoglobinemia and Heinz body hemolytic anemia. In: Kirk RW, Bonagura J, eds. Current veterinary therapy XII, Philadelphia: Saunders, 1995:443–446.

Harvey JW, Dahl M, High ME. Methemoglobin reductase deficiency in a cat. J Am Vet Med Assoc 1994;205:1290–1291.

Harvey JW, King RR, Berry CR, Blue JT. Methaemoglobin reductase deficiency in dogs. Comp Haematol Int 1991;1:55–59.

Author John W. Harvey
Consulting Editor Susan M. Cotter

MONOCYTOSIS

BASICS

DEFINITION
Absolute number of circulating monocytes greater than the reference range: dogs, $> 1.3 \times 10^9$/L or > 1300/µL or mm^3; cats, $> 0.9 \times 10^9$/L or 900/µL or mm^3

PATHOPHYSIOLOGY
• Monocytes are derived from hematopoietic stem cells named CFU-GM, which (with the appropriate stimulus) differentiate into monoblasts (or myeloblasts) and then into monocytes.
• The production, differentiation, and release of monocytes are regulated by a variety of substances derived from macrophages, T lymphocytes, endothelial cells, and fibroblasts.
• Monocytopoiesis is stimulated by substances such as IL-3, IL-11, GM-CSF, monocytopoietin, an MS-CSF, and a macrophage-derived factor that increases the mitotic activity of monocyte precursors in the bone marrow.
• Monocyte production is inhibited by PGE$_1$, PGE$_2$, and corticosteroids.
• Production to release of monocytes normally takes 36–60 hr, although with disease, production time can be shortened to a minimum emergence time of about 6 hr.
• The bone marrow lacks a reserve of monocytes because newly formed monocytes are released immediately to the circulation.
• Monocytes have a circulating half-life of about 8 hr before exiting the circulation to reside in various tissues; this process triggers another stage of differentiation, involving changes in ultrastructure, cell receptors, and metabolism; these transformed cells are referred to as macrophages, or histiocytes, and are part of the mononuclear phagocyte system.
• Fixed macrophages can be found in most tissues, including lymph nodes, bone marrow, spleen, liver (Kupffer cells), bone (osteoclasts), lamina propria of the intestinal tract, and the CNS (microglial cells).

• Free macrophages—found primarily in the pleural, peritoneal, and synovial cavities; lungs (alveolar macrophages); and inflammatory sites; can migrate through the lymphatic system into another tissue.
• Several macrophages may fuse to form multinucleated giant cells, a common response to fungi, mycobacteria, syncytial virus, and foreign material.
• There are far more tissue macrophages than circulating monocytes, perhaps owing to their long life span of several days to months.
• Most macrophages in a region originate from circulating monocytes; but under specific microenvironmental stimuli, they can be derived from local production; accumulation of monocytes in an area of acute or chronic inflammation is caused by chemotactic factors that attract monocytes to these specific foci. Functions of the Mononuclear Phagocyte System
• Phagocytic removal of damaged or aged cells or debris, tumor cytolysis, and microbicidal activity
• Regulation of the immune system via antigen processing and presentation and by secretion of interleukins responsible for promoting granulopoiesis, lymphocyte proliferation, and lymphokine production
• Vital in controlling certain pathogens, including intracellular bacteria (e.g., *Mycobacterium, Listeria,* and *Brucella*), mycotic agents, protozoa, and viruses
• Involved in regulation of coagulation, fibrinolysis, healing, and bone repair.

SYSTEMS AFFECTED
• Respiratory—alveolar macrophages
• Hemic/Lymph/Immune—lymph nodes (histiocytic proliferation), spleen (mononuclear phagocyte system proliferation), and bone marrow
• Hepatobiliary—Kupffer cells
• Musculoskeletal—osteoclasts
• Nervous system—microglial cells
• Thoracic and abdominal cavities—macrophage proliferation

SIGNALMENT
Dogs and cats

SIGNS
Related to primary cause

CAUSES

General
Any process that stimulates neutrophilia, because monocytes and neutrophils share the same stem-cell precursor CFU-GM

Glucocorticoids
• Corticosteroids stimulate absolute monocytosis in dogs and less frequently in cats.
• Monocytosis develops within hours of steroid exposure and resolves within 24 hr after removing the corticosteroid stimulus.
• Glucocorticoid treatment, stress of disease, and hyperadrenocorticism.

Inflammation
• Infectious—mycotic (e.g., *Aspergillus* and *Blastomycosis*), protozoal (e.g., *Toxoplasma*), viral (e.g., FIP and FIV), bacterial (e.g., *Mycobacterium* and *Brucella*); unlike most infectious diseases in which monocytosis is accompanied by neutrophilia, in some animals with bacterial endocarditis monocytosis is the only leukogram abnormality.
• Noninfectious—foreign material, necrotic tissue, malignant tumor, hemolytic anemia, trauma, immune-mediated disease, and hemorrhage

Bone Marrow Disease
• Marrow recovery from leukopenia—because of the rapid induction of monocytes and their uniquely short marrow transit time, monocytosis is often the earliest sign of marrow recovery and can exceed 20,000/µL.
• Monocytic or myelomonocytic leukemia—neoplastic proliferation of the monocyte cell line or a combined myeloid and monocyte cell line produces monocytosis; immature, bizarre cells are present in the circulation.
• Canine cyclic hematopoiesis (silver-gray collies)—cyclic neutropenia occurs at 10–14-day intervals, lasts 2–4 days, and is soon followed by a monocytosis; a "rebound" neutrophilia appears 2–4 days later.

• Canine granulocytopathy syndrome (Irish setters)—a defect in neutrophil intracellular bactericidal activity resulting in recurrent bacterial infection, marked neutrophilia, and variable monocytosis
• Leukocyte surface glycoprotein deficiency—abnormality reported in one Irish setter cross-bred dog with a history of recurrent bacterial infection associated with marked neutrophilia and variable monocytosis; this deficiency in adhesion molecules resulted in impaired granulocyte aggregation and adhesion.

RISK FACTORS
N/A

DIAGNOSIS

DIFFERENTIAL DIAGNOSIS
• Severely stressed or ill dogs—consider endogenous glucocorticoids
• Concurrent alopecia, potbelly, thin skin, and muscle atrophy—consider hyper-adrenocorticism
• Fever of undetermined origin—consider endocarditis and immune-mediated disease
• Draining cutaneous wound—consider mycotic infection and foreign body
• Splenomegaly, hepatomegaly, or lymphadenopathy—consider leukemia and malignant histiocytosis

LABORATORY FINDINGS

Drugs That May Alter Laboratory Results
None

Disorders That May Alter Laboratory Results
None

Valid If Run in Human Laboratory?
• Yes, but certain automated techniques for counting monocytes can yield errors.
• Mechanical blood-spreading devices shift larger cells, such as monocytes, into the "counting area," with absolute, artifactual monocytosis reported.
• Incorrect identification of metamyelocytes, other immature neutrophils, or toxic neutrophils can result in erroneous monocytosis.

CBC/BIOCHEMISTRY/URINALYSIS
• Severe monocytosis (e.g., $> 20,000/\mu L$)—consider leukemia or rebound phase of cyclic hematopoiesis
• Immature, bizarre, and abnormal cells in circulation—consider monocytic leukemia and myelomonocytic leukemia
• Mature neutrophilia, lymphopenia, and eosinopenia—consider stress and hyperadrenocorticism
• Neutrophilia—consider chronic inflammation or inherited neutrophil dysfunction
• Anemia—consider immune-mediated hemolytic anemia

OTHER LABORATORY TESTS
None

IMAGING
N/A

DIAGNOSTIC PROCEDURES
None

TREATMENT
Treatment directed at the underlying cause of monocytosis

MEDICATIONS

DRUGS OF CHOICE
N/A

CONTRAINDICATIONS
N/A

PRECAUTIONS
N/A

POSSIBLE INTERACTIONS
N/A

ALTERNATIVE DRUGS
N/A

FOLLOW-UP

PATIENT MONITORING
N/A

POSSIBLE COMPLICATIONS
N/A

MISCELLANEOUS

ASSOCIATED CONDITIONS
• Other diseases that effect the mononuclear phagocyte system but do not cause consistent monocytosis.
• Malignant and systemic histiocytosis—although Bernese mountain dogs have a predilection for this solid histiocytic neoplasm, it has been reported in other breeds as well as in a few cats; occasionally, abnormal macrophages can be found in the circulation.
• Lysosomal storage diseases

AGE-RELATED FACTORS
None

ZOONOTIC POTENTIAL
None

PREGNANCY
N/A

SYNONYMS
N/A

SEE ALSO
None

ABBREVIATIONS
• CFU-GM = colony-forming unit–granulocyte, monocyte
• FIP = feline infectious peritonitis
• FIV = feline immunodeficiency virus
• GM-CSF = granulocyte-monocyte colony-stimulating factor
• IL-3, IL-11 = interleukin 3, interleukin 11
• MS-CSF = monocyte-specific colony-stimulating factor
• PGE_1, PGE_2 = prostaglandin E_1, prostaglandin E_2

Suggested Reading
Giger U, Boxer LA, Simpson PJ, et al. Deficiency of leukocyte surface glycoproteins Mo1, LFA-1 and Leu M5 in a dog with recurrent bacterial infections. Blood 1987; 69:1622–1630.
Renshaw HW, Davis WC. Canine granulocytopathy syndrome. Am J Pathol 1979; 95:731–744.
Author Joyce S. Knoll
Consulting Editor Susan M. Cotter

NEUTROPENIA

BASICS

DEFINITION
• Neutrophil count < 2900 neutrophils/μL in dogs and < 2500 neutrophils/μL in cats
• Can develop alone or as a component of pancytopenia
• Often accompanied by a left shift and toxic change (e.g., cytoplasmic basophilia, cytoplasmic vacuolation, Döhle bodies, and toxic granulation)

PATHOPHYSIOLOGY
• Results from one of three mechanisms—(1) deficient neutrophil production in the bone marrow, (2) cells shifting from the circulating neutrophil pool to the marginal neutrophil pool in the blood, and (3) reduced neutrophil survival because of excessive tissue demand or immune-mediated destruction of cells
• Most commonly associated with infection, because emigration of neutrophils from the blood into the tissues exceeds the rate at which the bone marrow can replace them.

SYSTEMS AFFECTED
• Predisposes the patient to systemic infection by a variety of pathogens
• Many body systems can be affected in any combination, depending on the site(s) of infection.

SIGNALMENT
• Nothing specific for generalized infection
• Giant schnauzers with inherited vitamin B$_{12}$ malabsorption
• Gray collies and possibly border collies with cyclic neutropenia

SIGNS
• Signs of localized or systemic infection
• Pyrexia

CAUSES

Deficient Neutrophil Production
Stem Cell Death or Inhibition
• Infectious agents—dogs and cats, parvoviruses and bacterial-induced myelonecrosis; cats, FeLV and FIV; dogs, *Ehrlichia canis*

• Drugs, chemicals, and toxins—dogs and cats, chemotherapy agents and cephalosporins; cats, T-2 mycotoxin ingestion, chloramphenicol and benzene-ring compounds, and griseofulvin; dogs, estrogen, phenylbutazone, trimethoprim-sulfadiazine, Noxzema ingestion, thiacetarsamide administration (idiosyncratic)
• Lack of trophic factors—inherited malabsorption of vitamin B$_{12}$ (giant schnauzers); ionizing radiation

Reduced Hematopoietic Space Secondary to Myelophthisis
• Bone marrow necrosis
• Myelofibrosis
• Osteopetrosis
• Disseminated neoplasia, leukemia, and myelodysplastic syndrome
• Disseminated granulomatous disease (histoplasmosis)

Cyclic Stem Cell Proliferation
• Inherited cyclic hematopoiesis (gray collies)
• Cyclophosphamide treatment
• Idiopathic disease
• Immune-mediated suppression of granulopoiesis
• Poorly documented in dogs and cats

Neutrophil Migration
A shift in neutrophils from the circulating neutrophil pool (where they can be quantitated by the WBC count) to the marginal neutrophil pool (where they cannot be counted) occurs in patients with endotoxemia.

Reduced Survival
• Severe bacterial infection (most common cause)—pneumonia, peritonitis, and pyothorax
• Immune-mediated destruction
• Drug-induced destruction
• Hypersplenism (sequestration)
• Paraneoplastic syndrome (precise mechanism unknown)

RISK FACTORS
• Inherited disease—cyclic hematopoiesis in gray collies and possibly border collies; neutropenia in giant schnauzers
• Drug and chemical exposure—estrogen overdose in dogs (pancytopenia) and chloramphenicol and benzene-ring compounds in cats
• Exposure to various infectious agents—dogs and cats, overwhelming bacterial infection; dogs, acute *Ehrlichia canis* infection and parvovirus infection; cats, FeLV infection
• Middle-aged and old animals are less effective at repopulating the bone marrow after a severe toxic insult.

DIAGNOSIS

DIFFERENTIAL DIAGNOSIS
• Breed of dog may promote suspicion of inherited disease (e.g., cyclic hematopoiesis in gray collies and neutropenia in giant schnauzers)
• History should include information concerning drugs, toxins, and radiation exposure.

LABORATORY FINDINGS

Drugs That May Alter Laboratory Results
None

Disorders That May Alter Laboratory Results
• Failure to properly mix the blood specimen before sampling for CBC (laboratory error)
• Obtaining blood specimen from an IV catheter used for fluid administration (diluted specimen)
• Partial clotting of the blood specimen with neutrophil entrapment or aggregation (poor anticoagulation)

Valid If Run in Human Laboratory?
Automated neutrophil counts are valid; however, technicians identify too many bands in animal blood (left shift).

CBC/BIOCHEMISTRY/URINALYSIS
• Diagnosis is verified by CBC and leukocyte differential counts.
• Multiple CBC necessary to confirm or exclude a diagnosis of cyclic hematopoiesis

OTHER LABORATORY TESTS
• Serologic test—exclude ehrlichiosis in dogs and FeLV and FIV infections in cats
• Demonstration of antineutrophil antibodies—essential for diagnosing immune-mediated neutropenia
• Consider microbiological culture of putative sites(s) of bacterial infection or empirical antibiotic administration if occult infection is suspected.

IMAGING
Survey radiography and ultrasonography may help locate occult sites of infection not apparent during physical examination.

DIAGNOSTIC PROCEDURES

• Examination of a bone marrow aspirate and core biopsy—to evaluate neutrophil production and exclude myelophthisis, myelonecrosis, myelofibrosis, and osteopetrosis
• Provocative exposure to parenteral vitamin B_{12} should reverse anemia, neutropenia, and neutrophil hypersegmentation in affected giant schnauzers.
• Cytologic examination of preparations—to document excess tissue demand for neutrophils, verify sequestration of neutrophils in body cavities or between tissue planes, confirm bacterial infection, and identify sites of insensible or occult loss of neutrophils from mucous membranes or skin lesions.

 TREATMENT

• Primary concern is development of secondary infection
• In the absence of pyrexia, broad-spectrum antibiotics should be given prophylactically on an outpatient basis (especially if the count is < 1000 neutrophils/µL).
• Pyrexia—indicates current infection; treated more aggressively; inpatient treatment recommended for administration of parenteral medications until the infection is contained
• Transfusion may be indicated in patients with severe anemia (PCV < 15%).

 MEDICATIONS

DRUGS OF CHOICE

• Nonfebrile (dogs and cats)—trimethoprim-sulfadiazine (14 mg/kg PO q12h)
• Febrile(dogs and cats)—ampicillin (20 mg/kg IV q6–8h) and gentamicin sulfate (1–2 mg/kg IV q6–8h)
• rcG-CSF (dogs and cats)—5 µg/kg/day; may be of benefit in minimizing the duration; effective in dogs for prolonged periods and in cats for 42+ days; this drug not commercially available
• rhG-CSF—may be effective short term; however, development of antibodies to the protein takes place in 14–21 days
• Neutrophilia subsides within 5 days after G-CSF is discontinued.

CONTRAINDICATIONS

Adequately controlled safety studies of rcG-CSF and rhG-CSF have not been performed in dogs and cats (including pregnant animals); high-dose administration (80 µg/kg/day) of rhG-CSF in pregnant rabbits was associated with fetal resorption, abortion, and increased genitourinary tract hemorrhage.

Pregnant Animals

• Drugs listed should be used only if the benefits supersede the inherent risks.
• Sulfa drugs cross the placenta and can cause jaundice, hemolytic anemia, and kernicterus.
• Trimethoprim crosses the placenta; no harm accompanies drug administration in early pregnancy; however, this drug should not be used near term because of folic acid inhibition.
• Gentamycin sulfate crosses the placenta and may be associated with fetal ototoxicity.

PRECAUTIONS

• Maintain hydration when administering sulfa drugs to prevent renal crystallization.
• Gentamycin sulfate may be nephrotoxic and ototoxic.
• Risk of nephrotoxicity higher in dehydrated and overdosed animals

POSSIBLE INTERACTIONS

N/A

ALTERNATIVE DRUGS

Enrofloxacin or orbifloxacin can be substituted for gentamycin.

 FOLLOW-UP

PATIENT MONITORING

• Periodic CBC; improvement denoted by a rising leukocyte or neutrophil count, resolution of left shift, and disappearance of toxic change.
• Rebound neutrophilic leukocytosis expected during recovery from neutropenia.

POSSIBLE COMPLICATIONS

Secondary infections

 MISCELLANEOUS

ASSOCIATED CONDITIONS

Secondary infection

AGE-RELATED FACTORS

Repopulation of bone marrow with hematopoietic cells is more difficult in middle-aged and old animals because of age-related reduction in stem cell numbers.

ZOONOTIC POTENTIAL

None

PREGNANCY

N/A

SYNONYMS

None

SEE ALSO

• Ehrlichiosis
• Estrogen Toxicity
• Feline Immunodeficiency Virus
• Feline Leukemia Virus Infection
• Feline Panleukopenia
• Parvovirus Infection—Dogs

ABBREVIATIONS

• FeLV = feline leukemia virus
• FIV = feline immunodeficiency virus
• PCV = packed cell volume
• rcG-CSF = recombinant canine granulocyte colony-stimulating factor
• rhG-CSF = recombinant human granulocyte colony-stimulating factor

Suggested Reading

August JR. Consultations in feline internal medicine. 2nd ed. Philadelphia: Saunders, 1994.
Duncan JR, Prasse KW, Mahaffey EA. Veterinary laboratory medicine. 3rd ed. Ames: Iowa State University Press, 1994.
Ettinger SJ, Feldman EC. Textbook of veterinary internal medicine. 4th ed. Philadelphia: Saunders, 1995.
Sherding RG. Cat diseases and clinical management. New York: Churchill Livingstone, 1989.

Author Kenneth S. Latimer
Consulting Editor Susan M. Cotter

DIAGNOSTICS—LAB

NEUTROPHILIA

BASICS

DEFINITION
• Abnormally high absolute number of circulating neutrophils
• In adult dogs and cats, neutrophil counts > 12,000–13,000/μL
• The most common cause of leukocytosis

PATHOPHYSIOLOGY
• Neutrophils are produced in the bone marrow, released into the blood, circulate briefly, and migrate into tissue spaces and onto epithelial surfaces.
• CSFs govern the proliferation and maturation of immature neutrophils in the marrow.
• Injury or bacterial invasion of tissue results in the production and release of CSFs, which increase proliferation and maturation of neutrophilic progenitor cells in the bone marrow; other mediators of inflammation stimulate bone marrow release and promote margination and adhesion of neutrophils to vascular endothelium at the site of inflammation.
• Transit time for bone marrow granulopoiesis is 4–6 days.
• Neutrophils circulate for about 10 hr and are compartmentalized into a CNP and an MNP; neutrophils in the CNP circulate with other blood cells and are measured in the CBC; neutrophils in the MNP are intermittently adherent to endothelium, especially in small veins and capillaries.
• Migration of neutrophils into the tissues occurs randomly and is unidirectional.
• Neutrophils are also destroyed in spleen, liver, and bone marrow.
• Number of circulating neutrophils is affected by the rate of bone marrow production and release, the rate of exchange between the CNP and the MNP, and the rate of migration into tissue; changes in these rates can favor an increase in circulating neutrophils.
• Results when one or more of the following occurs—(1) rates of marrow production and release increase, (2) neutrophils demarginate from the MNP into the CNP, (3) tissue demand for neutrophils increases, and (4) granulocytic neoplasia develops.

SYSTEMS AFFECTED
Hemic/Lymph/Immune–a hematologic abnormality and is the result of a systemic response or disease rather than a cause thereof.

SIGNALMENT
N/A

SIGNS
• Vary with cause
• History and clinical findings evaluated for evidence of inflammation or sepsis as a cause; once eliminated, other causes explored

CAUSES

Physiologic Neutrophilia
• Fear, excitement, vigorous exercise, and seizure activity, which lead to epinephrine release
• Neutrophils demarginate from the MNP into the CNP, resulting in transient (1-hr), mature neutrophilia.
• In cats, marked lymphocytosis (6,000–15,000/μL) occurs concurrently.

Corticosteroid- or Stress-induced
• Endogenous release or exogenous administration of corticosteroids increases bone marrow release of mature neutrophils, demargination into the CNP, and diminished tissue migration.
• Leukocytosis (15,000–35,000/μL) and neutrophilia occur 4–8 hr after corticosteroid administration and return to normal 1–3 days after treatment.
• In dogs, lymphopenia, eosinopenia, and monocytosis occur concurrently.
• Pain, traumatic injury, boarding, transport, or other stressful conditions

Acute Inflammation
• Inflammation, sepsis, necrosis, or immune-mediated disease cause an increase in tissue demand and bone marrow release of segmented and band neutrophils.
• Leukocytosis (15,000–35,000/μL), neutrophilia with left shift, toxic neutrophils, lymphopenia, eosinopenia, and variable monocytosis are usual responses.
• Surgical removal or drainage of septic focus may increase neutrophilia.

Chronic Inflammation
• Chronic suppuration (e.g., pyometra, abscesses, pyothorax, and pyoderma) and some neoplasms cause marrow granulocytic hyperplasia, resulting in severe leukocytosis (50,000–120,000/μL), neutrophilia with a left shift, variable numbers of toxic neutrophils, monocytosis, and hyperglobulinemia.
• Anemia of chronic disease may be noted.
• Leukemoid response—describes inflammatory neutrophilia with WBC counts > 100,000/μL, which is as high as in patients with chronic granulocytic leukemia.

Hemolytic or Hemorrhagic Anemias
• Neutrophilia with a left shift can occur in dogs with immune-mediated hemolytic anemia.
• Mature neutrophilia occurs within 3 hr after acute hemorrhage.

Chronic Granulocytic Leukemia
• Hematologic response in dogs similar to neutrophilia of chronic inflammation
• Severe neutrophilic leukocytosis (> 80,000/μL), disordered left shift, and variable degrees of thrombocytopenia and anemia are observed.
• Splenomegaly and hepatomegaly may be pronounced.

Other Causes
• Granulocytopathy
• Cyclic hematopoiesis

RISK FACTORS
N/A

DIAGNOSIS

DIFFERENTIAL DIAGNOSIS
• Animals with inflammatory neutrophilia usually have historical or clinical evidence of septic or nonseptic inflammatory disease, such as pyrexia, weight loss, anorexia, and specific organ system involvement.
• Stress neutrophilia occurs frequently in dogs and cats examined because of noninflammatory disorders.
• Physiologic neutrophilia with concurrent lymphocytosis occurs in young healthy animals, especially apprehensive cats.

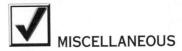
LABORATORY FINDINGS

Drugs That May Alter Laboratory Results
• Corticosteroid administration causes stress-induced neutrophil response.
• Neutrophilia subsides with long-term therapy but lymphopenia persists.

Disorders That May Alter Laboratory Results
• Falsely high electronic WBC counts—caused by large platelets, platelet clumps, and Heinz bodies
• Falsely low electronic WBC counts—caused by leukocyte clumping

Valid If Run in Human Laboratory?
• Yes, but some human laboratories overestimate the number of band cells at the expense of mature neutrophils.
• Normal animals will appear to have left shifts.

CBC/BIOCHEMISTRY/URINALYSIS
• Assessment of sequential leukograms—important because the number of segmented and band neutrophils can change dramatically in a few hours; trends important in diagnosis and prognosis
• Toxic neutrophils—observed in patients with neutrophilia caused by inflammation, especially those associated with toxemia; observed in blood and bone marrow characterized by diffuse cytoplasmic basophilia, foamy vacuolated cytoplasm, Döhle bodies, and giant forms with bizarre nuclear shapes
• Animals with acute sepsis and neutrophilia can become hypoglycemic.

OTHER LABORATORY TESTS
• Blood culture
• Bacterial or fungal culture of urine, tissue samples, and body fluids
• Serologic tests for fungi, protozoa, or rickettsia, especially *Blastomyces, Histoplasma, Coccidioides, Actinomyces, Nocardia, Toxoplasma, Hepatozoon,* and *Rickettsia*
• Coombs' test, antinuclear antibody test, or rheumatoid factor test is indicated if immune-mediated disease suspected.
• Tests of neutrophil adhesion, chemotaxis, and bactericidal activity are indicated if granulocytopathy is suspected.

IMAGING
Radiography and ultrasonography of abdomen, thorax, soft tissue, or skeleton—inflammatory or neoplastic lesions (e.g., abscess, granulomatous lesion, effusions, foreign body, and organomegaly)

DIAGNOSTIC PROCEDURES
• Cytologic examination of suspect tissues or fluids for bacteria, fungi, protozoa, or neoplasia
• Aspiration of bone marrow and spleen if chronic granulocytic leukemia suspected

TREATMENT
• Varies with the identity and severity of underlying cause
• Animals with acute sepsis or hemolytic anemia require aggressive intervention.
• Animals with inflammatory neutrophilia caused by localized sites of suppuration may require surgical removal or drainage of affected tissues.
• Animals with chronic granulocytic leukemia require chemotherapy.

MEDICATIONS

DRUGS OF CHOICE
Appropriate antimicrobial therapy for septic inflammation decided after identification of causative agent and sensitivity testing

CONTRAINDICATIONS
Corticosteroids should be avoided if fungal or protozoal infection is suspected.

PRECAUTIONS
N/A

POSSIBLE INTERACTIONS
N/A

ALTERNATIVE DRUGS
N/A

FOLLOW-UP

PATIENT MONITORING
Animals with inflammatory neutrophilia, especially those of acute onset, may require daily or twice-daily hematologic assessment.

POSSIBLE COMPLICATIONS
• Animals with acute inflammatory neutrophilia may become neutropenic if neutrophil migration into the inflamed tissue exceeds the bone marrow production rate.
• If neutropenia develops, prognosis is grave.

✓ MISCELLANEOUS

ASSOCIATED CONDITIONS
N/A

AGE-RELATED FACTORS
N/A

ZOONOTIC POTENTIAL
Some causes of neutrophilia

PREGNANCY
N/A

SYNONYMS
None

SEE ALSO
• Cyclic Hematopoiesis—Dogs
• Hyperadrenocorticism (Cushing Disease)
• Infectious disease topics
• Lymphocytosis
• Myeloproliferative Disorders

ABBREVIATIONS
• CNP = circulating neutrophil pool
• CSF = colony-stimulating factor
• MNP = marginal neutrophil pool

Suggested Reading
Latimer KS. Leukocytes in health and disease. In: Ettinger SJ, Feldman EC, eds. Textbook of veterinary internal medicine. Philadelphia: Saunders, 1995:1892–1929.
Tvedten H. Leukocyte disorders. In: Willard MD Tvedten H, Turnwald GH, eds. Small animal clinical diagnosis by laboratory methods. Philadelphia: Saunders, 1994:53–79.
Author Peter S. MacWilliams
Consulting Editor Susan M. Cotter

OSMOLARITY, HYPEROSMOLARITY

BASICS

DEFINITION
• Osmolarity—expressed in mOsm/L; represents the number of solute particles per liter of solution
• Osmolality—expressed in mOsm/kg; represents the number of solute particles per kilogram of solution
• Hyperosmolarity—a high concentration of solute particles per liter of solution
• Serum concentrations > 310 mOsm/L in dogs and > 330 mOsm/L in cats are usually considered hyperosmolar.

PATHOPHYSIOLOGY
• Serum sodium is responsible for most of the osmotically active particles that contribute to serum osmolarity; serum glucose and urea also contribute to serum osmolarity.
• Anything that causes water loss increases concentrations of solutes in plasma or serum, thereby increasing serum osmolarity.
• Blood volume, hydration status, and ADH are intimately involved in controlling extracellular fluid volume.
• Low circulating blood volume stimulates carotid and aortic baroreceptors to respond to changes in blood pressure, causing ADH secretion.
• Hyperosmolarity affects the osmoreceptors in the hypothalamus and stimulates ADH secretion from the neurohypophysis; the hypothalamic thirst center is also stimulated and causes an increase in water consumption to counteract serum hyperosmolarity by solute dilution.
• Rapid increases in serum osmolarity cause water movement along its concentration gradient from intracellular to extracellular spaces, resulting in neuronal dehydration, cell shrinkage, and cell death; cerebral vessels may weaken and hemorrhage.

SYSTEMS AFFECTED
• Nervous—excessive thirst may be the first sign of hyperosmolarity.
• Cardiovascular—hypotension and decreased ventricular contractility
• Renal/Urologic—low urine output

SIGNALMENT
• Dogs and cats
• Hypodipsia and hyperosmolarity have been reported in young female miniature schnauzers.

SIGNS

General Comments
• Primarily neurologic or behavioral
• Severity is related more to how quickly hyperosmolarity occurs than to the absolute magnitude of change.
• Most likely to occur if serum osmolarity is >350 mOsm/L and usually severe if >375 mOsm/L

Historical Findings
Anorexia, lethargy, vomiting, weakness, disorientation, ataxia, seizures, and coma; polydipsia followed by hypodipsia

Physical Examination Findings
• Normal, or abnormalities may reflect underlying disease
• In addition to historical findings, dehydration, tachycardia, hypotension, weak pulses, and fever may be detected.

CAUSES

Increased Solutes
Hypernatremia, hyperglycemia, severe azotemia, ethylene glycol toxicosis, salt poisoning, sodium phosphate enemas in cats and small dogs, mannitol, radiographic contrast solution, administration of ethanol, aspirin toxicosis, shock, lactate in patients with lactic acidosis, acetoacetate and β-hydroxybutyrate in patients with ketoacidosis, liquid enteral nutrition, and parenteral nutrition solutions

Decreased Extracellular Fluid Volume
Dehydration—gastrointestinal loss, cutaneous loss, third space loss, low water consumption, and polyuria without adequate compensatory polydipsia

RISK FACTORS
• Medical conditions that predispose—renal failure, diabetes insipidus, diabetes mellitus, hyperadrenocorticism, hyperaldosteronism, and heat stroke
• Therapeutic hyperosmolar solutions—hypertonic saline, sodium bicarbonate, sodium phosphate enemas in cats and small dogs, and mannitol
• High environmental temperatures
• Fever

DIAGNOSIS

DIFFERENTIAL DIAGNOSIS
• Primary CNS disease and neoplasia may be characterized by altered mentation, but serum osmolarity is usually normal.
• Physical evidence or history of injury usually helps to rule out CNS depression caused by cranial trauma.
• Perform a thorough physical examination to assess hydration status and obtain information regarding previous therapy that may have included sodium-containing fluids or hyper-osmolar solutions.

LABORATORY FINDINGS

Drugs That May Alter Laboratory Results
Excessive administration of sodium-containing fluids or hyperosmolar solutions increase serum osmolarity.

Disorders That May Alter Laboratory Results
N/A

Valid If Run in Human Laboratory?
Yes

CBC/BIOCHEMISTRY/URINALYSIS
• High PCV, hemoglobin, and plasma proteins in dehydrated patients; serum electrolytes may also be increased.
• Hyperosmolarity is an indication to evaluate serum sodium and glucose concentrations.
• Without the presence of excessive unmeasured osmoles, estimated serum osmolarity may be calculated from serum chemistries as follows:

$$\frac{1.86(Na + K) + BUN + glucose}{2.8 \times 18}$$

- Normally, calculated osmolarity should not exceed measured osmolarity; if it is, consider laboratory error.
- If measured osmolarity exceeds the calculated osmolarity, determine the osmolar gap.
- Osmolar gap = measured osmolarity − calculated osmolarity.
- High measured osmolarity and normal calculated osmolarity with a high osmolar gap indicate the presence of unmeasured solutes (not Na, K, glucose, BUN).
- High measured osmolarity and high calculated osmolarity with a normal osmolar gap usually indicate that the hyperosmolarity is caused by hyperglycemia or hypernatremia.
- Serum sodium concentration may be artificially low in patients with severe hyperglycemia and hyperosmolarity.
- Fasting hyperglycemia and glucosuria support a diagnosis of diabetes mellitus.
- Numerous calcium oxalate crystals in the urine suggest ethylene glycol toxicosis.
- High urinary specific gravity rules out diabetes insipidus.
- Low urinary specific gravity, especially hyposthenuria, suggests diabetes insipidus.

OTHER LABORATORY TESTS
Urinary osmolarity lower than serum osmolarity suggests diabetes insipidus; concentrated urine rules out diabetes insipidus.

IMAGING
Renal ultrasonography may reveal bright, hyperechoic kidneys in patients with ethylene glycol toxicosis.

DIAGNOSTIC PROCEDURES
N/A

TREATMENT
- Mild hyperosmolarity without clinical signs may not warrant specific treatment, but diagnose and treat underlying diseases.

- Hospitalize patients with moderate-to-high osmolarity (>350 mOsm/L) and patients exhibiting clinical signs and gradually lower serum osmolarity with intravenous fluids while a definitive diagnosis is pursued.
- Administer D_5W or 0.45% saline slowly IV.
- Initially, 0.9% saline may be used to restore normal hemodynamics and replace dehydration deficits; replace one-half of dehydration deficits over 12 h and the remainder over 24 h; then switch to D_5W or 0.45% saline.

MEDICATIONS

DRUGS OF CHOICE
Seizures can be controlled with diazepam, phenobarbital, or pentobarbital.

CONTRAINDICATIONS
Hypertonic saline and hyperosmolar solutions

PRECAUTIONS
- May use normal saline initially, but rapid administration may worsen neurologic signs.
- Rapid administration of hypotonic fluids (e.g., D5W and 0.45% saline) may also cause cerebral edema and worsen neurologic signs.

POSSIBLE INTERACTIONS
N/A

ALTERNATIVE DRUGS
N/A

FOLLOW-UP

PATIENT MONITORING
- Hydration status; avoid overhydration.
- Bladder size, urine output, and breathing patterns during IV fluid administration.
- Anuria and irregular breathing patterns may be signs of deterioration.

POSSIBLE COMPLICATIONS
Altered consciousness and abnormal behavior

MISCELLANEOUS

ASSOCIATED CONDITIONS
Hypernatremia and hyperglycemia

AGE-RELATED FACTORS
N/A

ZOONOTIC POTENTIAL
N/A

PREGNANCY
N/A

SYNONYMS
Hyperosmolality

SEE ALSO
- Sodium, Hypernatremia
- Glucose, Hyperglycemia
- Diabetes Mellitus, Nonketotic Hyperosmolar Syndrome

ABBREVIATIONS
ADH = antidiuretic hormone

Suggested Reading
DiBartola SP, ed. Fluid therapy in small animal practice. Philadelphia: Saunders, 1992.
DiBartola SP, Green RA, Autran de Morais HS. Osmolality and osmolal gap. In: Willard MD, Tvedten H, Turnwald GH eds. Small animal clinical diagnosis by laboratory methods. 2nd ed. Philadelphia: Saunders, 1994:106–107.
Riley JH, Cornelius LM. Osmolality. In: Loeb WF, Quimby FW, eds. The clinical chemistry of laboratory animals. New York: Pergamon Press, 1989:395–397.
Author Margaret R. Kern
Consulting Editor Deborah S. Greco

PANCYTOPENIA

BASICS

DEFINITION
Concurrently low peripheral blood concentrations of WBCs, RBCs, and platelets

PATHOPHYSIOLOGY
• Pathophysiologic mechanisms are destruction, excessive use, loss, sequestration, and reduced production of WBCs, RBCs, and platelets; these mechanisms may act alone or together.
• Reduced production occurs when pluripotent, multipotent, or committed stem cells are destroyed; their proliferation or differentiation is suppressed; or the maturation of differentiated cells is delayed or arrested.
• If pluripotent stem cells are affected, pancytopenia develops; if committed stem cells are affected, cytopenia of the cell type affected develops.
• Destruction, use, or loss of mature WBCs, RBCs, and platelets in excess of their production; WBC, RBC, and platelet production can markedly increase in response to demand; about 2 days are required before increased production begins to have an effect on the peripheral blood counts, and peak output usually takes about 1 week; thus the rate of destruction necessary to cause cytopenia is not as great during the first few days of disease as later.
• Sequestration of WBC, RBC, or platelets in the microcirculation, especially that of the spleen, intestine, and lungs, can cause cytopenia of the sequestered cell type.

SYSTEMS AFFECTED
Hemic/Lymph/Immune—bone marrow, spleen, lymph nodes, and lymphoid tissues; depending on the cause, these organs can be affected by cellular depletion, degeneration, necrosis, hyperplasia, dysplasia, or dyscrasia; changes may occur alone or in combination.

SIGNALMENT
Dogs and cats

SIGNS

Historical Findings
• History reflects the underlying cause.
• Lethargy or pallor owing to anemia
• Petechial hemorrhage or mucosal bleeding owing to thrombocytopenia
• Repeated febrile episodes or frequent or persistent infection owing to leukopenia

Physical Examination Findings
• Lethargy
• Pale mucous membranes
• Mucosal hemorrhage (e.g., hematuria, hemoptysis, melena, and epistaxis)
• Fever or other evidence of infection

CAUSES

Infectious Diseases (Most Common)
• FeLV infection*
• FIV infection
• Ehrlichiosis
• FIP
• Feline and canine parvovirus
• Infectious canine hepatitis virus
• Histoplasmosis
• Endotoxemia and septicemia (especially that caused by the gram-negative organisms or tularemia)

Drugs, Chemicals, and Toxins
• Estrogen* (Sertoli cell tumor, interstitial cell tumor, and prescribed estrogen compounds)
• Phenylbutazone
• Griseofulvin
• Methimazole (cats)
• Chloramphenicol
• Trimethoprim-sulfadiazine
• Albendazole
• Captopril
• Second-generation cephalosporins
• Chemotherapeutics
• Thallium
• Toxins (e.g., *Fusarium* T-2 toxin)
• Ionizing radiation

Proliferative and Infiltrative Diseases
• Hematopoietic neoplasia* (leukemia, myelodysplasia)
• Myelofibrosis
• Severe diffuse infiltration of the bone marrow by metastatic tumor cells
• Myelophthisis

Immune-Mediated disease
Aplastic anemia

RISK FACTORS
Varies with individual cause

DIAGNOSIS

DIFFERENTIAL DIAGNOSIS
• Extremely rapid onset with severe clinical signs—more consistent with conditions that cause necrosis, destruction, or sequestration of cells
• Slow, insidious onset—more consistent with conditions that cause bone marrow suppression

LABORATORY FINDINGS

Drugs That May Alter Laboratory Results
Glucocorticoids often increase the neutrophil count by two times or more and can, therefore, obscure an otherwise low neutrophil count.

Disorders That May Alter Laboratory Results
Poor phlebotomy technique may cause platelet clumping and hemolysis, leading to spuriously low platelet counts and spuriously low PCV, respectively.

Valid If Run in Human Laboratory?
• Varies with laboratory
• Check that the laboratory has validated their hematology instruments for dog and cat specimens.

CBC/BIOCHEMISTRY/URINALYSIS
• WBC, RBC, and platelet counts—low
• Anemia—usually nonregenerative
• Blood smear evaluation—may reveal infectious organisms (e.g., *Ehrlichia* spp. and *Histoplasma capsulatum*)
• Rapid, sudden onset and toxic changes in leukocytes—suggest bone marrow injury (e.g., parvovirus and chemical agents), septicemia, or endotoxemia
• Atypical or blastic leukocytes, rubricytes, and megakaryoblasts—suggest myeloproliferative disease
• High ALT, AST, ALP, and GGT activities—suggest myeloproliferative or lymphoproliferative disease with bone marrow and hepatic involvement

OTHER LABORATORY TESTS
• Reticulocyte count—determine if bone marrow is regenerative; a regenerative response to the anemia suggests cause is destruction, use, or sequestration; a nonregenerative response suggests cause is bone marrow suppression and merits examination of a bone marrow aspirate or punch biopsy.
• Serologic testing—detect suspected infectious agents (e.g., FIV, FeLV, and *Ehrlichia* spp.)

IMAGING
N/A

OTHER DIAGNOSTIC PROCEDURES

Bone Marrow Examination
- Indicated when the cause cannot be determined
- Hypercellular bone marrow associated with myelodysplasia, myelophthisis, and the recovery phase of parvovirus infection
- Hypocellular bone marrow associated with bone marrow necrosis (e.g., toxins and parvovirus), fibrosis, and suppression (e.g., drugs, hormones, and aplastic anemia)
- If the bone marrow is unaspirable, fibrosis or necrosis of the bone marrow should be considered; bone marrow necrosis is usually associated with rapid onset of severe clinical signs, often including emesis and diarrhea.

TREATMENT

- Supportive treatment depends on the clinical situation and includes aggressive antibiotic therapy, blood transfusion, and transfusion of platelet-rich plasma.
- Treat the underlying condition.

MEDICATIONS

DRUGS OF CHOICE
Treatment should be appropriate for the clinical situation (e.g., the degree to which each cell population is low, whether the patient has fever or infection, and established or suspected specific diagnoses); see specific causes.

CONTRAINDICATIONS
- Drugs known to suppress hematopoiesis (see Causes)
- Aspirin or other drugs known to interfere with platelet function

PRECAUTIONS
Because of the patient's compromised immune status, glucocorticoids and other immuno-suppressive drugs should be used only when absolutely necessary and with extreme care.

POSSIBLE INTERACTIONS
N/A

ALTERNATIVE DRUGS

Recombinant Growth Factors
- rhG-CSF—5 μg/kg/day
- rhEPO—initial dosage, 50–100 U/kg SC 3 times/week; used in an attempt to stimulate erythropoiesis

FOLLOW-UP

PATIENT MONITORING
- Daily physical examination, including frequent monitoring of body temperature
- Periodic CBC—the frequency of hematologic testing depends on the severity of the cytopenias, age and general physical condition of the patient, and underlying cause.

POSSIBLE COMPLICATIONS
- Hemorrhage
- Infection, usually bacterial

MISCELLANEOUS

ASSOCIATED CONDITIONS
Infection in patients with leukopenia

AGE-RELATED FACTORS
N/A

ZOONOTIC POTENTIAL
- Tularemia
- The owner can contract histoplasmosis from the same source as the patient.

PREGNANCY
Associated stress can cause abortion; see respective topics for the effects of different causes on pregnancy.

SYNONYMS
None

SEE ALSO
- Anemia, Nonregenerative
- Anemia, Regenerative
- Anemia, Aplastic
- Neutropenia
- Specific causes of pancytopenia
- Thrombocytopenia

ABBREVIATIONS
- ALP = alkaline phosphatase
- ALT = alanine aminotransferase
- AST = aspartate aminotransferase
- FeLV = feline leukemia virus
- FIP = feline infectious peritonitis
- FIV = feline immunodeficiency virus
- GGT = γ-glutamyltransferase
- PCV = packed cell volume
- rhEPO = recombinant human erythropoietin
- rhG-CSF = recombinant human granulocyte colony-stimulating factor

Suggested Readings
Baldwin CJ, Ledet, AE. Pancytopenia. In: August JR, ed. Consultations in feline internal medicine. 2nd ed. Philadelphia: Saunders, 1993:495–502.

Hollan M, Stobie D, Shapiro W. Pancytopenia associated with administration of captopril to a dog. J Am Vet Med Assoc 1996;208:1683–1686.

Shelly SM. Causes of canine pancytopenia. Compend Contin Ed Pract Vet 1988;10:9–16.

Tvedten H. Erythrocyte disorders. In: Willard MD, Tvedten H, Turnwald GH, eds. Small animal clinical diagnosis by laboratory methods. 2nd ed. Philadelphia: Saunders, 1994:31–51.

Author Gregory O. Freden
Consulting Editor Susan M. Cotter

PARAPROTEINEMIA

 BASICS

DEFINITION
• An immunoglobulin produced by a clone of neoplastic immune cells, either plasma cells in patients with multiple myeloma or macroglobulinemia or lymphocytes in patients with lymphoma.
• In any single patient, the paraprotein will be a single class and subclass of immunoglobulin with a single light chain class.

PATHOPHYSIOLOGY
• Primary signs relate to the effects of the underlying tumor in the bone and bone marrow or to the primary effects of the paraproteins.
• The abnormal immunoglobulin also can produce a variety of effects.

SYSTEMS AFFECTED
• Musculoskeletal—bone lysis by the neoplastic cells can cause lameness
• Nervous—bone lysis of the axial skeleton can cause neurologic signs; if the paraprotein reaches a sufficient concentration, hyperviscosity syndrome develops, usually causing neurologic signs.
• Hemic/Lymph/Immune—myelophthisis may cause anemia, leukopenia, or thrombocytopenia; hemostasis may be compromised by paraprotein interference with platelet and coagulation factor function.

SIGNALMENT
• Dogs and cats
• Middle-aged to old dogs more frequently affected
• No sex predilection

SIGNS
• Lameness
• Paresis
• Weakness
• Weight Loss
• Epistaxis
• Gingival bleeding
• Petechia
• Ecchymoses
• Melena

CAUSES
• No carcinogenic agent has been associated with multiple myeloma, macroglobulinemia, or lymphoproliferative disorders in dogs.
• FeLV causes lymphosarcoma in cats.

RISK FACTORS
N/A

 DIAGNOSIS

DIFFERENTIAL DIAGNOSIS
• Other causes of narrow-based gammopathy resembling paraprotein or monoclonal gammopathy are ehrlichiosis, acute-phase reactants in the α_2-region, leishmaniasis, amyloidosis, plasmacytic gastroenterocolitis, and benign monoclonal gammopathy.
• Bleeding disorders occurring concurrently can be assumed to be caused by the paraproteinemia; primary bleeding disorders probably do not need to be initially considered.

LABORATORY FINDINGS
Drugs That May Alter Laboratory Results
None

Disorders That May Alter Laboratory Results
None

Valid If Run in Human Laboratory?
Yes

CBC/BIOCHEMISTRY/URINALYSIS
• Total protein and globulin—usually high in patients with disease severe enough to cause clinical signs
• Proteinuria caused by light chains (i.e., Bence-Jones protein)—not detected by routine tests; immunoassay or electrophoresis of a urine sample that has been concentrated in the laboratory more likely to result in detection; not seen in patients with pseudoparaproteinemia
• Hypercalcemia—in some patients; generally correlated with bone lysis

OTHER LABORATORY TESTS
• Viscosimetry—may help define hyperviscosity syndrome but not usually necessary
• Serologic tests—rule out *Ehrlichia canis*

IMAGING
Radiography of affected bones indispensable to identify lytic bone lesions and sometimes a site for aspiration.

OTHER DIAGNOSTIC PROCEDURES
• Bone marrow biopsy with examination of bone marrow aspirate reveals > 5% plasma cells, often with criteria of malignancy; the distribution of multiple myeloma is patchy; aspiration and examination of a lytic lesion may be necessary to detect malignant plasma cells.
• Cytologic or histopathologic examinations of affected organs may identify lymphoproliferative diseases that cause true paraproteinemia and other diseases that cause narrow-based gammopathies, which are not true paraproteinemias.

TREATMENT

• Supportive treatment varies depending on the manifestations of disease and the organ systems affected.
• Hyperviscosity syndrome may present as a neurologic emergency.
• Plasmapheresis can be life-saving even if done by removal of whole blood, manual centrifugation, and replacement with fluid and the retrieved cells.
• Chemotherapy for myeloma

MEDICATIONS

DRUGS OF CHOICE
• Patients are probably immunocompromised and may need aggressive antibiotic therapy.
• See Multiple Myeloma.

CONTRAINDICATIONS
N/A

PRECAUTIONS
N/A

POSSIBLE INTERACTIONS
N/A

ALTERNATIVE DRUGS
N/A

FOLLOW-UP

PATIENT MONITORING
• Observe clinical signs and repeat abnormal laboratory tests and radiographs at 2–4-week intervals.
• Animals that respond will improve clinically before radiographs and laboratory tests show improvement.

POSSIBLE COMPLICATIONS
Vertebral involvement associated with fracture and severe neurologic compromise.

MISCELLANEOUS

ASSOCIATED CONDITIONS
Immunologic incompetence

AGE-RELATED FACTORS
None

ZOONOTIC POTENTIAL
None

PREGNANCY
N/A

SYNONYMS
• Monoclonal gammopathy
• M protein

SEE ALSO
• Lymphosarcoma—Cats
• Lymphosarcoma—Dogs
• Multiple myeloma

ABBREVIATION
FeLV = feline leukemia virus

Suggested Reading

Breitschwerdt EB, Woody BJ, Zerbe CA, et al. Monoclonal gammopathy associated with naturally occurring canine ehrlichiosis. J Vet Int Med 1987;1:2–9.
Font A, Closa JM, Mascort J. Monoclonal gammopathy in a dog with visceral leishmaniasis. 1994;8:233–235.
Matus RE, Leifer CE. Immunoglobulin-producing tumors. Vet Clin North Am Small Anim Pract 1985;15:741–752.
Matus RE, Leifer CE, MacEwen EG, Hurvitz AI. Prognostic factors for multiple myeloma in the dog. J Am Vet Med Assoc 1986;188:1288–1292.

Author G. Daniel Boon
Consulting Editor Susan M. Cotter

PHOSPHORUS, HYPERPHOSPHATEMIA

 BASICS

DEFINITION
• Serum total phosphorus > 5.5 mg/dL (dogs)
• Serum total phosphorus > 6.0 mg/dL (cats)

PATHOPHYSIOLOGY
• Control of phosphorus is complex and is influenced by the actions of PTH and vitamin D and the interaction of these hormones with the gut, bone, kidneys, and parathyroid glands.
• High serum phosphorus results from excessive gastrointestinal absorption of phosphorus, excessive bone resorption of phosphorus, and reduced renal excretion of phosphorus.

SYSTEMS AFFECTED
• Renal
• Endocrine
• Metabolic

SIGNALMENT
• Dog and cat
• Any age, but commonly young, growing animals or old animals with renal insufficiency

SIGNS

Historical Findings
• Depend on the underlying cause of hyperphosphatemia
• No specific signs directly attributable to hyperphosphatemia
• Acute hyperphosphatemia causes hypocalcemic tetany and/or vascular collapse.

Physical Examination Findings
Chronic hyperphosphatemia causes calcification of soft tissues, resulting in chronic renal failure and tumoral calcinosis.

CAUSES
• Reduced glomerular filtration rate
• Prerenal azotemia
• Renal azotemia
• Postrenal azotemia
• Hyperphosphatemia secondary to excessive bone resorption or muscle breakdown
• Young growing dogs
• Hypoparathyroidism
• Hypersomatotropism
• Hyperphosphatemia caused by excessive gastrointestinal absorption of phosphorus
• Osteolysis
• Disuse osteoporosis
• Osseous neoplasia
• Hyperthyroidism
• Phosphorus-containing enemas
• Vitamin D toxicosis
• Phosphorus dietary supplementation
• Nutritional secondary hyperparathyroidism

RISK FACTORS
Use of phosphorus-containing enemas to small animals such as cats

 DIAGNOSIS

DIFFERENTIAL DIAGNOSIS
• Hypoparathyroidism—also characterized by clinical signs of hypocalcemia such as seizures and tetany
• Prerenal azotemia as a cause of hyperphosphatemia—associated with disease states that result in low cardiac output such as congestive heart failure, dehydration, hypoadrenocorticism and shock
• Renal insufficiency, either acute or chronic renal failure—attended by azotemia and abnormal findings on urinalysis (low urinary specific gravity)
• Young, growing animals—can have serum phosphorus concentrations twice those of adults
• Vitamin D intoxication—history of vitamin D supplementation or ingestion of rodenticides (Rampage)
• Nutritional secondary hyperparathyroidism—history of dietary calcium–phosphorus imbalance
• Hyperthyroidism in cats—clinical signs of weight loss, polyphagia, and polydipsia and polyuria
• Hypersomatotropism—attended by a history of progesterone administration in dogs and insulin-resistant diabetes mellitus in cats
• Nonazotemia tumoral calcinosis—observed in human beings as an autosomal dominant disorder; rare cause of hyperphosphatemia associated with large bone lesions
• Jasmine toxicity—history of plant ingestion
• Factitious

LABORATORY FINDINGS

Drugs That May Alter Laboratory Results
• Phosphorus-containing enemas
• Intravenous KPO_4
• Anabolic steroids
• Furosemide
• Hydrochlorothiazide
• Minocycline

Disorders That May Alter Laboratory Results
• Hemolysis and lipemia can falsely raise phosphorus concentrations.
• Collection in citrate, oxalate, or EDTA

Valid If Run in Human Laboratory?
Valid

CBC/BIOCHEMISTRY/URINALYSIS
• Serum phosphorus > 6.0 mg/dL
• Low serum calcium in patients with primary hypoparathyroidism
• High serum calcium in patients with vitamin D intoxication
• Azotemia and isosthenuria help define degree of renal impairment.
• Hyperkalemia and hyponatremia suggest hypoadrenocorticism.

OTHER LABORATORY TESTS
- Serum PTH measurement—intact molecule and two-site assay methods have the greatest specificity; high-normal or high concentrations suggest primary hyperparathyroidism; low concentrations suggest neoplasia.
- Thyroxine concentrations—indicated in cats with hyperphosphatemia and clinical signs consistent with hyperthyroidism
- Insulin-like growth factor I (IGF-1) concentrations—indicated in dogs or cats with unexplained hyperphosphatemia and clinical signs consistent with acromegaly; IGF-1 concentrations are elevated in animals with hypersomatotropism.
- Vitamin D assays are not readily available.

IMAGING
- Abdominal radiography to assess renal size and symmetry
- Renal ultrasonography to detect soft-tissue mineralization
- Thyroid scan to rule out hyperthyroidism
- Radiography of long bones to detect osteoporosis or neoplasia

DIAGNOSTIC PROCEDURES
- ACTH stimulation testing to confirm hypoadrenocorticism
- Serum thyroxine to confirm hyperthyroidism
- Renal biopsy

 TREATMENT

- Inpatient, because of the deleterious effects of hyperphosphatemia and the need for fluid therapy; consider severe hyperphosphatemia a medical emergency.
- Restrict dietary phosphorus.
- Normal saline is the fluid of choice.

 MEDICATIONS

DRUGS OF CHOICE
Acute Hyperphosphatemia
- Dextrose (1g/kg IV) and insulin (0.5 U/kg IV)
- Avoid phosphorus-containing fluids.

Chronic Hyperphosphatemia
Oral administration of phosphorus binders (Amphojel)

CONTRAINDICATIONS
N/A

PRECAUTIONS
N/A

POSSIBLE INTERACTIONS
N/A

ALTERNATIVE DRUGS
N/A

 FOLLOW-UP

PATIENT MONITORING
- Serum calcium every 12 h
- Renal function tests—urine output must be monitored, particularly if oliguric renal failure is suspected, in which case urine output should be measured carefully; oliguria cannot be determined unless the patient is fully hydrated.
- Hydration status—indicators of overhydration include increased body weight, increased central venous pressure, and edema (pulmonary or subcutaneous).

POSSIBLE COMPLICATIONS
- Hypophosphatemia resulting in hemolysis
- Soft-tissue mineralization

 MISCELLANEOUS

ASSOCIATED CONDITIONS
Hypocalcemia

AGE-RELATED FACTORS
Mild elevations in phosphorus may be normal in growing animals.

ZOONOTIC POTENTIAL
N/A

PREGNANCY
N/A

SYNONYMS
None

SEE ALSO
- Hypoparathyroidism
- Renal Failure (Chronic or Acute)

ABBREVIATIONS
- ACTH = adrenocorticotropin
- IGF-1 = insulin-like growth factor I
- PTH = parathyroid hormone

Suggested Reading
Aurbach GD, Marx SJ, Spiegel AM. Parathyroid hormone, calcitonin, and the calciferols. In: Wilson JD, Foster DW, eds. Williams textbook of endocrinology. 7th ed. Philadelphia: Saunders, 1985:1208–1209.
Willard MD, Tvedten H, Turnwald GH. Clinical diagnosis by laboratory methods. Philadelphia: Saunders, 1989.
Author Deborah S. Greco
Consulting Editor Deborah S. Greco

DIAGNOSTICS—LAB

PHOSPHORUS, HYPOPHOSPHATEMIA

 BASICS

DEFINITION

Serum phosphorus concentration < 2.5 mg/dL

PATHOPHYSIOLOGY

• A low phosphorus concentration can be caused by shifts of phosphorus from the extracellular fluid into body cells, reduced intestinal absorption of phosphorus, or reduced renal phosphorus reabsorption.
• Because phosphorus is an important component of ATP, low serum phosphorus concentration can cause ATP depletion and affect cells that are high energy users, including RBCs, skeletal muscle cells, and brain cells.

SYSTEMS AFFECTED

• Hemic/Lymphatic/Immune—hemolysis
• Musculoskeletal—weakness and respiratory paralysis
• Nervous—seizures

SIGNALMENT

Dog and cat

SIGNS

Historical Findings

Consistent with the primary disease responsible for the hypophosphatemia rather than relating to the phosphate concentration itself

Physical Examination Findings

• Pallor from hemolytic anemia (severe hypophosphatemia)
• Red or dark-colored urine due to hemoglobinuria—severe hypophosphatemia
• Tachypnea, dyspnea, and anxiety secondary to hypoxia
• Muscle weakness
• Mental depression
• Rapid, shallow respirations because of poor respiratory muscle function

CAUSES

• Laboratory error
• Mannitol administration
• Transcellular shift (maldistribution)—enteral nutrition and total parenteral nutrition; diabetes mellitus; carbohydrate loading with insulin administration; respiratory alkalosis
• Reduced intestinal absorption of phosphorus—phosphorus-poor diet; vitamin D deficiency; phosphate-binding agent; malabsorption syndrome
• Reduced renal phosphate reabsorption—primary hyperparathyroidism; renal tubular defects (e.g., Fanconi's syndrome); hyperadrenocorticism; proximal tubular diuretics (e.g., carbonic anhydrase inhibitors); hypocalcemic tetany (eclampsia); sodium bicarbonate administration

RISK FACTORS

• Undiagnosed or poorly regulated diabetes mellitus
• Prolonged anorexia, starvation, or malnutrition

 DIAGNOSIS

DIFFERENTIAL DIAGNOSIS

• Severe hypophosphatemia (<1.0 mg/dL) is seen most often as a complication of diabetic ketoacidosis; monitor severely ill diabetics closely during the first few days of treatment for the development of hypophosphatemia.
• Patients with prolonged anorexia, starvation, or severe intestinal malabsorption may develop hypophosphatemia if given hyperalimentation, especially if the formulas have marginal phosphorus content.

LABORATORY FINDINGS

Drugs That May Alter Laboratory Results

Mannitol interferes with analysis, falsely lowering serum phosphorus concentration.

Disorders That May Alter Laboratory Results

Hemolysis, hyperlipidemia, and hyperproteinemia may falsely elevate serum phosphorus.

Valid If Run in Human Laboratory?

Valid

CBC/BIOCHEMISTRY/URINALYSIS

• Concurrent findings of hyperglycemia, glucosuria, ketonuria, and a high anion gap metabolic acidosis confirm that the hypophosphatemia is a complication of diabetic ketoacidosis.
• Hypercalcemia in association with hypophosphatemia suggests primary hyperparathyroidism.
• Hypocalcemia with hypophosphatemia is reported in patients with eclampsia.
• Moderate hypophosphatemia with high serum alkaline phosphatase activity suggests hyperadrenocorticism.
• Panhypoproteinemia suggests an intestinal malabsorption disorder.
• Hypophosphatemia in association with glucosuria, normoglycemia, isosthenuria, or azotemia suggests a renal tubular defect such as Fanconi's syndrome.

OTHER LABORATORY TESTS

• PTH assay—useful to diagnose primary hyperparathyroidism
• Measurement of vitamin D metabolites, particularly cholecalciferol—useful to diagnose vitamin D deficiency

IMAGING

Radiology may reveal poor bone quality or pathologic fractures in patients with disorders of calcium, phosphorus, and vitamin D.

DIAGNOSTIC PROCEDURES

Exploratory surgery of the cervical region confirms hyperparathyroidism.

TREATMENT

• Hospitalize patients with severe hypophosphatemia (phosphorus concentration < 1.5 mg/dL) to observe for hemolysis and provide treatment as needed.
• If the condition is caused by initiation of insulin therapy or hyperalimentation, suspend these treatments until phosphate has been administered for a few hours.
• Obtain fresh whole blood in case a transfusion is required.
• Can evaluate patients with moderate hypophosphatemia (1.5–2.5) as outpatients if other conditions are stable
• If the serum phosphorus is < 1.5 mg/dL, administer a balanced electrolyte solution IV (e.g., 0.9 % saline, lactated Ringer solution, Normosol-R, or Plasma-Lyte), supplemented with either sodium or potassium phosphate.

MEDICATIONS

DRUGS
• Potassium phosphate for injection has 3 mmol of phosphate and 4.4 mEq of potassium per milliliter; the dose of phosphate is 0.01–0.03 mmol/kg/h for 6 h; however, many cats with diabetic ketoacidosis who develop hypophosphatemia require higher dosages and a longer duration of therapy; a rate of 0.06–0.12 mmol/kg/h for 6–24 h is typical.
• Oral supplementation of phosphate may benefit animals with moderate hypophosphatemia; sodium and potassium phosphate powders and tablets are commercially available, but current dosing in veterinary medicine is empirical.

CONTRAINDICATIONS
• Avoid diuretics, especially carbonic anhydrase inhibitors.
• Avoid phosphate-poor enteral feeding formulas and total parenteral nutrition solutions in patients with hypophosphatemia and patients with predisposing disorders.

• Avoid intravenous supplementation of phosphate in hypercalcemic patients; precipitation of calcium and phosphate causes soft tissue mineralization and renal damage.

PRECAUTIONS
Oversupplementation, especially in patients with renal impairment or inadequate hydration, can cause hyperphosphatemia; acute hyperphosphatemia can result in hypocalcemia.

ALTERNATIVE DRUGS
If an oral or parenteral phosphate supplement is unavailable, skim or low-fat milk may be administered; this will be insufficient in severely affected patients.

FOLLOW-UP

PATIENT MONITORING
• Measure serum phosphorus every 12–24 h until the concentration is stable within the normal range.
• If hyperphosphatemia develops, stop all supplementation and provide intravenous fluid diuresis until the phosphorus returns to normal.
• Administer calcium gluconate intravenously *only* if tetany from hypocalcemia develops.
• Monitor hyperphosphatemic animals for acute renal failure.
• Check the serum potassium concentration daily until stable.

POSSIBLE COMPLICATIONS
• Hemolysis from hypophosphatemia may be acute and severe, requiring transfusion; fresh blood is preferred over stored blood products because stored RBCs may use serum phosphate and exacerbate the condition.
• Cardiac arrest and respiratory failure are life-threatening complications of severe hypophosphatemia.
• Respiratory support with positive pressure ventilation is an option.
• See Patient Monitoring for other complications.

MISCELLANEOUS

ASSOCIATED CONDITIONS
Hypokalemia is often concurrent, especially in patients with diabetic ketoacidosis.

AGE-RELATED FACTORS
N/A

ZOONOTIC POTENTIAL
N/A

PREGNANCY
• Hypophosphatemia in the periparturient animal may be associated with hypocalcemia caused by secretion of PTH to mobilize calcium for neonatal bone growth and lactation.
• PTH promotes phosphaturia and hypophosphatemia.

SYNONYMS
N/A

SEE ALSO
• Diabetes Mellitus, Ketoacidotic
• Hyperparathyroidism

ABBREVIATIONS
• ALP = alkaline phosphatase
• PTH = parathyroid hormone

Suggested Reading

DiBartola SP. Disorders of phosphorus: hypophosphatemia and hyperphosphatemia. In: DiBartola SP, ed. Fluid therapy in small animal practice. Philadelphia: Saunders, 1992:177–191.
Forrester SD, Moreland RJ. Hypophosphatemia: causes and clinical consequences. J Vet Intern Med 1989;3:149–159.
Willard MD, Zerbe CA, Schall WD, et al. Severe hypophosphatemia associated with diabetes mellitus in six dogs and one cat. J Am Vet Med Assoc 1987;190:1007–1010.

Author Melissa S. Wallace
Consulting Editor Deborah S. Greco

POLYCYTHEMIA

 BASICS

DEFINITION
Higher than reference range values for PCV, hemoglobin concentration, and RBC count because of a relative or absolute increase in the number of circulating RBC

PATHOPHYSIOLOGY
• Number of circulating RBCs affected by changes in plasma volume, rate of RBC destruction or loss, splenic contraction, EPO secretion, and rate of bone marrow production.
• Erythropoiesis also affected by hormones from the adrenal cortex, thyroid gland, ovary, testis, and anterior pituitary gland; normal PCV maintained by an endocrine loop

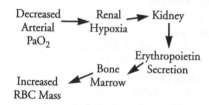

• Classified as relative, transient, or absolute
• Relative—develops when a decrease in plasma volume, usually caused by dehydration, produces a relative increase in circulating RBCs.
• Transient—caused by splenic contraction, which injects concentrated RBCs into the circulation; because splenic contraction is a momentary response to epinephrine, this type not usually a major diagnostic consideration.
• Absolute—characterized by an absolute increase in the circulating RBC mass as a result of an increase in bone marrow production; either primary or secondary to an increase in the production of EPO
• Primary absolute (polycythemia rubra vera)— a myeloproliferative disorder characterized by the uncontrolled but orderly production of excessive numbers of mature RBCs
• Secondary absolute—caused by a physiologically appropriate release of EPO resulting from chronic hypoxemia or by an inappropriate and excessive production of EPO or an EPO-like substance in an animal with normal SaO_2.

SYSTEMS AFFECTED
• Cardiovascular, Respiratory, Nervous, Renal/Urologic—hyperviscosity and poor perfusion and oxygenation of tissues, which are related directly to the high PCV, especially values > 60%
• Animals with absolute polycythemia have expanded blood volume, whereas those with relative polycythemia (dehydration) have decreased volume; both types can compromise tissue perfusion and oxygenation.

SIGNALMENT
• Reference values for PCV, hemoglobin, and RBC count vary with geographic location and breed.
• Animals at altitudes > 6000 ft have higher values than those at sea level.
• Brachycephalic breeds have higher PCV values than do normocephalic breeds.
• Large, excitable breeds are prone to splenic contraction.
• Greyhounds typically have high PCV; normal range is 50–65%

SIGNS

General Comments
Vary with the degree of polycythemia

Historical Findings
• Transient—excitement or vigorous exercise
• Absolute—lethargy, anorexia, epistaxis, seizures, or stunted growth

Physical Examination Findings
• Relative—dehydration caused by vomiting, diarrhea, or lack of water intake and oliguria
• Absolute—lethargy, low exercise tolerance, behavioral change, brick red or cyanotic mucous membranes, sneezing, bilateral epistaxis, large size and tortuosity of retinal and sublingual vessels, and cardiopulmonary impairment
• Primary absolute—variable degrees of splenomegaly, hepatomegaly, thrombosis, and hemorrhage; occasional seizure
• Secondary absolute caused by tissue hypoxia—clinical signs of hypoxemia caused by chronic pulmonary disease, cardiac disease or anomaly with right to left shunting, or hemoglobinopathy.
• Secondary absolute caused by inappropriate EPO secretion—signs associated with neoplasia, space-occupying renal lesion, or endocrine disorder

CAUSES
• Relative (common)—vomiting, diarrhea, diminished water intake, diuresis, hyper-ventilation, renal disease, and shift of plasma water to interstitium or gastrointestinal lumen
• Transient—excitement, anxiety, seizures, and restraint
• Primary absolute—rare myeloproliferative disorder
• Secondary absolute caused by tissue hypoxia—chronic pulmonary disease, cardiac disease or anomaly with right to left shunting, high altitude, brachycephalic breed conformation, methemoglobinemia, and impairment of renal blood supply
• Secondary absolute caused by inappropriate EPO secretion (rare)—renal cyst or tumor, hydronephrosis, hyperadrenocorticism, hyperthyroidism, pheochromocytoma, nasal fibrosarcoma, hepatic neoplasia, and hyperandrogenism

RISK FACTORS
None

 DIAGNOSIS

DIFFERENTIAL DIAGNOSIS
• Moderately high PCV and total plasma protein with concurrent dehydration— suggest relative polycythemia
• Secondary absolute—caused by diseases that produce chronic hypoxemia or by space-occupying lesions of the kidney, endocrine disorders, and neoplasms that produce EPO or an EPO-like substance independent of hypoxia
• Polycythemia vera—diagnosed by elimination of other causes

LABORATORY FINDINGS

Drugs That May Alter Laboratory Results
Dilutional effect of fluid therapy on PCV and total plasma protein

Disorders That May Alter Laboratory Results
Concurrent anemia, hypoproteinemia, or dehydration can affect interpretation of PCV and total plasma protein values.

Valid If Run in Human Laboratory?
Yes.

CBC/BIOCHEMISTRY/URINALYSIS
Assessment begins with CBC and total plasma protein measurement; additional tests selected as indicated

Mechanism	Relative Dehydration	Absolute Primary Myeloprо- liferative	Absolute Secondary Hypoxemia	Absolute Secondary Excess EPO
PCV	Inc	Marked Inc > 60%	Marked Inc > 60%	Marked Inc > 60%
TPP	Inc	N	N	N
SaO₂		N > 90%	Dec << 90%	N > 90%
EPO		N/Dec	Inc	Inc
Bone marrow		----------Erythroid Hyperplasia----------		
Other	Prerenal Azotemia	Inc WBC Inc Plat		

OTHER LABORATORY TESTS
• PaO₂ and EPO determinations—diagnose absolute polycythemia
• Hormone assays—assessment of endocrine dysfunction; EPO samples can be sent to a human testing laboratory; control sample from a normal animal (not a blood donor) should also be submitted
• Extensive overlap in EPO values exists between normal and affected animals; in some animals with secondary absolute polycythemia, low or normal EPO values have been reported.

IMAGING
Radiography and ultrasonography to detect cardiopulmonary disease and space-occupying lesions of the kidneys

DIAGNOSTIC PROCEDURES
Pulse oximetry to determine oxygen saturation of the blood

TREATMENT
• Relative—rehydration with IV fluids appropriate for the primary cause; assessment of renal function, gastrointestinal system, acid–base status, and electrolyte balance important to the selection of the fluid
• Absolute—phlebotomy recommended (20 mL/kg over one to several days) to reduce the RBC mass to a PCV of 55%; blood volume should be replaced concurrently with isotonic fluids to prevent hypotension, cardiovascular collapse, and thrombosis.
• Secondary caused by inappropriate EPO production—phlebotomy and removal of the EPO source
• Secondary caused by hypoxemia—the high PCV is an appropriate compensatory response; thus phlebotomy may be dangerous; if indicated, remove blood at a slower rate (5 mL/kg); a higher PCV (60–65%) may be necessary to sustain life until the cause of hypoxemia can be corrected.
• Polycythemia vera—phlebotomy (20 mL/kg) and hydroxyurea; frequency of bleeding and dosage adjusted to maintain a PCV of 55% in dogs and 45% in cats

MEDICATIONS
DRUG OF CHOICE
Polycythemia vera—hydroxyurea (30–50 mg/kg PO q24h, dogs; 30 mg/kg q24h, cats)

CONTRAINDICATIONS
Phlebotomy may be contraindicated in patients with hypoxemia.

PRECAUTIONS
Removal of blood at a rapid rate can cause hypotension and cardiovascular collapse.

POSSIBLE INTERACTIONS
None

ALTERNATIVE DRUGS
Polycythemia vera—chlorambucil (0.2 mg/kg PO q24h, dogs and cats) or busulfan (2.0–4.0 mg/m² PO q24h, dogs)

FOLLOW-UP
PATIENT MONITORING
• PCV, total plasma protein, urine output, and body weight 2–3 times daily in severely dehydrated animals until normal hydration is maintained
• Patients being treated for polycythemia vera by chemotherapy—monitor weekly for changes in PCV, neutrophil count, and platelets during the initial treatment; then monthly for adjustment of chemotherapy and periodic phlebotomy

POSSIBLE COMPLICATIONS
• Hyperviscosity in patients with absolute polycythemia, especially polycythemia vera, may lead to thrombosis, infarction, or hemorrhage.
• Chemotherapy may cause bone marrow suppression.

MISCELLANEOUS
ASSOCIATED CONDITIONS
None

AGE-RELATED FACTORS
None

ZOONOTIC POTENTIAL
None

PREGNANCY
N/A

SYNONYM
Erythrocytosis

SEE ALSO
• Hyperviscosity Syndrome
• Polycythemia Vera

ABBREVIATIONS
• EPO = erythropoietin
• PCV = packed cell volume
• SaO₂ = arterial oxygen saturation
• TPP = total plasma protein
• RBC = red blood cell

Suggested Reading
Cook SM, Lothrop CD. Serum erythropoietin concentrations measured by radioimmunoassay in normal, polycythemic, and anemic dogs and cats. J Vet Int Med 1994;8:18–25.
Hasler AH, Giger U. Serum erythropoietin values in polycythemic cats. J Am Anim Hosp Assoc 1996;12:294–301.
Morrison WB. Polycythemia. In: Ettinger SJ, Feldman EC, eds. Textbook of veterinary internal medicine. Philadelphia: Saunders, 1995:197–199.

Author Peter S. MacWilliams
Consulting Editor Susan M. Cotter

POTASSIUM, HYPERKALEMIA

BASICS

DEFINITION
Serum potassium concentration higher than the testing laboratory's upper limit of normal, generally > 5.7 mEq/L (mmol/L)

PATHOPHYSIOLOGY
• Potassium is primarily intracellular; serum concentrations do not accurately reflect tissue concentrations.
• Hyperkalemia is often associated with cellular injury (e.g., trauma and ischemia) and other causes of translocation of potassium out of the intracellular space (e.g., acidosis).
• Potassium is eliminated in the kidneys and elimination is enhanced by aldosterone; conditions that inhibit renal elimination of potassium will cause hyperkalemia.

SYSTEMS AFFECTED
• Cardiovascular—potassium affects cardiac conduction, and changes are reflected on the ECG; as potassium rises, the T waves become tall and spiked with a narrow base, the QRS complexes widen, and the P-R intervals lengthen; the P waves become smaller and wider and, in animals with severe hyperkalemia, disappear (atrial standstill); higher concentrations of potassium cause fusion of the QRS-T, which causes a wide, complex idioventricular rhythm followed by ventricular fibrillation or asystole; ECG changes in animals with hyperkalemia vary and are diminished by hypernatremia, hypercalcemia, and alkalosis.
• Nervous—neuromuscular function affected

SIGNALMENT
• Dogs and cats
• Pseudohyperkalemia in akita

SIGNS

Historical Findings
• Weakness
• Collapse
• Flaccid paralysis
• Death

Physical Examination Findings
In addition to historical findings, arrhythmias, especially bradyarrhythmias, in some animals

CAUSES
• Pseudohyperkalemia—some blood cells (i.e., platelets, WBCs, and RBCs in akita), contain high concentrations of potassium; if the blood sample is not analyzed or separated promptly, this intracellular potassium is released into the serum, causing the potassium concentration to be artificially high (pseudohyperkalemia).
• Low potassium elimination—anuric or oliguric renal failure; ruptured bladder; administration of potassium-sparing diuretics, ACE inhibitors, nonsteroidal antiinflammatory drugs, or heparin (causing hypoaldosteronism); and urinary tract rupture or urethral obstruction
• Translocation of potassium—acidosis, muscle trauma, severe digitalis overdose, infusion of mannitol, and hyperglycemia causing hyperosmolality
• High potassium intake—oral or parenteral potassium supplements
• Miscellaneous—pleural effusion and ascites

RISK FACTORS
• Akita breed—pseudohyperkalemia
• Fluid therapy with potassium supplementation
• Administration of potassium-sparing diuretics and ACE inhibitors
• Conditions associated with acidosis
• Trauma
• Renal disease
• Lower urinary tract disease in male cats
• Cystic calculi in male dogs

DIAGNOSIS

DIFFERENTIAL DIAGNOSIS
• Waxing and waning history of gastrointestinal complaints, weakness, collapse—consider hypoadrenocorticism.
• Straining to urinate or low urine output—consider urinary obstruction or oliguric/anuric renal failure

LABORATORY FINDINGS

Drugs That May Alter Laboratory Results
None

Disorders That May Alter Laboratory Results
• Thrombocytosis (>1,000,000 cells/mm³), leukocytosis (>200,000 cells /mm³), and abnormal (leukemic) leukocytes can cause release of large amounts of potassium into the serum if not separated quickly.

Valid If Run in Human Laboratory?
Yes

CBC/BIOCHEMISTRY/URINALYSIS
• In patients with Na:K ratio < 27, consider hypoadrenocorticism; some patients with nonspecific diarrhea and metabolic acidosis may also have a low Na:K ratio.
• In patients with azotemia, consider hypoadrenocorticism, anuric or oliguric renal failure, and ruptured or obstructed urinary tract.
• In patients with high creatine kinase, aspartate aminotransferase, and lactic dehydrogenase, consider muscle injury.
• In patients with severe thrombocytosis or leukocytosis or if the patient is an akita, consider pseudohyperkalemia.

OTHER LABORATORY TESTS
ACTH response test to rule out hypoadrenocorticism

IMAGING
Radiographic contrast studies or ultrasound to rule out urinary tract rupture or obstruction.

DIAGNOSTIC PROCEDURES
None

TREATMENT
• Varies, depending on the underlying cause of hyperkalemia
• Aggressiveness is dictated by patient's appearance and severity of ECG abnormalities.
• Initiate supportive measures to lower potassium while pursuing definitive diagnosis.
• Saline (0.9%) is the fluid of choice for lowering potassium concentrations and blunting the effects of hyperkalemia on cardiac conduction; if the patient is dehydrated or hypotensive, fluids can be administered rapidly (dogs, up to 90 mL/kg/h; cats, 60 mL/kg/h or faster with monitoring of central venous pressure).

MEDICATIONS

DRUGS OF CHOICE
• Can administer sodium bicarbonate to patients with severe hyperkalemia to induce translocation of potassium into cells; if blood pH and base deficit cannot be determined, administer 1–2 mEq/kg slowly IV; to calculate bicarbonate dose more accurately

$$\text{dogs, } 0.3 \times \text{body weight (kg)} \times (21 - \text{patient HCO}_3^-)$$

$$\text{cats, } 0.3 \times \text{body weight (kg)} \times (19 - \text{patient HCO}_3^-)$$

Administer half of dose and reevaluate
• Can administer dextrose and regular insulin to patients with severe hyperkalemia to induce translocation of potassium into cells (regular insulin, 0.5 U/kg IV with 50% dextrose, 1 g/kg IV); dextrose can also be used without insulin
• For patients with life-threatening hyperkalemia, administer calcium gluconate (0.5–1 mL/kg slowly IV over 10 min) while monitoring the ECG; calcium antagonizes the effect of potassium on the conduction system without lowering the potassium concentration.

CONTRAINDICATIONS
• Avoid potassium-containing fluids and fluids that cause hyponatremia, acidosis, or hypocalcemia.
• Avoid drugs that contain potassium or interfere with potassium elimination (e.g., ACE inhibitors and potassium-sparing diuretics).

PRECAUTIONS
Kayexalate and sodium bicarbonate cause a sodium load that may lead to fluid retention

in patients with cardiac or renal failure.

POSSIBLE INTERACTIONS
N/A

ALTERNATIVE DRUGS
Sodium polystyrene sulfonate (Kayexalate) per os or rectum binds potassium within the intestinal tract, limiting absorption and reabsorption; rarely used in veterinary practice.

 FOLLOW-UP

PATIENT MONITORING
• Recheck potassium at frequency dictated by the underlying disease.
• Check ECG frequently until rhythm disturbances resolve.

POSSIBLE COMPLICATIONS
Death of animals with severe hyperkalemia

 MISCELLANEOUS

ASSOCIATED CONDITIONS
N/A

AGE-RELATED FACTORS
N/A

ZOONOTIC POTENTIAL
N/A

PREGNANCY
N/A

SYNONYMS
N/A

SEE ALSO
• Acidosis, Metabolic
• Atrial Standstill
• Hypoadrenocorticism
• Renal Failure, Acute

• Urinary Tract Obstruction

ABBREVIATION
ACE = angiotensin converting enzyme

Suggested Reading
DiBartola SP, Autran de Morais HS. Disorders of potassium: hypokalemia and hyperkalemia. In: DiBartola SP, ed. Fluid therapy in small animal practice. Philadelphia: WB Saunders, 1992:89-115.

Willard MD. Electrolyte and acid-base abnormalities. In: Willard MD, Tvedten H, Turnwald GH, eds. Small animal clinical diagnosis by laboratory methods. Philadelphia: WB Saunders, 1989.

Author Francis W. K. Smith, Jr.
Consulting Editors Deborah S. Greco

K> 5.7 mEq/ml

↓

History: R/O potassium supplementation or treatment with any drugs that can elevate potassium (ACE inhibitors, potassium sparing diuretics, nonsteroidal antiinflammatory drugs, digitalis, mannitol, succinylcholine)

↓

Physical Examination: R/O urethral obstruction and evaluate for possibility of urinary tract rupture

↓

Is value > 7.0 or patient showing signs or ECG changes consistent with hyperkalemia

YES → Evaluate CBC, serum chemistry profile and urinalysis

NO → Repeat with lithium heparin plasma to rule out pseudohyperkalemia (Akita, severe thrombocytosis or leukocytosis) and lab error → K > 5.7 mEq/ml → Evaluate CBC, serum chemistry profile and urinalysis

Evaluate CBC, serum chemistry profile and urinalysis branches to:

- **Elevated CK, AST, LDH** → R/O muscle trauma, tumor lysis syndrome, reperfusion post thrombolysis → Depressed response: R/O Addison's disease or prior corticosteroid therapy

- **Na/K < 27 or unexplained hyperkalemia** → ACTH response test → Normal or exagerated response: R/O gastrointestinal disease (recheck when signs resolve), primary hypoaldosteronism → Measure aldosterone following ACTH stimulation → Decreased aldoserone: R/O primary hypoldosteronism

- **None of these** → R/O Pleural or abdominal effusion, hyperosmolality (hyperglycemia) psedohypoadrenocorticism, hyperkalemic periodic paralysis → Recheck after effusions resolved, Recheck after hyperosmolality corrected, Challenge with low-dose oral KCl

- **Azotemia** → Check urine specific gravity → specific gravity > 1.029 (dog) or 1.034 (cat) R/O prerenal causes and post renal obstruction or tear

- **Hypercholoremic acidosis (normal anion gap)** → R/O translocation secondary to acidosis → specific gravity < 1.029 (dog) or 1.034 (cat) R/O Addisons disease, oliguric or anuric renal failure

POTASSIUM, HYPOKALEMIA

 BASICS

DEFINITION
Serum potassium concentration < 3.5 mEq/L

PATHOPHYSIOLOGY
• Potassium is the major intracellular cation and thereby largely responsible for maintenance of intracellular volume.
• The ratio of intracellular to extracellular potassium concentration is important in determining the cellular membrane potential. Rapid alterations in extracellular potassium concentration alter this ratio and predispose an animal to arrhythmias and conduction disturbances in excitable tissues (e.g., heart, nerve, and muscle)
• Hypokalemia can be caused by excessive potassium loss via the gastrointestinal tract or kidneys or movement of potassium from the extracellular fluid compartment into cells (i.e., translocation).

SYSTEMS AFFECTED
• Endocrine/Metabolic—carbohydrate intolerance
• Neuromuscular—skeletal muscle weakness and intestinal ileus
• Cardiovascular—arrhythmias
• Renal/Urologic—hyposthenuria and renal failure

SIGNALMENT
Burmese cats 4–12 months old; recurrent episodes of hypokalemic periodic paralysis

SIGNS
• Historical complaints are often referable to the disease or factors contributing to the hypokalemia
• Weakness
• Lethargy
• Anorexia
• Polyuria
• Polydipsia
• Vomiting
• Ventroflexion of the neck (cats)
• Stilted gait in the forelimbs (cats)

CAUSES
Urinary Potassium Loss
• Chronic renal railure
• Renal tubular acidosis
• Diuretic administration (other than potassium sparing diuretics)
• Postobstructive diuresis
• Dialysis
• Intravenous fluid diuresis
• Mineralcorticoid excess
• Administration penicillins
• Administration amphoteracin B

Gastrointestinal Potassium Loss
• Vomiting
• Diarrhea

Insufficient Potassium Intake
• Anorexia
• Potassium deficient diet
• Potassim free fluids
Translocation (Extracellular Fluid to Intracellular Fluid)
• Insulin and glucose administration
• Sodium bicarbonate administration
• Catecholamine administration
• Alkalemia
• Hypokalemic periodic paralysis

RISK FACTORS
Feeding cats acidifying diet that is marginal in potassium.

 DIAGNOSIS

DIFFERENTIAL DIAGNOSIS
• Azotemia, isosthenuria, and historical PU/PD—rule out chronic renal failure and hypokalemic nephropathy.
• Glucosuria, hyperglycemia, and historical PU/PD—rule out diabetes mellitus
• Metabolic acidosis and urine pH > 6.5—rule out renal tubular acidosis
• Metabolic alkalosis, and hypochloremia—rule out upper gastrointestinal obstruction and severe vomiting.
• Young Burmese cat with episodes of severe musele weakness—rule out hypokalemic periodic paralysis
• Historical urethral obstruction—rule out postobstructive diuresis

LABORATORY FINDINGS
Drugs That May Alter Laboratory Results
Excessive volume of K_3EDTA raises plasma potassium concentration.

Disorders That May Alter Laboratory Results
• Hemolysis in dogs with high RBC potassium (e.g., Akitas) and phosphofructokinase deficiency in the English springer spaniel can cause falsely high potassium concentration.
• Thrombocytosis increases serum potassium due to release from platelets during clot formation.

Valid If Run in Human Laboratory?
Yes

CBC/BIOCHEMISTRY/URINALYSIS
• Results may reveal normocytic normochromic nonregenerative anemia in patients with chronic renal failure.
• High BUN and creatinine (with or without phosphate) in patients with chronic renal failure or hypokalemic nephropathy.
• Low total CO_2 in patients with renal tubular acidosis or renal failure.
• High total CO_2 in patients with metabolic alkalosis.
• High glucose in patients with diabetes mellitus.
• Glucosuria in patients with diabetes mellitus
• pH > 6.5 in patients with renal tubular acidosis
• Isosthenuria in patients with chronic renal

failure or hypokalemic nephropathy

OTHER LABORATORY TESTS
• Aldosterone measurement to diagnose primary hyperaldosteronism.
• ACTH stimulation or Low Dose Dexamethasone Suppression Test to diagnose hyperadrenocoritcism (cause of mineralcorticoid excess).
• Urinary fractional excretion of K+ is elevated in chronic renal failure and hypokaelmic nephropathy.

IMAGING
• Ultrasonography may reveal an adrenal tumor—R/O hyperaldosteronism or hyperadrenocorticism.
• Radiographs and ultrasonography—useful in chronic renal failure work-up.
• Upper G.I. barium studies—to diagnose upper G.I. disorders (anatomic or functional) causing metabolic alkalosis

OTHER DIAGNOSTIC PROCEDURES
Gastroscopy is useful in diagnosis of upper G.I. disorders resulting in metabolic alkalosis, such as pyloric hyopertrophy or gastric neoplasia.

TREATMENT
• Animals with mild hypokalemia (potassium 3.0–3.5) can be treated as outpatients by oral supplementation
• Severely affected patients should be hospitalized; these animals are at risk of respiratory muscle paralysis and cardiac arrhythmias and should be handled with minimal stress.

MEDICATIONS

DRUGS AND FLUIDS
• Oral supplementation—potassium gluconate (Tumil-K, Kaon) is an effective treatment, and is the only treatment required in mildly affected animals (initial dosage, 1–3

mEq/kg/day divided q8h).
• Once serum potassium has normalized, administer a maintenance dosage (1.0 mEq/kg/day divided q12h).
• Parenteral supplementation—in patients with anorexia or vomiting, parenteral supplementation is required. Potassium chloride is added to maintenance fluid therapy according to the schedule below and is adjusted according to the patient's response. *Do not exceed an intravenous rate of 0.5 mEq/kq/hr.* At high rates of supplementation, an infusion pump is required to avoid overdosage.

SERUM K+ SUPPLEMENT (MEQ/L)

3.5–4.5	20
3.0–3.5	30
2.5–3.0	40
2.0–2.5	60
< 2.0	80

CONTRAINDICATIONS
Avoid sodium bicarbonate, insulin, and glucose (if possible) in patients with severe hypokalemia.

PRECAUTIONS
See above

POSSIBLE INTERACTIONS
Potassium supplementation in conjunction with ACE inhibitor, potassium-sparing diuretic, prostaglandin inhibitor, or beta blocker may cause hyperkalemia.

ALTERNATE DRUGS
Potassium phosphate is used in patients with concurrent hypophosphatemia. Dosage is based on phosphate content (see Phosphorus, Hypophosphatemia).

FOLLOW-UP

PATIENT MONITORING
Serum potassium with the frequency dictated by the degree of hypokalemia and the severity of clinical signs

POSSIBLE COMPLICATIONS

Arrhythmias

MISCELLANEOUS

ASSOCIATED CONDITIONS
• Hypomagnesemia
• Hypophosphatemia

AGE RELATED FACTORS
N/A

ZOONOTIC POTENTIAL
N/A

PREGNANCY
N/A

SYNONYMS
N/A

SEE ALSO
See Causes

ABBREVIATIONS
ECF = extracellular fluid
ICF = intracellular fluid
PU/PD = polyuria/polydipsia
ACE = angiotensin converting enzyme

References
DiBartola SP, Autran de Morais HS. Disorders of potassium: hypokalemia and hyperkalemia. In: DiBartola SP, ed. Fluid therapy in small animal practice. Philadelphia: WB Saunders Co., 1992:89–115.
DiBartola SP, Green RA, Autran de Morais HS. Electrolytes and acid-base. In: Willard MD, Tvedten H, Turnwald GH, eds. Small animal clinical diagnosis by laboratory methods. 2nd ed. Philadelphia: WB Saunders Co., 1994:97–113.
Willard MD. Disorders of potassium homeostasis. Vet Clin North Am Small Anim Pract 1989;19:241–263.

Author Melissa S. Wallace
Consulting Editor Deborah S. Greco

PROTEINURIA

BASICS

DEFINITION
A subjective increase in urinary protein detected by dipstick analysis; objectively, a urinary protein:creatinine ratio > 1 or a 24-h urinary protein content > 20 mg/kg

PATHOPHYSIOLOGY
• Greater than normal delivery of low-molecular-weight plasma proteins to the glomerulus
• Excessive leakage of proteins across the glomerular basement membrane secondary to altered permselectivity of the glomerulus
• Reduced tubular reabsorptive capacity for proteins, or exudation of blood or serum into the lower urinary tract

SYSTEMS AFFECTED
• Renal/Urologic—damaging to the renal tubules; longstanding proteinuria causes tubular damage with subsequent isosthenuria and renal failure.
• Cardiovascular—circulating plasma volume can be reduced if proteinuria is large enough to lower serum albumin concentrations rapidly; this can lead to sodium retention, which results in the formation of edema and hypertension; severe proteinuria can lead to a hypercoagulable state that is brought about by several mechanisms, including hyper-fibrinogenemia, platelet abnormalities, and loss of antithrombin III.

SIGNALMENT
• Dogs and cats
• Familial renal diseases associated with proteinuria occur in soft-coated wheaten terrier, Lhasa apso, shih tzu, bull terrier, English cocker spaniel, samoyed, Doberman pinscher, standard poodle, basenji, Norwegian elkhound, dalmatian, and Chinese shar pei.

SIGNS
• Vary with severity of proteinuria and the underlying cause
• None directly attributed to proteinuria

CAUSES

Preglomerular proteinuria
• Functional proteinuria—strenuous exercise, fever, hypothermia, seizures, or venous congestion
• Poorly documented as a cause of proteinuria in dogs and cats
• Overload proteinuria—tubular resorptive capacity exceeded by large amounts of low-molecular-weight plasma proteins in the glomerular filtrate (e.g. neoplastic production of paraproteins or Bence-Jones proteinuria and excessive hemolysis or rhabdomyolysis)

Glomerular Proteinuria
• Glomerulonephritis
• Amyloidosis
• Glomerulosclerosis
• In general, amyloidosis results in the heaviest proteinuria, although dogs with glomerulonephritis can also have massive proteinuria.

Postglomerular Proteinuria
• Hemorrhage or inflammation of the urogenital tract
• Tubular dysfunction resulting in failure of tubular protein reabsorption can cause mild-or-moderate postglomerular proteinuria.

RISK FACTORS
• Many chronic inflammatory (e.g. infectious and immune-mediated) and neoplastic diseases can lead to development of glomerulonephritis and perhaps amyloidosis, including dirofilariasis, ehrlichiosis, borelliosis, chronic bacterial infections (e.g. endocarditis), pyometra, FIV, hyperadrenocorticism, and systemic lupus erythematosus.
• Hematuria and pyuria
• Multiple myelomas can produce paraproteins resulting in Bence-Jones proteinuria.

DIAGNOSIS

DIFFERENTIAL DIAGNOSIS
• Need to differentiate preglomerular, glomerular, and postglomerular causes
• Patients with glomerular proteinuria are frequently asymptomatic or have signs attributable to an underlying disease process; many have vague signs of weight loss and lethargy; some have signs of uremia, hypertension, edema, ascites, and/or thromboembolism.
• Patients with lower urinary tract disorders and postglomerular proteinuria may have dysuria, pollakiuria, inappropriate urination, and/or hematuria.

LABORATORY FINDINGS

Drugs That May Alter Laboratory Results
• Contamination with quarternary ammonium compounds causes false-positive urine dipstick colorimetric (tetrabromphenol blue) test results.
• Results of the sulfosalicylic acid (SSA) turbidimetric test (Bumintest Tabs) are falsely increased by radiographic contrast media, penicillins, cephalosporins, sulfa drugs, or the urine preservative thymol.

Disorders That May Alter Laboratory Results
• False-positive urine dipstick test results occur when urine is highly alkaline (pH > 8–9).
• SSA test results are falsely decreased by very alkaline or dilute urine and increased by uncentrifuged urine.

Valid If Run in Human Laboratory?
Yes

CBC/BIOCHEMISTRY/URINALYSIS
• The urine dipstick and SSA tests allow qualitative and semiquantitative assessment of urine protein content, respectively. These screening tests are quick and inexpensive; however, results of both are affected by urine concentration and must be interpreted in light of urinary specific gravity. Low urinary protein (trace or 1+) may be normal in a concentrated urine sample. These methods may not detect high protein in dilute urine; if it is detected by these methods, the urine sediment should be evaluated for hematuria, pyuria, or bacteriuria.
• Repeat the urinary protein screening test in dogs and cats that initially have a normal urinary sediment examination or have been treated for urinary tract inflammation or hemorrhage. If proteinuria is transient and the

urine sediment is normal, consider functional proteinuria or false-positive test results.

OTHER LABORATORY TESTS
• Urinary protein should be quantified by urinary protein:creatinine ratio or 24-h urinary protein determination in dogs and cats that have hypoalbuminemia or repeatedly positive urine dipstick or SSA tests in the absence of lower urinary tract hemorrhage or inflammation.
• Suspect glomerular disease if the urinary protein:creatinine ratio or 24-h urine protein content is abnormal, concurrent hypoalbumi-nemia is detected, little evidence supports primary tubular disease, or a large amount of albuminuria has been detected by electrophor-esis. In such dogs, make aggressive attempts to identify an underlying disease (e.g. neoplasia, ehrlichiosis, dirofilariasis, systemic lupus erythematosus, hyperadrenocorticism, and chronic bacterial infection).

IMAGING
Ultrasound and radiographs may identify an underlying infectious, inflammatory, or neoplastic disease process. Ultrasound may provide information about structural changes suggesting primary renal disease (e.g., loss of corticomedullary distinction, hyperecho-genicity, and irregular surface margin).

DIAGNOSTIC PROCEDURES
Renal biopsy is needed to differentiate glomerulosclerosis, glomerulonephritis, and amyloidosis when an underlying disease cannot be identified or proteinuria has persisted for several months following treatment of the underlying disease.

TREATMENT
• Patients do not need hospitalization or their activity altered if proteinuria is the only laboratory abnormality.
• If glomerular disease is suspected, feed a diet moderately reduced in protein.

MEDICATIONS
DRUGS OF CHOICE
See chapters describing azotemia and uremia, nephrotic syndrome, glomerulonephritis, amyloidosis.

CONTRAINDICATIONS
N/A

PRECAUTIONS
Drugs that are highly bound to albumin may have an altered effect if proteinuria is severe enough to cause hypoalbuminemia. Lower dosages of Coumadin may be required for effective anticoagulation. Higher doses of furosemide may be required to mobilize edema effectively. See Hypoalbuminemia.

POSSIBLE INTERACTIONS
N/A

ALTERNATIVE DRUGS
See chapters describing azotemia and uremia, nephrotic syndrome, glomerulonephritis, and amyloidosis.

FOLLOW-UP
PATIENT MONITORING
• The urinary protein:creatinine ratio or 24-h urine protein content should be assessed for months after resolution of any treatable underlying disease.
• Protein quantitation—can use to assess progression of glomerular disease and response to treatment
• Monitor serum creatinine concurrently; in some patients reduced proteinuria may reflect deteriorating renal function.
• Assess disease progression and subsequent therapeutic changes on the basis of trends noted in repeat urinary protein:creatinine ratio or 24-h urinary protein content rather than on one or two data points.

POSSIBLE COMPLICATIONS
• Edema
• Thromboembolism
• Systemic hypertension
• Poor wound healing

MISCELLANEOUS
ASSOCIATED CONDITIONS
Heavy proteinuria can be associated with hypoalbuminemia, hypoglobulinemia (rare), hypercholesterolemia, low antithrombin III, thrombocytosis, and hyperfibrinogenemia.

AGE-RELATED FACTORS
N/A

ZOONOTIC POTENTIAL
N/A

PREGNANCY
Some drugs used in the treatment of diseases associated with proteinuria may be contraindicated in pregnancy. See specific sections.

SYNONYMS
N/A

SEE ALSO
• Albumin, Hypoalbuminemia
• Amyloidosis
• Creatinine and Blood Urea Nitrogen (BUN) —Azotemia and Uremia
• Glomerulonephritis
• Hematuria
• Nephrotic Syndrome
• Pyuria

ABBREVIATIONS
• FIV = feline immunodeficiency virus
• SSA = sulfosalicylic acid

Suggested Reading
Hurley K, Vaden SL. Proteinuria in dogs and cats —a diagnostic approach. In: Bonagura JD, ed. Kirk's current veterinary therapy XII. Philadelphia, Saunders, 1995:937–940.
Lulich JP, Osborne CA. Interpretation of urine protein-creatinine ratios in dogs with glomerular and nonglomerular disorders. Comp Cont Ed Pract Vet 1990; 12:59–72.
Author Shelly L. Vaden
Consulting Editors Larry G. Adams and Carl A. Osborne

PYURIA

BASICS

DEFINITION
• WBCs (i.e., neutrophils, eosinophils, monocytes, lymphocytes, or plasma cells) in urine
• More than five WBCs per high-power field is generally considered abnormal, but the number of WBCs found in urinary sediment depends on method of collection, sample volume and concentration, degree of cellular destruction after collection, and laboratory technique.

PATHOPHYSIOLOGY
• Large numbers of WBCs in voided urine samples indicate active inflammation somewhere along the urogenital tract. • Can be associated with any pathologic process (infectious or noninfectious) that causes cellular injury or death; tissue damage evokes exudative inflammation characterized by evidence of leukocytic extravasation (pyuria) and increased vascular permeability (hematuria and proteinuria)

SYSTEMS AFFECTED
• Renal/Urologic—urethra, urinary bladder, ureters, and kidneys • Genital—prepuce, prostate, vagina, and uterus

SIGNALMENT
Dogs and cats

SIGNS

General Comments
Inflammation can cause clinical signs localized to the site(s) of injury or may be accompanied by systemic manifestations. Historical and physical examination findings depend on the underlying cause, organ(s) affected, degree of organ dysfunction, and magnitude of systemic inflammatory responses. Nonobstructive lesions confined to the urinary bladder, urethra, vagina, or prepuce rarely cause systemic signs of inflammation. Systemic signs may accompany generalized inflammatory lesions of the kidneys, prostate, or uterus.

Physical Examination Findings
Local Effects of Inflammation
• Erythema of mucosal surfaces—e.g., redness of vaginal or preputial mucosa • Tissue swelling—e.g., renomegaly, prostatomegaly, mural thickening of urinary bladder or urethra
• Exudation of leukocytes and protein-rich fluid—e.g., pyuria, purulent urethral or vaginal discharges, pyometra, and prostatic abscess
• Pain—e.g. adverse response to palpation, dysuria, pollakiuria, stranguria • Loss of function—e.g. polyuria, dysuria, pollakiuria, urinary incontinence
Systemic Effects of Inflammation
• Fever • Depression • Anorexia • Dehydration

CAUSES

Kidney
• Pyelonephritis—e.g., bacterial, fungal, parasitic, and mycoplasmal • Nephrolith(s)
• Neoplasia • Trauma • Immune • mediated
• Ureter • Ureteritis—e.g., bacterial • Ureterolith(s) • Neoplasia

Urinary Bladder
• Cystitis—e.g., bacterial, mycoplasmal, fungal, and parasitic • Urocystolith(s) • Neoplasia • Trauma • Overdistension—urethral obstruction • Pharmacologic—cyclophosphamide

Urethra
• Urethritis—e.g., bacterial, fungal, and mycoplasmal
• Urethrolith(s)
• Neoplasia
• Trauma
• Foreign body

Prostate
• Prostatitis/abscess—e.g., bacterial and fungal
• Neoplasia

Penis/Prepuce
• Balanoposthitis
• Neoplasia
• Foreign body

Uterus
Pyometra/metritis—e.g., bacterial

Vagina
• Vaginitis—bacterial, mycoplasmal, viral, or fungal
• Neoplasia
• Foreign body
• Trauma

RISK FACTORS
• Any disease process, diagnostic procedure, or therapy that alters normal host urinary tract defenses and predisposes to infection
• Any disease process, dietary factor, or therapy that predisposes to formation of metabolic uroliths

DIAGNOSIS

DIFFERENTIAL DIAGNOSIS

Voided Specimens
• Rule out vaginitis—signs include vaginal discharge, erythema of vaginal mucosa, licking of vulva, and attracting male dogs.
• Rule out pyometra, metritis—signs include vaginal discharge, large uterus, pyrexia, depression, anorexia, polyuria, polydipsia, and a recent history of estrus, parturition, or progestin administration.
• Rule out balanoposthitis—signs include preputial discharge, erythema of preputial or penile mucosa, and licking of prepuce.

• Rule out prostatitis, prostatic abscess, or prostatic neoplasia—signs include urethral discharge, prostatomegaly, pyrexia, depression, dysuria, tenesmus, caudal abdominal pain, and stiff gait.
• Rule out urethritis, urethroliths, urethral neoplasms—signs include dysuria, pollakiuria, stranguria, and/or palpable uroliths or mass lesions in the urethra.
• Rule out inflammatory disorders of urinary bladder and kidneys.

Specimens Collected by Cystocentesis
• Rule out urethral obstruction—signs include stranguria, anuria, and a large overdistended urinary bladder.
• Rule out prostatic and urethral disorders (see previous text); purulent prostatic or urethral exudates can reflux into the urinary bladder.
• Rule out cystitis, urocystoliths, and urinary bladder neoplasia—signs may include dysuria, pollakiuria, stranguria, and/or palpable uroliths or mass lesions in the urinary bladder.
• Rule out pyelonephritis—signs may include pyrexia, depression, anorexia, polyuria, polydipsia, renal pain, and renomegaly.
• Rule out posttraumatic pyuria—signs may include history of trauma, including iatrogenic

LABORATORY FINDINGS

Drugs That May Alter Laboratory Results
• WBCs lyse rapidly in hypotonic or alkaline urine. Administration of alkalinizing agents (e.g., sodium bicarbonate, potassium citrate, chlorothiazide, or acetazolamide) or agents that produce hypotonic urine (e.g., diuretics and glucocorticoids) may falsely decrease urine WBC numbers.
• Nitrofurantoin, cephalosporins, and gentamicin can cause false-positive leukocyte esterase reactions with reagent strip (dipstick) methods.
• Urinary WBC concentrations can be low in patients with inflammatory disorders who have been given steroidal or nonsteroidal antiinflammatory drugs.

Disorders That May Alter Laboratory Results
• Disorders associated with diminished WBC function or absolute neutropenia can artificially lower values.
• Disorders associated with production of hypotonic urine or alkaline urine artificially lower values.

Miscellaneous Factors That May Alter Lab Results
• False-negative leukocyte esterase reaction in dogs when urine is tested by the reagent strip (dipstick) method
• False-positive and false-negative leukocyte esterase reaction in cats when urine is tested by the reagent strip (dipstick) method

Valid If Run in Human Laboratory?

Valid if urinary sediment is examined microscopically; invalid if only leukocyte esterase reagent strip (dipstick) method is used.

CBC/BIOCHEMISTRY/URINALYSIS

• Pyuria in specimens collected by voiding, manual compression, or catheterization indicates an inflammatory lesion involving at least the urinary or genital tracts.
• Pyuria in specimens collected by cystocentesis localizes the site of inflammation to at least the urinary tract, but does not exclude the urethra and genital tract. Reflux of prostatic exudates into the urinary bladder may result in pyuria in patients with prostatic disease.
• Pyuria associated with WBC casts is unequivocal evidence of renal parenchymal inflammation.
• Generalized renal injury may be associated with concomitant leukocytosis, isosthenuria, and azotemia.
• Pyuria associated with bacteria, fungi, or parasite ova in sufficient numbers to be seen by microscopic sediment examination indicates that the inflammatory lesion was caused or complicated by urinary tract infection.
• Pyuria associated with neoplastic cells indicates neoplasia. Diagnosis of urinary tract neoplasia by cytologic examination of urine may be complicated by epithelial cell hyperplasia and atypia caused by urinary tract inflammation or the physiochemical properties of urine (pH and tonicity).

OTHER LABORATORY TESTS

• Perform quantitative urine culture on all patients with pyuria; it provides the most definitive means of identifying and characterizing bacterial urinary tract infection.
• Negative urine culture results suggest a noninfectious cause of inflammation (e.g. uroliths, neoplasia) or inflammation associated with urinary tract infection caused by fastidious organisms (e.g., mycoplasmas and viruses).
• Cytologic evaluation of urinary sediment, prostatic fluid, urethral or vaginal discharges, or biopsy specimens obtained by catheter or needle aspiration may help evaluate patients with localized urinary or genital tract disease. Cytologic examination may establish a definitive diagnosis of urinary tract neoplasia, but negative cytologic findings do not rule out neoplasia.

IMAGING

Survey abdominal radiography, contrast urethrocystography and cystography, urinary tract ultrasonography, and excretory urography are important means of identifying and localizing underlying causes.

DIAGNOSTIC PROCEDURES

• Urethrocystoscopy—indicated in patients with persistent lesions of the lower urinary tract for which a definitive diagnosis has not been established by other, less invasive, means
• Light microscopic evaluation of tissue specimens—indicated in patients with lesions of the urinary or genital tracts for which a definitive diagnosis has not been established by other, less invasive, means; tissue specimens may be obtained by catheter biopsy, cystoscopy and pinch biopsy, or exploratory laparotomy; aspiration and punch biopsy techniques may be used to evaluate the prostate gland.

TREATMENT

• Treatment varies, depending on the underlying cause and specific organs involved.
• Pyuria associated with systemic signs of illness (i.e., pyrexia, depression, anorexia, vomiting, dehydration, leukocytosis, polyuria, and polydipsia) or urinary obstruction warrants aggressive diagnostic evaluation and initiation of specific, supportive, and/or symptomatic treatment.

MEDICATIONS

DRUGS OF CHOICE
N/A

CONTRAINDICATIONS
• Avoid glucocorticoids or other immuno-suppressive agents in patients suspected of having urinary or genital tract infection.
• Avoid potentially nephrotoxic drugs (e.g., gentamicin) in febrile, dehydrated, or azotemic patients and those suspected of having pyelonephritis, septicemia, or preexisting renal disease.

PRECAUTIONS
N/A

POSSIBLE INTERACTIONS
N/A

ALTERNATIVE DRUGS
N/A

FOLLOW-UP

PATIENT MONITORING
Response to treatment by serial urinalyses, including examination of urine sediment; collect specimens from most patients by cystocentesis to avoid contamination by preputial or vaginal exudates; perform transurethral catheterization if the expected benefits outweigh the risk of bacterial urinary tract infection.

POSSIBLE COMPLICATIONS
• Infectious and noninfectious inflammatory disorders of the urinary tract can cause primary renal failure, urinary obstruction, uremia, septicemia, and death. • Pyuria is a potential risk factor for formation of matrix or matrix-crystalline urethral plugs and subsequent urethral obstruction in male cats.

MISCELLANEOUS

ASSOCIATED CONDITIONS
Hematuria, proteinuria, and bacteriuria

AGE-RELATED FACTORS
N/A

ZOONOTIC POTENTIAL
N/A

PREGNANCY
N/A

SYNONYMS
Leukocyturia

SEE ALSO
• Dysuria and Pollakiuria • Hematuria
• Lower Urinary Tract Infection • Proteinuria
• Pyelonephritis

ABBREVIATIONS
N/A

Suggested Reading

Lulich JP, Osborne CA. Bacterial infections of the urinary tract. In: Ettinger SJ, Feldman EC, eds. Textbook of veterinary internal medicine. 4th ed. Philadelphia: Saunders, 1995:1775–1788.

Lulich JP, Osborne CA, Bartges JW, et al. Canine lower urinary tract disorders. In: Ettinger SJ, Feldman EC, eds. Textbook of veterinary internal medicine. 4th ed. Philadelphia: Saunders, 1995:1833–1861.

Osborne CA, Kruger JM, Lulich JP, et al. Feline lower urinary tract diseases. In: Ettinger SJ, Feldman EC, eds. Textbook of veterinary internal medicine. 4th ed. Philadelphia: Saunders, 1995:1805–1832.

Osborne CA, Stevens JB, Lulich JP, et al. A clinician's analysis of urinalysis. In: Osborne CA, Finco DR, eds. Canine and feline nephrology and urology. 2nd ed. Baltimore: Williams & Wilkins, 1995:136–205.

Polzin D, Osborne C, O'Brien T. Diseases of the kidneys and ureters. In: Ettinger SJ, Feldman EC, eds. Textbook of veterinary internal medicine. 4th ed. Philadelphia: Saunders, 1995:1962–2046.

Authors John M. Kruger, Carl A. Osborne, and Cheryl L. Swenson
Consulting Editors Larry G. Adams and Carl A. Osborne

SODIUM, HYPERNATREMIA

 BASICS

DEFINITION

Serum sodium concentration >158 mEq/L in dogs or >165 mEq/L in cats

PATHOPHYSIOLOGY

• Sodium is the most abundant cation in the extracellular fluid, so hypernatremia usually reflects hyperosmolality.
• Common causes of hypernatremia include renal or gastrointestinal loss of water in excess of sodium loss and low water intake.

SYSTEMS AFFECTED

• Endocrine/Metabolic
• Nervous

SIGNALMENT

Dogs and cats

SIGNS

• Polydypsia
• Disorientation
• Coma
• Seizures
• Other findings depend on underlying cause
• Severity of signs usually correlates to the degree of hypernatremia

CAUSES

• Total body sodium high—oral ingestion (rare); IV administration of NaCl during cardiovascular resuscitation; hyperaldosteronism (rare)
• Total body sodium normal plus water deficit—low water intake (e.g., no access to water and adipsia or hypodipsia); high urinary water loss (e.g., diabetes insipidus); high insensible water loss (e.g., panting and hyperthermia)
• Total body sodium low and hypotonic fluid loss (i.e., loss of fluid containing sodium without adequate water replacement)—urinary loss (e.g., diabetes mellitus, osmotic diuresis, and diuresis after acute urinary obstruction); gastrointestinal sodium loss (e.g., administration of osmotic cathartic, vomiting, and diarrhea)

RISK FACTORS

N/A

 DIAGNOSIS

DIFFERENTIAL DIAGNOSIS

• Diabetes insipidus
• Hyperosmolar nonketotic syndrome
• Hypertonic dehydration
• Salt ingestion—rare

LABORATORY FINDINGS

Drugs That May Alter Laboratory Results

A wide variety of drugs interfere with renal capacity to concentrate urine, leading to water loss in excess of sodium and high serum sodium concentration; these drugs include lithium, demeclocycline, and amphotericin.

Disorders That May Alter Laboratory Results

Lipemia or hyperproteinemia (>11 g/dL) can artifactually raise sodium concentration when the flame photometry method is used.

Valid If Run in a Human Laboratory?

Yes

CBC/BIOCHEMISTRY/URINALYSIS

• High serum sodium concentration
• Diabetes insipidus—polyuria, low urinary specific gravity, and low urinary sodium concentration
• Hyperosmolar nonketotic syndrome—high blood glucose, low urine output, and high urinary specific gravity (usually >1.025)
• Hypertonic dehydration—low urinary sodium concentration and high urinary specific gravity (usually >1.030)

OTHER LABORATORY TESTS

• Modified water deprivation test (see Appendix for test protocol) to differentiate diabetes insipidus from other causes of polyuria and polydipsia; performed after results of CBC, biochemical analysis, urinalysis, and endocrine testing are evaluated to rule out hyperadrenocorticism
• After water restriction, patients with diabetes insipidus have little or no increase in urinary specific gravity or osmolality.
• After ADH or DDAVP administration, patients with nephrogenic diabetes insipidus have <10% increase in urinary specific gravity; those with central diabetes insipidus have a 10–800% increase.

IMAGING
CT scan or MRI in patients with diabetes insipidus to rule out pituitary tumor

DIAGNOSTIC PROCEDURES
N/A

TREATMENT
• After resolution of the hypernatremia, consider a sodium-restricted diet (especially in patients with nephrogenic diabetes insipidus).
• Water must be available at all times for patients with diabetes insipidus.

MEDICATIONS

DRUGS OF CHOICE
• If hypovolemia is severe—replace volume with isotonic saline (i.e., lactated Ringer or normal saline) or isotonic fluids (i.e., 5% dextrose with half-normal saline)
• Hypernatremia—administer hypotonic fluids (e.g., 5% dextrose in water) to reduce serum sodium by 0.5 mEq/h or by no more than 20 mEq/L/day; supplement with potassium and phosphate if needed.
• Central diabetes insipidus—DDAVP (1–2 drops in subconjunctival sac q12–24h)
• Nephrogenic diabetes insipidus—chlorothiazide (10–40 mg/kg PO q12h)

CONTRAINDICATIONS
Refer to manufacturer's literature.

PRECAUTIONS
• Rapid correction of hypernatremia can cause pulmonary edema.
• Hypocalcemia may develop during correction of hypernatremia.

POSSIBLE INTERACTIONS
N/A

ALTERNATE DRUGS
N/A

FOLLOW-UP

PATIENT MONITORING
• Acute setting—electrolytes, urine output, and body weight
• Diabetes insipidus—water intake

POSSIBLE COMPLICATIONS
• CNS thrombosis or hemorrhage
• Hyperactivity
• Seizures
• Serum sodium >180 mEq/L often associated with residual CNS damage
• Many patients recover, but possibility of neurologic damage is high.

MISCELLANEOUS

ASSOCIATED CONDITIONS
N/A

AGE-RELATED FACTORS
N/A

ZOONOTIC POTENTIAL
N/A

PREGNANCY
N/A

SYNONYMS
None

SEE ALSO
• Diabetes Insipidus
• Hyposthenuria

ABBREVIATIONS
• ADH = antidiuretic hormone
• DDAVP = brand name of desmopressin, a synthetic ADH preparation

Suggested Reading
DiBartola SP. Fluid therapy in small animal practice. Philadelphia: Saunders, 1992.
Ross DB Clinical physiology of acid-base and electrolyte disorders. 3rd ed. New York: McGraw-Hill, 1989.
Author Rhett Nichols
Consulting Editor Deborah S. Greco

DIAGNOSTICS—LAB

SODIUM, HYPONATREMIA

 BASICS

DEFINITION
Serum sodium concentration below the lower limit of normal. Usually associated with low total body sodium.

PATHOPHYSIOLOGY
Sodium is the most abundant cation in the extracellular fluid and, therefore, hyponatremia usually reflects hypoosmolality. Either solute loss or water retention can theoretically cause hyponatremia. Most solute loss occurs in isoosmotic solutions (e.g., vomit and diarrhea) and, as a result, water retention in relation to solute is the underlying cause in almost all patients with hyponatremia. In general, hyponatremia occurs only when a defect in renal water excretion is present.

SYSTEMS AFFECTED
Nervous—severe neurologic dysfunction is not usually seen until serum sodium concentration falls below 110–115 mEq/L. Overly rapid correction of hyponatremia can also cause neurologic damage.

SIGNALMENT
Dogs and cats.

SIGNS
• Lethargy
• Seizures
• Obtundation
• Coma
• Other findings depend on the underlying cause.

CAUSES

Disorders Associated with Normal Renal Water Excretion
• Primary polydipsia
• Reset osmostat

Disorders Associated with Reduced Renal Water Excretion
• Low effective circulating volume—gastrointestinal losses, renal losses (including mineralocorticoid deficiency), skin losses, and edematous states (e.g., heart failure, end stage liver disease, and nephrotic syndrome)
• Diuretic administration
• Renal failure
• ADH excess with normovolemia—syndrome of inappropriate ADH secretion, hypocortisolemia, and hypothyroidism
• Low solute intake

RISK FACTORS
N/A

 DIAGNOSIS

DIFFERENTIAL DIAGNOSIS
N/A

LABORATORY FINDINGS

Drugs That May Alter Lab Results
Mannitol can cause pseudohyponatremia.

Disorders That May Alter Lab Results.
Hyperlipidemia, hyperglycemia, and hyperproteinemia can cause pseudohyponatremia.

Valid If Run In A Human Lab?
Yes

CBC/BIOCHEMISTRY/URINALYSIS
• Low serum sodium concentration.
• Other abnormalities may point to the underlying cause.

OTHER LABORATORY TESTS
• Plasma osmolality is low; if plasma osmolality is normal or high, exclude renal failure or causes of pseudohyponatremia (e.g., hyperlipidemia, hyperglycemia, hyperproteinemia, and mannitol administration).
• Urine osmolality < 100–150 mosmol/kg indicates primary polydipsia or reset osmostat. Urine osmolality > 150–200 mosmol/kg indicates impaired renal water excretion.
• Urine sodium concentration < 15–20 mEq/L indicates low effective circulating volume, pure cortisol deficiency, primary polydipsia with high urine output. Urine sodium concentration > 20 to 25 mEq/L indicates syndrome of inappropriate ADH secretion, adrenal insufficiency, renal failure, reset osmostat, diuretic administration, or vomiting with marked bicarbonate loss.

IMAGING
N/A

DIAGNOSTIC PROCEDURES
N/A

GROSS AND HISTOPATHOLOGIC FINDINGS
N/A

 TREATMENT

INPATIENT VERSUS OUTPATIENT
Depends on severity of hyponatremia, associated neurologic dysfunction, and the underlying disorder

DIET
N/A

CLIENT EDUCATION
Depends on the underlying disorder

SURGICAL CONSIDERATIONS
N/A

MEDICATIONS

DRUGS AND FLUIDS

Treatment consists of increasing the serum sodium concentration and treating the underlying cause. Hyponatremia is corrected by administering NaCl if the patient has hypovolemia (e.g., volume depletion, adrenal insufficiency, and diuretic administration) and by restricting water if the patient has normovolemia or edema (e.g., renal failure, SIADH, primary polydipsia, and edematous states). Hypertonic saline administration is usually indicated if the patient has clinical signs or serum sodium concentration < 105–110 mEq/L. The sodium deficit is estimated by 0.5 × lean BW (kg) × (120 - serum sodium concentration). If the patient has no to mild clinical signs, increase sodium concentration at a rate of 0.5 mEq/L per hour until sodium concentration is 120–125 mEq/L, then discontinue hypertonic saline and normalize serum sodium concentration over several days with isotonic saline or water restriction as dictated by the cause of hyponatremia. If the patient has seizures or coma, a rate of 1–1.5 mEq/L per hour for the first 10 mEq/L may be indicated. True volume depletion must also be corrected. In edematous patients with symptomatic hyponatremia, administration of a loop diuretic in addition to hypertonic saline may be necessary. Other medications are dictated by the underlying cause.

CONTRAINDICATIONS

N/A

PRECAUTIONS

Overly rapid correction of hyponatremia can result in neurologic damage (demyelination); avoid increasing serum sodium concentration by more than 25 mEq/L in the first 48 hours.

POSSIBLE INTERACTIONS

N/A

ALTERNATE DRUGS

N/A

FOLLOW-UP

PATIENT MONITORING

Serum electrolyte concentrations as needed to assure appropriate response to NaCl and other indicated therapies.

PREVENTION/AVOIDANCE

Depends on the underlying disorder

POSSIBLE COMPLICATIONS

Depends on the underlying disorder

EXPECTED COURSE/PROGNOSIS

Depends on the underlying disorder

MISCELLANEOUS

ASSOCIATED CONDITIONS

Other electrolyte and acid–base abnormalities are often associated with the clinical disorders that cause hyponatremia.

AGE RELATED FACTORS

Depends on the underlying cause

ZOONOTIC POTENTIAL

N/A

PREGNANCY

N/A

SYNONYMS

N/A

SEE ALSO

N/A

ABBREVIATIONS

ADH = antidiuretic hormone

REFERENCES

Rose DB. Clinical physiology of acid–base and electrolyte disorders. 3rd ed. New York: McGraw-Hill, 1989.

DiBartola SP. Fluid therapy in small animal practice. Philadelphia: WB Saunders, 1992.

Author Peter P. Kintzer

Consulting Editor Rhett Nichols

THROMBOCYTOPENIA

BASICS

DEFINITION
- Platelet count below the lower limit of the reference range
- Purdue University Teaching Hospital reference range—200,000–900,000/μL, dogs; 300,000–700,000/μL, cats

PATHOPHYSIOLOGY
- Platelets are produced by megakaryocytes in the bone marrow, released into bloodstream, and circulate for a few to several days.
- In the normal state, the platelet count remains stable, because production of platelets is equivalent to the removal of platelets from the circulation and the spleen holds a fairly large reserve.
- Caused by decreased production, sequestration, increased destruction, or increased use of platelets.

SYSTEMS AFFECTED
- If the platelet count is low enough (< 40,000/μL), hemorrhage can occur into any organ system.
- Hemorrhage is commonly recognized in the Skin/Exocrine, Gastrointestinal, Renal/Urologic, and Respiratory systems; more difficult to document in the Nervous and Cardiovascular systems

SIGNALMENT
- Dogs and cats
- Primary immune-mediated thrombocytopenia more common in female dogs than in male dogs and cats
- Primary immune-mediated thrombocytopenia more common in poodles, Old English sheepdogs, cocker spaniels, and possibly German shepherds than in other breeds
- Non-immune-mediated thrombocytopenia more common in Doberman pinschers than in other breeds
- Idiopathic asymptomatic thrombocytopenia with macroplatelets described in Cavalier King Charles spaniels

SIGNS

General Comments
Signs typically do not develop until the platelet count is < 40,000/μL.

Historical Findings
- Spontaneous and inappropriate mucous membrane, cutaneous, nasal, urinary, and gastrointestinal bleeding
- Weakness and collapse
- Dyspnea

Physical Examination Findings
- Petechial and ecchymotic hemorrhages in the skin and mucous membranes
- Epistaxis
- Melena, hematochezia, and/or hematemesis
- Hematuria
- Scleral hemorrhages, retinal hemorrhages, and hyphema
- Pale mucous membranes
- Lethargy, weakness, and collapse
- Dyspnea
- Heart murmur
- Neurologic signs

CAUSES
- Decreased production—infectious agents, neoplasia, drugs, and immune-mediated
- Increased sequestration—splenomegaly or hepatomegaly
- Increased use—DIC, vasculitis, and blood loss; blood loss alone does not lead to severe thrombocytopenia.
- Increased destruction—primary or secondary immune-mediated thrombocytopenia (i.e., immune-mediated hemolytic anemia, SLE, drugs, infectious agents, and neoplasia)
- Miscellaneous—infectious agents (e.g., distemper, *Ehrlichia*, FeLV, FIV, Rocky Mountain spotted fever, and dirofilariasis), idiopathic asymptomatic thrombocytopenia in Cavalier King Charles spaniels

RISK FACTORS
- Potentially any drug; but gold compounds, cephalosporins, trimethoprim/sulfonamide, and estrogens have been associated with immune-mediated thrombocytopenia in dogs
- Recent vaccination

DIAGNOSIS

DIFFERENTIAL DIAGNOSIS
- Splenomegaly or hepatomegaly and mild thrombocytopenia—consider sequestration of platelets
- Blood loss associated with traumatic even—consider increased use of platelets
- Exposure to vitamin K antagonist—consider increased use of platelets
- Vasculitis—consider Rocky Mountain spotted fever
- Multisystemic failure—consider DIC
- Drug history—consider secondary immune-mediated thrombocytopenia
- Mass—consider neoplasia-associated secondary immune-mediated thrombocytopenia, often lymphoproliferative disorders or hemangiosarcoma
- Polyarthritis, dermatitis, polymyositis, and glomerulonephritis—consider SLE
- Primary immune-mediated thrombocytopenia diagnosed by exclusion of other causes

LABORATORY FINDINGS

Drugs That May Alter Laboratory Results
None

Disorders That May Alter Laboratory Results
- Poor venipuncture technique can cause clumping of platelets in vitro and may provide a falsely low platelet count.
- Difficult to obtain accurate platelet count in cats with automated blood analyzers

Valid If Run in Human Laboratory?
Because of the large size of cat platelets, they are not measured accurately by most automated hematology analyzers.

CBC/BIOCHEMISTRY/URINALYSIS
- If results reveal anemia and leukopenia—consider decreased production caused by neoplastic infiltration, and immune-mediated, chemically induced, or infectious causes (e.g., ehrlichiosis, FeLV, and FIV)

- Results reveal anemia with spherocytosis with or without agglutination—consider immune-mediated hemolytic anemia with secondary immune-mediated thrombocytopenia
- Results reveal anemia, leukopenia or leukocytosis, and proteinuria—consider SLE
- Eosinophilia—consider heartworm disease
- Morulae detected in platelets—consider *E. platys*
- Morulae detected in neutrophils—consider granulocytic ehrlichiosis
- Morulae detected in monocytes—consider *E. canis*

OTHER LABORATORY TESTS
- Canine heartworm antigen test—rule out dirofilariasis
- FeLV and FIV tests—rule out viral infections
- Serum titers—rule out ehrlichiosis and Rocky Mountain spotted fever
- Coagulation profile (e.g., activated clotting time, APTT, and PT)—normal clotting times rule out DIC and exposure to vitamin K antagonists.
- Antiplatelet antibody test or antimegakaryocyte antibody—evaluate immune-mediated mechanism
- ANA test—screen for SLE
- Coombs test—help document concurrent immune-mediated hemolytic anemia

IMAGING
Radiography or ultrasonography to identify splenomegaly, hepatomegaly, internal bleeding, and internal neoplasms

DIAGNOSTIC PROCEDURES
Bone marrow aspirate—rule out primary bone marrow disease

TREATMENT
- If animal is severely affected, restrict activity to prevent fatal bleed
- Minimize bleeding associated with diagnostic procedures (e.g., minimize or eliminate jugular venipuncture and apply extended pressure after venipuncture; bone marrow aspiration is safe)
- Once stabilized, treat as outpatient
- If anemia owing to blood loss is severe, give blood transfusion

MEDICATIONS

DRUGS OF CHOICE
- Immune-mediated—prednisolone (2.2 mg/kg PO q12h for at least 2 weeks or until marked improvement in platelet count is seen) and other immunosuppressive drugs; see Thrombocytopenia, Primary Immune-Mediated
- Rickettsial diseases—doxycycline (5mg/kg q12h PO for 14 days) or tetracycline (20 mg/kg, q8h PO for 21 days); see Ehrlichiosis and Rocky Mountain Spotted Fever
- DIC—heparin (70 U/kg SC q8h); see Disseminated Intravascular Coagulation

CONTRAINDICATIONS
NSAIDs that interfere with platelet function

PRECAUTIONS
None

POSSIBLE INTERACTIONS
None

ALTERNATIVE DRUGS
None

FOLLOW-UP

PATIENT MONITORING
- Amount of bleeding
- Platelet counts daily until patient is stable, then weekly until platelets return to normal range
- Serial coagulation profiles if DIC suspected

POSSIBLE COMPLICATIONS
Excessive bleeding, which can be fatal

MISCELLANEOUS

ASSOCIATED CONDITIONS
Immune-mediated hemolytic anemia

AGE-RELATED FACTORS
None

ZOONOTIC POTENTIAL
None

PREGNANCY
- Treatment of pregnant animals with immune-mediated thrombocytopenia by administration of corticosteroids should be done with caution.
- Treatment of animals with rickettsial diseases by administration of tetracycline or doxycycline can cause fetal abnormalities.

SYNONYMS
None

SEE ALSO
- Anemia, Immune-Mediated
- Distemper—Dogs
- Ehrlichiosis
- Feline Immunodeficiency Virus
- Feline Leukemia Virus Infection
- Lupus Erythematosus, Systemic (SLE)
- Rocky Mountain Spotted Fever
- Thrombocytopenia, Primary Immune-Mediated

ABBREVIATIONS
- APTT = activated partial thromboplastin time
- DIC = disseminated intravascular coagulation
- FeLV = feline leukemia virus
- FIV = feline immunodeficiency virus
- PT = prothrombin time
- SLE = systemic lupus erythematosus

Suggested Reading
Grindem CB, Breischwerdt EB, Corbett WT, Jans HE. Epidemiologic survey of thrombocytopenia in dogs: a report of 987 cases. Vet Clin Pathol 1991;20:38–43.

Lewis DC, Myers KM. Canine idiopathic thrombocytopenia purpura. J Vet Int Med 1996;10:207–218.

Reagan WJ, Rebar AH. Platelet disorders. In: Ettinger SL, Feldman EC, eds. Textbook of veterinary internal medicine. 4th ed Philadelphia: Saunders, 1995:1964-1976

Thompson JP, Immunologic diseases. In: Ettinger SL, Feldman EC, eds. Textbook of veterinary internal medicine. 4th ed Philadelphia: Saunders, 1995:2002-2029

Williams DA, Maggio-Price L. Canine idiopathic thrombocytopenia: clinical observations and long-term follow-up in 54 cases. J Am Vet Med Assoc 1984;185:660–663.
Author William J. Reagan
Consulting Editor Susan M. Cotter

THROMBOCYTOSIS

 BASICS

DEFINITION
• A platelet count above the upper end of the reference range
• Purdue University Teaching Hospital reference ranges—dogs, 200,000–900,000/µL; cats, 300,000–700,000/µL

PATHOPHYSIOLOGY
• Can be caused by overproduction of platelets, decreased clearance of platelets, and decreased sequestration of platelets.
• Overproduction occurs secondary to bone marrow stimulation by thrombopoietin and factors such as IL-1, IL-3, IL-6, and IL-11.
• For most associated diseases, the exact mechanisms are not well documented.

SYSTEMS AFFECTED
• Usually does not cause systemic abnormalities
• Thrombosis not commonly observed; if the patient has concurrent altered blood flow and endothelial cell damage, thrombosis can develop and cause organ dysfunction.
• Bleeding not commonly observed; if the patient has concurrent platelet functional defect, hemorrhage can occur and cause organ dysfunction.

SIGNALMENT
Excitement-induced thrombocytosis more common in cats, especially kittens, than in dogs.

SIGNS
Usually none directly attributed to the thrombocytosis

CAUSES
• Primary thrombocytosis
• Essential thrombocythemia
• Secondary thrombocytosis
• Chronic hemorrhage
• Iron deficiency
• Neoplasia, of both bone marrow and non–bone marrow origin*

• Inflammatory diseases—pancreatitis, hepatitis, gingivitis, colitis*
• Endocrine disorders—diabetes mellitus, hyperadrenocorticism, hypothyroidism
• Rebound thrombocytosis in patients with immune-mediated disorders such as immune-mediated hemolytic anemia, immune-mediated thrombocytopenia, SLE
• Splenic contraction
• Drugs—corticosteroids, chemotherapeutics, and antibiotics
• Fractures or soft tissue trauma
• Myelofibrosis
• Splenectomy

RISK FACTORS
None

 DIAGNOSIS

DIFFERENTIAL DIAGNOSIS
• Mass—consider thrombocytosis associated with neoplasia
• Diarrhea and vomiting—consider associated inflammatory conditions of the gastrointestinal tract
• Polydipsia and polyuria—consider associated hyperadrenocorticism and diabetes mellitus
• Weight gain, bilateral alopecia, and dry hair coat—consider associated hypothyroidism
• Gastrointestinal or integumentary chronic blood loss—consider associated iron deficiency
• Polyarthritis, dermatitis, polymyositis, and glomerulonephritis—consider SLE
• Splenectomy—consider reduced sequestration of platelets
• Drug therapy (e.g., corticosteroids, vincristine, antibiotics, and antineoplastic drugs)—consider drug-induced thrombocytosis

• Bone fracture or soft tissue trauma—consider thrombocytosis associated with trauma
• Excited patients during venipuncture—consider excitement-induced splenic contraction
• Essential thrombocytosis diagnosed by ruling out other causes of thrombocytosis

LABORATORY FINDINGS
Drugs That May Alter Laboratory Results
None

Disorders That May Alter Laboratory Results
Excessively large platelets, such as in cats or in cats and dogs with a myeloproliferative disorder, may disallow an accurate platelet count by an automated hematology analyzer.

Valid If Run in Human Laboratory?
Because of the large size of cat platelets, an accurate count may not be attainable.

CBC/BIOCHEMISTRY/URINALYSIS
• Mild normocytic normochromic nonregenerative anemia—consider hypothyroidism or neoplasia
• Inflammatory leukogram—consider secondary thrombocytosis associated with an inflammatory response
• High hepatocellular and cholestatic liver enzymes with or without high bilirubin—consider hepatic disease
• High lipase and amylase—consider pancreatitis
• Stress leukogram, fasting hyperglycemia, high liver enzyme activity, including alkaline phosphatase—consider hyperadrenocorticism
• Fasting hyperglycemia and glucosuria—consider diabetes mellitus
• Regenerative anemia with spherocytosis with or without agglutination—consider immune-mediated hemolytic anemia.
• Microcytic hypochromic anemia—consider iron deficiency
• Concurrent neutrophilia and lymphocytosis—consider excitement-induced thrombocytosis

• Concurrent hyperkalemia—consider release of intracellular potassium of platelets during clotting
• Severe nonregenerative anemia with or without dacryocytes and with or without neutropenia—consider myelofibrosis
• Blast cells or bone marrow precursor cells in the circulation—consider myeloproliferative disorders, including megakaryoblastic leukemia and basophilic leukemia
• Extremely high platelet count, macroplatelets, hypogranulation or hypergranulation with or without basophilia—consider the myeloproliferative disorder essential thrombocythemia; diagnosis made by ruling out all other causes of thrombocytosis.

OTHER LABORATORY TESTS
• Serum T_4 concentration with or without TSH and free T_4 concentration—hypothyroidism
• ACTH stimulation or low-dose dexamethasone-suppression test—hyperadrenocorticism
• Serum iron, ferritin, and total iron-binding capacity—iron deficiency
• FIV and FeLV tests in cats with myeloproliferative disorders

IMAGING
To detect internal neoplasm, organomegaly, and inflammatory disease

DIAGNOSTIC PROCEDURES
• Examination of bone marrow aspirate and core biopsy—myeloproliferative disorder, iron deficiency, and myelofibrosis
• Endoscopy—gastrointestinal disease
• Biopsy of any internal or external mass

TREATMENT
• Usually no specific treatment is necessary.
• Excitement-induced thrombocytosis is usually transient.
• Treat underlying disease, and platelet count will return to normal.

MEDICATIONS

DRUGS OF CHOICE
• Immediate treatment not necessary to correct laboratory abnormality

CONTRAINDICATIONS
If platelet function is abnormal, do not use NSAIDs.

PRECAUTIONS
None

POSSIBLE INTERACTIONS
None

ALTERNATIVE DRUGS
None

FOLLOW-UP

PATIENT MONITORING
• CBC as needed to monitor the underlying disease process
• Thrombocytosis will resolve once the primary disease is eliminated.

POSSIBLE COMPLICATIONS
Bleeding abnormality may be noted owing to concurrent platelet function defect.

MISCELLANEOUS

ASSOCIATED CONDITIONS
• Hyperkalemia, caused by release of potassium from platelets during clotting in vitro, sometimes associated with severe thrombocytosis
• Plasma potassium should be normal.

AGE-RELATED FACTORS
Excitement-induced thrombocytosis more common in cats, especially kittens, than in dogs

ZOONOTIC POTENTIAL
None

PREGNANCY
N/A

SYNONYM
Thrombocythemia

SEE ALSO
• Anemia, Iron Deficiency
• Hyperadrenocorticism (Cushing's Disease)
• Hypothyroidism

ABBREVIATIONS
• FeLV = feline leukemia virus
• FIV = feline immunodeficiency virus
• IL = interleukin
• SLE = systemic lupus erythematosus
• TSH = thyroid-stimulating hormone

Suggested Reading
Hammer AS. Thrombocytosis in dogs and cats: a retrospective study. Comp Haematol Int 1991;1:181–186.
Jain NC. The platelets. In: Jain NC, ed. Essentials of veterinary hematology. Philadelphia: Lea & Febiger, 1993:105–132
Reagan WJ, Rebar AH. Platelet disorders. In: Ettinger SL and Feldman EC, eds. Textbook of veterinary internal medicine. 4th ed Philadelphia: Saunders, 1995:1964–1967
Author William J. Reagan
Consulting Editor Susan M. Cotter

DIAGNOSTICS–LAB

THYROID HORMONES

 BASICS

DEFINITION
Serum concentrations of T_4, T_3, free thyroxine, or endogenous canine TSH outside the normal range

PATHOPHYSIOLOGY
• The thyroid gland regulates basal metabolism; two molecules, *tyrosine* and *iodine,* are important for thyroid hormone synthesis.
• The tyrosyl ring can accommodate two iodide molecules; if one iodide attaches, it is called *monoiodotyrosine* (MIT); if two iodide molecules attach to the tyrosyl ring, it is called *diiodotyrosine* (DIT).
• Two DIT molecules form T_4; one MIT coupled with one DIT molecule forms T_3.
• T_4 is the major storage form of thyroid hormone; T_3 is the active form of the hormone; most T_3 is formed outside the thyroid gland by deiodination of T_4.
• Another type of T_3 is formed when an iodide molecule is removed from the inner phenolic ring of T_4; this compound is called *reverse* T_3 and increases in nonthyroidal illness.
• Thyrotropin, or TSH, is the most important regulator of thyroid activity.
• TSH secretion is regulated by thyroid hormones via negative feedback inhibition of the synthesis of TRH at the level of the hypothalamus and by inhibition of the activity of TSH at the level of the pituitary.
• With thyroid gland failure, the pituitary gland senses decreases in serum free thyroxine (FT_4) and TT_4, resulting in increased serum endogenous TSH concentration.

• The use of endogenous TSH alone is not recommended as a method of assessing thyroid function.
• FT_4 concentrations are measured by equilibrium dialysis (gold standard) or analogue immunoassays.

SYSTEMS AFFECTED
• Ophthalmic
• Nervous
• Endocrine/Metabolism
• Gastrointestinal
• Hepatobiliary
• Cardiovascular
• Renal
• Reproductive

SIGNALMENT
Dog and cat

SIGNS
Historical Findings
See Hypothyroidism and Hyperthyroidism.
Physical Examination Findings
See Hypothyroidism and Hyperthyroidism.

CAUSES
See Hypothyroidism and Hyperthyroidism.

RISK FACTORS
Greyhounds have approximately half the normal TT_4 and FT_4 concentrations of other dogs.

 DIAGNOSIS

DIFFERENTIAL DIAGNOSIS
N/A

LABORATORY FINDINGS
Sample Handling
• Collect blood samples for TT_4, cTSH, and TT_3 and spin and freeze serum for submission; It should be mailed and arrive at laboratory cool; ice is not necessary.
• Plasma and serum samples for FT_4 by

dialysis should arrive at laboratory frozen; may require the use of dry ice
Drugs That May Alter Laboratory Results
• Anesthetics
• Phenobarbital
• Primidone
• Diazepam
• Trimethoprim-sulfas
• Quinidine
• Phenylbutazone
• Salicylates
• Glucocorticoids

Disorders That May Alter Laboratory Results
• Any nonthyroidal illness
• Hyperadrenocorticism
• Renal failure
• Diabetes mellitus
• Liver disease
• Pregnancy

Valid If Run in Human Laboratory?
• Serum concentrations of thyroid hormone (TT_4) are much lower in dogs than in human beings; therefore, TT_4 assays must be run in a veterinary diagnostic endocrine laboratory.
• Endogenous TSH is species–specific; therefore, TSH assays do not cross-react with canine or feline TSH.

CBC/BIOCHEMISTRY/URINALYSIS
• Normocytic, normochromic anemia resulting from erythropoietin deficiency, decreased bone marrow activity, and decreased serum iron and iron-binding capacity are observed in about 25–30% of hypothyroid dogs; clinicopathologic features of hyperthyroidism include erythrocytosis and excitement leukogram (neutrophilia, lymphocytosis).
• Hypercholesterolemia is seen in approximately 75% of hypothyroid dogs because of altered lipid metabolism, decreased fecal excretion of cholesterol, and decreased conversion of lipids to bile acids.

• Hyponatremia, a common finding in human beings with hypothyroidism, is observed as a mild decrease in serum sodium in about 30% of hypothyroid dogs.
• Increased serum CPK, possibly as a result of hypothyroid myopathy.
• Hyperthyroid cats may exhibit increased BUN.
• Serum activities of liver enzymes (ALT, AST) increase in most hyperthyroid cats.

OTHER LABORATORY TESTS
• The antithyroglobulin autoantibody test (ATAA)—the presence of antithyroglobulin antibodies theoretically presages the onset of hypothyroidism in dogs with autoimmune thyroiditis.
• TSH stimulation test—was considered the gold standard for diagnosis of hypothyroidism in dogs; does not differentiate between early hypothyroid dogs and those with "euthyroid-sick" syndrome, nor does it identify dogs with secondary or tertiary hypothyroidism; exogenous bovine TSH is no longer commercially available.
• TRH stimulation test
• FT_4 by dialysis (along with TT_4)
• Dynamic endocrine testing (see T_3 suppression test)

IMAGING
Thyroid scan with Technetium-99m

DIAGNOSTIC PROCEDURES
Thyroid biopsy

TREATMENT
See Hypothyroidism and Hyperthyroidism.

MEDICATIONS
N/A

DRUGS OF CHOICE
N/A

CONTRAINDICATIONS
N/A

PRECAUTIONS
N/A

POSSIBLE INTERACTIONS
N/A

ALTERNATIVE DRUGS
N/A

FOLLOW-UP

PATIENT MONITORING
See Hypothyroidism and Hyperthyroidism.

POSSIBLE COMPLICATIONS
N/A

MISCELLANEOUS

ASSOCIATED CONDITIONS
• "Euthyroid-sick" syndrome is characterized by decreased serum TT_4 and increased reverse T_3 (see above).
• Concurrent illnesses such as diabetes mellitus, CRF, hepatic insufficiency, and infections can cause euthyroid-sick syndrome, resulting in decreased serum TT_4 concentrations.

AGE-RELATED FACTORS
• Puppies exhibit serum TT_4 concentrations 2–5 times those of adult dogs.
• There is an age-related decline in serum TT_4 concentrations and response to TSH stimulation in dogs.

ZOONOTIC POTENTIAL
N/A

PREGNANCY
May affect serum total T_4 concentrations because of changes in protein binding

SYNONYMS
N/A

SEE ALSO
• Canine Hypothyroidism
• Feline Hyperthyroidism

ABBREVIATIONS
• ATAA = antithyroglobulin autoantibody test
• CPK = creatine phosphokinase
• DIT = diiodotyrosine
• eTSH = endogenous canine thyroid stimulating hormone
• FT_4 = free thyroxine, unbound to serum protein
• FT_3 = free triiodothyronine
• MIT = monoiodotyrosine
• T_4 = thyroxine
• T_3 = triiodothyronine

Selected Reading
Moncrieff JC, Nelson RW, Bruner JM, et al. Comparison of serum concentrations of thyroid-stimulating hormone in healthy dogs, hypothyroid dogs, and euthyroid dogs with concurrent disease. J Am Vet Med Assoc 1998;212:387–391.
Peterson ME, Melian C, Nichols R. Measurement of serum total thyroxine, triiodothyronine, free thyroxine and thyrotropin concentrations for diagnosis of hypothyroidism in dogs. J Am Vet Med Assoc 1997;211:1396–1402.
Author Deborah S. Greco
Consulting Editor Deborah S. Greco

TRYPSIN-LIKE IMMUNOREACTIVITY (TLI)

BASICS

DEFINITION
• Markedly subnormal serum TLI—a highly sensitive and specific indicator of EPI secondary to loss of pancreatic acinar cells, the only cells that synthesize trypsinogen in dogs and cats
• Above–normal serum TLI concentration in the face of normal or near–normal renal function—inflammatory or other disease of the exocrine pancreas is causing increased release of this pancreatic acinar cell specific marker.

PATHOPHYSIOLOGY
• Trypsinogen is synthesized and stored only in pancreatic acinar cells, and a small proportion of the trypsinogen synthesized each day normally leaks into the blood, where low concentrations can be detected using sensitive and specific TLI immunoassays.
• Serum TLI concentration decreases when the mass of pancreatic acinar cells is decreased by pancreatic disease, most commonly by pancreatic acinar atrophy in dogs and by end-stage CP in cats; both disease processes may lead to EPI.
• Serum TLI concentration increases with pancreatic inflammatory disease, most commonly AP in dogs and CP in cats.

SYSTEMS AFFECTED
• Gastrointestinal—chronic diarrhea, weight loss, polyphagia (EPI); vomiting, anorexia, fever, abdominal pain, lethargy, depression (AP, CP)
• Skin—poor haircoat condition (EPI)
• Musculoskeletal—weight loss, cachexia (EPI)

SIGNALMENT
• Dogs and cats
• Pancreatic acinar atrophy is most common in German shepherd dogs between 1 and 5 years of age (although any age and breed of dog can be affected).

• AP is reportedly particularly common in miniature schnauzers, but many other breeds are affected too.

SIGNS

Historical Findings
• Chronic diarrhea, weight loss, polyphagia, anorexia, vomiting (EPI)
• Anorexia, depression, vomiting (AP, CP)
• Many cats with CP also have concurrent inflammatory bowel disease.

Physical Examination Findings
• Weight loss, poor haircoat (EPI)
• Depression, abdominal discomfort (AP, CP)

CAUSES
• Pancreatic acinar atrophy
• AP
• CP
• Pancreatic atrophy/hypertrophy in cats

RISK FACTORS
Hyperlipidemia and some drugs (tetracyclines, l-asparaginase, azathioprine, doxorubicin, others) and toxins (cholinesterase inhibitors) may predispose to AP.

DIAGNOSIS

DIFFERENTIAL DIAGNOSIS
• Serum TLI decreases very specifically only when pancreatic acinar cell mass decreases.
• Serum TLI increases when release from the pancreas increases as in pancreatitis and when clearance from the plasma decreases because of a decreased glomerular filtration rate in severe renal disease.
• Mild renal dysfunction does not significantly increase serum TLI.

LABORATORY FINDINGS
• Serum TLI determined only by highly species-specific immunoassays
• A radioimmunoassay for canine TLI is available commercially and is used by many veterinary laboratories.

• At the time of writing, feline TLI assay is available only through the author's laboratory at Texas A&M University.
• Lipemia, hemolysis, icterus, and delayed separation of serum do not affect serum TLI assay.
• Serum TLI is very stable and is unaffected by storage for up to 7 days at 37°C.

Drugs That May Alter Laboratory Results
N/A

Disorders That May Alter Laboratory Results
N/A

Valid If Run in Human Laboratory?
No

CBC/BIOCHEMISTRY/URINALYSIS
• Consider abnormalities in patients with EPI as indicating coexistent disease.
• Patients with AP often have neutrophilic leukocytosis (sometimes left-shifted), hyperlipidemia, hyperglycemia, hypocalcemia, elevated alkaline phosphatase, and sometimes hyperbilirubinemia.

OTHER LABORATORY TESTS
• Cats with EPI, and, to a lesser extent, dogs, almost always have markedly subnormal serum cobalamin (vitamin B_{12}) concentrations.
• Cats with EPI also often have subnormal serum folate, reflecting coexistent inflammatory bowel disease.
• Dogs with EPI often have above-normal serum folate reflecting a coexistent enteropathy associated with overgrowth of folate-synthesizing bacteria in the upper small intestine.
• Amylase and lipase do not decrease in the serum of dogs and cats with EPI.
• Serum amylase and lipase may increase along with TLI in dogs with AP or CP, but do not increase in cats with AP or CP.

TRYPSIN-LIKE IMMUNOREACTIVITY (TLI)

IMAGING
Abdominal ultrasonography and (to a lesser extent) radiography may be helpful in AP, but findings are unremarkable in EPI.

DIAGNOSTIC PROCEDURES
Histologic examination of pancreatic biopsy specimens obtained at laparoscopy or exploratory laparotomy may be required to define the underlying pathology fully.

TREATMENT
• Patients with EPI can be treated by pancreatic enzyme replacement as outpatients. Patients with subnormal serum cobalamin or folate may require parenteral or oral supplementation, respectively, to respond optimally to enzyme replacement.
• Avoid diets containing large amounts of fiber; some fiber binds pancreatic enzymes and inhibits their activity.
• Patients with AP usually require hospitalization for supportive care (fluid therapy, temporary cessation of oral food intake, enteral or parenteral nutrition) and may experience life-threatening complications (pulmonary edema, DIC, shock).

MEDICATIONS

DRUGS OF CHOICE
• Patients with EPI require supplementation of food with pancreatic extract containing digestive enzymes (1 tsp pancreatic enzyme powder/l0 kg body weight, mixed well with food).
• Patients with AP may require treatment for specific complications (e.g., antibiotic therapy for infections, plasma transfusion to reverse hypoalbuminemia, and depletion of plasma protease inhibitors).

CONTRAINDICATIONS
N/A

PRECAUTIONS
• Give corticosteroids to patients with severe AP only when in acute shock; these drugs may impair removal of toxic digestive enzymes from the blood and impair recovery.
• Patients with CP, especially feline patients with coexistent inflammatory bowel disease, can usually be given corticosteroid therapy without apparent exacerbation of pancreatitis.

POSSIBLE INTERACTIONS
N/A

ALTERNATIVE DRUGS
N/A

FOLLOW-UP

PATIENT MONITORING
• Patients with EPI—monthly, to ensure resolution of diarrhea and return to normal body weight and condition
• Patients with AP and CP—do not feed high-fat-content diet.

POSSIBLE COMPLICATIONS
Vitamin deficiency (cobalamin, tocopherol, vitamin K)—may develop over months to years despite apparent resolution of weight loss and diarrhea; consider in patients with unexplained anorexia, neuromuscular or retinal disease, or bleeding disorders.

MISCELLANEOUS

ASSOCIATED CONDITIONS
Patients with EPI often have concurrent small intestinal abnormalities (small intestinal bacterial overgrowth in dogs and inflammatory bowel disease in cats) that may impair the response to pancreatic enzyme replacement alone.

AGE-RELATED FACTORS
N/A

ZOONOTIC POTENTIAL
None

PREGNANCY
N/A

SYNONYMS
N/A

SEE ALSO
• Serum Cobalamin and Folate
• Pancreatitis

ABBREVIATIONS
• AP = acute pancreatitis
• CP = chronic pancreatitis
• EPI = exocrine pancreatic insufficiency
• TLI = trypsin-like immunoreactivity

Suggested Reading
Steiner JM, Williams DA. Feline trypsin-like immunoreactivity in feline exocrine pancreatic disease. Compend Contin Educ Pract Vet 1996;18:543–547.
Steiner JM, Williams DA. Feline exocrine pancreatic disorders. Vet Clin North Am 1999;29:551–575.
Williams DA. Exocrine pancreatic disease. In: Thomas DA, Simpson JW, Hall EJ, eds. Manual of canine and feline gastroenterology. BSAVA Publications, 1996:171–190.
Williams DA. The pancreas. In: Strombeck DR, Guilford WG, Center SA, et al., eds. Small animal gastroenterology. 3rd ed. Philadelphia: Saunders, 1996:381–410.
Author David A. Williams
Consulting Editors Brett M. Feder and Mitchell A. Crystal

DIAGNOSTICS—LAB

URINE CORTISOL:CREATININE RATIO

BASICS

DEFINITION
• To measure a urine cortisol:creatinine ratio (UCCR), a single midstream free-catch urine sample is used.; cortisol and creatinine are both measured and the concentrations converted into the same units; the UCCR is simply the ratio of the two values.
• A normal UCCR is less than approximately 10–30 × 10^{-6} depending on the laboratory; this value has no units and is typically reported without the scientific notation, e.g. 10 × 10^{-6} would be reported as 10.

PATHOPHYSIOLOGY
• A UCCR is used to screen for spontaneous hyperadrenocorticism (Cushing's syndrome).
• Urine cortisol excretion increases as a reflection of augmented adrenal secretion of the hormone; this can be due either to excess stimulation by a pituitary adrenocorticotropin (ACTH)-secreting tumor (i.e. pituitary-dependent hyperadrenocorticism, PDH) or by an autonomously functioning adrenal tumor (AT).
• Since creatinine excretion is relatively constant while kidney function is stable, dividing the urine cortisol concentration by the creatinine concentration negates the effect of urine volume in interpreting urine cortisol concentration.
• The finding of an elevated UCCR is a sensitive marker of hyperadrenocorticism, being present in 90–100% of affected animals.
• An elevated UCCR can also be due to nonadrenal illness and nonspecific activation of the hypothalamic-pituitary-adrenal axis in dogs and cats.
• The chance of a false-positive is great since only about 25–30% of dogs with an elevated UCCR actually have Cushing's syndrome while the other 70–75% have non-adrenal illness.

SYSTEMS AFFECTED
• Organ systems are not affected by an abnormal UCCR *per se;* they are affected by excess cortisol secreted in Cushing's syndrome.
• See Hyperadrenocorticism.

SIGNALMENT
Dog and cat

SIGNS

General comments
• No historical or physical examination findings are specifically due to abnormal UCCR; they will be due to Cushing's syndrome.
• See Hyperadrenocorticism.

Historical Findings
N/A

Physical Examination Findings
N/A

CAUSES
• Cushing's syndrome
• Nonadrenal illness

RISK FACTORS
N/A

DIAGNOSIS

DIFFERENTIAL DIAGNOSIS
• Historical findings of hyperadrenocorticism include polyuria/polydipsia, alopecia or failure to regrow hair; abdominal enlargement, polyphagia, obesity, panting, lethargy, muscle weakness, anestrus, heat intolerance.
• Physical examination findings of hyperadrenocorticism include thin skin, abdominal enlargement, bilaterally symmetrical alopecia, hepatomegaly, pyoderma, seborrhea, cutaneous hyperpigmentation, muscle wasting of extremities, calcinosis cutis, bruising, testicular atrophy.
• Historical and physical examination findings vary depending on which non-adrenal illness present.

LABORATORY FINDINGS

Drugs That May Alter Laboratory Results
Prednisone, prednisolone and hydrocortisone will cross-react on a radioimmunoassay and cause an artifactual increase in measured cortisol concentration; the ratio will be elevated as well.

Disorders That May Alter Laboratory Results
An elevated UCCR may be seen in dogs with non-adrenal illness; this is a highly sensitive but non-specific test for Cushing's syndrome; the specificity is approximately 25 to 30%.

Valid If Run In Human Laboratory?
Yes, if assay validated for dogs and cats.

CBC/BIOCHEMISTRY/URINALYSIS
• CBC: With hyperadrenocorticism, a mature leukocytosis, neutrophilia, lymphopenia, eosinopenia or mild polycythemia.
• Biochemistry: Increased alkaline phosphatase (ALP, elevation may be extreme), alanine aminotransferase (ALT), cholesterol, fasting blood glucose and lipase can be seen with hyperadrenocorticism. Lipemia and decreased BUN may also be noted.
• Urinalysis: Dilute urine (e.g. urine specific gravity < 1.015) and bacteriuria with or without pyuria have been associated with Cushing's syndrome.

OTHER LABORATORY TESTS
• An elevated UCCR is consistent with but *not* diagnostic for hyperadrenocorticism.
• An ACTH response test, a low-dose dexamethasone suppression test (LDDST) or a combined high dose dexamethasone suppression/ACTH response test must be done to confirm the diagnosis.
• If nonadrenal illness is present, the ACTH response test may be preferred as it is more specific, and normal findings would suggest an elevated UCCR is due to non-adrenal illness.

URINE CORTISOL:CREATININE RATIO

IMAGING
• Abdominal radiography and ultrasonography can be used to differentiate PDH from AT.
• CT and MRI can reveal a pituitary tumor.

DIAGNOSTIC PROCEDURES
• With hyperadrenocorticism, a urine protein: creatinine ratio and systemic blood pressure may be mildly elevated, but neither are specific findings.
• A skin biopsy can confirm the diagnosis of calcinosis cutis, a pathognomonic finding for hyperadrenocorticism; oither skin biopsy changes may be suggestive of an endocrinopathy but are not specific.
• A liver biopsy can show changes consistent with steroid hepatopathy, a sensitive but non-specific marker of Cushing's syndrome.

TREATMENT
• Lack of suppression itself does not need to be treated.
• If the test result is due to nonadrenal illness, therapy should be directed toward resolution of that disease.
• If Cushing's syndrome is believed to be present, therapy is directed toward management of hyperadrenocorticism; unless a complication of Cushing's syndrome is present that requires hospitalization (e.g. pulmonary thromboembolism), patients can be treated as outpatients.

MEDICATIONS

DRUG(S) OF CHOICE
• Lack of suppression does not need to be treated while completing all tests for the diagnosis.

CONTRAINDICATIONS
Glucocorticoids

PRECAUTIONS
N/A

POSSIBLE INTERACTIONS
N/A

ALTERNATIVE DRUGS
N/A

FOLLOW-UP

PATIENT MONITORING
• If hyperadrenocorticism is present, follow-up is done depending on the type of therapy chosen (see Hyperadrenocorticism).
• If nonadrenal illness is present and believed possibly to be the cause of the abnormal UCCR results, the illness should be treated; once the animal is stable, the UCCR should be repeated or an ACTH response test should be performed after 4–8 weeks.

POSSIBLE COMPLICATIONS
Untreated hyperadrenocorticism can lead to development of all classical signs if not already present (e.g. polyuria, polydipsia, panting, polyphagia) as well as life-threatening complications such as pulmonary thromboembolism or diabetes mellitus.

MISCELLANEOUS

ASSOCIATED CONDITIONS
None related to elevated ratio *per se.*

AGE-RELATED FACTORS
• Nonadrenal illness can occur in an animal of any age.
• Hyperadrenocorticism is typically a disease of middle-aged to older cats and dogs, although it has been reported in dogs one-year old.

ZOONOTIC POTENTIAL
N/A

PREGNANCY
N/A

SYNONYMS
N/A

SEE ALSO
• Hyperadrenocorticism
• ACTH response test
• Low-dose dexamethasone suppression test

ABBREVIATIONS
ACTH = adrenocorticotropic hormone
ALP = alkaline phosphatase
AT = adrenal tumor
LDDST = low-dose dexamethasone suppression test
PDH = pituitary-dependent hyperadrenocorticism
UCCR = urine cortisol:creatinine ratio

Suggested Reading
Galac S, Kooistra HS, Teske E, Rijnberk A. Urinary corticoid/creatinine ratios in the differentiation between pituitary-dependent hyperadrenocorticism and hyperadrenocorticism due to adrenocortical tumour in the dog. Vet Quarterly 1997;19:17–20.
Henry CJ, Clark TP, Young DW, Spano JS. Urine cortisol:creatinine ratio in healthy and sick cats. J Vet Int Med 1996;10:123–6.
Jensen AL, Iversen L, Koch J, Hoier R, Petersen TK. Evaluation of the urinary cortisol:creatinine ratio in the diagnosis of hyperadrenocorticism in dogs. J Small Anim Pract 1997;38:99–102.
Kaplan AJ, Peterson ME, Kemppainen RJ. Effects of disease on the results of diagnostic tests for use in detecting hyperadrenocorticism in dogs. J Am Vet Med Assoc 1995;207:445–451.
Smiley LE, Peterson ME. Evaluation of a urine cortisol:creatinine ratio as a screening test for hyperadrenocorticism in dogs. J Vet Int Med 1993;7:163–168.
Authors Ellen N. Behrend and Robert J. Kemppainen
Consulting Editor Deborah S. Greco

URINE ELECTROLYTES AND URINE COMPOSITION

BASICS

DEFINITIONS
• Quantitative determination of urinary electrolyte excretion requires collection of all urine produced during a specified time period. A minimum of 24 h is usually recommended. Urine electrolyte concentrations are generally reported as total milligrams or total milliequivalents per kg of body weight per 24 h.
• Urinary FE of analytes is defined as the fraction of filtered analytes that is not reabsorbed by renal tubules and therefore appears in urine.
• In medical literature, both FE and fractional clearance have been used to describe the fraction of filtered analytes appearing in urine.
• Traditional method for measurement of FE of analytes requires measuring glomerular rate (GFR) and plasma and urine concentrations of analytes being evaluated. The formula for calculation of FE is

$$FE = \frac{U\ (mL/min) \times U\ (\text{concentration of electrolyte})}{GFR\ (mL/min) \times P\ (\text{concentration of electrolyte})}$$

where U = urine and P = plasma.
• Alternate method for measurement of FE (also known as "spot" method) eliminates the need to measure analytes in timed urine collections. Instead, the ratio of urine:plasma creatinine concentrations is used to account for renal tubular water absorption. The urine: plasma ratio is also used for analyte concentrations to determine FE. The formula for this method of FE is

$$FE = \frac{U\ (\text{analyte conc.}) \times P(\text{creatinine conc.})}{U\ (\text{creatinine conc.}) \times P(\text{analyte conc.})}$$

where U = urine and P = plasma.
• In dogs and cats, "spot" determination of FE for many analytes (e.g., sodium, uric acid, carnitine) is unreliable as an index for evaluating 24-h electrolyte excretion concentrations.

PATHOPHYSIOLOGY
The kidneys help maintain homeostasis by selectively reabsorbing and/or secreting electrolytes, such as sodium, potassium, chloride, inorganic phosphate, calcium, magnesium, bicarbonate, and protons (H^+). As a result, blood concentrations of these analytes are maintained in a steady state in blood.

SYSTEMS AFFECTED
• Renal/Urologic
• Cardiovascular—cardiac arrhythmias and dysfunction can occur with retention of some electrolytes, such as potassium and protons, and excessive loss of others, such as magnesium.
• Neuromuscular—weakness occurs with excessive loss of some electrolytes, such as potassium, calcium, and magnesium.
• Respiratory—excessive retention or loss of bicarbonate and/or protons can cause changes in respiratory rate and pattern.

SIGNALMENT
Dogs and cats

SIGNS
Clinical signs vary with the analyte in question and the magnitude of the abnormality. For specific clinical signs associated with each analyte, refer to the specific sections listed elsewhere in this book.

CAUSES
• Urinary excretion of analytes is affected by dietary intake, hydration status, endogenous production, status of renal function, hormonal activity, circadian rhythm, pharmacologic agents, and parenteral fluid therapy.
• Laboratory reference values are influenced by samples collected during fasting or nonfasting conditions and the composition of diets being consumed. Altered excretion of analytes associated with metabolic diseases often overlaps with "normal reference ranges"; thus determination of urine concentration and FE of analytes is of limited diagnostic usefulness unless comparisons are made using a standardized diet for both normal animals and patients.

• Consider measuring urinary analyte excretion in patients with serum or plasma electrolyte abnormalities with no obvious cause. For example, hypokalemia associated with mineralocorticoid excess secondary to primary hyperaldosteronism or hyperadrenocorticism (especially of adrenal origin) may result in increased urinary loss of potassium. Evaluation of urinary electrolyte excretion may also be of value in dogs with suspected Fanconi's syndrome.

RISK FACTORS
N/A

DIAGNOSIS

DIFFERENTIAL DIAGNOSIS
N/A

LABORATORY FINDINGS

Drugs That May Alter Laboratory Results
• Loop diuretics such as furosemide—increase renal excretion of sodium, potassium, chloride, calcium, magnesium, hydrogen, and bicarbonate
• Thiazide diuretics (chlorothiazide, hydrochlorothiazide)—increase renal excretion of sodium, chloride, potassium, magnesium, and phosphorus, and tubular reabsorption of calcium
• Amphotericin B—increases renal excretion of potassium
• Angiotensin-converting enzyme (ACE) inhibitors (captopril, enalapril)—reduce renal excretion of potassium
• Potassium-sparing diuretics (spironolactone)—reduce renal excretion of potassium and phosphorus; increase renal excretion of sodium and chloride
• Glucocorticoids—increase renal excretion of potassium and calcium; decrease excretion of sodium and chloride

Disorders That May Alter Laboratory Results
Hematuria (RBC and plasma) may alter test results.

URINE ELECTROLYTES AND URINE COMPOSITION

Valid If Run in Human Laboratory?
• Yes, if normal ranges have been established
• Serum noncreatinine chromogens may be present in plasma but are not excreted in urine. Either the kinetic or regular Jaffe method of measuring plasma creatinine concentration may spuriously elevate plasma creatinine concentrations because of noncreatinine chromogens, which may cause in errors in determining FE in spot urine samples.

CBC/BIOCHEMISTRY/URINALYSIS
• Inappropriate increases in urine pH associated with metabolic acidosis are the hallmark of distal renal tubular acidosis (RTA).
• Hyperchloremic metabolic acidosis and normal GFR in patients with acidic urine should prompt an investigation for proximal RTA.
• Hyperchloremic metabolic acidosis may also occur in patients with Fanconi's syndrome.
• Normal or low urine specific gravity values associated with glucosuria and normal blood glucose concentration may occur in association with acute renal failure, Fanconi's syndrome, or primary renal glucosuria or during early stages of diabetes mellitus. Renal clearance studies to identify reabsorptive defects for electrolytes and amino acids may help differentiate Fanconi's syndrome from primary renal glucosuria.
• Hypokalemia without an obvious cause (e.g., parental administration of potassium-deficient fluids or renal failure) may be associated with mineralocorticoid excess secondary to primary hyperaldosteronism.

OTHER LABORATORY TESTS
• Measurement of serum aldosterone concentrations may help in evaluating patients with serum sodium or potassium abnormalities.
• Serum intact parathyroid hormone concentrations may be helpful in patients with calcium and/or phosphorus abnormalities.
• ACTH stimulation test may be helpful in patients with potassium and sodium abnormalities.

IMAGING
Abdominal radiography and ultrasonography may help localize disorders to the kidneys and adrenal glands.

DIAGNOSTIC PROCEDURES
N/A

TREATMENT
Refer to specific disorders listed elsewhere in this textbook.

MEDICATIONS

DRUGS OF CHOICE
Vary with underlying disease process

CONTRAINDICATIONS
Vary with the underlying disease process

PRECAUTIONS
Vary with the underlying disease process

POSSIBLE INTERACTIONS
Vary with the underlying disease process

ALTERNATIVE DRUGS
Vary with the underlying disease process

FOLLOW-UP

PATIENT MONITORING
Varies, depending on the underlying disease process

POSSIBLE COMPLICATIONS
N/A

MISCELLANEOUS

ASSOCIATED CONDITIONS
N/A

AGE-RELATED FACTORS
Renal excretion of analytes by immature patients may differ from that in mature patients.

ZOONOTIC POTENTIAL
N/A

PREGNANCY
N/A

SYNONYMS
In medical literature, both FE and fractional clearance have been used to describe the fraction of filtered analytes appearing in urine.

SEE ALSO
N/A

ABBREVIATIONS
• ACE = angiotensin-converting enzyme
• FE = urinary fractional excretion
• GFR = glomerular filtration rate
• RTA = renal tubular acidosis

Suggested Reading
Autran de Morais HS, Chew DJ. Use and interpretation of serum and urine electrolytes. Semin Vet Med Surg 1992;7:262–274.
Finco DR. Evaluation of renal functions. In: Osborne CA, Finco DR, eds. Canine and feline nephrology and urology. Baltimore: Williams & Wilkins, 1995:216–229.
Finco DR, Barsanti JA, Brown SA. Solute fractional excretion rates. In: Kirk RW, Bonagura JD, eds. Current veterinary therapy XI. Philadelphia: WB Saunders, 1992:818–820.
Finco DR, Brown SA, Barsanti JA, et al. Reliability of using random urine samples for "spot" determination of fractional excretion of electrolytes in cats. Am J Vet Res 1997;58:1184–1187.
Vaden SL, Babineau C, Ford RB. Comparison of methods to evaluate urine electrolyte concentrations in normal dogs (abstract). J Vet Int Med 1989;3:138.

Authors Sherry L. Sanderson, Carl A. Osborne, and Jody P. Lulich
Consulting Editors Larry G. Adams and Carl A. Osborne

DIAGNOSTICS—LAB

DIAGNOSTICS–
ELECTROCARDIOGRAPHY

ATRIAL FIBRILLATION AND ATRIAL FLUTTER

 BASICS

DEFINITION
• Atrial fibrillation—rapid, irregularly irregular supraventricular rhythm. Two forms recognized: primary atrial fibrillation, a rare disease that occurs in large dogs with no or mild underlying cardiac disease, and secondary atrial fibrillation, which occurs in dogs and cats secondary to severe underlying cardiac disease. • Atrial flutter—fast supraventricular tachycardia (SVT)

ECG FEATURES
Atrial Flutter
• Atrial rhythm usually regular; rate approximately 300–400 bpm • P waves usually discerned as either discrete P waves or a "saw-toothed" baseline • Ventricular rhythm and rate generally depend on the atrial rate and AV nodal conduction, but are generally regular. • Conduction pattern to the ventricles is variable—in some cases every other atrial depolarization produces a ventricular depolarization (2:1 conduction ratio), giving a regular ventricular rhythm; other times the conduction pattern appears random, giving an irregular ventricular rhythm that can mimic atrial fibrillation.

Secondary Atrial Fibrillation
• No P waves present—baseline may be flat or may have small irregular undulations ("f" waves); some undulations may look like P waves. • Ventricular rate high—usually 180–240 bpm in dogs and >220 bpm in cats. • Interval between QRS complexes is irregularly irregular; QRS complexes usually appear normal, not wide and bizarre.

Primary Atrial Fibrillation
• Similar to secondary atrial fibrillation except ventricular rate usually 100–140 bpm.

PATHOPHYSIOLOGY
• Atrial fibrillation—caused by numerous small reentrant pathways creating a rapid (>500 depolarizations/min) and disorganized depolarization pattern in the atria; results in cessation of atrial contraction. Depolarizations continuously bombard the AV junctional tissue, which acts as a filter and does not allow all depolarizations to conduct to the ventricles. Many atrial depolarizations activate only a part of the atria because the rapid rate renders portions of the atria refractory, and thus they cannot reach the AV junction. Other atrial impulses penetrate into the AV junctional tissue but are not robust enough to penetrate the entire length. Blocked impulses affect the conduction properties of the AV junctional tissue and alter conduction of subsequent electrical impulses; electrical impulses are conducted through the AV junction irregularly, producing an irregular ventricular rhythm. • Atrial flutter—probably originates from one site of reentry that moves continuously throughout the atrial myocardium and frequently and regularly stimulates the AV node. When the atrial rate becomes sufficiently fast, the refractory period of the AV node exceeds the cycle length (P to P interval) of the SVT, and some atrial depolarizations are blocked from traversing the AV node (functional second-degree AV block).

SYSTEMS AFFECTED
Cardiovascular
Loss of atrial systolic contraction results in decreased stroke volume and cardiac output; high heart rate results in deterioration in myocardial function.

GENETICS
No breeding studies available

INCIDENCE AND PREVALENCE
N/A

GEOGRAPHIC DISTRIBUTION
N/A

SIGNALMENT
Species
Dogs and cats
Breed Predilections
Large and giant–breed dogs are more prone to primary atrial fibrillation.
Mean Age and Range
N/A
Predominant Sex
N/A

SIGNS
General Comments
Generally relate to the underlying disease process and/or CHF rather than the arrhythmia itself
Historical Findings
• Coughing/dyspnea/tachypnea • Exercise intolerance • Rarely syncope • Dogs with primary atrial fibrillation are typically asymptomatic.
Physical Examination Findings
• On auscultation, patients with atrial fibrillation have an erratic heart rhythm that sounds like "tennis shoes in a dryer." • First heart sound intensity in atrial fibrillation is variable; second heart sound only heard on beats with effective ejection, not on every beat. • Third heart sounds (gallop sounds) may be present. • Patients with atrial fibrillation have pulse deficits and variable pulse intensity. • Signs of CHF often present (e.g., cough, dyspnea, cyanosis)

CAUSES
• Chronic valvular disease • Cardiomyopathy • Congenital heart disease • Digoxin toxicity • Idiopathic • Ventricular pre–excitation (atrial flutter)

RISK FACTORS
• Heart disease • Digoxin administration

 DIAGNOSIS

DIFFERENTIAL DIAGNOSIS
• Frequent atrial (supraventricular) premature depolarizations • Supraventricular tachycardia with AV block

CBC/BIOCHEMISTRY/URINALYSIS
N/A

OTHER LABORATORY TESTS
N/A

IMAGING
• Echocardiography and radiography may characterize type and severity of the underlying cardiac disease; moderate to severe left atrial enlargement common • Typically normal in patients with primary atrial fibrillation, although mild left atrial enlargement may accompany the hemodynamic alterations imposed by the arrhythmia.

DIAGNOSTIC PROCEDURES
N/A

PATHOLOGIC FINDINGS
N/A

 TREATMENT

APPROPRIATE HEALTH CARE
• Patients with fast (secondary) atrial fibrillation are treated medically to slow the ventricular rate. Converting the atrial fibrillation to sinus rhythm would be ideal, but such attempts in patients with severe underlying heart disease or left atrial enlargement are futile because of a low success rate and high rate of recurrence. Consider quinidine or electrical cardioversion to sinus rhythm for a dog with primary atrial fibrillation. • Electrical (DC) cardioversion—application of a transthoracic electrical shock at a specific time in the cardiac cycle; it requires special equipment and trained personnel; general anesthesia is required to avoid patient discomfort. A small (10 joules) electrical shock may suffice, but most require higher power (50–150 joules).

NURSING CARE
As indicated for CHF

ACTIVITY
Restrict activity until tachycardia is controlled.

DIET
Sodium restriction if CHF

CLIENT EDUCATION

• Secondary atrial fibrillation is usually associated with severe underlying heart disease; goal of therapy is to lower heart rate and control clinical signs. • Conversion to sinus rhythm is unlikely with secondary atrial fibrillation.

SURGICAL CONSIDERATIONS

N/A

 MEDICATIONS

DRUGS OF CHOICE

Digoxin, β-adrenergic blockers, and calcium channel blockers (diltiazem) are frequently used to slow conduction through the AV node; definition of an adequate heart rate response varies among clinicians, but in dogs is generally 140–160 bpm.

Dogs

• Digoxin—maintenance oral dose 0.005–0.01 mg/kg PO q12h; to achieve a therapeutic serum concentration more rapidly, the maintenance dose can be doubled for the first day. If digoxin is administered alone and the heart rate remains high, check the digoxin level and adjust the dose to bring the level into the therapeutic range. If the heart rate remains high, consider adding a calcium channel blocker or a β-adrenergic blocker. • Propranolol—initially administered at a dose of 0.1–0.2 mg/kg PO q8h, then titrated upward until an adequate response is obtained. We do not exceed a dose of 0.5 mg/kg PO q8h. • Diltiazem—initially administered at a dose of 0.5 mg/kg PO q8h, then titrated up to a maximum of 1.5 mg/kg PO q8h or until an adequate response is obtained. • Either high-dose oral quinidine or electrical cardioversion can be used to convert primary atrial fibrillation into sinus rhythm. Quinidine doses as high as 20 mg/kg PO q2h

can be used safely; doses lower than 12.5 mg/kg q6h are generally ineffective.

Cats

• Diltiazem (1–2.5 mg/kg PO q8h) or atenolol (6.25–12.5 mg/cat PO q12–24h) are the drugs of choice in most cats. • If the heart rate is not sufficiently slowed with these drugs or if myocardial failure is present, digoxin (0.005 mg/kg PO q24–48h) can be added.

CONTRAINDICATIONS

• Digoxin, diltiazem, propranolol, and atenolol should not be used in patients with preexisting AV block. • Use of calcium channel blockers in combination with β-blockers should be avoided because clinically significant bradyarrhythmias and/or AV block can develop.

PRECAUTIONS

• Calcium channel blockers and β-adrenergic blockers, both negative inotropes, should be used cautiously in animals with myocardial failure. • Using high-dose oral quinidine for conversion into sinus rhythm carries a risk of quinidine toxicity (e.g., weakness, ataxia, and seizures)—administration of diazepam intravenously controls seizures; other signs abate within several hours of discontinuing quinidine administration.

POSSIBLE INTERACTIONS

Quinidine raises the digoxin level, generally necessitating a digoxin dose reduction.

ALTERNATIVE DRUGS

N/A

 FOLLOW-UP

PATIENT MONITORING

Monitor heart rate and ECG closely.

POSSIBLE COMPLICATIONS

Worsening of cardiac function with onset of arrhythmia

PREVENTION/AVOIDANCE

N/A

EXPECTED COURSE AND PROGNOSIS

• Secondary atrial fibrillation—associated with severe heart disease, so a guarded-to-poor prognosis • Primary atrial fibrillation with normal ultrasound findings—guarded-to-good prognosis; some of these animals develop dilated cardiomyopathy later in life.

 MISCELLANEOUS

ASSOCIATED CONDITIONS

N/A

AGE-RELATED FACTORS

N/A

ZOONOTIC POTENTIAL

N/A

PREGNANCY

N/A

SYNONYMS

N/A

SEE ALSO

N/A

ABBREVIATIONS

• SVT = supraventricular tachycardia
• AV = atrioventricular

Suggested Reading

Kittleson MD. Electrocardiography. In: Kittleson MD, Kienle RD, eds. Small animal cardiovascular medicine. St Louis: Mosby, 1998:72–94.

Author Richard D. Kienle
Consulting Editors Larry P. Tilley and Francis W. K. Smith, Jr.

DIAGNOSTICS—ECG

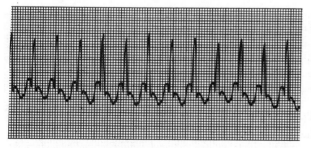

Figure 1.

Atrial flutter with 2:1 conduction at ventricular rate of 330/min in a dog with an atrial septal defect. This supraventricular tachycardia was associated with a Wolff-Parkinson-White pattern. (From: Tilley LP. Essentials of canine and feline electrocardiography, 3rd ed. Baltimore: Williams & Wilkins, 1992, with permission.)

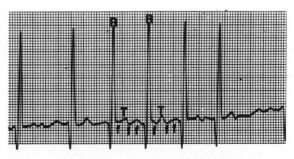

Figure 2.

"Coarse" atrial fibrillation in a dog with patent ductus arteriosus. The f waves are prominent. (From: Tilley LP. Essentials of canine and feline electrocardiography, 3rd ed. Baltimore: Williams & Wilkins, 1992, with permission.)

ATRIAL PREMATURE COMPLEXES (APCs)

BASICS

DEFINITION
• Premature atrial beats that originate outside the sinoatrial node and disrupt the normal sinus rhythm for one or more beats

ECG Features
• Heart rate usually normal; rhythm irregular due to the premature P wave (called a P′ wave) that disrupts the normal P wave rhythm (Fig 2). • Ectopic P′ wave—premature; configuration differs from that of the sinus P waves and may be negative, positive, biphasic, or superimposed on the previous T wave. • QRS complex—premature; configuration usually normal (same as that of the sinus complexes). If the P′ wave occurs during the refractory period of the AV node, ventricular conduction does not occur (nonconducted APCs), so no QRS complex follows the P′ wave. If there is partial recovery in the AV node or intraventricular conduction systems, the P′ wave is conducted with a long P′-R interval or with an abnormal QRS configuration (aberrant conduction). The more premature the complex, the more marked the aberration. • In the P–QRS relationship, the P′-R interval is usually as long as, or longer than, the sinus P–R interval. • A noncompensatory pause—when the R–R interval of the two normal sinus complexes enclosing an APC is less than the R–R intervals of three consecutive sinus complexes—usually follows an APC (Fig 2). The ectopic atrial impulse discharges the sinus node and resets the cycle.

PATHOPHYSIOLOGY
• Mechanisms—an increase in automaticity of atrial myocardial fibers or a single reentrant circuit • May be normal finding in aged dogs; commonly seen in dogs with atrial enlargement secondary to chronic mitral valvular insufficiency; may also be observed in dogs or cats with any atrial disease • May not cause hemodynamic problems; the clinical significance relates to their frequency, timing relative to other complexes, and to the underlying clinical problems. • Can presage more serious rhythm disturbances (e.g., atrial fibrillation, atrial flutter, or atrial tachycardia)

SYSTEMS AFFECTED
Cardiovascular

GENETICS
N/A

INCIDENCE/PREVALENCE
Not documented

GEOGRAPHIC DISTRIBUTION
N/A

SIGNALMENT
Species
Dogs and cats

Breed Predilections
Small breed dogs

Mean Age and Range
Geriatric animals, except those with congenital heart disease

Predominant Sex
N/A

SIGNS
Historical Findings
• No signs • CHF
• Coughing and dyspnea • Exercise intolerance
• Syncope

Physical Examination Findings
• Irregular heart rhythm • Cardiac murmur
• Gallop rhythm • Signs of CHF

CAUSES & RISK FACTORS
• Chronic valvular disease* • Congenital heart disease • Cardiomyopathy* • Atrial myocarditis • Electrolyte disorders • Neoplasia • Hyperthyroidism • Toxemias • Drug toxicity (e.g., digitalis) • Normal variation in aged animals

Risk Factors
Same as causes

DIAGNOSIS

DIFFERENTIAL DIAGNOSIS
• Marked sinus arrhythmia • Ventricular premature complexes when aberrant ventricular conduction follows an APC

CBC/BIOCHEMISTRY/URINALYSIS
N/A

OTHER LABORATORY TESTS
N/A

IMAGING
Echocardiography and Doppler ultrasound may reveal the type and severity of the underlying heart disease.

DIAGNOSTIC PROCEDURES
Electrocardiography

PATHOLOGIC FINDINGS
Atrial enlargement; other features vary depending on underlying cause.

TREATMENT

APPROPRIATE HEALTH CARE
• Treat animal as inpatient or outpatient.
• Treat the underlying CHF, cardiac disease, or other causes.

NURSING CARE
Usually not necessary; varies with underlying cause

ACTIVITY
Restrict if symptomatic.

DIET
No modifications unless required for management of underlying condition (i.e., low-salt diet)

CLIENT EDUCATION
APCs may not cause hemodynamic abnormalities; may be precursors of serious arrhythmias

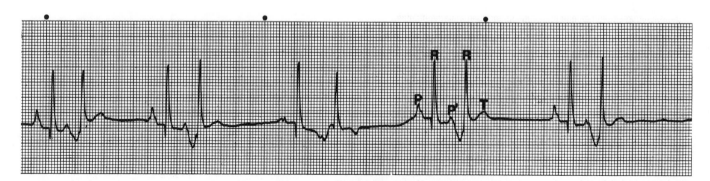

Figure 1.

APC in a dog. P′ represents the premature complex. The premature QRS resembles the basic QRS. The upright P′ wave is superimposed on the T wave of the preceding complex. APC. (From: Tilley LP. Essentials of canine and feline. 3rd ed. Philadelphia: Lea & Febiger, 1992, with permission.)

ATRIAL PREMATURE COMPLEXES (APCs)

SURGICAL CONSIDERATIONS
N/A

MEDICATIONS

DRUGS OF CHOICE
Treat CHF and correct any electrolyte or acid/base imbalances.

Dogs
• Digoxin (0.005–0.01 mg/kg PO q12h, maintenance dosage), diltiazem (0.5–1.5 mg/kg PO q8h), propranolol (0.2–1 mg/kg PO q8h), or atenolol (0.25–1 mg/kg PO q12h) are used to treat clinically significant arrhythmia. • Digoxin—treatment of choice; also indicated to treat the cardiac decompensation that is usually present • CHF is treated with appropriate dosage of diuretic and angiotensin converting enzyme inhibitor; appropriate management of CHF may reduce APC frequency.

Cats
• Cats with hypertrophic cardiomyopathy—diltiazem (1–2.5 mg/kg PO q8h) or atenolol (6.25–12.5 mg PO q12–24h) • Cats with dilated cardiomyopathy—digoxin (1/4 of a 0.125 mg digoxin tablet q24h or q48h)

CONTRAINDICATIONS
Negative inotropic agents (e.g., propranolol) should be avoided in animals with CHF.

PRECAUTIONS
Use digoxin, diltiazem, atenolol, or propranolol cautiously in animals with underlying atrioventricular block or hypotension.

POSSIBLE INTERACTIONS
N/A

ALTERNATIVE DRUGS
N/A

FOLLOW-UP

PATIENT MONITORING
Monitor heart rate and rhythm with serial ECG.

PREVENTION/AVOIDANCE
N/A

POSSIBLE COMPLICATIONS
Frequent APCs may further diminish cardiac output in patients with underlying heart disease and worsen clinical symptoms.

EXPECTED COURSE AND PROGNOSIS
Even with optimal antiarrhythmic drug therapy some animals have an increased frequency of APCs or deteriorate to more severe arrhythmia as the underlying disease progresses.

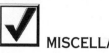

MISCELLANEOUS

ASSOCIATED CONDITIONS
None

AGE-RELATED FACTORS
Typically occurs in geriatric dogs

ZOONOTIC POTENTIAL
N/A

PREGNANCY
N/A

SYNONYMS
Atrial extrasystoles, atrial premature contractions, atrial premature impulses

SEE ALSO
Supraventricular tachycardia

ABBREVIATIONS
APCs = atrial premature complexes
AV = atrioventricular
CHF = congestive heart failure

Suggested Reading
Tilley LP, Goodwin, J. eds. Manual of canine and feline cardiology. 3rd ed. Philadelphia: WB Saunders, 2000.

Authors Larry P. Tilley and Naomi L. Burtnick

Consulting Editors Larry P. Tilley and Francis W. K. Smith, Jr.

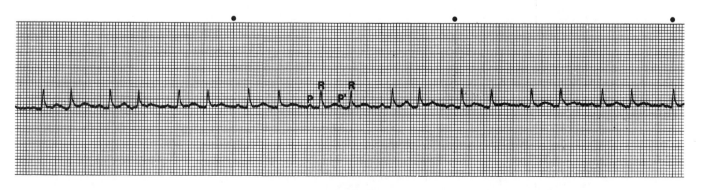

Figure 2.

APCs in bigeminy in a cat under general anesthesia. The second complex of each pair is an APC, where the first is a sinus complex. The abnormality in rhythm disappeared after the anesthetic was stopped. (From: Tilley L.P. Essentials of canine and feline electrocardiography. 3rd ed. Baltimore: Williams & Wilkins, 1992, with permission.)

ATRIAL STANDSTILL

BASICS

DEFINITION
ECG rhythm characterized by absence of P waves; condition can be temporary (e.g., associated with hyperkalemia or drug-induced), terminal (e.g., associated with severe hyperkalemia or dying heart), or persistent

ECG Features
PAS
- P waves absent (Figure 1)
- Heart rate usually slow (<60 bpm)
- Rhythm regular with supraventricular type QRS complexes
- Heart rate does not increase with atropine administration.
Hyperkalemic atrial standstill
- Heart rate normal or slow
- Rhythm regular or irregular
- QRS complexes tend to be wide and become wider as the potassium level rises; with severe hyperkalemia (potassium >10 mEq/mL), the QRS complexes are replaced by a smooth biphasic curve (Fig 2)

PATHOPHYSIOLOGY
PAS
Caused by an atrial muscular dystrophy; skeletal muscle involvement common

Hyperkalemic Atrial Standstill
Generally occurs with serum potassium levels > 8.5 mEq/L; value influenced by serum sodium and calcium levels and acid–base status. Hyperkalemic patients with atrial standstill have sinus node function, but impulses do not activate atrial myocytes; thus, the associated rhythm is termed a sinoventricular rhythm. Since the sinus node is functional, an irregular rhythm may be due to sinus arrhythmia.

SYSTEMS AFFECTED
Cardiovascular

GENETICS
N/A

INCIDENCE/PREVALENCE
Rare rhythm disturbance

GEOGRAPHIC DISTRIBUTION
N/A

SIGNALMENT
Species
Dog and cat

Breed Predisposition
PAS—most common in English springer spaniels; other breeds occasionally affected; hypoadrenocorticism more common in females

Mean Age and Range
Most animals with PAS are young; animals with hypoadrenocorticism are usually young to middle–aged.

SIGNS
Historical Findings
- Vary with underlying cause
- Lethargy common; syncope may occur.
- Patients with PAS may show signs of congestive heart failure (CHF).

Physical Examination Findings
- Vary with underlying cause
- Bradycardia common
- Patients with PAS may have skeletal muscle wasting of the antebrachium and scapula.

CAUSES
- Hyperkalemia
- Atrial disease, often associated with atrial distension (cats with cardiomyopathy)
- Atrial myopathy (PAS)

RISK FACTORS
Hyperkalemic Atrial Standstill
- Hypoadrenocorticism
- Conditions leading to obstruction or rupture of the urinary tract
- Oliguric or anuric renal failure

DIAGNOSIS

DIFFERENTIAL DIAGNOSIS
- Slow atrial fibrillation
- Sinus bradycardia with small P waves lost in the baseline

CBC/BIOCHEMISTRY/URINALYSIS
PAS
Normal

Hyperkalemic Atrial Standstill
- Hyperkalemia
- Hyponatremia and sodium:potassium ratio <27 if atrial standstill secondary to hypoadrenocorticism
- Azotemia and hyperphosphatemia with hypoadrenocorticism, renal failure, and rupture or obstruction of the urinary tract

OTHER LABORATORY TESTS
ACTH stimulation test if hypoadrenocorticism suspected

IMAGING
Echocardiogram and electromyography if PAS suspected—cardiomegaly and depressed contractility may be seen.

DIAGNOSTIC PROCEDURES
Skeletal muscle biopsy in animals with PAS

PATHOLOGIC FINDINGS
PAS
- Greatly enlarged and paper-thin atria; usually biatrial involvement, although one case of only left atrial involvement was reported

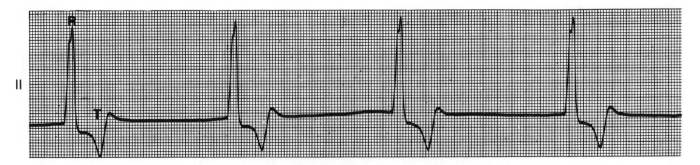

Figure 1.

Persistent atrial standstill in English Springer Spaniel. No P waves are present on any of the leads (also including chest leads and intracardiac electrocardiogram, not shown here). The regular bradycardia is either junctional in origin, with pathologic involvement of the left bundle branch block (wide positive QRS complexes), or ventricular. (From: Tilley LP: Essentials of canine and feline electrocardiography. 3rd ed. Baltimore: Williams & Wilkins, 1992, with permission.)

ATRIAL STANDSTILL

• Severe scapular and brachial muscle wasting in some dogs
• Marked fibrosis, fibroelastosis, chronic mononuclear cell inflammation, and steatosis throughout the atria and interatrial septum

TREATMENT

APPROPRIATE HEALTH CARE

PAS
Not life-threatening condition; animal can be treated as an outpatient

Hyperkalemic Atrial Standstill
Potentially life-threatening; often requires aggressive treatment

NURSING CARE
Aggressive fluid therapy with 0.9% saline often required to correct hypovolemia and lower serum potassium levels (see *potassium, hyperkalemia*) in patients with hyperkalemic atrial standstill

ACTIVITY
Restrict activity in patients with PAS and signs of CHF or syncope.

DIET
N/A

CLIENT EDUCATION

PAS
Clinical signs generally improve after pacemaker implantation; signs of CHF may develop, and weakness and lethargy may persist even after heart rate and rhythm are corrected with the pacemaker.

SURGICAL CONSIDERATIONS

PAS
Implant permanent ventricular pacemaker to regulate rate and rhythm.

Hyperkalemic Atrial Standstill
Hyperkalemia secondary to urinary tract obstruction or rupture may require surgery.

MEDICATIONS

DRUGS OF CHOICE

PAS
Treat with diuretics, digoxin (after pacemaker is implanted), and ACE inhibitor if CHF develops.

Hyperkalemic Atrial Standstill
• Treat the underlying cause (e.g., oliguric renal failure, hypoadrenocorticism).
• Aggressive fluid therapy with 0.9% saline and possibly insulin: dextrose or sodium bicarbonate as discussed under *Potassium, Hyperkalemia.*
• Calcium gluconate—counters the effects of hyperkalemia; can be used in life-threatening situations to reestablish a sinus rhythm while instituting treatment to lower potassium concentration

CONTRAINDICATIONS
Avoid potassium-containing fluids or medications that increase potassium concentration in hyperkalemic patients.

PRECAUTIONS
Diuretics lower preload and may worsen weakness in dogs with PAS and CHF unless a pacemaker has been implanted.

POSSIBLE INTERACTIONS
N/A

ALTERNATIVE DRUGS
N/A

FOLLOW-UP

PATIENT MONITORING
• Monitor ECG during treatment of hyperkalemia and periodically in animals with a permanent ventricular pacemaker.
• Monitor electrolytes in patients with hyperkalemic atrial standstill.
• Monitor patients with PAS for signs of CHF.

PREVENTION/AVOIDANCE
N/A

POSSIBLE COMPLICATIONS
CHF in patients with PAS

EXPECTED COURSE AND PROGNOSIS

PAS
Clinical signs generally improve after pacemaker implantation; signs of CHF may develop, and weakness and lethargy persist even after heart rate and rhythm are corrected with the pacemaker; persistence of signs related to muscular dystrophy

Hyperkalemic Atrial Standstill
Long-term prognosis excellent if underlying cause can be corrected and hyperkalemia reversed.

MISCELLANEOUS

ASSOCIATED CONDITIONS
Diseases causing hyperkalemia (e.g., hypoadrenocorticism, urethral obstruction or urinary tract tear, acidosis, and drugs)

AGE-RELATED FACTORS
PAS—usually diagnosed in young animals; hypoadrenocorticism—usually diagnosed in young to middle-aged animals

ZOONOTIC POTENTIAL
N/A

PREGNANCY
N/A

SYNONYMS
N/A

SEE ALSO
• Potassium, Hyperkalemia
• Digoxin Toxicity
• Hypoadrenocorticism
• Urinary Tract Obstruction

ABBREVIATIONS
• ACE = angiotensin-converting enzyme
• CHF = congestive heart failure
• PAS = persistent atrial standstill

Suggested Reading
Tilley LP. Essentials of canine and feline electrocardiograph. 3rd ed. Philadelphia: Lea & Febiger, 1992.
Author Francis W. K. Smith, Jr.
Consulting Editors Larry P. Tilley and Francis W. K. Smith, Jr.

ATRIOVENTRICULAR BLOCK, COMPLETE (THIRD-DEGREE)

BASICS

DEFINITION
• All atrial impulses are blocked at the AV junction; atria and ventricles beat independently. A secondary "escape" pacemaker site (junctional or ventricular) stimulates the ventricles. • Atrial rate normal • Idioventricular escape rhythm slow

ECG Features
• Ventricular rate slower than the atrial rate (more P waves than QRS complexes)—ventricular escape rhythm (idioventricular) usually <40 bpm; junctional escape rhythm (idiojunctional) 40–60 in dogs and 60–100 in cats • P waves—usually normal configuration (Figure) • QRS complex—wide and bizarre when pacemaker located in the ventricle, or in the lower AV junction in a patient with bundle branch block; normal when escape pacemaker in the lower AV junction (above the bifurcation of the bundle of His) in a patient without bundle branch block • No conduction between the atria and the ventricles; P waves have no constant relationship with QRS complexes; P-P and R-R intervals relatively constant (except for a sinus arrhythmia)

PATHOPHYSIOLOGY
Slow ventricular escape rhythms (<40 bpm) result in low cardiac output and eventual heart failure, often when animal is excited or exercised, since demand for greater cardiac output is not satisfied. As the heart fails, signs increase with mild activity.

SYSTEMS AFFECTED
Cardiovascular

GENETICS
Can be an isolated congenital defect

INCIDENCE/PREVALENCE
Not documented

GEOGRAPHIC DISTRIBUTION
N/A

SIGNALMENT

Species
Dogs and cats

Breed Predilections
• Cocker spaniels—can have idiopathic fibrosis • Pugs and Doberman pinschers—can have associated sudden death, AV conduction defects, and bundle of His lesions.

Mean Age and Range
Geriatric animals, except congenital heart disease patients

Predominant Sex
N/A

SIGNS

Historical Findings
• Exercise intolerance • Weakness or syncope • Occasionally, CHF

Physical Examination Findings
• Bradycardia • Variable third and fourth heart sounds • Variation in intensity of the first heart sounds • Signs of CHF • Intermittent "cannon" A waves in jugular venous pulses

CAUSES
• Isolated congenital defect • Idiopathic fibrosis • Infiltrative cardiomyopathy (amyloidosis or neoplasia) • Hypertrophic cardiomyopathy in cats* • Digitalis toxicity • Myocarditis • Endocarditis • Electrolyte disorder • Myocardial infarction • Other congenital heart defects • Lyme disease

RISK FACTORS
Same as Causes

DIAGNOSIS

DIFFERENTIAL DIAGNOSIS
• Advanced second-degree AV block • Atrial standstill • Accelerated idioventricular rhythm

CBC/BIOCHEMISTRY/URINALYSIS
• Abnormal serum electrolytes (e.g., hyperkalemia, hypokalemia) possible • High WBC with left shift in animals with bacterial endocarditis

OTHER LABORATORY TESTS
• High serum digoxin concentration if AV block is due to digoxin toxicity • Lyme titer and accompanying clinical signs if AV block due to Lyme disease

IMAGING
Echocardiography and Doppler ultrasound to assess cardiac structure and function

DIAGNOSTIC PROCEDURES
• Electrocardiography • His bundle electrogram to determine the site of the AV block • Long-term (Holter) ambulatory recording if AV block is intermittent

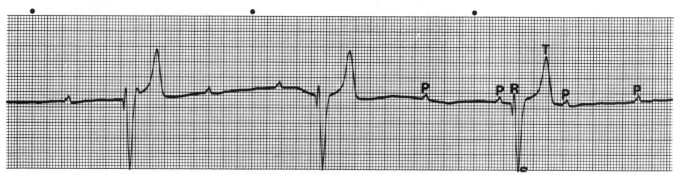

Figure 1.

Complete heart block. The P waves occur at a rate of 120, independent of the ventricular rate of 50. The QRS configuration is a right bundle branch block pattern. The regular rate and stable QRS indicate that the rescuing focus is probably near the AV junction. (From: Tilley LP: Essentials of canine and feline electrocardiography. 3rd ed. Baltimore: Williams & Wilkins, 1992, with permission.)

ATRIOVENTRICULAR BLOCK, COMPLETE (THIRD-DEGREE)

PATHOLOGIC FINDINGS
Degeneration or fibrosis of the AV node and its bundle branches, associated with endocardial and myocardial fibrosis and organized endomyocarditis

TREATMENT

APPROPRIATE HEALTH CARE
• Temporary or permanent cardiac pacemaker—only effective treatment in symptomatic patients • Carefully monitor asymptomatic patients without a pacemaker for development of clinical signs.

NURSING CARE
Cage rest prior to pacemaker implantation; when the pulse generator is put into a subcutaneous pocket, a nonconstricting bandage is required around the ventral neck or abdomen for 3–5 days to prevent seroma formation or pacemaker movement.

ACTIVITY
Restrict if symptomatic.

DIET
No modifications unless required to manage underlying condition (e.g., low-salt diet)

CLIENT EDUCATION
• Temporary or permanent cardiac pacemaker—only effective treatment in symptomatic patients • Asymptomatic patients without a pacemaker—must be carefully monitored for development of clinical signs

SURGICAL CONSIDERATIONS
• Most patients—at high anesthetic cardiopulmonary risk; usually paced preoperatively with a temporary external pacemaker system • The small size of cats makes pacemaker implantation more difficult than in dogs.

MEDICATIONS

DRUGS OF CHOICE
• Treatment with drugs—usually of no value. Traditionally used to treat complete AV block: atropine, isoproterenol, theophylline, and corticosteroids • Intravenous isoproterenol infusion may help increase the rate of the ventricular escape rhythm to stabilize hemodynamics. • If CHF—diuretic and vasodilator therapy may be needed before pacemaker implantation

CONTRAINDICATIONS
Avoid digoxin, xylazine, acepromazine, β-blockers (e.g., propranolol and atenolol), and calcium channel blockers (e.g., verapamil and diltiazem); ventricular antiarrhythmic agents are dangerous because they suppress lower escape foci.

PRECAUTIONS
Vasodilators—may cause hypotension in animals with complete AV block; monitor closely if used, especially prior to pacemaker implantation.

POSSIBLE INTERACTIONS
N/A

ALTERNATIVE DRUGS
N/A

FOLLOW-UP

PATIENT MONITORING
• Monitor—pacemaker function with serial ECGs • Radiographs—following pacemaker implantation, to confirm the position of the lead and generator

PREVENTION/AVOIDANCE
N/A

POSSIBLE COMPLICATIONS
Pulse generators—broad range of clinical life; pacemaker replacement necessary when battery is depleted, pulse generator malfunction occurs, or exit block develops; pacemaker leads can become dislodged and infected.

EXPECTED COURSE AND PROGNOSIS
Poor long-term prognosis if no cardiac pacemaker implanted, especially when the animal has clinical signs.

✓ MISCELLANEOUS

ASSOCIATED CONDITIONS
None

AGE-RELATED FACTORS
N/A

ZOONOTIC POTENTIAL
N/A

PREGNANCY
N/A

SYNONYMS
None

SEE ALSO
Atrioventricular Dissociation

ABBREVIATIONS
• AV = atrioventricular
• CHF

Suggested Reading
Tilley LP, Goodwin J, eds. Manual of canine and feline cardiology. 3rd ed. Philadelphia: WB Saunders, 2000.

Authors Larry P. Tilley and Naomi L. Burtnick

Consulting Editors Larry P. Tilley and Francis W. K. Smith, Jr.

DIAGNOSTICS—ECG

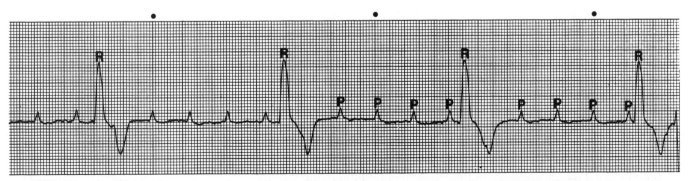

Figure 2.

Complete heart block in a cat. The P waves rate is 240/min, independent of the ventricular rate of 48/min. QRS configuration is a left bundle branch block pattern. (From: Tilley LP: Essentials of canine and feline electrocardiography. 3rd ed. Baltimore: Williams & Wilkins, 1992, with permission.)

ATRIOVENTRICULAR BLOCK, FIRST-DEGREE

BASICS

DEFINITION
Refers to a delay in conduction that occurs between atrial and ventricular activation

ECG Features
- Rate and rhythm—usually normal
- Regularly occurring normal P waves and QRS complexes (Figures 1 and 2)
- Prolonged, consistent PR intervals—dogs, >0.13 sec; cats, >0.09 sec

PATHOPHYSIOLOGY
- Virtually never causes clinical signs
- May become a more severe AV conduction disturbance in some animals
- PR interval tends to shorten with rapid heart rates.

SYSTEMS AFFECTED
Cardiovascular

GENETICS
N/A

INCIDENCE/PREVALENCE
Common

GEOGRAPHIC DISTRIBUTION
N/A

SIGNALMENT

Species
Dogs and cats

Breed Predilections
American cocker spaniels, dachshunds

Mean Age and Range
- May occur in young, otherwise healthy dogs as a manifestation of high vagal tone
- May be noted in aged patients with degenerative conduction system disease, particularly cocker spaniels and dachshunds
- Also seen in immature cats with hypertrophic cardiomyopathy

SIGNS

Historical Findings
- Most animals are asymptomatic
- If drug–induced, may see signs of drug toxicity—anorexia, vomiting, and diarrhea with digoxin; weakness with calcium channel blockers or β-adrenergic antagonists

Physical Examination Findings
Normal—unless also signs of more generalized myocardial disease or extracardiac disease

CAUSES
- May occur in normal animals
- Enhanced vagal stimulation resulting from noncardiac diseases—usually accompanied by sinus arrhythmia, sinus arrest, and/or Mobitz type I second-degree AV block
- Pharmacologic agents (e.g., digoxin, β-adrenergic antagonists, calcium channel blocking agents, α_2-adrenergic agonists, or severe procainamide or quinidine toxicity)
- Degenerative disease of the conduction system
- Hypertrophic cardiomyopathy
- Myocarditis (especially Trypanosoma cruzi, Borrelia burgdorferi, Rickettsia rickettsii)
- Infiltrative diseases (tumors, amyloid)
- Atropine administered intravenously may briefly prolong the PR interval

RISK FACTORS
Any condition or intervention that raises vagal tone

DIAGNOSIS

DIFFERENTIAL DIAGNOSIS
- P waves superimposed upon preceding T waves because of first-degree AV block should be differentiated from bifid T waves.
- Hypokalemia may predispose to first-degree block

OTHER LABORATORY TESTS
- Serum digoxin concentration—may be high
- T. cruzi, B. burgdorferi, R. rickettsii titers—may be high

IMAGING
Echocardiographic examination—may reveal hypertrophic or infiltrative myocardial disorder

DIAGNOSTIC PROCEDURES
May be needed to identify causes of high vagal tone—upper airway disease, cervical and thoracic masses, gastrointestinal disorders, and high intraocular pressure

PATHOLOGIC FINDINGS
Variable—depends on underlying cause

TREATMENT

APPROPRIATE HEALTH CARE
- Usually unnecessary
- Remove or treat underlying cause(s)
- Hospitalization may be necessary to manage the underlying cause (e.g., cardiomyopathy, gastrointestinal disease, airway disease)

NURSING CARE
N/A

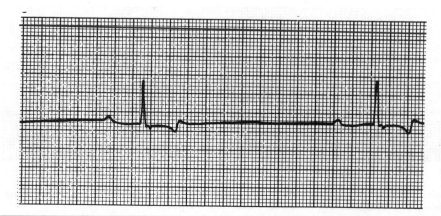

Figure 1.
Lead II ECG rhythm strip recorded from a dog being treated with digoxin and showing first-degree AV block (PR interval = 0.26 sec) (paper speed = 50 mm/sec) (From: Tilley LP, Miller MS, Smith FWK Jr. Canine and feline cardiac arrhythmias: self-assessment. Baltimore: Williams & Wilkins, 1993, with permission.)

ATRIOVENTRICULAR BLOCK, FIRST-DEGREE

ACTIVITY
Unrestricted

DIET
No modifications or restrictions unless required to manage an underlying condition

CLIENT EDUCATION
Generally unnecessary

SURGICAL CONSIDERATIONS
None unless required to manage an underlying condition

 MEDICATIONS

DRUG OF CHOICE
Medications—only if needed to manage an underlying condition

CONTRAINDICATIONS
Hypokalemia—increases sensitivity to vagal tone; may potentiate AV conduction delay

PRECAUTIONS
Drugs with vagomimetic action (e.g., digoxin, bethanechol, physostigmine, pilocarpine) may potentiate first-degree block.

POSSIBLE INTERACTIONS
N/A

ALTERNATIVE DRUGS
N/A

 FOLLOW-UP

PATIENT MONITORING
Except in healthy, young animals, monitor ECG to detect any progression in conduction disturbance.

PREVENTION/AVOIDANCE
N/A

POSSIBLE COMPLICATIONS
N/A

EXPECTED COURSE AND PROGNOSIS
N/A

 MISCELLANEOUS

ASSOCIATED CONDITIONS
N/A

AGE-RELATED FACTORS
PR interval—tends to lengthen with advancing age

ZOONOTIC POTENTIAL
None

PREGNANCY
N/A

SYNONYMS
None

SEE ALSO
• Atrioventricular Block, Second-degree, Mobitz Type I
• Atrioventricular Block, Second-degree, Mobitz Type II
• Atrioventricular Block, Complete (Third-degree)

ABBREVIATION
• AV = atrioventricular

Suggested Reading

Miller MS, Tilley LP, Smith FWK, Fox PR. Electrocardiography. In: Fox PR, Sisson D, Moise NS, eds. Textbook of canine and feline cardiology. Philadelphia: Saunders, 1999:67–106.

Podrid PJ, Kowey PR. Cardiac arrhythmia—mechanisms, diagnosis, and management. Baltimore: Williams & Wilkins, 1995.

Smith FWK, Hadlock DJ. Electrocardiography. In: Miller MS, Tilley LP, eds. Manual of canine and feline cardiology. 2nd ed. Philadelphia: Saunders, 1995:47–74.

Tilley LP. Essentials of canine and feline electrocardiography. 3rd ed. Baltimore: Williams & Wilkins, 1992.

Author Janice McIntosh Bright
Consulting Editors Larry P. Tilley and Francis W. K. Smith, Jr

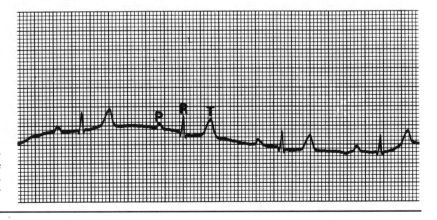

Figure 2.

First-degree AV block in a cat with hyperkalemia (serum potassium, 7.5 mEq/L). The P-R interval is 0.12 sec (6 boxes). Note the large T waves. (From: Tilley LP, Miller MS, Smith FWK Jr. Canine and feline cardiac arrhythmias: self-assessment. Baltimore: Williams & Wilkins, 1993, with permission.)

ATRIOVENTRICULAR BLOCK, SECOND-DEGREE, MOBITZ TYPE I

BASICS

DEFINITION
Occurs when AV transmission is progressively delayed prior to a nonconducted P wave

ECG Features
• PR interval—becomes progressively longer prior to the appearance of a P wave not followed by a QRS complex (Figures 1 and 2)
• Heart rate and QRS morphology—usually normal
• Often cyclical

PATHOPHYSIOLOGY
• Frequently associated with high resting vagal tone and sinus arrhythmia in dogs
• Generally not hemodynamically significant

SYSTEMS AFFECTED
Cardiovascular

GENETICS
N/A

INCIDENCE/PREVALENCE
Studies using radiotelemetry found that this arrhythmia occurs in 64% of healthy adult dogs and 100% of healthy puppies 8–12 weeks of age

GEOGRAPHIC DISTRIBUTION
N/A

SIGNALMENT
Species
Dogs; uncommon in cats

Breed Predilections
May be hereditary in pugs

Mean Age and Range
• May occur in young, otherwise healthy dogs as a manifestation of high vagal tone
• Rarely noted in old dogs with degenerative conduction system disease

SIGNS
Historical Findings
• Most animals—asymptomatic
• If drug–induced may see signs of drug toxicity—anorexia, vomiting, and diarrhea with digoxin; weakness with calcium channel blockers or β-adrenergic antagonists
• If heart rate is abnormally slow—syncope or weakness may occur.

Physical Examination Findings
• May be normal unless signs of more-generalized myocardial disease or extracardiac disease
• First heart sound may become progressively softer, followed by a pause.

CAUSES
• Occasionally noted in normal animals
• Enhanced vagal stimulation resulting from noncardiac diseases—usually accompanied by sinus arrhythmia, sinus arrest
• Pharmacologic agents—digoxin, β-adrenergic antagonists, calcium channel blocking agents, α₂-adrenergic agonists, opioids

RISK FACTORS
Any condition or intervention that enhances vagal tone

DIAGNOSIS

DIFFERENTIAL DIAGNOSIS
• Nonconducted P waves from supraventricular premature impulses or supraventricular tachycardias should be distinguished from pathologic AV block.
• Type II second-degree AV block (no variation in PR intervals)

CBC/BIOCHEMISTRY/URINALYSIS
Hypokalemia may predispose to AV conduction disturbances.

OTHER LABORATORY TESTS
Serum digoxin concentration—may be high

IMAGING
N/A

DIAGNOSTIC PROCEDURES
• May be needed to identify causes of enhanced vagal tone (e.g., upper airway disease, cervical and thoracic masses, gastrointestinal disorders, and high intraocular pressure)
• Atropine response test—administer 0.04 mg/kg atropine IM and repeat ECG in 20–30 min; may be used to determine whether AV block is due to vagal tone; loss of AV block with atropine supports vagal cause.

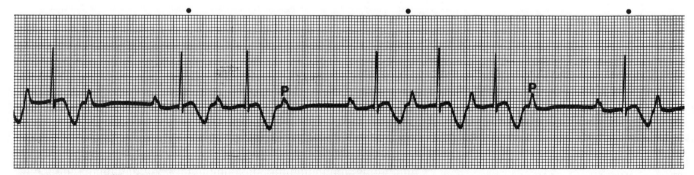

Figure 1.

Typical Wenckebach phenomenon (Mobitz type I) for the first labeled nonconducted P wave. The longest P-R interval precedes this nonconducted P wave. The P-R intervals preceding the second labeled nonconducted P wave are variable, an atypical form of Mobitz type I. (From: Tilley LP: Essentials of canine and feline electrocardiography. 3rd ed. Baltimore: Williams & Wilkins, 1992, with permission.)

ATRIOVENTRICULAR BLOCK, SECOND-DEGREE, MOBITZ TYPE I

PATHOLOGIC FINDINGS
• Generally, no gross or histopathologic findings
• Old dogs may have focal mineralization of the interventricular septal crest visible grossly, with chondroid metaplasia of the central fibrous body and increased fibrous connective tissue in the AV bundle noted microscopically.

TREATMENT

APPROPRIATE HEALTH CARE
• Treatment usually unnecessary
• Treat or remove underlying cause(s)

NURSING CARE
Generally unnecessary

ACTIVITY
Unrestricted

DIET
Modifications or restrictions only to manage an underlying condition

CLIENT EDUCATION
Explain that any treatment is directed toward reversing or eliminating an underlying cause.

SURGICAL CONSIDERATIONS
N/A except to manage an underlying condition

MEDICATIONS

DRUG OF CHOICE
N/A except to manage an underlying condition)

CONTRAINDICATIONS
Drugs with vagomimetic action (e.g., digoxin, bethanechol, physostigmine, pilocarpine) may potentiate block.

PRECAUTIONS
Hypokalemia increases the sensitivity to vagal tone and may potentiate AV conduction delay.

POSSIBLE INTERACTIONS
N/A

ALTERNATIVE DRUGS
N/A

FOLLOW-UP

PATIENT MONITORING
Unless the conduction disturbance resulted from normal vagal tone, the ECG should be monitored to detect progression to a more significant conduction disturbance.

PREVENTION/AVOIDANCE
N/A

POSSIBLE COMPLICATIONS
N/A

EXPECTED COURSE AND PROGNOSIS
N/A

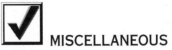

MISCELLANEOUS

ASSOCIATED CONDITIONS
N/A

AGE-RELATED FACTORS
N/A

ZOONOTIC POTENTIAL
N/A

PREGNANCY
N/A

SYNONYMS
Wenckebach phenomenon

SEE ALSO
• Atrioventricular Block, First-degree
• Atrioventricular, Second-degree Mobitz Type II
• Atrioventricular Block, Complete (Third-degree)

ABBREVIATION
AV = atrioventricular

Suggested Reading

Branch CE, Robertson BT, Williams JC. Frequency of second-degree atrioventricular heart block in dogs. Am J Vet Res 1975;36:925–929.

Miller MS, Tilley LP. Electrocardiography in canine and feline cardiology. Fox PR, ed. New York: Churchill Livingstone, 1988.

Podrid PJ, Kowey PR. Cardiac arrhythmia—mechanisms, diagnosis, and management. Baltimore: Williams & Wilkins, 1995.

Tilley LP. Essentials of canine and feline electrocardiography. 3rd ed. Baltimore: Williams & Wilkins, 1992.

Author Janice McIntosh Bright
Consulting Editors Larry P. Tilley and Francis W. K. Smith, Jr.

DIAGNOSTICS—ECG

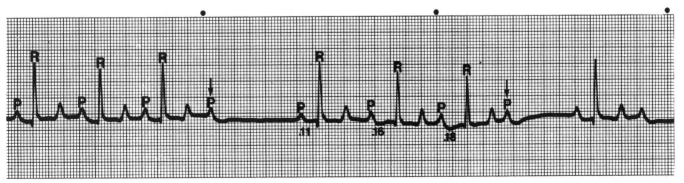

Figure 2.

Mobitz type I AV block (typical Wenckebach phenomenon) in a dog with digoxin toxicity. Note the progressive lengthening of P-R interval from the first sinus complex to the third complex. The P wave (arrow) that follows is blocked. The R-R interval becomes shorter. (From: Tilley LP: Essentials of canine and feline electrocardiography. 3rd ed. Baltimore: Williams & Wilkins, 1992, with permission.)

ATRIOVENTRICULAR BLOCK, SECOND-DEGREE, MOBITZ TYPE II

BASICS

DEFINITION
Occurs when one or more P waves are blocked without a preceding progressive delay in AV transmission.

ECG Features
• One or more P waves not followed by a QRS complex, and PR intervals of conducted beats are consistent (Figure 1)
• Ventricular rate—usually slow • Fixed ratio of P waves to QRS complexes may occur (e.g., 2:1, 3:1, 4:1 AV block).
• QRS complexes may appear normal but are often wide or have an abnormal morphology due to aberrant intraventricular conduction or to ventricular enlargement.
• Abnormally wide QRS complexes (type B) generally indicates serious, extensive cardiac disease.

PATHOPHYSIOLOGY
• Rare in healthy animals
• May be hemodynamically important when ventricular rate is abnormally slow
• Frequently progresses to complete AV block, particularly when accompanied by wide QRS complexes

SYSTEMS AFFECTED
• Cardiovascular
• Central nervous system if inadequate cerebral blood flow

GENETICS
May be heritable in pugs

INCIDENCE/PREVALENCE
Unknown

GEOGRAPHIC DISTRIBUTION
N/A

SIGNALMENT

Species
Dogs and cats

Breed Predilections
• American cocker spaniels and dachshunds
• Pugs

Mean Age and Range
Often occurs in older animals

Predominant Sex
N/A

SIGNS

Historical Findings
• Presenting complaint may be syncope, collapse, weakness, or lethargy
• Some animals are asymptomatic.

Physical Examination Findings
• May be weakness
• Bradycardia common
• May be intermittent pauses in the cardiac rhythm • An S4 may be audible in lieu of the normally expected heart sounds (i.e., S1,S2) when the block occurs.
• If associated with digoxin intoxication; may be vomiting, anorexia, and diarrhea

CAUSES
• Heritable in pugs • Enhanced vagal stimulation from noncardiac diseases
• Degenerative change within the cardiac conduction system—replacement of AV nodal cells and/or Purkinje fibers by fibrotic and adipose tissue in old cats and dogs*
• Pharmacologic agents (e.g., digoxin, β-adrenergic antagonists, calcium channel blocking agents, α₂-adrenergic agonists, muscarinic cholinergic agonists, or severe procainamide or quinidine toxicity)
• Infiltrative myocardial disorders (neoplasia, amyloid)
• Endocarditis (particularly involving the aortic valve)
• Myocarditis (viral, bacterial, parasitic, idiopathic)

• Atropine administered intravenously may cause a brief period of first- or second-degree heart block before increasing the heart rate.

RISK FACTORS
Any condition or intervention that enhances vagal tone

DIAGNOSIS

DIFFERENTIAL DIAGNOSIS
• Advanced form (i.e., persistent block of two or more consecutive P waves) distinguished from complete AV block
• Nonconducted P waves arising from refractoriness of the conduction system during supraventricular tachycardias differentiated from pathologic conduction block

CBC/BIOCHEMISTRY/URINALYSIS
Electrolyte abnormalities (e.g., severe hypokalemia or hypercalcemia) may predispose to AV block.

OTHER LABORATORY TESTS
• Serum digoxin concentration—may be high
• High T₄ in cats—if associated with hyperthyroidism
• High arterial blood pressure in cats—if associated with hypertensive heart disease
• Positive *Borrelia, Rickettsia,* or *Trypanosome cruzi* titers—if associated with one of these infectious agents
• Blood cultures may be positive in patients with vegetative endocarditis.

IMAGING
Echocardiographic examination may reveal structural heart disease (e.g., endocarditis, neoplasia, or left ventricular hypertrophy)

DIAGNOSTIC PROCEDURES
• Atropine response test—administer 0.04 mg/kg atropine IM and repeat ECG in 20–30 min; may be used to determine whether AV

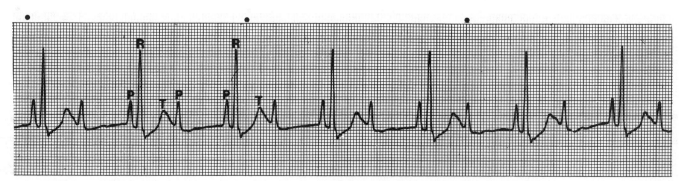

Figure 1.

Second-degree 2:1 AV block (Mobitz type II), as well as probable right atrial enlargement (P waves, 0.8 mv or 8 boxes). Because the QRS complexes are normal, the conduction failure is probably within the AV node. (From: Tilley LP: Essentials of canine and feline electrocardiography. 3rd ed. Baltimore: Williams & Wilkins, 1992, with permission.)

ATRIOVENTRICULAR BLOCK, SECOND-DEGREE, MOBITZ TYPE II

block is due to high vagal tone.

PATHOLOGIC FINDINGS
• Variable—depend on underlying cause
• Old animals with degenerative change of the conduction system—may have focal mineralization of the interventricular septal crest visible grossly; chondroid metaplasia of the central fibrous body and increased fibrous connective tissue in the AV bundle noted histopathologically.

 TREATMENT

APPROPRIATE HEALTH CARE
• Treatment—may be unnecessary if heart rate maintains adequate cardiac output
• Positive chronotropic interventions indicated for symptomatic patients
• Treat or remove underlying cause(s)

NURSING CARE
Generally unnecessary

ACTIVITY
Cage rest advised for symptomatic patients

DIET
Modifications or restrictions only to manage an underlying condition

CLIENT EDUCATION
• Need to seek and specifically treat underlying cause
• Pharmacologic agents may not be effective long–term.

SURGICAL CONSIDERATIONS
Permanent pacemaker may be required for long-term management of symptomatic patients

 MEDICATIONS

DRUGS OF CHOICE
• Atropine (0.02–0.04 mg/kg IV, IM) or glycopyrrolate (0.005–0.01 mg/kg IV, IM) may be used short term if atropine response
• Chronic anticholinergic therapy (propantheline 0.5–2 mg/kg PO q8–12h)—indicated

for symptomatic patients if improved AV conduction with atropine response test
• Isoproterenol (0.04–0.09 µg/kg/min IV to effect) or dopamine (2–5 µg/kg/min IV to effect) may be administered in acute, life-threatening situations in attempt to enhance AV conduction and/or accelerate an escape focus

CONTRAINDICATIONS
• Drugs with vagomimetic action (e.g., digoxin, bethanechol, physostigmine, pilocarpine) may potentiate block • Avoid drugs likely to impair impulse conduction further or depress a ventricular escape focus (procainamide, quinidine, lidocaine, calcium channel blocking agents, β-adrenergic blocking agents)

PRECAUTIONS
Hypokalemia—increases sensitivity to vagal tone; may potentiate AV conduction delay

POSSIBLE INTERACTIONS
N/A

ALTERNATIVE DRUGS
N/A

 FOLLOW-UP

PATIENT MONITORING
Frequent ECG because often progresses to complete (third-degree) AV block

PREVENTION/AVOIDANCE
N/A

POSSIBLE COMPLICATIONS
Prolonged bradycardia may cause secondary congestive heart failure or inadequate renal perfusion.

EXPECTED COURSE AND PROGNOSIS
• Variable—depends on cause • If degenerative disease of the cardiac conduction system, often progresses to complete (third-degree) AV block

 MISCELLANEOUS

ASSOCIATED CONDITIONS
May be noted in cats with primary or secondary left ventricular hypertrophy

AGE-RELATED FACTORS
N/A

ZOONOTIC POTENTIAL
N/A

PREGNANCY
N/A

SYNONYMS
None

SEE ALSO
• Atrioventricular Block, Second-degree, Mobitz Type I
• Atrioventricular Block, Complete (Third-degree)

ABBREVIATION
• AV = atrioventricular

Suggested Reading

Edwards NJ. Bolton's handbook of canine and feline electrocardiography. 2nd ed. Philadelphia: Saunders, 1987.
Kittleson MD. Electrocardiography. In: Kittleson MD, Kienle RD, eds. Small animal cardiovascular medicine. St. Louis: Mosby, 1998:72–94.
Podrid PJ, Kowey PR. Cardiac arrhythmia—mechanisms, diagnosis, and management. Baltimore: Williams & Wilkins, 1995.
Tilley LP. Essentials of canine and feline electrocardiography. 3rd ed. Baltimore: Williams & Wilkins, 1992.

Author Janice McIntosh Bright
Consulting Editors Larry P. Tilley and Francis W. K. Smith, Jr.

ATRIOVENTRICULAR DISSOCIATION

BASICS

DEFINITION
Atrial and ventricular rhythms independent of each other—produced by many mechanisms; found in many arrhythmias; not an electrocardiographic diagnosis

ECG FEATURES
• Sinus P waves have no constant relationship to the QRS complexes (Figure 1).
• P waves—may precede, be in the middle of, or follow the QRS complex without changing their usually normal form
• P wave rate is usually slower than the QRS complex rate
• Ventricular capture complex—occasionally a P wave and QRS complex resemble the conducted sinus complexes during regular sinus rhythm; occurs whenever a sinus or ectopic supraventricular impulse arrives when the AV junctional and /or ventricular pathways have recovered from the preceding impulse; termed *incomplete AV dissociation*
• Ventricular fusion complex—occasionally appears as a premature complex during AV dissociation; always preceded by a P wave; the QRS complex of the fusion beat has a configuration intermediate to those of a normal sinus complex and a ventricular ectopic complex; termed *incomplete AV dissociation*

PATHOPHYSIOLOGY
• Possible causes—complete pathologic interruption of conduction between the atria and ventricles (complete AV block), temporary physiologic interruption, and variable AV conduction refractoriness
• Combination of two or three of the following mechanisms produces AV dissociation:

1. Depressed sinus node automaticity—allows an AV junctional or ventricular focus to escape and control the ventricles
2. Increased AV junctional or ventricular automaticity—ectopic focus controls the ventricles; sinus node controls the atria
3. Disturbed AV conduction—block at the AV node allows two independent rhythms, one in the atria and the other below the area of conduction delay
• Hemodynamic compromise due to reduced cardiac output may be evident with the slower junctional and ventricular escape rhythms or with tachyarrhythmia variations.

SYSTEMS AFFECTED
Cardiovascular

GENETICS
N/A

INCIDENCE/PREVALENCE
Not documented

GEOGRAPHIC DISTRIBUTION
N/A

SIGNALMENT
Species
Dogs and cats

Breed Predilections
N/A

Mean Age and Range
N/A

Predominant Sex
N/A

SIGNS
Historical Findings
• No signs
• CHF
• Exercise intolerance
• Syncope

Physical Examination Findings
• Jugular venous pulsations
• Regular or irregular rhythm
• Gallop rhythm
• Signs of CHF

CAUSES
• Digoxin toxicity
• Myocarditis • Cardiomyopathy • Chronic valvular insufficiency
• Congenital heart disease
• Halothane anesthesia in cats

RISK FACTORS
Same as causes

DIAGNOSIS

DIFFERENTIAL DIAGNOSIS
• Atrial or ventricular premature complexes
• Ventricular tachycardia
• Complete AV block—atrial rate more rapid than AV junctional or ventricular rate; in AV dissociation the atrial rate is slower than the AV junctional rate

CBC/BIOCHEMISTRY/URINALYSIS
N/A

OTHER LABORATORY TESTS
N/A

IMAGING
Echocardiography and Doppler ultrasound to assess cardiac structure and function.

DIAGNOSTIC PROCEDURES
Electrocardiography

PATHOLOGIC FINDINGS
Variable—depend on underlying cause

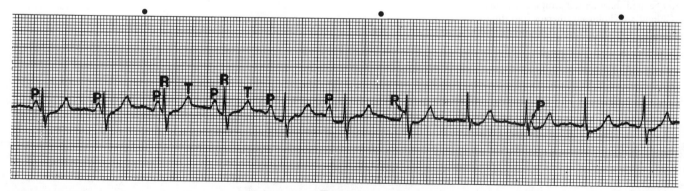

Figure 1.

AV dissociation between the SA node and the AV junction, probably from an accelerated AV junctional focus. The P waves travel away from, then toward, and finally merge with the QRS complexes. This dog had severe digitalis intoxication. (From: Tilley LP: Essentials of canine and feline electrocardiography. 3rd ed. Baltimore: Williams & Wilkins, 1992, with permission.)

ATRIOVENTRICULAR DISSOCIATION

 TREATMENT

APPROPRIATE HEALTH CARE
• Inpatient or outpatient—depends on severity of clinical signs
• Treat underlying CHF or other causes.
• Not an ECG diagnosis; describes a phenomenon secondary to various types of electrical abnormalities that require different treatments (e.g., if AV dissociation is due to AV block, treatment may be a pacemaker; if it is due to an accelerated junctional rhythm, the animal may be reacting to digoxin or have myocarditis)

NURSING CARE
Varies with underlying cause

ACTIVITY
Restrict if symptomatic.

DIET
Only modifications required to manage underlying condition (eg., low-salt diet for CHF)

CLIENT EDUCATION
• Further diagnostics may be necessary to determine the cause and appropriate therapy.

SURGICAL CONSIDERATIONS
If AV dissociation is due to AV block, treatment may be pacemaker implantation.

 MEDICATIONS

DRUGS OF CHOICE
• Correct electrolyte and acid–base disturbances.
• Treat the underlying cardiac disease appropriately.
• See treatment sections for complete AV block and ventricular tachycardia.

CONTRAINDICATIONS
N/A

PRECAUTIONS
N/A

POSSIBLE INTERACTIONS
N/A

ALTERNATIVE DRUGS
N/A

 FOLLOW-UP

PATIENT MONITORING
Heart rate and rhythm—serial ECGs

PREVENTION/AVOIDANCE
N/A

POSSIBLE COMPLICATIONS
N/A

EXPECTED COURSE AND PROGNOSIS
N/A

 MISCELLANEOUS

ASSOCIATED CONDITIONS
None

AGE-RELATED FACTORS
N/A

ZOONOTIC POTENTIAL
N/A

PREGNANCY
N/A

SYNONYMS
• Complete AV dissociation
• Incomplete AV dissociation

SEE ALSO
• Idioventricular Rhythm
• Atrioventricular Block, Complete
• Ventricular Tachycardia

ABBREVIATIONS
• AV = atrioventricular
• CHF = congestive heart failure

Suggested Readings
Tilley LP. Essentials of canine and feline electrocardiography. 3rd ed. Baltimore: Williams & Wilkins, 1992.
Authors Larry P. Tilley and Naomi L. Burtnick
Consulting Editors Larry P. Tilley and Francis W. K. Smith, Jr.

DIAGNOSTICS—ECG

IDIOVENTRICULAR RHYTHM

BASICS

DEFINITION
If conduction of sinus node pacemaker impulses to the ventricles is blocked or the impulses decrease in frequency, the lower regions of the heart automatically take over the role of pacemaker for the ventricles, which results in ventricular escape complexes (Figure 1) or an idioventricular rhythm (Figure 2).

ECG Features
• A series of ventricular escape beats with a heart rate < 65 bpm in dogs and less than 100 bpm in cats; heart rates of 65–100 in dogs and 100–160 in cats are often termed *accelerated idioventricular rhythms.*
• P waves may be absent or may precede, be hidden within, or follow, the ectopic QRS complex.
• P waves are unrelated to the QRS complexes • QRS configuration—wide and bizarre; similar to that of a ventricular premature complex

PATHOPHYSIOLOGY
• May be hemodynamically important with slow ventricular rates
• Does not occur in healthy animals
• Subsidiary pacemakers seem to discharge more rapidly in cats than in dogs.

SYSTEMS AFFECTED
Cardiovascular

GENETICS
N/A

INCIDENCE/PREVALENCE
Unknown

GEOGRAPHIC DISTRIBUTION
N/A

SIGNALMENT

Species
Dogs and cats

Breed Predilections
• Atrial standstill in English springer spaniels and Siamese cats
• Pugs, miniature schnauzers, and dalmatians prone to conduction abnormalities

Mean Age and Range
N/A

Predominant Sex
N/A

SIGNS

Historical Findings
• Some animals asymptomatic
• Weakness
• Lethargy
• Exercise intolerance
• Syncope
• Heart failure

PHYSICAL EXAMINATION FINDINGS
• Irregular rhythm associated with pulse deficits
• Variation in heart sounds
• Possible intermittent "cannon" waves in the jugular venous pulses (with atrioventricular [AV] block)

CAUSES
• Not a primary disease—a secondary result of a primary disease
• The escape rhythm is a safety mechanism to maintain cardiac output.

Causes of Sinus Bradycardia and Sinus Arrest
• Increased vagal tone (high intracranial pressure, high ocular pressure)

• Drugs—digoxin, tranquilizers, propranolol, quinidine, and anesthetics
• Addison's disease
• Hypoglycemia
• Renal failure
• Hypothermia
• Hyperkalemia
• Hypothyroidism

Causes of AV Block
• Congenital
• Neoplasia
• Fibrosis
• Lyme disease

RISK FACTORS
N/A

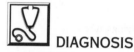

DIAGNOSIS

DIFFERENTIAL DIAGNOSIS
• Ventricular tachycardia—dogs have a cardiac rate > 100 bpm; cats > 150 bpm
• Slow heart rate in animals with right bundle branch block, left bundle branch block, or left anterior fascicular block; animals with these disturbances have the P waves associated with the QRS complexes.

CBC/BIOCHEMISTRY/URINALYSIS
• No specific findings
• Complete blood testing may suggest a metabolic abnormality.

OTHER LABORATORY TESTS
• Drug toxicity
• Lyme's titer in animals with complete AV block

IMAGING
Echocardiogram may show structural heart disease.

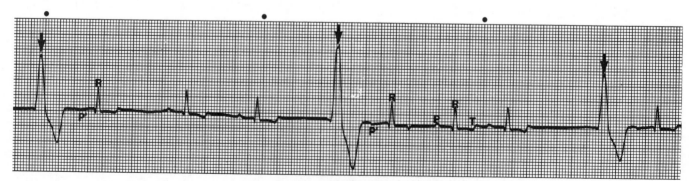

Figure 1.

Ventricular escape complexes (arrows) during various phases in the dominant sinus rhythm in a dog during anesthesia. The sinus rate increased (not shown) after anesthesia was stopped; ¹/₂ cm = 1 mv. (From: Tilley LP: Essentials of canine and feline electrocardiography. 3rd ed. Baltimore: Williams & Wilkins, 1992, with permission.)

IDIOVENTRICULAR RHYTHM

DIAGNOSTIC PROCEDURES
Electrocardiography

PATHOLOGIC FINDINGS
Depend on underlying cause

 TREATMENT

APPROPRIATE HEALTH CARE
• Rhythm is an escape or safety mechanism for maintaining cardiac output; do *not* direct treatment toward suppressing this escape rhythm, but toward the primary disease process that allows the escape rhythm to assume pacemaker control of the heart.
• Symptomatic treatment is directed toward increasing the heart rate.

NURSING CARE
May be required for underlying disease

ACTIVITY
Symptomatic animals may require cage rest.

DIET
No modifications or restrictions unless required for management of the underlying condition.

CLIENT EDUCATION
Inform of the need to seek and specifically treat an underlying cause.

SURGICAL CONSIDERATIONS
Pacemaker implantation may be necessary.

 MEDICATIONS

DRUGS OF CHOICE
• Atropine or glycopyrrolate usually indicated to block vagal tone or increase the heart rate
• If those drugs are ineffective, isoproterenol, dopamine, dobutamine, or artificial pacing may be needed.

CONTRAINDICATIONS
Lidocaine, procainamide, quinidine, propranolol, diltiazem, or any other drug that slows the cardiac rate or reduces contractility

PRECAUTIONS
Atropine is briefly vagotonic immediately postinjection and can temporarily exacerbate the condition.

POSSIBLE INTERACTIONS
N/A

ALTERNATIVE DRUGS
N/A

 FOLLOW-UP

PATIENT MONITORING
• Serial ECG may show clearing of the lesion or progression to complete heart block.
• Serial blood profiles may be needed to monitor progress of the primary disease process.
• Serial echocardiograms may show improvement or progressive changes in cardiac structure.

PREVENTION/AVOIDANCE
N/A

POSSIBLE COMPLICATIONS
Prolonged bradycardia may cause secondary congestive heart failure or inadequate renal perfusion.

EXPECTED COURSE AND PROGNOSIS
• Arrhythmia may abate when the primary disorder is corrected.
• Guarded if condition is associated with cardiac or metabolic disorder; poor if the rate is not increased pharmacologically or underlying cause cannot be identified and treated

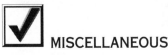 **MISCELLANEOUS**

ASSOCIATED CONDITIONS
N/A

AGE-RELATED FACTORS
N/A

ZOONOTIC POTENTIAL
N/A

PREGNANCY
N/A

SYNONYMS
None

SEE ALSO
• Atrioventricular Dissociation
• Atrial Standstill
• Atrioventricular Block, Complete

ABBREVIATION
AV = atrioventricular

Suggested Readings
Tilley LP. Essentials of canine and feline electrocardiography. 3rd ed. Baltimore: Williams & Wilkins, 1992:152, 222.
Authors Larry P. Tilley and Naomi L. Burtnick
Consulting editors Larry P. Tilley and Francis W. K. Smith, Jr.

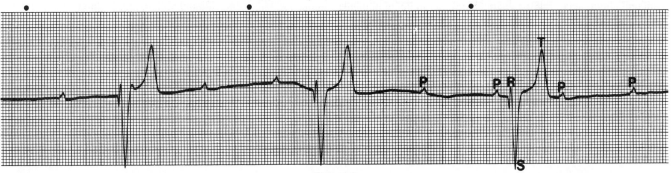

Figure 2.

Complete heart block. The P waves occur at a rate of 120, independent of the ventricular rate of 50. The QRS configuration is a right bundle branch block pattern. The regular rate and stable QRS indicate that the rescuing focus is probably near the AV junction. (From: Tilley LP: Essentials of canine and feline electrocardiography. 3rd ed. Baltimore: Williams & Wilkins, 1992, with permission.)

LEFT ANTERIOR FASCICULAR BLOCK

BASICS

DEFINITION
• Conduction delay or block in the anterior fascicle of the left bundle branch (Figures 1 and 2)
• Left ventricle activation then altered or delayed toward the blocked fascicle and corresponding papillary muscle

ECG Features
• QRS complex—normal duration
• Left axis deviation—dogs, $< +40°$; cats, $< 0°$
• Small q waves and tall R waves in leads I and aVL—small q not essential
• Deep S waves (exceeding the R waves) in leads II, III, and aVF

PATHOPHYSIOLOGY
• Anatomic basis still speculative—anterior fascicle vulnerable because it has a single blood supply, is long and thin, and is located in the turbulent outflow tract of the left ventricle
• No hemodynamic compromise

SYSTEMS AFFECTED
Cardiovascular

GENETICS
N/A

INCIDENCE/PREVALENCE
• Most commonly described form of bundle branch block in cats
• Uncommon in dogs

GEOGRAPHIC DISTRIBUTION
N/A

SIGNALMENT

Species
Dogs and cats

Breed Predilections
N/A

Mean Age and Range
N/A

Predominant Sex
N/A

SIGNS

Historical Findings
• Signs usually associated with the underlying cause
• Usually an incidental ECG finding

Physical Examination Findings
No associated signs or hemodynamic compromise

CAUSES
• Hypertrophic cardiomyopathy (cats)*
• Left ventricular hypertrophy (e.g., mitral insufficiency, aortic stenosis, aortic body tumor, hypertension, and hyperthyroidism)
• Hyperkalemia (e.g., urethral obstruction, acute renal insufficiency, and Addison's disease)
• Ischemic cardiomyopathy (e.g., arteriosclerosis of the coronary arteries, myocardial infarction, and myocardial hypertrophy that obstructs coronary arteries)
• Surgical repair of a cardiac defect (e.g., ventricular septal defect or aortic valvular disease)
• Restrictive cardiomyopathy (cats)
• Fibrosis

RISK FACTORS
N/A

DIAGNOSIS

DIFFERENTIAL DIAGNOSIS
• Left ventricular enlargement—absence of left ventricular enlargement on thoracic radiograph or cardiac ultrasound supports a diagnosis of left anterior fascicular block.
• Right bundle branch block—deep, wide S-waves in leads I, II, III and aVF causing a right axis deviation; in patients with left anterior fascicular block, leads I and aVL are positive and leads II, III, and aVF have deep S waves resulting in a left axis deviation.
• Altered position of the heart within the thorax—thoracic radiographs help identify mass or foreign body that may be displacing the heart.
• Suspect hyperkalemia if signs of urethral obstruction, renal insufficiency, or hypoadrenocorticism (Addison's disease); determine serum potassium concentration.

CBC/BIOCHEMISTRY/URINALYSIS
Hyperkalemia possible

OTHER LABORATORY TESTS
N/A

IMAGING
• Echocardiogram may show structural heart disease.
• Thoracic and abdominal radiographs may show mass, pulmonary metastatic lesion, foreign body, or abnormal cardiac position.

DIAGNOSTIC PROCEDURES
• Electrocardiography
• Long-term ambulatory monitoring (Holter) may reveal intermittent bundle branch block.

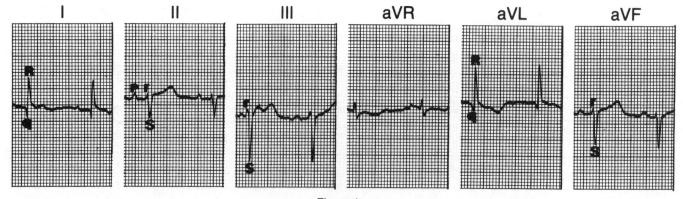

| I | II | III | aVR | aVL | aVF |

Figure 1.

Left anterior fascicular block in a cat with hypertrophic cardiomyopathy. Severe left axis deviation (2608) with a qR pattern in leads I and aVL and an rS pattern in leads II, III, and aVF. The QRS complexes are of normal duration. (From: Tilley LP: Essentials of canine and feline electrocardiography. 3rd ed. Baltimore: Williams & Wilkins, 1992, with permission.)

LEFT ANTERIOR FASCICULAR BLOCK

PATHOLOGIC FINDINGS

Possible lesions or scarring on endocardial surface in the path of the bundle branches; applying Lugol's iodine to the endocardial surface within 2 h postmortem enables clear visualization of the conduction system.

TREATMENT

APPROPRIATE HEALTH CARE
• Treatment unnecessary
• Treat underlying cause.

NURSING CARE
Unnecessary

ACTIVITY
Unrestricted unless indicated by underlying condition

DIET
No modifications unless indicated by underlying condition

CLIENT EDUCATION
Fascicular block per se does not cause hemodynamic compromise; combined with right bundle branch block it may develop into second- or third-degree AV block, making treatment essential; need to treat underlying cause

SURGICAL CONSIDERATIONS
N/A

MEDICATIONS

DRUGS OF CHOICE
Treatment directed toward the underlying primary disease (e.g., drugs to lower the serum potassium in hyperkalemia)

CONTRAINDICATIONS
N/A

PRECAUTIONS
N/A

POSSIBLE INTERACTIONS
N/A

ALTERNATIVE DRUGS
N/A

FOLLOW-UP

PATIENT MONITORING
ECG regularly.

PREVENTION/AVOIDANCE
N/A

POSSIBLE COMPLICATIONS
Causative lesion could progress and lead to a more serious arrhythmia or complete heart block.

EXPECTED COURSE AND PROGNOSIS
No hemodynamic compromise

MISCELLANEOUS

ASSOCIATED CONDITIONS
N/A

AGE-RELATED FACTORS
N/A

ZOONOTIC POTENTIAL
N/A

PREGNANCY
N/A

SYNONYMS
None

SEE ALSO
• Right Bundle Branch Block
• Left Bundle Branch Block
• Atrioventricular Block, First-degree
• Atrioventricular Block, Second-degree
• Atrioventricular Block, Complete

ABBREVIATION
AV = atrioventricular

Suggested Readings
Tilley LP. Essentials of canine and feline electrocardiography. 3rd ed. Baltimore: Williams & Wilkins, 1992
Authors Larry P. Tilley and Naomi L. Burtnick
Consulting Editors Larry P. Tilley and Francis W. K. Smith, Jr.

DIAGNOSTICS—ECG

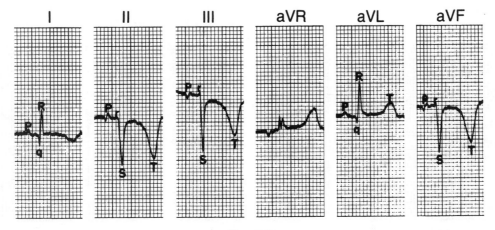

I   II   III   aVR   aVL   aVF

Figure 2.

Left anterior fascicular block in a dog with hyperkalemia (serum potassium, 5.3 mEq/L). There is abnormal left axis deviation (−60°) with a qR pattern in leads *I* and *aVL* and an rS pattern in leads *II, III,* and *aVF.* The large T waves are compatible with hyperkalemia. (From: Tilley LP: Essentials of canine and feline electrocardiography. 3rd ed. Baltimore: Williams & Wilkins, 1992, with permission.)

LEFT BUNDLE BRANCH BLOCK

BASICS

DEFINITION
Conduction delay or block in both the left posterior and left anterior fascicles of the left bundle (Figures 1 and 2); a supraventricular impulse activates the right ventricle first through the right bundle branch; the left ventricle is activated late, causing the QRS to become wide and bizarre.

ECG Features
• QRS prolonged—dogs, >0.08 sec, cats, >0.06 sec
• QRS wide and positive in leads I, II, III, and aVF
• Block can be intermittent or constant.

PATHOPHYSIOLOGY
• Because the left bundle branch is thick and extensive, the lesion causing the block must be large.
• Usually an incidental ECG finding—does not cause hemodynamic abnormalities

SYSTEMS AFFECTED
Cardiovascular

GENETICS
N/A

INCIDENCE/PREVALENCE
Uncommon in cats and dogs. In cats with hypertrophic cardiomyopathy, left bundle branch block is not as commonly seen as left anterior fascicular block.

GEOGRAPHIC DISTRIBUTION
N/A

SIGNALMENT

Species
Cats and dogs

Breed Predilections
N/A

Mean Age and Range
N/A

Predominant Sex
N/A

SIGNS

Historical Findings
• Usually an incidental ECG finding—does not cause hemodynamic abnormalities
• Signs usually associated with the underlying condition

Physical Examination Findings
Does not cause signs or hemodynamic compromise

CAUSES
• Cardiomyopathy*
• Direct or indirect cardiac trauma (e.g., hit by car and cardiac needle puncture)
• Neoplasia
• Subvalvular aortic stenosis
• Fibrosis • Ischemic cardiomyopathy (e.g., arteriosclerosis of the coronary arteries, myocardial infarction, and myocardial hypertrophy that obstructs coronary arteries)

RISK FACTORS
N/A

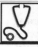

DIAGNOSIS

DIFFERENTIAL DIAGNOSIS
• Left ventricular enlargement
• No left ventricular enlargement on thoracic radiograph or cardiac ultrasound studies supports diagnosis of isolated left bundle branch block.
• Can also be confused with ventricular ectopic beats, but the PR interval is usually constant and left bundle branch block has no pulse deficits

CBC/BIOCHEMISTRY/URINALYSIS
N/A

OTHER LABORATORY TESTS
N/A

IMAGING
• Echocardiography may reveal structural heart disease; absence of left heart enlargement supports a diagnosis of left bundle branch block.
• Thoracic and abdominal radiographs may show masses or pulmonary metastatic lesions; traumatic injuries could result in localized or diffuse pulmonary densities.

DIAGNOSTIC PROCEDURES
• Electrocardiography
• Long-term ambulatory monitoring (Holter) may reveal intermittent left bundle branch block.

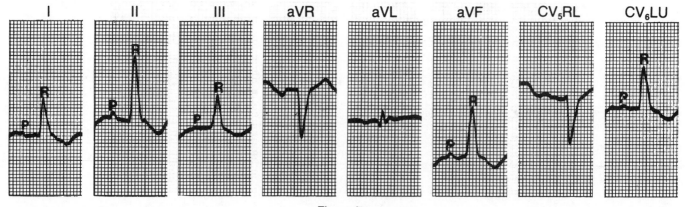

Figure 1.

Left bundle branch block in a cat with hypertrophic cardiomyopathy. The QRS complex is of 0.07-sec duration and is positive in leads I, II, III, aVF. Neither a Q wave nor an S wave occurs in these leads. The QRS complex is inverted in leads aVR. (From: Tilley LP. Essentials of canine and feline electrocardiography. 3rd ed. Baltimore: Williams & Wilkins, 1992, with permission.)

LEFT BUNDLE BRANCH BLOCK

PATHOLOGIC FINDINGS

Possible lesions or scarring on endocardial surface in the path of the bundle branches; applying Lugol's iodine to the endocardial surface within 2 h postmortem enables clear visualization of the conduction system.

TREATMENT

APPROPRIATE HEALTH CARE
Directed toward the underlying cause

NURSING CARE
Generally not necessary

ACTIVITY
Unrestricted unless required for management of underlying condition

DIET
No modifications unless required for management of underlying condition

CLIENT EDUCATION
• Left bundle branch block per se does not cause hemodynamic abnormalities.
• Lesion causing the block could progress, leading to more serious arrhythmias or complete heart block.

SURGICAL CONSIDERATIONS
N/A

MEDICATIONS

DRUGS OF CHOICE
N/A (unless required for management of underlying condition)

CONTRAINDICATIONS
N/A

PRECAUTIONS
N/A

POSSIBLE INTERACTIONS
N/A

ALTERNATIVE DRUGS
N/A

FOLLOW-UP

PATIENT MONITORING
Serial ECG may show clearing or progression to complete heart block.

PREVENTION/ AVOIDANCE
N/A

POSSIBLE COMPLICATIONS
• Causative lesion could progress, leading to a more serious arrhythmia or complete heart block.
• First- or second-degree AV block may indicate involvement of the right bundle branch.

EXPECTED COURSE AND PROGNOSIS
No hemodynamic compromise

MISCELLANEOUS

ASSOCIATED CONDITIONS
N/A

AGE-RELATED FACTORS
N/A

ZOONOTIC POTENTIAL
N/A

PREGNANCY
N/A

SYNONYMS
N/A

SEE ALSO
• Atrioventricular Block, Complete
• Atrioventricular Block, First-degree
• Atrioventricular Block, Second-degree
• Left Anterior Fascicular Block
• Right Bundle Branch Block

ABBREVIATIONS
AV = atrioventricular

Suggested Readings
Tilley LP. Essentials of canine and feline electrocardiography. 3rd ed. Baltimore: Williams & Wilkins, 1992.
Authors Larry P. Tilley and Naomi L. Burtnick
Consulting Editors Larry P. Tilley and Francis W. K. Smith, Jr.

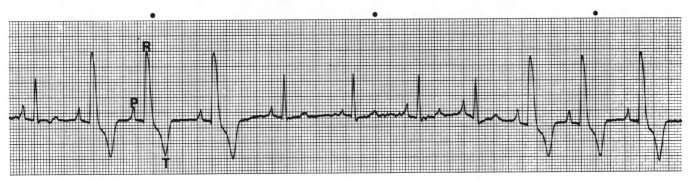

Figure 2.

Intermittent left bundle branch block in a Chihuahua. QRS complexes are wider (0.07–0.08 sec) in the second, third and fourth complexes and in the last three complexes. Consistent P-R interval confirms a sinus origin for the abnormal-appearing QRS complexes (lead II, 50 mm/sec, 1 cm = 1 mV). (From: Tilley LP. Essentials of canine and feline electrocardiography. 3rd ed. Baltimore: Williams & Wilkins, 1992, with permission.)

RIGHT BUNDLE BRANCH BLOCK

 BASICS

DEFINITION
Conduction delay or block in the right bundle branch resulting in late activation of the right ventricle; the block can be complete or incomplete. (Figures 1 and 2)

ECG Features
• A right axis deviation and wide QRS (≥ 0.08 sec in dogs; ≥ 0.06 in cats) in most patients
• Large, wide S waves in leads I, II, III, and aVF

PATHOPHYSIOLOGY
• The right bundle branch is anatomically vulnerable to injury because it is a thin strand of tissue and has a long undivided course.
• No hemodynamic compromise

SYSTEMS AFFECTED
Cardiovascular

GENETICS
N/A

INCIDENCE/PREVALENCE
• Dogs—most frequent form of intraventricular conduction defect
• Cats—not as frequent as left anterior fascicular block

GEOGRAPHIC DISTRIBUTION
N/A

SIGNALMENT

Species
Dogs and cats

Breed Predilections
In beagles, incomplete right bundle branch block can result from a genetically determined localized variation in right ventricular wall thickness.

Predominant Sex
N/A

SIGNS

Historical Findings
• Usually an incidental ECG finding—does not cause hemodynamic abnormalities
• Observed signs are usually associated with the underlying condition.

Physical Examination Findings
• Splitting of heart sounds because of asynchronous activation of ventricles in some patients
• Does not cause signs or hemodynamic compromise

CAUSES
• Occasionally seen in normal and healthy dogs and cats
• Congenital heart disease
• Chronic valvular fibrosis
• After surgical correction of a cardiac defect
• Trauma caused by cardiac needle puncture to obtain blood sample
• Trauma from other causes
• Chronic infection with *Trypanosoma cruzi* (Chagas' disease)
• Neoplasia
• Heartworm disease
• Acute thromboembolism
• Cardiomyopathy
• Hyperkalemia (most commonly in cats with urethral obstruction)

RISK FACTORS
N/A

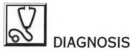 DIAGNOSIS

DIFFERENTIAL DIAGNOSIS
• Right ventricular enlargement—absence of right ventricular enlargement on thoracic radiographs or echocardiogram supports a diagnosis of right bundle branch block.
• Can also be confused with ventricular ectopic beats (especially if the block is intermittent), but consistent PR intervals and no pulse deficits with right bundle branch block

CBC/BIOCHEMISTRY/URINALYSIS
• None specific
• Serum potassium may be extremely high in cats with urethral obstruction.

OTHER LABORATORY TESTS
• Occult heartworm test may be positive in dogs or cats.
• Chagas' indirect fluorescent antibody test, direct hemagglutination, and complement fixation test may be positive in dogs.

IMAGING
• Echocardiogram may show structural heart disease; absence of right heart enlargement supports the diagnosis.
• Thoracic and abdominal radiographs may show masses or pulmonary metastatic lesions; traumatic injuries could cause localized or diffuse pulmonary densities.

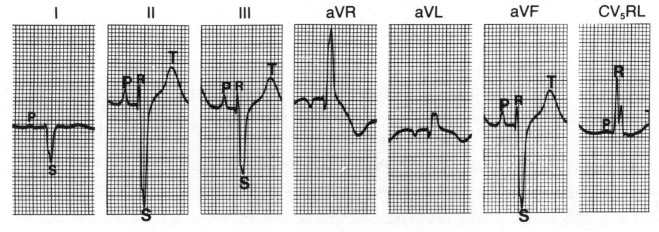

| I | II | III | aVR | aVL | aVF | CV₅RL |

Figure 1.

Right bundle branch block in a dog. The electrocardiographic features include QRS duration of 0.08 sec; positive QRS complex in aVR, aVL, and CV5RL (M shaped); and large wide S waves in leads I, II, III, and aVF. There is a right axis deviation (approximately −110°) (50 mm/sec, 1 cm = 1 mV). (From: Tilley LP. Essentials of canine and feline electrocardiography. 3rd ed. Baltimore: Williams & Wilkins, 1992, with permission.)

DIAGNOSTIC PROCEDURES
- Electrocardiography
- Echocardiography

PATHOLOGIC FINDINGS
Possible lesions or scarring on endocardial surface in the path of the bundle branches; applying Lugol's iodine to the endocardial surface within 2 h postmortem gives clear visualization of the conduction system.

 TREATMENT

APPROPRIATE HEALTH CARE
Direct treatment toward the underlying cause.

NURSING CARE
N/A

ACTIVITY
Unrestricted

DIET
No modifications unless required to manage underlying condition

CLIENT EDUCATION
- Does not cause hemodynamic abnormalities itself
- The lesion causing the block could progress, leading to more serious arrhythmias or complete heart block.

SURGICAL CONSIDERATIONS
N/A

 MEDICATIONS

DRUGS OF CHOICE
Not required unless needed to manage underlying condition

CONTRAINDICATIONS
N/A

PRECAUTIONS
N/A

POSSIBLE INTERACTIONS
N/A

ALTERNATIVE DRUGS
N/A

 FOLLOW-UP

PATIENT MONITORING
Serial ECG may show resolution of the lesion or progression to complete heart block.

PREVENTION/AVOIDANCE
N/A

POSSIBLE COMPLICATIONS
- The causative lesion could progress, leading to a more serious arrhythmia or complete heart block.
- First- or second-degree AV block may indicate involvement of the left bundle branch.

EXPECTED COURSE AND PROGNOSIS
No hemodynamic compromise

 MISCELLANEOUS

ASSOCIATED CONDITIONS
N/A

AGE-RELATED FACTORS
N/A

ZOONOTIC POTENTIAL
N/A

PREGNANCY
N/A

SYNONYMS
None

SEE ALSO
- Left Bundle Branch Block
- Left Anterior Fascicular Block
- Atrioventricular Block, First-degree
- Atrioventricular Block, Second-degree
- Atrioventricular Block, Complete

ABBREVIATIONS
AV = atrioventricular

Suggested Readings
Tilley LP. Essentials of canine and feline electrocardiography. 3rd ed. Baltimore: Williams & Wilkins, 1992.
Authors Larry P. Tilley and Naomi L. Burtnick
Consulting Editors Larry P. Tilley and Francis W. K. Smith, Jr.

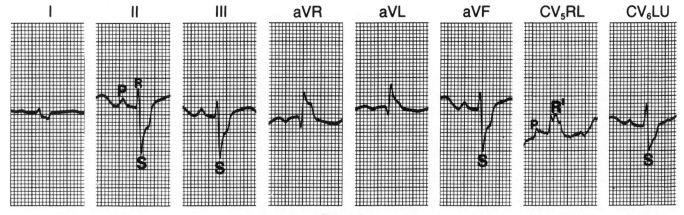

Figure 2.

Right bundle branch block in a cat with the dilated form of cardiomyopathy. The QRS duration is 0.08 sec (4 boxes). Large and wide S waves are present in leads *I, II, III, aVF,* and *CV₆LU.* The QRS in *CV₅RL* has a wide R wave (M-shaped). There is a marked axis deviation (approximately −90°). (From: Tilley LP: Essentials of canine and feline electrocardiography. 3rd ed. Baltimore: Williams & Wilkins, 1992, with permission.)

SICK SINUS SYNDROME

 BASICS

DEFINITION
A disorder of impulse formation within, and conduction out of, the sinus node; it also affects subsidiary pacemakers and the specialized conduction system of the atria, AV node, His bundle, and bundle branches.

ECG Features
• Arrhythmias noted with SSS include any or all of the following: inappropriate sinus bradycardia, sinus arrest, sinoatrial exit block, or alternating periods of sinus bradyarrhythmias and SVT (Figures 1 and 2)
• Paroxysms of SVT may alternate with prolonged periods of sinus node inertia and often AV nodal inertia as well, producing tachycardia–bradycardia syndrome, a variant of SSS
• P waves and QRS complexes are usually normal.

PATHOPHYSIOLOGY
• ECG manifestations may preceed development of clinical signs.
• Clinical signs usually result from the failure of subsidiary pacemakers to generate escape rhythms when sinus node dysfunction occurs.
• The common clinical manifestations reflect transient decreases in organ perfusion, particularly reduced cerebral perfusion.
• Rarely, congestive heart failure develops

SYSTEMS AFFECTED
• Cardiovascular
• Nervous, musculoskeletal, and renal systems may be secondarily affected because of hypoperfusion.

GENETICS
May be heritable in miniature schnauzers

INCIDENCE/PREVALENCE
N/A

GEOGRAPHIC DISTRIBUTION
N/A

SIGNALMENT
Species
Dogs

Breed Predilections
• Miniature schnauzers (may be heritable)
• Noted commonly in cocker spaniels, dachshunds, and pugs

Mean Age and Range
Most dogs > 6 years old

Predominant Sex
Female

SIGNS
Historical Findings
• Clinical signs vary from asymptomatic to weakness, syncope, collapse, and/or seizures.
• Sudden death is infrequent.

Physical Examination Findings
• Heart rate may be abnormally rapid or abnormally slow.
• Pauses may be noted.
• Some patients appear normal.

CAUSES
• Idiopathic
• Familial in miniature schnauzers
• Metastatic disease
• Ischemic disease

RISK FACTORS
N/A

 DIAGNOSIS

DIFFERENTIAL DIAGNOSIS
• Healthy dogs may exhibit sinus bradycardia (rate as low as 30 beats/min) and sinus pauses (as long as 3 sec) normally during sleep.
• Bradycardia and sinus arrest due to normal or enhanced vagal tone
• Drug-induced (digitalis, β-adrenergic antagonists, α_2-adrenergic agonists, calcium channel antagonists, cimetidine, opioids, amiodarone)
• Seizures or syncope due to noncardiac disease

• Atrial standstill secondary to hyperkalemia or atrial disease
• Weakness due to neurologic, musculoskeletal, or metabolic diseases

CBC/BIOCHEMISTRY/URINALYSIS
Normal

OTHER LABORATORY TESTS
N/A

IMAGING
N/A

DIAGNOSTIC PROCEDURES
• Atropine response testing—indicated in dogs with sinus bradycardia, sinus arrest, and sinoatrial exit block. Administer atropine (0.04 mg/kg IM), and evaluate the ECG 20–30 min later. A normal (positive) response is > 50% increase in heart rate with abolishment of pauses; dogs with SSS generally have no response or an incomplete response to atropine.
• Electrophysiologic testing of sinus node recovery time and sinoatrial conduction time
• 24-hr ambulatory ECG (Holter) or event monitoring to correlate clinical signs with arrhythmia

PATHOLOGIC FINDINGS
Vary with cause

 TREATMENT

APPROPRIATE HEALTH CARE
• Hospitalization rarely necessary except for electrophysiologic testing or pacemaker implantation
• Do not treat asymptomatic animals.

NURSING CARE
N/A

ACTIVITY
Avoid vigorous exercise and stressful situations.

DIET
Modifications unnecessary

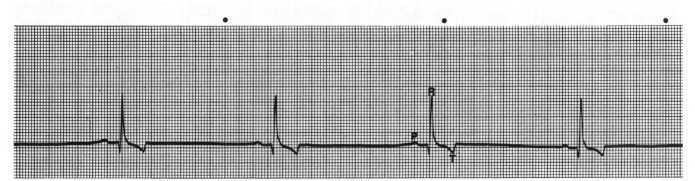

Figure 1.

Sinus bradycardia (approx. 60 beats/min) in a miniature schnauzer with fainting. Paper speed = 50 mm/sec. (From: Tilley LP: Essentials of canine and feline electrocardiography. 3rd ed. Baltimore: Williams & Wilkins, 1992, with permission.)

CLIENT EDUCATION
Owner should be aware that medical management is often ineffective.

SURGICAL CONSIDERATIONS
• Permanent pacemaker necessary for dogs failing to respond to medical treatment and those exhibiting unacceptable medication side effects
• Permanent pacemaker usually required for dogs with bradycardia–tachycardia syndrome

MEDICATIONS

DRUGS OF CHOICE
• Do not treat asymptomatic animals.
• Symptomatic dogs are grouped into those showing primarily bradycardia, sinus arrest, and/or sinoatrial exit block and those with supraventricular tachycardia followed by sinus arrest
• Atropine-responsive symptomatic dogs with bradycardia or sinus arrest—anticholinergic agents (propantheline: small dogs, 3.75–7.5 mg PO q8–12h; medium dogs, 15 mg PO q8h; large dogs, 30 mg PO q8h)
• Dogs with bradycardia and sinus arrest—may try theophylline (Theo-Dur, 20 mg/kg PO q12h) or terbutaline (0.2 mg/kg PO q8–12h) if anticholinergic drugs are ineffective
• Dogs with bradycardia-tachycardia whose clinical signs are due to tachycardia or tachycardia-induced sinus arrest—can give digoxin (0.005 mg/kg PO q12h) or atenolol (0.5–1.0 mg/kg PO q12–24h) in attempt to suppress the SVT (monitor closely for exacerbation of bradycardia)

CONTRAINDICATIONS
Avoid drugs that may worsen sinus node dysfunction (e.g., β-adrenergic antagonists, calcium channel blocking agents, phenothiazines, class I and III antiarrhythmic agents, opioids, cimetidine, α$_2$-adrenergic agonists)

PRECAUTIONS
• Attempts to manage bradycardia-tachycardia syndrome medically without prior pacemaker implantation carry significant risk because drugs used to control SVT may worsen the bradyarrhythmias, and vice versa.
• Adverse effects of anticholinergic medication (constipation, difficulty voiding, keratoconjunctivitis sicca, emesis) occur commonly.

POSSIBLE INTERACTIONS
N/A

ALTERNATIVE DRUGS
N/A

FOLLOW-UP

PATIENT MONITORING
• ECG in asymptomatic patients—to detect progression of disease
• ECG in patients treated medically or with pacemaker implantation

PREVENTION/AVOIDANCE
N/A

POSSIBLE COMPLICATIONS
Rarely, reduced cerebral or renal perfusion results in chronic renal dysfunction or CNS damage.

EXPECTED COURSE AND PROGNOSIS
• Good, following pacemaker implantation in animals without congestive heart failure
• Medical management—often ineffective; initial beneficial effects often not sustained

MISCELLANEOUS

ASSOCIATED CONDITIONS
None

AGE-RELATED FACTORS
N/A

ZOONOTIC POTENTIAL
N/A

PREGNANCY
N/A

SYNONYMS
• Bradycardia-tachycardia syndrome
• Tachycardia-bradycardia syndrome

SEE ALSO
• Sinus Arrest or Sinoatrial Block
• Supraventricular Tachycardia
• Sinus Bradycardia

ABBREVIATIONS
• AV = atrioventricular
• SSS = sick sinus syndrome
• SVT = supraventricular tachycardia

Suggested Reading
Belic N, Talano JV. Current concepts in sick sinus syndrome: I. Anatomy, physiology, and pharmacologic causes. Arch Intern Med 1985;145:521–523.
Belic N, Talano JV. Current concepts in sick sinus syndrome: II. ECG manifestation and diagnostic and therapeutic approaches. Arch Intern Med 1985;145:722–726.
Hamlin RL, Smetzer DK, Breznock EM. Sinoatrial syncope in miniature schnauzers. J Am Vet Med Assoc 1972;161:1022–1028.
Reiffel JA. Normal sinus rhythm and its variants. In: Podrid PJ, Kowey PR, eds. Cardiac arrhythmia—mechanisms, diagnosis, and management. Baltimore: Williams & Wilkins, 1995:752–767.
Tilley LP. Essentials of canine and feline electrocardiography. 3rd ed. Baltimore: Williams & Wilkins, 1992.
Author Janice McIntosh Bright
Consulting Editors Larry P. Tilley and Francis W. K. Smith, Jr.

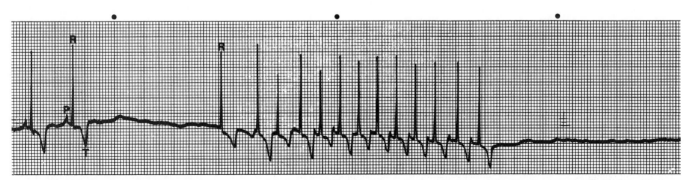

Figure 2.

Sick sinus syndrome (paper speed, 25 mm/sec), a bradycardia-tachycardia pattern. Note the two long periods of SA block. The first period is followed by a junctional escape complex and a rapid supraventricular tachycardia. The continuous bombardment of the SA node by these impulses suppresses its automaticity, causing another long pause. (From: Tilley LP: Essentials of canine and feline electrocardiography. 3rd ed. Baltimore: Williams & Wilkins, 1992, with permission.)

SINUS ARREST OR BLOCK

BASICS

DEFINITION
• Sinus arrest—a disorder of impulse formation caused by slowing or cessation of spontaneous sinus nodal automaticity; the SA node fails to initiate an impulse at the expected time.
• Sinus block—a defect in impulse conduction; an impulse formed within the sinus node fails to depolarize the atria or does so with delay; the basic rhythmicity of the sinus node is not disturbed; the duration of the pause is a multiple of the basic P-P interval.

ECG Features
• A normal P wave exists for each QRS complex with a pause equal to or greater than twice the normal P-P interval; rhythm is regularly irregular or irregular with pauses (Figure 1).
• Junctional or ventricular escape beats—may occur if pauses significantly prolonged.
• Surface ECG cannot differentiate sinus arrest from sinus block in the dog because of normal R-R interval variation (sinus arrhythmia).

PATHOPHYSIOLOGY
• Sympathetic and parasympathetic influences can alter spontaneous sinus node depolarization; vagal stimulation of acetylcholine, which binds to SA nodal receptor sites, can slow automaticity of the sinus node by reducing the slope of phase 4 depolarization; sympathetic stimulation releases norepinephrine that binds to β_1 receptors on the SA node, enhancing spontaneous SA nodal discharge rate.
• Intrinsic disease of the sinus node may affect the balance between the parasympathetic and sympathetic efferent traffic to the SA node and its spontaneous discharge rate.

SYSTEMS AFFECTED
Cardiovascular—clinical signs of weakness or syncope may appear if sinus arrest or block with resultant absence of atrial depolarization causes sufficiently long periods of ventricular asystole with no escape beats initiated by latent pacemakers.

GENETICS
• Seen in purebred pugs with hereditary stenosis of the bundle of His.
• Seen in female miniature schnauzers predisposed to sick sinus syndrome (SSS)
• Congenitally deaf Dalmatian coach hounds often have abnormal SA node and multiple atrial arteries.

INCIDENCE/PREVALENCE
• Normal incidental finding in brachycephalic breeds of dogs in which inspiration causes a reflex increase in vagal tone
• Common in dog breeds predisposed to SSS.
• Uncommon in cats

GEOGRAPHIC DISTRIBUTION
N/A

SIGNALMENT

Species
Dogs and cats

Breed Predilections
• Brachycephalic breeds
• Breeds predisposed to SSS (e.g., miniature schnauzers, dachshunds, cocker spaniels, pugs and West Highland white terriers)

Mean Age and Range
If associated with SSS, generally older animal

Predominant Sex
In association with SSS, older females

SIGNS

Historical Findings
• Usually none
• Signs of low cardiac output (e.g., weakness and syncope) may occur with failure of the SA node to fire on time if no lower pacemaker focus takes over the rhythm.
• Sudden death is possible with prolonged periods of ventricular asystole.

Physical Examination Findings
• May be normal.
• Heart sounds following a pause may be louder than usual because the ventricles had longer to fill and eject a larger amount of blood.
• Extremely slow heart rate if arrest or block is prolonged or frequent
• With significant pathologic cardiac disease—may be findings consistent with poor cardiac output (e.g. prolonged perfusion time, pale mucous membranes, weak femoral pulses)

CAUSES

Physiologic
• Vagal stimulation secondary to coughing, pharyngeal irritation
• Ocular or carotid sinus pressure

Pathologic
• Degenerative heart disease (fibrosis)
• Dilatory heart disease
• Acute myocarditis
• Neoplastic heart disease
• SSS
• Irritation of vagus nerve secondary to thoracic or cervical neoplasia
• Electrolyte imbalance
• Drug toxicity (e.g., digoxin)

RISK FACTORS
• Certain drugs, including digitalis, quinidine, propranolol, xylazine, acepromazine
• Respiratory tract disease
• Vagal maneuvers

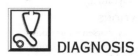

DIAGNOSIS

DIFFERENTIAL DIAGNOSIS
• Marked sinus arrhythmia and sinus bradycardia

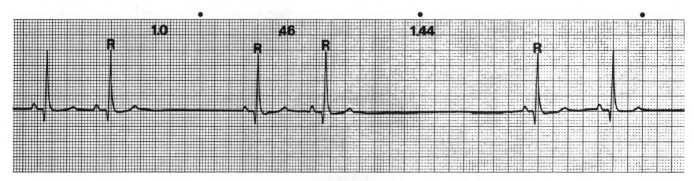

Figure 1.

Intermittent sinus arrest in a brachycephalic breed with an upper respiratory disorder and episodes of fainting. The pauses (1 and 1.44 sec) are greater than twice the normal R-R interval (0.46). (From: Tilley LP: Essentials of canine and feline electrocardiography. 3rd ed. Baltimore: Williams & Wilkins, 1992, with permission.)

• Not always possible to differentiate sinus arrest from block without direct recordings of sinus node discharge; pauses that are precise multiples of the dominant beat interval suggest sinus block.

CBC/BIOCHEMISTRY/URINALYSIS
Serum electrolyte abnormalities in some animals, especially hyperkalemia (serum K^+ > 5.7 mEq/L)

OTHER LABORATORY TESTS
N/A

IMAGING
• Thoracic radiographs if neoplastic or cardiac disease suspected
• Cardiac ultrasound if structural or neoplastic heart disease suspected

DIAGNOSTIC PROCEDURES
• Provocative atropine response test to assess sinus node function. Administer 0.04 mg/kg atropine IM; evaluate ECG lead II rhythm strip 30 min later for response. Resolution of the arrhythmia with atropine administration suggests high vagal tone as the underlying cause.
• Ambulatory monitoring may reveal prolonged periods of failure of impulses from the SA node if signs of weakness or syncope.
• In people, a period of sinus arrest following right carotid massage that lasts longer than 3 sec suggests inappropriate sinus responsiveness.

PATHOLOGIC FINDINGS
Histologic study of the SA node may reveal necrosis, fibrosis, and/or degenerative changes in the sinus node.

TREATMENT

APPROPRIATE HEALTH CARE
Asymptomatic sinus arrest or block does not require therapy. If clinical signs, therapeutic approach depends on underlying cause and severity of symptoms. Any indicated treatment may be outpatient unless pacemaker implantation is necessary, which necessitates hospital management.

NURSING CARE
Correct any electrolyte abnormalities that may be contributing.

ACTIVITY
Unrestricted unless signs of weakness, syncope, or CHF develop

DIET
N/A

CLIENT EDUCATION
An artificial pacemaker may be necessary when patient is symptomatic and non-responsive to medical management.

SURGICAL CONSIDERATIONS
Implantation of an artificial demand pacemaker in animals with clinical signs nonresponsive to therapy

MEDICATIONS

DRUGS OF CHOICE
• If patient is symptomatic, consider atropine (0.02 mg/kg IV, 0.04 mg/kg IM), glycopyrrolate (0.005–0.01 mg/kg IV, IM), or isoproterenol (10 μg/kg IM, SC q6h or dilute 1 mg in 500 mL of 5% dextrose or Ringer solution, and infuse IV 0.5–1 mL/min [1–2 μg/min] or to effect); dosages for both dog and cat
• If responsive to injectable anticholinergic drugs (e.g. atropine)—can prescribe oral propantheline bromide for at–home management; bronchodilator therapy with aminophylline, theophylline, albuterol, or terbutaline can also be considered for oral therapy.

CONTRAINDICATIONS
If patient is symptomatic secondary to prolonged pauses, discontinue any drugs that may be causative (e.g. digitalis, β-blockers, calcium channel blockers).

PRECAUTIONS
Avoid drugs that depress SA node function when indicated.

POSSIBLE INTERACTIONS
N/A

ALTERNATIVE DRUGS
If medical therapy does not resolve signs, consider a ventricular demand artificial pacemaker.

FOLLOW-UP

PATIENT MONITORING
When indicated, periodic serial ECG evaluation to assess therapeutic efficacy and possible progression to a more serious dysrhythmia.

PREVENTION/AVOIDANCE
N/A

POSSIBLE COMPLICATIONS
If associated with primary cardiac disease, CHF may develop and necessitate appropriate therapies.

EXPECTED COURSE AND PROGNOSIS
If cause is SSS, symptomatic patient may respond well to medical intervention; if poorly responsive, permanent pacemaker implantation would improve prognosis markedly.

MISCELLANEOUS

ASSOCIATED CONDITIONS
• SSS
• Sinus arrhythmia
• Sinus bradycardia

AGE-RELATED FACTORS
N/A

ZOONOTIC POTENTIAL
N/A

PREGNANCY
N/A

SYNONYMS
• Sinus block
• Sinus pause
• Sinus or Sinoatrial (SA) exit block types I and II
• Type I (Wenckebach)—P-P interval progressively shortens prior to pause; duration of the pause is less than two P-P cycles
• Type II—duration of pause is a multiple of the basic P-P interval.

SEE ALSO
• Sick Sinus Syndrome
• Sinus Bradycardia
• Sinus Arrhythmia

ABBREVIATIONS
• CHF = congestive heart failure
• SA = sinoatrial
• SSS = sick sinus syndrome

Suggested Reading
Braunwald E, ed. Heart disease. 5th ed. Philadelphia: Saunders, 1997.
Fox PR, ed. Canine and feline cardiology. New York: Churchill Livingstone, 1988.
Tilley LP, Goodwin J, eds. Manual of canine and feline cardiology. 3rd ed. Philadelphia: Saunders, 2000.
Tilley LP, ed. Essentials of canine and feline electrocardiography. 3rd ed. Baltimore: Williams & Wilkins, 1992.
Author Deborah J. Hadlock
Consulting Editors Larry P. Tilley and Francis W. K. Smith, Jr.

SINUS ARRHYTHMIA

BASICS

DEFINITION
Normal sinus impulse formation with irregular R-R interval that has more than 10% variation in sinus cycle length (Figure 1).

ECG Features
- P wave for every QRS complex
- P-R interval relatively constant
- P wave morphology may vary (wandering pacemaker) as P-P intervals vary.

PATHOPHYSIOLOGY
- Sinus node discharge rate depends on the two opposing influences of the autonomic nervous system. Vagal stimulation decreases spontaneous sinus nodal discharge rate and predominates over sympathetic stimulation. During inspiration, feedback from the respiratory and cardiac centers in the medulla produces cardiac acceleration by decreasing vagal restraint on the sinus node; the opposite occurs during exhalation. The genesis of sinus arrhythmia (SA) also depends on reflexes involving stretch receptors in the lung, pressure-volume sensory receptors in the heart (Bainbridge, baroreceptor), blood vessels, and chemical factors of the blood.
- Respiratory SA—P-P interval cyclically shortens during inspiration resulting from reflex inhibition of vagal tone and slows during expiration; nonrespiratory SA—phasic variation in P-P interval unrelated to the respiratory cycle

SYSTEMS AFFECTED
Cardiovascular—generally no hemodynamic consequence, but marked SA may produce a long enough sinus pause to produce syncope if not accompanied by an escape rhythm

GENETICS
N/A

INCIDENCE/PREVALENCE
Most frequent form of arrhythmia in the dog.

GEOGRAPHIC DISTRIBUTION
N/A

SIGNALMENT

Species
- Common and normal in dogs
- Uncommon, usually abnormal in cats

Breed Predilections
- Brachycephalic breeds predisposed
- Dogs—bulldogs, Lhasa apsos, Pekingese, pugs, shar-peis, shih tzus, boxers
- Cats—Persians, Himalayans

Mean Age and Range
N/A

Predominant Sex
N/A

SIGNS

General Comments
Uncommon, but weakness may develop if pauses between beats are excessively long; syncope can occur if long pauses are not followed by a junctional or ventricular escape rhythm.

Historical Findings
- Respiratory SA—none
- Nonrespiratory SA—may be findings related to underlying disease

Physical Examination Findings
- May be normal
- Irregular rhythm on auscultation
- May be findings related to specific disease accentuating vagal tone (e.g., stertor and stridor in a patient with brachycephalic airway syndrome)

CAUSES
- Normal cyclic change in vagal tone associated with respiration in the dog; heart rate increases with inspiration and decreases with expiration
- Underlying conditions that increase vagal tone—high intracranial pressure, gastrointestinal disease, respiratory disease, cerebral disorders, digitalis toxicity
- Carotid sinus massage or ocular pressure

(vagal maneuver) may accentuate

RISK FACTORS
- Brachycephalic conformation
- Digoxin therapy
- Any disease that increases vagal tone

DIAGNOSIS

DIFFERENTIAL DIAGNOSIS
- Auscultation of SA is often confusing; ECG helps differentiate normal SA from true pathologic arrhythmia.
- Wandering pacemaker frequently associated. Site of impulse formation shifts within the sinoatrial node or to an atrial focus or AV node, changing the configuration of the P wave.
- Important to differentiate normal SA from other pathologic arrhythmias including atrial premature complexes, sinus bradycardia-sinus tachycardia syndrome (SSS), slow atrial fibrillation, and AV dissociation

CBC/BIOCHEMISTRY/URINALYSIS
N/A

OTHER LABORATORY TESTS
- Serum digoxin concentration, if applicable; assay 6–8 hr postpill; therapeutic serum concentrations typically are 0.8–1.5 ng/mL.
- Cats with chronic respiratory disease may be positive for feline leukemia or feline immunodeficiency virus.

IMAGING
Radiographs of head and neck to assess for abnormal anatomic conformation that might predispose to airway problems

DIAGNOSTIC PROCEDURES
- Pharyngoscopy/laryngoscopy if upper airway disease suspected
- Atropine challenge test (administer atropine 0.04 mg/kg IM followed by ECG in 30 min) if associated with sinus bradycardia and primary dysfunction of sinus node is suspected

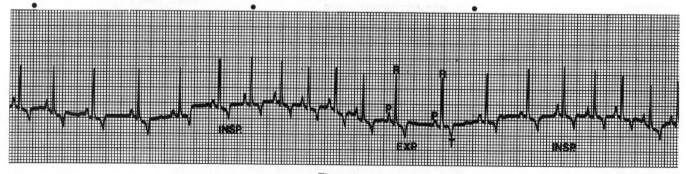

Figure 1.

Respiratory sinus arrhythmia with an average rate of 120/min (paper speed, 25 mm/sec; 6 complexes between one set of time lines × 20). The rate increases during inspiration (*INSP*) and decreases during expiration (*EXP*). The fluctuation of the baseline correlates with the movement of the electrodes by the thoracic cavity. (From: Tilley LP: Essentials of canine and feline electrocardiography. 3rd ed. Baltimore: Williams & Wilkins, 1992, with permission.)

PATHOLOGIC FINDINGS
See specific disease

TREATMENT

APPROPRIATE HEALTH CARE
Generally, specific treatment required only when associated with symptomatic sinus bradycardia; if not related to respiration, underlying cause is treated. If patient is suffering respiratory distress, appropriate inpatient management indicated until patient is stable.

NURSING CARE
None unless associated with underlying disease (see also below)

ACTIVITY
Not restricted unless associated with specific disease; (e.g., brachycephalic animals may need to limit exercise, especially in high ambient temperatures)

DIET
Caloric restriction for obese animals with airway compromise

CLIENT EDUCATION
None unless associated with specific disease

SURGICAL CONSIDERATIONS
None unless associated with specific disease

MEDICATIONS

DRUGS OF CHOICE
• Generally no therapy indicated; this is a normal rhythm.
• Infectious respiratory diseases require appropriate antibiotic therapy.

• If associated with symptomatic sinus bradycardia or sinus arrest or block, anticholinergics may be indicated—atropine (0.04 mg/kg IM, SC) or glycopyrrolate (0.01 mg/kg IM, SC)

CONTRAINDICATIONS
Stop administering digoxin if toxicity is a problem.

PRECAUTIONS
Avoid atropine in patients with respiratory disease; it dehydrates respiratory secretions.

POSSIBLE INTERACTIONS
N/A

ALTERNATIVE DRUGS N/A

FOLLOW-UP

PATIENT MONITORING
Only if associated with specific disease (see also)

PREVENTION/AVOIDANCE
N/A

POSSIBLE COMPLICATIONS
N/A

EXPECTED COURSE AND PROGNOSIS
N/A

MISCELLANEOUS

ASSOCIATED CONDITIONS
• SSS
• Brachycephalic airway syndrome
• Asthma
• Chronic obstructive pulmonary disease

AGE-RELATED FACTORS
Generally more pronounced in young adult.

ZOONOTIC POTENTIAL
N/A

PREGNANCY
Increased incidence of arrhythmias

SYNONYMS
• Respiratory SA = phasic SA
• Nonrespiratory SA = nonphasic SA; sinus irregularity.
• Ventriculophasic SA—form of nonphasic SA in which atrial cycles containing ventricular complexes are shorter than those in which they are absent (ex: advanced AV block).

SEE ALSO
• Sick Sinus Syndrome
• Sinus Arrest and Block
• Brachycephalic Airway Syndrome

ABBREVIATIONS
• SA = sinus arrhythmia
• AV = atrioventricular
• SSS = sick sinus syndrome

Suggested Reading
Berne RM, Levy MN. Cardiovascular physiology. 6th ed. St. Louis: Mosby Year Book, 1992.
Braunwald E, ed. Heart disease. 5th ed. Philadelphia: Saunders, 1997.
Fox PR, ed. Canine and feline cardiology. New York: Churchill Livingstone, 1988.
Tilley LP, Goodwin J. eds. Manual of canine and feline cardiology. 3rd ed. Philadelphia: Saunders, 2000.
Author Deborah J. Hadlock
Consulting Editors Larry P. Tilley and Francis W. K. Smith, Jr.

SINUS BRADYCARDIA

BASICS

DEFINITION
Sinus rhythm in which impulses arise from the sinoatrial node at a slower than normal rate

ECG Features
• Dogs—sinus rate < 70 bpm (< 60 bpm in giant breeds) • Cats—sinus rate < 120 bpm at home or < 150 bpm at the clinic • Rhythm regular, often with a slight variation in R-R interval; may be irregular if bradycardia due to high vagal tone • Normal P wave for each QRS complex • P-R interval constant

PATHOPHYSIOLOGY
• May represent normal physiologic response to athletic training; may result from enhanced cardiac parasympathetic tone or decreased sympathetic tone as well as from intrinsic changes in the sinus node; changes in sinoatrial nodal discharge frequency are usually produced by the cardiac autonomic nerves, • May represent pathophysiologic response due to high vagal tone, change in blood pH, PCO_2, PO_2, or serum electrolyte derangements

SYSTEMS AFFECTED
Cardiovascular—may be beneficial by producing a longer period of diastole and increased ventricular filling time; can be associated with syncope if due to abnormal reflex (neurocardiogenic) or intrinsic disease of sinus node

GENETICS
Female miniature schnauzers predisposed to SSS, which may cause bradycardia

INCIDENCE/PREVALENCE
Common in the dog, less common in cats

GEOGRAPHIC DISTRIBUTION
N/A

SIGNALMENT

Species
Dogs and cats

Breed Predilections
If SSS causes the bradycardia—miniature schnauzers, cocker spaniels, dachshunds, pugs, and West Highland white terriers

Mean Age and Range
• Decreased prevalence with advancing age unless associated with intrinsic disease of SA node • SSS typically seen in geriatric patients

Predominant Sex
With SSS, older females

SIGNS

General Comments
Importance depends on cause, insignificant or serious, depending upon signs and underlying cause.

Historical Findings
• May be none • Lethargy • Exercise intolerance • Syncope • Episodic ataxia • Seizures

Physical Examination Findings
• Pulse rate slow • Hypothermia may occur.

CAUSES

Physiologic
• Athletic conditioning • Hypothermia • Intubation

Pathophysiologic
High vagal tone associated with gastrointestinal, respiratory, neurologic, and pharyngeal diseases

Pathologic
• High intracranial pressure • Hyperkalemia • Hypercalcemia • Hypocalcemia • Hypermagnesemia • Hypoxemia • Hypothyroidism • May precede cardiac arrest • SSS • Feline dilated cardiomyopathy • Sinoatrial block • Neurocardiogenic • Vasovagal • Carotid sinus hyperactivity • Situational (micturition, defecation, cough, swallowing)

Pharmacologic
• General anesthesia • Phenothiazines • β-Blockers • Digitalis • Calcium channel blockers • Xylazine

RISK FACTORS
• Any situation or disease that may increase parasympathetic tone • Oversedation • Hypoventilation under anesthesia

DIAGNOSIS

DIFFERENTIAL DIAGNOSIS
• Often coexists with sinus arrhythmia • Persistent and marked (SB) should raise possibility of SSS. • Clinical signs may mimic cerebral dysfunction.

CBC/BIOCHEMISTRY/URINALYSIS
• Hyperkalemia, hypercalcemia, hypocalcemia, or hypermagnesemia possible • CBC and serum chemistry profile may reveal changes associated with metabolic disease such as renal failure.

OTHER LABORATORY TESTS
• Serum T_4 and T_3, free T_4 (FT_4), and TSH assay if hypothyroidism suspected • Measure serum digoxin concentration 8–10 h after last dose; normal therapeutic serum concentration should be 0.8–1.5 ng/mL.

IMAGING
Survey radiographs and ultrasound may reveal evidence of cardiac, renal, or other organ abnormalities.

DIAGNOSTIC PROCEDURES
• Provocative atropine response test to assess sinus node function—administer atropine 0.04 mg/kg IM; follow-up ECG 30 min post–atropine administration; lower doses of atropine have increased tendency to cause initial accentuation of sinus bradycardia and first- or second-degree AV block because of centrally mediated increase in vagal tone. • 24-h Holter monitoring or ECG event recorder useful if transient bradyarrhythmia is suspected cause for clinical signs

PATHOLOGIC FINDINGS
Depends on primary disease, if any

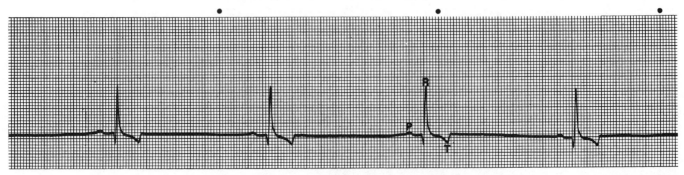

Figure 1.

Sinus bradycardia at a rate of 75 beats/min in a cat during anesthetic complications during surgery. (From: Tilley LP: Essentials of canine and feline electrocardiography. 3rd ed. Baltimore: Williams & Wilkins, 1992, with permission.)

TREATMENT

APPROPRIATE HEALTH CARE
• Many animals exhibit no clinical signs and require no treatment. In dogs without structural heart disease, heart rates as low as 40–50 bpm generally provide normal cardiac output at rest. • Therapeutic approaches—vary markedly; depend on the mechanism for SB, the ventricular rate, and severity of clinical signs • Inpatient or outpatient management—depends on underlying cause and clinical status of patient

NURSING CARE
• Provide general supportive therapy including intravenous fluid therapy for hypothermic and hypovolemic patients. • Discontinue any causative drug. • Correct any serious electrolyte imbalance with appropriate fluid therapy.

ACTIVITY
No restrictions unless patient has symptomatic SB related to structural heart disease; then exercise restriction recommended until effective medical and/or surgical therapy.

DIET
Special considerations may be indicated if cause is associated with electrolyte imbalance secondary to renal disease.

CLIENT EDUCATION
• Discuss importance of complying with daily medical management when treating underlying disease. • Advise that persistent symptomatic bradycardia may necessitate permanent pacemaker implantation for reliable long-term management.

SURGICAL CONSIDERATIONS
• If progressive bradycardia occurs during anesthesia and is attributed to hypoventilation, immediately discontinue inhalation anesthetics and provide adequate ventilation; atropine is generally ineffective in this situation. • If surgical manipulation triggering vagal reflexes (eye, vagus nerve, larynx) is anticipated, pretreatment with atropine (0.04 mg/kg IM, SC) or glycopyrrolate (0.005–0.01 mg/kg IM, SC) may prevent bradycardia. • Severe bradycardia may precipitate cardiopulmonary arrest; identify the causative agent or condition for effective management.

MEDICATIONS

DRUGS OF CHOICE
• If patient is hypothyroid, supplement with L-thyroxine • For severe hypocalcemia (< 6 mg/dL) administer 10% calcium gluconate (0.5–1.5 mL/kg IV) slowly over 15–30 min; monitor with ECG.
• For symptomatic drug-induced bradycardias,

disorders causing excessive vagal tone, and initial management of bradycardia associated with SSS, administer atropine (0.02 mg/kg IV) or glycopyrrolate (0.005–0.01 mg/kg IV); anticholinergic therapy may be continued short-term using atropine (0.04 mg/kg IM, SC q6–8 h) or glycopyrrolate (0.01 mg/kg IM, SC q6–8h). • Consider propantheline bromide (0.5–2 mg/kg PO q8–2h), theophylline (Theo-Dur 20 mg/kg PO q12h, dogs; 25 mg/kg PO q24h, cats), and/or terbutaline (0.2 mg/kg PO q8h, dogs; 0.625 mg/cat PO, cats) to manage bradycardia associated with SA node disease. • For temporary management of symptomatic persistent bradycardia until pacing can be accomplished, consider continuous IV infusion of isoproterenol (1–2 μg/min or to effect) or dobutamine (2.5–20 μg/kg/min IV infusion, dogs; 1–5 μg/kg/min IV infusion, cats).

CONTRAINDICATIONS
Parasympatholytic agents contraindicated for acidotic, hypercarbic patients under anesthesia (hypoventilation); bradycardia in this setting may protect the myocardium by decreasing oxygen consumption.

PRECAUTIONS
• Close ECG monitoring recommended when administering calcium solutions for treatment of hypocalcemia; if QT interval shortening or bradycardia, stop administration temporarily. • In patients with heart disease, a lower initial dose of L-thyroxine is advised to allow adaptation to higher metabolic rate. • Administer atropine selectively; rapid IV administration may predispose to ventricular arrhythmias by altering autonomic balance.

POSSIBLE INTERACTIONS
N/A

ALTERNATIVE DRUGS
• Bradycardia associated with structural heart disease is most reliably treated by permanent pacemaker implantation. • Glycopyrrolate may have longer vagal blocking effect and cause less frequent ventricular ectopic beats than atropine.

FOLLOW-UP

PATIENT MONITORING
• Assess postpill serum T_4 4–6 hr after dose, 30 and 60 days after starting treatment.
• Addison's disease—assess electrolytes every 3–4 months after patient is stable. • ECG check of pacemaker function and pacing rate is recommended during each follow-up examination.

PREVENTION/AVOIDANCE
• Maintain normal PAO_2 under anesthesia with proper ventilation; monitor with pulse oximetry or blood gases. • Avoid hypothermia intraoperatively.

POSSIBLE COMPLICATIONS
Malfunctioning pacemaker

EXPECTED COURSE AND PROGNOSIS
• Signs, if present, should resolve with correction of causative metabolic or endocrine problem. • Treatment of symptomatic SB with a permanent pacemaker generally offers a good prognosis.

MISCELLANEOUS

ASSOCIATED CONDITIONS
• SSS • Heart block

AGE-RELATED FACTORS
N/A

ZOONOTIC POTENTIAL
N/A

PREGNANCY
Postparturient hypocalcemia usually develops 1–4 weeks postpartum, but can occur at term, prepartum, or late lactation.

SYNONYMS
N/A

SEE ALSO
• Calcium, Hypercalcemia • Calcium, Hypocalcemia • Digoxin Toxicity • Eclampsia • Hypothermia • Hypothyroidism • Magnesium, Hypermagnesemia • Organophosphate and Carbamate Toxicity • Potassium, Hyperkalemia • SSS

ABBREVIATIONS
• SA = sinoatrial
• SSS = sick sinus syndrome
• SB = sinus bradycardia
• T_4 = thyroxine
• T_3 = triiodothyronine
• TSH = thyroid stimulating hormone

Suggested Reading
Miller MS, Tilley LP, Smith FWK, Fox PR. Electrocardiography. In: Fox PR, Sisson D, Moise NS, eds. Textbook of canine and feline cardiology. Philadelphia: Saunders, 1999:67–106.

Moses BL. Cardiopulmonary resuscitation. In: Murtaugh RJ, Kaplan PM, eds. Veterinary emergency and critical care medicine. St. Louis: Mosby Year Book, 1992:508–525.

Smith FWK, Hadlock DJ. Electrocardiography. In: Miller MS, Tilley LP, eds. Manual of canine and feline cardiology. 2nd ed. Philadelphia: Saunders, 1995:47–74.

Tilley LP, ed. Essentials of canine and feline electrocardiography. 3rd ed. Baltimore: Williams & Wilkins, 1992.

Author Deborah J. Hadlock
Consulting Editors Larry P. Tilley and Francis W. K. Smith, Jr.

SINUS TACHYCARDIA

 BASICS

DEFINITION
Disturbance of sinus impulse formation; acceleration of the sinoatrial node beyond its normal discharge rate. (Figure 1)

ECG Features
- Dogs—HR > 160 bpm (toy breeds HR > 180 bpm; giant breeds HR > 140 bpm; puppies HR > 220 bpm)
- Cats—HR > 240 bpm
- ECG shows a regular rhythm with possible slight variation in R-R interval
- Normal P wave (may be peaked) for each QRS complex with constant P-R interval
- P waves may be partially or completely fused with preceding T waves.
- Rate change in ST is usually gradual, not paroxysmal.

PATHOPHYSIOLOGY
Enhanced adrenergic effect or cholinergic inhibition results in high rate of sinus impulse formation; changes in heart rate usually involve a reciprocal action of the parasympathetic and sympathetic divisions of the autonomic nervous system.

SYSTEMS AFFECTED
Cardiovascular—cardiac output = heart rate × stroke volume. Changes in heart rate affect preload, afterload, and contractility, which determine stroke volume; severe tachycardia can compromise cardiac output. Rapid rates shorten diastolic filling time, and particularly in diseased hearts, the increased heart rate can fail to compensate for decreased stroke volume, resulting in decreased cardiac output and coronary blood flow. Chronic tachycardias can cause cardiac dilation.

GENETICS
N/A

INCIDENCE/PREVALENCE
- Most common arrhythmia in the dog and cat
- Most common rhythm disturbance in the postoperative patient

GEOGRAPHIC DISTRIBUTION
N/A

SIGNALMENT

Species
Dogs and cats

Breed Predilections
N/A

Mean Age and Range
N/A

Predominant Sex
N/A

SIGNS

General Comments
Often no clinical signs because condition is a natural response to a variety of physiologic or pathophysiologic stresses

Historical Findings
Weakness, exercise intolerance, or possible collapse if associated with primary cardiac disease or extracardiac disorder

Physical Examination Findings
- High HR
- May otherwise be normal if not associated with a pathologic condition
- Pale mucous membranes if associated with anemia or CHF
- Fever may be present.
- Signs of CHF (e.g., dyspnea, cough, cyanosis, ascites) when ST is associated with primary cardiac disease

CAUSES

Physiologic
- Exercise
- Pain
- Restraint
- Excitement

Pathologic
- Fever
- CHF
- Hyperthyroidism
- Shock
- Anemia
- Infection
- Hypoxia
- Pulmonary thromboembolism
- Hypotension
- Hypovolemia
- Functional pheochromocytoma

Pharmacologic
- Atropine
- Epinephrine
- Ketamine
- Quinidine
- Xanthine bronchodilators
- β-Agonists
- Light anesthesia

RISK FACTORS
- Thyroid medications
- Primary cardiac diseases
- Inflammation
- Pregnancy

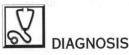 **DIAGNOSIS**

DIFFERENTIAL DIAGNOSIS
Must differentiate from atrial tachycardia, atrial flutter with 2:1 AV block, and AV junctional tachycardia; as sinus rate increases, the P wave appears closer to the T wave of the previous beat, and at very rapid rates, it becomes difficult to distinguish this condition from other pathologic supraventricular tachycardias.

CBC/BIOCHEMISTRY/URINALYSIS
- Low PCV if patient is anemic
- Leukocytosis with left shift if inflammation or infection is causative

OTHER LABORATORY TESTS
- High serum T_4 or free T_4 concentration (cats) if secondary to hyperthyroidism
- T_3 suppression test or TRH response test if T_4 values are normal and hyperthyroidism is suspected
- 24-hr urine sample collection for catecholamine assay and their metabolites in diagnosis

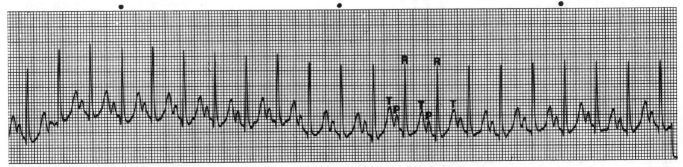

Figure 1.

Sinus tachycardia at a rate of 272/min in a dog in shock. The rhythm is sinus because the P waves are normal, the P-R relationship is normal, and the rhythm is regular. (From: Tilley LP: Essentials of canine and feline electrocardiography. 3rd ed. Baltimore: Williams & Wilkins, 1992, with permission.)

of pheochromocytoma; provocative testing to induce hypertension with histamine and glucagon or hypotension with phentolamine may be useful but is not practical.

IMAGING
• Thoracic radiographs to evaluate for evidence of primary cardiac disease
• Echocardiogram to evaluate for any structural cardiac disease
• Thyroid scan to evaluate for hyperthyroidism
• Abdominal ultrasound and angiography to evaluate for adrenal mass

DIAGNOSTIC PROCEDURES
• Consider nonpharmacologic vagal maneuver to differentiate from other supraventricular tachyarrhythmias; carotid sinus or ocular pressure may terminate ectopic supraventricular tachycardias. With ST, vagal maneuvers produce gradual, transient slowing of the HR if any. Less commonly, varying degrees of AV block (usually first-degree or Wenckebach) may occur transiently. ECG monitoring is recommended during these vagal maneuvers.
• Serial arterial blood pressure measurement may document hypertension in patients with hyperthyroidism, pheochromocytoma, or renal disease.

PATHOLOGIC FINDINGS
• None if associated with physiologic or pharmacologic cause
• Pathologic findings depend on the primary disease process.

TREATMENT

APPROPRIATE HEALTH CARE
• Identify and correct underlying cause whenever possible.
• Whether inpatient or outpatient depends on clinical status of patient and primary disease, if any (e.g., if CHF, treat as outpatient unless animal is dyspneic or severely hypotensive).

NURSING CARE
Depends on whether associated with a specific disease

ACTIVITY
Exercise restriction recommended if symptomatic cardiac disease

DIET
Sodium restriction generally advised in hypertension and CHF.

CLIENT EDUCATION
Discuss importance of managing any primary disease appropriately, with medical or surgical intervention.

SURGICAL CONSIDERATIONS
• Thyroidectomy recommended for hyperthyroidism (cats)
• Tumor removal is the definitive treatment for patients with pheochromocytoma.

MEDICATIONS

DRUGS OF CHOICE
• Establish underlying cause and treat appropriately; specific antiarrhythmic therapy is generally limited to patients in CHF or those with secondary cardiac disease due to hyperthyroidism or hypertension.
• Dogs—if CHF is the cause, administer digoxin along with a diuretic and angiotensin-converting enzyme (ACE) inhibitor. If ST persists despite digoxin, consider adding a β-blocker (e.g., atenolol 0.25–1.0 mg/kg PO q12–24h) or calcium channel blocker (e.g., diltiazem at 0.5–1.5 mg/kg PO q8h) after congestion is controlled.
• Cats—if ST is associated with hyperthyroidism without CHF, a β-blocker (e.g., atenolol 6.25–12.5 mg/cat PO q24h) may lower the HR. Consider digoxin (0.0312 mg PO q24h, average-size cat, tablet preferred) if chronic hyperthyroidism with CHF or for treatment of primary dilated cardiomyopathy. If ST associated with hypertrophic cardiomyopathy, administer diltiazem (1.75–2.4 mg/kg PO q8h) or use sustained-release form of diltiazem (XR or CD 10 mg/kg PO q24h).

CONTRAINDICATIONS
Avoid drugs such as atropine or catecholamines (epinephrine) that may further increase the HR.

PRECAUTIONS
β-Blockers and calcium channel antagonists can worsen signs of congestion and lower cardiac output in patients with systolic dysfunction.

POSSIBLE INTERACTIONS
See manufacturer's insert for specific drug.

ALTERNATIVE DRUGS
• If associated with pericardial effusion, avoid drug therapy and perform pericardiocentesis.
• If associated with a certain drug (e.g., hydralazine, bronchodilators), discontinue the medication or adjust the dose.

FOLLOW-UP

PATIENT MONITORING
Depends on specific disease—for CHF, serial ECG, thoracic radiographs, BUN, creatinine and serum electrolytes; for hyperthyroidism, serial serum T_4, CBC, and biochemistry

PREVENTION AVOIDANCE
Minimize stress, exercise, and dietary sodium, if heart disease.

POSSIBLE COMPLICATIONS
• Weakness or syncope if associated with low cardiac output • Development of CHF if persistent ST associated with heart disease

EXPECTED COURSE AND PROGNOSIS
• Arrhythmia usually resolves with correction of the underlying cause.
• Poor despite treatment if arrhythmia is associated with CHF
• Favorable for remission of ST when hyperthyroidism is controlled medically, surgically, or by radioactive iodine.

MISCELLANEOUS

ASSOCIATED CONDITIONS
N/A

AGE-RELATED FACTORS
N/A

ZOONOTIC POTENTIAL
N/A

PREGNANCY
• Increase in cardiac output in late pregnancy (third trimester) largely due to an accelerated HR • Pregnancy of multiple fetuses in humans associated with an even higher HR; increased susceptibility to arrhythmias, including ST

SYNONYMS
N/A

SEE ALSO
• Atrial Fibrillation and Flutter • Congestive Heart Failure, Left-sided • Congestive Heart Failure, Right-sided • Hyperthyroidism • Pheochromocytoma • Supraventricular Tachycardia

ABBREVIATIONS
• AV = atrioventricular • CHF = congestive heart failure • HR = heart rate • ST = sinus tachycardia • T_4 = thyroxine • T_3 = triiodothyronine • TRH = thyrotropin-releasing hormone

Suggested Reading
Berne RM, Levy MN. Cardiovascular physiology. 6th ed. St. Louis: Mosby Year Book, 1992.
Braunwald E, ed. Heart disease. 5th ed. Philadelphia: Saunders, 1997.
Miller MS, Tilley LP, Smith FWK, Fox PR. Electrocardiography. In: Fox PR, Sisson D, Moise NS, eds. Textbook of canine and feline cardiology. Philadelphia: Saunders, 1999:67–106.
Smith FWK, Hadlock DJ. Electrocardiography. In: Miller MS, Tilley LP, eds. Manual of canine and feline cardiology. 2nd ed. Philadelphia: Saunders, 1995:47–74.
Author Deborah J. Hadlock
Consulting Editors Larry P. Tilley and Francis W. K. Smith, Jr

SUPRAVENTRICULAR TACHYCARDIA

BASICS

DEFINITION
Repetitive supraventricular premature depolarizations that usually originate from a site other than the sinus node, such as the atrial myocardium or atrioventricular junctional tissue

ECG Features
• Heart rate—rapid, 150–350 bpm in dogs
• Rhythm usually very regular (R-R interval is constant) and may be sustained, but there can be frequent or infrequent short runs of supraventricular tachycardia (SVT), so-called paroxysmal SVT. Rarely, the rhythm during the tachycardia will be irregular, suggesting abnormal automaticity.
• Usually the QRS complexes are typical of normal sinus complexes, narrow and upright in lead II. In some cases a coexisting bundle branch block or aberrant ventricular conduction makes it difficult, if not impossible, to differentiate an SVT from a ventricular tachycardia by examining the ECG.
• P waves can be positive or negative in lead II and typically differ in configuration from the sinus P waves. P waves may be buried in the previous T wave and therefore not visualized.
• Atrioventricular conduction is usually normal (1:1), but various levels of functional second-degree AV block may occur at higher atrial rates (2:1, 3:1, 4:1, etc.).

PATHOPHYSIOLOGY
• May result from a reentrant mechanism or from abnormal automaticity in an ectopic focus. Reentrant SVT produces a very regular rhythm; SVT due to an automatic focus in atrial myocardium can be irregular.
• Most cases in dogs respond to drugs that specifically alter conduction and refractoriness in the AV junctional tissue, suggesting AV junctional reentry as the mechanism.
• Recent electrophysiologic studies revealed that some SVT in dogs is related to a congenital accessory pathway between the atria and ventricles that allows the electrical impulses to travel freely between the atria and ventricles (usually in either direction) without traversing the AV node and without conduction delay; in these patients, the SVT is caused by reentry through the accessory pathway.

SYSTEMS AFFECTED

Cardiovascular
Rarely CHF develops secondary to progressive myocardial failure associated with a chronically high heart rate.

Neuromuscular
Syncope or generalized episodic weakness due to reduced cardiac output and oxygen delivery

GENETICS
Labrador retrievers suspected on the basis of clinical data to have a genetic predisposition to one form

SIGNALMENT

Species
Dogs and less commonly cats.

Breed Predilections
Labrador retrievers are overrepresented in the literature.

SIGNS

General Comments
• Clinical signs may relate to the underlying cause.
• Dogs with slow SVT exhibit no clinical signs.
• Dogs with fast SVT (heart rate usually > 300 bpm) generally exhibit weakness or collapse.

Historical Findings
• Owners are generally unaware of the arrhythmia.
• Coughing or breathing abnormalities in dogs with CHF
• Possible episodes of weakness or collapse

Physical Examination Findings
• Rapid, usually regular heart rhythm
• May have evidence of poor peripheral perfusion—pale mucous membranes, a prolonged capillary refill time, and weak pulses
• May have no signs other than the rapid heart rate
• Findings may reflect an underlying cardiac condition (e.g., heart murmur).

CAUSES
• Chronic valvular disease
• Cardiomyopathy
• Congenital heart disease
• Cardiac neoplasia
• Systemic disorders
• Ventricular preexcitation
• Electrolyte imbalances
• Digoxin toxicity
• Idiopathic

RISK FACTORS
Heart disease

DIAGNOSIS

DIFFERENTIAL DIAGNOSIS
• Sinus tachycardia
• Atrial flutter
• Atrial fibrillation
• Ventricular tachycardia (SVT with right bundle branch block or aberrant conduction can look like ventricular tachycardia; resolution of arrhythmia after lidocaine administration usually confirms ventricular tachycardia)

IMAGING
• Echocardiography (including Doppler studies) may help characterize the type and severity of underlying cardiac disorders.
• When viewed on an echocardiogram during bursts of SVT, the left ventricle has a normal end-systolic diameter and a small end-diastolic diameter, resulting in a decreased shortening fraction because of inadequate filling.
• Usually left or right atrial enlargement in dogs with SVT secondary to other cardiac disorders

DIAGNOSTIC PROCEDURES
• Long-term ambulatory (Holter) recording of the ECG may detect paroxysmal SVT in cases of unexplained syncope; Holter monitors may also help characterize the rate and frequency of sustained SVT and are useful in evaluating therapy.
• Sustained SVT must be distinguished from sinus tachycardia because the two arrhythmias have different implications and treatment. A precordial thump may help differentiate sinus tachycardia from SVT when the heart rate is in the 150–250 bpm range; it will usually stop an SVT for at least 1 or 2 beats, while a sinus tachycardia will not slow. A vagal maneuver (e.g., ocular pressure or carotid sinus massage) may break an SVT abruptly but only gradually slows sinus tachycardia.

PATHOLOGIC FINDINGS
N/A

TREATMENT

APPROPRIATE HEALTH CARE
• Asymptomatic patients can be managed on an out-patient basis; patients with a sustained SVT or signs of heart failure should be hospitalized until stable.
• SVT is a medical emergency in dogs that exhibit weakness and collapse; nondrug interventions that may break an SVT include vagal maneuvers, precordial thump, and electrical cardioversion
• Vagal maneuvers are often unsuccessful but may be used initially because of their ease of administration and noninvasive nature.
• Delivering a precordial thump very successfully (>90% of the time) terminates an SVT in dogs, but, this maneuver may only break the rhythm for a brief period. At other times the rhythm remains converted. To perform a precordial thump, the dog is placed on its right side and the left apex beat is located. This region is then "thumped" with a fist while recording the ECG. Electrical cardioversion or intracardiac electrophysiologic pacing methods may be considered in extreme cases.

NURSING CARE
Treat CHF and correct any underlying electrolyte or acid/base disturbances.

ACTIVITY
Restrict until arrhythmia has been controlled

DIET
Sodium restriction if in CHF

CLIENT EDUCATION
Owners should observe patients closely for signs of low cardiac output such as weakness and collapse.

SURGICAL CONSIDERATIONS
Consider transvenous catheter ablation for patients with accessory pathways

MEDICATIONS

DRUGS OF CHOICE

Emergency Therapy
Administer one of the following drugs:
• Calcium channel blockers—verapamil (0.05 mg/kg boluses IV over 3–5 min up to 3 times) or diltiazem (0.05–0.25 mg/kg IV over 5–15 min)
• β-Adrenergic blockers—propranolol (0.02 mg/kg slow IV boluses up to a total dose of 0.1 mg/kg) or esmolol (0. 25–0.5 mg/kg slow IV bolus administration followed by a constant-rate infusion of 50–200 μg/kg/min); moderate-to-severe myocardial failure is a relative contra-indication to the administration of these drugs at these doses.

Long-term Therapy
• Digoxin—administer at either a maintenance oral dose or double the maintenance dose for the first day to produce a therapeutic serum concentration more rapidly; contraindicated in patients with accessory pathways
• β-Adrenergic blocker—propranolol or atenolol can be administered at doses of 0.5–2.0 mg/kg as long as the patient does not have underlying moderate-to-severe myocardial failure.

• Diltiazem is the calcium channel blocker of choice for long-term control of SVT. The dosage required to control SVT has not been reported in the dog. Diltiazem is used more frequently to control the ventricular rate in patients with atrial fibrillation at a dosage of 0.5–1.5 mg/kg PO q8h. In our clinic, we generally start in this dosage range but almost always need to increase the dose to 2.0–3.0 mg/kg PO q8h to effect control.
• Class I antiarrhythmic agents such as quinidine and procainamide can be tried when the aforementioned drugs are ineffective or when the SVT is thought to be due to an automatic, rather than a reentrant, rhythm. SVT caused by an automatic atrial focus may produce an irregular rhythm and may be refractory to conventional drug therapy.

CONTRAINDICATIONS
Avoid use of calcium channel blockers in combination with β-blockers; clinically significant bradyarrhythmias can develop.

PRECAUTIONS
Calcium channel blockers and β-adrenergic blockers have negative inotropic properties and should be used cautiously in dogs with documented myocardial failure.

POSSIBLE INTERACTIONS
N/A

ALTERNATIVE DRUGS
Emergency treatment—intravenous adenosine (1–12 mg IV rapidly) or digoxin (0.01 mg/kg IV slowly). Adenosine is very expensive and short-lived; intravenous digoxin therapy is not recommended because of the risk of overdose.

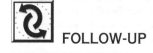

FOLLOW-UP

PATIENT MONITORING
Serial ECG

POSSIBLE COMPLICATIONS
Syncope and CHF

EXPECTED COURSE AND PROGNOSIS
Most is controlled effectively with medication.

MISCELLANEOUS

ASSOCIATED CONDITIONS
Accessory pathways in some patients

AGE-RELATED FACTORS
In young dogs without evidence of structural heart disease, suspect a reentrant tachycardia involving an accessory pathway.

SYNONYMS
Atrial tachycardia, junctional tachycardia

SEE ALSO
Atrial Fibrillation and Atrial Flutter

ABBREVIATIONS
• CHF = congestive heart failure
• SVT = supraventricular tachycardia

Suggested Reading
Atkins CE, Wright KN. Supraventricular tachycardia associated with accessory path-ways in dogs. In: Bonagura JD, ed. Current veterinary therapy XII. Philadelphia: WB Saunders, 1995:807–810.
Wright KN. Assessment and treatment of supraventricular tachyarrhythmias. In: Bonagura JD, ed. Kirk's current veterinary therapy XIII. Philadelphia: WB Saunders. 1999:726–730.
Author Richard D. Kienle
Consulting Editors Larry P. Tilley and Francis W. K. Smith, Jr.

DIAGNOSTICS—ECG

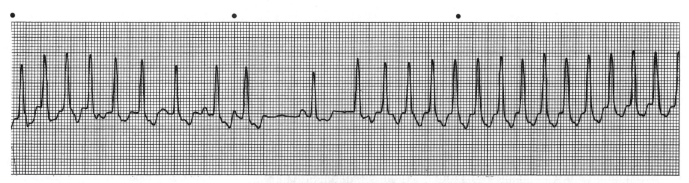

Figure 1.

Sinus with an atrial premature complex and paroxysmal supraventricular tachycardia. Abrupt initiation and termination of the tachycardia help distinguish it from sinus tachycardia (lead II, 50 mm/sec, 1 cm = 1 mV). (From: Tilley LP: Essentials of canine and feline electrocardiography. 3rd ed. Baltimore: Williams & Wilkins, 1992, with permission.)

VENTRICULAR FIBRILLATION

 BASICS

DEFINITION
Ventricular rhythm associated with loss of organized ventricular activity resulting in cardiac muscle fibrillation

ECG Features
• Rapid, chaotic, irregular rhythm with bizarre waves or oscillations (Figures 1 and 2)
• No P waves
• No QRS complexes
• Oscillations may be large (coarse fibrillation) or small (fine fibrillation)

PATHOPHYSIOLOGY
Loss of organized ventricular activity results in acute and profound drop in cardiac output, usually followed by death.

SYSTEMS AFFECTED
• Cardiovascular
• All organ systems affected by loss of perfusion

GENETICS
N/A

INCIDENCE/PREVALENCE
Unknown

GEOGRAPHIC DISTRIBUTION
None

SIGNALMENT

Species
Dogs and cats

Breed predisposition
None

Mean age and range
Unknown, but probably more common in old animals

SIGNS

Historical Findings
• Severe systemic illness or cardiac disease in many patients
• Previous cardiac arrhythmias in some patients

Physical Examination Findings
• Cardiac arrest
• Collapse
• Death

CAUSES
• Anoxia
• Aortic stenosis
• Autonomic imbalances, especially high sympathetic tone or administration of catecholamines
• Cardiac surgery
• Drug reactions—e.g., anesthetic agents, especially halothane and ultrashort-acting barbiturates, digoxin
• Electrical shock
• Electrolyte and acid–base imbalances
• Hypothermia
• Myocardial injury
• Myocarditis
• Shock

RISK FACTORS
Any severe systemic illness or heart disease

 DIAGNOSIS

DIFFERENTIAL DIAGNOSIS
Rule out ECG artifact. Reapply ECG clips and ensure good skin contact and adequate alcohol applied to leads.

CBC/BIOCHEMISTRY/URINALYSIS
Abnormalities generally relate to the underlying metabolic problem that causes ventricular fibrillation

OTHER LABORATORY TESTS
N/A

IMAGING
N/A

DIAGNOSTIC PROCEDURES
N/A

PATHOLOGIC FINDINGS
N/A

 TREATMENT

APPROPRIATE HEALTH CARE
• Rapidly fatal rhythm requiring immediate, aggressive treatment
• Patient will probably die without electrical cardioversion.

Cardioversion Technique
• External countershock—50–100 watt-sec (small patients); 100–360 watt-sec (large patients)
• Internal countershock—10–25 watt-sec (small patients); 25–100 watt-sec (large patients)
• Repeat twice if first attempts fail.
• Start at the low end and increase power with each shock.
• If no access to electrical defibrillator, administer a precordial thump. Apply a sharp blow with your open fist to the chest wall over the heart. Rarely successful, but you have nothing to lose.

NURSING CARE
Treat any problems such as hypothermia, hyperkalemia, and acid–base disorders.

ACTIVITY
N/A

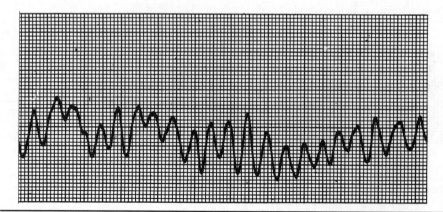

Figure 1.

Coarse ventricular fibrillation. (From: Tilley LP: Essentials of canine and feline electrocardiography. 3rd ed. Baltimore: Williams & Wilkins, 1992, with permission.)

VENTRICULAR FIBRILLATION

DIET
N/A

CLIENT EDUCATION
If the patient is converted back to a sinus rhythm, warn the owner that the patient is at high risk for recurrence of the arrhythmia in the immediate postresuscitation period.

SURGICAL CONSIDERATIONS
N/A

MEDICATIONS

DRUGS OF CHOICE
• Institute CPCR.
• Epinephrine (0.2 mg/kg IV, IT, IL; double the dose and dilute with equal volume of saline for IT administration)—may change fine fibrillation to coarse fibrillation and increase the chances of electrical cardioversion
• Once animal is successfully converted, administer lidocaine to lower the risk of refibrillation or development of ventricular tachycardia.

CONTRAINDICATIONS
None

PRECAUTIONS
Lidocaine raises the fibrillation threshold, but makes defibrillation more difficult.

POSSIBLE INTERACTIONS
Bretylium is recommended in humans to treat recurrent ventricular fibrillation, but in dogs and cats this drug may precipitate ventricular arrhythmias, including ventricular fibrillation.

ALTERNATIVE DRUGS
Chemical conversion can be attempted if no access to electrical defibrillator. Administer 1.0 mEq potassium/kg and 6.0 mg acetylcholine/kg IC; rarely successful

FOLLOW-UP

PATIENT MONITORING
• CBC, urinalysis, biochemistry profile, arterial blood gases, and acid–base status.
• If primary cardiac disease is suspected—echocardiogram and thoracic radiographs
• Monitor ECG closely and frequently.

PREVENTION/AVOIDANCE
Careful monitoring of critically ill patients to prevent and correct acid–base disturbances, hypotension, and hypoxemia

POSSIBLE COMPLICATIONS
• Death
• DIC and multiorgan failure

EXPECTED COURSE AND PROGNOSIS
Most patients die because of either the arrhythmia or the underlying disease.

MISCELLANEOUS

ASSOCIATED CONDITIONS
None

AGE-RELATED FACTORS
None

ZOONOTIC POTENTIAL
None

PREGNANCY
N/A

SYNONYMS
None

SEE ALSO
Cardiopulmonary Arrest

ABBREVIATIONS
• DIC = disseminated intravascular coagulation
• IC = intracardiac
• IL = intralingual
• IT = intratracheal

Suggested Reading
Crowe DT, Fox PR, Devey JJ, Spreng D. Cardiopulmonary and cerebral resuscitation. In: Fox PR, Sisson D, Moise NS, eds. Textbook of canine and feline cardiology. 2nd ed. Philadelphia: WB Saunders. 1999:427–454.
Tilley LP. Essentials of canine and feline electrocardiography. 3rd ed. Baltimore: Williams & Wilkins. 1992.
Author Francis W. K. Smith, Jr.
Consulting Editors Larry P. Tilley and Francis W. K. Smith, Jr.

DIAGNOSTICS—ECG

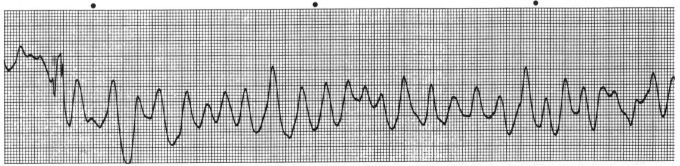

Figure 2.

Ventricular flutter-fibrillation in a cat with severe myocardial damage from an 11-story fall. The complexes are very wide, bizarre, tall, and rapid. (From: Tilley LP: Essentials of canine and feline electrocardiography. 3rd ed. Baltimore: Williams & Wilkins, 1992, with permission.)

VENTRICULAR PREMATURE COMPLEXES

 BASICS

DEFINITION
Single cardiac impulse initiated within the ventricles instead of the sinus node

ECG Features
• QRS complexes typically wide and bizarre (Figures 1 and 2)
• P waves dissociated from the QRS complexes

PATHOPHYSIOLOGY
Mechanisms include increased automaticity, reentry, and delayed afterdepolarizations.

SYSTEMS AFFECTED
Cardiovascular—secondary effects on other systems because of poor perfusion

GENETICS
N/A

INCIDENCE/PREVALENCE
Unknown

GEOGRAPHIC DISTRIBUTION
N/A

SIGNALMENT

Species
Dog and cat

Breed Predisposition
• Common in large-breed dogs with cardiomyopathy, especially boxers and Doberman pinschers
• Common in cats with cardiomyopathy; occasionally seen in cats with hyperthyroidism

Mean Age and Range
Seen in all age groups

SIGNS

Historical Findings
• Weakness
• Exercise intolerance
• Syncope
• Sudden death
• Often asymptomatic

Physical Examination Findings
• Irregular rhythm associated with pulse deficits; may auscult splitting of the first or second heart sound
• May be normal if arrhythmia is intermittent and absent during examination
• May observe signs of CHF (e.g., cough, dyspnea) or murmur, depending on the cause of arrhythmia

CAUSES
• Cardiomyopathy
• Congenital defects (especially subaortic stenosis)
• Chronic valve disease
• Gastric torsion/volvulus
• Traumatic myocarditis (dogs)
• Digitalis toxicity
• Hyperthyroidism (cats)
• Cardiac neoplasia
• Myocarditis

RISK FACTORS
• Hypokalemia
• Hypomagnesemia
• Acid–base disturbances
• Hypoxia

 DIAGNOSIS

DIFFERENTIAL DIAGNOSIS
Supraventricular premature beats with bundle branch block
• Look for P waves associated with the wide QRS complexes; an atrial premature complex with aberrant conduction has an associated P wave.
• An atrial premature complex is usually followed by a noncompensatory pause (Fig. 2)
• A ventricular premature complex is usually followed by a compensatory pause (Fig. 1).

CBC/BIOCHEMISTRY/URINALYSIS
• Hypokalemia and hypomagnesemia predispose animals to ventricular arrhythmias and blunt the response to class 1 antiarrhythmic drugs (e.g., lidocaine, procainamide, and quinidine).
• High amylase and lipase if condition is secondary to pancreatitis

OTHER LABORATORY TESTS
High T_4 (cats) if condition is secondary to hyperthyroidism

IMAGING
Echocardiography may reveal structural heart disease.

DIAGNOSTIC PROCEDURES
Long-term ambulatory (Holter) recording of the ECG to detect transient ventricular arrhythmias in patients with unexplained syncope or weakness

PATHOLOGIC FINDINGS
Varies with underlying cause

 TREATMENT

APPROPRIATE HEALTH CARE
Generally outpatient basis

NURSING CARE
Varies with underlying cause

ACTIVITY
Restrict if the arrhythmia is accompanied by clinical signs or evidence of structural heart disease.

DIET
N/A

CLIENT EDUCATION
Alert owner to potential for the arrhythmia worsening and syncope or sudden death.

SURGICAL CONSIDERATIONS
• Continuous ECG monitoring recommended while anesthetized
• Premedicating the patient with acepromazine (0.02–0.05 mg/kg) raises the threshold for ventricular fibrillation.
• Mask inductions not recommended; sympathetic release during mask induction can aggravate arrhythmia.

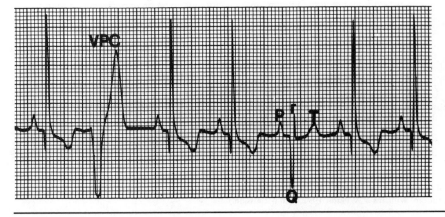

Figure 1.

VPC and a fusion complex (fifth complex) in a dog with myocarditis from a pancreatitis. A fusion complex is the simultaneous activation of the ventricle by impulses coming from the SA node and the ventricular ectopic foci. The QRS complex is intermediate in form. (From: Tilley LP: Essentials of canine and feline electrocardiography. 3rd ed. Baltimore: Williams & Wilkins, 1992, with permission.)

VENTRICULAR PREMATURE COMPLEXES

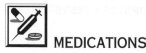

MEDICATIONS

DRUGS OF CHOICE

General Comments
- Correct any hypokalemia or hypomagnesemia.
- Drug therapy in the absence of clinical signs—controversial; studies in humans with asymptomatic VPCs and myocardial infarctions demonstrated a high incidence of sudden death when treatment is initiated with class 1 antiarrhythmic agents; no similar studies in veterinary patients
- The author generally does not prescribe antiarrhythmic drugs unless there is evidence of clinical signs of low cardiac output (e.g. episodic weakness or syncope) or the belief that the patient is at high risk of sudden death, based on presence of R on T phenomenon or breed association with VPCs and sudden death (e.g., boxers and Doberman pinschers).
- If antiarrhythmic therapy is initiated in an attempt to lower the risk of sudden death, the author usually chooses a β-blocker; no studies have been done to confirm efficacy of β-blockers for prevention of sudden death in dogs or cats.

Dogs
- Patient not in CHF or hypotensive—initiate therapy with a β-blocker such as propranolol (0.2–1 mg/kg PO q8h), atenolol (0.2–1 mg/kg q12h), or metoprolol (0.2–1 mg/kg PO q8–12h).
- Patient in CHF or hypotensive—initiate therapy with a class I antiarrhythmic agent such as procainamide (8–20 mg/kg PO q6–8h) or mexiletine (5–8 mg/kg PO q8h).
- Combine a class I antiarrhythmic drug with a β-blocker if important arrhythmia persists.

Cats
Propranolol (2.5–5 mg PO q8h) or atenolol (6.25 mg PO q12h)

CONTRAINDICATIONS
Avoid atropine, catecholamines (e.g., epinephrine and dopamine) until arrhythmia is controlled.

PRECAUTIONS
- Use β-blockers cautiously in animals with CHF; they initially depress myocardial contractility.
- Use digoxin cautiously; it can potentially aggravate ventricular arrhythmias.

POSSIBLE INTERACTIONS
Quinidine and amiodarone raise serum digoxin levels.

ALTERNATIVE DRUGS
- Consider sotalol or amiodarone for refractory arrhythmias in dogs (generally reserved for ventricular tachycardia).
- Consider procainamide for cats that do not tolerate β-blockers.

FOLLOW-UP

PATIENT MONITORING
- Holter monitoring preferred for monitoring severity of the arrhythmia and efficacy of antiarrhythmic therapy; the goal of antiarrhythmic therapy is to reduce the frequency of ventricular ectopy by > 75%.
- Serial ECGs and telemetry can be used, but are not as useful as Holter monitoring as VPCs; paroxysmal ventricular tachycardia can occur sporadically through the day.
- Serum digoxin levels in patients receiving that medication

PREVENTION/AVOIDANCE
Correct predisposing factors such as hypokalemia, hypomagnesemia, myocardial hypoxia, and digoxin toxicity.

POSSIBLE COMPLICATIONS
Syncope, sudden death

EXPECTED COURSE AND PROGNOSIS
- If cause is metabolic—condition may resolve with good prognosis.
- If condition is associated with cardiac disease—prognosis is guarded; VPCs may increase the risk of sudden death.

MISCELLANEOUS

ASSOCIATED CONDITIONS
N/A

AGE-RELATED FACTORS
N/A

ZOONOTIC POTENTIAL
N/A

PREGNANCY
N/A

SYNONYMS
N/A

SEE ALSO
- Digoxin Toxicity
- Myocarditis
- Trypanosomiasis (Chagas' Disease)
- Ventricular Tachycardia

ABBREVIATIONS
- bpm = beats per minute
- CHF = congestive heart failure
- VPC = ventricular premature complex

Suggested Reading
Calvert CA. Diagnosis and management of ventricular arrhythmias in Doberman pinschers with cardiomyopathy. In: Bonagura JD, ed. Current veterinary therapy XII. Philadelphia: Saunders, 1995:799–806.
Moise NS, Gilmour RF Jr. Inherited sudden cardiac death in German shepherds. In: Kirk RW, Bonagura JD, eds. Current veterinary therapy XI. Philadelphia: Saunders, 1992:749–751.
Tilley LP. Essentials of canine and feline electrocardiography. 3rd ed. Baltimore: Williams & Wilkins, 1992.

Author Francis W. K. Smith, Jr.
Consulting Editors Larry P. Tilley and Francis W. K. Smith, Jr.

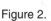
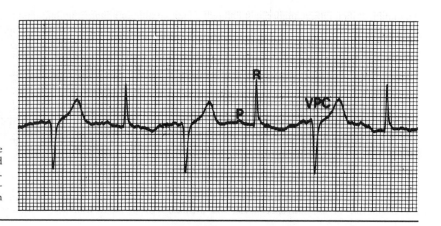

Figure 2.

Ventricular bigeminy. Every other complex is a VPC from the same focus. Each is coupled (interval the same between it and the adjacent sinus complex) to the preceding normal complex. (From: Tilley LP: Essentials of canine and feline electrocardiography. 3rd ed. Baltimore: Williams & Wilkins, 1992, with permission.)

VENTRICULAR STANDSTILL (ASYSTOLE)

 ## BASICS

DEFINITION
Absence of ventricular complexes on the ECG or absence of ventricular activity (electrical–mechanical dissociation)

ECG Features
Ventricular asystole—can result from severe sinoatrial block or arrest or by third-degree AV block (Figure 1) without a junctional or ventricular escape rhythm
• P waves present if patient has complete AV block
• P waves absent during asystole if patient has severe sinoatrial block or arrest
• No QRS complexes
• Electrical-mechanical dissociation—a recorded ECG cardiac rhythm (P-QRS-T) and no effective cardiac output or palpable femoral pulse

PATHOPHYSIOLOGY
Ventricular asystole represents cardiac arrest; if the ventricular rhythm is not restored in 3–4 min, irreversible brain injury can occur

SYSTEMS AFFECTED
• Cardiovascular
• All organ systems affected by loss of perfusion

GENETICS
N/A

INCIDENCE/PREVALENCE
Unknown

GEOGRAPHIC DISTRIBUTION
None

SIGNALMENT

Species
Dogs and cats

Breed Predisposition
none

Mean Age and Range
Unknown

SIGNS

Historical Findings
• Severe systemic illness or cardiac disease in many patients
• Other cardiac arrhythmias in some
• Syncope

Physical Examination Findings
• No ventricular pulse can be palpated.
• Cardiac arrest
• Collapse
• Death

CAUSES
• Complete AV block with absence of ventricular or junctional escape rhythm
• Severe sinus arrest or block
• Hyperkalemia (Figure 2)

RISK FACTORS
• Any severe systemic illness (e.g., severe acidosis and hyperkalemia) or heart disease
• Hypoadrenocorticism causing hyperkalemia
• Urinary tract rupture of obstruction, resulting in hyperkalemia

 ## DIAGNOSIS

DIFFERENTIAL DIAGNOSIS
Rule out ECG artifact; reapply ECG clips and make sure skin contact is good and adequate alcohol is applied to leads.

CBC/BIOCHEMISTRY/URINALYSIS
Severe hyperkalemia possible cause

OTHER LABORATORY TESTS
N/A

IMAGING
N/A

DIAGNOSTIC PROCEDURES
Systemic blood pressure—readable pressure absent

PATHOLOGIC FINDINGS
N/A

 ## TREATMENT

APPROPRIATE HEALTH CARE
• Potentially fatal rhythm requiring immediate aggressive treatment
• Artificial pacing with a transvenous pacemaker may succeed if myocardium is mechanically responsive.
• DC electrical conversion is not effective unless the rhythm can first be converted to ventricular fibrillation with medications.

NURSING CARE
Treat any treatable problems such as hypothermia, hyperkalemia, and acid–base disorders.

ACTIVITY
N/A

DIET
N/A

CLIENT EDUCATION
None

SURGICAL CONSIDERATIONS
None

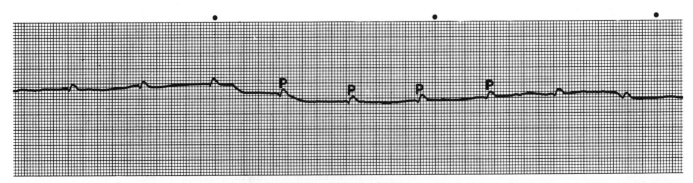

Figure 1.

Ventricular asystole in a dog with severe complete AV block. Only P wages (atrial activity) are present; there is no ventricular activity. (Lead II, 50 mm/sec, 1 cm = 1 mV) (From: Tilley LP: Essentials of canine and feline electrocardiography. 3rd ed. Baltimore: Williams & Wilkins, 1992, with permission.)

VENTRICULAR STANDSTILL (ASYSTOLE)

 MEDICATIONS

DRUGS OF CHOICE
• Institute cardiopulmonary resuscitation.
• Epinephrine—0.2 mg/kg IV, IT, or IL (double the dose for IT administration and deliver with equal volume of saline)
• Atropine—0.05 mg/kg IV, IT, or IL (double the dose for IT administration and deliver with equal volume of saline)
• Sodium bicarbonate—1 mEq/kg IV for each 10 min of cardiac arrest
• Dexamethasone and dopamine may be helpful in patients with electrical-mechanical dissociation

CONTRAINDICATIONS
Drugs that depress sinus node or AV node conduction in patients with sinus arrest or heart block (e.g., β-blockers, calcium channel blockers, digoxin)

PRECAUTIONS
None

POSSIBLE INTERACTIONS
None

ALTERNATIVE DRUGS
Calcium gluconate—patients with ventricular standstill and hyperkalemia.

 FOLLOW-UP

PATIENT MONITORING
• If animal is resuscitated—evaluate CBC, biochemical analysis, and urinalysis
• If animal survives and primary cardiac disease is suspected—an echocardiogram and thoracic radiographs
• ECG—closely and frequently

PREVENTION/AVOIDANCE
Careful monitoring of critically ill patients to prevent and correct acid–base disturbances, hypotension, and hypoxemia

POSSIBLE COMPLICATIONS
• Death
• DIC and multiorgan failure

EXPECTED COURSE AND PROGNOSIS
Patients that arrest frequently have recurrent arrest.

 MISCELLANEOUS

ASSOCIATED CONDITIONS
None

AGE-RELATED FACTORS
None

ZOONOTIC POTENTIAL
None

PREGNANCY
None

SYNONYMS
Ventricular asystole

SEE ALSO
• Cardiopulmonary arrest
• Atrioventricular block, complete
• Sinus arrest or block

ABBREVIATIONS
• AV = antrioventricular
• DC = direct current
• DIC = disseminated intravascular coagulation
• IL = intralingual
• IT = intratracheal

Suggested Reading
Tilley LP. Essentials of canine and feline electrocardiography 3rd ed. Baltimore: Williams & Wilkins, 1992.
Author Francis W. K. Smith, Jr.
Consulting Editors Larry P. Tilley and Francis W. K. Smith, Jr.

DIAGNOSTICS—ECG

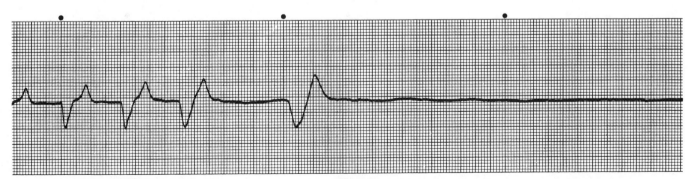

Figure 2.

Ventricular asystole in a cat with severe hyperkalemia (11 mEq/L) from urethral obstruction. No P waves or QRS complexes are seen after four wide and bizarre QRS complexes (atrial standstill with delayed ventricular conduction). (Lead II, 50 mm/sec, 1 cm = 1 mV) (From: Tilley LP: Essentials of canine and feline electrocardiography. 3rd ed. Baltimore: Williams & Wilkins, 1992, with permission.)

VENTRICULAR TACHYCARDIA

 BASICS

DEFINITION

ECG Features
• Three or more ventricular premature contractions in a row
• May be intermittent (paroxysmal) or sustained; heart rate > 150 bpm with a regular rhythm
• QRS complexes—typically wide and bizarre.
• If P waves—dissociated from the QRS complexes (Figure 1).

PATHOPHYSIOLOGY
Potentially life-threatening arrhythmia, usually signifying myocardial disease or metabolic derangement; mechanisms include increased automaticity, reentry, and delayed afterdepolarizations

SYSTEMS AFFECTED
Cardiovascular system, with secondary effects on other systems because of poor perfusion

GENETICS
Ventricular arrhythmias and sudden cardiac death hereditary in German shepherds, but mode of inheritance not determined. Arrhythmogenic boxer cardiomyopathy—probably inherited

INCIDENCE/PREVALENCE
Common arrhythmia in dogs, uncommon in cats

GEOGRAPHIC DISTRIBUTION
None

SIGNALMENT

Species
Dogs and cats

Breed predisposition
• German shepherds with sudden cardiac death
• Commonly seen in large-breed dogs with cardiomyopathy, especially boxers and Doberman pinschers

Mean Age and Range
• All age groups
• German shepherds with sudden cardiac death—usually present at 4–6 months of age
• Boxers with arrhythmogenic cardiomyopathy—usually present at 4–6 years of age.
• Doberman pinschers with occult cardiomyopathy typically develop ventricular arrhythmias beginning at 3–6 years of age, but can be much earlier; frequency and severity of the arrhythmia usually increases over time.

SIGNS

Historical Findings
• Weakness
• Exercise intolerance
• Syncope
• Sudden death
• May be asymptomatic

Physical Examination Findings
• Paroxysmal or sustained tachycardia
• May be normal if arrhythmia is paroxysmal and absent during examination
• Signs of congestive heart failure (CHF) or murmur may be present, depending on cause of arrhythmia

CAUSES
• Cardiomyopathy
• Congenital defects (especially subaortic stenosis)
• Chronic valve disease
• Gastric dilation and volvulus
• Traumatic myocarditis (dogs)
• Digitalis toxicity
• Hyperthyroidism (cats)
• Cardiac neoplasia
• Myocarditis
• Pancreatitis

RISK FACTORS
• Hypokalemia
• Hypomagnesemia
• Acid–base disturbances
• Hypoxemia

 DIAGNOSIS

DIFFERENTIAL DIAGNOSIS
Supraventricular tachycardia with bundle branch block. If P waves can be identified, look for association between P waves and QRS complexes. If there is a consistent P-R interval, then the rhythm is supraventricular with bundle branch block. If no association between P waves and QRS complexes, the rhythm is probably ventricular tachycardia. If P waves cannot be identified, use response to lidocaine to differentiate. Termination of arrhythmia after administration of lidocaine supports ventricular tachycardia.

CBC/BIOCHEMISTRY/URINALYSIS
• Hypokalemia and hypomagnesemia predispose animal to ventricular tachycardia and blunt response to class 1 antiarrhythmic drugs (e.g., lidocaine, procainamide, and quinidine).
• High amylase and lipase if arrhythmia is secondary to pancreatitis

OTHER LABORATORY TESTS
High T_4 (cats) if arrhythmia is secondary to hyperthyroidism

IMAGING
Echocardiography may reveal structural heart disease.

DIAGNOSTIC PROCEDURES
Long-term ambulatory (Holter) recording of the ECG—detection of transient ventricular arrhythmias in patients with unexplained syncope or weakness

PATHOLOGIC FINDINGS
Vary with underlying cause

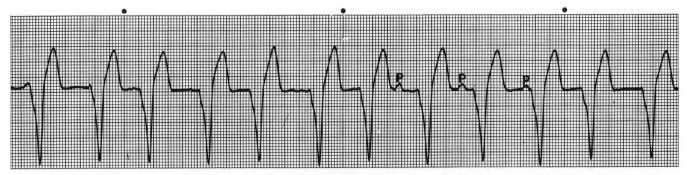

Figure 1.

Ventricular tachycardia. The wide and bizarre QRS complexes occur at a rate of 160 beats/min, with no relationship to the P waves. There are more QRS complexes than P waves. Ventricular tachycardia should be treated as soon as possible. Acid-base and electrolyte abnormalities should always be corrected. (From: Tilley LP: Essentials of canine and feline electrocardiography. 3rd ed. Baltimore: Williams & Wilkins, 1992, with permission.)

VENTRICULAR TACHYCARDIA

 TREATMENT

APPROPRIATE HEALTH CARE
Treat as inpatient until arrhythmia is controlled and patient is hemodynamically stable.

NURSING CARE
Varies with underlying cause

ACTIVITY
Restrict

DIET
N/A

CLIENT EDUCATION
Alert the owner to the potential for sudden death.

SURGICAL CONSIDERATIONS
• Continuous ECG while anesthetized—recommended
• Should be controlled prior to inducing general anesthesia
• Premedication with acepromazine (0.02–0.05 mg/kg) raises the threshold for ventricular fibrillation.
• Mask inductions not recommended in patients with ventricular arrhythmias; sympathetic release during mask induction can aggravate the arrhythmia.

 MEDICATIONS

DRUGS OF CHOICE
Correct any hypokalemia or hypomagnesemia

Dogs
• Administer lidocaine slowly in 2 mg/kg IV boluses (up to 8 mg/kg total) to convert to sinus rhythm; follow with lidocaine infusion 25–75 µg/kg/min.
• If lidocaine fails—administer procainamide slowly in 2 mg/kg IV boluses (up to 20 mg/kg total) to convert to sinus rhythm; follow with procainamide infusion at 20–50 µg/kg/min or 8–20 mg/kg IM q6h.
• If lidocaine and procainamide fail to convert the rhythm—administer magnesium sulfate diluted in normal saline or D_5W at 25–30 mg/kg IV over 5–10 min. If the arrhythmia improves, administer the same dosage in intravenous fluids over the next 4–8 h.
• If the patient does not respond to lidocaine, procainamide or magnesium—administer slow IV boluses of esmolol (a short-acting β-blocker) at 0.05–0.1 mg/kg q5min to cumu-

lative dose of 0.5 mg/kg; or 50–200 µg/kg/min constant rate infusion
• When the patient is stable, give procainamide (8–20 mg/kg PO q6–8h), quinidine (6–20 mg/kg PO q6–8h), mexiletine (5–8 mg/kg PO q8h), or sotalol (1–2 mg/kg PO q12h)
• Combine previous drugs (except sotalol) with a β-blocker (e.g., propranolol or atenolol) if arrhythmia persists.

Cats
• Use lidocaine cautiously and only for sustained ventricular tachycardia; neurotoxicity is common in cats. Use one-tenth of the dosage for dogs.
• Propranolol (2.5–5 mg PO q8h) or atenolol (6.25–12.5 mg PO q12h) is preferred in cats.

CONTRAINDICATIONS
• Avoid atropine, catecholamines (e.g., epinephrine, dopamine), and digoxin until arrhythmia is controlled.

PRECAUTIONS
Use β-blockers cautiously in animals with CHF.

POSSIBLE INTERACTIONS
Quinidine and amiodarone raise digoxin levels.

ALTERNATIVE DRUGS
• Consider amiodarone for refractory arrhythmias in dogs.
• Consider procainamide for refractory arrhythmias in cats.

 FOLLOW-UP

PATIENT MONITORING
• Holter monitoring is preferred for monitoring severity of the arrhythmia and efficacy of antiarrhythmic therapy; the goal of antiarrhythmic therapy is to reduce the frequency of ventricular ectopy by > 75%.
• Serial ECGs and telemetry can be used—not as useful as Holter monitoring because ventricular premature complexes and paroxysmal ventricular tachycardia can occur sporadically through the day.
• Serum digoxin levels in patients receiving that medication.

PREVENTION/AVOIDANCE
Correct predisposing factors such as hypokalemia, hypomagnesemia, myocardial hypoxia, and digoxin toxicity.

POSSIBLE COMPLICATIONS
• Syncope
• Sudden death

EXPECTED COURSE AND PROGNOSIS
• If cause is metabolic—condition may resolve with good prognosis.
• If condition is associated with cardiac disease—prognosis guarded; ventricular tachycardia may increase the risk of sudden death.
• Approximately 50% of German shepherds with ventricular tachycardia and inherited sudden death syndrome die acutely within the first year of life.

 MISCELLANEOUS

ASSOCIATED CONDITIONS
N/A

AGE-RELATED FACTORS
N/A

ZOONOTIC POTENTIAL
None

PREGNANCY
N /A

SYNONYMS
None

SEE ALSO
• Digoxin Toxicity
• Myocarditis
• Trypanosomiasis (Chagas' Disease)
• Ventricular Premature Complexes

ABBREVIATION
• bpm = beats per minute
• CHF = congestive heart failure

Suggested Reading
Calvert CA. Diagnosis and management of ventricular arrhythmias in Doberman pinschers with cardiomyopathy. In Bonagura JD, ed. Current veterinary therapy XII. Philadelphia: Saunders, 1995:799–806.
Moise NS, Gilmour RF Jr. Inherited sudden cardiac death in German shepherds. In: Kirk RW, Bonagura JD, eds. Current veterinary therapy XI. Philadelphia: Saunders, 1992:749–751.
Tilley LP. Essentials of canine and feline electrocardiography. 3rd ed. Baltimore: Williams & Wilkins, 1992.
Author Francis W. K. Smith, Jr.
Consulting Editors Larry P. Tilley and Francis W. K. Smith, Jr

DIAGNOSTICS—ECG

WOLFF-PARKINSON-WHITE SYNDROME

BASICS

DEFINITION
• Ventricular preexcitation occurs when impulses originating in the sinoatrial node or atrium activate a portion of the ventricles prematurely through an accessory pathway without going through the AV node; the remainder of the ventricles is activated normally through the usual conduction system.
• WPW syndrome consists of ventricular preexcitation with episodes of paroxysmal supraventricular tachycardia. (Figures 1 and 2)

ECG Features of Ventricular Preexcitation
• Normal heart rate and rhythm
• Normal P waves
• Short P-R interval (dogs, < 0.06 sec; cats, < 0.05 sec)
• Widened QRS (small dogs, > 0.05 sec; large dogs, > 0.06 sec; cats, > 0.04 sec), often with slurring or notching of the upstroke of the R wave (delta wave)

ECG Features of Ventricular Preexcitation with WPW Syndrome
• Extremely rapid heart rate (dogs, often > 300 bpm; cats, approaching 400–500 bpm)
• P waves may be difficult to recognize.
• QRS complexes may be normal, wide with delta wave, or very wide and bizarre, depending on the circuit
• Conduction is usually 1:1 (i.e., one P wave for every QRS complex).

PATHOPHYSIOLOGY
• Can be associated with congenital or acquired cardiac defects in dogs or cats
•

May be associated with hypertrophic cardiomyopathy in cats
• Hemodynamic compromise during episodes of supraventricular tachycardia with WPW syndrome

SYSTEMS AFFECTED
Cardiovascular

GENETICS
N/A

INCIDENCE/PREVALENCE
Unknown

GEOGRAPHIC DISTRIBUTION
N/A

SIGNALMENT

Species
Dogs and cats

Breed Predilections
N/A

Mean Age and Range
N/A

Predominant Sex
N/A

SIGNS

Historical Findings
• None in patients with ventricular preexcitation
• Syncope in patients with WPW syndrome

Physical Examination Findings
• None in animals with ventricular preexcitation
• Rapid heart rate in animals with WPW syndrome

CAUSES

Congenital heart disease
• Congenital defect limited to the conduction system*
• Atrial septal defect in dogs or cats
• Tricuspid valvular dysplasia in dogs

Acquired heart disease
Hypertrophic cardiomyopathy in cats

RISK FACTORS
N/A

DIAGNOSIS

DIFFERENTIAL DIAGNOSIS
• Ventricular preexcitation—differentiate from other causes of short P-R intervals (e.g., fever, hyperthyroidism, and anemia); these conditions do not cause delta waves.
• Narrow complex WPW syndrome—differentiate from other supraventricular arrhythmias (e.g., atrial tachycardia, atrial flutter, and atrial fibrillation); WPW syndrome is most easily recognized after conversion to normal heart rate and rhythm.
• Alternating WPW syndrome should not be confused with ventricular bigeminy.
• Wide complex WPW syndrome must be differentiated from ventricular tachycardia.
• Short PR interval may be correlated with a normal QRS complex if the anomalous pathway bypasses the AV node and connects to the bundle of His (i.e., Lown-Ganong-Levine syndrome).

CBC/BIOCHEMISTRY/URINALYSIS
N/A

OTHER LABORATORY TESTS
N/A

IMAGING
Echocardiography may show structural heart disease.

DIAGNOSTIC PROCEDURES

Electrocardiography
• Pathologic findings vary with underlying cause.
• Possibility of no organic heart lesions

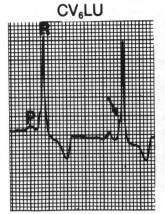

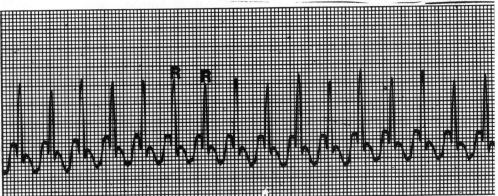

Figure 1.

Wolff-Parkinson-White syndrome (canine). Ventricular preexcitation represented by the short P-R interval, wide QRS complex, and delta wave (arrow) in CV6LU. Paroxysms of supraventricular tachycardia are represented in the long lead II rhythm strip. (From: Tilley LP: Essentials of canine and feline electrocardiography. 3rd ed. Baltimore: Williams & Wilkins, 1992, with permission.)

WOLFF-PARKINSON-WHITE SYNDROME

TREATMENT

APPROPRIATE HEALTH CARE
• Ventricular preexcitation without tachycardia—no treatment needed
• WPW syndrome requires conversion by ocular or carotid sinus pressure, direct current shock (the most effective treatment), or drugs.

NURSING CARE
N/A

ACTIVITY
May need to be limited with WPW until supraventricular tachycardias are controlled

DIET
N/A

CLIENT EDUCATION
WPW—explain the need to identify and treat the underlying cause in addition to therapy for supraventricular tachycardia.

SURGICAL CONSIDERATIONS
Catheter ablation with radiofrequency current—a relatively recent technique that allows accessory pathways to be destroyed or ablated by a transvenous catheter positioned at the site of the pathway; can be preferred alternative to lifelong therapy with drugs

MEDICATIONS

DRUGS OF CHOICE
• A variety of drugs are used in humans; opinions differ on agents of choice.
• Lidocaine IV bolus (2 mg/kg) followed by IV drip (25–75 µg/kg/min CRI—dogs only)
• Procainamide (8–20 mg/kg q8h—dogs only)
• Propranolol (cats, 2.5–5 mg PO q8–12h; dogs, 0.2–1.0 mg/kg PO q8h) or atenolol (cats, 6.2–12.5 mg PO q24h; dogs, 0.25–1.0 mg/kg PO q12h)
• Diltiazem may be effective (cats, 1–2.5 mg/kg PO q8h; dogs, 0.5–1.5 mg/kg PO q8h).

CONTRAINDICATIONS
• Digitalis, verapamil, and propranolol may be contraindicated—by slowing conduction through the AV node, these drugs may favor conduction through the anomalous pathways.
• Cats—propranolol and atenolol are the drugs of choice.

PRECAUTIONS
N/A

POSSIBLE INTERACTIONS
N/A

ALTERNATIVE DRUGS
N/A

FOLLOW-UP

PATIENT MONITORING
Serial ECG

PREVENTION/AVOIDANCE
N/A

POSSIBLE COMPLICATIONS
None expected

EXPECTED COURSE AND PROGNOSIS
Depends on severity of the underlying cause; most WPW patients respond to therapy for supraventricular tachycardia—favorable prognosis

MISCELLANEOUS

ASSOCIATED CONDITIONS
N/A

AGE-RELATED FACTORS
N/A

ZOONOTIC POTENTIAL
N/A

PREGNANCY
N/A

SYNONYMS
None

SEE ALSO
N/A

ABBREVIATIONS
• AV = atrioventricular
• bpm = beats per minute
• WPW = Wolff-Parkinson-White

Suggested Readings
Al-Khatib SM, Pritchett ELC. Clinical features of Wolff-Parkinson-White syndrome. Am Heart J 1999;138:403–413.
Hill BL, Tilley LP. Ventricular preexcitation in seven dogs and nine cats. J Am Vet Med Assoc 1985;187:1026–1031.
Tilley LP. Essentials of canine and feline electrocardiography. 3rd ed. Baltimore: Williams & Wilkins, 1992.
Wright KN. Assessment and treatment of supraventricular tachyarrhythmisas. In: Bonagura JD, ed. Kirk's current veterinary therapy XIII. Philadelphia: Saunders, 2000:726–729.
Authors Larry P. Tilley and Naomi L. Burtnick
Consulting Editors Larry P. Tilley and Francis W. K. Smith, Jr.

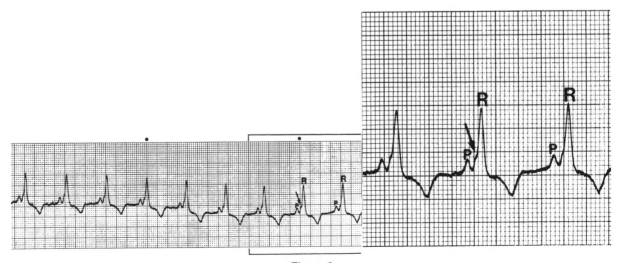

Figure 2.

Ventricular pre-excitation in a cat with episodes of fainting. The P waves are normal, the P-R interval is short, and the QRS complex is wide; delta waves (arrow) are present. (From: Tilley LP: Essentials of canine and feline electrocardiography. 3rd ed. Baltimore: Williams & Wilkins, 1992, with permission.)

DISEASES AND
CLINICAL SYNDROMES

ABSCESSATION

 BASICS

DEFINITION
An abscess is a localized collection of purulent exudate contained within a cavity.

PATHOPHYSIOLOGY
• Bacteria are often inoculated under the skin via a puncture wound; the wound surface then seals.
• When bacteria and/or foreign objects persist in the tissue, purulent exudate forms and collects.
• Accumulation of purulent exudate—if not quickly resorbed or discharged to an external surface, stimulates formation of a fibrous capsule; may eventually lead to abscess rupture
• Prolonged delay of evacuation—formation of a fibrous abscess wall; to heal, the cavity must be filled with granulation tissue from which the causative agent may not be totally eliminated; may lead to chronic or intermittent discharge of exudate from a draining sinus tract

SYSTEMS AFFECTED
• Skin/Exocrine—percutaneous (cats > dogs); anal sac (dogs > cats)
• Gastrointestinal—pancreas (dogs > cats)
• Reproductive—prostate gland (dogs > cats); mammary gland
• Ophthalmic—periorbital tissues
• Hepatobiliary—liver parenchyma

GENETICS
N/A

INCIDENCE/PREVALENCE
N/A

GEOGRAPHIC DISTRIBUTION
N/A

SIGNALMENT
Species
Cats and dogs
Breed Predilections
N/A
Mean Age and Range
N/A
Predominant Sex
Mammary glands (female); prostate gland (male)

SIGNS
General Comments
• Determined by organ system and/or tissue affected
• Associated with a combination of inflammation (pain, swelling, redness, heat, and loss of function), tissue destruction, and/or organ system dysfunction caused by accumulation of exudate

Historical Findings
• History of traumatic insult or previous infection
• A rapidly appearing painful swelling with or without discharge, if affected area is visible

Physical Examination Findings
• Determined by the organ system or tissue affected
• A discrete mass may be detectable.
• Inflammation and discharge from a fistulous tract may be visible if the abscess is superficial and has ruptured to an external surface.
• A variably sized, painful mass of fluctuant to firm consistency attached to surrounding tissues may be palpable.
• Fever if abscess is not ruptured and draining
• Sepsis occasionally, especially if abscess ruptures internally

CAUSES
• Foreign objects
• Pyogenic bacteria—*Staphylococcus* spp.; *Escherichia coli;* β-hemolytic *Streptococcus* spp.; *Pseudomonas; Mycoplasma* and *Mycoplasma*-like organisms (L-forms); *Pasteurella multocida; Corynebacterium; Actinomyces* spp.; *Nocardia*
• Obligate anaerobes—*Bacteroides* spp.; *Clostridium* spp.; *Peptostreptococcus; Fusobacterium*

RISK FACTORS
• Anal sac—impaction; anal sacculitis
• Brain—otitis interna sinusitis oral infection
• Liver—omphalophlebitis sepsis
• Lung—foreign object aspiration bacterial pneumonia
• Mammary gland—mastitis
• Periorbital—dental disease; chewing of wood or other plant material
• Percutaneous—fighting
• Prostate gland—bacterial prostatitis
• Immunosuppression—FeLV/FIV infection, immunosuppressive chemotherapy, acquired or inherited immune system dysfunctions, underlying predisposing disease (e.g., diabetes mellitus, chronic renal failure, hyperadrenocorticism)

 DIAGNOSIS

DIFFERENTIAL DIAGNOSIS
Mass Lesions
• Cyst—less or only transiently painful; slower growing
• Fibrous scar tissue—firm; nonpainful
• Granuloma—less painful; slower growing; generally firmer without fluctuant center
• Hematoma/seroma—variable pain (depends on cause); nonencapsulated; rapid initial growth but slow increase once full size is attained; unattached to surrounding tissues; fluctuant and fluid-filled initially but more firm with organization

• Neoplasia—variable growth; consistent; painful
Draining Tracts
• Mycobacterial disease
• Mycetoma—botryomycosis, actinomycotic mycetoma, eumycotic mycetoma
• Neoplasia
• Phaeohyphomycosis
• Sporotrichosis
• Systemic fungal infection—blastomycosis, coccidioidomycosis, cryptococcosis, histoplasmosis, trichosporosis

CBC/BIOCHEMISTRY/URINALYSIS
• CBC—normal or neutrophilia with or without regenerative left shift. Neutropenia and degenerative left shift if sepsis present
• Urinalysis and serum chemistry profile—depend on system affected
• Prostatic—pyuria
• Liver and/or pancreatic—high liver enzymes and/or total bilirubin
• Pancreatic (dogs)—high amylase/lipase
• Diabetes mellitus—persistent hyperglycemia and glucosuria

OTHER LABORATORY TESTS
• FeLV and FIV—for cats with recurrent or slow healing abscesses
• CSF evaluation—increase in cellularity and protein expected with brain abscess
• Adrenal function—evaluate for hyperadrenocorticism

IMAGING
• Radiography—soft tissue density mass in affected area; may reveal foreign body
• Ultrasonography—determine if mass is fluid filled or solid; determine organ system affected; reveal flocculent-appearing fluid characteristic of pus; may reveal foreign object
• Echocardiography—helpful for diagnosis of pericardial abscess
• CT or MRI—helpful for diagnosis of brain abscess

DIAGNOSTIC PROCEDURES
Aspiration
• Reveals a red, white, yellow, or green liquid
• Protein content—> 2.5–3.0 g/dL
• Nucleated cell count—3,000–100,000 (or more) cells/μL; primarily degenerative neutrophils with lesser numbers of macrophages and lymphocytes
• Pyogenic bacteria—may be seen in cells and free within the fluid
• If the causative agent is not readily identified with a Romanovsky-type stain, specimens should be stained with an acid-fast stain to detect mycobacteria or *Nocardia* and PAS stain to detect fungus.

Biopsy
• Sample should contain both normal and abnormal tissue in the same specimen.
• Impression smears—stained and examined
• Tissue—submit for histopathologic examination and culture
• Contact the diagnostic laboratory for specific instructions.

Culture
• Affected tissue and/or exudate—aerobic and anaerobic bacteria and fungus
• Blood and/or urine—isolate bacterium responsible for possible sepsis
• Bacterial sensitivity

PATHOLOGIC FINDINGS
• Pus-containing mass lesion accompanied by inflammation
• Palpable—variably firm or fluctuant mass
• Ruptured—may see pus draining directly from the mass or an adjoining tract
• Exudate—large numbers of neutrophils in various stages of degeneration; other inflammatory cells; necrotic tissue
• Surrounding tissue—congested; fibrin; large number of neutrophils; variable number of lymphocytes; plasma cells; macrophages
• Causative agent variably detectable

TREATMENT

APPROPRIATE HEALTH CARE
• Depends on location of abscess and treatment required
• Outpatient—bite-induced abscesses
• Inpatient—sepsis; extensive surgical procedures; treatment requiring extended hospitalization
• Establish and maintain adequate drainage
• Surgical removal of nidus of infection or foreign object(s) if necessary
• Institution of appropriate antimicrobial therapy

NURSING CARE
• Depends on location of abscess
• Apply hot packs to inflamed area as needed.
• Use protective bandaging and/or Elizabethan collars as needed.
• Accumulated exudate—drain abscess; maintain drainage by medical and/or surgical means.
• Sepsis or peritonitis—aggressive fluid therapy and support

ACTIVITY
Restrict until the abscess has resolved and adequate healing of tissues has taken place.

DIET
• Sufficient nutritional intake to promote a positive nitrogen balance
• Depends on location of abscess and treatment required

CLIENT EDUCATION
• Discuss need to correct or prevent risk factors.
• Discuss need for adequate drainage and continuation of antimicrobial therapy for an adequate period of time.

SURGICAL CONSIDERATIONS
• Appropriate débridement and drainage—may need to leave the wound open to an external surface; may need to place surgical drains
• Early drainage—to prevent further tissue damage and formation of abscess wall
• Remove any foreign objects(s), necrotic tissue, or nidus of infection.

MEDICATIONS

DRUGS OF CHOICE
• Antimicrobial drugs—effective against the infectious agent; gain access to site of infection
• Broad-spectrum agent—bactericidal and with both aerobic and anaerobic activity; until results of culture and sensitivity are known; dogs and cats: amoxicillin (11–22 mg/kg PO q8–12h); amoxicillin/clavulanic acid (12.5–25 mg/kg PO q12h); clindamycin (5 mg/kg PO q12h); and trimethoprim/sulfadiazine (15 mg/kg PO IM q12h); cats with *Mycoplasma* and l-forms: doxycycline (3–5 mg/kg PO q12h)
• Aggressive antimicrobial therapy—sepsis or peritonitis

CONTRAINDICATIONS
N/A

PRECAUTIONS
N/A

POSSIBLE INTERACTIONS
N/A

ALTERNATIVE DRUGS
N/A

FOLLOW-UP

PATIENT MONITORING
Monitor for progressive decrease in drainage, resolution of inflammation, and improvement of clinical signs

PREVENTION/AVOIDANCE
• Percutaneous abscesses—prevent fighting
• Anal sac abscesses—prevent impaction; consider anal saculectomy for recurrent cases
• Prostatic abscesses—castration possibly helpful

• Mastitis—prevent lactation (spaying)
• Periorbital abscesses—do not allow chewing on foreign object(s)

POSSIBLE COMPLICATIONS
• Sepsis
• Peritonitis/pleuritis if intra-abdominal or intrathoracic abscess ruptures
• Compromise of organ function
• Delayed evacuation may lead to chronically draining fistulous tracts.

EXPECTED COURSE AND PROGNOSIS
Depend on organ system involved and amount of tissue destruction

MISCELLANEOUS

ASSOCIATED CONDITIONS
• FeLV or FIV infection
• Immunosuppression

AGE-RELATED FACTORS
N/A

ZOONOTIC POTENTIAL
• Minimal for pyogenic bacteria
• Mycobacteria and systemic fungal infections carry some potential.

PREGNANCY
Teratogenic agents—avoid use in pregnant animals.

SEE ALSO
• Actinomycosis
• Bacterial Infections, Anaerobic
• Colibacillosis
• Mycoplasma
• Nocardiosis
• Sepsis and Bacteremia

ABBREVIATIONS
• CSF = cerebrospinal fluid
• FeLV = feline leukemia virus
• FIV = feline immunodeficiency virus
• PAS = periodic acid-Schiff

Suggested Reading
Birchard SJ, Sherding RG, eds. Saunders manual of small animal practice. Philadelphia: Saunders, 1994.
DeBoer DJ. Nonhealing cutaneous wounds. In: August JR, ed. Consultations in feline internal medicine. Philadelphia: Saunders, 1991:101-106.
McCaw D. Lumps, bumps, masses, and lymphadenopathy. In: Ettinger SJ, Feldman EC, eds. Textbook of veterinary internal medicine. 4th ed. Philadelphia: Saunders, 1995:219-222.
Author Johnny D. Hoskins
Consulting Editor Stephen C. Barr

DISEASES

ACETAMINOPHEN TOXICITY

BASICS

DEFINITION
Results from owners overdosing the patient with over-the-counter acetaminophen-containing analgesic and antipyretic medications

PATHOPHYSIOLOGY
When the normal biotransformation mechanisms for detoxification (glucuronidation and sulfation) are diminished, cytochrome P450–mediated oxidation produces a toxic metabolite (N-acetyl benzoquinoneimine) that is electrophilic, conjugates with glutathione, and toxicologically binds to liver proteins.
Dogs
• Receipt of ≥ 150–200 mg/kg—sufficient electrophilic metabolite generated through the cytochrome P450 pathway that RBC glutathione binding produces methemoglobinemia and attacks liver proteins
• Causes hepatotoxicity in a dose-dependent fashion
Cats
• Lower ability to glucuronidate; more limited capacity for acetaminophen elimination than dogs
• Saturate glucuronidation and sulfation biotransformation routes
• Develop toxic cytochrome P450 metabolite at much lower doses than dogs
• Poisoned by as little as 50–60 mg/kg (often as little as one-half tablet); leads to rapid RBC glutathione depletion that produces rapidly developing methemoglobinemia, because of the unique feline hemoglobin molecule with eight sulfhydryl groups sensitive to oxidation
• Slower-developing hepatotoxicosis may not be fully expressed before development of fatal methemoglobinemia.

SYSTEMS AFFECTED
• Hemic/Lymph/Immune—RBCs are damaged by glutathione depletion allowing oxidation of hemoglobin to methemoglobin
• Hepatobiliary—liver necrosis
• Cardiovascular (cats)—edema of the face, paws, and (to a lesser degree) forelimbs through an undefined mechanism

GENETICS
• Cats—genetic deficiency in the glucuronide conjugation pathway makes them vulnerable.

INCIDENCE/PREVALENCE
• Most common drug toxicity in cats; considerably less frequent in dogs
• Over-the-counter medications—fourth most common cause of poison exposures in small animals

GEOGRAPHIC DISTRIBUTION
N/A

SIGNALMENT
Species
Cats more often than dogs
Breed Predilections
N/A
Mean Age and Range
N/A
Predominant Sex
N/A

SIGNS
General Comments
Relatively common—owing to increasing use in humans
Historical Findings
• Depression
• Rapid breathing
• Darkened mucous membranes
• Owner may recall warnings about acetaminophen in cats after dosing the pet.
Physical Examination Findings
• May develop 1–4 hr after dosing
• Progressive depression
• Salivation
• Vomiting
• Abdominal pain
• Tachypnea and cyanosis—reflect methemoglobinemia
• Edema—face, paws and possibly forelimbs; after several hours
• Chocolate-colored urine—hematuria and methemoglobinuria; especially in cats
• Death

CAUSES
Acetaminophen overdosing

RISK FACTORS
• Nutritional deficiencies of glucose and/or sulfate
• Simultaneous administration of other glutathione-depressing drugs

DIAGNOSIS

DIFFERENTIAL DIAGNOSIS
• Nitrites
• Phenacetin
• Nitrobenzene
• Phenol and cresol compounds
• Sulfites
• History of exposure—important for differentiating from methemoglobin-forming drugs

CBC/BIOCHEMISTRY/URINALYSIS
• Methemoglobinemia and progressively rising serum activities of liver enzymes—characteristic
• Heinz bodies (cats)—prominent in RBCs
• Hematuria and/or hemoglobinuria

OTHER LABORATORY TESTS
• Acetaminophen serum concentration—maximally elevated 1–3 hr after ingestion; decay dose-dependent in cats (approximately 1/10 the plasma elimination rate of dogs)
• Blood glutathione level—low

IMAGING
N/A

DIAGNOSTIC PROCEDURES
N/A

PATHOLOGIC FINDINGS
• Methemoglobinemia
• Pulmonary edema
• Liver and kidney congestion
• Dogs—centrilobular necrosis of the liver; icterus in chronic cases

TREATMENT

APPROPRIATE HEALTH CARE
• With methemoglobinemia—must evaluate promptly
• With dark or bloody colored urine or icterus—inpatient

NURSING CARE
• Gentle handling—imperative for clinically affected patients
• Emesis and gastric lavage—useful within 4–6 hr of ingestion
• Anemia, hematuria, or hemoglobinuria—may require whole blood transfusion

• Fluid therapy—maintain hydration and electrolyte balance
• Drinking water—available at all times
• Food—offered 24 hr after initiation of treatment

ACTIVITY
Restricted

DIET
N/A

CLIENT EDUCATION
• Warn client that treatment in clinically affected patients may be prolonged and expensive.
• Inform client that patients with liver injury may require prolonged and costly management.

SURGICAL CONSIDERATIONS
N/A

MEDICATIONS

DRUGS OF CHOICE
• Activated charcoal—2 g/kg PO; immediately after completion of emesis or gastric lavage
• N-acetylcysteine (Mucomyst)—140 mg/kg loading dose PO, IV; then 70 mg/kg PO, IV, q4h for five to seven treatments

CONTRAINDICATIONS
Drugs that contribute to methemoglobinemia or hepatotoxicity

PRECAUTIONS
Drugs requiring extensive liver metabolism or biotransformation—use with caution; expect their half-lives to be extended.

POSSIBLE INTERACTIONS
Drugs requiring activation or metabolism by the liver have reduced effectiveness.

ALTERNATIVE DRUGS
• Other sulfur donor drugs—if N-acetylcysteine not available; sodium sulfate (50 mg 1.6% solution/kg IV q4h for six treatments); effective use requires conscientious management.
• A 1% methylene blue solution—8.8 mg/kg IV q2–3h for two to three treatments; combats methemoglobinemia without inducing a hemolytic crisis
• Ascorbic acid—125 mg/kg PO q6h for six treatments; only slowly reduces methemoglobinemia

FOLLOW-UP

PATIENT MONITORING
• Continual clinical monitoring of methemoglobinemia—vital for effective management; laboratory determination of methemoglobin percentage every 2–3 hr
• Serum liver enzyme activities (ALT, ALP)—determined every 12 hr; monitor liver damage
• Blood glutathione level—provide evidence of the effectiveness of sulfhydryl-replacement therapy

PREVENTION/AVOIDANCE
• Never give acetaminophen to cats
• Give careful attention to the acetaminophen dose in dogs.

POSSIBLE COMPLICATIONS
Liver necrosis and resulting fibrosis—may compromise long-term liver function in recovered patients

EXPECTED COURSE AND PROGNOSIS
• Rapidly progressive methemoglobinemia—serious sign
• Methemoglobin concentrations > 50%—grave prognosis
• Progressively rising serum liver enzymes 12–24 hr after ingestion—serious concern
• Expect clinical signs to persist 12–48 hr; death owing to methemoglobinemia possible at any time
• Dogs and cats receiving prompt treatment that reverses methemoglobinemia and prevents excessive liver necrosis—may recover fully
• Dogs—death as a result of liver necrosis may occur in a few days.
• Cats—death as a result of methemoglobinemia occurs 18–36 hr after ingestion.

MISCELLANEOUS

ASSOCIATED CONDITIONS
N/A

AGE-RELATED FACTORS
Young and small dogs and cats—greater risk from owner-given single-dose acetaminophen medications

ZOONOTIC POTENTIAL
N/A

PREGNANCY
Imposes additional stress and higher risk on exposed animals.

SYNONYMS
• Paracetamol
• Tylenol

SEE ALSO
Poisoning (Intoxication)

ABBREVIATIONS
• ALP = alkaline phosphatase
• ALT = alanine aminotransferase

Suggested Reading

Hjelle JJ, GF Grauer. Acetaminophen-induced toxicosis in dogs and cats. J Am Vet Med Assoc 1986;188:742–746.

Oehme FW. Aspirin and acetaminophen. In: Kirk RW, ed., Current veterinary therapy IX. Small animal practice. Philadelphia: Saunders, 1986:188–189.

Rumbeiha WK, Oehme FW. Methylene blue can be used to treat methemoglobinemia in cats without inducing Heinz body hemolytic anemia. Vet Hum Toxicol 1992;34:120–122.

Savides MC, Oehme FW, Leipold HW. Effects of various antidotal treatments on acetaminophen toxicosis and biotransformation in cats. Am J Vet Res 1985;46:1485–1489.

Savides MC, Oehme FW, Nash SL, Leipold HW. The toxicity and biotransformation of single doses of acetaminophen in dogs and cats. Toxicol Appl Pharmacol 1984;74:26–34.

Author Frederick W. Oehme
Consulting Editor Gary D. Osweiler

DISEASES

BASICS

OVERVIEW
• Some animals have a single episode; many have a lifelong recurrent problem; for a few, the disease process is continual; frequency and severity of each occurrence varies with the individual.
• Involves the chin and lower lip
• Cause unknown

SIGNALMENT
• Cats
• Any sex, age, and breed

SIGNS
• Comedones, mild erythematous papules, and serous crusts develop on the chin and less commonly on the lips.
• Sometimes swelling of the chin.
• More severe cases—nodules, hemorrhagic crusts, pustules, severe erythema, alopecia, and pain.
• Pain indicates furunculosis.

CAUSES & RISK FACTORS
• Poor grooming
• Abnormalities in keratinization, sebum production, or immune-barrier function

DIAGNOSIS

DIFFERENTIAL DIAGNOSIS
• Demodicosis
• *Malassezia* infection
• Feline leprosy
• Dermatophytosis
• Neoplasia of the sebaceous glands and other follicular and epidermal neoplasia
• Allergy (including eosinophilic granuloma complex)

CBC/BIOCHEMISTRY/URINALYSIS
N/A

OTHER LABORATORY TESTS
N/A

IMAGING
N/A

DIAGNOSTIC PROCEDURES
• Biopsy—rarely needed but sometimes necessary in selected cases
• Histopathologic examination—differentiate acne from other diseases such as demodicosis, dermatophytosis, and rarely neoplasia

PATHOLOGIC FINDINGS
• Mild disease—follicular distention with keratin (comedo), hyperkeratosis, and follicular plugging
• More severe disease—mild to severe folliculitis and perifolliculitis with follicular pustule formation
• Follicular rupture of keratin and hair into the dermis—leads to furunculosis, which is manifested by neutrophils and numerous macrophages surrounding the keratin debris; bacteria and *Malassezia* in these lesions are considered secondary invaders and not causative agents.

TREATMENT
• Initial treatment—one or a combination of the drugs listed below until all lesions have resolved
• Discontinue treatment by tapering medication over a 2–3-week period.
• Recurrent episodes—once the recurrence rate is determined, an appropriate maintenance protocol can be designed for each individual
• Continual episodes—lifelong treatment twice per week is necessary

MEDICATIONS

DRUGS
• Systemic antibiotics—amoxicillin with clavulanate, or enrofloxacin alone, or cephalosporin alone

• Shampoo—one or twice a week with antiseborrheic (sulfur–salicylic acid, benzoyl peroxide, or ethyl lactate) products
• Topical cleansing agents—benzoyl peroxide, salicylic acid
• Topical antibiotic cream—mupirocin
• Other topicals—clindamycin or erythromycin solution or ointment
• Combination topicals—benzoyl peroxide–antibiotic gels (e.g., Benzamycin)
• Topical retinoids (Retin-A 0.01% gel); tretinoin (vitamin A acid, retinoic acid)

CONTRAINDICATIONS/POSSIBLE INTERACTIONS
• Benzoyl peroxide and salicylic acids—can be irritating
• Systemic isotretinoin—use with caution, if animal will not allow application of topical medications; **CAUTION:** inform owners that it can have potential deleterious side effects in humans (drug interactions and teratogenic) if taken by mistake; container should be labeled for animal use only and kept separate from human medications to avoid accidental use.

FOLLOW-UP
• After medication is discontinued, monitor for relapses.
• Maintenance cleansing programs can be used between relapses to extend the time between episodes.

MISCELLANEOUS

PREGNANCY
Systemic isotretinoin should not be used on breeding animals.

Suggested Reading
Scott DW. Feline dermatology 1900–1978. A monograph. J Am Anim Hosp Assoc 1980;16:331–459.
Author David Duclos
Consulting Editor Karen Helton Rhodes

BASICS

OVERVIEW
• Chronic inflammatory disorder of the chin and lips of young animals
• Characterized by folliculitis and furunculosis
• Recognized almost exclusively in short-coated breeds
• Once thought that hormones played a triggering role; now speculated that genetic predisposition plays a more important role

SIGNALMENT
• Dogs
• Predisposed short-coated breeds—boxers, Doberman pinschers, English bulldogs, great Danes, weimaraners, mastiffs, rottweilers, and German short-haired pointers

SIGNS
• The area may be minimally to markedly swollen with numerous erythematous papules.
• Advanced stages—lesions may be exudative and indicate a secondary deep bacterial infection.
• Lesions may be painful on palpation.
• Chronic resolved lesions may be scarred and lichenified.

CAUSES & RISK FACTORS
Some short-coated breeds appear to be genetically predisposed to follicular keratosis and secondary bacterial infection.

DIAGNOSIS

DIFFERENTIAL DIAGNOSIS
• Dermatophytosis
• Demodicosis
• Foreign body
• Contact dermatitis

CBC/BIOCHEMISTRY/URINALYSIS
N/A

OTHER LABORATORY TESTS
N/A

IMAGING
N/A

DIAGNOSTIC PROCEDURES
• Bacterial culture and sensitivity testing—in patients with suppurative folliculitis and furunculosis that are responsive to initial antibiotic selection
• Biopsy—histologic confirmation for cases in which diagnosis is in question

PATHOLOGIC FINDINGS
• Clinical signs and histopathologic findings are diagnostic.
• Initial lesions—hairless follicular papules; characterized histopathologically by marked follicular keratosis, plugging, dilatation, and perifolliculitis
• Bacteria—in the early stages: not seen and cannot be isolated from lesions; as disease progresses: papules enlarge and rupture, promoting a suppurative folliculitis and furunculosis.

TREATMENT

• Depends on the severity and chronicity of the disease
• Reduce behavioral trauma to the chin (e.g., rubbing on the carpet, chewing bones that increase salivation)
• Frequent cleaning with benzoyl peroxide shampoo or gel or mupirocin ointment to reduce the bacterial numbers on the surface of the skin
• Instruct owners to avoid expressing the lesions, which may cause internal rupture of the papule and massive inflammation

MEDICATIONS

DRUGS
Topical
• Benzoyl peroxide shampoo or gel (antibacterial)
• Mupirocin ointment (antibacterial-staph)
• Isotretinoin (Retin-A) or tretinoin (vitamin A acid, retinoic acid gel)—may reduce follicular keratosis
• Corticosteroids—may be necessary to reduce inflammation

Systemic
• Antibiotics appropriate for deep bacterial infection—especially cephalosporins (Cephalexin, 22 mg/kg PO q8h for 6–8 weeks)
• May need to perform bacterial culture and sensitivity test.

CONTRAINDICATION/POSSIBLE INTERACTIONS
• Benzoyl peroxide—may bleach carpets and fabrics; may be irritating
• Mupirocin ointments—greasy
• Topical retinoids—may be drying and irritating
• Topical steroids—may cause adrenal suppression with repeated use

FOLLOW-UP
Long-term topical treatment required

MISCELLANEOUS

Suggested Reading
Scott DW, Miller WH, Griffin CE. Bacterial skin diseases. In: Kirk's small animal dermatology. 5th ed. Philadelphia: Saunders, 1995:304–305.
Author Karen Helton Rhodes
Consulting Editor Karen Helton Rhodes

DISEASES

ACRAL LICK DERMATITIS

BASICS

OVERVIEW
A firm, raised, ulcerative, or thickened plaque that is usually located on the dorsal aspect of the carpus, metacarpus, tarsus, or metatarsus

SIGNALMENT
- Primarily dogs
- Most common in large-breeds—especially Doberman pinschers, Labrador retrievers, Great Danes, Irish and English setters, golden retrievers, akitas, Dalmatians, shar peis, and Weimaraners
- Age at onset—varies with the cause
- Sex predilection—some sources suggest more common in males; others indicate no preference

SIGNS
- Excessive licking and chewing of the affected area
- Occasionally a history of trauma to the affected area
- Alopecic, ulcerative, thickened, and raised firm plaques, usually located on the dorsal aspect of the carpus, metacarpus, tarsus or metatarsus
- Lesions often occur singly, although they may occur in more than one location.

CAUSES & RISK FACTORS
Associated diseases—staphylococcal furunculosis, allergy, endocrinopathy, demodicosis, dermatophytosis, foreign body reaction, neoplasia, trauma, and psychogenic and sensory nerve dysfunction.

DIAGNOSIS

DIFFERENTIAL DIAGNOSIS
- Allergic animals often have multiple lick granulomas and other areas of pruritus compatible with the specific allergy.
- Endocrinopathies, demodicosis, and dermatophytosis—determined on the basis of laboratory test results

CBC/BIOCHEMISTRY/URINALYSIS
Normal except in cases of hyperadrenocorticism

OTHER LABORATORY TESTS
- Low thyroid levels—suggests hypothyroidism
- Abnormal ACTH-stimulation test or abnormal LDDST—suggests hyperadrenocorticism

IMAGING
Radiology—neoplasia; some forms of trauma; radiopaque foreign bodies; bony proliferation may be seen secondary to the chronic irritation.

DIAGNOSTIC PROCEDURES
- Examine skin scrapings, dermatophyte culture, and Tzanck preparations—rule out demodicosis, dermatophytosis, or a bacterial infection
- Bacterial culture and sensitivity (if indicated)—determine appropriate antibiotics
- Food-elimination diet—determine food allergy
- Intradermal allergy testing—helpful for atopic animals
- Biopsy—to rule out neoplasia, if necessary

PATHOLOGIC FINDINGS
Histopathology—ulcerative, hyperplastic epidermis with mild perivascular dermatitis; varying degrees of fibroplasia

TREATMENT

- Affected animal must get plenty of attention and exercise.
- Diet—no modification unless an allergy is suspected
- Difficult to treat, especially if no underlying cause is found; warn owner that patience and time are necessary.
- Surgery—do not consider until all other therapies have been exhausted; will often cause increased licking and attention to the affected area, resulting in poor wound closure; if underlying causes are not addressed, recurrence is likely.

MEDICATIONS

DRUGS

Antibiotics
• Based on bacterial culture and sensitivity
• Give until infection is completely resolved, often at least 6 weeks.

Systemic
• Hydroxyzine HCl (1–2 mg/kg PO q8h)
• Chlorpheniramine (4–8 mg/dog q12h PO; maximum of 0.5 mg/kg q12h)
• Naltrexone (2.2 mg/kg PO q12–24h)
• Amitriptyline HCl (1.1–2.2 mg/kg PO q12h); used at the lower dosage for 10 days; if no improvement, use at the higher dosage for 10 days
• Doxepin may also be tried (3–5 mg/kg PO q12h; maximum 150 mg q12h).
• CAUTION: none of these medications should be used concurrently.

Topical
• Flunixin meglumine and fluocinolone in dimethyl sulfoxide (combined), mupirocin, topical 5% benzoyl peroxide, and capsalcin products
• Intralesional corticosteroids may be used in early or very small lesions; rarely of any use in chronic lesions
• Topical medications should be applied with gloves.
• Animals should be kept from licking the area for 10–15 min.

Other
• After all other underlying diseases have been ruled out or treated, therapies for psychogenic dermatoses may be tried.
• Psychotropic drugs—fluoxetine hydrochloride (1 mg/kg PO q24h) or clomipramine hydrochloride (1–3 mg/kg PO q24h)
• Physical restraints—Elizabethan collars and bandaging; short-term use

CONTRAINDICATIONS/POSSIBLE INTERACTIONS
• Doxepin—do not use with monoamine oxidase inhibitors, clonidine, anticonvulsants, oral anticoagulants, steroid hormones, antihistamines, or aspirin.
• Antihistamines—do not use more than one at a time.

 FOLLOW-UP

• Monitor level of licking and chewing closely.
• Treat underlying disease to prevent recurrence.
• If no underlying disease is detected, suspect psychogenic causes (obsessive-compulsive or self-mutilation disorder); prognosis is guarded.
• Animals receiving tricyclic antidepressants—CBC, chemistry profile, ECG every 1–2 months, because of potential for cardiotoxicity and hepatotoxicity.

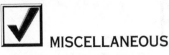 **MISCELLANEOUS**

AGE-RELATED FACTORS
Dogs > 5 years old—strongly consider allergy

ZOONOTIC POTENTIAL
Transmitted to humans only if dermatophytosis is the underlying cause; exceedingly rare

ABBREVIATION
LDDST = low-dose dexamethasone-suppression test

Suggested Reading
Shanley K, Overall K. Psychogenic dermatoses. In: Kirk RW, Bonagura JD, eds. Current veterinary therapy XI. Philadelphia: Saunders, 1992:552–557.

Authors Karen A. Kuhl and Jean S. Greek
Consulting Editor Karen Helton Rhodes

DISEASES

ACROMEGALY—CATS

BASICS

OVERVIEW
• A clinical syndrome resulting from growth hormone (somatotropin) hypersecretion by tumorous somatotrophs in the anterior pituitary of adult cats
• Clinical signs are a consequence of growth hormone's direct catabolic and indirect anabolic effects.
• The anabolic effects are mediated by somatomedin C (insulin-like growth factor I), which is secreted by the liver in response to growth hormone stimulation; somatomedin C promotes protein synthesis and growth in a variety of tissues; in juvenile animals, somatomedin C is essential for normal growth and development; in adult animals, excessive somatomedin C levels cause abnormal growth of bone (particularly membranous bone), cartilage, soft tissues, and visceral organs.
• The bony and soft tissue changes are most prominent in the head and neck region and distal extremities.
• Abnormalities in articular cartilage growth and metabolism alter normal joint biomechanics, which can lead to degenerative joint disease.
• Many organs undergo hypertrophy and/or hyperplasia without significant alterations in function, but cardiac hypertrophy frequently results in congestive heart failure; the clinical signs and cardiac pathology are very similar to those seen with idiopathic feline hypertrophic cardiomyopathy.
• The catabolic actions of growth hormone result from insulin antagonism; growth hormone causes a postreceptor defect in insulin activity and promotes lipolysis and hepatic glucose formation, actions that lead to persistent hyperglycemia, hyperinsulinemia, and eventually pancreatic B cell exhaustion; the resultant diabetes mellitus is permanent and resistant to insulin therapy; insulin-resistant diabetes mellitus was found in all reported cases of feline acromegaly.

SIGNALMENT
• A rare disease of middle-aged and older male cats
• The average age of affected cats is 10 years; reported range is 8–14 years
• Over 90% of the reported cases have been in males.

SIGNS

General Comments
• Patients are initially presented for clinical signs related to unregulated diabetes mellitus.
• As the disease progresses, clinical signs of heart failure, renal failure, or CNS abnormalities caused by tumor expansion frequently develop.

Historical/Physical Examination Findings
• Polyuria, polydipsia, and polyphagia have been presenting complaints in all reported cases.
• Weight loss is common at presentation; over time many patients gain weight and have increased body size.
• Weight gain is due to increased bone and soft tissue mass, not from increased adipose tissue.
• Weight gain in an unregulated diabetic cat strongly suggests acromegaly.
• Often, patients gradually develop broadening of the facial features and prognathia inferior.
• Abdominal palpation may detect organ enlargement.
• Systolic heart murmurs develop commonly; ~50% of acromegalic cats have congestive heart failure; signs are usually consistent with left heart failure, but a few have exhibited signs consistent with right heart failure or biventricular failure.
• As the pituitary tumor expands dorsally, some cats may develop seizures or other CNS signs very late in the disease process.

CAUSES & RISK FACTORS
• Caused by growth hormone hypersecretion by an anterior pituitary acidophil adenoma
• Progesterones, endogenous or exogenous, do not cause growth hormone secretion and acromegaly in cats, unlike in dogs.

DIAGNOSIS

DIFFERENTIAL DIAGNOSIS
• Diabetes mellitus, hyperthyroidism, hyperadrenocorticism, pancreatic exocrine insufficiency, and renal failure all cause clinical signs resembling those seen in acromegalic cats.
• Insulin-resistant diabetes mellitus (>2.0 U of insulin/kg/dose)—found in all reported cases of feline acromegaly; the insulin resistance tends to increase over time, requiring ever-increasing dosages of insulin; requirements of 20–130 U/day (average dose, 9.8 U/kg/day) have been reported in acromegalic cats.
• A presumptive diagnosis of feline acromegaly is reached by ruling out other causes of insulin-resistant diabetes mellitus.

CBC/BIOCHEMISTRY/URINALYSIS
• Most laboratory abnormalities are caused by unregulated diabetes mellitus.
• Since ~50% of reported patients eventually developed renal failure, laboratory evidence of renal failure may become evident in the later stages of the disease.
• Reported abnormalities include hyperglycemia (100%), hyperproteinemia with normal pattern of distribution on serum electrophoresis (~50%), hyperphosphatemia without azotemia (~50%), hypercholesterolemia (~50%), and azotemia (~50%).
• Glucosuria has been present in all cats diagnosed with acromegaly; ketonuria is unusual.
• Proteinuria has been present in >50% of affected cats and in all that go on to develop renal failure.

OTHER LABORATORY TESTS
- Demonstration of elevated basal serum growth hormone levels in a cat with insulin-resistant diabetes mellitus is diagnostic for acromegaly; unfortunately, no validated growth hormone assay is currently available.
- A radioimmunoassay for plasma somatomedin C is available at Michigan State University; a significant elevation in plasma somatomedin C levels in a cat with insulin-resistant diabetes mellitus strongly supports a diagnosis of acromegaly.

IMAGING
Radiography
- Mild-to-moderate cardiomegaly is found in most affected cats; cardiac enlargement tends to worsen over time.
- May find radiographic evidence of pulmonary edema in patients that develop left-sided congestive heart failure
- Marked vertebral spondylosis is common.
- Radiographic evidence of degenerative arthropathy is common.

Echocardiography
The interventricular septum and/or left ventricular free wall (>5 mm) is usually thickened.

Computed Tomography or Magnetic Resonance Imaging
Identified a pituitary mass in most acromegalic cats that have been scanned

DIAGNOSTIC PROCEDURES
N/A

TREATMENT
- Therapy is usually palliative, not curative.
- Aim medical treatment at controlling or ameliorating the secondary diseases (i.e., diabetes mellitus, heart failure, and kidney failure) that develop following prolonged growth hormone hypersecretion.

- Cobalt radiotherapy was used in a small number (7) of acromegalic cats—6 of them showed permanent or transient resolution of insulin resistance following therapy; in 4 cats, insulin therapy was discontinued 4–16 months after cobalt radiotherapy, but 2 of them eventually became diabetic again; 1 cat had resolution of CNS signs following therapy; plasma growth hormone or somatomedin C levels decreased following therapy in 5 of the treated cats.
- Cobalt radiotherapy shows promise as a palliative and, in some instances, a definitive treatment.
- Surgical removal of small, noninvasive pituitary adenomas is frequently curative in humans with acromegaly; most affected cats have exhibited large tumors, which would markedly decrease the chance for complete surgical tumor removal; surgical removal has not been described in cats.
- Cryohypophysectomy was described in one acromegalic cat—plasma somatomedin C slowly returned to normal over a period of months, and the cat's diabetes mellitus resolved ~2 months after cryosurgery; the cat did not develop hypoadrenocorticism, hypothyroidism, or central diabetes mellitus, as occurs when surgical hypophysectomy is performed.

MEDICATIONS
- In humans, dopamine agonists and the long-acting somatostatin analogue, octreotide, have been used with variable success to inhibit pituitary growth hormone secretion; dopamine agonists have not been used in cats with acromegaly, and octreotide therapy has not been effective.
- Diabetes mellitus is treated with insulin; goals of insulin therapy are to prevent ketoacidosis and to minimize clinical signs associated with diabetes mellitus; high-dose (>2.2 U/kg/dose), twice-daily insulin therapy is usually required to meet those treatment objectives.

- Patients with heart failure have responded well to diuretic therapy; concurrent or alternative therapy with diltiazem, propranolol, and/or an angiotensin-converting enzyme inhibitor (e.g., enalapril) may be appropriate, based on clinical signs, cardiac ultrasound, or electrocardiogram abnormalities.

FOLLOW-UP
PROGNOSIS
- Patients are usually euthanized or die because of congestive heart failure, renal failure, and/or progressive CNS signs.
- Reported survival times following diagnosis vary between 4 and 42 months; median survival time is 20 months.

MISCELLANEOUS
ASSOCIATED CONDITIONS
- Diabetes mellitus
- Hypertrophic cardiomyopathy
- Glomerulonephropathy
- Renal failure

Suggested Reading
Peterson ME, Taylor RS, Greco DS, et al. Acromegaly in 14 cats. JVIM 1990;4:192–201.
Author John W. Tyler
Consulting Editor Deborah S. Greco

ACTINOMYCOSIS

BASICS

OVERVIEW
• An infectious disease caused by gram-positive, branching, pleomorphic, rod-shaped bacteria of the genus *Actinomyces*
• *A. viscosus*—most commonly identified; survives in microaerophilic or anaerobic conditions
• Rarely found as the single bacterial agent in a lesion; more commonly, it is a component of a polymicrobial infection.
• There may be synergism between *Actinomyces* and other organisms.

SIGNALMENT
• Dogs and cats
• Especially common in young male dogs of sporting breeds

SIGNS
• Infections—usually localized; may be disseminated; cervicofacial area commonly involved
• Cutaneous swellings or abscesses with draining tracts—yellow granules ("sulfur granules") may be seen in associated exudates.
• Pain and fever
• Exudative pleural or peritoneal effusions
• Retroperitonitis—in one study, *Actinomyces* was identified in 3 of 34 affected dogs
• Osteomyelitis of vertebrae or long bones—probably secondary to extension of cutaneous infection; lameness or a swollen extremity may develop
• Motor and sensory deficits—reported with spinal cord compression by granulomas

CAUSES & RISK FACTORS
• *Actinomyces* spp.—normal inhabitants of the oral cavity of dogs and cats
• Loss of normal protective barriers (mucosa, skin), immunosuppression, or change in the bacterial microenvironment could predispose animals; thought to occur as an opportunistic infection
• Specific risk factors—trauma (bite wound), migrating foreign body (foxtail in the western U.S.), and periodontal disease

DIAGNOSIS

DIFFERENTIAL DIAGNOSIS
• Nocardiosis—primary differential diagnosis; *Actinomyces* not reliably distinguished from *Nocardia* spp. by gram staining, cytology, or clinical signs
• Other causes of chronic draining tracts and pleural or peritoneal effusions must be addressed.

CBC/BIOCHEMISTRY/URINALYSIS
• Leukocytosis with a left shift and monocytosis—common
• Nonregenerative anemia—may develop
• Hypoglycemia and hyperglobulinemia—common

OTHER LABORATORY TESTS
N/A

IMAGING
Radiographs of infected bone—periosteal new bone production, reactive osteosclerosis, and osteolysis

DIAGNOSTIC PROCEDURES
• Pus or osteolytic bone fragments submitted in anaerobic specimen containers for culture—see Anaerobic Infections; provides

the only definitive diagnosis; inform the lab to check for actinomycosis
• Fresh smears—gram staining, cytology, and acid-fast staining; staining does not preclude the need for culture; *Actinomyces* does not stain acid-fast; *Nocardia* is variable.

PATHOLOGIC FINDINGS
Histopathologic examination—not reliable for distinguishing actinomycosis from nocardiosis; useful diagnostic tool, especially with sulfur granules; may demonstrate pyogranulomatous or granulomatous cellulitis with colonies of filamentous bacteria

 TREATMENT

• Drain abscesses and lavage for several days; leave lesions open for continued drainage; Penrose drains may be needed.
• Bony involvement—May need to débride or remove bone
• Surgical resection of tissue—not needed in all cases

 MEDICATIONS

DRUGS
• Important to distinguish between *Actinomyces* and *Nocardia* for appropriate antimicrobial selection
• Antibiotics—a retrospective study suggests administration for a minimum of 3–4 months after resolution of all signs; may need to be directed against other associated microbes
• Penicillin G—considered to be reliable; specific recommendations for duration of therapy are not determined; try 65,000 U/kg q8h
• Metronidazole—avoid use; actinomycosis unlikely to respond
• Aminoglycosides—do not use; ineffective against anaerobic infections
• *A. hordeovulneris*—cell-wall deficient variant (L-phase); does not usually respond well to penicillin; consider clindamycin, erythromycin, and chloramphenicol

CONTRAINDICATIONS/POSSIBLE INTERACTIONS
N/A

 FOLLOW-UP

• Redevelopment of infection at the initial site may be expected in about half of all cases.
• Monitor patients closely, recurrence in the months after discontinuation of therapy.

 MISCELLANEOUS

Suggested Reading
Edwards DF. Actinomycosis and nocardiosis. In: Greene CE, ed. Infectious diseases of the dog and cat. Philadelphia: Saunders, 1998:303–313.
Author Sharon K. Fooshee
Consulting Editor Stephen C. Barr

ACUTE RESPIRATORY DISTRESS SYNDROME (ARDS)

BASICS

DEFINITION
• An acute, life-threatening, respiratory failure caused by heterogenous acute lung injury and increased capillary permeability–induced (noncardiogenic) pulmonary edema • Progression (dogs)—appears to result from amplification of the response to lung injury and subsequent ongoing disease • Characterized by normal PCWP; impaired pulmonary compliance; refractory hypoxemia; radiographic findings consistent with diffuse bilateral pulmonary infiltration; in severely affected patients, acute pulmonary arterial hypertension

PATHOPHYSIOLOGY
• No single mechanism responsible • Initially, noncardiogenic pulmonary edema develops after pulmonary capillary endothelial injury; fluid and proteins leak into gas exchange areas of the lung, causing stiff, noncompliant lungs with low functional and residual capacity, impaired respiratory compliance, and severe hypoxemia. • Inflammatory mediators injure the alveolar–capillary membrane, causing exudation of proteins that can inactivate surfactant and damage type II pneumocytes; surfactant deficiency decreases lung compliance and leads to atelectasis, causing maldistribution of ventilation and right-to-left shunting with areas of low ventilation to perfusion. • Vasoconstriction and widespread occlusion of pulmonary microvasculature cause pulmonary hypertension, which may lead to right ventricular dysfunction. • Death—refractory hypoxemia; frequently secondary sepsis or multiple organ dysfunction or failure

SYSTEMS AFFECTED
• Respiratory—acute respiratory distress • Other systems—depend on inciting cause and development of multiple organ dysfunction

GENETICS
Unknown

INCIDENCE/PREVALENCE
Unknown; 19 cases reported in 1996

GEOGRAPHIC DISTRIBUTION
N/A

SIGNALMENT

Species
Dogs and presumably cats

Breed Predilections
N/A

Mean Age and Range
Report of 19 dogs—median age, 3.5 years; range, 2 months to 10 years

Predominant Sex
N/A

SIGNS

General Comments
Four stages common: (1) gradual onset of tachypnea, shallow breathing related to decreased functional residual capacity, and pulmonary compliance; (2) apparent stabilizing, mild atelectasis, may see early signs of diffuse interstitial pulmonary infiltrates on thoracic radiographs; (3) signs of respiratory insufficiency characterized by hyperventilation, tachycardia, and pulmonary crackles; (4) persistent, severe hypoxemia (despite administration of 100% oxygen), tachypnea, and cyanosis

Historical Findings
• Dyspnea—most of 19 affected dogs; range of onset, 0.5–48 hr (median, 4.5 hr) before clinical evaluation • Lethargy, anorexia, evidence of trauma, collapse, seizures and tremors, vomiting and diarrhea, retching, and distended abdomen—may be seen, depending on the inciting cause

Physical Examination Findings
• Severe respiratory distress—tachypnea, dyspnea, cyanosis, and shallow breathing • Crackles and harsh bronchovesicular lung sounds on auscultation • Occasionally coughing • Others, depending on cause

CAUSES
• Bacterial septicemia—especially gram-negative • Viral infection—parvoviral enteritis • Other severe infection • Aspiration pneumonia* • Massive trauma; lung contusion • Hypotension • Thromboembolic disease • Burns • Pancreatitis • Massive transfusion • Uremia • Eclampsia • CNS disease • Radiation • Smoke or noxious gas inhalation • High inspired oxygen fractions—oxygen toxicity • Near–drowning • Pulmonary infection—viral, bacterial, mycoplasma, or fungal • Drug ingestion—acetylsalicylic acid; heroin; methadone; barbiturates; propoxyphene • Paraquat ingestion • Peritonitis

RISK FACTORS
• Sepsis syndrome • Circulating endotoxin and increased TNF • Sustained shock • Organ torsion—gastric dilatation volvulus and splenic torsion; lung lobe torsion • Upper airway obstruction—strangulation • Thrombocytopenia • Aspiration of gastric contents • Microbial pneumonia • Lung contusion; thoracic trauma • Multiple transfusions • Multiple fractures

DIAGNOSIS
Presumed diagnosis—serious underlying disease (particularly trauma or sepsis) with respiratory distress, refractory hypoxemia, and radiographic alveolar and interstitial infiltrates in the absence of heart disease

DIFFERENTIAL DIAGNOSIS
• Cardiogenic pulmonary edema • Pneumonitis • Pulmonary contusion or hemorrhage

CBC/BIOCHEMISTRY/URINALYSIS
• Variable abnormalities—depend on the inciting cause • Early stages—neutropenia and thrombocytopenia caused by sequestration into the lungs

OTHER LABORATORY TESTS
Alveolar–arterial oxygen gradient—widened, > 30 mm Hg on room air; normal, < 10 mm Hg

Arterial Blood Gas Analysis
• Reveals persistent, severe hypoxemia despite oxygen administration • Hypercapnia—late in disease; ominous prognostic sign • Metabolic acidosis—common and persistent finding in dogs despite fluid treatment and careful attention to tissue perfusion*

IMAGING

Radiography
• Clinical signs usually precede radiographic changes by as much as 12–24 hr. • Findings may correlate poorly with physiologic status. • Early findings—fine interstitial infiltrates, which may progress to diffuse alveolar and interstitial infiltrates • Cardiac silhouette—usually normal

Echocardiography
• Rules out cardiogenic pulmonary edema • May reveal moderately decreased shortening fraction in patients with septicemia-induced disease

DIAGNOSTIC PROCEDURES
• Cardiac catheterization—high pulmonary artery pressure with normal or low PCWP • PPV—high peak and plateau pressures

PATHOLOGIC FINDINGS
• Depend on the primary cause • Lungs—usually deep red; firm, heavy, and wet in appearance; ooze a clear, sometimes pinkish fluid on cut surface; severe interstitial and alveolar edema with a membrane of proteinaceous material in the alveoli • Lung tissue specimens—infiltrates of WBCs (mainly neutrophils) and RBCs; hyaline membranes; proliferation of type II alveolar cells often detected

TREATMENT
• Resolution and survival—contingent on the ability to maintain adequate tissue oxygenation, providing time for reversal of the primary disease process and repair of pulmonary endothelial and epithelial defects • Treat the underlying cause(s). • Prevent or treat infection.

APPROPRIATE HEALTH CARE
• Mechanical ventilation—recommended;

PEEP of 5–15 cm H_2O offers the greatest potential to reverse alveolar flooding and ventilation-perfusion mismatching by opening poorly ventilated regions of the lung; goal is to achieve adequate oxygenation ($PaO_2 > 60$ mm Hg) at the lowest possible inspired oxygen concentration (< 0.6 FIO_2) to prevent oxygen toxicosis. • If PPV cannot be provided, give supplemental oxygen by oxygen cage or nasal canula. • To optimized oxygen delivery, maintain hemoglobin at normal values by packed RBCs or whole blood transfusion.

NURSING CARE
• Supportive care for underlying causes—necessary • Pulmonary toilet • Frequent positional changes • Physical therapy • Coupage for patients receiving PPV • Fluids (crystalloid and colloid)—administer to maintain proper fluid balance and oxygen delivery; avoid hypervolemia and hypovolemia. • Balloon-tip pulmonary artery catheter (e.g., Swan-Ganz)—optimal for monitoring fluid administration

ACTIVITY
Cage confinement to reduce oxygen requirements

DIET
• Nutritional support—extremely important for restoring positive nitrogen balance, enhance respiratory muscle strength, and reduce susceptibility to pulmonary infection • Enteral feeding—preferred over parenteral • Avoid diets high in carbohydrates; may increase carbon dioxide production and cause progressive hypercapnia and respiratory acidosis

CLIENT EDUCATION
• Discuss the necessity for advanced medical care. • Warn client about the high cost of therapy and the grave prognosis.

SURGICAL CONSIDERATIONS
Surgery—may be indicated, depending on inciting cause (e.g., repair of trauma and removal of foci of infection)

MEDICATIONS

DRUGS OF CHOICE
• Anti-inflammatory drugs (corticosteroids)—controversial; benefits not documented; increase morbidity and mortality in affected humans; do not prevent development in susceptible human patients* • Positive inotropes (e.g., dopamine or dobutamine)—often needed to enhance cardiac output, particularly in septic patients • Intravenously administered furosemide and vasodilator (e.g., nitroprusside)—may cautiously give if PCWP is high; little effect on permeability-related edema and atelectasis; furosemide shown to dilate pulmonary vessels in nonedematous lung units, thereby improving

gas exchange* • Broad-spectrum antimicrobial therapy—for bacterial infection

CONTRAINDICATIONS
N/A

PRECAUTIONS
• Increased PEEP (> 15 cm H_2O)—results in increased intrathoracic pressure and decreased venous return, causing decreased cardiac output; along with high airway pressures, increased incidence of barotrauma and subsequent pneumothorax • Excessive diuretic use—may decrease blood volume and cardiac output • Intravenously infused vasodilators—usefulness limited because effects are not limited to the pulmonary vasculature (systemic hypotension is an unwanted side effect); may also increase intrapulmonary shunting by dilating vessels to areas of poor ventilation, lowering PaO_2

POSSIBLE INTERACTIONS N/A

ALTERNATIVE DRUGS N/A

FOLLOW-UP

PATIENT MONITORING
• Closely observe for changes in body temperature, pulse rate and character, ECG, and respiratory rate and character. • Arterial blood gas analyses—required frequently; assess adequacy of oxygenation, ventilation, and fluid therapy; monitor progression of disease • Alveolar–arterial oxygen gradients and hypoxemia scores (PaO_2/FIO_2)—repeat; monitor progression or improvement in oxygenation • Monitor pressures—pulmonary artery, central venous, PCWP (by a pulmonary artery catheter, if available), and arterial blood • Monitor urine output and calculate "ins and outs"—may prevent overhydration • Pulse oximetry—may use for continuous monitoring of hemoglobin oxygen saturation • Capnography—may used for continuous monitoring of ventilation • Monitor for multiple organ dysfunction—jaundice, gastrointestinal hemorrhage, or signs of DIC • Repeat biochemical and coagulation profiles—may detect early organ failure

PREVENTION/AVOIDANCE
• Early and aggressive treatment for sepsis syndrome • Use of in-line micropore filters when large volumes of stored blood are administered • Proper immobilization of long bone fractures—may decrease incidence of fat embolization • Carefully monitor all trauma patients for clinical signs of progressive hypoxia for at least 24–48 hr.

POSSIBLE COMPLICATIONS
Sepsis—frequently a secondary complication

EXPECTED COURSE AND PROGNOSIS
• Study of 19 dogs—all died despite aggressive treatment (12 euthanatized; 7 cardio-

pulmonary arrest); death attributed solely to respiratory failure in 8 (42%) patients; remaining patients most likely died of sepsis, shock, or severe organ failure of nonpulmonary origin. • Humans—mortality rates, 16%–90%; unfavorable prognostic factors: sepsis, sepsis with thrombocytopenia ($< 100,000$ platelets/μL), multiple organ dysfunction syndrome, renal failure, acidemia despite mechanical ventilation, requiring $> 50\%$ inspired oxygen concentration to maintain adequate oxygenation, pulmonary hypertension, and low diastolic blood pressure

MISCELLANEOUS

ASSOCIATED CONDITIONS
• DIC • Shock • Multiple organ dysfunction syndrome

AGE-RELATED FACTORS
Unknown

ZOONOTIC POTENTIAL N/A

PREGNANCY N/A

SYNONYMS
• Shock lung • Traumatic wet lung • Post-traumatic pulmonary insufficiency • Stiff lung • Adult pulmonary distress syndrome • Acute lung injury • Noncardiogenic pulmonary edema • Posttraumatic atelectasis • Post-traumatic massive pulmonary collapse • Congestive atelectasis • Adult hyaline membrane disease • Capillary leak syndrome • Post-transfusion lung • Microembolism syndrome

SEE ALSO
• Pulmonary Edema, Noncardiogenic • Dyspnea, Tachypnea, and Panting

ABBREVIATIONS
• DIC = disseminated intravascular coagulation • PCWP = pulmonary capillary wedge pressure • PEEP = positive end-expiratory pressure • PPV = positive pressure ventilation • TNF = tumor necrosis factor

Suggested Reading

Frevert CW, Warner AE. Respiratory distress resulting from acute lung injury in the veterinary patient. J Vet Intern Med 1992;6:154–165.

Parent C, King LG, Van Winkle TJ, Walker LM. Respiratory function and treatment in dogs with acute respiratory distress syndrome: 19 cases (1985–1993). J Am Vet Med Assoc 1996;208:1428–1433.

Parent C, King LG, Walker LM, Van Winkle TJ. Clinical and clinicopathologic findings in dogs with acute respiratory distress syndrome: 19 cases (1985–1993). J Am Vet Med Assoc 1996;208:1419–1427.

Author Cynthia C. Ramsey
Consulting Editor Eleanor C. Hawkins

DISEASES

ADENOCARCINOMA, ANAL SAC/PERIANAL/RECTAL

BASICS

DEFINITION
• Anal sac carcinoma—malignant neoplasm derived from apocrine glands of the anal sac; the most common malignant tumor arising from the perianal area in dogs
• Perianal gland tumors—arise from modified sebaceous glands of the skin; often benign (adenoma); may be malignant (adenocarcinoma)

PATHOPHYSIOLOGY
• Anal sac carcinoma—may be hormonally influenced because it occurs primarily in females
• Perianal gland tumors—may be caused by androgen stimulation because they occur predominantly in males; may be the result of combined androgenic and estrogenic influences because spayed females are more commonly affected than are intact females

SYSTEMS AFFECTED
Renal/Urologic—hypercalcemia (paraneoplastic syndrome); adversely affects renal function in some patients
Skin/Exocrine
• Anal sac carcinoma—invades surrounding tissues; metastasizes to the regional lymph nodes
• Perianal gland tumors (e.g., adenoma)—affect the skin at the site of origin, around the anus
• Adenocarcinoma—invades locally; causes distant metastasis

GENETICS
N/A

INCIDENCE/PREVALENCE
Perianal gland tumors—4.8% of all tumors in dogs

GEOGRAPHIC DISTRIBUTION
N/A

SIGNALMENT

Species
Dogs most commonly affected; rare in cats

Breed Predilections
Perianal gland tumors—dachshunds, cocker spaniels, German shepherds, beagles, English bulldogs, Samoyeds

Mean Age and Range
• Dogs > 8 years old most commonly affected
• One large study—median age, 11 years; range, 6–16 years

Predominant Sex
• Anal sac carcinoma—female (intact or spayed)
• Perianal gland tumors—intact male

SIGNS

Historical Findings
• Anal sac carcinoma—development of a mass; difficult defecation; anorexia; polyuria and polydipsia
• Perianal gland tumors—development of a mass (often multiple); licking at the anal region; scooting

Physical Examination Findings
Anal Sac Carcinoma—mass originating in the anal sac; sublumbar lymphadenopathy (metastasis) common
Perianal Gland Tumors
• Adenomas—usually nonfixed, encapsulated masses in the skin around the anus; may be seen along dorsal midline beginning at the neck, tail, and ventral midline, especially on the prepuce, ending at the umbilicus; may become ulcerated secondary to self-trauma
• Adenocarcinomas—fixed to the underlying tissues; dogs: may metastasize, often to sublumbar lymph nodes and distant organs; cats: metastasis uncommon

CAUSES
Hormonal role hypothesized

RISK FACTORS
N/A

DIAGNOSIS

DIFFERENTIAL DIAGNOSIS
• Tumors of other glands in the perineum—dermal sebaceous, apocrine, and merocrine anal glands
• Cutaneous malignant lymphoma
• Squamous cell carcinoma
• Mast cell tumor
• Anal sac abscess
• Perineal hernias

CBC/BIOCHEMISTRY/URINALYSIS
• Anal sac carcinoma—high serum calcium; occasionally concurrent hypophosphatemia; secondary renal failure may develop with hypercalcemia.
• Perianal gland tumors—usually normal

OTHER LABORATORY TESTS
N/A

IMAGING
• Abdominal radiography—evaluate sublumbar lymph nodes
• Thoracic radiography—perform, but pulmonary metastasis uncommon

DIAGNOSTIC PROCEDURES
• Cytologic examination—fine-needle aspirate; rule out conditions other than anal sac or perianal tumors; differentiation of benign versus malignant seldom possible
• Surgical biopsy—required for a definitive diagnosis; perform whenever possible

PATHOLOGIC FINDINGS

Gross
• Anal sac carcinoma—infiltrative tumor; 0.5–10 cm in diameter; may be unilateral or bilateral
• Perianal gland tumors—often multiple; adenomas: encapsulated, occasionally ulcerated, confined to the skin, 0.5–5 cm in diameter; adenocarcinomas: frequently fixed to the underlying tissues; ulcerated

Histopathology
• Anal sac tumors—areas of both acinar formation and solid lobules of carcinoma cells
• Perianal tumors—adenomas: characterized by cells that resemble hepatocytes; malignant: may have characteristic morphology of either adenocarcinoma or carcinoma

TREATMENT

APPROPRIATE HEALTH CARE
• Outpatient—for diagnosis; unless hypercalcemia and resultant renal failure dictates hospitalization
• Inpatient—for biopsy or surgical resection; until the postoperative status of patient is stable

NURSING CARE
As needed

ACTIVITY
• Unrestricted
• May need a side brace or Elizabethan collar to prevent licking

DIET
• Normal, unless patient has hypercalcemia-induced renal failure

CLIENT EDUCATION

Anal Sac Carcinoma
• Warn client of the poor prognosis.
• Inform client that metastasis at the time of initial surgery is associated with a shortened survival time.

Perianal Gland Tumors
• Inform client that prognosis for adenomas is good after castration.
• Warn client that estrogen administration may be complicated by pancytopenia.
• Inform client that adenomas also respond well to radiotherapy.

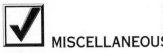

• Warn client that adenocarcinomas have a poor prognosis and are not likely to respond to hormonal manipulation.

• If resection is impossible for adenocarcinomas, advise client to consider radiotherapy.

SURGICAL CONSIDERATIONS

• Excisional biopsy—when possible

• Abdominal surgery and resection of affected nodes—consider for metastasis to the sublumbar lymph nodes

• Multiple or large perianal adenomas (males)—recommend castration and observation for 4–6 weeks before attempting aggressive surgery; orchiectomy alone often leads to complete remission.

• Cryosurgery—no advantage over conventional surgery

• Fecal incontinence—may develop if > 50% of the anal sphincter is resected or destroyed by freezing; transient likely (approximately 1 week) if < 50% is resected or frozen

MEDICATIONS

DRUGS OF CHOICE

Anal Sac Carcinoma

• Hypercalcemia—saline diuresis (200 mL/kg/day if possible) and furosemide (1–2 mg/kg PO q6–12h); reduce serum calcium

• Inoperable—consider cisplatin (60 mg/m² IV every 21 days)

Perianal Gland Adenomas

If castration of male dogs is rejected, consider treatment with estrogen.

CONTRAINDICATIONS

None

PRECAUTIONS

• Estrogen—use with caution because of risk of bone marrow suppression and pancytopenia.

• Cisplatin—may cause acute gastrointestinal disturbances, bone marrow suppression, and renal failure

• Chemotherapy—may be toxic; seek advice if you are unfamiliar with cytotoxic drugs.

POSSIBLE INTERACTIONS

None

ALTERNATIVE DRUGS

N/A

FOLLOW-UP

PATIENT MONITORING

Anal Sac Carcinoma

• Complete resection—physical examination, abdominal radiography, and biochemical analysis 1, 3, 6, 9, and 12 months after surgery

• Incomplete resection—measure tumor to determine response to treatment; necessary to carefully monitor serum calcium and renal function

Perianal Gland Tumors

• Evaluate 4 weeks after castration.

• No orchiectomy—monitor males for additional tumor development.

• Estrogen—perform CBC and platelet count monthly.

PREVENTION/AVOIDANCE

Perianal gland tumors—castration in males

POSSIBLE COMPLICATIONS

• Metastasis of malignant tumors

• Fecal incontinence after surgery

• Hypercalcemia and secondary renal failure

EXPECTED COURSE AND PROGNOSIS

Anal Sac Carcinoma

• Prognosis for cure poor

• Local progression and metastasis to sublumbar lymph nodes—common; negative prognostic factor

• Life expectancy—seldom > 1 year without treatment; quality of life may be good if hypercalcemia does not cause renal failure

• Hypercalcemia—negative prognostic factor

• Chemotherapy—may be useful in selected patients; many drugs have been used without improving survival beyond that with surgery alone (e.g., cisplatin, carboplatin, doxorubicin, melphalan, mitoxantrone, actinomycin, chlorambucil, piroxicam, and epirubicin).

Perianal Gland Tumors

• Adenomas—good prognosis after castration

• Adenocarcinomas—prognosis guarded to poor; progressive disease and metastasis to sublumbar lymph nodes and other organs likely

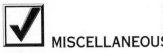

MISCELLANEOUS

ASSOCIATED CONDITIONS

Perianal gland adenomas—with recurrence in castrated males or in females, consider adrenal glands (e.g., hyperadrenocorticism) as a possible source of testosterone.

AGE-RELATED FACTORS

Old dogs (> 8 years old)

ZOONOTIC POTENTIAL

None

PREGNANCY

N/A

SYNONYMS

• Anal sac carcinoma—anal sac tumor; anal sac adenocarcinoma; apocrine gland tumor of the anal sac

• Perianal gland tumors—perianal adenomas; circumanal gland adenomas; hepatoid gland tumors; perianal adenocarcinomas

SEE ALSO

Calcium, Hypercalcemia

Suggested Reading

Chun R, Jakovljevic S, Morrison WB, et al. Apocrine gland adenocarcinoma and pheochromocytoma in a cat. J Am Anim Hosp Assoc 1997;33:33–36.

Meuten DJ, Cooper BJ, Capen CC, et al. Hypercalcemia associated with adenocarcinoma derived from the apocrine glands of the anal sac. Vet Pathol 1981;18:454–471.

Thomas RC, Fox LE. Tumors of the skin and subcutis. In: Morrison WB, ed. Cancer in dogs and cats: medical and surgical management. Baltimore: Williams & Wilkins, 1998:489–510.

Williams LE. Response to chemotherapy in dogs with adenocarcinomas of the perineum: retrospective study 1985–1995. Paper presented at the annual meeting of the Veterinary Cancer Society, Chicago, IL, 1997.

Author Ralph C. Richardson
Consulting Editor Wallace B. Morrison

DISEASES

ADENOCARCINOMA, LUNG

BASICS

OVERVIEW
- Makes up 75% of primary pulmonary tumors in dogs and cats
- Primary pulmonary tumors rare in dogs and cats
- Solitary tumors more prevalent than multi-lobed tumors
- May metastasize

SIGNALMENT

Dogs
- Makes up 1% of all tumors
- Mean age of affected animals 10 years
- No sex predilection
- Reports that boxers or brachycephalics predisposed

Cats
- More rare than in dogs
- Mean age of affected animals 11 years
- No breed predilection
- Some studies suggest females are over-represented.

SIGNS

Historical Findings
- Nonproductive cough
- Dyspnea
- Tachypnea
- Lethargy
- Anorexia
- Weight loss
- Hemoptysis
- Pain—pleural involvement
- Lameness—bone metastasis or hypertrophic osteopathy
- Polyuria or polydipsia—hypercalcemia or hyperadrenocorticism from ectopic production of ACTH
- Weakness or muscle wasting—polyneuropathy; polymyopathy

Physical Examination Findings
- May be none referable to respiratory system
- Tachypnea and dyspnea
- Fever
- Limb swelling
- Ascites
- Anterior vena cava syndrome

CAUSES & RISK FACTORS
- Some evidence correlates risk to urban environment; controversial
- Exposure to passive cigarette smoke unproven

DIAGNOSIS

DIFFERENTIAL DIAGNOSIS
- Granulomatous lesion
- Pulmonary abscess
- Other primary lung tumor—squamous cell carcinoma
- Metastatic lung tumor
- Pneumonia
- Asthma
- Congenital cyst
- Parasitic lesion

CBC/BIOCHEMISTRY/URINALYSIS
No specific abnormalities

OTHER LABORATORY TESTS
N/A

IMAGING
- Thoracic radiography—usually demonstrate a focal, solitary, well-circumscribed mass
- Ultrasonography—may help assess hilar or mediastinal lymphadenopathy; may help with obtaining an aspirate or biopsy specimen

DIAGNOSTIC PROCEDURES
- Thoracocentesis with cytologic examination—if pleural effusion noted
- Transtracheal lavage—limited diagnostic value
- Cytology—transthoracic fine-needle aspiration
- Percutaneous tissue biopsy—use Tru-Cut instrument
- Open lung biopsy—specimen via thoracotomy

PATHOLOGIC FINDINGS
- Adenocarcinoma—classified according to location (bronchial, bronchiolar, bronchiolar-alveolar, or alveolar) and degree of differentiation
- Undifferentiated tumors—more invasive and more likely to metastasize than well-differentiated tumors; sites of metastasis include lymph nodes, bones, pleura, eyes, and CNS.

TREATMENT
- Surgery—partial or complete lobectomy; mainstay
- Radiotherapy—may be of some benefit (mediastinal lymphadenomegaly); reports are only anecdotal.

MEDICATIONS

DRUGS
- Chemotherapy—no standard protocol; may be palliative
- Doxorubicin, cisplatin, carboplatin, and/or vindesine—rational choices for palliation
- Chemotherapy can be toxic; seek advice if unfamiliar with cytotoxic drugs.

CONTRAINDICATIONS/POSSIBLE INTERACTIONS
- Doxorubicin—monitor patients with underlying cardiac disease carefully; consider pretreatment and serial echocardiograms and ECG.
- Cisplatin—do not give to cats (fatal); do not use in dogs with pre-existing renal disease; never use without appropriate and concurrent diuresis.

FOLLOW-UP

PATIENT MONITORING
- Serial thoracic radiographs—consider every 3 months; administer a minimum of two cycles of chemotherapy before evaluating response to treatment.
- Perform CBC (doxorubicin, cisplatin, carboplatin, and vindesine), biochemical analysis (cisplatin), and urinalysis (cisplatin) before each chemotherapy treatment.

POSSIBLE COMPLICATIONS
- Anemia
- DIC
- Hemoptysis
- Spontaneous pneumothorax
- Hypercalcemia
- Hypertrophic osteopathy

EXPECTED COURSE AND PROGNOSIS
- Metastasis to the tracheobronchial lymph nodes—single best prognostic indicator; median survival without metastasis approaches 1 year and with metastasis, 60 days.
- Prognostic factors after surgery—ability to achieve complete cytoreduction; size of the primary tumor; metastasis; degree of cell differentiation
- Patients with well-differentiated adenocarcinomas have a better prognosis that those with undifferentiated tumors.

MISCELLANEOUS

PREGNANCY
Chemotherapy is not advised in pregnant animals.

ABBREVIATION
DIC = disseminated intravascular coagulation

Suggested Reading
Fox LE, King RR. Cancers of the respiratory system. In: Morrison WB, ed. Cancer in dogs and cats: medical and surgical management. Baltimore: Williams & Wilkins 1998:521-536.
Ogilvie GK, Weigel RM, Haschek WM, et al. Prognostic factors for tumor remission and survival in dogs after surgery for primary lung tumor: 76 cases (1975–1985). J Am Vet Med Assoc 1989;195;109–112.
Author Renee Al-Sarraf
Consulting Editor Wallace B. Morrison

ADENOCARCINOMA, NASAL

 BASICS

OVERVIEW
• Slow, progressive local invasion of the nasal and paranasal sinuses by neoplastic epithelial and glandular epithelial cells
• Most begin as unilateral but progress to bilateral by the time of examination.
• Approximately 20% arise from the frontal sinuses.
• In dogs and cats, more common than fibrosarcoma, squamous cell carcinoma, chondrosarcoma, and others.
• Prevalence of epithelial nasal neoplasia (dogs and cats)—0.3%–8% of all tumors

SIGNALMENT
• Median age (dogs and cats)—10 years (range, 18 months to 18 years)
• Medium to large breeds affected more commonly than are small breeds

SIGNS
Historical Findings
• Intermittent and progressive history of unilateral to bilateral epistaxis (median duration, 3 months)
• Epiphora
• Sneezing
• Halitosis
• Anorexia
• Seizures secondary to cranial invasion

Physical Examination Findings
• Noninfectious nasal discharge
• Facial deformity or exophthalmia
• Pain with nasal or paranasal sinus examination
• Obstructed nares (unilateral or bilateral)

CAUSES & RISK FACTORS
Urban environment suspected in dolichocephalic dogs secondary to pollutant exposure

 DIAGNOSIS

DIFFERENTIAL DIAGNOSIS
• Bacterial sinusitis—uncommon
• Viral infection—cats
• Aspergillosis
• Cryptococcosis—cats
• Foreign body
• Trauma
• Tooth root abscess
• Oronasal fistula
• Coagulopathy

CBC/BIOCHEMISTRY/URINALYSIS
Usually normal

OTHER LABORATORY TESTS
Cytologic and bacterial examination—rarely helpful

IMAGING
• Survey skull radiography—shows typical pattern of asymmetrical destruction of caudal turbinates with superimposition of a soft tissue mass; may see fluid density in the frontal sinuses secondary to outflow obstruction
• Thoracic radiography—evaluate for lung metastasis (uncommon)
• CT or MRI—best method for observing integrity of cribriform plate or orbital invasion

DIAGNOSTIC PROCEDURES
• Rhinoscopy—visual observation poor; soft, friable, fleshy masses that may be papillary, tubular, or solid and well formed; avoid progressing caudally into the cribriform plate
• Tissue biopsy—necessary for definitive diagnosis
• Bacterial culture—often positive

 TREATMENT

• Surgery alone ineffective
• Turbinectomy—may do before external (teletherapy) or internal (brachytherapy) irradiation
• Inpatient radiotherapy (with or without surgery)—best clinical control in dogs

 MEDICATIONS

DRUGS
• Chemotherapy—good option in some patients
• Cisplatin (dogs)—60–70 mg/m² IV once every 3 weeks; median survival after therapy 22 weeks; may provide marked palliation of clinical signs; **caution:** nephrotoxic; use with saline diuresis (18.3 mL/kg/hr IV over 6 hr; give cisplatin after 4 hr)
• Butorphanol—0.4 mg/kg IM; before and after cisplatin to reduce emesis

CONTRAINDICATIONS/POSSIBLE INTERACTIONS
• Chemotherapy can be toxic; seek advice before initiating treatment if unfamiliar with cytotoxic drugs.
• Cisplatin—never use in cats.

 FOLLOW-UP

• Untreated—median survival 3–5 months
• Radiotherapy—median disease-free interval 8–25 months in dogs and 1–36 months in cats; 1-year survival rate 38%–57% (dogs and cats); 2-year survival rate 30%–48% (dogs and cats)
• Brain involvement—poor prognostic sign
• Survey skull radiography, CT, MRI—when clinical signs recur

 MISCELLANEOUS

Suggested Reading

Cox NR, Brawner WR, Powers RD, Wright JC. Tumors of the nose and paranasal sinuses in cats: 32 cases with comparison to a national database (1977 through 1987). J Am Anim Hosp Assoc 1991;27:339–347.

Hahn KA, Knapp DW, Richardson RC, Matlock CL. Clinical response of nasal adenocarcinoma to cisplatin chemotherapy in 11 dogs. J Am Vet Med Assoc 1992;200: 355–357.

Theon AP, Peaston AE, Madewell BR, Dungworth DL. Irradiation of nonlymphoproliferative neoplasms of the nasal cavity and paranasal sinuses in 16 cats. J Am Vet Med Assoc 1994;204:78–83.
Author Kevin A. Hahn
Consulting Editor Wallace B. Morrison

DISEASES

ADENOCARCINOMA, PANCREAS

BASICS

OVERVIEW
• Malignant tumor of ductal or acinar origin
• Usually metastatic by the time of diagnosis

SIGNALMENT
• Rare in dogs—0.5%–1.8% of all tumors
• Rare in cats—2.8% of all tumors
• Older female dogs and Airedale terriers at higher risk than others
• Median age (dogs)—9.2 years

SIGNS
• Nonspecific—fever; vomiting; weakness; anorexia; icterus; maldigestion; weight loss
• Abdominal pain—variable
• Metastasis to bone and soft tissue common
• Pathologic fractures secondary to metastasis reported
• Diabetes insipidus secondary to pituitary metastasis reported in one dog
• Abdominal mass

CAUSES & RISK FACTORS
Unknown

DIAGNOSIS

DIFFERENTIAL DIAGNOSIS
• Primary pancreatitis; may be concurrent and complicate or delay early diagnosis
• Other causes of vomiting and icterus

CBC/BIOCHEMISTRY/URINALYSIS
• Usually nonspecific changes (e.g., mild anemia and neutrophilia)
• Hyperamylasemia less reliable than hyperlipasemia
• Lipase concentration often markedly high

OTHER LABORATORY TESTS
N/A

IMAGING
• Abdominal radiographs—may reveal a mass or loss of contrast associated with concurrent pancreatitis
• Ultrasonography—may reveal a mass or concurrent pancreatitis (mixed echogenicity, large pancreas, hyperechoic peripancreatic fat)

DIAGNOSTIC PROCEDURES
Surgical biopsy—definitive diagnosis

TREATMENT

• None reported successfully curative
• Palliation of pain and intestinal and biliary obstruction—surgery, if necessary
• Partial or total pancreatectomy

MEDICATIONS

DRUG(S)
N/A

CONTRAINDICATIONS/POSSIBLE INTERACTIONS
N/A

FOLLOW-UP

POSSIBLE COMPLICATIONS
• Intestinal obstruction
• Biliary obstruction
• Pancreatic abscess
• Peritonitis

EXPECTED COURSE AND PROGNOSIS
Usually a rapid progression to death, because no successful curative treatment available

MISCELLANEOUS

ASSOCIATED CONDITIONS
Gastrin-secreting pancreatic carcinoma—reported in dogs and cats; clinical signs also caused by hypergastrinemia, which results in inappropriate HCl secretion by the stomach, leading to gastroduodenitis

Suggested Reading
Harari J, Lincoln J. Surgery of the exocrine pancreas. In: Slatter D, ed., Textbook of small animal surgery. Philadelphia: Saunders, 1993:678–691.
Morrison WB. Primary cancers and cancer-like lesions of the liver, biliary epithelium, and exocrine pancreas. In: Morrison WB, ed., Cancer in dogs and cats: medical and surgical management. Baltimore: Williams & Wilkins 1998:559–568.
Author Wallace B. Morrison
Consulting Editor Wallace B. Morrison

BASICS

OVERVIEW
• A malignant tumor that develops in both neutered and intact male dogs
• Represents < 1% of all canine malignancies, but is the most common prostatic disorder in neutered male dogs
• Metastases to regional lymph nodes, lungs, and lumbosacral skeleton common

SIGNALMENT
• Medium to large-breed, intact or neutered male dogs
• Median age, 9–10 years
• Rare in cats

SIGNS
Historical Findings
• Tenesmus—with the production of ribbon-like stool
• Weight loss
• Stranguria and dysuria
• Rear limb lameness
• Weakness
• Lethargy
• Exercise intolerance

Physical Examination Findings
• Firm, asymmetrical, and immobile prostate gland
• Prostatomegaly common
• Pain—may be elicited in response to abdominal or rectal palpation
• May note caudal abdominal mass, cachexia, pyrexia, and dyspnea

CAUSES & RISK FACTORS
• Hormonal cause theorized
• Castration appears to have no protective effect against the development of this tumor.

DIAGNOSIS

DIFFERENTIAL DIAGNOSIS
• Other primary neoplasia—squamous cell carcinoma
• Metastatic or locally invasive neoplasia—transitional cell carcinoma
• Acute or chronic prostatitis, benign prostatic hypertrophy, and prostatic cysts—possible in intact male dogs; unlikely in neutered dogs

CBC/BIOCHEMISTRY/URINALYSIS
• Inflammatory leukogram possible
• Alkaline phosphatase—may be high
• Postrenal azotemia if urethral obstruction exists
• Evaluate urine samples taken by cystocentesis and free-catch technique—hematuria, pyuria, and malignant epithelial cells may be seen in free-catch samples but are unusual in cystocentesis samples.

OTHER LABORATORY TESTS
Serum and seminal plasma markers (e.g., acid phosphatase, prostate specific antigen, and canine prostate-specific esterase)—not high with prostatic adenocarcinoma

IMAGING
• Thoracic radiography—metastasis may appear as pulmonary nodules or increased interstitial markings.
• Abdominal radiography—sublumbar lymphadenomegaly, mineralization of the prostate, and lytic lesions to the lumbar vertebrae or pelvis
• Ultrasonography—focal to multifocal hyperechogenicity with asymmetry and irregular prostatic outline, with or without prostatic mineralization
• Contrast cystography—may help differentiate prostatic from urinary bladder disease

DIAGNOSTIC PROCEDURES
• Examination of prostatic aspirate (percutaneous or transrectal) or prostatic wash
• Prostatic biopsy—take specimen either percutaneously or during surgery.

TREATMENT

• Prostatectomy—local disease; success depends on the skill of the surgeon and the extent of disease.
• Radiotherapy—some therapeutic benefit; median survival after intraoperative radiotherapy, 114 days
• Castration—however, most tumors are not androgen responsive

MEDICATIONS

DRUGS
• Chemotherapy—carboplatin, cisplatin, or doxorubicin; may offer short-term benefit
• Pain relief—NSAID and opioid drugs
• Stool softeners—relieve tenesmus

CONTRAINDICATIONS/POSSIBLE INTERACTIONS
N/A

FOLLOW-UP

PATIENT MONITORING
• Ability to urinate and defecate
• Pain secondary to skeletal metastases
• Quality of life

PREVENTION/AVOIDANCE
Castration does not prevent disease.

POSSIBLE COMPLICATIONS
• Urethral obstruction
• Metastasis to regional lymph nodes, skeleton, and lungs

EXPECTED COURSE AND PROGNOSIS
• Grave prognosis
• Survival 1–3 months

MISCELLANEOUS

ABBREVIATION
NSAID = nonsteroidal anti–inflammatory drug

Suggested Reading
Bell FW, Klausner JS, Hayden DW, et al. Clinical and pathologic features of prostatic adenocarcinoma in sexually intact and castrated dogs: 31 cases (1970–1987). J Am Vet Med Assoc 1991:1623–1630
Morrison WB. Cancers of the reproductive tract. In: Morrison WB, ed. Cancer in dogs and cats: medical and surgical management. Baltimore: Williams & Wilkins 1998:581–590.
Author Ruthanne Chun
Consulting Editor Wallace B. Morrison

DISEASES

ADENOCARCINOMA, RENAL

BASICS

OVERVIEW
• Accounts for < 1% of all reported neoplasms in dogs
• Tend to be highly metastatic, locally invasive, and often bilateral
• Renal cystadenocarcinoma—German shepherds prone; an apparently heritable syndrome; less aggressive and has a better long-term prognosis than does renal adenocarcinoma

SIGNALMENT
• Adenocarcinoma–old (8–9 years) dogs; male:female ratio 1.6:1; no breed predilection
• Cystadenocarcinoma—German shepherds; often female
• Cats—rare

SIGNS
• Adenocarcinoma—may be insidious with nonspecific signs (e.g., weight loss, inappetence, lethargy, hematuria, and pale mucous membranes)
• Cystadenocarcinoma—may resemble nodular dermatofibrosis (a syndrome of painless, firm, fibrous lesions of the skin and subcutaneous tissues)

CAUSES & RISK FACTORS
• Adenocarcinoma—unknown
• Cystadenocarcinoma—appears to be heritable in German shepherds

DIAGNOSIS

DIFFERENTIAL DIAGNOSIS
• Other primary neoplasia—lymphosarcoma; nephroblastoma
• Metastatic neoplasia—hemangiosarcoma
• Renal adenoma or cyst
• Pyelonephritis

CBC/BIOCHEMISTRY/URINALYSIS
• CBC—may note paraneoplastic polycythemia, leukocytosis, or anemia
• Biochemistry—may be normal; may reveal azotemia
• Urinalysis—may show hematuria, proteinuria, bacteriuria, or casts

OTHER LABORATORY TESTS
Urine culture and sensitivity

IMAGING
• Thoracic radiographs—metastatic disease reported in up to 34% of patients
• Abdominal radiographs—mass visualized in 81% of patients
• Intravenous pyelography or abdominal ultrasonography—identify and stage disease

DIAGNOSTIC PROCEDURES
Renal biopsy—ultrasound-guided or surgical; definitive diagnosis

TREATMENT
• Unilateral adenocarcinoma or cystadeno-carcinoma—aggressive surgical excision is the treatment of choice.
• Renal failure—supportive management may be necessary.

MEDICATIONS

DRUGS
Chemotherapeutic management—success has not been described for either disease.

CONTRAINDICATIONS/POSSIBLE INTERACTIONS
N/A

FOLLOW-UP

PATIENT MONITORING
• Renal failure—measure serum urea nitrogen and creatinine; urinalysis
• Metastasis—imaging studies
• Quality of life—bilateral or otherwise nonsurgical disease

PREVENTION/AVOIDANCE
N/A

POSSIBLE COMPLICATIONS
• Renal failure
• Metastatic disease
• Anemia or polycythemia
• Invasion of local vital structures—vena cava; aorta

EXPECTED COURSE AND PROGNOSIS
• Long-term prognosis—poor, even with apparently localized disease
• Adenocarcinoma—patients who survive the first 21 days postsurgery have a mean survival of 6–10 months.
• Cystadenocarcinoma—better long-term prognosis, survival of 12 months or longer with no definitive treatment

MISCELLANEOUS

ASSOCIATED CONDITIONS
• Paraneoplastic syndromes—hypertrophic osteopathy, polycythemia, and neutrophilic leukocytosis reported in isolated cases
• Renal failure—may develop
• Nodular dermatofibrosis and uterine leiomyoma—commonly associated with cystadenocarcinoma

Suggested Reading
Morrison WB. Cancers of the urinary tract. In: Morrison WB, ed. Cancer in dogs and cats: medical and surgical management. Baltimore: Williams & Wilkins 1998:569–579
Author Ruthanne Chun
Consulting Editor Wallace B. Morrison

ADENOCARCINOMA, SALIVARY GLAND

 BASICS

OVERVIEW
• Tumor arising from major (e.g., parotid, mandibular, sublingual, or zygomatic) or minor glands
• Parotid gland—most frequently affected
• Locally invasive
• Metastasis—regional lymph node common; distant reported but may be slow to develop
• Other salivary gland neoplasms—carcinoma; squamous cell carcinoma; fibrosarcoma; mixed neoplasia
• Epithelial malignancies—constitute roughly 85% of salivary gland tumors

SIGNALMENT
• Dogs and cats
• Mean age, 10–12 years
• Spaniel dogs—may be at relatively higher risk
• No other breed or sex predilection has been determined.

SIGNS
Unilateral, firm, painless swelling of the upper neck (mandibular and sublingual), ear base (parotid), upper lip or maxilla (zygomatic), or mucous membrane of lip (accessory or minor salivary tissue)

CAUSES & RISK FACTORS
Unknown

 DIAGNOSIS

DIFFERENTIAL DIAGNOSIS
• Mucocele
• Abscess
• Lymphosarcoma

CBC/BIOCHEMISTRY/URINALYSIS
Results normal

OTHER LABORATORY TESTS
N/A

IMAGING
• Regional radiographs—usually normal; may see periosteal reaction on adjacent bones or displacement of surrounding structures
• Thoracic radiographs—roughly 33% of patients have lung metastases.

DIAGNOSTIC PROCEDURES
• Cytologic examination of aspirate—differentiate salivary adenocarcinoma from mucocele and abscess
• Needle core or wedge biopsy—definitive diagnosis

 TREATMENT

• Aggressive surgical resection—when possible; most are invasive and difficult to excise
• Radiotherapy—good local control and prolonged survival in three reported cases
• Clinical experience in a limited number of patients—suggests that aggressive local resection (usually histologically incomplete) followed by adjuvant radiation can achieve permanent local control and long-term survival

 MEDICATIONS

DRUGS
Chemotherapy—largely unreported

CONTRAINDICATIONS/POSSIBLE INTERACTIONS
N/A

 FOLLOW-UP

• Evaluations—dictated by tumor growth; every 3–6 months reasonable
• Long-term prognosis—unknown

 MISCELLANEOUS

Suggested Reading
Carberry CA, Flanders JA, Harvey HJ, et al. Salivary gland tumors in dogs and cats: a literature and case review. J Am Anim Hosp Assoc 1988;24:561–567.
Morrison WB. Cancers of the head and neck. In: Morrison WB, ed. Cancer in dogs and cats: medical and surgical management. Baltimore: Williams & Wilkins, 1998:511–519.
Author James P. Thompson
Consulting Editor Wallace B. Morrison

ADENOCARCINOMA, SKIN (SWEAT GLAND, SEBACEOUS)

BASICS

OVERVIEW
Malignant growth originating from sebaceous and apocrine sweat glands within the skin

SIGNALMENT
• Sebaceous gland—rare in dogs and cats
• Apocrine sweat gland—rare in dogs and cats; occurs more frequently in cats than does sebaceous gland adenocarcinoma
• Both types—more common in old patients

SIGNS
• Appear as solid, firm, raised lesions
• May be ulcerated and bleeding and accompanied by inflammation of the surrounding tissue
• Apocrine sweat gland—often poorly circumscribed; very invasive into underlying tissue
• Sebaceous gland—cats (rare) may have inflammation and swelling of multiple digits owing to metastasis of multicentric ungual adenocarcinoma from a distant cutaneous site.

CAUSES & RISK FACTORS
Unknown

DIAGNOSIS

DIFFERENTIAL DIAGNOSIS
• Any other skin tumor
• Cellulitis

CBC/BIOCHEMISTRY/URINALYSIS
Normal

OTHER LABORATORY TESTS
N/A

IMAGING
Thoracic radiographs and cytologic examination or biopsy of regional lymph nodes—required at the time of diagnosis; rule out metastatic disease

DIAGNOSTIC PROCEDURES
• Histopathologic examination—essential to confirm diagnosis
• Apocrine sweat gland—typically invasive into the underlying stroma and blood vessels; has poorly demarcated borders and a high mitotic index

TREATMENT

• Aggressive surgical excision required for both types
• Entire tissue specimen must be evaluated histologically to assess completeness of resection
• Radiotherapy—recommended for local control when complete surgical excision not possible

MEDICATIONS

DRUGS
Apocrine sweat gland—chemotherapy after surgery recommended, particularly in cats; carboplatin most effective agent in author's experience

CONTRAINDRATIONS/POSSIBLE INTERACTIONS
None

FOLLOW-UP

• Sebaceous gland—little known about the metastatic potential; prognosis good if complete surgical excision is achieved, particularly in dogs
• Apocrine sweat gland—associated with a very guarded prognosis; aggressive surgical resection required for local tumor control; postoperative chemotherapy recommended to delay or prevent development of metastasis

MISCELLANEOUS

Suggested Reading

Carpenter JL, Andrews LK, Holzworth J. Tumors and tumor like lesions. In: Holzworth J, ed. Diseases of the cat. Medicine and surgery. Philadelphia: Saunders, 1987; 406–596.

Thomas RC, Fox LE. Tumors of the skin and subcutis. In: Morrison WB, ed. Cancer in dogs and cats: medical and surgical management. Baltimore: Williams & Wilkins, 1998:489–510.

Author Robyn Elmslie
Consulting Editor Wallace B. Morrison

ADENOCARCINOMA, STOMACH, SMALL AND LARGE INTESTINE, RECTAL

 BASICS

OVERVIEW
• Uncommon tumor arising from the epithelial lining of the gastrointestinal tract
• Prognosis usually poor

SIGNALMENT
• Dogs more commonly affected than cats
• Middle-aged to old (> 6 years) animals; age range 3–13 years
• No breed predisposition
• More common in males than females

SIGNS

Historical Findings
• Clinical history often vague
• Owners complain of quality of life issues rather than specific clinical signs.
• Stomach—anorexia, weight loss, vomiting, hematemesis, and melena
• Small intestine—vomiting, weight loss, borborygmus, flatulence, and melena
• Large intestine and rectum—mucous and blood-tinged feces and tenesmus

Physical Examination Findings
• Stomach—nonspecific
• Small intestine—midabdominal mass; may see distended, painful loops of small bowel, melena
• Large intestine and rectum—palpable mass per rectum, forming a "napkin ring," or multiple nodular lesions protruding into the colon; bright red blood on feces

CAUSES & RISK FACTORS
• Unknown
• Nitrosamines—reported as causative agent in experimental literature

 DIAGNOSIS

DIFFERENTIAL DIAGNOSIS
• Foreign body
• Lymphosarcoma
• Leiomyoma
• Leiomyosarcoma
• Pancreatitis

CBC/BIOCHEMISTRY/URINALYSIS
• Stomach and small intestine—microcytic; hypochromic anemia
• Large intestine and rectum—no characteristic changes

OTHER LABORATORY TESTS
Fecal occult blood—positive after feeding nonmeat diet for 3 days

IMAGING
• Ultrasound—may reveal a thickened stomach or bowel wall; may see mass in the gastrointestinal tract
• Positive contrast radiography—may reveal a filling defect (stomach); may note intraluminal space-occupying or annular constriction (small bowel); gastric neoplasm most often found in distal two thirds of stomach
• Double contrast radiography—large intestine and rectum; may reveal polypoid or annular space-occupying masses

DIAGNOSTIC PROCEDURES
Endoscopic biopsy—may be nondiagnostic because tumors are frequently deep in the mucosal surface; thus surgical biopsy frequently required

 TREATMENT

• Surgical resection—treatment of choice; seldom curative
• Gastric—usually nonresectable
• Small intestine—remove by resection and anastomosis; metastasis to regional lymph nodes and the liver common
• Large intestine and rectal—may occasionally be resected by a pull-through surgical procedure; metastasis common; transcolonic debulking may provide palliation of obstruction.

 MEDICATIONS

DRUGS
• Chemotherapy—usually unsuccessful
• 5-Fluorouracil—200 mg/m^2 IV for 7 days; one case of partial remission in a dog

CONTRAINDICATIONS/POSSIBLE INTERACTIONS
• 5-Fluorouracil—cats: do not use, lethal; dogs: occasionally may cause seizures
• Seek advice before initiating treatment if you are unfamiliar with cytotoxic drugs.

 FOLLOW-UP

• Physical examination and abdominal and thoracic radiographs—at 1, 3, 6, 9. and 12 months postsurgery
• Instruct clients to watch for melena.

✓ **MISCELLANEOUS**

Suggested Reading

Morrison WB. Nonlymphomatous cancers of the esophagus, stomach, and intestines. In: Morrison WB., ed. Cancer in dogs and cats: medical and surgical management. Baltimore: Williams & Wilkins, 1998:551–558.

Takiguchi M, Yasuda J, Hashimoto A, et al. Esophageal/gastric adenocarcinoma in a dog. J Am Anim Hosp Assoc 1997;33:42–44.

Author Ralph C. Richardson
Consulting Editor Wallace B. Morrison

ADENOCARCINOMA, THYROID—DOGS

 BASICS

DEFINITION
Malignant neoplasm arising from the thyroid gland

PATHOPHYSIOLOGY
• Tumors rarely produce excess thyroid hormone.
• Locally invasive and moderately to highly metastatic, usually to regional lymph nodes and lungs

SYSTEMS AFFECTED
• Respiratory—dogs may be dyspneic owing to a space-occupying mass adjacent to the trachea; metastasis to the lungs common
• Endocrine/metabolic—affected dogs may be hypothyroid, euthyroid, or hyperthyroid; hypercalcemia may be seen as a paraneoplastic syndrome or secondary to concurrent parathyroid hyperplasia or parathyroid adenocarcinoma.
• Cardiovascular—hyperthyroid dogs usually tachycardic and may have systemic hypertension; may see anemia and DIC in advanced disease

GENETICS
Unknown

INCIDENCE/PREVALENCE
• Represents 1.2–3.7% of all tumors in dogs
• Represents 10–15% of all primary head and neck tumors

GEOGRAPHIC DISTRIBUTION
May be more common in iodine-deficient areas

SIGNALMENT

Species
Dogs

Breed Predilections
• Beagles, boxers, and golden retrievers—reported to be at higher risk than other breeds
• Any breed may be affected.

Mean Age and Range
• Mean—approximately 9 years
• Range—4–18 years

Predominant Sex
None

SIGNS

General Comments
• Usually not diagnosed until a large mass is palpable
• Approximately 65% are unilateral, 35% are bilateral.

Historical Findings
• Common—dyspnea; large ventral cervical mass; dysphagia; weight loss
• Less common—dysphonia; regurgitation; polydipsia; polyuria
• Hyperthyroid patients—large appetites; weight loss; polydipsia; polyuria; tachypnea; episodes of collapse
• Hypothyroid patients—poor-quality hair coats; lethargy

Physical Examination Findings
• Firm, nonpainful ventral cervical mass, moveable or fixed
• Usually unilateral
• Hyperthyroid patients—may be tachycardic, perhaps with irregular rhythms; tachypneic; emaciated

CAUSES
Unknown

RISK FACTORS
• Breed predilection
• Iodine deficiency

 DIAGNOSIS

DIFFERENTIAL DIAGNOSIS
• Other primary neoplasms—lymphosarcoma; soft tissue sarcoma; salivary gland adenocarcinoma; parathyroid carcinoma; carotid body tumor
• Secondary tumors—metastatic oral squamous cell carcinoma; oral melanoma
• Inflammatory—abscess or granuloma
• Salivary mucocele

CBC/BIOCHEMISTRY/URINALYSIS
• Usually normal
• May see nonregenerative anemia of chronic disease
• Rare—hypercalcemia; isosthenuria; DIC

OTHER LABORATORY TESTS
• T_4 and/or free T_4 concentration
• Endogenous canine TSH concentration
• TSH stimulation test—with suspected hypothyroidism

IMAGING
• Thoracic radiographs (three views)—rule out pulmonary metastasis
• Cervical radiographs—evaluate displacement of normal structures
• Cervical ultrasound—determine degree of encroachment on adjacent structures
• Thyroid gland scintigraphy—identify location of primary tumor and possible metastatic foci
• Radioiodine studies—may provide information about the tumor's ability to produce thyroid hormone

DIAGNOSTIC PROCEDURES

Biopsy
Tru-Cut not recommended owing to high risk of hemorrhage; open biopsy usually required

Cytology
• Examination of fine–needle aspirate from tumor and palpable regional lymph nodes
• Specimen almost always heavily contaminated with blood owing to highly vascular nature of tumor
• Homogeneous population of epithelial cells, sometimes with colloid—common
• Unable to differentiate malignant from benign thyroid cells; but almost all thyroid neoplasms in dogs are malignant.

PATHOLOGIC FINDINGS

Gross
• Characterized by high vascularity with areas of hemorrhage and necrosis
• Usually poorly encapsulated; often invade adjacent tissues (e.g., trachea and esophagus); may adhere to the jugular vein, carotid artery, and vagosympathetic trunk

Histopathology
• Three main types—follicular, papillary, and compact (solid); mixed follicular and solid tumors most common in dogs
• C-cell (e.g., parafollicular, medullary) carcinomas rare

 TREATMENT

APPROPRIATE HEALTH CARE
• Usually outpatient
• Inpatient—hyperthyroid patients after episodes of collapse

NURSING CARE
Varies with signs on examination

ACTIVITY
Restrict activity if dyspneic

DIET
N/A

CLIENT EDUCATION
Warn owners of the importance of controlling heart rate and rhythm in hyperthyroid patients and of the possibility of episodes of collapse.

SURGICAL CONSIDERATIONS
• Complete surgical excision—clearly treatment of choice for nonattached tumors
• Examine regional lymph nodes for staging and prognosis.
• Preoperative radiotherapy—consider for shrinking tumor
• Contralateral gland may be involved.

Risks
• Marked hemorrhage—tumors highly vascular; may need blood transfusion and intensive postoperative care
• Laryngeal paralysis—owing to trauma to recurrent laryngeal nerve
• Damaged parathyroid glands—may occur during surgery

 MEDICATIONS

DRUGS OF CHOICE
• Cisplatin (60 mg/m^2 every 3 weeks) and doxorubicin (30 mg/m^2 every 3 weeks)—reported to effect partial remission in approximately 50% of cases
• Cisplatin—nephrotoxic; must use with saline diuresis (18.3 mL/kg/hr IV over 6 hr; give cisplatin after 4 hr)
• Butorphanol—0.4 mg/kg IM before and after cisplatin to reduce emesis
• Thyroxine—maintenance doses to decrease TSH production have been recommended; some tumors contain TSH receptors; value of hormone-replacement therapy in affected dogs not determined
• Methimazole—5 mg PO q8h for medium to large dogs; may be beneficial for hyperthyroid patients
• β-blockers—may be indicated for tachycardia or hypertension

CONTRAINDICATIONS
• Doxorubicin—decreased myocardial function, usually determined by measuring fractional shortening by cardiac ultrasound
• Cisplatin—decreased renal function; monitored via BUN, creatinine, and urine specific gravity

PRECAUTIONS
• Doxorubicin and cisplatin—myelosuppressive
• Chemotherapy can be toxic; consult with an oncologist before initiating treatment.

POSSIBLE INTERACTIONS
Verapamil—may potentiate doxorubicin-induced cardiotoxicity

ALTERNATIVE DRUGS
• Radioactive iodine—may be useful for tumors that produce excess thyroid hormone
• External beam radiation therapy—may be beneficial to shrink tumors before surgery or to prevent local tumor recurrence after surgery; may be used palliatively to temporarily relieve signs caused by a space-occupying mass

 FOLLOW-UP

PATIENT MONITORING
• Serum calcium concentration—if bilateral thyroidectomy was performed; signs of hypocalcemia: agitation, panting, muscle tremors, tetany, and seizures; treatment: 10% calcium gluconate (1.0–1.5 mL/kg IV over 10–20 min)
• ECG—during IV administration of calcium; may use subcutaneous injection or intravenous constant-rate infusion until patient is stable enough to start dihydrotachysterol (vitamin D) orally
• Thyroid hormone concentration—treatment with thyroxine may be necessary after bilateral thyroidectomy
• Site of primary tumor—physical examination; thoracic radiographs every 3–4 months to detect pulmonary metastasis

PREVENTION/AVOIDANCE
Unknown

POSSIBLE COMPLICATIONS
• Tumor—anemia; thrombocytopenia; hypercalcemia; DIC; respiratory distress
• Chemotherapy—dilated cardiomyopathy; renal failure; pancreatitis; sepsis
• Surgery—hemorrhage; hypothyroidism; hypoparathyroidism leading to hypocalcemia; laryngeal paralysis
• Radiotherapy—pharyngeal mucositis; esophagitis; hair loss, and skin or coat color change (at radiation site)

EXPECTED COURSE AND PROGNOSIS
• Prognosis—related to size and resectability of primary tumor (small, nonattached tumors have best prognosis), involvement of regional lymph nodes, and occurrence of distant (usually pulmonary) metastases
• Approximately one third of patients have detectable metastasis at the time of diagnosis, usually to the regional lymph nodes or lungs.

 MISCELLANEOUS

ASSOCIATED CONDITIONS
• Nonthyroidal malignancies common
• Multiple endocrine neoplasia reported

AGE-RELATED FACTORS
None

ZOONOTIC POTENTIAL
None

PREGNANCY
Do not use chemotherapy in pregnant animals.

SYNONYMS
Thyroid carcinoma

ABBREVIATIONS
• DIC = disseminated intravascular coagulation
• TSH = thyroid-stimulating hormone

Suggested reading
Adams WH, Walker MA, Daniel GB, et al. Treatment of differentiated thyroid carcinoma in 7 dogs utilizing ^{131}I. Vet Radiol Ultrasonogr 1994;36:417–424.

Fineman LS, Hamiltion TA, de Gortari A, et al. Cisplatin chemotherapy for treatment of thyroid carcinoma in dogs: 13 cases. J Am Anim Hosp Assoc 1998;34;109–112.

Jeglum KA, Whereat A. Chemotherapy of canine thyroid carcinoma. Compend Contin Educ Pract Vet 1983;5:96–98.

Klein MK, Powers BE, Withrow SJ, et al. Treatment of thyroid carcinoma in dogs by surgical resection alone: 20 cases (1981–1989). J Am Vet Med Assoc 1995;206:1007–1009.

Waters CB, Scott-Moncrieff JCR. Cancer of endocrine origin. In: Morrison WB, ed. Cancer in dogs and cats: medical and surgical management. Baltimore: Williams & Wilkins, 1998:599–637.

Author Linda S. Fineman
Consulting Editor Wallace B. Morrison

AFLATOXIN TOXICOSIS

BASICS

OVERVIEW
- Result of a fungal toxin that affects the liver of dogs
- Rarely reported; possible in hot, humid climates where grain-based foods are exposed to moisture or if contaminated grains are used in production of feeds
- Clinical signs and lesions—dose and time dependent

SIGNALMENT
- Dogs
- Not reported in cats
- Young males and pregnant females—probably more susceptible

SIGNS
- Sudden death
- Anorexia
- Weight loss
- Icterus
- Ascites
- Hemorrhage

CAUSES & RISK FACTORS
- Grain-based feeds contaminated with *Aspergillus flavus, A. parasiticus,* or *Penicillium puberulum*
- Feeds exposed to elements with obvious mold spoilage
- Outside dogs at more risk

DIAGNOSIS

DIFFERENTIAL DIAGNOSIS
- Other causes of subacute to chronic liver disease and associated DIC
- No differentiating tests

CBC/BIOCHEMISTRY/URINALYSIS
- Thrombocytopenia
- High ALT and SAP
- Hypoalbuminemia
- High blood ammonia
- Hyperbilirubinemia

OTHER LABORATORY TESTS
- PT and APTT—prolonged; reduction in absolute concentrations and/or reduction in activated liver–produced clotting factors

- High FDP
- Hypofibrinogenemia

IMAGING
N/A

DIAGNOSTIC PROCEDURES
- Liver biopsy—not definitive

PATHOLOGIC FINDINGS
- Fatty change
- Icterus
- Ascites
- Mottled liver
- Biliary proliferation
- Hepatocellular necrosis
- Cholestasis
- Cholecystic edema

TREATMENT
- Aimed at reducing liver stress
- Diet—high-quality protein; dietary glucose source (e.g., corn syrup)
- Intravenous fluid therapy
- Possibly heparin and antithrombin III—with DIC

MEDICATIONS

DRUG(S)
No specific therapy

CONTRAINDICATIONS/ POSSIBLE INTERACTIONS
- Avoid drugs metabolized by the liver for activation.
- Do not expose patient to organophosphates or strong pyrethroid insecticides.

FOLLOW-UP

PREVENTION/AVOIDANCE
- Avoid using feedstuff that is obviously moldy.
- Store feed in clean dry area.
- Clean feed dispensers and feed bowls regularly.

POSSIBLE COMPLICATIONS
- With significant liver damage—persistent liver dysfunction
- Nephropathy—liver induced

EXPECTED COURSE AND PROGNOSIS
Prognosis—poor, even with treatment

MISCELLANEOUS

PREGNANCY
- Indirect effects on uterus
- Potentially teratogenic
- Pregnant animals may be more susceptible to toxicosis.

ABBREVIATIONS
- ALT = alanine aminotransferase
- APTT = activated partial thromboplastin time
- DIC = disseminated intravascular coagulation
- FDP = fibrin degradation products
- PT = prothrombin time
- SAP = serum alkaline phosphatase

Suggested Reading

Nicholson SS. Mycotoxicosis. In: Kirk RW, ed. Current veterinary therapy IX. Small animal practice. Philadelphia: Saunders, 1986:225–226.

Author George H. D'Andrea
Consulting Editor Gary D. Osweiler

AMELOBLASTOMA

 ## BASICS

OVERVIEW
• Oral tumor of odontogenic (tooth structure) origin
• Called adamantinoma in the older literature
• Most are benign, but rare malignant (highly invasive) forms occur.

SIGNALMENT
• Middle-aged and old dogs
• Uncommon in dogs compared to epulides
• Rare in cats

SIGNS
Smooth, firm, gingival mass that is usually nonulcerated

CAUSES & RISK FACTORS
N/A

 ## DIAGNOSIS

DIFFERENTIAL DIAGNOSIS
• Epulis
• Malignant oral tumor
• Gingival hyperplasia

CBC/BIOCHEMISTRY/URINALYSIS
Unaffected

OTHER LABORATORY TESTS
N/A

IMAGING
Radiographs of skull—often show bone lysis deep to the superficial mass

DIAGNOSTIC PROCEDURES
Deep tissue biopsy—necessary for definitive diagnosis

 ## TREATMENT

Radical surgical excision—mandibulectomy/ maxillectomy; at least 1–2-cm margins to ensure complete excision

 ## MEDICATIONS

DRUGS
N/A

CONTRAINDICATIONS/POSSIBLE INTERACTIONS
N/A

 ## FOLLOW-UP

Careful oral examination—1, 3, 6, 9, and 12 months after definitive treatment

 ## MISCELLANEOUS

Many histologic subtypes exist and all have similar invasive behavior.

Suggested Reading
Morrison WB. Cancers of the head and neck. In: Morrison WB, ed. Cancer in dogs and cats: medical and surgical management. Baltimore: Williams & Wilkins, 1998:511–519.
Richardson RC, Jones MA, Elliott GS. Oral neoplasms in the dog: a diagnostic and therapeutic dilemma. Compend Contin Educ Small Anim Pract 1983;5:441–446.
Author Wallace B. Morrison
Consulting Editor Wallace B. Morrison

DISEASES

AMITRAZ TOXICOSIS

BASICS

OVERVIEW
• Amitraz—formamidine acaricide; applied topically to control ticks, mites, and lice
• Amitraz-containing products (for dogs)—formulated as a 19.9% emulsifiable concentrate in 10.6-mL bottles for dilution and application as a topical pour on and as a 9.0% impregnated 25-in. 27.5 g collar • Systems affected—nervous; endocrine/metabolic (β cells of the pancreas); gastrointestinal
• Clinical signs—most associated with α_2-adrenoreceptor agonist
• After high-dose oral administration (dogs)—peak plasma concentration reached at approximately 6 hr; elimination half-life as long as 24 hr; metabolites excreted in the urine
• Ingestion of sustained-release-impregnated collars—constant release and continued systemic exposure until collar segments have passed in the stool
• Toxicosis—generally occurs when impregnated collars are ingested, when improperly diluted solutions are applied topically, or when solutions are taken orally
• Idiosyncratic reactions may occur.

SIGNALMENT
• Thorough history—usually identifies use topically or as a collar
• Dogs—common, owing to more common use
• Cats and other species—rarely reported
• Predilection for old animals

SIGNS

Historical Findings
• Develop acutely after exposure

Physical Examination Findings
• Minor to severe depression
• Weakness
• Ataxia
• Recumbency
• Bradycardia
• Hypothermia • Vomiting
• Diarrhea • Polyuria
• Abdominal pain
• Death

CAUSES & RISK FACTORS
• Ingestion of impregnated collar or pieces of collar
• Inappropriate direct application
• Ingestion of undiluted product
• After application of properly diluted and applied solutions—less common
• Elderly, sick, or debilitated animals—may be predisposed

DIAGNOSIS

Depends on clinical signs, history of exposure, or evidence of exposure and elimination of other causes

DIFFERENTIAL DIAGNOSIS
• Recreational and prescription drugs—marijuana; opioids; barbiturates; benzodiazepines; phenothiazines; antihypertensive medications; skeletal muscle relaxants; other depressant drugs or chemicals
• Ivermectins, avermectins, milbemycins—generally very high dose or exceptionally sensitive breed
• Alcohols—ethanol; ethylene glycol (antifreeze); methanol (windshield washer fluid); isopropyl alcohol (rubbing alcohol)
• Tick paralysis, botulism, cranial trauma, diabetes, hyperadrenocorticism, hypothyroidism, severe anemia, cardiac failure, and anaphylactic shock—marked depression or weakness

CBC/BOCHEMISTRY/URINALYSIS
• Hyperglycemia—common
• Elevated liver enzymes—uncommon

OTHER LABORATORY TESTS
N/A

IMAGING
Abdominal radiography—may reveal a collar buckle in the gastrointestinal tract

DIAGNOSTIC PROCEDURES
• Identify amitraz on hair or in gastrointestinal contents—analytical methods described; useful only to prove exposure; no data available correlating concentration with clinical signs

PATHOLOGIC FINDINGS
High-dose, prolonged exposure—increased liver weight; slight enlargement of hepatocytes; thinning of the zonae fasciculata and reticularis; slight hyperplasia of the zona glomerulosa of the adrenal glands

TREATMENT

• Inpatient—severely affected patients
• Mild sedation after correctly applied sponge-on solutions—often transient; may require no treatment
• Mild signs after topical application—scrub with a hand dish-washing detergent; rinse with copious amounts of warm water; institute nonspecific supportive therapy (e.g., intravenous fluids, maintenance of normal body temperature, and nutritional support); monitor 1–2 days until improvement is noted.
• Ingestion of collar possible—endoscopic retrieval of the collar—removal of large segments from the stomach may be beneficial; usually numerous small pieces are located throughout the gastrointestinal tract, making removal unrealistic.

MEDICATIONS

DRUGS

Collar Ingestion, Asymptomatic Patient
• Emetic—3% USP hydrogen peroxide (2.2 mL/kg PO; maximum 45 mL after feeding a moist meal); apomorphine and especially xylazine not recommended
Activated charcoal (2 g/kg PO) containing sorbitol as an osmotic cathartic—administer by stomach tube; re-administer every 4 hr until pieces of collar are noted in the stool and the patient is markedly improved.

Marked Depression
• May require pharmacologic reversal of the α_2-adrenergic effects
• Yohimbine (Yobine)—0.11 mg/kg IV, administered slowly; reverses depression and bradycardia within minutes; objective is to keep the patient in a state of low-level depression with normal heart rate, body temperature, and blood glucose concentrations
• Collar ingestions—monitor for recurrence of symptoms; may need additional yohimbine until collar segments appear in the stool
• Atipamezole (Antisedan)—0.05 mg/kg, IM; reported to reverse poisoning within 10 min; repeated as needed; an alternative when yohimbine is unavailable
• Yohimbine and atipamezole—may require initial repeated administration every 4–8 hr, because half-life in dogs is shorter than in other species and elimination half-life of amitraz is longer

CONTRAINDICATIONS/POSSIBLE INTERACTIONS

Yohimbine and atipamezole—excessive administration may result in apprehension, CNS stimulation, and rarely seizures.

FOLLOW-UP

• Body temperature, serum glucose, and heart rate—important parameters • Close observation for recurrence of clinical signs—required for 24–72 hr
• Yohimbine and atipamezole—requires re-administration in severe cases, because reversal effects subside before collar segments have passed or before amitraz has been eliminated from the body
• No long-term adverse effects expected

MISCELLANEOUS

Elderly, sick, or debilitated animals may take longer to fully recover.

Suggested Reading

Grossman MR. Amitraz toxicosis associated with ingestion of an acaricide collar in a dog. J Am Vet Med Assoc 1993:203:55–57.
Hugnet C, Buronfosse F, Pineau X, et al. Toxicity and kinetics of amitraz in dogs. Am J Vet Res 1996;57:1506–1510.
Author Steven R. Hansen
Consulting Editor Gary D. Osweiler

AMYLOIDOSIS

 BASICS

DEFINITION
A group of conditions of diverse cause in which extracellular deposition of insoluble fibrillar proteins (amyloid) in various organs and tissues compromises their normal function

PATHOPHYSIOLOGY
• Patients usually affected by systemic reactive amyloidosis; tissue deposits contain AA, which is a fragment of an acute–phase reactant called SAA • Phases of amyloid deposition

Predeposition phase: SAA concentration is high but without amyloid deposits; colchicine administration during this phase may prevent development of the disease.
Deposition phase (rapid portion): amyloid deposits increase rapidly; colchicine administration delays but does not prevent tissue deposition of amyloid; DMSO may promote resolution of amyloid deposits and a persistent decrease in SAA concentration.
Deposition phase (plateau portion): net deposition of amyloid changes little; neither DMSO or colchicine is beneficial.

• Clinical signs in dogs and cats usually are associated with amyloid deposition in the kidneys. • Dogs—amyloid deposits usually found in the glomeruli leading to proteinuria and nephrotic syndrome. • Cats—amyloid deposits usually found in the medullary interstitium but may occur in glomeruli.
• Some Chinese shar pei dogs with familial amyloidosis have medullary amyloidosis without glomerular involvement.

SYSTEMS AFFECTED
Renal/Urologic—predilection for renal AA deposition; liver, spleen, adrenal glands, pancreas, and gastrointestinal tract also may be affected.

GENETICS
No genetic involvement is clearly established; familial amyloidosis occurs in Chinese shar pei, English foxhound, and beagle dogs, and in Abyssinian, Oriental shorthair, and Siamese cats.

INCIDENCE/PREVALENCE
Uncommon disease in domestic animals; occurs most commonly in dogs; rare in cats, except Abyssinians

GEOGRAPHIC DISTRIBUTION
N/A

SIGNALMENT
Species
Dogs and cats

Breed Predilections
• Dogs—Chinese shar pei, beagle, collie, pointer, English foxhound, and walker hound; German shepherd dog and mixed breeds are at lower risk. • Cats: Abyssinian, Oriental shorthair, and Siamese

Mean Age and Range
• Most affected dogs and cats are more than 5 years old. • Dogs—mean age at diagnosis is 9 years; range, 1–15 years • Cats—mean age at diagnosis 7 years; range, 1–17 years • Prevalence increases with age. • Abyssinian cats—range < 1–17 years • Chinese shar pei dogs—usually <6 years of age when signs of renal failure develop; range, 1.5–6 years • Siamese cats with familial amyloidosis of the liver and thyroid gland usually develop signs of liver disease when 1–4 years old.

Predominant Sex
Dogs and Abyssinian cats—females appear to be at a slightly higher risk (< 2:1).

SIGNS
General Comments
• Depend on the organs affected, the amount of amyloid, and the reaction of the affected organs to amyloid deposits • Usually caused by renal involvement; occasionally, hepatic involvement may cause signs in Chinese shar pei dogs and Oriental shorthair and Siamese cats.

Historical Findings
• No clear history of a predisposing disorder in most (˜75%) cases • Anorexia, lethargy, polyuria and polydipsia, weight loss, vomiting, and diarrhea (uncommon) • Ascites and peripheral edema in animals with nephrotic syndrome
• Chinese shar pei dogs may have a history of previous episodic joint swelling and high fever that resolves spontaneously within a few days.
• Beagle dogs with juvenile polyarteritis may have a history of fever and neck pain that persist for 3–7 days.

Physical Examination Findings
• Related to renal failure—oral ulceration, emaciation, vomiting, and dehydration; kidneys usually small, firm, and irregular in affected cats; they may be small, normal-sized, or slightly enlarged in affected dogs. • Signs of nephrotic syndrome (e.g., ascites, subcutaneous edema) • Related to the primary inflammatory or neoplastic disease process • Thromboembolic phenomena—may occur in up to 40% of affected dogs; signs vary with the location of the thrombus; patients may develop pulmonary thromboembolism (e.g., dyspnea) or iliac or femoral artery thromboembolism (e.g., caudal paresis). • Chinese shar pei dogs and Oriental shorthair and Siamese cats may have signs of hepatic disease (e.g., jaundice, cachexia, and spontaneous hepatic rupture with intraperitoneal bleeding).

CAUSES
• Chronic inflammation—systemic mycoses (e.g., blastomycosis, coccidioidomycosis), chronic bacterial infections (e.g., osteomyelitis, bronchopneumonia, pleuritis, steatitis, pyometra, pyelonephritis, chronic suppurative dermatitis, chronic suppurative arthritis, chronic peritonitis, nocardiosis, chronic stomatitis), parasitic infections (e.g., dirofilariasis, leishmaniasis, hepatozoonosis), and immune-mediated diseases (e.g., systemic lupus erythematosus) • Neoplasia (e.g., lymphosarcoma, plasmacytoma, multiple myeloma, mammary tumors, testicular tumors) • Familial (e.g., Chinese shar pei, English foxhound and beagle dogs; Abyssinian, Siamese, and Oriental shorthair cats) • Others—cyclic hematopoiesis in gray collies; juvenile polyarteritis in beagles

RISK FACTORS
• Chronic inflammation or neoplasia • Family history in certain breeds

 DIAGNOSIS

DIFFERENTIAL DIAGNOSIS
• Dogs—glomerulonephritis is the main differential diagnosis; proteinuria tends to be more severe in dogs with glomerular amyloidosis than those with glomerulonephritis.
• Cats and Chinese shar pei dogs with medullary amyloidosis—consider other causes of medullary renal disease (e.g., pyelonephritis, chronic interstitial disease). • Renal biopsy—necessary for definitive diagnosis

CBC/BIOCHEMISTRY/URINALYSIS
• Nonregenerative anemia is found in some dogs and cats with amyloid-induced renal failure. • Dogs—may see hypercholesterolemia (>85%), azotemia (>70%), hypoalbuminemia (70%), hyperphosphatemia (>60%), hypocalcemia (50%), and metabolic acidosis • Hypercholesterolemia—common finding in cats with renal disorders (>70% of cats with renal disease in one study) but does not reliably predict glomerular disease • Hypoproteinemia—more common than hyperproteinemia (24 vs. 8.5%) in dogs with amyloidosis; hyperglobulinemia common in cats • Proteinuria—with an inactive sediment common in dogs; mild or absent in animals with medullary amyloidosis without glomerular involvement (most mixed-breed cats, at least 25% of Abyssinian cats, and at least 33% of Chinese shar pei dogs). • Isosthenuria, and hyaline, granular, and waxy casts in some patients

OTHER LABORATORY TESTS
Proteinuria—quantify by 24-h urinary protein excretion or urinary protein:creatinine ratio

IMAGING

Abdominal Radiographic Findings
• Kidneys usually small in affected cats • Kidneys small, normal-sized, or large in affected dogs

Abdominal Ultrasonographic Findings
Kidneys usually hyperechoic and small in affected cats; may be small, normal-sized, or large in affected dogs

DIAGNOSTIC PROCEDURES
Renal biopsy needed to differentiate amyloidosis from glomerulonephritis. In dogs other than Chinese shar pei, amyloidosis is primarily a glomerular disease and diagnosis can be obtained by renal cortical biopsy. In most domestic cats, some Abyssinian cats, and some Chinese shar pei dogs, medullary amyloidosis can occur without glomerular involvement; obtain medullary tissue to make the diagnosis.

PATHOLOGIC FINDINGS
• Small kidneys in cats; small, normal, or large kidneys in dogs • Amyloid deposits appear homogeneous and eosinophilic when stained by hematoxylin and eosin and viewed by conventional light microscopy. They demonstrate green birefringence after Congo red staining when viewed under polarized light. Evaluation of Congo red–stained sections before and after permanganate oxidation permits presumptive diagnosis of AA amyloidosis (versus other types) because AA amyloidosis loses its Congo red affinity after permanganate oxidation.

TREATMENT

APPROPRIATE HEALTH CARE
• Hospitalize patients with chronic renal failure and dehydration for initial medical management. • Can manage stable patients and those with asymptomatic proteinuria as outpatients

NURSING CARE
Correct dehydration with 0.9% NaCl solution or lactated Ringer's solution; patients with severe metabolic acidosis may require bicarbonate supplementation (see Acidosis, Metabolic).

ACTIVITY
Normal

DIET
• Patients with chronic renal failure—restrict phosphorus and moderately restrict protein. • Patients with hypertension—restrict sodium.

CLIENT EDUCATION
• Discuss progression of the disease. • Discuss familial predisposition in susceptible breeds. • Discuss potential complications (e.g., hypertension, thromboembolism).

SURGICAL CONSIDERATION
N/A

MEDICATIONS

DRUGS OF CHOICE
• Identify underlying inflammatory and neoplastic processes and treat if possible. • Manage renal failure according to the principles of conservative medical treatment (see Renal Failure, Acute and Chronic). • Normalize blood pressure in patients with hypertension (see Hypertension, Systemic). • Patients with thromboembolic syndrome and nephrotic syndrome caused by glomerular amyloidosis usually have a low plasma concentration of antithrombin III; thus heparin is relatively ineffective. Aspirin (0.5 mg/kg q12h) has been suggested for dogs with glomerular disease; this low dosage is as effective in preventing platelet aggregation as is 10 mg/kg q24h. • DMSO—may help patients by solubilizing amyloid fibrils, reducing serum concentration of SAA, and reducing interstitial inflammation and fibrosis in the affected kidneys; may cause lens opacification in dogs. Perivascular inflammation and local thrombosis may occur if undiluted DMSO is administered intravenously. Subcutaneous administration of undiluted DMSO may be painful. The authors have used 90% DMSO diluted 1:4 with sterile water subcutaneously at a dosage of 90 mg/kg three times per week in dogs. Whether or not DMSO treatment benefits renal amyloidosis in dogs remains controversial. • Colchicine—impairs release of SAA from hepatocytes; prevents development of amyloidosis in humans with familial Mediterranean fever (a familial amyloidosis) and stabilizes renal function in patients with nephrotic syndrome but without overt renal failure; no evidence of benefit once the patient develops renal failure; may cause vomiting, diarrhea, and idiosyncratic neutropenia in dogs

CONTRAINDICATIONS
Avoid use of nephrotoxic drugs (e.g., aminoglycosides).

PRECAUTIONS
• Dosage of drugs excreted by the kidneys may need adjustment in patients with renal failure. • Use nonsteroidal antiinflammatory drugs cautiously in patients with medullary amyloidosis; they can decrease renal blood flow in dehydrated patients.

POSSIBLE INTERACTIONS
None

ALTERNATIVE DRUGS
None

FOLLOW-UP

PATIENT MONITORING
• Appetite and activity level daily by the owner; body weight weekly • Serum albumin, creatinine, and BUN concentrations every 2–6 months in stable patients • Can assess degree of proteinuria serially by urine protein: creatinine ratios

PREVENTION/AVOIDANCE
Do not breed affected animals.

POSSIBLE COMPLICATIONS
• Renal failure • Nephrotic syndrome • Systemic hypertension • Hepatic rupture causing intraperitoneal hemorrhage • Thromboembolic disease

EXPECTED COURSE AND PROGNOSIS
This is a progressive disease that is usually advanced at the time of diagnosis. Survival for dogs with glomerular amyloidosis varied from 3 to 20 months in one study; some dogs may occasionally live longer. Cats with renal failure because of amyloidosis usually survive < 1 year. Mildly affected cats may not develop renal failure and have an almost normal life expectancy.

MISCELLANEOUS

ASSOCIATED CONDITIONS
• Urinary tract infection • Polyarthritis in Chinese shar pei dogs • Polyarteritis in beagle dogs

AGE-RELATED FACTORS
N/A

ZOONOTIC POTENTIAL
None

PREGNANCY
High risk in affected animals

SYNONYMS
N/A

SEE ALSO
• Renal Failure, Acute and Chronic • Glomerulonephritis • Nephrotic Syndrome • Proteinuria

ABBREVIATIONS
• AA = amyloid A protein • SAA = serum amyloid A protein • DMSO = dimethylsulfoxide

Suggested Reading
DiBartola SP. Renal amyloidosis. In: Osborne CA, Low D, Finco DR, eds. Canine and feline urology. 2nd ed. Philadelphia: Saunders, 1995:400–415.

DiBartola SP, Tarr MJ, Webb DM, et al. Renal amyloidosis in related Chinese shar pei dogs. J Am Vet Med Assoc 1990;197:483–487.

Authors Helio Autran de Morais and Stephen P. DiBartola

Consulting Editors Larry G. Adams and Carl A. Osborne

ANAEROBIC INFECTIONS

BASICS

OVERVIEW
- Caused by bacteria requiring low oxygen tension
- Most commonly found genera—*Bacteroides, Fusobacterium, Actinomyces, Clostridium,* and *Peptostreptococcus*
- Individual organisms vary in their potential to withstand oxygen exposure.
- A number of injurious toxins and enzymes may be elaborated by the organisms, leading to extension of the infection into adjacent, healthy tissue.

SIGNALMENT
Dogs and cats

SIGNS

General Comments
- Determined by the body system involved
- Certain areas of the body are more commonly associated with anaerobic infection, perhaps because of proximity to mucosal surfaces.
- It is possible to overlook the potential for anaerobes to be involved in an infectious process, leading to confusion in interpreting culture results and in selecting inappropriate antimicrobials.

Physical Examination Findings
- A foul odor associated with a wound or exudative discharge
- Gas in the tissue or associated exudate
- Peritonitis, pyothorax, or pyometra
- Severe dental disease
- Wounds or deep abscesses that do not heal as anticipated

CAUSES & RISK FACTORS
- Usually caused by normal flora of the body; a break in protective barriers allows bacterial invasion.
- Predisposing factors—bite wounds, dental disease, open fractures, abdominal surgery, and foreign bodies

DIAGNOSIS

DIFFERENTIAL DIAGNOSIS
- Wounds that fail to respond to appropriate medical therapy—aerobic cultures may be negative; suspect anaerobic organisms
- Cats with nonhealing wounds—test for FeLV and FIV.

- Middle-aged and old animals—tumor invasion (e.g., in the gastrointestinal tract) may be responsible for establishing infection.

CBC/BIOCHEMISTRY/URINALYSIS
- Neutrophilic leukocytosis and monocytosis common
- Biochemical abnormalities depend on specific organ involvement.

OTHER LABORATORY TESTS
N/A

IMAGING
None required, except perhaps with bone infection

DIAGNOSTIC PROCEDURES
- Appropriate samples—pus (1–2 mL in stoppered syringe) and tissue (minimum 1g sample)
- Proper handling of samples—minimize exposure to air when collecting and transporting; appropriate transport devices should be on hand before the sample is collected and include screw-top glass vials with media that accept a Culturette swab and syringes evacuated of all air and capped with a rubber stopper.

PATHOLOGIC FINDINGS
N/A

TREATMENT
- Thoracic drainage—important with pyothorax (see specific chapter)
- Hyperbaric oxygen—some potential use; may be limited in availability

SURGERY
- Should not be delayed when anaerobes are suspected
- Generally indicated for all except pyothorax and CNS infections
- Combined with systemic antimicrobial therapy—the best chance of a positive outcome
- Usually indicated when anaerobic organisms complicate pyometra, osteomyelitis, and peritonitis
- Cleanse the wound of toxins and devitalized tissue
- Enhance drainage of pus
- Improve local blood flow
- Increase oxygen tension

MEDICATIONS

DRUGS
- Antimicrobial therapy alone—unlikely to be successful; poor drug penetration into exudates
- Antibiotic selection—largely empiric, owing to the difficulty of isolating anaerobes and the delay in return of culture results; cytology and Gram staining of exudates may aid in selecting the initial antibiotic.
- Although most anaerobic infections are polymicrobial, antibiotic therapy targeted against the anaerobes is more likely to be successful than selecting multiple antibiotics because of the symbiotic nature of the infection.
- Penicillin G—considered the antibiotic of choice (except for *Bacteroides* strains)
- Amoxicillin—comparable to penicillin G in spectrum of activity; convenient and accessible; may be useful to combine with clavulanic acid for *Bacteroides*
- Cefoxitin—the only cephalosporin with reliable activity against anaerobes; expensive
- Clindamycin—may be especially useful for respiratory tract infections
- Chloramphenicol—good tissue penetration; but bacteriostatic
- Metronidazole—useful against all clinically significant anaerobes (except *Actinomyces*)
- Aminoglycoside—uniformly ineffective against anaerobes
- Trimethoprim-sulfa combinations—ineffective; poor penetration into purulent exudates

CONTRAINDICATIONS/POSSIBLE INTERACTIONS
N/A

FOLLOW-UP
Long-term antibiotic therapy may be required.

MISCELLANEOUS

ABBREVIATIONS
- FeLV = feline leukemia virus
- FIV = feline immunodeficiency virus

Suggested Reading
Hirsh DC, Jang SS. Anaerobic infections. In: Greene CE, ed. Infectious diseases of the dog and cat. Philadelphia: Saunders, 1998:258–263

Author Sharon K. Fooshee
Consulting Editor Stephen C. Barr

BASICS

OVERVIEW
• Dogs—three types (impaction, sacculitis, and abscess), which are probably stages of the same disease process
• Cats—rare; impaction occasionally noted

SIGNALMENT
• Dogs
• Rarely cats
• Small breeds—miniature poodles, toy poodles, and Chihuahuas reportedly predisposed
• No age or sex predispositions

SIGNS
• Scooting
• Tenesmus
• Perianal pruritus
• Tail chasing
• Perianal discharge, if abscess ruptures
• Behavioral changes
• Pyotraumatic dermatitis

CAUSES & RISK FACTORS
• Unknown
• Possible predisposing factors—chronically soft feces, recent diarrhea, excessive glandular secretions, and poor muscle tone
• Retained secretions may lead to infection and abscess formation.

DIAGNOSIS

DIFFERENTIAL DIAGNOSIS
• Erythema and swelling of the perineum—anal sac neoplasia
• Perianal pruritus—food hypersensitivity, flea allergy dermatitis, atopy, tapeworms, tail fold pyoderma, and seborrheic skin disorders affecting the perineum
• Anal sac abscesses must be differentiated from perianal fistulas.

CBC/BIOCHEMISTRY/URINALYSIS
N/A

OTHER LABORATORY TESTS
N/A

IMAGING
N/A

DIAGNOSTIC PROCEDURES
• History and digital palpation examination—establish diagnosis; if easily palpated through the skin, sacs are considered enlarged.
• Normal anal sacs—clear or pale yellow-brown secretion
• Impaction—thick, pasty brown secretion
• Anal sacculitis—creamy yellow or thin green-yellow secretion
• Abscessed—red-brown exudate, fever, swelling, and erythema over the anal sacs
• Ruptured—discharging sinus
• Cytology of anal sac contents—number of leukocytes and bacteria indicate infection
• Bacterial culture and sensitivity—may help for animals with chronic or recurrent anal sac infections

TREATMENT
• Express contents for impaction or sacculitis.
• Instill an antibiotic/corticosteroid ointment for infected anal sacs.
• If necessary, establish drainage in abscesses; clean and flush anal sacs.
• Recurrent abscesses—consider anal sac excision.

MEDICATIONS

DRUGS
Abscesses systemic and topical antibiotics

CONTRAINDICATIONS/POSSIBLE INTERACTIONS
N/A

FOLLOW-UP

Abscesses—examine after 3–7 days of therapy.

MISCELLANEOUS

Suggested Reading
Burrows CF, Ellison GW. Recto-anal diseases. In: Ettinger SJ, ed. Textbook of veterinary internal medicine. 3rd ed. Philadelphia: Saunders, 1989:1570–1572.
Author Jon D. Plant
Consulting Editor Karen Helton Rhodes

DISEASES

ANEMIA OF CHRONIC RENAL DISEASE

BASICS

DEFINITION
Low PCV, RBC count, and hemoglobin and hypoplasia of erythroid elements of the bone marrow are associated with progressive or end-stage renal failure. Anemia is normocytic, normochromic, nonregenerative, and proportional to the severity of the azotemia. Principal cause is bone marrow failure secondary to inadequate production of erythropoietin by the diseased kidneys. Shortened RBC life span, uremic inhibitors of erythropoiesis, blood loss, nutritional deficiencies, and marrow fibrosis may contribute.

SIGNALMENT
Middle-aged to old dogs and cats mostly affected; also seen in young animals with heritable, congenital, or acquired chronic renal failure

SIGNS
• Anemia contributes to development of anorexia, weight loss, fatigue, lethargy, depression, weakness, apathy, cold intolerance, and behavior and personality changes characterizing chronic renal failure.
• Syncope and seizures (rare)
• Pallor of the mucous membranes
• Tachycardia
• Systolic murmur

CAUSES & RISK FACTORS
• Inherited, congenital, and acquired forms of chronic renal failure (e.g., pyelonephritis, glomerulonephritis, amyloidosis, and lymphoma)
• Exacerbated by iron deficiency, inflammatory or neoplastic disease, gastrointestinal blood loss, hemolysis, and myeloproliferative disorder

DIAGNOSIS

DIFFERENTIAL DIAGNOSIS
• Anemia of chronic infectious, inflammatory, or neoplastic disease; myeloproliferative disease; chronic blood loss; aplastic anemia; endocrine disease; drug reaction; and immune-mediated or parasitic hemolytic anemia
• Regenerative anemia excludes diagnosis of anemia of chronic renal failure.

CBC/BIOCHEMISTRY/URINALYSIS
• Normocytic, normochromic, *nonregenerative* anemia (anemia may be masked by dehydration)
• Reticulocytes—low corrected indices and absolute counts
• High BUN, creatinine, and phosphorus; variably high calcium; variably low bicarbonate and potassium
• High BUN:creatinine ratio may predict concurrent gastrointestinal blood loss.
• Impaired urine-concentrating ability, mild to moderate proteinuria, and variably active sediment

OTHER LABORATORY TESTS
• Serum iron—normal or variably low (≤60 mg/dL)
• Transferrin saturation—normal or variably low (=15%)
• FeLV and FIV testing (cats) to exclude virus-induced myelodyscrasia
• Serum erythropoietin—normal (inappropriately) or low

IMAGING
Small, irregular kidneys with loss or disruption of renal architecture on radiographs

DIAGNOSTIC PROCEDURES
Cytologic examination of bone marrow—erythroid hypoplasia; myeloid:erythroid ratio normal or high; stainable iron normal or variably low

TREATMENT
• Increase RBC mass if patient is symptomatic for anemia (dogs, PCV = 25%; cats, =20).
• Stabilize azotemia in patients in uremic crisis (i.e., acute decompensation).
• Establish appropriate nitrogen, caloric, vitamin, and iron intake to reduce uremic inhibitors and bleeding tendency and lengthen life span of RBC.
• Ensure that iron is not deficient.
• Correct gastrointestinal ulceration and blood loss by administrating cimetidine, ranitidine, or sucralfate.
• Correct systemic hypertension.

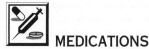

MEDICATIONS

DRUG AND FLUIDS

Erythropoietin Replacement
• r-HuEPO—a replica of human erythropoietin available as epoetin alfa (brands, Epogen and Procrit) and epoetin beta (brand, Marogen); provides consistent, rapid, and

long-term correction of anemia in dogs and cats with chronic renal failure
• Target PCV—dogs, 37–45%; cats, 30–40%
• Initial dosage—50–100 U/kg SC thrice weekly until PCV reaches 37% in dogs or 30% in cats (2–8 weeks), then decrease to twice weekly
• Maintenance dosage—50–100 U/kg SC once or twice weekly to maintain target PCV; individualize to each patient; life-long treatment required
• If PCV exceeds target, discontinue until upper target range achieved, then decrease previous dosage by 25–50% or increase dosage interval.
• Serum iron and transferrin saturation should be normalized before initiating and during r-HuEPO administration. Give ferrous sulfate (dogs, 100–300 mg PO q24h; cats, 50–100 mg PO q24h) if deficiencies are documented.

Blood Transfusion
• Short-term or rapid correction (PCV ≤ 20%)—give compatible whole blood or packed RBCs.
• Target PCV 25–30%.
• May be given intermittently for prolonged management

Anabolic Steroids
Little or no efficacy or indication for use

 FOLLOW-UP

PATIENT MONITORING
• PCV—weekly–semimonthly for 3 months, then monthly to bimonthly
• Blood pressure—semimonthly to monthly
• Iron and transferrin saturation—at 1, 3, and 6 months, then semiannually
• Discontinue erythropoietin if patient develops evidence of polycythemia, local or systemic sensitivity, anti-r-HuEPO antibody formation, or refractory hypertension.

POSSIBLE COMPLICATIONS

Erythropoietin–related
• Development of anti-r-HuEPO antibodies, polycythemia, seizures, hypertension, iron depletion, injection pain, and mucocutaneous reactions
• Anti-r-HuEPO antibodies neutralize r-HuEPO and native erythropoietin causing severe anemia in 20–30% of animals; reversible with cessation of treatment
• Signs associated with production of anti-r-HuEPO antibodies while the patient is receiving erythropoietin include decreasing PCV, erythroid hypoplasia, and myeloid:erythroid ratio ≥ 8.
• Use r-HuEPO cautiously or withhold if hypertension or iron deficiency develops; treatment can be reinstituted once hypertension and iron deficiency are corrected.

Transfusion–related
• Incompatibility reaction
• Circulatory or iron overload
• Transmissible infection

EXPECTED COURSE AND PROGNOSIS
• Disease correction increases appetite, activity, grooming, affection and playfulness, weight gain, and cold tolerance, and decreases sleeping.
• Although highly effective, use of r-HuEPO in dogs and cats requires careful assessment of the risks and benefits for individual patients.
• Short-term prognosis depends on the severity of the renal failure. Long-term prognosis is guarded to poor because of the underlying chronic renal failure.

 MISCELLANEOUS

ABBREVIATIONS
• FeLV = feline leukemia virus
• FIV = feline immunodeficiency virus
• PCV = packed cell volume
• r-HuEPO = recombinant human erythropoietin

Suggested Reading
Cowgill LD. Pathophysiology and management of anemia in chronic progressive renal failure. Semin Vet Med Surg 1992;7:175–182.
Author Larry D. Cowgill
Consulting Editors Larry G. Adams and Carl A. Osborne

BASICS

OVERVIEW
- A disorder of hematopoietic precursor cells characterized by impaired bone marrow function and inadequate production of granulocytes, erythrocytes, and platelets that results in pancytopenia in the peripheral blood
- The profound deficit in hematopoietic stem cells is most frequently caused by direct hematopoietic injury, e.g., cytotoxic chemotherapy and radiotherapy.
- Immune-mediated mechanisms often suspected
- Hemic/Lymph/Immune systems affected

SIGNALMENT
Dogs and cats

SIGNS
- Pale mucous membranes
- Lethargy
- Mucosal hemorrhages
- hematuria
- hemoptysis
- melena
- Fever

CAUSES & RISK FACTORS
- Rarely identified

Infectious agents
- FeLV*
- Canine and feline parvovirus
- *Ehrlichia canis*

Drugs and chemicals
- Estrogen*
- Sertoli cell tumor
- Interstitial cell tumor
- Methimazole (cats)
- Azathioprine
- Trimethoprim-sulfadiazine
- Griseofulvin
- Phenylbutazone
- Albendazole
- Captopril
- Second-generation cephalosporins
- Meclofenamic acid
- Quinidine gluconate
- Ionizing radiation

DIAGNOSIS

DIFFERENTIAL DIAGNOSIS
Causes of pancytopenia (e.g., infectious agents, myelosuppressive drugs, and toxins)

CBC/BIOCHEMISTRY/URINALYSIS
- Normocytic normochromic, nonregenerative anemia
- Leukopenia
- Thrombocytopenia

OTHER LABORATORY TESTS
- Serologic test for infectious disease (e.g., FeLV and *E. canis*)
- Serologic test for anti-erythrocyte antibodies (Coombs test)

IMAGING
N/A

DIAGNOSTIC PROCEDURES
- Bone marrow examination—frequently a specimen cannot be obtained by aspiration or a fatty specimen with very few hematopoietic cells is obtained.
- Core biopsy reveals markedly low cellularity in all cell lines.

TREATMENT

Supportive treatment or transfusions appropriate to clinical condition

MEDICATIONS

DRUGS
- Cyclosporine A—10–17 mg/kg PO q24h (dogs); 10 mg/kg PO q12h (cats)
- rhG-CSF—5 μg/kg/day
- Drugs to destroy T cells or block T-cell function
- Androgen and corticosteroid administrations have been largely unsuccessful.

CONTRAINDICATIONS/POSSIBLE INTERACTIONS
N/A

ALTERNATIVE DRUGS
- Antibiotics to treat secondary infection if fever is present
- Whole or component blood transfusion if indicated

FOLLOW-UP

PATIENT MONITORING
- Daily physical examination
- CBC every 3–5 days to weekly

PREVENTION/AVOIDANCE
- Castration of cryptorchid males
- Careful periodic monitoring of CBC in cancer patients receiving chemotherapeutic drugs

POSSIBLE COMPLICATIONS
- Sepsis
- Hemorrhage

EXPECTED COURSE AND PROGNOSIS
- Guarded to poor
- Recovery of hematopoiesis may take weeks to months.
- Spontaneous recovery occasionally occurs, especially in young dogs.

MISCELLANEOUS

SEE ALSO
Pancytopenia

ABBREVIATIONS
- PCV = packed cell volume
- rhG-CSF = recombinant human granulocyte colony–stimulating factor

Suggested Reading
Young NS, Maciejewski J. The Pathophysiology of acquired aplastic anemia New Engl J Med 1997;336:1365–1372.

Author Gregory O. Freden
Consulting Editor Susan M. Cotter

BASICS

OVERVIEW
• Hemolytic anemia caused by RBC inclusions called Heinz bodies, which are clumps of oxidized, denatured hemoglobin that cause splenic entrapment or lysis of RBCs.
• Caused by ingestion or administration of chemical or dietary oxidants
• New methylene blue stain used to identify Heinz bodies
• Sometimes accompanied by methemo-globinemia
• Treatment includes removing the offending oxidant and providing supportive care.

SIGNALMENT
• Dogs and cats
• More common in cats, which have oxidant-sensitive hemoglobin
• No sex, breed, or age disposition

SIGNS
Historical Findings
• Exposure to oxidant drug, plant, or chemical
• Sudden onset of weakness, anorexia, and fever
• Reddish brown urine (hemoglobinuria), if hemolysis is severe

PHYSICAL EXAMINATION FINDINGS
• Pale or icteric mucous membranes
• Cyanosis, if concurrent methemoglo-binemia

CAUSES & RISK FACTORS
• Acetaminophen (cats)
• Phenacetin (cats)
• Phenazopyridine
• Methylene blue
• Onions (i.e., raw, cooked, dehydrated, and powdered)
• Vitamin K_3 (not vitamin K_1)
• Zinc toxicity
• D,L-methionine (cats)
• Benzocaine (topical)
• Naphthalene (moth ball) ingestion
• Propylene glycol, fish-based diets, propofol anesthesia, diabetes mellitus, and other systemic diseases can cause Heinz bodies in cats, but oxidation is not severe enough to cause hemolytic anemia.

DIAGNOSIS

DIFFERENTIAL DIAGNOSIS
Other causes of regenerative, hemolytic anemia (e.g., immune-mediated and RBC organisms such as *Haemobartonella*)

CBC/BIOCHEMISTRY/URINALYSIS
• PCV and reticulocyte count indicate regenerative, mild to severe anemia (**REMEMBER:** not all cats with Heinz bodies have hemolytic anemia).
• Mean corpuscular hemoglobin concen-tration and automated WBC count—may be falsely high because of interference from Heinz bodies
• Heinz bodies may be visible on a routine blood smear as pale, spherical inclusions that protrude from RBCs.
• Dogs have fragmented RBCs and eccentro-cytes.
• Hyperbilirubinemia and bilirubinuria are possible.
• Hemoglobinemia and hemoglobinuria—uncommon but may occur if hemolysis is severe

OTHER LABORATORY TESTS
• Supravital new methylene blue stain—Heinz bodies stain blue for easy visibility and quantitation.
• Heinz bodies—can be present in up to 100% of RBCs; usually small and multiple in dogs; single and large in cats; normal cats have Heinz bodies in < 5% of RBCs.
• Methemoglobin test if animal is cyanotic
• Serum zinc concentration if indicated

IMAGING
Abdominal radiographs if zinc toxicity suspected

DIAGNOSTIC PROCEDURES
None

TREATMENT

APPROPRIATE HEALTH CARE
Identify and remove the source of oxidant (may be enough for recovery).

NURSING CARE
Provide supportive care for anemia (e.g., transfusion, oxygen, and quiet).

MEDICATIONS

DRUGS OF CHOICE
• Acetaminophen toxicity—*N*-acetylcysteine (140 mg/kg q8h PO or IV, or 140 mg/kg loading dose PO or IV followed by 70 mg/kg q4h for 5 doses)
• Methemoglobinemia—methylene blue (1.0–1.5 mg/kg IV once, slowly)

ALTERNATIVE DRUGS
Acetaminophen toxicity—sodium sulfate (50 mg/kg q8h IV)

CONTRAINDICATIONS/POSSIBLE INTERACTIONS
Methylene blue is an oxidant in high doses; use with caution.

FOLLOW-UP
• Monitor PCV, reticulocytes, and percentage of Heinz bodies.
• Document disappearance of Heinz bodies and regeneration of RBCs.
• Counsel clients on potential causes of the disorder and how to avoid exposing their pets.
• Prognosis is good once the hemolytic crisis is over.

MISCELLANEOUS

SEE ALSO
• Acetaminophen Toxicity
• Anemia, Regenerative
• Zinc Toxicity

ABBREVIATION
PCV = packed cell volume

Suggested Reading
Weiser MG. Erythrocyte responses and disor-ders. In: Ettinger SJ, ed. Textbook of veteri-nary internal medicine. 4th ed. Philadel-phia: Saunders, 1995:1864–1891.
Author Mary M. Christopher
Consulting Editor Susan M. Cotter

DISEASES

ANEMIA, IMMUNE–MEDIATED

BASICS

DEFINITION
Accelerated destruction or removal of RBC because of anti-RBC antibodies with or without complement

PATHOPHYSIOLOGY
• Anti-RBC antibodies form against normal (primary IMHA) or altered (secondary IMHA) RBC membrane antigens. • Infectious organisms, exposure of previously unexposed antigens, or adsorption of preformed antigen–antibody complexes to the RBC membrane can alter RBC membrane antigens • Antibodies can be warm type (reactive at body temperature, usually IgG) or cold type (reactive at subnormal body temperature, usually IgM). • Immunoglobulin (IgG or IgM, with or without complement) deposits on the RBC membrane, causing either direct intravascular hemolysis, intravascular agglutination of RBCs, or accelerated removal by the reticuloendothelial system in the spleen and/or liver (extravascular hemolysis). • Intravascular hemolysis occurs when adsorbed antibodies (usually IgG) activate complement; in vivo agglutination of RBCs occurs when IgM or high titers of IgG molecules cause bridging of RBCs. • Removal of RBCs occurs in the spleen and/or liver and is considered a type of extravascular hemolysis. • A form of nonregenerative IMHA is believed to be caused by immune-mediated destruction of RBC precursors in the bone marrow.

SYSTEMS AFFECTED
• Hemic/Lymphatic/Immune—immune-mediated destruction or removal of RBCs • Hepatobiliary—hemolysis leads to hyper-bilirubinemia and icterus when hepatic function is overwhelmed; hypoxia may cause centrilobular necrosis. • Cardiovascular—hypoxia leads to tachycardia; low blood viscosity and turbulent blood flow cause low-grade heart murmurs; high-output heart failure with chronic anemia. • Respiratory—hypoxia causes tachypnea. • Renal/urologic—hypoxia causes renal tubular necrosis. • Skin/Exocrine—cold-type IMHA may cause necrosis of extremities and ear tips because of capillary sludging.

GENETICS
• Isolated families of dogs have been documented to be affected (Viszla, Scottish terrier). • No genetic basis has been established.

INCIDENCE/PREVALENCE
Unknown

GEOGRAPHIC DISTRIBUTION
Secondary IMHA may have a higher prevalence in areas endemic to associated infectious diseases.

SIGNALMENT
Species
• Dogs • Rarely cats

Breed Predilections
Old English sheepdogs, cocker spaniels, poodles, Irish setters, English springer spaniels, collies

Mean Age and Range
• Mean age, 5–6 years • Reported range, 1–13 years

Predominant Sex
Females

SIGNS
General Comments
The remaining discussion focuses on primary IMHA.

Historical Findings
• Collapse • Weakness • Lethargy • Anorexia • Exercise intolerance • Dyspnea • Tachypnea • Vomiting • Diarrhea • Occasionally polyuria and polydipsia

Physical Examination Findings
• Pale mucous membranes, tachycardia, and tachypnea • Splenomegaly and hepatomegaly • Icterus and pigmenturia (hemoglobin or bilirubin) • Fever and lymphadenomegaly • Systolic murmur and S_3 gallop • Petechia, ecchymoses, or melena possible in animals with concurrent thrombocytopenia or DIC • Skin lesions possible in animals with cold-type IMHA • Other systemic signs possible (e.g., joint pain and glomerulonephritis) if IMHA a component of SLE

CAUSES
Primary IMHA (Normal RBC Membrane Antigens)
• Autoimmune hemolytic anemia • SLE • Neonatal isoerythrolysis • Dysregulated immune system (e.g., depressed suppressor T cell activity, high production of immuno-globulins) • Shared antigenic determinants (e.g., infectious agents and drugs) • Idiopathic

Secondary IMHA (Altered RBC Membrane Antigens)
• Infectious causes (e.g., *Haemobartonella, Babesia, Leptospira, Ehrlichia,* FeLV, and other viral agents) • Exposure of previously unexposed antigens • Microangiopathic hemolytic anemia (e.g., heartworm disease, vascular or gastrointestinal neoplasia, vasculitis, and DIC) • Adsorption of antigen–antibody complexes to RBC membrane • Drugs (e.g., sulfa drugs, cephalosporins, heparin, quinidine, propylthiouracil, and methimazole) • Type III hypersensitivity reactions (e.g., Arthus reaction)

RISK FACTORS
Exposure to infectious agents or drugs known to cause IMHA

DIAGNOSIS

DIFFERENTIAL DIAGNOSIS
Dogs
• Hemorrhage • Pyruvate kinase deficiency • Phosphofructokinase deficiency • Heinz body anemia • Zinc toxicity • Splenic torsion • Chronic progressive hepatitis in Bedlington terriers

Cats
• Hemorrhage • Heinz body anemia • Acetaminophen toxicity • Severe hypophosphatemia • Methemoglobin reductase deficiency • Congenital feline porphyria • Cytauxzoonosis

CBC/BIOCHEMISTRY/URINALYSIS
• CBC—anemia, high MCV (3–5 days posthemolytic episode), spherocytes, anisocytosis, polychromasia, nucleated RBC, and leukocytosis with neutrophilic left shift • Serum biochemistry–hyperbilirubinemia, hemoglobinemia, high ALT • Urinalysis—hemoglobinuria, bilirubinuria

OTHER LABORATORY TESTS
• Positive direct antiglobulin (Coombs') test—positive in 60% of animals with IMHA • Spontaneous autoagglutination in saline • Reticulocytosis—absolute count > 60,000/µl in dogs and > 50,000/µl in cats • Thrombocytopenia in animals with Evan's syndrome and DIC • Prolonged APTT and PT in animals with DIC • Positive ANA titer and LE cell test in animals with SLE • Positive serologic titers for infectious causes • Evidence of hematologic parasites in blood smears of capillary blood • Expanded RBC distribution width • High RBC osmotic fragility (may be useful in cats)

IMAGING
• Radiographs—hepatomegaly and splenomegaly; thorax usually within normal limits; may see evidence of pulmonary thromboembolism, cardiomegaly, or evidence of heart failure if animal has chronic anemia. • Echocardiography—generalized cardio-megaly, eccentric hypertrophy, and hyper-dynamic state in animals with chronic anemia • Abdominal ultrasonography—hepatomegaly and splenomegaly; liver and spleen can be mottled and hyperechoic or hypoechoic.

DIAGNOSTIC PROCEDURES
• Examination of bone marrow aspirate usually reveals hyperplasia of the erythroid series. • In animals with nonregenerative IMHA, may see maturation arrest or low numbers erythroid precursors. • In animals with chronic IMHA, myelofibrosis may be seen.

PATHOLOGIC FINDINGS
• Hepatosplenomegaly • Splenic and hepatic extramedullary hematopoiesis • Reactive lymphadenomegaly • Signs of congestive heart failure (e.g., pulmonary edema, cardiomegaly, and hepatic congestion), pulmonary thromboembolism, and DIC

TREATMENT

APPROPRIATE HEALTH CARE
• Inpatient during the acute hemolytic crisis;

outpatient when PCV has stabilized, ongoing hemolysis has been controlled, and clinical signs of anemia have resolved. • Inpatient if animal has complications such as DIC, pulmonary thromboembolism, thrombocytopenia, gastrointestinal bleeding, and heart failure and/or the need for multiple transfusions. • Chronic, low-grade, extravascular hemolysis can be treated on an outpatient basis if the patient is not exhibiting clinical signs secondary to anemia.

NURSING CARE
Fluids to maintain vascular volume and correct dehydration; exercise caution with chronic anemia patients because volume overload is a concern.

ACTIVITY
Cage rest until stable

DIET
N/A

CLIENT EDUCATION
• IMHA and its complications (e.g., DIC and pulmonary thromboembolism) can be fatal. • Life-long treatment may be needed, and the disease may recur. • Side effects of treatment may be severe.

SURGICAL CONSIDERATIONS
Splenectomy can be considered if medical management fails to control the disease after 4–6 weeks of treatment.

MEDICATIONS

DRUGS OF CHOICE
• Address underlying cause (e.g., infection and drugs) if secondary IMHA • Cross-matched, packed RBCs (6–10 mL/kg) or oxyhemoglobin (30 mL/kg at 10 mL/kg/hr) for severe anemia • Supportive treatment for animals with DIC • Corticosteroids—prednisone, 2 mg/kg/day divided BID 2–4 weeks; if PCV stable, decrease to 1 mg/kg/day for 2–4 weeks; then, if PCV stable, decrease to 1 mg/kg every other day for 2–4 weeks; then, if PCV stable, gradually discontinue over another 2–4 weeks • Cytotoxic drugs if autoagglutination or peracute hemolysis exists or if there is a poor response to prednisone after 14–21 days • Azathioprine— dogs, 50 mg/m² (2 mg/kg/day) 1–2 weeks; then 1 mg/kg PO every other day; cats, 1.5– 3.125 mg PO q48h (CAUTION: severe bone marrow suppression may develop) • Cyclophosphamide—50 mg/m²/day (2 mg/kg/day) 4 consecutive days; then skip 3 days; repeat up to 6–8 weeks; studies have shown no increased efficacy with combination therapy of cyclophosphamide and prednisone vs. prednisone alone

CONTRAINDICATIONS
None

PRECAUTIONS
• Caution with administration of azathioprine to cats; dosage of 2 mg/kg has produced severe bone marrow toxicity. • Check blood type

before any transfusion in cats, • Prednisone can cause Cushing syndrome, pulmonary thromboembolism, pancreatitis, secondary infection, gastric ulcers (consider misoprostol [2–5 μg/kg PO q8–12h] to prevent ulcers) • Cytotoxic drugs can cause bone marrow suppression, secondary infection, pancreatitis (azathioprine), cystitis (cyclophosphamide).

POSSIBLE INTERACTIONS
Azathioprine and prednisone can cause pancreatitis.

ALTERNATIVE DRUGS
• Dexamethasone (0.3–0.9 mg/kg/day) can be used instead of prednisone; follow similar tapering schedule • Chlorambucil—for cats, 2 mg PO q48–72h • Danazol—5–10 mg/kg PO q2h; taper to 5 mg/kg/day when patient is in remission; then gradually discontinue over 3 to 4 months (studies have shown no less severity of disease or mortality with this drug) • Human γ-globulin—0.5–1.5 g/kg over 12 hr, single IV infusion • Cyclosporine—10–20 mg/kg/day IM or PO • Eicosapentaenoic acid • Plasmapheresis

FOLLOW-UP

PATIENT MONITORING
• Monitor heart rate, respiratory rate, and temperature frequently during hospitalization. • Monitor for adverse reactions to treatment (e.g., transfusion reactions and overhydration). • If pulmonary thromboembolism is suspected, monitor thoracic radiographs and arterial blood gases frequently. • During the first month of treatment, check the PCV weekly until stable and then every 2 weeks for 2 months; if still stable, recheck PCV monthly for 6 months and then 2–4 times per year; rechecks may need to be more frequent if patient on long-term medication. • A CBC should be rechecked at least monthly during treatment, especially if cytotoxic drugs are used; if the neutrophil count falls < 3000 cells/mL, discontinue cytotoxic drugs until the count recovers; reinstitute at a lower dosage. • Reticulocyte count and Coombs tests can be monitored if the PCV is not rising as expected.

PREVENTION/AVOIDANCE
N/A

POSSIBLE COMPLICATIONS
• Pulmonary and multiorgan thromboembolism (up to 44% of all cases) • Portal vein thrombosis • DIC • Cardiac arrhythmias, centrilobular hepatic necrosis, and renal tubular necrosis secondary to hypoxia • Secondary infection and endocarditis

EXPECTED COURSE AND PROGNOSIS
• Peracute disease usually caused by autoagglutination or intravascular hemolysis. • Acute disease usually caused by intravascular or extravascular hemolysis. • Chronic disease usually caused by extravascular hemolysis or cold-reacting antibodies. • Hyperbilirubinemia > 10 mg/dL and low reticulocyte count

associated with a poor prognosis • Overall mortality 33.3% • Autoagglutination associated with up to 50% mortality • Peracute, fulminating hemolytic disease associated with up to 80% mortality • Warm-type IMHA has a guarded prognosis; of patients who survive hospitalization (up to 71%), long-term prognosis relatively good. • Cold-type IMHA more resistant to immunosuppressive drugs than warm type. • Response to treatment may take weeks to months; nonregenerative IMHA may have a more gradual onset than typical IMHA and may be slower to respond to treatment. • Hemolysis may recur despite previous or current therapy.

MISCELLANEOUS

ASSOCIATED CONDITIONS
• Evan's syndrome • SLE

AGE-RELATED FACTORS
None

ZOONOTIC POTENTIAL
None

PREGNANCY
Cytotoxic drugs should not be used in pregnant animals.

SYNONYMS
Autoimmune hemolytic anemia

SEE ALSO
• Anemia, Regenerative • Chapters on various causes of secondary IMHA • Cold Agglutinin Disease • Disseminated Intravascular Coagulation (DIC)

ABBREVIATIONS
• ALT = alanine aminotransferase • ANA = antinuclear antibody • APTT = activated partial thromboplastin time • DIC = disseminated intravascular coagulation • FeLV = feline leukemia virus • IMHA = immune mediated hemolytic anemia • LE = lupus erythematosus • MCV = mean cell volume • PCV = packed cell volume • PT = prothrombin time • SLE = systemic lupus erythematosus

Suggested Reading
Bucheler J, Cotter S. Canine immune-mediated hemolytic anemia. In: Bonagura J, Kirk R, eds. Current veterinary therapy XII. Philadelphia: Saunders, 1995:152–157.

Klag A, Giger U, Shofer F. Idiopathic immune-mediated hemolytic anemia in dogs: 42 cases (1986–1990). J Am Vet Med Assoc 1993;202:783–788.

Stewart A, Feldman B. Immune-mediated hemolytic anemia. Part I. An overview. Comp Cont Ed Pract Vet 1993;15:372–381.

Stewart A, Feldman B. Immune-mediated hemolytic anemia. Part II. Clinical entity, diagnosis, and treatment theory. Comp Cont Ed Pract Vet 1993;15:1479–1491.

Author Cathryn M. Calia
Consulting Editor Susan M. Cotter

ANEMIA, IRON-DEFICIENCY

 BASICS

OVERVIEW

- In adults, caused by hemorrhage
- Develops when erythrocytes are produced under the condition of limited iron availability
- Characteristic changes include erythrocyte microcytosis and hypochromic appearance caused by thin cell geometry.
- Important to recognize—leads clinician to the underlying disease problem, which is chronic external blood loss
- Most common site of blood loss is the gastrointestinal tract.

SIGNALMENT

- Fairly common in adult dogs
- Rare in adult cats
- Transient, neonatal iron-deficiency anemia occurs at 5–10 weeks of age in about 50% of kittens.

SIGNS

- Signs of anemia (e.g., lethargy, depression, weakness, anorexia, and tachypnea)
- Melena with gastrointestinal blood loss
- Possible heavy blood-sucking parasite load (e.g., fleas and hookworms)

CAUSES & RISK FACTORS

- Any form of chronic external blood loss
- Blood loss most often occurs through the gastrointestinal tract
- Common causes—lymphoma,* hookworm infestation,* stomach or intestinal neoplasia
- Less common sites—skin (e.g., flea infestation) and urinary tract
- Overuse of blood donors

 DIAGNOSIS

DIFFERENTIAL DIAGNOSIS

- Any cause of anemia, especially hemorrhage
- Specific features of the hemogram used to identify iron deficiency

CBC/BIOCHEMISTRY/URINALYSIS

- PCV usually low, generally 10–40% in dogs
- Anemia, either regenerative or nonregenerative
- Microcytosis—indicated by low normal or low MCV, often accompanied by high-volume heterogeneity, detected by erythrocyte histogram widening or high RBC distribution width value
- Changes in erythrocytes seen on the blood film—hypochromia (indicated by marked central pallor) oxidative lesions (e.g., keratocytes), fragmentation
- Thrombocytosis
- Hypoproteinemia—consistent finding if the blood loss is sustained; both albumin and globulin fractions are low normal or low.

OTHER LABORATORY TESTS

- Hypoferremia (serum iron < 70 μg/dL)and low transferrin saturation (< 15%) support the diagnosis.
- Serum iron values may be normal, even in animals with hematologic features of iron deficiency, if blood loss has ceased and the animal is undergoing iron repletion.
- Fecal flotation to rule out hookworms
- Fecal examination for occult blood or gross melena to detect gastrointestinal bleeding

IMAGING

Radiographic or ultrasonographic studies—gastrointestinal disease that accounts for blood loss

DIAGNOSTIC PROCEDURES

Cytologic examination of bone marrow specimen stained with Prussian blue—reveals absence of iron particles (hemosiderin); indicated only when documentation of the diagnosis is difficult; best performed on a core biopsy specimen of marrow.

 TREATMENT

- Identify and correct cause of chronic external blood loss.
- Administer iron until hematologic features of iron deficiency resolve.
- If unusually severe (i.e., PCV < 12%), transfusion may be required to treat life-threatening condition; administer whole blood (10–20 mL/kg IV) or packed red blood cells.

MEDICATIONS

DRUGS

Iron Supplementation
• Animals with severe iron deficiency have impaired intestinal absorption of iron, making oral supplementation of little value until partial iron repletion has occurred.
• Follow parenterally injected iron with oral iron supplementation for 1–2 months, or until features of iron deficiency have resolved.
• Kittens undergo spontaneous recovery and iron repletion beginning at 5–6 weeks of age, coinciding with intake of solid food.
Parenteral Iron Supplementation
• Iron dextran—a slowly released form of injectable iron; 1 injection (10–20 mg/kg IM) followed by oral supplementation

Oral iron supplements
• Ferrous sulfate powder—place in food or drinking water (100–300 mg PO q24h)
• Ferrous gluconate—1 (325-mg) tablet PO q24h
• Iron and vitamins—Visorbin, liquid iron and multiple vitamin supplement (1 tsp PO q24h)

CONTRAINDICATIONS/POSSIBLE INTERACTIONS
Oral iron supplementation is associated with unexplained death in kittens and should be avoided.

 FOLLOW-UP
• Monitor CBC every 1–4 weeks; if the anemia is severe, monitor more frequently to follow the animal through recovery from a life-threatening illness.
• Effectiveness of iron supplementation can be monitored less frequently.
• Effective treatment associated with an increase in MCV
• Erythrocyte histogram—effective treatment associated with movement to the right as new, normal cells are produced; subpopulation of microcytes produced under conditions of iron deficiency slowly disappear, as these cells complete their survival time; may take a few months in some animals to establish a normal histogram

 MISCELLANEOUS

ABBREVIATIONS
• MCV = mean cell volume
• PCV = packed cell volume

Suggested Reading
Weiser MG. Erythrocyte responses and disorders. In: Ettinger SJ and Feldman EC, eds. Textbook of veterinary internal medicine. 4th. ed. Philadelphia: Saunders, 1995:1864–1891.
Author Glade Weiser
Consulting Editor Susan M. Cotter

DISEASES

ANEMIA, METABOLIC (ANEMIAS WITH SPICULATED RED CELLS)

 BASICS

OVERVIEW
- Sometimes occurs concomitantly with diffuse diseases of the liver and kidney
- In most animals with liver disease, spiculated cells have 2–10 elongated, blunt, finger-like projections from their surfaces and are classified as acanthocytes.
- Acanthocytic anemias can be associated with renal disease; anemias of renal disease more often have oval red cells with irregular or ruffled membranes (burr cells).
- Pathogenesis not entirely clear; abnormal lipid metabolism with free cholesterol loading of RBC membranes is most frequently implicated as cause.
- Dogs with disseminated abdominal hemangiosarcoma with liver involvement often have acanthocytes.

SIGNALMENT
Dogs and cats (infrequently)

SIGNS
- None in most animals (usually mild to moderate condition)
- Detection of spiculated RBC on peripheral blood film can be first marker for liver or kidney disease.
- In large-breed dogs with vague signs or large spleen, suggests possibility of splenic or hepatic hemangiosarcoma

CAUSES & RISK FACTORS
- Any disease of the liver or kidneys
- The likelihood of RBC morphologic abnormalities parallels the severity of organ involvement.
- Hemangiosarcoma involving the liver is a frequent cause.
- Observed in cats with fatty liver syndrome

 DIAGNOSIS

DIFFERENTIAL DIAGNOSIS
Determination of renal or hepatic causes based on results of biochemistry profile and urinalysis

CBC/BIOCHEMISTRY/URINALYSIS
- Mild to moderately low PCV, RBC count, and hemoglobin
- Normal mean corpuscular volume and mean corpuscular hemoglobin concentration in most animals
- Normocytic, normochromic, and nonregenerative
- Polychromasia on blood films only with accompanying blood loss (as with hepatic hemangiosarcoma)
- WBC changes variable, based on underlying cause of hepatic or renal pathology
- Inflammatory conditions likely to be accompanied by inflammatory leukogram
- Variable findings in liver and kidney function tests (serum biochemistry and urinalysis)

Hepatic Diseases
- High ALT, ALP, and γ-glutamyl transferase
- High bile acids
- Possibly low albumin and serum urea nitrogen
- Bilirubinuria

Renal Diseases
- High serum urea nitrogen, creatinine, and phosphorus
- Highly variable urinalysis findings, including isosthenuria (urine specific gravity 1.008–1.025 in dogs; 1.008–1.035 in cats)
- Tubular and/or protein casts
- Pyuria
- Proteinuria
- Hematuria

OTHER LABORATORY TESTS
None

IMAGING
Abdominal radiographs and ultrasound—evaluate hepatic and renal structure

DIAGNOSTIC PROCEDURES
Liver or kidney biopsy if indicated

 TREATMENT

Focus treatment on diagnosis and treatment of underlying hepatic or renal disease.

 MEDICATIONS

DRUGS
Variable according to underlying cause

CONTRAINDICATIONS/POSSIBLE INTERACTIONS
Variable according to underlying cause

 FOLLOW-UP

Monitor CBC periodically while treating the underlying condition.

 MISCELLANEOUS

SEE ALSO
- Anemia of Chronic Renal Disease
- Hemangiosarcoma, spleen and liver

ABBREVIATIONS
- ALP = alkaline phosphatase
- ALT = alanine aminotransferase
- PCV = packed cell volume

Suggested Reading
Rebar AH, Lewis HB, DeNicola DB, Halliwell WH, Boon GD. Red blood cell fragmentation in the dog: an editorial review. Vet Pathol 1981;18:415–426.

Weiser EG. Erythrocyte responses and disorders. In: Ettinger SJ, Feldman EC, eds. Textbook of veterinary internal medicine. 4th ed. Philadelphia: Saunders, 1995: 1864–1891.

Author Alan H. Rebar
Consulting Editor Susan M. Cotter

ANEMIA, NUCLEAR MATURATION DEFECT (ANEMIA, MEGALOBLASTIC)

BASICS

OVERVIEW
• Nonregenerative anemia characterized by arrested development of the nuclei of RBC precursors (as a result of interference with DNA synthesis) while the cytoplasm develops normally (nuclear-cytoplasmic asynchrony)
• Affected RBC precursors fail to divide normally and thus are larger than corresponding normal precursors with the same degree of cytoplasmic maturity (hemoglobinization); because their nuclei are deficient in chromatin (DNA), they have a distinctive open and stippled appearance; these giant precursors with atypical, immature nuclei are known as megaloblasts.
• Although these asynchronous changes are most prominent in RBC precursors, WBC and platelet precursors are similarly affected.

SIGNALMENT
• Dogs and cats
• Spontaneous, clinically unimportant occurrence in toy poodles (occasional)
• No breed or sex predilection
• Defect usually acquired

SIGNS
• Generally mild, usually not clinically important
• In cats with FeLV-associated nuclear maturation anemia, FeLV-related signs can be anticipated.

CAUSES & RISK FACTORS
• Infectious—FeLV and FIV; retroviral infection the most common cause of megaloblastic anemia in cats
• Nutritional—folic acid and vitamin B_{12} deficiencies
• Toxic—phenytoin (Dilantin) toxicity and methotrexate toxicity (folate antagonist)
• Congenital—toy poodles

DIAGNOSIS

DIFFERENTIAL DIAGNOSIS
• All other mild to moderate nonregenerative anemias, including anemia of inflammatory disease, renal disease, and lead poisoning
• Differentiation based on the distinctive CBC and bone marrow findings listed

CBC/BIOCHEMISTRY/URINALYSIS
• Mild to moderate anemia (PCV: in dogs, 30–40%; in cats, 25–38%)
• Anemia classically macrocytic (high mean corpuscular volume) and normochromic (normal mean corpuscular hemoglobin concentration)
• Large, fully hemoglobinized RBC; occasional to numerous megaloblasts, particularly at the feather edge; no polychromasia
• Mild panleukopenia (common)
• Mild thrombocytopenia (common)
• In cats with FeLV, anemia may occur in association with a myelodysplastic syndrome or in conjunction with leukemia of a different cell line.

OTHER LABORATORY TESTS
FeLV and FIV test

IMAGING
N/A

OTHER DIAGNOSTIC PROCEDURES
Bone Marrow Biopsy
• Hyperplastic, often in all cell lines
• Maturation arrest with nuclear and cytoplasmic asynchrony in all cell lines
• Many megaloblastic RBC precursors may be observed.
• Macrophagic hyperplasia with active phagocytosis of nucleated RBCs and megaloblasts (common)

TREATMENT
• Treat by targeting the underlying cause, if possible.
• Except for that occurring with FeLV in cats, megaloblastic anemia is a relatively mild condition.
• Treat most patients on an outpatient basis.

MEDICATIONS

DRUGS
• In animals with drug toxicity, discontinue the offending drug.
• In all animals, consider supplementation with folic acid (4–10 mg/kg/day) or vitamin B_{12} (dogs, 100–200 mg/day PO; cats, 50–100 mg/day PO).
• Giant schnauzers with inherited cobalamin

malabsorption require parenteral treatment with vitamin B_{12} (0.5–1.0 mg IM weekly to every few months).

CONTRAINDICATIONS/POSSIBLE INTERACTIONS
Drugs known to cause megaloblastic anemia (e.g., methotrexate and phenytoin) should be avoided in patients whose condition results from other causes.

FOLLOW-UP
• Monitor response to treatment by CBC (weekly) and occasional bone marrow collection and evaluation.
• Closely monitor FeLV-positive cats for evidence of onset of other signs of hematopoietic dyscrasia in the peripheral blood and bone marrow.
• Prognosis—depends on underlying cause; in FeLV-positive cats, prognosis guarded; in animals with drug-associated anemia, prognosis good when use of offending drug is interrupted

MISCELLANEOUS

SEE ALSO
• Anemia, Nonregenerative
• Feline Immunodeficiency Virus
• Feline Leukemia Virus Infection

ABBREVIATIONS
• FeLV = feline leukemia virus
• FIV = feline immunodeficiency virus
• PCV = packed cell volume

Suggested Reading
Weiser MG. Erythrocyte responses and disorders. In: Ettinger SJ, Feldman EC, eds. Textbook of veterinary internal medicine. Philadelphia: Saunders, 1995:1864–1891.
Author Alan H. Rebar
Consulting Editor Susan M. Cotter

DISEASES

ANTEBRACHIAL GROWTH DEFORMITIES

 BASICS

DEFINITION
Abnormally shaped forelimbs and/or mal-alignments of the elbow or antebrachial carpal joints that result from abnormal development of the radius or ulna in the growing animal

PATHOPHYSIOLOGY
• Antebrachium—predisposed to deformities resulting from continual growth of one bone after premature growth cessation or decreased growth rate of the paired bone
• Decreased rate of elongation in one bone behaves as a retarding strap; the growing paired bone must twist and bow away from the short bone or overgrow at the elbow or carpus; causes joint malalignment
• Normal growth—bones elongate through the process of endochondral ossification, which occurs in the physis; physis closure occurs when the germinal cell layer stops producing new cartilage and the existing cartilage hypertrophies, ossifies, and is remodeled into bone.
• Hereditary—premature closure of distal ulnar physis reported as recessive trait in Skye terriers; may be a component of common elbow joint malalignment in many chondrodysplastic breeds (basset hounds and Lhasa apsos)
• Osteochondrosis or dietary oversupplementation—possibly associated with retardation of endochondral ossification in giant-breed dogs
• Trauma—most common cause; if chondro-proliferative layer of the physis is crushed (Salter V fracture), new cartilage production and bone elongation are stopped.

SYSTEMS AFFECTED
Musculoskeletal

GENETICS
• Skye terriers—reported as a recessive inheritable trait
• Chondrodysplastic breeds (dogs)—predisposed to elbow malalignment

INCIDENCE/PREVALENCE
• Traumatic—may occur after forelimb injuries in up to 10% of actively growing animals; uncommon in cats
• Elbow malalignment syndrome (chondrodysplastic dog breeds)—fairly common
• Nutritionally induced—incidence decreasing as nutritional standards are improved.
• Congenital agenesis of the radius (cats)—occasionally seen; results in severely bowed antebrachium and carpal subluxation

GEOGRAPHIC DISTRIBUTION
N/A

SIGNALMENT

Species
Dogs and cats

Breed Predilections
• Skye terriers—recessive inheritable form
• Chondrodysplastic and toy breeds (especially basset hounds, dachshunds, Lhasa apsos, Pekingese)—may be predisposed to elbow malalignments
• Giant breeds (e.g., Great Danes, wolfhounds)—may be induced by rapid growth owing to excessive or unbalanced nutrition

Mean Age and Range
• Traumatic—anytime during the active growth phase
• Elbow malarticulations—during growth; may not be recognized until secondary arthritic changes become severe, occasionally at several years of age

Predominant Sex
N/A

SIGNS

General Comments
• Longer-limbed dogs—angular deformities generally more common
• Shorter-limbed dogs—tend to develop more severe joint malalignments
• Age at the time of premature closure—affects relative degree of deformity and joint malarticulation; perhaps because of the variation in stiffness of bone with age and the duration of altered growth until maturity

Historical Findings
• Traumatic—progressive limb angulation or lameness 3–4 weeks after injury; owner may not be aware of causative event.
• Developmental elbow malalignments—insidious onset of lameness in one or both forelimbs; most apparent after exercise

Physical Examination Findings
Premature Distal Ulnar Closure
• Three deformities of the distal radius—lateral deviation (valgus), cranial bowing (curvus), and external rotation (supination)
• Relative shortening of limb length compared to the contralateral normally growing limb
• Caudolateral subluxation of the radial carpal joint and malarticulation of the elbow joint—may occur; causes lameness and painful joint restriction
Premature Radial Physeal Closure
• Affected limb—significantly shorter than the normal contralateral
• Severity of lameness—depends on degree of joint malarticulation

• Complete symmetrical closure of distal physis—may note straight limb with a widened radial carpal joint space; may note caudal bow to radius and ulna
• Asymmetrical closure of medial distal physis—varus angular deformity; occasionally inward rotation
• Closure of lateral distal physis—valgus angular deformity; external rotation
• Closure of proximal radial physis with continued ulnar growth—malarticulation of the elbow joint; widened radial to humeral space and humeral to anconeal space

CAUSES
• Trauma
• Developmental basis
• Nutritional basis

RISK FACTORS
• Forelimb trauma
• Excessive dietary supplementation

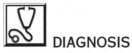 DIAGNOSIS

DIFFERENTIAL DIAGNOSIS
• Elbow dysplasia
• Fragmented medial coronoid process
• Un-united anconeal process
• Panosteitis
• Flexor tendon contracture

CBC/BIOCHEMISTRY/URINALYSIS
N/A

OTHER LABORATORY TESTS
N/A

IMAGING
• Damage to growth potential of the physis—cannot be seen at the time of trauma; usually 2–4 weeks before radiographically apparent
• Standard craniocaudal and mediolateral radiographic views—include entire elbow joint; proximally extend to midmetacarpal level distally; take same series for normal comparison of contralateral limb.
• Degree of angular deformities and relative shortening—determined by comparing relative lengths of radius and ulna within the deformed pair to the normal contralateral pair
• Elbow and carpal joints—evaluate for malalignment (treated surgically) and arthritis (e.g., osteophytes; influences prognosis)
• Elbow joint—evaluate for associated un-united anconeal process and fragmented medial coronoid process

DIAGNOSTIC PROCEDURES
N/A

PATHOLOGIC FINDINGS
Cartilage of prematurely closed physis replaced with bone

ANTEBRACHIAL GROWTH DEFORMITIES

TREATMENT

APPROPRIATE HEALTH CARE
• Genetic predisposition—cannot be treated
• Traumatic physeal damage—not seen at time of injury; revealed 2–4 weeks later
• Surgical treatment is recommended as soon as possible following diagnosis

NURSING CARE
N/A

ACTIVITY
Exercise restriction—reduces joint malalignment damage; slows arthritic progression

DIET
• Decrease nutritional supplementation in giant breed dogs—slows rapid grow; may reduce incidence
• Avoid excess weight—helps control arthritic pain resulting from joint malalignment and overuse

CLIENT EDUCATION
• Discuss heritability in Skye terriers and chondrodysplastic breeds.
• Explain that damage to physeal growth potential is not apparent at time of forelimb trauma and that the diagnosis is often made at 2–4-weeks following an injury.
• Discuss the importance of joint malalignment and resultant arthritis as primary causes of lameness.
• Emphasize that early surgical treatment leads to a better prognosis.

SURGICAL CONSIDERATIONS
• Premature distal ulnar physeal closure in a patient < 5–6 months of age (significant amount of radial growth potential remaining)—treated with a segmental ulnar ostectomy, valgus deformities ≤ 25°—often spontaneously correct and may not require additional surgery, young patients and those with more severe deformities—often require a second definitive correction after maturity
• Radial or ulnar physeal closure in a mature patient (limited or no growth potential) requires deformity correction, joint realignment, or both.
• Deformity correction—may be accomplished with a variety of osteotomy techniques; may be stabilized with several different fixation devices; must correct both rotational and angular deformities; performed at the point of greatest curvature
• Joint malalignment (particularly elbow)—must correct to minimize arthritic development (primary cause of lameness); obtain optimal joint alignment via dynamic proximal ulnar osteotomy (uses triceps muscle traction and joint pressure).

• Significant limb length discrepancies—distraction osteogenesis; osteotomy of the shortened bone is progressively distracted at the rate of 1 mm/day with an external fixator system to create new bone length.

MEDICATIONS

DRUGS OF CHOICE
Anti-inflammatory drugs—symptomatic treatment of arthritis

CONTRAINDICATIONS
Corticosteriods—do not use owing to potential systemic side affects and cartilage damage seen with long-term use.

PRECAUTIONS
Warn client of possible gastrointestinal upset associated with chronic anti-inflammatory therapy.

POSSIBLE INTERACTIONS
N/A

ALTERNATIVE DRUGS
Neutrapheuicals (e.g., glycosamines)—may help minimize cartilage damage and arthritis development; may be anti-inflammatory and analgesic

FOLLOW-UP

PATIENT MONITORING
• Postoperative—depends on surgical treatment
• Periodic checkups—evaluate arthritic status and anti-inflammatory therapy

PREVENTION/AVOIDANCE
Avoid dietary oversupplementation in rapidly growing giant-breed dogs.

POSSIBLE COMPLICATIONS
N/A

EXPECTED COURSE AND PROGNOSIS
• Generally, best results seen with early diagnosis and surgical treatment—minimizes arthritis
• Premature ulnar closure—tends to be easier to manage; yields better results
• Limb lengthening by distraction osteogenesis—requires extensive postoperative management by the veterinarian and owner; high rate of complications

MISCELLANEOUS

ASSOCIATED CONDITIONS
Osteochondrosis

AGE-RELATED FACTORS
• The younger the age at the time of traumatically induced physeal closure, the more severe the deformity and malarticulation.

ZOONOTIC POTENTIAL
N/A

PREGNANCY
N/A

SYNONYMS
Radius curvus

Suggested Reading
Forrell EB, Schwarz PD. Use of external skeletal fixation for treatment of angular deformity secondary to premature distal ulnar physeal closure. J Am Anim Hosp Assoc 1993;29:460–465.
Gilson SD, Piermattei DL, Schwarz PD. Treatment of humeroulnar subluxation with a dynamic proximal ulnar osteotomy: a review of 13 cases. Vet Surg 1989;18:114–122.
Henney LH, Gambardella PC. Premature closure of the ulnar physis in the dog: a retrospective clinical study. J Am Anim Hosp Assoc 1989;25:573–581.
Johnson AL. Correction of radial and ulnar growth deformities resulting from premature physeal closure. In: Bojrab MJ, ed. Current techniques in small animal surgery. 3rd ed. Philadelphia: Lea & Febiger, 1990:793–801.
Johnson KA. Retardation of endochondral ossification at the distal ulnar growth plate in dogs. Austral Vet J 1981;57:474–478.
Lau RE. Inherited premature closure of the distal ulnar physis. J Am Anim Hosp Assoc 1978;14:690–697.
Yanoff SR, Hulse DA, Palmer RH, Herron MR. Distraction osteogenesis using modified external fixation devices in five dogs. Vet Surg 1992;21:480–486.
Author Erick L. Egger
Consulting Editor Peter D. Schwarz

ANTERIOR CROSSBITE

 BASICS

OVERVIEW
Common malocclusion of incisors in dogs

SIGNALMENT
• Occurs in dogs at eruption of permanent dentition; temporary dentition is usually spaced far enough apart that the problem does not occur.
• Can be seen where relationship of other teeth and mandible to maxilla is considered normal—dental malocclusion
• Can be seen where relationship of other teeth and mandible to maxilla is not considered normal—skeletal malocclusion

SIGNS
• One or more incisors are in version to corresponding teeth in the opposing jaw— palatally displaced maxillary incisors and/or labially displaced mandibular incisors
• Skeletal relationship of mandible to maxilla may or may not be normal—undershot, scissor bite, or overshot
• Often associated with open or partially open bite or overcrowding of teeth in dental arch space

CAUSES & RISK FACTORS
Commonly caused by retained deciduous teeth

 DIAGNOSIS

DIFFERENTIAL DIAGNOSIS
• Malocclusion may be skeletal or dental in origin, or a combination of factors may be present.
• Evaluate alignment of incisors, premolars, and carnassials, as well as maxilla to mandible; if only the incisors are malaligned, the problem is of dental origin.
• Determine if the bite is open or partially open, and assess arch space discrepancies; an open bite and crowded arch space indicate that the problem is of skeletal origin.

CBC/BIOCHEMISTRY/URINALYSIS
N/A

OTHER LABORATORY TESTS
N/A

IMAGING
Oral radiographs to evaluate root anatomy— look for supernumerary, bifurcated, geminated, or retained deciduous teeth.

DIAGNOSTIC PROCEDURES
• Ask about litter mates and stud history to see if prevalent in breed or line.
• Check breed standard—it may be acceptable in some breeds.

 TREATMENT

• Treat to prevent contact trauma or abnormal wear to teeth in pet dogs.
• Show dogs—if treated they should not subsequently be shown; the breed society should be notified.
• Tipping is the most common movement to correct malocclusion and may need to be combined with extrusion in cases of open bite; treatment tends not to work long-term unless there is self-retention of occlusion.
• Arch crowding may require shaving the side cusps of teeth to allow room for movement.
• Can achieve movement by lingual maxillary arch bar with finger spring, elastic ligature ties, labial maxillary arch bar with elastics, mandibular or maxillary incline plane, maxillary expansion screw appliance, or mandibular brackets and elastic chains

MEDICATIONS

DRUGS

If correcting with appliances, use oral hygiene products (e.g., 0.2% chlorhexidine rinse) during treatment.

CONTRAINDICATIONS/POSSIBLE INTERACTIONS

N/A

FOLLOW-UP

PATIENT MONITORING

Need self-retention of occlusion or tends to revert to malocclusion; check weekly for 4 weeks postappliance, then monthly for 3 months.

EXPECTED COURSE AND PROGNOSIS

• Can take 3–8 weeks to move teeth, depending on severity and if extrusion is needed.
• Good prognosis in most patients
• If malocclusion is not corrected, more-frequent dental care may be needed than if occlusion were normal.

MISCELLANEOUS

• Need to ascertain owner's reasons for treating/correction of malocclusion
• Do not correct in show dogs to obtain unfair advantage in show ring.
• Common malocclusion in certain breeds in Australia where desirable breed "type" has changed over last 30 years to narrower maxilla, causing overcrowding (e.g., Staffordshire bull terrier and Doberman pinschers)

Suggested Reading

Wiggs BW, Loprise HB. Veterinary dentistry—principles and practice. Philadelphia: Lippincott-Raven, 1997:457–463.
Author Stephen Coles
Consulting Editor Jan Bellows

ANTERIOR UVEITIS—CATS

 BASICS

DEFINITION
Inflammation of the iris and/or ciliary body

PATHOPHYSIOLOGY
• Common theme from all causes—tissue destruction secondary to breakdown of the blood–aqueous barrier
• Increased vascular permeability—mediated by histamine, serotonin, prostaglandins, and leukotrienes; results in the extravasation of fluids, plasma proteins, and cells
• Associated with cellular infiltration, iridal congestion, aqueous flare, hypopyon, keratic precipitates, and corneal edema

SYSTEMS AFFECTED
• Ophthalmic
• Others—if cause is a systemic disease

GENETICS
N/A

INCIDENCE/PREVALENCE
• Common
• True incidence unknown

GEOGRAPHIC DISTRIBUTION
N/A

SIGNALMENT
Species
Cats

Breed Predilections
None

Mean Age and Range
• Mean—8–9 years of age
• Range—several weeks to 21 years of age

Predominant Sex
• Idiopathic—marked predilection for males
• Patients for which a definitive diagnosis is made—even sex distribution
• With FIV infection—strong predilection for old males

SIGNS
General Comments
Related to the severity and range from low intraocular pressure to hyphema with blindness

Historical Findings
• Usually owner complains of a change in appearance of the affected eye(s).
• Pain and secondary conjunctival hyperemia—generally less pronounced than in dogs

Physical Examination Findings
• Ocular discomfort—suggested by photophobia, blepharospasm, and epiphora

• Conjunctival hyperemia—common; nonspecific indication of ocular irritation
• Aqueous flare—increased turbidity of aqueous humor; common; can see a continuous beam of light in the anterior chamber (Tyndall phenomenon) owing to light scattering from particles
• Fibrinous exudation—severe disease; may cause fibrin clot formation within the anterior chamber
• Intraocular pressure—commonly low; depends on severity and duration of disease; may be high with severe disease and secondary glaucoma
• Miosis—pupillary constriction; subtle miosis best observed in a darkened room by simultaneously examining both eyes with retroillumination.
• Iridal swelling, nodules, and congestion—may be observed
• Pupil—often slow to dilate after installation of a short-acting mydriatic (1% tropicamide)
• Keratic precipitates—seen on the corneal endothelial surface; indicates active or previous disease
• Ciliary flush—may be observed in the limbal region; result of hyperemia of the perilimbal anterior ciliary vessels; along with conjunctival hyperemia, may contribute to red eye
• Corneal edema—not as common as in dogs
• Hyphema (accumulation of RBCs in the anterior chamber) and hypopyon (accumulation of WBCs in the anterior chamber)—develop with extreme breakdown of blood–aqueous barrier; cellular components typically settle homogeneously in the ventral anterior chamber; hyphema is common with intraocular tumors and systemic hypertension.

CAUSES
• Metabolic—systemic hypertension
• Neoplastic—primary (melanoma most common); secondary (lymphoma most common); post-traumatic sarcoma
• Immune mediated—lens trauma (rupture of lens capsule); vasculitis; thrombocytopenia
• Infectious—bacterial (any systemic bacterial disease); fungal (*Blastomyces dermatitidis; Candida albicans; Coccidioides immitis; Cryptococcus neoformans; Histoplasma capsulatum*); protozoan (*Toxoplasma gondii*); viral (coronavirus of FIP, FeLV, and FIV)
• Traumatic—blunt or penetrating injuries
• Idiopathic
• Miscellaneous—coagulopathy; ulcerative keratitis of any cause; periarteritis nodosa

RISK FACTORS
None

 DIAGNOSIS

DIFFERENTIAL DIAGNOSIS
• Other causes of red eye (see Red Eye)
• Conjunctivitis—clinical signs (hyperemia, chemosis, follicles, ocular discharge, and pain) vary, depending on the duration and severity; normal intraocular pressure and intraocular examination
• Glaucoma—pupil usually dilated; clinical signs may be identical; must measure intraocular pressure to distinguish
• Nonulcerative keratitis—intraocular examination usually normal
• Ulcerative keratitis—may be accompanied by anterior uveitis
• Horner syndrome—may have similar appearance because the pupil is miotic and upper lid ptosis creates the impression of blepharospasm; normal intraocular pressure; no aqueous flare; conjunctiva not or mildly injected

CBC/BIOCHEMISTRY/URINALYSIS
• CBC and urinalysis—usually unremarkable
• Serum biochemistry—high concentration of plasma proteins caused by high globulin concentration common; elevation is usually lower than that observed with FIP.

OTHER LABORATORY TESTS
• Serologic testing for feline infectious diseases—indicated if standard laboratory tests fail to reveal abnormalities
• Antigen for FeLV or cryptococcus; antibody titer FIP; *Toxoplasma gondii* (both IgM and IgG concentration); FIV
• High or rising titer for FIP—supports diagnosis of FIP; test lacks specificity because of cross-reactivity with the enteric coronavirus; high titers in patients with clinical signs of anterior uveitis are important.

IMAGING
• Thoracic radiographs—rule out neoplastic and fungal diseases
• Abdominal radiographs and ultrasound—for palpable abdominal mass
• Ocular ultrasonography—for trauma; rule out penetrating wounds and foreign bodies not obviously visible; when the ocular media are too opaque to allow complete examination of the eye

DIAGNOSTIC PROCEDURES
• Blood pressure—high with systemic hypertension
• Aqueous humor paracentesis—seldom helpful
• Tonometry—usually reveals low intraocular pressure unless secondary glaucoma has developed

PATHOLOGIC FINDINGS
- Eye—conjunctival hyperemia; ciliary flush; aqueous flare; miosis; variable vision
- Iris and ciliary body (idiopathic disease)—diffusely infiltrated with primarily lymphocytes and plasma cells
- Iridal nodules—composed of accumulations of lymphocytes and plasma cells

 TREATMENT

APPROPRIATE HEALTH CARE
- Inpatient—severe disease and/or high intraocular pressure; for initial diagnostic workup and medical management
- Outpatient—mild to moderate disease

NURSING CARE
N/A

ACTIVITY
No restrictions

DIET
No restrictions

CLIENT EDUCATION
- Discuss the need for early aggressive medical management and a thorough diagnostic workup to identify the cause.
- Warn client of the adverse sequelae, including blindness, cataracts, endophthalmitis or panophthalmitis, lens luxation, phthisis bulbi, posterior synechiae with iris bombé, and secondary glaucoma.
- Inform client that patients with infectious causes of uveitis (e.g., FeLV, FIV, and FIP) may be contagious to other cats.

SURGICAL CONSIDERATIONS
None

 MEDICATIONS

DRUGS OF CHOICE

Topically Applied Agents
- Frequency of treatment depends on the severity of disease.
- Corticosteroids—1% prednisolone acetate or 0.1% dexamethasone; q1–2h initially, then q4–8h with severe disease
- NSAIDs—0.03% flurbiprofen (Ocufen) or 1% suprofen (Profenal); q6h daily with severe disease
- Mydriatic-cycloplegic drugs—1% atropine; q6–12h (ointment may produce less salivation than solution); indicated for acute disease

Subconjunctivally Applied Corticosteroids
- Administered as an adjunct to topical agents in severe disease
- Betamethasone—0.75–1.5 mg/eye
- Dexamethasone—4.0–8.0 mg/eye
- Methylprednisolone acetate—4.0–8.0 mg/eye
- Triamcinolone acetonide—4.0–8.0 mg/eye

Systemically Administered Corticosteroids
- Indicated for moderate to severe disease when systemic infectious disease has been ruled out
- Prednisone—1.0–2.0 mg/kg/day for 7 days, then gradually decrease dosage

Antibiotics
Clindamycin HCl—25 mg/kg PO divided twice daily for 14–21; for patients with high *Toxoplasma gondii* titers.

CONTRAINDICATIONS
Steroids—avoid topical or subconjunctival administration with corneal ulcers.

PRECAUTIONS
- Topical atropine—may cause salivation; occasional vomiting
- Topical NSAIDs—safety in cats not determined

POSSIBLE INTERACTIONS
N/A

ALTERNATIVE DRUGS
N/A

 FOLLOW-UP

PATIENT MONITORING
- Complete ocular examination—repeated 5–7 days after initiation of treatment for severe disease
- Intraocular pressure—monitored for secondary glaucoma
- Re-evaluation—every 2–3 weeks, depending on response to treatment

PREVENTION/AVOIDANCE
N/A

POSSIBLE COMPLICATIONS
- Adverse sequelae—blindness; cataracts; endophthalmitis or panophthalmitis; iris atrophy; lens luxation; phthisis bulbi; rubeosis iridis; posterior synechiae with iris bombé; secondary glaucoma
- Secondary glaucoma—frequent complication; tends to be recalcitrant to medical treatment
- Idiopathic disease—may be so insidious that buphthalmia is the presenting complaint

EXPECTED COURSE AND PROGNOSIS
- Regardless of the initial response to treatment, treat for at least 2 months with decreasing frequency because the blood–aqueous barrier remains disrupted for about 8 weeks after an insult.
- Secondary to a systemic disease—prognosis usually determined by the systemic disease rather than by the anterior uveitis
- Prognosis for resolution of inflammation without deleterious sequelae—depends on severity of the disease at initial examination and on the response to aggressive medical treatment

 MISCELLANEOUS

ASSOCIATED CONDITIONS
N/A

AGE-RELATED FACTORS
Patients with serologically confirmed infectious disease tend to be younger (mean, 5.0 years) than patients with idiopathic disease (mean, 9.3 years) or ocular melanoma (mean, 9.0 years).

ZOONOTIC POTENTIAL
None

PREGNANCY
- Systemic steroids—do not use in pregnant cats if at all avoidable
- Topical steroids—use with caution; systemic absorption occurs with more than twice-a-day treatment.

SYNONYM
Iridocyclitis

SEE ALSO
Red Eye

ABBREVIATIONS
- FeLV = feline leukemia virus
- FIP = feline infectious peritonitis
- FIV = feline immunodeficiency virus

Suggested Reading
Davidson MG, Nasisse MP, English RV, et al. Feline anterior uveitis: a study of 53 cases. J Am Anim Hosp Assoc 1991;27:77–83.
Glaze MB, Gelatt KN. Feline ophthalmology. In: Gelatt KN, ed. Veterinary ophthalmology. 3rd ed. Philadelphia: Lippincott Williams & Wilkins, 1999:997–1052.
Slatter D. Fundamentals of veterinary ophthalmology. 2nd ed. Philadelphia: Saunders, 1990.

Author Michael J. Ringle
Consulting Editor Paul E. Miller

DISEASES

ANTERIOR UVEITIS—DOGS

BASICS

DEFINITION
Inflammation of the iris and/or ciliary body

PATHOPHYSIOLOGY
• Common theme from all causes—tissue destruction secondary to breakdown of the blood–aqueous barrier
• Increased vascular permeability—mediated by histamine, serotonin, prostaglandins, and leukotrienes; results in the extravasation of fluids, plasma proteins, and cells
• Associated with cellular infiltration, iridal congestion, aqueous flare, hypopyon, keratic precipitates, and corneal edema

SYSTEMS AFFECTED
• Ophthalmic
• Others—if cause is a systemic disease

GENETICS
N/A

INCIDENCE/PREVALENCE
• Common
• True prevalence unknown

GEOGRAPHIC DISTRIBUTION
Depends on underlying cause, e.g. the deep fungals; *Rickettsia, spirochetes*

SIGNALMENT
Species
Dogs

Breed Predilections
None

Mean Age and Range
Any

Predominant Sex

None

SIGNS
General Comments
Related to severity and may range from low intraocular pressure to hyphema with blindness

Historical Findings
• Pain—exhibited as photophobia, blepharospasm, or epiphora
• Redness—owing to conjunctival hyperemia or hyphema
• Blue or white cornea—from edema
• Blindness

Physical Examination Findings
• Ocular discomfort—suggested by photophobia, blepharospasm, and epiphora; not specific for the condition

• Conjunctival hyperemia—common Intraocular pressure—commonly low; depends on the severity and duration of disease; may be high with severe disease and secondary glaucoma
• Miosis—pupillary constriction; subtle miosis best observed in a darkened room by simultaneously examining both eyes with retroillumination.
• Iridal swelling—may be noted
• Pupil—often slow to dilate after installation of a short-acting mydriatic (1% tropicamide)
• Corneal edema—often noted
• Ciliary flush—may be observed in the limbal region; result of hyperemia of the perilimbal anterior ciliary vessels; along with conjunctival hyperemia, may contribute to red eye
• Aqueous flare—excess turbidity of aqueous humor; can see a continuous beam of light in the anterior chamber (Tyndall phenomenon) owing to light scattering from particles
• Fibrinous exudation—severe disease; may cause fibrin clot formation within the anterior chamber
• Hyphema (accumulation of RBCs in the anterior chamber) and hypopyon (accumulation of WBCs in the anterior chamber)—develop with extreme breakdown of blood–aqueous barrier; cellular components typically settle homogeneously in the ventral anterior chamber; hyphema is common with intraocular tumors.
• Keratic precipitates—seen on the corneal endothelial surface; indicates active or previous disease

CAUSES
• Metabolic—diabetes mellitus (lens-induced uveitis); hyperlipidemia; systemic hypertension
• Neoplastic—primary (melanoma most common); secondary (lymphoma most common); hyperviscosity syndrome
• Immune mediated—cataracts (lens-induced uveitis); lens trauma (rupture of lens capsule); Vogt-Koyanagi-Harada-like syndrome; vasculitis; thrombocytopenia
• Infectious—algal (*Prototheca* spp.); bacterial (*Brucella canis, Borrelia burgdorferi, Leptospira* spp.; any systemic bacterial disease); fungal (*Blastomyces dermatitidis, Coccidioides immitis, Cryptococcus neoformans, Histoplasma capsulatum*); parasitic (*Baylisascaris* spp., *Diptera* spp., *Dirofilaria immitis, Toxocara* spp.); protozoan (*Leishmania donovani, Toxoplasma gondii*); rickettsial (*Ehrlichia canis, Ehrlichia platys, Rickettsia rickettsii*); viral (adenovirus, distemper)

• Traumatic—blunt or penetrating injuries
• Miscellaneous—coagulopathy; secondary to episcleritis or scleritis; idiopathic; radiation therapy; ulcerative keratitis from any cause

RISK FACTORS
Exposure to causative organisms

DIAGNOSIS

DIFFERENTIAL DIAGNOSIS
• Other causes of red eye (see Red Eye)
• Conjunctivitis—clinical signs (hyperemia, chemosis, ocular discharge, and pain) vary, depending on duration and severity; normal intraocular pressure and intraocular examination
• Episcleritis and scleritis—may be nodular, diffuse, and infiltrative or necrotizing; in uncomplicated disease, only the fibrous tunic of the globe is involved; may note anterior uveitis because of extension of the inflammation to adjacent tissues
• Glaucoma—pupil usually dilated; clinical signs may be identical must measure intraocular pressure to distinguish
• Nonulcerative keratitis—intraocular examination usually normal
• Ulcerative keratitis—may be accompanied by anterior uveitis
• Horner syndrome—may have similar appearance because the pupil is miotic and upper lid ptosis creates the false impression of blepharospasm; normal intraocular pressure; no aqueous flare; conjunctiva not or only mildly injected

CBC/BIOCHEMISTRY/URINALYSIS
• Usually normal
• Abnormalities reflect the underlying systemic disease—neutropenia or neutrophilia with systemic bacterial or fungal disease; high serum glucose concentration with diabetes mellitus; thrombocytopenia with hyphema; high triglycerides with hyperlipidemia

OTHER LABORATORY TESTS
• Serum titers for infectious agents—toxoplasmosis, ehrlichiosis, and the deep fungals; may be performed in appropriate geographic locations; high titers in patients with clinical signs of anterior uveitis are usually important.
• Clotting profile—indicated for hyphema of undetermined cause

IMAGING
• Thoracic radiographs—rule out neoplastic and fungal disease
• Abdominal radiographs and ultrasound—for palpable abdominal mass

• Ocular ultrasonography—for trauma; rule out penetrating wounds and radiolucent foreign bodies not obviously visible; when the ocular media are too opaque to allow complete examination of the eye

DIAGNOSTIC PROCEDURES
• Blood pressure—high with systemic hypertension
• Aqueous humor paracentesis—seldom helpful
• Tonometry—usually reveals low intraocular pressure unless secondary glaucoma has developed

PATHOLOGIC FINDINGS
• Eye—conjunctival hyperemia; ciliary flush; corneal edema; aqueous flare; miosis; variable vision
• Iris and ciliary body—infiltrated with a mixture of inflammatory or neoplastic cell types, depending on the cause and chronicity of the disease

 TREATMENT

APPROPRIATE HEALTH CARE
• Inpatient—severe disease and/or high intraocular pressure; for initial diagnostic workup and medical management
• Outpatient—mild to moderate disease

ACTIVITY
No restrictions

DIET
N/A

CLIENT EDUCATION
• Discuss the need for early aggressive medical management and a thorough diagnostic workup to identify the cause.
• Warn client of the adverse sequelae, including blindness, cataracts, endophthalmitis and panophthalmitis, lens luxation, phthisis bulbi, posterior synechia with iris bombé, and secondary glaucoma

SURGICAL CONSIDERATIONS
None

 MEDICATIONS

DRUGS OF CHOICE

Topically Applied Agents
• Frequency of treatment depends on the severity of disease.
• Corticosteroids—1% prednisolone acetate or 0.1% dexamethasone; q1–2h initially, then q4–8h with severe disease

• NSAIDs—0.03% flurbiprofen (Ocufen) or 1% suprofen (Profenal); q6h with severe disease
• Mydriatic-cycloplegic drugs—1% atropine q4–6h initially for severe disease, then q6–12h times daily; to dilate the pupil, minimize posterior synechia, paralyze the ciliary muscle (cycloplegia); reduces ocular pain

Subconjunctivally Applied Corticosteroids
Administered as an adjunct to topical agents in severe disease
• Betamethasone—0.75–1.5 mg/eye
• Dexamethasone—4.0–8.0 mg/eye
• Methylprednisolone acetate—4.0–8.0 mg/eye
• Triamcinolone acetonide—4.0–8.0 mg/eye

Systemically Administered Corticosteroids
• Indicated for moderate to severe disease when systemic infectious disease has been ruled out
• Prednisone—1.0–2.0 mg/kg/day for 7 days, then gradually decrease dosage

Immunosuppressive Drugs
• For patients unresponsive to conventional therapy
• Azathioprine (Imuran)—1–2 mg/kg/day for 3–7 days, then taper. Perform a CBC, platlet count and liver enzyme screen every 1–2 weeks for 8 weeks then periodically

Antibiotics or Antifungal Drugs
Rarely indicated unless a susceptible infectious agent (e.g., *Ehrlichia* spp., *Toxoplasma gondii*, deep fungals) has been identified

CONTRAINDICATIONS
• Corneal ulcer—do not use steroids.
• Diabetes mellitus—do not use systemic steroids; use topical steroids with caution (may alter insulin requirements); may try topical nonsteroidal agents

PRECAUTIONS
Azathioprine—myelosupressive and hepatotoxic.

POSSIBLE INTERACTIONS
N/A

ALTERNATIVE DRUGS
N/A

 FOLLOW-UP

PATIENT MONITORING
• Complete ocular examination—repeated 5–7 days after initiation of treatment for severe disease
• Intraocular pressure—monitored for secondary glaucoma

• Re-evaluation—every 2–3 weeks. depending on response to treatment

PREVENTION/AVOIDANCE
N/A

POSSIBLE COMPLICATIONS
Adverse sequelae—blindness; cataracts; endophthalmitis and panophthalmitis; iris atrophy; lens luxation; phthisis bulbi; rubeosis iridis; posterior synechia with iris bombé; secondary glaucoma

EXPECTED COURSE AND PROGNOSIS
• Regardless of the initial response to treatment, treat for at least 2 months with decreasing frequency because the blood–aqueous barrier remains disrupted for about 8 weeks after an insult.
• Secondary to a systemic disease—prognosis usually determined by underlying condition
• Prognosis for resolution of inflammation without deleterious sequelae—depends on severity at initial examination and on the response to aggressive medical treatment

 MISCELLANEOUS

ASSOCIATED CONDITIONS
None

AGE-RELATED FACTORS
None

ZOONOTIC POTENTIAL
Depends on underlying cause—*Brucella canis, leptospirosis,* and *Blastomyces dermatitidis* (rare)

PREGNANCY
• Systemic steroids—do not use in pregnant dogs if at all avoidable
• Topical steroids—use with caution; systemic absorption occurs with more than twice-a-day treatment.

SYNONYM
Iridocyclitis

SEE ALSO
Red Eye

Suggested Reading
Collins BK, Moore CP. Diseases and surgery of the canine anterior uvea. In: Gelatt KN, ed., Veterinary ophthalmology. 3rd ed. Philadelphia: Lippincott Williams & Wilkins. 1999:755–775.
Slatter D. Fundamentals of veterinary ophthalmology. 2nd ed. Philadelphia: Saunders, 1990:304–337.

Author Michael J. Ringle
Consulting Editor Paul E. Miller

DISEASES

AORTIC STENOSIS

BASICS

DEFINITION
Narrowing of the left ventricular outflow tract of the heart, most commonly seen as a congenital or perinatal disease. Defect can be valvular, subvalvular (most common in dogs), or supravalvular (most common in cats). As a congenital anomaly in dogs, the obstruction is usually caused by fibrous tissue proximal to the valve, and the disease is referred to as subaortic stenosis (SAS).

PATHOPHYSIOLOGY
Marked aortic obstruction compels the left ventricle to increase intraventricular pressure to maintain forward blood flow and systemic blood pressure. The myocardium compensates by hypertrophy of myocytes leading to thickening of the heart walls. Coronary artery disease, relative cardiac ischemia, arrhythmias, aortic or mitral regurgitation, left-sided congestive heart failure (CHF), and diminished systemic blood flow may result.

SYSTEMS AFFECTED
• Cardiovascular—pressure overload of the left ventricle. • Pulmonary–if pulmonary edema develops. • Multisystemic signs may develop secondary to CHF or low cardiac output. If bacterial endocarditis is the cause of the stenosis, the patient may have multisystemic signs due to septic embolization.

GENETICS
Inherited trait in Newfoundland dogs. Polygenic transmission exhibiting pseudodominance; a major dominant gene with modifiers may be involved.

INCIDENCE/PREVALENCE
Approximately 1.5 to 2.0 per 1000 dogs admitted to veterinary teaching institutions; SAS is probably the second most common congenital heart defect in dogs. Approximately 0.2 per 1000 cats admitted to veterinary teaching institutions. In one study, aortic stenosis accounted for 6% of congenital cardiac defects in cats.

SIGNALMENT
Species: Dogs and cats

Breed Predilections
Most common in Newfoundland, German shepherd, golden retriever, Rottweiler, and boxer. Samoyed, English bulldog, and Great Dane also at higher risk than other breeds

Mean Age and Range
SAS develops postnatally over the first weeks to months of life. Onset of clinical signs can occur at any age depending on the severity of obstruction. Signs may be seen on physical examination without any historical evidence of disease.

SIGNS

Historical Findings
• Related to the severity of obstruction; range from none to CHF, syncope, and sudden death. • Genetic history of affected litters from same sire or bitch.

Physical Examination Findings
• Systolic ejection murmur loudest near the left, fourth intercostal space at the heart base to costochondral junction, which may radiate to the thoracic inlet, carotid arteries, and, if very loud, even to the cranium. Radiation to the left apex and right cranial thorax is common. • Thrill at the left heart base to costochondral junction in some animals. • Diastolic murmur may be heard at the left apex, if aortic regurgitation develops. • Holosystolic murmur at the left apex may be present, if mitral regurgitation develops • Dyspnea, tachypnea, and crackles with the onset of left-sided CHF. • Femoral pulses typically weakened and late rising (pulsus tardus) in animals with disease severe enough to affect hemodynamics. • A left ventricular 'heave' (i.e., prolonged and pronounced cardiac impulse palpated on the thorax) in animals with left ventricular hypertrophy. • Arrhythmias.

CAUSES
• Congenital disease • Secondary to bacterial endocarditis of the aortic valve in some dogs. • In cats with hypertrophic cardiomyopathy, functional stenosis (e.g., muscular or subvalvular) is common but significance unknown. • 'Dynamic' subaortic stenosis reported in dogs in which muscular hypertrophy can contribute to narrowing of the aortic outflow tract.

RISK FACTORS
• Familial history of subaortic stenosis. • Aortic endocarditis is predisposed by immunosuppression, systemic infection, bacteremia, and abnormal intracardiac blood flow.

DIAGNOSIS

DIFFERENTIAL DIAGNOSIS
• A systolic ejection murmur may represent an innocent murmur in a young animal; anemia, pain, fever, excitement. Systolic murmurs on the left thorax are commonly caused by patent ductus arteriosus (usually a continuous murmur, but diastolic component may be localized), pulmonic stenosis, mitral regurgitation, ventricular septal defect, atrial septal defect, or tetralogy of Fallot in dogs. Some of these conditions may coexist with SAS. • Weakened pulses may occur in animals with other cardiac conditions in which stroke volume is limited (e.g., pulmonic stenosis and cardiomyopathy) or in animals with aortic obstruction distal to the outflow tract (e.g.,

aortic coarctation, aortic interruption, and aortic thromboembolism).

CBC/BIOCHEMISTRY/URINALYSIS
Typically normal

IMAGING

Thoracic Radiographic Findings
• May be subtle because myocardial hypertrophy from pressure overload may not increase the size of the cardiac silhouette. • Left-sided heart enlargement, which may appear on lateral radiographs as straightening of the caudal border of the heart. Normal lung fields unless CHF develops causing pulmonary venous distention and interstitial or alveolar pulmonary infiltrates. Mediastinum may be widened and cranial waist of the cardiac silhouette filled as a result of post-stenotic dilation of the aorta.

Echocardiographic Findings
• Spectrum of findings depending on the severity of disease. • Thickening of the left ventricular wall and interventricular septum. • Echogenic ridge and gross narrowing of the left ventricular outflow tract may be visible proximal to the aortic valve in SAS. • The mitral valve is adjacent to the outflow tract, and its anterior leaflet may also be thickened and echogenic. • Post-stenotic dilation of the aorta in some animals. • Increased echogenicity of the myocardium in some animals, particularly the subendocardial zone and papillary muscles. • 'Premature closure' of the aortic valve often seen on M-mode echocardiography.

Doppler echocardiographic Findings
• Stenosis leads to high peak ejection velocity (> 2 m/s), which may be delayed to a later time in ejection; flow acceleration proximal to the obstruction, and a jet of turbulent blood flow distal to the valve recognized as a wide range of measured velocities ('spectral broadening'). • Transvalvular pressure gradient can be estimated from the flow velocity (pressure gradient = 4 × flow velocity squared) with variable accuracy. Color-flow Doppler allows direct visualization of the turbulent jet distal to the obstruction and "flow convergence" proximal.

Angiocardiographic Findings/Cardiac Catheterization
• Contrast radiography shows thickening of the left ventricular wall and septum, narrowing of the left ventricular outflow tract, and post-stenotic dilation of the aorta. Cardiac catheterization allows determination of the transvalvular pressure gradient. Pressure gradients < 50 mm Hg suggest mild disease, 50–75 mm Hg, moderate, 75–100 mm Hg, severe, and > 100 mm Hg, very severe disease. Pressure gradients are greater with increased ejection volume and, therefore, must be interpreted in light of other aspects of cardiac function. Anesthesia depresses myocardial function, so

these gradients may underestimate the actual ones (unanesthetized). • Angiocardiography and cardiac catheterization allow characterization of uncommon types of stenosis including valvular, supravalvular, and 'tunnel outflow tract' and evaluation of concurrent defects.

DIAGNOSTIC PROCEDURES

Electrocardiographic Findings
• ECG may show signs of left ventricular hypertrophy such as a tall R wave in lead II (> 3.0 mv in dogs), CV6LL (> 3.0 mv in dogs), and others (leads I, III, aVF, CV6LU). • Widening of the QRS complex (> 0.06 sec in dogs) may also be evident. • Mean electrical axis may be shifted to the left (< 40 degrees in dogs) but is typically normal. • Slurring of ST segment consistent with left ventricular hypertrophy ischemia; ST-segment deviation after mild exercise strongly suggests coronary insufficiency. • Ventricular tachyarrhythmias may occur in severely affected cases and are a potential cause for clinical signs and sudden death. Holter 24-hour ECG monitoring is appropriate in symptomatic or severely affected animals.

TREATMENT

APPROPRIATE HEALTH CARE
Management recommendations for small animals are controversial and vary among experts.
Inpatient management appropriate for complications including arrhythmias, episodes of syncope, and CHF

ACTIVITY
Restricted in animals with more than mild disease. Syncope, collapse, or sudden death may be brought on by exertion in animals with severe disease.

DIET
Restricted sodium in animals with overt or impending CHF

CLIENT EDUCATION
• Affected animals should be neutered or otherwise not permitted to breed. • Evaluate closely related dogs for evidence of clinical disease. • Alert owners to potential complications (e.g., sudden death and CHF) in severely affected animals.

SURGICAL CONSIDERATIONS
• Definitive treatment requires open heart surgery and is rarely practical in small animals for economic and technical reasons. • Balloon dilation of the outflow tract during cardiac catheterization results in acute reduction of transvalvular gradients and improvement of clinical signs in some symptomatic dogs. Long-term benefits have not been adequately studied in dogs and the procedure is not entirely benign.

MEDICATIONS

DRUGS OF CHOICE
• Medical management is, at best, palliative and empirical; no data have been published supporting a specific treatment. • Beta adrenergic blockers have been advocated for dogs with subaortic stenosis with a history of syncope or collapse, a transvalvular pressure gradient > 75 mm Hg, or when ventricular arrhythmias or ST-segment changes are evident on a postexercise ECG. Potential benefits include limitation of myocardial oxygen requirements, protection from ventricular arrhythmias, and slowing of the heart rate. Beta blockers are always given to effect which depends on the state of the autonomic system of the individual. Therapy should be initiated with caution at low dosages and titrated upwards over days to weeks. Propranolol (dogs, 0.2–1.0 mg/kg PO q8h; cats, 2.5–5.0 mg/cat PO q8h–q12h) is the prototype beta blocker. • Specific treatment for ventricular arrhythmias, atrial fibrillation, or left-sided CHF may also be required. Requires careful monitoring (see precautions). • Affected animals are at risk of developing bacterial endocarditis. Meticulous treatment of infections is recommended as is chemoprophylaxis for dental or genitourinary procedures.

CONTRAINDICATIONS
Beta blockers in animals with overt CHF or bronchoconstrictive disorders; discontinue if these complications develop

PRECAUTIONS
• Beta blockers limit the ability of the dysfunctional heart to increase cardiac output, which occurs primarily by an increase in heart rate. • With SAS, the incompliant myocardium is dependent on adequate filling pressure (preload), and overzealous use of diuretics or venodilators may cause a precipitous drop in cardiac output. • Marked reduction of systemic blood pressure by ACE inhibitors, calcium channel blockers, or arteriolar dilators may worsen outflow obstruction or coronary insufficiency. • Digitalis glycosides and positive inotropes may exacerbate outflow obstruction or ventricular arrhythmias. • Anesthetic agents and sedatives with marked hypotensive, arrhythmogenic, or cardiac depressant side effects should be avoided. A narcotic (e.g., butorphanol or oxymorphone) with diazepam for sedation can be combined with low inspired concentrations of isofluorane for anesthesia if necessary.

ALTERNATIVE DRUGS
• Metoprolol tartrate (0.5–1.0 mg/kg PO q8–12h for dogs; 2–15 mg/cat PO q8h), nadolol (0.25–0.5 mg/kg PO q12h), and atenolol (0.25–1.0 mg/kg PO q12h for dogs;

6.25–12.5 mg/cat PO q12–24h) are alternative beta blockers. • Diltiazem (dogs, 0.5–2.0 mg/kg PO q8h for dogs; 7.5–15.0 mg/cat PO q8h) may have similar theoretical benefits in this disease.

FOLLOW-UP

PATIENT MONITORING
Monitor by ECG, thoracic radiography, two-dimensional and Doppler echocardiography. Treatment of complications (e.g., CHF and arrhythmias) necessitates careful monitoring to detect renal/electrolyte, proarrhythmic, negative inotropic, and hypotensive side effects of drugs.

POSSIBLE COMPLICATIONS
CHF, arrhythmias, myocardial infarction, aortic regurgitation, mitral regurgitation, sudden death, bacterial endocarditis

EXPECTED COURSE AND PROGNOSIS
• Mildly affected dogs may live a normal life span without treatment. • Severe disease typically limits longevity. • CHF suggests severe disease and an ominous prognosis.

MISCELLANEOUS

ASSOCIATED CONDITIONS
Other cardiac defects

AGE RELATED FACTORS
Murmur typically not present at birth in SAS; develops in the first weeks to months postnatally along with development of stenotic lesion

PREGNANCY
Contraindicated

SEE ALSO
• Endocarditis, bacterial • Congestive heart failure, left-sided • Cardiomyopathy, Hypertrophic—Cats and Dogs

Suggested Reading
Lehmkuhl LB and Bonagura JD. CVT Update: Canine subvalvular aortic stenosis. In Bonagura JD, Kirk RW, eds. Kirk's current veterinary therapy XII. Philadelphia: WB Saunders, 1995.
Sisson D. Fixed and dynamic subvalvular aortic stenosis in dogs. In: Kirk RW, Bonagura JD, eds. Current veterinary therapy XI. Philadelphia: WB Saunders, 1992.
Author Donald J. Brown
Consulting Editors Larry P. Tilley and Francis W. K. Smith, Jr.

AORTIC THROMBOEMBOLISM

BASICS

DEFINITION
Aortic thromboembolism (ATE) results from a thrombus or blood clot that is dislodged within the aorta, causing severe ischemia to the tissues served by that segment of aorta. It is one of the most devastating complications associated with myocardial diseases in cats.

PATHOPHYSIOLOGY
• ATE is most commonly associated with myocardial disease in cats, including hypertrophic, restrictive, and dilated cardiomyopathy. Although the exact etiology of ATE has not been determined, it is theorized that abnormal blood flow (stasis) and a hypercoaguable state contribute to the formation of the thrombus within the left atrium. The blood clot is then embolized distally to the aorta. The most common site of embolization is the caudal aorta trifurcation (hind legs). Other less common sites include the front leg, kidneys, gastrointestinal tract, or cerebrum.
• Rarely, aortic thromboembolism occurs in dogs. ATE in dogs typically is associated with neoplasia, sepsis, Cushing's disease, protein-losing nephropathy, or other hypercoaguable states.

SYSTEMS AFFECTED
• Cardiovascular-the majority of affected cats have advanced heart disease and left heart failure. • Nervous/musculoskeletal-severe ischemia to the muscles and nerves served by the segment of occluded aorta causes variable pain and paresis. Gait abnormalities or paralysis results in the leg or legs involved.

GENETICS:
N/A

INCIDENCE/PREVALENCE
• Although ATE is a well-recognized complication of myocardial disease in cats, the exact prevalence of ATE is not known in the general population of cats. In one study of cats with hypertrophic cardiomyopathy, 12% presented with signs of ATE. In a retrospective study of 100 cats with ATE, only 11% of cats had previous evidence of heart disease. Therefore, it is usually the initial sign of cardiovascular disease in most cases. • Rare in dogs.

GEOGRAPHIC DISTRIBUTION
N/A

SIGNALMENT
Species
Cats, rarely dogs

Breed Predilections
None

Mean Age and Range
Age distribution is 1–20 years. The median age is 10.5 years; the mean age is 7.7 years.

Predominant Sex
Males are more commonly affected than females (2:1).

SIGNS
Historical Findings
• Acute onset paralysis and pain are the most common complaints. • Lameness or a gait abnormality. • Tachypnea or respiratory distress is common. • Vocalization and anxiety are common.

Physical Examination Findings
• Usually paraparesis or paralysis of the rear legs. Less commonly, monoparesis of a front leg. • Pain upon palpation of the legs. • Gastrocnemius muscle often becomes firm several hours after embolization. • Absent or diminished femoral pulses. • Cyanotic or pale nail beds and foot pads. • Cardiac murmur or gallop sound. • Tachypnea or dyspnea. • Cardiac arrhythmias.

CAUSES
• Hypertrophic cardiomyopathy • Restrictive cardiomyopathy • Dilated cardiomyopathy • Neoplasia • Sepsis • Hyperadrenocorticism (dogs) • Protein-losing nephropathy (dogs)

RISK FACTORS
Although clear risk factors have not been defined, it is theorized that an enlarged left atrium or spontaneous echo contrast (smoke) observed on an echocardiographic examination may be risk factors.

DIAGNOSIS

DIFFERENTIAL DIAGNOSIS
Hind limb paresis secondary to other causes such as spinal neoplasia, trauma, myelitis, fibrocartilaginous infarction, or intervertebral disk protrusion. These conditions resulting in spinal cord injury present with signs of upper motor neuron disease, whereas ATE patients present with signs of lower motor neuron disease.

CBC/BIOCHEMISTRY/URINALYSIS
• High creatine kinase as a result of muscle injury.
• High aspartate aminotransferase and alanine aminotransferase as a result of muscle and liver injury.
• Hyperglycemia secondary to stress.
• Mild increases in blood urea nitrogen and creatinine as a result of possible dehydration and renal emboli.
• CBC and urinalysis changes are nonspecific.

OTHER LABORATORY TESTS
Coagulation profile typically does not reveal significant abnormalities because the hypercoagulability results from hyperaggregable platelets. Coagulation profile may be helpful

to titrate heparin and possibly warfarin dosages.

IMAGING
Radiographic Findings
• Cardiomegaly is seen in 85–90% of cats.
• Pulmonary edema and/or pleural effusion is seen in approximately 66% of cats.

Echocardiographic Findings
• The majority of cats will have hypertrophic cardiomyopathy characterized by left ventricular hypertrophy, nondilated left ventricular lumen, large left atrium, and hypercontractility.
• The second most common echocardiographic diagnosis is restrictive cardiomyopathy.
• Dilated cardiomyopathy also can be seen.
• Regardless of the type of myocardial disease present, the majority (> 50%) have severe left atrial enlargement, i.e., a left atrial to aortic ratio of 2.0 or greater.
• Occasionally, a left atrial thrombus or spontaneous echo contrast (smoke) may be seen.

Abdominal Ultrasonographic Findings
An experienced sonographer may be able to identify the thrombus in the caudal aorta. However, this imaging modality typically is not necessary to reach a diagnosis.

Angiographic Findings
Nonselective angiography should identify a negative filling defect in the caudal aorta representing the thrombus. As with abdominal sonography, this test may not be necessary to reach a diagnosis.

DIAGNOSTIC PROCEDURES
Electrocardiography
• The most common rhythm diagnoses are sinus rhythm and sinus tachycardia. Less common rhythm disturbances include atrial fibrillation, ventricular arrhythmias, supraventricular arrhythmias, and sinus bradycardia.
• Left ventricular enlargement pattern and left ventricular conduction disturbances (left anterior fascicular block) are commonly noted.

PATHOLOGIC FINDINGS
• Thrombus typically is identified at the caudal aortic trifurcation.
• Occasionally, a left atrial thrombus is seen.
• Emboli of the kidneys, gastrointestinal tract, cerebrum, and other organs also may be seen.

TREATMENT

APPROPRIATE HEALTH CARE
Initially, cats with ATE should be treated as inpatients because most have concurrent congestive heart failure and require injectable drugs.

NURSING CARE
• Fluid therapy is rarely necessary in the initial stages as most cats are in congestive heart failure.
• Supplemental oxygen therapy or thoracocentesis may be beneficial if in congestive heart failure.
• Initially, the affected legs should be minimally handled. However as reperfusion occurs, physical therapy (passive extension and flexion of the legs) may speed full recovery.
• No venipuncture should be performed on the affected legs.
• Initially, these cats may have difficulty posturing to urinate and may need to have their bladders expressed periodically to prevent over-distention of the bladder or urine scald.

ACTIVITY
Activity should be restricted. The cat should be kept quiet and stress-free.

DIET
• Initially, most cats are anorexic. Tempt these cats with any type of diet. It is important to keep these cats eating to avoid hepatic lipidosis.
• Chronic dietary management usually involves sodium restriction.

CLIENT EDUCATION
• Owners should be aware of the poor short- and long-term prognosis.
• Most cats will re-embolize. Most cats that survive an initial episode will be on some type of anticoagulant therapy that may require frequent reevaluations and an indoor lifestyle.
• Typically, most cats that survive an initial episode will recover complete function to the legs; however, neurologic deficits may persist.

SURGICAL CONSIDERATIONS
Surgical embolectomy typically is not recommended because these patients are high risks for surgery as a result of their heart disease.

MEDICATIONS

DRUG (S) OF CHOICE
• Thrombolytic therapy such as streptokinase and tissue plasminogen activator is used extensively in humans and infrequently in cats. These drugs are prohibitively expensive and carry a significant risk for bleeding complications and thus are rarely used in general practice.
• Heparin is the preferred drug in general practice. It has no effect on the established clot; however, it prevents further activation of the coagulation cascade. An initial dose of 100–200 units/kg is given intravenously and then followed with 200–300 units/kg SQ q8h. The dose is then titrated to prolong the activated partial thromboplastin time (APTT) approximately twofold.
• Aspirin is theoretically beneficial during and after an episode of thromboembolism because of its antiplatelet effects. The dose is an 81-mg tablet PO every second or third day.
• Butorphenol may be used for its analgesic effects at a dose of 0.5–1.0 mg SQ or IV q6h–q8h.
• Acepromazine may be used for its sedative and vasodilatory properties at a dose of 0.1–0.5 mg SQ q 8–12 h.
• Warfarin, a vitamin K antagonist, is the anticoagulant most widely used in humans and has recently been proposed for prevention of reembolization in cats surviving an initial episode. The initial dose is 0.25–0.5 mg PO q24h. It should be overlapped with heparin therapy for 3 days. The dose is then adjusted to prolong the prothrombin time (PT) approximately two times its baseline value or to attain an international normalized ratio (INR) of 2.0–4.0.
• Treatment of the patient's heart disease should be addressed.

CONTRAINDICATIONS
N/A

PRECAUTIONS
• Anticoagulant therapy with heparin, warfarin, or the thrombolytic drugs may cause severe bleeding complications.
• Avoid a nonselective beta-blocker such as propranolol as it may enhance peripheral vasoconstriction.

POSSIBLE INTERACTIONS
Warfarin may interact with other drugs, which may enhance its anticoagulant effects.

ALTERNATIVE DRUGS
N/A

FOLLOW-UP

PATIENT MONITORING
• Daily examination of the legs should be performed to assess clinical response to therapy. Initially, APTT should be performed once daily to titrate the heparin dose. • If warfarin is used, PT or INR is measured approximately 3 days after initiation of therapy and then weekly until the desired anticoagulant effect is reached. Thereafter, it could be measured 3–4 times yearly or when drug regimen is altered.

PREVENTION/AVOIDANCE
Because of the high rate of re-embolization after surviving an initial episode, prevention with either chronic aspirin or warfarin is strongly recommended.

POSSIBLE COMPLICATIONS
• Bleeding complications may arise with the anticoagulant therapy. • Permanent neurological deficits or muscular abnormalities in the hind limbs may arise in cats with prolonged ischemia. • Recurrence of ATE is common. • Recurrent congestive heart failure or sudden death are other possible complications of this disease syndrome.

EXPECTED COURSE AND PROGNOSIS
• Expected course is days to weeks for full recovery of function to the legs. • Prognosis in general is poor. In one study of 100 cats, approximately 60–70% of cats were euthanized or died during the initial thromboembolic episode. Long-term prognosis varies between 2 months to several years; however, the average is approximately 11 months with treatment.

MISCELLANEOUS

ASSOCIATED CONDITIONS
See causes and risk factors.

AGE RELATED FACTORS
N/A

ZOONOTIC POTENTIAL
N/A

PREGNANCY
N/A

SYNONYMS
Saddle thromboembolism
Systemic thromboembolism

SEE ALSO
Hypertrophic Cardiomyopathy-Cats
Restrictive Cardiomyopathy
Dilated Cardiomyopathy

ABBREVIATION
ATE = aortic thromboembolism

Suggested Reading
Flanders JA. Feline aortic thromboembolism. Compend Cont Ed Pract Ved 1986;8:473–484.
Laste NJ, Harpster NK. A retrospective study of 100 cats with feline distal aortic thromboembolism: 1977–1993. J Am An Hosp Assoc 1995;31:492–500.
Miller WP, Sisson DD. Myocardial diseases. In: Ettinger SJ, Feldman EC, eds. Textbook of Veterinary Internal Medicine. 4th ed. Philadelphia: WB Saunders, 1995.
Author Teresa C. DeFrancesco
Consulting Editors Larry P. Tilley and Francis W. K. Smith, Jr.

BASICS

OVERVIEW

• Tumors of endocrine cells that are capable of amine precursor uptake and decarboxylation (APUD) and secretion of peptide hormones; the tumors are named after the hormone they secrete.
• APUD cells are generally found in the gastrointestinal tract and CNS.
• Gastrin- and pancreatic polypeptide-secreting tumors are discussed here; insulinoma and glucagonoma are discussed separately.
• Hypergastrinemia from gastrin-secreting tumors causes gastritis and duodenal hyperacidity, which can cause gastric ulceration, esophageal dysfunction from chronic reflux, and intestinal villous atrophy.
• High concentration of pancreatic polypeptide also causes gastric hyperacidity and its consequences.

SIGNALMENT

• Gastrinoma—rare in dogs and cats; age range 3–12 years, mean 7.5 years (dogs)
• Pancreatic polypeptide—extremely rare in dogs

SIGNS

• Vomiting
• Weight loss
• Anorexia
• Diarrhea
• Lethargy, depression
• Polydipsia
• Melena
• Abdominal pain
• Hematemesis
• Hematochezia
• Fever

CAUSES & RISK FACTORS

Unknown

DIAGNOSIS

DIFFERENTIAL DIAGNOSIS

Other conditions associated with hypergastrinemia, gastric hyperacidity, and gastrointestinal ulceration
• Uremia
• Hepatic failure
• Drug-induced ulceration (e.g., NSAIDs or steroids)
• Inflammatory gastritis
• Stress-induced ulceration
• Mast cell disease

CBC/BIOCHEMISTRY/URINALYSIS

• Normal or reflect the chronic effects of general disease
• Iron-deficiency anemia secondary to gastrointestinal bleeding
• Increased BUN secondary to gastrointestinal bleeding
• Hypoproteinemia
• Electrolyte abnormalities with chronic vomiting

OTHER LABORATORY TESTS

• Serum gastrin concentration normal or high normal in patients with gastrinoma
• Provocative test of gastrin secretion—increased gastrin concentration after intravenous calcium gluconate or secretin administration suggests gastrinoma; see Appendix for protocol and interpretation.

IMAGING

Abdominal ultrasound sometimes demonstrates a pancreatic mass but is usually normal.

DIAGNOSTIC PROCEDURES

• Endoscopy with gastric and duodenal biopsy
• Aspirate any detectable masses because of suspicion of mast cell disease.
• If no detectable masses exist, examine a buffy coat smear for mast cells.

PATHOLOGIC FINDINGS

• Endoscopic biopsy reveals gastrointestinal ulceration.
• Histopathologic examination of pancreatic tumors reveals findings consistent with islet cell tumor but not specific for hormone type.
• Immunocytochemical staining can aid in the specific diagnosis.
• Histopathologic examination also can reveal metastasis to liver and regional lymph nodes.

TREATMENT

• Tell owner that most APUDomas are malignant and have metastasized by the time of diagnosis and that long-term control is often difficult.
• Aggressive medical management can sometimes palliate signs for months to years.
• Surgical exploration and excisional biopsy of a pancreatic mass is important both diagnostically and therapeutically.
• Medical management is useful for gastric hyperacidity.

MEDICATIONS

DRUGS

• Histamine H_2-receptor antagonists—cimetidine, ranitidine, and famotidine; decrease acid secretion by gastric parietal cells
• Omeprazole—a proton pump inhibitor; the most potent inhibitor of gastric acid secretion available; highly effective and expensive
• Sucralfate—adheres to ulcerated gastric mucosa and protects it from acid; promotes healing by binding pepsin and bile acids and stimulating local prostaglandins

CONTRAINDICATIONS/POSSIBLE INTERACTIONS

None

FOLLOW-UP

PATIENT MONITORING

• Physical examination and clinical signs are the most useful measures of treatment effectiveness and disease progression.
• Gastroscopy can monitor progression of gastritis, but it is not necessary.
• Abdominal radiography or ultrasound may detect development of abdominal masses.

PROGNOSIS

• Difficult to predict
• Patients with gastrinoma have been controlled on medical management for months to years.
• No cure available

MISCELLANEOUS

SEE ALSO

Gastric Erosions and Ulcerations

ABBREVIATION

• APUD = amine precursor uptake and decarboxylation

Suggested Reading

Zerbe CA. Islet cell tumors secreting insulin, pancreatic polypeptide, gastrin, or glucagon. In: Kirk RW, Bonagura JD, eds. Current veterinary therapy XI. Philadelphia: Saunders, 1992:368–375.

Author Thomas K. Graves
Consulting Editor Deborah S. Greco

BASICS

OVERVIEW
• Caused by herbicides, insecticides, wood preservatives, and treatments for blood parasites
• Leads to disruption of many important metabolic reactions
• Exposure—oral most common; percutaneous may cause systemic toxicosis.

SIGNALMENT
Cats and dogs

SIGNS

Acute Exposure
• Abdominal pain
• Vomiting
• Weakness
• Diarrhea
• Hematochezia
• Rapid weak pulse
• Prostration
• Subnormal temperature
• Collapse
• Death

Subchronic to Chronic Oral Exposure
• Anorexia
• Weight loss

CAUSES & RISK FACTORS
• Oral, percutaneous, or therapeutic exposure to arsenic-containing compounds
• Toxicity varies greatly.
• Weak and debilitated animals more susceptible

DIAGNOSIS

DIFFERENTIAL DIAGNOSIS
• Heavy metal toxicosis
• Ingestion of caustic agents
• Ingestion of irritating plants
• Canine or feline parvovirus

CBC/BIOCHEMISTRY/URINALYSIS
Serum biochemical analysis—liver and renal damage

OTHER LABORATORY TESTS
Arsenic concentration—urine, vomitus or stomach content (acute poisoning), kidney, liver (subacute), hair (chronic); decreases dramatically in urine, kidney, and liver 1–2 days after exposure; unreliable in blood

IMAGING
N/A

DIAGNOSTIC PROCEDURES
N/A

PATHOLOGIC FINDINGS
• Peracute poisoning—death without lesions
• Gastrointestinal tract lesions—common and severe; reddening of the gastric mucosa and proximal small intestine; watery gastrointestinal content; blood and sloughed mucosa in feces
• Liver—soft, yellow liver
• Lungs—congested; edematous lungs
• Skin lesions (cutaneous exposure)—blistering; edema; cracking; bleeding; secondary infections

TREATMENT
• Remove arsenic source
• Gastric lavage—if vomiting has not occurred
• Promote excretion.
• Dialysis—renal failure
• Appropriate fluid therapy
• Kaolin-pectin—soothe gastrointestinal tract.
• Keep patient warm and comfortable.
• Diet—when patient is able to keep food down, provide small amounts of high-quality food; increase as tolerated

MEDICATIONS

DRUGS

Dimercaprol (BAL)
• Give 2.5–5 mg/kg in oil by deep IM injection q4h for 2 days; q8h on day 3; q12h for up to 10 days; 5 mg/kg in only acutely affected patients on day 1
• Signs of toxicosis—vomiting; tremors; convulsions; subside as BAL is excreted over 3–4 hr
• Releases arsenic, which may worsen signs; give additional BAL.

Other
• DMSA—less toxic than BAL; children, 10 mg/kg q8h; effective in laboratory animals and humans
• Emetics
• Strong cathartics
• Parasympathomimetic drugs

FOLLOW-UP
• Prognosis grave with high-dose exposure, unless the diagnosis is made and treatment is started early
• Monitor closely for signs of BAL toxicosis.

MISCELLANEOUS

SEE ALSO
Poisoning (Intoxication)

ABBREVIATIONS
• BAL = British anti-Lewisite
• DMSA = 2,3-dimercaptosuccinic acid

Suggested Reading
Hatch RC. Poisons causing abdominal distress of liver or kidney damage. In: Booth NH, McDonald LE, eds. Veterinary pharmacology and therapeutics. 6th ed. Ames: Iowa State University Press, 1988:1102–1125.

Author Regg D. Neiger
Consulting Editor Gary D. Osweiler

DISEASES

ARTERIOVENOUS FISTULA

BASICS

OVERVIEW
An abnormal, low resistance connection between an artery and vein. A large arteriovenous fistula allows a significant fraction of the total cardiac output to bypass the capillary bed. The resulting increase in cardiac output may lead to 'high output' congestive heart failure (CHF). Location of arteriovenous fistula varies. Reported sites include the head, neck, ear, tongue, limbs, flank, spinal cord, cerebrum, lung, liver, vena cava, and gastrointestinal tract. Usually seen as an acquired lesion.

SIGNALMENT
• Dogs and cats (rare in both).
• No specific age, breed, or sex predilections known

SIGNS

Historical Findings
• Animals with acquired disease often have a history of trauma to the affected area.
• Owner may notice a warm, nonpainful swelling at the site.
• History consistent with impending or overt CHF is possible depending on shunt size and duration.
• Other historical findings depend on the location of the lesion. The shunt may cause local organ dysfunction.

Physical Examination Findings
• Vary and depend on location of the arterio-venous fistula.
• Signs of CHF (e.g., coughing, dyspnea, tachypnea, and exercise intolerance) may develop in animals with long-standing disease and high blood flow.
• Bounding pulses are present in some animals because of high ejection volume and rapid runoff through the arteriovenous fistula.
• Continuous murmur (bruit) at the site caused by blood flow through the lesion.
• Cautious compression of the artery proximal to the lesion abolishes the bruit. When blood flow is high, this compression may also elicit an immediate reflex decrease in heart rate (Branham's sign).
• Edema, ischemia, and congestion of organs and tissues caused by high venous pressure in the proximity of the lesion.
• If the lesion is on a limb, pitting edema, lameness, ulceration, scabbing, and gangrene may result.
• Lesion near vital organs may cause signs associated with organ failure such as ascites (liver), seizures (brain), paresis (spinal cord), and dyspnea (lung).

CAUSES & RISK FACTORS
• Rarely, a congenital lesion.
• Acquired arteriovenous fistula typically results from local damage to vasculature secondary to trauma, surgery, venipuncture, perivascular injection (e.g., barbiturates), or tumor.

DIAGNOSIS

DIFFERENTIAL DIAGNOSIS
• The lesion may look like an aneurysm or false aneurysm.
• Bizarre clinical findings, depending on location of arteriovenous fistula, may suggest other disease processes; arteriovenous fistula may be a late diagnostic consideration.

CBC/BIOCHEMISTRY/URINALYSIS
May reflect damage to systems in the vicinity of the lesion. i.e. biochemical abnormalities suggesting hepatic, renal, or other organ dysfunction are possible.

OTHER LABORATORY TESTS
N/A

IMAGING

Thoracic Radiographic Findings
Cardiac enlargement and pulmonary over-circulation in some animals with hemody-namically significant arteriovenous fistula.

Echocardiographic Findings
• May allow imaging of the arteriovenous fistula depicting its cavernous nature.
• Doppler ultrasound may demonstrate high velocity, turbulent flow within the lesion.

Angiography
Selective angiography outlines the lesion, may be necessary for definitive diagnosis, and is highly desirable for presurgical evaluation. Placement of the catheter close to the lesion and rapid injection is necessary; high volume blood flow dilutes the contrast medium quickly.

DIAGNOSTIC TESTS
N/A

TREATMENT

• Definitive treatment requires surgery to divide and remove abnormal vascular connections. Surgery is recommended in animals with clinical signs related to the arteriovenous fistula, since lesions may increase in size.
• Surgery can be difficult and labor intensive and may require blood transfusion; delineation of lesion before surgery by angiography is advised.
• Although surgery is often successful, arteriovenous fistula may recur. In some animals, amputation of the affected part may be necessary.

MEDICATIONS

DRUGS

• Concurrent medical treatment depends on the site of the arteriovenous fistula and secondary clinical features.
• Medical treatment for congestive heart failure may be required before surgery.

CONTRAINDICATIONS/POSSIBLE INTERACTIONS

Avoid excessive fluid administration; animals with arteriovenous fistula are volume overloaded.

FOLLOW-UP

Postoperative reevaluation is needed to determine whether arteriovenous fistula recurred.

MISCELLANEOUS

SEE ALSO

Congestive Heart Failure, Left-sided

Suggested Reading

Suter PF, Fox PR. Peripheral vascular disease. In: Ettinger SJ, Feldman EC, eds. Textbook of veterinary internal medicine. 4th ed. Philadelphia: WB Saunders, 1995.

Author Donald J. Brown

Consulting Editors Larry P. Tilley and Francis W. K. Smith, Jr.

ARTHRITIS (OSTEOARTHRITIS)

 BASICS

DEFINITION
• Progressive deterioration of articular cartilage found in diarthrodial joints
• Degenerative joint disease—more appropriate term in veterinary medicine; two broad classes: primary (idiopathic) and secondary

PATHOPHYSIOLOGY
• Usually categorized as noninflammatory, but mild inflammation plays an important role
• Adverse stimuli—cause release of inflammatory mediators from leukocytes, chondrocytes, and synoviocytes; lead to loss of proteoglycans from the extracellular matrix of articular cartilage, owing to increased destruction and decreased production
• Breakdown and loss of collagen and chondrocytes—as disease progresses; lead to irreversible change

SYSTEMS AFFECTED
Musculoskeletal—diarthrodial joints

GENETICS
• Generally not assumed to be associated with hereditary factors
• Primary—associated with a colony of beagles
• Secondary—may be hereditary (e.g., hip dysplasia and osteochondrosis)

INCIDENCE/PREVALENCE
• Probably the most common skeletal disease encountered in dogs
• Actual incidence unknown

GEOGRAPHIC DISTRIBUTION
N/A

SIGNALMENT

Species
Dogs and cats

BREED PREDILECTIONS
None

Mean Age and Range
• Hereditary or developmental disorders (e.g., osteochondrosis, elbow dysplasia, hip dysplasia)—immature animals
• Trauma induced—any age

Predominant Sex
None

SIGNS

General Comments
• Vary greatly among
• Radiographic severity often does not correlate with clinically severity.

Historical Findings
• Dogs—intermittent lameness or stiff gait that slowly becomes more severe and frequent; may have history of previous joint trauma (fracture, ligament injury, dislocation), osteochondral disease, or developmental disorder (patellar luxation, fragmented medial coronoid, un-united anconeal process, hip dysplasia)
• May be exacerbated by exercise, long periods of recumbency, and weather changes (cold weather)

PHYSICAL EXAMINATION FINDINGS
• Stiffness of gait
• Lameness
• Decreased range of motion
• Crepitus
• Joint swelling, and pain
• Joint instability (ligament tear, subluxation), depending on the duration of disease

CAUSES
• Primary—thought to be the result of long-term use combined with aging; associated with a known predisposing cause
• Secondary—much more common; results from an initiating cause: joint instability, trauma, osteochondral defects, joint incongruity

RISK FACTORS
• Working, athletic, and obese dogs—place more stress on their joints and thus are more likely to incur injury and degenerative changes than other dogs
• Cushing disease or diabetes mellitus (dogs)—may also be more prone owing to catabolic processes

 DIAGNOSIS

DIFFERENTIAL DIAGNOSIS
• Immune-mediated arthritis
• Infectious arthritis
• Neoplasia

CBC/BIOCHEMISTRY/URINALYSIS
N/A

OTHER LABORATORY TESTS
• Coombs, ANA, and rheumatoid factor tests—help rule out immune-mediated arthritis
• Serum titers for *Borrelia, Ehrlichia,* and *Rickettsia*—evaluate for infectious arthritis

IMAGING
Radiographic changes—joint capsular distension; osteophytosis; enthesiophytosis; soft tissue thickening; narrowed joint spaces; subchondral sclerosis (severely affected patients)

DIAGNOSTIC PROCEDURES
• Arthrocentesis and synovial fluid analysis—support the diagnosis; slight increase in mononuclear cells (generally < 2000 cells/mL); large numbers of neutrophils likely the result of underlying immune-mediated or infectious arthritis
• Bacterial culture and sensitivity—synovial fluid
• Biopsy of synovial tissue—helps rule out other arthritides or neoplasia

PATHOLOGIC FINDINGS
• Erosion of articular cartilage
• Eburnation and sclerosis of subchondral bone
• Full-thickness cartilage loss in chronic cases
• Thickening and fibrosis of the joint capsule
• Synovial fluid—grossly normal; usually increased volume
• Osteophytes and enthesiophytes—at joint capsular attachments and adjacent to the joint

TREATMENT

APPROPRIATE HEALTH CARE
• Includes medical or surgical options
• Medical—usually tried initially; wide variety of pharmaceuticals that inhibit prostaglandins, leukotrienes, serine proteases, metalloproteases, interleukins, and tumor necrosis factor; other drugs (e.g., chondroprotective agents) to inhibit inflammatory mediators and stimulate metabolic activity of synoviocytes and chondrocytes
• Surgical options—if inadequate response to medical management

NURSING CARE
Physical therapy—very beneficial in enhancing good limb function and general well-being; range-of-motion exercises, massage, combination heat and cold therapy, and swimming

ACTIVITY
Limited to a level that minimizes aggravation of clinical signs

DIET
• Weight reduction for obese patients—decreases stress placed on affected joints
• Reduced caloric intake—recommended because of decreased activity as a result of disease and aging

CLIENT EDUCATION
• Inform client that medical therapy is palliative and the condition is likely to progress.
• Discuss treatment options, activity level, and diet.

SURGICAL CONSIDERATIONS

• Arthrotomy—often used to treat underlying causes (e.g., fragmented medial coronoid process, osteochondral diseases, un-united anconeal process)
• Reconstructive procedures—to eliminate joint instability; correct anatomic deficiencies

Arthroplasty Procedures

• Commonly performed for hip
• THR—may give excellent results; recommended for dogs that can accommodate the implants
• Femoral head ostectomy—for smaller dogs and cats; selected patients that cannot afford THR

Arthrodesis

• Selected chronic cases and for joint instability
• Complete or partial—based on the location of condition or instability
• Carpus—generally yields excellent results
• Shoulder, elbow, stifle, or hock—less predictable results

MEDICATIONS

DRUGS OF CHOICE

NSAIDs

• Work by inhibiting prostaglandin synthesis
• Aspirin (25 mg/kg PO q12h) and phenylbutazone (3–7 mg/kg PO q8h)—most commonly used agents in dogs
• Meclofenamic acid—0.5 mg/kg PO q12h; may also be given
• Carprofen (2.2 mg/kg PO q12h) and etodolac (10–15 mg/kg PO q24h)—less ulcerogenic and irritating to the gastrointestinal system
• Cats—limited to aspirin (10 mg/kg PO every 3 days)

Chondroprotective Agents

• Inhibition of various destructive enzymes and prostaglandins
• Chondrostimulation—associated with increased production of proteoglycan, hyaluronate, and collagen
• GAGPs (Adequan)—gaining popularity for use in dogs; recent clinical study of dogs with hip dysplasia found the greatest improvement in orthopedic scores at 4.4 mg/kg (2 mg/lb) IM every 3 to 5 days for eight injections.

CONTRAINDICATIONS

• NSAIDs and chondroprotective agents—avoid or use cautiously in dogs with disorders of hemostasis; may inhibit platelets and coagulation

• NSAIDs and GAGPs—simultaneous use not recommended; potential additive inhibition of hemostasis

PRECAUTIONS

• NSAIDs—use cautiously owing to potential for gastric ulceration
• Naproxen, piroxicam, flunixin meglumine, and ibuprofen—although many references suggest dosages, their use is discouraged because of increased ulcerogenic potential.

POSSIBLE INTERACTIONS

None known

ALTERNATIVE DRUGS

Nutraceuticals

• Classified as nutritional supplements rather than pharmaceuticals
• Little controlled experimental or clinical research substantiate efficacy in dogs
• Oral glycosaminoglycan products—contain varying amounts of chondroitin sulfates
• Cosequin—provides raw materials needed for glycosaminoglycan synthesis; contains glucosamine, chondroitin sulfate, mixed glycosaminoglycans, and manganese ascorbate
• Methyl sulfonyl methane—derivative of DMSO; promoted as reducing pain, inflammation, and free radicals

Free-Radical Scavengers

• Oral superoxide dismutase—controversial; lack of controlled clinical studies evaluating efficacy; questions regarding bioavailability after ingestion; efficacy of subcutaneous administration unproven
• Topical DMSO—may provide short-term relief in dogs

Corticosteroids

• Glucocorticoids—inhibit inflammatory mediators and cytokines; seem to be ideal treatment; however, chronic use delays healing and initiates damage to articular cartilage; potential systemic side effects documented; goal is low-dose (dogs, 0.5–2.0 mg/kg; cats, 2.0–4.0 mg/kg), alternate-day therapy.
• Prednisone—initial dose of 1–2 mg/kg PO q24h for dogs and 4 mg/kg PO q24h for cats
• Triamcinolone hexacetonide—intra-articular injection of 5 mg in dogs showed a protective and therapeutic effect in one model.

FOLLOW-UP

PATIENT MONITORING

Clinical deterioration—indicates need to change drug selection or dosage; may indicate need for surgical intervention

PREVENTION/AVOIDANCE

Early identification of predisposing causes and prompt treatment—help reduce progression of secondary condition

POSSIBLE COMPLICATIONS

N/A

EXPECTED COURSE AND PROGNOSIS

• Slow progression of disease likely
• Some form of medical or surgical treatment usually allows a good quality of life.

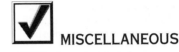

MISCELLANEOUS

ASSOCIATED CONDITIONS

N/A

AGE-RELATED FACTORS

N/A

ZOONOTIC POTENTIAL

N/A

PREGNANCY

N/A

SYNONYMS

Degenerative joint disease

ABBREVIATIONS

• ANA = antinuclear antibody
• DMSO = dimethyl sulfoxide
• GAGPs = glycosaminoglycan polysulfate esters
• THR = total hip replacement

Suggested Reading

Beale BS. Arthropathies. In: Bloomberg MS, Taylor RT, Dee JF, eds. Canine sports medicine and surgery. Philadelphia: Saunders, 1998:517–532.
Beale BS, Goring RL. Degenerative joint disease. In: Bojrab MJ, ed. Disease mechanisms in small animal surgery. Philadelphia: Lea & Febiger, 1993:727–736.
Pedersen NC. Joint diseases of dogs and cats. In: Ettinger SJ, ed. Textbook of veterinary internal medicine. 3rd ed. Philadelphia: Saunders, 1989:2329–2377.
Todhunter RJ, Lust G. Polysulfated glycosaminoglycan in the treatment of osteoarthritis. J Am Vet Med Assoc 1994;204:1245–1251.

Author Brian S. Beale
Consulting Editor Peter D. Schwarz

ARTHRITIS, SEPTIC

 BASICS

DEFINITION
Pathogenic microorganisms within the closed space of one or more synovial joints

PATHOPHYSIOLOGY
• Usually caused by the hematogenous spread of microorganisms from a distant septic foci, contamination associated with traumatic injury (e.g., a direct penetrating injury such as bite and gunshot wounds), the extension of a primary osteomyelitis, or a contaminated surgery
• Lack of a basement membrane—may predispose the synovium to bacterial seeding
• Sources of infection—skin; dental disease; gastrointestinal system; prostate; anal sacs

SYSTEMS AFFECTED
Musculoskeletal system—usually affects one joint

GENETICS
N/A

INCIDENCE/PREVALENCE
Relatively uncommon cause of monoarticular arthritis in dogs and cats

GEOGRAPHIC DISTRIBUTION
May be an increased incidence in Lyme disease–endemic areas.

SIGNALMENT
Species
• Most common in dogs
• Rare in cats

Breed Predilections
Medium to large breeds—most commonly German shepherds, Dobermans, and Labrador retrievers

Mean Age and Range
Any age; usually between 4 and 7 years

Predominant Sex
Male

SIGNS
General Comments
Always consider the diagnosis in patients monoarticular lameness associated with soft tissue swelling, heat, and pain.

Historical Findings
• Lameness—acute onset common; be mild with a gradual onset
• Lethargy
• Anorexia
• May report previous trauma—dog bite, penetrating injury

Physical Examination Findings
• Monoarticular lameness
• Joint pain and swelling—commonly carpus, stifle, hock, shoulder, or cubital joint
• Localized joint heat
• Decreased range of motion
• Fever

CAUSES
• Aerobic bacterial organisms—most common: staphylococci, streptococci, coliforms, and *Pasteurella*
• Anaerobic organisms—most common: *Propionibacterium, Peptostreptococcus, Fusobacterium,* and *Bacteroides*
• Spirochete—*Borrelia burgdorferi*
• Mycoplasma
• Fungal agents—*Blastomyces,* cryptococcus, and *Coccidiodes*
• *Ehrlichia*
• Leishmania

RISK FACTORS
• Predisposing factors for hematogenous infection—diabetes mellitus; Addison disease; immunosuppression
• Penetrating trauma to the joint

 DIAGNOSIS

DIFFERENTIAL DIAGNOSIS
• Immune-mediated arthropathy
• Postvaccinal transient polyarthritis
• Greyhound polyarthritis
• Crystal-induced joint disease
• Synovial cell sarcoma

CBC/BIOCHEMISTRY/URINALYSIS
• Hemogram—inflammatory left shift
• Other results normal

OTHER LABORATORY TESTS
Serologic testing for specific pathogens

IMAGING
Radiography
• Early disease—may reveal thickened and dense of periarticular tissues; may see evidence of synovial effusion
• Late disease—reveals bone destruction, osteolysis, irregular joint space, discreet erosions, and periarticular osteophytosis

DIAGNOSTIC PROCEDURES
Synovial Fluid Analysis
• Increased volume
• Turbid fluid
• Decreased mucin clot reaction
• Elevated WBC count—predominate neutrophils > 40,000/mm³; (normal joint fluid < 10% neutrophils)
• Bacteria in the synovial fluid or within neutrophils—show chromatolysis, nuclear swelling, and loss of segmentation

Synovial Fluid Culture
• Must be collected aseptically; requires heavy sedation or general anesthesia
• Place fluid sample in aerobic and anaerobic Culturettes and in blood culture medium
• Culturette samples—cultured immediately upon arrival to the laboratory
• Blood culture medium—reculturing after 24 hr of incubation increases accuracy by 50%.

Other
• A synovial fluid glucose level below a paired serum glucose level strongly suggests sepsis.
• Synovial biopsy—to rule out immune-mediated joint disease; no more effective than culturing incubated blood culture medium

PATHOLOGIC FINDINGS
• Synovium—thickened; discolored; often very proliferative
• Histology—evidence of hyperplastic synviotocytes
• Increased numbers of neutrophils, macrophages, and fibrinous debris

TREATMENT

APPROPRIATE HEALTH CARE
• Inpatient—initial stabilization; perform open arthrotomy and/or place irrigation catheter (ingress/egress) to lavage joint as soon as possible to minimize intra-articular injury.
• Outpatient—long-term management

NURSING CARE
Alternating heat and cold packing—beneficial in promoting increased blood flow and decreased swelling

ACTIVITY
Restricted until resolution of symptoms

DIET
N/A

CLIENT EDUCATION
• Discuss probable cause.
• Warn client about the need for long-term antibiotics and the likelihood of residual degenerative joint disease.

SURGICAL CONSIDERATIONS
• Acute disease with minimal radiographic changes—place an irrigation catheter (ingress/egress) to lavage the joint.
• Chronic disease—requires open arthrotomy with débridement of the synovium and copious lavage; place an irrigation catheter (ingress/egress) to lavage the joint postoperatively.
• Lavage—use warmed physiologic saline (2–4 mL/kg q8h) until effluent is clear.
• Effluent fluid—cytologically monitored daily for existence and character of bacteria and neutrophils
• Removal of catheters—when effluent fluid has no bacteria and the neutrophils are cytologically healthy

MEDICATIONS

DRUGS OF CHOICE
• Pending culture susceptibility data—first-generation cephalosporin and ampicillin-clavulanic acid

• Choice of antimicrobial drugs—primarily depends on in vitro determination of susceptibility of microorganisms; toxicity, frequency, route of administration, and expense also considered; most penetrate the synovium well; need to be given for a minimum of 4–8 weeks
• NSAIDs—may help decrease pain and inflammation

CONTRAINDICATIONS
Avoid quinolones in pediatric patients; they induce cartilage lesions experimentally

PRECAUTIONS
Failure to respond to conventional antibiotic therapy—may indicate anaerobic disease or other unusual cause (fungal, spirochete)

POSSIBLE INTERACTIONS
N/A

ALTERNATIVE DRUGS
N/A

FOLLOW-UP

PATIENT MONITORING
• Drainage and irrigation catheters—may be pulled after 4–6 days or after reassessment of synovial fluid cytology
• Duration of antibiotic therapy—4–8 weeks or longer; depends on clinical signs and pathogenic organism
• Persistent synovial inflammation without viable bacterial organisms (dogs)—may be caused by antigenic bacterial fragments or antigen antibody deposition
• Systemic corticosteroid therapy and aggressive physical therapy—may be needed to maximize normal joint dynamics

PREVENTION/AVOIDANCE
N/A

POSSIBLE COMPLICATIONS
• Chronic disease—severe degenerative joint disease
• Recurrence of infection
• Limited joint range of motion
• Generalized sepsis
• Osteomyelitis

EXPECTED COURSE AND PROGNOSIS
• Acutely diagnosed disease—responds well to antibiotic therapy
• Delayed diagnosis or resistant or highly virulent organisms—guarded to poor prognosis

MISCELLANEOUS

ASSOCIATED CONDITIONS
N/A

AGE-RELATED FACTORS
N/A

ZOONOTIC POTENTIAL
N/A

PREGNANCY
N/A

SYNONYMS
• Infectious arthritis
• Joint ill

SEE ALSO
• Osteomyelitis
• Polyarthritis, Erosive Immune-Mediated
• Polyarthritis, Nonerosive Immune-Mediated

Suggested Reading
Bennett D, Taylor DJ. Bacterial infective arthritis in the dog. J Sm Anim Pract 1988;29:207–230.
Ellison RS. The cytologic examination of synovial fluid. Semin Vet Med Surg Sm Anim 1988;3:133–139.
Hodgin EC, Michaelson F, Howerth EW. Anaerobic bacterial infections causing osteomyelitis/arthritis in a dog. J Am Vet Med Assoc 1992;201:886–888.
Montgomery RD, Long IR, Milton JL. Comparison of aerobic Culturette, synovial membrane biopsy, and blood culture medium in detection of canine bacterial arthritis. Vet Surg 1989;18:300–303.
Author Robert A. Taylor
Consulting Editor Peter D. Schwarz

DISEASES

ASPERGILLOSIS

BASICS

OVERVIEW
• An opportunistic fungal infection caused by *Aspergillus* spp., common molds that are ubiquitous in the environment, forming numerous spores in dust, straw, grass clippings, and hay
• Two types of infections—disease localized to the nasal cavity and frontal sinuses and disseminated disease; do not appear to be related, but a report of a dog that developed fungal osteomyelitis 6 months after treatment of nasal aspergillosis raises the possibility
• Nasal cavity—*A. fumigatus* most frequently involved; *A. flavus, A. niger,* and *A. nidulans* also isolated; presumably acquired through direct inoculation of the nasal mucosa
• Disseminated disease—usually *A. terreus; A. deflectus* and *A. fumigatus* also associated; portal of entry not definitively established, but possibly through the respiratory or gastrointestinal tract with subsequent hematogenous spread

SIGNALMENT
Dogs
• Both forms—more common in dogs than in cats
• Nasal—more common in young adult dolichocephalic and mesaticephalic breeds
• Disseminated—more common in German Shepherds, but not confined to this breed; reported average age of affected dogs 3 years, with a range of 1–9 years; slight bias toward females

Cats
• Persians—marginally increased incidence
• A total of 40 cases documented; majority involved disseminated disease affecting the lungs and/or gastrointestinal tract
• Nasal—2 cases with frontal sinus involvement reported
• Disseminated—associated with a high incidence of concurrent disease or long-term use of corticosteroids or antibiotics

SIGNS
Dogs
Nasal
• Chronic unilateral or bilateral serous, mucopurulent, or more commonly profuse sanguinopurulent nasal discharge unresponsive to antibiotics
• Nasal pain and depigmentation or ulceration around the external nares—common
• Sneezing and intermittent epistaxis—sometimes reported

• External nasal distortion or swelling—uncommon
• Invasion of the cribriform plate infrequently leads to signs of CNS involvement.
Disseminated
• May develop acutely or slowly over a period of months
• Often associated with spinal pain owing to fungal diskospondylitis or lameness owing to fungal osteomyelitis
• Neurologic—spinal cord damage
• Polyuria/polydipsia and hematuria—renal involvement
• Uveitis—ocular involvement
• Nonspecific—fever, weight loss, vomiting, lymphadenopathy, and anorexia

Cats
• Nasal—associated with nasal discharge and stertor
• Disseminated—most commonly associated with nonspecific signs (e.g., lethargy and depression or vomiting and diarrhea)

CAUSES & RISK FACTORS
• Nasal—more common in outdoor dogs and farm dogs; young adult dolichocephalic and mesaticephalic dogs
• Disseminated—German shepherds most commonly but not exclusively affected
• Immune deficiency—may be a factor because the organism is widespread but the disease is uncommon; breed-related immune defect proposed in German shepherds and their crosses
• Geographical/environmental conditions—may be a factor because some regions have a higher incidence than others (e.g., California, Louisiana, Michigan, Georgia, Florida, and Virginia in the U.S.; Western Australia, Barcelona, and Milan).
• Cats—associated with FIP, FePLV, FeLV, diabetes mellitus, and chronic corticosteroid or antibiotic administration

DIAGNOSIS

DIFFERENTIAL DIAGNOSIS
• Nasal—nasal neoplasia; bacterial rhinitis/sinusitis; penicilliosis; foreign body; nasal mites; nasopharyngeal polyps (cats); nasal cryptococcosis (cats)
• Disseminated—bacterial osteomyelitis/diskospondylitis; spinal neoplasia; intervertebral disk disease; skeletal neoplasia; bacterial pyelonephritis; bacterial pneumonia; other causes of uveitis (see Uveitis)

CBC/BIOCHEMISTRY/URINALYSIS
Nasal—may see neutrophilic leukocytosis and monocytosis reflecting chronic inflammation

Disseminated
• Variable
• Dogs—often have mature neutrophilic leukocytosis and lymphopenia
• Cats—may have nonregenerative anemia and leukopenia
• Biochemistry changes—may see high globulins, creatinine, phosphate, and BUN
• Urinalysis—may see isosthenuria, hematuria, pyuria, and possibly fungal hyphae in the sediment; detection of fungal hyphae in sediment can be improved by allowing the sample to incubate at room temperature for 24–48 hr; sediment samples may be examined unstained as wet preparations or may be air-dried and stained with Diff-Quick (the branching hyphae stain purple).

OTHER LABORATORY TESTS
• Positive fungal serology (agar gel double diffusion, counterimmunoelectrophoresis, and ELISA)—support the diagnosis; false positives and cross-reactivity with *Penicillium* spp. reported
• Cats—test for FeLV and FIV because they affect prognosis

IMAGING
Nasal
• Radiography—open-mouth ventrodorsal view and skyline views of the frontal sinuses most useful; reveal an increase in radiolucency in the affected rostral and maxillary nasal turbinate areas owing to turbinate lysis; mixed density may be seen as a result of a combination of turbinate destruction and soft tissue dense fungal granulomas and/or nasal discharge; fungal disease changes are typically more rostral than those seen in nasal neoplasia; affected frontal sinuses have an increase in opacity owing to the soft tissue density of the fungal elements and accumulation of associated inflammatory fluid; may see frontal sinus lysis
• CT and MRI—define the extent of disease more accurately; allow assessment of the integrity of the cribriform plate (which may be of concern before performing nasal flushing in dogs showing CNS signs)

Disseminated
Radiography—spinal views may show end plate lysis, attempted bony intervertebral bridging, and lysis of vertebral bodies consistent with diskospondylitis; bony proliferation and lysis and periosteal reaction typical of osteomyelitis of the diaphyseal region of long bones

DIAGNOSTIC PROCEDURES

Nasal
• Cytology of nasal swabs and flushes—usually nondiagnostic; findings reflect an inflammatory process; hyphae may be seen, especially if collected at rhinoscopy.
• Rhinoscopy—may allow direct visualization of the fungus on the nasal mucosa (grayish white plaques adherent to inflamed mucosa); destructive nature can be appreciated (nasal cavity takes on a vast cavernous appearance in severe cases); excellent tool for collecting samples for culture, cytology, and histology.
• Fungal cultures of nasal exudate—not accurate for obtaining a definitive diagnosis; may give false-positive or false-negative results; the organism is a common laboratory contaminant; positive culture should be confirmed by histopathology or supported by the history and radiographic and serologic testing.

PATHOLOGIC FINDINGS
Histopathologic examination of tissue—most likely to render a definitive diagnosis; special stains may be required; granulomas and multiple organ infarcts noted with disseminated disease (kidneys, spleen, and vertebrae)

 ## TREATMENT

Nasal (Dogs)
Clotrimazole
• Systemic antifungal agents—limited success
• Local administration into both nasal cavities under general anesthesia via the nares—treatment of choice
• Place a well-fitted, cuffed endotracheal tube to prevent aspiration of the drug (which may irritate the esophageal mucosa)
• Important to ensure that the caudal nasopharynx is well occluded—use a Foley catheter and sponges placed dorsal to the soft palate; sponges or gauze swabs may be placed by first passing a length of heavy suture material (sometimes assisted by a red rubber feeding tube) through the nasal cavity until it feeds out through the caudal nares; then attach the gauze swabs to the suture material and pull rostrally to firmly wedge in the caudal nares.
• Position the patient in dorsal recumbency with its head at right angles to the table.
• Fill the nasal passages with 1% clotrimazole for 1 hr; intermittently top off the passages as the solution is absorbed into the gauze and redistributed to the sinuses; average dog requires 50–60 mL for each side.

• Then place patient in sternal recumbency to allow the solution to drain out via gravity.
• Remove the gauze swabs and Foley catheter; gently flush the pharynx with saline to remove any residual solution.
• Carefully monitor recovery from anesthesia; some dogs may develop stridor if laryngeal edema occurs (treated with corticosteroids).

Disseminated (Dogs)
• Difficult to eliminate infection; rare cures have been reported
• Halt progression of clinical signs rather than eliminate the infection.
• Itraconazole—most effective
• Combination of flucytosine and subcutaneous infusion of amphotericin B in 4.5% saline and 2.5% dextrose—used to successfully treat disseminated cryptococcosis; may prove to have some use to treat aspergillosis (no published reports)
• Fluid therapy—indicated by the degree of renal compromise and azotemia

Cats
• Nasal—might be managed successfully using the same techniques used in dogs but no reports are published
• Disseminated—likely difficult to treat; data are limited.

 ## MEDICATIONS

DRUGS

Nasal
• 1% clotrimazole—50–60 mL instilled into each nasal cavity for 1 hr; treatment of choice
• Enilconazole—10% solution diluted 50:50 with water immediately before administration; 10 mg/kg q12h instilled into the nasal sinuses via surgically implanted frontal sinus catheters for 14 days
• Oral azoles—much lower rates of cure than topical treatment; thiabendazole (10 mg/kg q12h), ketoconazole (5 mg/kg q12h), or itraconazole (5 mg/kg q24h)

Disseminated
• Itraconazole—10 mg/kg daily (can be divided); drug of choice; dogs unlikely to be cured, though the disease may be contained with continued use
• Combination therapy with flucytosine and amphotericin B—may prove successful

CONTRAINDICATIONS/POSSIBLE INTERACTIONS
Amphotericin B—contraindicated in dogs with pre-existing renal compromise or failure

 ## FOLLOW-UP
• Nasal—discharge should be well reduced 2 weeks after treatment and eliminated by 4 weeks; if still significant discharge, re-treat; consider antibiotics, because bacterial infection can be a problem owing to damage sustained to nasal mucosa and turbinates.
• Disseminated—monitor serial radiographs every 1–2 months, renal function, and urine fungal cultures

 ## MISCELLANEOUS

ZOONOTIC POTENTIAL
None

ABBREVIATIONS
• ELISA = enzyme-linked immunoadsorbent assay
• FeLV = feline leukemia virus
• FePLV = feline panleukopenia virus
• FIP = feline infectious peritonitis
• FIV = feline immunodeficiency virus

Suggested Reading
Davidson A, Pappagianis D. Treatment of nasal aspergillosis with topical clotrimazole. In: Bonagura J, Kirk R, eds. Current veterinary therapy XII. Philadelphia: Saunders, 1995:899–901.
Kelly SE, Shaw SE, Clark WT. Long-term survival of four dogs with disseminated *Aspergillus terreus* treated with itraconazole. Aust Vet J 1995;72:311–313.
Author Tania N. Davey
Consulting Editor Stephen C. Barr

DISEASES

ASPIRIN TOXICITY

 BASICS

OVERVIEW
• Given by owners to relieve minor pain and discomfort; less commonly used owing to increasing popularity of other over-the-counter pain-relieving drugs
• Gastric irritation and hemorrhage occur—10%–20% of cases
• Repeated doses may—produce gastro-intestinal ulceration and perforation
• Toxic hepatitis, suppression of bone marrow activity, and anemia—may occur, especially in cats

SIGNALMENT
Cats and less commonly dogs

SIGNS
• Depression
• Vomiting—vomitus may be blood-tinged.
• Tachypnea
• Fever
• Muscular weakness and ataxia
• Coma and death in 1 or more days

CAUSES & RISK FACTORS
• Owners employing human dosage guidelines to medicate cats—most common
• Deficiency in glucuronide conjugation capability (cats)
• Biological half-life—cats, 44.6 hr; dogs, 7.5 hr; responsible for higher risk in cats

 DIAGNOSIS

DIFFERENTIAL DIAGNOSIS
• Clinical signs—uncharacteristic
• History of aspirin ingestion or medication—important; within 5 days of signs should raise concern
• Pre-existing painful condition—question owner about aspirin administration.

CBC/BIOCHEMISTRY/URINALYSIS
• Cats—prone to Heinz body formation
• Hyponatremia and hypokalemia

OTHER LABORATORY TESTS
• Initial respiratory alkalosis followed by metabolic acidosis
• Salicylic acid concentrations in serum or urine
• High ketones and pyruvic, lactic, and amino acid levels
• Decreased sulfuric and phosphoric acid renal clearance

IMAGING
N/A

DIAGNOSTIC PROCEDURES
N/A

 TREATMENT

• Inpatient—following general principles of poisoning management
• Correction of acid–base balance—continuous intravenous fluids
• Induced gastric emptying—gastric lavage or induced emesis
• Peritoneal or hemodialysis or hemo-perfusion—heroic procedures

MEDICATIONS

DRUGS
• No specific antidote available
• Activated charcoal—2g/kg PO; decontaminate gut.
• Sodium bicarbonate—1 mEq/kg IV; alkalinize urine

CONTRAINDICATIONS/POSSIBLE INTERACTIONS
N/A

FOLLOW-UP
• Maintaining renal function and acid–base balance vital
• Severe acid–base disturbances, severe dehydration, toxic hepatitis, bone marrow depression, and coma—poor prognostic indicators

MISCELLANEOUS
Be sure that history of "aspirin" medication does not refer to other available pain medications.

Suggested Reading

Oehme FW. Aspirin and acetaminophen. In: Kirk RW, ed. Current veterinary therapy IX. Small animal practice. Philadelphia: Saunders, 1986:188–189.
Author Frederick W. Oehme
Consulting Editor Gary D. Osweiler

DISEASES

BASICS

DEFINITION
• Asthma—airway disorder characterized by bronchoconstrictive episodes that are reversible • Chronic bronchitis—a cough that persists for months to years

PATHOPHYSIOLOGY
• Airway narrowing—caused by thickening of the airway wall, mucus and cellular debris within the airway lumen, and bronchoconstriction; results in airflow obstruction that is greater on expiration than on inspiration • Bronchial wall changes—airway epithelial hyperplasia; metaplasia; erosion and ulceration; edema; infiltration with lymphocytes, neutrophils and eosinophils; airway goblet and submucosal gland hypertrophy; hyperplasia; lead to thickened airway wall and increased capacity for production of more and thicker mucus • Altered viscosity and greater volume of mucus produced in conjunction with a less functional ciliary apparatus—create obstruction and plugging within the airways • Bronchial smooth muscle—controlled by the parasympathetic, sympathetic, and nonadrenergic–noncholinergic nervous systems; stimulation of various receptors causes either bronchodilation or bronchoconstriction.

SYSTEMS AFFECTED
• Respiratory—obstruction of airflow • Cardiovascular—may lead to cor pulmonale

GENETICS
No clear basis

INCIDENCE/PREVALENCE
Approximately 1% of adult cats

GEOGRAPHIC DISTRIBUTION
N/A

SIGNALMENT

Species
Cats

Breed Predilections
• Siamese • Himalayans

Mean Age and Range
• Any age • Signs of asthma may have a younger age at onset than those of bronchitis.

Predominant Sex
N/A

SIGNS

General Comments
• Cough—most common • Chronic bronchitis—no episodes of acute and severe respiratory distress caused by bronchoconstriction seen with asthma; severely affected patients may develop chronic bronchial wall and lung changes causing persistent tachypnea, lethargy, and anorexia with subsequent and severe weight loss.

Historical Findings
• Paroxysmal cough—variable frequency; may be associated with periods of respiratory difficulty, wheezing, and tachypnea; often follows exposure to dusty, fragranced, smoky, or polluted air • Patient usually normal between episodes. • Duration of cough—may have only a short history and present in status asthmaticus; may have occurred for months (owners notice an increase in frequency, duration, or violence) • Owners may confuse cough with hairball problems.

Physical Examination Findings
• Variable; depend on severity and stage of disease • Patient often normal between episodes; may have no obvious respiratory abnormality at the time of examination • Symptomatic patient—may show signs of respiratory distress, cyanosis, open-mouth breathing, gastric distention, abdominal effort, and frantic facial expression • Auscultation—varies from wheeze and crackles to almost absent breath sounds • Expiratory phase of respiration—may be prolonged and forced • Tracheal sensitivity and sneezing—may be noted

CAUSES
• None proven • Environmental influences—suspected; when eliminated, condition resolves

RISK FACTORS
• Air pollutants • Fragrant sprays • Powders • Cleaning solutions • Dust • Smoke—cigar, pipes, cigarettes, fireplaces

 DIAGNOSIS

DIFFERENTIAL DIAGNOSIS
• Congestive heart failure—heart murmur; diastolic gallop; cardiomegaly; cardiac arrhythmia; pleural effusion; pulmonary edema; rarely cough • Pulmonary parasites—ova or larva in tracheal wash findings (*Aelurostrongylus, Capillaria*); pulmonary artery enlargement; positive heartworm serology if *Dirofilaria immitis* is noted • Pleural disorders—fluid, air, or abdominal contents detected in pleural spaces • Pulmonary neoplasia—diffuse interstitial opacity; solid or cavitated nodular opacity; opacities with irregular contour • Foreign body aspiration—pulmonary infiltrate or foreign object • Infectious tracheitis, bronchitis, or pneumonitis—usually history of exposure; oral, nasal, and ocular involvement; fever and malaise, if viral • Pneumonia—patchy alveolar densities

CBC/BIOCHEMISTRY/URINALYSIS
• Neutrophilia—noted in moderately affected patients • Neutrophilia and monocytosis—seen in severely affected patients • Eosinophilia—reported in 57% of severely affected

patients and 20% mildly affected • Eosinophilia—steroids and stress lower blood number; absence does not rule out asthma; occurrence does not confirm diagnosis • Hypergammaglobulinemia—may be mild to moderate with chronic airway disease

OTHER LABORATORY TESTS
Fecal analyses and heartworm serology—help rule out parasites

IMAGING

Thoracic Radiography
• Bronchial thickening—donuts and tramlines • Right middle lung lobe collapse—resorption atelectasis • Small nodular densities—may indicate mucus plugs within the airway • Aerophagia • Overexpanded lung field, flattened diaphragm, and peripheral lung field hyperlucency—indicate trapping of air within the lungs owing to airway narrowing and obstruction • Minimal changes—do not exclude lower airway disease

Echocardiography
Indicated with heart murmur, diastolic gallop, cardiac arrhythmia, or cardiac enlargement and for evaluation of heartworms or cor pulmonale

DIAGNOSTIC PROCEDURES
• Tracheal washes, bronchoalveolar lavage, and bronchoscopy—sample airways (and interstitium) for cytologic analysis and culture • Abundance of mucus and lack of ova and larva—expected • Bronchitis—predominance of neutrophils • Asthma—typically more eosinophils. Remember that patients without signs of airway disease may have eosinophils in the washings. • Bronchoalveolar lavage—consider if tracheal wash results are nonconclusive, if response to treatment based on tracheal wash findings is poor, or with suspected interstitial diseases • Bronchoscopy—help rule out causes of cough such as endobronchial masses • Positive culture results from tracheal washings—interpret carefully; the trachea and major airways of normal cats are populated with a mixed population of aerobic bacterial similar to the oropharyngeal flora • *Mycoplasma* isolated from cats—only found with airway disease; found in as many as 25% of such patients • Pulmonary function testing—blood gas analysis; measurement of lung resistance, compliance, and tidal breathing flow volume loops

PATHOLOGIC FINDINGS
• Gross—lungs poorly deflate; atelectatic right middle lung lobe; right ventricular enlargement; pulmonary artery thickening • Histopathologic—see Pathophysiology

 TREATMENT

APPROPRIATE HEALTH CARE

• Usually outpatient • Inpatient—short hospital stay if tracheal washes need to be performed • Emergency and intensive care management—indicated for respiratory distress

NURSING CARE
Oxygen therapy—with respiratory distress, tachypnea, cyanosis, or marked blood gas abnormalities

ACTIVITY
• Most patients will limit their own activity when they experience difficulty breathing. • Stop, prevent, or discourage any specific activity that routinely triggers signs.

DIET
Restrict calories in obese patients

CLIENT EDUCATION
• Explain that a cure is unlikely and that both diseases require chronic and possibly life-long medical attention and home care. • Inform client that inflammation of the airways plays a key role in the disorder's progression. • Teach client how to give subcutaneous injections of terbutaline for asthmatic patients when severe bronchoconstriction occurs suddenly; instruct client to concurrently increase the dose of steroids

SURGICAL CONSIDERATIONS
N/A

MEDICATIONS

DRUGS OF CHOICE

Bronchodilators
• Choices—methylxanthines (e.g., aminophylline, theophylline) and the β_2-adrenergic agonist terbutaline • Methylxanthines—most widely used and studied; aminophylline (6.6 mg/kg PO q12h); sustained-release theophylline (Theo-Dur; 25–50 mg/cat PO at night) more convenient; ideally, maintain plasma concentration of theophylline at 10–20 µg/mL (may need to increase dose to 50–100 mg/cat).

Glucocorticoids
• Anti-inflammatory—essential for lower airway disease • Increase the affinity for and number of receptors for β_2-adrenergic drugs thus promoting bronchodilation • Prednisone or prednisolone—agent of choice; 1–2 mg/kg PO q24h; then taper 50% each week until a maintenance dose of 1.25–2.5 mg/cat 3 times a week; if cough, wheeze, or tachypnea return while tapering or while on maintenance, immediately increase to 1–2 mg/kg PO q24h • If increased dose is not sufficient to control signs, use a different bronchodilator or add an antibiotic. • If these steps fail to control signs, re-evaluate (possibly repeat thoracic radiographs and tracheal washing). • Change the glucocorticoid—may be next logical step;

triamcinolone (Vetalog) at 0.25–0.5 mg PO q24h, tapering to 0.25 mg PO 1–2 times a week; methylprednisolone acetate (Depo Medrol) at 10–20 mg SC, IM every 6–8 weeks

Antibiotics
• Use with suspected or confirmed secondary bacterial infection; selection based on tracheal washing cultures and sensitivity testing • Duration—10–14 days • Trial dose—acceptable when washing or rewashing is not possible

Emergency Treatment of Asthma
• When possible, give an intravenous, rapidly acting glucocorticoid—prednisolone sodium succinate (Solu-Delta Cortef) at 50–100 mg IV or dexamethasone sodium phosphate at 1 mg/kg IV preferred; give same dose intramuscularly if intravenous administration not possible. • Bronchodilator—administer; terbutaline at 0.01 mg/kg IV, IM, SC; hypotension noted if given intravenously; second choice: injectable aminophylline injectable (25 mg/mL) at 1–3 mg/kg IM or 1–2 mg/kg IV slowly; **CAUTION:** toxic levels may be reached if the patient recently received the oral preparation at home or is given a rapid intravenous bolus. • Most patients respond within 20 min; nonresponsive patients: give epinephrine (1:1,000 injection solution, 1mg/mL) at 0.1 mL/kg SC. • On rare occasions atropine (0.02–0.04 mg/ kg IV, IM, SC) may be indicated. • Oxygen—administer; oxygen cage least stressful; delivery by mask or hood acceptable if it does not stress patient

CONTRAINDICATIONS
• β-antagonists—do not give with bronchoconstrictive airway diseases. • β-agonists—contraindicated with left-ventricular outflow obstructions

PRECAUTIONS
• Daily glucocorticoid use—diabetes mellitus; chronic immune suppression • Chronic bacterial infections especially of the urinary tract—treat and follow appropriately.

POSSIBLE INTERACTIONS
• β_2-agonists seem to work synergistically with glucocorticoids; may try a lower dose of glucocorticoids • Fluoroquinolones—decrease metabolism of methylxanthines

ALTERNATIVE DRUGS
• None shows a consistent positive response when bronchodilators, glucocorticoids, and antibiotics fail. • Suggested possible alternative mediations—cyproheptadine (Periactin) at 1–2 mg/cat PO q12h and cyclosporin A • Antihistamines—not effective

FOLLOW-UP

PATIENT MONITORING
• Instruct client to report any increased frequency, violence, or duration of cough; leth-

argy; rapid respirations; wheezing; weight loss or gain; and polyuria or polydipsia. • Usually adjustment in medications is all that is needed to improve the respiratory tract signs. • Persistent or worsening wheeze or tachypnea—advise client that the patient should be seen immediately. • Blood tests and urinalysis—indicated for polyuria or polydipsia • Re-examine every 4–6 months; blood tests and thoracic radiographs not indicated if patient is stable and findings do not change

PREVENTION/AVOIDANCE
Eliminate any identified environmental triggers from the patient's surroundings.

POSSIBLE COMPLICATIONS
Asthma—potential life-threatening condition

EXPECTED COURSES AND PROGNOSIS
• Successful treatment—requires a close working association between an observant and compliant owner and the veterinarian • Generally patient does well for long periods. • If owner stops giving medications, signs will return as the inflammatory changes in the airways progress.

MISCELLANEOUS

ASSOCIATED CONDITIONS
Some asthmatic patients also have allergic dermatitis and rhinitis.

AGE-RELATED FACTORS
N/A

ZOONOTIC POTENTIAL
N/A

PREGNANCY
Use glucocorticoids and β_2-adenergic agonists with caution in pregnant cats.

SYNONYMS
• Eosinophilic bronchitis • Allergic bronchitis • Chronic obstructive airway disease • Chronic obstructive pulmonary disease • Asthmatic bronchitis • Allergic asthma • Bronchitis with emphysema

SEE ALSO
• Heartworm Disease—Cats • Paragonimiasis • Respiratory Parasites

Suggested Reading
Dye JA, McKiernan BC, Rozanski EA, et al. Bronchopulmonary disease in the cat: historical, physical, radiographic, clinicopathologic, and pulmonary functional evaluation of 24 affected and 15 healthy cats. J Vet Intern Med 1996;10:385–400.
Henik RA, Yeager AE. Bronchopulmonary diseases. In: Sherding RG, ed. The cat—diseases and clinical management. New York: Churchill Livingstone, 1994:979–1051.
Author Kathleen E. Noone
Consulting Editor Eleanor Hawkins

DISEASES

ASTROCYTOMA

BASICS

OVERVIEW
- Glial cell neoplasm of the brain
- Most common primary intracranial neoplasm of dogs; rarely diagnosed in cats
- Biologic behavior depends on the degree of anaplasia (graded I–IV, from best to worst prognosis)

SIGNALMENT
- Dogs—often brachycephalic breeds > 5 years of age; no sex predilection reported
- Cats—usually old (> 9 years); no sex or breed predilection reported

SIGNS
- Depend on tumor location
- Seizures
- Behavioral changes
- Disorientation
- Loss of conscious proprioception
- Cranial nerve abnormalities
- Upper motor neuron tetraparesis

CAUSES & RISK FACTORS
Unknown

DIAGNOSIS

DIFFERENTIAL DIAGNOSIS
- Other primary or metastatic CNS tumors
- Granulomatous meningoencephalitis
- Trauma
- Cerebrovascular accident
- Meningitis

CBC/BIOCHEMISTRY/URINALYSIS
Usually normal

OTHER LABORATORY TESTS
CSF analysis—may show albuminocytologic dissociation (high protein with few cells)

IMAGING
- MRI or CT (brain)—ideal
- Radionuclide imaging—may show area of increased activity at the tumor site
- Radiography (skull)—rarely aids in detection

DIAGNOSTIC PROCEDURES
EEG—may localize lesion

TREATMENT
Surgery or radiotherapy

MEDICATIONS

DRUGS

Seizure Control
- Status epilepticus—diazepam (0.5–1.0 mg/kg IV given up to 3 times to achieve effect); if no response to diazepam, use pentobarbital (5–15 mg/kg IV slowly to effect)
- Long-term management—phenobarbital (1–4 mg/kg PO q12h)

Tumor Control
- Chemotherapy—lomustine (90 mg/m^2 PO every 3 weeks) or carmustine (50 mg/m^2 IV every 6 weeks) reported to achieve partial and complete remissions
- Prednisone—0.5–1.0 mg/kg q24h; may be effective in controlling peritumoral edema

CONTRAINDICATIONS/POSSIBLE INTERACTIONS
- Prednisone and phenobarbital—polyphagia; polydipsia; polyuria
- Phenobarbital—may cause sedation for up to 2 weeks after initiation of treatment
- CBC and platelet count—must perform 7–10 days after chemotherapy and immediately before each dose of chemotherapy to monitor myelosuppression
- Carmustine—cumulative doses of 1400 mg/m^2 may cause pulmonary toxicity
- Chemotherapy may be toxic; seek advice before initiating treatment if unfamiliar with cytotoxic drugs.

FOLLOW-UP

PATIENT MONITORING
- Blood phenobarbital concentration—after 7–10 days of treatment; modify dosage as needed.
- CT or MRI—after every other chemotherapy treatment; monitor response

EXPECTED COURSE AND PROGNOSIS
- Long-term prognosis—guarded
- Survival time with no treatment—2 months
- Median survival after chemotherapy plus medical management—up to 7 months
- Median survival after radiotherapy—may be as high as 12 months

MISCELLANEOUS

PREGNANCY
Do not breed animals undergoing chemotherapy.

SEE ALSO
- Seizures (Convulsions, Status Epilepticus)—Cats
- Seizures (Convulsions, Status Epilepticus)—Dogs

ABBREVIATIONS
- CSF = cerebrospinal fluid
- EEG = electroencephalogram

Suggested Reading
Frenier SL, Kraft SL, Moore MP, et. al. Canine intracranial astrocytomas and comparison with the human counterpart. Compend Contin Educ Pract Vet 1990;12: 1422–1433.

Morrison WB. Cancer affecting the nervous system. In: Morrison WB, ed. Cancer in dogs and cats: medical and surgical management. Baltimore: Williams & Wilkins 1998:655–665.

Author Ruthanne Chun
Consulting Editor Wallace B. Morrison

BASICS

OVERVIEW
An uncommon intestinal viral infection characterized by enteritis and diarrhea

SIGNALMENT
• Cats
• No known breed, sex, or age predilection

SIGNS
Diarrhea

CAUSES & RISK FACTORS
• A small, nonenveloped, RNA virus of the genus *Astrovirus*
• Details of the incidence, prevalence, and predisposing factors unknown

DIAGNOSIS

DIFFERENTIAL DIAGNOSIS
• Many causes of gastroenteritis
• Food allergy
• Toxin ingestion
• Inflammatory bowel disease
• Neoplasia
• Intestinal parasites
• Viral infections—panleukopenia, rotavirus, enteric coronavirus, enteric calicivirus
• Bacterial infections—salmonellosis, coliforms
• Protozoal infections—*Giardia,* cryptosporidiosis

CBC/BIOCHEMISTRY/URINALYSIS
N/A

OTHER LABORATORY TESTS
• Electron microscopy of feces—identify *Astrovirus* particles
• Difficult to isolate in the laboratory

IMAGING
N/A

DIAGNOSTIC PROCEDURES
None

PATHOLOGIC FINDINGS
None described; similar to mild enteritis, rotavirus, or coronavirus enteritis

TREATMENT

• Control diarrhea.
• Re-establish fluid and electrolyte balance.

MEDICATIONS

DRUG(S)
No specific antiviral drugs

CONTRAINDICATIONS/POSSIBLE INTERACTIONS
None

FOLLOW-UP

PATIENT MONITORING
Monitor fluid and electrolytes.

PREVENTION/AVOIDANCE
Isolate infected cats during acute disease.

POSSIBLE COMPLICATIONS
Secondary intestinal viral and bacterial infections

EXPECTED COURSE AND PROGNOSIS
• Illness usually < 1 week
• Mortality—appears low
• Prognosis—good

MISCELLANEOUS

ZOONOTIC POTENTIAL
• Unknown
• Produces enteritis in many species, including sheep and humans

Suggested Reading
Barr MC, Olsen CW, Scott FW. Feline viral diseases. In: Ettinger SJ, Feldman EC, eds. Veterinary internal medicine. Philadelphia: Saunders, 1995:409–439.
Author Fred W. Scott
Consulting Editor Stephen C. Barr

DISEASES

ATHEROSCLEROSIS

BASICS

OVERVIEW
Thickening of the inner arterial wall in association with lipid deposits. Chronic arterial change characterized by loss of elasticity, luminal narrowing, and proliferating and degenerative lesions of the intima and media

SIGNALMENT
- Rare in dogs
- Not described in cats
- Higher prevalence in miniature schnauzer, Doberman pinscher, poodle, and Labrador retriever
- Geriatric patients (> 9 years)

SIGNS
Historical Findings
- None in some animals
- Lethargy
- Anorexia
- Weakness
- Dyspnea
- Collapse
- Vomiting
- Diarrhea

Physical Examination Findings
- Dyspnea
- Irregular rhythm
- Heart failure
- Disorientation
- Blindness
- Circling
- Coma

CAUSES & RISK FACTORS
- Severe hypothyroidism
- Increasing age
- Hyperlipidemia in miniature schnauzers
- Male gender (male dogs may have predisposition)
- High total cholesterol

DIAGNOSIS

DIFFERENTIAL DIAGNOSIS
Arteriosclerosis

CBC/BIOCHEMISTRY/URINALYSIS
- Hypercholesterolemia
- Hyperlipidemia
- High BUN and creatinine
- High liver enzymes

OTHER LABORATORY TESTS
- Low T_3 and T_4
- High values for alpha-2 and beta fractions on protein electrophoresis

IMAGING
Radiography
Thoracic and abdominal radiographs may reveal cardiomegaly and hepatomegaly.

DIAGNOSTIC PROCEDURES
Electrocardiography
- Conduction abnormalities and notched QRS complexes
- Atrial fibrillation
- ST segment elevation or depression with myocardial infarction

TREATMENT
- Treat the underlying disorder and clinical signs (e.g., dyspnea if congestive heart failure develops).
- Diet—low-fat diet, weight loss program, and high soluble fiber intake to control hyperlipidemia.

MEDICATIONS

DRUGS
- Treat conduction disturbances and arrhythmias if clinically indicated
- Thyroid replacement if hypothyroidism is confirmed
- Antihypertensive therapy if hypertension is documented (e.g., enalapril—0.5 mg/kg PO q12h–q24h or benazepril—0.5 mg/kg PO q24h)
- Blood cholesterol reducing medications (e.g., Niacin, Lopid) if hyperlipidemic.

CONTRAINDICATIONS/POSSIBLE INTERACTIONS
N/A

FOLLOW-UP
- Monitor T_4 concentration 4–6 hours post-administration after the first 6 weeks of treatment and adjust dosage accordingly.
- Monitor blood triglyceride and cholesterol levels.
- Monitor ECG for conduction disturbances and ST segment changes.

MISCELLANEOUS

ASSOCIATED CONDITIONS
Hypothyroidism

AGE RELATED FACTORS
Geriatric patients (> 9 years)

SEE ALSO
Myocardial Infarction

Suggested Reading
Drost WT, Bahr RJ, Henay GA, Campbell GA. Aortoiliac thrombus secondary to a mineralized arteriosclerotic lesion. Vet Rad Ultrasound 1999; 40:262–266.

Hamlen HJ. Sinoatrial node arteriosclerosis in two young dogs. J Am Vet Med Assoc 1994;204:751.

Liu SK, Tilley LP, Tappe JP, Fox PR. Clinical and pathologic findings in dogs with artheriosclerosis: 21 cases (1970–1983). J Am Vet Med Assoc 1986;189:227–232.
Authors Larry P. Tilley
Consulting Editors Larry P. Tilley and Francis W. K. Smith, Jr.

ATLANTOAXIAL INSTABILITY

 BASICS

OVERVIEW
• Results from malformation or disruption of the articulation between the first two cervical vertebrae (atlas and axis); causes spinal cord and nerve root compression
• Usually owing to a congenital anomaly of the dens (aplasia, hypoplasia, or deviation of the dens) and its ligamentous attachments
• May be a consequence of traumatic injury, particularly fracture of the dens
• Spinal cord compression at the junction between the atlas and axis—may cause neck pain and/or upper motor neuron tetraparesis to paralysis

SIGNALMENT
• Congenital—toy breed dogs (poodles, Chihuahuas, Pekingese)
• Age at onset—usually before 12 months of age
• Uncommon in larger-breed dogs, dogs > 1 year old, and cats
• No sex predilection

SIGNS
• Intermittent or progressive tetraparesis, usually with neck pain—most common
• Episodes of collapse—may occur
• May see proprioceptive deficits to complete paralysis, depending on degree of spinal cord compression
• Spinal reflexes—normal to exaggerated in all four limbs
• May lead to catastrophic, acute spinal cord trauma, respiratory arrest, and death

CAUSES & RISK FACTORS
• Usually caused by abnormal formation of the dens
• Fracture of the dens
• Clinical signs—may be exacerbated by activity, especially flexion of the neck
• Toy-breed dogs—at risk for congenital malformation of the dens

 DIAGNOSIS

DIFFERENTIAL DIAGNOSIS
• Disk herniation
• Fibrocartilaginous embolism
• Neoplasia
• Trauma
• Seizures
• With exercise intolerance—myasthenia gravis; hypoglycemia; hypoxia; cardiac abnormalities
• Diagnosis based on thorough physical examination and imaging

CBC/BIOCHEMISTRY/URINALYSIS
Normal

IMAGING
• Cervical spine radiographs—made with patient under general anesthesia; lateral view reveals increase in dorsal atlantoaxial space; lateral and ventrodorsal views reveal absence or fracture of dens.
• Do not hyperflex the neck during radiography; may cause severe spinal cord trauma and even death
• Myelography—seldom necessary for diagnosis

 TREATMENT

Conservative—reserved for patients with neck pain alone; includes neck brace and cage confinement for several weeks; recurrence common

Surgery
• Definitive; always indicated for neck pain with neurologic signs; dorsal and ventral approaches
• Dorsal—use wire or synthetic suture material to fix the dorsal spinous process of the axis to the dorsal arch of the atlas; common and serious postoperative complication: breakage of the dorsal arch of the atlas by the wire or suture
• Ventral—cancellous bone grafting and transarticular pinning; more stable; use polymethyl methacrylate to lock together the ventral tips of the pins to prevent pin migration; may use lag screws instead

 MEDICATIONS

DRUGS
Methylprednisolone sodium succinate—30 mg/kg; for acute paralysis and perioperatively

CONTRAINDICATIONS/POSSIBLE INTERACTIONS
• Glucocorticoids—use caution when given in conjunction with conservative treatment; may reduce pain, resulting in increased activity and spinal cord trauma
• Avoid NSAIDs in combination with glucocorticoids in all patients—increases risk of life-threatening gastrointestinal hemorrhage

 FOLLOW-UP

• Conservative treatment—re-evaluated weekly until clinical signs have resolved; often see recurrence, necessitating surgery
• Surgical treatment—usually no recurrent episodes; success influenced by the expertise and experience of the surgeon; intraoperative and immediately postoperative complications possible
• Untreated—may lead to catastrophic, acute spinal cord trauma, respiratory arrest, and death

 MISCELLANEOUS

Suggested Reading
Fossum TW, Hedlund CS, Johnson AL, et al. Small animal surgery. St. Louis: Mosby Year Book, 1997.
Author Mary O. Smith
Consulting Editor Peter D. Schwarz

DISEASES

ATOPY

BASICS

DEFINITION
Predisposition to become allergic to normally innocuous substances, such as pollens (grasses, weeds, and trees), molds, house dust mites, epithelial allergens, and other environmental allergens

PATHOPHYSIOLOGY
• Susceptible animals become sensitized to environmental allergens by producing allergen-specific IgE, which binds to receptor sites on cutaneous mast cells; further allergen exposure (inhalation, percutaneous absorption) causes mast cell degranulation, which is a type I immediate hypersensitivity reaction, and results in the release of histamine, proteolytic enzymes, cytokines, chemokines, and many other chemical mediators. • Non-IgE antibodies (IgGd) and a late-phase reaction (8–12 hr) may also be involved.

SYSTEMS AFFECTED
• Skin/Exocrine—pruritus, xerosis, or generalized dryness of the skin; recurrent superficial pyoderma and yeast infections; recurrent bilateral otitis externa • Ophthalmic—recurrent bilateral conjunctivitis • Respiratory, Reproductive, and Gastrointestinal—reported, but not well documented

GENETICS
• Canine—although there is an inherited predisposition, the mode of inheritance is unknown and other factors may also be important. • Feline—unclear

INCIDENCE/PREVALENCE
• Canine—true incidence unknown; estimated at 3%–15% of the canine population; reported to be the second most common allergic skin disease
• Feline—unknown; generally believed to be much lower than that for dogs

GEOGRAPHIC DISTRIBUTION
Canine—recognized worldwide; local environmental factors (temperature, humidity, and flora) influence the seasonality, severity, and duration of signs.

SIGNALMENT

Species
Dogs and cats

Breed Predilections
• Canine—any breed, including mongrels; because of genetic predisposition, it may be recognized more frequently in certain breeds or families, which can vary geographically.
• In the United States (canine)—Boston terriers, Cairn terriers, dalmatians, English bulldogs, English setters, Irish setters, Lhasa apsos, miniature schnauzers, pugs, Sealyham terriers, Scottish terriers, West Highland white terriers, wire-haired fox terriers, and golden retrievers
• Feline—none reported

Mean Age and Range
Canine—mean age at onset 1–3 years; range 3 months–6 years; signs may be so mild the first year that they are not noted but are usually progressive and clinically apparent before 3 years of age.

Predominant Sex
• Both sexes are probably affected equally.

SIGNS

General
• Hallmark sign—pruritus (itching, scratching, rubbing, licking)
• Primary lesions may occur, but most cutaneous changes are believed to be produced by self-induced trauma.

Historical Findings
• Facial, pedal, or axillary pruritus
• Early onset
• Family history of atopy
• May be seasonal
• Recurring skin or ear infections
• Temporary response to glucocorticoids
• Symptoms progressively worsen with time

Physical Examination Findings
• Areas most commonly affected—interdigital spaces, carpal and tarsal areas, muzzle, periocular region, axillae, groin, and pinnae
• Lesions—vary from none to broken hairs or salivary discoloration to erythema, papular reactions, crusts, alopecia, hyperpigmentation, lichenification, excessively oily or dry seborrhea, and hyperhidrosis (apocrine sweating)
• Secondary bacterial and yeast skin infections (common)
• Chronic relapsing otitis externa
• Conjunctivitis may occur.

CAUSES
• Airborne pollens (grasses, weeds, and trees)
• Mold spores (indoor and outdoor)
• House dust mite
• Animal danders
• Insects (controversial)

RISK FACTORS
• Temperate environments with long allergy seasons and high pollen and mold spore levels
• Concurrent pruritic dermatoses, such as flea allergy dermatitis and food hypersensitivity (summation effect)

DIAGNOSIS

DIFFERENTIAL DIAGNOSIS
• Food hypersensitivity—may cause identical lesion distribution and physical examination findings but should be nonseasonal; may occur concurrently with atopy; differentiation is made by noting response to hypoallergenic diet.
• Flea bite hypersensitivity—most common cause of seasonal pruritus in many geographical regions; may occur concurrently with atopy; differentiation is made by noting lesion distribution, response to flea control, and results of intradermal skin testing.
• Sarcoptic mange—often occurs in young or recently stray dogs; usually causes severe pruritus of the ventral chest, lateral elbows, lateral hocks, and pinnal margins; multiple skin scrapings and/or complete response to a trial of miticidal therapy are indicated to rule out sarcoptic mange.
• Secondary pyoderma—usually caused by *Staphylococcus intermedius;* characterized by follicular papules, pustules, crusts, and epidermal collarettes
• Secondary yeast infections—usually caused by *Malassezia* pachydermatis; characterized by erythematous, scaly, crusty, greasy, and very malodorous body folds and intertriginous areas; demonstration of numerous budding yeast organisms by skin cytology and obtaining a favorable response to antifungal therapy are diagnostic.
• Contact dermatitis (allergic or irritant)—may cause severe erythema and pruritus of the feet and thinly haired areas of the ventral abdomen; history of exposure to a known contact sensitizer or irritant, response to a change of environment, and patch testing may be diagnostic; thought to be rare in dogs and cats.

CBC/BIOCHEMISTRY/URINALYSIS
Eosinophilia—rare in dogs without concurrent flea infections; common in cats

OTHER LABORATORY TESTS

Serologic Allergy Tests
• Tests to measure the amount of allergen-specific IgE antibody in the patient's serum are commercially available.
• Advantages over IDST—availability; large areas of hair do not have to be shaved
• Disadvantages—frequent false-positive reactions; limited number of allergens tested; inconsistent assay validation and quality control (may vary with the laboratory used)
• Reliability in cats is unknown.

IMAGING
N/A

DIAGNOSTIC PROCEDURES

IDST
• Small amounts of test allergens are injected intradermally and wheal formation is measured.
• Most accurate method of identifying offending allergens for possible avoidance or inclusion in an immunotherapy prescription.
• Results are sometimes difficult to interpret in cats owing to the relatively small wheals

produced.

PATHOLOGIC FINDINGS
• Gross lesions—see Physical Examination Findings
• Skin biopsy—may help rule out other differential diagnoses; results are usually not pathognomonic.
• Dermatohistopathologic changes—acanthosis, mixed mononuclear superficial perivascular dermatitis, sebaceous gland metaplasia, and secondary superficial pyoderma

TREATMENT

APPROPRIATE HEALTH CARE
Outpatient

NURSING CARE
N/A

ACTIVITY
Avoid offending allergens when possible.

DIET
Essential fatty acid supplementation may be beneficial in some cases.

CLIENT EDUCATION
• Explain the progressive nature of the condition.
• Inform client that it rarely goes into remission and cannot be cured.
• Inform client that some form of therapy may be necessary for life.

SURGICAL CONSIDERATIONS
N/A

MEDICATIONS

DRUGS OF CHOICE

Immunotherapy (Hyposensitization)
• Administration (usually SC injections) of gradually increasing doses of the causative allergens to affected patients in an attempt to reduce their sensitivity
• Allergens selected—based on allergy test results, patient history, and knowledge of local flora
• Indicated when it is desirable to avoid or reduce the amount of corticosteroids required to control signs, when signs last longer than 4–6 months per year, or when nonsteroidal forms of therapy are ineffective
• Successfully reduces pruritus in 60–80% of dogs and cats
• The response is usually slow, often requiring 3–6 months and up to 1 year.

Corticosteroids
• May be given for short-term relief and to break the itch–scratch cycle
• Should be tapered to the lowest dosage that adequately controls pruritus

• Best choices—prednisone suspension (0.5 to 1.0 mg/kg SC or IM); prednisone or methylprednisolone tablets (0.2 to 0.5 mg/kg PO q48h)
• Repository injectable corticosteroids should be avoided in dogs.
• Cats may require methylprednisolone acetate treatment (4 mg/kg SC or IM).

Antihistamines
• Less effective than are corticosteroids
• Efficacy as a sole treatment is probably in the 10%–20% range.
• May act synergistically with essential fatty acid supplements
• Corticosteroid therapy can often be avoided or given at a reduced dosage when used concurrently.
• Dogs—hydroxyzine (1–2 mg/kg PO q8h), chlorpheniramine (0.2–0.4 mg/kg PO q12h), diphenhydramine (2.2 mg/kg PO q8h), and clemastine (0.04–0.10 mg/kg PO q12h)
• Cats—chlorpheniramine (0.5 mg/kg PO q12h); efficacy estimated at 10%–50%

CONTRAINDICATIONS
N/A

PRECAUTIONS
• Corticosteroids—use judiciously in dogs to avoid iatrogenic hyperglucocorticism and associated problems, aggravation of pyoderma, and induction of demodicosis.
• Antihistamines—can produce drowsiness, anorexia, vomiting, diarrhea, and even increased pruritus; use with caution in patients with cardiac arrhythmias.

POSSIBLE INTERACTIONS
The antihistamine astemizole have been associated with life-threatening cardiac arrhythmias in humans when administered concomitantly with imidazole antifungal drugs.

ALTERNATIVE DRUGS
• Frequent bathing in cool water with antipruritic shampoos can be beneficial.
• Supplementation with ω-3 and ω-6 fatty acids helps some pruritic patients; some studies have indicated that ω-3 (eicosapentaenoic acid 66 mg/kg/day) may be more effective than ω-6 (linoleic acid 130 mg/kg/day); other studies suggest that a 5:1 ratio of ω-6:ω-3 in the diet is indicated.
• Tricyclic antidepressants (doxepin 1.0–2.0 mg/kg PO q12h; or amitriptyline 1.0–2.0 mg/kg PO q12h) have been given to dogs as antipruritics but their overall effectiveness and mode of action is unclear; not extensively studied in the cat

FOLLOW-UP

PATIENT MONITORING
• Examine patient every 2–8 weeks when a new course of therapy is started • Monitor

pruritus, self-trauma, pyoderma, and possible adverse drug reactions • Once an acceptable level of control is achieved, examine patient every 3–12 months • CBC, serum chemistry profile, and urinalysis—recommended every 6–12 months for patients on chronic corticosteroid therapy

PREVENTION/AVOIDANCE
• If the offending allergens have been identified through allergy testing, the owner should undertake to reduce the animal's exposure as much as possible. • Minimizing other sources of pruritus (e.g., fleas, food hypersensitivity, and secondary skin infections) may reduce the level of pruritus enough to be tolerated by the animal.

POSSIBLE COMPLICATIONS
Secondary pyoderma and concurrent flea allergy dermatitis

EXPECTED COURSE AND PROGNOSIS
• Not life-threatening unless intractable pruritus results in euthanasia • If left untreated, the degree of pruritus worsens and the duration of signs last longer each year of the animal's life. • Only rare cases spontaneously resolve.

MISCELLANEOUS

ASSOCIATED CONDITIONS
• Flea allergy dermatitis • Food hypersensitivity • Pyoderma • Otitis externa

AGE-RELATED FACTORS
Severity worsens with age.

ZOONOTIC POTENTIAL
None

PREGNANCY
• Corticosteroids—contraindicated during pregnancy • Antihistamines—safety during pregnancy has not been established.

SYNONYMS
• Canine allergic inhalant dermatitis • Canine atopic dermatitis • Canine atopic disease

SEE ALSO
• Fleas and Flea Control • Food Reactions (dermatologic) • Otitis Externa and Media • Pyoderma

ABBREVIATION
IDST = intradermal skin test

Suggested Reading
Reedy LM, Miller WH, Willemse T. Allergic skin diseases of dogs and cats. 2nd ed. Philadelphia: Saunders, 1997.
Authors Jon D. Plant and Lloyd M. Reedy
Consulting Editor Karen Helton-Rhodes

DISEASES

ATRIAL SEPTAL DEFECT

BASICS

OVERVIEW
- Congenital cardiac anomaly allowing communication between the atria through a defect in the interatrial septum (Figure 1)
- Defects occur in one of three locations: ostium primum defect, lower atrial septum; ostium secundum defect, near fossa ovalis; and sinus venous defect, craniodorsal to fossa ovalis.
- Blood usually shunts into the right atrium causing volume overload to the right atrium, right ventricle, and pulmonary vasculature.
- If right-sided pressures are high, shunting may occur right to left, causing generalized cyanosis.
- Uncommon congenital defect—1.3% of congenital heart defects in dogs and 4% of congenital heart defects in cats.

SIGNALMENT
- Dogs and cats
- Genetic basis suggested for Old English sheepdog
- Doberman pinscher, boxer, and samoyed may be overrepresented.

SIGNS

General
If defect is small, maybe none

Historical Findings
Variable degrees of exercise intolerance, syncope, and dyspnea the first year of life

Physical Examination Findings
- Soft systolic murmur over the pulmonic valve and tricuspid valve
- Splitting of the second heart sound

CAUSES & RISK FACTORS
Unknown; genetic basis not documented

DIAGNOSIS

DIFFERENTIAL DIAGNOSIS
Pulmonic stenosis—murmur of pulmonic stenosis usually harsh and loud

CBC/BIOCHEMISTRY/URINALYSIS
Polycythemia in some patients with right-to-left shunt

OTHER BLOOD TESTS
N/A

IMAGING

Radiographic Findings
- None in patients with small defects
- Right-sided heart and pulmonary vessel enlargement in patients with large defects

Echocardiographic Findings
- Right atrial and right ventricular dilation
- May reveal the defect—septal dropout
- Doppler useful in documenting flow through the defect and high ejection velocity through the pulmonary artery

OTHER DIAGNOSTIC PROCEDURES
- Electrocardiography
- Right ventricular enlargement pattern on ECG in some patients with large defects

TREATMENT
- Hospitalize patients with congestive heart failure (CHF) until stable.
- Restrict activity
- A low-sodium diet may be of value.
- Surgical correction is prohibitively expensive for most owners.
- Pulmonary artery banding may be palliative in patients with severe disease.

MEDICATIONS

DRUGS AND FLUIDS
- CHF—diuretics; aggressiveness of therapy proportional to the degree of pulmonary edema (furosemide, 1–2 mg/kg PO q6–12h)
- Vasodilators may help reduce signs (e.g., enalapril, 0.5 mg/kg PO q12–24h or benazepril 0.5 mg/kg PO q24h).

CONTRAINDICATIONS/POSSIBLE INTERACTIONS
N/A

FOLLOW-UP

PATIENT MONITORING
Recheck when decompensation or other clinical signs develop.

EXPECTED COURSE AND PROGNOSIS
- Depend on size of the defect and coexisting abnormalities; small, isolated defects unlikely to cause signs or to progress
- Progressive, right-sided CHF expected if the defect is large

MISCELLANEOUS

ASSOCIATED CONDITIONS
Pulmonic stenosis and tricuspid dysplasia

SEE ALSO
Congestive Heart Failure, Right-sided

ABBREVIATIONS
CHF = congestive heart failure

Suggested Reading
Bonagura JD, Darke P. Congenital heart disease. In: Ettinger SJ, Feldman EC, eds. Textbook of veterinary internal medicine. 4th ed. Philadelphia: WB Saunders, 1995: 892–943.

Author John-Karl Goodwin
Consulting Editors Larry P. Tilley and Francis W. K. Smith, Jr.

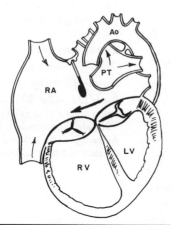

Figure 1.
Atrial septal defect. Defect involves the lowermost part of the arial septum, known as ostium primum defect. Note the left dominant left-to-right shunt. RV = right ventricle, LV = left ventricle, RA = right atrium, Ao = aorta, PT = pulmonary trunk. From Roberts W. Adult congenital heart disease. Philadelphia: FA Davis Co., 1987, with permission.

BASICS

OVERVIEW

• Split in the endocardial surface or complete tear (rupture) in the atrial wall when the left atrium is distended beyond its elastic limits; if the split is incomplete, fibrin may seal the defect temporarily; this either heals as a depression in the atrial surface or subsequently ruptures completely.
• When a tear is complete, bleeding occurs into the pericardial sac and cardiac tamponade quickly ensues; if the interatrial wall is affected, an acquired atrial septal defect may form.
• Death occurs quickly in most patients.

SIGNALMENT

• Dogs and rarely cats
• No breed, age, or sex predilections

SIGNS

Historical Findings

• Acute onset of weakness and collapse that may progress quickly to death
• Long-standing cardiac disease in most patients, so other signs of congestive heart failure may have been observed

Physical Examination Findings

• Pale mucous membranes
• Tachycardia
• Weak arterial pulses
• Collapse
• Signs of right heart failure (e.g., ascites and jugular venous distension) in some patients
• Some patients show other signs of cardiac disease (e.g., murmur, gallop rhythm, arrhythmia, and dyspnea).
• If a murmur was heard before the atrial wall tear occurred, it may not be as loud.
• Muffled heart sounds

CAUSES & RISK FACTORS

• Mitral valve endocardiosis—chronic valvular heart disease
• Dilated cardiomyopathy
• Patent ductus arteriosus
• Cardiac neoplasia
• Chest trauma

DIAGNOSIS

DIFFERENTIAL DIAGNOSIS

Other causes of acute cardiovascular collapse
• Pericardial effusion from other causes (e.g., neoplastic and idiopathic)
• Severe cardiac arrhythmias
• Myocardial infarction
• Pulmonary thromboembolism
• Other causes of hypotension

CBC/BIOCHEMISTRY/URINALYSIS

• Anemia is uncommon since volume of blood loss is relatively small.
• Prerenal azotemia in some patients

IMAGING

Radiographic Findings

• Comparison with previous thoracic radiographs may show rounding of cardiac silhouette; however, the spherical cardiac silhouette seen in patients with pericardial effusion is often not observed.
• Ascites and large caudal vena cava in some patients

Echocardiographic Findings

• Pericardial effusion is seen as an echo-free space between the heart and pericardial sac; the heart may swing in the pericardial sac.
• Left atrium often remains large; may see a clot in the left atrium or pericardial sac

DIAGNOSTIC PROCEDURES

Electrocardiographic Findings

• Arrhythmias
• Tachycardia
• Dampened QRS complex
• Electrical alternans
• ST-segment abnormalities
• May reveal heart enlargement pattern

TREATMENT

• If a left atrial tear is strongly suspected, perform pericardiocentesis only if the effusion is considered life-threatening; further hemorrhage into the pericardial sac or exsanguination may occur.
• If a fibrin clot forms over the defect, the patient may stabilize; if pericardiocentesis is performed, remove only enough fluid to improve clinical signs.

• Strict cage rest
• Surgical exploration may be considered if hemorrhage persists or recurs.
• Administer fluids IV to expand the intravascular space and maintain cardiac output.

MEDICATIONS

DRUGS

Combination of fluids and dobutamine has improved hemodynamic status in models of cardiac rupture.

CONTRAINDICATIONS/POSSIBLE INTERACTIONS

Preload (e.g., diuretics and venous dilators) and afterload reducers (e.g., arterial vasodilators) are not indicated in the treatment of left atrial rupture, because they may further diminish cardiac output; if necessary to treat concomitant congestive heart failure, use sparingly.

FOLLOW-UP

• Prognosis is poor; even if the tear seals, the patient is prone to further tears because of underlying cardiac disease.
• If the patient survives, follow-up examination with echocardiography helps determine resolution of pericardial effusion and resorption of an atrial or pericardial clot.

MISCELLANEOUS

SEE ALSO

Pericardial Effusion

Suggested Reading

Allen DG. Small animal medicine. Philadelphia: Lippincott, 1991.
Author Patti S. Snyder
Consulting Editors Larry P. Tilley and Francis W. K. Smith, Jr.

ATRIOVENTRICULAR VALVE DYSPLASIA

 BASICS

DEFINITION
A congenital malformation of either the mitral valve apparatus or the tricuspid valve apparatus

PATHOPHYSIOLOGY
• Atrioventricular valve dysplasia (AVD) causes insufficiency of the affected valve; depending on the type of malformation, various degrees of valvular stenosis may occur as well.
• Mitral valve dysplasia—mild-to-severe mitral regurgitation with corresponding dilation of the left atrium and rise in pulmonary venous pressure; left-sided congestive heart failure (CHF) may develop
• Tricuspid valve dysplasia—right atrial dilation subsequent to tricuspid regurgitation, which may lead to signs of right-sided CHF; high right atrial pressure may maintain a patent foramen ovale, allowing right-to-left shunting of blood at the atrial level
• Cardiac arrhythmias (especially atrial fibrillation) may occur secondary to atrial dilation.

SYSTEMS AFFECTED
• Cardiovascular—volume overload
• Respiratory—if pulmonary edema or cyanosis

GENETICS
Genetic basis likely in some breeds but not confirmed

INCIDENCE/PREVALENCE
One of the most common cardiac congenital anomalies in cats (17% of reported congenital cardiac defects in one study); infrequently diagnosed in dogs

GEOGRAPHIC DISTRIBUTION
N/A

SIGNALMENT

Species
Dogs and cats

Breed Predilections
• Great Dane, German shepherd, Afghan hound—mitral valve dysplasia
• Labrador retriever, Old English sheepdog—tricuspid valve dysplasia

Mean Age and Range
Most patients develop clinical signs within the first year of life.

Predominant Sex
Male

SIGNS

General Comments
Progression and severity of clinical signs correlate with severity of the valvular insufficiency.

Historical Findings
• Classic signs of left-sided CHF (i.e., cough, dyspnea, and exercise intolerance) are usually found in patients with moderate-to-severe mitral valve dysplasia.
• Stunted growth, exercise intolerance, and ascites usually occur in patients with moderate-to-severe tricuspid valve dysplasia.

Physical Examination Findings
Mitral valve dysplasia
• Prominent holosystolic murmur heard over the mitral valve area (left apex), often associated with a precordial thrill; an S3 in some patients with severe disease
• Tachypnea and abnormally loud respiratory sounds in animals with left-sided CHF
Tricuspid valve dysplasia
• Prominent holosystolic murmur heard over the tricuspid valve area (right apex), often associated with a precordial thrill.
• Prominent jugular pulsations in most patients
• Ascites in patients with right-sided CHF; peripheral edema in some
• Variable degrees of generalized cyanosis in patients with right-to-left shunting through a patent foramen ovale or coexisting atrial septal defect

CAUSES
Unknown; possible genetic basis

RISK FACTORS
N/A

 DIAGNOSIS

DIFFERENTIAL DIAGNOSIS
• Degenerative valve disease (especially if AVD is present in an old dog)
• Other defects causing a systolic murmur, especially ventricular septal defect

• Tricuspid dysplasia may be a variant of Ebstein's anomaly
• Mitral and tricuspid stenosis share some features with mitral and tricuspid dysplasia; they differ in that the stenotic valve lesions cause a diastolic murmur.

CBC/BIOCHEMISTRY/URINALYSIS
Usually normal

OTHER LABORATORY TESTS
N/A

IMAGING

Thoracic Radiographic Findings
Mitral valve dysplasia
• Left-sided cardiomegaly, with a prominent left atrium on both lateral and ventrodorsal views
• An alveolar-interstitial pattern in patients with left-sided failure
Tricuspid valve dysplasia
• Severe right-sided cardiomegaly (right atrial enlargement) in most patients
• Enlargement of the caudal vena cava in some patients

Echocardiographic Findings
Mitral valve dysplasia
• Moderate-to-severe left atrial dilation with abnormal-appearing mitral valve leaflets—hallmark findings; malposition of the leaflets or chordae tendineae in some patients
• Moderate-to-severe left ventricular dilation in most patients
• Fractional shortening usually normal, but may be reduced if myocardial failure develops
• Doppler echocardiography demonstrates mitral regurgitation; high transmitral flow in patients with valvular stenosis
Tricuspid valve dysplasia
• Moderate-to-severe right atrial dilation with abnormal-appearing tricuspid valve leaflets—hallmark findings; malposition of the leaflets or chordae tendineae in some patients
• Right ventricle diminished in size, may be hypoplastic
• Doppler echocardiography demonstrates tricuspid regurgitation; high transtricuspid flow in patients with valvular stenosis.

Cardiac Catheterization
• Can be used to confirm the diagnosis
• Infrequently used because of invasiveness and the ability of echocardiography to confirm the diagnosis

ATRIOVENTRICULAR VALVE DYSPLASIA

Mitral valve dysplasia
• Left ventriculogram shows various degrees (usually severe) of mitral insufficiency and severe left atrial dilation.
• Selective catheterization of the left ventricle required
• Pressure measurements demonstrate high left atrial pressure.
Tricuspid valve dysplasia
• Right ventriculogram demonstrates various degrees (usually severe) of tricuspid insufficiency and severe right atrial dilation.
• Contrast within the left atrium immediately after a right-sided injection indicates a patent foramen ovale or coexisting atrial septal defect.
• Selective catheterization of the right ventricle required
• Pressure measurements demonstrate high right atrial pressure.

DIAGNOSTIC PROCEDURES

Electrocardiographic Findings
• Evidence of atrial enlargement in some patients—P-pulmonale (tall P waves) for right atrial enlargement, and P-mitrale (widened P waves) for left atrial enlargement
• Chamber enlargement in some patients—right bundle branch block often occurs in those with tricuspid valve dysplasia
• Arrhythmias common, especially atrial premature complexes or atrial fibrillation

PATHOLOGIC FINDINGS
• Valvular abnormalities may include leaflet thickening, notching, rolling, and shortening; fusion, thickening, or aplasia of the chordae tendineae; dysplastic and malpositioned papillary muscles.
• Dilation of the affected chambers
• Evidence of congestion—pulmonary (mitral dysplasia) or systemic (tricuspid dysplasia)

TREATMENT

APPROPRIATE HEALTH CARE
Inpatient if CHF

NURSING CARE
N/A

ACTIVITY
Restricted

DIET
Restrict sodium for patients with CHF.

CLIENT EDUCATION
• Defect may be inherited—advise against breeding
• Signs of CHF probably progressive

SURGICAL CONSIDERATIONS
Impractical—by-pass requirement and remarkable expense

MEDICATIONS

DRUGS OF CHOICE
• Diuretics—indicated in patients with CHF; aggressiveness of therapy proportional to the degree of pulmonary edema; furosemide (1–3 mg/kg PO q6–8h)
• Vasodilators—may reduce clinical signs; enalapril (0.5 mg/kg PO q12–24h)
• Specific antiarrhythmic therapy may be warranted—digoxin (0.005–0.010 mg/kg PO q12h) is most often used to manage atrial arrhythmias

CONTRAINDICATIONS
Fluids in patients with severe CHF

PRECAUTIONS
Standard patient monitoring for cardiac medication side effects (e.g., digitalis toxicity and azotemia)

POSSIBLE INTERACTIONS
N/A

ALTERNATIVE DRUGS
N/A

FOLLOW-UP

PATIENT MONITORING
Recheck when decompensation or other clinical signs occur.

PREVENTION/AVOIDANCE
Do not breed affected animals.

POSSIBLE COMPLICATIONS
• Left heart failure—mitral
• Right heart failure—tricuspid
• Arrhythmias

EXPECTED COURSE AND PROGNOSIS
• Guarded to poor, depending on severity of defect
• Refractory heart failure develops in most patients.

MISCELLANEOUS

ASSOCIATED CONDITIONS
May accompany other cardiac defects, especially endocardial cushion defects (cats) and atrial septal defect (dogs)

AGE-RELATED FACTORS
Clinical signs usually evident in young animals, but onset of signs may be delayed until maturity

ZOONOTIC POTENTIAL
N/A

PREGNANCY
Likely to cause CHF

SYNONYMS
N/A

SEE ALSO
• Congestive Heart Failure, Left-Sided
• Congestive Heart Failure, Right-Sided

ABBREVIATIONS
• AVD = atrioventricular valve dysplasia
• CHF = congestive heart failure

Suggested Reading
Bonagura JD. Cardiovascular diseases. In: Sherding RG, ed. The cat—diseases and clinical management. New York: Churchill Livingstone, 1989.
Kittleson MD, Kienle RD, eds. Small animal cardiovascular medicine, St. Louis: Mosby, 1998.
Author John-Karl Goodwin
Consulting Editors Larry P. Tilley and Francis W. K. Smith, Jr.

ATRIOVENTRICULAR VALVE ENDOCARDIOSIS

BASICS

DEFINITION
A chronic degenerative disease affecting the mitral and tricuspid valves, leading to valvular insufficiency and heart failure

PATHOPHYSIOLOGY
• Proliferation and deposition of mucopolysaccharide within the subendothelial spongiosa layer leads to thickening, distortion, and stiffening of the AV valves; initially, swellings are nodular, but coalescence occurs until the entire valve and often the attached chordae are involved. • AV valve incompetence causes regurgitation, high atrial pressure, reduced cardiac output, activation of compensatory mechanisms (sympathetic nervous system, renin-angiotensin-aldosterone system, and atrial natruretic factor), and CHF. • Volume overload leads to progressive ventricular dilation, advancing ventricular stiffness, and impaired ventricular function; congestive and low-output (forward) failure result. • With atrial tear, acute cardiac tamponade may result. • Degenerative changes in the chordae tendineae lead to distortion, weakening, and rupture, causing valvular instability and increased regurgitation.

SYSTEMS AFFECTED
• Cardiovascular—both AV valves are affected, but Buchanan (1979) found the distribution in necropsy specimens to be mitral alone, 62%; tricuspid alone, 1%; and both, 33%. • Respiratory—if edema develops • Renal/Urologic—prerenal azotemia • Hepatobiliary—passive congestion of the liver

GENETICS Not established

INCIDENCE/PREVALENCE
Chronic valvular disease increases from about 5% in middle-aged dogs (5–7 years) to >35% in old dogs (=12 years).

GEOGRAPHIC DISTRIBUTION N/A

SIGNALMENT

Species
Predominantly dogs, but may be seen in old cats

Breed Predilections
• Typically small breeds • Highest prevalence—Cavalier King Charles spaniel, Chihuahua, miniature schnauzer, Maltese, Pomeranian, cocker spaniel, Pekingese, fox terrier, Boston terrier, miniature poodle, toy poodle, miniature pinscher, and whippet

Mean Age and Range
Heart failure onset at 10–12 years, although may detect a murmur several years earlier; Cavalier King Charles spaniels are typically affected much earlier (6–8 years)

Predominant Sex
Males—male:female ratio, 1.5:1

SIGNS

General Comments
For treatment purposes, the International Small Animal Cardiac Health Council (ISACHC) divides patients into those with mild-to-moderate heart failure and those with severe heart failure.

Asymptomatic Valve Disease
• Systolic murmur heard best at the left fifth intercostal space (mitral) or right fourth intercostal space (tricuspid). • Murmurs may vary from a low-frequency, holosystolic, band-shaped sound to a shorter, high-frequency, midsystolic murmur; occasionally only a midsystolic click is detected. • As the disease progresses, the murmur typically gets louder and radiates more widely; with severe disease, the volume of regurgitation becomes so large that the murmur may decrease in frequency and loudness.

Mild Heart Failure
Coughing, exercise intolerance, and dyspnea with exercise

Moderate Heart Failure
Coughing, exercise intolerance, and dyspnea at all times

Severe Heart Failure
Severe dyspnea, profound weakness, abdominal distension, productive coughing (i.e., pink, frothy fluid), orthopnea, cyanosis, and syncope; occasionally, syncope may be the only owner complaint.

CAUSES Idiopathic

RISK FACTORS N/A

DIAGNOSIS

DIFFERENTIAL DIAGNOSIS
• Dilated cardiomyopathy • Congenital heart disease • Chronic airway or interstitial lung disease • Pneumonia • Pulmonary embolism • Pulmonary neoplasia • Heartworm disease

CBC/BIOCHEMISTRY/URINALYSIS
• Prerenal azotemia secondary to impaired renal perfusion; urinary specific gravity is high unless complicated by underlying renal disease or previous diuretic administration • High liver enzyme activity in many patients with passive congestion

OTHER LABORATORY TESTS
N/A

IMAGING

Radiographic Findings
• Heart size ranges from normal to left-sided or generalized cardiomegaly. • Left atrial enlargement in the lateral projection exhibits elevation of the distal fourth of the trachea and splitting of the mainstem bronchi; dorsoventral projection shows accentuation of the angle between the mainstem bronchi, a double shadow at the six o'clock position, where the caudal edge of the atrium extends beyond the left ventricle, and bulging of the left atrial appendage in the one to three o'clock position. • Left-sided heart failure—the pulmonary vein is larger than the associated pulmonary artery; air bronchograms are typical of, but not pathognomic for, cardiogenic pulmonary edema; initially, congestion and edema are perihilar, with all lung fields eventually showing changes. The right lung may be affected before the left.

Echocardiographic Findings
• Thickening and distortion of the mitral valve; septal leaflet is most severely affected. • Elongation and rupture of the chordae tendineae, causing mitral valve prolapse • Large left atrium • The left ventricle may be distended and is hyperdynamic if the regurgitant flow is high and myocardial function intact; as the ventricle becomes more grossly distended, it may become hypodynamic due to myocardial failure. • Pericardial effusion in some patients • Doppler studies document a jet of regurgitation into the left atrium and the area of the regurgitant jet on color flow. • Doppler has been used to assess severity.

DIAGNOSTIC PROCEDURES
• Abdominocentesis/pleurocentesis—a modified transudate is characteristic of CHF. • Arterial/venous blood gases—has been used to quantify hypoxemia and monitor treatment response

Electrocardiographic Findings
• Sinus tachycardia is common in animals with CHF. • May show evidence of left atrial enlargement (P mitrale) or left ventricular enlargement (tall and wide R waves) • Atrial arrhythmias (e.g., atrial premature complexes, atrial tachycardia, and atrial fibrillation) or ventricular arrhythmias may develop.

PATHOLOGIC FINDINGS
• Gross valvular changes are divided into four types—type I shows only a few discrete nodules at the line of closure; type IV shows gross distortion of the valve by gray-white nodules and plaques causing contraction of the cusps and rolling of the free edge; the chordae are irregularly thickened with regions of tapering and rupture. • Jet lesions—irregular thickening and opacity of the atrial endocardium • Recent and healed left atrium splits or tears in some patients; full-thickness tears lead to hemopericardium (free wall) or acquired atrial septal defect (septum). • Left atrium and left ventricle dilation in many patients • The degree of left ventricular hypertrophy may only be apparent on weighing the heart. • Small thrombi in the left atrium are rare in dogs—more common and extensive in cats • Histopathologic examination reveals thickening of the valve

spongiosa due to fibroblast proliferation, deposition of mucopolysaccharide and edema (myxomatous degeneration), and degeneration of the fibrosa.

TREATMENT

APPROPRIATE HEALTH CARE
Treat patients that need oxygen support as inpatients; if stable, patients may be less stressed at home.

NURSING CARE
Oxygen therapy as needed for hypoxemia

ACTIVITY
• Absolute exercise restriction recommended for symptomatic patients • Stable patients receiving medical treatment—restrict exercise to leash walking; avoid sudden, explosive exercise.

DIET
• A salt-restricted diet recommended, if tolerated, for a patient in heart failure; close monitoring of sodium concentration is recommended. • Hyponatremia may develop as CHF progresses and in patients fed severely sodium-restricted diets in conjunction with loop diuretics and angiotensin-converting enzyme (ACE) inhibitors; signs of hyponatremia include weakness. • If hyponatremia develops, switch to a less sodium-restricted diet—diet prepared for management of renal disease or the geriatric patient

CLIENT EDUCATION
• Discuss the progressive nature of the disease. • Emphasize the importance of consistent dosing of all medications and diet and exercise management. • Highlight the signs of digoxin toxicity, and advise the owner to stop treatment and notify the veterinarian immediately should any develop.

SURGICAL CONSIDERATIONS
Surgical valve replacement and purse-string suture techniques to reduce the area of the mitral valve orifice have been used; experience with these techniques is limited, but surgical repair may be an option when access to a cardiovascular surgeon and cardiopulmonary bypass is available.

MEDICATIONS

DRUGS OF CHOICE
Recommended treatment depends on the stage of the disease; these recommendations follow the guidelines set by the ISACHC.

Asymptomatic Patients
• If no cardiac enlargement, no treatment is recommended. • Administering ACE inhibitors to asymptomatic patients showing progressive cardiomegaly may slow progres-

sion; this hypothesis is, as yet, unsubstantiated.

Mild or Moderate CHF
• Diuretics—furosemide (1–2 mg/kg q8–12h) • ACE inhibitors (vasodilators)—enalapril (0.5 mg/kg q12–24h), benazepril 0.25–0.5 mg/kg q24h • Nitroglycerine (venodilator)—2% percutaneous ointment (0.125–1 inch q6h until patient is stable) • Digoxin—especially if supraventricular arrhythmias, including atrial fibrillation, are documented (0.005 mg/kg or 0.22 mg/m2 PO q12h) • Sodium restriction if tolerated • Antiarrhythmics—as needed • Calcium channel blockers—to treat atrial arrhythmias • β-Blockers—to treat atrial and ventricular arrhythmias • Class 1 antiarrhythmics—procainamide, quinidine, mexiletine, and tocainide; to treat ventricular arrhythmias • Class III antiarrhythmics—sotalol, amiodarone for intractable arrhythmias

Severe Congestive Heart Failure
• Oxygen—40% in O_2 cage (can go as high as 100%) up to 24h; use nasal O_2 in large-breed dogs, 50–100 mL/kg/min through humidifier • Diuretics—furosemide (Lasix, 2–4 mg/kg IV q4–8h)

Vasodilators
• Benazepril (0.25–0.5 mg/kg q24h) • Enalapril (0.5 mg/kg q12h-q24h) • Hydralazine (0.5 mg/kg q12h titrated up to 2 mg/kg if necessary)—used in acute stages to decrease afterload rapidly; may cause hypotension • Nitroglycerine—ointment (1/4 inch/5 kg up to 2 inches percutaneously) or injectable (1–5 µg/kg/min CRI • Sodium nitroprusside (1–10 µg/kg/min—monitor blood pressure

Positive Inotropes
• Digoxin (0.005 mg/kg or 0.22 mg/m² PO q12h) • Dobutamine (dogs, 1–10 µg/kg/min; cats, 1–5 mg/kg/min)—may cause seizures • Dopamine (1–10 µg/kg/min) • Agents with β-blocking properties (e.g., carvedilol) are being investigated for their ability to upregulate β-receptors in patients with severe myocardial dysfunction.

CONTRAINDICATIONS N/A

PRECAUTIONS
• Use digoxin, diuretics, and ACE inhibitors with caution in patients with renal disease. • Nitrate tolerance may develop if appropriate 12-h nitrate-free intervals are omitted from the dosing schedule.

POSSIBLE INTERACTIONS
Monitor digoxin concentration in patients receiving concurrent calcium channel blockers or quinidine.

ALTERNATIVE DRUGS
• Diuretics—add thiazide and potassium-sparing diuretic (e.g., spironolactone) in refractory animals. • Bumetanide is an alternative to furosemide. • Vasodilators—other ACE inhibitors include lisinopril; isosorbide dinitrate can be used in place of

nitroglycerin ointment in patients requiring long-term nitrate administration.

FOLLOW-UP

PATIENT MONITORING
• Take a baseline radiograph when a murmur is first detected and every 6–12 months thereafter to document progressive cardiomegaly. • After an episode of CHF, check patients weekly during the first month of treatment; may repeat thoracic radiographs and an ECG at the first weekly checkup and on subsequent visits if any changes are seen on physical examination. • Monitor BUN and creatinine when diuretics and ACE inhibitors are used in combination.

PREVENTION/AVOIDANCE
N/A

POSSIBLE COMPLICATIONS
Endocarditis because of bacterial colonization of the diseased mitral valve

EXPECTED COURSE AND PROGNOSIS
Progressive degeneration of both valve changes and myocardial function occurs, necessitating increasing drug dosages; long-term prognosis depends on response to treatment and stage of heart failure.

MISCELLANEOUS

ASSOCIATED CONDITIONS N/A

AGE-RELATED FACTORS N/A

ZOONOTIC POTENTIAL N/A

PREGNANCY N/A

SYNONYMS
Degenerative valve disease, chronic valve disease, acquired valvular insufficiency, and valve fibrosis

SEE ALSO
• Congestive Heart Failure, Left-sided and Right-sided • Atrial Wall Tear

ABBREVIATIONS
• ACE = angiotensin-converting enzyme • AV = atrioventricular • CHF = congestive heart failure

Suggested Reading
Atkins CE. Acquired valvular insufficiency. In: Miller MS, Tilley LP, eds. Manual of canine and feline cardiology. Philadelphia: Saunders, 1995:129–143.
Keene BW. Chronic valvular disease in the dog. In: Fox PR, ed. Canine and feline cardiology. New York: Churchill Livingstone, 1988:409–418.
Author Andrew Beardow
Consulting Editors Larry P. Tilley and Francis W. K. Smith, Jr.

DISEASES

ATRIOVENTRICULAR VALVULAR STENOSIS

BASICS

OVERVIEW
- AV valvular stenosis is a pathologic narrowing of the mitral or tricuspid valve orifice; ventricular filling in clinically significant disease requires a persistent, diastolic pressure gradient between atrium and ventricle.
- Rarely diagnosed in dogs and cats.
- Concomitant valvular regurgitation is common.
- The increased atrial pressure can lead to atrial dilation, venous congestion, or CHF.
- The foramen ovale may remain patent in patients with tricuspid stenosis, allowing right-to-left shunting with signs of cyanotic heart disease.
- Cardiac output and exercise capacity are limited; with mitral stenosis, exertional dyspnea and left-sided CHF are common.

SIGNALMENT
- Mitral stenosis is a condition of uncertain genetic basis; bull terriers and Newfoundlands may be overrepresented, but the condition is also seen in other breeds.
- Of the three reported cats with mitral stenosis, two were Siamese.
- Tricuspid stenosis has been reported most often in Old English sheepdogs and Labrador retrievers.
- Most patients are presented at a young age, though exceptions do occur, especially in cats.

SIGNS

Historical Findings
- Exercise intolerance
- Syncope
- Exertional dyspnea or tachypnea
- Cough—mitral stenosis
- Cyanosis—tricuspid stenosis
- Abdominal distension—tricuspid stenosis

- Acute posterior paresis—cats with mitral stenosis
- Stunted growth

Physical Examination Findings
- Soft diastolic murmur with point of maximal intensity over the left apex (mitral stenosis) or right hemithorax (tricuspid stenosis)
- Holosystolic murmur of mitral or tricuspid regurgitation is common, especially with mitral stenosis.
- Crackles, dyspnea with mitral stenosis
- Jugular distension, jugular pulses, ascites, hepatomegaly with tricuspid stenosis
- Cyanosis from right to left shunt with tricuspid stenosis

CAUSES & RISK FACTORS
- AV valvular stenosis is most likely due to congenital valve dysplasia; supravalvular lesions (a membrane with central perforation or a fibrous ring) have been described.
- Bacterial endocarditis and intracardiac neoplasia are potential causes of acquired AV valvular stenosis.

DIAGNOSIS

DIFFERENTIAL DIAGNOSIS
Must differentiate from the more common causes of mitral and tricuspid regurgitation in the absence of stenosis

CBC/BIOCHEMISTRY/URINALYSIS
May be normal or reflect changes related to CHF or drug therapy for heart failure

OTHER LABORATORY TESTS
N/A

IMAGING

Thoracic Radiography
- Atrial enlargement is the most consistent and outstanding feature.
- May see generalized cardiomegaly

- If the patient is in left-sided CHF, may see patchy alveolar opacities of pulmonary edema
- Tricuspid stenosis—may be hepatomegaly; diameter of the caudal vena cava may be increased.

Echocardiography
- Diagnostic test of choice
- Two-dimensional echocardiography reveals a markedly dilated atrium with attenuated valve excursion during diastole, often with thickened irregular AV valve leaflets evident; mobile, but fused, valve leaflets may appear to "dome" during diastole.
- May see shortened chordae tendineae or an anomalous papillary muscle; may see some subtle tethering of the mitral valve in some asymptomatic breeds at risk (e.g., bull terrier, mastiff)
- M-mode studies show an enlarged atrium with concordant motion of the AV valve leaflets; both leaflets move together during diastole, indicating commisural fusion; the E-to-F slope is decreased.
- Color-flow imaging reveals a turbulent diastolic jet that originates at the stenotic valve and projects toward the apex of the ventricle; a turbulent jet of AV valve regurgitation is often present as well.
- Pulsed-wave and continuous-wave Doppler studies—increased, diastolic transvalvular flow velocities; prolonged calculated pressure half-time is a hallmark feature; E-wave/A-wave amplitude reversal may be seen.

Angiography
- Atrial injection demonstrates a markedly dilated atrium; with tricuspid stenosis and a patent foramen ovale, opacification of the left atrium may be observed following right atrial injection.
- Often see delayed opacification of the ventricle and great vessels; one may visualize thickened, irregular valve leaflets or a stenotic valve funnel; ventricular injection typically reveals valvular regurgitation.

ATRIOVENTRICULAR VALVULAR STENOSIS

Cardiac Catheterization
• A diastolic pressure gradient exists between the atrium and ventricle.
• High left atrial, pulmonary capillary wedge, and pulmonary artery pressures occur in mitral stenosis.
• High right atrial and central venous pressures are present in tricuspid stenosis.
• Ventricular pressure may be normal in the absence of concurrent defects.

DIAGNOSTIC PROCEDURES

Electrocardiography
May be variable enlargement patterns (atrial and ventricular); ectopic rhythms, especially of atrial origin, are often observed.

PATHOLOGIC FINDINGS
• Usually the atrioventricular valve is abnormal, with thickened leaflets and fused commissures.
• Many patients also have evidence of valve dysplasia with abnormal chordae tendineae and papillary muscles.
• Atrial dilation and hypertrophy are common.
• Concurrent cardiac defects are not uncommon, especially a patent foramen ovale in tricuspid stenosis (due to increased right atrial pressure) and subaortic stenosis in cases of mitral stenosis.

TREATMENT
• Hospitalization and diuresis for patients in overt CHF
• Surgical valve replacement or repair is the therapy of choice; this requires cardiopulmonary bypass or hypothermia; cost and availability are limiting factors.
• Balloon valvuloplasty is an alternative referral treatment to decrease the diastolic gradient between the atrium and ventricle.
• Use medical therapy for CHF; feed a low-sodium diet to patients with over CHF.
• The diastolic pressure gradient increases exponentially at higher heart rates, and the

ability to increase cardiac output is limited; exercise restriction is recommended for patients with exercise intolerance, exertional dyspnea, and CHF.

MEDICATIONS

DRUGS

CHF
• Digoxin—dogs, 0.01–0.015 mg/kg divided q12h; cats, 1/4 of a 0.125-mg tablet q48h
• Furosemide—dogs, 2–6 mg/kg IV, IM, SC, PO q8–24h; cats, 1–4 mg/kg IV, IM, SC, PO q8–24h
• Enalapril—dogs, 0.5 mg/kg PO q12–24h; cats, 0.25–0.5 mg/kg PO q12–48h; see below.

Atrial Tachyarrhythmias
• Digoxin as above
• β-Blocker (atenolol: dogs, 6.25–12.5 mg/dog q12h; cats, 6.25–12.5 mg/cat q24h) or calcium channel blocker (diltiazem: dogs, 0.5–1.5 mg/kg PO q8h; Dilacor XR or Cardizem CD: cats, 10 mg/kg q24h) for heart rate control

CONTRAINDICATIONS/POSSIBLE INTERACTIONS
Use ACE inhibitors or other vasodilators judiciously in patients with AV valvular stenosis and CHF; cardiac output is limited and vasodilation may induce hypotension; monitor arterial blood pressure.

FOLLOW-UP

PATIENT MONITORING
• Digoxin level—check 7–10 days following institution of therapy; 8- to 12-h trough should be 0.8–1.5 ng/mL.
• Renal function, electrolyte status (especially potassium), and arterial blood pressure when on diuretic and/or ACE inhibitor

POSSIBLE COMPLICATIONS
• CHF
• Atrial fibrillation
• Syncope
• Aortic thromboembolism—cats

EXPECTED COURSE AND PROGNOSIS
• Morbidity is high; except for mild cases, prognosis is generally poor.
• Surgical intervention or balloon valvuloplasty may alter course of disease, but data are limited.

MISCELLANEOUS

ASSOCIATED CONDITIONS
Concurrent congenital defects are common (e.g., subaortic stenosis in mitral stenosis, patent foramen ovale in tricuspid stenosis).

SEE ALSO
• Atrioventricular Valve Dysplasia
• Endocarditis, Bacterial
• Cardiac Neoplasia

ABBREVIATIONS
• ACE = angiotensin converting enzyme
• AV = atrioventricular
• CHF = congestive heart failure

Suggested Reading
Sisson DD, Thomas WP, Bonagura JD. Congenital heart disease. In: Ettinger SJ, Feldman EC, eds. Textbook of veterinary internal medicine, 5th edition. Philadelphia: WB Saunders, 2000;737–787.
Authors Lora S. Hitchcock and John D. Bonagura
Consulting Editor Larry P. Tilley and Francis W. K. Smith, Jr.

DISEASES

BASICS

OVERVIEW
• RBC destruction and anemia caused by *Babesia* spp. of intracellular protozoa
• *B. cani*—a large (4–7 mm-long), pear-shaped parasite of canine RBCs; in the U.S., strains generally cause mild or inapparent disease in adults (unless immunosuppressed), but severe disease in pups; South African strains cause severe disease and death in some adult dogs.
• *B. gibsoni*—a small (2.5 mm), ring-shaped organism that causes severe disease in most infected adult dogs; rare in the U.S. but common in Africa and Asia; organisms can be difficult to see in stained blood films.
• *B. felis*—a very small (1 mm), ring-shaped organism that occurs in cats in Africa and southern Asia; of similar size and morphology to *Cytauxzoon felis,* which occurs in cats in the U.S.

SIGNALMENT
• Dogs in many countries, including the U.S.
• Cats in Africa and southern Asia

SIGNS
• Signs and laboratory findings similar in cats and dogs
• Vary with age of the animal and the species and strain of *Babesia*
• Course of disease may be acute and fulminating, subclinical, or chronic
• Dogs—lethargy, anorexia, pale mucous membranes, fever, emesis, amber to brown urine, splenomegaly, icterus, weight loss, tachycardia, and tachypnea
• Cats—lethargy, anorexia, rough hair coat, pale mucous membranes, tachycardia, tachypnea, and occasionally icterus (fever not reported)

CAUSES & RISK FACTORS
• Caused by *B. canis* and *B. gibsoni* in dogs and *B. felis* in cats; additional *Babesia* spp. in African wild cats may be transmitted to domestic cats.
• Can be transmitted by ticks and blood transfusions
• Risk of disease increased by splenectomy and immunosuppression

DIAGNOSIS

DIFFERENTIAL DIAGNOSIS
• Other causes of hemolytic anemia, including autoimmune hemolytic anemia, hemobartonellosis, cytauxzoonosis (cats only), Heinz body hemolytic anemia, microangiopathic hemolytic anemia, pyruvate kinase deficiency, and phosphofructokinase deficiency (dogs only)
• Difficult to differentiate from autoimmune hemolytic anemia if parasites are not recognized in blood; both may be Coombs test positive
• New methylene blue stains used to identify Heinz bodies
• Enzyme assays or specialized DNA tests used to identify pyruvate kinase or phosphofructokinase deficiencies
• *C. felis* infection differentiated from *B. felis* infection by schizonts in tissues of cats with cytauxzoonosis, which are not seen in cats with babesiosis

CBC/BIOCHEMISTRY/URINALYSIS
• Anemia with evidence of a regenerative response (reticulocytosis) unless a precipitous decrease in PCV occurs early in the course of disease
• A peracute form of disease, resulting in DIC and death before anemia is severe, has been reported in dogs in South Africa.
• Differential leukocyte counts variable and provide little diagnostic assistance; mild lymphocytosis may occur in dogs.
• Mild to severe thrombocytopenia often present
• Bilirubinemia and anemic hypoxia demonstrated in biochemical profiles of some animals
• Bilirubinuria in many dogs; prominent hemoglobinuria rarely recognized in dogs in the U.S.

OTHER LABORATORY TESTS
• Definitive diagnosis made by identification of protozoal organisms in stained blood films
• IFA—tests for *B. canis* and *B. gibsoni* demonstrate antibodies in serum directed against these organisms, but some cross-reactivity occurs between *Babesia* spp.; high titers suggest current infection; tests may be negative in acutely infected animals, especially pups.
• Direct Coombs' test positive in some animals
• Prolonged coagulation times (i.e., APTT, PT, ACT) and positive fibrin degradation product test in some animals with severe DIC
• Metabolic acidosis in some severely affected animals secondary to tissue hypoxia and shock

IMAGING
N/A

DIAGNOSTIC PROCEDURES
N/A

TREATMENT
• None required in adult animals with mild anemia and clinical signs, although these animals can be reservoirs of infection for other animals
• Life-threatening anemia—IV blood transfusions necessary
• Shock—use IV fluids with added bicarbonate.

MEDICATIONS

DRUGS

• Dogs—diminazene aceturate (3.5 mg/kg SC or IM, single injection) *or* imidocarb dipropionate (5 mg/kg SC, single injection) *or* phenamidine (15 mg/kg SC on 2 consecutive days) may be efficacious in treating babesiosis; these drugs are not approved for use in the U.S.; thus an ECINAD exemption from the FDA is required before drugs can be obtained from suppliers.

• Cats—primaquine phosphate (1 mg/kg IM, single injection); not approved for use in cats in the U.S.

CONTRAINDICTIONS/POSSIBLE INTERACTIONS

Antibabesial drugs potentially dangerous and can cause neuromuscular signs and liver or kidney injury

 ## FOLLOW-UP

• Animals may relapse after completion of treatment; more likely to occur in dogs with *B. gibsoni* infection than in those with *B. canis* infection

• Many treated and untreated animals remain carriers of disease.

• Organisms not usually seen in blood films of recovered carrier animals

 ## MISCELLANEOUS

ABBREVIATIONS

• ACT = activated clotting time
• APTT = activated partial thromboplastin time
• DIC = disseminated intravascular coagulation
• ECINAD = emergency compassionate investigational new animal drug
• IFA = indirect fluorescent antibody
• PCV = packed cell volume
• PT = prothrombin time

Suggested Reading

Breitschwerdt E. Babesiosis. In: Greene CE, ed. Infectious diseases of the dog and cat. Philadelphia: Saunders, 1990:796–805.

Author John W. Harvey
Consulting Editor Susan M. Cotter

BARTONELLOSIS—CAT SCRATCH DISEASE

BASICS

OVERVIEW
• Human syndrome—typified by regional lymphadenopathy after a cat scratch or bite distal to the involved lymph node
• Agents—small curved, argyrophilic, gram-negative rod *Bartonella henselae* (formerly *Rochalimaea henselae*) in majority of cases; *B. clarridgeiae* and *Afipia felis* also reported
• Worldwide occurrence
• Estimated > 25,000 cases/year in U.S.; > 2,000 cases require hospitalization; almost no fatalities

SIGNALMENT
• More males than females (1.2:1)
• Majority of patients (80%) < 21 years
• Seasonal; more cases reported between July and January

SIGNS
Human
• Erythematous papule at inoculation site (scratch, bite); then unilateral regional lymphadenopathy (painful, often suppurative) in 3–10 days (> 90%)
• Mild fever
• Chills—infrequent
• Malaise
• Anorexia
• Myalgia
• Nausea
• Atypical manifestations—encephalopathy (7%); palpebral conjunctivitis (3–5%); meningitis; osteolytic lesions; granulomatous hepatitis; pneumonia

Cats
• No signs of illness
• Between 5 and 60% seropositive, depending on geographical area
• Lymphoid hyperplasia—sometimes

CAUSES & RISK FACTORS
• Contact with domestic kittens and cats (> 90%), particularly young cats with fleas
• Scratched by cat—up to 83%
• Up to 95% of cats residing in households of affected humans are seropositive
• Other members of household likely exposed to *B. henselae*

DIAGNOSIS

DIFFERENTIAL DIAGNOSIS
• Benign adenopathy in human children and young adults—most common cause
• History of contact with a cat
• Formation of a papule at the site of primary inoculation (scratch or bite)
• Compatible clinical picture—unilateral regional lymphadenitis
• Exclusion of other identifiable causes
• Characteristic histopathological findings
• Serologic tests—indirect fluorescent antibody for *B. henselae*
• Positive skin test no longer used
• Other causes of lymphadenopathy—lymphogranuloma venereum; syphilis; typical or atypical tuberculosis; other forms of bacterial adenitis; sporotrichosis; tularemia; brucellosis; histoplasmosis; sarcoidosis; toxoplasmosis; infectious mononucleosis; and benign or malignant tumors

CBC/BIOCHEMISTRY/URINALYSIS
Noncontributory

OTHER LABORATORY TESTS
• Indirect fluorescent antibody test
• Enzyme immunoassay—IgG antibodies to *B. henselae* (Specialty Laboratories, Santa Monica, CA)
• Culture—on enriched (blood-containing) media in presence of 5% carbon dioxide at 35–37°C; fastidious and slow growing; requires 14–30 days
• PCR amplification of bacterial DNA from lesions

DIAGNOSTIC PROCEDURES
N/A

IMAGING
N/A

PATHOLOGIC FINDINGS
• Histopathology of lymph nodes—nonspecific inflammatory reaction, including granuloma, microabscess, and necrosis
• Warthin-Starry silver stain—bacilli

TREATMENT
• Supportive treatment—bed rest; heat on swollen lymph nodes; needle aspiration of suppurative nodes
• Thoroughly cleanse all cat scratches or bites.
• Prevent cats from contacting open wounds.

MEDICATIONS

DRUGS
• Specific antimicrobials—not efficacious
• Most cases spontaneously resolve in few weeks or months.
• Severe cases—antibiotic therapy (gentamicin, doxycycline, erythromycin) based on the antimicrobial susceptibility of *B. henselae* may be appropriate.

CONTRAINDICATIONS/POSSIBLE INTERACTIONS
N/A

FOLLOW-UP
One episode appears to confer lifelong immunity.

PREVENTION/AVOIDANCE
Immunocompromised persons should avoid young cats.

POSSIBLE COMPLICATIONS
Uncommon

MISCELLANEOUS
• Bacillary angiomatosis—vascular proliferative disease of the skin; may also be caused by *B. henselae;* responds to antimicrobial drugs (bartonellosis rarely does)
• Natural host of *B. henselae* is unknown; a related species, *B. quintana,* is spread by lice and causes trench fever in humans.

ZOONOTIC POTENTIAL
Uncertain for *Bartonella* infections in dogs and cats

ABBREVIATION
PCR = polymerase chain reaction

Suggested Reading
Schwartzman W. Bartonella infections: beyond cat scratch. Annu Rev Med 1996;47:355–364.
Author J. Paul Woods
Consulting Editor Stephen C. Barr

BASICS

OVERVIEW
- Tumor that originates from the basal epithelium of the skin
- Includes benign (e.g., basal cell epithelioma and basaloid tumor) and malignant (e.g., basal cell carcinoma) tumors

SIGNALMENT
- Common—makes up 3%–12% and 15%–18% of all skin tumors in dogs and cats, respectively
- Age—dogs: 6–9 years; cats: 5–18 years (mean, 10.8 years)
- Cocker spaniels, poodles, and Siamese cats—more commonly affected than other breeds

SIGNS
- Solitary, well-circumscribed, formed, hairless, intradermal raised mass, typically located on the head, neck, or shoulders
- Variable in size—0.2–10 cm in diameter
- Masses (cats)—often heavily pigmented, cystic, and occasionally ulcerated

CAUSES & RISK FACTORS
Unknown

 DIAGNOSIS

DIFFERENTIAL DIAGNOSIS
- Other skin tumors—mast cell tumor; melanoma; hemangioma; hemangiosarcoma
- Intradermal cysts

CBC/BIOCHEMISTRY/URINALYSIS
Normal

OTHER LABORATORY TESTS
N/A

IMAGING
N/A

DIAGNOSTIC PROCEDURES
Histopathologic examination—definitive diagnosis

PATHOLOGIC FINDINGS
- Histologic cellular patterns—vary from solid to cystic to ribbon appearance
- Tumor cells—may contain melanin pigmentation; may have a fine eosinophilic stroma

 TREATMENT

Surgical excision—treatment of choice; generally curative

 MEDICATIONS

DRUGS
N/A

CONTRAINDICATIONS/POSSIBLE INTERACTIONS
N/A

 FOLLOW-UP

- Tumors—< 10% malignant
- Complete surgical excision—usually curative

 MISCELLANEOUS

Suggested Reading
Holzworth J. Diseases of the cat: medicine and surgery. Philadelphia: Saunders, 1987.
Thomas RC, Fox LE. Tumors of the skin and subcutis. In: Morrison WB. ed. Cancer in dogs and cats: medical and surgical management. Baltimore: Williams & Wilkins, 1998:489–510.
Author Robyn Elmslie
Consulting Editor Wallace B. Morrison

BASE NARROW MANDIBULAR CANINE TEETH

BASICS

OVERVIEW
• Common malocclusion of mandibular canines of dogs
• Occurs at eruption of temporary and/or permanent dentition; if it occurs in temporary dentition, it almost always occurs in permanent dentition if no corrective steps instituted
• Can be unilateral or bilateral..

SIGNALMENT
• Dogs
• Seen in many breeds; most commonly in German shepherds, Doberman pinschers, Staffordshire bull terriers, and Rottweilers
• Anecdotally much increased prevalence in certain breeds is associated with change of type from large head and wide maxilla to fine head and narrow maxilla.
• No sex predilection
• Not known if direct genetic basis

SIGNS
• Linguoversion of temporary or permanent mandibular canines; displacement can be unilateral or bilateral
• May be mesiodistal displacement of mandibular canines
• Tips of mandibular canines touch maxillary hard palate lingual to normal contact point, which is just labial to diastema between lateral incisor and maxillary canine; premature contact with soft issue causes damage to soft tissue, remodeling, and possibly discomfort.
• May be food impaction in remodeled soft tissue
• Oronasal fistula may ultimately develop.

CAUSES & RISK FACTORS
• Retained deciduous canines are proposed as main cause.
• Narrow mandibles can also cause base narrow malocclusion.

DIAGNOSIS

DIFFERENTIAL DIAGNOSIS
Diagnosis is made by physical examination of dental occlusion.

CBC/BIOCHEMISTRY/URINALYSIS
N/A

OTHER LABORATORY TESTS
N/A

IMAGING
Check if retained temporary roots or other dental abnormalities.

DIAGNOSTIC PROCEDURES
Ask about litter mates and stud history to see if prevalent in breed or line.

TREATMENT

• To prevent contact trauma, pain and discomfort, and oronasal fistulae
• If performed in show dogs, they should not subsequently be shown and the breed society should be notified.
• If associated with the temporary dentition, remove the mandibular temporary canines immediately; this may allow enough room for the permanent mandibular canines to erupt more labially into a normal position.
• Puppies and adult dogs given rubber balls for extended periods may act as an orthodontic device to help correct problem.
• If the malocclusion in the permanent dentition is very mild (i.e., very little linguoversion) then a gingivectomy of the gingival diastema may suffice to prevent contact and subsequent trauma.
• Moderate-to-severe malocclusion in the permanent dentition is an indication for orthodontic movement; tipping is the most common movement to correct malocclusion.
• Tipping can be performed by a number of different appliances—acrylic inclined plane, expansion screws, W springs, cast metal incline planes

MEDICATIONS

DRUGS
If correcting with appliances, use oral hygiene products (e.g., 0.2% chlorhexidine rinses) during treatment.

CONTRAINDICATIONS/POSSIBLE

INTERACTIONS
N/A

FOLLOW-UP

PATIENT MONITORING
Check monthly posttreatment for 3 months to see if desired outcome is stable.

EXPECTED COURSE AND PROGNOSIS
• Can take 2–5 weeks for canines to move
• Good prognosis in most patients; should be self-retaining once movement has occurred.
• If malocclusion is not corrected, more-frequent dental care may be needed than for a dog with normal occlusion.

MISCELLANEOUS

• May or not be associated with mesiodistal discrepancies of occlusion
• Synonyms include linguoversion of mandibular canines and inverted canines (sic)
• Ascertain owner's reasons for correction of malocclusion; should not be corrected in show dogs to obtain unfair advantage in the show ring

Suggested Reading
Wiggs BW, Loprise HB. Veterinary dentistry principles and practice. Philadelphia: Lippincott-Raven, 1997;464.

Author Stephen Coles
Consulting Editor Jan Bellows

BASICS

OVERVIEW
- Age-related pathologic change in the prostate gland making it nonpainfully large
- Occurs in two phases, glandular and complex
- Glandular phase characterized by high number of large prostatic cells and a symmetrically large prostate gland
- Complex phase characterized by glandular hyperplasia, glandular atrophy, small cyst formation, chronic inflammation, and squamous metaplasia of epithelium

SIGNALMENT
- Observed initially in intact male dogs 1–2 years old
- Prevalence increases linearly; 60% of male dogs are affected by 6 years of age and 95% of male dogs are affected by 9 years of age

SIGNS

Historical Findings
- None in most dogs
- Bloody urethral discharge
- Hematuria
- Blood in ejaculate
- Straining to defecate
- Ribbon-like stools
- Dysuria

Physical Examination Findings
- Symmetric, nonpainfully large prostate gland
- Prostatic pain in dogs with complication of bacterial infection or prostatic carcinoma

CAUSES & RISK FACTORS
- Testosterone and 5-α-dihydrotestosterone
- Estrogens
- Prostatic stroma
- Aging
- Risk eliminated by castration

DIAGNOSIS

DIFFERENTIAL DIAGNOSIS
- Acute bacterial prostatitis—typically associated with fever, depression, pain on rectal palpation, neutrophilia, pyuria, and bacteriuria; may occur concurrently with benign prostatic hyperplasia

- Chronic bacterial prostatitis—typically associated with recurrent lower urinary tract infections; may occur concurrently with benign prostatic hyperplasia.
- Prostatic adenocarcinoma—typically associated with poor appetite, weight loss, hind limb weakness, dysuria, hematuria, and dyschezia; may see carcinoma cells in urine sediment
- Prostatic and paraprostatic cysts—can cause palpable abdominal cystic mass filled with yellow to orange fluid

CBC/BIOCHEMISTRY/URINALYSIS
- CBC and biochemistry—normal
- Urinalysis—may be normal or reveal hematuria; pyuria and bacteriuria are absent unless dog has concurrent bacterial infection

OTHER LABORATORY TESTS
- Prostatic fluid obtained by ejaculation or prostatic massage is clear or hemorrhagic; RBC count high; WBC count normal; culture reveals <10,000 bacteria/mL unless the dog has concurrent bacterial infection
- Serum concentration of prostatic esterase is high in some dogs.

IMAGING

Radiography
- Abdominal radiographs reveal prostatomegaly.
- Retrograde urethrocystography may be normal or reveal narrowing of prostatic urethra or reflux of contrast media into the prostate gland.

Ultrasonography
Reveals large prostate gland with uniform prostatic parenchymal echogenicity; small, fluid-filled cysts in some dogs

DIAGNOSTIC PROCEDURES
N/A

TREATMENT
- Frequently not required
- Castration—most effective and prevents recurrence; if benign prostatic hyperplasia is complicated by acute bacterial prostatitis, delay until the infection is resolved

MEDICATIONS

DRUGS
If castration is not acceptable, the following drugs may temporarily shrink the prostate gland:
- Finasteride (0.5 mg/day)
- Megestrol acetate (0.11 mg/kg PO daily for 3 weeks)
- Medroxyprogesterone (3 mg/kg SC)

CONTRAINDICATIONS/POSSIBLE INTERACTIONS
- Avoid estrogens because of possible hematologic toxicity and development of squamous metaplasia of the prostate.
- Long-term administration of megestrol acetate or medroxyprogesterone may result in development of diabetes mellitus.

FOLLOW-UP
Castration will result in rapid involution of the enlarged prostate.

MISCELLANEOUS

ASSOCIATED CONDITIONS
- Bacterial prostatitis and prostatic carcinoma
- Prostatomegaly in a castrated dog strongly suggests prostatic carcinoma

SEE ALSO
- Prostatic Cysts
- Prostatitis and Prostatic Abscess
- Prostatomegaly

Suggested Reading

Barsanti JA, Finco DR. Prostatic diseases. In: Ettinger SJ, Feldman EC, eds. Textbook of veterinary internal medicine. Philadelphia: WB Saunders, 1995:1662–1685.

Author Jeffrey S. Klausner

Consulting Editors Larry G. Adams and Carl A. Osborne

BILE DUCT CARCINOMA

 BASICS

OVERVIEW
• Most common hepatic neoplasia in cats; second-most common hepatic malignancy in dogs
• Intrahepatic bile duct origin more frequently reported than extrahepatic bile duct or gallbladder origin in cats and dogs

SIGNALMENT
• Dogs and cats > 10 years of age
• Female predisposition may exist.
• No reported breed predilection

SIGNS

Historical Findings
• Anorexia
• Lethargy
• Polydipsia and polyuria
• Vomiting
• Advanced disease—icterus; abdominal distension

Physical Examination Findings
• Hepatomegaly
• Ascites
• Abdominal distension
• Icterus
• Palpable abdominal mass uncommon

CAUSES & RISK FACTORS
• Possible association with liver fluke and other parasitic infestations
• Environmental exposure to carcinogens implicated

 DIAGNOSIS

DIFFERENTIAL DIAGNOSIS
• Gross pathologic—hepatocellular adenoma; hepatocellular adenocarcinoma; nodular hyperplasia; cirrhosis; chronic active hepatitis; hepatic myelolipoma; hepatobiliary cysta-denoma; cholangiocellular adenoma
• Histopathology—easily distinguished from hepatocellular carcinoma

CBC/BIOCHEMISTRY/URINALYSIS
• Leukocytosis and bilirubinemia—inconsistent findings
• High serum enzyme (e.g., ALP, ALT, and AST) activity—not specific for neoplastic disease; high ALP less common in cats because of the enzyme's short half-life

OTHER LABORATORY TESTS
• α-Fetoprotein concentration—may differentiate neoplastic from nonneoplastic lesions in dogs
• Coagulation profile—perform before biopsy or any surgical procedure
• No known association with FeLV in cats

IMAGING
• Abdominal radiographs—may localize a mass to the liver; may show loss of detail in patients with ascites
• Thoracic radiographs—may identify pulmonary metastases
• Abdominal ultrasound—assess location of lesion; echogenicity; may guide biopsy

DIAGNOSTIC PROCEDURES
• Abdominocentesis and cytologic evaluation—with ascites
• Neoplastic tissue examination—obtain by percutaneous biopsy, laparoscopy, or laparotomy; definitive diagnosis

PATHOLOGIC FINDINGS
• Massive (most common), nodular, or diffuse
• Benign lesions—usually cystic and multi-nodular
• Malignant tumors—often involve multiple lobes
• Histological classification—not prognostic

 TREATMENT
• Surgical excision—treatment of choice
• Up to 80% of the liver can be resected if the remaining liver tissue is functional.

MEDICATIONS

DRUGS
No reported effective chemotherapy

CONTRAINDICATIONS/POSSIBLE INTERACTIONS
• Medications requiring metabolism by the liver—use with caution in patients with hepatopathies
• Hepatotoxicity caused by chemotherapeutics—appears to be of little or no importance in small animals

 FOLLOW-UP

EXPECTED COURSE AND PROGNOSIS
• Aggressive; high rate of metastasis (67%–88%)
• Common metastatic sites—lungs; hepatic lymph nodes; peritoneum
• Other metastatic sites—thoracic lymph nodes; diaphragm; spleen; urinary bladder; intestine, bone
• Complete surgical resection—unlikely owing to multifocal or diffuse involvement of the liver

 MISCELLANEOUS

ASSOCIATED CONDITIONS
Unlike in humans, no association with biliary calculi reported

PREGNANCY
• Chemotherapy drugs may be carcinogenic and mutagenic.

SYNONYMS
• Cholangiocellular carcinoma
• Cholangiocarcinoma

ABBREVIATIONS
• ALP = alkaline phosphatase
• ALT = alanine aminotransaminase
• AST = aspartate aminotransaminase
• FeLV = feline leukemia virus

Suggested Reading

Hammer AS, Sikkema DA. Hepatic neoplasia in the dog and cat. Vet Clin North Am Small Anim Pract 1995;25:419–435.

Morrison WB. Primary cancers and cancer-like lesions of the liver, biliary epithelium, and exocrine pancreas. In: Morrison WB, ed. Cancer in dogs and cats: medical and surgical management. Baltimore: Williams & Wilkins, 1998:559–568.

Author Sue Downing
Consulting Editor Wallace B. Morrison

BILE DUCT OBSTRUCTION

BASICS

DEFINITION
Cholestasis caused by obstruction of the biliary tree at the level of the common extrahepatic bile duct or at the level of the hepatic ducts (may involve one, several, or all, depending on the causal disorder in the porta hepatis)

PATHOPHYSIOLOGY
• Serious hepatobiliary injury—may occur within just a few weeks; derived from inflammatory mediators (e.g., eicosanoids) and oxidative damage
• Bile—may become colorless (white bile) owing to reduced secretion of bilirubin pigments and increased production of mucin
• Bacterial infection of biliary structures—possible owing to impairment of the normal biliary–enteric bacterial circulation and elimination

SYSTEMS AFFECTED
Hepatobiliary

SIGNALMENT

Species
Dogs and cats

Breed Predilections
Animals predisposed to pancreatitis—hyperlipidemic breeds (e.g., miniature schnauzers, Shetland sheepdogs)

Age and Age Range
Usually affects middle-aged to old animals

Predominant Sex
None

SIGNS

Historical Findings
• Depend on underlying disorder
• Progressive lethargy
• Intermittent illness
• Jaundiced mucous membranes
• Pale (acholic) stools
• Polyphagia—if complete obstruction and nutrient malassimilation
• Bleeding tendencies

Physical Examination Findings
• Depend on underlying disorder
• Weight loss
• Severe jaundice
• Hepatomegaly
• Cranial mass lesion—some small dogs and cats (gallbladder)
• Acholic feces—unless melena
• Bleeding tendencies
• Orange urine

CAUSES
• Associated with a number of diverse disorders
• Cholelithiasis
• Choledochitis
• Neoplasia

• Malformation of ducts—choledochal cysts, polycystic hepatobiliary disease
• Parasitic infestation—flukes
• Extrinsic compression—lymph nodes, pancreatic mass, entrapment in diaphragmatic hernia
• Duct fibrosis—trauma, peritonitis, pancreatitis
• Duct stricture—blunt trauma, iatrogenic from surgical handling or procedures

RISK FACTORS
See Causes

DIAGNOSIS

DIFFERENTIAL DIAGNOSIS
• Mass lesions—primary hepatic tumors; metastatic hepatic tumors; tumors in adjacent viscera
• Diffuse infiltrative liver disease—inflammatory; neoplastic; amyloid; hepatic lipidosis (cats)
• Biliary cysts—cystadenoma; choledochal cyst; hepatobiliary cystic disease
• Pancreatitis
• Fulminant hepatic failure
• Infectious hepatitis—bacteria; viral; flukes
• Decompensated chronic active hepatitis
• Copper storage hepatopathy—acute crisis
• End-stage cirrhosis
• Hepatic lipidosis—cats
• Cholangitis or cholangiohepatitis—cats; sclerosing form

CBC/BIOCHEMISTRY/URINALYSIS

CBC
• Anemia—mild nonregenerative (chronic disease) or regenerative (significant gastro-intestinal bleeding owing to propensity for gastroduodenal ulcerations)
• Microcytosis—uncommon
• Leukogram—may show neutrophilic leukocytosis
• Plasma—markedly jaundiced

Biochemistry
• Liver enzymes—variable; marked increases in ALP and GGT typical; markedly increased transaminases
• Serum total bilirubin—moderately to markedly high; often lower than that observed with hemolysis and hepatic lipidosis
• Albumin—usually within the normal range except when condition is > 6 weeks old (established biliary cirrhosis); values decline with chronicity owing to synthetic failure.
• Globulins—normal
• Glucose—usually normal, unless biliary cirrhosis develops (may note hypoglycemia) or sepsis syndrome occurs (acquired biliary tree infection)
• Hypercholesterolemia—common

Urinalysis
• Bilirubinuria
• Bilirubin crystals
• Absence of urobilinogen—unreliable marker

OTHER LABORATORY TESTS
• Serum bile acids—always markedly increased; do not add diagnostic information
• Coagulation abnormalities—develop after 3 weeks; linked to vitamin K deficiency (PIVKA and PT clotting times most sensitive); may note DIC owing to active pancreatitis or tumor necrosis

Fecal Examination
• Acholic stools—suggest complete obstruction; masked by small-volume melena
• Trematode eggs—suggest fluke infestation

IMAGING
• Abdominal radiography—hepatomegaly; may suggest mass lesion in area of gallbladder; may demonstrate signs of pancreatitis (e.g., duodenal ileus, mass lesion in right cranial abdominal quadrant, ill-defined right kidney silhouette, cranial displacement of the transverse colon, saponification of peripancreatic fat); rarely mineralized cholelith(s)
• Cholecystography—rarely provides additional information, because contrast competes with bilirubin for accumulation in the biliary tree and requires bile flow
• Abdominal ultrasonography—evidence of obstruction may be noted within 72 hr (distended tortuous extrahepatic bile duct, distended intrahepatic bile ducts); may note evidence of underlying or primary disease (e.g,. pancreatitis, cystic lesions, mass lesions, choleliths)
• Biliary scintigraphy—may assist in detection when combined with ultrasonography; usually unnecessary

DIAGNOSTIC PROCEDURES
• Hepatic aspiration cytology—indicated only when imaging reveals a mass lesion and surgery is based on a mass that is not highly malignant
• Needle biopsy—strongly contraindicated; leads to bile peritonitis
• Laparotomy—advised for tissue biopsy; perform biliary decompression; be prepared to excise mass lesions, remove choleliths or inspissated bile, and create a biliary–enteric anastomosis.

PATHOLOGIC FINDINGS
• Gross—distended and tortuous bile duct; distended gall bladder; cause is usually obvious; obstruction > 2 weeks old: large, dark green or mahogany colored liver; chronic complete: white or clear bile
• Microscopic—early: biliary epithelial hyperplasia and bile ductule proliferation; chronic: distention of the biliary structures; devitalized biliary epithelium; necrotic debris

and suppurative inflammation within bile ducts; periportal accumulations of neutrophils, lymphocytes, and plasma cells; periportal edema; and multifocal parenchymal necrosis

TREATMENT

APPROPRIATE HEALTH CARE
Inpatient—surgical intervention for suspected obstruction

NURSING CARE
• Fluid therapy—depends on underlying condition (see Pancreatitis); rehydrate and provide maintenance fluids before general anesthesia and surgical intervention; judiciously supplement polyionic fluids with potassium chloride, depending on electrolyte status
• Water-soluble vitamins—provide parenterally in intravenous fluids; B complex (2 mL/L polyionic fluids)

ACTIVITY
Depends on patient's condition and bleeding tendencies

DIET
• Maintain nitrogen balance.
• Restrict fat—fat malassimilation caused by lack of enteric bile acids

CLIENT EDUCATION
• Inform client that surgical biliary decompression is essential, because obstruction will progress to biliary cirrhosis within 6 weeks.
• Warn client that success of surgical treatment is contingent on the underlying cause and the results of the liver biopsy and tissue and bile cultures.

SURGICAL CONSIDERATIONS
• Surgical exploration—imperative for treatment and determination of underlying cause
• Excise masses and remove any choleliths and inspissated bile.
• Resect gallbladder—with necrotizing cholecystitis
• Biliary–enteric anastomosis—with uncorrectable occlusion, fibrosing pancreatitis, or neoplasia; anastomotic stoma must be at least 2.5 cm wide
• Hypotension and bradycardia—may occur when biliary tree is manipulated; ensure volume expansion; administer colloid administration, if appropriate, place intravenous catheter; ensure availability of emergency drugs (anticholinergics).
• Tissue and bile—submit for aerobic and anaerobic cultures, histology, and cytology; look for bacterial infection or fluke eggs
• Bacterial organisms observed on Wright-Giemsa-type stain—use gram stain to characterize organism and guide antimicrobial selection.

• Sclerosing cholangitis (cats)—may appear like an obstruction; will not respond as expected to biliary decompression; tissue biopsy important for diagnosis

MEDICATIONS

DRUG(S) OF CHOICE
• Antibiotics—before surgery; broad-spectrum antimicrobials for any suppurative infectious process within the biliary structures must be present when surgical manipulations open biliary drainage and damage microcirculation, permitting bacteremia; initially select empirically
• Vitamin K_1—must provide 12–36 hr before surgery (0.5–1.5 mg/kg IM, SC; **CAUTION:** IV may cause anaphylaxis)
• Ursodeoxycholic acid—10–15 mg/kg PO per day; required for postsurgical choleresis; maintain adequate hydration; will not improve fat maldigestion or malabsorption
• Gastrointestinal protectants—agents to reduce gastric acidity, omeprazole (pump inhibitor) or famotidine (H_2-blocker), combined with sucralfate for local cytoprotection if oral medications are tolerated
• Antioxidants—vitamin E (α-tocopherol) at 10–100 IU/kg PO (larger dose for chronic obstruction and suspected vitamin deficiency); for uncorrected chronic condition, use water-soluble vitamin E (acetate form).

CONTRAINDICATIONS
Ursodeoxycholic acid—never use without first providing biliary decompression; a powerful choleretic that could potentiate biliary tree rupture

PRECAUTIONS
N/A

ALTERNATIVE DRUGS
N/A

FOLLOW-UP

PATIENT MONITORING
• Depends on underlying condition
• Total bilirubin values—assess biliary decompression; decline to near normal within 10 days if adequate
• Liver enzyme activities—decline more slowly than does total bilirubin
• CBC—repeat every few days initially; characterize systemic response
• Bile peritonitis—evaluate abdominal girth and abdominal fluid accumulation (palpation, ultrasound preferred, appropriate abdominocentesis)
• Determine necessity for oral treatment with pancreatic enzymes—based on site of biliary–enteric anastomosis; patients with

cholecystojejunostomies more likely to benefit from exogenous enzyme supplementation; cannot rely on trypsin-like immunoactive substance values; evaluate body weight, condition, and feces; steatorrhea suggests fat malassimilation (suspend feces in a small amount of water and examine microscopically for lipid globules; relevant only if patient is on a normal fat content diet).

PREVENTION/AVOIDANCE
N/A

POSSIBLE COMPLICATIONS
• Bile peritonitis
• Re-stenosis of bile duct—if not bypassed at surgery
• Stenosis of biliary–enteric anastomosis stoma
• Severe gastrointestinal hemorrhage during obstruction—from ulceration
• Hemorrhage during surgery
• Pathologic hypotension and bradycardia—vagovagal response during surgery

EXPECTED COURSE AND PROGNOSIS
• Depend on underlying disease
• Prognosis good if fibrosing pancreatitis and pancreatic inflammation resolve; bile duct patency may be restored and biliary–enteric anastomosis may spontaneously close.

MISCELLANEOUS

ASSOCIATED CONDITIONS
• See Causes

AGE-RELATED FACTORS
N/A

ZOONOTIC POTENTIAL
N/A

PREGNANCY
N/A

SEE ALSO
• Cholangitis/Cholangiohepatitis
• See Causes

ABBREVIATIONS
• ALP = alkaline phosphatase
• DIC = disseminated intravascular coagulation
• GGT = gamma–glutamyltransferase
• PIVKA = proteins invoked by vitamin K absence or antagonism
• PT = prothrombin time

Suggested Reading
Center SA. Diseases of the gallbladder and biliary tree. In: Guilford WG, Center SA, Strombeck DR, et al., eds. Strombeck's small animal gastroenterology. 3rd ed. Philadelphia, Saunders 1996:860–888.
Author Sharon A. Center
Consulting Editor Sharon A. Center

BILIOUS VOMITING SYMDROME

 BASICS

OVERVIEW
• Clinical entity associated with chronic intermittent vomiting of bile caused by bile reflux into the stomach
• Normal gastric motility and pressure gradients prevent or quickly remove any refluxed bile before gastric mucosal irritation occurs.
• Bile in the gastric lumen subsequently causes gastric mucosal damage.
• Bile reflux is suspected to be secondary to alterations in normal gastrointestinal motility.
• Clinical signs usually occur early in the morning, suggesting that fasting or inactivity may modify normal motility patterns, resulting in duodenal reflux.

SIGNALMENT
• Commonly observed in dogs; rarely in cats
• Most patients are middle-aged or older.
• No breed, age, or sex predisposition

SIGNS
• Chronic intermittent vomiting of bile associated with an empty stomach
• Generally occur late at night or early in the morning
• May occur daily, but usually are more intermittent
• Between episodes, the patient appears normal in all other respects.
• Results of physical examination are usually unremarkable.

CAUSES & RISK FACTORS
• Cause unknown
• Primary gastric hypomotility suspected to be the underlying cause.
• Conditions causing gastritis or duodenitis are also responsible for altered motility and may cause bile reflux; investigate *Giardia* and inflammatory bowel disease as possible causes.

 DIAGNOSIS

DIFFERENTIAL DIAGNOSIS
• Many gastrointestinal and nongastrointestinal disorders can cause chronic vomiting.
• Exclude *Giardia*—the signs of this disease may mimic those of bilious vomiting.
• Inflammatory bowel disease can cause bile reflux.
• Rule out intestinal obstruction or partial obstructions.

CBC/BIOCHEMISTRY/URINALYSIS
Usually normal

OTHER LABORATORY TESTS
Fecal examination to detect *Giardia* or other parasites

IMAGING
Liquid barium contrast study may reveal delayed gastric emptying or depressed gastric contractions.

DIAGNOSTIC PROCEDURES
• Endoscopic findings are frequently normal.
• Some patients show evidence of bile in the stomach or gastritis in the antral region.
• Endoscopy is useful to rule out structural or inflammatory disease of the stomach and duodenum.

 TREATMENT

• Not a serious debilitating disorder; treat patient symptomatically on an outpatient basis.
• Feeding a late evening meal often resolves clinical signs; food possibly buffers the refluxed bile or may enhance gastric motility.
• If diet modification fails, consider medical treatment.

BILIOUS VOMITING SYMDROME

 MEDICATIONS

DRUGS
- Choices include agents for gastric mucosal protection against the refluxed bile or gastric prokinetic agents to improve motility; often a single evening dose of medication prevents clinical signs.
- Drugs for gastric mucosal protection include cimetidine (5 mg/kg PO), ranitidine (2 mg/kg PO), or sucralfate (1 g/25 kg PO).
- Gastric prokinetic agents include metoclopramide (0.2–0.4 mg/kg PO) and cisapride (0.1 mg/kg PO).
- Erythromycin (1–5 mg/kg PO) also promotes gastric motility and may resolve signs; this drug is inexpensive.

CONTRAINDICATIONS/POSSIBLE INTERACTIONS
- Do not administer gastric prokinetic agents to patients with gastrointestinal obstruction.
- Do not give metoclopramide with concurrent phenothiazine or narcotic administration or to animals with epilepsy; metoclopramide can cause nervousness, anxiety, or depression.
- Cisapride can cause vomiting, diarrhea, or abdominal cramping.
- Erythromycin can cause vomiting.

 FOLLOW-UP

Most patients respond to one of the above treatments, and a clinical response supports the diagnosis; failure to respond suggests another underlying or causative factor.

 MISCELLANEOUS

ASSOCIATED CONDITIONS
Gastroesophageal reflux

SEE ALSO
- Gastric Motility Disorders
- Gastroesophageal Reflux

Suggested Reading

Hall JA, Twedt DC, Burrows CF. Gastric motility in dogs. Part 2. Disorders of gastric motility. Compend Small Anim Med Pract Vet 1990;12:1373–1390.

Author David C. Twedt
Consulting Editors Brett M. Feder and Mitchell A. Crystal

DISEASES

BLASTOMYCOSIS

 BASICS

DEFINITION
A systemic, mycotic infection caused by the soil organism *Blastomyces dermatitidis*

PATHOPHYSIOLOGY
• A small spore (conidia) is shed from the mycelial phase of the organism growing in the soil and inhaled, entering the terminal airway
• At body temperature, the spore becomes a yeast, which initiates the infection in the lungs.
• From this focus of mycotic pneumonia, the yeast disseminates hematogenously throughout the body.
• The immune response to the invading organism produces a pyogranulomatous infiltrate to control the organism.
• The result is organ dysfunction.

SYSTEMS AFFECTED
• Respiratory—85% of affected dogs have lung disease
• Eyes, skin, lymphatic system, and bones—commonly affected
• Brain, testes, prostate, mammary gland, nasal cavity, gums, and vulva—less commonly affected

GENETICS
• No genetic predisposition identified
• Large breeds of dogs most often affected

INCIDENCE/PREVALENCE
• Depends on environmental and soil conditions that favor growth of *Blastomyces*
• Some areas of Wisconsin—incidence in dogs reaches 1,420/100,000 annually

GEOGRAPHIC DISTRIBUTION
Most common along the Mississippi, Ohio, and Tennessee River basins

SIGNALMENT

Species
• Dogs
• Occasionally cats

Breed Predilection
Large breed dogs weighing ≤ 25 kg, especially sporting breeds; may reflect exposure rather than susceptibility

Mean Age and Range
• Dogs—most common 2–4 years of age; uncommon after 7 years of age
• Cats—young to middle-aged

Predominant Sex
Dogs—males

SIGNS

Historical Findings
• Weight loss
• Depressed appetite
• Cough and dyspnea
• Eye inflammation and discharge
• Lameness
• Draining skin lesions

Physical Examination Findings

DOGS
• Fever up to 104.0°F (40°C)—approximately 50% of patients
• Harsh, dry lung sounds associated with increased respiratory effort—common
• Generalized or regional lymphadenopathy with or without skin lesions
• Uveitis with or without secondary glaucoma and conjunctivitis, ocular exudates, and corneal edema
• Lameness—common owing to fungal osteomyelitis
• Testicular enlargement and prostatomegaly—occasionally seen

Cats
• Increased respiratory effort
• Granulomatous skin lesions

CAUSES
Inhaling fungal spores

RISK FACTORS
• Wet environment—fosters growth of the fungus; banks of rivers, streams, and lakes or in swamps; most affected dogs live within 400 m of water.
• Exposure to recently excavated areas

 DIAGNOSIS

DIFFERENTIAL DIAGNOSIS
• Respiratory signs—bacterial pneumonia, neoplasia, heart failure, or other fungal infection
• Lymph node enlargement—similar to lymphosarcoma
• The combination of respiratory disease with eye, bone, and skin involvement in a young dog suggests the diagnosis.

CBC/BIOCHEMISTRY/URINALYSIS
• CBC changes reflect mild to moderate inflammation.
• High serum globulins with borderline low albumin concentrations in dogs with chronic infections
• Hypercalcemia in some dogs secondary to the granulomatous changes
• Blastomyces yeasts can be found in the urine of dogs with prostatic involvement.

OTHER LABORATORY TESTS
AGID—useful for making a diagnosis if organisms cannot be found on cytology or histopathology; positive test strongly supports diagnosis, with a specificity of > 90%; negative tests common in dogs with early infection

IMAGING

Radiographs
• Lungs—essential for diagnosis and prognosis
• Generalized interstitial to nodular infiltrate
• Tracheobronchial lymphadenopathy—common
• Changes—inconsistent with bacterial pneumonia; may resemble metastatic tumors, especially hemangiosarcoma
• Focal bone lesions—lytic and proliferative; can be mistaken for osteosarcoma

DIAGNOSTIC PROCEDURES
• Cytology of lymph node aspirates, tracheal wash fluid, or impression smears of draining skin lesions—best method for diagnosis
• Histopathology of bone biopsies or enucleated blind eyes—identify the organism
• Organisms—usually plentiful in the tissues; may be scarce in tracheal washes if there is no productive cough

PATHOLOGIC FINDINGS
• Lesions—pyogranulomatous with many thick walled, budding yeast; occasionally very fibrous with few organisms found
• Lungs with large amounts of inflammatory infiltrate do not collapse when the chest is opened.
• Special fungal stains—facilitate finding the organisms

 TREATMENT

APPROPRIATE HEALTH CARE
Usually outpatient with oral itraconazole treatment

NURSING CARE
Severely dyspneic dogs—require an oxygen cage for a minimum of 1 week before lung improvement is sufficient for comfort in room air; many have worsening of lung disease during the first few days of treatment, owing to an increase in the inflammatory response after the *Blastomyces* organisms die and release their contents.

ACTIVITY
Patients with respiratory compromise must be restricted.

DIET

Palatable and high-quality to stimulate the appetite

CLIENT EDUCATION

Inform owner that treatment is costly and requires a minimum of 60–90 days.

SURGICAL CONSIDERATIONS

Removal of an abscessed lung lobe may be required when medical treatment cannot resolve the infection.

MEDICATIONS

DRUGS OF CHOICE

Itraconazole

• Dogs—5 mg/kg PO q12h with a fat-rich meal, such as canned dog food, for the first 3 days to achieve a therapeutic blood concentration as soon as possible; then reduce to once a day
• Cats—5 mg/kg PO q12h; open the 100-mg capsules containing pellets and mix with palatable food
• Treat for a minimum of 60 days or for 1 month after all signs of disease have disappeared.

CONTRAINDICATIONS

Corticosteroids—usually contraindicated because the anti-inflammatory effects allow uninhibited proliferation of the organisms; patients with previous steroid therapy require a longer duration of treatment; for dogs with life-threatening dyspnea, dexamethasone (0.2 mg/kg daily) may be lifesaving when given in conjunction with itraconazole treatment; discontinue steroids as soon as possible

PRECAUTIONS

Itraconazole Toxicity

• Anorexia—most common sign; attributed to liver toxicity; monitor serum ALT monthly for duration of treatment or when anorexia occurs; temporarily discontinue drug for patients with anorexia and ALT activities > 200; after appetite improves, restart at half the previously used dose.
• Ulcerative dermatitis—seen in some dogs; the result of vasculitis; dose-related condition; temporarily discontinue drug; when ulcers have resolved, restart at half the previously used dose.

POSSIBLE INTERACTIONS

For humans, itraconazole is contraindicated with terfenadine and cisapride.

ALTERNATIVE DRUGS

• Amphotericin B—0.5 mg/kg IV every other day in dogs that cannot take oral medication or that do not respond to itraconazole (see Histoplasmosis); use the lipid complex for dogs with renal dysfunction that cannot take itraconazole
• Ketoconazole—10 mg/kg PO q12h; cheaper alternative to itraconazole; lower response rate and higher recurrence rate

FOLLOW-UP

PATIENT MONITORING

Serum chemistry—monthly to monitor for hepatic toxicity or if anorexia develops

Thoracic Radiographs

• Determine duration of treatment
• Considerable permanent changes in the lungs after the infection has resolved may occur, making determination of persistent active disease difficult.
• At 60 days of treatment—if active lung disease is seen, continue treatment for 30 days
• At 90 days of treatment—if the same as day 60, changes are residual effects of inactive disease; if better than day 60, continue treatment for 30 days, if worse than day 60, continue treatment for 30 days more, then re-radiograph.
• At 120 days of treatment—re-radiograph. If worse, continue treatment for further 30 days and then re-radiograph. If inactive disease, continue treatment for 30 more days and then stop.

PREVENTION/AVOIDANCE

• Location of environmental growth of *Blastomyces* organisms unknown; thus difficult to avoid exposure; restricting exposure to lakes and streams could be done but is not very practical.
• Dogs that recover from the infection are probably immune to reinfection.

POSSIBLE COMPLICATIONS

Death

EXPECTED COURSE AND PROGNOSIS

• Death—25% of dogs die during the first week of treatment; early diagnosis improves chance of survival.
• Severity of lung involvement and invasion into the brain affect prognosis
• Recurrence—about 20% of dogs; usually within 3–6 months after completion of treatment, even with 60–90 days of treatment; may occur up to 15 months after treatment; a second course of itraconazole treatment will cure most patients; drug resistance to itraconazole has not been observed

✓
MISCELLANEOUS

ASSOCIATED CONDITIONS

N/A

AGE-RELATED FACTORS

N/A

ZOONOTIC POTENTIAL

• Not spread from animals to people, except through bite wounds; inoculation of organisms from dog bites has occurred.
• Avoid cuts during necropsy of infected dogs and avoid needle sticks when aspirating lesions.
• Warn clients that blastomycosis is acquired from an environmental source and that they may have been exposed at the same time as the patient; common source exposure has been documented in duck and coon hunters; the incidence in dogs is 10 times that in humans
• Encourage clients with respiratory and skin lesions to inform their physicians that they may have been exposed to blastomycosis.

PREGNANCY

No teratogenic effects of itraconazole at therapeutic doses in rats and mice; embryotoxicity found at high doses; no dog or cat studies; one dog started on itraconazole halfway through her pregnancy delivered a normal litter.

SYNONYM

N/A

SEE ALSO

N/A

ABBREVIATIONS

• AGID = agar gel immunodiffusion
• ALT = alanine transferase

Suggested Reading

Krawiec DR, McKiernan BC, Twardock AR, et al. Use of amphotericin B lipid complex for treatment of blastomycosis in dogs. J Am Vet Med Assoc 1996;209:2073–2075.

Legendre AM, Rohrbach BW, Toal RL, et al. Treatment of blastomycosis with itraconazole in 112 dogs. J Vet Intern Med 1996;10:365–371.

Legendre AM. Blastomycosis. In: Greene CE, ed., Infectious diseases of the dog and cat. Philadelphia: Saunders, 1998:371–377.

Author Alfred M. Legendre
Consulting Editor Stephen C. Barr

BLEPHARITIS

 BASICS

DEFINITION
• Inflammation of the outer (skin) and middle portion (muscle, connective tissue, and glands) of the eyelid, usually with secondary inflammation of the palpebral conjunctiva
• Chronic—anterior or posterior, based on the site of predominant involvement • Anterior—most commonly associated with bacterial infection or self-trauma • Posterior—disorders of the meibomian glands

PATHOPHYSIOLOGY
• Same as virtually every condition that affects the skin in general • Mechanisms of inflammation—immune mediated, infectious, endocrine mediated, self- and external trauma, parasitic, radiation, and nutritional.
• Inflammatory response often exaggerated because eyelid conjunctiva is rich in mast cells and densely vascularized • Meimbomian gland dysfuncion—common; bacterial lipases alter meimbomian lipids so they plug the gland, they also produce irritating fatty acids, enhance bacterial growth and destabilize the tear film.

SYSTEMS AFFECTED
Ophthalmic

SIGNALMENT
See Causes

SIGNS
• Serous, mucoid, or mucopurulent ocular discharge • Blepharospasm • Eyelid hyperemia, edema, and thickening • Pruritus • Excoriation • Depigmentation—skin; hair • Alopecia • Swollen, cream-colored meibomian glands • Elevated, pinpoint meibomian gland orifices • Abscesses • Scales and crusts • Papules or pustules • Single or multiple nodular hyperemic swellings • Concurrent conjunctivitis or keratitis

CAUSES
Congenital
• Eyelid abnormalities—may promote self-trauma or moist dermatitis • Prominent nasal folds and medial trichiasis lower lid entropion—shih tzus, Pekingese, English bulldogs, lhasa apsos, pugs, Persian and Himalayan cats • Distichia— shih tzus, pugs, golden retrievers, Labrador retrievers, poodles, English bulldogs • Ectopic cilia • Lateral lid entropion—various dog breeds (shar peis and chow chows); adult cats (rare) • Lagophthalmos—brachycephalic dogs; Persian, Himalayan, and Burmese cats • Deep medial canthal pockets—dolichocephalic dogs • Dermoids—rottweilers, dachshunds, and others; Burmese cats

Allergic
• Type I (immediate)—atopy; food; insect bite; inhalant; staph hypersensitivity • Type II (cytotoxic)—pemphigus; pemphigoid; drug eruption • Type III (immune complex)—SLE; staph hypersensitivity; drug eruption • Type IV (cell mediated)—contact and flea bite hypersensitivity; drug eruption

Bacterial
• Hordeolum—localized abscess of eyelid glands, usually staphylococcal; may be external (sty in young dogs, involving glands of Zeis) or internal (in old dogs, involves one or more meibomian glands) • Generalized bacterial blepharitis and meibomianitis—usually staph or strep • Pyogranulomas • Staph hypersensitivity—young and old dogs

Neoplastic
• Sebaceous adenomas and adenocarcinomas—originate from meibomian gland • Squamous cell carcinoma—white cats • Mast cell—may masquerade as swollen, hyperemic lesion

Other
• External trauma—eyelid lacerations; thermal or chemical burns • Mycotic—dermatophytosis; systemic fungal granulomas • Parasitic—demodicosis; sarcoptic mange; *Cuterebra* and *Notoedres cati* • Chalazia (singular, chalazion)—usually sterile, yellow-white, painless eyelid swellings caused by a granulomatous inflammatory response to escape of meibum into the surrounding eyelid tissue • Nutritional—zinc-responsive dermatosis (Siberian huskies, Alaskan malamutes, puppies); fatty acid deficiency • Endocrine—hypothyroidism (dogs); hyperadrenocorticism (dogs); diabetic dermatosis • Viral—chronic blepharitis secondary to FHV-1 • Irritant—topical ocular drug reaction; nicotine smoke in environment; after parotid duct transposition • Familial canine dermatomyositis—collies and Shetland sheepdogs • Nodular granulomatous episclerokeratitis—fibrous histiocytoma and collie granuloma; collies; may affect the eyelids, cornea or conjunctiva • Eosinophilic granuloma—cats; may affect eyelids, cornea, or conjunctiva • Eyelid contact with purulent exudate (tear burn), conjunctivitis, keratitis, dry eye, dacryocystitis, and orbital disease after radiotherapy • Idiopathic—particularly in cats with chronic idiopathic conjunctivitis

RISK FACTORS
• Breed predisposition to congenital eyelid abnormalities eg. entropion, ectropion etc.
• Outdoor animals—traumatic
• Hypothyroidism—may promote chronic bacterial disease in dogs
• Canine seborrhea—may promote chronic generalized meibomianitis

 DIAGNOSIS

DIFFERENTIAL DIAGNOSIS
Clinical signs are diagnostic.

CBC/BIOCHEMISTRY /URINALYSIS
Usually nondiagnostic unless metabolic cause (e.g., diabetic dermatosis)

OTHER LABORATORY TESTS
• Indicated for suspected systemic disorder
• Consider tests for hypothyroidism.

DIAGNOSTIC PROCEDURES
If possible, avoid topical anesthetic or fluorescein before obtaining culture.
• Cytology—deep skin scrapings; conjunctival scrapings; expressed exudate from meibomian glands and pustules • Dermatophyte culture—deep skin scrapings • Wood's light evaluation—skin • KOH preparation—skin scrapings • Aerobic bacterial culture and sensitivity—exudate from skin; conjunctiva; expressed exudate from meibomian glands and pustules; often will not recover staph from patients with chronic meibomianitis and suspected staph hypersensitivity • IFA or PCR for FHV-1 and chlamydia—conjunctival scrapings from cats with primary conjunctivitis or keratitis • Eye examination—potential inciting cause; corneal ulcer; foreign body; distichia; ectopic cilia; dry eye • Ancillary ocular tests—fluorescein application; Schirmer tear test. • Thorough medical history and dermatologic examination—help identify generalized dermatologic disease • Full-thickness wedge biopsy of eyelid—histologic evaluation • Special tests—direct immuno-fluorescence (autoimmune disease); intradermal skin testing (hypersensitivity-induced disease); RAST and ELISA (atopy); food-elimination diet (allergy)

PATHOLOGIC FINDINGS
• Routine histopathology often nondiagnostic in chronic disease • Wedge biopsy—may be unrewarding; carefully select patients based on history, ophthalmic exam, and response to medical therapy.

 TREATMENT

APPROPRIATE HEALTH CARE
See Nursing Care

NURSING CARE
• Secondary disease—treat primary disease
• Suspected self-trauma—elizabethen collar
• Topical gentamicin, neomycin, terramycin, antiviral medication (e.g., trifluridine solution), and most ointments—may cause an irritant blepharoconjunctivitis (rare); withdrawal of agent may resolve condition

• Cleanse eyelids—to remove crusts; warm compresses applied for 5–15 min 3–4 times daily avoiding ocular surfaces; saline, lactated Ringer solution, or a commercial ocular cleansing agent (e.g., Eye Scrub); must clip periocular hair short

DIET
Only with food allergy–induced disease

CLIENT EDUCATION
• Warn client that most patients cannot be cured but that the condition often can be controlled medically. • Inform client that there is no cure for FHV-1 and that clinical signs often recur when the animal is stressed. • Instruct owner to keep the restraint collar on at all times.

SURGICAL CONSIDERATIONS
• Temporary everting eyelid sutures—spastic entropion; or in puppies before permanent surgical correction • Repair eyelid lacerations • Lancing—large abscesses only; lance and curette hordeola that are resistant to medical treatment and chalazia that have hardened and come to a point causing keratitis; manually express infected meibomian secretions.

MEDICATIONS

DRUGS OF CHOICE

Antibiotics
• Systemic—generally required for effective treatment of bacterial eyelid infections; may try amoxicillin–clavulanic acid, or cephalexin; 20 mg/kg q8h • Topical—may try neomycin, polymyxin B, and bacitracin or chloramphenicol

Congenital
• Topical antibiotic ointment—q6–12h; until surgery is performed; prevent frictional rubbing of eyelid hairs or cilia on the ocular surface • Saline, lactated Ringer solution, or ocular irrigant—regularly flush deep medial canthal pocket debris

External Trauma
• Topical antibiotic ointment—q6–12h; for spastic entropion secondary to pain and blepharospasm; reduce friction until entropion is surgically relieved • Systemic antibiotics indicated

Allergic
• Staph hypersensitivity blepharitis—systemic broad-spectrum antibiotics and systemic corticosteroids (prednisolone, 0.5 mg/kg q12h for 3–5 days, then taper); many patients respond to systemic corticosteroids alone. • Affected meibomian glands—oral tetracycline (15–20 mg/kg PO q8h) or doxycycline (3–5 mg/kg PO q12h) for at least 3 weeks (lipophilic and cause decreased production of bacterial lipases and irritating fatty acids); topical polymyxin B

and neomycin with 0.1% dexamethasone (q6–8h to the eye) • Failure of treatment—may try injections of homologous or commercial *Staphylococcus aureus* bacterin (Staphage Lysate) • *Propionibacterium acnes* immunotherapy—investigational; of unknown value • Eyelid lesions associated with puppy strangles—usually benefit from treatment of the generalized condition

Bacterial
• Based on culture and sensitivity testing • While results are pending—topical polymyxin B and neomycin with 0.1% dexamethasone ointment (q4–6h); plus a systemic broad-spectrum antibiotic

Mycotic
Microsporium canis infection—usually self-limiting; treatment includes 2% miconazole cream, 1% clotrimazole cream, or diluted povidone-iodine solution (1 part to 300 parts saline) applied q12–24h for at least 6 weeks; do not use lotions.

Parasitic
• Demodicosis—localized disease, diluted amitraz (1 part amitraz to 9 parts mineral oil; Mitaban) once every 3 days for 4–8 weeks; fairly safe around the eyes (see Demodicosis) • Notoedres infection—lime sulfur dips • Sarcoptic mange—same as for generalized disease

Idiopathic
Clinical signs often controlled with topical polymyxin B and neomycin with 0.1% dexamethasone (q8–24h or as needed); occasionally may also need systemic prednisolone (0.5 mg/kg q12h for 3–5days, then taper) and/or a systemic antibiotic

CONTRAINDICATIONS
• Topical corticosteroids—do not use with corneal ulceration • Cats—many patients with presumed idiopathic blepharoconjunctivitis actually have FHV-1 infection; topical and systemic corticosteroids may exacerbate the infection • Oral tetracycline and doxycycline—do not use in puppies and kittens

PRECAUTIONS
Ectoparasitism—wear gloves; do not contact ocular surfaces with the drug; apply artificial tear ointment to the eye for protection.

POSSIBLE INTERACTIONS
Staphylococcal bacterin for staph hypersensitivity—anaphylactic reaction (rare)

FOLLOW-UP

PATIENT MONITORING
• Depends on cause • Bacterial—treated with systemic and topical treatment for at least 3 weeks; should notice improvement within 3–7 days • Most common causes of treatment

failure—use of subinhibitory antibiotic concentrations; failure to correct one or more predisposing factors; stopping medications too soon

PREVENTION/AVOIDANCE
Depend on cause

POSSIBLE COMPLICATIONS
• Cicatricial lid contracture—results in trichiasis, ectropion, or lagophthalmos • Spastic entropion—because of blepharospasm and pain • Inability to open eyelids—owing to matting of discharge and hair • Qualitative tear film deficiency—result of loss of proper meibum secretion • Recurrence of bacterial infection or FHV-1 blepharoconjunctivitis

EXPECTED COURSE AND PROGNOSIS
Depends on cause

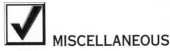

MISCELLANEOUS

ZOONOTIC POTENTIAL
• Dermatophytosis • Sarcoptic mange

SEE ALSO
• Conjunctivitis—Cats • Conjunctivitis—Dogs • Epiphora • Keratitis Nonulcerative • Keratitis, Ulcerative • Red Eye

ABBREVIATIONS
• ELISA = enzyme-linked immunoadsorbent assay • FHV-1 = feline herpesvirus type 1 • PCR = polymerase chain reaction • RAST = radioallergosorbent test • SLE = systemic lupus erythematosus

Suggested Reading
Bedford PCG. Diseases and surgery of the canine eyelid. In: Gelatt KN, ed. Veterinary ophthamology, 3rd ed. Philadelphia: Lippincott Williams and Wilkins 1995:535–568

Author Terri L. McCalla

Consulting Editor Paul E. Miller

BLOOD TRANSFUSION REACTIONS

BASICS

OVERVIEW
• Classified as acute or delayed, immune mediated or not immune-mediated
• Severe reactions usually occur during or shortly after transfusion.

SIGNALMENT
• Dogs and cats
• No sex predilection
• All ages affected

SIGNS

Acute Hemolytic Reaction
• Restlessness
• Fever
• Tachycardia
• Vomiting
• Tremors
• Weakness
• Incontinence
• Collapse
• Shock
• Oliguria
• Loss of transfusion efficacy

Delayed Hemolytic Reaction
Loss of transfusion efficacy—usually no clinical signs

Acute Nonhemolytic Reaction
• Anaphylactic reaction—fever, urticaria, erythema, and pruritus
• Transfusion of contaminated blood—acute septicemia, fever, and shock
• Circulatory overload/rapid transfusion—vomiting, distended jugular veins, dyspnea, cough, cyanosis, and congestive heart failure
• Citrate toxicity—hypocalcemia, myocardial depression, and weakness
• Hyperammonemia—encephalopathy
• Hypothermia—shivering and impaired platelet function

CAUSES & RISK FACTORS
Purebred cats and previously transfused dogs have a higher risk of severe transfusion reaction than other animals.

Acute Hemolysis
• Blood group mismatch
• Transfusion of damaged and hemolyzed RBCs (after excessive heating, freezing, or mechanical damage)

Delayed Hemolysis
Immune reaction to minor red cell antigens; occurs after 3–14 days

Acute Nonhemolytic Reaction
• Anaphylaxis and immune reaction to donor leukocytes, major histocompatibility complex antigens, or plasma antigens, resulting in release of inflammatory mediators and pyrogens
• Transfusion of contaminated blood—lack of aseptic collection and storage conditions
• Circulatory overload—rapid transfusion; excessive volume of blood in small animal or in animal with heart failure or oliguric renal failure
• Citrate toxicity—after circulatory overload, particularly in small animal or in animal with hepatopathy
• Hyperammonemia—high ammonia concentration in stored blood; important only for animal with hepatopathy
• Hypothermia—rapid transfusion of refrigerated blood to small or already hypothermic animal

Delayed Nonhemolytic Reaction
Transmission of blood-borne disease—use of infected donor

DIAGNOSIS

DIFFERENTIAL DIAGNOSIS
• Hemolysis—rule out ongoing fulminant hemolytic disease and use of hemolyzed blood
• Fever, hypotension—rule out underlying infectious and inflammatory diseases

CBC/BIOCHEMISTRY/URINALYSIS
Hemoglobinemia, leukocytosis, bilirubinemia, hemoglobinuria, and bilirubinuria

OTHER LABORATORY TESTS
• Repeat cross-match to confirm incompatibility.
• Bacterial culture or gram staining of contaminated blood may reveal organism.

IMAGING
N/A

DIAGNOSTIC PROCEDURES
N/A

TREATMENT
• Immediately discontinue transfusion.
• Administer fluids to maintain blood pressure and renal blood flow; for severe hypotension, use lactated Ringer's solution (50–90 mL/kg/h to effect).
• Additional supportive therapy for DIC, shock, or thromboembolism (see appropriate chapters)

BLOOD TRANSFUSION REACTIONS

MEDICATIONS

DRUGS
• For hemolysis—rapid-acting corticosteroid, such as prednisolone sodium succinate (10–30 mg/kg once) or dexamethasone sodium phosphate (6–15 mg/kg once); heparin (75 U/kg SC q6h; not for use in bleeding animals)
• For urticaria, fever—diphenhydramine (1–2 mg/kg); prednisolone (2–4 mg/kg); continue transfusion afterward, if clinically indicated.
• For septicemia—broad-spectrum IV antibiotics while bacterial culture results are pending (e.g., cephalothin/gentamycin); heparin

CONTRAINDICATIONS/POSSIBLE INTERACTIONS
None

FOLLOW-UP

PATIENT MONITORING
• Check attitude, temperature, vital signs, lung sounds, PCV/total solids, and plasma color before, during, and after transfusion.
• If pulmonary thromboembolism is suspected, check chest radiographs and arterial blood gases frequently

PREVENTION/AVOIDANCE
• Carefully record any transfusion reaction in the patient's medical file.
• Adhere to standard transfusion protocols (e.g., blood typing; cross-matching; use of healthy donors; and appropriate collection, storage, and administration techniques).

POSSIBLE COMPLICATIONS
• Fulminant hemolysis may cause acute renal failure, pulmonary thromboembolism, multiorgan thromboembolism, DIC, and cardiac arrhythmias.
• Volume overload may cause heart failure.
• Cardiac arrest

EXPECTED COURSE AND PROGNOSIS
• Acute course in most animals
• Prognosis good in stable animals, guarded in severely ill animals or when not recognized early
• Cats with type B blood receiving mismatched blood have the worst prognosis

MISCELLANEOUS

ABBREVIATIONS
• DIC = disseminated intravascular coagulation
• PCV = packed cell volume

Suggested Reading
Stone MS, Cotter SM. Practical guidelines for transfusion therapy. In: Kirk RW, Bonagura JD, eds. Current veterinary therapy XI. Philadelphia, Saunders: 1992:475–479.
Author Jörg Bücheler
Consulting Editor Susan M. Cotter

BORDETELLOSIS—CATS

BASICS

OVERVIEW
A contagious bacterial disease of cats that primarily causes respiratory abnormalities

SIGNALMENT
• Most severe in kittens < 6 weeks old and kittens living in less than ideal hygienic conditions
• Occurs at all ages and often with pre-existing, subclinical airway disease (e.g., feline herpesvirus and calicivirus infections)
• No breed or gender predilection recognized

SIGNS
• May be or nonexistent, mild, or severe (e.g., kittens with life-threatening pneumonia); usually begin about 5 days after exposure to infecting agent
• Bacterial agent—spreads rapidly from seemingly healthy cats to others in the same environment
• Fever, sneezing, nasal discharge, mandibular lymphadenopathy, and spontaneous or induced cough—characteristic of uncompli-cated disease

Severe Disease
• May note constant, low-grade, or fluctuating fever (39.4–40°C; 103–104°F)
• Appetite—severely affected
• Cough—may be noted; moist and productive
• Nasal discharge
• Lethargy
• Anorexia
• Dyspnea
• Lung sounds—often normal; may detect increased intensity of normal sounds, crackles, or (less frequently) wheezes

CAUSES & RISK FACTORS
• *Bordetella bronchiseptica*—a small, aerobic gram-negative coccobacillus
• Coexisting subclinical airway disease—congenital anomalies; chronic bronchitis

DIAGNOSIS

DIFFERENTIAL DIAGNOSIS
• Specific diagnosis difficult; clinical signs mimic those seen with other respiratory disease agents.
• Several agents may be involved concur-rently, which adds to the confusion of signs.
• See Cough

CBC/BIOCHEMISTRY/URINALYSIS
• Neutrophilic leukocytosis with a left shift—frequently found with severe pneumonia
• Serum chemistry profile and urinalysis—usually normal

OTHER LABORATORY TESTS
• Oropharyngeal swab specimens—identify *B. bronchiseptica* infection
• Isolation of the bacterium—with active clinical disease, relatively easy; with chronic carrier state, often few organisms are shed.

IMAGING
Thoracic radiographs—unremarkable with uncomplicated disease; useful for ruling out noninfectious causes; may demonstrate an interstitial and alveolar lung pattern with a cranioventral distribution typical of bacterial pneumonia, a diffuse interstitial lung pattern typical of viral pneumonia, or a mixed lung pattern (combination of alveolar, interstitial, and peribronchial lung patterns)

DIAGNOSTIC PROCEDURES
Endotracheal tracheal wash or tracheobronchial lavage via bronchoscopy—suspected severe disease; identify antimicrobial sensitivity pattern; helps develop an effective treatment plan

TREATMENT
• Outpatient—strongly recommended for uncomplicated disease
• Inpatient—strongly recommended for complicated disease and/or pneumonia
• Fluid therapy—with complicated disease and/or pneumonia
• Enforced rest—for at least 14–21 days with uncomplicated disease; for at least the duration of radiographic evidence of pneumonia

MEDICATIONS

DRUGS
• Tetracycline (10 mg/kg PO q8h), doxycycline (3–5 mg/kg PO, IV q12h or 10 mg/kg PO q24h), or amoxicillin/clavulanic acid (62.5 mg/cat PO q12h) for 10–14 days
• Antimicrobial therapy—may continue for at least 10 days beyond radiographic resolution

CONTRAINDICATIONS/POSSIBLE INTERACTIONS
Tetracycline and related drugs—may induce a drug fever

FOLLOW-UP

PATIENT MONITORING
• Uncomplicated disease—should respond to treatment in 10–14 days; question diagnosis of uncomplicated disease if respiratory signs exist 14 days or more after initiating treatment
• Severe disease—repeat thoracic radiography until at least 14 days beyond resolution of all clinical signs

PREVENTION/AVOIDANCE
• Shedding of *B. bronchiseptica* in respiratory secretions of asymptomatic carriers—accounts for the persistence of disease in catteries, animal shelters, boarding facilities, and veterinary hospitals
• Bacterial vaccine

POSSIBLE COMPLICATIONS
N/A

EXPECTED COURSE AND PROGNOSIS
• Uncomplicated disease without treatment—natural course, 10–14 days
• Severe disease—typical course, 2–6 weeks
• Death—severe pneumonia that affects multiple lung lobes
• Seroconversion of kittens in infected environments—at 7–10 weeks of age
• Affected cats may shed *B. bronchiseptica* for at least 19 weeks after infection.

MISCELLANEOUS

Suggested Reading
Coutts AJ, Dawson S, Binns S, et al. Studies on natural transmission of *Bordetella bron-chiseptica* in cats. Vet Microbiology 1996;48:19–27.
Hoskins JD, Williams J, Rohde KR, et al. The prevalence of feline *Bordetella bron-chiseptica* in the respiratory tract. (abst) J Vet Intern Med 1997;11:133.
Jacobs AA, Chalmers WS, Pasman J, et al. Fe-line bordetellosis: challenge and vaccine studies. Vet Rec 1993;133:260–263.
Author Johnny D. Hoskins
Consulting Editor Eleanor Hawkins

BASICS

OVERVIEW
• Results from the ingestion of the preformed *Clostridium botulinum* type C neurotoxin contained in carrion and spoiled foodstuff (e.g., raw meat)
• Botulinal neurotoxin inhibits acetylcholine release at neuromuscular junctions and autonomic cholinergic synapses, resulting in diffuse neuromuscular blockade and autonomic dysfunction

SIGNALMENT
• Dogs
• Cats—susceptible experimentally; no natural cases reported

SIGNS

Historical Findings
• Onset of signs appear a few hours to 6 days after toxin ingestion.
• Other dogs of the household, neighborhood, or kennel may be affected.
• Acute hind limb weakness that rapidly ascends to the trunk, front limbs, neck, and muscles innervated by the cranial nerves
• Gait—may appear stiff and short-strided (but not ataxic) until recumbency develops (usually within 12–24 hr)

Physical Examination Findings
• Generalized lower motor neuron weakness to tetraplegia—hypotonia or atonia; hyporeflexia or areflexia
• Tail—tone and movements (wagging) preserved
• Patient remains alert with normal pain perception.
• Cranial nerve dysfunction—dysphagia with pseudoptyalism; weak voice; droopy face with poor eyelid closure; poor jaw and tongue tone; megaesophagus with regurgitation
• Autonomic—mydriasis with decreased pupillary light reflexes; ileus or constipation; urine retention or frequent voiding of small volumes; decreased lacrimation
• Muscle atrophy—may be marked after 5–7 days

CAUSES & RISK FACTORS
Amount of ingested toxin determines severity of disease, from mild paraparesis to tetraplegia with respiratory muscle paralysis.

DIAGNOSIS

DIFFERENTIAL DIAGNOSIS
• Coonhound paralysis (idiopathic polyradiculoneuritis)—may follow a raccoon bite, systemic illness, or vaccination; cause often unknown; cranial nerve involvement usually limited to facial and pharyngeal/laryngeal paresis; no autonomic signs; diffuse hyperesthesia may be present; lumbar CSF protein may be high; diffuse denervation potentials on electromyography (after 5–7 days)
• Tick bite paralysis—in U.S.: cranial nerve involvement unusual or mild; no autonomic signs; rapid recovery after tick removal or insecticide treatment (within 24–72 hr); in Australia: cranial nerve and autonomic involvement; more severe signs that may continue after tick removal
• Myasthenia gravis—exercise-induced weakness leading to collapse; rapid improvement after a short period of rest; megaesophagus common but other cranial nerve involvement limited to moderate facial and pharyngeal/laryngeal paresis; normal spinal reflexes if patient is ambulatory

CBC/BIOCHEMISTRY/URINALYSIS
Usually normal

OTHER LABORATORY TESTS
Identify organism—in ingested material, serum, vomit, and feces; by neutralization test in small rodents or in vitro tests (measure toxin antigenicity rather than toxicity)

IMAGING
Thoracic radiographs—may reveal megaesophagus and aspiration pneumonia

DIAGNOSTIC PROCEDURES
EMG—usually no or few denervation potentials (more numerous during the recovery phase); reduced amplitude of motor unit; evoked potentials

PATHOLOGIC FINDINGS
None

TREATMENT
• Respiratory difficulties—intensive care with maximal monitoring capabilities
• Swallowing difficulties—alimentation by nasogastric tube; ensure presence of peristalsis
• Turn patient frequently and use good padding to prevent pressure sores.
• Passive and active physiotherapy—minimize tendon contraction and muscle atrophy

MEDICATIONS

DRUGS
• Type C or polyvalent containing type C antitoxin—may not be available; not effective after toxin has penetrated the nerve endings but could prevent further binding if absorption is still occurring
• Laxative and enemas—if recent ingestion
• Antibiotics—no benefit; gastrointestinal colonization does not occur.
• Neuromuscular potentiators (e.g., 4-aminopyridine, diaminopyridine, guanidine) and anticholinesterase (e.g., neostigmine) have not been proven to be effective or safe.

CONTRAINDICATIONS/POSSIBLE INTERACTIONS
Aminoglycosides, procaine penicillin, tetracyclines, phenothiazines, and magnesium—may potentiate neuromuscular blockade

FOLLOW-UP

PATIENT MONITORING
• Monitor intensively during progressive stage to assist patient with developing respiratory difficulties.
• Meticulously manage the airway in patients with ventilatory support.

PREVENTION/AVOIDANCE
• Prevent access to carrion.
• Thoroughly cook food fed to dogs.

POSSIBLE COMPLICATIONS
• Respiratory failure and death in severe cases
• Aspiration pneumonia from regurgitation or false deglutition
• Keratoconjunctivitis sicca
• Prolonged recumbency—pulmonary atelectasia and infection; decubital sores; urine scalding

EXPECTED COURSE AND PROGNOSIS
• Maximum severity of signs usually reached within 12–24 hr
• Signs disappear in the reverse order in which they appeared.
• Complete recovery occur within 1–3 weeks

MISCELLANEOUS

SEE ALSO
• Coonhound Paralysis (Idiopathic Polyradiculoneuritis)
• Myasthenia Gravis
• Tick Bite Paralysis

ABBREVIATIONS
• CSF = cerebrospinal fluid
• EMG = electromyography

Suggested Reading
Barsanti JA. Botulism. In: Greene CE, ed. Infectious diseases of the dog and cat. 2nd ed. Philadelphia: Saunders, 1998:263–267.
Author Andrée D. Quesnel
Consulting Editor Joane M. Parent

DISEASES

BRACHIAL PLEXUS AVULSION

BASICS

OVERVIEW
• Trauma with traction and/or abduction of the forelimb causes avulsion of nerve rootlets from their spinal cord attachment.
• Ventral (motor) roots are more susceptible than are dorsal (sensory) roots.
• Most common forelimb neurologic injury of small animals
• Rule out nerve root avulsion in traumatized animals not able to bear weight on a forelimb, especially before surgical repair of orthopedic injuries.

SIGNALMENT
• Dogs and cats
• No age, sex, or breed predilection

SIGNS
• Depend on the extent and distribution of rootlet damage
• Motor signs—weakness to complete paralysis (ventral root avulsion)
• Sensory signs—decreased to absent pain perception (dorsal root avulsion)
• Muscle atrophy—begins within a week of injury
• Complete—spinal nerves C5 to T2; most common; combines cranial and caudal avulsion deficits
• Cranial—spinal nerves C5 to C7; causes loss of shoulder movements, elbow flexion (dropped elbow), and analgesia of the craniodorsal scapula and medial forearm; if roots C8 to T2 preserved: weight-bearing remains almost normal; hemiplegia of the diaphragm may be seen by fluoroscopy (phrenic nerve roots C5 to C7).
• Caudal—spinal nerves C7 to T2; causes inability to bear weight, with knuckling over of the dorsum of the paw; if C5 to C7 spared: limb held in a flexed position and analgesia distal to the elbow (except for a small area on medial aspect of forearm); T1 to T2 involvement: causes an ipsilateral partial Horner syndrome (anisocoria only) and lack of ipsilateral contraction of the cutaneous trunci reflex (contraction present contralaterally)
• Bilateral—rarely encountered after a significant fall with sternal landing

CAUSES & RISK FACTORS
Trauma—road accident; hung by foot; fall

DIAGNOSIS

DIFFERENTIAL DIAGNOSIS
• Brachial plexus trauma without avulsion—rare; temporary deficit owing to root contusion
• Brachial plexus tumor—usually chronic onset
• Brachial plexus neuritis—rare, bilateral deficits
• Focal lateralized spinal cord tumor or ischemic myelopathy owing to fibrocartilaginous emboli—mild deficits of the ipsilateral hindlimb and contralateral forelimb
• Pure radial nerve paralysis caused by fracture of the humerus or first rib—no nerve root sign

CBC/BIOCHEMISTRY/URINALYSIS
Usually normal

OTHER LABORATORY TESTS
N/A

IMAGING
High-definition CT or MRI scan—visualize lesion; rarely needed for diagnosis

DIAGNOSTIC PROCEDURES
• Clinical—history of trauma with sudden onset of typical neurologic deficits
• Define involved spinal nerve roots—map motor and sensory deficits; note signs of Horner syndrome; determine cutaneous trunci reflex
• Electrophysiology (EMG)—shows denervation in affected muscles 5–7 days post-injury; with nerve-conduction studies, may help further define deficits

PATHOLOGIC FINDINGS
• Ventral and dorsal root avulsions—intradurally at the level of root–spinal cord junction (most fragile area, because it lacks protective perineurium)
• Neuroma formation—on the pial surface of the spinal cord

TREATMENT

APPROPRIATE HEALTH CARE
• No specific treatment
• Outcome depends on initial damage.
• Amputation of limb—advisable for patients showing complications and no improvement
• Carpal fusion (arthrodesis) and transposition of the biceps muscle tendon—consider only with adequate function of the triceps muscle and musculocutaneous

NURSING CARE
• Use protective wrapping or boot when patient walks on rough surfaces, because of increased skin fragility and lack of protective reflexes in the affected limb.
• Physical therapy—crucial for keeping joints and muscles mobile during recovery of reversible injuries
• Monitor noncomplicated cases for 4–6 months before considering amputation.

MEDICATIONS

DRUG
Prednisolone (prednisone)—initial anti-inflammatory course for 1 week; may decrease edema and favor healing of reversible components of injury

CONTRAINDICATIONS/POSSIBLE INTERACTIONS
N/A

FOLLOW-UP

PATIENT MONITORING
Serial clinical and electrophysiologic monitoring—assess improvement

PREVENTION/AVOIDANCE
Avoid free roaming.

POSSIBLE COMPLICATIONS
• Skin excoriation with secondary infection of the digit(s)—from rubbing the paw on the ground
• Trophic ulcers—on thin, traumatized skin, especially over arthrodesis sites
• Self-mutilation—frequent and often devastating; result of paresthesia

EXPECTED COURSE AND PROGNOSIS
• Pain sensation (dorsal roots intact)—less severe injury to the ventral nerve roots
• Cranial—better prognosis because sensation to the distal limb and ability to bear weight are spared
• Complete—very poor prognosis
• Rarely, mild cases may resolve after 2–3 months.

MISCELLANEOUS

SEE ALSO
Peripheral Neuropathies (Polyneuropathies)

ABBREVIATION
EMG = electromyography

Suggested Reading
Bailey CS. Patterns of cutaneous anesthesia associated with brachial plexus avulsions in the dog. J Am Vet Med Assoc 1984;185:889–899.

Author Christine Berthelin-Baker
Consulting Editor Joane M. Parent

DISEASES

BRACHYCEPHALIC AIRWAY SYNDROME

BASICS

DEFINITION
• Partial upper airway obstruction caused by the conformation of short-head breeds of dogs and cats
• Obstruction may include any of the following airway passages—nasal (stenotic nares), pharyngeal (overlong soft palate), laryngeal (everted laryngeal ventricles, laryngeal collapse), and tracheal (hypoplastic trachea)
• Both stertor and stridor—usually occur

PATHOPHYSIOLOGY
• Compressed, narrowed air passages—characteristic of animals selectively bred for a flat face, round head, and short, thick neck
• Respiratory muscles must generate more force to produce airflow than in normal animals—may result in barotrauma to the soft tissues lining the airways, causing edema, inflammation, and even inward collapse that further narrows the airways
• Extreme cases—respiratory muscles become fatigued; may result in ventilatory failure

SYSTEMS AFFECTED
• Respiratory
• Gastrointestinal—secondary effects from aerophagia and the high forces used to breathe, which compress abdominal contents
• Others—with hypoxia

GENETICS
Appears to be linked to anatomic features that result from selective breeding; no reported experimental data reported that identify the underlying genetics.

INCIDENCE/PREVALENCE
• Within affected breeds—common
• Various reports that virtually all English bulldogs suffer from some degree of upper airway obstruction

GEOGRAPHIC DISTRIBUTION
N/A

SIGNALMENT
Species
• Dogs and cats of brachycephalic breeds
• Cats—rarely severe enough to recommend surgery

Breed Predilections
• Dogs—English bulldogs most commonly require surgery; other bulldogs, Lhasa apsos, Pekingese, shar peis, shih tzus, and boxers
• Cats—Persian and Himalayan breeds have the most extreme conformation.

Mean Age and Range
• Young adults—1–2 years of age; most surgical patients
• Old adults—surgical patients may be as old as 9–10 years; the search for an exacerbating cause in these patients is particularly important.

Predominant Sex
None

SIGNS
General Comments
• Virtually all brachycephalic animals—some degree of stertorous or stridorous breathing
• Dogs—to relieve high upper airway resistance, breathe with mouth open, pant even in cool ambient temperatures, and snore; owners may not consider noisy or rapid breathing as abnormal unless there has been a sudden or dramatic increase in severity.

Historical Findings
Collapse, exercise intolerance, and gastrointestinal signs (e.g., vomiting, regurgitation, or dysphagia)—presenting complaints

Physical Examination Findings
• Stertor arising from the pharynx and stridor arising from the nasal and laryngeal areas—most, if not all, brachycephalic animal; usually audible without a stethoscope; careful auscultation may help locate point of origin.
• Stenotic nares—readily noticeable
• Recruitment of accessory muscles (e.g., nasolabial elevators, strap muscles of the ventral neck during inspiration, and abdominal muscles during expiration)—with abnormally increased force to overcome increased upper airway resistance; readily seen or felt
• Paradoxical respiratory movements—soft tissues surrounding the chest cavity (thoracic inlet, intercostal spaces, and abdomen) collapse during inspiration and puff during expiration; appearance of increased effort or abdominal breathing; represent wasted work for the respiratory muscles
• With aerophagia—stomach may be grossly dilated with air.

CAUSES
• Brachycephalic head and neck conformation
• Underlying congenital obstruction—may become clinical as a result of a number of exacerbating factors

RISK FACTORS
• Underlying conformation
• Environmental—exercise; high ambient temperature; stimuli causing excitement, anxiety, or fear
• Respiratory—pulmonary disease (e.g., infection or edema); conditions that further narrow the airway (foreign body, tumor, or fat accumulation)
• Metabolic—any condition that increases metabolic rate (e.g., fever or hyperthyroidism)
• Neuromuscular—condition affecting upper airway muscle (e.g., myasthenia gravis, polyneuropathy, or polymyopathy)
• State of consciousness—sleep (severe snoring and obstruction); sedation; anesthesia
• Endocrine—acromegaly

DIAGNOSIS

DIFFERENTIAL DIAGNOSIS
• Brachycephalic animal exhibiting stertor or stridor and paradoxical movements—makes diagnosis
• Carefully search for additional contributing factors and risk factors to anticipate, prevent, and/or treat complications.

CBC/BIOCHEMISTRY/URINALYSIS
N/A

OTHER LABORATORY TESTS
N/A

IMAGING
• Lateral radiographs (head and neck)—useful for suggesting an overlong soft palate; diagnostic for hypoplastic trachea
• Hypoplastic trachea (dogs)—calculate the ratio of the tracheal diameter at the thoracic inlet to the distance from the sternum to the ventral surface of T1; normal, > 0.16; brachycephalic, averages 0.13; ratio does not correlate well with clinical signs.

DIAGNOSTIC PROCEDURES
Pharyngoscopy or laryngoscopy—diagnose overlong soft palate, laryngeal collapse, and everted laryngeal ventricles

PATHOLOGIC FINDINGS
• Tracheal cartilages—may be thick and noncompliant; may find only a narrow strip of dorsal tracheal membrane at necropsy
• Edema—seen in palate tissue resected for a palate clip

TREATMENT

APPROPRIATE HEALTH CARE
• Respiratory distress because of obstruction—evaluate for surgery
• No treatment—when owner believes patient is not compromised; provide appropriate owner education.

NURSING CARE
Requires vigilant nursing care by owners or professional for signs of upper airway obstruction, hypoventilation, and complications

ACTIVITY
• Patient often restricts its own activity.
• Instruct owners not to force patient to exercise and especially to limit exertion in high ambient temperatures to the absolute minimum.

DIET
Obesity—may worsen the condition; fat accumulation may further narrow the airway; may compromise chest wall movements; make every effort to keep patient lean.

CLIENT EDUCATION
• It may be difficult to communicate to the client that the pet's congenital conformation is a risk factor for serious, even fatal, respiratory distress.
• Make client aware of the risk factors that may trigger a serious episode.
• Advise client to keep the pet from becoming overweight; to limit its exercise, especially in high ambient temperatures; and to be cautious when considering sedation or anesthesia.
• Alert owners to exacerbating factors such as infectious respiratory disease.
• Discuss these precautions even if surgical correction has been attempted; resection of the soft tissue cannot alleviate the bony or cartilaginous abnormalities that narrow the nasal turbinates, larynx, and trachea.

SURGICAL CONSIDERATIONS
• Surgical resection of the soft tissues that narrow the airway—most appropriate treatment for uncomplicated condition
• Procedures—open up the stenotic nares; remove excessive tissue at the caudal edge of the soft palate; remove everted laryngeal ventricles.
• Conditions not relieved by surgery—collapsed larynx; hypoplastic trachea; pulmonary or cardiovascular factors (may dramatically increase the risk of the anesthesia)
• Careful postoperative monitoring—required both short-term and long-term

MEDICATIONS

DRUGS OF CHOICE
N/A

CONTRAINDICATIONS
N/A

PRECAUTIONS
• Sedatives—use with extreme caution, although anxiety or fear may be factors.
• Atropine—avoid; dehydrates respiratory secretions

POSSIBLE INTERACTIONS
N/A

ALTERNATIVE DRUGS
N/A

FOLLOW-UP

PATIENT MONITORING
• Postoperative period—observe continuously until completely recovered from anesthesia.
• Monitor closely for airway obstruction resulting from postoperative inflammation or edema.
• For several days, watch for aspiration while the patient is eating.
• Lifelong avoidance of all risk factors necessary

PREVENTION/AVOIDANCE
• Prevention—presumably requires that breeders refrain from selecting animals with this conformation; no other rational advice, because no evidence that families within affected breeds vary in severity of the condition
• To prevent severe obstruction, avoid all risk factors.

POSSIBLE COMPLICATIONS
• Patients that have been through an obstructive event may aspirate.
• Airway obstruction—may lead to noncardiogenic pulmonary edema, which may progress to ARDS, which has a high mortality rate

EXPECTED COURSE AND PROGNOSIS
• Compensation—increased activity of the upper airway dilating muscles
• Decompensation—appears to occur after a prolonged period of compensation; may be a result of further narrowing of the airways caused by inward collapse or inflammation and edema, respiratory muscle fatigue leading to ventilatory failure, or myopathy of the chronically hyperactive upper airway dilating muscles

• Patients that do not undergo surgery—often reduce their own activity; may survive for several years; will not have a normal life; if exposed to risk factors, usually will decompensate and become severely obstructed
• Patients that undergo resection of obstructing soft tissue—usually improve, even if they are still far from normal; long-term outcome studies not available

MISCELLANEOUS

ASSOCIATED CONDITIONS
N/A

AGE-RELATED FACTORS
N/A

ZOONOTIC POTENTIAL
N/A

PREGNANCY
• The large additional abdominal contents tend to compromise the movement of the diaphragm; dams may become noticeably worse during the late stages of pregnancy.
• Effect of chronic or intermittent respiratory distress on small litter sizes typical of brachycephalic breeds—matter for speculation

SEE ALSO
Stertor and Stridor

ABBREVIATION
ARDS = acute respiratory distress syndrome

Suggested Reading
Harvey CE. Soft palate resection of brachycephalic dogs. J Am Anim Hosp Assoc 1982;18:535–537.
Hendricks JC. Brachycephalic airway syndrome. Vet Clin North Am Small Anim Pract 1992;22:1145–1153.
Petrof BJ, Pack AI, Kelly AM, et al. Pharyngeal myopathy of loaded upper airway in dogs with sleep apnea. J Appl Physiol 1994;76:1746–1752.
Authors Joan C. Hendricks and Tricia Mullane
Consulting Editor Eleanor C. Hawkins

BRAIN INJURY (HEAD TRAUMA AND HYPOXIA)

BASICS

DEFINITION
• Primary—direct result of the initial insult; complete at the time of presentation; cannot be altered • Secondary—alteration of brain tissue; anatomic or physiologic; occurs after a primary injury; can be prevented or ameliorated with optimal supportive care

PATHOPHYSIOLOGY
• Brain—high oxygen and glucose requirements; minimal storage of oxygen; few recruitable capillaries; consumes oxygen at a constant rate; stage is set for hypoxic injury • Secondary—from bleeding, cerebral edema, or vasospasms; causes elevation in ICP • Elevated ICP—vicious circle occurs when high ICP leads to low cerebral perfusion and blood flow, leading to further ischemia and brain swelling; may result in brain shift or herniation; slow, progressive rise better tolerated than a small acute increase • Hypotension and hypoxia—the major contributors to ICP elevation and secondary brain injury; at the cellular level: high energy substrates depleted and anaerobic glycolysis results in lactic acid production and intracellular acidosis

SYSTEMS AFFECTED
• Nervous—secondary brain injury and interruption of function • Ophthalmic—potential changes in eye position, eye movements, pupillary light reflexes, and vision • Cardiovascular—arrhythmias caused by dysfunction of central cardiovascular centers • Respiratory—abnormal breathing patterns caused by dysfunction of regulatory centers • Musculoskeletal—possible postural and/or gait abnormalities caused by lesions of the central motor pathways

GENETICS N/A

INCIDENCE/PREVALENCE N/A

GEOGRAPHIC DISTRIBUTION N/A

SIGNALMENT
• Dogs and cats • No breed, age, or sex predilections

SIGNS

Historical Findings
• Determine possible cause—trauma; cardiac arrest; prolonged syncopal episodes; severe heart failure; thromboembolic episodes; coagulopathies with intracranial bleeding; prolonged severe respiratory compromise • Decline in the level of consciousness—implies progression of secondary brain injury from intracranial bleeding or cerebral edema • Seizure activity—localizes lesion to the cerebral cortex or diencephalon • Trauma—associated with secondary brain injury from either bleeding or cerebral edema • Ischemia—

associated with secondary brain injury from cerebral edema

Physical Examination Findings
• Look for external and internal evidence of trauma. • Hypoxia or cyanosis, ecchymosis or petechiations, or cardiac or respiratory insufficiency—metabolic causes • Retinal hemorrhages or distended vessels—hypertension or coagulopathy • Papilledema—cerebral edema • Retinal detachment—infectious, neoplastic, or hypertensive causes • Sustained bradycardia with normal potassium—midbrain, pontine, or medullary lesion • Blood from the ears or nose—severe trauma with intracranial bleeding • Palpation of the skull—reveals fractures that require surgical decompression • Ischemic causes—examine carefully for cardiovascular, respiratory, or hemorrhagic problems.

Neurologic Examination Findings
• Can worsen dramatically during resuscitative efforts owing to hypertension and intracranial bleeding • Determine level of consciousness and whether patient is arousable. • Oculocephalic reflex—perform if cervical manipulation is possible; loss of physiologic vestibular nystagmus: brainstem involvement • Postural changes—decerebrate rigidity: midbrain lesion • Absence of lateralizing signs—suggests diffuse cerebrocortical involvement
Pupillary Light Reflexes
• Miotic responsive pupils—cerebral or diencephalic lesion • Dilated unresponsive pupils (unilateral or bilateral) or midpoint fixed unresponsive pupils—midbrain lesion • Miotic or normal pupils—pontine or medullary lesion
Respiratory Patterns
• Cheyne-Stokes—severe diffuse cerebral or diencephalic pathology • Hyperventilation—midbrain pathology • Ataxic or apneustic—pontine or medullary pathology
Cranial Nerves
• Normal—cerebrum-diencephalon lesion • Cranial nerve III deficit—midbrain lesions • Cranial nerves V–XII—pons or medulla lesions

CAUSES
• Head trauma* • Prolonged hypoxia or ischemia

RISK FACTORS
• Free roaming—trauma • Coexisting cardiac or respiratory disease

DIAGNOSIS

DIFFERENTIAL DIAGNOSIS
• Other causes of brain disease—neoplasia; inflammation; immune-mediated processes; infection; congenital problems • Systemic causes of altered states of consciousness—

narcolepsy; syncope; metabolic disease; toxins; drugs; infection; nutrition • Other causes of brainstem signs—tentorial herniation after progression of cerebral edema

CBC/BIOCHEMISTRY/URINALYSIS
Reflect systemic effects of trauma or hypoxemia

OTHER LABORATORY TESTS
• Arterial blood gases—hypoxemia; severe pH changes; hypercarbia • Coagulogram—when intracranial bleeding or thrombosis may be cause

IMAGING
• Skull radiographs—fractures in trauma patients • CT scan—excellent for detecting acute hemorrhage within the calvaria; depressed fractures; penetrating foreign bodies

DIAGNOSTIC PROCEDURES
• Measure intracranial pressure—determine severity of ICP elevation and response to therapy • Evaluate brainstem auditory evoked potentials—determine brainstem function • ECG—detect arrhythmias

PATHOLOGIC FINDINGS
• Brain edema • Herniation • Hemorrhage • Laceration • Contusion • Hematomas • Skull fracture

TREATMENT

APPROPRIATE HEALTH CARE
• Head position—level with the body or elevated to a 20° angle; never lower than the body to avoid significant elevations in ICP • $PaCO_2$—maintain at 35–45 mm Hg; with suspected elevated ICP: hyperventilation to 25–30 mm Hg may reduce cerebral blood flow and ICP. • PaO_2—must be > 50 mm Hg to maintain cerebral blood flow autoregulation • Avoid cough or sneeze reflex during intubation or oxygen supplementation by nasal cannula—may severely elevate ICP; give lidocaine (dogs, 0.75 mg/kg IV) before intubation to blunt the gag and cough reflexes. • Use peripheral veins, leaving the jugular vein blood flow unobstructed; shifting of blood volume into the jugular veins is an important compensatory mechanism during ICP elevation.

NURSING CARE
• Meticulous nursing care prevents secondary complications of recumbency. • Maintain unobstructed airways; use suction and humidify if intubated. • Lubricate the eyes. • Turn the patient every 2 hr to avoid hypostatic pulmonary congestion. • Prevent fecal or urine soiling. • Maintain core body temperature at normal or mildly hypothermia; avoid hyperthermia. • Maintain hydration with a balanced electrolyte crystalloid solution.

BRAIN INJURY (HEAD TRAUMA AND HYPOXIA)

ACTIVITY
Restricted

DIET
Maintain nutrition during recovery, compensating for elevated metabolic demands of brain injury.

CLIENT EDUCATION
• Inform client that the extent of neurologic recovery may not be evident for several days in the acute phase, and possibly > 6 months for residual neurologic deficits. • Inform client that there may be serious systemic abnormalities that could contribute to the instability of the nervous system.

SURGICAL CONSIDERATIONS
Worsening of neurologic signs, increased ICP not responsive to medical therapy, midbrain signs with history of cerebral trauma or bleed, depressed skull fracture, or penetrating foreign body—seriously consider surgical decompression and exploration

MEDICATIONS

DRUGS OF CHOICE

Poor Perfusion
• Resuscitate with a minimal amount of crystalloids, because these contribute to brain edema. • Small-volume resuscitation—combination of crystalloids with large molecular weight colloids (hetastarch at 5 mL/kg increments over 5–8 min; use minimal amount to maintain systolic blood pressure > 90 mm Hg) • Do not use colloids with intracranial hemorrhage

Systolic Arterial Blood Pressure
• Raise rapidly and maintain > 90 mm Hg using crystalloids and/or colloids. • Avoid hypertension.

Elevated ICP
• Lower by hyperventilation, drug therapy, drainage of CSF from the ventricles, or surgical decompression.
• Mannitol—0.1–0.5 g/kg IV bolus repeated at 2-hr intervals 3–4 times in dogs and 2–3 times in cats; repeated doses must be given on time; improves brain blood flow and lowers ICP; most commonly used in patients with hypoxic, ischemic, or traumatic brain injury and declining neurologic status or if surgical decompression is imminent; may exacerbate hemorrhage
• Furosemide—0.75 mg/kg IV; decreases CSF production; lowers ICP; preferably used in patients with hemorrhage, congestive heart failure, volume overload, and hyperosmolar or anuric renal failure; use before mannitol or as sole diuretic
• High-dose methylprednisolone—no benefit in the acute management of brain injury in

humans; no effect on reducing ICP; no effect on the volume–pressure response (a measure of brain elastance); no improvement on long-term outcome
• Barbiturate coma—for refractory ICP elevation; administer loading dose of pentobarbital to effect (up to 10 mg/kg IV over 30 min; maintain at 1 mg/kg/hr by constant rate infusion); must intubate patient and support blood pressure, oxygenation, and ventilation.

Other
• Cooling the patient down to 32–33°C (89–91°F) may provide cerebral protection when administered within 6 hr of global ischemia or severe brain injury.
• Glucose supplementation—as required for hypoglycemia

CONTRAINDICATIONS
• Drugs that cause hypertension
• Drugs that cause hyperexcitability
• Do not use colloids when there is intracranial hemorrhage.

PRECAUTIONS
• Avoid hypertension.
• Avoid intravascular volume overload.
• Do not allow head to lie below plane of body.
• Do not use the jugular veins.
• Mannitol and hypertonic saline—may worsen neurologic status when there is intracranial hemorrhage
• Hyperventilation—maintain PCO_2 > 25 mm Hg; do not perform for extended periods (> 48 hr).

POSSIBLE INTERACTIONS N/A

ALTERNATIVE DRUGS N/A

FOLLOW-UP

PATIENT MONITORING
• Neurologic examinations—detect deterioration of function that warrants aggressive therapeutic intervention • Blood pressure—keep fluid therapy adequate for perfusion but avoid hypertension • Blood gases—assess need for oxygen supplementation or ventilation; monitor PCO_2 when hyperventilation is required • Blood glucose—ensure adequate blood level to maintain brain functions and avoid hyperosmolality from high amounts • ECG—detect arrhythmias that may affect perfusion, oxygenation, and cerebral blood flow • ICP—to detect significant elevations; monitor success of therapeutics

PREVENTION/AVOIDANCE
Keep pets in a confined area with supervised activity.

POSSIBLE COMPLICATIONS
• Increasing ICP • Brain herniation • Intra-

cranial hemorrhage • Progression from cerebrocortical to midbrain signs • Seizures • Malnutrition • Hypostatic pulmonary congestion • Corneal desiccation • Urine scalding • Airway obstruction from mucus • Cardiac arrhythmias—usually bradyarrhythmias • Respiratory failure • Death

EXPECTED COURSE AND PROGNOSIS
• Minimal primary brain injury and secondary injury consisting of cerebral edema—best prognosis • No deterioration of neurologic status for 48 hr—better prognosis • Rapid resuscitation of systolic blood pressure to > 90 mm Hg—better neurologic outcome

MISCELLANEOUS

ASSOCIATED CONDITIONS N/A

AGE-RELATED FACTORS N/A

ZOONOTIC POTENTIAL N/A

PREGNANCY N/A

SYNONYMS
• Head trauma • Traumatic brain injury

SEE ALSO
Stupor and Coma

ABBREVIATIONS
• ICP = intracranial pressure
• CSF = cerebrospinal fluid

Suggested Reading
Bullock R. Mannitol and other diuretics in severe neurotrauma. N Horizons 1995;3:448–452.
Hayek DA, Veremakis C. Therapeutic options in brain resuscitation. In: Veremakis C, ed. Problems in critical care: resuscitation following acute brain injury. Philadelphia: Lippincott, 1991:156–186.
Kelly DF. Steroids in head injury. N Horizons 1995;3:453–455.
Wilberger JE, Cantella D. High-dose barbiturates for intracranial pressure control. N Horizons 1995;3:469–473.
Author Rebecca Kirby
Consulting Editor Joane M. Parent

DISEASES

BRONCHIECTASIS—DOGS

 BASICS

OVERVIEW
- Condition seen primarily in dogs, characterized by an irreversible dilatation of the bronchi with accumulation of pulmonary secretions
- Diseases that lead to condition—those associated with ciliostasis, which disrupts the normal defense mechanisms within the lung and delays clearance of bacteria and mucus
- Pro-duction of cytokines and destructive enzymes by WBCs or bacteria and prolonged contact of inflammatory mediators with pulmonary tissue—lead to damage of supporting struc-tures within the lung
- The airways are pulled open by surrounding lung tissue; further pooling of secretions occurs, which perpetuates lung damage and colonization by bacteria.

SIGNALMENT
- Primarily dogs and rarely cats
- Cocker spaniels—seem predisposed
- In the U.K.—reported higher incidence in large-breed dogs
- Young animals (< 1 year)—secondary to primary ciliary dyskinesia
- Middle-aged to old dogs with chronic pulmonary disease

SIGNS
- Chronic cough—usually moist and productive; observant owners may notice hemoptysis.
- Recurrent fever • Exercise intolerance
- Tachypnea or dyspnea
- Crackles and moist rales; loud expiratory lung sounds
- Tracheal hypersensitivity
- Chronic nasal discharge or sinusitis, particularly with primary ciliary dyskinesia

CAUSES & RISK FACTORS
- Primary ciliary dyskinesia
- Inadequately treated infectious or inflammatory lung conditions—may lead to severe inflam-mation, tissue destruction, and irreversible lung damage
- Smoke inhalation, aspiration pneumonia, radiation injury, and inhalation of environmental toxins—may predispose animal to airway injury and colonization by bacteria
- Chronic bronchial obstruction—development of bronchiectasis distal to the obstructed region common, owing to accumulation of inflammatory mediators and bacterial colonization

 DIAGNOSIS

DIFFERENTIAL DIAGNOSIS
- Recurrent bacterial bronchopneumonia
- Fungal pneumonia
- Chronic bronchitis
- Infectious or parasitic bronchitis
- Con-gestive heart failure
- Neoplasia
- Tracheal collapse

CBC/BIOCHEMISTRY/URINALYSIS
- Neutrophilia and monocytosis
- Hyper-globulinemia owing to chronic antigenic stimulation
- Proteinuria—may be seen with secondary amyloidosis, glomerulonephritis, or sepsis

OTHER LABORATORY TESTS
Arterial blood gas analysis—hypoxemia; high alveolar–arterial gradient

IMAGING
- Radiography—dilatation of the lobar bronchi with lack of normal tapering in the periphery; mixed bronchial, interstitial, and alveolar pattern; diffuse thickening of bronchial walls
- CT—abnormally dilated bronchi near the lung periphery; cystic dilatations of the bronchi with or without fluid

DIAGNOSTIC PROCEDURES
- Bronchoscopy—saccular or tubular dilatation of the airways; blunting of airway bifurcations and loss of the cylindrical shape to the lumen; airway hyperemia with or without mucosal irregularity and nodule formation; trapped secretions
- Airway sampling—cytologic examination of bronchoalveolar lavage fluid or transtracheal wash specimens; culture for aerobic and anaerobic bacteria; typically find suppurative inflammation with high numbers of neutrophils and monocytes; may culture a mixed population of bacteria; may appear to be sterile because of no growth of bacteria

PATHOLOGIC FINDINGS
- Diffuse peribronchial and alveolar inflammation and fibrosis
- Squamous metaplasia of bronchial epithelium
- Bronchiolar obliteration

 TREATMENT

- Inpatient—severe condition; intravenous fluids and antibiotics; oxygen administration
- Most patients benefit from airway humidification and coupage to facilitate removal of viscid pulmonary secretions.
- Encourage gentle activity, as much as the patient's condition allows; enhance clearance of secretions.
- Long-term antibiotic administration (2 months to lifelong)—may be needed; stress to owner importance of appropriate follow-up care.
- Single affected lung lobe or bronchial obstruction—may require lung lobectomy

MEDICATIONS

DRUGS
• Intravenous antibiotics—may be required initially; good choices: ampicillin (10–20 mg/kg IV q6–8h) and gentamicin (2–4 mg/kg IV q8–12h)
• Broad-spectrum agents with efficacy against both aerobes and anaerobes and that offer good penetration of pulmonary tissue—preferred; combination of enrofloxacin (2.5–10 mg/kg PO q12h) and clindamycin (5–11 mg/kg PO q12h)
• Long-term use of antibiotics—based on bacterial culture and sensitivity testing; may be required even if culture of airway specimens yield no growth
• Bronchodilators—may be beneficial, although animals usually have irreversible airflow limitation; Theo-Dur (10–20 mg/kg PO q12h), terbutaline (1.25–5.0 mg/dog PO q12h), or albuterol (0.03–0.05 mg/kg PO q8–12h)

CONTRAINDICATIONS/POSSIBLE INTERACTIONS
• Theophylline derivatives and fluoroquinolones—concurrent use causes high and possibly toxic plasma theophylline concentration.
• Furosemide—avoid; dries out airway secretions

 FOLLOW-UP

PATIENT MONITORING
• Body temperature—outpatient; by owner
• Serial CBC, blood gas analysis, and thoracic radiographs

PREVENTION/AVOIDANCE
Antibiotics—complete a full course of therapy in patients that appear to have parenchymal infection; short course (10–14 days) may predispose patient to infection by resistant bacteria.

POSSIBLE COMPLICATIONS
Chronic recurrent pulmonary infection likely

EXPECTED COURSE AND PROGNOSIS
• Patient may succumb to respiratory failure.
• Pulmonary hypertension and cor pulmonale may develop.
• Other organs may fail if bacteremia or glomerulonephritis develops.

 MISCELLANEOUS

ASSOCIATED CONDITIONS
• Primary ciliary dyskinesia
• Chronic sinusitis
• Chronic bronchitis
• Bacterial pneumonia
• Aspiration pneumonia
• Smoke inhalation

AGE-RELATED FACTORS
Evaluate young patients for primary ciliary dyskinesia.

SEE ALSO
• Ciliary Dyskinesia, Primary
• Pneumonia, Bacterial
• Smoke Inhalation

Suggested Reading
Nicotra MB. Bronchiectasis. Semin Respir Infect 1994;9:31–40.
Author Lynelle Johnson
Consulting Editor Eleanor C. Hawkins

DISEASES

BRONCHITIS, CHRONIC (COPD)

BASICS

DEFINITION
• Chronic coughing for 2 consecutive months that is not attributable to another cause (e.g., neoplasia and congestive heart failure) • Non-reversible and often slowly progressive condition, owing to the pathologic airway changes that accompany the process

PATHOPHYSIOLOGY
• Specific cause rarely determined • Recurrent airway inflammation (e.g., infection and inhaled irritant) suspected • Persistent tracheo-bronchial irritation—causes chronic coughing; leads to changes in the tracheobronchial epithelium and submucosal structures • Airway inflammation, epithelial edema, thickening, and metaplasia—prominent • Mucus production increased • Net effect of changes—narrow airways; increase lung resistance; decrease expiratory air flow rates

SYSTEMS AFFECTED
• Respiratory • Cardiovascular—pulmonary hypertension, cor pulmonale • Nervous—syncope

GENETICS
N/A

INCIDENCE/PREVALENCE
N/A

GEOGRAPHIC DISTRIBUTION
N/A

SIGNALMENT

Species
Dogs and cats

Breed Predilections
• Dogs—small and toy breeds common; also observed in large breeds • West Highland white terriers—develop a progressive disorder characterized by chronic coughing, respiratory distress, and crackles • Young to middle-aged cocker spaniels—bronchiectasis common after a long history of chronic bronchitis

Mean Age and Range
Most often affects middle-aged and old animals

Predominant Sex
N/A

SIGNS

Historical Findings
• Coughing—hallmark of tracheobronchial irritation; usually dry; posttussive gagging common (owners may misinterpret it as vomiting) • Exercise intolerance • Cyanosis and even syncope—may be noted

Physical Examination and Findings
• Patients usually bright, alert, and afebrile • Tracheal palpation—typically results in coughing because of tracheal sensitivity

• Small airway disease—assumed when an expiratory abdominal push (during quiet breathing) or end-expiratory wheezing is detected • Bronchovesicular lung sounds, end-inspiratory crackles, and wheezing—result of airways obstructed by secretions; may be heard • Cardiac auscultation—murmurs secondary to valvular insufficiency common but not always associated with congestive heart failure; chronic bronchitis usually results in a normal or slower than normal resting heart rate and pronounced sinus arrhythmia. • Obesity—common; important complicating factor

CAUSES
Chronic airway inflammation initiated by multiple causes

RISK FACTORS
• Recurrent bacterial infection • Long-term exposure to inhaled irritants • Obesity • Dental disease and laryngeal disease—result in bacterial showering of the lower airways

DIAGNOSIS

DIFFERENTIAL DIAGNOSIS
• Bacterial or fungal pneumonia • Bronchiectasis • Allergic lung disease • Foreign bodies • Heartworm disease • Neoplasia—metastatic more common than primary • Pulmonary parasites or parasitic larval migration • Pulmonary fibrosis • Pulmonary granulomatosis • Congestive heart failure–typically associated with a high resting heart rate

CBC/BIOCHEMISTRY/URINALYSIS
• Rarely diagnostic • Absolute eosinophilia—suggests but not diagnostic for allergic bronchitis; noted in < 50% of confirmed cases • Polycythemia secondary to chronic hypoxia—may be seen • SAP and ALT—may be high owing to passive congestion

OTHER LABORATORY TESTS
• Run routine fecal and heartworm tests. • Arterial blood gas analysis—collect, ice, and have analyzed at a local hospital; low PaO_2 but not high $PaCO_2$ common with severe condition

IMAGING

Thoracic Radiography
• Common features (in descending order of frequency)—bronchial thickening (classically doughnuts and tram lines); interstitial pattern; middle lung lobe consolidation;

atelectasis; hyperinflation and diaphragmatic flattening (primarily cats).

Echocardiography
• May confirm pulmonary hypertension • May reveal right heart enlargement • Helps rule out congestive heart failure as a cause of coughing

DIAGNOSTIC PROCEDURES

ECG
• Wandering atrial pacemaker, marked sinus arrhythmia, P pulmonale, and (occasionally) evidence of right ventricular hypertrophy—common • Estimate pulmonary hypertension via color flow Doppler echocardiography.

Evaluation of Airway Secretions
• From lower airways—establish underlying cause. • Throat swab cultures—not representative of lower airway flora • Transtracheal aspiration biopsy or bronchoalveolar lavage—collect specimens for cytologic examination and bacterial culture. • Cytology—inflammation primary finding; most cells neutrophils, eosinophils, or macrophages; evaluate for bacteria, parasites, and neoplastic cells. • Recurrent infections—implicated pathogenesis; positive cultures are not frequently reported (e.g., two recent studies noted positive aerobic cultures in 24% of cats and 17% of dogs); *Mycoplasma* discussed but rarely confirmed as a cause.

Bronchoscopy
• Preferred test for assessing the lower airways • Allows direct visualization of the structural and functional (dynamic) changes encountered; allows selected airway sampling (e.g., biopsy and lavage) • Gross changes—excess mucoid to mucopurulent secretions; epithelial edema or thickening and blunting of bronchial bifurcations; irregular or granular mucosa; (pathognomonic) mucosal polypoid proliferations; areas of pneumonia • Large airway caliber changes (e.g., dynamic airway collapse and bronchiectasis)—may detect as complicating problems

PATHOLOGIC FINDINGS
See Diagnostic Procedures—Bronchoscopy

TREATMENT

APPROPRIATE HEALTH CARE
• Usually outpatient • Inpatient—requires oxygen therapy, parenteral medication, or aerosol therapy; patients that owners cannot keep calm at home during recovery

NURSING CARE N/A

ACTIVITY

• Exercise—moderate (not forced) useful in clearing secretions; assists with weight loss
• Limit if exertion results in coughing.
• Use a harness instead of a collar.

DIET

Weight loss—marked improvement in PaO_2, cough frequency, attitude, and exercise tolerance in obese patients

CLIENT EDUCATION

• Warn client that chronic bronchitis is an incurable disease and complete suppression of all coughing is an unattainable goal.
• Stress that aggressive treatment—including weight control, avoiding risk factors, and medical treatment—minimizes the severity of the coughing episodes in most patients.

SURGICAL CONSIDERATIONS

Treat severe dental disease to minimize secondary bacterial complications.

MEDICATIONS

DRUGS OF CHOICE

Antitussives
• Indicated for nonproductive, paroxysmal, continuous, or debilitating cough
• Dogs—butorphanol (0.55 mg/kg PO q6–12h; 0.055–0.11 mg/kg SC); hydrocodone (2.5–5 mg/dog q6–24h PO); codeine (0.1–0.3 mg/kg q6–8h PO)

Antibiotics
• Select on the basis of sensitivity test results
• Bacterial culture results unavailable— choose an agent with a good gram-negative spectrum, with good tissue and secretion penetration, and that is bactericidal with minimal toxicity (e.g., enrofloxacilin, potentiated sulfa/trimethoprim, or amoxicillin/clavulanic acid).
• Associated chronic aspiration or dental disease—may prefer an anaerobic and gram-positive spectrum antibiotic

Corticosteroids
• Diminish airway inflammation and coughing regardless of the underlying cause
• Indicated with noninfectious condition
• With allergic or hypersensitivity reactions— require long-term administration; attempt to wean off steroids or determine lowest effective dosage.

Bronchodilators
• Beneficial effects (depend on drug)— bronchodilation; heightened mucociliary clearance; improvement in diaphragmatic contractility; lowered pulmonary artery pressure; increased CNS sensitivity to $PaCO_2$; and stabilization of mast cells
• β-agonists—terbutaline (1.25–5 mg/dog q8–12h; 0.625mg/cat q12h) and albuterol

(0.02–0.05 mg/kg q8–12h in dogs)
• Sustained-release theophylline—oral administration; dosages are product and species-specific; Theo-Dur tablets (not capsules) recommended at 20 mg/kg q12h (dogs) and 25 mg/kg q24 in the evening (cats); Slo-Bid Gyrocaps recommended at 25 mg/kg q12h (dogs) and 25 mg/kg q24h in the evening (cats); dosages designed to achieve theophylline therapeutic plasma concentrations between 5 and 20 µg/mL
• Aminophylline—immediate-release tablets or injectable; not recommended

CONTRAINDICATIONS

Lasix and atropine—do not use because of drying effects on tracheobronchial secretions.

PRECAUTIONS

• β-agonists (e.g., terbutaline and albuterol)—may cause tachycardia, nervousness, and muscle tremors; typically transient
• Methylxanthines (e.g., theophylline)—may cause tachycardia, restlessness, excitability, vomiting, and diarrhea; unlikely with sustained-release formula at recommended dosage; evaluate EDTA plasma sample, drawn 4–5 hr (dogs) or 10 hr (cats) after administration, for peak plasma concentration

POSSIBLE INTERACTIONS

Enrofloxacin decreases theophylline clearance in dogs; do not use concurrently.

ALTERNATIVE DRUGS

• Sustained-release theophylline—many products available; different bioavailabilities make dosages product specific; do not allow any substitution.
• Serotonin blockers (not leukotriene blockers)—shown to effectively block airway hyper-responsiveness in cats with experimentally induced airway disease
• Cyclosporin-induced immune suppression—shown to block changes associated with asthma in cats

FOLLOW-UP

PATIENT MONITORING

• Follow abnormalities revealed by physical examination and selected diagnostic tests— determine response to treatment • Monitor weight; arterial blood gases usually improve after marked weight loss

PREVENTION/AVOIDANCE

Avoid and address risk factors (see Risk Factors).

POSSIBLE COMPLICATIONS

• Syncope—frequent complication of chronic coughing, particularly in toy breed dogs
• Pulmonary hypertension and cor pulmonale—most serious complications

EXPECTED COURSE AND PROGNOSIS

• Progressive airway changes—syncopal episodes, chronic hypoxia, right ventricular hypertrophy, and pulmonary hypertension common • Acute exacerbations—common with seasonal changes, air quality changes, and development of secondary infection

MISCELLANEOUS

ASSOCIATED CONDITIONS

• Syncope—secondary to chronic coughing
• Increased susceptibility to airway infection, chronic hypoxia, pulmonary hypertension, and cor pulmonale

AGE-RELATED FACTORS N/A

ZOONOTIC POTENTIAL N/A

PREGNANCY

• Safety in pregnant animals not established for most of the recommended drugs

SYNONYMS

• Chronic obstructive pulmonary disease (COPD) • Chronic obstructive lung disease (COLD) • Bronchiolitis • Small airway disease

SEE ALSO

• Asthma, Bronchitis—Cats • Bronchiectasis
• Cough • Hypoxia • Tracheal Collapse— Dogs • Tracheobronchitis, Infectious—Dogs

ABBREVIATIONS

• ALT = alanine aminotransferase
• SAP = serum alkaline phosphatase

Suggested Reading

Bonagura JD. Bronchopulmonary disorders. In: Birchard SJ, Sherding RG, eds. Saunders manual of small animal practice. Philadelphia: Saunders, 1994:561–573.

Dye JA, McKiernan BC, Rozanski EA, et al. Bronchopulmonary disease in the cat. Historical, physical, radiographical, clinicopathologic and pulmonary functional evaluation of 24 diseased and 15 healthy cats. J Vet Intern Med 1996;10:385–400.

Johnson L. Bronchial disease. In: August JR, ed. Consultations in feline internal medicine. 3rd ed. Philadelphia: Saunders, 1997:303–309.

Padrid PA, Hornoff WJ, Kurpershoek CJ, Cross CE. Canine chronic bronchitis. J Vet Intern Med 1990;4:172–180.
Author Brendan C. McKiernan
Consulting Editor Eleanor Hawkins

BASICS

DEFINITION
• Contagious disease of dogs caused by *Brucella canis,* a small, intracellular, gram-negative organism
• Characterized by abortion and infertility in females and epididymitis and testicular atrophy in males

PATHOPHYSIOLOGY
B. canis—an intracellular parasite; has a propensity for growth in lymphatic, placental, and male genital (epididymis and prostate) tissues

SYSTEMS AFFECTED
• Reproductive—target tissues of gonadal steroids (gravid uterus, fetus, testes [epididymides], prostate gland)
• Hemic/Lymph/Immune—lymph nodes and spleen; bone marrow; mononuclear leukocytes
• Other tissues—intervertebral disks, anterior uvea, meninges (uncommon)

GENETICS
• No known genetic predisposition
• Occurs most commonly in beagles

INCIDENCE/PREVALENCE
• Incidence unknown
• Seroprevalence rates—not accurately defined; false-positive results common with agglutination tests
• Prevalence—relatively low (1–18%) in the U.S. and Japan; in the U.S., higher in rural areas of the south; in Mexico and Peru, 25–30% in stray dogs

GEOGRAPHIC DISTRIBUTION
Stray dogs, pets, and kennels—U.S. (mostly beagles), Mexico, Japan, and several South American countries; seen in Spain, Tunisia, China, and Bulgaria; individual outbreaks in Germany and the former Czechoslovakia (some traced to the importation of dogs)

SIGNALMENT

Species
Dogs and, infrequently, humans

Breed Predilections
• No evidence of breed susceptibility, but exceptionally high prevalence in beagles
• Infected Labrador retrievers and several other breeds found in commercial kennels ("puppy mills")

Mean Age and Range
• No age preference
• Most common in sexually mature dogs

Predominant Sex
• Both sexes are affected
• More common in females

SIGNS

General Comments
Suspect whenever female dogs experience abortions or reproductive failures or males have genital disease

Historical Findings
• Affected animals, especially females, may appear healthy or have vague signs of illness.
• Lethargy
• Loss of libido
• Swollen lymph nodes
• Back pain
• Abortion—commonly at 6–8 weeks after conception, although pregnancy may terminate at any stage

Physical Examination Findings
• Males—swollen scrotal sacs, often with scrotal dermatitis; enlarged and firm epididymides
• Chronic infection—unilateral or bilateral testicular atrophy; cloudy eyes (anterior uveitis with corneal edema); spinal pain; posterior weakness; ataxia
• Fever rare
• Enlarged superficial lymph nodes (e.g., retropharyngeal, external inguinal) common
• Vaginal discharge may last for several weeks after an abortion

CAUSES
B. canis—gram-negative coccobacillus; morphologically indistinguishable from other members of the genus; unlike other *Brucella* spp. (e.g., *B. abortus, B. suis,* and *B. melitensis*), can result in a high rate (50%) of false-positive reactions with commonly used tests

RISK FACTORS
• Breeding kennels and pack hounds
• Risk increases when popular breeding animals become infected.
• Contact with strays in endemic areas

DIAGNOSIS

DIFFERENTIAL DIAGNOSIS
• Abortions—maternal, fetal, or placental abnormalities
• Systemic infections—canine distemper, canine herpesvirus infection, *B. abortus* infection, hemolytic streptococci, *E. coli,* leptospirosis, and toxoplasmosis
• Inguinal hernias—may be provoked by epididymitis and scrotal edema; also caused by blastomycosis and other granulomatous infections, and Rocky Mountain spotted fever
• Diskospondylitis—fungal infections, actinomycosis, staphylococcal infections, nocardiosis, streptococci, or *Corynebacterium diphtheroids*

CBC/BIOCHEMISTRY/URINALYSIS
Generally normal in uncomplicated cases

OTHER LABORATORY TESTS
Serologic testing—most commonly used diagnostic method; subject to error; false-positive reactions to lipopolysaccharide antigens of several species of bacteria common with the RSAT and mercaptoethanol tube agglutination tests

RSAT
• Commercially available; simple and rapid
• Detects infected dogs 3–4 weeks after infection; accurate in identifying noninfected ("negative") dogs
• Suffers a high rate (50%) of false-positive reactions
• Results must be confirmed by other tests.

Mercaptoethanol Tube Agglutination Test
• Semiquantitative
• Generally performed by commercial diagnostic laboratories
• Provides information similar to the RSAT
• Suffers from lack of specificity

AGID Tests
• Cell wall antigen test—employs a lipopolysaccharide antigen derived from the cell walls of *B. canis;* highly sensitive; test conditions not standardized; frequent false positives
• Soluble antigen test—employs soluble antigens that consist of proteins extracted from the bacterial cytoplasm; antigens highly specific for antibodies against *Brucella* spp. (including *B. canis, B. abortus,* and *B. suis*); reactive antibodies appear 4–12 weeks after infection and persist for a long time; may give precipitin lines after other tests become equivocal or negative

IMAGING
Radiographic evidence of diskospondylitis—test for brucellosis

DIAGNOSTIC PROCEDURES

Isolation of Organism
• Blood cultures—when clinical and serologic findings suggest the diagnosis; *Brucella* are readily isolated from the blood of infected dogs if they have not received antibiotics; onset of bacteremia occurs 2–4 weeks after oral-nasal exposure and may persist for 8 months to 5.5 years.
• Cultures of vaginal fluids—after an abortion; usually give positive results
• Cultures of semen or urine—not practical for routine diagnosis, because overgrowth of contaminants is common
• Contaminated samples—media that contain antibiotics (e.g., Thayer-Martin medium) have proven useful.

Semen Quality
• Sperm motility, immature sperm, inflammatory cells (neutrophils)—with epididymitis
• Abnormalities—usually evident by 5–8 weeks postinfection; conspicuous by 20 weeks
• Aspermia without inflammatory cells—common with bilateral testicular atrophy

Lymph Node Biopsy
• Reveal lymphoid hyperplasia with large numbers of plasma cells
• If done in a sterile manner, tissues should be cultured on appropriate media.
• Intracellular bacteria—may be observed in macrophages with special stains (e.g., Brown-Brenn stain)
• Histopathological examination of the testes—often reveals necrotizing vasculitis, infiltration of inflammatory cells, and granulomatous lesions

PATHOLOGICAL FINDINGS
• Gross findings—lymph node enlargement; splenomegaly; males: enlarged and firm epididymides, scrotal edema, or atrophy of one or both testes; chronic infection: anterior uveitis and diskospondylitis
• Microscopic changes—relatively consistent; diffuse lymphoreticular hyperplasia; chronic infection: lymph node sinusoids with abundant plasma cells and macrophages that contain bacteria diffuse lymphocytic infiltration and granulomatous lesions in all genitourinary organs (especially prostate, epididymis, uterus, and scrotum); may be extensive inflammatory cell infiltration and necrosis of the prostate parenchyma and seminiferous tubules
• Ocular changes—granulomatous iridocyclitis; exudative retinitis; leukocytic exudates in the anterior chamber

 TREATMENT

APPROPRIATE HEALTH CARE
Outpatient

NURSING CARE
N/A

ACTIVITY
Restrict working dogs

DIET
N/A

CLIENT EDUCATION
• Client should be aware that the goal of treatment is the eradication of *B. canis* from the animal (seronegative status and no bacteremia for at least 3 months), but sometimes the result is persistent low antibody titers with no systemic infection.

• Inform client that antibiotic treatment, especially minocycline and doxycycline, is expensive, time-consuming, and controversial (because outcomes are uncertain).
• Treatment is not recommended for breeding or commercial kennels; it is recommended only for nonbreeding dogs or those who have been spayed or castrated.
• Before treatment is attempted for an intact household pet or breeding dog, the client must clearly agree that the animal must be neutered or destroyed if treatment fails.

SURGICAL CONSIDERATIONS
Neutering/spaying plus treatment—when euthanasia is unacceptable to an owner

 MEDICATIONS

DRUGS OF CHOICE
• Several therapeutic regimens have been evaluated, but results have been equivocal.
• Most successful—combination of a tetracycline (tetracycline hydrochloride, chlortetracycline, or minocycline at 25mg/kg PO q8h for 4 weeks) or doxycycline (10 mg/kg PO q12h for 4 weeks) and dihydrostreptomycin (10 mg/kg IM q8h during weeks 1 and 4)

CONTRAINDICATIONS
• Tetracyclines—do no use in immature pups
• Gentamicin—contraindicated with kidney disease

PRECAUTIONS
Gentamicin—monitor renal function closely.

POSSIBLE INTERACTIONS
N/A

ALTERNATIVE DRUGS
Gentamicin—3 mg/kg q12h; limited success; insufficient data on the efficacy combined with tetracycline

 FOLLOW-UP

PATIENT MONITORING
• Serologic tests—monthly for at least 3 months after completion of treatment; continuous, persistent decline in antibodies to negative status indicates successful treatment.
• Recrudescent infections (rise in antibody levels and recurrence of bacteremia after therapy)—re-treat, neuter and re-treat, or euthanize
• Blood cultures—negative for at least 3 months after completion of treatment

PREVENTION/AVOIDANCE
• Vaccine—none; would complicate serologic testing
• Testing—all brood bitches, before they come into estrus if a breeding is planned; males used for breeding, at frequent intervals
• Quarantine and test all new dogs twice at monthly intervals before allowing them to enter a breeding kennel.

POSSIBLE COMPLICATIONS
• Owners may be reluctant to neuter or destroy valuable dogs, regardless of treatment failure.
• Remind owners of ethical considerations and their obligation not to sell or distribute infected dogs.

EXPECTED COURSE AND PROGNOSIS
• Prognosis guarded
• Infected for < 3–4 months—likely to respond to treatment
• Chronic infections—males may fail to respond to therapy.
• Successfully treated (seronegative) dogs—fully susceptible to reinfection

 MISCELLANEOUS

ASSOCIATED CONDITIONS
N/A

AGE-RELATED FACTORS
N/A

ZOONOTIC POTENTIAL
Human infections—reported; usually mild; respond readily to tetracyclines

PREGNANCY
• Abortions at 45–60 days of gestation typical
• Pups from infected bitches may be infected or normal.

SYNONYMS
Contagious canine abortion

SEE ALSO
N/A

ABBREVIATIONS
• AGID = agar gel immunodiffusion
• RSAT = rapid 2-mercaptoethanol slide agglutination test

Suggested Reading

Carmichael LE. Brucella canis. In: Nielsen K, Duncan JR, eds. Animal brucellosis. Boca Raton, FL: CRC, 1990:335–350.
Carmichael LE, Greene CE. Canine brucellosis. In: Greene CE, ed. Infectious diseases of the dog and cat. Philadelphia: Saunders, 1990:573–585.
Johnson CA, Walker RD. Clinical signs and diagnosis of *Brucella canis* infection. Comp Contin Educ Prac Vet 1992:14:763–772.
Author Leland Carmichael
Consulting Editor Stephen C. Barr

DISEASES

CALICIVIRUS—CATS

 BASICS

DEFINITION
A common viral respiratory disease of domestic and exotic cats characterized by upper respiratory signs, oral ulceration, pneumonia, and occasionally arthritis

PATHOPHYSIOLOGY
Rapid cytolysis of infected cells with resulting tissue pathology and clinical disease

SYSTEMS AFFECTED
• Respiratory—rhinitis; interstitial pneumonia; ulceration of the tip of the nose
• Ophthalmic—acute serous conjunctivitis without keratitis or corneal ulcers
• Musculoskeletal—acute arthritis
• Gastrointestinal—ulceration of the tongue common; occasional ulceration of the hard palate and lips; infection occurs in intestines; usually no clinical disease

GENETICS
None

INCIDENCE/PREVALENCE
• Persistent infection common
• Clinical disease—common in multicat facilities and breeding catteries
• Routine vaccination—reduced incidence of clinical disease; has not decreased the prevalence of the virus

GEOGRAPHIC DISTRIBUTION
Worldwide

SIGNALMENT
Species
Cats

Breed Predilections
None

Mean Age and Range
• Young kittens > 6 weeks old—most common
• Cats of any age may show clinical disease.

Predominant Sex
None

SIGNS
General Comments
May present as an upper respiratory infection with eye and nose involvement, as an ulcerative disease primarily of the mouth, as pneumonia, as an acute arthritis, or any combination of these

Historical Findings
• Sudden onset
• Anorexia
• Ocular or nasal discharge, usually with little or no sneezing
• Ulcers on the tongue, hard palate, lips, tip of nose, or around claws
• Dyspnea from pneumonia
• Acute, painful lameness

Physical Examination Findings
• Generally alert and in good condition
• Fever
• Ulcers may occur without other signs.

CAUSES
• A small, nonenveloped single-stranded RNA virus
• Numerous strains exist in nature, with varying degrees of antigenic cross-reactivity.
• More than one serotype
• Relatively stable and resistant to many disinfectants

RISK FACTORS
• Lack of vaccination or improper vaccination
• Multicat facilities
• Concurrent infections with other pathogens (e.g., FHV-1 or FPV)
• Poor ventilation

 DIAGNOSIS

DIFFERENTIAL DIAGNOSIS
• Feline viral rhinotracheitis
• Chlamydiosis
• *Bordetella bronchiseptica*

CBC/BIOCHEMISTRY/URINALYSIS
No characteristic or consistent findings

OTHER LABORATORY TESTS
Serologic testing on paired serum samples—detect a rise in neutralizing antibody titers against the virus

IMAGING
Radiographs of the lungs—a consolidation of lung tissue in cats with pneumonia

DIAGNOSTIC PROCEDURES
• Cell cultures to isolating the virus—oral pharynx; lung tissue; feces; blood; secretions from the nose and conjunctiva
• Immunofluorescent assays of lung tissue—viral antigen

PATHOLOGIC FINDINGS
• Gross—upper respiratory infection; ocular and nasal discharge; pneumonia with consolidation of large portions of individual lung lobes; possible ulcerations on the tongue, lips, and hard palate
• Histopathologic—interstitial pneumonia of large portions of individual lung lobes; ulcerations on epithelium of the tongue, lips, and hard palate; mild inflammatory reactions in the nose and conjunctiva

 TREATMENT

APPROPRIATE HEALTH CARE
Outpatient, unless severe pneumonia occurs

NURSING CARE
• Clean eyes and nose as indicated
• Provide soft foods
• Oxygen—with severe pneumonia

ACTIVITY
Patients should be restricted from contact with other cats to prevent transmission of the disease.

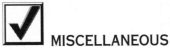
DIET
- No restrictions
- Special diets—perhaps to entice anorectic cats to resume eating
- Soft foods—if ulcerations restrict eating

CLIENT EDUCATION
Discuss the need for proper vaccination and the need to modify the vaccination protocol in breeding catteries to include kittens before they become infected (often at 6–8 weeks of age) from a carrier queen.

SURGICAL CONSIDERATIONS
None

MEDICATIONS

DRUGS OF CHOICE
- No specific antiviral drugs that are effective
- Broad-spectrum antibiotics—usually indicated (e.g., amoxicillin at 22 mg/kg PO q12h)
- Secondary bacterial infections of affected cats are not nearly as important as with FHV-1 infections.
- Antibiotic eye ointments—to reduce secondary bacterial infections of the conjunctiva
- Appropriate pain medication—for transient arthritis pain

CONTRAINDICATIONS
None

PRECAUTIONS
None

POSSIBLE INTERACTIONS
None

ALTERNATIVE DRUGS
None

FOLLOW-UP

PATIENT MONITORING
- Monitor for sudden development of dyspnea associated with pneumonia.
- No specific laboratory tests

PREVENTION/AVOIDANCE
- All cats should be vaccinated at the same time they are vaccinated against FHV-1; routine vaccination with either MLV or inactivated vaccines should be done at 8–10 weeks of age and repeated 3–4 weeks later.
- Breeding catteries—respiratory disease is a problem; vaccinate kittens at an earlier age, either with an additional vaccination at 4–5 weeks of age or with intranasal administration at 10–14 days of age; follow-up vaccinations at 6, 10, and 14 weeks of age
- Annual vaccines recommended; immunity undoubtedly lasts > 1 year
- American Association of Feline Practitioners—classifies FHV, FPV, and calicivirus as core vaccines; recommends vaccination of all cats with these three agents on the initial visit, after 12 weeks of age, and 1 year later; boosters for calicivirus should be given every 3 years.
- Vaccination will not eliminate infection in a subsequent exposure but will prevent clinical disease caused by most strains.

POSSIBLE COMPLICATIONS
- Interstitial pneumonia—most serious complication; can be life-threatening
- Secondary bacterial infections of the lungs or upper airways
- Oral ulcers and the acute arthritis usually heal without complications.

EXPECTED COURSE AND PROGNOSIS
- Clinical disease—usually appears 3–4 days after exposure
- Once neutralizing antibodies appear, about 7 days after exposure, recovery is usually rapid.
- Prognosis excellent, unless severe pneumonia develops
- Recovered cats—persistently infected for long periods; will continuously shed small quantities of virus in oral secretions

✓ MISCELLANEOUS

ASSOCIATED CONDITIONS
Affected cats may also be concurrently infected with FHV-1, especially in multicat and breeding facilities.

AGE-RELATED FACTORS
Usually occurs in young kittens whose maternally derived immunity has waned

ZOONOTIC POTENTIAL
None

PREGNANCY
Generally no problem, because most cats have been exposed or vaccinated before becoming pregnant

SYNONYMS
Feline picornavirus infection—originally classified as a picornavirus; older literature refers to the infection by this name; no known picornavirus that infects cats

SEE ALSO
- Bordetellosis—Cats
- Chlamydiosis—Cats
- Feline Rhinotracheitis Virus

ABBREVIATIONS
- FHV = feline herpesvirus
- FPV = feline parvovirus
- MLV = modified live vaccine

Suggested Readings

Barr MC, Olsen CW, Scott FW. Feline viral diseases. In: Ettinger SJ, Feldman EC, eds. Veterinary internal medicine. 4th ed. Philadelphia: Saunders, 1995:409–439.

Elston T, Rodan I, Flemming D, et al. 1998 report of the American Association of Feline Practitioners and Academy of Feline Medicine Advisory Panel on feline vaccines. J Am Vet Med Assoc 1998;212:227–241.

Ford RB, Levy JK. Infectious diseases of the respiratory tract. In: Sherding RG, ed. The cat: diseases and clinical management. New York: Churchill Livingstone, 1994:489–500.

Ford RB. Role of infectious agents in respiratory disease. Vet Clin North Am Sm Anim Pract 1993;23:17–35.

Pedersen NC. Feline calicivirus infection. In: Pratt PW, ed. Feline infectious diseases. Goleta, CA: American Veterinary, 1988:61–67.

Author Fred W. Scott
Consulting Editor Stephen C. Barr

DISEASES

CAMPYLOBACTERIOSIS

BASICS

OVERVIEW
• *Campylobacter jejuni*—fastidious, micro-aerophilic, gram-negative curved bacteria; often isolated from the gastrointestinal tract of healthy dogs, cats, and other mammals; may cause a superficial erosive enterocolitis
• Infection—fecal–oral route from contamination of food, water, fresh meat (poultry, beef), and the environment; localized in mucus-filled crypts of the intestine; darting motility (flagella) essential for colonization; produces enterotoxin, cytotoxin, cytolethal-distending toxin, and invasin
• Invasion of mucosa of gastrointestinal—hematochezia; leukocytes in feces; ulceration; edema; congestion of intestine; bacteremia; occasionally septicemia; bacteria shed in feces for weeks to months
• Up to 49% of dogs without diarrhea and 45% of normal cats carry *C. jejuni* and shed it in feces

SIGNALMENT
• Dogs and less commonly cats
• Prevalence—higher in puppies and kittens from birth to 6 months

SIGNS
• Diarrhea—ranges from mucous-like and watery to bloody or bile streaked; common; may be chronic
• Tenesmus common
• Fever (mild or absent), anorexia, and intermittent vomiting (3–15 days' duration) may accompany diarrhea.
• Young animals (up to 6 months of age)—clinical signs most severe; attributable to enterocolitis/diarrhea
• Adults—usually asymptomatic carriers

CAUSES & RISK FACTORS
• *C. jejuni*
• Kennels with poor sanitation and hygiene and fecal buildup in the environment
• Young animals—debilitated, immunosuppressed, or parasitized (e.g., *Giardia, Toxocara, Isospora*)
• Nosocomial infection may develop in hospitalized patients.
• Adults—concurrent gastrointestinal infections (e.g., *Salmonella*, parvovirus, hookworms)

DIAGNOSIS

DIFFERENTIAL DIAGNOSIS
• Signalment, history, physical examination, and fecal examination (direct smear and bacterial culture) enable diagnosis in most cases.
• Distinguish from other causes of acute enterocolitis.
• Bacterial enterocolitis—*Salmonella, Yersinia enterocolitica, Clostridium difficile*, and *Clostridium perfringens*
• Parasitic enterocolitis—helminths (particularly whipworms) and protozoa (e.g., *Giardia* and *Isospora*)
• Viral enterocolitis—enteric coronavirus and parvovirus; signs often more severe than with *Campylobacter*
• Dietary indiscretion or intolerance
• Drugs and toxins
• Acute pancreatitis
• Severely affected patients—also consider viral gastroenteritis, intussusception, and other causes of abdominal pain.
• Distinguish from other causes of chronic diarrhea.
• Primary intestinal disease

CBC/BIOCHEMISTRY/URINALYSIS
• Leukocytosis—if the strain is invasive and bacteremia develops
• Biochemistry abnormalities—effects of diarrhea and dehydration (e.g., azotemia, electrolyte disturbances)

OTHER LABORATORY TESTS
N/A

IMAGING
N/A

DIAGNOSTIC PROCEDURES
• Fecal leukocytes—in gastrointestinal tract and stool
• Fecal culture—microaerophilic at about 42°C for 48 hr on special *Campylobacter* blood agar plates

Direct Examination of Feces
• Gram stain—make a smear of watery stool on a glass slide; heat fix; use gram stain; leave counterstain (safranin) on for longer than usual.

• Wet mount—drop a small amount of stool (if not watery, mix with a small amount of saline or broth) on a glass slide; add a cover slip; view on phase or dark-field objective (40×); note large numbers of curved, highly motile bacteria (characteristic darting motility)

PATHOLOGIC FINDINGS
• Gross—diffuse colon thickening and congestion/edema; hyperemia of small intestine; enlarged mesenteric lymph nodes
• Histopathology—colon-mucosal thickening; exfoliation of brush border; goblet cells; cuboidal epithelium; reduced crypt height; crypt abscesses; RBCs and neutrophils in lamina propria and intestinal lumen

TREATMENT

Mild Enterocolitis
• Outpatient
• Usually self-limiting

Severe Enterocolitis
• Inpatient, especially neonatal and immature patients
• Severe neonatal disease—isolate; confine to cage; monitor; encourage rest
• NPO for 24 hr; then bland diet
• Mild dehydration—oral fluid therapy with an enteric fluid replacement solution
• Severe dehydration—intravenous fluid therapy with balanced polyionic isotonic solution (e.g., lactated Ringer's)
• Plasma transfusion may be required if serum albumin < 2.0 g/dL.
• Locally acting intestinal adsorbents and protectants

MEDICATIONS

DRUGS
• Antibiotics—recommended for signs of systemic illness (e.g., high fever or dehydration) when diarrhea or abnormal clinical signs persist > 7 days and in immune-suppressed patients
• Erythromycin—10–20 mg/kg PO q8h for 5 days; drug of choice
• Tylosin—11 mg/kg PO q8h for 7 days; may be effective
• Neomycin—10–20mg/kg PO q6–12h for 5 days; may be effective
• Penicillins and ampicillin—potentially ineffective
• Septicemia—parenteral antibiotics with an aminoglycoside (e.g., amikacin) and a cephalosporin may be initiated

CONTRAINDICATIONS/POSSIBLE INTERACTIONS
Antidiarrheal drugs that reduce intestinal motility are contraindicated.

 FOLLOW-UP

PATIENT MONITORING
Repeat fecal culture after completion of treatment.

PREVENTION/AVOIDANCE
• Good hygiene (hand washing)
• Routinely clean and disinfect runs, food, and water bowls

POSSIBLE COMPLICATIONS
Bacteremia and septicemia

EXPECTED COURSE AND PROGNOSIS
• Adults—usually self-limiting
• Juveniles with severe or persistent enterocolitis—treat with antibiotics

 MISCELLANEOUS

ASSOCIATED CONDITIONS
Concurrent infection with *Campylobacter* and other pathogenic bacteria, enteric parasites, or viruses

AGE-RELATED FACTORS
Young animals at greatest risk

ZOONOTIC POTENTIAL
High potential to infect humans

PREGNANCY
• Erythromycin—safe to use in early pregnancy
• Chloramphenicol and gentamicin—do not use in pregnant animals.

Suggested Reading
Fox JG. Enteric bacterial infections. In: Greene CE, ed. Infectious diseases of the dog and cat. Philadelphia: Saunders, 1998:226–229.
Authors Patrick L. McDonough and Kenneth W. Simpson
Consulting Editor Stephen C. Barr

DISEASES

CANDIDIASIS

 BASICS

OVERVIEW
• *Candida*—part of the normal flora of the mouth, nose, ears, and gastrointestinal and genital tracts of dogs and cats; recovery from mucosal surfaces does not imply disease; opportunistic, colonizing damaged tissues or invading normal tissues of immunosuppressed animals; pathogenic role determined by identifying a fungemia, infiltration of organisms into the tissues, or signs of organisms in presumed sterile sites (e.g., urinary bladder)
• Isolation—conditions that suppress the immune system increase the likelihood of isolation in asymptomatic animal; isolated from throat cultures five times more often in FIV-infected cats than in asymptomatic, non-FIV-infected cats of a similar age and sex
• Infection—rare; associated with neutropenia, diabetes mellitus, retrovirus-induced immunosuppression, chronic glucocorticoid treatment, and prolonged antibiotic treatment

SIGNALMENT
Cats and less commonly dogs

SIGNS
• Urinary bladder involvement—cystitis
• Ear infection—head shaking and scratching
• Oral cavity involvement—drooling

CAUSES & RISK FACTORS
• Skin damaged by burns, trauma, or necrotizing dermatitis
• Urinary tract—preferred site in diabetic cats and cats that have urinary retention owing to strictures secondary to urethrostomy; indwelling catheters
• Neutropenia secondary to parvovirus infection, FeLV, FIV, or bone marrow suppression from chemotherapy

 DIAGNOSIS

DIFFERENTIAL DIAGNOSIS
Considered whenever the primary condition does not respond as expected

CBC/BIOCHEMISTRY/URINALYSIS
• Reflect the underlying condition
• Urinalysis—may show yeast form or clumps of mycelial elements (pseudohyphae) accompanied by an increase in inflammatory cells; normal fat globules in cat urine may adhere, giving the appearance of budding yeast.
• Neutropenic patients—inflammatory response may be absent

OTHER LABORATORY TESTS
• Pyuria without bacterial growth—culture for fungi and *Mycoplasma*.

IMAGING
N/A

DIAGNOSTIC PROCEDURES
• Lesions—culture for histopathologic study to determine if *Candida* is truly a pathogen; requires demonstration of organisms penetrating the tissues
• Urine sample—obtain by cystocentesis; culture of a number of colonies of *Candida* strongly supports the diagnosis.
• Otitis (dogs)—culture of *Candida* or identification of yeast or mycelial elements on ear cytology suggests the diagnosis.

PATHOLOGIC FINDINGS
• White cheesy foci in the infected tissue may be noted.
• Usually large numbers of both yeast and pseudohyphae in the tissues surrounded by necrosis and a suppurative inflammatory reaction
• Response may be pyogranulomatous in more chronic sites of infection.

 TREATMENT
• Regulate diabetes mellitus.
• Remove indwelling catheters.
• Improve immune suppression, if possible.

 MEDICATIONS

DRUGS
• Fluconazole—5 mg/kg PO q12h (dogs and cats); very effective; excreted unchanged in the urine, achieving a high concentration in commonly infected sites
• Itraconazole—effective; use if the organism becomes resistant to fluconazole; not recommended for urinary tract infection because it is not excreted in the urine

CONTRAINDICATIONS/POSSIBLE INTERACTIONS
N/A

 FOLLOW-UP

PATIENT MONITORING
• Fluconazole and itraconazole—hepatic toxicity; monitor serum ALT monthly and check if patient becomes anorexic; withdraw drug if ALT > 200 U or with anorexia.
• After signs have resolved—reculture sites of infection; continue treatment for 2 weeks more; repeat cultures 2 weeks after completion of treatment and again if lesions recur.

EXPECTED COURSE AND PROGNOSIS
• Should resolve within 2–4 weeks of treatment
• Control of the underlying disease is necessary to prevent recurrence.

 MISCELLANEOUS

ZOONOTIC POTENTIAL
None

ABBREVIATIONS
• ALT = alanine transferase
• FeLV = feline leukemia virus
• FIV = feline immunodeficiency virus

Suggested Reading
Greene CE, Chandler FW. Candidiasis, torulopsosis, rhodotorulosis. In: Greene CE, ed. Infectious diseases of the dog and cat. Philadelphia: Saunders, 1998:414–417.
Lulich JP, Osborne CA. Fungal infections of the feline lower urinary tract. Vet Clin North Am 1996;26:309–315.
Author Alfred M. Legendre
Consulting Editor Stephen C. Barr

BASICS

OVERVIEW
• *Capillaria plica* is a parasite that invades the mucosa or submucosa of the bladder or (rarely) the renal pelvis and ureter, causing a mild inflammatory response.
• *C. plica* in dogs and cats and *C. feliscati* in cats have been uncommonly associated with signs of lower urinary tract disease.
• First stage in life cycle of *C. plica* is passage of bipolar ova in urine. After earthworms ingest embryonated ova, the parasite develops into the infective stage. Ingestion of infective earthworm results in a patent infection in dogs in 58–88 days.
• Details of life cycle of *C. feliscati* are poorly understood.

SIGNALMENT
• Dogs—no predilection reported
• Cats—affected cats almost always > 8 months old

SIGNS
• Usually none
• Pollakiuria, hematuria, stranguria, and dysuria in some animals, particularly those heavily infected

CAUSES & RISK FACTORS
Dogs
• High prevalence of infection (up to 50%) in the natural hosts, foxes and raccoons, in the southeastern United States may predispose animals in this geographic region.
• In kennels, high infection rates are associated with the use of soil surfaces.

Cats
Rare in United States; infection prevalence of 18–34% reported in Australia.

 DIAGNOSIS

DIFFERENTIAL DIAGNOSES
Consider other more common causes of lower urinary tract disease such as urolithiasis, urinary tract infection, trauma, and neoplasia.

CBC/BIOCHEMISTRY/URINALYSIS
• Bipolar ova in urine sediment are diagnostic.
• Consider the possibility of fecal contamination of urine with *Trichuris vulpis* ova if free-catch urine specimens are used or if inadvertent rectal puncture occurs during cystocentesis.
• Alternatively, in an affected animal, urine contamination of feces can produce false fecal examination findings.

OTHER LABORATORY TESTS
N/A

IMAGING
N/A

DIAGNOSTIC PROCEDURES
N/A

 TREATMENT

• Infection is usually self-limiting in both species; ova no longer detectable in the urine sediment of infected dogs in 10–12 weeks if isolated.
• Replacing soil surfaces with sand, gravel, or concrete may reduce prevalence of infection in kennels.

 MEDICATIONS

DRUGS
• Consider anthelmintic therapy if clinical signs are present; monitor therapeutic success by examining urine sediment for ova and observing clinical signs.
• Fenbendazole (50 mg/kg PO q24h for 5 days) has been reported to result in disappearance of ova from urine sediment in dogs and cats.
• Ivermectin (0.2 mg/kg SC once) has been suggested as an alternative therapy, but objective information on its efficacy in this disease is limited.

CONTRAINDICATIONS/POSSIBLE INTERACTIONS
N/A

 FOLLOW-UP

Monitor treatment success by examining urine sediment for ova and observing clinical signs.

✓ **MISCELLANEOUS**

Suggested Reading
Brown SA, Prestwood KA. Parasites of the urinary tract. In: Kirk RW, ed. Current veterinary therapy IX. Philadelphia: Saunders, 1986:1153–1155.
Authors Susan E. Little and Scott A. Brown
Consulting Editors Larry G. Adams and Carl A. Osborne

CARBON MONOXIDE POISONING

  BASICS

OVERVIEW

Carbon monoxide—odorless, colorless, nonirritating gas produced by inefficient combustion of carbonaceous fuels; absorbed into the blood, forming carboxyhemoglobin and reducing oxygen, which causes hypoxia of the brain and heart

SIGNALMENT

All animals

SIGNS

Historical Findings

Exposure to automobile exhaust or supplemental heating devices

Physical Examination Findings

Acute
- Drowsiness
- Lethargy
- Weakness
- Deafness
- Incoordination
- Reduced heart excitability
- Cherry red skin and mucous membranes
- Dyspnea
- Coma
- Terminal clonic spasms
- Acute death

Chronic
- Low exercise tolerance
- Disturbance of postural and position reflexes and gait

CAUSES & RISK FACTORS

- Incomplete combustion
- Automobile exhaust in a closed garage or faulty exhaust system
- Unvented or faulty furnaces, gas water heaters, or gas or kerosene space heaters
- Fires—carbon monoxide concentration may reach 10% in the atmosphere of a burning building
- Animals with impaired cardiac or pulmonary function—at higher risk than clinically normal animals

 DIAGNOSIS

DIFFERENTIAL DIAGNOSIS

Similar clinical signs—barbiturate, ethanol, cyanide, or hydrogen sulfide gas toxicosis

CBC/BIOCHEMISTRY/URINALYSIS

Creatine kinase—high because of muscle ischemia

OTHER LABORATORY TESTS

- Carboxyhemoglobin in whole blood—expressed as a percent of hemoglobin in the carboxyhemoglobin form
- Blood pH—lower than normal secondary to metabolic acidosis
- P_{AO_2}—normal; percent oxygen saturation low

IMAGING

N/A

DIAGNOSTIC PROCEDURES

ECG—consistent with anoxia and necrosis of single heart muscle fibers

 TREATMENT

- Restore adequate oxygen to brain and heart.
- Provide fresh air, maintain patent airway, and provide artificial respiration if necessary.
- Supplemental oxygen or hyperbaric oxygen—promotes recovery
- Supportive fluids

 MEDICATIONS

DRUG(S)

None

CONTRAINDICATIONS/POSSIBLE INTERACTIONS

Avoid respiratory depressants.

 FOLLOW-UP

- Significant response to therapy—should be observed in 1–4 hr, depending on cellular damage owing to hypoxia.
- Monitor cardiac, pulmonary, and neurologic function and limit physical activity for 2 weeks.
- Neurologic signs—may appear within a few days to as long as 6 weeks after apparent recovery
- Eliminate source of carbon monoxide; prevent re-exposure by using in-home carbon monoxide detectors.

✓ **MISCELLANEOUS**

PREGNANCY

Carbon monoxide—reduces oxygen-carrying ability of maternal blood; crosses the placenta, producing fetal hypoxia, abortion, or neurologic impairment of the fetus, even when the dam is asymptomatic

ZOONOTIC POTENTIAL

Humans in the same carbon monoxide–contaminated environment are at risk.

Suggested Reading

Ellenhorn MJ, Schonwald S, Ordog G, Wasserberger J . Ellenhorn's medical toxicology: diagnosis and treatment of human poisoning. 2nd ed. Baltimore: Williams & Wilkins, 1997:1465–1474.

Author Thomas L. Carson

Consulting Editor Gary D. Osweiler

BASICS

OVERVIEW
A familial cardiomyopathy of boxers characterized by ventricular and atrial arrhythmias, variable degrees of myocardial dysfunction, CHF, and sudden cardiac death. The first manifestations of the disease are transient ventricular arrhythmias. As the disease progresses, myocardial dysfunction occurs is approximately 30–40% of cases.

SIGNALMENT
• Dogs
• Occurs in all ages, most common in 4–8 year old boxers.
• A genetic basis is very likely.
• Incidence is slightly higher in males.

SIGNS

General Comments
Variable depending on stage and presence of myocardial dysfunction

Historical Findings
• In some boxers, the first sign of disease is sudden death.
• There may be a history of syncope or collapse.
• Relatives may be similarly affected.

Physical Examination Findings
• An irregular cardiac rhythm may be present in advanced cases.
• A systolic murmur is found in cases with mitral regurgitation and myocardial dysfunction.

CAUSES & RISK FACTORS
• Unknown, genetic basis likely

DIAGNOSIS

DIFFERENTIAL DIAGNOSIS
• Other causes of episodic weakness or collapse (hypoadrenocorticism, hypoglycemia)
• Dilated cardiomyopathy
• Viral myocarditis

CBC/BIOCHEMISTRY/URINALYSIS
Results usually normal

OTHER LABORATORY TESTS
N/A

IMAGING

Radiographic Findings
The cardiac silhouette is within normal limits unless there is accompanying myocardial dysfunction

Echocardiographic Findings
• There are no structural abnormalities until late in the course of disease.
• When myocardial dysfunction occurs, there is left ventricular and left atrial dilatation and a decrease in fractional shortening.

DIAGNOSTIC PROCEDURES

Electrocardiogram
May be within normal limits considering the transient arrhythmias typical of the disease. The hallmark is the occurrence of ventricular premature complexes with a left bundle branch block pattern (i.e., QRS complex in lead II positive, tall and wide).

Holter Monitoring
Continuous ambulatory electrocardiography for 24 hours (Holter monitoring) is currently the most sensitive diagnostic tool. The presence of ventricular premature complexes and ventricular tachycardia are common findings.

TREATMENT
• Patients with CHF should be hospitalized until stabilized
• Activity should be restricted if there is severe ventricular arrhythmia
• A low sodium diet is warranted if there are signs of congestive heart failure

MEDICATIONS

DRUGS
• Antiarrhythmic therapy is indicated when significant ventricular ectopy is definitively documented–atenolol at a dose of 12.5 to 25 mg PO q12h along with a class I antiarrhythmic (e.g., procainamide or mexiletine) are most commonly used. For refractory ventricular arrhythmias, sotalol at a dose of 1–3 mg/kg PO q12h can be substituted. Start with a dose at the low end of the range and titrate up to effect.

• Diuretics are indicated when CHF is present. The aggressiveness of diuretic therapy is proportional to the degree of pulmonary edema (furosemide 1–2 mg/kg PO q6–12h).
• Vasodilators may be beneficial in reducing clinical signs (enalapril—0.5mg PO q12–24h or benazepril 0.25–0.5 mg/kg PO q24h).
• Supplementation with l-carnitine may be of benefit (2 gm PO q8–12h) if there is myocardial dysfunction.

CONTRAINDICATIONS/POSSIBLE INTERACTIONS
N/A

FOLLOW-UP

PATIENT MONITORING
Frequent rechecks of the electrocardiogram are warranted when significant ventricular ectopy is detected and antiarrhythmic therapy used.

EXPECTED COURSE AND PROGNOSIS
• Control of syncope is often achieved with the use of antiarrhythmic medications
• Sudden cardiac death secondary to ventricular arrhythmia is common
• Boxers not succumbing to sudden death may develop signs of dilated cardiomyopathy

MISCELLANEOUS

PREGNANCY
• There may be an increase in ventricular arrhythmia associated with whelping and estrus
• Considering the familial nature, affected boxers should not be bred

ABBREVIATIONS
CHF = congestive heart failure

Suggested Reading
Goodwin JK, Cattiny G. Further characterization of boxer cardiomyopathy. Proc Thirteenth Annual Veterinary Medical Forum (ACVIM). 13:300–302, 1995.
Author John-Karl Goodwin
Consulting Editor Larry P Tilley and Francis W. K. Smith Jr.

DISEASES

CARDIOMYOPATHY, DILATED—CATS

BASICS

OVERVIEW
Dilated cardiomyopathy is a disease of the ventricular muscle characterized by systolic myocardial failure and an enlarged, volume overloaded heart that leads to signs of congestive heart failure or low cardiac output. Before 1987, dilated cardiomyopathy was one of the most commonly diagnosed heart diseases in cats. Most cats probably had secondary cardiomyopathy as a result of taurine deficiency. Primary idiopathic dilated cardiomyopathy is now an uncommon cause of heart disease in cats.

SIGNALMENT
Siamese, Abyssinian, and Burmese breeds have a reported increased incidence. Familial patterns have been identified in some families of cats.

SIGNS

Historical Findings
Signs related to low cardiac output
- Anorexia
- Weakness
- Depression
Signs related to congestive heart failure
- Dyspnea
- Tachypnea
Signs related to thromboembolism
- Sudden-onset pain
- Sudden onset of paraparesis

Physical Examination Findings
- Soft systolic heart murmur
- Weak left cardiac impulse
- Gallop rhythm
- Hypothermia
- Prolonged capillary refill time
- Quiet lung sounds (pleural effusion)
- Crackles (pulmonary edema)
- Hypokinetic femoral pulses
- Possibly posterior paresis and pain as a result of aortic thromboembolism.

CAUSES & RISK FACTORS
The underlying etiology of idiopathic dilated cardiomyopathy remains unknown, although a genetic predisposition has been identified in some families of cats. Taurine deficiency was a common cause of secondary myocardial failure before 1987.

DIAGNOSIS

DIFFERENTIAL DIAGNOSIS
- Taurine deficiency dilated cardiomyopathy. Because primary idiopathic dilated cardiomyopathy and taurine deficiency have similar clinical presentations, cats with myocardial failure should be assumed to have taurine deficiency until shown to be unresponsive to taurine.
- Myocardial failure secondary to longstanding congenital or acquired left ventricular volume overload diseases.

CBC/BIOCHEMISTRY/URINALYSIS
Many cats will have pre-renal azotemia related to low cardiac output.

OTHER LABORATORY TESTS
Plasma taurine concentrations less than 40 nmoles/L or whole blood taurine concentrations less than 250 nmoles/L are considered too low in cats. Taurine assays are performed at a limited number of institutions and require special handling.

IMAGING

Radiographic Findings
- Radiography often shows pleural effusion or pulmonary edema.
- The cardiac silhouette typically is enlarged in a globoid manner.

Echocardiographic Findings
- Echocardiography is the diagnostic modality of choice.
- Characteristic findings include thin ventricular walls, enlarged left ventricular end systolic and end diastolic dimensions, left atrial enlargement, and low fractional shortening.

DIAGNOSTIC TESTS

Electrocardiography
- Electrocardiography may be normal or may show left atrial or ventricular enlargement patterns.
- Both ventricular and supraventricular arrhythmias can be seen.

Pleural Effusion Analysis
Pleural effusion typically is a modified transudate with total protein less than 4.0 g/dl and nucleated cell counts of less than 2500/ml. Chylous effusion may also be present. Analysis of the pleural effusion is important to rule out other causes of pleural effusion such as pyothorax, infectious peritonitis, or lymphosarcoma.

PATHOLOGIC FINDINGS
• Heart to body ratio is increased.
• Ventricle walls are thin and the lumen is enlarged.
• Valve anatomy is normal.
• Histopathology shows myocyte atrophy and myocardial fibrosis.

TREATMENT
• These cats usually are in congestive heart failure and should be treated as inpatients.
• Thoracocentesis is both therapeutic and diagnostic.
• Supplemental oxygen therapy is beneficial for cats in congestive heart failure.
• If hypothermic, external heat (incubator or heating pad) is recommended.
• These cats typically are anorexic, thus tempting their appetite with many types of food may be necessary. Eventually, a low-sodium diet is recommended.

MEDICATIONS

DRUG(S)
• Furosemide is recommended at the lowest effective dose to eliminate pulmonary edema and pleural effusion. Recommended dose range is 1–3 mg/kg q8–12h. Initially, furosemide should be administered parenterally.
• Nitroglycerin (2% ointment) 0.25–0.5 inch applied topically can be used in conjunction with diuretics in the acute management of congestive heart failure to further reduce preload. Nitroglycerin will lower the dose of furosemide and is particularly useful in patients with hypothermia or dehydration.
• Enalapril at a dose of 0.25 to 0.5 mg/kg PO q24h is recommended to reduce afterload and preload.
• Digoxin is recommended to strengthen contractility at a dose of 0.03mg/cat (one quarter of a 0.125-mg tablet) or 0.01 mg/kg PO q48h.
• Taurine supplementation is recommended in all cats with myocardial failure at 250 mg PO q12h until it is demonstrated that the patient is unresponsive to taurine.
• Dobutamine at extremely low dosages can be given to a patient with severe signs of congestive heart failure and low cardiac output. Dose varies from 1–5 mcg/kg/min.
• See aortic thromboembolism chapter for therapeutic recommendations.

CONTRAINDICATIONS/POSSIBLE INTERACTIONS
• Unless needed for cardiac rhythm control, avoid drugs that reduce contractility such as calcium channel blockers or beta-adrenergic blockers.
• Overzealous diuretic therapy may cause dehydration and hypokalemia.
• Digoxin dose should be reduced if renal insufficiency is documented or suspected.
• Dobutamine may cause seizures and cardiac arrhythmias.

FOLLOW-UP
• Repeat thoracic radiographs within 1 week to determine efficacy of therapy.
• Periodically monitor electrolyte and renal parameters.
• Digoxin concentrations should be measured 2 weeks after initiating therapy. Therapeutic range is between 1–2 ng/dl 8–12 hours post-pill.
• Repeat echocardiogram in 3–6 months after initiating taurine supplementation to determine response to therapy.
• These cats have a poor prognosis despite intensive therapy.

MISCELLANEOUS

Suggested Reading
Pion PD, Kittleson MD, Rogers QR, et al. Myocardial failure in cats associated with low plasma taurine: A reversible cardiomyopathy. Science 1987; 237:764–768.
Author Teresa C. DeFrancesco
Consulting Editors Larry P. Tilley and Francis W. K. Smith, Jr.

CARDIOMYOPATHY, DILATED—DOGS

BASICS

DEFINITION
Characterized by left and right-sided dilatation, normal coronary arteries, normal (or minimally-diseased) atrioventricular valves, significantly decreased inotropic state, and myocardial dysfunction occurring primarily during systole

PATHOPHYSIOLOGY
• Myocardial failure leads to reduced cardiac output and CHF
• A-V annulus dilatation and altered papillary muscle function promote valvular insufficiency

SYSTEMS AFFECTED
• Cardiovascular
• Respiratory—pulmonary edema
• Renal/Urologic—pre-renal azotemia
• All organ systems are affected by reductions in cardiac output

GENETICS
Genetic cause or heritable susceptibility strongly suspected but as yet unproven

INCIDENCE/PREVALENCE
Estimated at 0.5–1.1%

GEOGRAPHIC DISTRIBUTION
N/A with the exception of Chagas' cardiomyopathy which is limited to the Southern United States

SIGNALMENT

Species
Dogs

Breed Predilections
• Doberman pinscher, boxer
• "Giant" breeds: Scottish deerhound, Irish wolfhound, Great Dane, Saint Bernards, Afghan hounds
• Cocker spaniels.

MEAN AGE AND RANGE
4–10 years.

PREDOMINANT SEX
Males > Females in most but not all breeds

SIGNS

Historical Findings
• Respiratory—tachypnea, dyspnea, coughing
• Weight loss
• Weakness, lethargy, anorexia
• Abdominal distension
• Syncope
• Some dogs are asymptomatic, having what is termed "occult dilated cardiomyopathy"

Physical Examination Findings
• Weakness, depression, possibly cardiogenic shock
• Hypokinetic femoral pulse from low cardiac output
• Pulse deficits with atrial fibrillation,

ventricular premature contractions, and paroxysmal ventricular tachycardia.
• Jugular pulses from tricuspid regurgitation, arrhythmias, or right-sided CHF
• Breath sounds are muffled if there is pleural effusion; crackles if there is pulmonary edema
• S_3 or summation gallops
• Mitral regurgitation and or tricuspid regurgitation murmurs are common but usually soft
• Auscultatory evidence of cardiac arrhythmia
• Slow capillary refill time, possible cyanosis
• Hepatomegaly with or without ascites

CAUSES
• Primary mechanism yet to be identified and is idiopathic in the vast majority of cases. Most authors believe that the majority of cases represent familial abnormalities of structural or contractile cardiac proteins
• Nutritional deficiencies (taurine and/or carnitine) have been documented in several breeds including golden retrievers, boxers, Doberman pinschers and Cocker spaniels
• Viral, protozoal, and immune-mediated mechanisms have been proposed

RISK FACTORS
N/A

DIAGNOSIS

DIFFERENTIAL DIAGNOSIS
• Endocardiosis
• Congenital heart disease
• Heartworm disease
• Bacterial endocarditis
• Cardiac tumors and pericardial effusion
• Airway obstruction: foreign body, neoplasm, laryngeal paralysis
• Primary pulmonary disease: bronchial disease, pneumonia, neoplasia, aspiration, vascular disease (e.g., heartworms)
• Pleural effusions (e.g., pyothorax, hemothorax, chylothorax)
• Trauma resulting in diaphragmatic hernia, pulmonary hemorrhage, pneumothorax

CBC/BIOCHEMISTRY/URINALYSIS
Routine hematologic tests and urinalysis are usually normal unless altered by severe heart failure (e.g. prerenal azotemia, high ALT, hyponatremia) , therapy for heart failure (e.g. hypokalemia, hypochloremia and metabolic alkalosis from diuresis) or concurrent disease

OTHER LABORATORY TESTS
N/A

IMAGING

Radiographic Findings
• Generalized cardiomegaly and signs of CHF are common
• Left ventricular enlargement and left atrial enlargement may be most evident in early cases

• Doberman Pinschers: marked LAE is a major finding; pulmonary edema is often patchy and diffuse
• Pleural effusion, hepatomegaly, ascites

Echocardiographic Findings
• "Gold Standard" for diagnosis
• Ventricular and atrial dilation
• Reduced myocardial systolic function (low FS%)
• Doppler studies may confirm low velocity and/or acceleration of transaortic flow as well as mitral regurgitation and/or tricuspid regurgitation.

DIAGNOSTIC TESTS

Electrocardiography
• Sinus rhythm or sinus tachycardia with isolated atrial or ventricular premature complexes
• Atrial fibrillation is common
• Ventricular tachycardia is very common in doberman pinschers and boxers
• Prolonged QRS (> 0.06 sec), possible increased voltages (R > 3.0 mV lead II) suggesting LV enlargement
• May have "sloppy" R wave descent with ST-T coving, suggesting myocardial disease or LV ischemia
• May have low voltages (pleural or pericardial effusion, concurrent hypothyroidism)

PATHOLOGIC FINDINGS
• Dilation of all chambers with thinning of the chamber walls
• Slightly thickened endocardium with pale areas within the myocardium (necrosis, fibrosis)
• Histopathologic changes are minimal: small areas of myocyte atrophy, myocytolysis, myocardial necrosis and fibrosis

TREATMENT

APPROPRIATE HEALTH CARE
With the exception of severely affected dogs, most therapy can be administered on an outpatient basis

NURSING CARE
N/A

ACTIVITY
Allow the dog to choose it's own level of activity

DIET
• Goal: reduce dietary sodium intake to < 12–15mg/kg/day
• Severe sodium restriction is not necessary when using potent vasodilators and diuretics
• Best to use commercially prepared diets

CLIENT EDUCATION
Emphasize potential signs associated with progression of disease and adverse side-effects of medication

SURGICAL CONSIDERATIONS
N/A

MEDICATIONS

DRUGS OF CHOICE
First identify patient problems: CHF (left or right-sided), arrhythmia, hypothermia, renal failure, shock
Initial Stabilization
• Treat hypoxemia with oxygen administration; prevent heat loss if hypothermic (warm environment); administer IV or SQ fluids (D_5W or 0.45% NaCl with 2.5% dextrose) only after pulmonary edema is controlled or pleural effusion has been aspirated
• If there is pulmonary edema: furosemide (2–4 mg/kg IM or IV then 1–2 mg/kg q8–12h for the first 2–3 days)
• 2% topical nitroglycerine for the first 24–48 hours for severe pulmonary edema—apply 1"-2" q8h
• Aminophylline (initial 24 hrs.) for bronchodilation (4–6 mg/kg, slowly IV q8h)
• If there is significant pleural effusion, drain each hemithorax with an 18–20 gauge butterfly catheter
• If there is severe heart failure and cardiogenic shock digoxin and dobutamine are indicated. These may predispose to malignant arrhythmias particularly in the hypoxic dog
• Digoxin—oral therapy (see below)
• Dobutamine: 5–10 mcg/kg/min infused for 24–72 hours with care
• If paroxysmal ventricular tachycardia is present, administer lidocaine slowly in 2 mg/kg boluses (up to 8 mg/kg total) to convert to sinus rhythm. Follow with lidocaine infusion (40–75 ug/kg/min)
• If lidocaine is ineffective administer procainamide slowly in 2 mg/kg/IV boluses (up to 20 mg/kg total) to convert to sinus rhythm. Follow with a 20–50 mcg/kg/min infusion or 8–20 mg/kg IM q6h
Maintenance Therapy
• Vasodilators, especially the ACE inhibitors (enalapril, benazepril, lisinopril) are considered a cornerstone of therapy for DCM
• Enalapril (0.25–0.5 mg/kg PO q12h), benazepril (0.5 mg/kg PO q24h), or lisinopril (0.5 mg/kg PO q24h) should be initiated early in the therapeutic regimen
• A daily maintenance dose of 0.375 to 0.75 mg of digoxin (divided q12h) is given to most giant breed dogs. Don't exceed 0.015 mg/kg/day and don't exceed 0.375 mg per day in doberman pinschers. If necessary, an oral loading dose (2× maintenance dose) can be given the first 24–48 hours to dogs with atrial fibrillation or cardiogenic shock (uncommonly needed)

• Furosemide 0.5–1 mg/kg/ PO q8–24h is used to control pulmonary edema, pleural effusion, or ascites.
• The role of carnitine and taurine in the therapy of DCM remains controversial. However, American cocker spaniels with dilated cardiomyopathy generally respond favorably to taurine supplementation. Those not responding to taurine will often respond to the addition of l-carnitine.
Arrhythmias
• In the case of atrial fibrillation, slowing of the ventricular rate response is achieved with chronic administration of digitalis combined with atenolol (0.75–1.5 mg/kg PO q12h) or diltiazem (1–1.5mg/kg PO q8h)
• Therapeutic goal is obtaining a ventricular rate between 100–140 bpm at rest.
• The above therapy merely controls the ventricular rate, by depressing A-V nodal conduction; it generally does not convert the rhythm from atrial fibrillation to sinus rhythm.
• Chronic oral therapy for ventricular tachycardia includes procainamide (8–20 mg/kg PO q6–8h), tocainide (10–20 mg/kg PO q8h), mexiletine (5–8 mg/kg PO q8h) or sotalol (2 mg/kg PO q12h)
• The procainamide, tocainide and mexiletine can be combined with a beta blocker if necessary

CONTRAINDICATIONS
Digoxin should be avoided in severe uncontrolled paroxysmal ventricular tachycardia

PRECAUTIONS
• Beta blockers and calcium channel blockers are negative inotropes and may have an acute adverse effect on myocardial function although recent human studies have suggested that chronic administration of beta blockers may be of benefit in DCM
• The combination of diuretics and ACE inhibitors my result in azotemia, especially in patients with severe heart failure or pre-existing renal dysfunction

POSSIBLE INTERACTIONS
• Both quinidine and verapamil will increase serum digoxin levels and predispose to digitalis intoxication
• Propranolol will decrease lidocaine excretion and predispose to toxicity
• Renal dysfunction, hypothyroidism and hypokalemia predispose to digitalis intoxication

ALTERNATIVE DRUGS
• Other vasodilators, including hydralazine and amlodipine, may be used instead of or in addition to an ACE inhibitor (beware of hypotension)
• Propranolol can be used instead of diltiazem or atenolol to help control ventricular response rate in atrial fibrillation
• The role of co-enzyme Q-10 remains to be determined

FOLLOW-UP

PATIENT MONITORING
• Serial clinical examinations, thoracic radiographs, and ECG are most helpful • Repeat echocardiography is rarely informative
• Serial evaluation of serum digoxin levels (therapeutic range=0.8–1.8 ng/ml) taken 6–8 hours post-pill and serum biochemistries may help prevent iatrogenic problems

PREVENTION/AVOIDANCE
N/A

POSSIBLE COMPLICATIONS
• Sudden death due to arrhythmias • Iatrogenic problems associated with medical management (see above)

EXPECTED COURSE AND PROGNOSIS
• Always fatal • Death usually occurs 6–24 month following diagnosis • Dobermans typically have a worse prognosis with survival generally less than 6month from the time of diagnosis. • Atrial fibrillation, paroxysmal ventricular tachycardia and markedly decreased FS% are probably markers for short survival and sudden death

MISCELLANEOUS

ASSOCIATED CONDITIONS
N/A

AGE RELATED FACTORS
Prevalence increases with age

ZOONOTIC POTENTIAL
N/A

PREGNANCY
N/A

SYNONYMS
• Congestive cardiomyopathy • Giant breed cardiomyopathy

SEE ALSO
• Carnitine deficiency • Taurine deficiency
• Ventricular tachycardia • Atrial fibrillation

ABBREVIATIONS
• DCM = dilated cardiomyopathy • FS% = percent fractional shortening

Suggested Reading
Sisson,DD, Thomas WP. Myocardial Diseases In Fox PR, Sisson DD and Moise NS (Editors) Canine and Feline Cardiology 2nd Ed. W.B. Saunders, Philadelphia, 1999
Author Matthew W. Miller
Consulting Editors Larry P. Tilley & Francis W. K. Smith Jr.

CARDIOMYOPATHY, HYPERTROPHIC—CATS

 BASICS

DEFINITION
Hypertrophic cardiomyopathy is characterized by inappropriate concentric hypertrophy of the ventricular free wall or the intraventricular septum of the nondilated left ventricle. The disease occurs independently of other cardiac or systemic disorders.

PATHOPHYSIOLOGY
• Diastolic dysfunction results from a thickened, noncompliant left ventricle. • High left ventricular filling pressure develops, causing left atrial enlargement. • Pulmonary venous hypertension causes pulmonary edema. Some cats develop biventricular failure (i.e., pulmonary edema, pleural effusion, and rarely ascites) • Stasis of blood in the large left atrium predisposes the patient to aortic thromboembolism. • Dynamic aortic outflow obstruction occurs in some cats.

SYSTEMS AFFECTED
• Cardiovascular—congestive heart failure (CHF), aortic thromboembolism, and arrhythmias • Pulmonary—dyspnea if CHF develops • Renal/urologic—azotemia due to poor perfusion

GENETICS
Some families of cats have been identified with a high prevalence of the disease, but the genetics have not been determined.

INCIDENCE/PREVALENCE
Unknown, but relatively common

GEOGRAPHIC DISTRIBUTION
N/A

SIGNALMENT
Species
Cats

Breed Predilections
A familial association has been documented in Maine coon cats and Persians

Mean Age and Range
5–7 years with reported ages of 6 months to 16 years

Predominant Sex
Male > female

SIGNS
Historical Findings
• Dyspnea • Anorexia • Exercise intolerance • Vomiting • Collapse • Sudden death • Coughing is uncommon in cats with cardiomyopathy and usually suggests pulmonary disease.

Physical Examination Findings
• Gallop rhythm (S3 or S4) heard best with the bell of the stethoscope in most animals • Systolic murmur in many animals • Apex heart beat may be exaggerated. • Muffled heart sounds, lack of chest compliance, and dyspnea characterized by rapid shallow respirations may be associated with pleural effusion. • Dyspnea and louder than normal lung sounds and crackles if pulmonary edema is present • Weak femoral pulse in many animals • Acute pelvic limb paralysis with cyanotic pads and nailbeds, cold limbs, and absence of femoral pulse in animals with aortic thromboembolism. Emboli rarely affect thoracic limbs • Arrhythmia in some animals

CAUSES
Unknown—probably multiple causes exist

Possible causes
• Abnormality of the contractile protein myosin or other sarcomeric proteins (e.g., troponin, myosin binding proteins, tropomyosin) • Abnormality affecting catecholamine influenced excitation-contraction coupling • Abnormal myocardial calcium metabolism • Collagen or other intercellular matrix abnormality • Growth hormone excess

RISK FACTORS
Offspring of animals with familial HCM

 DIAGNOSIS

DIFFERENTIAL DIAGNOSIS
• Hyperthyroidism • Aortic stenosis • Systemic hypertension • Acromegaly • Noncardiac causes of pleural effusion (e.g., pyothorax, chylothorax, neoplasia, diaphragmatic hernia)

CBC/BIOCHEMISTRY/URINALYSIS
• Results usually normal • Prerenal azotemia in some animals

OTHER LABORATORY TESTS
• In cats over 6 years old, check thyroid concentration to rule out hyperthyroidism. Hyperthyroidism causes myocardial hypertrophy that might be confused with HCM (hyperthyroidism does not cause HCM). • A validated growth hormone assay for cats is not currently available. Some cats with HCM have high growth hormone concentration.

IMAGING
Radiography
• Dorsal ventral radiographs often reveal a valentine-appearing heart because of biatrial enlargement and a left ventricle that comes to a point. • Pulmonary edema or pleural effusion or both in some animals • Radiographs may be normal in asymptomatic cats. • The different forms of cardiomyopathy can not be differentiated by radiography

Echocardiography
• Hypertrophy of the interventricular septum (IVS, diastolic diameter > 6 mm) • Hypertrophy of the left ventricular posterior wall (diastolic diameter > 6 mm) • Hypertrophy may be symmetric (affecting IVS and posterior wall) or asymmetric (affecting IVS or posterior wall, but not both) • Hypertrophy of the papillary muscles • Normal or high fractional shortening • Normal or reduced left ventricular lumen • Left atrial enlargement • Systolic anterior motion of the mitral valve (some animals) • Left ventricular outflow obstruction (some animals) • Thrombus in the left atrium (rare) • Note: There is some overlap between normal cats (especially ketaminized and dehydrated) and cats with mild HCM. Correlate echo findings with physical findings. Presence of left atrial enlargement favors HCM.

DIAGNOSTIC PROCEDURES
Electrocardiography
• Sinus tachycardia (HR > 240) is common in patients in heart failure; however, some cats with severe heart failure and hypothermia are bradycardic. • Atrial premature complexes and ventricular premature complexes occasionally seen • Atrial fibrillation is uncommon in cats; when it occurs, it is often associated with HCM or restrictive cardiomyopathy. • A left axis deviation is seen in many cats. • ECG can not differentiate different forms of cardiomyopathy or distinguish cardiomyopathy from hyperthyroidism. • Cats with HCM may have a normal ECG.

Systemic Blood Pressure
• Patients are normotensive or hypotensive. • Evaluate blood pressure in all patients with myocardial hypertrophy to rule out systemic hypertension as the cause or contributing factor.

PATHOLOGIC FINDINGS
• Nondilated left ventricle with hypertrophy of intraventricular septum or left ventricular free wall • Hypertrophy of papillary muscles • Left atrial enlargement • Mitral valve thickening • Myocardial hypertrophy with disorganized alignment of myocytes • Interstitial fibrosis • Myocardial scarring • Hypertrophy and luminal narrowing of intramural coronary arteries

 TREATMENT

APPROPRIATE HEALTH CARE
Cats with CHF should be hospitalized for initial medical management.

NURSING CARE
• Minimize stress • Oxygen if dyspneic • Warm environment if hypothermic

ACTIVITY
Restricted

DIET
Sodium restriction in animal's with CHF

CLIENT EDUCATION

• Many cats diagnosed while asymptomatic eventually develop CHF and may develop aortic thromboembolism and die suddenly.
• If cat is receiving warfarin, minimize potential for trauma and subsequent hemorrhage.

SURGICAL CONSIDERATIONS
N/A

MEDICATIONS

DRUGS OF CHOICE

Diltiazem
• Dosage—7.5–15 mg/cat PO q8h or 10 mg/kg PO q24h (Cardizem CD) or 30 mg/cat q12h (Dilacor XR) • Beneficial effects may include slower sinus rate, resolution of supraventricular arrhythmias, improved diastolic relaxation, coronary vasodilation, peripheral vasodilation, platelet inhibition.
• Reduces hypertrophy and left atrial dimensions in some cats with HCM • Superior to propranolol and verapamil according to one small study • Role in asymptomatic patients unresolved

Beta Blockers
• Dosage—propranolol (2.5–10 mg/cat PO q8h–q12h) or atenolol (6.25–12.5 mg/cat PO q12h) • Beneficial effects may include slowing of sinus rate, correcting atrial and ventricular arrhythmias, platelet inhibition. • More effective than diltiazem in controlling sinus tachycardia and dynamic outflow tract obstruction
• Role in asymptomatic patients unresolved

Aspirin
• Dosage—80 mg/cat q 2–3 days • Depresses platelet aggregation, hopefully minimizing the risk of thromboembolism • Warn owners that thrombi can still develop despite aspirin administration.

Furosemide
• Dosage—1–2 mg/kg PO, IM, IV q8h–q24h
• Critically dyspneic animals often require high dosage (4 mg/kg IV) to stabilize. This dose can be repeated in 1 hour if the cat is still severely dyspneic. Indicated to treat pulmonary edema, pleural effusion, and ascites. • Cats are sensitive to furosemide and prone to dehydration, prerenal azotemia, and hypokalemia. • Once pulmonary edema resolves, taper the dosage to the lowest that controls edema. • Not indicated in asymptomatic patients

Nitroglycerin Ointment
• Dosage—0.25–0.5 in/cat topically applied q6h–q8h or 2.5 mg/24-hr patch • Apply to a hairless area in the inguinal or axillary region or the inside of the pinna. If the pinna are cold, choose an alternate site. • Tolerance develops with frequent dosing, so use intermittently and with 12-hour dose-free interval between the last dose of one day and the first dose of the next day. • Venodilation lowers

atrial filling pressures thereby reducing pulmonary edema, and pleural effusion • Often used in the acute stabilization of cats with severe pulmonary edema or pleural effusion
• When used intermittently, it may be useful for long-term management.

CONTRAINDICATIONS
Avoid beta blockers in cats with emboli; these agents cause peripheral vasoconstriction. If beta blockers must be used in this setting for arrhythmia control, choose a beta-1 selective blocker like atenolol.

PRECAUTIONS
• Arterial vasodilators such as hydralazine may worsen or cause aortic outflow tract obstruction. • Use ACE inhibitors cautiously if the cat has renal disease.

POSSIBLE INTERACTIONS
N/A

ALTERNATIVE DRUGS

Enalapril
• Dosage—0.5 mg/kg PO q24h–q48h
• Indications in cats with HCM not well-defined—authors currently use for repeat bouts of CHF • Potential benefits include lowered angiotensin II concentration, lowered catecholamine concentration, minimizing of diuretic-induced potassium depletion.
• Angiotensin II is a potent stimulator of myocardial hypertrophy.

Warfarin
• Dosage—0.5 mg/cat PO q24h and then titrate to effect • Lowers risk of aortic thromboembolism • A procoagulant effect precedes the anticoagulant effect by several days. Use heparin (50–100 IU/kg SQ q8h) along with warfarin for the first 3–4 days of treatment.
• Raises risk of spontaneous hemorrhage, so requires careful and frequent monitoring

Beta Blocker Plus Diltiazem
• Cats that remain tachycardic on a single agent can be treated cautiously with a combination of a beta blocker and diltiazem. • Monitor closely for bradycardia and hypotension.

FOLLOW-UP

PATIENT MONITORING
• Observe closely for signs of dyspnea, lethargy, weakness, anorexia, and posterior paralysis. • If treating with warfarin, monitor prothrombin time (PT) frequently to avoid bleeding complications. Adjust warfarin dose to achieve a PT value that is 1.5–2 times the baseline value. International normalization ratios (INR) are recommended to minimize the effects of test kit variability on PT results. • If treating with enalapril, monitor renal function. • Repeat echocardiogram in 4 months to assess efficacy of treatment for hypertrophy. If a beta blocker

or diltiazem was prescribed in an asymptomatic animal and there is no evidence of improvement, consider discontinuing treatment or switch to another class of medications and recheck the patient 4 months later.

PREVENTION/AVOIDANCE
Avoid stressful situations that might precipitate CHF.

POSSIBLE COMPLICATIONS
• Left heart failure • Aortic thromboembolism and paralysis • Cardiac arrhythmias

EXPECTED COURSE AND PROGNOSIS
• Prognosis varies considerably, probably because there are multiple causes. Some animals have complete resolution and remain normal after medications are withdrawn. Others show poor response to medications and die shortly after examination. • In one study, cats that were asymptomatic at the time of diagnosis lived from 1 day to 6 years:
  median survival for cats with aortic thromboembolism was 61 days
  median survival for cats with heart failure was 92 days
  cats with a resting heart rate < 200 live longer than cats with rates > 200.

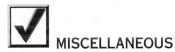

MISCELLANEOUS

ASSOCIATED CONDITIONS
Aortic thromboembolism

AGE RELATED FACTORS
N/A

ZOONOTIC POTENTIAL
N/A

PREGNANCY
• High risk of complications • Avoid aspirin

SYNONYMS
N/A

SEE ALSO
• Acromegaly • Congestive Heart Failure, Left-Sided • Murmurs, heart • Aortic Thromboembolism • Hypertension, Systemic
• Hyperthyroidism

ABBREVIATIONS
HCM = hypertrophic cardiomyopathy
IVS = intraventricular septum
PT = prothrombin time
PW = posterior wall

Suggested Reading
Atkins CE, Gallo AM, Kurman ID. A retrospective study of risk factors, presenting signs, and survival in 74 cases of feline idiopathic hypertrophic cardiomyopathy. J Vet Intern Med 1991;5:122.
Fox PR. Feline Cardiomyopathies. In Fox PR, Sisson D, Moise NS, eds. Textbook of Ca

CARDIOMYOPATHY, HYPERTROPHIC—DOGS

 BASICS

OVERVIEW

Hypertrophic cardiomyopathy is a rare disease in dogs characterized by left ventricular concentric hypertrophy (increased wall thickness). The primary disease process is confined to the heart and only affects other organ system when congestive heart failure is present. Increased LV wall thickness leads to impaired ventricular filling (due to lack of compliance) with a resultant increase in LV end-diastolic pressure and LA pressure. The LA usually enlarges in response to increased LV end-diastolic pressure. Mitral insufficiency and/or dynamic LV outflow tract obstruction commonly occur secondary to structural and/or functional changes of the mitral valve apparatus caused by papillary muscle mal-alignment secondary to the hypertrophy.

SIGNALMENT

The incidence of HCM in dogs is very low, such that, accurate accounts of signalment are lacking. Some authors have suggested that German shepherd dogs may be predisposed and recent reports suggest an increased incidence in the dalmation and pointer dogs.

SIGNS

Historical Findings
• Asymptomatic (usually)
• Left heart failure
• Syncope
• Sudden death (especially during anesthesia)

Physical Examination Findings
• Systolic heart murmur
• Cardiac gallop rhythm
• Signs of left heart failure (e.g., cough, dyspnea, cyanosis, exercise intolerance)

CAUSES & RISK FACTORS

The cause of hypertrophic cardiomyopathy is unknown. Genetic abnormalities in genes coding for myocardial contractile proteins have been documented in humans and in cats but not in dogs.

 DIAGNOSIS

DIFFERENTIAL DIAGNOSIS
• Systemic hypertension
• Infiltrative cardiac disorders
• Other causes of CHF
• Thyrotoxicosis

CBC/BIOCHEMISTRY/URINALYSIS
N/A

OTHER LABORATORY TESTS
N/A

IMAGING

Radiography
• May be normal.
• May show LA or LV enlargement.
• Pulmonary edema is present in dogs with left congestive heart failure.

Echocardiography
• Dogs with severe HCM usually have markedly thickened left ventricular walls, papillary muscle hypertrophy, and an enlarged left atrium. The hypertrophy can be global, affecting all areas of the left ventricular wall or can be more regional or segmental (asymmetric).
• Systolic anterior motion of the mitral valve, suggesting dynamic LV outflow tract obstruction, is common in dogs with HCM.

OTHER DIAGNOSTIC PROCEDURES

Electrocardiography
• May be normal.
• ST segment and T wave abnormalities have been reported.
• Atrial or ventricular ectopic arrhythmias may rarely occur.

Blood Pressure
Usually normal. Should be evaluated to rule out systemic hypertension as the cause of LV hypertrophy.

PATHOLOGIC FINDINGS
Abnormal heart : body weight ration. Left ventricular concentric hypertrophy. Left atrial enlargement.

 TREATMENT

Out patient management unless in congestive heart failure
Exercise restriction and sodium restriction are beneficial.

MEDICATIONS

DRUGS

• Treatment is generally only pursued if there is evidence of congestive heart failure.
• In patients with left congestive heart failure, diuretics and ACE inhibitor therapy are advocated.
• In dogs with high LV-Ao pressure gradients due to dynamic LV outflow obstruction, administration of a beta adrenergic blocker or calcium channel blocker has been advocated, however, benefit has not been proven.
• Beta adrenergic blockers or calcium channel blockers may also improve myocardial oxygenation, reduce heart rate, improve ventricular filling, and control arrhythmias and therefore may also be beneficial in dogs with left congestive heart failure.

CONTRAINDICATIONS/POSSIBLE INTERACTIONS

• Positive inotropic drugs should be avoided as they may worsen dynamic LV outflow obstruction.
• The use of a calcium channel blocker in combination with a beta blocker should be avoided as clinically significant bradyarrhythmias can develop.
• The use potent arteriolar dilators should be avoided in patients with dynamic LV outflow tract obstruction. However, the use of milder vasodilators such as ACE inhibitors in patients with congestive heart failure are generally well tolerated.

FOLLOW-UP

• Reevaluation depends on the severity of the clinical signs. Reevaluation with radiography and echocardiography may be useful to characterize disease progression and make appropriate medication adjustments.
• Due to the rarity of this condition in dogs, information regarding prognosis is lacking. In dogs with severe congestive heart failure or other complications, prognosis is generally guarded.

MISCELLANEOUS

ABBREVIATIONS

LV = left ventricle
LA = left atrium
HCM = hypertrophic cardiomyopathy
ACE = angiotensin converting enzyme

Suggested Reading

Kittleson MD, Kienle RD. eds. Small Animal Cardiovascular Medicine. St Louis: Mosby, 1998.
Author Richard D. Kienle
Consulting Editors Larry P. Tilley & Francis W. K. Smith Jr.

CARDIOMYOPATHY, RESTRICTIVE—CATS

 BASICS

OVERVIEW

• A poorly defined feline myocardial disease resulting from regional or diffuse ventricular myocardial or subendocardial fibrosis, sometimes referred to as "intermediate" or "intergrade" cardiomyopathy
• Myocardial fibrosis results in both systolic (pumping) and diastolic (filling) dysfunction, leading to congestive heart failure (CHF), arrhythmias and arterial thromboembolism
• May be "final common pathway" of more than one myocardial disease
• Usually diagnosed by recognition of "typical" clinical, radiographic and echocardiographic findings

SIGNALMENT

Cats

SIGNS

Historical Findings

If cat does not have CHF:
• Lethargy
• Poor appetite and weight loss
• Syncope (rare; usually indicates serious arrhythmia)
• Paresis or paralysis (i.e. signs of arterial thromboembolism)
• Some cats are asymptomatic
If cat has CHF, above signs plus the following:
• Dyspnea
• Tachypnea
• Open mouth breathing
• Cyanosis
• Abdominal distention

Physical Examination Findings

If cat does not have CHF:
• Depression
• Cachexia
• Tachycardia
• Arrhythmias,
• Gallop rhythm +/− systolic heart murmur
If cat has CHF, above signs plus the following:
• Tachypnea
• Dyspnea
• Panting
• Cyanosis
• Hepatomegaly or ascites with jugular venous distention
• Pulmonary crackles
• Muffled cardiac or respiratory sounds if cat has pleural effusion

• Paralysis or paresis with loss of femoral pulses; one or more extremities cold and painful (arterial thromboembolism)

CAUSES & RISK FACTORS

• True cause(s) unknown; often no "predisposing" disease can be documented
• Suspected initiating causes include myocarditis, endomyocarditis, eosinophilic myocardial infiltration, hypertrophic cardiomyopathy with myocardial infarction, diffuse "small vessel disease" and other causes of myocardial ischemia

 DIAGNOSIS

DIFFERENTIAL DIAGNOSIS

Other causes of signs of CHF (e.g. pulmonary edema, ascites, exercise intolerance):
• Hypertrophic cardiomyopathy
• Dilated cardiomyopathy
• Decompensated congenital cardiac abnormalities (e.g. aortic stenosis, ventricular septal defect, atrioventricular canal defect or excessive left ventricular moderator bands)
• CHF secondary to thyrotoxicosis or hypertensive heart disease
Other causes of syncope, collapse, weakness and lethargy:
• Arrhythmias associated with any other form of cardiac disease
• Arrhythmias associated with metabolic or neurologic disease
• Neurologic or musculoskeletal abnormality
• Metabolic disease or electrolyte disturbance
Other causes of paralysis or paresis (arterial thromboembolism):
• Any form of cardiac disease
• Neurologic or musculoskeletal abnormality

CBC/BIOCHEMISTRY/URINALYSIS

• Most laboratory testing does not contribute to diagnosis of restrictive cardiomyopathy
• Routine chemistry panel (with electrolytes) and urinalysis helpful to document concurrent or complicating conditions (e.g. pre-renal azotemia and potassium abnormality)

OTHER LABORATORY TESTS

• Plasma taurine levels low in some cats

IMAGING

Thoracic Radiographic Findings

• Cardiomegaly with disproportionate atrial enlargement

• Interstitial or alveolar infiltrates or pleural effusion with pulmonary venous distention if cat has CHF

Echocardiographic Findings

Note—"Typical" findings controversial; diagnosis of restrictive cardiomyopathy usually based on the following echocardiographic findings (see references):
• Mild or moderate right atrial and ventricular enlargement
• Left atrial enlargement inappropriate to the magnitude of hypertrophy, myocardial failure or mitral insufficiency
• Normal to slightly thickened left ventricular wall
• Small left ventricular lumen size or narrowing in midventricle caused by fibrosis or fibrous bands
• Dilation of the left ventricle immediately distal to the mitral valve
• Regional wall motion abnormalities or hypertrophy, hyperechoic subendocardial foci, moderator bands
• Normal to slightly decreased shortening fraction
• No or mild atrioventricular valve insufficiency by Doppler-echocardiography
• Pericardial effusion of variable severity
• Echodense intracardiac thrombi in atria or attached to atrial or ventricular wall in some cats

DIAGNOSTIC PROCEDURES

Electrocardiographic Findings

• Sinus tachycardia common
• Intraventricular conduction defects, including bundle branch blocks
• Isolated ectopy, paroxysmal or sustained supraventricular or ventricular tachycardias and atrial fibrillation
• Atrial or ventricular enlargement patterns

 TREATMENT

• Patients with acute, severe CHF are hospitalized for emergency care
• Mildly symptomatic or asymptomatic animals can be treated with outpatient medical management
• Severely dyspneic animals should receive oxygen via oxygen cage, nasal cannula or mask (beware of stress to patient)
• Life-threatening pleural effusions are reduced via thoracocentesis

• Low sodium fluids administered cautiously if dehydration occurs (beware of worsening CHF)
• Maintain a low stress environment to decrease patient anxiety (e.g. cage rest, minimize handling)
• Heating pad may be necessary for hypothermic patients
• Low salt diet chronically may decrease fluid retention but strict adherence to dietary changes should be avoided in acute CHF to maintain oral intake; handfeed as necessary

 MEDICATIONS

DRUG(S)

Acute CHF
• Parenteral administration of furosemide (0.5–2 mg/kg IV, IM, SC q8–q24h)
• Dermal application of nitroglycerin ointment (2%, 1/8–1/4 inch q12h)
• Oxygen delivered by cage, mask, nasal tube
• Thoracocentesis as necessary to relieve dyspnea due to pleural effusion
• Severe supraventricular arrhythmias may be treated with diltiazem (1.5–2.5 mg/kg PO q8h) or long-acting diltiazem (10 mg/kg PO q24h)
• Ventricular tachycardia may resolve with resolution of CHF
• Acute therapy of ventricular tachycardia may include lidocaine (0.25–0.5 mg/kg IV SLOWLY); monitor closely for neurologic signs of toxicity
• Beta blockers (propranolol [2.5–7.5 mg PO q8h], atenolol [6.25–12.5 mg PO q12h]) may be used to treat supraventricular or ventricular arrhythmias but not until CHF is treated (see contraindications)

Chronic Therapy
• Furosemide gradually decreased to lowest effective dose
• Chronic therapy with diltiazem decreases heart rate and improves supraventricular arrhythmias and may improve diastolic function
• Beta blockers may be used to slow heart rate and treat supraventricular or ventricular arrhythmias
• Enalapril (0.25–0.5 mg/kg PO q24h–48h) may reduce fluid retention and decrease need for diuretics

• Digoxin (0.01 mg/kg PO q48h) may be used if systolic function is impaired or atrial fibrillation is present
• Treat associated conditions (e.g., dehydration, hypothermia)
• Aspirin (80 mg PO q72h) may be administered to prevent thromboembolism, but efficacy is questionable
• Warfarin (0.5 mg PO q24 h) may be administered to prevent thromboembolism but is not recommended unless close monitoring and repeated measurement of prothrombin time are feasible

CONTRAINDICATIONS/POSSIBLE INTERACTIONS

Contraindications
• Beta-blocking drugs—atrioventricular block, untreated CHF, bradycardia, myocardial failure, and asthma (especially nonselective beta blockers, e.g. propranolol)
• Diltiazem—bradycardia, atrioventricular block, myocardial failure, and hypotension
• Digoxin—azotemia, atrioventricular block, and severe ventricular arrhythmias
• Furosemide—dehydration, hypokalemia, and azotemia
• Nitroglycerin ointment—hypotension
• Enalapril—azotemia, hypotension, and hyperkalemia

POSSIBLE INTERACTIONS
• Beta blockers and diltiazem should rarely be used together; combination may lead to bradycardia, hypotension, and severe atrioventricular block
• Use of enalapril in dehydrated or hyponatremic animals may result in hypotension, azotemia, and hyperkalemia
• Chronic aspirin therapy may increase risk of renal side effects of enalapril

 FOLLOW-UP

PATIENT MONITORING
• Frequent serial physical examinations (minimal stress to patient) to assess response to treatment and resolution of pulmonary edema and effusions
• Frequent assessment of hydration and renal function is important in first few days of therapy to avoid overdiuresis and azotemia

• Repeated thoracocentesis may be necessary to maintain effusions at level compatible with comfort
• Radiographs may be repeated in 12–24 hours to monitor pulmonary infiltrate resolution
• Electrolytes (especially creatinine and potassium) should be monitored closely during the first 3–5 days of therapy to detect dehydration, renal failure and hypokalemia (caused by diuretic administration and anorexia) or hyperkalemia (if enalapril is administered)
• Repeat physical examination and electrolyte analysis after approximately 10–14 days of treatment
• ECG and radiographs repeated at clinician's discretion
• Stable patients are reevaluated every 2–4 months, or more frequently if problems

Expected Course and Prognosis
• Most cats with restrictive cardiomyopathy and CHF live 3–12 months, some to 2 years

 MISCELLANEOUS

ASSOCIATED CONDITIONS
• Aortic thromboembolism

SEE ALSO
• Aortic thromboembolism
• Congestive heart failure, left-sided
• Congestive heart failure, right-sided

SYNONYMS
• Intermediate cardiomyopathy
• Intergrade cardiomyopathy

Suggested Reading
Pion PD, Kienle RD. Feline cardiomyopathy. In: Miller MS, Tilley LP, eds. Manual of canine and feline cardiology. 2nd ed. Philadelphia: WB Saunders, 1995.
Author Rebecca L. Stepien
Consulting Editors Larry P. Tilley and Francis W. K. Smith Jr.

DISEASES

CARNITINE DEFICIENCY

BASICS

OVERVIEW

L-carnitine is a quaternary amine that is an important part of the enzymes that transport fatty acids into mitochondria so that they can be oxidized to make energy available to the cell. In the heart and other organs that depend on the oxidation of fatty acids to supply their high energy requirements for contraction or other work, L-carnitine deficiency results in inadequate production of energy to meet those needs. Carnitine deficiency appears to complicate approximately 40% of cases of dilated cardiomyopathy in dogs. The presence of L-carnitine deficiency in association with cardiomyopathy does not mean that the deficiency is the sole cause of the myopathy, although correcting the deficiency (if possible) makes medical and physiologic sense. L-carnitine is not synthesized in heart or skeletal muscle, and must therefore be transported into those cells from plasma. In the dog, dietary carnitine intake influences plasma concentrations significantly, and oral carnitine supplementation is usually an effective means of raising plasma and subsequently muscle carnitine levels. The FDA has recently (1998) approved the addition of physiologic amounts of carnitine to commercial dog foods for the prevention of plasma (and subsequently muscle) carnitine deficiency. This action is prudent based on current knowledge regarding the lack of L-carnitine in most commercial dog food and the effect of those diets on canine carnitine plasma levels. It is not known whether this action will affect the prevalence of dilated cardiomyopathy or other manifestations of carnitine deficiency.

SIGNALMENT

• Dogs • Boxers, Doberman pinschers, Great Danes, Irish Wolfhounds, and other large and giant breed dogs appear to be most commonly affected with DCM.

• At least some American cocker spaniels with dilated cardiomyopathy are carnitine deficient, and a blinded, placebo controlled trial suggests showed that L-carnitine supplementation combined with taurine supplementation is beneficial in the medical management of these patients.

SIGNS

• Clinical signs of carnitine deficiency can be diverse, mitochondria in all tissues utilize L-carnitine to produce energy from fatty acids,

• Signs range from heart muscle failure and dilated cardiomyopathy (most frequently recognized) to skeletal muscle pain, weakness, exercise intolerance, and / or lethargy.

• See Cardiomyopathy, Dilated—Dogs

CAUSES & RISK FACTORS

• Some dogs with cardiomyopathy have been documented to have carnitine transport defects, where muscle carnitine is low even in the face of adequate plasma carnitine concentrations. In order to transport fatty acids or other compounds (such as acetyl Co-A) into or out of the mitochondria, free L-carnitine is esterified to the substance, forming a carnitine ester. In cases where a mitochondrial enzyme defect causes the accumulation of a metabolite to toxic levels within the mitochondria (e.g. multiple Co-A dehydrogenase defects), free L-carnitine is used to "scavenge" the potentially toxic excess metabolites, which appear harmlessly in the plasma and eventually the urine as carnitine esters. In these cases, the total amount of carnitine (free carnitine plus that esterified to other molecules) in the plasma or muscle may be normal or even high, but the ratio of free carnitine to esterified carnitine is decreased. This situation is known as carnitine insufficiency (because even though the concentration of free carnitine may be within the normal range, it is insufficient to meet the body's pathologically increased need for free carnitine). • Certain families of Boxers appear to be at especially high risk of developing symptomatic dilated cardiomyopathy in association with and probably caused by carnitine deficiency. A known first degree relative with cardiomyopathy should increase the index of suspicion.

DIAGNOSIS

DIFFERENTIAL DIAGNOSIS

See Cardiomyopathy, Dilated–Dogs

CBC/BIOCHEMISTRY/URINALYSIS

Normal

OTHER LABORATORY TESTS

Plasma carnitine concentrations appear to be a specific but insensitive indicator of myocardial or skeletal muscle carnitine deficiency. Plasma free carnitine concentrations of less than 8 micromoles/L are considered diagnostic of systemic carnitine deficiency. Plasma concentrations in the normal or supernormal range do not rule out myocardial carnitine deficiency or insufficiency.

IMAGING

See Cardiomyopathy, Dilated–Dogs

DIAGNOSTIC TESTS

Endomyocardial biopsy specimens must be blotted dry and snap frozen in liquid nitrogen. Measurement of free and esterified L-carnitine concentrations normalized to the amount of noncollagenous protein in the biopsy remains the only definitive diagnostic test. Myocardial free carnitine concentrations of less than 3.5 nanomoles/mg of non-collagenous protein are considered diagnostic of myocardial carnitine deficiency. Ratios of esterified to free carnitine greater than 0.4 are considered diagnostic of carnitine insufficiency.

TREATMENT

Treatment with L-carnitine does not replace conventional treatment for DCM, even in most dogs with carnitine deficiency. Some dogs, including some families of carnitine deficient boxers, fail to respond clinically to supplementation. While supplementation dramatically improves a small percentage (about 5% in the author's experience) of dogs with dilated cardiomyopathy, the overall efficacy of L-carnitine supplementation for the treatment of dilated cardiomyopathy is untested.

MEDICATIONS

DRUGS

Carnitine Supplementation
• Large breed dogs, 2g (approximately 1tsp. L-carnitine powder) q8h–q12h
• American Cocker Spaniels (in combination with Taurine) 1g (approximately 1/2tsp L-carnitine powder) q8h–q12h

CONTRAINDICATIONS/POSSIBLE INTERACTIONS
• None have been identified • Mild diarrhea has been associated with high doses of carnitine in some people

FOLLOW-UP

Repeat echocardiogram 3–6 months after initiating L-carnitine supplementation to assess the efficacy of treatment

MISCELLANEOUS

Suggested Reading

Keene BW, Panciera DP, Atkins CE, Regitz V, Schmidt MJ, Shug AL: Myocardial L-carnitine deficiency in a family of dogs with dilated cardiomyopathy. J Am Vet Med Assoc 201:647–50, 1991.
Keene BW, Kittleson MD, Rush JE, Pion PD, Atkins CE, DeLellis LD, Meurs KM and Shug AL: Myocardial carnitine deficiency associated with dilated cardiomyopathy in Doberman pinschers. J Vet Int Med 3:126, 1989 (Abstract)

Author Bruce W. Keene
Consulting Editor Larry P Tilley and Francis W. K. Smith Jr.

CATARACTS

 BASICS

DEFINITION
• Opacification of the lens
• Term *cataract*—may refer to an entire lens that is opaque or to a opacity within the lens; does not imply cause

PATHOPHYSIOLOGY
• Basic mechanism—thought to be cross-linking of lens protein
• Specific causes—genetic defects; nutritional deficiency; focal disruption of normal lens metabolism by adhesion to uveal tissue (synechia); radiation; elevated blood glucose; hypocalcemia; toxins; faulty embryogenesis; altered composition of the aqueous humor caused by uveitis
• Traditional terminology—immature (only part of the lens is involved); mature (entire lens is opaque); hypermature (lens liquefaction has occurred); implies progressive condition; but may note protein in each stage within the same lens
• Liquefaction—occurs more readily in young patients; with time will eventually occur to some degree in all patients

SYSTEMS AFFECTED
Ophthalmic

GENETICS
• Most are inherited.
• Most common mode of inheritance—simple autosomal recessive
• Some breeds—dominantly inherited

INCIDENCE/PREVALENCE
• Dogs—common; exact prevalence unknown; one of the most important causes of vision loss
• Cats—uncommon

GEOGRAPHIC DISTRIBUTION
N/A

SIGNALMENT
Species
Dogs and cats

Breed Predilections
• Many dog breeds are affected by hereditary cataracts; refer to general reference texts.
• Cataracts that typically progress to blindness—miniature poodles; American cocker spaniels; miniature schnauzers
• Other commonly affected breeds—golden retrievers; Boston terriers; Siberian huskies
• Cats—Persians; Birmans; Himalayans

Mean Age and Range
• Depend on cause

• Hereditary (dogs)—may be congenital; may be acquired anytime from several months to many years of age, depending on breed
• Hereditary (cats)—all reported to date have been congenital.

Predominant Sex
None

SIGNS
Historical Findings
• Related to the degree of vision impairment
• Occupy < 30% of the lens or affect only one eye—often go unnoticed
• Occupy > 60% of the lens—usually reported
• Caused by diabetes mellitus—polyuria, polydipsia, and weight loss
• Cloudiness noticed before vision impairment—usually sclerosis
• Associated progressive retinal degeneration (dogs)—difficulty seeing in dimly lighted conditions (nyctalopia)

Physical Examination Findings
• Opacification of lens
• Slit lamp biomicroscope—determine exact location (e.g., nuclear, cortical)
• Hypermature—minute crystals within the lens
• Liquefied lens material leaking from the lens—wrinkling of the lens capsule
• Associated with uveitis—typically see aqueous flare, synechia, and low intraocular pressure

Tapetal Reflection
• Easiest method of detection
• Obstruction of light by lenticular opacities (retroillumination)
• Appear as black or gray spots
• Cloudiness owing to sclerosis—will not detect discreet foci of tapetal obstruction

CAUSES
• Heredity
• Diabetes mellitus
• Spontaneous—age-related
• Advanced retinal degeneration—response to toxic dialdehydes
• Uveitis—secondary to synechia formation or altered aqueous humor composition
• Toxic substances—dinitrophenol; naphthalene
• Nutrition—milk-replacer diet
• Hypocalcemia
• Radiation
• Electric shock

RISK FACTORS
• Faulty heredity
• Multiple congenital ocular defects
• Any disease capable of causing uveitis

• Advanced retinal degeneration
• Systemic metabolic diseases—diabetes; diseases capable of causing hypocalcemia

 DIAGNOSIS

DIFFERENTIAL DIAGNOSIS
• Lenticular sclerosis—normal aging phenomenon; often mistaken for cataracts; does not cause vision loss; easily distinguished by retro-illumination (see Physical Examination Findings)
• Uveitis (dogs)—may cause or be caused by cataracts; distinction made on the basis of signalment, history, extent of cataract formation, and appearance of the cataract; assumed to be lens-induced until proven otherwise in pure breeds with concurrent complete cataracts; assumed to be secondary to the inflammation (especially in nonpure breeds) with concurrent incomplete cataracts
• Chronic uveitis (cats)—focal cataracts frequent sequelae

CBC/BIOCHEMISTRY/URINALYSIS
• Not routinely necessary; condition usually hereditary
• Routine hematology—screen for infectious diseases when associated with uveitis
• Blood chemistry profiles—rule out systemic metabolic disease (e.g., diabetes mellitus, hypocalcemia).

OTHER LABORATORY TESTS
Serologic Testing
• Non–lens-induced and associated with uveitis—routine
• Dogs—rule out systemic mycoses (e.g., histoplasmosis, coccidiomycosis, blastomycosis, cryptococcosis), rickettsial disease (e.g., *Ehrlichia canis, Borrelia burgdorferi, Rickettsia rickettsii*), and brucellosis.
• Cats with chronic uveitis and secondary cataracts—rule out toxoplasmosis, FeLV infection, and FIV infection.

IMAGING
• Ophthalmic ultrasonography—indicated for hypermature cataracts and anticipated surgery; associated retinal detachment
• Ultrasonographic—indicated for complete congenital cataracts; rule out other intraocular defects (e.g., persistent hyaloid artery, persistent primary vitreous, lenticonus).

DIAGNOSTIC PROCEDURES
Electroretinography—always done for anticipated surgery; evaluate the retina; rule out concurrent retinal degeneration.

PATHOLOGIC FINDINGS
- Lens fiber swelling
- Posterior migration of lens epithelium
- Liquefaction of lens material
- Lens epithelial fibrous metaplasia
- Lens mineralization

TREATMENT

APPROPRIATE HEALTH CARE
- Dogs undergoing surgery—inpatients or outpatients
- Hospitalization—rarely required > 48 hr

NURSING CARE
N/A

ACTIVITY
N/A

DIET
N/A

CLIENT EDUCATION
- Inform client that surgery can normally be done on any hereditary cataract that is causing or is anticipated to cause vision loss.
- Warn client that the prognosis for surgery is better if it is done early in the course of cataract development, before hypermaturity, lens-induced uveitis, and retinal detachment occur.
- It is not advisable to delay surgery until the patient is blind in both eyes.
- Discuss that surgery may or may not be indicated for nonhereditary cataracts.
- Point out that because of the high success rate of phacoemulsification, it is no longer appropriate to observe cataracts for possible resorption, even in young dogs.

SURGICAL CONSIDERATIONS
- Phacoemulsification—ultrasonic lens fragmentation; procedure of choice
- Prognosis for successful surgery—generally > 90%; depends on the stage of the cataract and other concurrent findings
- Intraocular lenses—may be safely implanted at the time of surgery, so patient will not suffer extreme farsightedness

MEDICATIONS

DRUGS OF CHOICE
1% prednisolone acetate—q6h; prevent and control lens-induced uveitis; indicated for progressing condition for which surgery is planned

CONTRAINDICATIONS
Chronic topical atropine therapy—avoid in dogs that will be undergoing surgery; causes parasympathetic receptor hyperplasia, thereby contributing to intraoperative miosis

PRECAUTIONS
N/A

POSSIBLE INTERACTIONS
N/A

ALTERNATIVE DRUGS
N/A

FOLLOW-UP

PATIENT MONITORING
- All patients—monitored carefully for progression
- Hereditary—condition may progress very quickly in young dogs.

PREVENTION/AVOIDANCE
Do not breed patients with known or suspected inherited condition.

POSSIBLE COMPLICATIONS
Complete cataracts—potential to cause lens-induced uveitis, secondary glaucoma, and retinal detachment

EXPECTED COURSE AND PROGNOSIS
- Rate of progression—depends on location within the lens, and patient's age
- Nuclear—may appear to become smaller because the nucleus compresses with age
- Cortical—almost always progress, except for specific hereditary types (e.g., posterior triangular cataracts in golden retrievers)
- Normal lens aging—lens protein becomes insoluble and sclerotic, inhibiting cataract progression; thus a small cataract in a 1-year-old cocker spaniel may enlarge and cause blindness within several months, whereas the same size cataract in 10-year-old poodle may cause blindness only after several years.
- Diabetes mellitus–induced—usually very rapid progress
- Surgical intervention—for hereditary or diabetes-caused cataracts: prognosis for good vision excellent; for other types of cataracts: depends on cause

✓ MISCELLANEOUS

ASSOCIATED CONDITIONS
See Causes.

AGE-RELATED FACTORS
- Development of nonhereditary cataracts in senile dogs—subject of debate, but seems to occur
- Age by itself is not a consideration when recommending surgery.

ZOONOTIC POTENTIAL
N/A

PREGNANCY
N/A

SEE ALSO
- Anterior Uveitis—Cats
- Anterior Uveitis—Dogs
- Blind Quiet Eye
- Diabetes Mellitus
- Retinal Degeneration

ABBREVIATIONS
- FeLV = feline leukemia virus
- FIV = feline immunodeficiency virus

Suggested Reading

Davidson MG, Nasisse MP, Jamieson VE, et al. Phacoemulsification and intraocular lens implantation: a study of results in 182 dogs. Prog Vet Compend Ophthalmol 1991;1:233–238.

Gelatt KN. The canine lens. In: Gelatt KN, ed. Veterinary ophthalmology. 2nd ed. Philadelphia: Lea & Febiger, 1992:429–460.

Glover TL, Constantinescu GM. Surgery for cataracts. Vet Clin North Am 1997;27:1143–1173.

Nasisse MP, Davidson MG, Jamieson VE, et al. Phacoemulsification and intraocular lens implantation: a study of technique in 182 dogs. Prog Vet Compend Ophthalmol 1991;1:225–232.

Nasisse MP. Innovations in cataract surgery. In: Kirk RW, ed. Current veterinary therapy XII. Philadelphia, Saunders, 1994:1261–1264.

van der Woerdt A, Wilkie DA, Myer W. Ultrasonic abnormalities in the eyes of dogs with cataracts. J Am Vet Med Assoc 1993;203:838–841.

Author Mark P. Nasisse
Consulting Editor Paul E. Miller

CECAL INVERSION

 BASICS

OVERVIEW
Cecal inversion or cecocolic intussusception causes partial-to-complete, intermittent obstruction of the ileocolic junction.

SIGNALMENT
• Reported more frequently in dogs, but has been reported in one cat.
• No age, sex, or breed predilection
• Age range, 1–15 years

SIGNS
Historical Findings
• Possibly weight loss
• Chronic intermittent hematochezia and soft stools
• Nonresponsive to administration of anthelmintics, protectants, and antibiotics, dietary adjustment, and motility modification

Physical Examination Findings
• Usually unremarkable
• Acute vomiting, depression, dehydration in patients with complete obstruction
• Painful midabdominal mass may be palpable.

CAUSES & RISK FACTORS
• Cause unknown
• Possible causes include parasitism (whipworms) and neoplasia.
• Intestinal lymphoma has been seen in patients with intussusception.

 DIAGNOSIS

DIFFERENTIAL DIAGNOSIS
• Consider diseases characterized by hematochezia and intermittent soft stool (e.g., intestinal parasitism, neoplasia, inflammatory bowel disease, ileocolic intussusception, infectious bowel diseases).
• Consider diseases that cause midabdominal palpable masses (e.g., neoplasia, abdominal lymphadenopathy)

CBC/BIOCHEMISTRY/URINALYSIS
• Usually normal or nonspecific
• Anemia or hypoalbuminemia associated with chronic blood loss is uncommon.

OTHER LABORATORY TESTS
Fecal flotation and direct examination are indicated.

IMAGING
Abdominal Radiography
Usually nonspecific unless the patient has gastrointestinal obstruction

Contrast Radiography
• Upper or lower gastrointestinal positive-contrast study—the inverted cecum may be seen in the proximal colon surrounded by contrast material.
• Pneumocolonography (negative-contrast study)—the inverted cecum may be seen in the proximal colon.

Abdominal Ultrasonography
Multiple intestinal wall layering may be seen in the area of the cecum/proximal colon.

DIAGNOSTIC PROCEDURES
• Flexible colonoscopy—allows direct visualization of a fingerlike projection protruding into the colon through the ileocolic junction
• Exploratory celiotomy on the basis of imaging or colonoscopic findings

 TREATMENT

• Inpatient surgical management
• Restore/address dehydration and any electrolyte abnormalities.
• Exploratory celiotomy and typhlectomy are indicated.
• If reduction can be achieved, perform the typhlectomy from the serosal surface.
• If reduction cannot be achieved, make an incision opposite the lesion on the antimesenteric border of the colon, and remove the cecum from the mucosal surface; in general, a two-layer closure is recommended for colonotomy and typhlectomy; surgical stapling has been described as appropriate for use in typhlectomy.
• Treat any underlying conditions (e.g., intestinal parasitism).

 MEDICATIONS

DRUGS
• Standard anesthetic protocols should be adequate.
• Perioperative antibiotics appropriate for colonic surgery (e.g., cefazolin sodium, 20–35 mg/kg IV or cefoxitin sodium, 30 mg/kg IV q6–8h) can be used as prophylaxis (during surgery q1.5–2.0h and for 12 h postoperatively).

CONTRAINDICATIONS/POSSIBLE INTERACTIONS
N/A

 FOLLOW-UP

PATIENT MONITORING
• Standard postoperative care for abdominal/GI surgery
• Suture removal 10–14 days

POSSIBLE COMPLICATIONS
• Potential for fecal staining with blood from typhlectomy site for 10–14 days
• Potential for colonic dehiscence in 5–7 days
• Potential for colonic stricture formation if colonotomy is required

 MISCELLANEOUS

Suggested Reading
Aronsohn M. Large intestine. In: Slatter DH, ed. Textbook of small animal surgery. 2nd ed. Philadelphia: Saunders, 1993:613–627.
Author Michelle J. Waschak
Consulting Editors Mitchell A. Crystal and Brett M. Feder

BASICS

OVERVIEW
• Progressive, breed-specific, and apparently genetically induced defect of unknown cause and pathogenesis; neonatal, postnatal, and (rare) adult onset; premature aging and death of cerebellar cortical neurons
• Occurs after in utero or neonatal viral infection in cats (feline panleukopenia) and dogs (canine herpesvirus)

SIGNALMENT
Nonprogressive
• Dogs and cats
• Irish setters, wire-haired fox terriers, Samoyeds, chow chows, rough-coated collies, border collies, bullmastiffs, Labrador retrievers, beagles—common; may be seen in other breeds of dogs and cats.
• Signs appear when patient is 3–5 weeks old.

Progressive
• Dogs and cats
• Kerry blue terriers (signs at 12–16 weeks), rough-coated collies in Australia, Finnish harriers, Bern running dogs, Irish setters, English pointers, Gordon setters (signs at 6–36 months), Brittany spaniels (signs at 7–13 years)—common
• Autosomal recessive mode of inheritance—probable in Gordon setters, Kerry blue terriers, and rough-coated collies
• X-linked mode of inheritance—probable in English pointers because only males affected
• Cerebellar degeneration and coat color dilution—reported in a family of Rhodesian ridgebacks
• Signs appear when patient is 6–16 weeks old.

SIGNS
• Dysmetria—frequently as hypermetria
• Broad-based stance
• Swaying of body
• Intention tremors
• Lack of menace responses with normal vision and facial muscle strength
• Head tilt and episodes of vestibular ataxia with resting or positional nystagmus
• Decerebellate posture—opisthotonos with extensor rigidity of the forelimbs and flexed hind limbs
• Alterations of mentation, proprioceptive deficits, and paresis are not features of this condition.
• Progression of signs varies

CAUSES & RISK FACTORS
• Feline panleukopenia or canine herpesvirus infection in utero or neonatally
• Poor vaccination history or exposure to modified live virus during gestation

• Breeding affected animals or those with a familial history and predisposition to cerebellar degeneration
• A syndrome of hepatocerebellar degeneration was described in a litter of Bernese mountain dogs.
• Paraneoplastic cerebellar degeneration has been reported in humans.

DIAGNOSIS

DIFFERENTIAL DIAGNOSIS
• Lysosomal storage diseases—diffuse diseases of the CNS; differentiate by signs related to other parts of the CNS besides the cerebellum
• Toxicity (e.g., hexachlorophene)—differentiate by history of exposure
• Inflammatory diseases (e.g., canine distemper and FIP)—frequently accompanied or preceded by systemic signs of illness; differentiate by CSF analysis
• Medulloblastoma (cerebellar tumor)—reported in dogs and cats < 1 year old; differentiate by imaging (MRI and CT) and CSF analysis
• Other primary and metastatic tumors in adult dogs—differentiate by imaging (MRI and CT) and CSF analysis

CBC/BIOCHEMISTRY/URINALYSIS
Usually normal

OTHER LABORATORY TESTS
N/A

IMAGING
MRI—cerebellum may be smaller than normal.

DIAGNOSTIC PROCEDURES
• CSF analysis—normal with nonprogressive disease; normal or high protein concentration and normal cell counts with progressive disease
• Cerebellar biopsy—may be only definitive means of antemortem diagnosis

TREATMENT
• None available that will alter the course of the disease.
• Outpatient—unless severe deficits preclude nursing care at home
• Restrict activity to safe areas; avoid stairs, swimming pools, etc.
• Diet—normal; restrict intake if vestibular episodes are accompanied by emesis (to avoid aspiration pneumonia).
• Nonprogressive disease—patient may show some improvement as it learns to compensate for disabilities.

MEDICATIONS

DRUG(S)
N/A

CONTRAINDICATIONS/POSSIBLE INTERACTIONS
N/A

FOLLOW-UP
• Neurologic status—examine at weekly to monthly intervals if progression of signs is uncertain; consider videotaping the patient to determine progression more objectively.
• Progression of signs—rate varies; depends on signalment; ranges from days to years
• Do not vaccinate pregnant animals with MLV.
• Do not breed animals with a familial history of cerebellar disease.

MISCELLANEOUS

ABBREVIATIONS
• CSF = cerebrospinal fluid
• FIP = feline infectious peritonitis

Suggested Reading
de Lahunta A. Comparative cerebellar disease in domestic animals. Compend Contin Educ Pract Vet 1980;8:8–19.
Summers BA, Cummings JF, de Lahunta A. Veterinary neuropathology. St. Louis: Mosby, 1995.
Author Richard J. Joseph
Consulting Editor Joane M. Parent

CEREBELLAR HYPOPLASIA

 BASICS

OVERVIEW
Caused by incomplete development of parts of the cerebellum owing to intrinsic (inherited) or extrinsic (infectious, toxic, or nutritional) factors

SIGNALMENT
• Symptoms visible when puppies and kittens begin to stand and walk (by age 6 weeks)
• Airedales, chow chows, Boston terriers, and bull terrier breeds—congenital

SIGNS
• Nonprogressive cerebellar—head bobbing; limb tremors; aggravated by movement or eating (intention tremors); disappear during sleep • Cerebellar ataxia with a wide-base stance
• Spastic gait
• Dysmetria and disequilibrium—falling, flipping over
• Slight improvement may occur as patient accommodates for its deficits.

CAUSES & RISK FACTORS
• Cats—usually transplacental or perinatal infection with panleukopenia virus (wild parvovirus or modified live virus), which selectively attacks rapidly dividing cells (e.g., external germinal layer of the cerebellum at birth and for 2 weeks postnatal)
• Dogs—congenital in some breeds (see Signalment)

 DIAGNOSIS

DIFFERENTIAL DIAGNOSIS
• Cerebellar abiotrophy—postnatal degeneration after normal development); slow progression of signs over weeks to months; neonatal onset (beagles, Samoyeds) or postnatal onset (Australian kelpies at 5–6 weeks; Kerry blue terriers at 9–16 weeks; rough-coated collies at 4–8 weeks)

• Neuroaxonal dystrophy—slowly progressive cerebellar signs starting around 5 weeks of age in cats and 7 weeks in Chihuahuas
• Cerebellar sequels of systemic canine herpesvirus infection—follow systemic illness
• Concomitant seizures or other cerebral symptoms—suggest multiple malformations, such as lissencephaly (wire-haired fox terriers and Irish setters) or hydrocephalus
• Age, breed, history, and typical nonprogressive symptoms—usually sufficient for tentative diagnosis
• Final diagnosis possible only at necropsy

CBC/BIOCHEMISTRY/URINALYSIS
Usually normal

OTHER LABORATORY TESTS
N/A

IMAGING
MRI scan—cerebellar atrophy or malformation (incomplete or asymmetrical filling of the caudal cranial fossa by the cerebellum); other malformations

PATHOLOGIC FINDINGS
• Cerebellum—normally very small in the newborn kitten or puppy, because development continues for up to 10 weeks postnatal; subtle to marked atrophy noted at necropsy performed weeks to months after birth; no sign of active inflammation
• Transverse fibers of the pons—decrease in size associated with marked cortical cerebellar atrophy • Hydrocephalus—may be noted; result of multifocal inflammation or multiple malformations (e.g., dandy walker syndrome)
• Microscopic—cellular depletion of cerebellar cortex

 TREATMENT

None

 MEDICATIONS

DRUG(S)
N/A

CONTRAINDICATIONS/POSSIBLE INTERACTIONS
N/A

 FOLLOW-UP

PATIENT MONITORING
N/A

PREVENTION/AVOIDANCE
N/A

POSSIBLE COMPLICATIONS
N/A

EXPECTED COURSE AND PROGNOSIS
• Some patients may be acceptable pets.
• Deficits—permanent; usually compatible with a normal life span
• Restrict environment to prevent injuries and road accidents—no climbing, falling, or escaping
• Euthanasia—severely affected animals that are unable to feed, groom, or be toilet trained

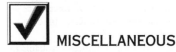 **MISCELLANEOUS**

Suggested Reading
Summers BA, Cummings JF, de Lahunta A. Veterinary neuropathology. St. Louis: Mosby, 1997.
Author Christine Berthelin-Baker
Consulting Editor Joane M. Parent

CERUMINOUS GLAND ADENOCARCINOMA, EAR

BASICS

OVERVIEW
• Primary malignant tumor of the external auditory meatus arising from coiled tubular apocrine sweat glands (e.g., ceruminous glands)
• May be locally invasive but has a low rate of distant metastasis

SIGNALMENT
• Rare but the most common malignant tumor of the ear canal in dogs and cats
• Cocker spaniel may be predisposed.
• Mean age—dogs, 8–11 years; cats, 10.5–13 years
• No known sex predisposition

SIGNS
• Similar to otitis externa
• Early appearance—pale pink, friable, ulcerative, bleeding nodular mass(es)
• Late appearance—large mass(es) filling the canal and invading through canal wall into surrounding structures
• Local lymphadenomegaly
• May see vestibular signs

CAUSES & RISK FACTORS
Chronic inflammation may play a role in tumor development.

DIAGNOSIS

DIFFERENTIAL DIAGNOSIS
• Nodular hyperplasia
• Pedunculated inflammatory polyps (cats)
• Squamous cell carcinoma
• Basal cell tumor
• Papilloma
• Sebaceous gland tumor
• Ceruminous gland adenoma

CBC/BIOCHEMISTRY/URINALYSIS
Usually normal

OTHER LABORATORY TESTS
N/A

IMAGING
• Skull radiography—determine involvement of tympanic bulla
• Thoracic radiography—evaluate for lung metastasis
• CT—useful before radiotherapy

DIAGNOSTIC PROCEDURES
• Cytologic examination of aspirate from large lymph nodes
• Biopsy

PATHOLOGIC FINDINGS
• Histopathologic characteristics—apocrine type differentiation from ceruminous glands and local invasion into stroma
• Tumor cells—show moderate to marked nuclear atypia with frequent mitosis

TREATMENT

• Ear canal ablation and lateral bulla osteotomy—preferred over lateral ear resection
• Radiotherapy—large or incompletely excised masses

MEDICATIONS

DRUGS
Chemotherapy not evaluated

CONTRAINDICATIONS/POSSIBLE INTERACTIONS
N/A

FOLLOW-UP

PATIENT MONITORING
Physical examination and thoracic radiography—at 1, 3, 6, 12, 16, and 24 months after treatment

POSSIBLE COMPLICATIONS
Permanent or transient Horner syndrome

EXPECTED COURSE AND PROGNOSIS
• Median survival after lateral ear resection (cats)—10 months (1-year survival, 33.3%)
• Median survival after ear ablation and lateral bulla osteotomy (cats)—42 months (1-year survival 75%)
• Median survival after radiotherapy (cats)—39.5 months (1-year survival 56%)
• Poor prognosis associated with extensive tumor involvement and neurologic signs

MISCELLANEOUS

ASSOCIATED CONDITIONS
• Otitis externa
• Peripheral vestibular disease

Suggested Reading
Marino DJ, MacDonald JM, Matthisen DT, et al. Results of surgery in cats with ceruminous gland adenocarcinoma. J Am Anim Hosp Assoc 1994;30:54–58.
Morrison WB. Cancers of the head and neck. In: Morrison WB, ed. Cancer in dogs and cats: medical and surgical management. Philadelphia: Williams & Wilkins, 1998:511–519.

Author Joanne C. Graham
Consulting Editor Wallace B. Morrison

DISEASES

CHAGAS DISEASE (AMERICAN TRYPANOSOMIASIS)

 BASICS

OVERVIEW
• Caused by the zoonotic hemoflagellate protozoan parasite *Trypanosoma cruzi* • Infection—infected feces of a vector (Triatominae, commonly called kissing or assassin bugs) are deposited in a wound (bite site of vector) or mucous membrane; dog eats an infected vector or infected host (opossum, raccoon, armadillo) in which the organism is sequestered in muscle; transmission by contaminated blood transfusion • After local multiplication at site of entry (5 days postinfection), hematogenous spread occurs to most organs but mainly the heart and brain. • Organisms become intracellular, multiply, then rupture out into the circulation to produce maximal parasitemias, associated particularly with acute myocarditis and less commonly with diffuse encephalitis (14 days postinfection). • Parasitemias wane (subpatient 30 days postinfection) • Antibody titers rise (detectable by 26 days postinfection) • Dog enters a protracted asymptomatic period (can last for months to years) if it survives the acute myocarditis; progressive and insidious development of myocardial degeneration; eventual dilative cardiomyopathy of unknown pathogenesis • South and Central America—endemic (in both humans and pets) • United States—most in Texas; also Louisiana, Oklahoma, South Carolina, and Virginia; infected vectors and reservoir hosts reported in the west (California, New Mexico), south (Florida, Georgia, North Carolina), and east (Maryland).

SIGNALMENT
• Young dogs—most common • Acute—dogs usually < 2 years • Chronic—old dogs • Hunting breeds—likely to contact vectors or reservoir hosts • More often males • Cats—can become infected; no case reported in North America

SIGNS
General Comments
• Two syndromes—acute (myocarditis or encephalitis in young dogs) and chronic (dilative cardiomyopathy in old dogs)

Historical Findings
Acute
• Sudden death • Lethargy • Depression • Anorexia • Diarrhea • Weakness • Exercise intolerance • Mild to severe CNS dysfunction (like distemper) • Ataxia, seizures
Chronic
• Weakness • Exercise intolerance • Syncope • Sudden death

Physical Examination Findings
Acute
• Generalized lymphadenopathy • Both left- and right-sided heart failure • Tachycardia with or without arrhythmias • Neurologic—weakness; ataxia; chorea; seizures (indistinguishable from distemper)
Chronic
Tachycardia—sustained or paroxysmal

CAUSES & RISK FACTORS
T. cruzi

 DIAGNOSIS

DIFFERENTIAL DIAGNOSIS
• Cardiomyopathy • Congenital cardiac defects • Traumatic myocarditis • Distemper • Toxoplasmosis • Neosporosis

CBC/BIOCHEMISTRY/URINALYSIS
Generally normal

OTHER LABORATORY TESTS
• Serology—positive titer confirms diagnosis available from the CDC's parasitology unit or from Dr. S. Barr, Department of Clinical Sciences, Cornell University (for research only) • Organism isolation—LIT culture; collect 50 mL heparinized blood • Examination above the buffy coat in a microhematocrit tube (spun down to read PCV) using 40× microscope objective—organisms during period of high parasitemia

IMAGING
• Radiography—acute: cardiomegaly, pulmonary edema, and (rarely) mild pleural effusion; chronic: cardiomegaly • Echocardiography—acute: rarely shows chamber or wall abnormalities; chronic: reduced ejection fraction, fractional shortening, and thinning of right and left ventricular free wall

DIAGNOSTIC PROCEDURES
Electrocardiography
• Acute—atrioventricular block; depression of R wave and QRS amplitude; right bundle branch block
• Chronic—low QRS amplitude; right bundle branch block; ventricular arrhythmias (initially unifocal VPC, becomes multiform, then degenerates into various forms of ventricular tachycardia)

 TREATMENT
• Medical therapy does not produce clinical cure.
• With poor prognosis and zoonotic potential, euthenasia is an option.

CLIENT EDUCATION
• Alert owner to possible zoonotic risk and potential for sudden death.
• Acute—invariably develops into the chronic form, which is usually fatal.
• Infected intact female—can transfer infection to offspring.

 MEDICATIONS

DRUGS
• Several drugs have limited efficacy during the acute stage; none produces a clinical cure; even treated animals progress to chronic disease.
• Nifurtimox (Lampit)—investigational drug available only from the Communicable Disease Center; 30 mg/kg PO q12h for 90–120 days
• Allopurinol—some efficacy in humans; use not reported in dogs; try 30 mg/kg PO q12h for 100 days
• Benzimidazole (Radamil)—5 mg/kg PO q24h for 60 days; markedly improves acute disease in humans
• Ketoconazole—little efficacy
• Verapamil (calcium channel blocker)—improves acute cardiac pathology and survival of *T. cruzi*–infected mice; use of the drug in dogs has not been as successful
• Cythioate (Proban)—3.3 mg/kg PO every other day; effective in reducing vector populations
• Supportive treatment of dilative cardiomyopathy (right and left cardiac failure) and ventricular arrhythmias

 FOLLOW-UP
• Cardiac disease—prognosis always guarded
• Chronic—prognosis guarded to hopeless

 MISCELLANEOUS

ZOONOTIC POTENTIAL
Exists; essentially incurable in humans, thus euthanasia of infected dogs is an option.

ABBREVIATIONS
• LIT = liver infusion tryptose • PCV = packed cell volume • VPC = ventricular premature complex

Suggested Reading
Barr SC. American trypanosomiasis. In: Greene CE, ed., Infectious diseases of the dog and cat. 2nd ed. Philadelphia: Saunders, 1998:445–449.
Author Stephen C. Barr
Consulting Editor Stephen C. Barr

BASICS

OVERVIEW
• Autosomal recessive inherited disorder of Persian cats characterized by abnormalities in cellular morphology and pigment formation
• Large intracytoplasmic granules in circulating leukocytes and melanocytes formed by fusion of pre-existing granules
• Storage pool deficiency of ADP, ATP, magnesium, and serotonin results from lack of platelet-dense granules.
• Prolonged bleeding from trauma, venipuncture, or minor surgery occurs because of impaired platelet aggregation and release reaction.
• Normal coagulation times
• Depressed chemotaxis
• No change in rates of infection
• Mildly depressed neutrophil count but within reference range

SIGNALMENT
• Persian cats with dilute smoke blue coat color and yellow-green irises (and white tigers)
• Does not occur in dogs
• Some Arctic foxes with blue or pearl hair coat color

SIGNS

Historical Findings
Prolonged bleeding from trauma, venipuncture, or minor surgery

Physical Examination Findings
• Red fundic reflex (lack of choroidal pigment)
• Dilute smoke-blue coat color and yellow-green irises
• Photophobia (blepharospasm and epiphora) in bright light

CAUSES & RISK FACTORS
Genetic disease

DIAGNOSIS

DIFFERENTIAL DIAGNOSIS
Dilute hair coat color

CBC/BIOCHEMISTRY/URINALYSIS
Romanowsky-stained blood smear—leukocytes, especially neutrophils, that contain pink to magenta cytoplasmic inclusions 2 mm in diameter

OTHER LABORATORY TESTS
None

IMAGING
N/A

DIAGNOSTIC PROCEDURES
None

TREATMENT
Provide ascorbic acid (vitamin C) to increase cGMP concentration and to improve cell and platelet function (no controlled studies in cats).

MEDICATIONS

DRUGS
Ascorbic acid (100 mg PO q8h)

CONTRAINDICATIONS/POSSIBLE INTERACTIONS
None

FOLLOW-UP

PATIENT MONITORING
None

PREVENTION/AVOIDANCE
• Advise owner of potential for prolonged bleeding after trauma, venipuncture, or minor surgery.
• Provide genetic counseling to eliminate Chediak-Higashi syndrome from animals used for breeding.
• Neuter affected and carrier animals or advise owner not to breed.

POSSIBLE COMPLICATIONS
Prolonged bleeding time

EXPECTED COURSE AND PROGNOSIS
Normal life span

MISCELLANEOUS

ABBREVIATION
cGMP = cyclic guanosine monophosphate

Suggested Reading
August JR. Consultations in feline internal medicine. 2nd ed. Philadelphia: Saunders, 1994.
Author Kenneth S. Latimer
Contributing Editor Susan M. Cotter

DISEASES

BASICS

OVERVIEW
Aortic body tumor in the heart-base region and carotid body tumor in the neck—two most common

SIGNALMENT
• Rare in cats
• Dogs—uncommon; 80%–90% are aortic body; age, 10–15 years old
• Boxers and Boston terriers—most commonly affected
• Aortic body—males predisposed
• Carotid body—no sex predilection

SIGNS
Aortic Body
• Similar to congestive heart failure
• Coughing
• Dyspnea

Carotid Body Tumor
• Regurgitation
• Dysphagia
• Neck mass
• Arteriovenous fistula in the neck

Both Types
• Acute hemorrhage from invaded blood vessels—may cause sudden death
• Distant metastasis with associated signs of organ dysfunction—up to 20% of patients
• Local invasion of blood vessels—up to 50% of patients

CAUSES & RISK FACTORS
Chronic hypoxemia—suspected risk factor; may explain predisposition of brachycephalic breeds

 DIAGNOSIS

DIFFERENTIAL DIAGNOSIS
• Congestive heart failure
• Megaesophagus
• Mediastinal lymphosarcoma
• Thyroid carcinoma

CBC/BIOCHEMISTRY/URINALYSIS
• Anemia from bleeding
• May see nucleated RBCs without anemia
• High liver enzymes, BUN, and creatinine—with metastasis to liver or kidneys

OTHER LABORATORY TESTS
N/A

IMAGING
Thoracic radiography (aortic body)—identify heart-base mass, lung metastasis, or vertebral invasion

DIAGNOSTIC PROCEDURES
Histopathologic examination—differentiate from other tumors

 TREATMENT

• Surgical removal—difficult because highly invasive
• Debulking—may be treatment of choice, especially if the masses are somewhat freely movable
• Radiotherapy—successful as adjuvant treatment to surgery in two dogs with carotid body tumor

 MEDICATIONS

DRUGS
• Chemotherapy—treatment not reported
• Doxorubicin and cyclophosphamide—for metastatic carotid body tumor; partial remission in one dog treated by the author; patient survived 15 months

CONTRAINDICATIONS/POSSIBLE INTERACTIONS
Doxorubicin—do not use with congestive heart failure

 FOLLOW-UP

• Thoracic radiography and physical examination—every 3 months; monitor for recurrence and metastasis
• Median survival time after surgery (dogs; carotid body)—23 months
• Survival after surgery and radiotherapy for two dogs—6 and 27 months

 MISCELLANEOUS

Suggested Reading

Morrison WB. Nonpulmonary intrathoracic cancer. In: Morrison WB, ed. Cancer in dogs and cats: medical and surgical management. Baltimore: Williams & Wilkins, 1998:537–550.

Obradovich JE, Withrow SJ, Powers BE, et al. Carotid body tumors in the dog: eleven cases (1978–1988). J Vet Intern Med 1992;6:96–101.

Author Terrance A. Hamilton
Consulting Editor Wallace B. Morrison

BASICS

OVERVIEW
• A highly contagious parasitic skin disease of dogs, cats, and rabbits, caused by infestation with *Cheyletiella* spp. mites
• Signs of scaling and pruritus can mimic other more common diseases.
• Often referred to as "walking dandruff," because of the large mite size and excessive scaling
• Prevalence varies by geographic region owing to mite susceptibility to common flea-control insecticides.
• Human (zoonotic) lesions can occur.

SIGNALMENT
• Dogs and cats
• More common in young animals
• Cocker spaniels, poodles, and long-haired cats are frequent asymptomatic carriers

SIGNS

Historical Findings
• Cats may exhibit bizarre behavioral signs or excessive grooming.
• Pruritus—none to severe, depending on the individual's response to infestation
• Infestation may be suspected after lesions in humans have developed.

Physical Examination Findings
• Scaling—most important clinical sign; diffuse or plaque-like; most severe in chronically infested and debilitated animals
• Lesions—dorsal orientation is commonly noted
• Underlying skin irritation may be minimal.
• Cats may exhibit bilaterally symmetrical alopecia.

CAUSES & RISK FACTORS
• Young animals and those in frequent contact with others are most at risk.
• Common sources of infestation—animal shelters, breeders, and grooming establishments.

 DIAGNOSIS

DIFFERENTIAL DIAGNOSIS
• Cheyletiellosis should be considered in every animal that has scaling, with or without pruritus.
• Also consider—seborrhea, flea allergic dermatitis, *Sarcoptes* spp. mite infestation, atopy, food hypersensitivity, and idiopathic pruritus

CBC/BIOCHEMISTRY/URINALYSIS
N/A

OTHER LABORATORY TESTS
N/A

IMAGING
N/A

DIAGNOSTIC PROCEDURES
• Examination of epidermal debris—very effective in diagnosing infestation
• Collection of debris—flea combing (most effective), skin scraping, and acetate tape preparation
• *Cheyletiella* mites are large and can be visualized with a simple handheld magnifying lens; scales and hair may be examined under low magnification; staining is not necessary.
• Response to insecticide preparations may be required to definitively diagnose suspicious cases in which mites cannot be identified.

 TREATMENT
• Must treat all animals in the household
• Clip long coats to facilitate treatment.
• Mainstay—6–8 weekly baths to remove scale, followed by rinses with an insecticide
• Lime-sulfur and pyrethrin rinses—cats, kittens, puppies, and rabbits
• Pyrethrin or organophosphates—dogs
• Routine flea sprays and powders—not always effective
• Environmental treatment with frequent cleanings and insecticide sprays—important for eliminating infestation
• Combs, brushes, and grooming utensils—discard or thoroughly disinfect before reuse
• Zoonotic lesions—self-limiting after eradication of the mites from household animals

 MEDICATIONS

DRUGS
• Alternatives (or additions) to topical therapy—amitraz and ivermectin
• Amitraz (Mitaban)—use on dogs (4 rinses at 2-week intervals)
• Ivermectin—highly effective (300 μg/kg SC 3 times at 2-week intervals); dogs, cats, and rabbits > 3 months old; pour-on forms have shown efficacy in cats (500 μg/kg 2 times at 2-week intervals).

CONTRAINDICATIONS/POSSIBLE INTERACTIONS
Ivermectin—not FDA-approved for this use in dogs, cats, or rabbits; client disclosure and consent are paramount before administration; several dog breeds (e.g., collies, shelties, Australian shepherds) have shown increased sensitivity and should not be treated.

 FOLLOW-UP
• Treatment failure necessitates re-evaluation for other causes of pruritus and scaling.
• Reinfestation may indicate contact with an asymptomatic carrier or the presence of an unidentified source of mites (e.g., untreated bedding).

 MISCELLANEOUS

ZOONOTIC POTENTIAL
A pruritic papular rash may develop in areas of contact with the pet.

Suggested Reading
Moriello KA. Cheyletiellosis. In: Griffin CE, Kwochka KW, MacDonald JM, eds., Current veterinary dermatology: the science and art of therapy. St. Louis: Mosby, 1993.
Author Alexander H. Werner
Consulting Editor Karen Helton Rhodes

DISEASES

CHLAMYDIOSIS—CATS

BASICS

DEFINITION
A chronic respiratory infection of cats caused by an intracellular bacterium, characterized by conjunctivitis, mild upper respiratory signs, and mild pneumonitis

PATHOPHYSIOLOGY
• *Chlamydia psittaci*—an obligate intracellular bacterium; replicates on the mucosa of the upper and lower respiratory epithelium; produces a persistent commensal flora that causes a local irritation with resulting mild upper and lower respiratory signs; can also colonize the mucosa of the gastrointestinal and reproductive tracts
• Incubation period—7–10 days; longer than that for other common respiratory pathogens of the cat

SYSTEMS AFFECTED
• Respiratory—mild rhinitis, bronchitis, and bronchiolitis
• Ophthalmic—chronic conjunctivitis, often unilateral but may be bilateral
• Gastrointestinal—cat: infection without clinical disease; other species: may have clinical gastroenteritis
• Reproductive—infection without clinical disease

GENETICS
None

INCIDENCE/PREVALENCE
• Incidence of clinical disease—sporadic; outbreaks of respiratory disease may occur, especially in multicat facilities
• Prevalence of *C. psittaci* in the feline population—not uncommon, 5–10% chronically infected

GEOGRAPHIC DISTRIBUTION
Worldwide

SIGNALMENT

Species
• Cats
• Humans

Breed Predilections
None

Mean Age and Range
Usually kittens 2–6 months of age; any age cat possible

Predominant Sex
None

SIGNS

General Comments
• Infection often subclinical
• Clinical disease—only as a co-infection by other organisms

Historical Findings
• Upper respiratory infection, with some sneezing, watery eyes, and coughing
• Sometimes difficult breathing
• Varying degrees of anorexia

Physical Examination Findings
• Conjunctivitis—often granular; initially unilateral, sometimes becoming bilateral
• Lacrimation, photophobia, and blepharospasm
• Rhinitis with nasal discharge—usually mild
• Pneumonitis—with the inflammatory process in the alveoli; bronchiolar tubes and airways give audible rales

CAUSE
C. psittaci

RISK FACTORS
• Concurrent infections with other respiratory pathogens
• Lack of vaccination
• Multicat facilities, especially adoption shelters and breeding catteries

DIAGNOSIS

DIFFERENTIAL DIAGNOSIS
• Feline viral rhinotracheitis—short incubation period (4–5 days); rapid bilateral conjunctivitis; severe sneezing; and ulcerative keratitis
• Feline calicivirus infection—short incubation period (3–5 days); ulcerative stomatitis; and severe pneumonia
• Feline reovirus infection—very mild upper respiratory infection; short incubation and duration
• Bronchial pneumonia caused by bacteria such as *Bordetella bronchiseptica*—localized areas of density within the lungs on radiographs

CBC/BIOCHEMISTRY/URINALYSIS
Leukocytosis

OTHER LABORATORY TESTS
None

IMAGING
Radiographs of lungs—helpful with pneumonitis

DIAGNOSTIC PROCEDURES
• Conjunctival scrapings stained with Giemsa stain—characteristic intracytoplasmic inclusions
• Swab samples taken from conjunctiva—isolation of the causative organism in cell cultures
• Smear samples taken from conjunctiva—immunofluorescence assay to detect chlamydial antigen

PATHOLOGIC FINDINGS
• Gross—evidence of chronic conjunctivitis with mucopurulent ocular discharge; minor rhinitis with nasal discharge; sometimes lung changes indicative of pneumonitis
• Histopathologic (conjunctiva)—an early intense infiltration of neutrophils; inflammatory response changes to lymphocytes and plasma cells; inclusions detected with special stains; inclusions invisible with routine H&E stains

TREATMENT

APPROPRIATE HEALTH CARE
Generally as outpatient

NURSING CARE
• Keep nostrils and eyes clean of discharge.
• Generally does not require other supportive therapy (e.g., fluids), unless complicated by concurrent infections

ACTIVITY
• Quarantine affected cats from contact with other cats.
• Do not allow affected cats to go outside.

DIET
Normal

CLIENT EDUCATION
Inform clients of the causative organism, the anticipated chronic course of disease, and the need to vaccinate other cats before exposure.

SURGICAL CONSIDERATIONS
None

MEDICATIONS

DRUG OF CHOICE
• Systemic—tetracycline (22 mg/kg PO q8h for 3–4 weeks)
• Ocular—ophthalmic ointments containing tetracycline (q8h)

CONTRAINDICATIONS
Tetracycline—may affect growing teeth of young kittens

PRECAUTIONS
Colonies—the entire colony may have to be treated; treatment may have to be continued for as long as 6 weeks.

POSSIBLE INTERACTIONS
None

ALTERNATIVE DRUGS
Other antibiotics are generally less effective than is tetracycline.

FOLLOW-UP

PATIENT MONITORING
Monitor for improved health as treatment proceeds.

PREVENTION/AVOIDANCE
Vaccines
• Both inactivated and modified live vaccines are available to reduce the severity of infection.
• None prevents infection but reduces severity and duration
• American Association of Feline Practitioners—classifies as noncore; give a single vaccination the initial visit; revaccinate 1 year later; then give annual revaccinations.

POSSIBLE COMPLICATIONS
Adverse vaccine reactions—mild clinical disease; small percentage of vaccinated cats

EXPECTED COURSE AND PROGNOSIS
• Tends to be chronic, lasting for several weeks or months, unless successful antibiotic treatment is given
• Prognosis good

MISCELLANEOUS

ASSOCIATED CONDITIONS
None

AGE-RELATED FACTORS
Primarily a disease of young cats

ZOONOTIC POTENTIAL
C. psittaci can infect humans; limited number of reports of mild conjunctivitis in humans transmitted from infected cats

PREGNANCY
Role of *C. psittaci* as a pathogen during pregnancy—unclear; can colonize the reproductive mucosa; severe conjunctivitis neonatorum can occur in neonatal kittens infected at or shortly after birth.

SYNONYMS
Feline pneumonitis

ABBREVIATIONS
H&E = hematoxylin and eosin

Suggested Reading
Elston T, Rodan I, Flemming D, et al. 1998 report of the American Association of Feline Practitioners and Academy of Feline Medicine Advisory Panel on feline vaccines. J Am Vet Med Assoc 1998;212:227–241.

Ford RB, Levy JK. Infectious diseases of the respiratory tract. In: Sherding RG, ed. The cat: diseases and clinical management. New York: Churchill Livingstone, 1994:489–500.

Ford RB. Role of infectious agents in respiratory disease. Vet Clin North Am Small Anim Pract 1993;23:17–35.

Gaskell RM. Upper respiratory disease in the cat (including *Chlamydia*): control and prevention. Feline Pract 1993;21:29–34.

Greene CE. Chlamydial infections. In: Greene CE, ed. Infectious diseases of the dog and cat. 2nd ed. Philadelphia: Saunders, 1998:172–174.

Hoover EA. Viral respiratory diseases and chlamydiosis. In: Holzworth J, ed. Diseases of the cat. Philadelphia: Saunders, 1987:214–237.

Author Fred W. Scott
Consulting Editor Stephen C. Barr

CHOCOLATE TOXICITY

 BASICS

DEFINITION
Acute gastroenteric, neurologic, and cardiac toxicosis caused by excessive intake of methylxanthine alkaloids, present in chocolate

PATHOPHYSIOLOGY
• Methylxanthine alkaloids—primarily theobromine and caffeine; inhibit adenosine receptors, leading to vasoconstriction, tachycardia, and CNS stimulation
• Inhibition of phosphodiesterase—increases cAMP, which potentiates catecholamine effects (increases its release)
• Combined effects—results in cerebral vasoconstriction, cardiac muscle contraction, and CNS stimulation and seizures

SYSTEMS AFFECTED
• Gastrointestinal—early onset of vomiting and diarrhea; may be mediated centrally; may result even from parenteral administration of methylxanthine alkaloids
• Nervous—stimulation; enhanced alertness and reflex hyperactivity; tremors; seizures
• Cardiovascular—increased myocardial contractility and tachyarrhythmias

GENETICS
N/A

INCIDENCE/PREVALENCE
• Dogs—among the 20 most common poisonings reported in recent literature, by the National Animal Poison Control Center, and by the Hennepin County (Minneapolis) Poison Control Center
• More common at holiday times—chocolate products and candies readily available
• Caffeine-containing stimulant tablets—occasional source

GEOGRAPHIC DISTRIBUTION
• Urban and indoor dogs—may be more at risk owing to close proximity to chocolate products

SIGNALMENT
Species
Dogs and rarely cats

Breed Predilections
Small dogs—may be more at risk (amount of chocolate available relative to body weight)

Mean Age and Range
Puppies and young dogs—may be more likely to ingest large amounts of unusual foods

Predominant Sex
N/A

SIGNS
Historical Findings
• Recent chocolate ingestion
• Vomiting and diarrhea—often the first reported; 2–4 hr after ingestion
• Early restlessness and enhanced activity
• Polyuria—may result from diuretic action
• Advanced signs—stiffness; excitement; seizures; hyperreflexia

Physical Examination Findings
• Hyperthermia
• Hyperreflexia
• Muscle rigidity
• Tachypnea
• Tachycardia
• Hypotension
• Advanced signs—lead to cardiac failure, weakness, coma, and death
• Death—12–36 hr after ingestion

CAUSES
• Usually some form of processed chocolate (used for candies and baking)—contain high concentrations of theobromine and caffeine

PRODUCTS WITH HIGH METHYLXANTHINE CONCENTRATIONS

Product	Methylxanthines (mg/g)
Cacao bean	14–53
Baking chocolate	16
Semisweet chocolate	9
Milk chocolate	2
Hot chocolate	0.4
White chocolate	0.05

• Minimum lethal dosage for caffeine and theobromine (dogs)—100–200 mg/kg
• Potentially lethal (dogs)—0.7 g baking chocolate or 60 g milk chocolate per kilogram of body weight; 450 g milk chocolate or 120 g baking chocolate in a 7-kg dog

RISK FACTORS
• Dogs—most commonly affected because they consume large amounts of unusual foods quickly
• Chocolate—highly palatable and attractive; often readily available and unprotected in homes and kitchens
• Methylxanthine alkaloids—readily and rapidly absorbed; only slightly bound (20%) to plasma proteins

 DIAGNOSIS

DIFFERENTIAL DIAGNOSES
• Convulsant or excitatory alkaloids—strychnine; amphetamine; nicotine; 4-aminopyridine
• Convulsant pesticides—cyclodiene-chlorinated hydrocarbons (e.g., chlordane, toxaphene, and lindane)
• Tremorogenic mycotoxins–penitrem A; aflatrem
• Acute psychogenic drugs—LSD; morning glory
• Fluoroacetate toxicosis
• Cardioactive glycosides—*Digitalis* spp.; *Nerium oleander*
• Hypomagnesemia and hypocalcemia

CBC/BIOCHEMISTRY/URINALYSIS
• Hypoglycemia—may note secondary to increased muscular activity
• Low urine specific gravity and proteinuria—occasionally

OTHER LABORATORY TESTS
• Stomach contents, plasma, and urine—analyzed chemically for methylxanthines
• Elimination half-life (dogs)—17.5 hr; detectable plasma or serum concentration should persist 3–4 days.

IMAGING
N/A

DIAGNOSTIC PROCEDURES
ECG—confirm tachycardia and ventricular tachyrhythmia

PATHOLOGIC FINDINGS
• Stomach contents—may note small or large amounts of chocolate
• Microscopic renal lesions—reported; characterized by hyaline droplets degeneration, pyknosis, and karyorrhexis

TREATMENT

APPROPRIATE HEALTH CARE
Reported by phone—attempt to determine type and amount of exposure; if not possible, recommend referral to hospital as a potential toxicologic emergency.

NURSING CARE
Fluid therapy—correct electrolyte disturbances caused by vomiting, as necessary.

ACTIVITY
Avoid stress and excitement—could precipitate hyperreflexia or seizures

DIET
• Acutely affected patient—do not feed.
• Convalescence—bland diet for several days to allow recovery from gastroenteritis

CLIENT EDUCATION
Warn client of the hazards of chocolate ingestion.

SURGICAL CONSIDERATIONS
N/A

MEDICATIONS

DRUGS OF CHOICE
• Induce emesis—*only if patient is not already seizing;* apomorphine (0.03 mg/kg IV); syrup of ipecac (1–2 mL/kg PO); hydrogen peroxide (1–5 mL/kg PO)
• Gastric lavage—only before onset of vomiting and other clinical signs, if emetics are not effective
• Vomiting controlled—activated charcoal (0.5–1.0 g/kg PO); adsorb remaining alkaloids in the gastrointestinal tract
• Osmotic cathartic—sodium sulfate (1 g/kg PO); promote gastrointestinal elimination of chocolate

• Hyperactivity and seizures—controlled with diazepam (0–5 mg/kg IV q10–20 min up to four times)
• Ventricular tachycardia (dogs)—lidocaine (without epinephrine; 1–2 mg/kg IV followed by 0.03–0.05 mg/kg/min IV drip)
• Serious refractory arrhythmias—metoprolol or propranolol (0.04–0.06 mg/kg IV; rate not > 1 mg/min); metoprolol preferred but may be difficult to obtain; may use oral therapy once patient is stable (metoprolol at 0.2–1.0 mg/kg PO q12h; propranolol at 0.2–1.0 mg/kg PO q8h); monitor ECG for hypotension (a sequela to this treatment).

CONTRAINDICATIONS
• Do not use epinephrine concurrent with lidocaine.
• Avoid erythromycin and corticosteroids—reduce the excretion of methylxanthines.
• Do not use lidocaine in affected cats.

PRECAUTIONS
• Effects may persist longer than the effective life of therapeutic drugs.
• Keep patient under observation until drug administration is no longer needed.
• Methylxanthines—cross the placenta; excreted in milk

POSSIBLE INTERACTIONS
N/A

ALTERNATIVE DRUGS
• Response to diazepam inadequate—consider phenobarbital (30 mg/kg IV administered over 5–10 min)
• Refractory seizures—pentobarbital (3–15 mg/kg IV slowly, as needed)

FOLLOW-UP

PATIENT MONITORING
• ECG—arrhythmias
• Watch for mild to moderate nephrosis in convalescent patients.

PREVENTION/AVOIDANCE
Warn owners about the toxicologic hazards of chocolate.

POSSIBLE COMPLICATIONS
Pregnant or nursing animals—risk for teratogenesis of newborns or stimulation of nursing neonates

EXPECTED COURSE AND PROGNOSIS
• Expected course—12–36 hr, depending on dosage and effectiveness of decontamination and treatment
• Successfully treated patients—usually recover completely
• Prognosis—good if oral decontamination occurs within 2–4 hr of ingestion; guarded with advanced signs of seizures and arrhythmias

MISCELLANEOUS

ASSOCIATED CONDITIONS
N/A

AGE-RELATED FACTORS
N/A

ZOONOTIC POTENTIAL
Not transmissible, but humans and dogs may access similar sources.

PREGNANCY
Methylxanthines—teratogens in laboratory animals

SEE ALSO
• Metaldehyde poisoning
• Poisoning (Intoxication)
• Strychnine Poisoning

Suggested Reading
Drolet P, Arendt TD, Stowe CM. Cacao bean shell poisoning in 2 dogs. J Am Vet Med Assoc 1984;185:902–904.
Glauberg A, Blumenthal HP. Chocolate toxicosis in a dog. J Am Anim Hosp Assoc 1983;19:246–248.
Hooser SB, Beasley VR. Methylxanthine poisoning (chocolate and caffeine toxicosis) In: Kirk RW, ed. Current veterinary therapy IX. Small animal practice. Philadelphia: Saunders, 1986.

Author Gary D. Osweiler
Consulting Editor Gary D. Osweiler

DISEASES

CHOLANGITIS/CHOLANGIOHEPATITIS

 BASICS

DEFINITION
• Cholangitis—inflammation of the biliary tree • Cholangiohepatitis—inflammation of the biliary structures and surrounding hepatocellular parenchyma • Cholangitis/cholangiohepatitis syndrome (CCHS)—occur together in cats; histologically classified as suppurative or nonsuppurative (lympho-plasmacytic, lymphocytic), pyogranulo-matous, or lymphoproliferative

PATHOPHYSIOLOGY
• Preceding or coexisting conditions—inflammation or obstruction of the extrahepatic biliary tree; pancreatitis; inflammatory bowel disease; chronic interstitial nephritis (cats) • Bacterial cholangitis—stasis of bile flow is permissive to development; may result in calcium deposition in biliary structures; stimulates biliary epithelial hyperplasia • Suppurative disease—often yields positive aerobic or anaerobic bacterial culture • Nonsuppurative disease—immune-mediated • Immune-mediated bile duct destruction—results in a ductopenia of small- and medium-sized bile ductules (sclerosing cholangitis) • Pyogranulo-matous disease—occurs secondary to infection or immune mechanisms; common in dogs • Lymphoproliferative disease—transition stage between inflammation and neoplasia

SYSTEMS AFFECTED
• Hepatobiliary—liver; bile ducts; gallbladder • Gastrointestinal—pancreas; intestine

GENETICS
N/A

INCIDENCE/PREVALENCE
Nonsuppurative disease—most common chronic liver disorder in cats

GEOGRAPHIC DISTRIBUTION
N/A

SIGNALMENT
Species
Cats and (uncommon) dogs
Breed Predilections
Possibly Himalayan, Persian, and Siamese cats
Mean Age and Range
• Suppurative disease—range, 0.4–16 years; mostly young to middle-aged cats • Nonsuppurative disease—range, 2–17 years; mostly middle-aged cats
Predominant Sex
• Suppurative disease—male cats • Nonsuppurative disease—none

SIGNS
General Comments
• Suppurative disease—most severe clinical manifestations; acute abdomen; acute febrile illness often < 5 days; highly associated with EHBDO • Nonsuppurative disease—illness ≥ 3 weeks (months to years)

Historical Findings
• Suppurative disease—rapid onset of acute illness; fever; anorexia; vomiting; collapse • Nonsuppurative disease—cyclic illness; chronic vague signs of lethargy, vomiting, anorexia, and weight loss • Ductopenia (cats)—polyphagic owing to reduced bile flow compromising nutrient assimilation

Physical Examination Findings
• Suppurative disease—fever; painful abdomen; anicteric or jaundiced; dehydration • Nonsuppurative—may have no physical abnormalities other than hepatomegaly; asymptomatic patients identified during routine health screen; jaundice common; thickened intestines with inflammatory bowel disease; abdominal effusion rare • Ductopenia (cats)—rough hair coat; intermittent acholic feces

CAUSES
Suppurative Disease
• Bacterial infection—most common in cats: *E. coli, Enterobacter,* β-hemolytic *Streptococcus, Klebsiella, Actinomyces, Clostridia,* and *Bacteroides* and may be associated with toxoplasmosis; reported in dogs: enteric organisms, *Campylobacter, Salmonella,* and *Leptospirosis* • Highly associated with EHBDO

Nonsuppurative Disease
Concurrent disorders—cholecystitis, cholelithiasis, pancreatitis, EHBDO, inflammatory bowel disease, chronic interstitial nephritis, infections elsewhere

RISK FACTORS
• Suppurative disease—EHBDO; cholestasis • Nonsuppurative disease—inflammatory bowel disease; pancreatitis; EHBDO

 DIAGNOSIS

DIFFERENTIAL DIAGNOSIS
• Hepatic lipidosis—may co-exist; typified by minimal increase in GGT activity with high ALP, AST, and ALT, and usually severe hyperbilirubinemia • EHBDO—marked jaundice, high ALP, GGT, ALT, AST, and cholesterol; gallbladder and bile duct distention with tortuosity of common bile duct noted on ultrasound • Pancreatitis—may be primary disorder; lipemic blood, high cholesterol, high trypsin-like immunoactive substance, inconsistently high lipase or amylase, and jaundice common; left quadrant signs of pancreatitis noted on ultrasound • Lymphoproliferative disease and lymphosarcoma involving intestines and portal tracts—same clinical features as CCHS; may have circulating blast cells; hepatic lesions differentiated on basis of histologic evaluations and immunohisto-chemistry of lymphocytes; thickened bowel wall • Jaundice associated with septicemia—high liver enzymes; sepsis • Polycystic hepatorenal disease (Himalayan and Persian cats)—minimally high enzymes; progressive severe peribiliary fibrosis; nonsuppurative disease around abnormal ducts

CBC/BIOCHEMISTRY/URINALYSIS
• Consistent findings—suppurative disease: left-shifted leukogram, toxic neutrophils; all forms: associated with high ALT, AST, ALP, and GGT • Variable findings—poikilocytosis, borderline nonregenerative anemia, leukocytosis, lymphocytosis (some cats with lymphocytic disease) • High bile acids, high bilirubin, variable cholesterol—depend on associated illnesses

OTHER LABORATORY TESTS
• Trypsin-like immunoactive substance—high with pancreatitis and enteritis • Vitamin B$_{12}$—low with malabsorption (inflammatory bowel disease) and malnutrition • Coagulation—normal or increased PT, APTT, and ACT; PIVKA more sensitive for vitamin K-induced coagulopathy • Aerobic and anaerobic bacterial culture—hepatic or biliary aspirations

IMAGING
• Survey radiography—nonsuppurative disease: hepatomegaly common; may find no abnormalities (especially suppurative disease); sternal lymphadenopathy common; mineralized biliary tree structures, radiodense microlithiasis, porcelain gallbladder, emphysematous hepatobiliary lesions, features consistent with pancreatitis, and abdominal effusion rare • Cholecystography or hepatobiliary scintigraphy—does not aid diagnosis • Abdominal ultrasonography—hepatomegaly; echogenic changes in the biliary tree; cholelithiasis; sludged bile; cholecystitis; rare parenchymal abscess; perihepatic and/or peripancreatic lymphadenopathy; mesenteric lymphadenopathy (inflammatory bowel disease); hepatic echogenicity (concurrent hepatic lipidosis); cysts (polycystic disease)

DIAGNOSTIC PROCEDURES
Fine-Needle Aspiration Cytology
• Hepatic aspiration—culture sample with suppurative disease; reveals bacterial organisms not visualized on histopathology; unreliable for detecting nonsuppurative disease; hepatocellular vacuolation with lipid common with chronically ill cats that are recently anorectic • Cholecystocentesis—use a 22-gauge spinal needle and a transhepatic approach under ultrasound guidance; may reveal suppuration, bacteria, trematode eggs, or neoplasia

Percutaneous Biopsy
• Ultrasound-directed core-needle biopsy—may misdiagnose condition • Requires a minimum of 15 portal triads for accurate categorization • Collect at least four,

preferably six, biopsies. • Postbiopsy complications and accidental biopsy of surrounding tissues (diaphragm, body wall, lung, stomach, bile duct, and gallbladder) may occur.

Laparoscopy

• Permits visualization of gallbladder, porta hepatis, pancreas, and perihepatic and peripancreatic lymph nodes and biopsy of liver and pancreas • EHBDO—not recommended; pursue laparotomy (biliary diversion) • Suspected nonsuppurative disease—couple with endoscopy (enteric biopsy); evaluate for concurrent inflammatory bowel disease

Laparotomy

• Suspected or probable EHBDO—recommended • Permits inspection of common bile duct, cystic duct, and gallbladder; removal of obstructing lesions (mass, cholelith, inspissated bile) or biliary enteric anastomosis (cholecystoenterostomy); and biopsy of liver, biliary tree, pancreas, intestines, and enlarged lymph nodes

PATHOLOGIC FINDINGS

Gross

• Suppurative disease—swollen liver with blunted margins; areas of focal discoloration; may note erythematous, necrotic, or thick-walled gallbladder with cholecystitis; peripancreatic steatonecrosis and fat saponification with pancreatic inflammation; perihepatic and peripancreatic lymphadenopathy; verification of EHBDO • Nonsuppurative disease—large, firm liver, rounded margins, and variable surface irregularity; yellow or pale in cats with hepatic lipidosis

Microscopic

• Severe ascending suppurative disease—thick extrahepatic biliary system; dilated intrahepatic bile ducts; periportal edema; periductal suppuration; intraductal exudate; variable periductal fibrosis and biliary hyperplasia • Nonsuppurative disease—periportal inflammation; bile duct hypertrophy or hyperplasia; small lymphocytes; connective tissue around and bridging between portal triads with chronic disease; ductopenia involving small- and medium-sized bile ducts; residual lipogranulomatous foci; new ductular elements on periphery of inflammatory nidus

TREATMENT

APPROPRIATE HEALTH CARE

Inpatient Management

• Suppurative disease with acute febrile illness, painful abdomen, and left-shifted leukogram—requires hydration support, best-guess bactericidal antimicrobials (aspiration cytology and gram staining initially); evaluate for EHBDO or cholecystitis requiring surgical intervention; continue antibiotic therapy for at least 8 weeks; choleretic therapy (urso-

deoxycholic acid) advised to thin bile secretions • Nonsuppurative symptomatic cats—fluid therapy; diagnostic evaluation; liver biopsy (24 hr before biopsy administer vitamin K_1 at 0.5–1.5 mg/kg IM) • Both forms (cats)—may require blood transfusion in association with surgery or biopsy

Outpatient Management

• Suppurative disease—after management of acute crisis • Nonsuppurative—after resolution of acute crisis; chronic (life-long) immunomodulatory therapy after diagnosis is confirmed

ACTIVITY

Restricted while symptomatic

DIET

Nutritional support—essential to avoid hepatic lipidosis; balanced high-protein, high-calorie feline stress ration with vitamins; antigens restricted with concurrent inflammatory bowel disease; fats restricted with severe ductopenia, fat malabsorption, or chronic pancreatitis

CLIENT EDUCATION

Emphasize the chronic nature of nonsuppurative disease and its requirement for life-long therapy.

SURGICAL CONSIDERATIONS

• Cholecystectomy—with cholecystitis
• Cholecystoenterostomy—with EHBDO
• Cholelith removal

MEDICATIONS

DRUGS OF CHOICE

Antibiotics

• Bactericidal—directed at enteric opportunists; clavamox or enrofloxacin combined with metronidazole (7.5 mg/kg PO BID) • Resistant enterococci—vancomycin • Modify initial empiric drug selection based on culture and sensitivity reports.

Immunomodulation

• Glucocorticoids—prednisolone (dogs: 2 mg/kg/day; cats: 4 mg/kg/day for 14–21 days; then slowly taper to lowest effective dose); plan on chronic therapy. • May try metronidazole combined with prednisolone (doses above) • Confirmed ductopenia (cats)—requires more aggressive therapy; poor response to azathioprine or chlorambucil; recent clinical work notes improved response with predisolone and metronidazole combined with methotrexate (0.4 mg PO total dose given at 7–10-day intervals; divide dose into 0.13-mg capsules given at 0, 12, and 24 hr for pulsatile therapy); evaluate CBC and adjust initial dosing strategy; combine with folate (0.25 mg/kg/day).
• Some cats require chemotherapy (e.g., as for lymphosarcoma).

Other

• Ursodeoxycholic acid (Actigall)—10–15 mg/kg PO daily given once or divided q12h; immunomodulatory, antifibrotic, and choleretic effects; nontoxic in cats with liver disease • Vitamin B supplementations • Vitamin E—antioxidant, aqueous α-tocopherol (10–100 IU/kg/day PO); use high dose with ductopenia.

CONTRAINDICATIONS

Adjust drug dosages based on liver function and cholestasis.

FOLLOW-UP

PATIENT MONITORING

Nonsuppurative disease—initially monitor at 7–14-day intervals to follow enzymes and bilirubin values; after remission, perform quarterly assessments of liver enzymes and bilirubin; sequential measurements of serum bile acids are complicated by ursodeoxycholic acid (detected by analyses).

PREVENTION/AVOIDANCE

Control inflammatory bowel disease

POSSIBLE COMPLICATIONS

• Suppurative disease—may progress to nonsuppurative disease and immune-mediated ductopenia • Diabetes mellitus—approximately 30% of cats with sclerosing lesion treated with prednisone • Hepatic lipidosis—with inadequate nutrition

EXPECTED COURSE AND PROGNOSIS

• Suppurative disease—may be cured by appropriate management • Nonsuppurative disease—chronic, long-term remission possible (> 8 years possible)

MISCELLANEOUS

ASSOCIATED CONDITIONS

• Pancreatitis • Hepatic lipidosis • Polycystic liver disease • Lymphosarcoma • Lymphoproliferative disease • Cholangiocarcinoma—some cats with chronic nonsuppurative disease

ABBREVIATIONS

• ACT = activated clotting time • APTT = activated partial thromboplastin time • EHBDO = extrahepatic bile duct obstruction• PIVKA = proteins invoked by vitamin K absence or antagonism • PT = prothrombin time

Suggested Reading

Center SA. Diseases of the gallbladder and biliary tree. In: Guilford WG, Center SA, Strombeck DR, et al., eds. Strombeck's small animal gastroenterology. 3rd ed. Philadelphia: Saunders, 1996:860–888.
Author Sharon A. Center
Consulting Editor Sharon A. Center

DISEASES

CHOLECYSTITIS

BASICS

OVERVIEW
• Inflammation of the gallbladder, sometimes associated with cholelithiasis; often associated with obstruction and/or inflammation of the common bile duct and/or intrahepatic biliary system. • Severe disease—results in rupture of the gallbladder and subsequent bile peritonitis, necessitating combined surgical and medical treatment • Bile peritonitis—enhances transmural migration of enteric bacteria across the bowel wall and increases microvasculature permeability

SIGNALMENT
• Dogs and cats • No breed, sex, or age predilections • Necrotizing cholecystitis (dogs)—usually middle-aged or older • Hyperlipidemic dogs—seem to be predisposed; also predisposed to formation of rubbery bile concretions, causing cholestasis and cholecystitis

SIGNS
• Inappetence, depression, vomiting, and abdominal pain—sudden onset • Severe disease—shock owing to endotoxemia and hypovolemia • Mild to moderate jaundice and fever—common • Soft tissue mass in the right cranial abdominal quadrant—may develop subsequent to inflammation of the gallbladder and surrounding tissues

CAUSES & RISK FACTORS
• Usually attributed to coexisting impaired cystic duct flow and surface irritants (e.g., bacteria, sludged bile, lysolecithin, choleliths, liver flukes, pancreatic enzymes) • Anomalous development of the gallbladder—rarely implicated • Previous gastrointestinal disorders, trauma, or abdominal surgery—may be a contributing factor • Bacterial infection—common; retrograde invasion from the intestine or hematogenous spread • Toxoplasmosis and biliary coccidiosis—rarely reported causes • Necrotizing cholecystitis (dogs)—ruptured gallbladder common; cholelithiasis common; *Escherichia coli* common bacterial isolate • Emphysematous cholecystitis/choledochitis—associated with diabetes mellitus, traumatic ischemia of the gallbladder, and acute cholecystitis (with or without cholelithiasis); gasforming organisms (e.g., *Clostridia* and *E. coli*) usually cultured from bile or biliary structures

DIAGNOSIS

DIFFERENTIAL DIAGNOSIS
• Pancreatitis • Focal to diffuse peritonitis—owing to a variety of causes • Gastroenteritis with secondary biliary tract involvement • Bile peritonitis • Cholangiohepatitis • Hepatic necrosis • Hepatic abscessation • Septicemia

CBC/BIOCHEMISTRY/URINALYSIS
• Variable leukocytosis with toxic neutrophils and inconsistent left shift • Hyperbilirubinemia and bilirubinuria • High serum activity of ALT, AST, ALP, and GGT • Hypoalbuminemia—with peritonitis

OTHER LABORATORY TESTS
• Abdominocentesis—inflammatory cytology noted in abdominal effusion; bile indicates a ruptured biliary tract. • Bile culture (dogs)—*E. coli, Klebsiella* spp., *Pseudomonas* spp., and *Clostridium* spp. reported • Coagulation panels—abnormal with severe disease owing to vitamin K deficiency or DIC

IMAGING
• Abdominal radiography—may reveal focal to diffuse peritonitis, ileus, choleliths, or gas accumulation in the biliary tract; may note radiodense gallbladder if dystrophic mineralization has occurred • Ultrasonography—allows more discrete imaging of the gallbladder and adjacent structures; bilayer appearance of gallbladder common with inflammation, edema, ascites, hepatic inflammation, and hepatic congestion; failure to image the gallbladder may indicate that it or portions of the extrahepatic biliary structures are ruptured.

PATHOLOGIC FINDINGS
Histologic liver lesions—may note chronic active cholangiohepatitis, hepatic necrosis, hepatic fibrosis, or hepatic degeneration

TREATMENT
• Inpatient—usually required for critical care during diagnostic evaluations and presurgical preparation • Restoration of fluid and electrolyte balance and administration of colloids or plasma—usually indicated • Plasma—indicated with hypoalbuminemia attributed to protein sequestration in inflammatory abdominal effusions • Whole blood—indicated for surgical cases, especially with bleeding tendencies • Serum electrolytes—monitor frequently; used to guide potassium chloride fluid supplementation • Polyionic fluids—administer at one-third maintenance dose after volume expansion; concurrent administration of a synthetic colloid (e.g., hetastarch or vetaplasma at 20 mL/kg/day). • Dextrans—avoid; may impart bleeding tendencies • Urine output—monitor during surgery.

Surgery
• May involve cholecystectomy and/or biliary-enteric anastomosis • Manipulation of the biliary structures—may induce a vagovagal response (pathologic bradycardia, hypotension, and cardiac arrest); imperative to monitor for pathologic hypotension and to intervene as necessary.

MEDICATIONS

DRUGS
• Antibiotics—directed against enteric organisms; based on culture and sensitivity, if possible; good initial choices: combination of an aminoglycoside, metronidazole, or clindamycin and ampicillin or a fluorinated quinolone • Parenteral vitamin K_1—for associated cholestasis; 0.5–1.5 mg/kg, to a maximum of 3 parenteral doses over 36 hr • Ursodeoxycholic acid—choleretic agent; stimulates flow of watery bile; 10–15 mg/kg PO q24h

CONTRAINDICATIONS/POSSIBLE INTERACTIONS
Ursodeoxycholic acid—avoid if a biliary tree obstruction is possible.

FOLLOW-UP

PATIENT MONITORING
Physical examination and pertinent diagnostic testing—repeated every 2–4 weeks until signs and clinicopathologic abnormalities resolve

POSSIBLE COMPLICATIONS
Anticipate a protracted clinical course with ruptured biliary tract or peritonitis.

MISCELLANEOUS

ASSOCIATED CONDITIONS
• Cholelithiasis • Extrahepatic bile duct occlusion • Choledochitis

AGE-RELATED FACTORS
Congenital malformations of biliary structures do not predispose patients to cholecystitis.

ZOONOTIC POTENTIAL
• *Campylobacter* and *Salmonella* may cause cholecystitis in dogs.

ABBREVIATIONS
• ALP = alkaline phosphatase • ALT = alanine aminotransferase • AST = aspartate aminotransferase • DIC = disseminated intravascular coagulation • GGT = γ-glutamyltransferase

Suggested Reading
Center SA. Diseases of the gallbladder and biliary tree. In: Guilford WG, Center SA, Strombeck DR, et al., eds. Strombeck's small animal gastroenterology., Philadelphia: Saunders, 1996:860–888.
Author William E. Hornbuckle
Consulting Editor Sharon A. Center

BASICS

OVERVIEW
• Radiopaque or radiolucent calculi in the biliary tree or gallbladder
• May be asymptomatic or associated with signs attributed to sludged bile, OBTD, cholecystitis, cholangiohepatitis, or bile peritonitis
• Primary constituents of choleliths—mucin, calcium, and bilirubin; in dogs, usually lower cholesterol and calcium than in humans and cats
• Surgical and/or medical treatment—not recommended if there are no clinical or clinicopathologic signs

SIGNALMEN
• Cats and dogs
• Particularly miniature schnauzers and poodles
• Hyperlipidemic dogs—seemingly predisposed to developing thick mucinous biliary sludge, which may behave as choleliths

SIGNS
• May be asymptomatic
• When accompanied by infection or OBTD (with or without peritonitis)—vomiting; abdominal pain; fever; jaundice

CAUSES & RISK FACTORS
• Predisposing factors—conditions that cause stasis of bile flow, stone nidus formation (inflammatory debris, infection, tumor exfoliation), and supersaturation of bile (pigment, cholesterol); anatomic union of the pancreatic and biliary ducts (cats)
• Bile sludging and/or gallbladder distension—stimulate increased mucin production and coalescence of bile particles
• Inflammatory mediators and bacterial enzymes associated with cholecystitis—aggravate the condition; mucin production; subsequent stone formation
• Low-protein and low-taurine diet—lithogenic

DIAGNOSIS

DIFFERENTIAL DIAGNOSIS
• OBTD—attributed to inflammatory, infectious, or neoplastic conditions involving the liver or adjacent extrahepatic tissues in the porta hepatis; suggested by profound increases in cholesterol, ALP, and bilirubin
• Cholangiohepatitis
• Pancreatitis
• Bile peritonitis

CBC/BIOCHEMISTRY/URINALYSIS
• CBC—man be normal; abnormalities reflect bacterial infection, endotoxemia, biliary obstruction, or underlying causal factors; inflammatory leukogram
• Biochemistry—hyperbilirubinemia; variable elevations in serum ALP, GGT, ALT, and AST
• Urinalysis—bilirubinuria

LABORATORY PROCEDURES
• Bacterial culture—bile; aerobic and anaerobic bacteria common
• Coagulation profile—prolonged clotting time (especially PIVKA and PT); responsive to parenteral vitamin K administration, may be evident with chronic OBTD
• Histopathologic evaluation of underlying liver disease—prognostic significance

IMAGING
• Abdominal radiography—limited value in delineating gallbladder structure and content; choleliths often radiolucent
• Ultrasonography—may detect choleliths as small as 2 mm in diameter, thickening of the gallbladder wall, distension of the biliary tract, hepatocellular abnormalities, and extrahepatic tissue involvement; may facilitate collection of specimens for culture, cytology, and histopathology; may detect evidence of OBTD within 72 hr; sludged bile and a full gallbladder common ultrasonographic findings in anorectic patients do not mistake for cholelithiasis

TREATMENT

• Not indicated without clinical and clinicopathologic signs
• Supportive fluids—according to hydration status, electrolyte depletion, and acid–base balance
• Hyperlipidemia as a predisposing factor—prescribe a fat-restricted diet.
• Exploratory surgery and cholecystectomy—indicated for complicated cases
• Warn client that cholelithiasis is a chronic problem and that new stones may form even after surgical resection.

MEDICATION

DRUGS
• Antibiotics—based on biliary culture or directed against enteric organisms; initial treatment with Timentin, metronidazole, or clindamycin (anaerobic spectrum) combined with a fluoroquinolone, or ampicillin/gentamicin
• Ursodeoxycholic acid—10–15 mg/kg/day PO; induces choleresis, blunts hepatobiliary inflammation, and fibrogenesis; possibly assists in dissolving non–cholesterol-rich stones;

known to dissolve cholesterol-rich stones; must be used in the context of normal hydration; continued therapy may be necessary
• Vitamin K—parenterally; 0.5–1.5 mg/kg to a maximum of three doses in 36–48 hr

CONTRAINDICATIONS/POSSIBLE INTERACTIONS
• Ursodeoxycholic acid—contraindicated with OBTD until biliary decompression

FOLLOW-UP

PATIENT MONITORING
• Physical examination and pertinent diagnostic testing—every 2–4 weeks until clinical signs and clinicopathologic abnormalities resolve
• Periodic ultrasonography—assess cholelith status and integrity of biliary tract

POSSIBLE COMPLICATIONS
• Sudden onset of fever, abdominal pain, and depression—may signify bile peritonitis and/or sepsis from a breakdown in bile containment

EXPECTED COURSE AND PROGNOSIS
• May be asymptomatic
• Symptomatic disease—depend on existing infection, OBTD, cholecystitis, or bile peritonitis

MISCELLANEOUS

ASSOCIATED CONDITIONS
• Cholecystitis
• Choledochitis
• Biliary tree obstruction

SYNONYMS
• Gall stones

ABBREVIATIONS
• ALP = alkaline phosphatase
• ALT = alanine aminotransferase
• AST = aspartate aminotransferase
• GTT = γ-glutamyltransferase
• OBTD = obstructed biliary tract disease
• PIVKA = proteins invoked by vitamin K absence or antagonism
• PT = prothrombin time

Suggested Reading
Center SA. Diseases of the gallbladder and biliary tree. In: Guilford WG, Center SA, Strombeck DR, et al., eds. Strombeck's small animal gastroenterology. Philadelphia: Saunders, 1996:860–888.
Author William E. Hornbuckle
Consulting Editor Sharon A. Center

DISEASES

CHONDROSARCOMA, BONE

 BASICS

OVERVIEW
• Malignant neoplasm arising from cartilage and characterized histologically by anaplastic cartilage cells
• Second most common primary bone tumor in dogs; represents 5%–10% of all primary bone tumors
• More common in the axial skeleton
• Most common primary rib tumor
• Must differentiate from chondroblastic osteosarcoma
• Histologic grade and tumor location helpful for predicting survival
• High-grade tumors similar to osteosarcoma in respect to metastatic potential

SIGNALMENT
• Most common in large (not giant) dog breeds
• Uncommon in cats
• Mean age—8.7 years

SIGNS

Historical Findings
• Lameness
• Pain in affected limb
• Visible swelling at tumor site
• Nasal discharge

Physical Examination Findings
• Long-bone tumors
• Monostotic swelling in metaphyseal site
• Pain on palpation of tumor site
• May see pathologic fracture
• Rib tumors
• Asymptomatic palpable mass in thoracic wall
• May see pleural effusion secondary to intrathoracic extension of tumor

CAUSES & RISK FACTORS
Multiple cartilaginous exostosis

 DIAGNOSIS

DIFFERENTIAL DIAGNOSIS
• Osteosarcoma, fibrosarcoma, and hemangiosarcoma
• Metastatic bone lesion from another primary site
• Osteomyelitis—fungal or bacterial

CBC/BIOCHEMISTRY/URINALYSIS
Usually normal

OTHER LABORATORY TESTS
N/A

IMAGING
• Radiographs of primary lesion (lytic and/or productive lesions)—impossible to differentiate from other types of primary bone tumors; lesions in long bones usually located in metaphyseal sites
• Thoracic radiography—detects metastasis
• CT scan—may help determine local extent of disease in patients with rib tumor
• Nuclear bone scan or radiographic scan of entire skeleton—useful for staging

DIAGNOSTIC PROCEDURES
• Biopsy and histopathologic examination of bone tumor—as described for osteosarcoma
• Small specimens of osteosarcoma may be misdiagnosed as chondrosarcoma.

 TREATMENT

• Amputation or limb salvage—remove primary long bone tumor
• Chest wall resection—with rib tumor
• Hemipelvectomy—with tumor involving bones of the pelvis
• Radiotherapy—consider for palliation in patients with inoperable tumor

 MEDICATIONS

DRUGS
• Chemotherapy (dogs)—cisplatin; post-surgery for high-grade tumors, as recommended for osteosarcoma
• Doxorubicin-based protocols—may be useful

CONTRAINDICATIONS/POSSIBLE INTERACTIONS
• Cisplatin—contraindicated in cats; do not use with compromised renal function
• Doxorubicin—do not use with congestive heart failure

 FOLLOW-UP

• Thoracic radiography—monthly for 3 months and every 3rd month thereafter
• Low-grade tumor of long bones—prognosis excellent
• High-grade tumor of long bones—prognosis guarded to poor

 MISCELLANEOUS

Suggested Reading
Waters DJ, Cooley DM. Skeletal neoplasms. In: Morrison WB, ed. Cancer in dogs and cats: medical and surgical management. Baltimore: Williams & Wilkins, 1998:639–654.
Author Terrance A. Hamilton
Consulting Editor Wallace B. Morrison

CHONDROSARCOMA, LARYNX AND TRACHEA

BASICS

OVERVIEW
• Malignant, cartilage-producing tumors with progressive local invasion of the surrounding tissues
• Uncommon; slowly progressive (weeks)

SIGNALMENT
• Dogs and cats
• Middle-aged to old animals (5–15 years)
• No breed predilection
• Males affected slightly more than females

SIGNS

Historical Findings
• Change in voice; loss of bark or purr; or harsh, noisy breath
• Exercise intolerance
• Severe respiratory distress; open-mouth breathing; cyanosis; and acute collapse

Physical Examination Findings
• Inspiratory stridor
• Laryngeal mass
• Aspiration pneumonia secondary to laryngeal dysfunction

CAUSES & RISK FACTORS
None known

DIAGNOSIS

DIFFERENTIAL DIAGNOSIS
• Laryngeal paralysis
• Laryngeal spasm and collapse
• Laryngeal trauma and secondary inflammation
• Other laryngeal or tracheal malignancies—squamous cell carcinoma; oncocytoma (rhabdomyoma); mast cell tumor; lymphoma

CBC/BIOCHEMISTRY/URINALYSIS
Usually normal

OTHER LABORATORY TESTS
• Cytologic examination—tissue obtained by endoscopic bronchial brushing or fine-needle aspiration
• Biopsy—usually nondiagnostic

IMAGING
• Survey radiography—often not helpful
• Thoracic radiography—detect pulmonary metastasis

DIAGNOSTIC PROCEDURES
• Tissue biopsy—definitive diagnosis
• Careful cervical examination—regional lymphadenopathy

TREATMENT
• Inpatient
• Complete laryngectomy with a permanent tracheostomy—rarely performed in animals; does not offer any significant long-term palliation of clinical signs (< 15 weeks)
• Radiotherapy (with or without surgery)—rarely reported as effective

MEDICATIONS

DRUGS
Chemotherapeutic agent for local or systemic control—effective agent not reported

CONTRAINDICATIONS/POSSIBLE INTERACTIONS
N/A

FOLLOW-UP

PATIENT MONITORING
Survey radiography of the laryngeal region or laryngoscopy—may perform when clinical signs recur

EXPECTED COURSE AND PROGNOSIS
• Guarded prognosis because of advanced infiltrative disease at the time of diagnosis
• Local recurrence—common; with extension to regional lymph nodes
• Aspiration pneumonia—may occur secondary to laryngeal dysfunction or via tracheostomy site

MISCELLANEOUS

Suggested Reading
Flanders JA, Castleman W, Carberry CA, et al. Laryngeal chondrosarcoma in a dog. J Am Vet Med Assoc 1987;190:68–70.
Hahn KA, Anderson TA. Tumors of the respiratory tract. In: Bonagura JD, ed. Kirk's current veterinary therapy XIII. Philadelphia: Saunders, 1998:500–505.
Author Kevin A. Hahn
Consulting Editor Wallace B. Morrison

DISEASES

CHONDROSARCOMA, NASAL AND PARANASAL SINUS

 BASICS

OVERVIEW
• Slow, progressive invasion of neoplastic mesenchymal cells within the nasal and paranasal sinuses
• Usually begins as unilateral but progresses slowly to bilateral by the time the patient is examined
• Prevalence of nonepithelial nasal neoplasia in dogs and cats—0.3%–4.7% of all tumors

SIGNALMENT
• More common in dogs than cats (rare)
• Median age (dogs and cats)—7 years (range, 2–11 years)
• Tends to develop at a younger age than other nasal tumors (64% occur in dogs < 8 years old)

SIGNS
Historical Findings
• Intermittent and progressive history of unilateral to bilateral epistaxis (median duration, 3 months)
• Epiphora
• Sneezing
• Halitosis
• Anorexia
• Seizures secondary to cranial invasion

Physical Examination Findings
• Noninfectious nasal discharge
• Facial deformity or exophthalmia
• Pain on nasal or paranasal sinus examination

CAUSES & RISK FACTORS
Unknown

 DIAGNOSIS

DIFFERENTIAL DIAGNOSIS
• Bacterial sinusitis—uncommon
• Viral infection (cats)
• Aspergillosis
• Cryptococcosis (cats)
• Foreign body
• Trauma
• Tooth root abscess
• Oronasal fistula
• Coagulopathy

CBC/BIOCHEMISTRY/URINALYSIS
Usually normal

OTHER LABORATORY TESTS
Cytologic and bacterial examination—rarely helpful

IMAGING
• Survey radiography (skull)—shows typical pattern of asymmetrical destruction of caudal turbinates with superimposition of a soft tissue mass; may see fluid density in the frontal sinuses secondary to outflow obstruction
• Thoracic radiography—detect lung metastasis (uncommon)
• CT or MRI—best for observing integrity of cribriform plate or orbital invasion

DIAGNOSTIC PROCEDURES
• Rhinoscopy (visual observation poor)—chondrosarcoma may be firm, hard mass or soft, friable, fleshy mass; avoid progressing caudally into the cribriform plate.
• Tissue biopsy—necessary for definitive diagnosis
• Bacterial culture—often positive

 TREATMENT

• Surgery alone—ineffective
• Turbinectomy—may be done before external (teletherapy) or internal (brachytherapy) irradiation
• Inpatient radiotherapy (with or without surgery)—60–80 Gy; best clinical control in dogs

 MEDICATIONS

DRUGS
Chemotherapy—good option in some animals; doxorubicin (30 mg/m² IV once every 2 weeks for 5 treatments in dogs weighing > 10 kg; 1 mg/kg for dogs < 10 kg and for cats); median survival (dogs) 18 weeks; may provide marked palliation of clinical signs

CONTRAINDICATIONS/POSSIBLE INTERACTIONS
Chemotherapy can be toxic; seek advice before initiating treatment if you are unfamiliar with cytotoxic drugs.

 FOLLOW-UP

PATIENT MONITORING
Survey radiography (skull) and/or CT or MRI—may be performed when clinical signs recur

EXPECTED COURSE AND PROGNOSIS
• Median survival if left untreated—3-months
• Median disease-free interval after radiotherapy—dogs, 8–25 months; cats, 1–36 months
• Survival with radiotherapy (dogs and cats)—1-year survival, 38%–57%; 2-year survival, 30%–40%; some reports of shorter survival times with nonepithelial nasal tumors (8–16 months)
• Brain involvement—poor prognostic sign

 MISCELLANEOUS

Suggested Reading
Frazier DL, Hahn KA. Cancer chemotherapeutics. In: Hahn KA, Richardson RC, eds. Cancer chemotherapy—a veterinary handbook. Baltimore: Williams & Wilkins, 1995:77–150.
Patnaik AK. Canine sinonasal neoplasms: soft tissue tumors. J Am Anim Hosp Assoc 1989;25:491–497.
Author Kevin A. Hahn
Consulting Editor Wallace B. Morrison

BASICS

OVERVIEW
• Malignant, cartilage-producing tumor with progressive local invasion of the surrounding tissues
• Slowly progressive (months); adherent to bone; generally nonencapsulated with a smooth to slightly nodular surface (commonly mistaken as benign)
• Slow to metastasize; lung more common site than regional lymph nodes
• Death usually secondary to local recurrence and cachexia
• Uncommon in dogs and cats

SIGNALMENT
• Dogs and cats
• Dogs—usually middle-aged; more common in large breeds

SIGNS
Historical Findings
• Excessive salivation
• Halitosis
• Dysphagia
• Bloody oral discharge
• Weight loss

Physical Examination Findings
• Oral mass, most commonly located on the maxilla
• Loose teeth
• Facial deformity
• Occasional cervical lymphadenomegaly (reactive hyperplasia)

CAUSES & RISK FACTORS
None identified

DIAGNOSIS

DIFFERENTIAL DIAGNOSIS
Oral Malignancies
• Multilobular osteoma—appears radiographically as an osteoma arising from flat bones of the skull; highly metastatic; complete surgical excision uncommon
• Osteoma

• Multiple cartilaginous exostoses (osteochondromatosis)—condition of growing dogs; cartilage-capped bony growths from the surface of flat bones; growth ceases upon skeletal maturity; sessile or pedunculated painful bony mass; excise if growth continues beyond maturity; may transform to osteosarcoma or chondrosarcoma
• Undifferentiated oral malignancy

Oral Masses
• Epulis
• Abscess
• Benign polyp

CBC/BIOCHEMISTRY/URINALYSIS
Usually normal

OTHER LABORATORY TESTS
Cytologic evaluation—impression smear obtained by incisional biopsy (wedge); may yield diagnosis

IMAGING
• Skull radiography—evaluate for bone involvement deep to the mass
• Thoracic radiographs—evaluate lungs for metastasis

DIAGNOSTIC PROCEDURES
• A large, deep-tissue biopsy (down to bone)—required to sufficiently differentiate from other oral malignancies
• Carefully palpate regional lymph nodes (mandibular and retropharyngeal).

TREATMENT
• Radical excision—required (e.g., hemimaxillectomy); well-tolerated; margins of at least 2 cm necessary; survival rates after surgery limited, but the metastatic behavior of most chondrosarcomas is low (< 15%); survival improves when excisional margins are free of neoplastic cells.
• Cryosurgery—not indicated owing to invasive bony involvement
• Inpatient radiotherapy—results unreported; most chondrosarcomas poorly responsive
• Soft foods—may recommend to prevent ulceration of tumor or after radical oral excision

MEDICATIONS

DRUGS
• Chemotherapy—efficacy unreported; many mesenchymal-origin tumors poorly responsive
• Cisplatin—intralesionally administered; local control (palliation) reported

CONTRAINDICATIONS/POSSIBLE INTERACTIONS
Chemotherapy may be toxic; seek advice before initiating treatment if you are unfamiliar with cytotoxic drugs.

FOLLOW-UP
• Lymph node metastasis on examination common (dogs)
• Euthanasia—most dogs within 30 days of diagnosis; tumor growth progressive and uncontrolled, resulting in dysphagia and cachexia
• Survival rates after surgery limited

MISCELLANEOUS

Suggested Reading
Frazier DL, Hahn KA. Cancer chemotherapeutics. In: Hahn KA, Richardson RC, eds. Cancer chemotherapy—a veterinary handbook. Baltimore: Williams & Wilkins, 1995:77–150.
Oakes MG, Lewis DD, Hedlund CS, Hosgood G. Canine oral neoplasia. Compend Contin Educ Small Anim Pract 1993; 15:15–31.
Author Kevin A. Hahn
Consulting Editor Wallace B. Morrison

DISEASES

BASICS

DEFINITION
- Inflammation of the choroid and retina
- Also called posterior uvea
- Diffuse inflammation may result in frank retinal detachment (see Retinal Detachment).

PATHOPHYSIOLOGY
- Caused by infectious agents, neoplastic or immune cells, or immune complexes (immune-mediated diseases); hematogenous pathogenic factors, inducing choroidal inflammation, most common
- Choroid and retina—closely apposed; physiologically interdependent; inflammation of one usually results in inflammation of the other.
- May also occur as a retinochoroiditis—retinal inflammation preceding and inducing choroidal inflammation

SYSTEMS AFFECTED
- Ophthalmic
- Nervous
- Other systems if disease is systemic

GENETICS
N/A

INCIDENCE/PREVALENCE
- Fairly common
- Exact incidence unknown.

GEOGRAPHIC DISTRIBUTION
Depends on the prevalence of infectious cause (e.g., systemic mycoses, rickettsial disease)

SIGNALMENT
Species
Dogs and cats

Breed Predilections
- Systemic mycoses—more common in large hunting breed dogs
- Uveodermatologic syndrome—akitas, chows, Siberian huskies, and German shepherds predisposed

Mean Age and Range
Depend on underlying cause

Predominant Sex
Uveodermatologic syndrome—more common in young male dogs

SIGNS
- Not usually painful, except when anterior uvea is affected
- Vitreous abnormalities—may note exudates, hemorrhage, or syneresis (liquefaction)
- Interruption or alteration of the course of retinal blood vessels—owing to retinal elevation
- Ophthalmomyiasis (cats)—curvilinear tracts

from migrating larvae
- Others—related to underlying systemic disease

Lesions
- Indistinct margins; tapetal hyporeflectivity; white-gray color
- Alter course of retinal blood vessels
- Few, small—may note no apparent visual deficits
- Extensive, involving larger areas of the retina—blindness or reduced vision
- Inactive (scars)—discrete margins; hyper-reflective in the tapetum sometimes with hyperpigmented central areas; depigmented in the nontapetum and may have some surrounding or central hyperpigmentation

CAUSES
Dogs
- Viral—canine distemper; herpesvirus (rare, usually neonates); rabies
- Bacterial or rickettsial—septicemia or bacteremia; leptospirosis; brucellosis; pyometra (toxic uveitis); *Borrelia;* ehrlichiosis; Rocky Mountain spotted fever
- Fungal—aspergillosis; blastomycosis; coccidioidomycosis; histoplasmosis; cryptococcosis
- Algal—geotrichosis; prototothecosis
- Parasitic—ocular larval migrans (*Strongyles, Ascarids, Baylisascaris*); toxoplasmosis; leishmaniasis; *Neospora;* ophthalmomyiasis interna (Diptera larval migrans more common in cats)

Cats
- Viral—FeLV; FIV; FIP
- Bacterial—septicemia or bacteremia
- Fungal—cryptococcosis; histoplasmosis; blastomycosis; others
- Parasitic—toxoplasmosis; ophthalmomyiasis interna (Diptera); ocular larval migrans
- Protozoal—toxoplasmosis
- Autoimmune—periarteritis nodosa; SLE

Dogs and Cats
- Exogenous infection—trauma (perforating wound); intraocular surgery
- Endogenous or hematogenous infection—ocular manifestation of systemic disease; may extend from the CNS via the optic nerve
- Septicemia or bacteremia—diskospondylitis; endocarditis; pyometra; may result from primary infection or associated immune complex disease
- Neoplasia—primary or metastatic; with granulomatous meningoencephalitis, peri-papillary chorioretinal inflammation (around an inflamed optic nerve); lymphosarcoma most common; with early multiple myeloma, may

note multifocal chorioretinitis before frank bullous retinal detachment can be ruled out
- Immune mediated—may cause vasculitis or inflammation, resulting in exudative retinal detachment or chorioretinitis; exact cause usually undetermined; with thrombocytopenia, may see small multifocal or large retinal and/or vitreal hemorrhages with associated inflammation
- Autoimmune—target of Vogt-Koyanagi-Harada-like (uveodermatologic) syndrome is melanin pigment granule (abundant in uveal tissue), leading to severe anterior and posterior inflammation (affected dogs may also exhibit depigmentation of the skin, especially at mucocutaneous junctions); target of SLE is nuclear antigen.
- Idiopathic—common
- Toxicity—ethylene glycol; idiosyncratic drug reactions (e.g., trimethoprim sulfa)
- Trauma

RISK FACTORS
FeLV or FIV infection—may predispose cat to ocular toxoplasmosis and chorioretinitis

 DIAGNOSIS

DIFFERENTIAL DIAGNOSIS
- Ophthalmic examination—usually sufficient for diagnosis; may note a slow pupillary light reflex if large areas of the retina are affected
- Blindness or impaired vision—optic neuritis; CNS disease; diffuse retinal inflammation
- See Causes
- Retinal dysplasia—similar to inactive disease; bilateral, symmetrical folds or geographic clumps of pigment or altered fungus reflectivity; no associated signs inflammation in the eye; Labrador retrievers and springer spaniels predisposed

CBC/BIOCHEMISTRY/URINALYSIS
- Normal—problem confined to the eye
- Abnormal—depend on underlying systemic disease

OTHER LABORATORY TESTS
- Depend on suspected systemic problem
- Protein electrophoresis
- Documentation of Bence-Jones protein in urine
- Skin biopsy—SLE; uveodermatologic syndrome
- Coagulation profile
- Bacterial culture of ocular or body fluids
- Serologic testing—infectious disease (see Causes)

IMAGING
• Thoracic radiography—lymphadenopathy; metastatic disease; infiltrates consistent with infectious agents
• Spinal radiography—bony changes consistent with diskospondylitis or multiple myeloma
• Ocular ultrasound—retinal detachments; intraocular masses; especially helpful if the ocular media are not clear

DIAGNOSTIC PROCEDURES
• Indirect ophthalmoscopy—screens a large area of the retina
• Direct ophthalmoscopy—facilitates examination of suspicious areas
• CSF tap—indicated for signs of CNS disease or optic neuritis
• Vitreocentesis or subretinal fluid aspirate—may perform if other diagnostic tests fail to yield a causal agent or for suspected infectious agent or neoplasia; vitreocentesis may aggravate inflammation or induce hemorrhage, lessening the chance for retinal reattachment and restoration of vision.

PATHOLOGIC FINDINGS
• Masses or retinal or choroidal exudates
• Fungal organisms—in exudates and inflammatory cells
• Perivascular inflammation—vasculitis; FIP
• Inactive lesions—retinal and choroidal atrophy (thinning); may note RPE hyperpigmentation and tapetal destruction

TREATMENT

APPROPRIATE HEALTH CARE
• Depends on physical condition of patient
• Usually outpatient

NURSING CARE
Fluid or other therapy for systemic disease

ACTIVITY
N/A

DIET
N/A

CLIENT EDUCATION
• Inform client that chorioretinitis may be a sign of systemic disease, so diagnostic testing is important.
• Warn client that immune-mediated disease requires lifelong therapy for controlling inflammation.
• Inform client that dogs with uveodermatologic syndrome may also have anterior uveitis and secondary glaucoma, which require treatment.

SURGICAL CONSIDERATIONS
N/A

MEDICATIONS

DRUGS OF CHOICE
• Identify and definitely treat any underlying systemic disease (e.g., itraconazole for systemic mycosis).
• Topical medications—may not reach effective concentrations in dogs with intact lenses
• Systemic therapy—required
• Systemic prednisone at anti-inflammatory doses—0.5 mg/kg PO, then taper; when systemic mycosis has been ruled out or is being treated with appropriate systemic antifungal therapy; avoid use, unless large areas of the retina are affected and vision is severely threatened.
• Prednisone at immunosuppressive doses—2 mg/kg divided q12 for 3–10 days (ideal), then taper very slowly over months; for immune-mediated disease; may facilitate retinal reattachment
• Topical corticosteroids (1% prednisolone acetate or 0.1% dexamethasone give TID to QID) and parasympatholytics (1% atropine given at a frequency that dilates the pupil and reduces pain)—for panuveitis (concurrent anterior uveitis)
• Anti-glaucoma therapy—as appropriate for secondary glaucoma

CONTRAINDICATIONS
Systematically administered corticosteroids—do not use unless systemic mycosis is ruled out or is being definitively treated.

PRECAUTIONS
N/A

POSSIBLE INTERACTIONS
N/A

ALTERNATIVE DRUGS
• Neoplastic conditions (lymphosarcoma or multiple myeloma)—chemotherapeutic agents
• Uveodermatologic syndrome—may require azathioprine (see Retinal Detachment) and steroids (control inflammation)

FOLLOW-UP

PATIENT MONITORING
• As appropriate for underlying cause and type of medical treatment
• CBC platlet count and liver enzymes—if giving azathioprine
• IOP—for anterior uveitis

PREVENTION/AVOIDANCE
N/A

POSSIBLE COMPLICATIONS
• Permanent blindness
• Cataracts
• Glaucoma
• Chronic ocular pain
• Death—secondary to systemic disease

EXPECTED COURSE AND PROGNOSIS
• Prognosis for vision—guarded to good, depending on amount of retina affected; visual deficits or blindness if large areas of the retina were destroyed; focal and multifocal disease do not markedly impair vision but do leave scars.
• Prognosis for life—guarded to good, depending on underlying cause

MISCELLANEOUS

ASSOCIATED CONDITIONS
Several systemic diseases

AGE-RELATED FACTORS
N/A

ZOONOTIC POTENTIAL
Toxoplasmosis—may be transmitted to humans if patient is shedding oocysts in feces

PREGNANCY
N/A

SYNONYMS
Retinochoroiditis

SEE ALSO
• Retinal Degeneration
• Retinal Detachment

ABBREVIATIONS
• CSF = cerebrospinal fluid
• FeLV = feline leukemia virus
• FIP = feline infectious peritonitis
• FIV = feline immunodeficiency virus
• IOP = intraocular pressure
• RPE = retinal pigment epithelium
• SLE = systemic lupus erythematosus

Suggested Reading

Narfström K, Ekesten B. Diseases of the canine ocular fundus. In: Veterinary opthalmology 3rd ed. Philadelphia: Lippincott Williams and Wilkins 1999:869–993.
Millichamp NJ, Dziezyc J,. Small animal ophthalmology. Vet Clin North Am Small Anim Prac 1990;20:564–877.
Author Patricia J. Smith
Consulting Editor Paul E. Miller

DISEASES

CHYLOTHORAX

BASICS

DEFINITION
• A collection of chyle in the pleural space
• Chyle—lymphatic fluid arising from the intestine and, therefore, containing a high quantity of fat
• Thoracic lymphangiectasia—the tortuous, dilated lymphatics found in many animals with chylothorax
• Fibrosing pleuritis—condition in which pleural thickening leads to constriction of the lung lobes; when severe, results in marked restriction of ventilation; may be caused by any chronic pleural exudate but is most commonly associated with chylothorax and pyothorax

PATHOPHYSIOLOGY
• Abnormal flows or pressures within the thoracic duct are thought to lead to exudation of chyle from intact, but dilated, thoracic lymphatic vessels in most animals.
• Lymphangiectasia—may result from increased lymphatic flows, decreased lymphatic drainage into the venous system because of high venous pressures, or both factors acting simultaneously
• May be caused by any disease or process that increases systemic venous pressures, including right heart failure, mediastinal neoplasia, and cranial vena cava thrombi or granulomas
• Thoracic duct rupture, as from trauma—uncommon cause in dogs and cats

SYSTEMS AFFECTED
Respiratory—chylous effusion or fibrosing pleuritis interferes with the ability of the lungs to expand.

GENETICS
Unknown

INCIDENCE/PREVALENCE
Unknown

GEOGRAPHIC DISTRIBUTION
Worldwide

SIGNALMENT

Species
Dogs and cats

Breed Predilections
• Dogs—Afghan hounds and Shiba Inus
• Cats—Asian breeds (e.g., Siamese and Himalayan) appear to have a higher prevalence than other breeds.

Mean Age And Range
• Any age may be affected
• Cats—old animals may be more likely to develop condition than young cats; may indicate an association with neoplasia
• Afghan hounds—develop when middle-aged
• Shiba Inus—develop when young (< 1–2 years of age)

Predominant Sex
None identified

SIGNS

General Comments
• Vary, depending on the underlying cause, rapidity of fluid accumulation, and volume of fluid
• Usually not exhibited until there is marked impairment of ventilation
• Many patients appear to have condition for prolonged periods before diagnosis; they probably reabsorb chyle at a rate that prevents obvious respiratory impairment.

Historical Findings
• Usually examined because of evaluation of dyspnea or coughing
• Coughing—may have been present for months before examination
• Many patients will have been treated with antibiotics for presumed respiratory infection before diagnosis
• Tachypnea
• Depression
• Anorexia and weight loss
• Exercise intolerance

Physical Examination Findings
• Muffled heart and lung sounds
• Increased bronchovesicular sounds, particularly in the dorsal lung fields
• Cyanosis
• Pale mucous membranes
• Arrhythmia
• Murmur
• Jugular pulses in association with right-sided heart failure
• Decrease in the compressibility of the anterior chest—common in cats with a cranial mediastinal mass and pleural effusion

CAUSES
• Anterior mediastinal masses—mediastinal lymphosarcoma; thymoma
• Heart disease—cardiomyopathy; pericardial effusion; heartworm infection; tetralogy of Fallot; tricuspid dysplasia; cor triatriatum dexter
• Fungal granuloma
• Venous thrombus
• Congenital abnormality of the thoracic duct
• Idiopathic—most patients

RISK FACTORS
Unknown

DIAGNOSIS

DIFFERENTIAL DIAGNOSIS
• Consider any cause of respiratory distress or coughing.
• Once pleural effusion has been identified—diseases causing exudative pleural effusion (e.g., pyothorax, FIP, and neoplastic effusion)
• Pseudochylous effusion—misused in the veterinary literature to describe an effusion that looks like chyle but in which a ruptured thoracic duct is not found; reserve term for effusions in which fluid cholesterol is higher than serum cholesterol and fluid triglyceride is lower than serum triglyceride

CBC/BIOCHEMISTRY/URINALYSIS
• Often normal
• Lymphopenia and hypoalbuminemia—may be found

OTHER LABORATORY TESTS

Fluid Analysis
• Characteristics—usually milky white and opaque, may range from yellow to pink, depending on diet and the occurrence of concurrent hemorrhage
• Protein content—inaccurate owing to interference of the refractive index by the high lipid content of the fluid
• Total nucleated cell count—usually < 10,000 cells/μL

Cytology
• Primarily small lymphocytes or neutrophils
• Nondegenerative neutrophils—may predominate with prolonged loss of lymphocytes, with chronicity, or when multiple therapeutic thoracocenteses have induced inflammation
• Abnormal lymphocytes—may indicate underlying neoplasia

OTHER LABORATORY TESTS
• Compare fluid and serum triglyceride concentrations—true chyle if higher in the fluid
• Sudan III stain—lipid droplets
• Ether clearance test—not quantitative

IMAGING

Thoracic Radiography
• Dyspnea—dorsoventral and standing lateral views
• No dyspnea—ventrodorsal and lateral recumbent views
• Pleural effusion—repeat studies after removal of most of the pleural fluid; if collapsed lung lobes do not appear to re-expand after pleural fluid is removed; suspect underlying pulmonary parenchymal or pleural disease (e.g., fibrosing pleuritis); if dyspnea persists with only minimal fluid, consider fibrosing pleuritis

Ultrasonography
• Perform before removing fluid—fluid acts as an acoustic window, enhancing visualization of thoracic structures.
• Detect abnormal cardiac structure and function, pericardial disease, and mediastinal masses

PATHOLOGIC FINDINGS

• Lymphatics (including the thoracic duct)—difficult to identify at necropsy
• Fibrosing pleuritis—lungs appear shrunken; pleura (visceral and parietal) are diffusely thickened.
• Fibrosing pleuritis—characterized histologically by diffuse, moderate to marked thickening of the pleura by fibrous connective tissue with moderate infiltrates of lymphocytes, macrophages, and plasma cells

TREATMENT

APPROPRIATE HEALTH CARE

• Dyspneic patients with suspected pleural effusion—immediate thoracentesis; removal of even small amounts of pleural effusion may markedly improve ventilation.
• Identify and treat the underlying cause, if possible.
• Medical management—usually outpatient with intermittent thoracentesis as necessary to prevent dyspnea
• Chest tubes—place only in patients with suspected chylothorax secondary to trauma (very rare), with rapid fluid accumulation, or after surgery
• Unsuccessful medical management (try 2–3 months)—consider surgery (see Surgical Considerations).

NURSING CARE

• Patients may become debilitated if thoracentesis is performed frequently; attention to diet (see below) is important.
• Chest taps—perform under aseptic conditions to reduce the risk of iatrogenic infection; antibiotic prophylaxis generally unnecessary if proper technique is used

ACTIVITY

Patients will usually restrict their own exercise as the pleural fluid volume increases or if they develop fibrosing pleuritis.

DIET

• Low-fat—may decrease the amount of fat in the effusion, which may improve the patient's ability to resorb fluid from the thoracic cavity; not a cure; may help in management by facilitating reabsorption
• Medium-chain triglycerides—once thought to be absorbed directly into the portal system, bypassing the thoracic duct; actually transported via the thoracic duct of dogs; thus less useful than previously believed; no longer recommended by the author

CLIENT EDUCATION

• Inform client that no treatment will stop the effusion in all patients with the idiopathic form of the disease.
• Inform client that the condition may spontaneously resolve in some patients after several weeks or months

SURGICAL CONSIDERATIONS

Thoracic Duct Ligation

• Recommended initially in patients who do not respond to medical management
• The duct usually has multiple branches in the caudal thorax where ligation is performed; failure to occlude all branches results in continued pleural effusion.
• Always perform in conjunction with catheterization of a mesenteric lymphatic for lymphangiography or injection of dye; methylene blue injected in the mesenteric catheter greatly facilitates visualization and complete occlusion of all branches.

Other

• Thoracic duct ligation not successful—may consider pleuroperitoneal or pleurovenous shunts
• Extensive fibrosing pleuritis—poor surgical candidate; very grave prognosis

MEDICATIONS

DRUG OF CHOICE

Rutin—50 mg/kg PO q8h; preliminary findings by the author suggest that complete resolution of effusion was achieved 2 months after initiation in at least 25% of patients; further study is required to determine whether resolution occurred spontaneously or in response to drug therapy.

CONTRAINDICATIONS

Severe fibrosing pleuritis—poor prognosis; medical or surgical treatment unlikely to offer benefit

PRECAUTIONS

N/A

POSSIBLE INTERACTIONS

N/A

ALTERNATIVE DRUGS

N/A

FOLLOW-UP

PATIENT MONITORING

• Monitor closely for dyspnea; perform thoracentesis as needed.
• Resolution (spontaneously or postsurgery)—periodically re-evaluate for several years to detect recurrence

PREVENTION/AVOIDANCE

N/A

POSSIBLE COMPLICATIONS

• Fibrosing pleuritis—most common serious complication of chronic disease

• Immunosuppression—caused by lymphocyte depletion; may develop in patients undergoing repeated and frequent thoracentesis
• Hyponatremia and hyperkalemia—documented in affected dogs undergoing multiple thoracentesis

EXPECTED COURSE AND PROGNOSIS

• May resolve spontaneously or after surgery
• Untreated or chronic disease—may result in severe fibrosing pleuritis and persistent dyspnea
• Euthanasia—frequently performed in patients that do not respond to surgery or medical management

MISCELLANEOUS

ASSOCIATED CONDITIONS

Diffuse lymphatic abnormalities (e.g., intestinal lymphangiectasia, hepatic lymphangiectasia, pulmonary lymphangiectasia, and chylous ascites)—may be noted; may worsen the prognosis

AGE-RELATED FACTORS

Young patients may have a better prognosis than old animals because of the association of neoplasia with advanced age.

ZOONOTIC POTENTIAL

N/A

PREGNANCY

N/A

ABBREVIATION

FIP = feline infectious peritonitis

Suggested Reading

Fossum TW, Birchard SJ, Jacobs RM. Chylothorax in thirty-four dogs. J Am Vet Med Assoc 1986;188:1315–1318.
Fossum TW, Evering WN, Miller MW, et al. Severe bilateral fibrosing pleuritis associated with chronic chylothorax in dogs and cats. J Am Vet Med Assoc 1992;201:317–324.
Fossum TW, Miller MW, Rogers KS, et al. Chylothorax associated with right-sided heart failure in 5 cats. J Am Vet Med Assoc 1994;204:84–89.
Kerpsack SJ, McLoughlin MA, Birchard SJ, et al. Evaluation of mesenteric lymphangiography and thoracic duct ligation in cats with chylothorax: 19 cases (1987–1992). J Am Vet Med Assoc 1994;205:711–715.
Author Theresa W. Fossum
Consulting Editors Eleanor C. Hawkins

DISEASES

CILIARY DYSKINESIA, PRIMARY

BASICS

OVERVIEW
- Congenital disorder caused by ciliary dysfunction
- Cilia—complex structures lining various organs including the upper and lower respiratory tracts, auditory tubes, ventricles of the brain, spinal canal, oviducts, and efferent ducts of the testes; sperm flagellum a modified cilium
- Ciliary beating—normally coordinated by an intricate mechanochemical interaction of numerous proteins contained within each cilium; characteristically uncoordinated (dyskinetic) or absent in affected dogs; cilia often, but not invariably, have structural lesions.
- Clinical signs predominate in ciliated organs—lack of mucociliary clearance in the respiratory tract (recurrent bacterial rhinosinusitis, bronchopneumonia) and auditory canal (secretory otitis media); chronic inflammation and obstruction of the airways (bronchiectasis); male infertility (live but immotile or hypomotile spermatozoa; may also see unexplained oligospermia and azoospermia)
- Hydrocephalus and situs inversus—common but variable features; genesis of these lesions not determined
- Diagnosis—confirmed by demonstrating the absence of tracheal mucociliary clearance and the presence of a specific ultrastructural lesion in respiratory cilia or sperm flagella; established in patients without ultrastructural ciliary lesions by in vitro analysis of ciliary function
- Dogs with chronic respiratory tract disease and situs inversus (e.g., Kartagener syndrome)—in all probability have primary ciliary dyskinesia and do not warrant an extensive workup

SIGNALMENT
- Genetic disease—probable autosomal recessive mode of inheritance
- Signs typically develop at an early age (days to 5 weeks); dogs have remained asymptomatic for prolonged periods (6 months to 10 years).
- Reported only in purebred dogs—Bichon Frises, border collies, Chihuahuas, shar peis, chow chows, Dalmatians, Doberman pinschers, English pointers, English setters, English springer spaniels, golden retrievers, Gordon setters, miniature poodles, old English sheepdogs, Newfoundlands, and rottweilers

- Kartagener syndrome—unpublished observation in a Norwegian elkhound and a domestic shorthair cat

SIGNS

Historical Findings
- Young purebred dog
- Chronic sneezing and coughing—may produce copious amounts of mucoid to mucopurulent material
- Despite dramatic response to antibiotics, patients have continuous serous to mucoid nasal discharge and relapse after treatment is stopped.
- Family history—large litters tend to have > 1 affected animal; progeny from prior matings of the dam and sire may have been affected.
- Fertility—females fertile; males characteristically not

Physical Examination Findings
- Bilateral, mucopurulent nasal discharge
- Moist, productive cough that can be elicited by exercise or tracheal palpation
- Tachypnea, dyspnea, and cyanosis—may be seen
- Diffuse increase in lung sounds of variable intensity—typically auscated; sounds from the ventral thorax diminish with more advanced lung disease (consolidation).
- Heart sounds—may be inaudible with severe bronchopneumonia; loudest on the right side of thorax with situs inversus totalis (Kartagener syndrome)
- Hydrocephalus—common; but clinical signs (e.g., dome-shaped calvarium and CNS dysfunction) rarely observed

CAUSES & RISK FACTORS
- Genetic disease
- Inbreeding

DIAGNOSIS

DIFFERENTIAL DIAGNOSIS
- Congenital (e.g., neutrophil dysfunction and immunoglobulin deficiency) or acquired disease (e.g., canine distemper) that develops in young dogs and produces chronic rhinosinusitis and bronchopneumonia
- Recurrent aspiration pneumonia
- Chronic bacterial pneumonia—caused by resident organisms, inadequate antimicrobial therapy, foreign body, abscess, or other persistent nidus of infection
- Bronchoesophageal fistula

CBC/BIOCHEMISTRY/URINALYSIS
- Mature neutrophilic leukocytosis and normal or high numbers of lymphocytes—common
- Lymphocyte numbers—help distinguish from canine distemper viral infection, which typically produces marked lymphopenia
- With severe bronchopneumonia—may see left shift and toxic change in the blood neutrophils
- Old dogs—may note hyperglobulinemia
- With chronic hypoxemia—may see polycythemia

OTHER LABORATORY TESTS
- Blood gas analysis—may reveal hypoxemia and normocapnia or hypocapnia
- Transtracheal lavage—typically recovers a mucoid to mucopurulent material characterized cytologically as a purulent exudate; one or more bacterial species commonly cultured
- *Mycoplasma* spp. and *Pasteurella multocida*—most common isolates; *Mycoplasma* too small to see in a cytologic specimen and require special culture medium to recover

IMAGING

Radiography
- Changes consistent with bronchopneumonia and sometimes bronchiectasis
- Mirror image reversal of viscera (situs inversus) involving the thorax or abdomen or both body cavities—common
- Thickened tympanic bullae or sclerotic (secretory otitis media) and radiopaque rhinoliths—may note in old patients

Mucociliary Scintigraphy
- Tracheal mucus clearance—determined with radiopharmaceuticals (^{99m}Tc-macroaggregated albumin) and γ camera imaging; no clearance observed in patients
- Mucociliary clearance—determine before ultrastructural analysis of cilia (avoids unnecessary use of electron microscopy); normal results exclude the diagnosis.

MRI
Moderate to severe dilation of the lateral cerebral ventricles—found in many patients

DIAGNOSTIC PROCEDURES

Electron Microscopy
- Ultrastructural lesions in the cilia—most patients; identify by pinch biopsy of the nasal mucosa; dynein arm deficiency, abnormal microtubular patterns, and random orientation common

• Diagnostic significance—specific lesion must be found in a high percentage of cilia; same defect must be found in cilia from multiple locations (e.g., nasal and bronchial cilia and sperm flagella) and from affected litter mates
• Acquired ultrastructural lesions—common in humans (and presumably dogs) with chronic respiratory tract infection; vary; typically involve < 5% of cilia
• Dogs with primary ciliary dyskinesia but no ultrastructural ciliary lesions have been described.

Other
• In vitro analysis of ciliary beat frequency and synchrony—confirms diagnosis in patients with no ultrastructural lesions
• Electrocardiogram—inversion of lead I and transposition of leads II and III in patients with thoracic situs inversus or isolated dextrocardia

PATHOLOGIC FINDINGS

Upper Respiratory Tract
• Chronic bacterial rhinitis—characterized by a mucoid to mucopurulent exudate overlaying an inflamed mucosa
• Histologic—mucosa infiltrated with plasma cells and neutrophils and has mucous gland hyperplasia; may note hypoplastic nasal turbinates, atresia of the frontal sinuses, frontal sinusitis, nasal polyps, and rhinoliths

Lower Respiratory Tract
• Lesions—vary with severity of bronchopneumonia and chronicity of disease
• Mucoid to mucopurulent material—observed throughout the airways
• Gross lung lesions—atelectasis, bronchiectasis, and subpleural emphysema; most pronounced in the ventral aspect of the cranial and middle lung lobes and in the cranioventral portion of the caudal lung lobes
• Histologic—bronchitis, bronchiolitis, and bronchiectasis

Miscellaneous
• Severe dilatation of the lateral cerebral ventricles—may be noted
• Situs inversus of thoracic viscera or abdominal viscera or both—situs inversus totalis; may occur
• Impaction of one or both middle ears with a sterile gelatinous material—secretory otitis media; may be seen

TREATMENT
• Airway secretions—cleared by the shear force produced by expiration and coughing
• Routine exercise—may enhance mucous clearance by increasing respiration and inducing coughing
• Daily positioning of patient in dorsal recumbency—may promote postural drainage of mucus from dependent airways; may facilitate expectoration
• Supplemental oxygen therapy—may be needed during acute episodes of life-threatening bronchopneumonia

MEDICATIONS

DRUGS
• Antibiotics—for respiratory infections; selected on the basis of bacterial culture and sensitivity testing; duration varies with the severity of infection; continuous therapy often rendered ineffective by colonization with resistant bacteria

CONTRAINDICATIONS/POSSIBLE INTERACTIONS
• Radiographic contrast medium used for bronchography—patient cannot clear it; may eventually elicit a pyogranulomatous inflammatory reaction

Anesthesia
• Patients have impaired gas exchange and, therefore, have increased risk of complications.
• Goal—minimize respiratory depression and recovery time
• Preanesthetic medication with narcotics—contraindicated
• Anticholinergics—increase dead air space by bronchodilatation; give only at induction.
• Nitrous oxide—do not use if obstructed bullae are noted in the lungs.
• Assisted or controlled ventilation—adjust ventilator to provide a long expiratory phase to prevent air trapping.
• Suction endotracheal tube and trachea intermittently during prolonged periods of anesthesia.
• Patients positioned on their backs are at greater risk for complications; because of small airway obstruction, atelectasis, and pulmonary fibrosis in the dependent portions of the lung, a severe ventilation–perfusion mismatch may develop.
• Postanesthesia—keep patient in sternal recumbency until it is fully recovered.

FOLLOW-UP

POSSIBLE COMPLICATIONS
• High ambient temperature—may produce hyperthermia and potential heat stroke because of reduced capacity for evaporative heat loss through the lungs
• Subpleural cysts—bronchiectatic cysts, interstitial cysts, and emphysematous bullae; may develop from prolonged air entrapment; may rupture, producing pneumothorax
• Chronic hypoxemia in association with a small pulmonary vascular bed—may precipitate pulmonary artery hypertension, cor pulmonale, and right-sided heart failure
• Persistent bacterial infections in the airways—may result in systemic reactive amyloidosis

EXPECTED COURSE AND PROGNOSIS
• The clinical course of disease and longevity of patients—highly variable
• Appropriate antibiotic treatment and pulmonary physical therapy—may result in prolonged survival; reactive systemic amyloidosis and cor pulmonale potential sequelae of chronic bacterial infection of the airways
• Patients < 1 year old—may develop chronic rhinosinusitis or bronchopneumonia with periodic exacerbations that can be life-threatening
• Patients > 1 year old—clinical disease varies considerably; despite persistent lack of mucociliary clearance, may become virtually asymptomatic for respiratory disease; may continue to have mucoid to mucopurulent nasal discharge, sneezing, and coughing but with less frequent acute exacerbations of bronchopneumonia
• Symptomatic patients who survive several years develop progressive pulmonary disease characterized by ventral consolidation of the lungs and bronchiectasis.
• Appropriate treatment may result in a normal life span; patients may, however, die during the acute episodes of bronchopneumonia.

MISCELLANEOUS

SEE ALSO
Pneumonia, Bacterial

Suggested Reading
Edwards DF, Patton CS, Kennedy JR. Primary ciliary dyskinesia in the dog. Probl Vet Med 1992;4:291–319.
Author David F. Edwards
Consulting Editor Eleanor C. Hawkins

DISEASES

CIRRHOSIS/FIBROSIS OF THE LIVER

BASICS

DEFINITION
• Fibrosis—accumulation of extracellular matrix containing excessive collagen • Cirrhosis—hepatic fibrosis, regenerative nodules, and irreparably altered hepatic architecture

PATHOPHYSIOLOGY
• Fibrosis—develops after repeated injury or inflammation; may be idiopathic in young dogs • Cirrhosis—irreversible sequela of chronic liver damage • Fibrosis and regenerative nodules—augment self-perpetuating injury by impairing hepatic blood and bile flow; lead to increased vascular resistance, causing portal hypertension, acquired portosystemic shunts, hepatic encephalopathy, and ascites • Sinusoidal collagenization and capillarization and loss of hepatic mass—impair hepatocellular functions

SYSTEMS AFFECTED
• Gastrointestinal—liver failure, portal hypertension causes ascites and altered splanchnic circulation, leading to gastric and duodenal erosions and ulcers; fat malabsorption from portal hypertension and abnormal bile acid circulation • Nervous—hepatic encephalopathy • Respiratory—tachypnea secondary to tense ascites; pulmonary edema (rare) • Skin/Exocrine—necrolytic migratory erythema (hepaticocutaneous syndrome); severe hyperkeratotic ulcerative epidermal lesions on pressure points and mucocutaneous junctions; edema and anasarca owing to hypoalbuminemia; water and sodium retention • Hemic/Lymphatic/Immune—RBC microcytosis mild anemia (acquired portosystemic shunts); bleeding tendencies; DIC • Renal/Urologic—ammonium biurate urolithiasis; renal failure as part of the hepatorenal syndrome (rare)

GENETICS
• Familial predisposition for chronic active hepatitis—Doberman pinchers; cocker spaniels; Labrador retrievers • Copper storage hepatopathy—autosomal recessive trait; Bedlington terriers • Juvenile idiopathic fibrosis—German shepherds; standard poodles • Uncertain disorders—West Highland white terriers; Skye blue terriers

INCIDENCE/PREVALENCE
High in dogs with chronic liver disease

GEOGRAPHIC DISTRIBUTION N/A

SIGNALMENT
Species
Dogs and cats (biliary cirrhosis)
Breed Predilection
• Any breed • Some breeds predisposed—see Genetics

Mean Age and Range
• Cirrhosis (dogs)—any age; signs most common in the middle-aged to old; Bedlington terriers young • Cirrhosis, biliary (cats)—with chronic cholangiohepatitis > 7 years of age • Idiopathic fibrosis (dogs)—< 2 years of age
Predominant Sex
• Cocker spaniels—males two to eight times more common than females • Doberman pinchers and Labrador retrievers—females more common than males • Bedlington terriers (idiopathic fibrosis)—none

SIGNS
General Comments
• Initially vague • Later—relate to portal hypertension, ascites, hepatic encephalopathy
Historical Findings
• Chronic history of waxing and waning lethargy, anorexia, loss of body condition • Vomiting • Diarrhea or constipation • Melena • Polydipsia and polyuria • Late onset—ascites; jaundice; bleeding tendencies; hepatic encephalopathy • Cats—ascites not common until very advanced disease; ptyalism with hepatic encephalopathy
Physical Examination Findings
• Lethargy • Poor body condition • Ascites • Jaundice • Hepatic encephalopathy • Cirrhosis—ascites, jaundice, and hepatic encephalopathy • Bleeding tendencies, cutaneous lesions of the hepaticocutaneous syndrome, obstructive uropathy owing to ammonium urate calculi—rare • Anasarca—initially rare; may develop after overzealous fluid therapy • Microhepatia—common in dogs • Liver size—often normal in cats

CAUSES
• Hepatic copper toxicosis • Chronic inflammatory or idiopathic immune-mediated chronic active hepatitis • Chronic inflammatory bowel disease causing portal triad inflammation • Chronic hypoxia • Drug- and toxin-induced liver injury—anticonvulsants; azole antifungals; mebendazole; oxidbendaxole-diethycarbamazine; trimethoprim sulfa • Viral infections—end-stage acidophil cell hepatitis (rare); infectious hepatitis (canine adenovirus 1; rare) • Leptospirosis—grippotyphosa • Cholangiohepatitis complex leading to biliary cirrhosis (cats) • EHBDO of > 6 weeks' duration • Single episode of massive hepatic necrosis—postnecrotic cirrhosis; rare

RISK FACTORS
• Breed associations • Chronic hepatobiliary inflammation • Hepatic copper or iron accumulation • EHBDO

DIAGNOSIS

DIFFERENTIAL DIAGNOSIS

• Chronic hepatitis—common in dogs • Cholangiohepatitis—common in cats • Chronic EHBDO • Chronic fibrosing pancreatitis • Hepatic neoplasia • Metastatic neoplasia or carcinomatosis • Congenital portosystemic shunt • Right-sided heart failure • Hemolytic anemia • Cats—hepatic lipidosis; FIP; toxoplasmosis

CBC/BIOCHEMISTRY/URINALYSIS
CBC
• Microcytic or normocytic, normochromic nonregenerative anemia • Mild thrombocytopenia—rare
Biochemistry
• Hyperbilirubinemia • Liver enzyme activities—high (mostly ALP and ALT); noted before clinical signs appear; with end-stage disease, may be normal or only mildly high • Hypoalbuminemia • Hyperglobulinemia • Low cholesterol—end-stage disease or acquired portosystemic shunts • Low BUN—with reduced urea cycle activity, acquired portosystemic shunts, or protein-restricted diet • Hypoglycemia—dogs; rarely in cats • Hypokalemia—predisposes patient to hepatic encephalopathy
Urinalysis
• Isosthenuria—with polydipsia and polyuria • Ammonium biurates

OTHER LABORATORY TESTS
• Ascitic fluid—pure or modified transudate • Coagulation tests—prolonged PT, APTT, ACT, and/or buccal mucosal bleeding time • Serum bile acids—markedly high before jaundice • Hyperammonemia

IMAGING
• Radiographic findings—small liver (dogs); normal to large liver (cats); ascites may obscure abdominal detail; radiolucent urate calculi may be visible if complexed with calcium-containing mineral. • Ultrasonographic findings—image may be hyperechoic or have mixed echogenicity; may note nodular pattern, abdominal effusion, splenomegaly, and multiple acquired portosystemic shunts; ascites • Doppler—evaluate portal hypertension

DIAGNOSTIC PROCEDURES
• Fine-needle aspirate cytology—may reveal hyperplastic or reactive hepatocytes, bile ductule epithelia, and canalicular cholestasis; vacuolated hepatocytes common in chronically ill dogs, dogs treated with glucocorticoids, and recently anorectic cats • Laparoscopy—confirm diffusely nodular liver • Biopsy—surgical, laparoscopic, or ultrasound-guided needle; tissue necessary for definitive diagnosis; needle sample possibly insufficient for an accurate diagnosis because only regenerative nodules may be sampled

PATHOLOGIC FINDINGS
• Gross—fibrosis: small and firm liver with an

irregular to finely nodular contour; cirrhosis: firm liver with an irregular contour and prominent nodules • Histopathology—idiopathic fibrosis: noninflammatory; characterized as central perivenous, diffuse, pericellular, or periportal; cirrhosis: inflammation, necrosis, fibrosis, and nodular regeneration with marked architectural distortion

 ## TREATMENT

APPROPRIATE HEALTH CARE
• Outpatient—patients that appear normal and are eating • Inpatient—evaluation; treatment or dehydration, anorexia, or neurologic disorders; diagnostic tests

NURSING CARE
• Fluid—avoid lactated Ringer's solution with severe hepatic failure avoid 0.9% NaCl with ascites. • B complex vitamins—2 ml/L fluids; advised • Glucose—for hypoglycemia; initiate with 2.5% dextrose combined with half-strength polyionic solutions; for persistent hypoglycemia, increase concentration to avert neuroglycopenia; must administer into a large central vein • Potassium chloride—as appropriate for electrolyte balance

ACTIVITY
Limit

DIET
• High-quality, normal-content protein—except with hepatic encephalopathy or ammonium urate crystalluria • Geriatric diet—suitable for most patients • Hepatic encephalopathy—see Hepatic Encephalopathy • Ascites—restrict sodium

CLIENT EDUCATION
• Warn client that treatment is palliative and symptomatic once cirrhosis is established. • Inform client that dehydration, infection, hypokalemia, high-protein diet, enteric parasitism, gastrointestinal bleeding, and certain catabolic drugs may predispose the patient to hepatic encephalopathy. • Advise client that survival is directly related to the severity of the pathologic changes.

SURGICAL CONSIDERATIONS
• Cirrhosis—high anesthetic risk; avoid certain drugs or use with special considerations (barbiturates, phenothiazines, benzodiazepines); predisposes patient to bacterial infection • Gas anesthetics (e.g., isoflurane) best • Coagulation abnormalities—may lead to severe hemorrhagic complications from even minor surgical procedures • Postoperative intensive care—critical for avoiding hepatic encephalopathy; maintain hydration and euglycemia; administer antibiotics to avoid iatrogenic sepsis • Perioperative interval—lactulose advised

 ## MEDICATIONS

DRUGS OF CHOICE
• No specific therapy; no controlled drug studies in dogs and cats • Tailor to the patient; see Copper Hepatopathy, Hepatitis, Chronic Active, and/or Hepatic Encephalopathy • Prednisone—lowest effective level; often 0.25 mg/kg on alternate days; Doberman pinschers: often controlled with 20–40 mg PO q24–48h in combination with ursodeoxycholic acid. • Azathioprine—combine with prednisone; 1 mg/kg PO q48h • Ursodeoxycholic acid—10–15 mg/kg PO q24h or divided q12h • Colchicine—reserved for idiopathic fibrosis; 0.03 mg/kg PO q24h • Zinc acetate—see Copper Hepatopathy • D-Penicillamine—copper chelator; reduces fibrosis; 10–15 mg/kg PO q12h • Gastroprotectants (sucralfate) or gastric-acid inhibitors—enteric bleeding is leading cause of hepatic encephalopathy; eliminate enteric parasites.

Specific Conditions
• Ascites—diuretics; spironolactone (1–2 mg/kg PO q12h) combined with furosemide (1–2 mg/kg PO q12h); perform therapeutic abdominocentesis if patient fails to respond within 10–14 days of titrated doses of diuretics; increase spironolactone every four to six days by 1 mg/kg to a maximum dose of 4 mg/kg PO q12h; increase Lasix to a maximal dose of 2 mg/kg PO q12h. • Hemorrhage—fresh whole blood transfusion; fresh frozen plasma as second choice; avoid stored blood (may contain high ammonia concentrations and less viable cells, causing an encephalopathic challenge). • Oxidative damage—vitamin E (α-tocopherol): 10 IU/kg PO q24h; S-adenosylmethionine: 10–20 mg/kg PO q24h

CONTRAINDICATIONS N/A

PRECAUTIONS
• Diuretics—may worsen hepatic encephalopathy • Glucocorticoids—increase susceptibility to infections • Avoid drugs that depend on first-pass hepatic extraction and drugs that rely solely on hepatic conjugation or biotransformation for elimination; if use is necessary, empirically reduce the dose. • Tetracycline, NSAIDs, barbiturates, lidocaine, theophylline, propranolol, captopril, benzodiazepines, and methionine—avoid if possible • Metronidazole—reduce the dose with hepatic encephalopathy; 7.5 mg/kg PO q8–12h

POSSIBLE INTERACTIONS N/A

ALTERNATIVE DRUGS
• Dexamethasone—instead of prednisone, which may worsen ascites owing to mineralocorticoid activity; use a comparable dose; lacks mineralocorticoid activity; administer every three to four days (long duration of action).

 ## FOLLOW-UP

PATIENT MONITORING
• Liver enzymes, albumin, BUN, and cholesterol—monthly or quarterly, depending on patient's condition • Serial bile acid values—does not add prognostic or diagnostic information • Body condition and muscle mass—prognostic indicators of nutritional intake and nitrogen balance • With azathioprine—monitor for possible short- or long-term bone marrow toxicity via sequential CBC.

PREVENTION/AVOIDANCE N/A

POSSIBLE COMPLICATIONS
• Hepatic encephalopathy, septicemia, and bleeding—may be life-threatening • DIC—may be a terminal event

EXPECTED COURSES AND PROGNOSIS
• Idiopathic fibrosis (dogs)—reported survival of up to 4 years • Cirrhosis (dogs and cats)—possible survival of 3 years • Severe fibrosis associated with cholangiohepatitis (cats)—survival of > 7 years

 ## MISCELLANEOUS

ASSOCIATED CONDITIONS
Many types of liver disease

AGE-RELATED FACTORS N/A

ZOONOTIC POTENTIAL
Dogs with leptospirosis-associated chronic liver disease (rare) may shed infectious organisms.

SEE ALSO
• Copper Hepatopathy • Hepatic Encephalopathy • Hepatitis, Chronic Active

ABBREVIATIONS
• ACT = activated clotting time • APPT = activated partial thromboplastin time • DIC = disseminated intravascular coagulation • EHBDO = extrahepatic bile duct occlusion; • FIP = feline infectious peritonitis • PT = prothrombin time

Suggested Reading
Center SA. Chronic hepatitis, cirrhosis, breed-specific hepatopathies, copper storage hepatopathy, suppurative hepatitis, granulomatous hepatitis, and idiopathic hepatic fibrosis. In: Guilford WG, Center SA, Strombeck DR, et al., eds. Strombeck's small animal gastroenterology. Philadelphia: Saunders, 1996:705–765.

Author David C. Twedt
Consulting Editor Sharon A. Center

DISEASES

CLOSTRIDIAL ENTEROTOXICOSIS

BASICS

DEFINITION
A syndrome characterized by large bowel diarrhea due to enterotoxin production by certain strains of enteric *Clostridium perfringens* (CP)

PATHOPHYSIOLOGY
• CP is a common enteric inhabitant generally found in the vegetative form living in a symbiotic relationship with the host.
• Certain strains of CP (type A) are genetically capable of producing enterotoxin that binds to the enteric mucosa, alters cell permeability, and results in cell damage and or subsequent cell death.
• Enterotoxin production is associated with enteric sporulation of CP.
• A number of intrinsic host-related factors appear to influence enterotoxin production and pathogenicity of CP.

SYSTEMS AFFECTED
Gastrointestinal

GENETICS
N/A

INCIDENCE/PREVALENCE
• Unknown; suspected to be associated with up to 15–20% of cases of chronic large bowel diarrhea in dogs
• Less common in cats

GEOGRAPHIC DISTRIBUTION
N/A

SIGNALMENT
Species
Dogs and cats

Breed Predilections
N/A

Mean Age and Range
• May occur in any age animal
• Most patients that develop chronic clinical signs tend to be middle-aged or older.

Predominant Sex
N/A

SIGNS
General Comments:
• Clinical syndromes are associated with either an acquired, acute, self-limiting large bowel diarrhea lasting 5–7 days; chronic intermittent large bowel diarrhea; or signs associated in conjunction with other gastrointestinal or nongastrointestinal disease.
• Chronic signs—often intermittent episodes occurring every 2–4 weeks that may persist for months to years
• May be a nosocomial (hospital acquired) disease with signs precipitated during or shortly following hospitalization or boarding at a kennel

Historical Findings
• Most common—large bowel diarrhea with fecal mucus, small amounts of fresh blood, small scant stools, and tenesmus with an increased frequency of stools
• Occasionally dogs have small bowel diarrhea characterized by a large volume of watery stool.
• Other signs include vomiting, flatulence, abdominal discomfort, or generalized unthriftiness.

Physical Examination Findings
• Evidence of systemic illness or debilitation is rare.
• Abdominal discomfort may be detected on palpation.
• May be evidence of blood or mucus in the feces; fever is uncommon.

CAUSES
• Not known if enterotoxigenic CP is a true acquired infection or an opportunistic pathogen
• Only certain strains of CP can produce enterotoxin, and certain animals are affected clinically.
• Disease may be associated with small intestinal bacterial overgrowth.

RISK FACTORS
• Stress factors to the gastrointestinal tract, dietary change, concurrent disease, or hospitalization
• CP pathogenicity may depend on the metabolic, mucosal, and immunologic integrity of the colon.
• Possibly IgA deficiency
• An alkaline intestinal lumen environment promotes CP sporulation.
• Primary intestinal bacterial overgrowth

DIAGNOSIS

Patients with chronic intermittent clinical signs—always evaluate during the onset of episodes.

DIFFERENTIAL DIAGNOSIS
• Consider all causes of large bowel diarrhea, including systemic or metabolic disease, as well as specific intestinal disorders.
• Gastrointestinal parasites, inflammatory bowel disease, chronic idiopathic colitis, and nervous or irritable bowel syndrome may resemble CP enterotoxicosis.

CBC/BIOCHEMISTRY/URINALYSIS
Usually normal

OTHER LABORATORY TESTS
Fecal flotation to rule out intestinal parasites

Microbiology
• Anaerobic fecal cultures generally find high concentrations of CP organisms, but occasionally are negative.
• Specific fecal spore cultures detect high concentrations of clostridial spores ($>10^6$ spores/g of feces) in affected animals, but are rarely done.

Enterotoxin Assay
• Identification of fecal CP enterotoxin in conjunction with clinical signs supports CP as a contributing pathogen.
• Enterotoxin analysis—fecal ELISA (Tech Labs, Blacksburg, VA) or reverse passive latex agglutination assay (RPLA, Oxoid USA, Columbia, MO); enterotoxin is not species-specific, and these tests are valid for use in the dog and cat; assay requires 1 g (small pea-size sample) of feces; enterotoxin is quite stable, and feces can be refrigerated or frozen prior to analysis.
• Assay results do not always correlate with clinical disease; false-positive results are observed in a number of asymptomatic dogs, suggesting inherent resistance to pathogenicity of the enterotoxin; interfering substances in the feces or samples taken during the recovery period may give false-negative results.

Fecal Cytology
• Large numbers of CP spores in the feces in a patient with evidence of clinical disease correlates well with fecal enterotoxin assay; more than five spores per high power oil immersion field is considered abnormal.

CLOSTRIDIAL ENTEROTOXICOSIS

• Cytology—make a thin fecal smear on a microscope slide, air-dry or heat fix, and stain with Diff-Quick or Wright's stain or use malachite green, a specific spore stain.
• CP spores have a "safety-pin" appearance—an oval structure with a dense body at one end of the spore wall
• Examine for spores shortly after onset of clinical signs.

IMAGING
N/A

DIAGNOSTIC PROCEDURES
Colonoscopy helps rule out concurrent intestinal disease.

PATHOLOGIC FINDINGS
• Colon biopsy specimens taken during asymptomatic periods are usually normal.
• Patients may have colonoscopic evidence of hyperemic or ulcerated mucosa.
• Histology may show catarrhal or suppurative colitis; mild inflammatory bowel disease is occasionally present.

TREATMENT

APPROPRIATE HEALTH CARE
• Most are outpatients.
• May need hospitalization when diarrhea or vomiting is severe, resulting in dehydration and electrolyte imbalance

NURSING CARE
May need fluid and electrolyte therapy to replace losses from diarrhea (uncommon)

ACTIVITY
Restrict during acute disease.

DIET
• Dietary manipulation important in the treatment and management of chronic reoccurring disease
• Diets high in both soluble and insoluble fiber yield clinical improvement by reducing enteric clostridial numbers and acidifying the distal intestine, thus limiting CP sporulation and enterotoxin production.
• Prescribe commercial high-fiber diets and supplement with psyllium (1/2–2 tsp/day) as a source of soluble fiber.
• Supplement low-fiber diets with coarse bran (1–3 tbs/day) as a source of insoluble fiber; add psyllium as a source of soluble fiber.

CLIENT EDUCATION
Acute disease is often self-limiting; chronic disease may require prolonged therapy.

SURGICAL CONSIDERATIONS
N/A

MEDICATIONS

DRUGS OF CHOICE

Antibiotics
• Acute, self-limiting disease usually requires a 5- to 7-day antibiotic course.
• Most patients respond well to appropriate antibiotic therapy (e.g., oral ampicillin or amoxicillin, clindamycin, metronidazole, or tylosin).
• Patients with chronic disease often require prolonged antibiotic therapy.
• Tylosin at a dosage of 10–20 mg/kg q12–24h (~1/8 tsp/25 kg), mixed with the food, is suggested for long-term management.
• Administering oral antibiotics at submicrobial inhibitory concentrations appears effective in chronic patients.
• Low antibiotic levels may not actually reduce enteric CP numbers but may change the ecological microenvironment and prevent sporulation and enterotoxin production.

CONTRAINDICATIONS
N/A

PRECAUTIONS
N/A

POSSIBLE INTERACTIONS
N/A

ALTERNATIVE DRUGS
N/A

FOLLOW-UP

PATIENT MONITORING
Response to therapy supports the diagnosis; repeat diagnostics are rarely necessary.

PREVENTION/AVOIDANCE
• Infection is associated with environmental contamination; disinfection is difficult.
• Feeding high-fiber diets may decrease the incidence of nosocomial diarrhea.

POSSIBLE COMPLICATIONS
N/A

EXPECTED COURSE AND PROGNOSIS
• Most animals respond well to therapy; chronic patients may require lifelong therapy.
• Failure to respond suggests concurrent disease; further diagnostic evaluation is indicated.

MISCELLANEOUS

ASSOCIATED CONDITIONS
Frequently other enteric disease (e.g., parvovirus or inflammatory bowel disease)

AGE-RELATED FACTORS
N/A

ZOONOTIC POTENTIAL
Unknown

PREGNANCY
Antibiotic therapy may be contraindicated.

SYNONYMS
Idiopathic chronic colitis

SEE ALSO
• Colitis and Proctitis
• Small Intestinal Bacterial Overgrowth

ABBREVIATIONS
• CP = *Clostridium perfringens*
• ELISA = enzyme-linked immunosorbent assay
• tbs = tablespoon
• tsp = teaspoon

Suggested Reading

Foley J, Hirsh DC, Pedersen NC: An outbreak of Clostridium perfringens enteritis in a cattery of Bengal cats and experimental transmission to specific pathogen free cats. Feline Pract 1996;24(6):31–35.

Kirth SA, Prescott JF, Welch MK, et al. Nosocomial diarrhea associated with enterotoxigenic Clostridium perfringens infection in dogs. J Am Vet Med Assoc 1989;195:331.

McClane BA, Hanna PC, Wnek AP. Clostridium perfringens enterotoxin. Microb Pathog 1988;4:317.

Twedt DC. Clostridium perfringens associated enterotoxicosis in dogs. In: Kirk RW, Bonagura JD, eds. Current veterinary therapy XI. Philadelphia: Saunders, 1992: 602–604.

Author David C. Twedt
Consulting Editors Brett M. Feder and Mitchell A. Crystal

COAGULOPATHY OF LIVER DISEASE

BASICS

OVERVIEW
• Many patients with liver disease have a measurable hemostatic defect, but few exhibit clinical bleeding. • Coagulation factors—liver primary site of synthesis and posttranslational modification, except factor VIII, von Willebrand factor, and most of the major coagulation inhibitors • Causes of impaired hemostasis—reduced synthesis of clotting factors; synthesis of abnormal clotting proteins; vitamin K deficiency; high concentrations of fibrin degradation productions and other anticoagulants; thrombocytopenia or thrombocytopathy; reduced synthesis of normal coagulation inhibitors; enhanced fibrinolysis; DIC • AT III—primarily produced in the liver; binds to and inactivates activated factors (II, VII, IX, X, XI, and XII), plasmin, and kallikrein • Vitamin K deficiency—may occur with obstruction to bile flow (especially EHBDO) and fat malabsorption • Hemorrhagic complications—usually arise from local injuries (e.g., gastroduodenal ulceration, gastritis, tumor, or invasive procedures)

SIGNALMENT
Dogs and cats of any age

SIGNS
• Usually no obvious signs of bleeding • Gastrointestinal blood loss—melena; hematemesis; hematochezia • Prolonged bleeding—venipuncture; biopsy sites; surgical wounds • Spontaneous bruising or hematomas—uncommon

CAUSES & RISK FACTORS
• Fulminant hepatic failure • Acute viral liver disease • Cirrhosis • Portosystemic vascular anomalies • EHBDO • Chronic liver disease—usually no bleeding until cirrhosis develops or with EHBDO • Concurrent small bowel disease (e.g., cats with the cholangiohepatitis complex) may predispose the patient to vitamin K deficiency

DIAGNOSIS

DIFFERENTIAL DIAGNOSIS
• Vitamin K antagonism—rodenticides • Primary coagulation defects • DIC • Immune-mediated thrombocytopenia • Vitamin K–related coagulopathy—Devon rex cats • Hepatic amyloidosis—fractured liver lobe hemorrhage

CBC/BIOCHEMISTRY/URINALYSIS
• CBC—may be normal; regenerative anemia with severe bleeding lasting for several days; thrombocytopenia (rare unless DIC noted) • Biochemistry—high liver enzyme activities with acquired liver disease; low albumin with synthetic failure, accompanied by hypoglobulinemia with extracorporeal blood loss

• Urinalysis—microhematuria; gross blood

OTHER LABORATORY TESTS
• Prolonged PT, APTT, and ACT • Decreased platelet aggregation • High-fibrin degradation products • Low AT III • May note low concentrations of individual clotting factors • Prolonged PIVKA and PT

IMAGING
N/A

DIAGNOSTIC TESTS
Prolonged mucosal bleeding time

TREATMENT

• Not usually necessary unless invasive procedures are planned or extensive spontaneous hemorrhage occurs • Spontaneous bleeding—indicates severe liver dysfunction; initiate treatment • Fresh whole blood—for anemia; before invasive procedures • Fresh frozen plasma (5–10 mL/kg) or cryoprecipitate—supplies enough clotting factors and AT III for immediate effect • Platelet transfusion—rarely beneficial

Biopsy
• Fine-needle aspiration for cytologic interpretation—not contraindicated with coagulopathy • Mucosal bleeding time, PIVKA, PT, APTT, or ACT prolonged by > 50% or thrombocytopenia < 50,000/uL—increased likelihood of bleeding • Iatrogenic hemorrhage—grave risk with spontaneous bleeding for which a cause cannot be identified and eliminated • Liver—must provide hemostasis for postprocedure hemorrhage • Ultrasound-guided core—most risky; observe site for 15 min and again several hours after procedure • Laparoscopic—affords visibility and hemostasis (Gelfoam, cautery) • Laparotomy—wedge biopsy; ill-advised with overt bleeding tendencies

MEDICATIONS

DRUGS
• Parenteral vitamin K_1—0.5–1.5 mg/kg/day IM, SC; with significant cholestasis or concurrent malabsorptive disease • Chronic administration of vitamin K—every 7–28 days; may be appropriate with chronic hepatopathies and prolonged PIVKA but normal PT and APTT; titrate frequency based on sequential PIVKA results. • DDAVP—0.3 μg/kg IV in saline; may increase factors VII, VIII, IX, IX, and XII; may shorten the mucosal bleeding time, PT, and APTT; may reduce bleeding tendencies • Heparin—50–75 U/kg SC q8h along with AT III via transfusion; may be necessary with DIC • Mini-dose aspirin—0.5 mg/kg PO q12–24h; for DIC; as antithrombotic with AT III depletion

CONTRAINDICATIONS/POSSIBLE INTERACTIONS
• Whole blood transfusion—may precipitate hepatic encephalopathy, especially if using stored blood • Vitamin K (cats)—too much causes Heinz body hemolytic anemia and oxidant liver injury • Aspirin—may reduce renal prostaglandin synthesis, worsen ascites, and predispose patient to renal failure • Citrated blood—large-volume infusions may result in citrate overload and spurious coagulopathy. • Avoid using jugular catheters in patients with bleeding tendencies.

FOLLOW-UP

PATIENT MONITORING
• PIVKA and mucosal bleeding time; if no improvement within 48 hr after vitamin K injection, unlikely that subsequent injections will be beneficial. • Heart rate, peripheral blood pressure, mucous membrane color and refill, PCV, and total solids—with suspected active bleeding • Biopsy site—observe immediately and sequentially (ultrasound imaging) for evidence of hemorrhage. • Sample accumulating abdominal effusion—determine if patient is hemorrhaging

PREVENTION/AVOIDANCE
• Well-balanced diet replete with vitamins • Consider possibility of impaired vitamin K availability or synthesis owing to chronic oral antimicrobial therapy. • Invasive procedures—anticipate bleeding tendencies; be prepared for blood component therapy (intravenous catheter, blood components); administer DDAVP within 20 min of anticipated iatrogenic trauma (biopsy); pretreat patient with vitamin K_1. • Ensure enteric parasitism is appropriately treated.

POSSIBLE COMPLICATIONS DIC

EXPECTED COURSE/PROGNOSIS
Spontaneous hemorrhage—poor prognostic sign

MISCELLANEOUS

ABBREVIATIONS
• ACT = activated clotting time • APTT = activated partial thromboplastin time • AT III = antithrombin III • EHBDO = extrahepatic bile duct obstruction • PIVKA = proteins invoked by vitamin K absence or antagonism • PT = prothrombin time

Suggested Reading
Center SA. Pathophysiology of liver disease: normal and abnormal function. In: Guilford WG, Center SA, Strombeck DR, et al., eds. Strombeck's small animal gastroenterology. 3rd ed. Philadelphia: Saunders, 1996:553–632.

Author Joseph Taboada
Consulting Editor Sharon A. Center

COBALAMIN MALABSORPTION IN GIANT SCHNAUZERS AND BORDER COLLIES

BASICS

OVERVIEW
• Congenital anomaly involving selective malabsorption of cobalamin (vitamin B_{12})
• Occurs secondary to absence of the receptor for intrinsic factor–cobalamin complex in the ileal brush border in Giant schnauzers; very rare

SIGNALMENT
• Inherited as a simple autosomal recessive trait in the Giant schnauzer
• Signs appear at 6–12 weeks of age in giant schnauzers but at 4–6 months of age in Border collies.

SIGNS
• Anorexia
• Lethargy
• Failure to gain weight

CAUSES & RISK FACTORS
The disease is inherited.

DIAGNOSIS

DIFFERENTIAL DIAGNOSIS
• Other congenital metabolic diseases
• Gastrointestinal parasitism

CBC/BIOCHEMISTRY/URINALYSIS
• Mild-to-severe neutropenia (1760–4440/mm³)
• Chronic nonregenerative anemia (PCV 21–33%)

OTHER LABORATORY TESTS
• Serum cobalamin concentrations are very low (<100 ng/L; normal, >225 ng/L).
• Serum and urinary methylmalonic acid concentrations are above normal.

IMAGING
Not useful

DIAGNOSTIC PROCEDURES
N/A

TREATMENT

Outpatient medical treatment is warranted (long-term parenteral administration of cobalamin).

MEDICATIONS

DRUGS
Cyanocobalamin (0.5–1.0 mg IM q24h for 7 days, then q3–6months).

CONTRAINDICATIONS/POSSIBLE INTERACTIONS
N/A

FOLLOW-UP
Periodic parenteral administration of cobalamin

MISCELLANEOUS

SEE ALSO
Serum Cobalamin and Folate

Suggested Reading
Fyfe JC, Giger U, Hall CA, et al. Inherited selective intestinal cobalamin malabsorption and cobalamin deficiency in dogs. Pediatr Res 1991;29:24–31.
Outerbridge CA, Myers SL, Giger U. Hereditary cobalamin deficiency in collie dogs. J Vet Int Med 996; (Abstract) 10.
Author David A. Williams
Consulting Editors Brett M. Feder and Mitchell A. Crystal

COCCIDIOIDOMYCOSIS

 BASICS

DEFINITION
A systemic mycosis caused by the inhalation of infective arthroconidia of the soil borne fungus Coccidioides immitis

PATHOPHYSIOLOGY
• Inhalation of infective arthroconidia is the primary route of infection. Fever, lethargy, inappetence, coughing, and joint pain or stiffness may be noticed. Dissemination may occur within 10 days of exposure resulting in signs related to the organ system involved. Asymptomatic infections may occur, and most animals develop immunity without onset of clinical signs. The majority of animals become solidly immune after initial infection. • Skin lesions are usually associated with dissemination, but penetrating wounds have rarely been associated with skin lesions. • Fewer than 10 inhaled arthrospores are sufficient to cause disease in susceptible animals. "Susceptible" refers to the animals in which extrapulmonary dissemination occurs. Signs of dissemination may not be evident for several months after the initial infection.

SYSTEMS AFFECTED
• Respiratory—the site of initial infection
• Extrapulmonary spread may occur to long bones and joints, eyes, skin, liver, kidneys, CNS, cardiovascular system (pericardium and myocardium), and testes.

GENETICS
N/A

INCIDENCE/PREVALENCE
An uncommon disease, even in endemic areas. It occurs more commonly in dogs, and rarely in cats.

GEOGRAPHIC DISTRIBUTION
Coccidioides immitis is found in the southwestern United States in the geographic Lower Sonoran life zone. It is more common in Southern California, Arizona and southwest Texas and is less prevalent in New Mexico, Nevada, and Utah

SIGNALMENT
Species
Dogs and cats

Breed Predilections
None

Mean Age and Range
Most patients are young animals < 4 years of age.

Predominant Sex
None

SIGNS
Historical Findings
• Anorexia • Coughing • Fever unresponsive to antibiotics • Lameness • Weakness, paraparesis, back and neck pain • Seizures • Visual changes • Weight loss

Physical Examination Findings
Dogs

Signs with pulmonary involvement
• Coughing • Dyspnea • Fever

Signs with disseminated disease
• Bone swelling, joint enlargement and lameness • Cachexia • Lethargy • Lymphadenomegaly • Neurologic dysfunction caused by dissemination to both the central and peripheral CNS • Skin ulcers and draining tracts • Uveitis, keratitis

Cats
• Cachexia • Draining skin lesions • Dyspnea • Lameness caused by bone involvement • Uveitis

CAUSE
Coccidioides immitis grows several inches deep in the soil, where it survives high ambient temperatures and low moisture. After a period of rainfall, the organism returns to the soil surface where it sporulates releasing many arthroconidia that are disseminated by wind and dust storms.

RISK FACTORS
• Aggressive nosing about in soil and underbrush may expose susceptible animals to large doses of the fungus in contaminated soil.
• Dust storms after the rainy season. Increased incidences are noted after earthquakes. • Land development where much earth disruption occurs may lead to increased exposure.

 DIAGNOSIS

DIFFERENTIAL DIAGNOSIS
• Pulmonary lesions may resemble those of other systemic mycoses (e.g, histoplasmosis, blastomycosis). • Lymphadenomegaly may be seen in lymphosarcoma, other systemic mycoses, and localized bacterial infections. • Bone lesions may resemble those caused by primary or metastatic bone tumors or bacterial osteomyelitis. • Skin lesions must be differentiated from routine abscesses or other bacterial disease processes.

CBC/BIOCHEMISTRY/URINALYSIS
• Hemogram—mild nonregenerative anemia, neutrophilic leukocytosis, monocytosis • Serum chemistry profile—hyperglobulinemia, hypoalbuminemia, azotemia with renal involvement • Urinalysis—low urine specific gravity and proteinuria with inflammatory glomerulonephritis

OTHER LABORATORY TESTS
Serologic tests for antibody to C. immitis by a laboratory proficient in handling the tests may provide a presumptive diagnosis and aid in monitoring response to therapy.

IMAGING
Radiography of lung (interstitial infiltrates) and bone (osteolysis) lesions may aid in diagnosis.

DIAGNOSTIC PROCEDURES
• Microscopic identification of the large spherule form of C. immitis in lesion or biopsy material is the definitive method of diagnosis. Lymph node aspirates and impression smears of skin lesions or draining exudate may, in some patients, yield organisms. • Caution should be used if culturing draining lesions suspected of being infected with C. immitis, as the mycelial form is highly contagious. • Biopsy of infected tissue often is preferred to avoid false-negative results. Tissues involved, however, are not readily accessible and serologic testing is a more logical approach.

PATHOLOGIC FINDINGS
• Granulomatous, suppurative or pyogranulomatous inflammation present in many tissues. • Presence of the characteristic spherule forms in affected tissues. In some patients, the numbers of spherules present may be small.

 TREATMENT

APPROPRIATE HEALTH CARE
Generally treated as outpatients. Patients treated with amphotericin B, however, will require hospitalization several times a week during their treatment period. Concurrent clinical symptoms (eg: seizures, pain, coughing) should be treated appropriately.

NURSING CARE
N/A

ACTIVITY
Restrict activity until clinical signs begin to subside.

DIET
Feed a high quality palatable diet to maintain body weight.

CLIENT EDUCATION
The necessity and expense of long-term therapy of a serious illness with the possibility of treatment failure should be reviewed. In addition, the client should be made aware of the possible side effects of the drugs used.

SURGICAL CONSIDERATIONS
In cases of focal granulomatous organ involvement (eg. consolidated pulmonary lung lobe, eye, kidney) surgical removal of the affected organ may be indicated.

 MEDICATIONS

DRUGS OF CHOICE
Coccidioidomycosis is considered the most severe and life-threatening of the systemic

mycoses. Treatment of disseminated disease requires at least one year of aggressive antifungal therapy.

Dogs
Several oral medications in the azole family of drugs are currently available for the treatment of coccidioidomycoses.
• Ketoconazole (KTZ) is dosed at 5–10 mg/kg PO q12h. The medication may be given with food, and there is some belief that co-administration of high doses of vitamin C may improve the absorption of the drug. Treatment should be continued for 1 year. • Itraconazole (ITZ) is dosed at 5 mg/kg PO q12h. The drug is administered similarly as KTZ. It has been reported to have a higher penetration rate than ketoconazole, but a better clinical response has not been observed. • Fluconazole (FCZ) is dosed at 5 mg/kg PO q12h has been noted to greatly increase the success of treatment, especially in neurologic infections. The drug is extremely expensive, and the client should be prepared for the expense. After extended use, the frequency of dosing in some cases may be lowered to once a day.
• Amphotericin B (AMB) is less commonly recommended because of the high risk of renal damage with amphotericin B and the availability of effective oral medications. Amphotericin B can be administered at a dosage of 0.5 mg/kg IV 3 times a week, for a total cumulative dosage of 8–10 mg/kg. It is given IV either as a slow infusion (in dogs that are gravely ill) or as a rapid bolus (in fairly healthy dogs). For slow infusion, add AMB to 250–500 ml of 5% dextrose solution and administer as a drip over a period of 4–6 hours. For a rapid bolus, add AMB to 30 ml of 5% dextrose solution and administer over a period of 5 minutes through a butterfly catheter. To lessen the adverse renal effects of AMB, give 0.9% NaCl (2 ml/kg/hr) for several hours before initiating AMB therapy. • A combination of AMB and KTZ may be used in dogs that have not responded to either drug alone or have exhibited significant toxicity. It is not clear that combination therapy is any more effective than single drug therapy in the treatment of coccidioidomycoses. For combination chemotherapy, administer AMB as described to a total cumulative dosage of 4–6 mg/kg, together with KTZ at 10 mg/kg PO divided daily for at least 8–12 months.

Cats
• Any of the following azoles may be used in cats:

> Ketoconazole 50 mg total dose PO q12h
> Itraconazole 25–50 mg total dose PO q12h
> Fluconazole 25–50 mg total dose PO q12h

• Alternatively, AMB can be administered by rapid IV bolus at a dosage of 0.25 mg/kg, 3 times a week, for a total cumulative dosage of 4 mg/kg. This can then be followed by long-term KTZ therapy, depending on the clinical response.

CONTRAINDICATIONS
• Drugs metabolized primarily by the liver should not be administered along with ketoconazole. • Drugs metabolized primarily by the kidneys should not be administered along with AMB.

PRECAUTIONS
• Side effects of azoles include inappetence, vomiting, and hepatotoxicity. The drugs may be stopped until signs abate, and restarted at a lower dose which may be slowly increased to the recommended dose if the animal is able to tolerate the drug. The newer azoles (ITZ and FCZ) have fewer side effects. • Side effects of AMB therapy can be severe and include renal dysfunction, fever, inappetence, vomiting, and phlebitis.

POSSIBLE INTERACTIONS
N/A

ALTERNATIVE DRUGS
N/A

 FOLLOW-UP

PATIENT MONITORING
• Serologic titers should be monitored every 2–3 months. Animals should be treated until their titers fall to less than 1:2. Animals displaying poor response to therapy should have a 2–4 hour post pill drug level measured to assure adequate absorption of the drug. • BUN and urinalysis should be monitored in all animals treated with AMB. Treatment should be temporarily discontinued if the BUN rises above 50 mg/dl or granular casts are noted in the urine.

PREVENTION/AVOIDANCE
• No vaccine is available for dogs or cats. • Contaminated soil in endemic areas should be avoided, particularly during dust storms after the rainy season

POSSIBLE COMPLICATIONS
• Pulmonary disease resulting in severe coughing may temporarily worsen after therapy is begun due to inflammation in the lungs. Low dose short-term oral prednisone and cough suppressants may be required to alleviate the respiratory signs. • Hepatotoxicity may result from KTZ therapy. • Nephrotoxicity may result from AMB therapy.

EXPECTED COURSE AND PROGNOSIS
• The prognosis is guarded to grave. Many dogs will improve following oral therapy; however, relapses may be seen especially if therapy is shortened. The overall recovery rate has been estimated at 60%, but some report a 90% response to fluconazole therapy. • The prognosis for cats is not well documented, but rapid dissemination requiring long term therapy should be anticipated. • Serologic testing every 3–4 months after completion of therapy is recommended to monitor the possibility of relapse. • Spontaneous recovery from disseminated coccidioidomycosis without treatment is extremely rare

 MISCELLANEOUS

ASSOCIATED CONDITIONS
N/A

AGE-RELATED FACTORS
N/A

ZOONOTIC POTENTIAL
The spherule form of the fungus, as found in animal tissues, is not directly transmissible to people or other animals. Under certain rare circumstances, however, there could be reversion to growth of the infective mold form of the fungus on or within bandages placed over a draining lesion or in contaminated bedding. Draining lesions can lead to contamination of the environment with arthrospores. Care should exercised whenever handling an infected draining lesion. Special precautions should be recommended to households where the owners may be immunosuppressed.

PREGNANCY
• KTZ should be used in pregnant animals only if the potential benefit justifies the potential risk to offspring. • Teratogenic effects of AMB have not been identified.

SYNONYMS
San Joaquin Valley fever, valley fever, desert rheumatism (in humans)

SEE ALSO
N/A

ABBREVIATIONS
• KTZ = ketoconazole • ITZ=itraconazole • FCZ=fluconazole • AMB = amphotericin B

Suggested Reading
Armstrong PJ, DiBartola SP. Canine coccidioidomycosis: a literature review and report of eight cases. J Am Anim Hosp Assoc 1983;19:937–945.
Greene RT. Coccidioidomycosis. In: Greene CE, ed. Infectious diseases of the dog and cat. 2nd ed. Philadelphia: Saunders, 1998:391–398.
Legendre AM. Coccidioidomycosis. In: Sherding RG, ed. The cat: diseases and clinical management. 2nd ed. New York: Churchill Livingstone, 1994:561–562.
Stevens DA. Coccidioidomycosis. N Engl J Med 1995;332:1077–1082.
Author Nita Kay Gulbas
Consulting Editor Stephen C. Barr

DISEASES

COCCIDIOSIS

BASICS

OVERVIEW
- An enteric infection, traditionally associated with *Isospora canis* (dogs) and *Isospora felis* (cats) as potential pathogens; other species of *Isospora* may be present.
- Strictly host-specific (i.e., no cross-transmission)
- *Eimeria* spp. are not parasitic for dogs or cats.
- *Toxoplasma gondii* in cats and *Cryptosporidium parvum* in neonatal pups and kittens are coccidians in a nontraditional sense.
- *Toxoplasma* infection in cats may cause clinical signs similar to those with *Isospora* infections; oocysts shed in the environment may potentially cause a public health problem.
- *Cryptosporidium* is still being assessed as an acute, life-threatening coccidiosis (cryptosporidiosis) of neonatal pups and kittens.
- Voluminous watery diarrhea is characteristic; autoinfection and continuing recycling within the intestinal tract result in a rapid loss of mucosal lining.

SIGNALMENT
Dogs and cats (especially pups and kittens)

SIGNS
- Watery-to-mucoid, sometimes blood-tinged, diarrhea
- Weak pups and kittens

CAUSES & RISK FACTORS
- Infected dogs or cats contaminating environment with oocysts of *Isospora* spp. or *Cryptosporidium*
- Stress

DIAGNOSIS

DIFFERENTIAL DIAGNOSIS
Enteric viral infections and other intestinal parasites

CBC/BIOCHEMISTRY/URINALYSIS
Usually normal; may be hemoconcentrated if dehydrated

OTHER LABORATORY TESTS
N/A

IMAGING
N/A

DIAGNOSTIC PROCEDURES
- Fecal examination for oocysts; special staining such as acid-fast for *Cryptosporidium*
- *Isospora* oocysts should be 40 μm long; cysts of *Cryptosporidium* approximately 5 μm diameter

TREATMENT
- Usually treated as an outpatient
- Inpatient if debilitated
- Fluid therapy if dehydrated

MEDICATIONS

DRUGS
- Sulfadimethoxine—55 mg/kg PO on the first day, then 27.5 mg/kg for 4 days or until dog is asymptomatic for *Isospora* and fecal examination is negative for oocysts
- On an extralabel use basis, albendazole for *Isospora*—25 mg/kg PO q12h for 2 days
- None known for *Cryptosporidium,* although pyrimethamine has been used experimentally

CONTRAINDICATIONS/POSSIBLE INTERACTIONS
N/A

FOLLOW-UP
Fecal examination for oocysts 1–2 weeks following treatment

MISCELLANEOUS

AGE-RELATED FACTORS
More severe disease in young patients

SEE ALSO
- Toxoplasmosis
- Cryptosporidiosis

Suggested Reading
Bowman DD, ed. Georgi's parasitology for veterinarians, 6th ed. Philadelphia: WB Saunders, 1994:95, 97.

Author Robert M. Corwin

Consulting Editors Brett M. Feder and Mitchell A. Crystal

BASICS

OVERVIEW
• A rare type II autoimmune disorder in which antierythrocyte antibodies have enhanced activity at temperatures < 99°F (37.2°C) and usually < 88°F (31.1°C)
• Cold agglutinins are typically IgM, although IgG and IgG-IgM mixed have been reported.
• Cold agglutinins with low thermal amplitude usually associated with direct erythrocyte agglutination at low body temperatures in the peripheral microvasculature and with acrocyanotic disease or other peripheral vaso-occlusive phenomena, all initiated or intensified by cold exposure
• Fixation of complement and hemolysis is a warm reactive process occurring at high body temperatures; therefore, patients may have very high titers of cold agglutinins, but these antibodies may be unable to hemolyze erythrocytes at temperatures achieved in the bloodstream.
• Most cold agglutinins cause little or no shortening of erythrocyte life span.
• High thermal amplitude cold agglutinins (rare)—may cause sustained hemolysis; resulting anemia is often mild and stable, but exposure to cold may greatly augment the binding of cold agglutinins and complement-mediated intravascular hemolysis.

SIGNALMENT
• Rare disorder in dogs and cats
• Low titer of naturally occurring cold agglutinins (usually 1:32 or less) may be found in healthy dogs and cats; this is without clinical significance.
• Genetic basis, mean age and range, breed and sex predilections unknown
• More likely to occur in colder climates

SIGNS
• Often a history of cold exposure
• Acrocyanosis associated with sludging of erythrocyte agglutinates in cutaneous microvasculature
• Erythema
• Skin ulceration with secondary crusting
• Dry, gangrenous necrosis of ear tips, tail tip, nose, and feet
• Affected areas may be painful.
• Anemia may or may not be an important feature; clinical signs include pallor, weakness, tachycardia, tachypnea, icterus, pigmenturia, mild splenomegaly, and soft heart murmur

CAUSES & RISK FACTORS
• Primary disease—idiopathic
• Secondary disease—associated with upper respiratory infection (cats), neonatal isoerythrolysis, and lead intoxication (dogs)
• Cold exposure a risk factor

DIAGNOSIS

DIFFERENTIAL DIAGNOSIS
• Diagnosis made by historical findings (cold exposure), results of physical examination, and by demonstrating cold agglutination in vitro
• Skin lesions—cutaneous vasculitis, hepato-cutaneous syndrome, erythema multiforme, toxic epidermic necrolysis, dermatomyositis, DIC, SLE, lymphoreticular neoplasms, frostbite, lead poisoning, and pemphigus
• Anemia—warm antibody hemolytic anemia; other causes of anemia
• Macroscopic hemagglutination in vitro—dysproteinemias may lead to rouleaux formation, mimicking erythrocyte agglutination on a glass slide.

CBC/BIOCHEMISTRY/URINALYSIS
• Autoagglutination at room temperature
• Laboratory abnormalities secondary to hemolysis

OTHER LABORATORY TESTS
• Cold agglutinins should be suspected when blood in heparin or EDTA on a glass slide agglutinates spontaneously at room temperature with enhancement at 39°F (3.9°C), and the erythrocytes disperse again upon warming to 99°F (37.2°C)
• If no agglutination can be induced in vitro, it is inconceivable for it to occur in vivo in extremities.
• Doubtful cases can be confirmed by Coombs test at 39°F and 99°F
• Coombs test at 99°F—cold agglutinins usually not detected because they may be eluted off the erythrocytes during washing; thus test requires the use of anti-c′ sera.
• Coombs test at 39°F—incidence of a positive result in healthy dogs has been reported to be > 50%, which may be caused by unspecific binding of the reagent itself or by binding of naturally occurring nonpathogenic low-titer cold agglutinins.
• The globulin class can be established by immunoelectrophoresis of a concentrated eluate of the patient's erythrocytes, which is important for prognosis and treatment.

IMAGING
N/A

DIAGNOSTIC PROCEDURES
None

PATHOLOGIC FINDINGS
• Dermal necrosis
• Ulceration with secondary features of opportunistic infections
• Vascular thrombosis with evidence of ischemic necrosis

TREATMENT
• The patient should be hospitalized in a warm environment until the disease is nonprogressive.
• Supportive care and wound management depend on clinical signs; if necrosis involving the tail tip or feet is severe, amputation may be required.
• Splenectomy of little assistance in patients with IgM-mediated hemolytic disorders, but may be helpful in those with therapy-resistant IgG-mediated hemolytic anemia
• Inform the client to keep the patient in a warm environment at all times to prevent relapse.

MEDICATIONS

DRUGS

IgM Cold Agglutinins
• Immunosuppressive therapy is not very effective against IgM-mediated disorders but should be tried (i.e., corticosteroids, cyclophosphamide, or azathioprine).
• Plasmapheresis

IgG Cold Agglutinins
Immunosuppressive therapy

CONTRAINDICATIONS/POSSIBLE INTERACTIONS
• Monitor patient for signs of infection secondary to immunosuppressive therapy.
• Do not use cold IV fluids.

FOLLOW-UP
• A patient with known cold agglutinin disease should be kept in warm environments at all times.
• Cold agglutinin disease usually characterized by acute onset and rapid progression
• Prognosis guarded to fair
• Recovery may take weeks.

MISCELLANEOUS

SEE ALSO
Anemia, Immune-mediated

ABBREVIATIONS
• DIC = disseminated intravascular coagulation
• SLE = systemic lupus erythematosus SLE

Suggested Reading
Dickson NJ. Cold agglutinin disease in a puppy associated with lead intoxication. J Small Anim Pract 1990;31:105–108.
Author Jörg Bücheler
Consulting Editor Susan M. Cotter

DISEASES

COLIBACILLOSIS

 BASICS

DEFINITION
• *Escherichia coli*—gram-negative member of the Enterobacteriaceae; normal inhabitant of the intestine of most mammals; along with other infectious agents, may increase the severity of parvovirus infections
• Acute infection of puppies and kittens in the first week of life; characterized by septicemia and multiple organ involvement
• Isolation from stool of young animals—inconclusive evidence of pathogenic potential because it is normal flora
• Isolation from blood cultures or internal organs—good evidence of causality
• Infection of old dogs and cats—documented; individual strains poorly characterized in regard to virulence attributes

Pathophysiology
• Virulence factors—not well defined; likely *E. coli* as a cause of septicemia in neonatal dogs and cats has more to do with the immunologic immaturity of the host than with the virulence of a particular strain
• ETEC, EPEC, uropathogenic *E. coli,* and CNF+ *E. coli* strains—recovered from dogs
• EPEC, VTEC, and uropathogenic *E. coli* strains—isolated from cats
• Intestinal strains colonize and multiply in the small intestine; ETEC then elaborates *E. coli* K99 or other uncharacterized adhesins and enterotoxins; the attaching and effacing factor of ETEC (EAE+) or VTEC (EAE+) produces SLT.
• Many strains of *E. coli* from dogs and cats are hemolytic.

SYSTEMS AFFECTED
• Neonates—small intestine (enteritis); multiple body systems (septicemia)
• Puppies/kittens and adults—small intestine (enteritis); urogenital (cystitis, endometritis, pyelonephritis, prostatitis); mammary gland (mastitis)

GENETICS
N/A

INCIDENCE/PREVALENCE
• Few statistics available
• More common in neonatal puppies and kittens < 1 week old that have not received any or adequate amounts of colostrum
• Problem in overpopulated kennels and catteries
• Sporadic accounts in old dogs and cats (mainly diarrhea and urogenital problems)

Dogs
• ETEC—2.7–29.5% of diarrheic dogs; strains: K99+/−, Sta/STb+/−, and CNF+ isolated from diarrheic dogs along with hemolysin
• *E. coli* (usually β-hemolytic)—major cause of septicemia in newborn puppies exposed in utero, during birth, or from mastitic milk

Cats
EPEC/VTEC—diarrheic cats; strains: EAE+, SLT+, hemolytic, aerobactin+, serum resistant, and CNF+

GEOGRAPHIC DISTRIBUTION
Worldwide

SIGNALMENT

Species
Dogs and cats

Breed Predilections
None

Mean Age and Range
• Neonatal infections common (diarrhea, septicemia) up to 2 weeks of age
• Puppies/kittens and adult animals—sporadic disease often associated with other infectious agents

Predominant Sex
None

SIGNS

General Comments
E. coli—one of the most common causes of septicemia and death in puppies and kittens

Historical Findings
• Neonates—sudden-onset vomiting, weakness/lethargy, diarrhea, cold skin; one or more animals affected in a litter
• Puppies/kittens and adults—vomiting and diarrhea

Physical Examination Findings
• Neonates—acute depression, anorexia, vomiting, tachycardia, weakness, hypothermia, cyanosis, watery diarrhea
• Puppies/kittens and adults—ETEC associated with acute vomiting, diarrhea, anorexia, rapid dehydration, fever

CAUSES
• *E. coli*—member of the endogenous microbial flora of the adult's gastrointestinal tract, prepuce, and vagina
• Many strains isolated from case material are poorly characterized in regard to virulence factors.
• Often found in old dogs and cats concurrently with other infectious agents

RISK FACTORS

Neonates
• Bitch/queen in poor health and nutritional status—unable to provide good care and colostrum to offspring

• Lack of colostrum or insufficient colostrum
• Dirty birthing environment
• Difficult or prolonged labor and birth
• Crowded facilities—build up of feces in environment, greater chance for fecal–oral spread of infection

Puppies/Kittens and Adults
• Concurrent disease—parvovirus; heavy parasitism
• Antimicrobial drugs—upset microbial flora of gastrointestinal tract
• Immunosuppression

 DIAGNOSIS

DIFFERENTIAL DIAGNOSIS
• Infectious enteritis—viral: feline panleukopenia, FeLV, FIV, enteric coronavirus, canine parvovirus, rotavirus, canine distemper; bacterial: *Salmonella, E. coli, Campylobacter jejuni, Yersinia enterocolitica;* bacterial overgrowth syndrome, *Clostridium difficile, Clostridium perfringens;* parasitic: hookworms, ascarids, whipworms, *Strongyloides, Giardia,* coccidia, *Cryptosporidia; Rickettsiae* (salmon poisoning)
• Dietary-induced enteritis—overeating; abrupt changes; starvation; thirst; food intolerance or allergy; indiscretions (e.g., foreign material or garbage)
• Drug- or toxin-induced enteritis—antimicrobial agents; antineoplastic agents; anthelminthics; heavy metals; organophosphates
• Extraintestinal disorders or metabolic diseases—acute pancreatitis; hypoadrenocorticism; liver or kidney disease; pyometra; peritonitis
• Functional or mechanical ileus—gastric-dilatation volvulus; intussusception; electrolyte disorder; gastrointestinal foreign body
• Neurologic disorders—vestibular disease; psychogenic such as fear; excitement, pain
• Fading neonates

CBC/BIOCHEMISTRY/URINALYSIS
• Few abnormalities noted, owing to rapidity of death in puppies
• Adults with enteritis may show chemistry abnormality, depending on the state of dehydration.

OTHER LABORATORY TESTS
N/A

IMAGING
N/A

DIAGNOSTIC PROCEDURES
• Antimicrobials—produce false-negative results if used before obtaining bacterial cultures

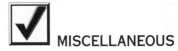

• Routine bacterial culture and identification of *E. coli* from blood (antemortem) or necropsy tissue (bone marrow, heart blood, liver/spleen, brain, mesenteric lymph node) required
• Appropriate testing of strains—identify adhesins and toxins (by DNA colony hybridization, PCR) in ETEC and VTEC strains.

PATHOLOGIC FINDINGS
• Acute enteritis
• Mucosal inflammation of small intestine
• Petechia and hemorrhagic lesions on serosa surface of gastrointestinal mucosae and all body cavities
• Fibrin on abdominal wall
• Necrosis of liver/spleen

TREATMENT

APPROPRIATE HEALTH CARE
Acutely ill puppies/kittens—inpatients; good nursing care

NURSING CARE
• Balanced parenteral polyionic isotonic solution (lactated Ringer's)—restore fluid balance
• Oral hypertonic glucose solution—for secretory diarrhea, as required

ACTIVITY
Acutely ill immature puppies/kittens (bacteremic/septicemic)—restricted activity, cage rest, monitoring, and warmth

DIET
Puppies—likely to still be nursing when affected; good nursing care needed with bottle-feeding and/or IV nutrients

CLIENT EDUCATION
Neonates—life-threatening with poor prognosis

SURGICAL CONSIDERATIONS
N/A

MEDICATIONS

DRUGS OF CHOICE
• Antimicrobial therapy—septicemia
• Guided by culture and susceptibility (MIC) testing of *E. coli;* empiric therapy until results available
• Trimethoprim-sulfa—dogs, 30 mg/kg PO q12–24h; cats, 30 mg/kg PO or SC q12–24h
• Chloramphenicol—dogs, 50 mg/kg PO, IM, IV, or SC q8h; cats, 12.5–20 mg/kg PO, IV, IM, or SC q12h
• Amoxicillin—dogs and cats, 10–20 mg/kg PO q8–12h

CONTRAINDICATIONS
Fluoroquinolones—do not use in immature dogs and cats

PRECAUTIONS
Chloramphenicol and trimethoprim-sulfa—use with caution in neonates; monitor

POSSIBLE INTERACTION
N/A

ALTERNATIVE DRUGS
• Adult—fluoroquinolones: in dogs only (enrofloxacin, 2.5–5 mg/kg PO q12h); avoid use in pregnant, neonatal, or growing animals (medium-sized dogs < 8 months of age; large or giant breeds < 12–18 months of age) because of cartilage lesions.
• Immature—third-generation cephalosporin class drugs

FOLLOW-UP

PATIENT MONITORING
• Blood culture—puppies/kittens with fever and/or diarrhea
• Monitor temperature—with signs of lethargy and/or depression
• Monitor behavior—eating, drinking, and/or nursing; adequate weight gain

PREVENTION/AVOIDANCE
• Bitch/queen—good health; vaccinated; good nutritional status
• Clean and disinfect parturition environment (1:32 dilution of bleach); clean bedding after birth frequently.
• Ensure adequate colostrum intake of all litter mates.
• Separate mother with nursing litter from other cats or dogs.
• Keep the density low in kennel or cattery rooms.
• Wash hands and change clothes and shoes after handling other cats/dogs and before dealing with neonates.

POSSIBLE COMPLICATIONS
N/A

EXPECTED COURSE AND PROGNOSIS
• Neonates—life-threatening; prognosis often poor; neonate may rapidly succumb; quick treatment with supportive care essential for survival
• Adults—self-limiting with supportive care, depending on the degree of dehydration and existence of other diseases

MISCELLANEOUS

ASSOCIATED CONDITIONS
N/A

AGE-RELATED FACTORS
Neonates—greatest risk of infection and subsequent septicemia

ZOONOTIC POTENTIAL
• Little documented information of the virulence potential of *E. coli* strains from dogs or cats for humans
• Always wash hands after handling animals (especially patients with diarrhea) because of the risk of acquiring other infectious agents (e.g., salmonellae, *Giardia*)
• **CAUTION:** keep children and immunosuppressed persons away from pets with diarrhea

PREGNANCY
N/A

SYNONYMS
• Neonatal enteritis
• *E. coli* septicemia

ABBREVIATIONS
• CNF = cytotoxic necrotizing factor
• EAE = experimental autoimmune encephalomyelitis
• EPEC = enteropathogenic *E. coli*
• ETEC = enterotoxigenic *E. coli*
• FeLV = feline leukemia virus
• FIV = feline immunodeficiency virus
• MIC = minimal inhibitory concentration
• PCR = polymerase chain reaction
• SLT = Shiga-like toxin
• VTEC = verocytotoxigenic *E. coli*

Suggested Reading

Gyles CL. *Escherichia coli*. In: Gyles CL, Thoen CO, eds. Pathogenesis of bacterial infections in animals. 2nd ed. Ames: Iowa State University Press, 1993:164–187.

Kruth SA. Gram-negative bacterial infections. In: Greene CE, ed. Infectious diseases of the dog and cat. Philadelphia: Saunders, 1998:217–222.

Peeters JE. *Escherichia coli* infections in rabbits, cats, dogs, goats and horses. In: Gyles CL, ed., *Escherichia coli* in domestic animals and humans. United Kingdom: Wallingford: Commonwealth Agricultural Bureaux, 1994:261–283.

Authors Patrick L. McDonough and Kenneth W. Simpson

Consulting Editor Stephen C. Barr

DISEASES

COLITIS AND PROCTITIS

BASICS

DEFINITION
• Colitis—inflammation of the colon
• Proctitis—inflammation of the rectum

PATHOPHYSIOLOGY
• Inflammation of the colon causes accumulation of inflammatory cytokines, disrupts tight junctions between epithelial cells, stimulates colonic secretion, stimulates goblet cell secretion of mucus, and disrupts motility.
• These mechanisms reduce the ability of the colon to absorb water and store feces; which causes frequent diarrhea, often with mucus or blood.

SYSTEMS AFFECTED
Gastrointestinal

GENETICS
Breed predisposition to histiocytic ulcerative colitis in young boxers

INCIDENCE/PREVALENCE
Approximately 30% of dogs with chronic diarrhea examined at the University of Florida Veterinary Medical Teaching Hospital; prevalence not well documented

GEOGRAPHIC DISTRIBUTION
• Generally N/A, but pythiosis is seen in Gulf Coast and southeast United States
• Histoplasmosis is seen in the Midwest and, to a lesser extent, eastern United States

SIGNALMENT

Species
Dogs and cats

Breed Predilections
Boxer (histiocytic ulcerative colitis)

Mean Age and Range
Any age; boxers usually symptomatic by 2 years old.

Predominant Sex
None

SIGNS

Historical Findings
• Feces vary from semiformed to liquid
• High frequency of defecation with small fecal volume
• Often demonstrate prolonged tenesmus after defecation
• Chronic diarrhea often with mucus or blood; cats may have formed feces with hematochezia.
• Vomiting in some (~30%) dogs
• Weight loss is rare.

Physical Examination Findings
Usually normal

CAUSES
• Infectious—*Trichuris vulpis, Ancylostoma caninum, Entamoeba histolytica, Balantidium coli, Giardia* spp., *Trichomonas* spp., *Cryptosporidium* spp., *Salmonella* spp, *Clostridium* spp., *Campylobacter* spp., *Yersinia enterocolitica, Escherichia coli, Prototheca, Histoplasma capsulatum,* and pythiosis/phycomycosis
• Traumatic—foreign body and abrasive material
• Uremia
• Segmental—secondary to chronic pancreatitis (transverse colitis)
• Allergic—dietary protein and possibly bacterial protein
• Inflammatory/immune—lymphoplasmacytic, eosinophilic, granulomatous, and histiocytic

RISK FACTORS
N/A

DIAGNOSIS

DIFFERENTIAL DIAGNOSIS
• Neoplasia—lymphoma and adenocarcinoma
• Irritable bowel syndrome
• Rectocolonic polyps
• Cecal inversion
• Ileocecocolic intussusception

CBC/BIOCHEMISTRY/URINALYSIS
• Results usually normal; neutrophilia with a left shift is possible; eosinophilia occasionally observed in eosinophilic colitis, parasitism, and pythiosis/phycomycosis
• Mild microcytic, hypochromic anemia may occur in some patients with persistent bleeding.
• Rare hyperglobulinemia in some patients (especially cats) with chronic disease.

OTHER LABORATORY TESTS
• Examination of fecal floatation, direct fecal smear, bacterial culture, or fungal culture *(Pythium)* may reveal an infectious cause.
• Feces may test positive for *Clostridium perfringens* toxin.

IMAGING
• Abdominal radiographs—usually normal
• Barium enema—may reveal mucosal irregularities or filling defects in severely affected patients, but this procedure is time-consuming and not cost-effective
• Abdominal ultrasonography—may reveal masses, diffuse thickening, or altered architecture; can perform guided biopsies or fine-needle aspiration

OTHER DIAGNOSTIC PROCEDURES
• Colonoscopy with biopsy—technique of choice for diagnosis; may see disappearance of submucosal blood vessels, granular appearance of mucosa, hyperemia, excessive mucus, ulceration, pinpoint hemorrhage (small ulcerations), or mass
• Always take multiple biopsy specimens because the extent of mucosal change does not necessarily reflect severity or absence of disease.

PATHOLOGIC FINDINGS
• Gross findings as described
• Histopathologic findings depend on the histologic type of colitis—lymphoplasmacytic, eosinophilic, granulomatous, or histiocytic; hyperplastic mucosa may be seen with irritable bowel syndrome; various infectious agents may be seen with special stains.

TREATMENT

APPROPRIATE HEALTH CARE
Outpatient medical management unless diarrhea is severe enough to cause dehydration.

NURSING CARE
Give dehydrated patients balanced electrolyte solution with potassium, intravenously, subcutaneously, or orally.

ACTIVITY
N/A

DIET
• Patients with acute colitis can be fasted for 24–48 h.
• Try a hypoallergenic diet in patients with inflammatory colitis; use a commercial or home-prepared diet that contains a protein to which the dog or cat has not been exposed.
• Fiber supplementation with poorly fermented fiber (e.g., bran and α-cellulose) is recommended to increase fecal bulk, improve colonic muscle contractility, and bind fecal water to produce formed feces.
• Some fermentable fiber (e.g., psyllium or a diet containing beet pulp or fructooligosaccharides) may be beneficial—short-chain fatty acids produced by fermentation may help the colon heal and restore normal colonic bacterial flora.

CLIENT EDUCATION
• Treatment may be intermittent and long-term in patients with inflammatory/immune colitis, and repeated recurrence is seen in some cases, especially those with the histiocytic and granulomatous forms.
• Granulomatous and histiocytic colitis, pythiosis/phycomycosis, and protothecal colitis respond poorly to medical treatment; surgery may be necessary.

SURGICAL CONSIDERATIONS
Segments of colon severely affected by fibrosis from chronic inflammation and subsequent stricture formation may need surgical excision, especially in patients with the granulomatous

form of the disease; cecal inversion, ileocecocolic intussusception require surgical intervention; pythiosis/phycomycosis often requires surgical excision or debulking.

 MEDICATIONS

DRUGS OF CHOICE

Antimicrobial Drugs
• *Trichuris, Ancylostoma,* and *Giardia*—fenbendazole (50 mg/kg PO q24h for 3 days, repeat in 3 months)
• *Entamoeba, Balantidium, Giardia,* and *Trichomonas*—metronidazole (25 mg/kg PO q12h for 5–7 days)
• *Salmonella*—treatment is controversial because a carrier state can be induced; in patients with systemic involvement, choose the antibiotic on the basis of bacterial culture and sensitivity testing (e.g., enrofloxacin, chloramphenicol, or trimethoprim-sulfa).
• *Clostridium*—metronidazole (10–15 mg/kg PO q12h for 5–14 days) or tylosin (10–15 mg/kg PO q12h for 7 days)
• *Campylobacter*—erythromycin (30–40 mg/kg PO q24h for 5 days) or tylosin (45 mg/kg PO q24h for 5 days)
• *Yersinia* and *E. coli*—choose the drug on the basis of bacterial culture and sensitivity testing
• *Prototheca*—no known treatment
• *Histoplasma*—itraconazole (dogs, 5 mg/kg PO q24h; cats, 5 mg/kg PO q12 h; several months of therapy is necessary); amphotericin B (0.25–0.5 mg/kg slow IV q48h up to cumulative dose of 4–8 mg/kg) in advanced cases
• Pythiosis/phycomycosis—ABLC (dilute in 5% dextrose to 1 mg/mL, give 3 mg/kg IV Monday-Wednesday-Friday for 9 treatments)

Antiinflammatory and Immunosuppressive Drugs for Inflammatory/Immune Colitis
• Sulfasalazine (dogs, 25–40 mg/kg PO q8h for 2–4 weeks; cats, 20 mg/kg PO q12h for 2 weeks)
• Corticosteroids—prednisone (dogs, 1–2 mg/kg PO q24h; cats, 2–4 mg/kg PO q24h; taper dosage slowly over 4–6 months once clinical remission is achieved)
• Azathioprine (dogs, 1 mg/kg PO q24h for 2 weeks followed by alternate-day administration; cats, 0.3 mg/kg PO q24h for 3–4 months)
• Sulfasalazine—drug of choice for plasmacytic lymphocytic colitis
• Prednisone and azathioprine are indicated only in eosinophilic colitis and *severe* plasmacytic lymphocytic colitis that does not respond to sulfasalazine
• Reexamine the diagnosis carefully in dogs that do not respond to sulfasalazine treatment in 4 weeks; the need for chronic maintenance

therapy means that an underlying cause (e.g., *C. perfringens* infection) may have been missed.

Motility Modifiers (Symptomatic Relief Only)
• Loperamide (0.1 mg/kg PO q8–12h)
• Diphenoxylate (0.1–0.2 mg/kg PO q8h)
• Paregoric (0.06 mg/kg PO q8–12h)
• Propantheline bromide (0.25–0.5 mg/kg PO q8h) if colonic spasm is contributing to clinical signs

CONTRAINDICATIONS
Anticholinergics

PRECAUTIONS
• Monitor patients on sulfasalazine for signs of keratoconjunctivitis sicca.
• Monitor patients on azathioprine for bone marrow suppression—CBC every 2–3 weeks; stop treatment or go to alternative-day if WBC count falls below 3000 cells/µL.
• Amphotericin B and ABLC are nephrotoxic and require renal assessment and monitoring.

POSSIBLE INTERACTIONS
N/A

ALTERNATIVE DRUGS
Albendazole (25 mg/kg PO q12h for 2 days) to treat giardiasis if fenbendazole or metronidazole are ineffective

 FOLLOW-UP

PATIENT MONITORING
Infrequent recheck examinations or client communication by phone

PREVENTION/AVOIDANCE
• Avoid exposure to infectious agents (e.g., other dogs, contaminated foods, moist environments).
• Avoid abrupt dietary changes.

POSSIBLE COMPLICATIONS
• Recurrence of signs without treatment, when treatment is tapered, and with progression of disease
• Stricture formation due to chronic inflammation

EXPECTED COURSE AND PROGNOSIS
• Most infections—excellent with treatment (cure)
• Prototheca—grave; no known treatment except excision
• *Histoplasma*—poor in moderate-to-advanced or disseminated disease; mild cases may respond to therapy.
• Pythiosis/phycomycosis—guarded to poor; poorly responsive to treatment; some dogs have fair results with excision and ABLC
• Traumatic, uremic, and segmental—good, if underlying cause is treatable

• Cecal inversion, ileocecocolic intussusception, and polyps—good with surgical removal
• Inflammatory—good with treatment in patients with lymphoplasmacytic and eosinophilic disease; most patients with lymphoplasmacytic colitis respond to sulfasalazine therapy within 2–4 weeks of treatment.
• Reexamine the diagnosis if signs persist; prognosis poor in patients with granulomatous and histiocytic disease in the short term and worsens with recurrence or poor response to treatment.

 MISCELLANEOUS

ASSOCIATED CONDITIONS
Inflammatory/immune disease and infectious agents may also affect the small intestine.

AGE-RELATED FACTORS
N/A

ZOONOTIC POTENTIAL
Entamoeba, Balantidium, Giardia, Salmonella, Clostridium, Campylobacter, Yersinia, and *E. coli; Prototheca, Histoplasma* in immunosuppressed individuals

PREGNANCY
Caution with drug use—corticosteroids, azathioprine, antifungals, and antibiotics

SYNONYMS
• Large bowel diarrhea
• Inflammatory bowel disease

SEE ALSO
• Inflammatory Bowel Disease
• Colitis, Histiocytic Ulcerative
• Individual infectious and parasitic agents

ABBREVIATIONS
ABLC = Amphotericin B Lipid Complex

Suggested Reading
Burrows CF. Canine colitis. Comp Cont Ed Pract Vet 1992;10:1347–1354.
Leib MS, Matz ME. Diseases of the large intestine. In: Ettinger SJ, Feldman EC, eds., Textbook of veterinary internal medicine. Philadelphia: Saunders, 1995:1232–1260.
Sherding RG, Burrows CF. Diarrhea. In: Anderson NV, ed., Veterinary gastroenterology. Philadelphia: Lea & Febiger, 1992:455–477.
Authors Colin F. Burrows and Lisa E. Moore
Consulting Editors Mitchell A. Crystal and Brett M. Feder

DISEASES

COLITIS, HISTIOCYTIC ULCERATIVE

BASICS

OVERVIEW
• Rare disease characterized by colonic mucosal ulceration and inflammation with periodic acid–Schiff (PAS) positive histiocytes
• Etiologic and pathogenic mechanism unknown

SIGNALMENT
• Dogs; primarily affects young boxers, usually less than 2 years of age
• Reported in a French bulldog
• Possible genetic basis, but unknown

SIGNS
• Bloody, mucoid diarrhea with increasing frequency of defecation
• Tenesmus
• Weight loss and debilitation may develop late in the disease process

CAUSES & RISK FACTORS
No known cause or predisposing factors

DIAGNOSIS

DIFFERENTIAL DIAGNOSIS
• Other causes of colitis—nonhistiocytic IBD, infectious colitis, parasitic colitis, allergic colitis
• Cecal inversion
• Ileocolic intussusception
• Neoplasia—lymphoma, adenocarcinoma
• Foreign body
• Rectocolonic polyps
• Irritable bowel syndrome
• Differentiate by examination of fecal flotations, direct smears, bacterial culture for pathogens, abdominal imaging, and colonoscopy and biopsy

CBC/BIOCHEMISTRY/URINALYSIS
• Usually normal
• Neutrophilia and mild anemia in some patients

OTHER LABORATORY TESTS
N/A

IMAGING
N/A

DIAGNOSTIC PROCEDURES
Colonoscopy reveals patchy red foci (pinpoint ulcerations), overt ulceration, thick mucosal folds, areas of granulation tissue, and strictures; take multiple biopsy specimens.

PATHOLOGIC FINDINGS
• Thickening of the lamina propria and infiltration of the mucosa and submucosa with histiocytes, lymphocytes, and plasma cells; ulceration with neutrophil infiltration in some animals
• Histiocytes are PAS positive.

TREATMENT
• Outpatient medical management
• Change diet to include fiber supplementation
• Advise owner of progressive nature, possibility of recurrence, and ultimate inability to control disease

MEDICATIONS

DRUGS

Antiinflammatory/Immunosuppressive Drugs
• Corticosteroids—prednisone (1–2 mg/kg PO q24h until clinical remission, then taper slowly over 4–6 months)
• Sulfasalazine (25–40 mg/kg PO q8h)
• Azathioprine (dogs, 1 mg/kg q24h for 2 weeks followed by alternate-day administration)

Antimicrobials
• Metronidazole (25 mg/kg PO q12h)
• Tylosin (45 mg/kg PO q24h)

CONTRAINDICATIONS/POSSIBLE INTERACTIONS
• Avoid anticholinergics
• Monitor for keratoconjunctivitis sicca sometimes seen with sulfasalazine therapy
• Monitor for immunosuppression (CBCs) sometimes seen with azathioprine

FOLLOW-UP

PATIENT MONITORING
Clinical signs and body weight every week to 2 weeks initially

PREVENTION/AVOIDANCE
N/A

POSSIBLE COMPLICATIONS
• Progressive, uncontrollable disease
• Colonic stricture

EXPECTED COURSE AND PROGNOSIS
Patient may initially respond to treatment if begun early in course of disease; eventually, the disease usually progresses over months; prognosis is guarded.

MISCELLANEOUS

PREGNANCY
• Caution with drug use—corticosteroids, azathioprine
• Patients probably should not be bred, because of the potential for inheritance.

SEE ALSO
Colitis and Proctitis

ABBREVIATIONS
• PAS = periodic acid-Schiff
• IBD = inflammatory bowel disease

Suggested Reading
Hall EJ, Rutgers HC, et al. Histiocytic ulcerative colitis in boxer dogs in the U.K. J Small Anim Pract 1994;35:509–515.
Sherding RG, Burrows CF. Diarrhea. In: Anderson NV, ed. Veterinary gastroenterology. Philadelphia: Lea & Febiger, 1992:465–466.
Authors Lisa E. Moore and Colin F. Burrows
Consulting Editors Mitchell A. Crystal and Brett M. Feder

BASICS

OVERVIEW
• Congenital, autosomal recessive condition minimally consisting of temporal to superio-temporal choroidal hypoplasia and excessive tortuosity of primary retinal vessels
• Possible accompanying defects indicating more severe manifestations—optic nerve coloboma; staphylomas; retinal detachment; intraocular hemorrhage
• Always bilateral; may note disparate severity between the eyes
• Potential for blindness because of retinal detachment
• Associated anomalies not directly part of syndrome—enophthalmia; microphthalmia; retinal folds; mineralization of the anterior corneal stroma
• Approximately 85% of collies in North America are homozygously affected or heter-ozygous carriers.
• Less than 10% of collies in Europe are affected or carriers.

SIGNALMENT
• Dogs
• Present at birth
• Seen in both smooth and rough-coated collies
• Similar condition affects Shetland sheep-dogs, Australian Shepherds, and border collies

SIGNS
• None to partial or complete blindness
• Minimal ophthalmoscopic findings necessary for diagnosis—increased retinal vessel tortuosity and choroidal hypoplasia
• Vessels tortuous and disorganized (radiating pattern normal)
• Choroidal hypoplasia—a focal to diffuse area of anomalous choroidal vasculature; reduced number of vessels; temporal or superior-temporal to the optic disk; may extend more nasally with severe disease
• Overlying tapetum—usually focally absent; allows visualization of the underlying choroid
• Underlying sclera—may be seen between choroidal vessels
• May note optic nerve coloboma (pitting of the optic nerve head), retinal detachment, and intraocular hemorrhage

CAUSES & RISK FACTORS
• Autosomal recessive trait; occurs only from mating between affected or carrier animals

DIAGNOSIS

DIFFERENTIAL DIAGNOSIS
• Excessive tortuosity of retinal vessels with no choroidal hypoplasia—not classified as collie eye anomaly
• Merling of the coat—usually associated with lack of pigment in the pigmented epithelial layer of the retina, allowing visualization of normal choroidal vasculature; differentiated by normal, regular, radiating choroidal vessels
• Optic nerve colobomata and retinal detach-ment independent of choroidal hypoplasia—not classified as collie eye anomaly

CBC/BIOCHEMISTRY/URINALYSIS
N/A

OTHER LABORATORY TESTS
N/A

IMAGING
N/A

DIAGNOSTIC PROCEDURES
N/A

TREATMENT
• None for reversal of condition
• Cryosurgery or laser surgery around the area of the optic nerve coloboma—may prevent retinal detachment; may be used to help reattach a retina

MEDICATIONS

DRUG(S)
None

CONTRAINDICATIONS/POSSIBLE INTERACTIONS
N/A

FOLLOW-UP

PATIENT MONITORING
Patients with colobomata—monitor during first year of life for secondary retinal detach-ment; after 1 year, retinal detachments rarely occur.

PREVENTION/AVOIDANCE
• Breed only genotypically normal dogs
• Breeding of minimally affected dogs to other minimally affected or carrier dogs may result in minimally affected offspring; how-ever, any level of severity can be produced by such breedings.

EXPECTED COURSE AND PROGNOSIS
• Does not progress, except colobomata that leads to retinal detachment after birth
• Some patients with minor areas of choroidal hypoplasia may develop pigment across the affected area but appear phenotypically normal; thus early examination (in the first 6–8 weeks of life) is highly recommended.

MISCELLANEOUS

ASSOCIATED CONDITIONS
• Microphthalmia
• Enophthalmia
• Retinal folds
• Anterior corneal stromal mineralization

SYNONYM
Scleral ectasia syndrome

Suggested Reading
Roberts SR. The collie eye anomaly. J Am Vet Med Assoc 1969:155:859–864.
Author Stephanie L. Smedes
Consulting Editor Paul E. Miller

CONGENITAL OCULAR ANOMALIES

BASICS

DEFINITION
Solitary or multiple abnormalities that affect the globe or its adnexa that may be observed in young dogs and cats at birth or within the first 6–8 weeks of life

PATHOPHYSIOLOGY
• Breed-related inherited defects—most common; include colobomas (segmental areas that fail to develop properly) of the fundus in collie eye anomaly • Spontaneous malformations—colobomas of the anterior segment, resulting in notch-like defects of the iris or lens • In utero systemic infections and inflammations, exposure to toxic compounds, and lack of specific nutrients in pregnant dams or bitches

SYSTEMS AFFECTED
Ophthalmic—entire eye or any part; unilateral or bilateral

GENETICS
• Suspected genetic background for several causal diseases, some with a unknown mode of inheritance • PPM in basenjis—simple autosomal dominant trait • PHTVL and PHPV in Doberman pinschers—autosomal dominant allele with variable expression • Multifocal retinal dysplasia in English springer spaniels—autosomal simple recessive trait • Collie eye anomaly—autosomal recessive trait • Retinal dystrophy in briards—simple autosomal recessive allele • Photoreceptor dysplasia in collies and Irish setters—autosomal recessive trait; nonallelic disease • Other photoreceptor dysplasias in dogs—recessively inherited • Photoreceptor dysplasia in Abyssinians and domestic shorthair cats—postulated autosomal dominant trait

INCIDENCE/PREVALENCE
• Incidence in dogs and cats—low in the general population; somewhat higher in dogs than cats • Collie eye anomaly—affects collies and Shetland sheepdogs; most common; worldwide prevalence > 50%

SIGNALMENT
• Dogs and cats • See Genetics.

SIGNS
General Comments
• Depend on defect • May cause no signs of disease and may be an incidental finding in a thorough ophthalmic examination.

Historical Findings
• Ranges from none to severe visual impairment or blindness.

Physical Examination Findings
• Microphthalmos—a congenitally small eye; found in different degrees; easily noted by comparing the eyes; more difficult to detect if bilateral; often associated with other hereditary defects (e.g., corneal opacities, PPM, cataract, detachment, and retinal dysplasia) • Anophthalmos—congenital lack of the globe; often associated with other hereditary defects (e.g., corneal opacities, PPM, cataract, detachment, and retinal dysplasia) • Cryptophthalmos—a small globe that is concealed by other adnexal defects; often associated with other hereditary defects (e.g., corneal opacities, PPM, cataract, detachment, and retinal dysplasia) • Eyelid agenesis or colobomas of the eyelids—often result in congenitally open eyelids; considered hereditary in Burmese cats; usually affect the temporal portion of the upper eyelid; may note blepharospasm and epiphora • Dermoids—congenital, tumor-like, islands of aberrant skin tissue involving either eyelids, conjunctiva, or cornea; sometimes affect more than one structure; may note blepharospasm and epiphora • Congenital atresia and imperforate puncta of the lacrimal system—affects cats and dogs; imperforate puncta: common in several dog breeds (e.g., cocker spaniels); results in a tear streak at the nasal canthus and on the side of the nose; usually not associated with other ocular findings • Congenital KCS—may occur sporadically in any dog or cat breed; may be hereditary in Yorkshire terriers; usually unilateral; affected eye often appears smaller than the normal eye; results in a thick mucoid discharge from a red and irritated eye • PPM—remnants of the pupillary membrane that extend from the iris collarette to the corneal endothelium, the anterior lens capsule, or just across the pupil; may coexist with a variety of iris defects, cataracts, and uveal colobomata; affects any species; recorded in numerous dog breeds; shown to be hereditary in basenjis • Iris cysts—circular, pigmented or nonpigmented ball-like structures that float freely in the anterior chamber or are attached to the iris or corneal endothelium • Congenital glaucoma with buphthalmos—affects dogs and cats; rare; often note increased tearing and an enlarged, red, and painful eye • Congenital pupillary abnormalities—polycoria (more than one pupil); ancoria (no pupil); aniridia (lack of iris); dyscoria (abnormally shaped pupil) • Congenital cataracts—primary, often inherited (e.g., cavalier King Charles spaniels) or secondary to other developmental defects; often associated with other congenital anomalies of the lens, including microphakia (a small lens), lenticonus or lentiglobus (a protrusion of the lens capsule, most often posteriorly), and coloboma (notching of the lens equator, which may also include defects in the zonules and ciliary body); associated leukocoria common • PHTVL and PHPV—hereditary defect; affects Doberman pinschers and Staffordshire bull terriers; persistence of parts of the hyaloid vasculature; developmental aberrations of the vitreous, lens, and lens capsule; may note a cataract and leukocoria or a reddish sheen from the pupillary area in conjunction with intralenticular bleeding (unusual) or vascular abnormalities on the posterior lens capsule • Retinal dysplasia—affects a variety of dog breeds; occurs sporadically in cats; affect on neural retinal structure depends on severity; ranges from focal folds to geographic focal detachment to complete retinal detachment • Coloboma of the posterior segment—found in conjunction with hereditary collie eye anomaly; occurs sporadically in other dog breeds; typically seen in the optic nerve head, usually at the 6 o'clock position; may also be noted in other locations in the fundus, usually in the vicinity of the optic nerve head • Photoreceptor dysplasia—hereditary anomaly in dogs and cats; rods, cones, or both may be affected from birth; direct and indirect pupillary light reflexes may be abnormal and may react sluggishly when the patient opens its eyes • Rod and cone dysplasias of dogs—rods and cone dysplasia affects Irish setters (*rcd1*) and collies (*rcd2*); rod dysplasia and early rod degeneration affects the Norwegian elkhound; cone degeneration or hemeralopia affects Alaskan malamutes. • Rod–cone dysplasia of cats—affects Persians, Abyssinians, and American mixed-breeds; may show pupillary dilation at 2–3 weeks, nystagmus at 4–5 weeks, ophthalmoscopic signs of retinal degeneration at 8 weeks, and night and day blindness some weeks later • Retinal dystrophy—congenital disease; found in briards; affects retinal pigment epithelium and photoreceptors • Retinal detachment—seen in conjunction with the hereditary diseases (e.g., retinal dysplasia); mainly found in Labrador retrievers, Bedlingtons, and Sealyham terriers and with collie eye anomaly; may be seen with other ocular syndromes in which several other eye defects are involved; may note a widely dilated pupil that is unresponsive to light stimuli; may be seen in the pupil as a funnel-shaped curtain; complete detachment results in blindness. • Optic nerve hypoplasia—occurs sporadically as a congenital ocular defect in dogs and cats; believed to have a hereditary background in miniature and toy poodles; often results in blindness

CAUSES
• Hereditary factors • Spontaneous malformations
• Infections and inflammations during pregnancy—congenital cataracts; syndromes with multiple defects • Toxicity during pregnancy
• Nutritional deficiencies

DIAGNOSIS

DIFFERENTIAL DIAGNOSIS
• Early-onset infectious and inflammatory processes of the adnexal structures—may mimic and even mask congenital abnormalities, such as congenital KCS • Cataracts induced at an early age and especially those that progress quickly (e.g., after trauma or with diabetes mellitus)—may seem to be congenital • Postinflammatory ophthalmic lesions resulting in synechia—may be confused with PPM • Tumors of the anterior segment of the eye—may be confused with iris cysts • Generalized retinopathy of inflammatory origin—may appear to be photoreceptor dysplasia with retinal atrophy; usually unilateral • Retinal detachment as result of trauma or uveitis in young dogs—may appear to be a congenital abnormality of the neural retina (e.g., postinflammatory neuroretinal folding as opposed to multifocal retinal dysplasia) • Optic nerve atrophy owing to an inflammatory process—may be difficult to differentiate from congenital optic nerve hypoplasia

IMAGING

Ultrasound—diagnosis of abnormalities of the lens and the posterior segment of the eye, abnormalities of the position of the lens or configuration of its capsule, and abnormalities in the vitreous and retina (e.g., congenital retinal detachment)

DIAGNOSTIC PROCEDURES

• Penlight examination—usually permits the diagnosis of complete cataract or retinal detachment • Evaluation of tear production (using Shirmer tear strips)—perform routinely with chronic adnexal inflammatory and infectious processes • Direct and/or indirect ophthalmoscope and slitlamp biomicroscopy—necessary to diagnose most abnormalities of the internal structures (e.g., multifocal retinal dysplasia and PHTVL/PHPV); examine after pupil dilation (check pupillary light reflexes before dilating); difficult to perform in patients younger than 5 weeks • Electroretinography and visually evoked potentials—objective evaluation and differentiation of retinal and optic nerve function; usually performed in patients aged 7–12 weeks; electroretinography diagnostic for photoreceptor dysplasias and retinal dystrophy of briards

PATHOLOGIC FINDINGS

• Depend on type and severity of defect; range from solitary defects of specific structures to involvement of the whole globe, such as severe microphthalmos • Congenital KCS—usually a severe keratitis with corneal neovascularization, scarring, and pigmentation; inflammatory changes of the conjunctiva; may note abnormally developed or atrophied lacrimal glands • Congenital glaucoma—buphthalmos common, sometimes with secondary lens luxation and always neuroretinal thinning; collapse of the iridocorneal filtration angle • PHTVL and PHPV—range of defects; retrolental darkly pigmented dots and plaques to complete strands of vascular tissue passing from the optic nerve head to the posterior lens capsule; often malformations of the posterior lens capsule (e.g., lenticonus) and some degree of cataract formation • Retinal dysplasia—some degree of abnormality and folding of the retina; with multifocal defect, often see rosettes of abnormal neuroretinal tissue along the major blood vessels in the central tapetal fundus; with geographical defect, usually find a large, abnormal area where the retina is slightly elevated and the surrounding tissue is hyperpigmented and scarred; may note an abnormal and completely detached retina • Photoreceptor dysplasia—abnormalities in the rods and/or cones; thin inner and outer segment layers; dropout of photoreceptor nuclei in the outer nuclear layer • Retinal dystrophy (briards)—large lipoid-like inclusions in the retinal pigment epithelium • Colobomas—a notch in the tissue with anterior defect (e.g., lens or iris); thinning of the neural retina, either in the region of the optic nerve head or near its border with posterior defect; may be rather large and extend far back as an outpouching of the sclera • Retinal detachment—neural retina detached from the retinal pigment epithelium; usually attached only around the optic nerve

head • Optic nerve hypoplasia—avascular, dark, abnormally small, and circular optic nerve head

TREATMENT

APPROPIATE HEALTH CARE

• Patients are usually referred to an ophthalmologist for a complete evaluation, especially if abnormality affects the internal structures of the eye or vision is impaired. • No medical treatment for most congenital abnormalities, except possibly symptomatic treatment (e.g., congenital KCS)

NURSING CARE

Inhibit self-mutilation after surgical procedures by using an Elizabethan collar or by directly bandaging the paws or eye.

ACTIVITY

Usually unaltered

CLIENT EDUCATION

• Discuss visual capacity, possible progression, and sequelae. • Inform client that blind animals may need direct supervision when exposed to a potentially hazardous environment. • Congenital KCS—discuss medical treatment versus surgical intervention; inform client that if the eye is medicated on a regular basis, the patient will do fine, especially if there is some tear production; if client cannot or will not medicate, recommend surgery.

SURGICAL CONSIDERATIONS

• Depend on specific abnormality • Adnexal abnormalities (e.g., dermoids or severe malformations of the eyelids)—perform surgery as soon as possible. • If undesirable sequelae will not result, it may be advantageous to wait until the patient has clearly reached adult size to avoid overcorrecting the defect. • Imperforate puncta—surgically corrected as soon as anesthesia is safe • Congenital KCS—warn client of increased tearing in conjunction with parotid duct transposition. • Cataract extraction—not always successful in conjunction with congenital lens opacifications, because there may be other aberrations in back of the lens that could not be detected preoperatively (e.g., PHTVL and PHPV with large functional vessels in back of the lens that cause surgical complications) • Congenital glaucoma—enucleation usually treatment of choice; consider euthanasia if bilateral.

MEDICATIONS

DRUGS OF CHOICE

• Congenital KCS—tear substitutes (Tears Naturale and Visco-Tears), possibly in combination with antibiotics (drops or gel); cyclosporin ophthalmic (Optimmune) ointment BID may be advantageous. • Congenital cataracts—cyclosporin may be advantageous; when involving the nuclear region of the lens, mydriatics may be used to increase visual capability.

FOLLOW-UP

PATIENT MONITORING

• Depends on defect • Congenital KCS—requires frequent monitoring of tear production and the status of the external eye structures • Congenital cataracts and severe PHTVL and PHPV—regular checkups, usually on a 6-month basis, to monitor possible progression • Large colobomatous defects of the fundus and geographical retinal dysplasia—yearly checkups to monitor possible complete retinal detachment

PREVENTION/AVOIDANCE

• Depend on type and severity of defect • Restrict breeding of affected animals and of known carriers of documented hereditary defects.

POSSIBLE COMPLICATIONS

• Depend on defect • Untreated eyelid agenesis, dermoids, and congenital KCS—recurrent problems with conjunctivitis and keratitis • Congenital glaucoma—painful, blind eye in conjunction with buphthalmos; often a dry, pigmented cornea • Large colobomas of the optic nerve head—may cause retinal detachment • Retinal detachment—may cause intraocular primarily vitreal hemorrhage

EXPECTED COURSE AND PROGNOSIS

• Depend on defect and type of medical and/or surgical treatment provided • Adnexal abnormalities—good prognosis with surgical treatment • Congenital KCS—rather poor prognosis with medical treatment only; somewhat better prognosis with surgical treatment • Congenital cataract—usually good prognosis with surgical treatment.

MISCELLANEOUS

ASSOCIATED CONDITIONS

Retinal dysplasia—described with chondrodysplastic skeletal abnormalities in field-trial Labradors

Suggested Reading

Gelatt KN, ed. Veterinary ophthalmology. 2nd ed. Philadelphia: Lea & Febiger, 1991.

Peiffer RL, Petersen-Jones SM. Small animal ophthalmology: a problem-oriented approach. London, Saunders, 1997.

Petersen-Jones SM, Crispin SM. Manual of small animal ophthalmology. Gloucestershire, UK: British Small Animal Veterinary Association, 1993.

Slatter D. Fundamentals of veterinary ophthalmology. Philadelphia, Saunders, 1990.

Author Kristina Narfström

Consulting Editor Paul E. Miller

CONGESTIVE HEART FAILURE, LEFT-SIDED

BASICS

DEFINITION
Failure of the left side of the heart to advance blood at a sufficient rate to meet the metabolic needs of the patient or to prevent blood from pooling within the pulmonary venous circulation

PATHOPHYSIOLOGY
• Low cardiac output causes lethargy, exercise intolerance, syncope, and prerenal azotemia. • High hydrostatic pressure causes leakage of fluid from pulmonary venous circulation into pulmonary interstitium and alveoli. When fluid leakage exceeds ability of lymphatics to drain the affected areas, pulmonary edema develops.

SYSTEMS AFFECTED
• All organ systems can be affected by poor delivery of blood. • Respiratory because of edema • Cardiovascular

GENETICS
• Some congenital heart defects have a genetic basis in certain breeds.

INCIDENCE/PREVALENCE
• Common syndrome in clinical practice

GEOGRAPHIC DISTRIBUTION
• Seen everywhere, but prevalence of causes varies with location.

SIGNALMENT
Species Dogs and cats
Breed Predilections Varies with cause
Mean Age and Range Varies with cause
Predominant Sex Varies with cause

SIGNS

General Comments
Signs vary with underlying cause and between species

Historical Findings
• Weakness, lethargy, exercise intolerance. • Coughing (dogs) and dyspnea. Respiratory signs often worsen at night and can be relieved by assuming a standing, sternal, or "elbows abducted" position (orthopnea). • Cats rarely cough.

Physical Examination Findings
• Tachypnea • Coughing, often soft in conjunction with tachypnea • Inspiratory and expiratory dyspnea when animal has pulmonary edema • Pulmonary crackles and wheezes • Prolonged capillary refill time • Possible murmur or gallop • Weak femoral pulses

CAUSES
Pump (Muscle) Failure of Left Ventricle
• Idiopathic dilated cardiomyopathy (DCM) • Trypanosomiasis (rare) • Doxorubicin cardiotoxicity (dogs) • Hypothyroidism (rare)

• Hyperthyroidism (rarely causes pump failure; more commonly causes high output failure)

Pressure Overload to Left Heart
• Systemic hypertension • Subaortic stenosis • Coarctation of the aorta (rare; airdales predisposed) • Left ventricular tumors (rare)

Volume Overload of the Left Heart
• Mitral valve endocardiosis • Mitral valve dysplasia • PDA • Ventricular septal defect

Impediment to Filling of Left Heart
• Pericardial effusion with tamponade • Restrictive pericarditis • Restrictive cardiomyopathy • Hypertrophic cardiomyopathy • Left atrial masses (e.g., tumors and thrombus) • Pulmonary thromboembolism • Mitral stenosis (rare)

Rhythm Disturbances
• Bradycardia (AV block) • Tachycardia (e.g., atrial fibrillation, atrial tachycardia, and ventricular tachycardia)

RISK FACTORS
Diseases requiring high cardiac output (eg, hyperthyroidism, anemia, and pregnancy)

DIAGNOSIS

DIFFERENTIAL DIAGNOSIS
Must differentiate from other causes of coughing, dyspnea, and weakness; generally requires a complete diagnostic work-up.

CBC/BIOCHEMISTRY/URINALYSIS
• CBC usually normal; may be stress leukogram • Mild to moderately high alanine transaminase, aspartate transaminase, and serum alkaline phosphatase; Bilirubin generally normal. • Prerenal azotemia (high BUN +/– high creatinine with normal urine concentrating ability) in some animals

OTHER LABORATORY TESTS
Thyroid disorders may be detected.

IMAGING

Radiographic Findings
• Left heart and pulmonary veins enlarged • Pulmonary edema, often hilar, initially; may be patchy, especially in cats; usually symetrical, but may begin in right caudal lung lobe

Echocardiography
• Findings vary markedly with cause, but left atrial enlargement a relatively consistent finding in congested animals • Diagnostic test of choice for documenting congenital defects, cardiac masses, and pericardial effusion

DIAGNOSTIC PROCEDURES

Electrocardiographic Findings
• Atrial or ventricular arrhythmias • Evidence of left heart enlargement (eg, wide P waves, tall and wide QRS complexes, and left axis orientation) • May be normal

PATHOLOGIC FINDINGS
Cardiac findings vary with disease

TREATMENT

APPROPRIATE HEALTH CARE
• Usually treat as outpatient unless animal is dyspneic or severely hypotensive • Identify and correct underlying cause whenever possible. • Minimize handling of critically dyspneic animals. Stress can kill!

NURSING CARE
• Oxygen is life saving in critically dyspneic patients; administer in an oxygen cage, by oxygen mask, or by nasal catheter.

ACTIVITY
Restrict activity

DIET
Initiate moderately sodium-restricted diet. Severe sodium restriction indicated in animals with advanced disease.

CLIENT EDUCATION
• With few exceptions (ie, animals with thyroid disorders, arrhythmias, idiopathic pericardial effusion); left congestive heart failure (L-CHF) is not curable.

SURGICAL CONSIDERATIONS
• Surgical intervention or balloon valvuloplasty may benefit selected patients with congenital defects such as PDA and subaortic stenosis. Response to these interventions varies. • Pericardiocentesis in animals with pericardial effusion

MEDICATIONS

DRUGS OF CHOICE

Diuretics
• Furosemide (1–2 mg/kg q8h–q24h) or other loop diuretic is the initial diuretic of choice; diuretics indicated to remove pulmonary edema • Critically dyspneic animals often require high doses (4–8 mg/kg) given IV to stabilize; this dose can be repeated in 1 hour if animal is still severely dyspneic. • Predisposes the patient to dehydration, prerenal azotemia, and electrolyte disturbances. • Once edema resolves, taper the diuretic to the lowest effective dosage.

Digoxin
• Digoxin (dogs, 0.22 mg/M2 q12h; cats, 0.01 mg/kg q48h) is used in animals with myocardial failure (e.g., dilated cardiomyopathy). • Digoxin also indicated to treat supraventricular arrhythmias (e.g., sinus tachycardia, atrial fibrillation, and atrial or junctional tachycardia) in patients with CHF

Venodilators

• Nitroglycerin ointment (0.25 in/5 kg q6h–q8h) causes venodilation, lowering left atrial filling pressures. • Used for acute stabilization of patients with severe pulmonary edema and dyspnea. Apply to the gums, a hairless area in the inguinal or axillary region, or the inside of the pinna. If the pinna are cold, choose an alternate site. • May be useful in animals with chronic L-CHF when used intermittently. To avoid tolerance, use intermittently and with 12-hour, dose-free interval between the last dose of one day and the first dose of the next day.

ACE Inhibitors

• ACE inhibitor such as enalapril (0.5 mg/kg q12h–q24h) indicated in animal with L-CHF secondary to degenerative mitral valve disease and in dog with DCM. In such patients, ACE inhibitor improves survival and quality of life. • ACE inhibitor may also be of benefit in selected animals with congenital defects (eg, mitral valve dysplasia and ventral septal defect). • May be helpful in cats with cardiomyopathy and signs of CHF.

Positive Inotropes

• Dopamine (dogs, 2.5–10 mcg/kg/min; cats, 1–5 mcg/kg/min) and dobutamine (dogs, 2.5–10 mcg/kg/min; cats, 2–10 mcg/kg/min) are potent positive inotropic agents that may provide valuable short-term support of a heart failure patient with poor cardiac contractility. • These agents are arrhythmogenic, and dopamine can cause hypertension at high infusion rates. Careful monitoring is required.

Antiarrhythmic Agents

Treat arrhythmias if clinically indicated.

CONTRAINDICATIONS

• Avoid vasodilators in patients with pericardial effusion or fixed outflow obstruction.

PRECAUTIONS

• ACE inhibitor and arterial dilators must be used with caution in patients with possible outflow obstruction. • Patients with pulmonary hypertension and hypoxia are at high risk for digoxin toxicity. • ACE inhibitor and digoxin must be used cautiously in patients with renal disease. • Use dobutamine cautiously in cats. • Hypothyroidism predisposes animal to digoxin toxicity, while hyperthyroidism diminishes effects of digoxin.

POSSIBLE INTERACTIONS

• Combination of high-dose diuretics and ACE inhibitor may alter renal perfusion, and cause azotemia, especially in animals with severe sodium restriction. • Combination diuretic therapy adds to risk of dehydration and electrolyte disturbances. • Combination vasodilator therapy predisposes animal to hypotension.

ALTERNATIVE DRUGS

Arterial Dilators

• Hydralazine (1–2 mg/kg PO q12h) can be substituted for an ACE inhibitor in patients that do not tolerate the drug or have advanced renal failure, or if the cost is prohibitive. Monitor for hypotension and reflex tachycardia. Add digoxin if sinus tachycardia develops. Can be used with an ACE inhibitor in animals with refractory L-CHF. • Nitroprusside (1–10 mcg/kg/min) is a potent arterial dilator. Usually reserved for short-term support of patients with life-threatening edema.

Calcium Channel Blockers

• Diltiazem (0.5–1.5 mg/kg PO q8h) is frequently used in L-CHF patients for rate control in animals with supraventricular arrhythmias not controlled by digoxin and in cats with hypertrophic cardiomyopathy.

Beta Blockers

• Propranolol, atenolol, and metoprolol are used for rate control in animals with supraventricular tachycardia, hypertrophic cardiomyopathy, and hyperthyroidism. • Used alone or with a class 1 antiarrhythmic drug for control of ventricular arrhythmias. These drugs depress contractility (negative inotropes), so use cautiously in patients with myocardial failure. • On basis of human studies, may enhance survival in animals with idiopathic DCM. Treatment best initiated under the guidance of a cardiologist, starting with very low dosage and gradually increasing the dosage. • Patients unresponsive to furosemide, vasodilator, and digoxin (if indicated) may benefit from combination diuretic therapy by adding spironolactone (1–2 mg/kg PO q12h) and/or a thiazide diuretic to furosemide.

Nutritional Supplements

• Potassium supplementation if hypokalemia is documented. Use potassium supplements cautiously in animals receiving ACE inhibitor or spironolactone. • Taurine supplementation in cats with DCM and dogs with DCM and taurine deficiency (e.g., American cocker spaniels) • L-carnitine supplementation may help some dogs with DCM. • Coenzyme Q_{10} of potential value based on the results of small trials in humans with DCM.

 FOLLOW-UP

PATIENT MONITORING

• Monitor renal status, electrolytes, hydration, respiratory rate and effort, heart rate, body weight, and abdominal girth (dogs). • If azotemia develops, reduce the dosage of diuretic. If azotemia persists and the animal is also on an ACE inhibitor, reduce or discontinue the ACE inhibitor. Use digoxin with caution if azotemia develops. • Monitor ECG if arrhythmias are suspected. • Check digoxin concentration periodically. Normal range is 1–2 ng/ml, 8–10 hours after a dose.

PREVENTION/AVOIDANCE

• Minimize stress, exercise, and sodium intake in patients with heart disease. • Prescribing an ACE inhibitor early in the course of heart disease in patients with mitral valve disease and DCM may slow the progression of heart disease and delay onset of CHF. Consider this in asymptomatic animals if they have DCM or if they have mitral valve disease and radiographic or echocardiographic evidence of left heart enlargement.

POSSIBLE COMPLICATIONS

• Syncope • Aortic thromboembolism (cats) • Arrhythmias • Electrolyte imbalances • Digoxin toxicity • Azotemia and renal failure

EXPECTED COURSE AND PROGNOSIS

Prognosis varies with underlying cause

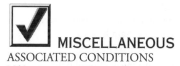 MISCELLANEOUS

ASSOCIATED CONDITIONS
N/A

AGE-RELATED FACTORS

• Congenital causes seen in young animals • Degenerative heart conditions and neoplasia generally seen in old animals

ZOONOTIC POTENTIAL
N/A

PREGNANCY
N/A

SYNONYMS
N/A

SEE ALSO

• Diseases Causing L-CHF • Pulmonary Edema

ABBREVIATIONS

• ACE = angiotensin converting enzyme • DCM = dilated cardiomyopathy • L-CHF = left-sided congestive heart failure • PDA = patent ductus arteriosus

Suggested Reading

Keene BW, Bonagura JD. Therapy of heart failure. In: Bonagura JD, ed. Current Veterinary Therapy XII. Philadelphia: WB Saunders, 1995.

Authors Francis W. K. Smith, Jr. and Bruce W. Keene

Consulting Editors Larry P. Tilley and Francis W. K. Smith, Jr.

DISEASES

CONGESTIVE HEART FAILURE, RIGHT-SIDED

BASICS

DEFINITION
• Failure of the right side of the heart to advance blood at a sufficient rate to meet the metabolic needs of the patient or to prevent blood from pooling within the systemic venous circulation

PATHOPHYSIOLOGY
• High hydrostatic pressure leads to leakage of fluid from venous circulation into the pleural and peritoneal space and interstitium of peripheral tissue.
• When fluid leakage exceeds ability of lymphatics to drain the affected areas, pleural effusion, ascites, and peripheral edema develop.

SYSTEMS AFFECTED
All organ systems can be affected by either poor delivery of blood or the effects of passive congestion from backup of venous blood.

GENETICS
Some congenital cardiac defects have a genetic basis in certain breeds.

INCIDENCE/PREVALENCE
Common syndrome in clinical practice

GEOGRAPHIC DISTRIBUTION
Syndrome seen everywhere, but prevalence of various causes varies with location

SIGNALMENT
Species Dogs and cats
Breed Predilections Vary with cause
Mean Age and Range Vary with cause
Predominant Sex Varies with cause

SIGNS

General Comments
• Signs vary with underlying cause and between species
• Pleural effusion without ascites and hepatomegaly is rare in dogs with R-CHF (right-sided congestive heart failure).
• Ascites without pleural effusion is rare in cats with R-CHF.

Historical Findings
• Weakness
• Lethargy
• Exercise intolerance.
• Abdominal distension
• Dyspnea, tachypnea

Physical Examination Findings
• Jugular venous distention
• Hepatojugular reflex
• Jugular pulse in some animals
• Hepatomegaly
• Ascites common in dogs and rare in cats with R-CHF

• Possible regurgitant murmur in tricuspid valve region or ejection murmur at left heart base (pulmonic stenosis)
• Muffled heart sounds if animal has pleural or pericardial effusion
• Weak femoral pulses
• Rapid, shallow respiration if animal has pleural effusion or severe ascites
• Peripheral edema (infrequent)

CAUSES

Pump (Myocardial) Failure of Right Ventricle
• Idiopathic dilated cardiomyopathy (DCM)
• Trypanosomiasis
• Doxorubicin cardiotoxicity

Pressure Overload to Right Ventricle
• Heartworm disease
• Chronic obstructive pulmonary disease
• Pulmonary thromboembolism
• Pulmonic stenosis
• Tetralogy of Fallot
• Right ventricular tumors
• Primary pulmonary hypertension

Impediment to Right Ventricular Filling
• Pericardial effusion
• Restrictive pericarditis
• Right atrial or caval masses (caval syndrome and tumors)
• Tricuspid stenosis
• Cortriatriatum dexter

Rhythm Disturbances
• Bradycardia, generally atrioventricular block
• Tachyarrhythmias, generally supraventricular tachycardia

RISK FACTORS
• No heartworm prophylaxis
• Offspring of animal with right-sided congenital cardiac defect
• Diseases that augment demand for cardiac output (e.g., hyperthyroidism, anemia, pregnancy)

DIAGNOSIS

DIFFERENTIAL DIAGNOSIS
• Must differentiate from other causes of pleural effusion and ascites; generally requires a complete diagnostic work-up to include CBC, biochemistry profile, heartworm test, thoracentesis or abdominocentesis with fluid analysis and cytologic examination and, sometimes, thoracic and abdominal ultrasound
• Animals with ascites or pleural effusion due to heart failure should have jugular venous distension.

CBC/BIOCHEMISTRY/URINALYSIS
• CBC usually normal; animal with heartworm disease may have eosinophilia

• Mild to moderately high alanine aminotransferase, aspartate aminotransferase, serum alkaline phosphatase because of passive congestion of the liver; bilirubin generally normal
• Prerenal azotemia in some animals

OTHER LABORATORY TESTS
Heartworm test may be positive

IMAGING

Thoracic Radiographic Findings
• Right heart enlargement in some animals
• Dilated caudal vena cava (diameter greater than the length of the vertebra directly above the heart)
• Pleural effusion (especially cats)
• Hepatosplenomegaly and possible ascites (especially dogs)

Echocardiography
• Findings vary with underlying cause. Especially useful for documenting congenital defect, cardiac mass, and pericardial effusion.
• Abdominal ultrasound reveals hepatomegaly with hepatic vein dilation and, possibly, ascites.

DIAGNOSTIC PROCEDURES

Electrocardiographic Findings
• Small complexes if animal has pericardial or pleural effusion
• Electrical alternans or elevated ST segment in animal with pericardial effusion
• Evidence of right heart enlargement (e.g., tall P waves in lead II, deep S waves in leads I, II, aVF, and right axis deviation)
• Atrial or ventricular arrhythmias
Note: ECG may be normal in patients with R-CHF

Abdominocentesis
• Analysis of ascitic fluid in patients with R-CHF generally reveals modified transudate with a TP>2.5 mg/dl.

Thoracentesis
• Cats with pleural effusion associated with R-CHF may have transudate, modified transudate, or chylous effusion.
• Dogs with pleural effusion and R-CHF may have transudate or modified transudate.

Central Venous Pressure
Central venous pressure is high (> 9 cm H_2O)

PATHOLOGIC FINDINGS
• Cardiac findings vary with disease
• Hepatomegaly in animals with centrolobular necrosis (chronic condition)

TREATMENT

APPROPRIATE HEALTH CARE
Most animals treated as outpatient unless dyspneic

CONGESTIVE HEART FAILURE, RIGHT-SIDED

NURSING CARE
Thoracentesis and abdominocentesis may be required periodically for patients no longer responsive to medical management or for those with severe dyspnea due to pleural effusion or ascites.

ACTIVITY
Restrict activity.

DIET
Restrict sodium moderately; severe sodium restriction is indicated for animals with advanced disease.

CLIENT EDUCATION
• With few exceptions (e.g., heartworm disease, arrhythmias, and idiopathic pericardial effusion), R-CHF is not curable.
• Most patients improve with initial treatment but often have recurrent failure.

SURGICAL CONSIDERATIONS
• Surgical intervention or balloon valvuloplasty indicated to treat certain congenital defects such as pulmonic stenosis.
• Pericardiocentesis or pericardectomy if animal has pericardial effusion.

MEDICATIONS

DRUGS OF CHOICE
Drugs should be administered only after a definitive diagnosis is made.

Diuretics
• Furosemide (1–2 mg/kg q8h–q24h) or other loop diuretic is the initial diuretic of choice. Diuretics are indicated to remove excess fluid accumulation (i.e., ascites or pleural effusion).
• Predisposes the patient to dehydration, prerenal azotemia, and electrolyte disturbances.
• Contraindicated in animals with pericardial disease

Digoxin
• Digoxin (dogs, 0.22 mg/M^2 q12h; cats, 0.01 mg/kg q48h) is used in animals with myocardial failure (eg, dilated cardiomyopathy).
• Digoxin is also indicated in animals with CHF that have supraventricular arrhythmias (e.g., sinus tachycardia, atrial fibrillation, and atrial or junctional tachycardia).

ACE Inhibitors
ACE inhibitors such as enalapril (0.5 mg/kg q12h–q24h) or benazepril (0.5 mg/kg q24h) may be helpful, especially if R-CHF results from L-CHF.

CONTRAINDICATIONS
Avoid vasodilators in patients with pericardial effusion or fixed outflow obstructions.

PRECAUTIONS
• ACE inhibitors and arterial dilators must be used with caution in patients with possible outflow obstructions.
• Patients with pulmonary hypertension and hypoxia are at higher risk than others for digoxin toxicity.
• ACE inhibitors and digoxin must be used cautiously in patients with renal disease.
• Animals with hypothyroidism are predisposed to digoxin toxicity, while hyperthyroidism diminishes digoxin effects.

POSSIBLE INTERACTIONS
• Combination of high-dose diuretics and ACE inhibitor may alter renal perfusion and cause azotemia.
• Combination diuretic therapy promotes risk of dehydration and electrolyte disturbances.
• Combination vasodilator therapy predisposes animal to hypotension—monitor closely in hospital when initiating treatment with a second vasodilator

ALTERNATIVE DRUGS
• Patients unresponsive to furosemide, vasodilator, and digoxin (if indicated) may benefit from combination diuretic therapy by adding spironolactone.
• Potassium supplementation if animal has hypokalemia; use potassium supplements cautiously in animals receiving ACE inhibitor or spironolactone.
• Treat arrhythmias if clinically indicated.
• Taurine supplementation in cats with DCM and dogs with DCM and taurine deficiency
• Carnitine supplementation may help some dogs with DCM (e.g., cocker spaniels and boxers).

FOLLOW-UP

PATIENT MONITORING
• Monitor renal status, electrolytes, hydration, respiratory rate and effort, body weight, and abdominal girth (dogs).
• If azotemia develops, reduce the diuretic dosage. If azotemia persists and the animal is also on an ACE inhibitor, reduce or discontinue this drug. If azotemia develops, reduce the digoxin dosage to avoid toxicity.
• Monitor ECG periodically to detect arrhythmias.
• Monitor digoxin concentrations. Normal values are 1–2 ng/ml for a serum sample obtained 8–10 hours after a dose is administered.

PREVENTION/AVOIDANCE
N/A

POSSIBLE COMPLICATIONS
• Pulmonary thromboembolism
• Arrhythmias
• Electrolyte imbalances
• Digoxin toxicity
• Azotemia and renal failure

EXPECTED COURSE AND PROGNOSIS
Prognosis varies with underlying cause.

MISCELLANEOUS

ASSOCIATED CONDITIONS
N/A

AGE RELATED FACTORS
• Congenital causes seen in young animals
• Degenerative heart conditions and neoplasia generally seen in old animals

ZOONOTIC POTENTIAL
N/A

PREGNANCY
N/A

SYNONYMS
N/A

SEE ALSO
• Diseases causing R-CHF
• Ascites
• Pleural Effusion
• Chylothorax

ABBREVIATIONS
ACE = angiotensin converting enzyme
DCM = dilated cardiomyopathy
L-CHF = left-sided congestive heart failure
R-CHF = right-sided congestive heart failure

Suggested Reading
Keene BW, Bonagura JD. Therapy of heart failure. In: Bonagura JD, ed. Current Veterinary Therapy XII. Philadelphia: WB Saunders, 1995.
Smith TW, Braunwald E, Kelly RA. The management of heart failure. In: Braunwald E, ed. Heart disease. A textbook of cardiovascular medicine. 4th ed. Philadelphia: WB Saunders, 1992.
International Small Animal Cardiac Health Council. Recommendations for the diagnosis of heart disease and the treatment of heart failure in small animals. In: Miller MS, Tilley LP, eds. Manual of canine and feline cardiology. 2nd ed. Philadelphia: WB Saunders, 1995.

Authors Francis W. K. Smith, Jr. and Bruce W. Keene
Consulting Editors Larry P. Tilley and Francis W. K. Smith, Jr.

DISEASES

CONJUNCTIVITIS—CATS

 BASICS

DEFINITION
Inflammation of the conjunctiva, the vascularized mucous membrane that covers the anterior portion of the globe (bulbar portion) and lines the lids and third eyelid (palpebral portion)

PATHOPHYSIOLOGY
May be primary (e.g., infectious) or secondary to an underlying ocular or systemic disease (e.g., glaucoma, uveitis, immune-mediated disease, neoplasia)

SYSTEMS AFFECTED
Ophthalmic—ocular with occasional lid involvement (e.g., blepharoconjunctivitis)

GENETICS
N/A

INCIDENCE/PREVALENCE
Common

GEOGRAPHIC DISTRIBUTION
N/A

SIGNALMENT
Species
Cats

Breed Predilections
Infectious—purebred cats seem predisposed

Mean Age and Range
Infections—most commonly affects young animals

Predominant Sex
N/A

SIGNS
- Blepharospasm
- Conjunctival hyperemia
- Ocular discharge—serous, mucoid, or mucopurulent
- Chemosis
- Bulbar or palpebral conjunctiva—may be primarily involved
- Upper respiratory infection—possible

CAUSES
Viral
- FHV—most common infectious cause; only one that leads to corneal changes (e.g., dendritic or geographic ulcers)
- Calicivirus

Bacterial
- Primary condition (i.e., not secondary to another condition such as KCS)—rare, except for chlamydia and mycoplasma
- Neonatal—accumulation of exudates, often with a bacterial or viral component; seen before lid separation

Immune-mediated
- Eosinophilic
- Related to systemic immune-mediated diseases—pemphigus

Neoplastic, Pseudoneoplastic
Rare; lymphosarcoma and squamous cell carcinoma most common

Secondary to Adnexal Disease
- Aqueous tear film deficiency
- May develop KCS as a result of scarring (see Keratoconjunctivitis Sicca)
- Lid diseases (e.g., entropion)—may lead to clinical signs of conjunctivitis
- Secondary to obstruction of the outflow portion of the nasolacrimal system—obstructed nasolacrimal duct

Secondary to Trauma or Environmental Causes
- Conjunctival foreign body
- Irritation from dust, chemicals, or ophthalmic medications

Secondary to Other Ocular Diseases
- Ulcerative keratitis
- Anterior uveitis
- Glaucoma

RISK FACTORS
N/A

 DIAGNOSIS

DIFFERENTIAL DIAGNOSIS
- Primary—must distinguish from condition that is secondary to other ocular diseases
- Intraocular disease—involvement of the bulbar conjunctiva with minimal or no involvement of the palpebral conjunctiva
- Primary or allergic—involvement of mainly the palpebral conjunctiva, sparing the bulbar conjunctiva; consider primary and secondary causes if both surfaces are involved.
- Must differentiate between conjunctival vessels (freely mobile and will blanch with sympathomimetics) and episcleral (deep) vessels (immobile and do not blanch with sympathomimetics)—episcleral congestion indicates intraocular disease; conjunctival hyperemia may be a sign of primary conjunctivitis or intraocular disease.

CBC/BIOCHEMISTRY/URINALYSIS
Normal, except with systemic disease

OTHER LABORATORY TESTS
- Infectious—consider serologic tests for FeLV and FIV; rule out underlying immunocompromise.

IMAGING
N/A

DIAGNOSTIC PROCEDURES
- Complete ophthalmic examination—rule out underlying intraocular diseases (e.g., uveitis and glaucoma).
- Thorough adnexal examination—rule out lid abnormalities and foreign bodies in cul-de-sacs or under nictitans.
- Nasolacrimal flush—considered to rule out nasolacrimal disease
- Aerobic bacterial culture and sensitivity—with mucopurulent discharge; specimens ideally taken before anything is placed in the eye (e.g., topical anesthetic, fluorescein, and flush) to prevent inhibition or dilution of bacterial growth
- Conjunctival cytology—may reveal a cause (rare); eosinophils and basophils may help diagnose allergic and eosinophilic conjunctivitis but are rarely seen with allergic conjunctivitis except on biopsy; may see degenerate neutrophils and intracytoplasmic bacteria, which indicate bacterial infection; may see inclusion bodies with chlamydial or mycoplasmal infection; rarely see FHV inclusions
- Conjunctival scrapings for FHV—use PCR or an IFA technique; but may note false-positive results with chronic disease; PCR more sensitive and test of choice; may note false-positive result if fluorescein staining is done before IFA testing
- Conjunctival scrapings for *Chlamydia*—use special stains, which are fairly reliable
- Viral culture—may help diagnose FHV
- Conjunctival biopsy—may be useful with mass lesions and immune-mediated disease; may help with chronic disease for which a definitive diagnosis has not been made

PATHOLOGIC FINDINGS
- Biopsy—typical signs of inflammation (e.g., neutrophils and lymphocytes); possibly infectious agents
- Histopathologic features of mass lesions (e.g., squamous cell carcinoma and lymphosarcoma)—consistent with similar lesions elsewhere

 TREATMENT

APPROPRIATE HEALTH CARE
- Primary—often outpatient
- Secondary to other diseases (e.g., uveitis and ulcerative keratitis)—may need hospitalization while the underlying problem is diagnosed and treated

ACTIVITY
- Primary—no restriction for most patients
- Suspected contact irritant or acute allergic disease—prevent (if possible) contact with the offending agent
- Suspected FHV—minimizing stress recommended
- Do not expose patients to susceptible animals.

DIET
Suspected underlying skin disease and/or food allergy—food elimination diet recommended

CLIENT EDUCATION
• If copious discharge is noted, instruct the client to clean the eyes before giving treatment.
• If solutions and ointments are both prescribed, instruct the client to use the solution(s) should be before the ointment(s).
• If several solutions are prescribed, instruct the client to wait several minutes between treatments.
• Instruct the client to call for instructions if the condition worsens, which indicates that the condition may not be responsive or may be progressing or that the animal may be having an adverse reaction to a prescribed medication.

SURGICAL CONSIDERATIONS
• Nasolacrimal duct obstruction—difficult; treatment often not recommended (see Epiphora)
• Conjunctival neoplasia—may require only local resection; may involve excision followed by β-irradiation, cryotherapy, radiofrequency hyperthermia, enucleation, or exenteration, depending on the type of tumor and the extent of involvement
• Symblepharon—may require surgical resection once active conjunctival infection is controlled
• Corneal sequestration—keratectomy may be required

MEDICATIONS
DRUGS OF CHOICE
Herpetic
• Condition usually mild and self-limiting
• Antiviral treatment—indicated for herpetic keratitis, before keratectomy for corneal sequestrums suspected to be related to FHV, and for severe intractable conjunctivitis; drug penetration into the conjunctiva (vs. the cornea) poor; optional; treatment may be directed at only controlling secondary bacterial infection.
• Trifluridine—recommended hourly the first day and then 5 times a day

Chlamydia or Mycoplasmal
• Tetracycline—topical q6h; continue for several days past resolution of all clinical signs; recurrence or reinfection common; systemic treatment recommended by some authors for difficult cases

Bacterial
Based on bacterial culture and sensitivity results.

Neonatal
• Carefully open the lid margins (medial to temporal), establish drainage, and treat with topical antibiotic and an antiviral for suspected

FHV.
• Symblepharon (adhesions between the conjunctival surfaces and possibly the cornea)—common sequela; may require surgical intervention.

Eosinophilic
• Topical corticosteroids—usually treatment; 0.1% dexamethasone generally effective when used three or four times daily; taper to the lowest effective dose
• Oral megestrol acetate—may help resistant condition; consider possible systemic side effects

CONTRAINDICATIONS
• Topical corticosteroids—avoid with known or suspected herpetic conjunctivitis, evidence shows that agents predispose the patient to corneal sequestrum formation; avoid if corneal ulceration is noted.
• Topical cyclosporine—best to avoid with known or suspected herpetic conjunctivitis, unless a topically administered antiviral is used concurrently.

PRECAUTIONS
• Topical aminoglycosides and antiviral medication may be irritating.
• Monitor all patients treated with topical corticosteroids for signs of corneal ulceration; discontinue agent immediately if corneal ulceration occurs.

POSSIBLE INTERACTIONS
N/A

ALTERNATIVE DRUGS
• Other topical antiviral medications—adenine arabinoside and idoxuridine; some authors recommend oral lysine, interferon, and acyclovir for chronic herpetic conjunctivitis.
• Other corticosteroids—1% prednisolone acetate; betamethasone; hydrocortisone

FOLLOW-UP
PATIENT MONITORING
Recheck shortly after beginning treatment (at 5–7 days); then recheck as needed.

PREVENTION/AVOIDANCE
• Treat any underlying disease that may be exacerbating the ocular disease—allergic or immune-mediated skin disease; KCS
• Prevent re-exposure to source of infection.
• Minimize stress for patients with herpetic conjunctivitis.
• Isolate patients with infectious conjunctivitis to prevent spread.
• Vaccination against viral causes—recommended; infection is still possible if the cat was exposed to an infectious agent before being vaccinated (e.g., FHV infection from an infected queen).

POSSIBLE COMPLICATIONS
• Corneal sequestration
• Symblepharon
• KCS

EXPECTED COURSE AND PROGNOSIS
• FVH—most patients become chronic carriers; episodes less common as patient matures; may see repeated exacerbations; tend to note more severe clinical signs at times of stress or immunocompromise
• Bacterial conjunctivitis—usually resolves with appropriate administration of antibiotics; if an underlying disease is found (e.g., KCS), resolution may depend on appropriate treatment and resolution of the disease.
• Immune mediated diseases (e.g., eosinophilic)—control not cure; may require chronic treatment at the lowest level possible

MISCELLANEOUS
ASSOCIATED CONDITIONS
FeLV and FIV—may predispose patient to the chronic carrier state of FHV conjunctivitis

AGE-RELATED FACTORS
FHV—tends to be more severe in kittens and in old cats with waning immunity

ZOONOTIC POTENTIAL
Chlamydia psittaci—low

PREGNANCY
• Use systemic antibiotics and corticosteroids with caution, if at all, in pregnant animals.
• Absorption of topically applied medications should be considered a possibility, and the benefits of treatment should be weighed against the possible complications.

SEE ALSO
Keratoconjunctivitis Sicca (KCS)

ABBREVIATIONS
• FeLV = feline leukemia virus
• FHV = feline herpesvirus
• FIV = feline immunodeficiency virus
• IFA = immunofluorescent antibody test
• KCS = keratoconjunctivitis sicca
• PCR = polymerase chain reaction

Suggested Readings
Glazè MB, Gelett KN, Feline ophthalmology. In Gelatt KN, ed. Veterinary ophthalmology 3rd ed. Philadelphia: Lippincott Williams and Wilkins 1999:997–1052
Nasisse MP. Manifestations, diagnosis, and treatment of ocular herpesvirus infection in the cat. Compend Contin Educ Pract Vet 1982;4:962–971.
Nasisse MP, Weigler BJ. The diagnosis of ocular feline herpesvirus infection. Vet Comp Ophthalmol 1997;7:44–51
Author Erin S. Champagne
Consulting Editor Paul E. Miller

DISEASES

CONJUNCTIVITIS—DOGS

BASICS

DEFINITION
Inflammation of the conjunctiva, the vascularized mucous membrane that covers the anterior portion of the globe (bulbar portion) and lines the lids and third eyelid (palpebral portion)

PATHOPHYSIOLOGY
• Primary—allergic; infectious; environmental; KCS
• Secondary to an underlying ocular or systemic disease—glaucoma; uveitis; immune-mediated disease; neoplasia

SYSTEMS AFFECTED
Ophthalmic—ocular with occasional lid involvement (e.g., blepharoconjunctivitis)

GENETICS
N/A

INCIDENCE/PREVALENCE
Common

GEOGRAPHIC DISTRIBUTION
N/A

SIGNALMENT

Species
Dogs

Breed Predilections
Breeds predisposed to allergic or immune-mediated skin diseases (e.g., atopy)—tend to have more problems with allergic conjunctivitis or dry eye

Mean Age and Range
N/A

Predominant Sex
N/A

SIGNS
• Blepharospasm
• Conjunctival hyperemia
• Ocular discharge—serous, mucoid, or mucopurulent
• Chemosis
• Follicle formation
• Bulbar or palpebral conjunctiva—may be primarily involved

CAUSES

Bacterial
• Primary condition (i.e., not secondary to another condition such as KCS)—rare
• Neonatal—an accumulation of exudates, often with a bacterial or viral component; seen before lid separation

Viral
Canine distemper virus

Immune-mediated
• Allergic—especially in atopic patients
• Follicular conjunctivitis
• Plasma cell conjunctivitis—especially in German shepherds
• Related to systemic immune-mediated diseases (e.g., pemphigus)

Neoplastic, Pseudoneoplastic
• Tumors involving conjunctiva—rare; include melanoma, hemangioma, hemangiosarcoma, lymphosarcoma, papilloma, and mast cell
• Pseudoneoplastic—nodular episcleritis (also called fibrous histiocytoma, ocular nodular granuloma, and conjunctival pseudotumor); most commonly seen in collies and mixed collies; believed to be immune-mediated; pink mass, usually located at the temporal limbus

Secondary to Adnexal Disease
• Aqueous tear film deficiency (see Keratoconjunctivitis Sicca)
• Lid diseases (e.g., entropion, ectropion, exaggerated cul-de-sac) and lash diseases (e.g., distichiasis, ectopic cilia)—may lead to clinical signs of conjunctivitis
• Secondary to obstruction of the outflow portion of the nasolacrimal system (e.g., obstructed nasolacrimal duct and imperforate punctum)

Secondary to Trauma or Environmental Causes
• Conjunctival foreign body
• Irritation—dust, chemicals, or ophthalmic medications

Secondary to Other Ocular Diseases
• Ulcerative keratitis
• Anterior uveitis
• Glaucoma

RISK FACTORS
N/A

DIAGNOSIS

DIFFERENTIAL DIAGNOSIS
• Primary—must distinguish from condition that is secondary to other ocular diseases
• Intraocular disease—involvement of the bulbar conjunctiva with minimal or no involvement of the palpebral conjunctiva
• Primary or allergic—involvement of mainly the palpebral conjunctiva sparing the bulbar conjunctiva; consider primary and secondary causes if both surfaces are involved.
• Must differentiate between conjunctival vessels (freely mobile and will blanch with sympathomimetic) and episcleral (deep) vessels (immobile and do not blanch with sympathomimetics), because episcleral congestion indicates intraocular disease, whereas conjunctival hyperemia may be a sign of primary conjunctivitis or intraocular disease.

CBC/BIOCHEMISTRY/URINALYSIS
Normal, except with systemic disease

OTHER LABORATORY TESTS
N/A

IMAGING
N/A

DIAGNOSTIC PROCEDURES
• Complete ophthalmic examination (Schirmer tear test)—rule out KCS.
• Fluorescein stain—rule out ulcerative keratitis.
• Intraocular pressures—rule out glaucoma.
• Examine for signs of anterior uveitis (e.g., hypotony, aqueous flare, and miosis).
• Thorough adnexal examination—rule out lid abnormalities, lash abnormalities, and foreign bodies in cul-de-sacs or under nictitans.
• Consider a nasolacrimal flush—rule out nasolacrimal disease.
• Aerobic bacterial culture and sensitivity—consider with mucopurulent discharge; ideally specimens taken before anything is placed in the eye (e.g., topical anesthetic, fluorescein, and flush) to prevent inhibition or dilution of bacterial growth; not routinely indicated for KCS and a mucopurulent discharge (secondary bacterial overgrowth almost certain)
• Conjunctival cytology—may reveal a cause (rare); eosinophils and basophils may help diagnose allergic and eosinophilic conjunctivitis but are rarely seen with allergic conjunctivitis except on biopsy; may see degenerate neutrophils and intracytoplasmic bacteria, which indicate bacterial infection; may see inclusion bodies (intracytoplasmic with distemper virus)
• Conjunctival biopsy—may be useful with mass lesions and immune-mediated disease; may help with chronic disease for which a definitive diagnosis has not been made
• Intradermal skin testing—may be helpful with suspected allergic conjunctivitis

PATHOLOGIC FINDINGS

• Biopsy—typical signs of inflammation (e.g., neutrophils and lymphocytes); may note infectious agents
• Histopathologic features of mass lesions (e.g., papilloma and mast cell tumor)—consistent with similar lesions elsewhere

TREATMENT

APPROPRIATE HEALTH CARE

• Primary—often outpatient
• Secondary to other diseases (e.g., uveitis and ulcerative keratitis)—may require hospitalization while the underlying problem is diagnosed and treated

ACTIVITY

• Primary—usually no restriction
• Suspected contact irritant or acute allergic disease—prevent (if possible) contact with the offending agent.
• Do not expose patients to susceptible animals

DIET

Suspected underlying skin disease and/or food allergy—food elimination diet recommended

CLIENT EDUCATION

• If copious discharge is noted, instruct the client to clean the eyes before giving treatment.
• If solutions and ointments are both prescribed, instruct the client to use the solution(s) before the ointment(s).
• If several solutions are prescribed, instruct the client to wait several minutes between treatments.
• Instruct the client to call for instructions if the condition worsens, which indicates that the condition may not be responsive or may be progressing or that the animal may be having an adverse reaction to a prescribed medication.
• Inform client that an Elizabethan collar should be placed on the patient if self-trauma occurs.

SURGICAL CONSIDERATIONS

• Nasolacrimal duct obstruction—difficult; treatment often not recommended (see Epiphora)
• Conjunctival neoplasia—may require only local resection; may involve excision followed by β-irradiation, cryotherapy, radiofrequency hyperthermia, enucleation, or exenteration, depending on the type of tumor and the extent of involvement

MEDICATIONS

DRUGS OF CHOICE

Bacterial

• Based on bacterial culture and sensitivity results
• Initial treatment—broad-spectrum topical antibiotic or based on results of cytologic examination while waiting culture results; may try empirical treatment, performing a culture only if patient is refractory to treatment
• Topical triple antibiotic or chloramphenicol—cocci seen on cytologic examination
• Gentamicin or tobramycin—rods seen on cytologic examination
• Ciprofloxacin—q6–12h, depending on severity; limited bacterial resistance (some streptococci are resistant); may be useful for severe bacterial conjunctivitis
• Systemic antibiotics—occasionally indicated, especially for more generalized disease (e.g., pyoderma)

Neonatal

Carefully open the lid margins (medial to temporal), establish drainage, and treat with topical antibiotic.

Immune-mediated

• Depends on severity
• Topical corticosteroids—0.1% dexamethasone; improve clinical signs of allergic, follicular, and plasma cell conjunctivitis; improvement often temporary
• Treatment of any underlying disease (e.g., atopy) often improves clinical signs.

CONTRAINDICATIONS

Topical corticosteroids—avoid if corneal ulceration is noted.

PRECAUTIONS

• Topical aminoglycosides—may be irritating
• Topical corticosteroids—monitor all patients carefully for signs of corneal ulceration; discontinue agent immediately if corneal ulceration occurs.

POSSIBLE INTERACTIONS

N/A

ALTERNATIVE DRUGS

Other corticosteroids—1% prednisolone acetate; betamethasone; hydrocortisone

FOLLOW-UP

PATIENT MONITORING

Recheck shortly after beginning treatment (i.e., 5–7 days); then recheck as needed.

PREVENTION/AVOIDANCE

Treat any underlying disease that may be exacerbating the condition (e.g., allergic or immune-mediated skin disease; KCS).

POSSIBLE COMPLICATIONS

N/A

EXPECTED COURSE AND PROGNOSIS

• Bacterial—usually resolves with appropriate antibiotics; may depend on resolution of underlying disease (e.g., KCS)
• Immune-mediated disease—tend to be controlled and not cured; may require chronic treatment at the lowest level possible

MISCELLANEOUS

ASSOCIATED CONDITIONS

• Atopy
• Pyoderma

AGE-RELATED FACTORS

N/A

ZOONOTIC POTENTIAL

N/A

PREGNANCY

• Use systemic antibiotics and corticosteroids with caution, if at all, in pregnant animals.
• Consider absorption of topically applied medications; weigh benefits of treatment against possible complications.

SEE ALSO

• Keratoconjunctivitis Sicca (KCS)
• Red Eye

ABBREVIATION

KCS = keratoconjunctivitis sicca

Suggested Reading

Hendrix DVH, Diseases and surgery of the canine conjunctive. In: Gelatt KN, ed. Veterinary ophthalmology 3rd ed. Philadelphia: Lippincott Williams and Wilkins 1999: 619–634.

Author Erin S. Champagne
Consulting Editor Paul E. Miller

DISEASES

CONTACT DERMATITIS

 BASICS

OVERVIEW
• Irritant contact dermatitis (ICD) and allergic contact dermatitis (ACD)—two rare and distinctly different pathophysiologic syndromes with similar clinical signs • ICD—results from direct damage to keratinocytes by exposure to a particular compound; damaged keratinocytes induce an inflammatory response directed at the skin. • ACD—an immunologic event requiring sensitization, memory, and elicitation: Langerhans cells process antigens that penetrate the skin and present them to naive T cells within lymph nodes; sensitized T cell clones (memory cells) then proliferate and circulate throughout the body; Langerhans cells encounter the antigens again and present them to sensitized T cells, resulting in an immunologic response.

SIGNALMENT
• Dogs and cats • ICD—occurs at any age as a direct result of the irritant nature of the offending compound • ACD—rare in young animals; most animals are chronically exposed to the antigen; extremely rare in cats, except when exposed to D-limonene-containing insecticides • Predisposed to ACD—German shepherds • Increased risk to ACD (unsubstantiated)—French poodles, wire-haired fox terriers, Scottish terriers, West Highland white terriers, and golden retrievers

SIGNS

Lesions
• Location depends on the way in which the antigen is contacted; commonly limited to glabrous skin and regions frequently in contact with the ground (chin, ventral neck, sternum, ventral abdomen, inguinum, perineum, scrotum, and ventral contact regions of the tail and interdigital areas) • The thick hair coat of dogs is an effective barrier against contactants. • In classic cases, extreme erythroderma stops abruptly at the hairline. • Initially consist of erythema and swelling, leading to papules and plaques; vesicles are uncommon.

Others
• Reactions to topical medications (most often otic preparations) are usually localized; generalized reactions, resulting from shampoos or insecticide sprays, are less common. • Pruritus—moderate to severe; severe is most common. • A seasonal incidence may indicate that the offending antigen is a plant or outdoor compound.

CAUSES & RISK FACTORS
• Inflammatory dermatitis—may increase the penetration of antigens through the skin; thus may facilitate ACD. • Reported offending substances—plants, mulch, cedar chips; fabrics, rugs and carpets, plastics, rubber, leather, metal, concrete; soaps, detergents, floor waxes, carpet and litter deodorizers; herbicides, fertilizers, insecticides (including newer topical flea treatments), flea collars; topical preparations and medications

 DIAGNOSIS

DIFFERENTIAL DIAGNOSIS
• Atopy • Food allergy • Drug eruptions • Parasite hypersensitivity or infestation • Insect bites • Pyoderma • *Malassezia* dermatitis • Dermatophytosis • Demodicosis • Lupus erythematosus • Seborrheic dermatitis • Solar dermatitis • Thermal injuries • Trauma from rough surfaces

CBC/BIOCHEMISTRY/URINALYSIS
No abnormalities

OTHER LABORATORY TESTS
N/A

IMAGING
N/A

DIAGNOSTIC PROCEDURES
• Closed-patch testing—sometimes helpful (corticosteroids and NSAIDs must be discontinued 3–6 weeks before testing); use materials directly from the environment or a standard patch test kit for humans (Hermal, Oak Hill, NY) applied to the skin under a bandage for 48 hr. • Best diagnostic test—eliminate contact irritant or antigen, follow with provocative exposure testing • Bacterial cultures to define secondary pyoderma may be performed, if needed. • Because the hair coat can protect the skin from contact with antigen, clipping a patch of hair in a nonaffected region should result in development of a local reaction.

PATHOLOGIC FINDINGS
• Skin biopsies—intraepidermal vesiculation and spongiosis; superficial dermal edema with perivascular mononuclear cell infiltrate in ICD and ACD; polymorphonuclear cell infiltrate in ICD; leukocyte exocytosis common
• Histologic findings—vary with duration of antigen contact
• Primary changes—often obscured by secondary changes owing to pruritus and excoriation

 TREATMENT

• Eliminate offending substance(s).
• Bathe with hypoallergenic shampoos to remove antigen from the skin.
• Create mechanical barriers, if possible—socks, T-shirts, restriction from environment

MEDICATIONS

DRUGS
• Systemic corticosteroids—prednisone (0.25–0.5 mg/kg PO q24h for 3–5 days; then q48h for 2 weeks)
• Topical corticosteroids for focal lesions
• Recent studies report success in dogs with pentoxifylline (10 mg/kg PO q12h).

CONTRAINDICATIONS/POSSIBLE INTERACTIONS
Pentoxifylline—do not administer with alkylating agents, cisplatin, and amphotericin B; cimetidine may increase serum levels of pentoxifylline.

 FOLLOW-UP

PREVENTION/AVOIDANCE
Remove offending substances from the environment

EXPECTED COURSE AND PROGNOSIS

ICD
• Acute condition—may occur after only one exposure; can be manifested within 24 hr of exposure. • Steroids are rarely helpful.
• Lesions resolve 1–2 days after irritant removal.

ACD
• Requires months to years of exposure for the hypersensitivity to develop • Re-exposure results in the development of clinical signs 3–5 days following exposure; signs may persist for several weeks. • Responds well to corticosteroids; but the pruritus returns after discontinuation if the antigenic stimulus has not been removed. • Hyposensitization is disappointing. • Prognosis—good if the allergen is identified and removed; poor if the allergen is not identified, which may then require lifelong treatment

 MISCELLANEOUS

ABBREVIATIONS
• ACD = allergic contact dematitis • ICD = irritant contact dermatitis

Suggested Reading

Walder EJ, Conroy JD. Contact dermatitis in dogs and cats: pathogenesis, histopathology, experimental induction, and case reports. Vet Dermatol 1994;5:149–162.

Authors Alexander H. Werner and Margaret Swartout

Consulting Editor Karen Helton Rhodes

DISEASES

COONHOUND PARALYSIS (IDIOPATHIC POLYRADICULONEURITIS)

BASICS

DEFINITION
• Acute inflammation of multiple nerve roots and peripheral nerves in dogs, with or without a previous history of contact with a raccoon
• Proposed animal model for Guillain-Barré syndrome in humans

PATHOPHYSIOLOGY
• Largely unknown
• Suspected immune-mediated disease

SYSTEMS AFFECTED
Nervous
• PNS—most severe involvement in the ventral nerve roots and ventral root components of the spinal nerves
• Cranial nerves—in some patients; primarily nerves VII and X
• Respiratory paralysis—secondary to intercostal and phrenic nerve involvement in some patients

GENETICS
No proven basis

INCIDENCE/PREVALENCE
• Most commonly recognized polyneuropathy in dogs in North America
• Incidence low

GEOGRAPHIC DISTRIBUTION
• Coonhound paralysis—relative to the distribution of racoons (e.g., North and Central America; parts of South America)
• ACIP—worldwide

SIGNALMENT
Breed Predilections
• Coonhound paralysis—coonhounds; any breed in contact with raccoons susceptible
• ACIP—none

Mean Age and Range
N/A

Predominant Sex
N/A

SIGNS
General Comments
ACIP—neurologic signs and progression of disease same as listed, except for initial encounter with a racoon

Historical Findings
• Appear 7–14 days after contact with a raccoon
• Stiff-stilted gait in all four limbs—initially

• Rapid progression to a flaccid lower motor neuron tetraparesis to tetraplegia

Physical Examination Findings
• Usually symmetrical
• Generalized hyporeflexia to areflexia, hypotonia to atonia, and severe neurogenic muscle atrophy
• Pelvic limbs more severely affected than are thoracic limbs in a few patients
• Respiration—labored in severely affected dogs; occasional progression to respiratory paralysis; aphonia or dysphonia common
• Facial paresis—in a few patients
• Pain—sensation intact; hyperesthesia common, because of variable dorsal nerve root involvement
• Motor dysfunction—always predominates; even tetraplegic patient can usually wag its tail
• Appetite and water consumption—usually normal
• Urination and defecation—normal
• Initial progression—usually occurs over 4–5 days; maximum progression can take up to 10 days.

CAUSES
• Coonhound paralysis—contact with a raccoon; perhaps more important, contact with raccoon saliva
• ACIP—none proven; possibly previous respiratory or gastrointestinal viral or bacterial infection or vaccination

RISK FACTORS
• Coonhound paralysis—coonhounds tend to be predisposed primarily because of the nature of their activities; previous disease does not confer immunity and may increase risk of redevelopment; multiple bouts not uncommon
• ACIP—unknown

DIAGNOSIS

DIFFERENTIAL DIAGNOSIS
Other acute polyneuropathy
• Distal denervating disease
• Botulism
• Tick paralysis
• Generalized (diffuse) or multifocal myelopathy (involving both cervical and lumbosacral intumescences)

CBC/BIOCHEMISTRY/URINALYSIS
Usually normal

OTHER LABORATORY TESTS
• Serum immunoglobulins—high serum IgG but not IgM in some patients

• Immunologic—serum reaction to raccoon saliva on ELISA; dogs with coonhound paralysis have a strong positive reaction that decreases in intensity over time; dogs without disease but with racoon contact have a strong positive reaction; dogs with ACIP but with no raccoon contact have a negative reaction.

IMAGING
N/A

DIAGNOSTIC PROCEDURES
CSF Analysis
• Lumbar—high protein without an increase in leukocytes at all stages of disease
• Cerebellomedullary—mildly high protein in patients examined after the acute stages of disease
• Albumin leakage across a suspected disrupted blood–brain barrier is the primary cause of the protein increase.
• Most patients have no intrathecal production of immunoglobulin.

Electrodiagnostics
• Generalized spontaneous activity, the severity of which depends on the time of examination after disease onset and the severity of neurologic signs
• Markedly low compound muscle action potential amplitudes after motor nerve stimulation
• F waves—late waves that indicate proximal motor nerve and ventral nerve root function; common abnormalities: increased minimum latencies, increased ratio, low amplitudes
• Motor nerve conduction velocities—usually within normal range; severely affected patients may have mildly low values.
• Sensory nerve function—usually normal
• These abnormalities provide evidence of severe peripheral axonopathy, along with axonal involvement and demyelination in the ventral nerve roots.

PATHOLOGIC FINDINGS
• Ventral nerve roots and the ventral root components of the spinal nerves—develop the most severe lesions, consisting of various degrees of axonal degeneration, paranodal and segmental demyelination, and leukocyte infiltration (predominantly monocytes and macrophages, with scattered groups of lymphocytes and plasma cells)
• Peripheral nerves—similarly affected, although to a lesser degree
• Dorsal nerve roots—much less severely affected

COONHOUND PARALYSIS (IDIOPATHIC POLYRADICULONEURITIS)

TREATMENT

APPROPRIATE HEALTH CARE
• Inpatient—closely monitor patients in the progressive stage of the disease (especially during the first 4 days) for respiratory problems.
• Severe respiratory compromise—intensive care; ventilatory support, as required
• Intravenous fluid therapy—lactated Ringer solution; necessary only if patient is dehydrated because of an inability to reach water
• Outpatient—stabilized patient, after initial diagnostic confirmation of disease

NURSING CARE
• Patients are usually able to eat and drink if they can reach the food and water; often must be hand fed because of paralysis
• Intensive physiotherapy—important to decrease muscle atrophy
• Frequent turning and excellent padding—essential to prevent pressure sores

ACTIVITY
Encourage as much movement as possible; many patients are tetraplegic

DIET
• No restrictions
• Make sure patient is able to reach food and water.
• Cervical weakness—may need to hand feed patient

CLIENT EDUCATION
• Inform client that good nursing care is essential.
• Discuss the importance of preventing pressure sores and urine scalding and of limiting the degree of muscle atrophy by diligent physiotherapy (e.g., passive limb movement and swimming as the patient's strength begins to improve).
• Inform client that the patient needs soft, resilient bedding (straw is excellent) that must be kept clean and free of urine and feces, frequent turning (every 3–4 hr), frequent bathing, and adequate nutrition.

SURGICAL CONSIDERATIONS
N/A

MEDICATIONS

DRUGS OF CHOICE
• None proven effective
• Immunoglobulin—1 g/kg IV daily for 2 consecutive days or 0.4 g/kg IV daily for 4–5 consecutive days; given early may decrease severity and/or shorten recovery time

CONTRAINDICATIONS
Corticosteroids—do not improve clinical signs or shorten course of disease; may reduce survival in humans with Guillain-Barré syndrome

PRECAUTIONS
N/A

POSSIBLE INTERACTIONS
N/A

ALTERNATIVE DRUGS
N/A

FOLLOW-UP

PATIENT MONITORING
• Outpatient—keep in close contact with client regarding complications or changes in the patient's condition.
• Urinalysis—perform periodically to check for cystitis in tetraplegic or severely tetraparetic patients.
• Ideally, re-evaluate at least every 2–3 weeks.

PREVENTION/AVOIDANCE
• Coonhound paralysis—avoid contact with raccoons; often not feasible because of coonhounds' environment and primary use as raccoon hunters
• ACIP—none

POSSIBLE COMPLICATIONS
• Respiratory paralysis—in progressive stage of the disease
• Pressure sores, urine scalding, and cystitis—common in chronically recumbent dogs

EXPECTED COURSE AND PROGNOSIS
• Most recover fully.
• Mild residual neurologic deficits—duration of several weeks in mildly to moderately affected dogs; duration of 3–4 months with severe disease

MISCELLANEOUS

ASSOCIATED CONDITIONS
N/A

AGE-RELATED FACTORS
N/A

ZOONOTIC POTENTIAL
N/A

PREGNANCY
Unknown effect on the fetuses of an affected bitch

SYNONYM
• Coondog paralysis

SEE ALSO
• Botulism
• Peripheral neuropathies (Polyneuropathies)
• Tick Bite Paralysis

ABBREVIATIONS
• ACIP = acute canine idiopathic polyradiculoneuritis
• CSF = cerebrospinal fluid
• ELISA = enzyme-linked immunosorbent assay
• PNS = peripheral nervous system

Suggested Reading

Cuddon PA. Acute canine idiopathic polyradiculoneuropathy—electrophysiology, CSF analysis, and immunology. Paper presented at the eighth annual symposium of the European Society of Veterinary Neurologists, Limoges, France, 1994.

Cummings JF, Hass DC. Coonhound paralysis: an acute idiopathic polyradiculoneuritis resembling the Landry-Guillain-Barré syndrome. J Neurol Sci 1967;4:51–81.

Cummings JF, de Lahunta A, Holmes DF, Schultz RD. Coonhound paralysis: further clinical studies and electron microscopic observations. Acta Neuropathol 1982;56:167–178.

Northington JW, Brown MJ. Acute canine idiopathic polyneuropathy: a Guillain-Barré-like syndrome in dogs. J Neurol Sci 1982;56:259–273.

Author Paul A. Cuddon
Consulting Editor Joane M. Parent

DISEASES

COPPER HEPATOPATHY

BASICS

DEFINITION
• Hepatic accumulation of copper, causing chronic hepatitis and cirrhosis • Information presented is largely derived from affected Bedlington terriers.

PATHOPHYSIOLOGY
• Copper—absorbed in the small intestine; extracted and stored in the liver; excreted via the biliary system • Pathologic hepatic accumulation—owing to a genetic trait or secondary to cholestasis; causes oxidative damage to cell and organelle membranes, resulting in cell death • Episodic release—may cause acute severe hemolysis concurrent with fulminant hepatic necrosis

SYSTEMS AFFECTED
• Hepatobiliary—focal hepatitis leads to diffuse chronic hepatitis, culminating in cirrhosis. • Hemic/Lymphatic/Immune—hemolytic anemia (rare) with acute hepatocellular necrosis • Renal/Urologic—may note proximal renal tubular acidosis

GENETICS
• Bedlington terriers—autosomal recessive trait • West Highland white terriers—proposed; severity of accumulation does not correlate with age or severity of hepatic damage.

INCIDENCE/PREVALENCE
• Bedlington terriers—prevalence decreasing owing to vigilant testing; previously, two-thirds affected or carriers • Other dogs—occasionally develop condition as a presumed mutation • West Highland white terriers—prevalence of high hepatic copper; low incidence of disease

GEOGRAPHIC DISTRIBUTION
Bedlington terriers—worldwide

SIGNALMENT

Species
Dogs; very rare in cats

Breed Predilections
• Bedlington terriers • West Highland white terriers • Doberman pinchers and other breeds with chronic active hepatitis—accumulate hepatocellular copper as a sequela of cholestasis

Mean Age and Range
• Bedlington terriers—copper accumulates over time; peaks at about 6 years; may be clinically affected at any age; young may be asymptomatic or have acute or recurrent hepatic necrosis; middle-aged to old have progressive chronic hepatitis. • West Highland white terriers—maximum copper accumulation at 6 months; may develop liver disease at any age; may not develop disease

Predominant Sex
None

SIGNS

General Comments
Bedlington terriers—three clinical groups of patients: (1) young adults with peracute severe signs; (2) middle-aged to old adults with progressive clinical signs; (2) subclinically affected patients

Historical Findings
• Group 1—acute lethargy; anorexia; vomiting; rapidly deteriorating clinical signs, often culminating in death; may develop hemolytic crisis • Group 2—chronic history of waxing and waning lethargy, anorexia, weight loss, vomiting, diarrhea, and polydipsia or polyuria; later may note abdominal distention; jaundice; spontaneous bleeding; hepatic encephalopathy

Physical Examination Findings
• Group 1—lethargy; dehydration; hepatomegaly with or without jaundice; pale mucous membranes with anemia; hemoglobinuria with hemolytic crisis • Group 2—weight loss; ascites; jaundice; microhepatia; may note melena and bruising

CAUSES
• Abnormal hepatic copper binding or transport, leading to impaired biliary excretion • Cholestasis that impairs biliary copper excretion

RISK FACTORS
• High-copper diet • Chronic hepatobiliary disease

DIAGNOSIS

DIFFERENTIAL DIAGNOSIS

Acute Disease
• Infectious diseases affecting the liver—infectious canine adenovirus 1; Tyzzer disease; leptospirosis; bacterial septicemia • Acute hepatic necrosis • Hepatic abscess • Drug- or toxin-induced liver injury • Acute pancreatitis • Hepatic lymphoma • Autoimmune hemolytic anemia • Zinc intoxication

Chronic Disease
• Chronic hepatitis • Drug- or toxin-induced hepatic injury • Infectious hepatitis • Idiopathic chronic hepatitis • Cholangiohepatitis • Chronic biliary tract obstruction • Chronic fibrosing pancreatitis • Congenital portosystemic shunt • Hepatic neoplasia • Metastatic neoplasia or carcinomatosis • Lobular dissecting hepatitis

CBC/BIOCHEMISTRY/URINALYSIS

CBC
• May be normal • Acute hemolysis—regenerative anemia; leukocytosis, neutrophilia; left shift • Chronic progressive disease—microcytic or normocytic nonregenerative anemia

Biochemistry
• Bedlington terriers—suspect copper toxicity with high liver enzyme activities (e.g., ALT, AST, and ALP) but no clinical signs • Asymptomatic patients—normal liver enzymes in up to one-third • Chronically affected patients—may note hypoalbuminemia, hyperglobulinemia (β- and γ-globulins), low BUN, hypoglycemia, and hypokalemia

Urinalysis
• May be normal • Proximal renal tubular acidosis (Fanconi syndrome)—glucosuria • Hemolysis or hepatic necrosis—granular casts

OTHER LABORATORY TESTS
• High fasting and postprandial bile acids • Prolonged clotting times—PT, APTT, ACT, and/or buccal mucosal bleeding time • Blood copper concentration—no diagnostic value • Hepatic copper quantification—essential for definitive diagnosis; must be evaluated in light of histology • Microsatellite assay of DNA

IMAGING
• Radiography—hepatomegaly in acutely affected Bedlington terriers; microhepatia in chronically affected patients; poor abdominal detail with ascites; abdominal radiographs usually unremarkable • Ultrasonography—uniformly normal echogenic liver pattern with early disease; hyperechoic to mixed echogenic liver pattern in chronically affected patients; ascites

DIAGNOSTIC PROCEDURES

Hepatic Copper Determination
• Sample—fresh, formalin-fixed, or paraffin-embedded tissue (extracted); most laboratories can quantify copper in 1 g of tissue, some on a single full needle core biopsy • Concentration—must be expressed on a dry weight basis; normal: < 400 μg/g dry liver tissue; Bedlington terriers: 850–13,000 μg/g; with chronic hepatitis and cirrhosis: up to 3,000 μg/g; west Highland white terriers: up to 3,500 μg/g

Other
• Biopsy—same tissue submitted for copper quantification • Cytology—special histologic stains (rubeanic acid, rhodamine, Timms)—mark copper and its binding protein; may be used to estimate degree of hepatic retention • Fine-needle aspirate—may reveal abnormal hepatic copper stores that appear as small poorly stained, cytosolic inclusions on routine Wright-Giemsa preparations

PATHOLOGIC FINDINGS

Gross
• Peracute disease—may note enlarged, soft liver with large surface discoloration • Chronic disease—nodular surface contour and firm irregular texture • Cirrhosis—microhepatia and regenerative nodules

Histologic
• Asymptomatic disease—few changes; visible pink hepatocellular granules consistent with copper on routine H&E staining • Symptomatic disease—various degrees of hepato-

cellular and periportal inflammation and necrosis; focal hepatic necrosis progressing to chronic hepatitis and cirrhosis

TREATMENT

APPROPRIATE HEALTH CARE
• Usually outpatient • Inpatient—severely affected patients for supportive care

NURSING CARE
• Severe disease—fluids based on tolerance for sodium, need for chloride and potassium, and ability to regulate blood glucose • Ascites—do not use 0.9% NaCl. • Fulminant hepatic necrosis—do not use lactated Ringer, owing to diminished lactate metabolism • Hypophosphatemia (< 2 mg/dL)—must be corrected; intravenous potassium phosphate • Hypoglycemia (dogs)—initial administration of glucose as a 2.5% solution combined with half-strength polyionic fluids; then titrated • Hepatic encephalopathy—cleansing and retention enemas as necessary • B complex vitamins—2 mL/L fluids

ACTIVITY
Normal unless anemic

DIET
• Low-copper—initiate before clinical signs develop; balanced, homemade foods without copper-rich items (e.g., organ meats) or supplements containing copper; not always feasible • Protein—normal unless protein intolerance; with hepatic encephalopathy restricted and combined with lactulose, metronidazole, and/or neomycin

CLIENT EDUCATION
• Advise client to allow screening of all Bedlington terriers via DNA markers or liver biopsy; if DNA test is positive; advise client to allow blood testing and appropriate treatment with zinc acetate. • Advise client to allow screening of other high risk breeds with liver enzymes or liver biopsy. • Warn client that copper chelation is essential for several months, followed by lifelong zinc administration • Advise client to cull affected Bedlington terriers from breeding.

SURGICAL CONSIDERATIONS
• Tissue biopsy—only for Bedlington terriers that have not been tested for kindred satellite markers • Liver biopsy—establish severity of disease in chronically affected patients; demonstrate applicability of DNA satellite markers for a particular kindred; with severe disease, perform using the least invasive method (ultrasound guided or laparoscopic).

MEDICATIONS

DRUGS OF CHOICE
• Hepatic encephalopathy—lactulose (1 mL/kg PO q8h) and metronidazole (7.5 mg/kg PO q8–12h), or ampicillin (20 mg/kg q8h) or neomycin (22 mg/kg q8h) • D-penicillamine—chelates and promotes urinary excretion of copper; may have other protective effects; 10–15 mg/kg PO q12h; give 1 hr before feeding; use a minimum of 2 months in all affected Bedlington terriers and other patients with a copper concentration > 3000 μg/g dry liver weight; long-term, continuous use necessary to remove copper from the liver if chelation is the primary mode of therapy (removes 1000 μg/g dry weight per year) • 2,2,2 tetramine (trientine)—if patient is intolerant of D-penicillamine; used at a similar dosage; more avid copper chelator; difficult to acquire Zinc acetate (Bedlington terriers)—elemental zinc, 50–10 mg PO q12h; give 60 min before feeding to induce enteric metallothionein; irreversibly binds enteric metals; augments detoxification of hepatocellular copper; facilitates copper excretion in urine and bile; monitor serum concentrations to avoid toxicosis (see below); may not be effective in patients with high hepatic copper concentrations • Vitamin E—α-tocopherol, 10 IU/kg per day PO • S-adenosylmethionine—10–20 mg/kg PO per day (200–600 IU/day) • Ursodeoxycholic acid—10–15 mg/kg PO q24h or divided q12h

CONTRAINDICATIONS
• Compromised hepatic function—avoid drugs that rely on an enterohepatic circulation, require first-pass hepatic extraction, or biotransformation for activation or elimination • D-penicillamine—do not administer with zinc; combination makes each drug ineffective. • Avoid vitamin C (ascorbate)—known to promote oxidant damage owing to transition metals (iron and copper)

ALTERNATIVE DRUGS
2,3,2 tetramine—15 mg/kg PO q12h; a more potent chelator; not commercially available

FOLLOW-UP

PATIENT MONITORING
• Liver enzymes—quarterly • Body weight and condition—guide nitrogen intake • Hepatic copper concentration—sequential; assess treatment efficacy • Serum zinc concentration—every 2 weeks until stable; then quarterly (desirable range: 400–600 μg/dL); avoid approach to 1000 μg/dL (hemolytic)

PREVENTION/AVOIDANCE
Do not breed Bedlington terriers with the copper hematotoxicosis gene.

POSSIBLE COMPLICATIONS
• D-penicillamine—may cause anorexia and vomiting (avoid by introducing at the low end of the dosage for the first week); if vomiting occurs, reduce the dose and administer in a small piece of meat (reduces bioavailability by 50%); may rarely cause an autoimmune-like vesicular disorder of the mucocutaneous junctions (resolves with drug withdrawal) • Zinc—high serum concentrations (> 1000 μg/dL) may cause hemolytic anemia.

EXPECTED COURSE AND PROGNOSIS
• Acutely affected young patients with fulminant hepatic necrosis and in old dogs with cirrhosis—poor prognosis • Young dogs with mild to moderate hepatic necrosis—usually respond to symptomatic treatment and chelation • Detected and treated (chelation; then zinc acetate) before hepatic inflammation and necrosis develop—good prognosis

MISCELLANEOUS

ASSOCIATED CONDITIONS
• Proximal renal tubular transport defects • Hemolysis

AGE-RELATED FACTORS
• Tissue copper concentrations taken at 6 and 15 months—help decide need for chelation and lifelong zinc acetate • Homozygously affected Bedlington terriers—high copper at 6 months and higher at 15 months • Heterozygously affected Bedlington terriers—higher copper at 6 months than at 15 months • West Highland white terriers—highest concentration at 6 month; concentration not predictive of liver disease

ZOONOTIC POTENTIAL
None

PREGNANCY
N/A

SYNONYMS
• Bedlington hepatitis • Chronic active hepatitis • Chronic copper toxicity • Copper toxicosis

SEE ALSO
Hepatitis, Chronic Active

ABBREVIATIONS
• ALP = alkaline phosphatase • ALT = alanine transferase • APTT = activated partial thromboplastin time • AST = aspartate aminotransferase • H&E = hematoxylin and eosin • PT = prothrombin time

Suggested Reading
Center SA. Chronic hepatitis, cirrhosis, breed-specific hepatopathies, copper storage hepatopathy, suppurative hepatitis, granulomatous hepatitis, and idiopathic hepatic fibrosis. In: Guilford WG, Center SA, Strombeck DR, et al., eds. Strombeck's small animal gastroenterology. 3rd ed. Philadelphia: Saunders, 1996:705–765.
Author David C. Twedt
Consulting Editor Sharon A. Center

CORNEAL DEGENERATIONS AND INFILTRATIONS

 BASICS

OVERVIEW
• Corneal degeneration—secondary, non-inherited, unilateral or bilateral condition characterized by lipid or calcareous deposition within the corneal stroma and sometimes the epithelium
• Arcus lipoides corneae—bilateral, not necessarily symmetrical infiltration of lipid in the cornea associated with systemic hyper-lipoproteinemia

SIGNALMENT
• Degeneration—dogs; uncommon in cats; may affect any breed of any age
• Arcus lipoides corneae—middle-aged or old dogs; rare in cats; occurs most often in dogs that are hyperlipoproteinemic secondary to hypothyroidism

SIGNS
Degeneration or Infiltration
• Some degree of opacity of the cornea
• Usually some degree of inflammation, neo-vascularization, or pigmentation concurrent with the lipid and calcium deposits
• Deposits—gray or white; may be circular, band-shaped, irregular, or any combination thereof
• Cornea—may appear roughened
• Associated ocular conditions—corneal scars; KCS; exposure keratitis; chronic uveitis; phthisis bulbi

Arcus Lipoides Corneae
• Bilateral, silvery or blue-gray, and usually complete annulus (or ring) around the peripheral cornea
• Corneal vascularization—varies
• Clear area (or lucid interval) between the affected cornea and the limbus common

CAUSES & RISK FACTORS
Degeneration
• Hyperlipoproteinemia—may modify course once it has developed; may increase severity; alone not sufficient to cause corneal deposits
• External eye disease (dogs)—common in brachycephalic breeds; may be at higher risk

Arcus Lipoides Corneae
• Hyperlipoproteinemia—secondary to hypothyroidism increases risk; consider primary disease of miniature schnauzers; consider secondary to diabetes mellitus, pancreatitis, nephrotic syndrome, or liver disease
• Hypothyroidism—German shepherds may have a predilection.

 DIAGNOSIS

DIFFERENTIAL DIAGNOSIS
• Other causes of corneal opacity
• Corneal ulcer—retains fluorescein stain
• Uncomplicated scar—variably opaque; negative fluorescein stain retention; relatively smooth corneal surface
• Stromal lipid dystrophies—fluorescein negative; bilateral; often symmetrical foci of corneal lipid deposition, which are familial and not associated with ocular inflammation
• Edema—usually more homogenous; bluish white
• Inflammatory cell infiltrates—cytologic examination of a corneal scraping

CBC/BIOCHEMISTRY/URINALYSIS
• Degeneration—check fasting cholesterol, triglyceride, and calcium concentrations, because high concentrations may modify the corneal deposits although they do not usually cause the degeneration.
• Arcus lipoides corneae—hyperlipoproteinemia; high serum cholesterol and triglyceride concentrations

OTHER LABORATORY TESTS
Arcus lipoides cornea secondary to hypothyroidism—low thyroid hormone concentration and depressed response to TSH

IMAGING
N/A

DIAGNOSTIC PROCEDURES
Arcus lipoides corneae—may retain fluorescein stain if epithelial deposits are excessive

 TREATMENT

• Degeneration—treat the primary ocular disease.
• Arcus lipoides corneae—treat the systemic condition.
• Lipid and calcium deposits that impair vision, disrupt the corneal epithelium, or cause ulceration and ocular discomfort—may benefit from vigorous corneal scraping or superficial keratectomy followed by medical treatment
• Arcus lipoides corneae and possibly other lipid degenerations—may benefit from a low-fat diet

 MEDICATIONS

DRUGS
• Topical antibiotics (e.g., triple antibiotic)—indicated for ulcerated cornea

• Topical 1% atropine—q8–24h; may reduce pain associated with corneal ulceration when used to effect
• Topical EDTA solution—0.4%–1.38% q6h; may help minimize degeneration, but only if calcium deposits are noted; usually used after a procedure that removes most of the deposits and the epithelium (e.g., corneal scraping), to improve efficacy
• Artificial tear ointment—q6–12h; may prevent or reduce the frequency of recurrent corneal ulceration

CONTRAINDICATIONS/POSSIBLE INTERACTIONS
• Topical corticosteroids—questionable benefit for treating degeneration or infiltration; do not use with corneal ulceration.
• Topical atropine—contraindicated with glaucoma and lens luxation; relatively contra-indicated with KCS

 FOLLOW-UP

PATIENT MONITORING
Arcus lipoides cornea—monitor serum cholesterol and triglycerides to assess efficacy of dietary management or treatment of the primary systemic disease.

EXPECTED COURSE AND PROGNOSIS
• Corneal ulceration—may accompany progression of degeneration or arcus lipoides corneae
• Vision—not substantially affected, except with advanced degeneration and when primary disease has caused irreparable damage to the globe (e.g., chronic uveitis)
• Lipid and calcium deposits—may recur in patients that have undergone keratectomy surgery

 MISCELLANEOUS

SEE ALSO
• Keratitis, Ulcerative
• Corneal Dystrophies

ABBREVIATIONS
• KCS = keratoconjunctivitis sicca
• TSH = thyroid-stimulating hormone

Suggested Reading
Crispin SM, Barnett KC. Dystrophy, degeneration and infiltration of the canine cornea. J Small Anim Pract 1983;24:63–83.
Author B. Keith Collins
Consulting Editor Paul E. Miller

BASICS

OVERVIEW
• Primary, noninherited (or familial), bilateral, and often symmetrical condition of the cornea that is not associated with other ocular or systemic diseases
• Three types based on anatomic location—associated with abnormality of the epithelium or basement membrane; caused by lipid deposition within the corneal stroma; degenerative change of the corneal endothelium

SIGNALMENT
Usually dogs; rare in cats

Epithelial
• Shetland sheepdogs—sometimes before 1 year of age; slow progression throughout life
• Boxers—corneal erosions (see Keratitis, Ulcerative)

Lipid
• Usually affects young adult dogs
• Higher prevalence in females suggested for some breeds
• Affected breeds—Siberian huskies, Alaskan malamutes, Samoyeds, bearded collies, bichon frises, German shepherds, lhasa apsos, mastiffs, miniature pinschers, Weimaraners, whippets, cavalier King Charles spaniels, American cocker spaniels, beagles, rough collies, Afghan hounds, and Airedale terriers; inheritance pattern identified in only a few breeds

Endothelial
• Dogs—primarily affects Boston terriers and Chihuahuas; may affect other breeds; typically affects middle-aged or old animals; female predilection suggested
• Cats—affects young animals; described most often in domestic shorthairs; a similar condition that occurs without endothelial disease is inherited in Manx as an autosomal recessive disorder.

SIGNS
All cause some degree of opacity of the cornea.

Epithelial
Asymptomatic or blepharospasm—associated with corneal erosions

Lipid
• Usually asymptomatic with no associated ocular inflammation
• Vision—usually not affected; deficit is possible with advanced, diffuse, or annular disease
• Central—most common; gray, white, or silver oval to circular opacity of the central or paracentral cornea; on magnification may note multiple fibrillar to coalescing opacities that impart a crystalline or ground-glass appearance to the cornea (crystalline corneal dystrophy)

• Diffuse—affects Airedales; more diffuse opacity than with central dystrophy
• Annular—affects Siberian huskies; doughnut-shaped opacity of the paracentral or peripheral cornea

Endothelial
• Asymptomatic in the early stages
• Edema of the lateral or ventrolateral cornea that usually progresses to involve the entire cornea after months to years
• Corneal epithelial bullae (or bullous keratopathy) and subsequent corneal erosion or ulceration may develop.
• Pain caused by corneal ulceration and impaired visual acuity—with advanced disease

CAUSES & RISK FACTORS
• Epithelial—result of degenerative or innate abnormalities of the corneal epithelium or basement membrane
• Lipid—result of an innate abnormality or localized error in corneal lipid metabolism; may be affected by hyperlipoproteinemia (possibly increases opacity)
• Endothelial—result of degeneration of the endothelial cell layer, with corresponding loss of endothelial cell pump function and subsequent corneal edema

 DIAGNOSIS

DIFFERENTIAL DIAGNOSIS
• Other causes of corneal opacity—corneal degenerations; ulcers; scars; inflammatory cell infiltrates
• Endothelial—must distinguished from other causes of diffuse corneal edema, notably uveitis and glaucoma

CBC/BIOCHEMISTRY/URINALYSIS
Lipid—check cholesterol and triglyceride levels; high concentrations may modify the course of disease but are not the cause.

OTHER LABORATORY TESTS
N/A

IMAGING
N/A

DIAGNOSTIC PROCEDURES
• Lipid—usually does not retain fluorescein stain
• Epithelial or endothelial—may retain fluorescein stain, particularly with advanced disease

 TREATMENT
• Advanced epithelial or endothelial disease with ulceration (dogs)—may require treatment for ulcerative keratitis

• Lipid (dogs)—usually none required; may perform superficial keratectomy to remove lipid deposits, but is usually unnecessary and deposits may recur after surgery
• Inform client that some corneal dystrophies are inherited.
• Advanced endothelial dystrophy (dogs)—may benefit from penetrating keratoplasty surgery (e.g., corneal transplant); success rates vary.
• Other—debriding redundant corneal epithelial tags; therapeutic soft contact lenses; creating conjunctival flaps; thermokeratoplasty

 MEDICATIONS

DRUGS
• Topical antibiotics and possibly atropine—ulcerated cornea (see Keratitis, Ulcerative)
• Topical 5% sodium chloride ointment (Muro-128)—q6h; for endothelial dystrophy; palliative treatment; does not markedly clear cornea; may prevent progression and rupture of corneal epithelial bullae

CONTRAINDICATIONS/POSSIBLE INTERACTIONS
Topical corticosteroids—no benefit to lipid dystrophy; of questionable benefit to other forms of dystrophy

 FOLLOW-UP
• Reexamination—necessary only if ocular pain or corneal ulceration develop
• Corneal opacity—may wax and wane with lipid dystrophy; unlikely to resolve
• Corneal ulceration—may accompany progression of epithelial or endothelial disease
• Vision—not substantially affected, except with advance dystrophy

 MISCELLANEOUS

SEE ALSO
• Corneal Degenerations and Infiltrations
• Keratitis, Ulcerative

Suggested Reading
Crispin SM, Barnett KC. Dystrophy, degeneration and infiltration of the canine cornea. J Small Anim Pract 1983;24:63–83.
Author B. Keith Collins
Consulting Editor Paul E. Miller

DISEASES

CORONAVIRUS INFECTION—DOGS

BASICS

OVERVIEW
• CCV—sporadic outbreaks of vomiting and diarrhea in dogs; widely distributed throughout the world, including wild canids
• Infection—inapparent usual; mild to severe enteritis may occur, from which most dogs recover; death reported in young pups; restricted to the upper two-thirds of the small intestine and associated lymph nodes; unlike CPV-2 infection, crypt cells spared
• Simultaneous infection with CPV-2 may occur; more severe; often fatal
• No viremia or other manifestation of systemic disease

SIGNALMENT
• Only wild and domestic dogs are known to be susceptible to disease.
• CCV may cause inapparent infections in cats
• All ages and breeds

SIGNS
• Vary greatly
• Adults—most infections inapparent
• Puppies—may develop severe, fatal enteritis
• Incubation period—1–3 days
• Sudden-onset of vomiting, usually only once
• Diarrhea—may be explosive; yellow-green or orange; loose or liquid; typically malodorous (characteristic); may persist for a few days up tor > 3 weeks; may recur later
• Young pups—may suffer severe, protracted diarrhea and dehydration
• Anorexia and depression common
• Fever rare
• Mild respiratory effects

CAUSES & RISK FACTORS
• CCV—closely related to FIP virus, feline enteric coronavirus, and transmissible gastroenteritis virus of swine; pig and cat viruses not known to cause natural illness in dogs; readily inactivated by common disinfectants
• Stress (e.g., intensive training, crowding)—greatest risk; sporadic outbreaks have occurred in dogs attending shows and in kennels where introductions of new dogs are frequent; crowding and unsanitary conditions promote clinical illness
• Feces—primary source of infection; virus shed for about 2 weeks

DIAGNOSIS

DIFFERENTIAL DIAGNOSIS
• Infections caused by enteric bacteria, protozoa, or other viruses
• Food intoxication or intolerance

CBC/BIOCHEMISTRY/URINALYSIS
Normal

OTHER LABORATORY TESTS
• Serologic tests—available; not standardized
• Antibody titers—generally low; may not indicate recent infection because of high rate of asymptomatic infection

IMAGING
N/A

DIAGNOSTIC PROCEDURES
• Viral isolation—from feces in feline cell cultures at onset of diarrhea
• Immunofluorescent staining of frozen sections of the small intestine—fatal cases; may reveal viral antigen in cells lining the villus epithelium
• Electron microscopy—typical CCV particles; interpretation requires expertise.

PATHOLOGIC FINDINGS
• Necropsy reports limited, except experimental infections
• May be dilated loops of small intestine filled with gas and watery green-yellow material
• Gross—restricted to the small intestinal mucosa, which may be congested or hemorrhagic; mesenteric lymph nodes usually enlarged and edematous
• Typical microscopic changes—atrophy and fusion of intestinal villi; deepening of the crypts; increased cellularity of the lamina propria; flattening of epithelial cells with increased goblet cells
• Lesions—commonly obscured by postmortem autolysis

TREATMENT

• Most affected dogs recover without treatment.
• Supportive fluid and electrolyte treatment—indicated, especially in severe infections with dehydration

MEDICATIONS

DRUGS
Antibiotics—not usually indicated, except with enteritis, sepsis, or respiratory illness

CONTRAINDICATIONS/POSSIBLE INTERACTIONS
N/A

FOLLOW-UP

PATIENT MONITORING
Not usually required

PREVENTION/AVOIDANCE
• Vaccines—controversial; inactivated and live viral vaccines available; appear to be safe; efficacy unknown, except for brief periods (2–4 weeks) after vaccination
• Strict isolation and sanitation are essential in kennels.
• CCV—highly contagious; spreads rapidly

POSSIBLE COMPLICATIONS
Diarrhea—may persist 10–12 days; may reoccur

EXPECTED COURSE AND PROGNOSIS
• Prognosis—normally good, except severe infections of young pups
• Majority recover after a few days of illness.
• Fluid or soft stools may persist for several weeks.

MISCELLANEOUS

ASSOCIATED CONDITIONS
• Infection with canine parvovirus or other agent may occur concurrently.
• Infections by other enteric pathogens are believed to augment the disease.

AGE-RELATED FACTORS
• Young pups seem to be at risk.

ZOONOTIC POTENTIAL
N/A

ABBREVIATIONS
• CCV = canine coronavirus
• CPV = canine parvovirus
• FIP = feline infectious peritonitis

Suggested Reading
Hoskins JD. Canine viral enteritis. In: Greene, CE. Infectious diseases of the dog and cat. Philadelphia: Saunders, 1998.
Author Leland E. Carmichael
Consulting Editor Stephen C. Barr

BASICS

OVERVIEW
- A nonneoplastic, noninflammatory proliferative disease of the bones of the head
- Primary bones affected—mandibular rami; occipital and parietal; tympanic bullae; zygomatic portion of the temporal
- Bilateral symmetric involvement most common
- Affects musculoskeletal system

SIGNALMENT
- Scottish, cairn, and West Highland white terrier breeds—most common
- Labrador retrievers, Great Danes, Boston terriers, Doberman pinschers, Irish setters, English bulldogs, and boxers—may be affected
- Usually growing puppies 4–8 months of age
- No gender predilection
- Neutering may increase incidence.

SIGNS

Historical Findings
- Usually relate to pain around the mouth and difficulty eating
- Angular processes of the mandible affected—jaw movement progressively restricted
- Difficulty in prehension, mastication, and swallowing—may lead to starvation
- Lameness or limb swelling—may precede cranial involvement

Physical Examination Findings
- Temporal and masseter muscle atrophy—common
- Palpable irregular thickening of the mandibular rami and/or TMJ region
- Inability to fully open jaw, even under general anesthesia
- Intermittent pyrexia—40°C
- Bilateral exophthalmos

CAUSES & RISK FACTORS
- Believed to be hereditary—occurs in certain breeds and families
- West Highland white terriers—autosomal recessive trait
- Scottish terriers—possible predisposition
- Possible link to infection—pyrexia; histologic evidence of inflammation only at the periphery of the lesion
- Young terrier with periosteal long bone disease—monitor for disease.

 DIAGNOSIS

DIFFERENTIAL DIAGNOSIS
- Osteomyelitis—bones not symmetrically affected; generally not as extensive; lysis; lack of breed predilection; history of penetrating wound
- Traumatic periostitis—bones not symmetrically affected; generally not as extensive; history of trauma
- Neoplasia—mature patient; not symmetrically affected; more lytic bone reaction; metastatic disease

CBC/BIOCHEMISTRY/URINALYSIS
- Serum ALP and inorganic phosphate—may be high
- May note hypogammaglobulinemia or α_2-hyperglobulinemia

OTHER LABORATORY TESTS
Serology—rule out fungal agents; indicated in atypical cases

IMAGING
- Skull radiography—reveals uneven, bead-like osseous proliferation of the mandible or tympanic bullae (bilateral); extensive, periosteal new bone formation (exostoses) affecting one or more bones around the TMJ; may show fusion of the tympanic bullae and angular process of the mandible
- CT—may help evaluate osseous involvement of the TMJ

DIAGNOSTIC PROCEDURES
Bone biopsy and culture (bacterial and fungal)—necessary only in atypical cases; rule out neoplasia and osteomyelitis

PATHOLOGIC FINDINGS
- Bone biopsy—reveals normal lamellar bone being replaced by an enlarged coarse-fiber bone and osteoclastic osteolysis of the periosteal or subperiosteal region
- Bone marrow—replaced by a vascular fibrous-type stroma
- Inflammatory cells—occasionally seen at the periphery of the bony lesion

 TREATMENT
- Palliative only
- Surgical excision of exostoses—results in regrowth within weeks
- High-calorie, protein-rich gruel diet—help maintain nutritional balance
- Surgical placement of a pharyngostomy, esophagostomy, or gastrostomy tube—considered to help maintain nutritional balance

 MEDICATIONS

DRUGS
- Analgesics and anti-inflammatory drugs—palliative use warranted
- NSAIDs—may be used to minimize pain and decrease inflammation; may try buffered or enteric-coated aspirin (10–25 mg/kg PO q8h or q12h), caroprofen (2.2 mg/kg PO q12h), etodolac (10–15 mg/kg, PO, once daily), phenylbutazone (3–7 mg/kg PO q8h, total dose <800 mg/day), meclofenamic acid (0.5 mg/kg PO q12h), or piroxicam (0.3 mg/kg PO q24h for 3 days, then every other day)

CONTRAINDICATIONS/POSSIBLE INTERACTIONS
N/A

 FOLLOW-UP

PATIENT MONITORING
Frequent re-examinations—mandatory to ensure adequate nutritional balance and pain control

PREVENTION/AVOIDANCE
- Do not repeat dam–sire breedings that resulted in affected offspring.
- Discourage breeding of affected animals.

Expected Course and Prognosis
- Pain and discomfort may diminish at skeletal maturity (10–12 months of age); the exostoses may regress.
- Prognosis—depends on involvement of bones surrounding the TMJ
- Elective euthanasia may be necessary.

 MISCELLANEOUS

SYNONYMS
Lion jaw

ABBREVIATIONS
- ALP = alkaline phosphatase
- TMJ = temporomandibular joint

Suggested Reading
Watson ADJ, Adams WM, Thomas CB. Craniomandibular osteopathy in dogs. Compend Contin Educ Pract Vet 1995;17:911–921.

Author Peter D. Schwarz
Consulting Editor Peter D. Schwarz

DISEASES

CRUCIATE DISEASE, CRANIAL

BASICS

DEFINITION
The acute or degenerative injury of the CrCL, which results in partial to complete instability of the stifle joint

PATHOPHYSIOLOGY
• Function of the CrCL—constrain the stifle joint by limiting internal rotation and cranial displacement of the tibia relative to the femur; prevents hyperextension
• CrCL injury—from trauma (acute) or degenerative causes (chronic); breaking strength approximately equal to four times the body weight of the dog
• Acute rupture—<20% caused by exceeding the strength of the ligament in dogs; usually caused by hyperextension and excessive internal rotation with the stifle in partial flexion (20–50°); trauma most common cause in cats; a ligament weakened by degeneration is more easily ruptured than is a normal ligament.
• Degeneration—aging, conformational abnormalities, disuse related to sedentary habits or limb immobilization, and immune-mediated
• Aging and degeneration—related to size; dogs >15 kg show more changes and have a more significant change in CrCL strength than do smaller dogs; degenerative changes and a decrease in material properties have been shown consistently in dogs >5 years of age
• Conformational abnormalities—genu varum (bowlegged), genu valgum (knock-kneed), straight stifles and hock, caudal sloping of the tibial plateau, patella luxation, and narrowing of the intercondylar notch may predispose patient to rupture.
• Immune-mediated arthritis, lymphocytic–plasmocytic synovitis, and septic arthritis—may predispose patient to rupture
• Immune complexes—found in dogs with unilateral and bilateral rupture; unknown if they are a cause or a result of the rupture
• Partial rupture—accounts for 25–30% of stifle lameness cases
• Untreated rupture—degenerative changes within a few weeks; severe changes within a few months
• Medial meniscal (caudal horn) damage—from abnormal joint mechanics after CrCL injury; occurs in >50% of cases
• Cranial tibial thrust—may play an important role in CrCL rupture; theoretically, a cranially directed force is generated during weight bearing, based on the caudal slope of the tibial plateau and the tibial compression mechanism.

SYSTEMS AFFECTED
Musculoskeletal

GENETICS
• Unknown
• May be important in predisposing patient to DJD, degeneration of the CrCL, or conformation abnormalities

INCIDENCE/PREVALENCE
• CrCL rupture—one of the most common causes of hindlimb lameness in dogs; major cause of DJD in the stifle joint

GEOGRAPHIC DISTRIBUTION
N/A

SIGNALMENT

Species
• Dogs
• Uncommon in cats

Breed Predilections
• All susceptible
• Rottweilers and Labrador retrievers—increased incidence of CrCL rupture when <4 years of age

Mean Age and Range
• Dogs > 5 years of age
• Large breed dogs—between 1 and 2 years of age

Predominant Sex
Possibly female dogs

SIGNS

General Comments
Related to the degree of rupture (partial vs. complete), the mode of rupture (acute vs. chronic), the occurrence of meniscal injury, and the severity of inflammation and DJD

Historical Findings
• Athletic or traumatic events—generally precede acute injury, resulting in non-weight-bearing lameness with the affected limb held in flexion
• Normal activity resulting in acute lameness—suggests degenerative rupture
• Subtle to marked intermittent lameness (for weeks to months)—consistent with partial tears that are progressing to complete rupture

PHYSICAL EXAMINATION FINDINGS
• Demonstration of cranial drawer motion—diagnostic for rupture; often dramatic after acute injury; subtle, almost imperceptible motion that ends gradually as a result of tissue stretching consistent with chronic rupture or partial tears; tested in flexion, normal standing angle, and extension
• Cranial movement of tibia relative to the femur during the tibial compression test
• Joint effusion

• Palpable thickening of the joint capsule—especially on the medial aspect (medial buttress)
• Hindlimb muscle atrophy—especially the quadriceps muscle group
• No cranial drawer sign (or negative tibial compression test)—does not rule out rupture; may see false-negative results with chronic or partial tears and in painful or anxious patients that are not sedated or anesthetized

CAUSES
• Trauma
• Degenerative changes
• Conformation abnormalities
• Immune-mediated

RISK FACTORS
• Obesity
• Patella luxation
• Poor conformation
• Excessive caudal slope of tibial plateau
• Narrowed intercondylar notch

DIAGNOSIS

DIFFERENTIAL DIAGNOSIS
• Skeletally immature dogs and dogs with significant muscle atrophy—slight drawer motion that stops abruptly as the CrCL is stretched taut common
• Caudal cruciate ligament rupture—uncommon as an isolated occurrence
• Palpation—distinguish cranial from caudal rupture
• Patella luxation (medial or lateral)—alone or with CrCL rupture
• Stifle joint trauma
• Osteochondritis dissecans of the femoral condyle or patella
• Neoplasia (e.g., synovial cell sarcoma)—generally more painful than rupture

CBC/BIOCHEMISTRY/URINALYSIS
N/A

OTHER LABORATORY TESTS
N/A

IMAGING

Radiography
• Rarely diagnostic for rupture
• Extremely helpful in confirming intra-articular disease
• Common findings—joint effusion with capsular distention and compression of the infrapatellar fat pad; periarticular osteophytes; enthesiophytes; CrCL avulsion fractures; calcification of the CrCL

MRI
Graphically shows cruciate ligament and meniscal pathology

DIAGNOSTIC PROCEDURES
• Arthrocentesis—joint cytology to identify intra-articular disease and rule out sepsis and immune-mediated disease
• Arthroscopy—directly visualize the cruciate ligaments, menisci, and other intra-articular structures

PATHOLOGIC FINDINGS
• Varying degrees of cartilage fibrillation and erosion
• Periarticular osteophyte formation
• Meniscal damage
• Synovitis
• Ruptured fibers of the CrCL—hyalinization; fibrous tissue invasion; necrosis; loss of the parallel orientation of ligament bundles

TREATMENT

APPROPRIATE HEALTH CARE
• Dogs <15 kg—may treat conservatively as outpatients; 85% improve or are normal by 6 months
• Dogs >15 kg—treated with surgery; only 20% improve or are normal by 6 months
• Surgery—recommended for all dogs; speeds rate of recovery; prevents degenerative changes; enhances function

NURSING CARE
Postsurgery—physical therapy (e.g., ice packing, range-of-motion exercises, massage, and muscle electrical stimulation); important for improving mobility and strength

ACTIVITY
Restricted—with conservative treatment and after surgical stabilization; duration depends on method of treatment and progress of patient.

DIET
Weight control—important for decreasing the load and thus stress on the stifle joint

CLIENT EDUCATION
• Warn client that, regardless of the method of treatment, DJD is common.
• Inform client that return to complete athletic function is uncommon.
• Warn client that 20%–40% of dogs with unilateral CrCL rupture will experience rupture of the contralateral ligament within 17 months.

SURGICAL CONSIDERATIONS
No one technique has proven superior to the others.

Extra-articular Methods
• A wide variety of techniques that use a heavy-gauge implant to imbricate the joint and restore stability
• Implant material—placed in the approximate plane of the CrCL origin and insertion

Intra-articular Methods
• Designed to replace the CrCL anatomically
• Autografts (patella ligament, fascia), allografts (bone-tendon-bone), and synthetic materials—commonly used
• Femoral intercondylar notchplasty—recommended to minimize graft injury
• Arthroscopic replacement—recently described; long-term benefits unknown

Modified Extra-articular Methods
• Fibular head transposition or popliteal tendon transposition
• Realign and tension the lateral collateral ligament or popliteal tendon to restrict internal rotation and cranial drawer

Tibial Plateau Leveling Osteotomy
• Rotational osteotomy of the proximal tibia
• Levels tibial plateau and neutralizes cranial tibial thrust

MEDICATIONS

DRUGS OF CHOICE
• NSAIDs and analgesics—symptomatically treat associated synovitis and DJD; may use buffered or enteric-coated aspirin (10–25 mg/kg PO q8h or q12h), caroprofen (2.2 mg/kg PO q12h), etodolac (10–15 mg/kg PO q24h), phenylbutazone (3–7 mg/kg PO q8h, total dose <800 mg/day), meclofenemic acid (0.5 mg/kg PO q12h), or piroxicam (0.3 mg/kg PO q24h for 3 days, then every other day)

CONTRAINDICATIONS
Avoid corticosteroids—potential side effects; articular cartilage damage associated with long-term use

PERCAUTIONS
NSAIDs—may cause gastrointestinal irritation; may preclude use in some patients

POSSIBLE INTERACTIONS
N/A

ALTERNATIVE DRUGS
Chondroprotective drugs (polysulfated glycosaminoglycans, glucosamine, and chondroitin sulfate)—may help limit cartilage damage and degeneration

FOLLOW-UP

PATIENT MONITORING
• Depends on method of treatment
• Most techniques require 2–4 months of rehabilitation

PREVENTION/AVOIDANCE
Avoid breeding animals with conformation abnormalities.

POSSIBLE COMPLICATIONS
Second surgery—required in 10–15% of cases because of subsequent meniscal damage

EXPECTED COURSE AND PROGNOSIS
Regardless of surgical technique, the success rate is approximately 85%.

MISCELLANEOUS

ASSOCIATED CONDITIONS
Meniscal damage

AGE-RELATED FACTORS
See Pathophysiology

ZOONOTIC POTENTIAL
N/A

PREGNANCY
N/A

SEE ALSO
• Arthritis (Osteoarthritis)
• Patellar Luxation

ABBREVIATIONS
• CrCL = cranial cruciate ligament
• DJD = degenerative joint disease

Suggested Reading
Brinker WO, Piermattei DL, Flo GL. Rupture of the cranial cruciate ligament. In: Brinker WO, Piermattei DL, Flo GL, eds. Handbook of small animal orthopedics and fracture repair. 3rd ed. Philadelphia: Saunders, 1997:534–563.

Johnson JM, Johnson AL. Cranial cruciate ligament rupture: pathogenesis, diagnosis, and postoperative rehabilitation. Vet Clin North Am 1993;23:717–733.

Slocum B, Slocum TD. Treatment of the stifle for cranial cruciate ligament rupture. In: Bojrab MJ, ed. Current techniques in small animal surgery. 4th ed. Philadelphia: Lea & Febiger, 1998:1187–11215.
Author Peter D. Schwarz
Consulting Editor Peter D. Schwarz

DISEASES

CRYPTOCOCCOSIS

 BASICS

DEFINITION
A localized or systemic fungal infection caused by the environmental yeast *Cryptococcus neoformans*

PATHOPHYSIOLOGY
• *C. neoformans*—grows in bird droppings and decaying vegetation
• Dogs and cats inhale the yeast and a foci of infection is established, usually in the nasal passages; smaller dried, shrunken organisms may reach the terminal airways (uncommon)
• Dissemination—hematogenously from the nasal passages to the brain, eyes, lungs, and other tissues; by extension to the skin of the nose, the eye, retro-orbital tissues, and draining lymph nodes

SYSTEMS AFFECTED
• Cats—mainly the nose and sinuses; facial skin; nasal planum; nasopharynx; brain; eyes
• Dogs—mainly the head and brain, nasal passages, and sinuses; skin over the nose and sinuses; mucous membranes; draining lymph nodes; eyes; periorbital areas; occasionally lungs and abdominal organs

GENETICS
No known influence

INCIDENCE/PREVALENCE
• Dogs—rare in U.S.; prevalence 0.00013%
• Cats—7–10 times more common than in dogs

GEOGRAPHIC DISTRIBUTION
• Worldwide
• Some areas of southern California and Australia have an increased incidence
• Some *Cryptococcus* spp. grow well on eucalyptus trees.

SIGNALMENT
Species
Cats and dogs

Breed Predilection
• Dogs—American cocker spaniels, Doberman pinschers, and Labrador retrievers over-represented
• Cats—Siamese at increased risk

Mean Age and Range
• Most common 2–7 years of age (dogs and cats)
• May occur at any age

Predominant Sex
• Dogs—none
• Cats—males over-represented

SIGNS
Historical Findings
• Lethargy
• Vary depending on organ systems involved
Dogs
• Neurologic—seizures, ataxia, paresis, blindness
• Skin ulceration
• Lymphadenopathy
Cats
• Nasal discharge
• Granulomatous tissue seen at the nares
• Firm swellings over the bridge of the nose

Physical Examination Findings
• Mild fever—< 50% of patients
• Dogs—anorexia; nasal discharge
• Cats—increased respiratory noise; ulcerated crusty skin lesions on the head; lymphadenopathy; neurologic; ocular

CAUSES
Exposure to cryptococcal organisms and inability of the immune system to prevent colonization and invasion into tissues

RISK FACTORS
Cats concurrently infected with FeLV or FIV—higher risk; more extensive disease

 DIAGNOSIS

DIFFERENTIAL DIAGNOSIS
Dogs
• Other causes of focal or diffuse neurologic disease—distemper; bacterial meningo-encephalitis; brain tumors; rickettsial diseases; granulomatous meningoencephalomyelitis; other fungal diseases
• Nasal lesions, especially at the mucocutaneous junction—considered immune-mediated
• Lymphosarcoma—possible cause of the lymphadenopathy
• With chorioretinitis and optic neuritis—consider other fungal infections, distemper, and neoplasia

Cats
• Nasal lesions—similar to nasal tumors, chronic rhinitis, and chronic sinusitis
• Ulcerative skin changes—may be the result of bacterial infection, fights, or tumor (especially squamous cell carcinoma of the nasal planum)
• Ocular and brain signs—may be attributed to lymphosarcoma, FIP, and toxoplasmosis

CBC/BIOCHEMISTRY/URINALYSIS
• Mild anemia in some cats
• Eosinophilia occasionally seen
• Chemistries usually normal

OTHER LABORATORY TESTS
Latex agglutination or ELISA—detect cryptococcal capsular antigen in serum; few false-positive tests; most infected animals have measurable capsular antigen titers; magnitude of titer correlates with extent of infection

IMAGING
• Lateral radiographs of the nasopharynx—cryptococcal granuloma behind the soft palate
• Nasal radiographs (cats)—soft tissue–density material filling the nasal passage; occasional bone destruction of the nasal dorsum
• Thoracic radiographs—not indicated, unless signs of lower respiratory tract disease

DIAGNOSTIC PROCEDURES
Dogs with neurologic disease—additional procedures: cytologic examination and culture of CSF and measurement of CSF capsular antigen often make the diagnosis.

Cats
• Definitive diagnosis—aspirates of the mucoid material in the nasal passages or biopsy of the granulomatous tissue that protrudes from the nares
• Patients with upper respiratory obstruction or severe respiratory noise—granuloma in the nasopharynx; identify by pulling the soft palate forward with a spay hook to expose the mass
• Biopsy—skin lesions of the head; aspirates of involved lymph nodes; usually identifies organisms
• Cultures—confirm the diagnosis; determine drug susceptibility

PATHOLOGIC FINDINGS
• Gross lesions—gray, gelatinous mass produced by the polysaccharide capsule; usually found in the nose, sinuses, and nasopharynx of cats
• Neurologic lesions—usually seen in dogs; diffuse or fungal granulomas producing a mass in the brain
• Chorioretinitis with or without retinal detachment or optic neuritis—dogs and cats
• Histologic response—usually pyogranulomatous; inflammatory cell infiltrate may be mild because the polysaccharide capsule interferes with neutrophil migration.

 TREATMENT

APPROPRIATE HEALTH CARE
• Outpatient if stable
• Neurologic signs—may require inpatient supportive care until stable

NURSING CARE
Cats—nasal obstruction influences appetite; encourage patients to eat by offering palatable food

ACTIVITY
No restrictions in most cases

DIET
• No special foods
• Patients treated with itraconazole—give medication in fatty food (e.g., canned food) to improve absorption

CLIENT EDUCATION
• Inform client that this is a chronic disease that requires months of treatment.
• Reassure client that the infection is not zoonotic.

SURGICAL CONSIDERATIONS
Remove granulomatous masses in the nasopharynx to reduce respiratory difficulties.

MEDICATIONS

DRUGS OF CHOICE
• Triazole antifungal agents—expensive; itraconazole somewhat economical
• Fluconazole—preferred for ocular or CNS involvement because it is water-soluble and penetrates the nervous system better; cats, 50 mg PO q12h; dogs, 5 mg/kg PO q12h
• Itraconazole—give with a fatty meal to maximize absorption; cats, 10–15 mg/kg PO daily; dogs, 5 mg/kg PO q12h; pellets in the capsule can be mixed with food; no apparent adverse taste
• Flucytosine—100 mg/kg PO divided into 3–4 doses per day; in addition to Triazole; helpful when the infection does not respond well

CONTRAINDICATIONS
Avoid steroids

PRECAUTIONS
• Triazoles—hepatic toxicity; anorexia signals problems; monitor liver enzymes monthly.
• Itraconazole—ulcerative dermatitis (differentiate from the skin lesions of cryptococcosis); new skin lesions after the disease is much improved should be considered a drug reaction.
• Flucytosine—drug eruptions manifested as depigmentation of lips and nose, ulceration, exudation, and crusting of the skin; bone marrow suppression

POSSIBLE INTERACTIONS
Itraconazole—do not give with the antihistamines terfenadine and astemizole or with cisapride.

ALTERNATIVE DRUGS
Amphotericin B (intravenous) and flucytosine—dogs and cats that do not respond to a triazole; monitor BUN closely to avoid permanent renal damage

FOLLOW-UP

PATIENT MONITORING
• Monitor liver enzymes monthly in patients receiving a triazole antifungal agent
• Improvement in clinical signs, resolution of lesions, improvement in well-being, and return of appetite measure the response to treatment.
• Capsular antigen titers—determine response to and duration of treatment; after 2 months of treatment, the titers should decrease substantially if effective; if ineffective, try the other triazole, because organism can become resistant.

PREVENTION/AVOIDANCE
The organism is ubiquitous and cannot be avoided.

POSSIBLE COMPLICATIONS
Patients with neurologic disease may have seizures and permanent neurologic changes.

EXPECTED COURSE AND PROGNOSIS
• Treatment—anticipated duration 3 months to 1 year; patients with CNS disease require lifelong maintenance.
• Cats concurrently infected with FeLV or FIV—may have a worse prognosis
• Capsular antigen titers—measure every 2 months until 6 months after completion of treatment; continue treatment for 2 months after antigen is nondetectable, if possible; if patient maintains low titers for months after all signs of disease have resolved, continue treatment for at least 3 months after reduction in antigen levels and resolution of clinical signs; if titers then rise significantly, resume therapy.

MISCELLANEOUS

ASSOCIATED CONDITIONS
N/A

AGE-RELATED FACTORS
N/A

ZOONOTIC POTENTIAL
• Not considered zoonotic, but possibility of transmission through bite wounds
• Inform client that the organism was acquired from the environment and that he or she could be at increased risk, especially if immunosuppressed.

PREGNANCY
N/A

ABBREVIATIONS
• ELISA = enzyme-linked immunoadsorbent assay
• FeLV = feline leukemia virus
• FIP = feline infectious peritonitis
• FIV = feline immunodeficiency virus

Suggested Reading
Berthelin CF, Bailey CS, Kass PH, et al. Cryptococcosis of the nervous system in dogs. Part 1, Epidemiologic, clinical and neuropathologic features. Prog Vet Neurol 1994;5:88–97.
Berthelin CF, Legendre AM, Bailey CS, et al. Cryptococcosis of the nervous system in dogs. Part 2, Diagnosis, treatment, monitoring and prognosis. Prog Vet Neurol 1994;5:136–146.
Jacobs GJ, Medleau L, Clavert C, et al. Cryptococcal infection in cats: factors influencing treatment outcome, and results of sequential serum antigen titers in 35 cats. J Vet Internal Med 1997;11;1–4.
Malik R, Dill-Macky E, Maring P, et al. Cryptococcosis in dogs: a retrospective study of 20 consecutive cases. J Med Vet Mycol 1995;33:291–297.
Malik R, Martin P, Wigney DI, et al. Nasopharyngeal cryptococcosis. Aust Vet J 1997;75:483–488.
Malik R, Wigney DI, Muir DB, et al. Cryptococcosis in cats: clinical and mycological assessment of 29 cases and evaluation of treatment using orally administered fluconazole. J Med Vet Mycol 1992;30:133–144.
Medleau L, Jacobs GJ, Marks A. Itraconazole for the treatment of cryptococcosis in cats. J Vet Internal Med 1995;9:39–42.
Author Alfred M. Legendre
Consulting Editor Stephen C. Barr

DISEASES

CRYPTORCHIDISM

 BASICS

OVERVIEW
• The incomplete descent of one or both testes into the scrotum
• Inguinal—retained testis often palpable
• Abdominal—testis difficult to palpate or identify by radiology; may be imaged with ultrasound
• Descent to final scrotal position—expected to be complete by 2 months postpartum; may occur later in some breeds, but rarely after 4 months in any individual; presume the diagnosis if no palpable testes at 2 months
• Beagles—testes at the exterior inguinal ring by day 5 postpartum, between the inguinal ring and scrotum by day 15, and in the scrotum by day 40

SIGNALMENT
• Dogs—reported in almost all breeds; toy poodles, Pomeranians, Yorkshire terriers (especially toy and miniature breeds) at significantly higher risk; unilateral more common than bilateral (75:25); right testis retained twice as often as left
• Prevalence—dogs, 1.2%; cats, 1.7%
• Genetics—thought to be inherited; single autosomal recessive gene often assumed when owners of affected dogs are counseled; more than one gene probably involved

SIGNS
• Rarely associated with pain or other signs of disease
• Associated with other congenital defects—patellar subluxation and hypospadias

CAUSES & RISK FACTORS
• Removal of affected males from breeding lines—believed to cause a reduction in frequency; heritability thought to involve more than one gene
• Nonhereditary predisposing factors (e.g., birth weight)—identified in humans; not reported in dogs

 DIAGNOSIS

DIFFERENTIAL DIAGNOSIS
• Castration—differentiate bilateral condition from previous castration, previous castration of single scrotal testis with retained abdominal testis, or anorchidism (rare)
• Bilaterally cryptorchid cats may have urine odor and behavior of intact cats

CBC/BIOCHEMISTRY/URINALYSIS
N/A

OTHER LABORATORY TESTS
hCG stimulation—doubles blood testosterone with bilateral condition; doubles blood testosterone with unilateral condition in which only the scrotal testis has been removed; differentiates between cryptorchidism and castration; administration of 750IU hCG IV with sample collection pre- and 2-3hr post injection; castrated dogs have testosterone concentrations < 0.1 ng/ml

IMAGING
Ultrasound—locate testes

DIAGNOSTIC PROCEDURES
N/A

 TREATMENT

• None except castration of both retained and scrotal testes generally recommended
• Orchiopexy—surgical placement of a retained testis into the scrotum; considered unethical
• hCG or GnRH—anecdotal evidence of causing descent when given to dogs < 4 months old
• Warn client of the increased risk of testicular neoplasia in dogs with retained testes; encourage client to have dog castrated by 4 years of age; 53% of Sertoli cell tumors and 36% of seminomas occur in retained testes.

 MEDICATIONS

DRUGS
hCG (dogs)—100–1000 IU IM four times in a 2-week period before 16 weeks of age (dogs); after 16 weeks, generally unsuccessful

CONTRAINDICATIONS/POSSIBLE INTERACTIONS
N/A

 FOLLOW-UP

• Descent after 4 months is rare; after 6 months, unlikely
• Risk of testicular neoplasia thought to be approximately 10 times greater in affect dogs than in normal dogs.

 MISCELLANEOUS

ABBREVIATIONS
• GnRH = gonadotropin-releasing hormone
• hCG = human chorionic gonadotropin

Suggested Reading
England GCW, Allen WE, Porter DJ. Evaluation of the testosterone response to hCG and the identification of a presumed anorchid dog. J Sm Anim Pract 1989:441–443.
Feldman EC, Nelson RW. Canine and feline endocrinology and reproduction. Philadelphia: Saunders, 1987:697–699.
Romagnoli SE. Canine cryptorchidism. Vet Clin North Am Small Anim Pract 1991;21:533–544
Author Rolf E. Larsen
Consulting Editor Sara K. Lyle

BASICS

OVERVIEW
• *Cryptosporidium* spp.—coccidian protozoan; causes gastrointestinal disease in dogs, cats, humans, calves, and rodents; ubiquitous in nature; worldwide distribution; enteric life cycle
• Infection—when sporulated oocysts are ingested, sporozoites are released and penetrate intestinal epithelial cells; after asexual reproduction, merozoites are released to infect other cells.
• Prepatent period—cats, 5–10 days
• Immunocompetent animals—intestinal disease
• Immunocompromised animals—intestinal, liver, gallbladder, pancreatic, and respiratory infection

SIGNALMENT
• Dogs and cats
• No sex or breed predilection
• Dogs—virtually all clinical cases have occurred in animals ≤ 6 months of age; old dogs can excrete oocysts without clinical signs.
• Cats—no age predilection

SIGNS
• Most infections subclinical
• Principally small bowel diarrhea
• Large bowel diarrhea reported

CAUSES & RISK FACTORS
• *C. parvum*—acquired by ingestion of contaminated water or feces
• Immunosuppression—major risk factor: FeLV (cats), canine distemper virus (dogs), and intestinal lymphosarcoma (cats and dogs)

DIAGNOSIS

DIFFERENTIAL DIAGNOSIS
• Dietary indiscretion or intolerance
• Drugs—antibiotics
• Toxins—lead
• Parasites—giardiasis, trichuriasis
• Infectious agents—parvovirus, coronavirus, FIP, salmonella, *Campylobacter,* rickettsia, histoplasma
• Organ disease—cardiac, renal, hepatic, and pancreatic exocrine insufficiency
• Metabolic—hypoadrenocorticism, hyperthyroidism (cats)
• Neoplasia—intestinal lymphoma
• Infiltrative diseases—inflammatory bowel disease

CBC/BIOCHEMISTRY/URINALYSIS
Usually normal, unless an underlying immunosuppressive disease

OTHER LABORATORY TESTS
N/A

IMAGING
N/A

DIAGNOSTIC PROCEDURES
• Fecal antigen detection test (ProSpecT Cryptosporidium Microtiter Assay; Color-Vue Cryptosporidium)—available; not extensively evaluated using cat or dog feces
• Sugar and zinc sulfate flotation—specific gravity = 1.18; concentrate fecal oocysts (oocysts are 5 μm so routine salt flotation often fails); oocysts best visualized after staining with modified acid-fast stain
• Fluorescent antibody techniques—available in some laboratories
• Submitting feces to a laboratory—mix one part 100% formalin with nine parts feces to inactivate oocysts and decrease health risk to laboratory personal.
• Intestinal biopsy—cytologic and histopathologic identification of intracellular organisms; diagnostic but impractical; can produce false-negative results

PATHOLOGIC FINDINGS
• Gross lesions—enlarged mesenteric lymph nodes; hyperemic intestinal (particular ileum) mucosa; fix specimens in Bouin or formalin solution within hours of death because autolysis causes rapid loss of the intestinal surface containing the organisms.
• Microscopic lesions—villous atrophy; reactive lymphoid tissue; and inflammatory infiltrates (neutrophils, macrophages, lymphocytes) in the lamina propria; parasites may be found throughout the intestines but are usually most numerous in the distal small intestine.

TREATMENT

• Outpatient
• Food—may withhold 24–48 hr until diarrhea is under control
• Mild diarrhea—oral glucose–electrolyte solution (Entrolyte, SmithKline)
• Severe diarrhea with dehydration—parental fluids (isotonic with potassium added)

MEDICATIONS

DRUGS
• Paromomycin (Humatin)—125–165 mg/kg PO q12h for 5 days; aminoglycoside antibiotic; effective in treating acute intestinal patients
• Tylosin—11 mg/kg PO q12h for 28 days; effective in treating an affected cat that also had lymphocytic duodenitis

CONTRAINDICATIONS/POSSIBLE INTERACTIONS
N/A

FOLLOW-UP

• Monitor clinical improvement for treatment efficacy.
• Monitor oocyst shedding in the feces 2 weeks after completion of treatment or if signs persist.
• Prognosis excellent, if cause of immunosuppression can be overcome

MISCELLANEOUS

ZOONOTIC POTENTIAL
• Warn clients of potential zoonotic transmission from organisms in feces and that immunocompromised people (HIV infection, chemotherapy, systemic corticosteroids) are at great risk

ABBREVIATIONS
• FeLV = feline leukemia virus
• FIP = feline infectious peritonitis

Suggested Reading
Barr SC. Cryptosporidiosis. In: Greene CE, ed. Infectious diseases of the dog and cat. Philadelphia: Saunders, 1998:518–523.
Author Stephen C. Barr
Consulting Editor Stephen C. Barr

DISEASES

CUTANEOUS ASTHENIA

 BASICS

OVERVIEW
• Group of hereditary diseases characterized by abnormal skin hyperextensibility and fragility
• Also known as Ehlers-Danlos syndrome and dermatosparaxis
• Abnormal collagen synthesis or fiber formation is responsible for the skin fragility in most syndromes; however, the biochemical defects have been elucidated in only a few dogs and cats.
• Varying modes of inheritance have been suspected.

SIGNALMENT
• Congenital syndrome—patients are usually presented quite young.
• Dogs—beagles, dachshunds, boxers, St. Bernards, German shepherds, English springer spaniels, greyhounds, Manchester terriers, Welsh corgis, red kelpies, soft-coated wheaten terriers, Irish setters, Keeshonds, English setters, and mongrels.
• Cats—domestic shorthairs, domestic longhairs, and Himalayans

SIGNS
• Skin hyperextensibility
• Easily torn skin
• Diminished skin elasticity
• Scars from previous trauma
• Widening of the bridge of the nose
• Joint laxity
• Elbow hygromas
• Lens luxation
• Cataracts

CAUSES & RISK FACTORS
Even minor trauma to the skin can produce large skin tears.

 DIAGNOSIS

DIFFERENTIAL DIAGNOSIS
Clinically characteristic syndrome

CBC/BIOCHEMISTRY/URINALYSIS
N/A

OTHER LABORATORY TESTS
N/A

IMAGING
N/A

DIAGNOSTIC PROCEDURES
Skin extensibility index—identifies affected animals; calculated by dividing the maximal height of a dorsal lumbar skin fold by the body length (from the base of the tail to the occipital crest) and converting to a percentage; affected dogs >14.5% and affected cats > 19%

PATHOLOGIC FINDINGS
• Histopathologic examination of the skin—either normal dermal architecture or collagen abnormalities (disoriented, fragmented, abnormal tinctorial properties or abnormal organization)
• Electron microscopy—ascertain collagen abnormalities more precisely

 TREATMENT

• Because of poor prognosis, affected animals may be euthanatized.
• If the owner chooses to keep the animal—keep environment free of sharp corners and other animals; handle and restrain affected animal carefully to prevent large skin tears; keep resting areas well padded to prevent elbow hygromas.

 MEDICATIONS

DRUGS
No proven medical therapy.

CONTRAINDICATIONS/POSSIBLE INTERACTIONS
N/A

 FOLLOW-UP

Lacerations should be surgically repaired as they occur.

 MISCELLANEOUS

Suggested Reading
Scott DW, Miller WH, Griffin CE, eds. Congenital Hereditary Defects. In: Muller & Kirk's small animal dermatology. 5th ed. Congenital hereditary defects. Philadelphia: Saunders, 1995:785–789.
Author Jon D. Plant
Consulting Editor Karen Helton Rhodes

CUTANEOUS DRUG ERUPTIONS

BASICS

OVERVIEW
• A spectrum of diseases and clinical signs that vary markedly in clinical appearance and pathophysiology
• Likely that many mild drug reactions go unnoticed or unreported; thus incidence rates for specific drugs are unknown and most of the facts available on drug-specific reactivities have been extrapolated from reports in the human literature.

SIGNALMENT
• Dogs and cats
• Age, breed, and sex predispositions—unknown
• Some types of drug reactions appear to have a familial basis (e.g., rabies vaccine reactions in dogs have been diagnosed in litter mates).

SIGNS
• Pruritus—can be activated by a wide variety of compounds; most common symptom of drug eruption in humans
• Macular and papular rashes—commonly accompany pruritus as a nonspecific sign of inflammation
• Exfoliative erythroderma—a diffuse erythematous response caused by vasodilation; often leads to exfoliation (diffuse scaling)
• Urticaria/angioedema—results from an immediate (type I) hypersensitivity; requires prior sensitization; increased vascular permeability leads to fluid leakage into the interstitium.
• Hypersensitivity vasculitis—inflammation of cutaneous vasculature; results in poor blood flow and anoxic injury to recipient tissue; in most cases, thought to represent a type III hypersensitivity response
• EM—erythremic macules or plaques expand peripherally and may clear in the center, producing a bull's-eye appearance; multiple shapes/forms can be seen.
• TEN—extensive necrosis and sloughing of the epidermis in sheets; results in a moist and intensely inflamed skin surface
• Drug-induced pemphigus/pemphigoid—least common drug reaction in animals; can closely mimic the autoimmune (spontaneous) forms of these diseases

CAUSES & RISK FACTORS
• Drugs of any type
• Exfoliative erythroderma—most often associated with shampoos and dips
• Can occur after the first dose after weeks to months of administration of the same drug

DIAGNOSIS

DIFFERENTIAL DIAGNOSIS
• Pruritus, macular/papular rashes, and urticaria/angioedema—allergic diseases (atopy, food allergy, contact allergy) and reactions to ectoparasites (scabies, flea bite allergy, stinging insects)
• Exfoliative erythroderma—rule out cutaneous T cell lymphoma in old dogs and cats.
• Vasculitis—infectious, neoplastic, and autoimmune diseases; many cases of vasculitis are idiopathic.
• EM—rule out respiratory infections and internal neoplasms.
• Pemphigus/pemphigoid—consider drug reaction whenever these diseases are diagnosed; however, spontaneously occurring autoimmune disease is much more common.

CBC/BIOCHEMISTRY/URINALYSIS
When cutaneous vasculitis is suspected or diagnosed—potential for concurrent hepatic, renal, and gastrointestinal disease

OTHER LABORATORY TESTS
• Dogs with vasculitis—rickettsial serology, ANA
• Cats with vasculitis—FIV and FeLV serology
• Bacterial and fungal cultures and sensitivity testing—for vasculitis with pyogranulomatous inflammation

IMAGING
N/A

DIAGNOSTIC PROCEDURES
Skin biopsy for histopathology—mandatory for diagnosis of most drug-induced diseases (vasculitis, EM, TEN, pemphigus/pemphigoid)

PATHOLOGIC FINDINGS
Vary according to the specific disease process

TREATMENT

• Discontinue use of the offending drug.
• TEN—intensive supportive care and fluid/nutritional support because of fluid and protein exudation and risk of sepsis

MEDICATIONS

DRUG(S)
Varies according to the disease process if withdrawal of the offending drug alone is insufficient

CONTRAINDICATIONS/POSSIBLE INTERACTIONS
The offending drug or any other drug in the same class or family should be strictly avoided.

FOLLOW-UP

PATIENT MONITORING
• Inpatient—if debilitated
• Outpatient—regular rechecks, depending on physical condition

EXPECTED COURSE AND PROGNOSIS
• Some reactions appear to activate self-perpetuating immune responses.
• Some drug metabolites may persist for days to weeks and provoke a continued response.
• TENS—prognosis poor
• Vasculitis—prognosis guarded when there are systemic complications

MISCELLANEOUS

ASSOCIATED CONDITIONS
Cutaneous vasculitis—arthropathy, hepatitis, glomerulonephritis, and neuromuscular disorders, among others

SEE ALSO
• Pemphigus
• Vasculitis, Cutaneous

ABBREVIATIONS
• ANA = antinuclear antibody
• EM = erythema multiforme
• FeLV = feline leukemia virus
• FIV = feline immunodeficiency virus
• TEN = toxic epidermal necrolysis

Suggested Reading
Scott DW, Miller WH, Griffin GE, eds. In: Muller & Kirk's small animal dermatology. 5th ed. Philadelphia: Saunders, 1995:590–606.

Author Daniel O. Morris

Consulting Editor Karen Helton Rhodes

DISEASES

CYCLIC HEMATOPOIESIS—DOGS

BASICS

OVERVIEW
• Cyclic hematopoiesis in color-dilute gray collie pups is characterized by frequent episodes of infection with failure to thrive and early death; clinically, pups have diarrhea, conjunctivitis, gingivitis, pneumonia, skin infections, and carpal joint pain accompanied by fever; intussusception is a common cause of death.
• Episodes of illness, varying from inactivity accompanied by fever to life-threatening infection, repeat at 11–14-day intervals
• The pups are smaller than litter mates at birth, are weak, and are often abandoned by the bitch.
• The condition has been observed in many collie bloodlines throughout the U.S.; however, experienced collie breeders do not attempt to raise the pups; therefore, gray collie pups are not commonly seen.

SIGNALMENT
• Cyclic hematopoiesis has been observed only in color-dilute collies.
• Inherited as an autosomal recessive trait; thus it is possible to observe similar color-dilute pups with cyclic hematopoiesis in any mongrel litter from parents with collie parentage in their background.
• Clinical signs occur as early as 1–2 weeks of age and are always apparent by 8–12 weeks of age.
• Single cases of cyclic hematopoiesis have been reported in Pomeranians and cocker spaniels; the disease is not well characterized in these breeds.

SIGNS
Historical Findings
• Weakness
• Failure to thrive
• Conjunctivitis
• Gingivitis
• Diarrhea
• Pneumonia
• Skin infections
• Carpal joint pain

Physical Examination Findings
• Dilute coat color
• Color dilution on skin of the nose
• Smaller and weaker than normal-colored litter mates
• Fever
• Watery eyes, reddened gums, and diarrhea nearly always present during the phase of the hematopoietic cycle when clinical signs are evident; other signs vary depending on the site of sepsis.
• Painful carpal joints observed during the initial recovery phase of the disease cycle

CAUSES & RISK FACTORS
Inherited disease

DIAGNOSIS

DIFFERENTIAL DIAGNOSIS
• Coat color dilution pathognomonic for the disease
• Color dilution not associated with cyclic hematopoiesis also observed in collie pups
• Pups with other color variants—normal size; do not develop frequent episodes of infection; may attain normal coat color intensity by 6 months of age; normal color intensity on the nose
• Pups with cyclic hematopoiesis always have color dilution on the skin of the nose.

CBC/BIOCHEMISTRY/URINALYSIS
• Severe neutropenia, lasting 2–5 days and occurring at 11–14-day intervals with marginal normocytic to microcytic anemia
• Important to recognize that signs of infection are often minimal during the neutropenic episodes
• Local swelling, redness, and systemic signs of infection usually occur during the first days of the neutrophilic phase of the disease cycle; therefore, on initial examination, neutrophilia with moderate monocytosis is observed.
• CBC should be repeated at 2–3-day intervals to confirm the diagnosis.

OTHER LABORATORY TESTS
None

IMAGING
N/A

DIAGNOSTIC PROCEDURES
None

TREATMENT
• Advise clients not to attempt to raise the pup(s).
• Antibiotics and supportive therapy may extend the life of the pups for several years but at considerable cost.
• The disease cycle has been interrupted experimentally by bone marrow transplantation and by daily treatment with endotoxin, lithium carbonate (10 mg/kg PO q12h), or recombinant human colony-stimulating factor.

MEDICATIONS

DRUGS
Antibiotics and fluids as required

CONTRAINDICATIONS/POSSIBLE INTERACTIONS
None

MISCELLANEOUS

Suggested Reading
DiGiacomo RF, Hammond WP, Kunz LL, Cox PA. Clinical and pathologic features of cyclic hematopoiesis in grey collie dogs. Am J Pathol 1983;111:224–233.
Author John E. Lund
Consulting Editor Susan M. Cotter

BASICS

OVERVIEW
- Infection with the protozoan *Cytauxzoon felis*
- Affects vascular system of lungs, liver, spleen, kidneys, and brain; bone marrow; developmental stages of RBCs
- Uncommon
- Affects feral and domestic cats in south-central and southeastern U.S.

SIGNALMENT
- Feral and domestic cats of all ages
- No breed or sex predilection

SIGNS
- Severe illness at presentation
- Pale mucous membranes
- Depression
- Anorexia
- Dehydration
- High fever
- Icterus
- Splenomegaly
- Hepatomegaly

CAUSES & RISK FACTORS
- Bite of infected *Ixodid* tick
- Roaming in areas shared by reservoir hosts (bobcat, Florida panther)

DIAGNOSIS

DIFFERENTIAL DIAGNOSIS
Other causes of anemia—marked decrease in packed red cell volume beginning 5–6 days after infection

CBC/BIOCHEMISTRY/URINALYSIS
Reflect changes associated with the severe anemia, caused by combination of hemolysis and hemorrhage

OTHER LABORATORY TESTS
- Fresh blood smear—*Cytauxzoon* erythrocytic form; 1–2 μm in diameter; shape of a signet ring or safety pin or looks like tiny dots
- Splenic and bone marrow aspirate—best suited to demonstrate extraerythrocytic form

IMAGING
N/A

DIAGNOSTIC PROCEDURES
N/A

PATHOLOGIC FINDINGS
Organisms inside mononuclear cells in bone marrow aspirate and in dramatically enlarged endothelial cells of venules of lung, liver, spleen, kidney, and brain

TREATMENT
- Inpatient with supportive therapy
- Euthanasia

MEDICATIONS

DRUG(S)
No known chemotherapy—suggest supportive therapy or euthanasia

CONTRAINDICATIONS/POSSIBLE INTERACTIONS
N/A

FOLLOW-UP

EXPECTED COURSE AND PROGNOSIS
- Unfortunately, diagnosis usually made at postmortem
- All known infected cats have died within 2 weeks of presentation

MISCELLANEOUS

ZOONOTIC POTENTIAL
- No known risk to humans
- Cannot be directly transmitted to another cat except by blood or tissue inoculation

Suggested Reading

Kier AB, Greene CE. Cytauxzoonosis. In: Greene CE, ed. Infectious diseases of the dog and cat. 2nd ed. Philadelphia: Saunders, 1998:470–473.

Author Johnny D. Hoskins
Consulting Editor Stephen C. Barr

DISEASES

DANCING DOBERMAN DISEASE

 BASICS

OVERVIEW
• Syndrome characterized by the flexion of one rear limb when standing, progressing over months to years to involve the opposite pelvic limb
• Affected dog flexes and extends the limbs alternately, as in a dancing motion.
• A primary myopathy is suspected but not proven.
• Possible genetic predisposition

SIGNALMENT
• Dogs
• Doberman pinschers
• Age of onset 6 months to 7 years
• Males and females

SIGNS
• Affected dog holds one pelvic limb flexed while standing; the alternate limb usually becomes affected in 3–6 months.
• Hyperactive tendon reflexes with gastrocnemius muscle atrophy—early
• More extensive pelvic limb muscle atrophy—with progression
• Proprioceptive deficits—occasionally

CAUSES & RISK FACTORS
Unknown

 DIAGNOSIS

DIFFERENTIAL DIAGNOSIS
• Lumbosacral stenosis, intervertebral disk disease, and discospondylitis of the lower lumbar spine—usually painful
• Neoplasia of the lumbar spinal cord or nerve roots—progresses more rapidly; can be painful

CBC/BIOCHEMISTRY/URINALYSIS
• Usually normal

OTHER LABORATORY TESTS
N/A

IMAGING
N/A

DIAGNOSTIC PROCEDURES
• Electromyography—prolonged insertion activity; positive sharp waves; fibrillation potentials
• Motor and sensory nerve conduction velocity—normal
• Biopsy—gastrocnemius muscles; findings vary: some consistent with primary muscle disease, others suggest denervation

 TREATMENT

None effective at controlling clinical signs or altering progression

 MEDICATIONS

DRUGS
N/A

CONTRAINDICATIONS/POSSIBLE INTERACTIONS
N/A

 FOLLOW-UP

Several patients have been followed for > 5 years; all remain acceptable pets.

 MISCELLANEOUS

Suggested Reading
Chrisman CL. Dancing Doberman disease: clinical findings and prognosis. Prog Vet Neurol 1990;1:83–90.
Author Karen Dyer Inzana
Consulting Editor Joane M. Parent

BASICS

OVERVIEW
• Permanent teeth are formed by 11 weeks of age.
• Root development normally pushes the crown through the gingiva.
• Pressure from the erupting crown on root of temporary tooth causes resorption of root.
• Normally, loss of the primary tooth makes a pathway for the erupting permanent tooth.

SIGNALMENT
• Dogs and cats
• More common in small-breed dogs than in cats or large-breed dogs

SIGNS

Initial signs
• Two teeth of the same type (deciduous and permanent) occupying the same space (in the alveolus) at the same time
• Canine teeth—mandibular permanent canine tooth erupts lingual (medial) to the retained deciduous tooth; maxillary permanent canine tooth erupts mesial (rostral) to the retained deciduous canine tooth
• Incisors—permanent maxillary and mandibular incisors erupt palatal and lingual (respectively) to the retained deciduous incisors
• Premolars—permanent premolars erupt lingual (mandible) and palatal (maxilla) to the retained deciduous teeth, except the maxillary fourth premolar, which erupts buccal and slightly caudal (distal) to the last deciduous premolar

Halitosis
• Localized gingivitis
• Gingival recession and bone loss possible
• Sign when left untreated

Malocclusion
• Localized gingivitis
• Periodontal disease
• Oronasal fistula possible
Permanent lower canines erupt lingual to the retained deciduous teeth and will assume a vertical position in the mouth, resulting in impingement on the hard palate, which

creates pain, inflammation, and, long-term, an oronasal fistula if the teeth continue to erupt.

CAUSES & RISK FACTORS
• Cause unknown
• Small-breed dogs predisposed

DIAGNOSIS

DIFFERENTIAL DIAGNOSIS
N/A

CBC/BIOCHEMISTRY/URINALYSIS
N/A

OTHER LABORATORY TESTS
N/A

IMAGING
Intraoral radiographs to identify dental abnormalities prior to extraction; to identify retained root where crown is missing but opposite side retained; confirm absence of deciduous root after extraction.

DIAGNOSTIC PROCEDURES
N/A

PATHOLOGIC FINDINGS
Evidence of root resorption of the apex of the deciduous root

TREATMENT

SURGICAL CONSIDERATIONS
• Ideally, perform extraction as soon as the permanent tooth has erupted through the gingiva.
• Analgesia—butorphanol (0.22 mg/kg SC)
• General anesthesia with endotracheal tube in place and cuff inflated to prevent a foreign body (e.g., extracted tooth, dislodged piece of tartar) from entering upper airway

Extraction
• Sever epithelial attachment in gingival sulcus with a sharp blade (No. 15 or 150); elevate gingiva with a small surgical periosteal elevator.
• Sever periodontal ligament by placing a Luxator or elevator in the periodontal

ligament space (between the tooth and the bone of the socket) and gently move the instrument around the tooth.
• Advance the elevator as space allows, and apply even pressure for 30 sec to weaken the fibers and produce bleeding in the socket; the hemorrhage is space-occupying and facilitates extraction.

Extraction with Other Surgical Procedures
Extract the retained deciduous teeth of any patient undergoing anesthesia (e.g., spay/neuter).

Fractured and Retained Root Tips
If a fracture occurs during extraction, the retained root can deflect the permanent tooth's eruption and should be extracted; it may be necessary to make a full-thickness gingival flap and remove enough buccal bone to get good visualization.

MEDICATIONS

DRUGS
N/A

CONTRAINDICATIONS/POSSIBLE INTERACTIONS
N/A

FOLLOW-UP
Recheck patient within 1 week of surgery.

MISCELLANEOUS

Suggested Reading
Wiggs R, Lobprise H. Veterinary dentistry, principles and practice. Philadelphia: Lippincott-Raven, 1997.
Author Randi Brannan
Consulting Editor Jan Bellows

DEMODICOSIS

BASICS

DEFINITION
• An inflammatory parasitic disease of dogs and rarely cats that is characterized by an increased number of mites in the hair follicles, which often leads to furunculosis and secondary bacterial infection
• May be localized or generalized in dogs

PATHOPHYSIOLOGY
Dogs
• *Demodex canis*—a mite; part of the normal fauna of the skin; typically present in small numbers; resides in the hair follicles and sebaceous glands of the skin
• Pathology develops when numbers exceed that tolerated by the immune system.
• The initial proliferation of mites may be the result of a genetic or immunologic disorder.

Cats
• Poorly understood disorder
• Mites have been identified on the skin and within the otic canal.
• Two species: *D. cati* and an un-named species

SYSTEMS AFFECTED
Skin/Exocrine—dead and degenerate *D. canis* mites may be found in noncutaneous sites (e.g., lymph node, intestinal wall, spleen, liver, kidney, urinary bladder, lung, thyroid gland, blood, urine, and feces) and are considered to represent drainage to these areas by blood and/or lymph.

GENETICS
The initial proliferation of mites may be the result of a genetic disorder.

INCIDENCE/PREVALENCE
• Dogs—common
• Cats—rare

GEOGRAPHIC DISTRIBUTION
None

SIGNALMENT
Species
Dogs and rarely cats

Breed Predilections
Potential increased incidence in Siamese and Burmese cat breeds

Mean Age and Range
• Localized—usually in young dogs; median age 3–6 months
• Generalized—both young and old animals

Predominant Sex
None

SIGNS
Dogs
Localized
• Lesions—usually mild; consist of erythema and a light scale
• Patches—several may be noted; most common site is the face, especially around the perioral and periocular areas; may also be seen on the trunk and legs
Generalized
• Can be widespread from the onset, with multiple poorly circumscribed patches of erythema, alopecia, and scale
• As hair follicles become distended with large numbers of mites, secondary bacterial infections are common, often with resultant rupturing of the follicle (furunculosis).
• With progression, the skin can become severely inflamed, exudative, and granulomatous.

Cats
• Often characterized by partial to complete multifocal alopecia of the eyelids, periocular region, head, and neck
• Lesions—variably pruritic with erythema, scale, and crust; those caused by the un-named species are often quite pruritic.
• Ceruminous otitis externa has been reported.

CAUSES
• *Demodex canis*
• *Demodex cati*

RISK FACTORS
Dogs
• Exact immunopathologic mechanism unknown
• Studies indicate that dogs with generalized demodicosis have a subnormal percentage of IL-2 receptors on their lymphocytes and subnormal IL-2 production.
• Genetic factors, immunosuppression and/or metabolic diseases may predispose animal

Cats
• Often associated with metabolic diseases (e.g., FIV, systemic lupus erythematosus, diabetes mellitus)
• Unnamed species—short and blunted; rarely a marker for metabolic disease; individual reports indicate that it may be transferable from cat to cat within the same household.

DIAGNOSIS

DIFFERENTIAL DIAGNOSIS
Dogs
• Bacterial folliculitis/furunculosis
• Dermatophytosis
• Contact dermatitis
• Pemphigus complex
• Dermatomyositis
• Systemic lupus erythematosus

Cats
• Allergic dermatitis
• Scabies

CBC/BIOCHEMISTRY/URINALYSIS
• Nondiagnostic for *Demodex* sp.
• May be useful for identifying underlying metabolic diseases in cats

OTHER LABORATORY TESTS
FeLV and FIV serology—identify underlying metabolic diseases in cats

IMAGING
N/A

DIAGNOSTIC PROCEDURES
• Skin scrapings—diagnostic for finding large numbers of mites in the majority of cases
• Cutaneous biopsy—may be needed when lesions are chronic, granulomatous, and fibrotic (especially on the paw)

PATHOLOGIC FINDINGS
N/A

TREATMENT

APPROPRIATE HEALTH CARE
• Outpatient
• Localized—conservative; most cases (90%) resolve spontaneously with no treatment.
• Evaluate the general health status of dogs with either the localized or the generalized form.

NURSING CARE
N/A

ACTIVITY
N/A

DIET
N/A

CLIENT EDUCATION
• Localized—most cases resolve spontaneously
• Generalized (adult dog)—frequent management problem; expense and frustration with the chronicity of the problem are issues; many cases are medically controlled, not cured.

SURGICAL CONSIDERATIONS
N/A

MEDICATIONS

DRUGS OF CHOICE

Amitraz (Mitaban; Taktic-EC)
• A formamidine, which inhibits monamine oxidase and prostaglandin synthesis; an α_2-adrenergic agonist
• Use weekly (the label reads every other week) at 1/2 vial (5 mL)/gal water until resolution of clinical signs and no mites are found on skin scrapings; do not rinse off; let air-dry.
• Treat for one month following negative skin scrape
• Apply a benzoyl peroxide shampoo before application of the dip as a bactericidal therapy and to increase exposure of the mites to the miticide through follicular flushing activity.
• The efficacy is proportional to the frequency of administration and the concentration of the dip.
• May be mixed with mineral oil (3 mL amitraz to 30 mL mineral oil) for application to focal areas, such as pododemodicosis
• Success with the 9% amitraz collar has not been established, although there are positive anecdotal reports.
• Between 11% and 30% of cases will not be cured; may need to try an alternative therapy or control with maintenance dips every 2–8 weeks.

Ivermectin (Ivomec; Eqvalan Liquid)
• A macrocyclic lactone with GABA agonist activity.
• Daily oral administration of 0.3–0.6 mg/kg very effective, even when amitraz fails
• Treat for 60 days beyond negative skin scrapings (average 3–8 months).

Milbemycin (Interceptor)
• A macrocyclic lactone with GABA agonist activity
• Dosage of 1 mg/kg PO q24h cures 50% of cases; 2 mg/kg PO q24h cures 85% of cases.
• Treat for 60 days beyond multiple negative skin scrapings.

Cats
• Exact protocols are not defined.
• Topical lime-sulfur dips or amitraz solutions applied weekly for 4 treatments often lead to good resolution of clinical signs.

CONTRAINDICATIONS
Ivermectin—contraindicated in collies, Shetland sheepdogs, old English sheepdogs, other herding breeds, and crosses with these breeds; sensitive breeds appear to tolerate the acaricidal dosages of milbemycin (see above).

PRECAUTIONS

Amitraz
• Most common side effects—somnolence, lethargy, depression, anorexia seen in 30% of patients for 12–36 hr after treatment
• Other side effects—vomiting, diarrhea, pruritus, polyuria, mydriasis, bradycardia, hypoventilation, hypotension, hypothermia, ataxia, ileus, bloat, hyperglycemia, convulsions, death
• The incidence and severity of side effects do not appear to be proportional to the dose or frequency of use.
• Humans can develop dermatitis, headaches, and respiratory difficulty after exposure.
• Yohimbine at 0.11 mg/kg IV is an antidote.

Ivermectin and Milbemycin
Signs of toxicity—salivation, vomiting, mydriasis, confusion, ataxia, hypersensitivity to sound, weakness, recumbency, coma, and death

POSSIBLE INTERACTIONS
• Amitraz—may interact with heterocyclic antidepressants, xylazine, benzodiazepines, and macrocyclic lactones
• Ivermectin and milbemycin—cause elevated levels of monoamine neurotransmitter metabolites, which could result in adverse drug interactions with amitraz and benzodiazepines

ALTERNATIVE DRUGS
None

FOLLOW-UP

PATIENT MONITORING
Multiple skin scrapings and evidence of clinical resolution are used to monitor progress.

PREVENTION/AVOIDANCE
Avoid breeding animals with generalized form

POSSIBLE COMPLICATIONS
Secondary bacterial infections

EXPECTED COURSE AND PROGNOSIS
• Prognosis (dogs)—depends heavily on genetic, immunologic, and underlying diseases
• Localized—most cases (90%) resolve spontaneously with no treatment; < 10% progress to the generalized form
• Adult-onset (dogs)—often severe and refractory to treatment

MISCELLANEOUS

ASSOCIATED CONDITIONS
Adult-onset—sudden occurrence is often associated with internal disease, malignant neoplasia, and/or immunosuppressive disease; approximately 25% of cases are idiopathic over a follow-up period of 1–2 years.

AGE-RELATED FACTORS
Young dogs are often predisposed.

ZOONOTIC POTENTIAL
None

PREGNANCY
Do not breed animals with the generalized form.

SYNONYMS
Mange

SEE ALSO
• Amitraz toxicity
• Ivermectin toxicity

ABBREVIATIONS
• FeLV = feline leukemia virus
• FIV = feline immunodeficiency virus
• GABA = γ-aminobutyric acid
• IL = interleukin

Suggested Reading
Scott DW, Miller WH, Griffin CE, eds. Parasitic skin diseases. In: Muller & Kirk's small animal dermatology. 5th ed. Philadelphia: Saunders, 1995:417–432.
Author Karen Helton Rhodes
Consulting Editor Karen Helton Rhodes

DISEASES

DERMATOMYOSITIS

BASICS

DEFINITION
An inherited inflammatory condition of dogs that involves the skin and muscle and, occasionally, the blood vessels

PATHOPHYSIOLOGY
• Exact pathogenesis unknown
• Although it is well accepted that there is a genetic predisposition, some researchers suspect an infectious agent (i.e., a virus) triggers the clinical signs; others believe an immune-mediated or autoimmune process may be involved.

SYSTEMS AFFECTED
• Skin/Exocrine—initially, variable dermatitis on the face, ears, and tail tip and over the bony prominences of the distal extremities develops.
• Musculoskeletal—later, myositis, which can be subtle to severe, develops; usually the temporal and masseter muscles are involved; in more severe cases, generalized muscle disease and involvement of the esophageal muscles may occur; generally, the more severe the dermatitis, the more severe the myositis.

GENETICS
• Thought to be inherited as an autosomal dominant trait with variable expression in collies and Shetland sheepdogs

INCIDENCE/PREVALENCE
Unknown

GEOGRAPHICAL DISTRIBUTION
Probably worldwide

SIGNALMENT

Species
Dogs

Breed Predilection
• Collies, Shetland sheepdogs, and their crossbreeds
• Isolated reports—Australian cattle dogs, Welsh corgis, chow chows, German shepherds, and kuvaszes

Mean Age and Range
• Cutaneous lesions usually develop between 7 weeks and 6 months of age
• Mild disease—lesions may resolve in 3 months
• Moderate disease—lesions may persist for 6 months or more
• Severe disease—lesions usually persist throughout life
• Adult-onset disease—much less common

Predominant Sex
None

SIGNS

General Comments
The clinical signs vary from subtle skin lesions and subclinical myositis to severe skin lesions and generalized muscle atrophy.

Historical Findings
• Waxing and waning skin lesions—in dogs < 6 months old; around the eyes, lips, face, inner ear pinnae, tail tip, and bony prominences of distal extremities; healing may lead to residual scarring.
• Muscle atrophy of the masseter and/or temporal muscles may be evident.
• Severely affected dogs may have difficulty eating, drinking, and swallowing; have stunted growth, be lame, have widespread muscle atrophy, and be infertile
• Several litter mates may be affected, but the severity of the disease often varies significantly among the affected dogs.

Physical Examination Findings
• Skin lesions—characterized by papules and vesicles (rare); variable degrees of erythema; alopecia, scaling, crusting, ulceration, and scarring on the face, around the lips and eyes, in the inner ear pinnae, on the tail tip, and over bony prominences on the distal extremities
• Footpad and oral ulcers rare
• Myositis—vary from none to a bilateral symmetric decrease in the mass of the temporalis muscles to generalized symmetric muscle atrophy; lameness
• Aspiration pneumonia—with megaesophagus

CAUSES
• Hereditary*
• Infectious agents
• Immune-mediated

RISK FACTORS
• Trauma
• Sunlight
• Estrus
• Parturition
• Lactation

DIAGNOSIS

DIFFERENTIAL DIAGNOSIS
• Demodicosis
• Dermatophytosis
• Bacterial folliculitis
• Juvenile cellulitis
• Discoid lupus erythematosus
• Systemic lupus erythematosus
• Polymyositis

CBC/BIOCHEMISTRY/URINALYSIS
• Nonregenerative anemia may occur with severe disease.
• Serum creatine kinase may be normal or slightly high.

OTHER LABORATORY TESTS
ANA titers and lupus erythematosus tests negative

IMAGING
N/A

DIAGNOSTIC PROCEDURES
• EMG—abnormalities in affected muscles; fibrillation potentials; bizarre high frequency discharges; positive sharp waves
• Skin biopsy—choose papules, vesicles, or lesions that show alopecia and erythema; avoid infected and scarred lesions
• Muscle biopsy—difficult because pathologic changes may be mild, multifocal, or (in early states) absent; ideally, use EMG to select affected muscles; otherwise use atrophied muscles; if muscles appear clinically normal, random biopsies may not be diagnostic.

PATHOLOGIC FINDINGS

Skin Biopsy
• Scattered necrotic basal cells (colloid bodies) or vacuolated individual basal cells
• Occasionally, vesicles that contain small amounts of RBCs
• Superficial, mild, and diffuse dermal inflammatory infiltrates composed of lymphocytes and histiocytes with variable numbers of mast cells and neutrophils (especially perifollicularly)
• Usually, follicular basal cell degeneration and follicular atrophy
• Secondary epidermal ulceration and dermal scarring
• Combination of perifollicular inflammation, epidermal and follicular cell degeneration, and follicular atrophy strongly suggest the diagnosis.

Muscle Biopsy
• Variable multifocal accumulations of inflammatory cells, including lymphocytes, macrophages, plasma cells, neutrophils, and eosinophils
• Myofibril degeneration characterized by fragmentation, vacuolation, and increased eosinophilia of the myofibrils
• Myofiber atrophy and regeneration

TREATMENT

APPROPRIATE HEALTH CARE
• Most patients can be treated as outpatients.
• Severe myositis—may need hospitalized for supportive care

NURSING CARE
Nonspecific symptomatic therapy includes hypoallergenic shampoo baths, treating secondary pyoderma and demodicosis, and avoiding trauma and intense sunlight.

ACTIVITY
• Avoid activities that may traumatize the skin.
• Keep indoors during the day to avoid exposure to intense sunlight.

DIET
N/A

CLIENT EDUCATION
• Discuss the hereditary nature of the disease.
• Note that affected dogs should not be bred.
• Inform owner that the disease is not curable, although spontaneous resolution can occur.
• Discuss prognosis and possible complications, especially in severely affected dogs.
• Advise that medications may not help.

SURGICAL CONSIDERATIONS
Because estrus exacerbates the disease, neutering intact females is recommended.

MEDICATIONS

DRUGS OF CHOICE
• The therapeutic efficacy of medical treatment can be difficult to assess, because the disease tends to be cyclic and is often self-limiting.
• Vitamin E—100–400 IU PO q12–24h
• Prednisone—1–2 mg/kg PO q12h until remission; then alternate-day administration with the lowest dosage possible for long-term control
• Pentoxifylline (Trental)—400 mg PO with food q24h; human drug that increases microvascular blood flow and tissue oxygenation by lowering blood viscosity, inhibiting platelet aggregation, increasing RBC deformability, and reducing serum fibrinogen levels; sold as 400-mg tablets that should not be divided; beneficial in some dogs, but improvement may not be seen for 1–2 months

CONTRAINDICATIONS
Pentoxyifylline should not be used in dogs that are sensitive to methylxanthine derivatives (e.g., theophylline).

PRECAUTIONS
• Pentoxifylline—can cause gastric irritation; animals with prolonged clotting times and those receiving anticoagulant therapy should be monitored carefully.
• Glucocorticoids—discuss possible side effects with the owner.

POSSIBLE INTERACTIONS
See Precautions

ALTERNATIVE DRUGS
N/A

FOLLOW-UP

PATIENT MONITORING
N/A

PREVENTION/AVOIDANCE
• Minimize trauma and exposure to sunlight.
• Spay intact females to prevent estrus, parturition, and lactation (all precipitating causes of active dermatomyositis).
• Do not breed affected animals.

POSSIBLE COMPLICATIONS
• Secondary pyoderma and demodicosis
• Mild to moderate disease—residual foci of alopecia, hypopigmentation, and hyperpigmentation in areas of previously active skin lesions; occur most frequently on the bridge of the nose and around the eyes
• Severe disease—extensive scarring; trouble chewing, drinking, and swallowing if the masticatory and esophageal muscles are involved; megaesophagus may develop, predisposing the dog to aspiration pneumonia.
• Generalized myositis—growth may be stunted

EXPECTED COURSE AND PROGNOSIS
• Long-term prognosis—varies, depending on the severity
• Minimal disease—prognosis good; tends to spontaneously resolve with no evidence of scarring
• Mild to moderate disease—tends to eventually spontaneously resolve; usually with residual scarring
• Severe disease—poor prognosis for long-term survival; dermatitis and myositis are severe and life-long.

MISCELLANEOUS

ASSOCIATED CONDITIONS
Idiopathic ulcerative dermatosis of Shetland sheepdogs and collies—poorly understood disease; described in adult collies and Shetland sheepdogs; characterized by well-demarcated serpiginous ulcers in the intertriginous areas of the groin and axillae; may occur alone or concurrently with dermatomyositis; may be a subgroup of dermatomyositis

AGE-RELATED FACTORS
• Clinical signs are usually first seen in dogs < 6 months old.
• Adult-onset—rare; more commonly seen in dogs that had subtle lesions as puppies; more noticeable lesions develop as a result of some precipitating event (i.e., trauma, estrus).

ZOONOTIC POTENTIAL
None

PREGNANCY
• Do not breed affected dogs.
• Pregnancy exacerbates clinical symptoms.

SYNONYMS
• Familial canine dermatomyositis
• Canine familial dermatomyositis

SEE ALSO
• Lupus Erythematosus, Cutaneous (Discoid)
• Lupus Erythematosus, Systemic (SLE)

ABBREVIATIONS
• ANA = antinuclear antibody
• EMG = electromyography

Suggested Reading

Gross TL, Ihrke PJ, Walder E. Veterinary dermatopathology: a macroscopic and microscopic evaluation of canine and feline skin disease. St. Louis: Mosby, 1992.

Hargis AM, Mundell AC. Familial canine dermatomyositis. Comp Cont Ed 1992;14:855–864.

Hargis AM, Prieur DJ, Haupt KH, et al. Post-mortem findings in four litters of dogs with familial canine dermatomyositis. Am J Pathol 1986;123:480–496.

White SD, Shelton GD, Sisson A, et al. Dermatomyositis in an adult Pembroke Welsh corgi. J Am Anim Hosp Assoc 1992;28:398–401.

Authors Linda Medleau and Keith A. Hnilica
Consulting Editor Karen Helton Rhodes

DISEASES

DERMATOPHILOSIS

 BASICS

OVERVIEW
• A crusting skin disease in dogs and a nodular subcutaneous and oral disease in cats
• Reported infrequently
• *Dermatophilus congolensis*—causative agent; gram-positive, branching filamentous bacterium classified as an Actinomycete; common cause of crusting dermatoses in hoofed animals, causing crusted skin lesions of affected large animals and persists in their environment within crusts and other debris shed from infected hoof stock
• Dogs, cats, and humans can rarely be secondarily infected.

SIGNALMENT
• Dogs and cats
• No age, breed, or sex predilection

SIGNS
Historical Findings
• Association with farm animals or free-roaming lifestyle often reported
• Cats—episode of trauma; existence of a foreign body; lesions generally chronic; no systemic clinical signs, except when internal organs or large oral lesions develop

Physical Examination Findings
• Dogs—lesions: papular; crusted; mainly on the skin of the trunk or head; circular to coalescent; similar to those in superficial pyoderma caused by *Staphylococcus intermedius;* resemble dermatophilosis in horses (adherent thick, gray-yellow crusts that incorporate hair and leave a circular glistening shallow erosion when removed); pruritus variable
• Cats—subcutaneous, oral, or internal ulcerated and fistulated nodules or abscesses similar to lesions caused by other actinomycetes in this species

CAUSES & RISK FACTORS
• Dogs, cats, and humans can be exposed directly from lesions on large animals or from environmental exposure.
• Infectious stage—requires wetting for activation; probably cannot penetrate intact epithelium, thus antecedent minor trauma or mechanical transmission by biting ectoparasites required
• Deeper infections—presumably acquired by traumatic inoculation of infectious material

 DIAGNOSIS

DIFFERENTIAL DIAGNOSIS

Dogs
• Staphylococcal pyoderma
• Acute moist dermatitis
• Dermatophytosis
• Pemphigus foliaceus
• Keratinization disorder

Cats
• Actinomycosis and nocardiosis
• Atypical mycobacterial granuloma
• Sporotrichosis
• Other subcutaneous fungal infection
• Deep mycotic infection, especially *Cryptococcosis*
• Foreign body
• Chronic bite/wound abscess
• Bacterial L-form infection
• *Rhodococcus equi* infection
• Cutaneous or mucosal neoplasm, especially squamous cell carcinoma

CBC/BIOCHEMISTRY/URINALYSIS
Usually normal or neutrophilic leucocytosis in cats

OTHER LABORATORY TESTS N/A

IMAGING N/A

DIAGNOSTIC PROCEDURES

Dogs
• Cytologic examination of crusts—most important procedure; differentiates from more typical bacterial pyodermas
• Organism—distinctive morphology in cytologic and histologic preparations; resembles "railroad tracks" as the bacterium forms chains of small diplococci; chains often branching
• Cytologic diagnosis—from impression smears made of exudate from under crusts or by preparation of minced crusts; mince crusts finely in a drop of water and allow to macerate several minutes; then dry the preparation and stain with any Wright-Giemsa stain.
• Histopathologic specimens—from crusts

Cats
• Histopathologic examination—biopsy of ulcerated nodules; procedure of choice
• Cytologic examination—exudate obtained from aspiration or swabbing of a draining tract
• Culture of biopsy specimens—may yield the organism; facilitated if the laboratory is alerted to the possible presence of *Dermatophilus* (aerobic, relatively slow growing, and easily obscured by contamination)
• Culture from crusts—requires the use of special selective medium; generally employed to corroborate cytologic findings

PATHOLOGIC FINDINGS
• Dogs—crusting and superficial pustular dermatitis; palisading of the crusts with orthokeratotic and parakeratotic hyperkeratosis; organism visualized within the crusts, generally without the use of special bacterial stains
• Cats—pyogranulomatous inflammation; central necrosis; fistulous tract formation; organism visualized near the necrotic center of granulomas, especially with gram stain

TREATMENT

• Dogs—antibacterial shampoo and gentle removal (and disposal) of crusts; shampoo may contain benzoyl peroxide, ethyl lactate, chlorhexidine, or selenium disulfide; one or two applications suffice in most cases.
• Cats—for pyogranulomas and abscesses: surgical débridement; exploration for foreign body; establishment of drainage for exudate; maintain effective drainage and postoperative wound care.

MEDICATIONS

DRUGS
• Penicillin V—10 mg/kg PO q12h for 10–20 days; drug of choice
• Ampicillin—10–20 mg/kg PO q12h for 10–20 days
• Amoxicillin—10–20 mg/kg PO q12h for 10–20 days
• Tetracycline, doxycycline, or minocycline—standard dosage

CONTRAINDICATIONS/POSSIBLE INTERACTIONS
Penicillin and ampicillin—allergy

FOLLOW-UP

PATIENT MONITORING
• Dogs—re-examine after 2 weeks of treatment to ensure complete resolution of symptoms; give an additional 7 days of systemic therapy
• Cats—monitor biweekly for 1 month after apparent resolution of lesions, depending on their location

EXPECTED COURSE AND PROGNOSIS
• Dogs—excellent
• Cats—varies with the location of lesions and extent of surgical débridement; complete resolution can be achieved with timely diagnosis and appropriate surgical and medical therapy.

MISCELLANEOUS

ZOONOTIC POTENTIAL
• Veterinarians and animal care workers—very seldom infected, even after traumatic exposure when working with farm animals known to be infected
• Dogs and cats—very unlikely to serve as a source for human infection; caution is warranted for exposure of immuno-compromised individuals.

Suggested Reading
Greene CE. Dermatophilosis. In: Greene CE, ed. Infectious diseases of the dog and cat. Philadelphia: Saunders, 1998:326–327.
Author Carol S. Foil
Consulting Editor Stephen C. Barr

DISEASES

DERMATOPHYTOSIS

 BASICS

DEFINITION
• A cutaneous fungal infection affecting the cornified regions of hair, nails, and occasionally the superficial layers of the skin
• Most commonly isolated organisms—*Microsporum canis, Trichophyton mentagrophytes,* and *M. gypseum*

PATHOPHYSIOLOGY
• Exposure to or contact with a dermatophyte does not necessarily result in an infection.
• Infection may not result in clinical signs.
• Dermatophytes—grow in the keratinized layers of hair, nail, and skin; do not thrive in living tissue or persist in the presence of severe inflammation; incubation period: 1–4 weeks
• An affected animal that does not show signs may remain in this inapparent carrier state for a prolonged period of time; some animals never become symptomatic.
• Corticosteroids can modulate inflammation and prolong the infection.

SYSTEMS AFFECTED
Skin/Exocrine—keratinized layers of the hair, nails, and skin may harbor the hyphae and spores.

GENETICS
N/A

INCIDENCE/PREVALENCE
• Reliance on clinical signs and incorrectly interpreted Wood's lamp examination results in overdiagnosis.
• Infection rates vary widely, depending on the population studied.

GEOGRAPHIC DISTRIBUTION
Although ubiquitous, the incidence is higher in hot and humid regions.

SIGNALMENT
Species
Dogs and cats

Breed Predilections
Cats—more common in long-haired breeds

Mean Age and Range
Clinical signs—more common in young animals

Predominant Sex
None

SIGNS
Historical Findings
• Lesions may begin as alopecia or a poor hair coat.
• A history of previously confirmed infection or exposure to an infected animal or environment (e.g., a cattery) is a useful but not consistent finding.

Physical Examination Findings
• Vary from an inapparent carrier state to a patchy or circular alopecia
• Classic circular alopecia—common in cats; often misinterpreted in dogs
• Scales, erythema, hyperpigmentation, and pruritus—variable
• Paronychosis, granulomatous lesions, or kerions may occur.

CAUSES
• Cats—*M. canis* is by far the most common agent.
• Dogs—*M. canis, M. gypseum,* and *T. mentagrophytes;* incidence of each agent varies geographically.

RISK FACTORS
• Immunocompromising diseases or immunosuppressive medications
• High population density
• Poor nutrition
• Poor management practices
• Lack of an adequate quarantine period

 DIAGNOSIS

DIFFERENTIAL DIAGNOSIS
• Cats—miliary dermatitis and almost any other dermatitis
• Dogs—folliculitis, furunculosis, and most cases of alopecia
• Demodicosis and bacterial skin infection—epidermal collarettes more typical of a bacterial infection; grossly enlarged follicular ostia with furunculosis suggest demodicosis; these characteristics are not consistent; concurrent bacterial or mite infections can be seen with dermatophytosis; all three diseases can cause focal hyperpigmentation.
• Immune-mediated skin diseases—severe inflammation associated with dermatophytosis affecting the face or feet

CBC/BIOCHEMISTRY/URINALYSIS
Not useful for diagnosis

OTHER LABORATORY TESTS
N/A

IMAGING
N/A

DIAGNOSTIC PROCEDURES
Fungal Culture with Macroconidia Identification
• Best means of confirming diagnosis
• Hairs that exhibit a positive apple green florescence under Wood's lamp examination are considered ideal candidates for culture.
• Pluck hairs from the periphery of an alopecic area; do not use a random pattern.
• Use a sterile toothbrush to brush the hair coat of an asymptomatic animal to yield better results.
• Test media—change to red when they becomes alkaline; dermatophytes typically produce this color during the early growing phase of their culture; saprophytes, which also produce this color, do so in the late growing phase; thus it is important to examine the media daily.
• Microscopic examination of the macroconidia—necessary to confirm pathogenic dermatophyte and to identify genus and species; helps identify source of infection
• Positive culture—indicates existence of a dermatophyte; however, it may have been there only transiently, as commonly occurs when the culture is obtained from the feet, which are likely to come in contact with a geophilic dermatophyte.

Microscopic Examination of Hair
• Examination after using a clearing solution can help provide a rapid diagnosis.
• Time-consuming and often produces false-negative results
• Use hairs that fluoresce under Wood's lamp illumination to increase the likelihood of identifying the fungal hyphae associated with the hair shaft.
• Wood's lamp examination—not a very useful screening tool; many pathogenic dermatophytes do not fluoresce; false fluorescence is common; lamp should warm up for a minimum of 5 min and then be exposed to suspicious lesions for up to 5 min; a true positive reaction associated with *M. canis* consists of apple-green florescence of the hair shaft; keratin associated with epidermal scales and sebum will often produce a false-positive fluorescence.

Skin Biopsy
• Not usually needed
• Can be helpful in confirming true invasion and infection

PATHOLOGIC FINDINGS
• Folliculitis, perifolliculitis, or furunculosis
• Hyperkeratosis
• Intraepidermal pustules
• Pyogranulomatous reaction pattern
• Fungal hyphae may be observed in H&E-stained sections; special stains allow easier visualization of the organism.

TREATMENT

APPROPRIATE HEALTH CARE
• Most animals are treated as outpatients.
• Consider quarantine owing to the infective and zoonotic nature of the disease.

NURSING CARE
N/A

ACTIVITY
N/A

DIET
• A fatty meal improves absorption of griseofulvin.
• An acid meal (add tomato juice) enhances the absorption of ketoconazole.

CLIENT EDUCATION
• Inform owner that many short-haired cats in a single-cat environment and many dogs will undergo spontaneous remission.
• Advise that treatment can be both frustrating and expensive, especially in multianimal households or recurrent cases.
• Inform owner that environmental treatment, including fomites, is important, especially in recurrent cases; dilute bleach (1:10) is a practical and relatively effective means of providing environmental decontamination; concentrated bleach and formalin (1%) are more effective at killing spores, but their use is not as practical in many situations; chlorhexidine was ineffective in pilot studies.
• Inform owner that in a multianimal environment or cattery situation, treatment and control can be very complicated; referral to a veterinarian with expertise in this type of situation should be considered.

SURGICAL CONSIDERATIONS
N/A

MEDICATIONS

DRUGS OF CHOICE
• Griseofulvin—most widely prescribed systemic drug; microsized formulation: 25–60 mg/kg PO q12h for 4–6 weeks; ultra-microsized formulation: 2.5–5.0 mg/kg PO q12–24h; pediatric suspension: 10–25 mg/kg PO q12h; gastrointestinal upset is the most common side effect; alleviate by reducing the dose or dividing the dose for more frequent administration
• Ketoconazole—not labeled for use in dogs or cats in the U.S.; dose: 10 mg/kg PO q24h or divided twice per day for 3–4 weeks; anorexia is the most common side effect.

• Vaccination—product literature claims are based on clinical signs and Wood's lamp findings; may be useful as an adjuvant to systemic therapy; may be valuable for treating asymptomatic carriers, which can be frustrating to the client and veterinarian and can complicate the diagnosis and management; studies involving dermatophyte cultures as a measure of achieving a cure or prevention are necessary to ensure true efficacy.
• Topical therapy and clipping—once strongly advocated; may help prevent environmental contamination; often associated with an initial exacerbation of signs after the procedures are initiated; lime sulfur (1:16), enilconazole (bottle dilution), and miconazole shampoo are the most effective agents; lime sulfur is odiferous and can stain; enilconazole is not available in the U.S.

CONTRAINDICATIONS
Corticosteroids

PRECAUTIONS

Griseofulvin
• Bone marrow suppression (anemia, pancytopenia, and neutropenia) can occur as an idiosyncratic reaction or with prolonged therapy.
• Neutropenia—most common fatal reaction in cats; can persist after discontinuation of drug; weekly or biweekly CBC is recommended; can be life-threatening in cats with FIV infection
• Neurologic side effects
• Do not use during the first two trimesters of pregnancy; it is teratogenic.

Ketaconazole
• Hepatopathy has been reported and can be quite severe.
• Inhibits endogenous production of steroidal hormones in dogs

POSSIBLE INTERACTIONS
N/A

ALTERNATIVE DRUGS
Itraconazole—similar to ketoconazole but with fewer side effects; probably more effective; expensive; supplied as 100-mg capsules; dose: 10 mg/kg PO q24h or 5mg/kg PO q12h

FOLLOW-UP

PATIENT MONITORING
• Dermatophyte culture is the only means of truly monitoring response to therapy; many animals will clinically improve, but remain culture positive.
• Repeat fungal cultures toward the end of the treatment regimen and continue treatment until at least one culture result is negative.

• In resistant cases, the culture may be repeated weekly, using the toothbrush technique; continue treatment until 2–3 consecutive culture results are negative.

PREVENTION/AVOIDANCE
• Initiate a quarantine period and obtain dermatophyte cultures of all animals entering the household to prevent reinfection from other animals.
• Consider the possibility of rodents aiding in the spread of the disease.
• Avoid infective soil, if a geophilic dermatophyte is involved
• Consider using griseofulvin for 10–14 days as a prophylactic treatment of exposed animals.

POSSIBLE COMPLICATIONS
False-negative dermatophyte cultures

EXPECTED COURSE AND PROGNOSIS
• Many animals will "self-clear" a dermatophyte infection over a period of a few months.
• Treatment for the disease hastens clinical cure and helps reduce environmental contamination.
• Some infections, particularly in long-haired cats or multianimal situations, can be very persistent.

MISCELLANEOUS

ASSOCIATED CONDITIONS
N/A

AGE-RELATED FACTORS
N/A

ZOONOTIC POTENTIAL
Dermatophytosis is zoonotic.

PREGNANCY
• Griseofulvin is teratogenic.
• Ketoconazole can affect steroidal hormone synthesis, especially testosterone.

SYNONYMS
Ringworm

ABBREVIATIONS
• FIV = feline immunodeficiency virus
• H&E = hematoxylin and eosin

Suggested Reading
Moriello KA, DeBoer DJ. Dermatophytosis. In: August JR, ed. Consultations in feline internal medicine 2. Philadelphia: Saunders, 1994:219–225.
Scott DW, Miller WH, Griffin CE, eds. Fungal skin diseases. In: Muller & Kirk's small animal dermatology. 5th ed. Philadelphia: Saunders, 1995:332–350.
Author W. Dunbar Gram
Consulting Editor Karen Helton Rhodes

DISEASES

DIABETES INSIPIDUS

 BASICS

DEFINITION
DI is a disorder of water metabolism characterized by polyuria, urine of low specific gravity or osmolality (so-called insipid, or tasteless, urine), and polydipsia.

PATHOPHYSIOLOGY
• Central DI—deficiency in the secretion of ADH
• Nephrogenic DI—renal insensitivity to ADH

SYSTEMS AFFECTED
• Endocrine/Metabolic
• Renal/Urologic

GENETICS
N/A

INCIDENCE/PREVALENCE
• Central DI—rare
• Nephrogenic—rare

GEOGRAPHIC DISTRIBUTION
N/A

SIGNALMENT

Species
Dog and cat

Breed Predilections
None

Mean Age and Range
• Congenital forms <1 year
• Acquired forms (e.g., neoplastic, traumatic, and idiopathic), any age

Predominant Sex
None

SIGNS
• Polyuria
• Polydipsia
• Incontinence—occasional

CAUSES

Inadequate Secretion of ADH
• Congenital defect
• Idiopathic
• Trauma
• Neoplasia

Renal Insensitivity to ADH
• Congenital
• Secondary to drugs (e.g., lithium, demeclocycline, and methoxyflurane)
• Secondary to endocrine and metabolic disorders (e.g., hyperadrenocorticism, hypokalemia, pyometra, and hypercalcemia)
• Secondary to renal disease or infection (e.g., pyelonephritis, chronic renal failure, pyometra)

RISK FACTORS
N/A

 DIAGNOSIS

DIFFERENTIAL DIAGNOSIS

Polyuric Disorders
• Hyperadrenocorticism
• Diabetes mellitus
• Liver disease—portosystemic shunt
• Hyperadrenocorticism
• Pyometra
• Pyelonephritis
• Hyperthyroidism—cats
• Hypercalcemia
• Psychogenic polydipsia
• Renal failure

CBC/BIOCHEMISTRY/URINALYSIS
• Usually normal, hypernatremia in some patients
• Urinary specific gravity low (usually <1.012, often <1.008)

OTHER LABORATORY TESTS
Plasma ADH

IMAGING
MRI or CT scan if a pituitary tumor is suspected

DIAGNOSTIC PROCEDURES
• Modified water deprivation test (see Appendix for protocol)
• ADH supplementation trial—therapeutic trial with synthetic ADH (DDAVP); a positive response (water intake decreases by 50% in 3–5 days)
• Rule out all other causes of PU/PD before conducting an ADH trial.

PATHOLOGIC FINDINGS
Degeneration and death of neurosecretory neurons in the neurohypophysis (CDI)

 TREATMENT

APPROPRIATE HEALTH CARE
Patients should be hospitalized for the modified water deprivation test; the ADH trial is often performed as an outpatient procedure.

ACTIVITY
Not restricted

DIET
Normal, with free access to water

CLIENT EDUCATION
• Review dosage of DDAVP and administration technique.
• Importance of having water available at all times

SURGICAL CONSIDERATIONS
N/A

 MEDICATIONS

DRUGS OF CHOICE
• CDI—DDAVP (1–2 drops of the intranasal preparation in the conjunctival sac q12–24h to control PU/PD); alternatively, the intranasal preparation may be given SC (2–5 μg q12–24h).
• NDI—chlorothiazide (10–40 mg/kg PO q12h)

CONTRAINDICATIONS
None

PRECAUTIONS
Overdose of DDAVP can cause water intoxication.

ALTERNATIVE DRUGS
Chlorpropamide (Diabinese; 125–250 mg/day may reduce PU/PD in CDI)

 FOLLOW-UP

PATIENT MONITORING
• Adjust treatment according to the patient's signs; the ideal dosage and frequency of DDAVP administration is based on water intake.
• Laboratory tests such as PCV, total solids, and serum sodium concentration to detect dehydration (inadequate DDAVP replacement)—usually not necessary

PREVENTION/AVOIDANCE
Circumstances that might markedly increase water loss

POSSIBLE COMPLICATIONS
Anticipate complications of primary disease (pituitary tumor).

EXPECTED COURSE AND PROGNOSIS
• The condition is usually permanent, except in rare patients in which the condition was trauma induced.
• Prognosis is generally good, depending on the underlying disorder.
• Without treatment, dehydration can lead to stupor, coma, and death.

 MISCELLANEOUS

ASSOCIATED CONDITIONS
N/A

AGE-RELATED FACTORS
• Congenital CDI and NDI usually manifest before 6 months of age
• CDI related to pituitary tumors is usually seen in dogs >5 years old.

ZOONOTIC POTENTIAL
N/A

PREGNANCY
N/A

SYNONYMS
• Central diabetes insipidus
• Cranial diabetes insipidus
• ADH-responsive diabetes insipidus
• Nephrogenic diabetes insipidus

SEE ALSO
Hyposthenuria

ABBREVIATIONS
• ADH = antidiuretic hormone
• CDI = central diabetes insipidus
• DDAVP = brand name of desmopressin
• DI = diabetes insipidus
• MRI = magnetic resonance imaging
• NDI = nephrogenic diabetes insipidus
• PCV = packed cell volume
• PU/PD = polyuria/polydipsia

Suggested Reading
Feldman EC, Nelson RW. Canine and feline endocrinology and reproduction. Philadelphia: Saunders, 1997.
Author Rhett Nichols
Consulting Editor Deborah S. Greco

DIABETES MELLITUS, KETOACIDOTIC

 BASICS

DEFINITION
A true medical emergency secondary to absolute or relative insulin deficiency, characterized by hyperglycemia, ketonemia, metabolic acidosis, dehydration, and electrolyte depletion

PATHOPHYSIOLOGY
• Insulin deficiency causes an increase in lipolysis, which results in excessive ketone body production and acidosis; an inability to maintain fluid and electrolyte homeostasis causes dehydration, prerenal azotemia, electrolyte disorders, obtundation, and death.
• Many diabetic ketoacidosis patients have underlying conditions such as infection, inflammation, or heart disease that cause stress hormone (e.g., glucagon, cortisol, growth hormone, and epinephrine) secretion; this probably contributes to the development of diabetic ketoacidosis.

SYSTEMS AFFECTED
Endocrine/Metabolic

GENETICS
N/A

INCIDENCE/PREVALENCE
Unknown

GEOGRAPHIC DISTRIBUTION
N/A

SIGNALMENT
Species
Dogs and cats

Breed Predilections
• Dogs—miniature poodle and dachshund
• Cats—none

Mean Age and Range
• Dogs—mean age, 8.4 years
• Cats—median age, 11 years (range, 1–19 years)

Predominant Sex
• Dogs—females 1.5 times males
• Cats—males 2 times females

SIGNS
• Polyuria
• Polydipsia
• Diminished activity
• Anorexia
• Weakness
• Vomiting
• Lethargy and depression
• Muscle wasting
• Unkempt haircoat
• Dehydration
• Thin body condition
• Hypothermia
• Dandruff
• Thickened bowel loops
• Hepatomegaly

CAUSES
• Insulin-dependent diabetes mellitus
• Infection (e.g., skin, respiratory, urinary tract, and prostate gland)
• Concurrent disease (e.g., heart failure, renal failure, and pancreatitis)
• Idiopathic
• Medication noncompliance
• Stress
• Surgery

RISK FACTORS
• Any condition that leads to an absolute or relative insulin deficiency
• History of corticosteroid or β-blocker administration

 DIAGNOSIS

DIFFERENTIAL DIAGNOSIS
• Hyperosmolar nonketotic coma
• Acute hypoglycemic coma
• Uremia
• Lactic acidosis

CBC/BIOCHEMISTRY/URINALYSIS
• Leukocytosis with mature neutrophilia
• Hyperglycemia—blood glucose usually >250 mg/dL
• High liver enzyme activity
• Hypercholesterolemia
• Azotemia
• Hypochloremia
• Hypokalemia
• Hyponatremia
• Hypophosphatemia
• High anion gap—anion gap = (sodium + potassium) − (chloride + bicarbonate); normal is 16 ± 4.
• Glucosuria and ketonuria
• Variable urinary specific gravity with active or inactive sediment

OTHER LABORATORY TESTS
• Metabolic acidosis—venous TCO_2 < 15 mEq/L) caused by ketosis
• Hyperosmolarity
• Bacterial culture of urine and blood

IMAGING
N/A

DIAGNOSTIC PROCEDURES
ECG may help evaluate potassium status; prolonged Q-T interval in some patients with hypokalemia; tall, tented T waves in some patients with hyperkalemia

PATHOLOGIC FINDINGS
Pancreatic islet cell atrophy

 TREATMENT

APPROPRIATE HEALTH CARE
• If the animal is bright, alert, and well hydrated, intensive care and intravenous fluid administration are not required; start subcutaneous administration of insulin (short- or intermediate-acting insulin), offer food, and supply constant access to water; monitor closely for signs of illness (e.g., anorexia, lethargy, vomiting).
• Treatment of "sick" diabetic ketoacidotic dog or cat requires inpatient intensive care; this is a life-threatening emergency; goals are to correct the depletion of water and electrolytes, reverse ketonemia and acidosis, and increase the rate of glucose use by insulin-dependent tissues.

NURSING CARE
• Fluids—necessary to ensure adequate cardiac output and tissue perfusion and to maintain vascular volume; also reduce blood glucose concentration.
• IV administration of 0.9% saline supplemented with potassium is the initial fluid of choice.
• Volume determined by dehydration deficit plus maintenance requirements; replace over 24–48 h.

ACTIVITY
N/A

DIET
A low-fat, high-fiber, high-complex-carbohydrate diet recommended once the patient is stabilized

CLIENT EDUCATION
Serious medical condition requiring lifelong insulin administration in most patients

SURGICAL CONSIDERATIONS
N/A

MEDICATIONS

DRUGS OF CHOICE

Insulin
- Necessary to inhibit lipolysis, inhibit hepatic gluconeogenesis, and promote peripheral glucose uptake
- Regular insulin is the insulin of choice.
- Initial dosage—0.2 U/kg IM (or SC if hydration is normal)
- Subsequent dosage 0.1–0.2 U/kg given 3–6 h later—may be given hourly if patient is closely monitored; response to previous insulin dosage should be considered when calculating subsequent dosages. Ideally, glucose concentration should drop to 50–100 mg/dL/h
- Check blood glucose every 1–3 h with Chemstrip BG reagent strips and an automated test strip analyzer (Accu-Chek III, Boehringer Mannheim).
- Monitor urine glucose and ketones daily.
- Start administering longer-acting insulin (e.g., NPH, lente, and ultralente) when the patient is eating, drinking, and no longer receiving IV fluids and ketosis is resolved or greatly diminished; the dosage is based on that of short-acting insulin given in hospital.

Potassium Supplementation
- Total body potassium is depleted and treatment (e.g., fluids and insulin) will further lower serum potassium; potassium supplementation is always necessary.
- If possible, check potassium concentration before initiating insulin therapy, to guide supplementation dosage; if it is extremely low, insulin therapy may need to be delayed (hours) until serum potassium concentration increases.
- If potassium concentration is unknown, add potassium (40 mEq/L) to the IV fluids, obtain results of pretreatment biochemical analysis ASAP, and draw blood for follow-up biochemical analysis 24 h after treatment is initiated.

Dextrose Supplementation
- Must give insulin, regardless of the blood glucose concentration, to correct the ketoacidotic state
- Whenever blood glucose is < 200–250 mg/dL, 50% dextrose should be added to the fluids to produce a 2.5% dextrose solution (increase to 5% dextrose if needed). Discontinue dextrose once glucose is maintained above 250 mg/dL.
- Do not stop insulin therapy.

Bicarbonate Supplementation
- Controversial; consider if patient's venous blood pH is <7.0 or total CO_2 is <11 mEq/L; bicarbonate is of no benefit if the pH is >7.0.
- Dosage—body weight (kg) $\times$ 0.3 $\times$ base deficit (base deficit = normal serum bicarbonate − patient's serum bicarbonate); *slowly* administer one-quarter to one-half of the dose IV and give the remainder in fluids over 3–6 h.
- Recheck blood gas or serum TCO_2 before further supplementation.

Phosphorus Supplementation
- Pretreatment serum phosphorus usually is normal; however, treatment of ketoacidosis reduces phosphorus, and serum concentrations should be checked every 12–24 h once supplementation is initiated.
- Dosage—0.01–0.03 mmol/kg/h for 6–12 h in IV fluids (may need to increase dose to 0.03–0.06)

CONTRAINDICATIONS
If the patient is anuric or oliguric or if potassium is >5 mEq/L, do not supplement potassium until urine flow is established or potassium concentration decreases.

PRECAUTIONS
Use bicarbonate with caution in patients without normal ventilation because of their inability to excrete carbon dioxide created during treatment.

POSSIBLE INTERACTIONS
N/A

ALTERNATIVE DRUGS
N/A

FOLLOW-UP

PATIENT MONITORING
- Attitude, hydration, cardiopulmonary status, urine output, and body weight
- Blood sugar q1–3h initially; q6h once stable
- Electrolytes q4–8h initially; q24h once stable
- Acid–base status q8–12h initially; q24h once stable

PREVENTION/AVOIDANCE
Appropriate insulin administration

POSSIBLE COMPLICATIONS
- Hypokalemia
- Hypoglycemia
- Hypophosphatemia
- Cerebral edema
- Pulmonary edema
- Renal failure
- Heart failure

EXPECTED COURSE AND PROGNOSIS
Guarded

MISCELLANEOUS

ASSOCIATED CONDITIONS
- Pancreatitis
- Hyperadrenocorticism
- Diestrus
- Bacterial infection
- Electrolyte depletion

AGE-RELATED FACTORS
N/A

ZOONOTIC POTENTIAL
N/A

PREGNANCY
- Risk of fetal death may be relatively high.
- Glucose regulation is often difficult.

SYNONYMS
N/A

SEE ALSO
Diabetes Mellitus Uncomplicated

ABBREVIATIONS
None

Suggested Reading
Feldman EC, Nelson RW. Diabetic ketoacidosis. Canine and feline endocrinology and reproduction. 2nd ed. Philadelphia: Saunders, 1996.
MacIntire DK. Emergency treatment of diabetic crisis: insulin overdose, diabetic ketoacidosis and hyperosmolar coma. Vet Clin North Am Small Anim Pract 1995;25:639.
Nichols R, Crenshaw KL. Complications and concurrent disease associated with diabetic ketoacidosis and other severe forms of diabetes mellitus. In: Bonagura JB, ed. Small animal practice current veterinary therapy XII. Philadelphia: Saunders, 1995:384–386.
Author Kathy L. Crenshaw
Consulting Editor Deborah S. Greco

DIABETES MELLITUS, NONKETOTIC HYPEROSMOLAR SYNDROME

BASICS

DEFINITION
Disease characterized by severe hyperglycemia, hyperosmolarity, severe dehydration, lack of urine or serum ketones, lack of or mild-to-moderate metabolic acidosis, and CNS depression

PATHOPHYSIOLOGY
• Insulin deficiency causes reduced use of glucose and excessive glucose production.
• The resultant high extracellular blood glucose concentration causes a hyperosmolar state with a reduced extracellular fluid volume.
• Intracellular dehydration, azotemia, and uremia develop, and intracellular dehydration becomes more pronounced as the glomerular filtration rate decreases; tissue hypoxia ensues.
• Azotemia, hyperglycemia, and hyperosmolarity worsen as a result of glucose retention and glucose-induced osmotic diuresis.
• Although ketonemia and ketonuria usually are not features of this syndrome, anorexia (especially when prolonged) may cause mild ketoacidosis in some patients, but increased lactic acid is a major contributor to the metabolic acidosis that may develop in these patients.

SYSTEMS AFFECTED
• Renal/Urologic—prerenal and primary renal azotemia develop because of reduced extracellular fluid volume, reduced tissue perfusion, or diabetic glomerulonephropathy; urinary specific gravity is low because of osmotic diuresis, diabetic glomerulonephropathy, or concurrent renal insufficiency.
• Cardiovascular—hypotension because of low extracellular fluid volume, vascular collapse, and depressed myocardial contractility
• Nervous—depression, disorientation or mental confusion, seizures, and coma are caused by intracellular dehydration and hyperosmolarity; CNS dysfunction worsens as serum osmolarity rises.

GENETICS
N/A

INCIDENCE/PREVALENCE
Uncommon

GEOGRAPHIC DISTRIBUTION
N/A

SIGNALMENT
Species
Dogs and cats
Breed Predilections
N/A
Mean Age and Range
• Dogs—peak prevalence, 7–9 years of age
• Cats—any age; most >6 years old
Predominant Sex
• Dogs—female
• Cats—neutered males

SIGNS
Historical Findings
• Early signs—polydipsia, polyuria, polyphagia, and weight loss
• Late signs—weakness, vomiting, anorexia, depression, stupor, and coma
Physical Examination Findings
Dehydration, hypothermia, prolonged capillary refill time, cataracts, lethargy, depression, seizures (severe hyperosmolarity), and stupor or coma (severe hyperosmolarity)

CAUSES
Diabetes mellitus associated with severe hyperosmolarity, severe hyperglycemia, and severe dehydration

RISK FACTORS
• Concurrent problems such as heart disease, renal insufficiency, pneumonia, acute pancreatitis, and other severe diseases
• Drugs—anticonvulsants, glucocorticoids, and thiazide diuretics may precipitate or aggravate this syndrome.

DIAGNOSIS

DIFFERENTIAL DIAGNOSIS
• Uncomplicated diabetes mellitus—mentally alert with fasting hyperglycemia and glucosuria
• Ketoacidotic diabetes mellitus—fasting hyperglycemia with glucosuria, ketonuria, and metabolic acidosis
• Extreme lethargy and depression with severe hyperosmolality, severe hyperglycemia, severe dehydration without ketonemia and ketonuria usually differentiate diabetes mellitus nonketotic hyperosmolar syndrome from uncomplicated and ketoacidotic diabetes mellitus.

CBC/BIOCHEMISTRY/URINALYSIS
• Severe hyperglycemia—usually >600 mg/dL
• High BUN and creatinine concentration
• Normokalemia (despite total body potassium depletion) or hypokalemia
• Hyperkalemia is expected in patients with anuric or oliguric renal failure.
• Low TCO_2
• High anion gap
• Glucosuria
• Low urinary specific gravity

OTHER LABORATORY TESTS
• Severe hyperosmolarity—usually >350 mOsm/L
• High plasma lactate concentration may help confirm metabolic lactic acidosis in the absence of ketonemia and ketonuria.

IMAGING
N/A

DIAGNOSTIC PROCEDURES
N/A

PATHOLOGIC FINDINGS
Pancreatic islet cell atrophy

TREATMENT

APPROPRIATE HEALTH CARE
A life-threatening medical emergency requiring inpatient treatment

NURSING CARE
• Fluid therapy is a major component of medical management.
• Replace one-half the fluid deficits in the first 12 h and the remainder during the next 24 h.
• Administer normal saline (0.9%) IV if the patient is hypotensive or hyponatremic.
• Add potassium (20 mEq/L) to the initial fluids unless the patient has hyperkalemia.

DIABETES MELLITUS, NONKETOTIC HYPEROSMOLAR SYNDROME

• Switch to IV administration of 0.45% saline after restoration of normal blood pressure and urine output.
• Switch to 5% dextrose plus 0.45% saline when blood glucose < 250 mg/dL and continue until the patient is eating and drinking on its own.

ACTIVITY
N/A

DIET
A low-fat, high-fiber, high-complex carbohydrate diet is recommended once the patient is stabilized.

CLIENT EDUCATION
• Poor-to-guarded prognosis
• Intensive care and frequent monitoring are required during hospitalization.

SURGICAL CONSIDERATION
N/A

MEDICATIONS

DRUGS OF CHOICE
• Regular insulin for patients < 10 kg—initial dose is 2 U IM followed by 1 unit IM hourly until blood glucose is < 250 mg/dL.
• Regular insulin for patients >10 kg—initial dose is 0.25 U/kg IM followed by 0.1 U/kg I, hourly until blood glucose is < 250 mg/dL.
• Discontinue IM regular insulin when blood glucose is < 250 mg/dL.
• Monitor blood glucose hourly; aim is to drop concentration by 50–100 mg/dL/h; adjust insulin dosage accordingly.
• Discontinue hourly IM regular insulin when blood glucose is <250 mg/dL; switch to regular insulin (0.5 U/kg) IM q4–6h or SC q6–8h if blood glucose concentration remains between 150 and 250 mg/dL.
• A constant-rate infusion of regular insulin may be used in dogs at a dosage of 1.1 U/kg/24 h.
• Once the patient is stabilized (eating and drinking on its own without vomiting), discontinue fluids and regular insulin; NPH or Lente insulin can then be administered SC in a routine manner.
• Other concurrent diseases must be treated appropriately.

CONTRAINDICATIONS
N/A

PRECAUTIONS
Avoid rapid reduction of serum osmolarity and glucose because the brain will become hyperosmolar compared with serum; fluid may then shift from extracellular to intracellular spaces, resulting in cerebral edema and worsening of neurologic status.

POSSIBLE INTERACTIONS
N/A

ALTERNATIVE DRUGS
Once stable, oral hypoglycemics (e.g., glipizide, Glucotrol) may be tried; these agents are more likely to be efficacious in cats with type II (non–insulin-dependent diabetes mellitas) than in dogs.

FOLLOW-UP

PATIENT MONITORING
• Blood glucose concentrations, closely, to avoid hypoglycemia and abrupt, precipitous decreases
• Ideally, the blood glucose should drop 50–100 mg/dL/h until a concentration of 250 mg/dL is reached.
• Blood glucose hourly before administering the next dose of regular insulin IM during initial stabilization
• Urine output for early detection of acute renal failure
• Hydration status, ECG, CVP, serum electrolytes, BUN, and urine glucose every 2 h during the initial stabilization period
• Long-term glucose control by determining serum glycosylated hemoglobin and serum fructosamine concentrations
• For return of clinical signs such as polydipsia, polyuria, and polyphagia

PREVENTION/AVOIDANCE
• Inappropriate insulin therapy
• Avoid hypoglycemia, hypokalemia, and hyponatremia.

POSSIBLE COMPLICATIONS
• Irreversible coma and death are possible, especially in patients with renal insufficiency.
• Acute renal failure

EXPECTED COURSE AND PROGNOSIS
Clinical signs and laboratory values may improve within the initial 24 h of treatment, but these patients have a guarded prognosis.

MISCELLANEOUS

ASSOCIATED CONDITIONS
Congestive heart failure, renal disease, infection, gastrointestinal hemorrhage, and other serious illnesses

AGE-RELATED FACTORS
N/A

ZOONOTIC POTENTIAL
N/A

PREGNANCY
May encounter insulin resistance and thus poor glycemic in pregnant animals

SYNONYMS
• Diabetic coma
• Hyperosmolar coma

SEE ALSO
• Diabetes Mellitus, Uncomplicated
• Diabetes Mellitus, Ketoacidotic
• Osmolarity, Hyperosmolarity
• Glucose, Hyperglycemia

ABBREVIATIONS
• CVP = central venous pressure

Suggested Reading

Brody GM. Diabetic ketoacidosis and hyperosmolar hyperglycemic nonketotic coma. Topics Emerg Med 1992;14:12–22.

Chastain CB, Nichols CE. Low dose intramuscular insulin therapy for diabetic ketoacidosis in dogs. J Am Vet Med Assoc 1981;178:561–564.

Macintire DK. Treatment of diabetic ketoacidosis in dogs by continuous low dose intravenous infusion of insulin. J Am Vet Med Assoc 1993;202:1266–1272.

Melendez LD. Diabetes mellitus. In: Wingfield W, ed. Veterinary emergency medicine secrets. Philadelphia: Halnely and Belfus, 1997:253–258.

Murtaugh RJ, Kaplan PM. Veterinary emergency and critical care medicine. St. Louis: Mosby Year Book, 1992:253–254.

Author Margaret R. Kern
Consulting Editor Deborah S. Greco

DIABETES MELLITUS, UNCOMPLICATED

BASICS

DEFINITION
• Disorder of carbohydrate, fat, and protein metabolism caused by an absolute or relative insulin deficiency • Type I (insulin-dependent DM) is characterized by very low to absent insulin secretory ability; these patients die if not treated with insulin and are prone to ketoacidosis. • Type II (non-insulin-dependent DM) is characterized by inadequate or delayed insulin secretion relative to the needs of the patient; many of these patients live without exogenous insulin and are less prone to ketoacidosis.

PATHOPHYSIOLOGY
• Insulin deficiency impairs the ability of tissues (especially muscle, adipose tissue, and liver) to use carbohydrates, fats, and proteins. • Impaired glucose use and ongoing gluconeogenesis cause hyperglycemia. • Glucosuria develops, causing osmotic diuresis, polyuria, and compensatory weight loss; mobilization of free fatty acids to the liver causes both hepatic lipidosis and ketogenesis.

SYSTEMS AFFECTED
• Endocrine/Metabolic—electrolyte depletion and metabolic acidosis • Hepatobiliary—hepatic lipidosis; liver failure may develop, particularly in cats • Ophthalmic—cataracts in dogs • Renal/Urologic—urinary tract infection and osmotic diuresis • Nervous—peripheral neuropathy in cats

GENETICS
Familial associations in some breeds of dog

INCIDENCE/PREVALENCE
Prevalence in both dogs and cats varies between 1:400 and 1:500.

GEOGRAPHIC DISTRIBUTION
N/A

SIGNALMENT
Species
Dogs and cats

Breed Predilections
• Higher risk than other breeds—keeshond, puli, miniature pinscher, and Cairn terrier • Possibly higher risk than other breeds—poodle, dachshund, miniature schnauzer, and beagle • None in cats

Mean Age and Range
• Dogs—mean, ~8 years; range, 4–14 years (excluding rare juvenile form) • Cats—75% are 8–13 years; range, 1–19 years

Predominant Sex
• Dogs—female • Cats—male

SIGNS
• More often noticed in the early stages of disease in dogs than in cats • Early signs—polyuria and polydipsia (PU/PD), polyphagia, and weight loss • Later signs—anorexia, lethargy, depression, and vomiting • Obesity with recent weight loss is typical. • Dorsal muscle wasting and an oily coat with dandruff common in cats • Hepatomegaly in both species, but jaundice more prevalent in cats • Less common findings—cataracts in dogs; a plantigrade stance in cats (diabetic neuropathy)

CAUSES
• Genetic susceptibility • Infectious (viral) diseases • Immune-mediated β-cell destruction • Pancreatitis • Predisposing diseases (e.g., hyperadrenocorticism and acromegaly) • Drugs (e.g., glucocorticoids and progestogens)

RISK FACTORS
• Obesity for type II DM • Diestrus in the bitch • See Causes.

DIAGNOSIS

DIFFERENTIAL DIAGNOSIS
• Renal glucosuria—usually does not cause PU/PD, weight loss, or hyperglycemia • Stress hyperglycemia in cats—no PU/PD or weight loss; blood glucose concentration normal if sample taken when cat is not stressed.

CBC/BIOCHEMISTRY/URINALYSIS
• Results of hemogram usually normal • Glucose > 200 mg/dL in dogs; > 250 mg/dL in cats • High SAP, alanine aminotransferase (ALT), and aspartate aminotransferase (AST) activities, and hypercholesterolemia and lipemia common • Electrolytes vary, but hypernatremia, hypokalemia, and hypophosphatemia indicate severe decompensation. • Total CO_2 or HCO_3 is low if the patient has ketoacidosis or severe dehydration. • Glucosuria is a consistent finding. • Ketonuria is common. • Urinary specific gravity often is low.

OTHER LABORATORY TESTS
• Anion gap—high in patients with ketoacidosis • Plasma insulin—may help to differentiate type I from type II DM • Normal or high insulin concentration with hyperglycemia is found in patients with type II DM; low insulin concentration suggests type I DM but may be an incorrect diagnosis because persistent hyperglycemia can impair insulin secretory activity, even if functional β cells are present. • Glucose tolerance test—best way to differentiate types of DM, but impractical

IMAGING
• Radiography—useful to evaluate for concurrent or underlying disease (e.g., cystic or renal calculi, emphysematous cystitis or cholecystitis, and pancreatitis) • Ultrasonography—indicated in selected patients, particularly those with jaundice, to evaluate for hepatic lipidosis, cholangiohepatitis, and pancreatitis

DIAGNOSTIC PROCEDURES
Liver biopsy (percutaneous)—indicated in some jaundiced patients

PATHOLOGIC FINDINGS
• Usually no gross necropsy changes • Histopathologic findings may be normal or reveal vacuolar degeneration of the islets of Langerhans or low numbers of islet cells; immunohistochemical staining is necessary to show low numbers of β cells; in cats, usually see amyloid deposits in the islets

TREATMENT

APPROPRIATE HEALTH CARE
• Compensated dogs and cats can be managed as outpatients; they are alert, hydrated, and eating and drinking without vomiting. • For management of decompensated patients, see Diabetes Mellitus, Ketoacidotic.

NURSING CARE
• Fluid therapy—see Diabetes Mellitus, Ketoacidotic.

ACTIVITY
Strenuous activity may lower insulin requirement; a consistent amount of activity each day is helpful.

DIET
• Avoid soft, moist foods because they cause severe postprandial hyperglycemia. • Nonobese dogs and cats—feed a consistent diet that the pet will eat reliably; keep daily caloric intake constant. • Obese dogs and cats—gradual weight reduction improves insulin sensitivity and reverses diabetes in some cats with type II DM; either reduce the caloric intake to 70% (cats) or 60% (dogs) of the requirement for the animal's ideal body weight (technique 1) or feed a high-fiber, low-calorie food in an amount similar to what the pet is accustomed (technique 2); try to achieve the target weight over 2–4 months; rapid weight loss is inadvisable, especially in obese cats with DM, because they are prone to hepatic lipidosis. • Thin dogs and cats—avoid reduced-calorie diet; starvation exacerbates ketoacidosis and poor immune function. • Role of fiber—key role is in weight loss and obesity prevention; another benefit may be improved glycemic control; recommended diet is high in fiber, low in fat, and high in complex carbohydrates. • Feed the pet half its daily food every 12 h to coincide with twice-daily insulin injections or orally administered hypoglycemic agent; give animals on once-daily insulin injections half the food with the injection and the remainder in 8–10 h or at the time of peak insulin activity, if that is known; nibblers can be fed

dry food ad libitum and given two small meals of canned food as described.

CLIENT EDUCATION
• Discuss daily feeding and medication schedule, home monitoring, signs of hypoglycemia and what to do, and when to call or visit veterinarian.
• Clients are encouraged to keep a chart of pertinent information about the pet, such as urine dipstick results, daily insulin dose, and weekly body weight.

SURGICAL CONSIDERATIONS
Intact females should have an ovariohysterectomy when stable; progesterone secreted during diestrus makes management of DM difficult.

MEDICATIONS

DRUGS OF CHOICE
• Insulin—treatment of choice for all dogs and most cats
• Regular crystalline insulin—rapid bioavailability and short duration of action; can be given by any parenteral route; used for patients with anorexia, vomiting, or ketoacidosis; can mix with other insulins
• NPH (Isophane) insulin—intermediate duration; given SC q12h in all cats and most dogs; initial dosage: dogs, 0.5 U/kg; cats, 0.25–0.5 unit/kg; adjust the dosage according to individual response.
• Lente insulin—intermediate duration; given SC; initial dosage same as for NPH; often given q12h but q24h may be suitable for some patients
• Ultralente insulin—long-acting insulin; given SC, usually q24h; some animals require injections q12h.
• Insulin mixtures add rapid bioavailability to longer-duration insulins; the lente series can be mixed in any combination; NPH and regular insulin mixtures are commercially available; a combination of 25% regular and 75% ultralente can be used after it equilibrates in the vial for 24 h; most patients can be managed without insulin mixtures.
• Species of origin of the insulin may affect pharmacokinetics; beef, pork, beef/pork, and human recombinant insulin are options; animal-origin insulins are being phased out; keep the pet on the same type and species of insulin if possible; when changing from an animal origin to human recombinant insulin, lower the dosage and reregulate the animal.
• Oral administration of hypoglycemic agent—glipizide is useful with dietary therapy in some cats with type II DM; the cat should have uncomplicated DM and no history of ketoacidosis; initial dosage, 2.5 mg PO q12h; monitoring is the same as for patients on insulin; if hyperglycemia is not controlled, 5

mg q12h may be tried; potential side effects are hypoglycemia, hepatic enzyme alterations, icterus, and vomiting.

CONTRAINDICATIONS
N/A

PRECAUTIONS
• Glucocorticoids, megestrol acetate, and progesterone cause insulin resistance.
• Hyperosmotic agents (e.g., mannitol and radiographic contrast agents) if the patient is already hyperosmolar from hyperglycemia

POSSIBLE INTERACTIONS
Many drugs (e.g., NSAIDs, sulfonamides, miconazole, chloramphenicol, monoamine oxidase inhibitors, and β-blockers) potentiate the effect of hypoglycemic agents given orally; consult the product insert.

ALTERNATIVE DRUGS
Dietary therapy or oral administration of hypoglycemic agents or both can be tried if owners are unwilling or unable to give insulin; this is more successful in cats than dogs.

FOLLOW-UP

PATIENT MONITORING
• Glucose curve—best method of monitoring. The owner feeds the pet, injects the insulin, and then brings the patient to the hospital for serial blood glucose testing every 1–2 h, beginning about an hour after the injection. Animals receiving insulin q12h are followed for 12 h, and those on insulin q24h are followed for 24 h; the goal is to maintain blood glucose between 100 and 200 mg/100 mL for at least 20–22 h/day in dogs and between 100 and 300 mg/100 mL in cats; the curve is done every few weeks until the disease is regulated and then every few months or whenever a problem arises.
• Urinary glucose monitoring—urine is tested for glucose and ketones before the meal and insulin injection; to use this as a regulatory method, the pet must be allowed to have trace to 1/4% glucosuria to avoid hypoglycemia. Animals regulated by urine alone may be more hyperglycemic than ideal, and insulin overdose with rebound hyperglycemia is an inherent risk with this method. It is best to combine urine monitoring with intermittent glucose curves; owners should seek veterinary attention if ketonuria is detected.
• Clinical signs—owner can assess degree of PU/PD, appetite, and body weight; if these are normal, the disease is well regulated.

PREVENTION/AVOIDANCE
Prevent or correct obesity; avoid unnecessary use of glucocorticoids or megestrol acetate.

POSSIBLE COMPLICATIONS
• Cataracts (dogs) and diabetic neuropathy (cats) with poor glycemic control
• Seizure or coma with insulin overdose
• Anemia and hemoglobinemia with severe hypophosphatemia, which can occur after initial insulin therapy

EXPECTED COURSE AND PROGNOSIS
• Some cats recover but may relapse at a later time.
• Dogs have permanent disease.
• Prognosis with treatment is good; most animals have a normal life span.

MISCELLANEOUS

ASSOCIATED CONDITIONS
Urinary tract infection

AGE-RELATED FACTORS
Juvenile DM is rare and may be more difficult to manage.

ZOONOTIC POTENTIAL
N/A

PREGNANCY
• Diabetes mellitus can develop during pregnancy, in which case the pregnancy is difficult to maintain. • Exogenous insulin administration may cause fetal oversize and dystocia.
• Insulin resistance develops, making hyperglycemia difficult to control. • The pregnant bitch is prone to ketoacidosis; an emergency ovariohysterectomy may be necessary. • Do not breed dogs with DM.

SYNONYMS
N/A

SEE ALSO
Diabetes Mellitus, Ketoacidotic

ABBREVIATIONS
• ALT = alanine aminotransferase • AST = aspartate aminotransferase • DM = diabetes mellitus • NSAID = nonsteroidal anti-inflammatory drug • PU/PD = polyuria and polydipsia • SAP = serum alkaline phosphatase

Suggested Reading
Nelson RW. Diabetes mellitus. In: Ettinger SJ, Feldman EC, eds. Textbook of veterinary internal medicine. Philadelphia: Saunders, 1995:1510–1537.
Wallace MS, Kirk CA. The diagnosis and treatment of insulin-dependent and non-insulin-dependent DM in the dog and the cat. Probl Vet Med 1990;2:573–590.
Author Melissa S. Wallace
Consulting Editor Deborah S. Greco

DIAPHRAGMATIC HERNIA

BASICS

OVERVIEW
• Protrusion of an abdominal organ through an abnormal opening in the diaphragm either as an acquired injury or a congenital defect
• Traumatic—most common acquired cause; usually the result of automobile trauma but any forceful blow; sudden increase of pressure results in an abdominal–thoracic pressure gradient, causing a tear in the diaphragm, usually at a muscular portion
• Congenital—pleuroperitoneal or peritoneopericardial; may note other congenital defects (e.g., ventricular septal defect, aortic stenosis, portal caval shunt, and cranioventral abdominal wall defects)
• Mechanical and organic factors contribute to clinical signs
• Impaired normal lung expansion—because of lack of lung contact with parietal pleura
• Rib fractures—may contribute to hypoventilation because of pain or mechanical (flail chest) factors
• Accumulation of fluid or air or organ entrapment—prevents lung expansion and contributes to hypoventilation; fluid may be blood from a lung laceration or intercostal vessel tear, chyle from thoracic duct trauma, or transudate from abdominal organ entrapment, leading to transudation of fluid from venous stasis and increased hydrostatic pressure.

• Intrapulmonary changes (e.g., lung contusion, atelectasis, and capillary permeability changes causing edema)—contribute to poor gas exchange
• Myocardial trauma may result in various dysrhythmias—ventricular tachyarrhythmias: most common; may in turn cause low cardiac output and tissue hypoxia; dysrhythmias: most commonly seen within 24–72 hr after trauma; difficult to control with conventional treatment; commonly resolve within 5 days
• Various stages of shock—may cause multiple organ system failure

SIGNALMENT
• Dogs and cats
• Acquired—no breed predilection
• Congenital—Weimeraners and cocker spaniels may be predisposed; may be diagnosed at any age because clinical signs are variable and intermittent
• Young animals at higher risk

SIGNS
Traumatic
• May be acute, subacute, or chronic (with no history of trauma)
• Low-grade respiratory signs
• Vague history of gastrointestinal problems
• May be progressive
• Dyspnea—most common; acutely affected patients frequently in shock
• Arrhythmias—may detect
• Muffled heart and lung sounds along with intestinal sounds—may be auscultated in the thorax

• Abdomen may feel empty on palpation
• Acute incarceration of bowel—may cause vomiting, diarrhea, retching, bloating, pain, and acute collapse

Congenital
• May be asymptomatic; may become symptomatic late in life
• Referable to the respiratory, cardiac, or gastrointestinal system
• Dyspnea, muffled heart sounds, murmurs, and concurrent ventral abdominal wall defects—most common
• May be acute from strangulation of incarcerated bowel, liver, or spleen or rapid formation of pericardial effusions

CAUSES & RISK FACTORS
Traumatic—lack of confinement and exposure to automobiles; any blunt trauma; roaming animals and male dogs at higher risk than others

DIAGNOSIS

DIFFERENTIAL DIAGNOSIS
• See Dyspnea, Tachypnea, and Panting
• See Pleural Effusion

CBC/BIOCHEMISTRY/URINALYSIS
Nonspecific changes owing to ischemia or shock—may be noted

OTHER LABORATORY TESTS
N/A

IMAGING
• Radiography—most useful diagnostic test; may need prior thoracentesis for pleural effusion
• Positive-contrast celiography and/or ultrasonography—if definitive diagnosis not made

DIAGNOSTIC PROCEDURES
N/A

TREATMENT

TRAUMATIC
• Inpatient—treat shock; improve ventilation and cardiac output; manage concurrent injury; stabilize patient before surgery
• Surgery—intervention in the first 24 hr historically has resulted in a higher mortality rate; early intervention indicated with persistent hypotension despite adequate fluid therapy (including transfusion when needed), severe respiratory failure from excessive lung compression, severe liver failure secondary to organ entrapment, bowel rupture, or enlarging gas-filled bowel seen on radiographs; if patient cannot be stabilized, surgical repair will not necessarily improve cardiovascular and respiratory status,
• Intrathoracic gastric dilation—requires immediate decompression; use methods other than immediate surgery.

CONGENITAL
• Surgical repair—perform as early as possible to avoid adhesion formation and organ entrapment.
• Stabilize symptomatic patients before surgery.

MEDICATIONS

DRUGS
Antiarrhythmic agents—as indicated; cardiac arrhythmias often difficult to control

CONTRAINDICATIONS/POSSIBLE INTERACTIONS
Take care when treating for shock with concurrent severe pulmonary contusion; products such as hetastarch (Hespan) may be beneficial.

FOLLOW-UP

• Pneumothorax—may develop from excessive pressure on damaged lung tissue during anesthetic bagging or from failure to remove air from the chest cavity after diaphragmatic closure
• Pulmonary edema—may develop from excessive fluid administration in the face of low oncotic pressure from blood loss, capillary permeability changes secondary to inflammation in response to pulmonary contusion, or re-expansion
• Frequent electrocardiographic monitoring—advised; evaluate for arrhythmias
• Prognosis—always initially guarded; favorable after successful control of shock, elimination of any cardiac arrhythmias, successful surgery, and the lack of re-expansion pulmonary edema

MISCELLANEOUS

Suggested Reading
Boudrieau RJ, Muir WW. Pathophysiology of traumatic diaphragmatic hernia in dogs. Compend Contin Educ Pract Vet 1987;9:379–385.
Author Justin H. Straus
Consulting Editor Eleanor C. Hawkins

DIETARY INTOLERANCE

BASICS

DEFINITION
• Nonimmunologic reaction to food
• A syndrome in which adverse clinical signs are associated with the inability to digest, absorb, and/or utilize a foodstuff or with an untoward reaction to a diet
• Dietary allergies or allergic reactions to food are differentiated from dietary intolerance by the prominent immune component in the allergies.
• In a practical sense, dietary allergy and dietary intolerance may have similar signs, causes, diagnostics, and treatments and may not be easily distinguishable.

PATHOPHYSIOLOGY
• Dietary intolerance may be due to idiosyncratic reactions to dietary ingredients or additives, pharmacologic reactions to compounds in the diet, defects or deficiencies in the metabolic pathways needed to utilize the food, or a toxicity reaction to food ingredients or spoiled foodstuffs.
• Idiosyncratic reactions can produce local irritation to the intestinal lining and subsequent enteritis or such systemic signs as pruritus or urticaria.
• Pharmacologically active food ingredients can also produce local or systemic effects.
• Metabolic defects generally produce maldigestion of a dietary constituent and subsequent malabsorption, fermentation, and osmotic diarrhea.
• Toxic reactions to food may occur when a foodstuff is ingested in large amounts (e.g., onion poisoning).
• Food that is spoiled or that contains microorganisms or their toxins can produce a wide range of clinical signs and severity.

SYSTEMS AFFECTED
• Dermatologic
• Gastrointestinal
• Endocrine/Metabolic

GENETICS
• In general, no genetic basis has been shown.
• Gluten-sensitive enteropathy has been seen primarily in Irish setters.
• The specifics of a genetic basis are not well defined.

INCIDENCE/PREVALENCE
Common in cats and dogs

GEOGRAPHIC DISTRIBUTION
N/A

SIGNALMENT
• Cats and dogs of any age or breed and either sex can be affected.
• Irish setters seem predisposed to develop gluten-sensitive enteropathy; they tend to display clinical signs by 4–7 months of age.
• Juvenile dogs and cats have higher lactase activity and are less likely to display lactose intolerance, which is common in adults of both species.

SIGNS

General Comments
• Dietary intolerance commonly produces diarrhea (small or large bowel), vomiting, flatulence, anorexia, and abdominal discomfort.
• Dermatologic changes, poor weight gain, and failure to thrive may be seen in chronic dietary intolerance.

Historical Findings
• Acute dietary intolerance may accompany feeding a novel foodstuff, a new food source, or dietary change.
• The client may report cessation of clinical signs in the fasted state or with a dietary change.

Physical Examination Findings
The physical examination is generally nonspecific but may show abdominal discomfort, flatulence, gaseous bloating, or a poor body condition.

CAUSES
• Idiosyncratic reactions to food additives—colorings, preservatives (BHA, monosodium glutamate, sodium nitrate, sulfur dioxide, etc.), spices, propylene glycol, etc.
• Pharmacologic reactions—vasoactive substances (i.e., histamine), psychoactive agents, stimulants (i.e., theobromine, caffeine), etc.
• Metabolic defects or deficiencies—brush border enzyme defects (i.e., lactase deficiency), inborn errors of metabolism, aminopeptidase N (in gluten-sensitive enteropathy)
• Toxic reactions to foods or spoiled foods—spices, oxalate toxicity, lectin toxicity, N-propyl disulfide aflatoxicosis, ergotism, botulism, dietary indiscretion, etc.

RISK FACTORS
Young Irish setters susceptible to gluten-sensitive enteropathy may be at greater risk to develop the disease if exposed to gluten at an early age.

DIAGNOSIS

DIFFERENTIAL DIAGNOSIS
• Dietary allergies, inflammatory bowel disease, parasitism, exocrine pancreatic insufficiency, small intestinal bacterial overgrowth, and partial gastrointestinal obstruction can produce signs similar to those of dietary intolerance.
• Some of these disorders may occur with dietary intolerance, complicating diagnosis and treatment.
• Can make a presumptive diagnosis of dietary intolerance when dietary manipulation controls the clinical signs and other differentials are eliminated
• More-rigorous diagnosis requires demonstrating dietary sensitivity, with gastrointestinal histopathologic evaluation before and after a dietary challenge.
• Exclusion diet trials should use a novel protein source and not contain gluten (no wheat, barley, rye, buckwheat, or oats).
• Dietary trials should initially use home-cooked diets, or diets with minimal ingredients or additives.
• Clinical signs often improve within days; dietary allergies may require weeks to months of feeding before seeing improvement.
• Weight gain typically lags behind the resolution of other clinical signs.

CBC/BIOCHEMISTRY/URINALYSIS
No specific changes

OTHER LABORATORY TESTS
• Few diagnostic tests are specific.
• Diagnostics mostly aim to eliminate other differentials and treat complicating factors.
• Fasting serum folate and cobalamin levels are useful in evaluating for SIBO and small intestinal malabsorption.
• Rule out exocrine pancreatic insufficiency by a fasting serum trypsin-like immunoreactivity assay.
• In select patients, gastrointestinal permeability can be assessed with a differential sugar absorption test.
• Some specific enzyme activity assays are available in the research setting.
• Can use intradermal allergy testing and serologic RAST to assess dietary allergy, but their accuracy is not well accepted

IMAGING

Abdominal radiographs or ultrasound may be useful in eliminating differential diagnoses, but specific findings are not seen in dietary intolerance.

DIAGNOSTIC PROCEDURES

• Do fecal evaluation for parasites and empiric broad-spectrum deworming (e.g., fenbendazole 50 mg/kg PO q24h for 3 consecutive days; repeat in 3 weeks and 3 months) and anti-*Giardia* therapy (e.g., metronidazole 30–60 mg/kg PO q24h for 5 days) to rule out parasitism.
• Use dietary manipulation with an exclusion diet as outlined above when intolerance is suspected.
• Following improvement on an exclusion diet, use rigorous challenge exposure to sequential single ingredients to specifically identify a dietary intolerance.
• Practically, continuing an exclusion diet or avoiding suspected problem ingredients is often undertaken instead.
• Can use gastrointestinal endoscopy to assess the mucosa of the intestinal tract; can examine biopsy specimen and histopathology before and after a dietary challenge
• Evaluate for SIBO by bacterial quantification of samples of duodenal juice.
• Can perform IPEC with food antigens; this procedure is still being investigated in veterinary medicine.

PATHOLOGIC FINDINGS

Villous atrophy and lymphoplasmatic enteritis can be seen with dietary intolerance, but are not specific; thus pathologic evaluation must be done before and after provocation, to be useful.

TREATMENT

APPROPRIATE HEALTH CARE

• Patients with extreme and acute cases may need hospitalization for intravenous fluid therapy, antibiotics, and supportive care.
• Generally can treat on an outpatient basis

NURSING CARE

N/A

ACTIVITY

No restrictions

DIET

• Feed a diet free of the offending ingredient(s).

• If no specific ingredient has been identified, feed a nutritionally complete exclusion diet.
• Can use trial and error to find a commercial diet that does not cause dietary intolerance.
• If this approach is used, examination of the ingredients of the various diets is recommended to determine if any patterns exist that might help identify the offending ingredient(s).

CLIENT EDUCATION

Caution against feeding any scraps or varying from a set diet.

SURGICAL CONSIDERATIONS

N/A

MEDICATIONS

DRUGS OF CHOICE

• Generally no medications are used.
• Associated problems (e.g., bacterial overgrowth or inflammatory bowel disease) may require medical therapy as suggested in the sections specific to these problems.

CONTRAINDICATIONS

N/A

PRECAUTIONS

N/A

POSSIBLE INTERACTION

N/A

ALTERNATIVE DRUGS

N/A

FOLLOW-UP

PATIENT MONITORING

• Assess efficacy of treatment by observing improvement in clinical signs.
• Consider repeating evaluation for bacterial overgrowth or endoscopy and biopsy following dietary therapy.

PREVENTION/AVOIDANCE

• Avoiding the offending food ingredient(s) is recommended.
• If no specific ingredient has been identified, adherence to a set exclusion diet is recommended.

POSSIBLE COMPLICATIONS

SIBO and inflammatory bowel disease

EXPECTED COURSE AND PROGNOSIS

• Prognosis for a full recovery is excellent in most cases if diet is found that the patient tolerates.

• Occasionally, severe reactions are produced that require short-term, aggressive in-hospital therapy.

MISCELLANEOUS

ASSOCIATED CONDITIONS

SIBO and inflammatory bowel disease are frequently associated with chronic dietary intolerance.

AGE-RELATED FACTORS

The severity of gluten-sensitive enteropathy in susceptible Irish setter puppies may be reduced by avoiding gluten-containing cereals.

ZOONOTIC POTENTIAL

N/A

PREGNANCY

N/A

SYNONYMS

Food intolerance

SEE ALSO

• Chronic Diarrhea
• Acute Diarrhea
• Exocrine Pancreatic Insufficiency
• Dietary Allergy
• Gluten Enteropathy
• Inflammatory Bowel Disease
• Lymphocytic Plasmacytic Gastroenteritis
• Eosinophilic Gastroenteritis
• Small Intestinal Bacterial Overgrowth
• Trypsin-like Immunoreactivity (TLI)
• Cobalamin and Folate

ABBREVIATIONS

IPEC = intragastric provocation under endoscopic control
RAST = radioallergosorbent test
SIBO = small intestine bacterial overgrowth

Suggested Reading

Batt RM. Wheat-sensitive enteropathy in Irish setters. In: Kirk RW, ed. Current veterinary therapy IX. Philadelphia: Saunders, 1986:893–896.

Burrows CF, Batt RM, Sherding RG. Disease of the small intestine. In: Ettinger SJ, Feldman EC, eds. Textbook of veterinary internal medicine. Philadelphia: Saunders, 1995:1169–1232.

Guilford WG. Adverse reactions to food. In: Kirk RW, Bonagura JD, eds. Current veterinary therapy XI. Philadelphia: Saunders, 1992:587–592.

Author Derek S. Duval
Consulting Editors Brett M. Feder and Mitchell A. Crystal

DISEASES

DIGOXIN TOXICITY

 BASICS

OVERVIEW
Common in veterinary practice because of digoxin's narrow therapeutic index and prevalence of renal impairment in elderly patients with cardiac disease

SIGNALMENT
• Dogs and cats
• More common in geriatric patients

SIGNS

Historical Findings
• Anorexia
• Vomiting
• Diarrhea
• Lethargy
• Depression

Physical Examination Findings
Heart rate may range from severe bradycardia to severe tachycardia.

CAUSES & RISK FACTORS
• Renal disease—impairs digoxin elimination
• Chronic pulmonary disease—results in hypoxia and acid–base disturbances
• Obesity—if dosage not calculated on lean body weight
• Hypokalemia, hypercalcemia, hypomagnesemia, and hypoxia predispose to arrhythmias.
• Drugs and conditions that alter digoxin metabolism or elimination (e.g., quinidine and hypothyroidism)
• Rapid IV digitalization
• Overdosage or accidental ingestion of owner's medication
• Administration of diuretic leading to hypokalemia

 DIAGNOSIS

DIFFERENTIAL DIAGNOSIS
• Arrhythmias and conduction disturbances—may reflect structural heart disease not digoxin toxicity
• Anorexia—common in animals with heart failure

CBC/BIOCHEMISTRY/URINALYSIS
Animals with hypokalemia, hypercalcemia, hypomagnesemia, and renal failure are predisposed to toxicity.

OTHER LABORATORY TESTS
• Consider checking thyroid status.
• Obtain digoxin serum concentration 8–10 h after an oral dose—therapeutic range 0.8–1.5 ng/mL; not all patients with concentrations > 1.5 ng/mL have signs of toxicity; some with values in the normal range have signs of toxicity, especially if hypokalemic.

IMAGING
N/A

DIAGNOSTIC PROCEDURES

Electrocardiographic Findings
• Conduction disturbances—atrioventricular (AV) block), arrhythmias, and ST segment depression in some patients
• Digoxin—can cause any arrhythmia

 TREATMENT

• Discontinue digoxin until signs of toxicity resolve (24–72 h); reevaluate need for the medication; if necessary, resume treatment at a dosage based on the serum digoxin concentration.
• Maintain hydration and correct any electrolyte disturbance (especially hypokalemia) with parenteral fluid administration.
• Discontinue drugs that slow digoxin metabolism or elimination (e.g., quinidine, verapamil, amiodarone).
• Severe arrhythmias (ventricular tachycardia) and conduction disturbances—can be life threatening; require hospitalization for treatment and monitoring

MEDICATIONS

DRUGS
• Treat clinically important bradyarrhythmias with atropine or temporary transvenous pacemaker.
• Treat clinically important ventricular arrhythmias with lidocaine or phenytoin; phenytoin also reverses high-degree AV block.
• Digoxin-binding antibodies (Digibind) rapidly drop digoxin concentration in critically ill animals; the use of these products is limited in veterinary practice by their exorbitant cost.
• Thyroxin supplementation if hypothyroidism confirmed

CONTRAINDICATIONS/POSSIBLE INTERACTIONS
• Avoid or discontinue drugs that slow digoxin elimination or metabolism (e.g., quinidine, verapamil, and diltiazem).
• Avoid drugs that could worsen conduction disturbances (e.g., β-blockers and calcium channel blockers).
• Class 1A antiarrhythmic drugs (e.g., quinidine and procainamide) may enhance AV block.

 FOLLOW-UP

• Monitor renal function and electrolytes frequently in patients receiving digoxin; lower digoxin dose if renal disease develops.
• Monitor serum digoxin concentration periodically.
• Monitor ECG periodically to assess for arrhythmias or conduction disturbances that may suggest digoxin toxicity.
• Monitor body weight frequently; alter digoxin dosage accordingly; patients with congestive heart failure (CHF) often lose weight.

 MISCELLANEOUS

SEE ALSO
• AV block, complete
• AV block, first degree
• AV block, second degree, Mobitz type I
• AV block, second degree, Mobitz type II
• Ventricular tachycardia

ABBREVIATIONS
• AV = atrioventricular
• CHF = congestive heart failure

Suggested Reading

Marcus FI, Opie LH, Sonnenblick EH, Chatterjee K. Digitalis and acute inotropes. In: Opie LH, ed. Drugs for the heart. 4th ed. Philadelphia: Saunders, 1995:145–173.
Author Francis W. K. Smith, Jr.
Consulting Editors Larry P. Tilley and Francis W. K. Smith, Jr.

DISKOSPONDYLITIS

 BASICS

DEFINITION
A bacterial or fungal infection of the intervertebral disks and adjacent vertebral bodies

PATHOPHYSIOLOGY
• Hematogenous spread of bacterial or fungal organisms—most common cause
• Neurologic dysfunction—may occur; usually the result of spinal cord compression caused by proliferation of bone and fibrous tissue; less commonly owing to luxation or pathologic fracture of the spine, epidural abscess, or extension of infection to the meninges and spinal cord

SYSTEMS AFFECTED
• Musculoskeletal—infection and inflammation of the spine
• Nervous—compression of the spinal cord

GENETICS
• No definite predisposition identified
• An inherited immunodeficiency has been detected in a few cases.

INCIDENCE/PREVALENCE
Approximately 0.2% of dog hospital admissions

GEOGRAPHIC DISTRIBUTION
Grass awn migration and coccidiomycosis—more common in certain regions

SIGNALMENT
Species
Dogs; rare in cats
Breed Predilections
Large and giant breeds, especially German shepherds and Great Danes
Mean Age and Range
• Mean—4–5 years
• Range—5 months to 12 years
Predominant Sex
Males outnumber females by ~2:1

SIGNS
Historical Findings
• Onset usually relatively acute; some patients have mild signs for several months before examination.
• Pain—difficulty rising; reluctance to jump; stilted gait; most common
• Ataxia or paresis
• Weight loss and anorexia
• Lameness
• Draining tracts

Physical Examination Findings
• Focal or multifocal areas of spinal pain
• Any disk space may be affected; lumbosacral space is most commonly involved.
• Paresis or paralysis
• Fever
• Lameness

CAUSES
• Bacterial—*Staphylococcus aureus* and *Staphylococcus intermedius;* * *Brucella canis; Streptococcus* spp.; *Corynebacterium* spp.; *Escherichia coli; Proteus* spp.; *Pasteurella* spp.; *Actinomyces* spp.; *Bactericides* spp.
• Fungal—*Aspergillus* spp.; *Coccidioides immitis*
• Migrating plant material (e.g., grass awns)—may be a cause; tends to affect the L2 to L4 disk spaces and vertebral bodies
• Other causes—surgery; local soft tissue infection caused by bite wounds (cats)

RISK FACTORS
• Urinary tract infection
• Periodontal disease
• Bacterial endocarditis
• Dermatitis
• Immunodeficiency

 DIAGNOSIS

DIFFERENTIAL DIAGNOSIS
• Intervertebral disk protrusion—may cause similar clinical signs; differentiated on the basis of radiography and myelography
• Vertebral fracture or luxation—detected on radiographs
• Vertebral neoplasia—usually does not affect adjacent vertebral end plates
• Spondylosis deformans—rarely causes clinical signs; has similar radiographic features, including sclerosis, ventral spur formation, and collapse of the disk space; rarely causes lysis of the vertebral end plates
• Focal meningomyelitis—often identified by CSF analysis

CBC/BIOCHEMISTRY/URINALYSIS
• Hemogram—often normal; may see leukocytosis
• Urinalysis—may reveal pyuria and/or bacteriuria with concurrent urinary tract infections

OTHER LABORATORY TESTS
• Aerobic, anaerobic, and fungal blood cultures—identify the causative organism in up to 75% of cases; perform if available
• Sensitivity testing—indicated if cultures are positive
• Urine cultures—indicated; positive in about 25% of patients
• Organisms other than *Staphylococcus* spp.—may not be the cause
• Serologic testing for *Brucella canis*—indicated

IMAGING
• Spinal radiography—usually reveals lysis of vertebral end plates adjacent to the affected disk, collapse of the disk space, and varying degrees of sclerosis of the end plates and ventral spur formation; may not see lesions until 3–4 weeks after infection
• Myelography—indicated with substantial neurologic deficits; determine location and degree of spinal cord compression, especially if considering decompressive surgery; spinal cord compression caused by diskospondylitis typically displays an extradural pattern.

DIAGNOSTIC PROCEDURES
• CSF analysis—occasionally indicated to rule out meningomyelitis; usually normal or has mildly high protein
• Bone scintigraphy—occasionally useful for detecting early lesions; helps clarify if radiographic changes are infectious or degenerative (spondylosis deformans)
• Fluoroscopically guided fine-needle aspiration of the disk—valuable for obtaining tissue for culture when blood and urine cultures are negative and there is no improvement with empiric antibiotic therapy

PATHOLOGIC FINDINGS
• Gross—loss of normal disk space; bony proliferation of adjacent vertebrae
• Microscopic—fibrosing pyogranulomatous destruction of the disk and vertebral bodies

 TREATMENT

APPROPRIATE HEALTH CARE
• Outpatient—mild pain
• Inpatient—severe pain or progressive neurologic deficits

NURSING CARE
Nonambulatory patients—keep on a clean, dry, well-padded surface to prevent decubitus ulcers.

ACTIVITY
Restricted

DIET
Normal

CLIENT EDUCATION
• Explain that observation of response to treatment is very important in determining the need for further diagnostic or therapeutic procedures.
• Instruct the client to immediately contact the veterinarian if clinical signs progress or recur or if neurologic deficits develop.

SURGICAL CONSIDERATIONS
• Curettage of a single affected disk space—occasionally necessary for patients that are refractory to antibiotic therapy
• Goals—remove infected tissue; obtain tissue for culture and histologic evaluation
• Decompression of the spinal cord by hemilaminectomy or dorsal laminectomy—indicated for substantial neurologic deficits and spinal cord compression evident on myelography when there is no improvement with antibiotic therapy; also perform curettage of the infected disk space; it may be necessary to perform surgical stabilization if more than one articular facet is removed.

 MEDICATIONS

DRUGS OF CHOICE

Antibiotics
• Selection based on results of blood cultures and serology
• Negative culture and serology—assume causative organism is *Staphylococcus* spp.; treated with a cephalosporin (e.g., cefadroxil, dogs: 22 mg/kg PO q12h; cats: 22 mg/kg PO q24h)
• Acutely progressive signs or substantial neurologic deficits—initially be treated with parenteral antibiotics (e.g., cefazolin; dogs and cats: 20–35 mg/kg IV q8h); continued for at least 6 weeks
• Brucellosis—treated with tetracycline (dogs: 15 mg/kg PO q8h) and streptomycin (dogs: 3.4 mg/kg IM q24h) or enrofloxacin (dogs: 2.5–5.0 mg/kg PO q12h)

Analgesics
• Signs of severe pain—treated with an analgesic (e.g., oxymorphone; dogs: 0.05–0.2 mg/kg IV, IM, SC q4–6h)
• Taper dosage after 3–5 days to gauge effectiveness of antibiotic therapy.

CONTRAINDICATIONS
Glucocorticoids

PRECAUTIONS
Use NSAIDs and other analgesics cautiously—may cause a temporary resolution of clinical signs even when infection is progressing; when used, discontinue after 3–5 days to assess efficacy of antibiotic therapy.

POSSIBLE INTERACTIONS
None

ALTERNATIVE DRUGS
• Initial therapy—cephradine (dogs: 20 mg/kg PO q8h); cloxacillin (dogs: 10 mg/kg PO q8h)
• Refractory patients—clindamycin (dogs: 11 mg/kg PO q12h); enrofloxacin (dogs and cats: 2.5–5.0 mg/kg PO q12h)

 FOLLOW-UP

PATIENT MONITORING
• Re-evaluate after 5 days of therapy
• No improvement in pain, fever, or appetite—reassess therapy; consider a different antibiotic, percutaneous aspiration of the affected disk space, or surgery.
• Improvement—evaluate clinically and radiographically every 2–4 weeks.

PREVENTION/AVOIDANCE
Early identification of predisposing causes and prompt diagnosis and treatment—help reduce progression of clinical symptoms and neurologic deterioration

POSSIBLE COMPLICATIONS
• Spinal cord compression owing to proliferative bony and fibrous tissue
• Vertebral fracture or luxation
• Meningitis or meningomyelitis
• Epidural abscess

EXPECTED COURSE AND PROGNOSIS
• Recurrence is common if antibiotic therapy is stopped prematurely (before 6 weeks of treatment).
• Prognosis—depends on causative organism and degree of spinal cord damage
• Mild or no neurologic dysfunction (dogs)—usually respond within 5 days of starting antibiotic therapy
• Substantial paresis or paralysis (dogs)—prognosis guarded; may note gradual resolution of neurologic dysfunction after several weeks of therapy; treatment warranted
• *Brucella canis*—signs usually resolve with therapy; infection may not be eradicated; recurrence common

 MISCELLANEOUS

ASSOCIATED CONDITIONS
See Risk Factors

AGE-RELATED FACTORS
N/A

ZOONOTIC POTENTIAL
Brucella canis—human infection uncommon but may occur

PREGNANCY
N/A

SYNONYMS
• Intradiskal osteomyelitis
• Intervertebral disk infection
• Vertebral osteomyelitis
• Diskitis

SEE ALSO
Brucellosis

ABBREVIATION
CSF = cerebrospinal fluid

Suggested Reading
Fischer A, Mahaffey MB, Oliver JE. Fluoroscopically guided percutaneous disk aspiration in 10 dogs with diskospondylitis. J Vet Intern Med 1997;11:284–287.
Hurov L, Troy G, Turnwald G. Diskospondylitis in the dog: 27 cases. J Am Vet Med Assoc 1978;173:275–281.
Johnson RG, Prata RG. Intradiskal osteomyelitis: a conservative approach. J Am Anim Hosp Assoc 1983;19:743–750.
Kerwin SC, Lewis DD, Hribernik TN, et al. Diskospondylitis associated with *Brucella canis* infection in dogs: 14 cases (1989–1991). J Am Vet Med Assoc 1992;201:1253–1257.
Kornegay JN. Diskospondylitis. In: Kirk RW, ed. Current veterinary therapy IX. Philadelphia: Saunders, 1986:810–814.
Kornegay JN, Barber DL. Diskospondylitis in dogs. J Am Vet Med Assoc 1980;177:337–341.
Author William B. Thomas
Consulting Editor Peter D. Schwarz

DISEASES

DISSEMINATED INTRAVASCULAR COAGULATION (DIC)

BASICS

DEFINITION
A complex hemostatic defect with enhanced coagulation and fibrinolysis secondary to severe systemic disease

PATHOPHYSIOLOGY
• Occurs secondary to activation of coagulation and fibrinolysis; changes are induced in animals with diseases characterized by stasis of blood flow, vascular damage, activation and consumption of coagulation factors, reduced clearance of activated clotting factors by the liver, or release of tissue factors from damaged cells, tumors, or other tissues.
• Activation of fibrinolysis is a secondary response to clear fibrin thrombi in capillaries.
• Bleeding defect is complicated by thrombocytopenia related to consumption at sites of damaged endothelium and thrombi and by a platelet function defect induced by coating of platelets with FDP from the action of the fibrinolytic mechanism on fibrin or fibrinogen.

SYSTEMS AFFECTED
• Multisystemic
• Hemorrhages in many tissues
• Organ dysfunction related to obstruction of capillaries

GENETICS
N/A

INCIDENCE/PREVALENCE
• Associated with severe systemic disease
• Common in the terminal stages of several fatal diseases

GEOGRAPHIC DISTRIBUTION
N/A

SIGNALMENT
Species
Dogs and cats, but more commonly recognized in dogs

Breed Predilections
None

Mean Age and Range
Correlates with those of the severe systemic disease

Predominant Sex
None

SIGNS
• Usually relate to the primary disease
• Petechiae, abnormal bleeding from venipuncture sites, and other abnormal bleeding

CAUSES
• Malignancies
• Shock
• Pancreatitis
• Heatstroke
• Infectious canine hepatitis
• Other systemic infectious diseases (including gram-negative septicemia)
• Heart failure
• Hemorrhagic gastroenteritis
• Chronic active liver disease
• Splenic torsion
• Heartworm disease
• Snake venom
• Hemolysis
• Gastric dilatation-volvulus

RISK FACTORS
Vary with cause

DIAGNOSIS

DIFFERENTIAL DIAGNOSIS
• Immune-mediated or idiopathic thrombocytopenia
• Anticoagulant toxicity
• Coagulation factor deficiency
• Deficient production of clotting factors in severe liver disease
• Paraproteinemia
• Characterized by marked variation; diagnosis is usually based on the combination of at least three of the following: petechiae or abnormal bleeding from venipuncture sites, thrombocytopenia, prolonged PT, prolonged APTT, low antithrombin III, and high FDP.

CBC/BIOCHEMISTRY/URINALYSIS
• Thrombocytopenia is common, and macroplatelets provide evidence of enhanced thrombopoiesis.
• Schistocytes produced by mechanical fragmentation of erythrocytes on intraluminal fibrin strands.
• Biochemical analysis may reveal azotemia, acidosis, and high enzyme activities related to the primary disease and organ dysfunction or necrosis related to capillary obstruction.

OTHER LABORATORY TESTS
• PT and APTT may be prolonged secondary to the anticoagulant effects of FDP and consumption of coagulation factors, especially antithrombin III, factor VIII, and fibrinogen.
• Latex agglutination test for FDP (Thrombo-Wellcotest, Burroughs-Wellcome, Research Triangle Park, NC) reveals a high concentration.
• Practical assays to demonstrate depletion of clotting factors include fibrinogen and antithrombin III.

IMAGING
N/A

DIAGNOSTIC PROCEDURES
None

PATHOLOGIC FINDINGS
• Usually relate to the primary disease
• Petechiae common
• Fibrin thrombi may be dissolved by fibrinolysis during the postmortem interval.

TREATMENT

APPROPRIATE HEALTH CARE
Associated with severe disease, requiring intensive and inpatient treatment

NURSING CARE
• Most important is intensive treatment of the primary disease.
• Fluid therapy to correct deficits in plasma volume or acid–base imbalance reduces the potential for activation of clotting factors and enhances clearance of activated clotting factors by the mononuclear phagocyte system.

ACTIVITY
Not an issue because of the severity of the primary disease

DIET
N/A

DISSEMINATED INTRAVASCULAR COAGULATION (DIC)

CLIENT EDUCATION
• Inform the owner of the life-threatening nature of the associated processes.
• Prognosis is usually that associated with the primary disease.

SURGICAL CONSIDERATIONS
Related to primary disease

MEDICATIONS

DRUGS OF CHOICE
• Heparin administration is controversial but may be used to inhibit proteolytic activation of coagulation, preferably by continuous IV infusion sufficient to prolong the APTT to $1\frac{1}{2}$–2 times normal; low-dose heparin is safer and has been reported to produce beneficial results in some dogs when infused at 5–10 IU/kg/hr IV or at 75 IU/kg SC q8h.
• The anticoagulant effect of heparin is achieved by binding to antithrombin III, which may be depleted in these patients; therefore, it may be beneficial to transfuse with heparinized blood or heparinized plasma.

CONTRAINDICATIONS
• Although use of a high dosage of corticosteroids may be indicated to treat shock, the long-term use of corticosteroids should be considered carefully because of the inhibition of mononuclear phagocyte function, which might be important in clearance of activated coagulation factors.
• Inhibitors of fibrinolysis should not be used, because fibrinolysis is important in the clearance of thrombi.

PRECAUTIONS
High doses of heparin may cause bleeding episodes that could be life-threatening. If active bleeding, clotting factors should be replaced by plasma transfusion.

POSSIBLE INTERACTIONS
None

ALTERNATIVE DRUGS
None

FOLLOW-UP

PATIENT MONITORING
• Clinical improvement and the arrest of bleeding are positive indications of a response to treatment.
• Diminishing concentration of FDP is a positive sign.
• Platelet counts usually increase slowly over a period of days.

PREVENTION/AVOIDANCE
Related to primary disease

EXPECTED COURSE AND PROGNOSIS
Because of the serious nature of the primary diseases, these animals have a high rate of mortality.

✓ MISCELLANEOUS

ASSOCIATED CONDITIONS
See causes

AGE-RELATED FACTORS
N/A

ZOONOTIC POTENTIAL
N/A

PREGNANCY
Associated obstetric complications (e.g., dystocia, eclampsia, and retained fetuses) have been demonstrated in humans but are not well documented in dogs and cats.

SYNONYMS
• Consumption coagulopathy
• Intravascular coagulation-fibrinolysis syndrome

SEE ALSO
• Clotting Factor Deficiencies
• Thrombocytopenia

ABBREVIATIONS
• APTT = activated partial thromboplastin time
• FDP = fibrin degradation products
• PT = prothrombin time

Suggested Reading
Dodds WJ. Hemostasis. In: Kaneko JJ, Harvey JW, Bruss ML, eds., Clinical biochemistry of domestic animals. New York: Academic Press, 1997:241-283.

Feldman BF, Madewell BR, O'Neil S. Disseminated intravascular coagulation: antithrombin, plasminogen, and coagulation abnormalities in 41 dogs. J Am Vet Med Assoc 1981;179:151–154.

Slappendel RJ. Disseminated intravascular coagulation. In: Feldman BF, ed. Hemostasis. Vet Clin North Am 1988;18:169–184.

Slappendel RJ. Disseminated intravascular coagulation. In: Kirk RW, Bonagura JD, eds., Current veterinary therapy X. Philadelphia: Saunders, 1989:451–457.
Author Gary J. Kociba
Consulting Editor Susan M. Cotter

BASICS

DEFINITION
• An acute to subacute contagious febrile and often fatal disease with respiratory, gastrointestinal, and CNS manifestations
• Caused by CDV, a morbillivirus in the Paramyxoviridae family
• Affects many different species of the order Carnivora; mortality rate varies greatly among species.

PATHOPHYSIOLOGY
• Natural route of infection—airborne and droplet exposure; from the nasal cavity, pharynx, and lungs, macrophages carry the virus to local lymph nodes, where virus replication occurs; within 1 week, virtually all lymphatic tissues become infected; spreads via viremia to the surface epithelium of respiratory, gastrointestinal, and urogenital tracts and to the CNS
• Fever for 1–2 days and lymphopenia may be the only findings during initial period; further development depends on the virus strain and the immune response.
• Strong cellular and humoral immune response—may remain subclinical
• Weak immune response—subacute infection; may survive longer
• Failure of immune response—acute death within 2–4 weeks after infection; convulsions and other CNS disturbances frequent causes of death

SYSTEMS AFFECTED
• Multisystemic—all lymphatic tissues; surface epithelium in the respiratory, alimentary, and urogenital tracts; endocrine and exocrine glands
• Nervous—skin; gray and white matter in the CNS

GENETICS
N/A

INCIDENCE/PREVALENCE
• Dogs—restricted to sporadic outbreaks
• Wildlife (raccoons, skunks, fox)—fairly common

GEOGRAPHIC DISTRIBUTION
Worldwide

SIGNALMENT

Species
• Most species of the order Carnivora—Canidae, Hyaenidae, Mustelidae, Procyonidae, Viverridae
• Felidae families—recent; large cats in Californian zoos and in Tanzania

Breed Predilection
None

Mean Age and Range
Young animals are more susceptible than are adults.

Predominant Sex
None

SIGNS
• Fever—first peak 3–6 days after infection, may pass unnoticed; second peak several days later (and intermittent thereafter), usually associated with nasal and ocular discharge, depression, and anorexia
• Gastrointestinal and/or respiratory signs—follow, often enhanced by secondary bacterial infection
• CNS—many infected dogs; often, but not always, after systemic disease; depends on the virus strain; either acute gray matter disease (seizures and myoclonus with depression) or subacute white matter disease (incoordination ataxia, paresis, paralysis, and muscle tremors); meningeal signs of hyperesthesia and cervical rigidity may be seen in both.
• Optic neuritis and retinal lesions not uncommon; sometimes infected scleral blood vessels from anterior uveitis
• Hardening of the footpads (hyperkeratosis) and nose—some virus strains; now much less common than it once was
• Enamel hypoplasia of the teeth after neo-natal infection common

CAUSES
• CDV, a morbillivirus within the Paramyxoviridae family; closely related to measles virus, rinderpest virus of cattle, and phocine (seal) and dolphin distemper viruses
• Secondary bacterial infections frequently involve the respiratory and gastrointestinal systems.

RISK FACTORS
Contact of nonimmunized animals with CDV-infected animals (dogs or wild carnivores)

 DIAGNOSIS

DIFFERENTIAL DIAGNOSIS
• Kennel cough—can mimic the respiratory disease
• Enteric signs—differentiate from canine parvovirus and coronavirus infections, parasitism (giardiasis), bacterial infections, gastroenteritis from toxin ingestion, inflammatory bowel disease
• CNS form—confused with granulomatous meningoencephalomyelitis, protozoal encephalitis (toxoplasmosis, neosporosis), cryptococcosis or other infections (meningitis, ehrlichiosis, Rocky Mountain spotted fever), pug dog encephalitis, and lead poisoning
• Considered in any young unvaccinated dog with multifocal CNS disease with other organ involvement

CBC/BIOCHEMISTRY/URINALYSIS
Lymphopenia during early infection

OTHER LABORATORY TESTS
• Serology—limited value; positive antibody tests do not differentiate between vaccination and exposure to virulent virus; patient may die from acute disease before neutralizing antibody can be produced; IgM responses may be seen for up to 3 months after exposure to virulent virus and for up to 3 weeks after vaccination.
• CDV antibody in CSF—indicative, but not always diagnostic, of distemper encephalitis

IMAGING
• Radiographs—determine the extent of pneumonia
• CT and MRI—cannot typically detect brain changes

DIAGNOSTIC PROCEDURES
• Viral antigen or viral inclusions—in buffy coat cells and conjunctival or vaginal imprints; negative results do not rule out the diagnosis.
• PCR—on buffy coat and urine sediment cells; more sensitive
• CSF—test for cell and protein content, CDV-specific antibody, interferon, and viral antigen early in disease course.
• Postmortem diagnosis—histopathology, immunofluorescence and/or immuno-cytochemistry, virus isolation, and/or PCR; preferred tissues from lungs, stomach, urinary bladder, lymphs, and brain

PATHOLOGIC FINDINGS

Gross
• Thymus—in young animals greatly reduced in size; sometimes gelatinous
• Lungs—patchy consolidation as a result of interstitial pneumonia
• Footpads and nose—rarely hyperkeratosis
• Mucopurulent discharges—from eyes and nose, bronchopneumonia, catarrhal enteritis, and skin pustules; probably caused by secondary bacterial infections; commonly seen

Histologic
• Intracytoplasmic eosinophilic inclusion bodies—frequently found in epithelium of the bronchi, stomach, and urinary bladder; also seen in reticulum cells and leukocytes in lymphatic tissues
• Inclusion bodies in the CNS—glial cells and neurons; frequently intranuclear; can also be found in cytoplasm
• Staining by fluorescent antibody or immuno-peroxidase may detect viral antigen where inclusion bodies are not seen.

 TREATMENT

APPROPRIATE HEALTH CARE
Inpatients and in isolation, to prevent infection of other dogs

NURSING CARE
• Symptomatic
• Intravenous fluids—with anorexia and diarrhea
• Once fevers and secondary bacterial infections are controlled, patients usually begin to eat again.
• Clean away ocular discharges.

ACTIVITY
Limited

DIET
Depends on the extent of gastrointestinal involvement

CLIENT EDUCATION
• Inform client that mortality rate is about 50%.
• Inform client that dogs that appear to recover from early catarrhal signs may later develop fatal CNS signs.

SURGICAL CONSIDERATIONS
N/A

 MEDICATIONS

DRUGS OF CHOICE
• Antiviral drugs—none known to be effective
• Antibiotics—to reduce secondary bacterial infection, because CDV is highly immuno-suppressive
• Anticonvulsant therapy—phenobarbital, potassium bromide; to control less severe neurologic manifestations (e.g., myoclonus, seizures)

CONTRAINDICATIONS
Corticosteroids—do not use, because they augment the immunosuppression and may enhance viral dissemination; may provide short-term control of signs

PRECAUTIONS
Tetracycline and fluorinated quinolones—do not use for young and growing animals

POSSIBLE INTERACTIONS
N/A

ALTERNATIVE DRUGS
N/A

 FOLLOW-UP

PATIENT MONITORING
• Monitor for signs of pneumonia or dehydration from diarrhea in the acute phase of the disease.
• Monitor for CNS signs, because seizures generally follow.

PREVENTION/AVOIDANCE
• Avoid infection of pups by isolation to prevent infection from wildlife (e.g.,

raccoons, fox, skunks) or from CDV-infected dogs
• Recovered dogs are not carriers.

Vaccines
• MLV-CD—prevents infection and disease; two types available, each with advantages and disadvantages
• Canine tissue culture–adapted vaccines (e.g., Rockborn strain)—induce complete immunity in virtually 100% of susceptible dogs; rarely a postvaccinal fatal encephalitis develops 7–14 days after vaccination, especially in immunosuppressed animals
• Chick embryo–adapted vaccines (e.g., Onderstepoort, Lederle strain)—safer; postvaccinal encephalitis does not occur; only about 80% of susceptible dogs seroconvert
• Other species—chick embryo can safely be used in a variety of zoo and wildlife species (e.g., gray fox); Rockborn type fatal in these animals
• Killed vaccines—useful for species for which either MLV-CD is fatal (e.g., red panda, black-footed ferret)
• Canarypox recombinant CDV vaccine—recently available; being tested in other species

Maternal Antibody
• Important
• Most pups lose protection from maternal antibody at 6–12 weeks of age; give 2–3 vaccinations during this period.
• Heterotypic (measles virus) vaccination—recommended for pups that have maternal antibody; induces protection from disease but not from infection

POSSIBLE COMPLICATIONS
Possibility of occurrence of CNS signs for 2–3 months after catarrhal signs have subsided

EXPECTED COURSE AND PROGNOSIS
• Depend on the strain and the individual host response—subclinical, acute, subacute, fatal, or nonfatal infection
• Mild CNS signs (e.g., myoclonus)—patient may recover; myoclonus may continue for several months.
• Death—2 weeks to 3 months after infection; mortality rate approximately 50%
• Euthanasia—owner may elect if or when neurologic signs develop; indicated when repeated seizures occur
• Fully recovered dogs do not shed CDV.

 MISCELLANEOUS

ASSOCIATED CONDITIONS
• Persistent or latent toxoplasma infections—reactivated because of the immunosuppressive state

• Respiratory infections with *Bordetella bronchiseptica* (a major cause of kennel cough)

AGE-RELATED FACTORS
• Young pups—more susceptible; mortality rate is higher
• Nonimmunized old dogs—highly susceptible to infection and disease

ZOONOTIC POTENTIAL
• Possible that humans may become subclinically infected with CDV; immunization against measles virus also protects against CDV infection
• Speculated that CDV may cause MS; several studies have refuted this proposition; most compelling evidence: canine distemper became rare in dogs after the introduction of MLV-CD vaccines in the early 1960s, although the incidence of MS remained unchanged; incubation period of MS is usually < 30 years; thus CDV cannot be a factor.

PREGNANCY
In utero infection of fetuses—occurs in antibody-negative bitches; rare; may lead to abortion or to persistent infection; infected neonates appear but may develop fatal disease by 4–6 weeks of age.

SYNONYMS
• Canine distemper
• Maladie de Carré
• Hard pad disease
• Hundestaupe

SEE ALSO
Myoclonus

ABBREVIATIONS
• CDV = canine distemper virus
• CSF = cerebrospinal fluid
• MLV-CD = modified live virus of canine distemper
• MS = multiple sclerosis
• PCR = polymerase chain reaction

Suggested Reading
Appel MJG, Summers BA. Pathogenicity of morbilliviruses for terrestrial carnivores. Vet Microbiol 1995;44:187–191.
Greene CE, Appel MJ. Canine distemper. In: Greene CE, ed. Infectious diseases of the dog and cat. Philadelphia: Saunders, 1998:9–22.
Author Max J. G. Appel
Consulting Editor Stephen C. Barr

DISEASES

DOUBLE AORTIC ARCH

 ## BASICS

OVERVIEW
• Vascular ring anomaly caused by persistence of both sides of the fourth aortic arch
• The ascending aorta divides into a left branch (left and ventral to the esophagus) and a right branch (right and dorsal to the esophagus), which reunite to form the descending aorta.
• The two arches may constrict the esophagus.
• Both left and right branches are usually patent.

SIGNALMENT
• Dogs; rarely cats
• German shepherd predisposed

SIGNS

Historical Findings
• Regurgitation secondary to esophageal obstruction
• Failure to thrive

Physical Examination Findings
Stunted growth

CAUSES & RISK FACTORS
Unknown; genetic basis not documented

 ## DIAGNOSIS

DIFFERENTIAL DIAGNOSIS
• Right aortic arch—exploratory surgery required to differentiate
• Esophageal stenosis
• Esophageal hypoplasia

CBC/BIOCHEMISTRY/URINALYSIS
No consistent abnormalities

OTHER LABORATORY TESTS
N/A

IMAGING

Radiographic Findings
Esophageal dilatation cranial to heart

Angiographic findings
Diagnostic outline

DIAGNOSTIC TESTS

Electrocardiographic Findings
No consistent abnormalities

 ## TREATMENT

• Patients with aspiration pneumonia—hospitalize until stable.
• Surgical correction indicated—procedure similar to correction of persistent right aortic arch; the branch with the least blood flow is removed.

 ## MEDICATIONS

DRUGS
• Broad-spectrum antibiotics if animal has aspiration pneumonia
• No cardiac medications

CONTRAINDICATIONS/POSSIBLE INTERACTIONS
N/A

 ## FOLLOW-UP

• Clinical signs resolve after successful surgery.
• Very poor prognosis unless corrected
• Serious postoperative complications reported in one case (acute left heart failure)

 ## MISCELLANEOUS

ASSOCIATED CONDITIONS
Pulmonic stenosis and tricuspid dysplasia

SEE ALSO
Persistent Right Aortic Arch

Suggested Reading
Bonagura JD, Darke P. Congenital heart disease. In: Ettinger SJ, Feldman EC, eds. Textbook of veterinary internal medicine. 4th ed. Philadelphia: Saunders, 1995.

Author John-Karl Goodwin
Consulting Editors Larry P. Tilley and Francis W. K. Smith, Jr.

DYSAUTONOMIA (KEY-GASKELL SYNDROME)

BASICS

OVERVIEW
• Dysfunction of the autonomous nervous system
• Etiopathogenesis unknown

SIGNALMENT
• Mainly cats in Great Britain
• Rare in dogs and cats worldwide
• Most affected dogs and cats < 3 years old
• No breed or sex predilection
• No genetic basis

SIGNS
• Generally acute
• Depression
• Anorexia
• Constipation
• Dry external nares and mouth
• Reduced tear production
• Regurgitation owing to megaesophagus
• Dilated pupils with absent or depressed pupillary light reflexes
• Prolapsed third eyelids
• Bradycardia
• Less common—anal areflexia; fecal incontinence; dysuria or urinary incontinence
• Dog—diarrhea more common than constipation

CAUSES & RISK FACTORS
Unknown

DIAGNOSIS

DIFFERENTIAL DIAGNOSIS
• Dehydration secondary to a primary gastrointestinal disorder
• Most primary gastrointestinal diseases—differentiate by dilated, poorly responsive pupils, no tear production on Schirmer tear test, poor esophageal motility on contrast radiography

CBC/BIOCHEMISTRY/URINALYSIS
• Normal or indicate dehydration
• Heinz body anemia in some cats

OTHER LABORATORY TESTS
N/A

IMAGING
• Survey radiography of the thorax—often reveals megaesophagus
• Barium contrast radiography or fluoroscopy—demonstrates esophageal dysfunction; delayed gastric emptying and contrast retention in the colon common

DIAGNOSTIC PROCEDURES
• Schirmer tear test—usually < 5 mm/min
• Ophthalmic pharmacologic testing—phospholine iodide 0.06% has no miotic effect; pilocarpine 0.1% has an exaggerated miotic effect because of denervation hypersensitivity; testing is not 100% reliable: some patients do not respond as expected.
• Low plasma or urinary catecholamine concentration—confirms sympathetic insufficiency
• Intradermal histamine (1:1000) response test—fails to demonstrate the normal weal and flare reaction because of the defect in sympathetic innervation of blood vessels

TREATMENT
• Inpatient—initial treatment
• Warm isotonic fluids—intravenous administration; correct hypovolemia, hypothermia, hypoglycemia, and other electrolyte abnormalities
• Oral intake—temporarily withhold (especially dogs) to prevent aspiration pneumonia secondary to regurgitation.
• Nutrition—almost all patients require nasogastric tube, percutaneous gastrostomy tube, or total parenteral nutrition for weeks to months until regurgitation has subsided; percutaneous gastrostomy tube is generally best, because client can easily feed the patient at home.
• Outpatient—extensive nursing care; several months to 1 year for recovery; even with the best management, relapse and death common

MEDICATIONS

DRUGS
• Cisapride (dogs: 0.1–0.5 mg/kg PO q8–12h; cats: 2.5–5.0 mg/cat PO q8–12h) or metoclopramide (0.2–0.5 mg/kg IV, IM, PO q6–8h or 1–2 mg/kg continuous IV infusion daily) may reduce vomiting and improve gastrointestinal motility.
• Parasympathomimetic eye drops—pilocarpine (0.1%–1%) q8–12h; improve lacrimation
• Bethanechol—2.5–7.5 mg PO divided q8–12h; may improve gastrointestinal motility and bladder emptying

CONTRAINDICATIONS/POSSIBLE INTERACTIONS
Pilocarpine and bethanechol—use carefully; start with the lowest possible dosage; denervation hypersensitivity can cause arrhythmias and bradycardia

FOLLOW-UP
• Prognosis poor
• Only 20%–50% survive after several months to 1 year of slow recovery.
• Megaesophagus, constipation, fecal incontinence, and pupil dilation may persist.
• Aspiration pneumonia may cause death.

MISCELLANEOUS

Suggested Reading
Sharp NJH. Feline dysautonomia. Semin Vet Med Surg Small Anim 1990;5:67–71.
Author Allen Sisson
Consulting Editor Joane M. Parent

DYSRAPHISM, SPINAL

 BASICS

OVERVIEW
• Abnormal spinal cord development along the median plane leading to a variety of structural anomalies (e.g., hydromyelia, duplicated or absent central canal, syringomyelia, and aberrations in the dorsal median septum and ventral medial fissure)
• Thoracic and lumbar spinal segments most commonly affected
• The term *dysraphism* suggests an abnormality in closure of the neural tube, which is not the case; the term *myelodysplasia* may be preferable

SIGNALMENT
• Dogs and cats
• Weimaraners—hereditary
• English bulldogs, Samoyeds, Dalmatians, English setters, golden retrievers, mixed-breed dogs, and cats—reported
• No sex predilection

SIGNS
• Apparent by 3–6 weeks of age
• Do not progress
• Vary in severity
• Simultaneous flexion and extension of pelvic limbs (bunny hopping)
• Proprioceptive deficits, base wide stance, and crouched pelvic limb posture

CAUSES & RISK FACTORS
• Genetic—weimaraners; homozygous condition lethal; heterozygotes clinically affected
• In utero spinal cord damage caused by infection, trauma, and vascular compromise may cause syringomyelia (cavitation of the spinal cord).
• Idiopathic in isolated patients

 DIAGNOSIS

DIFFERENTIAL DIAGNOSIS
• Easily differentiated from common spinal cord diseases, because it is present at birth and nonprogressive
• Challenge is to define the malformations.

CBC/BIOCHEMISTRY/URINALYSIS
Usually normal

OTHER LABORATORY TESTS
N/A

IMAGING
• Survey and contrast spinal radiography—associated vertebral column anomalies and spinal cord compression in some patients
• Without sophisticated imaging techniques, an antemortem diagnosis may be impossible to make in dogs other than weimaraners.
• Weimaraner puppies—characteristic gait without evidence of microscopic abnormalities

OTHER DIAGNOSTIC PROCEDURES
N/A

TREATMENT
• None available
• Mildly affected animals—may be acceptable pets
• Severely affected animals—may benefit from a canine cart; consider euthanasia

 MEDICATIONS

DRUGS
Antibiotics—on basis of bacterial culture of urine and sensitivity test if the patient has secondary urinary tract infection

CONTRAINDICATIONS/POSSIBLE INTERACTIONS
N/A

 FOLLOW-UP

• Secondary urinary tract infection—seen in severely affected animals; owing to disorders of micturition
• Avoid decubitus ulcers and urine and fecal scalds by properly caring for recumbent patients.

 MISCELLANEOUS

ASSOCIATED CONDITIONS
Congenital vertebral arch (e.g., spina bifida) and vertebral body-disk malformation (e.g., hemivertebra and block vertebra)—alone often do not cause clinical signs

Suggested Reading
Bailey CS, Morgan JP. Congenital malformations. In: Moore MP, ed., Diseases of the spine. Vet Clin North Am Small Anim Pract 1992;22:985–1015.
Summers BA, Cummings JH, de Lahunta A. Veterinary pathology. St. Louis: Mosby, 1995.

Author Richard J. Joseph
Consulting Editor Joane M. Parent

BASICS

OVERVIEW
• *Otodectes cynotis* mites cause a hyper-sensitivity reaction that results in intense irritation of the external ear of dogs and cats.

SIGNALMENT
• Common in young dogs and cats, although it may occur at any age
• No breed or sex predilection

SIGNS
• Pruritus primarily located around the ears, head, and neck; occasionally generalized
• Thick, red-brown or black crusts—usually seen in the outer ear
• Crusting and scales may occur on the neck, rump, and tail.
• Excoriations on the convex surface of the pinnae often occur, owing to the intense pruritus.

CASES & RISK FACTORS
O. cynotis

DIAGNOSIS

DIFFERENTIAL DIAGNOSIS
• Flea bite hypersensitivity
• Pediculosis
• Pelodera dermatitis
• Sarcoptic mange
• Chiggers
• Allergic dermatitis

CBC/BIOCHEMISTRY/URINALYSIS
Normal

OTHER LABORATORY TESTS
N/A

IMAGING
N/A

DIAGNOSTIC PROCEDURES
• Skin scrapings—identify mites, if signs are generalized
• Ear swabs placed in mineral oil—usually a very effective means of identification

TREATMENT

• Outpatient
• Diet and activity—no alteration necessary
• Very contagious; important to treat all in-contact animals
• Thoroughly clean and treat the environment.

MEDICATIONS

DRUGS
• First clean the ears thoroughly with mineral oil or a commercial ear cleaner to remove debris.
• Rotenone-based products—treat ears twice per week initially; then decrease to weekly; continue for 2 weeks after clinical cure.
• Ivermectin—as an alternative; use systemically or topically; systemic: (bovine 1%) 300 µg/kg SC every 1–2 weeks for approximately 4 treatments was found to be effective; topical: place 500 µg directly in the ears every 1–2 weeks for approximately 5 weeks (associated with a higher incidence of recurrence); topical dosage not approved for use in dogs or cats in the U.S.; dogs with heartworm may exhibit a shock-like reaction, probably owing to dying microfilaria.
• Amitraz—topical; place 1 mL in 33 mL mineral oil directly into the ear; not approved for this use
• Pyrethrin-based flea spray—treat entire animal weekly for 4–6 weeks if not using systemic ivermectin.
• Environment—treat with a flea-type preparation two times, 2–4 weeks apart.

CONTRAINDICATIONS/POSSIBLE INTERACTIONS
• Ivermectin—do not use in collies, shelties, their crosses, or other herding breeds; use only if absolutely necessary in animals < 6 months of age, an increasing number of toxic reactions have been reported in kittens.
• Amitraz—reported to cause adverse reactions in cats when used topically for generalized infestations; thus use with caution

FOLLOW-UP

• An ear swab and physical examination should be done 1 month after therapy commences.
• For most patients, prognosis is good.
• Rarely, the infestation will be cleared only to find an underlying allergy that keeps the otitis externa active.

MISCELLANEOUS

ZOONOTIC POTENTIAL
The mites will also bite humans (rare).

Suggested Reading
Scott DW, Miller WH, Griffin CE. Muller & Kirk's small animal dermatology. 5th ed. Philadelphia: Saunders, 1995.
Author Karen A. Kuhl
Consulting Editor Karen Helton Rhodes

EBSTEIN'S ANOMALY

BASICS

OVERVIEW
• Atrialization of the right ventricle—apical displacement of the tricuspid valve complex into the right ventricle
• Accompanied by various degrees of tricuspid insufficiency
• Major pathophysiology related to the degree of tricuspid insufficiency
• An abnormal accessory pathway may lead to supraventricular tachycardias.

SIGNALMENT
• Very rare—occasionally encountered in dogs and cats
• No breed or sex predilection
• Congenital condition—murmur ausculted at young age

SIGNS
• Systolic regurgitant heart murmur with point of maximal intensity over the tricuspid valve region
• Animals with mild tricuspid insufficiency are asymptomatic.
• Animals with severe insufficiency have R-CHF with pleural effusion and/or ascites.

CAUSES & RISK FACTORS
N/A

DIAGNOSIS

DIFFERENTIAL DIAGNOSIS
Tricuspid dysplasia

CBC/BIOCHEMISTRY/URINALYSIS
Usually normal

OTHER LABORATORY TESTS
N/A

IMAGING

Thoracic Radiographic Findings
• Right atrial and ventricular enlargement
• Hepatomegaly

Echocardiography
Two-dimensional echocardiography—apically displaced tricuspid valve

DIAGNOSTIC PROCEDURES

Electrocardiography
• Simultaneous intracardiac pressure and ECG tracings may be needed to verify the diagnosis.
• Accessory conduction pathway (ventricular preexcitation) or supraventricular tachycardia

TREATMENT

• Medical management currently the only practical approach
• Restrict sodium intake if right heart failure develops

MEDICATIONS

DRUGS
• Patients with R-CHF—treat with furosemide (2–4 mg/kg PO q6–12h) and enalapril (0.5 mg/kg PO q12h) or benazepril (0.25–0.5 mg/kg PO q24h).

• Patients with supraventricular tachycardia (WPW syndrome)—procainamide (15 mg/kg PO q6–8h); if the WPW persists, consider a calcium channel blocker (i.e., verapamil or diltiazem) or a β-blocker (e.g., propranolol or atenolol).

CONTRAINDICATIONS/POSSIBLE INTERACTIONS
Do not use calcium channel blockers and β-blockers concurrently.

FOLLOW-UP

Monitor with serial echocardiograms, ECG, and radiographs.

MISCELLANEOUS

SEE ALSO
Tricuspid Valve Dysplasia

ABBREVIATIONS
• WPW = Wolff-Parkinson-White syndrome
• R-CHF = right-sided congestive heart failure

Suggested Reading
Bonagura JD, Lehmkuhl LB. Congenital heart disease. In: Fox PR, Sisson D, Moise NS, eds. Textbook of canine and feline cardiology. 2nd ed. Philadelphia: Saunders, 1999:471–535.

Author Carroll Loyer
Consulting Editors Larry P. Tilley and Francis W. K. Smith, Jr.

BASICS

OVERVIEW
• Postparturient hypocalcemia
• Usually develops 1–4 weeks postpartum; may occur at term, prepartum, or during late lactation
• Alters cell membrane potentials, causing spontaneous discharge of nerve fibers and tonoclonic contraction of skeletal muscles
• Life-threatening tetany and convulsions, leading to hyperthermia
• Cerebral edema possible

SIGNALMENT
• Dogs—postpartum bitch; most common in toy breeds; higher incidence with first litter
• Cats—rare

SIGNS
Historical Findings
• Restlessness, nervousness
• Panting, whining
• Ataxia, stiff gait
• Muscle tremors, tetany, convulsions
• Recumbency, extensor rigidity—usually seen 8–12 hr after onset of signs

Physical Examination Findings
• Hyperthermia
• Rapid respiratory rate
• Dilated pupils, sluggish pupillary light responses
• Muscle tremors, muscular rigidity, convulsions

CAUSES & RISK FACTORS
• Calcium supplementation during gestation
• Large litter size
• Poor prenatal nutrition

DIAGNOSIS

DIFFERENTIAL DIAGNOSIS
• Hypoglycemia—may be concurrent; muscular rigidity does not occur with hypoglycemia alone.

• Toxicosis—distinguished by signalment and history
• Epilepsy or other neurologic disorder—differentiated by signalment; calcium concentration diagnostic.

CBC/BIOCHEMISTRY/URINALYSIS
• Serum calcium < 7 mg/dL
• Hypoglycemia—may be concurrent

IMAGING
N/A

OTHER LABORATORY TESTS
N/A

DIAGNOSTIC PROCEDURES
ECG shows prolonged QT interval, bradycardia, tachycardia, or PVCs.

TREATMENT
• Emergency inpatient
• Hyperthermia—cool with cool water soak and fans; use caution with cool water enemas.
• Puppies—remove from dam to hand-raise; if owner refuses, remove pups from dam for 24 hr to spare her and provide supplementation for remainder of lactation.

MEDICATIONS

DRUGS
• Calcium gluconate—10% solution 1 mL/kg IV given slowly to effect over 5 min; monitor heart rate or ECG during administration; may give additional drug intramuscularly or subcutaneously
• Correct hypoglycemia.
• Diazepam—5 mg IV; for unresponsive seizures
• Cerebral edema—treat, if indicated.
• Calcium lactate, carbonate, or gluconate—30–100 mg/kg/day PO until lactation ends

CONTRAINDICATIONS/POSSIBLE INTERACTIONS
Corticosteroids—avoid; decrease intestinal

absorption of and increase renal excretion of calcium

FOLLOW-UP

PATIENT MONITORING
• Serum calcium concentration—monitor until it stabilizes in the normal range.
• Avoid calcium supplementation during gestation.
• Diet—maternal: ensure a calcium:phosphorus ratio of 1:1 or 1.2:1; avoid high-phytate foods (e.g., soybeans); puppies: supplement feeding for large litters.

POSSIBLE COMPLICATIONS
• Cerebral edema
• Death
• Hand-raising of puppies

EXPECTED COURSE AND PROGNOSIS
• Probably will recur with subsequent litters
• Prognosis—good with immediate treatment; poor with delayed treatment

MISCELLANEOUS

Suggested Reading
Kaufman J. Eclampsia in the bitch. In: Morrow DA, ed., Current therapy in theriogenology. 2nd ed. Philadelphia: Saunders, 1986:511–512.
Author: Joni L. Freshman
Consulting Editor: Sara K. Lyle

ECTOPIC URETERS

BASICS

OVERVIEW
• Congenital abnormality in which one or both ureters open into the urethra or vagina
• Dogs—the ureter may enter the bladder in the normal location, tunnel through the bladder wall, and bypass the trigone (intramural type).
• Less frequently, the ureter opens into the trigone and continues as a trough into the urethra.
• Cats—the ureter completely bypasses the bladder and enters the urethra (extramural type); this rarely occurs in dogs.

SIGNALMENT
• The following dog breeds are predisposed—Siberian husky, Newfoundland, bulldog, West Highland white terrier, fox terrier, and miniature and toy poodles
• Infrequently diagnosed in cats and male dogs

SIGNS
• Intermittent or continuous incontinence
• Normal voiding in some animals
• Vaginitis from urine scalding

CAUSES & RISK FACTORS
• Apparent breed predisposition
• Unknown mode of inheritance; bitches with ectopic ureters have had litters of puppies with no observed incontinence.

DIAGNOSIS

DIFFERENTIAL DIAGNOSIS
• Inappropriate urination—wrong place or time, but under voluntary control
• Urethral sphincter mechanism incompetence—use excretory urogram to exclude possibility of ectopic ureter; some dogs have ectopic ureters and urethral sphincter mechanism incompetence.
• Patent urachus—moist abdomen; radiographic contrast studies identify opening in ventral abdomen.

• Paradoxical incontinence—occurs secondary to urethral obstruction; pass catheter to identify calculi, stricture, or mass.
• Urinary tract infection—can cause pollakiuria that mimics incontinence
• Severe polyuria associated with renal failure caused by either congenital kidney disease or severe pyelonephritis—measure urine specific gravity to determine ability to concentrate urine; polyuria and polydipsia associated with low urine specific gravity

CBC/BIOCHEMISTRY/URINALYSIS
Urine specific gravity and serum creatinine or urea nitrogen concentration should be normal.

OTHER LABORATORY TESTS
Urine bacteriologic culture—collect by cystocentesis; often reveals concurrent urinary tract infection

IMAGING
Excretory urography and a pneumocystogram, followed by a vaginourethrogram (female) or urethrogram (male)—may be used to identify ectopic ureter(s); may also diagnose hydroureter; absent, small or misshapen kidneys; hydronephrosis; and tortuous or obstructed ureters

DIAGNOSTIC PROCEDURES
• Urethrocystoscopy—use for direct visualization of the opening of the ectopic ureter(s) into the urethra or vagina
• Urethral pressure profilometry—can detect concurrent urethral sphincter mechanism incompetence

TREATMENT
• Surgically create a new ureteral opening into the bladder or excise a hydronephrotic or severely infected kidney.
• Warn owners that incontinence may continue if dog also has urethral sphincter mechanism incompetence; some puppies with urethral sphincter mechanism incompetence become continent after their first heat cycle.
• Incontinent dogs should not be spayed before their first heat.

MEDICATIONS

DRUGS
N/A

CONTRAINDICATIONS/POSSIBLE INTERACTIONS
N/A

FOLLOW-UP
• Incontinence may persist after surgery.
• Incontinent dogs need repeat evaluation including excretory urogram, pneumocystogram, and vaginourethrogram.
• An intrapelvic bladder neck may contribute to urinary incontinence in dogs with urethral sphincter mechanism incompetence. Surgically advancing the bladder neck into an intraabdominal position using the colposuspension technique may correct the incontinence.
• If incontinence persists, try phenylpropanolamine (1.5 mg/kg PO q8h), an α-blocker, or imipramine (0.5–1 mg/kg PO q8h), a tricyclic antidepressor agent. Reproductive hormone therapy may increase the sensitivity of urethral α-adrenergic receptors to α-agonists.
• Diethylstilbestrol (1.0 mg q24h for 3–5 days, then no more than 1.0 mg/week) is administered orally to spayed bitches. In some dogs, a combination of estrogen therapy and phenylpropanolamine may be more effective.

MISCELLANEOUS

Suggested Reading
Stone EA, Barsanti JA. Urologic surgery of the dog and cat. Philadelphia: Lea & Febiger. 1992:201–211.
Author Elizabeth Arnold Stone
Consulting Editors Larry G. Adams and Carl A. Osborne

BASICS

OVERVIEW
• Eversion or rolling out of the eyelid margin, resulting in exposure of the palpebral conjunctiva
• Exposure and poor tear distribution—may predispose patient to sight-threatening corneal disease

SIGNALMENT
• Dogs, seldom cats
• Breeds with higher than average prevalence—sporting breeds (e.g., spaniels, hounds, and retrievers); giant breeds (e.g., St. Bernards and mastiffs); any breed with loose facial skin (especially bloodhounds)
• Developmental—genetic predisposition in listed breeds; may occur in dogs < 1 year old
• Acquired—noted in other breeds; occurs late in life secondary to age-related loss of facial musculature and developing skin laxity
• Intermittent—caused by fatigue; may be observed after strenuous exercise or when drowsy

SIGNS
• Eversion of the lower eyelid with lack of contact of the lower lid to the globe and exposure of the palpebral conjunctiva and third eyelid—usually obvious
• Facial staining caused by poor tear drainage—tears spill over onto the face instead of passing from the eye to the nose via the nasolacrimal ducts
• History of mucoid to mucopurulent discharge owing to conjunctival exposure
• Recurrent foreign body irritation
• History of bacterial conjunctivitis

CAUSES & RISK FACTORS
• Usually secondary to breed-associated alterations in facial conformation and eyelid support
• Marked weight loss or muscle mass loss about the head and orbits—may result in acquired disease
• Tragic facial expression in hypothyroid dogs
• Scarring of the eyelids secondary to injury or after overcorrection of entropion—may result in cicatricial disease

DIAGNOSIS

DIFFERENTIAL DIAGNOSIS
• Usually clinically obvious
• Look for any underlying disorder in non-predisposed breeds and patients with late-age onset.
• Loss of orbital or periorbital mass—may cause condition in patients with masticatory myositis
• Palpebral nerve paralysis—condition associated with lack of muscle tone of the orbicularis oculi muscles

CBC/BIOCHEMISTRY/URINALYSIS
N/A

OTHER LABORATORY TESTS
• Possible masticatory myositis—test for autoantibodies against type 2M muscle fibers.
• Palpebral nerve paralysis or tragic facial expression—consider testing for hypothyroidism.

IMAGING
N/A

DIAGNOSTIC PROCEDURES
• Palpebral nerve paralysis—full neurologic evaluation; potentially tested for hypothyroidism
• Secondary conjunctivitis—consider bacterial culture or cytologic examination to help select an appropriate topical antibiotic.
• Fluorescein or Rose Bengal staining of the cornea and conjunctiva—may document corneal ulcerations; may reveal severity of the exposure problem

TREATMENT
• Supportive care and good ocular and facial hygiene—sufficient for most mild disease
• Surgical treatment—eyelid shortening or radical facelift; necessary for severely affected patients that have chronic ocular irritation
• Intermittent, fatigue-induced condition—do not treat surgically.

MEDICATIONS

DRUGS
• Topical broad-spectrum ophthalmic antibiotics—bacterial conjunctivitis or corneal ulceration
• Lubricant eye drops and ointments—reduce conjunctival and corneal desiccation secondary to exposure
• Hypothyroid and masticatory myositis-induced conditions—may respond well to appropriate medical treatment of the underlying disease

CONTRAINDICATIONS/POSSIBLE INTERACTIONS
N/A

FOLLOW-UP
• May become more severe as patient ages
• Nonsurgically treated patient—monitor for signs of infectious conjunctivitis, exposure keratopathy, corneal ulceration, and facial dermatitis.

MISCELLANEOUS

ASSOCIATED CONDITIONS
• Hypothyroidism
• Masticatory myositis

AGE-RELATED FACTORS
Old animals more likely to have ectropion secondary to loss of facial muscle tone

SEE ALSO
• Hypothyroidism
• Myopathy, Masticatory Muscle Myositis

Suggested Reading
Slatter D. Eyelids. In: Fundamentals of veterinary ophthalmology. 2nd ed. Philadelphia: Saunders, 1990:147–203.
Author J. Phillip Pickett
Consulting Editor Paul E. Miller

EHRLICHIOSIS

BASICS

DEFINITION
Ehrlichia spp.—cause tick-borne rickettsial disease

Dogs
• Species divided into three groups
(1) *E. canis* (ehrlichiosis found intracytoplasmically in circulating leukocytes), *E. ewingii* (canine granulocytic ehrlichiosis), and *E. chaffeensis* (subclinical infections)
(2) *E. equi* and *E. phagocytophilia*
(3) *E. risticii* and *E. sennetsu* (not in the U.S.)
• *E. platys*—not fully characterized; causes infectious cyclic thrombocytopenia found in platelets
• Recent evidence suggests other as yet unidentified *Ehrlichia* species infect dogs.

Cats
• Extremely rare
• *E. risticii* and *E. equi*
• Serologic evidence suggests a species that cross-reacts with *E. canis* can cause illness

PATHOPHYSIOLOGY
E. canis
• *Rhipicephalus sanguineus*—brown dog tick; transmits disease to dogs in saliva; 1–3-week incubation period; 3 stages of disease
• Acute—spreads from bite site to the spleen, liver, and lymph nodes (causes organomegaly); then subclinical with mild thrombocytopenia; mainly endothelial cells affected; vasculitis; reduction in platelet survival time causing thrombocytopenia; variable leukopenia; mild anemia; severity depends on organism
• Subclinical—organism persists; antibody response increases (hyperglobulinemia); thrombocytopenia persists.
• Chronic—impaired bone marrow production (platelets, erythroid suppression); marrow becomes hypercellular with plasma cells.

SYSTEMS AFFECTED
• Multisystemic
• Bleeding tendencies—thrombocytopenia and vasculitis
• Lymphadenopathy
• Splenomegaly
• CNS, eyes (anterior uveitis), and lungs—rarely affected by vasculitis

INCIDENCE/PREVALENCE
• Occurs throughout the year; insidious
• Average duration from onset to presentation—usually > 2 months
• Prevalence varies, depending on geographic locality.

GEOGRAPHIC DISTRIBUTION
• Worldwide
• North America—mainly Gulf Coast and eastern seaboard; also the Midwest and California

SIGNALMENT

Species
• Dogs—can be infected with a number of species; *E. canis, E. platys,* and *E. ewingii* produce main disease entities.
• Cats—*E. risticii;* also serologic evidence suggests a species similar to *E. canis*

Breed Predilection
Chronic (*E. canis*)—seems more severe in Doberman pinschers and German shepherds

Mean Age and Range
• Average age—5.22 years
• Range—2 months to 14 years

Predominant Sex
None

SIGNS

General Comments
Duration of clinical signs from initial acute illness to presentation—usually > 2 months

Historical Findings
• Lethargy
• Depression
• Anorexia and weight loss
• Fever
• Spontaneous bleeding—sneezing, epistaxis
• Respiratory distress
• Ataxia
• Head tilt
• Ocular pain

Physical Examination Findings
Acute
• Bleeding diathesis (petechiation of mucous membranes as a result of thrombocytopenia) associated with fever (with depression, anorexia, weight loss) and generalized lymphadenopathy should raise suspicions.
• Ticks—found in 40% of cases
• Respiratory—dyspnea (even cyanosis); increased bronchovesicular sound
• Diffuse CNS disease
• Ataxia with upper motor neuron dysfunction
• Vestibular dysfunction
• Generalized or local hyperesthesia
• Most dogs recover without treatment and enter a subclinical state.
Chronic
• In nonendemic areas
• Spontaneous bleeding
• Anemia
• Generalized lymphadenopathy
• Scrotal and limb edema
• Splenomegaly
• Hepatomegaly
• Uveitis
• Hyphema
• Retinal hemorrhages and detachment with blindness
• Corneal edema
• Arthritis (rare)
• Seizures (rare)

RISK FACTORS
Concurrent infection with *Babesia, Haemobartonella, E. platys,* and *Hepatozoon canis*—worsens clinical syndrome

DIAGNOSIS

DIFFERENTIAL DIAGNOSIS
• Rocky Mountain spotted fever (*Rickettsia rickettsii*)—usually seasonal between March and October; serologic testing for diagnosis; responds to same treatment as ehrlichiosis
• Immune-mediated thrombocytopenia—not usually associated with fever or lymphadenopathy; serologic testing best distinguishes; may treat for both until results are known
• Systemic lupus erythematosus—ANA test usually negative with ehrlichiosis; serologic testing for diagnosis
• Multiple myeloma—serologic testing to differentiate and determine cause of hyperglobulinemia
• Chronic lymphocytic leukemia—differentiate by lymphocytosis and cytology of bone marrow
• Brucellosis—serologic testing for diagnosis and to determine cause of scrotal edema

CBC/BIOCHEMISTRY/URINALYSIS

Acute
• Thrombocytopenia—before onset of clinical signs
• Anemia
• Leukopenia—from lymphopenia and eosinopenia
• Leukocytosis and monocytosis—as disease becomes more chronic
• Morulae—intracytoplasmic inclusions in leukocytes rare
• Nonspecific changes—mild increases in ALT, ALP, BUN, creatinine, and total bilirubin (rare)
• Hyperglobulinemia—progressively increases 1–3 weeks postinfection
• Hypoalbuminemia—usually from renal loss
• Proteinuria—with or without azotemia; about have of patients

Chronic
• Pancytopenia—typical; monocytosis and lymphocytosis may be present.
• Hyperglobulinemia—magnitude of globulin increases correlates with duration of infection; usually polyclonal gammopathy, but monoclonal (IgG) gammopathies occur.
• Hypoalbuminemia
• High BUN and creatinine—from primary renal disease, owing to glomerulonephritis and renal interstitial plasmacytosis

OTHER LABORATORY TESTS

Serologic Testing
• Most clinically useful and reliable method for diagnosis

- IFA highly sensitive; low level of cross-reactivity exists between *E. canis* and *E. equi* but not between *E. canis* and *E. platys*
- Titers—reliable 3 weeks after infection; > 1:10 diagnostic
- Coombs-positive anemia—may be seen; may confuse the diagnosis
- PCR—proving to be more sensitive than IFA; not commercially available
- Test for other accompanying pathogens—*Babesiosis, Hemobartonellosis, E. platys,* and *Hepatozoon canis*

DIAGNOSTIC PROCEDURES

Bone Marrow Aspirate
- Acute—hypercellularity of megakaryocytic and myeloid series
- Chronic—often erythroid hypoplasia with increased M:E ratios and plasmacytosis
- Increased numbers of mast cells are occasionally seen on marrow smears.

PATHOLOGIC FINDINGS
- Acute—petechial hemorrhages on serosal and mucosal surfaces of most organs; generalized lymphadenopathy (brownish discoloration), splenomegaly, hepatomegaly, and red bone marrow (hypercellularity)
- Chronic—pale marrow (hypoplastic); subcutaneous edema; histologically, perivascular plasma cell infiltrate in numerous organs most characteristic; multifocal nonsuppurative meningoencephalitis with lymphoplasmacytic cell infiltrate into the meninges common

TREATMENT

APPROPRIATE HEALTH CARE
- Inpatient—initial medical stabilization for anemia and/or hemorrhagic tendency resulting from thrombocytopenia
- Outpatient—stable patients; monitor blood and response to medication frequently.

NURSING CARE
- Balanced electrolyte solution—indicated for dehydration
- Blood transfusion—indicated for anemia
- Platelet-rich plasma or a blood transfusion—indicated for hemorrhage resulting from thrombocytopenia

ACTIVITY
Restricted

CLIENT EDUCATION
- Acute—prognosis excellent with appropriate therapy
- Chronic—response may take 1 month; prognosis poor if the bone marrow is severely hypoplastic
- Progression from acute to chronic can be easily prevented by early, effective treatment; but many dogs remain seropositive and may relapse (even years later)

- German shepherds and Doberman pinschers—more chronic and severe form of disease

SURGICAL CONSIDERATIONS
If surgery is needed for other reasons, blood transfusion may be needed to correct anemia and/or thrombocytopenia.

MEDICATIONS

DRUGS OF CHOICE
- Doxycycline—5 mg/kg PO q12h or 10 mg/kg PO q24h for 14 days; give intravenously for 5 days if the dog is vomiting.
- Imidocarb dipropionate—5 mg/kg IM for 2 doses 14 days apart; effective against both *E. canis* and babesiosis; reasonable alternative to doxycycline
- Glucocorticoids—prednisolone or prednisone; 1–2 mg/kg PO q12h for 5 days; may be indicated when thrombocytopenia is life-threatening (thought to be a result of immune-mediated mechanisms); because immune-mediated thrombocytopenia is a principal differential diagnosis, may be indicated until results of serologic tests are available
- Androgenic steroids—to stimulate bone marrow production in chronically affected dogs with hypoplastic marrows; oxymetholone (2 mg/kg q24h PO until response) or nandrolone decanoate (1.5 mg/kg IM weekly)

CONTRAINDICATIONS
Tetracycline (and derivatives)—do not use in dogs < 6 months old (permanent yellowing of teeth occurs); do not use with renal insufficiency (try doxycycline because it can be excreted via the gastrointestinal tract)

PRECAUTIONS
Glucocorticoids—prolonged use at immuno-suppressive levels may interfere with the clearance and elimination of *E. canis* after use of tetracycline

ALTERNATIVE DRUGS
- Oxytetracycline and tetracycline—22 mg/kg PO q8h for 21 days; effective and less expensive
- Chloramphenicol—20 mg/kg PO q8h for 14 days; for puppies < 6 months of age; avoids yellow discoloration of erupting teeth caused by tetracyclines; warn client of public health risks, because it directly interferes with heme and bone marrow synthesis; avoid in dogs with thrombocytopenia, pancytopenia, or anemia

FOLLOW-UP

PATIENT MONITORING
- Platelet count—every 3 days after initiating antirickettsial agent until normal; improvement is rapid in acute cases.

- Serologic testing—repeat in 9 months; most dogs will become seronegative; positive titer suggests reinfection (prior infection does not imply protective immunity) or ineffective treatment (reinstitute treatment regimen)

PREVENTION/AVOIDANCE
- Control tick infestation—dips or sprays containing dichlorvos, chlorfenvinphos, dioxathion, propoxur, or carbaryl; flea and tick collars may reduce reinfestation but reliability unproven; avoid tick-infested areas.
- Removing ticks by hand—use gloves (see Zoonotic Potential); ensure mouth parts are removed to avoid a foreign body reaction

EXPECTED COURSE AND PROGNOSIS
- Acute—excellent prognosis with appropriate treatment
- Chronic—may take 4 weeks for a clinical response; prognosis poor with hypoplastic marrow

MISCELLANEOUS

ASSOCIATED CONDITIONS
- *Babesia* • *Haemobartonella* • *E. platys*

ZOONOTIC POTENTIAL
- Serologic evidence indicates that E. canis (or possibly a related species) occurs in people; probably not directly infected from dogs; tick exposure thought to be necessary; *R. sanguineus* probably not the vector in humans
- Most cases in the southern and south-central U.S. • Major clinical signs in humans—fever, headache, myalgia, ocular pain, and gastrointestinal upset • Treatment with tetracyclines results in rapid recovery.

SYNONYMS
- Tropical canine pancytopenia • Canine rickettsiosis • Canine hemorrhagic fever • Lahore canine fever • Canine typhus • Tracker dog disease • Nairobi bleeding disease

ABBREVIATIONS
- ALP = alkaline phosphatase • ALT = alanine transferase • ANA = antinuclear antibody • IFA = indirect fluorescent antibody • M:E = myeloid:erythroid ratio • PCR = polymerase chain reaction

Suggested Reading
Kordick DL, Lappin MR, Breitshwerdt EB. Feline rickettsial diseases. In: Bonagura JD, Kirk RW, eds. Current veterinary therapy XII. Philadelphia: Saunders, 1995:287–290.
Troy GC, Forrester SD. Canine ehrlichiosis. In: Greene CE, ed. Infectious diseases of the dog and cat. Philadelphia: Saunders, 1990:404–414.
Author Stephen C. Barr
Consulting Editor Stephen C. Barr

DISEASES

ELBOW DYSPLASIA

BASICS

DEFINITION
A series of four developmental abnormalities that lead to malformation and degeneration of the elbow joint

PATHOPHYSIOLOGY
• Four abnormalities—UAP, OCD, FMCP, and incongruity; may occur alone or in combination; may be seen in one or both elbows; bilateral disease common (50% of cases)
• UAP—characterized by failure of the anconeal process (which contains a separate ossification center) to unite with the proximal ulnar metaphysis (olecranon) by 5 months of age; may be the result of abnormal mechanical stress on the anconeal process
• OCD—affects the medial aspect of the humeral condyle; retention of articular cartilage owing to a disturbance in endochondral ossification and mechanical stress; leads to formation of a cartilage flap lesion; may be the result of abnormal mechanical stress on the medial aspect
• FMCP—chondral or osteochondral fragmentation or fissure of the medial coronoid process of the ulna; not considered a traumatic injury; a manifestation of osteochondrosis of the coronoid process; differs from the related pathology of the anconeal process because the coronoid does not have a separate ossification center; may be the result of abnormal mechanical stress on the medial coronoid process
• Incongruity—manifestation of malalignment and malformation of the elbow joint; asynchronous proximal growth between the radius and ulna may lead to abnormal load and wear and erosion of cartilage in the humeroulnar compartment; may be the result of malformation of the trochlear notch of the ulna; a slightly elliptical trochlear notch with a decreased arc of curvature is too small to articulate with the humeral trochlea, which results in major points of contact in areas of the anconeal process, coronoid process, and medial humeral condyle and little or no contact in other areas of the trochlea.

SYSTEMS AFFECTED
Musculoskeletal

GENETICS
• Inherited disease
• High heritability—heritability index ranges between 0.25 and 0.45.

INCIDENCE/PREVALENCE
• Most common cause for elbow pain and lameness
• One of the most common causes for forelimb lameness in large-breed dogs

GEOGRAPHIC DISTRIBUTION
N/A

SIGNALMENT

Species
Dogs

Breed Predilections
Large and giant breeds—Labrador retrievers; Rottweilers; golden retrievers; German shepherds; Bernese mountain dogs; chow chows; bearded collies; Newfoundlands

Mean Age and Range
• Age at onset of clinical signs—typically 4–10 months
• Age at diagnosis—generally 4–18 months
• Onset of symptoms related to DJD—any age

PREDOMINANT SEX
• FMCP—males predisposed
• UAP, OCD, incongruity—none established

SIGNS

General Comments
• Lameness—if no distinct abnormalities noted on physical examination or radiographs, repeat examination 4–8 weeks later.
• Not all patients are symptomatic when young.
• Acute episode of elbow lameness owing to advanced DJD changes in a mature patient—common

Historical Findings
Intermittent or persistent forelimb lameness—exacerbated by exercise; progressed from a stiffness seen only after rest

Physical Examination Findings
• Pain—elicited on elbow hyperflexion or extension; elicited when holding the elbow and carpus at 90° while pronating and supinating the carpus
• Affected limb—tendency to be held in abduction and supination
• Joint effusion and capsular distension—especially noted between the lateral epicondyle and olecranon
• Crepitus—may be palpated with advanced DJD
• Diminished range of motion

CAUSES
• Genetic
• Developmental
• Nutritional

RISK FACTORS
• Rapid growth and weight gain
• High-calorie diet

DIAGNOSIS

DIFFERENTIAL DIAGNOSIS
• Trauma
• Septic arthritis
• Panosteitis
• Avulsion or calcification of the flexor muscles
• Synovial cell sarcoma

CBC/BIOCHEMISTRY/URINALYSIS
N/A

OTHER LABORATORY TESTS
N/A

IMAGING

Radiography
• May need four views for diagnosis—mediolateral; mediolateral hyperflexed; 25° craniocaudal-lateromedial oblique; craniocaudal
• Image both elbows—high incidence of bilateral disease
• UAP—best diagnosed from the mediolateral hyperflexed view; may easily see lack of bony union
• OCD—best diagnosed from the craniocaudal and craniocaudal-lateromedial oblique views; reveals a radiolucent defect or flattening of the medial aspect of the humeral condyle
• FMCP—seldom visualized; diagnosis is presumptive based on DJD and the absence of UAP or OCD lesions; commonly see osteophyte formation on the proximal rim of the anconeal process, medial coronoid process, and cranial margin of the radial head and epicondyles (medial and lateral); also commonly see sclerosis of the ulna caudal to the coronoid process and trochlear notch and stairstep between the joint surface of the radius and lateral coronoid; may also see these changes with UAP, OCD, and incongruity

Other
CT, MRI, and linear tomography—accurately diagnose FMCP

DIAGNOSTIC PROCEDURES

• Joint tap and analysis of synovial fluid—confirm involvement of joint
• Synovial fluid—should be straw colored with normal to decreased viscosity; cytology reveals <10,000 nucleated cells/μL (>90% are mononuclear cells); normal results do not necessarily rule out the diagnosis.
• Arthroscopy—may use to diagnose UAP, FMCP, and OCD

PATHOLOGIC FINDINGS

• UAP—fibrous union between anconeal process and proximal ulnar metaphysis; fibrous tissue invasion and degeneration of the anconeal process; DJD
• OCD—chondral flap on medial humeral condyle; sclerosis of underlying subchondral bone with fibrous tissue invasion; erosive lesion on apposing coronoid cartilage; DJD
• FMCP—chondral or osteochondral fragmentation of the cranial tip or lateral margin of the medial coronoid; erosive lesion on cartilage of the apposing medial aspect of the humeral condyle; DJD
• Incongruity—erosive lesions involving part or all of medial coronoid process and the apposing articular cartilage of the medial aspect of the humeral condyle; DJD; linear striations in the articular cartilage

TREATMENT

APPROPRIATE HEALTH CARE

Surgery—controversial but recommended for all patients

NURSING CARE

• Cold packing the elbow joint—perform immediately postsurgery to help decrease swelling and control pain; perform at least 15–20 min q8h for 3–5 days.
• Range-of-motion exercises—beneficial until the patient can bear weight on the limb(s)

ACTIVITY

Restricted for all patients postoperatively

DIET

• Weight control—important for decreasing the load and stress on the affected joint(s)
• Restricted weight gain and growth in young dogs—may decrease incidence and severity

CLIENT EDUCATION

• Discuss the heritability of the disease.
• Discuss the potential for DJD progression.
• Discuss the influence of excessive intake of nutrients that promote rapid growth.

SURGICAL CONSIDERATIONS

• Severity of DJD and age of patient—negatively influence outcome
• UAP—four options: removal, lag screw fixation, dynamic proximal ulnar osteotomy, and lag screw fixation plus dynamic proximal osteotomy; base decision on degree of DJD, patient's age, and surgical expertise.
• OCD and FMCP—medial approach to elbow (diagnostic differentiation not necessary); removal of loose fragment(s)
• Incongruity—controversial; four options: no surgery, coronoidectomy, dynamic proximal ulnar osteotomy, intra-articular osteotomy; base decision on type of incongruity, degree of DJD, patient's age, and surgical expertise.
• Arthroscopic diagnosis and treatment—excellent option for FMCP, OCD, and incongruity; benefits: superior diagnostic capabilities, minimal invasiveness, decreased postoperative discomfort, and decreased postoperative morbidity

MEDICATIONS

DRUGS OF CHOICE

• None that promotes healing of osteochondral or chondral fragments
• NSAIDs—minimize pain, decrease inflammation, symptomatically treat associated DJD; may try buffered or enteric-coated aspirin (10–25 mg/kg PO q8h or q12h), caroprofen (2.2 mg/kg PO q12h), etodolac (10–15 mg/kg PO q24h), phenylbutazone (3–7 mg/kg PO q8h, total dose <800 mg/day), meclofenemic acid (0.5 mg/kg PO q12h), and piroxicam (0.3 mg/kg PO q24h for 3 days then q48h)

CONTRAINDICATIONS

Avoid corticosteroids—potential side effects; articular cartilage damage associated with long-term use

PRECAUTIONS

NSAIDs—gastrointestinal irritation may preclude use in some patients.

POSSIBLE INTERACTIONS

N/A

ALTERNATIVE DRUGS

Chondroprotective drugs (e.g., polysulfated glycosaminoglycans, glucosamine, and chondroitin sulfate)—may help limit cartilage damage and degeneration; may help alleviate pain and inflammation

FOLLOW-UP

PATIENT MONITORING

• Postsurgery—limit activity for a minimum of 4 weeks; encourage early, active movement of the affected joint(s).
• Yearly examinations—recommended to evaluate progression of DJD

PREVENTION/AVOIDANCE

• Discourage breeding of affected animals.
• Do not repeat dam–sire breedings that result in affected offspring.

POSSIBLE COMPLICATIONS

N/A

EXPECTED COURSE AND PROGNOSIS

• Progression of DJD—expected
• Prognosis—fair to good for all forms

MISCELLANEOUS

ASSOCIATED CONDITIONS

N/A

AGE-RELATED FACTORS

Middle-aged to old dogs with advanced DJD are not candidates for surgical intervention.

ZOONOTIC POTENTIAL

N/A

PREGNANCY

N/A

SYNONYMS

Elbow osteochondrosis

SEE ALSO

Osteochondrosis

ABBREVIATIONS

• DJD = degenerative joint disease
• FMCP = fragmented medial coronoid process
• OCD = osteochondritis dissecans
• UAP = un-united anconeal process

Suggested Reading

Olsson SE. Pathophysiology, morphology, and clinical signs of osteochondrosis in the dog. In: Bojrab MJ, ed. Disease mechanisms in small animal surgery. Philadelphia: Lea & Febiger, 1993:777–779.

Schwarz PD. Elbow dysplasia. In: Bonagura JD, Kersey R, eds. Current veterinary therapy XIII: Small animal practice. Philadelphia: Saunders, 2000:1004-1014.

Wind AP. Elbow incongruity and developmental elbow diseases in the dog: parts I and II. J Am Anim Hosp Assoc 1986;22:711–724.

Author Peter D. Schwarz
Consulting Editor Peter D. Schwarz

ENAMEL HYPOPLASIA/HYPOCALCIFICATION

BASICS

OVERVIEW
- Apparent defect in enamel surfaces, often pitted and discolored; focal or generalized
- Defects due to disruption of normal enamel formation
- Influences during enamel formation (distemper, fever, etc.) over an extended time may cause generalized changes; during a short time (focal, local; e.g., trauma, even from deciduous tooth extraction) they cause specific patterns or bands.
- Most cases are primarily esthetic; some patients can have extensive structural damage, even root involvement.
- A more correct description would be enamel hypocalcification, since the amount of enamel is adequate (not hypoplastic), but it has defects in calcification that lead to enamel defect.
- Teeth may be more sensitive with exposed dentin, and occasionally fractures of severely compromised teeth occur; usually they remain fully functional.

SIGNALMENT
- Dogs and cats (less common)
- Often apparent at time of tooth eruption (after 6 months of age) or shortly thereafter (with signs of wear)

SIGNS

Historical Findings
Discolored teeth

Physical Examination Findings
- Irregular, pitted enamel surface with discoloration of diseased enamel and potential exposure of underlying dentin (light brown).
- Early or rapid accumulation of plaque and calculus on roughened tooth surface; possible gingivitis and/or accelerated periodontal disease

CAUSES & RISK FACTORS
- Insult during enamel formation
- Canine distemper virus, fever, trauma (e.g., accidents, excessive force during deciduous tooth extraction)

DIAGNOSIS

DIFFERENTIAL DIAGNOSIS
- Enamel staining—discolored but smooth surface (tetracycline)
- Carious lesions—cavities with decay
- Amelogenesis imperfecta—genetic enamel disorder
- Erosive lesions—similar to those found in cats

CBC/BIOCHEMISTRY/URINALYSIS
Usually normal

OTHER LABORATORY TESTS
N/A

IMAGING
- Intraoral radiographs are necessary to determine viability of roots.
- Cases reported of abnormal root formation; no root formation, or separated crown and root

DIAGNOSTIC PROCEDURES
N/A

TREATMENT
- Treatment depends upon extent of lesions and equipment and materials available.
- Goal is to provide the smoothest surface possible.

Optimal Treatment
- Ideal treatment is to gently remove diseased enamel (enamel scrub) with white stone burs or finishing disks on high-speed handpiece (adequate water coolant); rotary burs can cause excessive damage and heat—handle with care!
- Take care not to damage the tooth—excess enamel/dentin removal; hyperthermic damage to pulp
- Focal defects may be amenable to composite or glass ionomer restoration, but long-term success is poor; metallic crown restoration is preferred; many restorative materials (bonding agents, composites) require use of light-curing units and appropriate skill levels.
- Bonding agent recommended to seal exposed dentinal tubules and protect surface.

Alternative Treatment
- Without a high-speed handpiece and appropriate attachments, treatment can be more challenging.
- The soft, diseased enamel can sometimes be removed with ultrasonic scalers, but take care to avoid damage and hyperthermia.
- A strong fluoride treatment (in-hospital, on a dry tooth surface; varnish or strong sodium fluoride paste) can be used to decrease sensitivity and enhance enamel strength.

MEDICATIONS

DRUGS
N/A

CONTRAINDICATION/POSSIBLE INTERACTIONS
N/A

 FOLLOW-UP

PATIENT MONITORING
Inform the owner that further degeneration of remaining enamel may occur, necessitating additional therapy in the future.

PREVENTION/AVOIDANCE
• Recommend regular professional dental cleaning and a routine home-care program (brushing); may include weekly application of stannous fluoride at home (minimize ingestion because of toxicity)
• Avoid excessive chewing on hard objects.

 MISCELLANEOUS

Suggested Reading
Wiggs BW, Loprise HB. Veterinary dentistry: principles and practice. Philadelphia: Lippincott-Raven, 1997.
Author Heidi Lobprise
Consulting Editor Jan Bellows

ENCEPHALITIS

BASICS

DEFINITION
Inflammation of the brain that may be accompanied by spinal cord and/or meningeal involvement

Pathophysiology
• Inflammation—caused by an infectious agent or by the patient's own immune system • Immune-mediated—cause of immune system derangement generally unknown

SYSTEMS AFFECTED
• Nervous • Multisystemic signs—may be noted in patients with infectious diseases

GENETICS
N/A

INCIDENCE/PREVALENCE
Unknown

GEOGRAPHIC DISTRIBUTION
Varies with the cause or agent implicated

SIGNALMENT

Species
Dogs and cats

Breed Predilections
• GME—mostly small-breed dogs, especially terriers and miniature poodles; large-breed dogs also affected • Pug encephalitis—pugs • PME—German short-haired pointers • Maltese encephalitis—Maltese • YNE—Yorkshire terriers

Mean Age and Range
N/A

Predominant Sex
N/A

SIGNS

Historical Findings
• Usually a peracute to acute onset of clinical signs that rapidly progresses • GME and fungal and protozoal encephalitis—sometimes signs are more chronically progressive

Physical Examination Findings
• Fever, lung disease, and/or gastrointestinal disturbances—usually precede encephalitis • With mycotic, rickettsial, viral, and prothothecal organisms—fundic lesions frequently seen

Neurologic Examination Findings
• Determined by the portion of the brain most affected • Rostral fossa—seizures; circling; pacing; personality change; decreasing level of responsiveness • Caudal fossa—abnormalities related to the brainstem (e.g., depression, head tilt, facial paresis/paralysis, incoordination) • Progression (e.g., anisocoria, pinpoint pupils, decreasing level of consciousness, and poor physiologic nystagmus)—suggests tentorial herniation

CAUSES

Dogs
• Idiopathic, immune-mediated—GME, pug encephalitis; Maltese encephalitis; YNE; EME • Viral—canine distemper virus; rabies; herpes; parvovirus; adenovirus; pseudorabies; Eastern and Venezuelan equine encephalomyelitis virus • Postvaccinal encephalomyelitis—canine distemper virus; rabies; canine coronavirus-parvovirus • Rickettsial—Rocky Mountain spotted fever; ehrlichiosis • Mycotic—cryptococcosis; blastomycosis; histoplasmosis; coccidioidomycosis; aspergillosis; phaeohyphomycosis • Bacterial—anaerobic and aerobic • Protozoal—toxoplasmosis; neosporosis; encephalitozoonosis • Spirochetes—borreliosis • Parasite migration— *Dirofilaria immitis; Toxocara canis; Ancylostoma caninum; Cuterebra;* cysticercosis • Migrating foreign body—plant awn; others • Prototothecosis • PME

Cats
• Idiopathic, immune-mediated—GME; EME • Idiopathic polioencephalomyelitis • Viral—FIP; rabies; FIV; pseudorabies; panleukopenia; rhinotracheitis • Mycotic—cryptococcosis; blastomycosis; phaeohyphomycoses • Bacterial—anaerobic and aerobic • Protozoal—toxoplasmosis • Parasite migration—*Dirofilaria immitis; Cuterebra*

RISK FACTORS
• Immunosuppressive drugs and FIV or FeLV infection—infectious encephalitides • Tick-infected areas—rickettsial and *Borrelia* infections • Travel history—mycotic infections

DIAGNOSIS

DIFFERENTIAL DIAGNOSIS
• Fungal encephalitides—frequently accompanied by systemic signs • Protozoal diseases—systemic; may have a chronic history • Rickettsial diseases—hemogram abnormalities common • FIP—patients usually < 3 years of age; protracted course; characteristic CSF analysis • Canine distemper virus—commonly seen as acute encephalitis with systemic signs in patients < 1 year old; can be difficult to confirm antemortem • Primary CNS neoplasia—signs may be similar to encephalitis. • Degenerative disorders—usually slow, insidiously progressive onset • Metabolic or toxic encephalopathy—bilateral, symmetrical neurologic abnormalities that relate to the cerebrum; confirm toxins by laboratory tests or serum assay.

CBC/BIOCHEMISTRY/URINALYSIS
• Hemogram—frequently normal; leukocytosis may be seen in diseases that produce systemic signs; may be lymphopenia in the early stages of canine distemper virus and rickettsial infection; rickettsial encephalitis may be accompanied by thrombocytopenia and anemia. • Serum chemistry—frequently normal; hyperproteinemia with polyclonal gammopathy often seen with FIP and chronic systemic infections; creatine kinase may be moderately high with *Neospora* infection (dogs).

OTHER LABORATORY TESTS
• Serology—available for fungal, protozoal, rickettsial, and viral diseases; helpful but must be interpreted with caution because a positive titer does not always indicate active disease (e.g., toxoplasma in cats) and a negative titer does not always rule out active disease (e.g., FIP) • Indirect fluorescent antibody—a single positive titer of 1:10 or greater confirms ehrlichiosis. • ELISA—a fourfold rise between acute and convalescent IgG titers when the first titer is > 1:128 confirms Rocky Mountain spotted fever; an IgM titer of > 1:256 suggests infection within the previous 16 weeks by *Toxoplasma gondii* and may indicate exacerbation of chronic infection. • Latex agglutination antigen—a single positive titer from serum or CSF confirms cryptococcus. • Agar-gel immunodiffusion—diagnose blastomycosis with a high degree of accuracy • Local production of canine distemper virus–specific antibody (IgG and IgM)—in CSF after virus infects the CNS • Positive *Neospora caninum* titer—correlates well with active disease • Positive FIP titer—indicates only infection with a coronavirus; may not be pathogenic • Positive *Borrelia burgdorferi* titer—indicates exposure to the organism, not necessarily active disease

IMAGING
• Thoracic radiographs—may confirm lung abnormalities • Skull radiographs—may confirm sinusitis/rhinitis in some cats with cryptococcosis • CT or MRI of the brain—may detect multifocal or single mass lesions

DIAGNOSTIC PROCEDURES
• CSF analysis—perform on all animals with clinical signs that suggest encephalitis; results almost always abnormal; normal results do not rule out acute viral encephalitis that is limited to the parenchyma; with pleocytosis, culture for bacteria (aerobic and anaerobic). • CNS reaction—neutrophils indicate an acute active inflammatory process; small lymphocytes indicate an antigenic response; eosinophils indicate an allergic response or a reaction to foreign material (tumor, parasite).

PATHOLOGIC FINDINGS
The lesions are a function of the brain response to the infectious agent or other cause.

TREATMENT

APPROPRIATE HEALTH CARE
Inpatient—diagnosis and initial therapy

NURSING CARE
• Symptomatic treatment—control brain edema and seizure activity as necessary. • Cerebral edema—give 20% mannitol (2.2 g/kg IV over 30–45 min); may repeat within 1–2 hr to achieve maximum response; limit parenteral fluids to prevent rebound cerebral edema; with mannitol, short-term (72 hr) corticosteroid treatment indicated for further control (dexamethasone sodium phosphate at 0.5 mg/kg IV q12h for 24 hr; then reduce to 0.25 mg/kg q12h for 48 hr) • Seizures—treat with antiepileptic drugs; control may be erratic until the encephalitis is treated; with boluses or constant-rate infusions, monitor closely for respiratory depression because the blood–brain barrier is altered.

ACTIVITY
As tolerated

DIET
With severe depression or vomiting—nothing by mouth until condition improves, to prevent aspiration

CLIENT EDUCATION
• Inform client that the condition is life-threatening if left untreated. • Inform client that relapse is possible with an idiopathic or immune-mediated encephalitis when therapy is discontinued.

SURGICAL CONSIDERATIONS
Brain biopsy—may be needed for specific diagnosis

MEDICATIONS

DRUGS OF CHOICE
• Apply specific therapy once diagnosis is reached or highly suspected. • Idiopathic and immune-mediated—respond to immunosuppressive dosage of prednisone • Rickettsial and borreliosis—doxycycline • Protozoal—clindamycin • Mycotic—requires treatment for 1–2 years; use itraconazole (5 mg/kg PO q12h with food) or fluconazole (6.25–12.5 mg/kg PO or IV q12h); corticosteroids often needed during the first 4–6 weeks to control cerebral edema • Viral and postvaccinal—none definitive; treated symptomatically • Bacterial—broad-spectrum antibiotics that penetrate the blood–brain barrier; if agent is unknown, try a combination of enrofloxacin (5 mg/kg PO or IV q12h) and ticarcillin-clavulanate (50 mg/kg IV q8h) or

amoxicillin-clavulanate (13.75 mg/kg PO q8h).

CONTRAINDICATIONS
• Bacterial and Rocky Mountain spotted fever—corticosteroids contraindicated • Puppies < 6 months of age with a rickettsial disease—avoid chloramphenicol (doxycycline-induced tooth discoloration) • Puppies < 8 months of age—eurofloxacin contraindicated (cartilage damage); use amoxicillin-clavulanate or ticarcillin-clavulanate alone. • CNS infections—do not use aminoglycosides and most cephalosporins because CNS penetration is poor.

PRECAUTIONS
• Administer mannitol intravenously 10 min before giving anesthesia for CSF collection, to decrease intracranial pressure. • Corticosteroids—observe closely for worsening signs that suggest an infectious cause.

POSSIBLE INTERACTIONS
• Chloramphenicol and cimetidine—do not use concurrently with phenobarbital, to avoid toxic serum phenobarbital levels secondary to interference with liver metabolism. • Corticosteroids alter the CSF for 12 hr or more.

ALTERNATIVE DRUGS
• Cyclosporine—2–3 mg/kg PO q12h; may be effective in maintaining remission in patients with immune-mediated diseases that repeatedly relapse when prednisone is withdrawn; Neoral is absorbed three times better orally than other forms of cyclosporine, lowering the dose by one-third and offering a considerable financial savings.

FOLLOW-UP

PATIENT MONITORING
• Frequent neurologic evaluations in the first 48–72 hr to monitor progress • Relapse as medication is withdrawn—repeat CSF analysis • Measure serum titer of cryptococcus capsular antigen every 3 months until negative.

PREVENTION/AVOIDANCE
A method of effective tick control should be used on animals that live in endemic areas.

POSSIBLE COMPLICATIONS
• Long-term corticosteroid therapy—signs of iatrogenic hyperadrenocorticism • CSF collection or natural course of the disease—tentorial herniation and death

EXPECTED COURSE AND PROGNOSIS
• Resolution of signs—generally gradual (2–8 weeks) • Viral and prototheal—almost always progress to death • Immune-mediated— fair prognosis for complete remission with aggressive immunosuppression • Rickettsial, mycotic, bacterial, protozoal, and spirochete

infections—fair chance of survival • Parasite migration, migrating foreign bodies, PME, YNE, and polioencephalomyelitis—usually fatal • Pug and Maltese encephalitis—generally fatal; course varies greatly; some patients respond to steroid treatment for long periods. • Postvaccinal encephalomyelitis—may resolve on its own; often permanent damage and death

MISCELLANEOUS

ASSOCIATED CONDITIONS
N/A

AGE-RELATED FACTORS
• Young (< 2 years) and old (> 8 years) animals—at more risk for infectious diseases • Dogs < 6 years of age—immune-mediated and idiopathic encephalitides

ZOONOTIC POTENTIAL
• Rabies—consider in endemic areas if the patient is an outdoor animal that has rapidly progressive encephalitis • Humans may be infected by the same vector tick that affected the patient. • Exudates from animals with mycosis can revert to the spore-forming, infectious mycelial stage. • Cultures are highly contagious and should be handled with great care.

PREGANCY
N/A

SYNONYMS
N/A

SEE ALSO
• See also Causes • Seizures (Convulsions, Status Epilepticus—Cats) • Seizures (Convulsions, Status Epilepticus—Dogs) • Stupor and Coma

ABBREVIATIONS
• CSF = cerebrospinal fluid • ELISA = enzyme-linked immunosorbent assay • EME = eosinophilic meningoencephalitis • FeLV = feline leukemia virus • FIP = feline infectious peritonitis • FIV = feline immunodeficiency virus • GME = granulomatous meningoencephalitis • PME = pyogranulomatous meningoencephalitis • YNE = Yorkshire terrier necrotizing encephalitis

Suggested Reading
Braund KG. Clinical syndromes in veterinary neurology. 2nd ed. St. Louis: Mosby, 1994.
Greene CE, ed. Infectious diseases of the dog and cat. Philadelphia: Saunders, 1990.
Summers BA, Cummings JF, de Lahunta A. Veterinary neuropathology. Baltimore: Mosby, 1995.
Author Allen Sisson
Consulting Editor Joane M. Parent

DISEASES

ENCEPHALITIS SECONDARY TO PARASITIC MIGRATION

 BASICS

OVERVIEW

- Aberrant migration of worms (helminthiasis) or fly larvae (myasis) into the CNS
- Parasites may normally affect another organ system of the same host (e.g., *Dirofilaria immitis, Taenia, Ancylostoma caninum, Angiostrongylus,* or *Toxocara canis*), or a different host species (e.g., raccoon roundworm, *Baylisascaris procyonis;* skunk roundworm, *B. columnaris; Coenurus* spp., or *Cysticercus cellulosae*).
- Access to CNS—generally: hematogenously (dirofilariasis) or through adjacent tissues; *Cuterebra* fly larvae: various routes, including through the middle ear, skull foramina, cribriform plate, or open fontanelles

SIGNALMENT

- Dogs and cats—rare and sporadic
- Dirofilariasis—adult animals
- Other parasites—young animals exposed to an outside environment

SIGNS

- Vary with the portion of CNS affected
- Likely asymmetrical
- May suggest a mass lesion or multifocal disease process
- Rat parasite, *Angiostrongylus cantonensis* (Australia)—lumbosacral syndrome (hindlimbs, tail, and bladder paralysis/paresis) in puppies which may ascend to thoracic limbs and cranial nerves

CAUSES & RISK FACTORS

Housing in a cage previously occupied by wildlife (raccoons, skunks)

 DIAGNOSIS

DIFFERENTIAL DIAGNOSIS

- Other causes of (focal) encephalopathy—infectious diseases (viral, bacterial, protozoan, or fungal); idiopathic granulomatous meningoencephalomyelitis; brain tumor; ischemic encephalopathy (cats)
- Diagnosis is usually made on necropsy, because the disease is difficult to diagnose antemortem.
- CSF analysis and brain imaging—often inconclusive

CBC/BIOCHEMISTRY/URINALYSIS

Normal unless the parasite also affects non-neural tissues

OTHER LABORATORY TESTS

CSF—may show an eosinophilic and neutrophilic-mononuclear pleocytosis (also found in protozoal, fungal, and protothecal encephalitides); may be normal in strictly intraparenchymal lesions

IMAGING

CT or MRI—brain; focal lesion or/and cerebral infarction from occlusion of cerebral vessels

PATHOLOGIC FINDINGS

- May be local to extensive necrosis, malacia, vascular rupture and hemorrhage, vascular emboli, granulomatous proliferation, or obstructive hydrocephalus
- *Dirofilaria immitis*—intravascular or extravascular
- Adult worms produce focal infarction or inflammation.

 TREATMENT

None effective

 MEDICATIONS

DRUGS

- Dirofilariasis and neural angiostrongylosis—anthelmintic treatments may cause worsening of signs and sometimes death.
- Mild neural angiostrongylosis—puppies with may recover with supportive care and corticosteroid therapy.

CONTRAINDICATIONS/INTERACTIONS

N/A

 FOLLOW-UP

PATIENT MONITORING

N/A

PREVENTION/AVOIDANCE

N/A

POSSIBLE COMPLICATIONS

N/A

EXPECTED COURSE AND PROGNOSIS

Usually progressive after acute or insidious onset

 MISCELLANEOUS

SEE ALSO

- Encephalitis
- Encephalitozoonosis
- Heartworm Disease—Cats
- Heartworm Disease—Dogs

ABBREVIATION

CSF = cerebrospinal fluid

Suggested Reading

Braund KG. Clinical syndromes in veterinary neurology. 2nd ed. St. Louis: Mosby, 1994.

Author Christine Berthelin-Baker
Consulting Editor Joane M. Parent

BASICS

OVERVIEW
• Infection with the protozoan *Cytauxzoon cuniculi*
• Involves lungs, heart, kidneys, and brain
• Uncommon in the U.S.

SIGNALMENT
• Dogs and cats
• No age, sex, or breed predilection

SIGNS

Neonates
• Appear a few weeks postpartum
• Stunted growth
• Unthriftiness
• Progress to renal failure
• Neurologic abnormalities

Adults
• Same as neonates
• May exhibit aggressive behavior, seizures, or blindness

CAUSES & RISK FACTORS
• Most likely route is oronasal from spore-contaminated urine
• Kennel housing is a risk factor.

DIAGNOSIS

DIFFERENTIAL DIAGNOSIS
• Rabies
• Canine distemper
• Neosporosis
• Toxoplasmosis

CBC/BIOCHEMISTRY/URINALYSIS
• Normochromic, normocytic anemia
• Lymphocytosis and monocytosis
• High serum ALT and ALP expected

OTHER LABORATORY TESTS
Serology—blood and CSF

IMAGING
May be contributory but not diagnostic

DIAGNOSTIC PROCEDURES
• Urinalysis—sediment stained with Gram or Ziehl-Neelsen; Gram-positive spores; birefringent
• Positive identification requires immunologic procedures.

PATHOLOGIC FINDINGS
• Nonsuppurative interstitial nephritis—consistent finding
• Hepatomegaly and petechiae throughout surfaces of multiple organs
• Swollen kidneys, hemorrhagic cystitis, renal cortical cysts, or infarcts
• Brain—if lesions present, thrombosis and encephalomalacia, cystic spaces in parenchyma

TREATMENT
• Inpatient with supportive therapy
• Euthanasia—when severe neurologic signs occur

MEDICATIONS

DRUGS
Chemotherapy—no known for dogs and cats; try benzimidazoles, particularly albendazole (50 mg/kg q8h for 7 days), because they work in mice and humans.

CONTRAINDICATIONS/POSSIBLE INTERACTIONS
N/A

FOLLOW-UP

PREVENTION/AVOIDANCE
Sanitation—important; accomplish with 70% ethanol

EXPECTED COURSE AND PROGNOSIS
A number of patients recover without further signs if neither the renal nor the cerebral manifestation becomes severe.

MISCELLANEOUS

ZOONOTIC POTENTIAL
Potential risks to humans, especially the immunosuppressed

ABBREVIATIONS
• ALP = alkaline phosphatase
• ALT = alanine transferase
• CSF = cerebrospinal fluid

Suggested Reading
Didier PJ, Didier ES, Snowden K, Shadduck JA. Encephalitozoonosis. In: Greene CE, ed., Infectious diseases of the dog and cat. 2nd ed. Philadelphia: Saunders, 1998:465–470.
Author Johnny D. Hoskins
Consulting Editor Stephen C. Barr

ENCEPHALOPATHY, ISCHEMIC—CATS

 BASICS

DEFINITION
Naturally occurring neurologic syndrome characterized by acute ischemic necrosis of brain tissue

Pathophysiology
• Underlying cause unknown
• Main lesion—often involves the middle cerebral artery on one side of the brain
• Unilateral lesions near the frontal lobe or rostral thalamus—often cause the patient to circle or turn toward the affected side; referred to as adversive syndrome
• Limbic system—involvement may cause behavioral changes and seizure activity.
• Vascular abnormalities (e.g., vascular thrombosis and vasculitis)—not consistently found
• Lesions are inconsistently found elsewhere, including in the heart.

SYSTEMS AFFECTED
Nervous—specifically the cerebrum; occasionally the brainstem; rarely the cerebellum

GENETICS
N/A

INCIDENCE/PREVALENCE
Unknown

GEOGRAPHIC DISTRIBUTION
N/A

SIGNALMENT

Species
Cats

Breed Predilections
N/A

Mean Age and Range
• Any age
• Kittens seem to be spared.

Predominant Sex
N/A

SIGNS

General Comments
Related to the severity and location of the ischemia

Historical Findings
• Acute onset
• Generalized or partial seizures—common
• Behavioral changes—aggression; depression; dementia; polyphagia; stupor
• Many affected cats are ambulatory but ataxic; may circle toward the side of the lesion (adversive syndrome)
• Blindness—may develop

Physical Examination Findings
• Consistent with a unilateral cerebral lesion—circling to the side of the lesion with contralateral motor and/or sensory deficits (e.g., reduced eyelid closure and lip retraction, reduced facial sensation, reduced menace response, impaired hemiwalking and hopping, and proprioceptive deficits)
• Behavioral changes—may be evident during examination
• Blindness—normal pupillary light reflexes imply a cerebral lesion; dilated, unresponsive pupils suggest an optic chiasm or mid-brain lesion.

CAUSES
• Unknown
• *Cuterebra*—larva migration has been incriminated; larva may cause a vasospasm, resulting in ischemia; may be toxic in nature in some cases

RISK FACTORS
• A history of recent upper respiratory infection has been observed in a few affected cats.
• Generally nonseasonal; one report of a higher prevalence in summer

 DIAGNOSIS

DIFFERENTIAL DIAGNOSIS
• Trauma and encephalitis—young to middle-aged cats
• Neoplasia, trauma, and encephalitis—old cats
• Distinguish by skull radiography (trauma), CSF analysis (encephalitis), and CT or MRI scans (neoplasia, trauma, and vascular disease); if tests are unavailable or non-diagnostic, note that clinical signs are usually nonprogressive with ischemia and trauma but progressive with neoplasia and encephalitis.

CBC/BIOCHEMISTRY/URINALYSIS
Usually normal

OTHER LABORATORY TESTS
FeLV and FIV tests—negative

IMAGING
• Radiography (skull)—normal; may reveal head trauma or bony neoplasia
• CT and MRI—may show edema and disruption of the blood–brain barrier in the acute stages; may reveal asymmetry of cerebral hemispheres and excessive CSF filling of subarachnoid space in chronic stages

DIAGNOSTIC PROCEDURES

CSF Analysis
• Normal or high protein or WBC count
• Primary cell type often mononuclear (e.g., lymphocytes and macrophages)
• Xanthochromia or erythrophagocytosis in some patients
• Cytology findings—may differ according to time of sampling in relation to onset of signs

Electroencephalogram
• May confirm brain dysfunction or help confirm a specific location
• Cannot distinguish among vascular disease, neoplasia, trauma, and infection

PATHOLOGIC FINDINGS
• With long duration of clinical signs—widened sulci and atrophy of the affected side
• Histologic—atrophy; degeneration; necrosis; astrocytosis; gliosis; phagocytic macrophages

ENCEPHALOPATHY, ISCHEMIC—CATS

 TREATMENT

APPROPRIATE HEALTH CARE
• Inpatient—at least 2 days for observation and treatment
• Hyperventilation (oxygen therapy)—may help reduce cerebral edema associated with ischemia
• Outpatient—if seizures are controlled and patient is able to eat and drink

NURSING CARE
Intravenous fluid administration—conservative to reduce risk of overhydration and worsening of cerebral edema

ACTIVITY
N/A

DIET
N/A

CLIENT EDUCATION
• About one-half of affected animals remain functional pets.
• Secondary (acquired) epilepsy—may develop as a result of ischemia

SURGICAL CONSIDERATIONS
N/A

 MEDICATIONS

DRUGS OF CHOICE
• Dexamethasone (0.5–1 mg/kg IV) or methylprednisolone sodium succinate (30 mg/kg IV bolus followed by 15 mg/kg IV 2 and 6 hr after initial dose) for edema and inflammation
• Diazepam—0.5–1.0 mg/kg IV; stop seizure activity
• Chronic oral administration of phenobarbital or diazepam—recommended for patients with seizures because of potential for acquired epilepsy; if patient remains seizure free for 6 months, wean from drug slowly (over 12 weeks).

CONTRAINDICATIONS
• Drugs that raise intracranial pressure
• Drugs that lower seizure threshold (e.g., acepromazine and amphetamines)

PRECAUTIONS
Overhydration with fluids can contribute to cerebral edema and worsen the clinical signs.

POSSIBLE INTERACTIONS
N/A

ALTERNATIVE DRUGS
N/A

 FOLLOW-UP

PATIENT MONITORING
Daily neurologic examination—determine if signs are stabilizing or improving

PREVENTION/AVOIDANCE
N/A

POSSIBLE COMPLICATIONS
• Status epilepticus
• Death—uncommon

EXPECTED COURSE AND PROGNOSIS
• Until it can be determined that the clinical signs are improving, prognosis guarded
• Steadily improving signs over 1–2 weeks—associated with favorable prognosis
• Permanent behavioral changes (especially aggression) and seizures—common sequelae

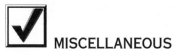 **MISCELLANEOUS**

ASSOCIATED CONDITIONS
N/A

AGE-RELATED FACTORS
N/A

ZOONOTIC POTENTIAL
N/A

PREGNANCY
N/A

SYNONYMS
• Feline cerebral infarct
• Feline stroke
• FIE

SEE ALSO
• Brain Injury (Head Trauma and Hypoxia)
• Seizures (Convulsions, Status Epilepticus)—Cats

ABBREVIATION
CSF = cerebrospinal fluid

Suggested Reading

Bernstein NM, Fiske RA. Feline ischemic encephalopathy in a cat. J Am Anim Hosp Assoc 1986;22:205–206.
De Lahunta A. Upper motor neuron system. In: Veterinary neuroanatomy and clinical neurology. 2nd ed. Philadelphia: Saunders, 1983:130–155.
Summers BA, Cummings JF, de Lahunta A. Veterinary neuropathology. St. Louis: Mosby, 1995.
Zaki FA, Nafe LA. Ischemic encephalopathy and focal granulomatous meningoencephalitis in the cat. J Small Anim Pract 1980;21:429–438.
Author Linda G. Shell
Consulting Editor Joane M. Parent

DISEASES

ENDOCARDITIS, BACTERIAL

BASICS

DEFINITION

PATHOPHYSIOLOGY
• Bacteremia develops from various portals of entry; bacteria invade and colonize the heart valves • Endocardial ulceration exposes collagen, causing platelet aggregation and clot formation; any valve can be affected—aortic and mitral valves most common • Vegetations on heart valves—vary in size, may affect more than one valve, and are covered by a layer of clotted blood • Valvular insufficiency develops in virtually all patients; aortic insufficiency almost invariably leads to intractable left-sided CHF within weeks to several months • CHF—less frequent and latent when only the mitral valve is affected

SYSTEM AFFECTED
• Cardiovascular—bacteremia • Respiratory—pulmonary edema • Renal/urologic—renal infarction • Musculoskeletal—septic or immune-mediated polyarthropathy

GENETICS
Genetic predisposition unlikely

INCIDENCE/PREVALENCE
Varies by geographic region and habitus

GEOGRAPHIC DISTRIBUTION
No well-documented patterns published; bacteremia and hence bacterial endocarditis may be more common in tropical and semitropical regions

SIGNALMENT
Species
Dogs; rarely cats

Breed Predilections
• Middle-sized to large • Those predisposed to subaortic stenosis

Mean Age and Range
Most affected dogs are 4–6 years of age; infection can occur at any age.

Predominant Sex
Most studies report male predominance—may be as great as 2:1

SIGNS
General Comments
• Depend on whether infection is subacute or chronic, and if CHF, renal failure, metastatic abscessation, or secondary immune complications • Most prevalent associated with sepsis and CHF

Historical Findings
• Infectious disease within the past weeks to several months in some patients • CHF (e.g., coughing, dyspnea, and exercise intolerance)

Physical Examination Findings
• Fever and general malaise • Dyspnea caused by CHF • Multiple single or shifting leg lameness in some patients • Systolic heart murmur • Diastolic heart murmur associated with aortic insufficiency—difficult to detect without careful auscultation of the right cranioventral precordium • Hyperdynamic femoral arterial pulses strongly suggest advanced aortic valve endocarditis. • Volume overload produces high systolic arterial pressure followed by a rapid, accentuated drop in diastolic pressure associated with blood "runoff" back into the left ventricle.

CAUSES
• Bacterial infection associated with the oral cavity, bone, prostate, and other sites • Invasive diagnostic or surgical procedures forcing bacteria into the bloodstream

RISK FACTORS
• Congenital subaortic stenosis • Immunosuppression from long-term or high-dose corticosteroid or cytotoxic drug administration

DIAGNOSIS

DIFFERENTIAL DIAGNOSIS
• Bacteremia of any cause produces identical hematologic abnormalities and similar clinical signs. • Polysystemic, immune-mediated disorders often difficult to differentiate from bacteremia and rickettsemia • Left-sided CHF caused by dilated cardiomyopathy or congenital subaortic stenosis

CBC/BIOCHEMISTRY/URINALYSIS
• Active, severe infection associated with an inflammatory leukogram (i.e., neutrophilia, left shift, and monocytosis)—patients with chronic, relatively inactive, or walled-off infection may have normal or nearly normal leukogram; those with chronic infection may have mature neutrophilia with monocytosis • Thrombocytopenia—variable severity; depends on duration and severity of infection, vasculitis, and DIC • Low-normal or low albumin, low-normal or low glucose, and high SAP activity are inconsistently associated with sepsis. • Proteinuria caused by bacteremia and septic embolization or infarction of the kidneys; hematuria, pyuria, and casts associated with pyelonephritis and glomerulonephritis

OTHER LABORATORY TESTS
• Blood culturing—three samples taken over 24 h; two should yield the same microbe; both aerobic and anaerobic cultures recommended; antibiotic removal systems available for diagnosis of patients given antibiotics • Catheter tips—culture

• Urine cultures—easy; often yield positive results; do not necessarily incriminate the urinary tract as the source of infection, but are not a substitute for blood cultures • Tests for prostate, kidney, and bone infection may be warranted. • Positive antinuclear antibody, lupus erythematosus, rheumatoid factor, and Coombs' test results occasionally found—nonspecific; tend to confound the diagnosis

IMAGING
Radiographic Findings
Cardiac chamber enlargement; rarely, calcification of one or more heart valves

Echocardiography
Vegetative endocarditis of the aortic valve is easily discerned; mitral valve infection is difficult to differentiate from myxomatous degeneration.

DIAGNOSTIC PROCEDURES
Joint taps for cytologic examination and culture—cytologic examination may not differentiate septic from immune-mediated arthritis; either can exist with bacterial endocarditis. Neutrophils usually nondegenerate regardless of cause; bacterial culture often negative

Electrocardiographic Findings
• ECG—may be normal; occasionally reflects left heart enlargement; often detects ventricular tachyarrhythmias; occasionally reveals heart block of variable severity • Heart block suggests aortic valve involvement with infection or infarction of the adjacent septum. • Intermittent heart rhythm disturbances often require extended ECG monitoring (Holter or cageside) for detection.

PATHOLOGIC FINDINGS
• Cardiac enlargement • Vegetative lesions and blood clot on one or more valves • Infection, hemorrhage, and infarction of adjacent myocardium • Renal infarcts • Primary or secondary sites of infection • Pulmonary hemorrhage or edema

TREATMENT

APPROPRIATE HEALTH CARE
Virtually all animals with suspected bacterial endocarditis should be hospitalized.

NURSING CARE
• Good hydration for septic patients, particularly those receiving an aminoglycoside • Aggressive fluid therapy—at least twice maintenance for patients with renal failure

• Overt or impending CHF limits fluid volumes that can be administered; this problem is virtually insurmountable in patients with concomitant renal failure.
• Imminent CHF—minimize fluid therapy; provide no more than maintenance volumes; alternate D5W with LRS (or 2.5% dextrose in half-strength LRS); potassium supplementation usually required

ACTIVITY
Variable—depends on whether or not CHF is present or imminent

DIET
Sodium restriction if CHF is present or imminent

CLIENT EDUCATION
Guarded prognosis if mitral valve only involved; grave prognosis if aortic valve involved

SURGICAL CONSIDERATIONS
Aortic valve endocarditis—almost always results in intractable left-sided CHF; aortic valve replacement indicated; procedure routinely performed in human medicine but rarely attempted in veterinary medicine because of lack of expertise and facilities, and high cost

MEDICATIONS

DRUGS OF CHOICE
Treatment variable—depends on severity of sepsis and presence or absence of CHF

Antibiotics
• Backbone of treatment but may not eradicate infection before irreversible valve damage occurs; more than minimal damage to the aortic valve is life threatening because aortic insufficiency tends to be a lethal complication.
• High-dose, IV administration is imperative; bactericidal antibiotics required because the bacteria are sequestered from the bloodstream; IV administration recommended for as long as feasible, followed by SQ administration.
• Oral administration—recommended only after at least 4 weeks of injectable therapy and at least 1 week after hematologic and clinical signs of infection and inflammation have disappeared; long-term (2–4 months) treatment required to eradicate the infection from sanctuary sites, principally the vegetations.
• Selection determined by both the urgency of septic complications and results of bacterial culture; coagulase-positive staphylococci and streptococci are most often incriminated, so choices can be logically made before culture results are obtained.
• Coagulase-positive staphylococci—usually

resistant to penicillin and ampicillin
• Streptococci—often resistant to aminoglycosides and fluoroquinalones
• Gram-negative bacteria—often sensitive to cephalosporins, fluoroquinalones, and aminoglycosides
• Cephalosporins—reasonable choice for stable patients until culture results are obtained
• Treat immediately life-threatening sepsis with drug combinations. Pending culture results, one of two regimens is recommended: either a penicillin, ampicillin, ticarcillin or cephalosporin is combined with an aminoglycoside. High doses of the latter cannot be administered, and good hydration with monitoring for nephrotoxicity is required; thus aminoglycosides are not good choices for animals with overt or impending CHF.
• Aminoglycosides recommended for 5–14 days only
• Gentamicin recommended at dosage of 2 mg/kg q8h.
• Clindamycin (5 to 10 mg/kg IV q8h) plus enrofloxacin (6 mg/kg q12h given slowly IV diluted 1:4 in D5W)
• Advanced-generation cephalosporins or ticarcillin-clavulonic acid (Timentin)—high dosages recommended for patients with resistant infections, normal dosages for patients with renal failure

Treatment of CHF
• Digoxin, angiotensin-converting enzyme inhibitor, and furosemide indicated for patients with chronic CHF
• Oxygen, nitroglycerin, high-dose furosemide (2–8 mg/kg IV), and possibly dobutamine (4–5 μg/kg/min CRI)—indicated for patients with acute, severe, pulmonary edema associated with aortic valve endocarditis

CONTRAINDICATIONS
Avoid antibiotics that cannot penetrate fibrin (e.g., sulfonamides).

PRECAUTIONS
Renal disease and digoxin, enalapril, and aminoglycoside administration

POSSIBLE INTERACTIONS
Concurrent use of aminoglycoside and furosemide raises the risk of nephrotoxicity and ototoxicity.

ALTERNATIVE DRUGS
N/A

FOLLOW-UP

PATIENT MONITORING
• Emergence of antibiotic resistance—relapsing fever and inflammatory leukogram; imperative; adjustment treatment on the basis

of culture results • Weekly examination and CBC after discharge • Repeat blood cultures 1 week after antibiotics are discontinued or if fever recurs.

PREVENTION/AVOIDANCE
• Indwelling catheters—restrict to appropriate indications; aseptic placement; replace within 3–5 days. • Administer antibiotics to animals undergoing dentistry—controversial except in animals with congenital heart defects and oral infections • Avoid careless use of corticosteroids.

POSSIBLE COMPLICATIONS
• CHF • Renal failure • Septic embolization of many tissues and organs • Persistent or latent immune-mediated polyarthropathy

EXPECTED COURSE AND PROGNOSIS
• Best prognosis associated with short history of bacteremia, rapid diagnosis, and aggressive treatment. • Mortality relatively higher in animals recently given corticosteroids.
• Grave prognosis for most patients with aortic valve endocarditis • Latent CHF may develop (months to years later) with mitral valve endocarditis.

MISCELLANEOUS

ASSOCIATED CONDITIONS
Congenital heart defects (usually subaortic stenosis) in some animals

AGE-RELATED FACTORS
N/A

ZOONOTIC POTENTIAL
NA

PREGNANCY
N/A

SYNONYMS
Infective endocarditis

SEE ALSO
• Congestive Heart Failure, Left-sided • Septicemia and Bacteremia • Discospondylitis • Prostatitis and Prostatic Abscess • Renal Failure, Acute

ABBREVIATIONS
• CHF = congestive heart failure • CRI = constant rate infusion

Suggested Reading
Miller MW, Sisson D. In Fox PR, Sisson D, Moise NS (eds): Textbook of Canine and Feline Cardiology. Philadelphia, WB Saunders, 1999: 567–580.
Author Clay A. Calvert
Consulting Editors Larry P. Tilley and Francis W. K. Smith, Jr.

ENDOMYOCARDIAL DISEASES—CATS

BASICS

OVERVIEW
• EMC—acute cardiopulmonary disease that typically develops following a stressful event; characterized by interstitial pneumonia and endomyocardial inflammation; pneumonia is usually severe and commonly causes death; one report recorded the incidence of EMC at postmortem to be equivalent to that of hypertrophic cardiomyopathy (HCM)
• Endocardial fibroelastosis—congenital heart disease in which severe fibrous endocardial thickening leads to heart failure secondary to diastolic and systolic failure

SIGNALMENT
• Cats
• EMC—predominantly males (62%) 1–4 years
• Endocardial fibroelastosis—early development of biventricular or left heart failure, usually prior to 6 months of age

SIGNS

Historical Findings
EMC
• Dyspnea following a stressful event in a young, healthy cat
• Respiratory signs usually occur 5–21 days after the stressor.
• In one report, 73% of cases presented between August and September.
Endocardial fibroelastosis
• Lethargy, weakness, collapse, syncope
• Poor appetite and weight loss
• Dyspnea
• Tachypnea
• Cyanosis

• Abdominal distention
• Paresis or paralysis, signs of thromboembolic disease

Physical Examination Findings
EMC
• Severe dyspnea
• Occasional crackles
• May be murmur or gallop; murmur may vary in intensity
• May be evidence of thromboembolic disease
• Typically no significant abnormalities prior to the stressful event
Endocardial fibroelastosis
• Gallop
• Systolic murmur, possible mitral regurgitation
• Dyspnea and increased lung sounds or crackles
• Paresis or paralysis with weak or absent femoral pulses
• Arrhythmias possible

CAUSES & RISK FACTORS
• Cause unknown for both diseases
• Risk factors for EMC include stressful incidents such as anesthesia (commonly associated with neutering or declawing), vaccination, relocation, or bathing.
• Endocardial fibroelastosis may be familial in Burmese and Siamese.

DIAGNOSIS

DIFFERENTIAL DIAGNOSIS

Other Causes of Cardiac Disease
HCM, RCM, DCM, congenital heart malformations

Other Causes of Dyspnea
• Other forms of cardiac disease, HCM, RCM, DCM, congenital malformations
• Primary respiratory disease

• Pleural space disease
• Mediastinal disorders, infection, trauma, neoplasia
• Hemoglobin disorders, anemia, methemoglobinemia, causes of central cyanosis

Other Causes of Collapse, Weakness, or Syncope
• Arrhythmias
• Neurologic or musculoskeletal disease
• Metabolic disease or electrolyte disorders
• Other forms of paresis or paralysis
• Arterial thromboembolism secondary to any form of cardiac disease or neoplasia
• Neurologic or musculoskeletal disease
• Neoplasia

CBC/BIOCHEMISTRY/URINALYSIS
Not diagnostic

OTHER LABORATORY TESTS
N/A

IMAGING

Thoracic Radiographic Findings for Both
• Cardiomegaly
• Interstitial or alveolar infiltrates or pleural effusion if congestion has developed

Echocardiographic Findings
Endomyocarditis
• Normal to mildly large left atrium
• Left ventricular wall thickness can be normal to mildly thick (0.6–0.7 cm).
• Hyperechoic endomyocardium reported—incidence seems to vary and is subjective; in one report it was as high as 86%.
Endocardial fibroelastosis
• Limited data available
• Reduced left ventricular function and enlarged left atrium

DIAGNOSTIC PROCEDURES

Electrocardiographic Findings
• EMC—sinus tachycardia common; ventricular premature complexes, atrial premature complexes, bundle branch block, and complete AV block reported

• Endocardial fibroelastosis—evidence for left-sided enlargement; sinus rhythm typically present, but various arrhythmias possible

PATHOLOGIC FINDINGS

EMC
• Interstitial pneumonia
• Left heart enlargement and opacity of the left ventricular endomyocardium with foci of hemorrhage; fibroplasia of the endocardium is striking.
• Varying degrees of endomyocardial inflammation with infiltrates of neutrophils, lymphocytes, plasma cells, histiocytes, and macrophages seen histologically

Endocardial Fibroelastosis
• Left ventricular and atrial dilation with severe diffuse white opaque thickening of the endocardium
• Diffuse hypocellular, fibroelastic thickening of the endomyocardium; prominent endomyocardial edema with dilation of lymphatics

 TREATMENT

EMC
• No one therapy protocol to date
• Small percentage of cats have survived; these cats are on no long-term therapy.
• Supportive care with oxygen and possibly ventilation

Endocardial fibroelastosis
• Oxygen therapy via cage delivery is least stressful.
• Thoracocentesis if pleural effusion

 MEDICATIONS

DRUGS OF CHOICE

EMC
Steroids, furosemide, and vasodilators have been tried, but efficacy is still unknown.

Endocardial fibroelastosis
Acute CHF
• Parenteral administration of furosemide, 0.5–1.0 mg/kg IV or IM, q1–6h
• Dermal application of 2% nitroglycerin ointment, 1/8 to 1/4 inch q4–6h
• Arrhythmias may resolve with stabilization. If rapid atrial fibrillation (heart rate > 200), a calcium channel blocker or β-blocker can be given to help control the ventricular response. If dilated cardiomyopathy, digoxin may be a better choice for controlling atrial fibrillation rate. For other supraventricular arrhythmias and ventricular arrhythmias, waiting for a response to heart failure therapy may be wise before starting antiarrhythmic therapy.
• Intractable edema—nitroprusside, 1–5 μg/kg/min, may be helpful
Chronic CHF
• Treat as other CHF, with furosemide and enalapril
• Digoxin can be added when patient is stable and eating.

CONTRAINDICATIONS/POSSIBLE INTERACTIONS
N/A

 FOLLOW-UP

EXPECTED COURSE AND PROGNOSIS
• Endomyocarditis—Poor, although some animals survive; consider the suggestion that EMC may progress to left ventricular endocardial fibrosis

• Endocardial fibroelastosis—medical treatment of CHF may prolong life, but recovery is unlikely.

 MISCELLANEOUS

ASSOCIATED CONDITIONS
• Aortic thromboembolism with both diseases
• May be a relationship between EMC and left ventricular endocardial fibrosis

SEE ALSO
• Aortic Thromboembolism
• CHF, Left Sided
• CHF, Right Sided
• Myocarditis

ABBREVIATIONS
• CHF = congestive heart failure
• DCM = dilated cardiomyopathy
• HCM = hypertrophic cardiomyopathy
• RCM = restrictive cardiomyopathy

Suggested Reading
Bossbaly MB, Stalis I, Knight D, Van Winkle T. Feline endomyocarditis: a clinical/pathological study of 44 cases. Proceedings of the 12th ACVIM Forum, 1994:975.
Stalis IH, Bossbaly MJ, Van Winkle TJ. Feline endomyocarditis and left ventricular endocardial fibrosis. Vet Pathol 1995;32(2):122–126.
Authors Carl D. Sammarco and Maribeth J. Bossbaly
Consulting Editors Larry P. Tilley and Francis W. K. Smith, Jr.

ENTROPION

 BASICS

OVERVIEW
• Inversion of part or all of the eyelid margin
• Frictional irritation of the cornea—because of contact by the eyelash or eyelid hair; may result in corneal ulceration or perforation or pigmentary keratitis
• Vision may be threatened.

SIGNALMENT
• Common in dogs; occasional in cats
• Cats—usually seen in brachycephalic breeds (e.g, Persian and Himalayan)
• Dogs—seen in chow chows, shar peis, Norwegian elkhounds, sporting breeds (e.g., spaniels retrievers), brachycephalic breeds (e.g., English bulldogs, pugs, Pekingese), toy breeds (e.g., poodles Yorkshire terriers), and giant breeds (e.g., mastiffs, St. Bernards, Newfoundlands)
• Age—seen in puppies 2–6 weeks old (especially chow chows and shar peis); usually identified in dogs < 1 year old

SIGNS
• Depend on type and degree of condition
• Mild, medial—chronic epiphora and medial pigmentary keratitis (toy dogs and brachycephalic dogs and cats)
• Mild, lateral—chronic mucoid to mucopurulent ocular discharge (giant-breed dogs)
• Upper lid, lower lid, or lateral canthal—severe blepharospasm, purulent discharge, pigmentary or ulcerative keratitis, and potential cornea rupture (chow chows, shar peis, and sporting breeds)

CAUSES & RISK FACTORS
• Primarily genetic predisposition in facial conformation and eyelid support
• Brachycephalic breeds (dogs and cats)—excessive tension on the ligamentous structures of the medial canthus coupled with nasal folds and facial conformation defects results in rolling inward of the medial aspects of the upper and lower eyelids and the medial canthus and upper and lower lids medially.
• Giant breeds and breeds with heavy facial skin (bloodhounds) or excessive facial folds (chow chows, shar peis)—laxity of the lateral canthal ligamentous structures allows for entropion of the upper and lower eyelids and the lateral canthus.

• Chronic infectious conjunctivitis or keratitis (cats)—may lead to functional entropion caused by chronic blepharospasm (spastic entropion)
• Predisposed breeds (dogs)—spastic entropion, if ocular irritation (e.g., distichia, ectopic cilia, trichiasis, foreign body, and irritant conjunctivitis) leads to excessive blepharospasm
• Nonpredisposed breeds—may be the result of a primary irritant causing secondary spastic entropion
• Severe weight loss or muscle atrophy caused by masticatory muscle myositis (dogs)—loss of orbital fat or periorbital musculature may lead to enophthalmos and entropion.

 DIAGNOSIS

DIFFERENTIAL DIAGNOSIS
• Usually obvious clinically—underlying causes of spastic entropion should be ruled out and corrected, if possible, before an attempt at surgical correction is made.
• Puppies—common for first-time breeders of chows and shar peis to mistakenly think that the eyelids have not opened at 4–5 weeks of age, when puppies actually have severe blepharospasm and entropion

CBC/BIOCHEMISTRY/URINALYSIS
N/A

OTHER LABORATORY TESTS
N/A

IMAGING
N/A

DIAGNOSTIC PROCEDURES
N/A

TREATMENT

PUPPIES
• Young (especially shar peis and chows)—do not initially perform skin resection surgery.
• Eyelid eversion suture technique—attempted to temporarily evert the eyelid margins to break the spasm-irritation-spasm cycle; if successful, permanent procedure is unnecessary.
• Permanent skin resection technique—postponed until patient's facial conformation matures (increases success)

DOGS AND CATS
Toy dog breeds and brachycephalic dogs and cats—medial canthal reconstruction, if medial condition and trichiasis cause pigmentary keratitis, chronic epiphora, or corneal scarring

MATURE DOGS
• Chronic entropion—requires some type of eyelid margin-everting surgery; simple Hotz-Celsus procedure or more radical lateral canthoplasty
• No history of previous entropion and clinical signs of acute condition—examine meticulously for cause of spastic condition and correct; may attempt a temporary eversion suture technique before performing permanent skin resection, if necessary

MEDICATIONS

DRUGS
Topical ophthalmic ointment—triple-antibiotic or antibiotic based on culture and sensitivity testing; q12–24h; may use postoperatively or as a presurgical lubricant

CONTRAINDICATIONS/POSSIBLE INTERACTIONS
NA

FOLLOW-UP

Temporary eversion suture technique—may revert when sutures are removed or spontaneously pull through the skin; repeated as necessary until the patient is mature enough to undergo a more permanent form of skin resection repair (approximately 6 months of age)

MISCELLANEOUS

Suggested Reading
Slatter D. Eyelids. Fundamentals of veterinary ophthalmology. 2nd ed. Philadelphia: Saunders, 1990; 147–203.
Author J. Phillip Pickett
Consulting Editor Paul E. Miller

EOSINOPHILIC GRANULOMA COMPLEX

 BASICS

DEFINITION
• Cats—often confusing term for three distinct syndromes: eosinophilic plaque, eosinophilic granuloma, and indolent ulcer; grouped primarily owing to their clinical similarities, their frequent concurrent development, and their positive response to corticosteroids
• Dogs—eosinophilic granulomas in dogs (EGD) rare; not part of disease complex; specific differences from cats are listed separately.

PATHOPHYSIOLOGY
• Eosinophilic plaque—hypersensitivity reaction, most often to insects (fleas, mosquitos); less often to food or environmental allergens
• Eosinophilic granuloma—multiple causes, including hypersensitivity and genetic predisposition
• Indolent ulcer—may have both hypersensitivity and genetic causes
• Eosinophil—major infiltrative cell for eosinophilic granuloma and eosinophilic plaque; leukocyte located in greatest numbers in epithelial tissues; most often associated with allergic or parasitic conditions, but has a more general role in the inflammatory reaction
• EGD—may have both a genetic predisposition and a hypersensitivity cause

SYSTEMS AFFECTED
• Skin/Exocrine—the integument is most often affected.
• Oral cavity—eosinophilic granuloma can affect the tongue, palatine arches, and palate.
• EGD—most often affects the tongue and palatine arches; reported cutaneous lesions on the prepuce and flanks

GENETICS
• Unknown
• Several reports of related affected individuals and a study of disease development in a colony of specific pathogen-free cats indicate that, in at least some individuals, genetic predisposition (perhaps resulting in a heritable dysfunction of eosinophilic regulation) is a significant component of the disease.

INCIDENCE/PREVALENCE
Unknown

GEOGRAPHIC DISTRIBUTION
Seasonal incidence in some geographical locations may indicate insect or environmental allergen exposure.

SIGNALMENT
Species
• Restricted to cats
• Eosinophilic granulomas occur in dogs and other species, but are not considered part of this disease complex.

Breed Predilections
• Cats—none
• EGD—Siberian huskies (76% of cases)

Mean Age and Range
• Eosinophilic plaque—2–6 years of age
• Genetically initiated eosinophilic granuloma—< 2 years of age
• Allergic disorder—> 2 years of age
• Indolent ulcer—no age predisposition reported
• EGD—usually < 3 years of age

Predominant Sex
• Cats—predilection for females has been reported only for the indolent ulcer.
• EGD—males (72% of cases)

SIGNS
General Comments
• Distinguishing among the syndromes depends on both clinical signs and histopathologic findings.
• Lesions of more than one syndrome may occur simultaneously.

Historical Findings
• Lesions of all three syndromes may develop spontaneously and acutely.
• Development of eosinophilic plaques can be preceded by periods of lethargy.
• A seasonal incidence is common.
• Waxing and waning of clinical signs is common in all three syndromes.

Physical Examination Findings
• Eosinophilic plaques—alopecic, erythematous, erosive patches and plaques; usually occur in the inguinal, perineal, lateral thigh, and axillary regions; frequently moist or glistening
• Eosinophilic granulomas—occur in a distinctly linear orientation (linear granuloma) on the caudal thigh, or as individual or coalescing plaques located anywhere on the body; ulcerated with a "cobblestone" or coarse pattern; white or yellow, possibly representing collagen degeneration; lip margin and chin swelling ("pouting"); footpad swelling, pain, and lameness; oral cavity ulcerations (especially on the tongue, palate, and palatine arches); cats with oral lesions may be dysphagic, have halitosis, and may drool.
• Lesion development may stop spontaneously in some cats, especially with the heritable form of eosinophilic plaque.
• Indolent ulcers—classically raised and indurated ulcerations confined to the upper lips adjacent to the philtrum
• EGD—lesions are ulcerated plaques and masses; dark or orange color

CAUSES
• Allergy—flea or insect, food hypersensitivity, and atopy
• A heritable dysfunction of eosinophil regulation has been proposed.

• EGD—unknown; a hypersensitivity reaction is often suspected.

RISK FACTORS
N/A

 DIAGNOSIS

DIFFERENTIAL DIAGNOSIS
• Includes the other diseases in the complex
• Unresponsive lesions—exclude pemphigus foliaceus, dermatophytosis and deep fungal infection, demodicosis, pyoderma, and neoplasia (especially metastatic adenocarcinoma and cutaneous lymphosarcoma)

CBC/BIOCHEMISTRY/URINALYSIS
• CBC—mild to moderate eosinophilia
• Biochemistry and urinalysis—usually normal

OTHER LABORATORY TESTS
FeLV and FIV—pruritic diseases have been associated with these viruses

IMAGING
N/A

DIAGNOSTIC PROCEDURES
• Impression smears from lesions—large numbers of eosinophils
• Comprehensive flea and insect control—assist in excluding flea or mosquito bite hypersensitivity
• Food-elimination trial—for all cases; feed a protein (e.g., lamb, pork, venison, or rabbit) to which the cat has never been exposed; use exclusively for 8–10 weeks; then reinstitute previous diet and observe for development of new lesions.
• Environmental allergy (atopy)—identified by intradermal skin testing (some cases); inject small amounts of dilute allergens intradermally; positive reaction (allergy) is indicated by the development of a hive or wheal at the injection site.
• In vitro serum tests—available for identifying allergy-specific serum in cats; tests have not been validated and are not recommended.

PATHOLOGIC FINDINGS
• Histopathologic diagnosis—required for distinguishing the syndromes
• Biopsy samples from indolent ulcers frequently fail to reveal eosinophils.
• Eosinophilic plaque—severe epidermal and follicular acanthosis with eosinophilic exocytosis and spongiosis; intense eosinophilic dermal infiltrate common; epidermis commonly eroded or ulcerated.
• Eosinophilic granuloma—distinct foci of eosinophilic degranulation and collagen degeneration similar to granuloma formation; epidermis may be eroded or ulcerated.
• Indolent ulcer—early lesions may be indistinguishable from those of eosinophilic

granuloma (eosinophilic infiltration and collagen degeneration); late-stage lesions characterized by fibrosis with perivascular neutrophilic and mononuclear infiltration
• EGD—foci of collagen degeneration with palisading granulomas; eosinophilic and histiocytic infiltration

TREATMENT

APPROPRIATE HEALTH CARE
• Most patients can be treated as outpatients unless severe oral disease prevents adequate fluid intake.
• Try to identify and eliminate offending allergen(s) before providing medical intervention.
• Hyposensitization of intradermal skin test–positive cats—may be successful in 60%–73% of cases; preferable to long-term corticosteroid administration

NURSING CARE
Discourage patient from damaging of lesions by excessive grooming.

ACTIVITY
No restrictions

DIET
No restrictions unless a food allergy is suspected

CLIENT EDUCATION
• Inform clients about the possible allergic or heritable causes.
• Discuss the waxing and waning nature of these diseases.
• Responsible clients may choose to postpone medical intervention, unless severe lesions develop.

SURGICAL CONSIDERATIONS
None

MEDICATIONS

DRUGS OF CHOICE

Eosinophilic Plaque
• Injectable methylprednisdone—20 mg/cat, repeat in 2 weeks (if needed); most common treatment
• Corticosteroids—ongoing treatment with prednisone (3–5 mg/kg q48h) rarely required to control lesions; steroid tachyphylaxis may occur and may be specific to the drug administered; may be useful to changing the formulation; other drugs: dexamethasone (0.1–0.2 mg/kg q24–72h) and triamcinolone (0.1–0.2 mg/kg q24–72h); higher induction dosages may be required but should be tapered as quickly as possible.

Eosinophilic Granuloma
• Injectable or oral corticosteroids—see

Eosinophilic Plaque (above); most common treatment
• Combination of oral corticosteroids and selective immunosuppressive agents—for severe lesions; e.g., chlorambucil (0.1–0.2mg/kg q24–48h)
• Chrysotherapy with aurothioglucose—1 mg/kg IM every 7 days; mixed results
• Cyclophosphamide—1 mg/kg q24h for 4 out of every 7 days; another alternative
• Antibiotics—may be beneficial if oral lesions are secondarily infected

Indolent Ulcer
• Injectable or oral corticosteroids—see Eosinophilic Plaque (above)
• α-interferon—30–60 U daily in cycles of 7 days on, 7 days off; limited success; side effects rare; no specific treatment monitoring required
• Antibiotics—trimethoprim-sulfadiazine (15 mg/kg PO q12h), cephalexin (22 mg/kg PO q12h), or amoxicillin trihydrate-clavulanate (12.5 mg/kg PO q12h); effective in some cases; preferable to long-term corticosteroid administration; response may be the result of the anti-inflammatory activity of these drugs rather than their primary bactericidal properties

Alternate Therapies
• Radiation, surgical excision, and immuno-modulation (e.g., levamisole, bacterin injections)—occasional reports of success
• CO_2 laser—newer treatment modality; may offer relief from individual or painful lesions, especially those in the mouth
• Topical—application of potent cortico-steroid ointments may help with isolated lesions but is rarely practical.

EGD
• Oral prednisone—0.5–2.2mg/kg/day initially; then taper gradually
• Cessation of therapy without recurrence is common.

CONTRAINDICATIONS
N/A

PRECAUTIONS
N/A

POSSIBLE INTERACTIONS
N/A

ALTERNATIVE DRUGS
Megestrol acetate—2.5–5 mg every 2–7 days; can be effective in rare cases; not recommended because of the severity of possible side effects

FOLLOW-UP

PATIENT MONITORING
• Corticosteroids—baseline and frequent hemograms, serum chemistry profiles, and urinalyses
• Selective immunosuppressant drugs—frequent hemograms (biweekly at first, then monthly or bimonthly as therapy continues)

to monitor for bone marrow suppression; routine serum chemistry profiles and urinalyses (monthly at first, then every 3 months) to monitor for complications (renal disease, diabetes mellitus, and urinary tract infection)

PREVENTION/AVOIDANCE
N/A

POSSIBLE COMPLICATIONS
N/A

EXPECTED COURSE AND PROGNOSIS
• If a primary cause (allergy) can be determined and controlled, lesions should resolve permanently, unless the animal re-encounters the offending allergen.
• Most lesions wax and wane, with or without therapy; thus an unpredictable schedule of recurrence should be anticipated.
• Drug dosages should be tapered to the lowest possible level (or discontinued, if possible) once the lesions have resolved.

MISCELLANEOUS

ASSOCIATED CONDITIONS
N/A

AGE-RELATED FACTORS
N/A

ZOONOTIC POTENTIAL
N/A

PREGNANCY
Systemic glucocorticoids and immuno-suppressive drugs should not be used during pregnancy.

SYNONYMS
• Eosinophilic granuloma—feline collagenolytic granuloma; feline linear granuloma
• Indolent ulcer—eosinophilic ulcer; rodent ulcer; feline upper lip ulcerative dermatitis

SEE ALSO
• Atopy
• Food Reactions (Dermatologic)

ABBREVIATIONS
EGD = eosmophilic granulomas in dogs

Suggested Reading
Power HT, Ihrke PJ. Selected feline eosinophilic skin diseases (eosinophilic granuloma complex). In: Kunkle G, ed. Feline dermatoses. Veterinary clinics of North America, small animal practice. Philadelphia: Saunders, 1995.
Rosenkrantz WS. Feline eosinophilic granuloma complex. In: Griffin CE, Kwochka KW, MacDonald JM, eds. Current veterinary dermatology: the science and art of therapy. St. Louis: Mosby, 1993.
Author Alexander H. Werner
Consulting Editor Karen Helton Rhodes

DISEASES

EPIDIDYMITIS/ORCHITIS

 BASICS

OVERVIEW
• Epididymitis—inflammation of the epididymis
• Orchitis—inflammation of the testis
• May be acute or chronic
• Direct trauma to the scrotum—most common cause of acute form

SIGNALMENT
• More common in dogs than cats
• No genetic basis

SIGNS
• Swollen testis
• Pain
• Licking of the scrotum—may lead to dermatitis
• Listlessness
• Anorexia
• Reluctance to walk
• Open wound or abscess

CAUSES & RISK FACTORS
• *Brucella canis*—predilection for infecting the tail of the epididymis
• Distemper
• Ascending infection—associated with prostatitis and cystitis
• Retrograde urine contamination of the ductus deferens—sequel to high intra-abdominal pressure as caused by automobile trauma
• Bite wounds and other puncture wounds—isolated from infected testes: *Staphylococcus, Streptococcus, Escherichia coli, Protcus,* and *Mycoplasma*
• Lymphocytic autoimmune thyroiditis and orchitis—familial in beagles

 DIAGNOSI

DIFFERENTIAL DIAGNOSIS
• Inguinoscrotal hernia
• Scrotal dermatitis
• Testicular neoplasia
• Prostatitis
• Cystitis

CBC/BIOCHEMISTRY/URINALYSIS
Leukocytosis—with acute or infectious orchitis

OTHER LABORATORY TESTS
B. canis antibodies—perform immediate testing.

IMAGING
• Ultrasonographic evaluation of the prostate—guided aspiration for cytologic examination and bacterial culture
• Ultrasonographic evaluation of the testes and epididymis—appearance and measurements; for future comparison

DIAGNOSTIC PROCEDURES
• Semen—collect if possible; cytological evaluation; bacterial culture
• Cytology (semen)—leukocytes; bacteria; spermatozoa with coiled tails, detached heads, and retained proximal and distal cytoplasmic droplets; head-to-head agglutination (*B. canis*)
• Prostatic massage—cytologic examination; bacterial culture; sample collected aseptically by urethral catheter
• Open wounds—bacterial culture

 TREATMENT

• Fertility not a concern—culture appropriate specimen; administer needed antibiotics; medically stabilize; castrate.
• Fertility a concern (unilateral orchitis)—unilateral castration when the patient's future as a sire must be maintained

MEDICATIONS

DRUGS

Antibiotics—continue for at least 3 weeks; initially oxacillin, trimethoprim-sulfonamide, aminoglycoside, or enrofloxacin; changed when results of culture and sensitivity testing are available

FOLLOW-UP

• Prognosis for fertility—guarded to poor, especially with bilateral orchitis
• Testicular heating causes testicular degeneration.
• Trauma or inflammation can cause obstruction of efferent tubules or epididymal duct, leading to spermatoceles or sperm granuloma
• Semen (dogs)—evaluate characteristics 3 months after treatment for orchitis is completed.

MISCELLANEOUS

Suggested Reading

Feldman EC, Nelson RW. Canine and feline endocrinology and reproduction. Philadelphia: Saunders, 1987:705–709

Author Rolf E. Larsen
Consulting Editor Sara K. Lyle

EPILEPSY, IDIOPATHIC, GENETIC, PRIMARY

BASICS

DEFINITION
• A brain disorder characterized by recurrent seizures in the absence of morphologic brain lesion
• The brain is structurally normal but not functionally normal.

PATHOPHYSIOLOGY
• Exact mechanism unknown
• Dysfunction may be biochemical or an intrinsic propensity to have seizures.

SYSTEMS AFFECTED
Nervous

GENETICS
• Genetic in many breeds
• Mode of inheritance unknown (several have been suggested)

INCIDENCE/PREVALENCE
• Between 0.5% and 2.3% of all dogs; higher for dogs in research colonies
• Highly prevalent; 40%–80% of dogs with seizure activity
• Cats—rare; poorly documented

GEOGRAPHIC DISTRIBUTION
Widespread

SIGNALMENT

Species
Dogs and rarely cats

Breed Predilections
Beagles; all shepherds (German, Australian, Belgian Tervuren); border collies; boxers; cocker spaniels; collies; dachshunds; golden retrievers; Irish setters; keeshonds; Labrador retrievers; poodles (all sizes); St. Bernards; shetlies; Siberian huskies; springer spaniels; Welsh corgis; wire-haired fox terriers

Mean Age and Range
• Range—6 months to 5 years
• Prevalence—6 months to 3 years

Predominant Sex
Male

SIGNS

General Comments
Seizures are generalized (bilateral and symmetrical) and usually convulsive.

Historical Findings
• Seizures—most occur while the patient is resting or asleep; often at night or in early morning; frequency tends to increase if left untreated; affected animal becomes stiff, chomps its jaw, salivates profusely, urinates, defecates, vocalizes, and paddles with all four limbs in varying combinations.

• Postseizure behavior—periods of confusion and disorientation; aimless, compulsive, blind pacing; frequent polydipsia and polyphagia; recovery immediate or may take up to 24 hr
• Dogs with established epilepsy experience cluster seizures at regular intervals of 1–4 weeks; particularly prevalent in large-breed dogs

Physical Examination Findings
• None; patient usually recovered
• Patient may be in the postictal phase of the seizure.

CAUSES
Likely genetic in some breeds, idiopathic in others

RISK FACTORS
Acepromazine—may cause seizures in otherwise normal dogs by lowering a subclinical seizure threshold

DIAGNOSIS

DIFFERENTIAL DIAGNOSIS
• Two most important factors—age at onset and pattern of seizures (type and frequency)
• First seizure—between 6 months and 5 years; the younger the animal, the more severe the epilepsy; as a rule, with an onset < 2 years, the condition has a good chance of becoming refractory to medication.
• Acute onset of cluster seizures or status epilepticus—unusual; indicates toxicity or structural brain disease
• More than two seizures within the first week at onset—consider a diagnosis other than idiopathic or genetic epilepsy.
• Seizures at < 6 months or > 5 years of age—may be metabolic or intracranial in origin
• Partial seizures or neurologic deficits—indicate structural intracranial disease

CBC/BIOCHEMISTRY/URINALYSIS
• Usually normal
• Perform before initiation of antiepileptic medication, to obtain baseline data.

OTHER LABORATORY TESTS
N/A

IMAGING
MRI and CT—only for suspected structural intracranial diseases

DIAGNOSTIC PROCEDURES
CSF analysis—for suspected structural intracranial diseases

PATHOLOGIC FINDINGS
• No primary lesion
• Secondary neuronal loss and gliosis from prolonged or repeated seizures

TREATMENT

APPROPRIATE HEALTH CARE
• Initiate treatment if there is more than one generalized seizure, acute cluster seizures, or acute status epilepticus.
• Inpatient—moderate to severe cluster seizures or status epilepticus; treat early and aggressively.
• Outpatient—recurrence of isolated seizures

NURSING CARE
• Inpatients with a seizure disorder require constant monitoring.

ACTIVITY
Avoid swimming to prevent drowning.

DIET
• Most dogs on chronic antiepileptic drugs become overweight; monitor closely; add a weight-reducing program as necessary.
• KBr treatment—patients should have steady levels of salt in their diet; an increase in salt causes an increase in bromide excretion preferentially over chloride, with subsequent decreased serum KBr levels; S/D prescription diets have higher chloride contents than do most diets.

CLIENT EDUCATION
• Inform client that animals do not die after a seizure; however, severe cluster seizures and status epilepticus are life-threatening emergencies that require immediate and aggressive medical attention.
• Advise client that he or she should prevent the patient from injuring itself on surrounding objects during a seizure.
• Encourage client to keep a calendar of the seizures, because it is the only objective way to assess response to treatment.
• Inform client that once treatment is instituted, the patient will require medication for life.

SURGICAL CONSIDERATIONS
Corpus callostomy—selected refractory patients

MEDICATIONS

DRUGS OF CHOICE

Phenobarbital and KBr
• Steady state—phenobarbital requires 12–15 days; KBr requires 3–4 months; if necessary, give both drugs at loading dosages to reach therapeutic levels rapidly (seizures may continue until steady state is reached).
• Both drugs combined—may produce a beneficial and synergistic effect
• Phenobarbital—traditional first-line drug; initial dosage: 2–5 mg/kg PO divided q12h;

evaluate serum levels 12–15 days after onset of treatment and after changes in dosage; levels decrease significantly in the first few weeks owing to activation of the lysosomal enzymes; evaluate levels again 4 weeks after initiation; optimal serum levels: 100–120 μmol/L or 23–28 μg/mL; increase dosage if needed and recheck levels until optimal therapeutic range
• KBr—alternative first-line drug; initial dosage: 30 mg/kg PO q24h or divided q12h; use same dosage as a substitute for or added to phenobarbital for patients started on PB that continue to have seizures at a frequency of more than one every 6–8 weeks; optimal serum levels: 15–20 mmol/L or 1.2–1.6 mg/mL
Loading Doses
• Sometimes desirable to reach the therapeutic range rapidly
• Phenobarbital—intravenous loading dose (total mg) = desired serum level (μg/mL) × body weight (kg) × 0.8 L/kg; oral loading dose: 5–10 mg/kg q12h for 2 days
• KBr—orally only; 500 mg/kg (dogs) to reach optimal range; large dose often creates gastric upset, which can be minimized by dividing dose into as many treatments as desired to reach the therapeutic level.

Diazepam
• Dogs with moderate to severe cluster seizures or status epilepticus
• Inpatient treatment—0.5–1.0 mg/kg IV bolus; repeat in 5 min if gross motor seizure activity persists; follow immediately with 0.5–1.0 mg/kg constant-rate infusion added to the maintenance fluids in an in-line burette (prepare only 1–2 hr of infusion at a time to avoid adsorption in the plastic tubing); if seizures continue, add pheno-barbital at 2–6 mg/dog/hr; once seizures have been controlled for at least 4–6 hr, slowly decrease the infusion rate, discontinuing over 4–12 hr
• Reinstate oral medications as soon as possible; increase the oral dosage to optimal ranges if the serum drug levels before emergency treatment were inadequate.
• Outpatient treatment—for cluster seizures; on the seizing day, insert 0.5–1.0 mg/kg injectable drug in the rectum via a teat cannula as soon as a seizure occurs; repeat 20 and 40 min later for a total of three insertions within 40 min; mimics intravenous infusion; given early in the course of ongoing seizures, in-creases the chance to abort subsequent seizures.

CONTRAINDICATIONS
Acepromazine, ketamine, and xylazine—do not administer; may cause seizure activity

PRECAUTIONS
• Phenobarbital and diazepam—use caution when combining for status epilepticus; they act synergistically; cardiac and respiratory depression may ensue.

• Phenobarbital—may cause polyphagia or polydipsia, which may disappear in a few weeks
• KBr—polyuria/polydipsia

POSSIBLE INTERACTIONS
• Cimetidine and chloramphenicol—interfere with the metabolism of phenobarbital; may lead to toxic levels of phenobarbital
• Whenever drugs must be given to affected animals on lifetime medication, refer to the manufacturer's drug profile or a pharmacist for interaction information.

ALTERNATIVE DRUGS
• Human antiepileptic drugs—many (e.g., phenytoin, valproic acid, and carbamazepine) cannot be used in dogs because of unsuitable pharmacokinetics.
• If phenobarbital and KBr fail, contact a veterinary neurologist.
• Other treatments—gabapentin, felbamate, clorazepam, and clonazepam

 FOLLOW-UP

PATIENT MONITORING
• Serum drug levels—essential to monitor; blood is usually drawn at trough and, if possible, at the same time for each sampling.
• Phenobarbital—measure 2 and 4 weeks after initiating therapy (when steady state is reached); adjust oral dose as needed; repeat until the optimal serum levels are reached; at these levels, hepatotoxicity is not as likely and the patients that are going to respond will have; with chronic use perform hemogram, serum chemistry profile, and drug levels every 6–12 months to monitor side effects; keep records of albumin, liver enzymes, and serum drug levels; drug essentially hepatotoxic and most dogs eventually develop hepatotoxicity
• KBr—elimination rate depends on concen-tration of salt in the food; measure serum levels (along with phenobarbital levels) 4–6 weeks after initiating (should be 8–12 mmol/L or 0.5–1.0 mg/mL); seems to enhance excretion or metabolism of phenobarbital, causing levels to drop; early measurements help keep dosage at the steady state

PREVENTION/AVOIDANCE
• Discuss with the client the possibility of inheritance and, for this reason, consider neutering.
• For humans and animals, unknown if estrogens decrease seizure threshold
• Abrupt discontinuation of oral medication may precipitate seizures.

POSSIBLE COMPLICATIONS
• Phenobarbital-induced high SAP (isoenzyme-steroid band)—occurs frequently; may be an early sign of hepatotoxicity but is of less concern if ALT is within reference range
• Phenobarbital-induced hepatotoxicity—

occurs after chronic treatment at serum levels in the middle to upper therapeutic range (> 140 μmol/L or > 33 μg/mL); may be insidious in onset; the only biochemical abnormality may be a decrease in albumin.
• Rare neutropenia may develop after onset of phenobarbital; discontinue use of the drug.
• KBr—when levels are > 22 mmol/L or > 1.8 mg/mL, owners frequently complain of patients' unsteadiness while managing stairs.

EXPECTED COURSE AND PROGNOSIS
• Antiepileptic treatment—decreases frequency, severity, and length of seizures; perfect control rarely achieved; goal is < 1 seizure/6–8 weeks.
• In many young, large-breed dogs, seizures may continue despite adequate treatment.
• Refractoriness may develop.
• Patient may develop status epilepticus and die.

 MISCELLANEOUS

ASSOCIATED CONDITIONS
N/A

AGE-RELATED FACTORS
• If onset is < 2 years of age, seizures are more likely to be difficult to control.
• If onset is > 2 years of age, generally seizures are adequately controlled or may not require treatment.

ZOONOTIC POTENTIAL
N/A

PREGNANCY
Avoid breeding affected animals.

SYNONYMS
Primary generalized epilepsy

SEE ALSO
Seizures (Convulsions, Status Epilepticus)—Dogs

ABBREVIATIONS
• ALT = alanine aminotransferase
• CSF = cerebrospinal fluid
• KBr = potassium bromide
• SAP = serum alkaline phosphatase

Suggested Reading
Oliver JE, Lorenz MD, Kornegay JN. Hand-book of veterinary neurology. 3rd ed. Philadelphia: Saunders, 1997.
Podell M. Canine epilepsy. In: Standards of care: emergency and critical care medicine. Vol. 1. Journal 1999:1–8.
Author Joane M. Parent
Consulting Editor Joane M. Parent

DISEASES

EPISCLERITIS

BASICS

OVERVIEW
• Focal or diffuse infiltration of the episclera and/or scleral stroma by a varying mix of inflammatory cells and fibroblasts
• Primary—affects only the eye; probably immune mediated; appears either as a peri-limbal episcleral/scleral nodule (nodular episcleritis) or as a diffuse thickening of the episclera (diffuse episcleritis); nodular form may affect cornea and third eyelid with similar appearing nodules
• Secondary—usually diffuse; from the spillover of inflammatory cells into the episclera from other ocular disorders (e.g., endophthalmitis and panophthalmitis); may affect virtually any other organ system

SIGNALMENT
• Dogs
• Young to middle-aged collies, Shetland sheepdogs

SIGNS
• Nodular—typically appears as a smooth, painless, localized, raised, pink-tan, firm episcleral/scleral mass.
• Diffuse—less common; appears as a diffuse reddening and thickening of the entire episclera/sclera; accompanied by variable amounts of ocular pain
• Secondary—uveitis often pronounced
• Conjunctiva—usually moves freely over the surface of the lesion
• Nodules—tend to be slowly progressive, bilateral, and prone to recurrence

CAUSES & RISK FACTORS
• Nodular and diffuse primary—idiopathic; believed to be immune mediated
• Secondary—may result from deep fungal or bacterial ocular infection, lymphosarcoma, systemic histiocytosis in Bernese mountain dogs, chronic glaucoma, and ocular trauma

DIAGNOSIS

DIFFERENTIAL DIAGNOSIS
• Other causes of a red eye—differentiated by careful ophthalmic examination and tonometry
• Other mass-like lesions—differentiated by biopsy or cytologic examination
• Neoplasia—lymphosarcoma; squamous cell carcinoma; extension of an intraocular mass; other tumors
• Granuloma—deep fungal infection; retained foreign body
• Granulation tissue—trauma; healing corneal ulcer; globe perforation with uveal prolapse

CBC/BIOCHEMISTRY/URINALYSIS
• Usually normal if the lesion is confined to eye or adnexa
• Secondary—may see abnormalities consistent with other systemic diseases (e.g., deep fungal or systemic histiocytosis)

OTHER LABORATORY TESTS
• Rheumatoid factor, antinuclear antibody, and lupus erythematosus cell preparations—usually not helpful
• Serologic testing—may help rule out deep fungal infection

IMAGING
• Thoracic and abdominal radiographs or abdominal ultrasound—may help rule out deep fungal infection or disseminated neoplasia
• Ocular ultrasound—may help reveal other ocular abnormalities if ocular media opacities prevent a thorough ocular examination

DIAGNOSTIC PROCEDURES
• Incisional biopsy and histopathologic examination of affected tissue
• Nodular—typified by varying numbers of histiocytes, lymphocytes, plasma cells, and fibroblasts
• For prominent uveitis—perform a uveitis workup (see Anterior Uveitis—Dogs).

TREATMENT
• Try to verify the diagnosis histologically or cytologically before treatment.
• Primary nodular—tends to have a benign course; observation alone may be appropriate with mild disease
• Outpatient—for ocular pain, diffuse scleral involvement, disruption of eyelid function, corneal encroachment, or a threat to vision

MEDICATIONS

DRUGS
• Progress down the list only if the previous modality was ineffective.
• Topically applied 1% prednisolone acetate—q4h for 1 week; then q6h for 2 weeks; then tapered
• Systemically administered prednisolone—1–2 mg/kg/day; tapered with improvement
• Systemically administered azathioprine—1–2 mg/kg/day for 3–7 days; then tapered to as low a dosage as possible
• Cryosurgery or attempt excision
• Alternative to listed drugs or surgery—may try a combination of tetracycline and niacinamide (q8h PO); 250 mg each for dogs < 10 kg; 500 mg each for dogs > 10 kg; may

not observe good clinical response for at least 8 weeks; side effects uncommon and primarily the result of gastrointestinal upset by niacinamide

CONTRAINDICATIONS/POSSIBLE INTERACTIONS
• Avoid systemic immunosuppressive drugs with deep fungal infections.
• Systemically administered prednisolone or azathioprine—may precipitate pancreatitis; potentially hepatotoxic
• Azathioprine—may induce potentially fatal myelosuppression
• Niacin—do not substitute for niacinamide.

FOLLOW-UP

PATIENT MONITORING
• Primary—monitor for nodule regression or reduction in episcleral thickening or reddening every 2–3 weeks for 6–9 weeks and then as needed; prognosis usually good; may require therapy for months to life
• Secondary—follow-up, prognosis, and complications usually depend on the primary disease.
• Azathioprine—repeat CBC, platelet count, and measurement of liver enzymes every 1–2 weeks for the first 8 weeks, then periodically.

POSSIBLE COMPLICATIONS
• Vision loss
• Chronic ocular pain
• Uveitis
• Secondary glaucoma

MISCELLANEOUS

SYNONYMS
• Collie granuloma
• Nodular granulomatous episcleritis
• Nodular fasciitis
• Fibrous histiocytoma
• Necrogranulomatous sclerouveitis
• Proliferative keratoconjunctivitis
• Limbal granuloma

Suggested Reading

Murphy CJ. Disorders of the cornea and sclera. In Kirk RW, ed., Current veterinary therapy XI. Philadelphia: Saunders, 1992:1101–1111.
Rothstein E, Scott DW, Riis RC. Tetracycline and niacinamide for the treatment of sterile pyogranuloma/granuloma syndrome in a dog. J Am Anim Hosp Assoc 1997;33:540–543.
Author Paul E. Miller
Consulting Editor Paul E. Miller

BASICS

OVERVIEW
• Categories of epulides are fibromatous, ossifying, and acanthomatous
• Tumors of nonodontogenic origin that arise from periodontal connective tissue stroma and do not metastasize
• Most tumors adhere to bone and are nonencapsulated, with a smooth to slightly nodular surface.

SIGNALMENT
• Dogs—fourth most common oral malignancy
• Cats—rare
• Most common in brachycephalic breeds
• Boxers have a higher incidence of fibromatous epuli
• Mean age, 7 years

SIGNS
Historical Findings
• Often none—incidental finding detected on routine physical examination
• Excessive salivation
• Halitosis
• Dysphagia
• Bloody oral discharge
• Weight loss

Physical Examination Findings
• Oral mass—in early cases, may appear as small pedunculated masses
• Acanthomatous epuli are most commonly found on the rostral mandible.
• Displacement of tooth structures due to the expansile nature of the mass
• Possible facial deformity due to asymmetry of the maxilla or mandible
• Occasionally cervical lymphadenopathy

CAUSES & RISK FACTORS
None identified

DIAGNOSIS

DIFFERENTIAL DIAGNOSIS
• Fibroma
• Benign polyp
• Ameloblastoma
• Malignant oral tumor
• Gingival hyperplasia
• Abscess
• Differentiated from other types of masses by excisional biopsy coupled with radiographic appearance

CBC/BIOCHEMISTRY/URINALYSIS
Results usually normal

OTHER LABORATORY TESTS
Cytologic preparations are rarely diagnostic.

IMAGING
• Determine tumor borders by intraoral radiographs.
• Radiographs of acanthomatous epuli typically demonstrate a well-defined area of lysis with margins that are distinct, smooth and sclerotic; fibromatous epuli do not have well-defined borders on radiographs; tooth structures are usually displaced, and resorption may occur unidirectionally along the lesion's edge in any epulis; ossifying epulis may have bony margins because of their osteoid component.
• CT scan may be necessary to detail the invasiveness of an acanthomatous epulis.

DIAGNOSTIC PROCEDURES
A large, deep tissue biopsy (down to bone) is required to differentiate from other oral malignancies—fibroma, fibrosarcoma, or low-grade fibrosarcoma

TREATMENT

DIET
Soft foods—may recommend to prevent tumor ulceration or after conservative or radical oral excision.

SURGICAL CONSIDERATIONS
• Fibromatous epulis—surgical excision with at least 1-cm margins is usually curative; these tumors are of periodontal ligament stromal origin, so extraction of affected teeth and curettage of the alveolar socket is indicated; more advanced cases may require en bloc tooth and bone excision; cryosurgery may be indicated for small lesions minimally adherent to bone.
• Ossifying epuli—characteristically have a bony matrix and excision is often more difficult; techniques are similar to those for the fibromatous epuli
• Acanthomatous epuli—because of the aggressiveness of this tumor, at least 2-cm margins are recommended; partial mandibulectomy or maxillectomy is often indicated by the location of the tumor.
• Radiotherapy offers long-term control in dogs with an acanthomatous epulis deemed inoperable; most radiotherapy plans attempt 40–60 Gy over 3–6 weeks.

MEDICATIONS

DRUGS
• Efficacy of outpatient chemotherapy is unreported most tumors of mesenchymal origin respond poorly.
• Local control (palliation) with intralesionally administered cisplatin has been reported.

• Bleomycin injected locally has been successful in treating acanthomaotus epuli.

CONTRAINDICATIONS/POSSIBLE INTERACTIONS
Chemotherapy can be toxic; seek advice before initiating treatment if you are unfamiliar with cytotoxic drugs.

FOLLOW-UP

PATIENT MONITORING
• Thorough oral, head, and neck examination 1, 2, 3, 6, 9, 12, 15, 18, and 24 months after treatment
• Periodic intraoral radiographs, especially for acanthomatous epuli

EXPECTED COURSE AND PROGNOSIS
• Epuli do not metastasize.
• Most epulides are cured when excisional margins are free of neoplastic cells; recurrence is likely if surgical margins do not include periodontal structures (i.e., excision includes normal bone).
• Mean survival time after surgery of acanthomatous epuli is 43 months (range, 6–134 months); mean survival times for patients with acanthomatous, ossifying, and fibromatous epulides are 52, 29, and 47 months, respectively.
• Mean survival after radiotherapy in dogs with acanthomatous epulis ranges from 1–102 months (median, 37 months); the 1-year survival rate is 85%; the 2-year survival rate is 67%.
• Malignant transformation of an acanthomatous epulis has been reported in up to 20% of irradiated patients years after treatment, suggesting that an acanthomatous epulis may be a precancerous lesion.
• Acanthomatous epulides are highly invasive to bone.

MISCELLANEOUS

Suggested Reading
Bjorling DE, Chambers JN, Mahaffey EA. Surgical treatment of epulides in dogs: 25 cases (1974–1984). J Am Vet Med Assoc 1987;190:1315–1318.
Thrall DE. Orthovoltage radiotherapy of acanthomatous epulides in 39 dogs. J Am Vet Med Assoc 1984;184:826–829.
Wiggs RB, Lobprise HB. Veterinary dentistry: principles and practice. Philadelphia: Lippincott-Raven, 1997.
Authors Thomas Klein
Consulting Editors Jan Bellows

DISEASES

ESOPHAGEAL DIVERTICULA

 BASICS

OVERVIEW
• An abnormal, circumscribed enlargement or dilatation of the esophagus producing a region for accumulation of ingesta
• Two types of esophageal diverticula exist.
• Pulsion (true) diverticula are associated with high intraluminal pressure leading to mucosal herniation through the muscularis; histologically, the cellular remnants are epithelium and connective tissue.
• Traction (false) diverticula are caused by the outward pull of connective tissue on the esophagus; all four cell layers (mucosa, submucosa, muscularis, and adventitia) remain intact.
• Approximately 50–70% of diverticula (especially epiphrenic pulsion types) are associated with other lesions of the esophagus or diaphragm.
• Organ systems affected include the gastrointestinal (regurgitation), musculoskeletal (weight loss), and respiratory (aspiration pneumonia).

SIGNALMENT
• Rare; more common in dogs than cats
• Congenital or acquired (no genetic basis proven)
• No important breed or sex predisposition

SIGNS
• Postprandial regurgitation, dysphagia, anorexia, coughing
• Weight loss, respiratory distress

CAUSES & RISK FACTORS
Congenital (Pulsion)
• Inherent weakness of the esophageal wall
• An abnormality of embryonic separation or eccentric vacuole formation in the esophageal wall

Acquired
Pulsion-type
• Caused by high intraluminal pressure and abnormal regional peristalsis
• Esophagitis
• Stricture
• Foreign body
• Neoplasia
• Vascular ring anomaly
• Megaesophagus
• Motility disturbance
Traction-type—inflammatory process associated with the trachea, lungs, hilar lymph nodes, or pericardium; causes fibrous tissue formation around the esophagus

 DIAGNOSIS

DIFFERENTIAL DIAGNOSIS
Esophageal Redundancy
• Contrast accumulation in the region of the thoracic inlet can occur normally in young dogs (especially brachycephalic breeds).
• Extension of the neck during esophagram eliminates the lesion.

Megaesophagus
Contrast esophagram or esophagoscopy should differentiate.

CBC/BIOCHEMISTRY/URINALYSIS
Usually within normal limits

OTHER LABORATORY TESTS
N/A

IMAGING
• Thoracic radiography—may show air or soft tissue density most commonly just cranial to the diaphragm (epiphrenic) or occasionally just cranial to the thoracic inlet
• Contrast esophagram—displays a focal dilated region of esophagus
• Fluoroscopy—useful to evaluate esophageal motility

DIAGNOSTIC PROCEDURES
Esophagoscopy is often useful for removing impacted ingesta and evaluating the mucosal surface.

 TREATMENT

• If the diverticulum is small and not causing significant clinical signs, treat conservatively with elevated feedings of a soft, bland diet followed by copious liquids.
• If the diverticulum is large or associated with significant clinical signs, surgical resection is recommended.
• Client education should include the importance of dietary management and the potential for aspiration pneumonia.
• Fluid therapy, antibiotics, and aggressive nursing, if concurrent aspiration pneumonia is present

MEDICATIONS

DRUGS
- No specific medication
- Give H$_2$ histamine antagonists (e.g., cimetidine 10 mg/kg PO q6–8h or ranitidine 2 mg/kg PO q12h) if the patient has concurrent esophagitis.
- Give broad-spectrum antibiotics if the patient has concurrent aspiration pneumonia; if severe pneumonia is present, base specific antibiotic selection on culture and sensitivity of samples obtained by transtracheal lavage, bronchoalveolar lavage, or transthoracic aspiration.

CONTRAINDICATIONS/POSSIBLE INTERACTIONS
It is best to avoid prokinetic agents (e.g., metoclopramide and cisapride) because of effects on the lower esophageal sphincter.

 FOLLOW-UP

PATIENT MONITORING
- Evaluate for evidence of fever, dyspnea, inflammatory leukogram, and sepsis.
- Maintain positive nutritional balance throughout disease process.

POSSIBLE COMPLICATIONS
Patients with diverticula and associated impaction are predisposed to development of perforation, fistula, stricture, and postoperative incisional dehiscence.

EXPECTED COURSE AND PROGNOSIS
Prognosis is guarded in patients with lesions that cause significant clinical signs.

 MISCELLANEOUS

Suggested Reading

Fingeroth J. Surgical diseases of the esophagus. In: Slatter D, ed. Textbook of small animal surgery. 2nd ed. Philadelphia: Saunders, 1993:534–561

Author James E. Williams, Jr.

Consulting Editors Brett M. Feder and Mitchell A. Crystal

DISEASES

ESOPHAGEAL FOREIGN BODIES

BASICS

DEFINITION
Ingestion of nondigestible foreign material or pieces of food too large to pass through the esophagus, with intraluminal entrapment

PATHOPHYSIOLOGY
N/A

SYSTEMS AFFECTED
• Gastrointestinal
• Respiratory—if aspiration pneumonia

GENETICS
N/A

INCIDENCE/PREVALENCE
Unknown

GEOGRAPHIC DISTRIBUTION
N/A

SIGNALMENT

Species
Due to the indiscriminate eating habits of many dogs, they have a higher incidence than cats.

Breed Predilection
More common in small-breed dogs; terrier breeds often overrepresented

Mean Age and Range
More common in young to middle-aged animals

Predominant Sex
N/A

SIGNS

General Comments
The pet may have been observed ingesting a foreign body.

Historical Findings
Most common include retching, gagging, lethargy, anorexia, ptyalism, regurgitation, restlessness, dysphagia, and persistent gulping.

Physical Examination Findings
• Most often unremarkable
• Occasionally discomfort when palpating the neck or cranial abdomen

CAUSES
Occurs most often with an object whose size, shape, or texture does not allow free movement through the esophagus, causing it to become lodged before it can pass

RISK FACTORS
N/A

DIAGNOSIS

DIFFERENTIAL DIAGNOSIS
• Esophagitis
• Esophageal stricture
• Esophageal neoplasia
• Megaesophagus
• Other esophageal disorders

CBC/BIOCHEMISTRY/URINALYSIS
• Usually normal
• Occasionally, electrolyte abnormalities, an inflammatory leukogram, and/or hemoconcentration, depending upon the severity of signs and degree of dehydration

OTHER LABORATORY TESTS
N/A

IMAGING

Thoracic Radiography
• Radiopaque foreign bodies are readily visualized.
• Esophageal distension with air may be visualized cranial to the foreign body.
• A contrast esophagram is required to identify radiolucent objects.
• Air and/or fluid in the mediastinum or pleural space suggests esophageal perforation; depending on severity, this can be an indication for surgery instead of esophagoscopy.
• Pulmonary infiltrates suggest aspiration pneumonia.

DIAGNOSTIC PROCEDURES
Esophagoscopy affords direct visualization of both the foreign object and the esophageal mucosa, allowing assessment of the extent of esophageal injury.

PATHOLOGIC FINDINGS
N/A

TREATMENT

APPROPRIATE HEALTH CARE
• Emergencies—treat as inpatients and perform endoscopy as soon as possible after diagnosis.
• If endoscopic retrieval of the foreign body succeeds *and* esophageal damage is minimal, the patient may be discharged the same day.

NURSING CARE
• If the procedure to remove the foreign body is atraumatic and the esophagus has sustained minimal damage, no special aftercare is needed.
• Severe mucosal trauma may require placing a gastrostomy tube for nutritional support during esophageal healing.

ACTIVITY
The patient may resume normal activity after a foreign body has been routinely removed.

DIET
No change needed

CLIENT EDUCATION
Discuss the possibility of complications and repeat offenders.

SURGICAL CONSIDERATIONS
• Endoscopy is much less traumatic and invasive than surgery.
• Surgery is indicated when

endoscopy failed to retrieve the foreign body; endoscopy enabled advancement of the object into the gastric lumen, but it is either not dissolvable or too sharp to pass comfortably through the rest of the gastrointestinal tract; a full-thickness esophageal perforation or large area of necrosis requires resection;
• It is often less traumatic to advance a bone foreign body into the stomach than to attempt retrieval.
• Most bone foreign bodies can be safely left to dissolve in the stomach without need for surgical removal.

MEDICATIONS

DRUGS OF CHOICE
If significant mucosal injury and esophageal ulceration, recommendations include:
• Analgesics (e.g., butorphanol 0.2–0.4 mg/kg IV, IM, SC q4h)
• Broad-spectrum antibiotics
• Sucralfate slurry (0.5–1 g/dog PO q8h) for mucosal protection and healing
• Short-term corticosteroids (prednisone 1 mg/kg PO q24h) decrease the risk of stricture formation by inhibiting fibroblasts; contraindicated if aspiration pneumonia
• H_2-antagonists (e.g., ranitidine 2 mg/kg PO, IV, SC q12h) for reflux esophagitis
• Metoclopramide (0.2–0.5 mg/kg IV, SC, PO q8h) for reflux esophagitis
• Percutaneous gastrostomy tube placement for nutrition during mucosal healing

CONTRAINDICATIONS
N/A

PRECAUTIONS
N/A

POSSIBLE INTERACTIONS
N/A

ALTERNATIVE DRUGS
N/A

FOLLOW-UP

PATIENT MONITORING
• Examine the esophagus closely for mucosal damage.
• Mild erythema/erosions are not uncommon, and tend to heal uneventfully.
• If an esophageal laceration/perforation—parenteral nutrition or gastrostomy tube feedings allow esophageal rest and healing.
• Advise postprocedural survey thoracic radiographs to assess for pneumomediastinum/pneumothorax.
• Monitor at least 2–3 months for evidence of stricture formation.
• Esophageal stricture—most common clinical sign is regurgitation; barium swallow and/or esophagoscopy may be indicated.

PREVENTION/AVOIDANCE
Carefully monitor the environment and what is fed to the pet.

POSSIBLE COMPLICATIONS
• Approximately 25% of patients with foreign bodies develop complications.
• Complications most frequently encountered include esophageal perforation, esophageal strictures, esophageal fistulas, and severe esophagitis.
• Pneumomediastinum, pneumothorax, pneumonia, pleuritis, mediastinitis, and bronchoesophageal fistulas can all occur secondarily to perforation.

EXPECTED COURSE AND PROGNOSIS
• Most of these patients do well and recover uneventfully.
• With complications, the prognosis is guarded.

MISCELLANEOUS

ASSOCIATED CONDITIONS
N/A

AGE-RELATED FACTORS
N/A

ZOONOTIC POTENTIAL
N/A

PREGNANCY
N/A

SYNONYMS
N/A

SEE ALSO
• Regurgitation
• Esophageal Diverticula

ABBREVIATIONS
N/A

Suggested Reading
Spielman BL, Shaker EH, Garvey MS. Esophageal foreign body in dogs: a retrospective study of 23 cases. J Am Anim Hosp Assoc 1992;28:570–574.
Twedt DC. Diseases of the esophagus. In: Ettinger SJ, Feldman EC, eds. Textbook of veterinary internal medicine. 4th ed. Philadelphia: Saunders, 1995:1124–1142.
Author Bari L. Spielman
Consulting Editors Brett M. Feder and Mitchell A. Crystal

ESOPHAGEAL STRICTURE

BASICS

DEFINITION
An abnormal narrowing of the esophageal lumen

PATHOPHYSIOLOGY
• Can occur secondary to severe esophagitis when the inflammation extends beyond the mucosa and into the submucosa and muscle layers, resulting in fibrosis
• Ingestion of acid or alkali, gastroesophageal reflux (especially secondary to general anesthetic procedures), or trauma from esophageal foreign bodies can result in severe esophagitis and consequent stricture formation.
• Can also be associated with esophageal surgery, esophageal neoplasia, and *Spirocerca lupi* granulomas

SYSTEMS AFFECTED
• Gastrointestinal—esophagus affected segmentally or diffusely
• Respiratory—aspiration pneumonia may develop secondary to regurgitation

GENETICS
No apparent genetic basis

INCIDENCE/PREVALENCE
Unknown; believed to be low

GEOGRAPHIC DISTRIBUTION
• *Spirocerca lupi* granulomatous strictures are occasionally seen in the southeastern United States.
• No specific geographic distribution for other causes

SIGNALMENT

Species
Dogs and cats

Breed Predilections
None reported

Mean Age and Range
Any age; neoplastic strictures tend to occur in middle-aged to old animals

Predominant Sex
None

SIGNS

General Comments
• Usually involve the entire circumference of the esophagus; can occur at any location or over any length of the esophagus
• Clinical signs are related to the severity and extent of stricture.

Historical Findings
• Regurgitation—usually of solid foods and observed shortly after feeding
• Affected animals may reingest the regurgitated meal.
• Liquid meals often tolerated better than solid meals.

• Dysphagia
• Salivation
• Howling/crying during swallowing (odynophagia) if active esophagitis
• Good appetite initially; eventually anorexia with progressive esophageal narrowing and inflammation
• Weight loss and malnutrition as the disease progresses
• May see aspiration pneumonia with progressive regurgitation and dysphagia

Physical Examination Findings
• Usually unremarkable
• Weight loss and cachexia in animals with chronic/advanced stricture
• May see ptyalism and/or pain on palpation of neck and esophagus in animals with concurrent esophagitis
• May detect pulmonary wheezes and coughing in animals with aspiration pneumonia

CAUSES
• Gastroesophageal reflux during anesthesia—most common
• Ingestion of chemical irritants
• Gastroesophageal reflux disease
• Esophageal foreign body
• Esophageal surgery
• Malignancies—intramural and extramural
• *Spirocerca lupi* granuloma

RISK FACTORS
• Poor preparation (not fasted) and poor positioning during anesthesia (abdomen positioned above thorax) place some patients at risk for gastroesophageal reflux, esophagitis, and subsequent stricture formation.
• Anesthesia—use of certain drugs prior to anesthesia (e.g., diazepam, atropine, pentobarbital, and phenothiazine-derivative tranquilizers) decrease the pressure of the lower esophageal sphincter and can result in gastroesophageal reflux.

DIAGNOSIS

DIFFERENTIAL DIAGNOSIS
• Vascular ring anomaly—important differential diagnosis in a young animal with midesophageal body stricture and proximal esophageal dilation; these animals are usually examined shortly after weaning.
• Esophagitis —patient may have clinical signs identical to those of esophageal stricture; differentiation requires barium contrast radiography or endoscopy.
• Esophageal foreign body —clinical signs may be identical to those of esophageal stricture; survey radiographs may identify an esophageal foreign body, although barium contrast radiography or endoscopy is often necessary.

• Intraluminal mass—rare condition, may be detected by radiography, but many require endoscopy; leiomyoma, squamous cell carcinoma, fibrosarcoma, and osteosarcoma are the most common esophageal malignancies.
• Extraluminal periesophageal mass—often detected by radiography, but may require thoracic ultrasonography; lymphoma, heart base tumors, and mediastinal abscessation are the most common causes of extraluminal esophageal compression.

CBC/BIOCHEMISTRY/URINALYSIS
Usually normal; patients with ulcerative esophagitis or aspiration pneumonia may have leukocytosis and neutrophilia.

OTHER LABORATORY TESTS
N/A

IMAGING
• Survey thoracic radiographs—usually normal
• Rarely, survey radiographs demonstrate dilation of the esophagus cranial to the stricture (retention of food may be seen in the dilated portion of the esophagus) or an intraluminal or extraluminal mass.
• Aspiration pneumonia may be evident in patients with dysphagia and frequent regurgitation.
• Barium contrast radiography—usually diagnostic; depending on stricture severity, liquid barium may pass unimpeded; barium paste or barium mixed with food is often necessary to identify the stricture; may see segmental or diffuse narrowing of the esophagus with some dilation proximal to the stricture
• Ultrasonography—not proved useful in diagnosing this disorder, unless an extramural compressive mass lesion is suspected

DIAGNOSTIC PROCEDURES
• Should perform endoscopy in all patients to confirm the site and severity of stricture and to exclude intraluminal malignancy
• Histopathology is sometimes necessary to differentiate neoplasia from nonneoplastic (i.e. fibrotic) stricture.

PATHOLOGIC FINDINGS
• Esophageal stricture
• Esophagitis in some patients
• Dilation and muscular hypertrophy proximal to the stricture
• Aspiration pneumonia

TREATMENT

APPROPRIATE HEALTH CARE
• Inpatient management initially
• May discharge patients from the hospital after addressing hydration needs, achieving dilation of the affected segment, and initiating any needed treatment for aspiration pneumonia and esophagitis

NURSING CARE
• May need intravenous fluids to correct hydration status
• Give medications parenterally following dilation procedures, to facilitate healing.
• Patients with severe concurrent aspiration pneumonia may need oxygen therapy.

ACTIVITY
Unrestricted

DIET
• Withhold oral feedings in patients with severe esophagitis and following dilation procedures.
• May place a temporary gastrostomy tube at the time of esophageal dilation as a means of providing continual nutritional support
• Use liquid meals when reinstituting oral feedings.

CLIENT EDUCATION
• Animals do not recover from untreated esophageal stricture.
• Benign strictures are best treated by esoph-ageal dilation.
• Patients with malignant stricture have a poor prognosis.
• Discuss the high probability of recurrence and common need for multiple dilation procedures.
• Discuss the possibility of improvement (decreased to absent regurgitation, ability to eat softened canned foods but not dry food) but not cure.

SURGICAL CONSIDERATIONS
• Best managed by mechanical dilation via a balloon dilation catheter under endoscopy or fluoroscopy
• Bougienage tube dilation is less effective.
• Balloon dilation under endoscopic or fluor-oscopic control is superior to bougienage, since applying radial forces rather than shearing forces results in less chance of esophageal perforation.
• Perform endoscopy after dilation to assess esophageal mucosal damage.
• Redilation at 1- to 2-week intervals may be necessary until stricture is resolved.
• Surgical resection of esophageal stricture reportedly has a <50% success rate and is often associated with substantial postoperative complications.
• Surgical methods described include esopha-gotomy, esophagectomy with anastamosis, jejunal interposition, and creation of a traction diverticulum.

 MEDICATIONS

DRUGS OF CHOICE
• Administer medications parenterally following dilation procedures and if severe esophagitis is present.

• When oral therapy is resumed, dissolve medications in water and give by syringe or give directly via gastrostomy tube to ensure that they reach the stomach.
• Antiinflammatory dosage of corticosteroids (e.g., prednisone 0.5–1.0 mg/kg PO q12h) may help prevent fibrosis and restricture during the healing phase.
• Sucralfate suspension 0.5–1.0 g PO q8h
• Gastric acid antisecretory agent—famotidine 0.5 mg/kg PO, IV q12–24h, ranitidine 1–4 mg/kg PO, IV, SC q8–12h, cimetidine 5–10 mg/kg PO, SQ, IV q8h, or omeprazole 0.7 mg/kg PO q24h
• May give the prokinetic agent cisapride (0.1–0.5 mg/kg PO q8–12h) to lower esophageal sphincter tone after resolution of the stricture
• May manage severe esophageal pain with lidocaine solution (0.5 mg/kg PO q4–6h)

CONTRAINDICATIONS
Emetic agents

PRECAUTIONS
None

POSSIBLE INTERACTIONS
• Cimetidine binds to hepatic cytochrome P450 enzyme and may interfere with metab-olism of other drugs.
• H$_2$ receptor antagonists prevent uptake of omeprazole by oxyntic cells.
• Sucralfate may inhibit the gastrointestinal absorption of other drugs (e.g., cimetidine, ranitidine, and omeprazole); this may not be clinically important.

ALTERNATIVE DRUGS
N/A

 FOLLOW-UP

PATIENT MONITORING
Repeat barium esophagrams or endoscopy every 2–4 weeks until clinical signs have resolved and adequate esophageal lumen size has been achieved.

PREVENTION/AVOIDANCE
• Proper patient preparation prior to anesthesia (12-hr preoperative fast) and proper patient positioning during anesthesia (prevent eleva-tion of abdomen above thorax) • Avoid certain drugs (diazepam, atropine, pentobarbital, mor-phine, phenothiazine derivative tranquilizers) prior to anesthesia. • If gastroesophageal reflux, owners should avoid late-night feedings—this tends to diminish gastroesophageal sphincter pressure during sleep • Prevent animals from ingesting caustic substances and foreign bodies.

POSSIBLE COMPLICATIONS
• Esophageal perforation—a life-threatening complication of esophageal stricture dilation;

usually occurs at the time of dilation, although it has been observed several days to weeks later
• Patients are at risk for aspiration pneumonia.

EXPECTED COURSE AND PROGNOSIS
• Generally, the longer the stricture, the more guarded the prognosis. • Patients with fibrosing esophageal strictures—generally fair-to-guarded prognosis; many of these strictures recur despite repeated esophageal dilation; improvement without cure is a more realistic goal (see Client Education above). • Patients with malignant stricture—poor prognosis

 MISCELLANEOUS

ASSOCIATED CONDITIONS
N/A

AGE-RELATED FACTORS
N/A

ZOONOTIC POTENTIAL
None

PREGNANCY
Patients with esophageal stricture and malnu-trition may have difficulty.

SYNONYMS
• Esophageal narrowing • Esophageal obstruction

SEE ALSO
• Esophagitis • Gastroesophageal Reflux
• Megaesophagus • Regurgitation • Esophageal Foreign Body • Dysphagia

ABBREVIATIONS
N/A

Suggested Reading
Burk RL, Zawie DA, Garvey MS. Balloon catheter dilation of intramural esophageal strictures in the dog and cat: a description of the procedure and a report of six cases. Semin Vet Med Surg 1987;2:241–247.
Guilford GW, Strombeck DR. Strombeck's small animal gastroenterology. 3rd ed. Philadelphia: Saunders, 1996.
Johnson, KA, Maddison, JE, Allan GS. Cor-rection of cervical esophageal stricture in a dog by creation of a traction diverticulum. J Am Vet Med Assoc 1992;201:1045–1048.
Twedt DC. Diseases of the esophagus. In: Et-tinger SJ, Feldman EC, eds. Textbook of veterinary internal medicine. Philadelphia: Saunders, 1994:1124–1142.
Zawie DA. Esophageal strictures. In: Kirk RW, ed. Current veterinary therapy X. Philadelphia: Saunders, 1989:904–906.
Authors Robert J. Washabau and Jocelyn Mott
Consulting Editors Mitchell A. Crystal and Brett M. Feder

DISEASES

ESOPHAGITIS

BASICS

DEFINITION
• Inflammation of the esophagus, typically the esophageal body and uncommonly the cricopharyngeal and gastroesophageal sphincters
• Varies from mild inflammation of the superficial mucosa to severe ulceration involving the submucosa and muscularis

PATHOPHYSIOLOGY
• Can be caused by gastroesophageal reflux of gastric and/or intestinal material; esophageal retention of pills or capsules; ingestion of caustic or irritating substances; gastroesophageal reflux due to anesthesia, hiatal hernia, vomiting, and/or infectious agents (calicivirus, pythiosis, *Candida*); esophageal foreign body; pharyngostomy, esophagostomy, or nasogastric feeding tubes; and/or esophageal or thoracic surgery
• The esophageal mucosa has several important barrier mechanisms to withstand caustic substances, including stratified squamous epithelium with tight intracellular junctions, mucous gel, and surface bicarbonate ions.
• Rapid esophageal clearance by peristalsis and neutralization of acid by bicarbonate-rich saliva are important defense mechanisms to prevent reflux esophagitis.
• Disruption of these barrier and defense mechanisms causes inflammation, erosion, and/or ulceration of the underlying structures.

SYSTEMS AFFECTED
• Gastrointestinal—esophageal body most commonly; occasionally the gastroesophageal sphincter
• Respiratory—aspiration pneumonia may develop with concurrent laryngitis and pharyngitis if regurgitation is severe.

GENETICS
N/A

INCIDENCE/PREVALENCE
Unknown; believed to be low

GEOGRAPHIC DISTRIBUTION
Esophagitis caused by *Pythium* spp.—usually regionally distributed in states that border the Gulf of Mexico

SIGNALMENT
Species
Dogs and cats

Breed Predilections
None reported

Mean Age and Range
Any age; young animals with congenital esophageal hiatal hernia may be at higher risk for reflux esophagitis.

Predominant Sex
None

SIGNS

General Comments
• Related to the type of chemical injury, the severity of inflammation, and the involvement of structures underlying the esophageal mucosa (e.g., muscularis)
• May be intermittent and are often more prominent after eating
• Patients with mild esophagitis show subtle or no clinical signs.

Historical Findings
• Regurgitation
• Ptyalism
• Howling/crying during swallowing (odynophagia)
• Extension of the head and neck during swallowing
• Dysphagia
• Avoidance of food
• Weight loss
• Coughing in animals with concurrent aspiration pneumonia

Physical Examination Findings
• Often unremarkable
• Oral and pharyngeal inflammation and/or ulceration if ingestion of caustic or irritating substances
• Fever and ptyalism in some patients with severe ulcerative esophagitis
• Pain on palpation of neck and esophagus
• Cachexia and weight loss with prolonged disease
• Pulmonary wheezes and coughing in patients with aspiration pneumonia

CAUSES
• Gastroesophageal reflux of gastric and/or intestinal juices
• Anesthesia resulting in gastroesophageal reflux
• Ingestion of chemical irritants
• Infectious agents—calicivirus, pythiosis, *Candida*
• Esophageal and/or thoracic surgery
• Nasogastric, esophagostomy, or pharyngostomy feeding tube
• Vomiting
• Esophageal retention of pills or capsules
• Esophageal foreign body

RISK FACTORS
• Hiatal hernias—increases risk for gastroesophageal reflux
• Anesthesia—use of certain drugs prior to anesthesia such as diazepam, atropine, pentobarbital, and phenothiazine-derivative tranquilizers decreases the pressure of the lower esophageal sphincter and can result in gastroesophageal reflux
• Poor preparation and poor positioning during anesthesia places some patients at risk for gastroesophageal reflux and esophagitis.

DIAGNOSIS

DIFFERENTIAL DIAGNOSIS
• Esophageal foreign body—usually detected by survey radiography or esophagoscopy
• Esophageal stricture—segmental narrowing revealed by barium contrast radiography or esophagoscopy
• Pharyngeal dysphagia—diagnosed by evaluating swallowing of barium under fluoroscopy
• Hiatal hernia—congenital form is usually recognized as a caudodorsal gas-filled opacity in the thoracic cavity; contrast studies may be required to document acquired hiatal hernia.
• Megaesophagus—survey radiography usually reveals diffuse dilation of the esophageal body.
• Esophageal diverticula—focal pouches detected by survey or contrast radiography or esophagoscopy
• Vascular ring anomaly—usually revealed by barium contrast radiography as a focal dilation of the proximal esophageal body

CBC/BIOCHEMISTRY/URINALYSIS
Usually normal; patients with severe ulcerative esophagitis or aspiration pneumonia may have leukocytosis and neutrophilia.

OTHER LABORATORY TESTS
N/A

IMAGING
• Survey thoracic radiographs—usually unremarkable
• Survey radiographs in patients with hiatal hernia may show increased density in the caudal esophagus.
• Aspiration pneumonia may be evident in the dependent portions of the lung.
• Barium contrast radiography may reveal an irregular mucosal surface, segmental narrowing, esophageal dilation, or diffuse esophageal hypomotility; stricture formation may be apparent in severely affected patients.
• Ultrasonography—not useful with this disorder

DIAGNOSTIC PROCEDURES
• Endoscopy and biopsy—most reliable means of diagnosing; in patients with severe esophagitis, the mucosa appears hyperemic and edematous with areas of ulceration and active bleeding.
• More mildly affected patients may appear endoscopically normal and require mucosal biopsy for confirmation of the diagnosis.
• Transtracheal aspiration for cytology and culture/sensitivity if aspiration pneumonia is suspected

PATHOLOGIC FINDINGS
• Esophageal inflammation and/or ulceration
• Aspiration pneumonia

TREATMENT

APPROPRIATE HEALTH CARE
Can manage mildly affected animals as outpatients; those with more severe esophagitis (e.g., complete anorexia, dehydration, and aspiration pneumonia) require hospitalization.

NURSING CARE
• Intravenous fluids to maintain hydration—more severe cases
• Give medications parenterally during hospitalization.
• Oxygen therapy—may be necessary in patients with severe aspiration pneumonia

ACTIVITY
N/A

DIET
• Withhold oral intake of food for 2–3 days in patients with mild esophagitis.
• Withhold food and water for 1–2 weeks in patients with severe esophagitis; maintain them by either gastrostomy tube feedings (preferably) or total parenteral nutrition.
• When patients can ingest food orally, give small, frequent, low-fat, high-protein meals of liquid or soft consistency.

CLIENT EDUCATION
• Discuss need to restrict food intake in patients with severe esophagitis.
• Discuss potential complications including aspiration pneumonia, esophageal stricture, esophageal perforation, and/or esophageal motility abnormalities.

SURGICAL CONSIDERATIONS
Percutaneous endoscopic gastrostomy or surgical gastrostomy tube placement is indicated in severe cases.

MEDICATIONS

DRUGS OF CHOICE
• Usually given parenterally (except for sucralfate) in severe cases; when administered enterally, dissolve in water and use oral (syringe, dropper, etc.) or gastrostomy tube delivery.
• Sucralfate suspension (0.5–1.0 g PO q8h) is more therapeutic than intact sucralfate tablets.
• Antibiotics—indicated if concurrent aspiration pneumonia or severe esophageal ulceration or esophageal perforation
• Gastric acid antisecretory agent (e.g., famotidine 0.5 mg/kg PO, SC, IV q12–24h, ranitidine 1–4 mg/kg PO, SC, IV q8–12h, cimetidine 5–10 mg/kg PO, SC, IV q8h, or omeprazole 0.7 mg/kg PO q24h)—useful to prevent occurrence of further irritation by gastroesophageal reflux

• May manage severe esophageal pain with lidocaine solution (0.5 mg/kg PO q4–6h)
• May administer antiinflammatory dosage of corticosteroids (prednisone 0.5–1.0 mg/kg PO q12h) to decrease the possibility of esophageal stricture formation in severe cases
• Gastric prokinetic drugs (metoclopramide 0.2–0.5 mg/kg PO, SC q8h) may help decrease gastroesophageal reflux.

CONTRAINDICATIONS
None

PRECAUTIONS
None

POSSIBLE INTERACTIONS
• Cimetidine binds to hepatic cytochrome P450 enzyme and may interfere with metabolism of other drugs.
• H_2 receptor antagonists prevent uptake of omeprazole by oxyntic cells.
• Sucralfate may inhibit gastrointestinal absorption of other drugs (e.g., cimetidine, ranitidine, and omeprazole).

ALTERNATIVE DRUGS
• Indomethacin—might be useful in refractory cases; use only for short periods because of its potential to cause gastrointestinal ulcers.
• Analogues of erythromycin—may be useful in treating cats with esophagitis secondary to gastroesophageal reflux disease

FOLLOW-UP

PATIENT MONITORING
• Patients with mild esophagitis do not necessarily require follow-up endoscopy; following clinical signs may suffice • Consider endoscopy in patients with ulcerative esophagitis and those at risk for esophageal stricture.

PREVENTION/AVOIDANCE
• Prevent animals from ingesting caustic substances and foreign bodies. • If gastroesophageal reflux is the cause of esophagitis, owners should avoid late-night feedings; this tends to diminish gastroesophageal sphincter pressure during sleep. • Proper patient preparation prior to anesthesia (fasting) and proper patient positioning during anesthesia (abdomen should not be elevated above thorax) decreases the risk of gastroesophageal reflux.

POSSIBLE COMPLICATIONS
• Stricture formation • Esophageal perforation • Aspiration pneumonia • Permanent esophageal motility dysfunction

EXPECTED COURSE AND PROGNOSIS
• Best results when patients are treated with a diffusion barrier (e.g., sucralfate) and gastric acid secretory inhibitor (e.g., famotidine, ranitidine, cimetidine, or omeprazole) • Patients with mild esophagitis—generally favorable

prognosis • Patients with severe or ulcerative esophagitis—guarded prognosis • Complete recovery is possible if the disorder is recognized and treated before serious complications develop.

MISCELLANEOUS

ASSOCIATED CONDITIONS
N/A

AGE-RELATED FACTORS
N/A

ZOONOTIC POTENTIAL
None

SYNONYMS
Esophageal inflammation

SEE ALSO
• Esophageal Stricture • Esophageal Diverticulum • Esophageal Foreign Body • Megaesophagus • Hiatal Hernia • Dysphagia • Regurgitation • Gastroesophageal Reflux

ABBREVIATIONS
None

Suggested Reading
Eastwood CL, Beck BD, Castell DO, et al. Beneficial effect of indomethacin on acid-induced esophagitis in cats. Dig Dis Sci 1981;26:601–608.
Eastwood CL, Castell DO, Higgs RH. Experimental esophagitis in cats impairs lower esophageal sphincter pressure. Gastroenterology 1975;69:146–153.
Greenwood B, Dieckman D, Kirst H, et al. Effects of LY267108, an erythromycin analogue derivative, on lower esophageal sphincter function in the cat. Gastroenterology 1994;106:624–628.
Katz PD, et al. Acid-induced esophagitis in cats is prevented by sucralfate but not synthetic prostaglandins. Dig Dis Sci 1988;33:217–224.
Twedt DC. Diseases of the esophagus. In: Ettinger SJ, Feldman EC, eds. Textbook of veterinary internal medicine. Philadelphia: Saunders, 1994:1124–1142.

Authors Robert J. Washabau and Jocelyn Mott

Consulting Editors Mitchell A. Crystal and Brett M. Feder

DISEASES

ESTROGEN TOXICITY

BASICS

OVERVIEW
• Dogs more sensitive to estrogen than other species but vary widely in their sensitivity
• Can cause pancytopenia, feminization of male animals, and estrus and pyometra in female animals
• In dogs, pancytopenia believed to result from the induction of a nonlymphoid, thymic-inhibitory, hematopoietic factor

SIGNALMENT
• Dogs
• Old, intact male and female animals at greater risk for developing estrogen-producing tumors, although cryptorchid males may be comparatively younger

SIGNS
• Exercise intolerance and pale mucous membranes because of anemia
• Hemorrhage—petechiae, hematuria, and melena caused by thrombocytopenia
• Fever associated with infection resulting from leukopenia
• Alopecia
• Estrus in females and feminization of males in some animals
• Abdominal masses, testicular masses, cryptorchidism in some animals

CAUSES & RISK FACTORS
• Endogenous estrogen from testicular Sertoli cell tumors and ovarian granulosa cell tumors
• Exogenous estrogen used in the management of benign prostatic hyperplasia, perianal adenoma, pregnancy prevention, urinary incontinence, and infertility
• Cryptorchid males at greater risk of developing Sertoli cell tumor

DIAGNOSIS

DIFFERENTIAL DIAGNOSIS
• Other causes of pancytopenia include toxins, drugs, infection, neoplastic, granulomatous, and immune-mediated diseases, and myelodysplasia.
• Important factors in the diagnosis include history of administration of estrogen, testicular or ovarian tumor, thin hair coat, evidence of estrus, and signs of feminization.

CBC/BIOCHEMISTRY/URINALYSIS

After Estrogen Overdosage
• Thrombocytosis occurs within 1 week, followed by thrombocytopenia within 2 weeks.
• Leukocytosis develops and persists until week 3.
• Normocytic, normochromic anemia develops insidiously.
• Pancytopenia occurs within 4 weeks.

OTHER LABORATORY TESTS
Blood culture may be considered in febrile, leukopenic patients.

IMAGING
Radiography and ultrasonography—locate and stage potential estrogen-producing tumors and help diagnose pyometra

DIAGNOSTIC PROCEDURES
• Examination of bone marrow aspirate—5–7 days after estrogen overdosage: suppression of megakaryocytopoiesis and erythropoiesis with concurrent stimulation of granulopoiesis; by day 10: all cell lines are affected; by day 20: granulopoiesis ceases completely while the other cell lines start to recover.
• Hematologic recovery can take 3 months; signs of marrow improvement are seen 3 days later in the peripheral blood.
• Abdominal laparotomy or laparoscopy and/or biopsy to locate and identify estrogen-producing tumors

TREATMENT
• Remove source of estrogen if possible.
• Severely affected animals may require extensive and prolonged supportive care, including transfusions of blood and platelet-rich plasma.
• Care should be taken with venipuncture and other invasive procedures to avoid bruising in severely thrombocytopenic patients.

MEDICATIONS
• Broad-spectrum antibiotics necessary in febrile, leukopenic patients; choice of antibiotic should be based on bacterial culture if possible.
• Although no reports have been published of their use to treat estrogen toxicity, growth factors such as recombinant human erythropoietin (100 IU/kg SC 3 times weekly) and rhG-CSF (2.5–5 μg/kg SC q24h) may be useful.

• Lithium carbonate (10 mg/kg PO q12h) has been used to treat estrogen-induced pancytopenia.

CONTRAINDICATIONS/POSSIBLE INTERACTIONS
Consider avoiding sulfonamides and cephalosporins, because they are occasionally associated with blood dyscrasia.

FOLLOW-UP
• Monitor the bleeding or febrile estrogen toxicity patient closely, including checking PCV 2–3 times daily; monitoring temperature, heart rate and rhythm, and respiratory rate; and checking for bleeding
• When PCV has stabilized or the temperature normalized, the patient may be monitored as an outpatient.
• CBC—biweekly or weekly, depending on the patient's progress; weekly in patients who have undergone surgical excision of an estrogen-producing tumor to check for progression of hematologic abnormalities
• The patient may require changes of antibiotics, multiple blood or platelet transfusions, and intermittent hospitalization.
• Complications include sepsis and hemorrhage into vital organs, such as the heart and CNS.
• Recovery may take as long as 3 months.
• Prognosis guarded

MISCELLANEOUS

SEE ALSO
• Anemia, Aplastic
• Anemia, Nonregenerative
• Leukopenia
• Ovarian Tumors
• Sertoli Cell Tumor

ABBREVIATIONS
• PCV = packed cell volume
• rhG-CSF = recombinant human granulocyte colony-stimulating factor

Suggested Reading
Hall EJ. Use of lithium for treatment of estrogen-induced bone marrow hypoplasia in a dog. J Am Vet Med Assoc 1992;200:814–816.
Author Orla M. Mahony
Consulting Editor Susan M. Cotter

BASICS

OVERVIEW
• Ethanol (CH$_2$OH)—short-chain aliphatic alcohol; highly miscible with water; soluble in aqueous systems; less volatile than comparable hydrocarbons (e.g., ethane); solvent for medications; major component of alcoholic beverages; metabolized to acetaldehyde

ALCOHOL CONTENT OF COMMON BEVERAGES

Beer	3–5%
Wines	9–12%
Whisky	50–90%

• Alcohol concentration—expressed as proof (twice the percentage concentration)
• Acute toxicity—5–8 mL/kg as pure alcohol; to calculate beverage volume that will cause toxicosis, consider the percentage of alcohol.
• Mechanism of action—effects lipids and proteins of the cell membrane; then reduces sodium and potassium conduction in nerve membranes

SIGNALMENT
• Most common in dogs
• No breed or sex predilections

SIGNS
• CNS—predominate; develop within 15–30 min after ingestion on an empty stomach or 1–2 hr on full stomach
• High dosages—ataxia; reduced reflexes; behavioral changes; excitement or depression
• Polyuria and/or incontinence
• Advanced signs—depression or narcosis; slowed respiratory rate; cardiac arrest; death

CAUSES & RISK FACTORS
• Accidental—access to spilled beverages or medications containing alcohol

• Intentional—given by owners or others; dogs may readily consume beer if offered.
• Fermented products—bread dough
• Dermal exposure—alcohol-containing products

DIAGNOSIS

DIFFERENTIAL DIAGNOSIS
• Other alcohols—methanol; isopropanol; butanol
• Abused drugs—marijuana
• Early stages of ethylene glycol (antifreeze) toxicosis
• Halogenated or aliphatic hydrocarbon solvents

CBC/BIOCHEMISTRY/URINALYSIS
Monitor for hypoglycemia.

OTHER LABORATORY TESTS
• Osmolal gap—increased
• Blood ethanol concentrations—clinical signs of toxicosis in puppies at > 0.6 mg/mL and in adults at > 1–4 mg/mL; available at human laboratories
• Blood gases and anion gap—evaluate potential acidosis

IMAGING
N/A

DIAGNOSTIC PROCEDURES
N/A

TREATMENT
• Depressed respiratory function—artificial ventilation
• Acidosis—treat.
• Cardiac arrest—cardiac therapy (see Cardiopulmonary Arrest)

MEDICATIONS

DRUGS
• Activated charcoal—2 g/kg PO; as soon as possible after exposure; gastrointestinal detoxication
• 4-Methyl pyrazole—possible inhibition of alcohol metabolism (see Ethylene Glycol Toxicity)
• Epinephrine and bicarbonate—cardiac arrest (see Cardiopulmonary Arrest)

CONTRAINDICATIONS/POSSIBLE INTERACTIONS
Do not administer other CNS depressive drugs.

FOLLOW-UP
• Monitor blood pH, blood gases, urine pH, and anion gap—evidence of acidosis
• Recovery from clinical signs—usually within 8–12 hr

MISCELLANEOUS

Suggested Reading
Valentine WM. Short chain alcohols. Vet Clin North Am 1990;20:515–523.
Author Gary D. Osweiler
Consulting Editor Gary D. Osweiler

ETHYLENE GLYCOL TOXICITY

 BASICS

DEFINITION
Results from ingesting substances containing ethylene glycol (e.g., antifreeze)

PATHOPHYSIOLOGY
• Ethylene glycol—rapidly absorbed from the gastrointestinal tract; food in the stomach delays absorption.
• Toxicity—initially causes CNS depression, ataxia, gastrointestinal irritation, and polyuria or polydipsia; rapidly metabolized by the liver enzyme ADH to glycoaldehyde, glycolic acid, glyoxalic acid, and oxalic acid leads to severe metabolic acidosis and renal epithelial damage.
• Minimum lethal dose—cats, 1.4 mL/kg; dogs, 6.6 mL/kg

SYSTEMS AFFECTED
• Nervous—inebriation from ethylene glycol and glycoaldehyde owing to inhibition of respiration, glucose metabolism, and serotonin metabolism and alteration of amine concentrations
• Gastrointestinal—irritated mucosa
• Renal/Urologic—initially, osmotic diuresis; later, metabolites are directly cytotoxic to renal tubular epithelium, resulting in renal failure; minor role for oxalate crystal deposition in causing renal tubular damage

GENETICS
N/A

INCIDENCE/PREVALENCE
• Common in small animals
• Highest fatality rate of all poisons; fatality rates higher for cats than dogs
• Incidence similar in cats and dogs

GEOGRAPHIC DISTRIBUTION
Higher incidence in colder areas where antifreeze is more commonly used

SIGNALMENT
Species
Dogs, cats, and many other species, including birds

Breed Predilections
N/A

Mean Age and Range
• Any age susceptible (3 months to 13 years)
• Mean—3 years

Predominant Sex
N/A

SIGNS
General Comments
• Dose-dependent
• Almost always acute
• Caused by unmetabolized ethylene glycol and its toxic metabolites (frequently fatal)

Physical Examination Findings
• Early—seen from 30 min to 12 hr postingestion in dogs; nausea and vomiting; mild to severe depression; ataxia and knuckling; muscle fasciculations; nystagmus; head tremors; decreased withdrawal reflexes and righting ability; polyuria and polydipsia
• Dogs—with increasing depression, patient drinks less but polyuria continues, resulting in dehydration; CNS signs abate transiently after approximately 12 hr, but recur later.
• Cats—usually remain markedly depressed; do not exhibit polydipsia
• Oliguria (dogs, 36–72 hr; cats, 12–24 hr) and anuria (72–96 hr postingestion)—often develop if untreated
• May note severe hypothermia
• Severe lethargy or coma
• Seizures
• Anorexia
• Vomiting
• Oral ulcers
• Salivation
• Kidneys—often swollen and painful, particularly in cats

CAUSES
Ingestion of ethylene glycol, the principal component (95%) of most antifreeze solutions

RISK FACTORS
Access to ethylene glycol—widespread availability; somewhat pleasant taste; small minimum lethal dose; lack of public awareness of toxicity

 DIAGNOSIS

DIFFERENTIAL DIAGNOSIS
• Acute (30 min to 12 hr postingestion)—ethanol toxicosis; ketoacidotic diabetes mellitus; pancreatitis; gastroenteritis
• Renal stage—acute renal failure by nephrotoxins (e.g., aminoglycoside antibiotics, amphotericin B, cancer chemotherapeutic drugs, cyclosporin, and heavy metals); tubulointerstitial nephritis; glomerular and vascular disease; renal ischemia (hypoperfusion)

CBC/BIOCHEMISTRY/URINALYSIS
• PCV and total protein—often high owing to dehydration
• Stress leukogram—common
• High BUN and creatinine—dog, 36–48 hr postingestion; cat, 12 hr postingestion
• Hypophosphatemia may occur transiently 3–6 hr postingestion, owing to phosphate rust inhibitors in the antifreeze, followed by hyperphosphatemia, owing to decreased glomerular filtration.
• Hyperkalemia
• Hypocalcemia—occurs in approximately half of patients, owing to chelation of calcium by oxalic acid; clinical signs infrequently observed because of acidosis
• Hyperglycemia—occurs in half of patients, owing to inhibition of glucose metabolism by aldehydes, increased epinephrine and endogenous corticosteroids, and uremia
• Isosthenuria—by 3 hr postingestion, owing to osmotic diuresis and serum hyperosmolality–induced polydipsia; continues in the later stages of toxicosis because of renal dysfunction
• Calcium oxalate crystalluria—consistent finding; as early as 3 hr postingestion in cats and 6 hr in dogs
• Urine pH—consistently decreases
• Inconsistent findings—hematuria; proteinuria; glucosuria
• May note granular and cellular casts, WBCs, RBCs, and renal epithelial cells

OTHER LABORATORY TESTS
Blood Gases
• Metabolites cause severe metabolic acidosis
• Total CO_2, plasma bicarbonate concentration, and blood pH—low by 3 hr postingestion; markedly low by 12 hr
• PCO_2—decreases, owing to partial respiratory compensation
• Anion gap—increased by 3 hr postingestion; peaks at 6 hr postingestion; remains increased for approximately 48 hr

Other
• Serum osmolality and osmolal gap—high by 1 hr postingestion, in parallel with serum ethylene glycol concentrations; dose-related; usually remain high for approximately 18 hr postingestion; ethylene glycol toxicosis most common cause of a high osmolal gap
• Ethylene glycol serum concentration—peaks 1–6 hr postingestion; usually not detectable in the serum or urine by 72 hr; commercial kits (EGT Test Kit) measure concentrations at > 50 mg/dL; estimate by multiplying the osmolal gap by 6.2.

IMAGING
Ultrasound—renal cortices may be hyperechoic as a result of crystals.

DIAGNOSTIC PROCEDURES
• Kidney biopsy—with anuria; confirm diagnosis
• Cytologic examination of kidney imprints—often diagnostic; numerous calcium oxalate crystals

PATHOLOGIC FINDINGS
Kidneys—often swollen

TREATMENT

APPROPRIATE HEALTH CARE
• Cats—usually inpatient
• Dogs—usually outpatient if < 5 hr postingestion and treated with fomepizole; inpatient if > 5 hr for intravenous fluids to correct dehydration, increase tissue perfusion, and promote diuresis

NURSING CARE
• Goals—prevent absorption; increase excretion; prevent metabolism
• Induction of vomiting and gastric lavage with activated charcoal—indicated within 1–2 hr of ingestion
• Intravenous fluids—correct dehydration, increase tissue perfusion, and promote diuresis; accompanied by bicarbonate given slowly intravenously to correct metabolic acidosis
• Monitor serial plasma bicarbonate concentrations—$0.3 - 0.5 \times$ body weight (kg) $\times$ (24 − plasma bicarbonate) = sodium bicarbonate needed (mEq)
• Monitor urine pH in response to therapy.
• Azotemia and oliguric renal failure (dogs)—most of the ethylene glycol has been metabolized; little benefit from inhibition of ADH; correct fluid, electrolyte, and acid–base disorders; establish diuresis; diuretics (particularly mannitol) may help; peritoneal dialysis may be useful; may need extended treatment (several weeks) before renal function is re-established

ACTIVITY
N/A

DIET
N/A

CLIENT EDUCATION
N/A

SURGICAL CONSIDERATIONS
Kidney transplantation—successfully employed in cats with ethylene glycol–induced renal failure

MEDICATIONS

DRUGS OF CHOICE
Dogs
• Fomepizole (4-methyl pyrazole; Antizol-Vet)—effective and nontoxic liver ADH inhibitor; more expensive than ethanol (initial cost offset by less time in intensive care); 5% (50 mg/mL) at 20 mg/kg IV initially; then 15 mg/kg IV at 12 and 24 hr; then 5 mg/kg IV at 36 hr

Cats
• Fomepizole—ineffective; not recommended, at least with dosage schedules used in dogs; clinical trials suggest much larger doses may be effective.
• Ethanol—therapy of choice; 20% at 5 mL/kg diluted in fluids and given in a IV drip over 6 hr for five treatments; then over 8 hr for four more treatments

CONTRAINDICATIONS
Avoid drugs that cause CNS depression.

PRECAUTIONS
• Competitive substrates (alcohols, such as ethanol)—contribute to CNS depression; monitor respiration
• Cats—usually become hypothermic; require an external heat source
• Other pyrazoles—may be toxic to the marrow and liver; do not substitute for fomepizole.

POSSIBLE INTERACTIONS
• Fomepizole—none
• Ethanol—contributes to CNS depression; further increases serum osmolality

ALTERNATIVE DRUGS
Ethanol, propylene glycol, and 1,3-butanediol—higher affinity for ADH than does ethylene glycol; effectively to inhibit ethylene glycol metabolism; may cause CNS depression and increase serum osmolality; constant serum ethanol concentrations of 100 mg/dL will inhibit most ethylene glycol metabolism.
• Ethanol—even in early stages requires hospitalization for approximately 3 days; constant intravenous infusion (ethanol and fluids); continuous monitoring for respiratory and acid–base status

FOLLOW-UP

PATIENT MONITORING
BUN, acid–base status, and urine output—monitored daily for the first few days

PREVENTION/AVOIDANCE
• Increasing client awareness of the toxicity—help prevent exposure; earlier treatment of patients
• Use of new antifreeze products containing propylene glycol (relatively nontoxic)

POSSIBLE COMPLICATIONS
• Without azotemia—usually no complications
• Urine concentrating ability—may be impaired with azotemia; patients recover.

EXPECTED COURSE AND PROGNOSIS
• Untreated—oliguric renal failure (dogs, 36–72 hr; cats, 12–24 hr); anuria by 72–96 hr postingestion

• Dogs treated < 5 hr postingestion—prognosis excellent with fomepizole treatment
• Dogs treated up to 8 hr postingestion—most recover
• Dogs treated up to 36 hr postingestion—may be of benefit to prevent metabolism of any remaining ethylene glycol
• Cats treated within 3 hr postingestion—prognosis good with ethanol treatment
• Patients with azotemia and oliguric renal failure—prognosis poor; almost all of the ethylene glycol will have been metabolized.

MISCELLANEOUS

AGE-RELATED FACTORS
Patients < 6 months of age with oliguric renal failure sometimes fully recover.

ZOONOTIC POTENTIAL
None

PREGNANCY
N/A

SYNONYMS
Antifreeze poisoning

SEE ALSO
• Osmolarity, Hyperosmolarity
• Renal Failure, Acute

ABBREVIATIONS
• ADH = alcohol dehydrogenase
• PCV = packed cell volume

Suggested Reading
Connally HE, Thrall MA, Forney SD, et al. Safety and efficacy of 4-methylpyrazole as treatment for suspected or confirmed ethylene glycol intoxication in dogs: 107 cases (1983–1995). J Am Vet Med Assoc 1996;209:1880–1883.

Dial SM, Thrall MA, Hamar DW. Comparison of ethanol and 4-methylpyrazole as therapies for ethylene glycol intoxication in the cat. Am J Vet Res 1994;55:1771–1782.

Dial SM, Thrall MA, Hamar DW. Efficacy of 4-methylpyrazole for treatment of ethylene glycol intoxication in dogs. Am J Vet Res 1994;55:1762–1770.

Thrall MA, Grauer GF, Dial SM. Antifreeze poisoning. In: Bonagura JD, ed. Kirk's current veterinary therapy XII. Small animal practice. Philadelphia: Saunders, 1995:232–237.

Authors Mary Anna Thrall, Gregory F. Grauer, and Sharon M. Dial
Consulting Editor Gary D. Osweiler

DISEASES

EXOCRINE PANCREATIC INSUFFICIENCY (EPI)

 BASICS

DEFINITION

Progressive loss of exocrine pancreatic acinar cells, causing failure of absorption because of inadequate production of digestive enzymes

PATHOPHYSIOLOGY

• Idiopathic pancreatic acinar atrophy—the most common cause in dogs
• Chronic pancreatitis, with resultant destruction of acinar tissue—much less common cause in dogs; most common cause in cats
• May rarely develop with adenocarcinoma and pancreatic duct obstruction
• Deficient exocrine pancreatic secretion results in maldigestion, nutrient malabsorption, and osmotic diarrhea.
• Malabsorption contributes to SIBO, which may cause secretory diarrhea.

SYSTEMS AFFECTED

• Gastrointestinal—duodenal mucosal disease (villus atrophy, inflammatory cellular infiltrates, and abnormal mucosal enzyme activities) and SIBO
• Nutritional—protein-calorie malnourishment

GENETICS

Assumed to be hereditary in the German shepherd dog and transmitted by an autosomal recessive trait

INCIDENCE/PREVALENCE

• Relatively common in the German shepherd dog; may be seen in all canine breeds
• Rare in cats

GEOGRAPHIC DISTRIBUTION

• Dogs—N/A
• Cats—may be seen with pancreatic fluke infestation (southeast United States)

SIGNALMENT

Species
Dogs and cats

Breed Predilections
German shepherd dogs

Mean Age and Range
• Pancreatic acinar atrophy in young dogs
• Chronic pancreatitis in old dogs
• Chronic pancreatitis or pancreatic fluke infestation in middle-aged and older cats

Predominant Sex
N/A

SIGNS AND SYMPTOMS

General Comments
• Consider in young German shepherd dogs with chronic diarrhea suggesting malassimilation.
• Severity—varies; depends on the time elapsed prior to diagnosis and therapy

Historical Findings
• Weight loss with a normal to increased appetite
• Chronic watery diarrhea of small bowel origin is common.
• Diarrhea—often resembles cow feces; may be continuous or intermittent
• Fecal volumes larger than normal; steatorrhea present
• Diarrhea generally decreases with a low-fat, highly digestible diet
• Flatulence and borborygmus—common
• May be coprophagia and pica
• May see polyuria/polydipsia with diabetes mellitus caused by chronic pancreatitis

Physical Examination Findings
• Thin body
• Decreased muscle mass
• "Unthrifty" appearance with a poor quality haircoat
• Cats with steatorrhea may have greasy "soiling" of the haircoat around the rectum.

CAUSES

• Pancreatic acinar atrophy
• Chronic relapsing pancreatitis
• Pancreatic adenocarcinoma
• Pancreatic fluke *(Eurytrema procyonis)* infection in cats

RISK FACTORS

• Breed—German shepherd dogs
• Any condition predisposing patients to recurrent pancreatitis

 DIAGNOSIS

DIFFERENTIAL DIAGNOSIS

• Exclude causes of malabsorption (small intestinal mucosal disease, lymphangiectasia) by intestinal mucosal biopsy
• Exclude chronic parasitism by performing multiple fecal examinations
• Exclude diabetes mellitus and feline hyperthyroidism by appropriate laboratory testing

CBC/BIOCHEMISTRY/URINALYSIS

Usually normal

OTHER LABORATORY TESTS

Direct/Indirect Fecal Examinations
Negative for parasites

Exocrine Pancreatic Function Tests—Trypsin-like Immunoreactivity (TLI)
• Diagnostic test of choice
• Theory of test—serum TLI can be detected by an assay that measures trypsinogen leaked directly into the blood from pancreatic acinar tissue; serum TLI is detected in all normal dogs and cats having functional exocrine pancreatic mass.
• Serum TLI concentrations—dramatically reduced with EPI
• Canine and feline TLI tests—differ; species-specific
• Advantages—simple; quick; single serum specimen (fasted) required; highly sensitive

Exocrine Pancreatic Function Tests—Others
• Bentiromide (BT-PABA) absorption test—indirectly assesses pancreatic enzyme activity in the small intestine; disadvantages include acquiring the agent, technical constraints, need for multiple sampling, and absence of proven benefit over assay of serum TLI
• Assays of fecal proteolytic activity using casein-based substrates—accurate means of diagnosing EPI in both dogs and cats; disadvantages include the need for collecting multiple fecal specimens over days and the lack of availability of the test.

Screening Tests for Malassimilation
Microscopic examination of feces for undigested food, assessment of fecal proteolytic activity by X-ray film digestion, and the plasma turbidity test—unreliable and *not* recommended

Cobalamin and Folate
• Often run as a panel with TLI
• Used to assess for SIBO and as a nonspecific indicator of moderate-to-advanced small intestinal malabsorption

IMAGING

Abdominal radiography and ultrasonography are unremarkable.

DIAGNOSTIC PROCEDURES

N/A

PATHOLOGIC FINDINGS

• Pancreatic acinar atrophy—marked atrophy/absence of pancreatic acinar tissue on gross inspection
• Pancreatitis—microscopically, acini and possibly islets are depleted and replaced by fibrous tissue.

TREATMENT

APPROPRIATE HEALTH CARE
• Outpatient medical management
• Patients with concurrent diabetes mellitus may initially require hospitalization for insulin regulation of hyperglycemia.

NURSING CARE
N/A

ACTIVITY
N/A

DIET
• Modification is a cornerstone of therapy in dogs.
• Ideally is highly digestible, low in fat, low in fiber, and nutritionally balanced
• High digestibility reduces nutrient availability for bacterial overgrowth
• Avoid high-fat diets—fat absorption remains impaired despite appropriate enzyme therapy.
• Avoid high-fiber diets—fiber inhibits the activity of pancreatic enzymes.
• Severely malnourished dogs may require supplementation with cobalamin, tocopherol, and fat-soluble vitamins A, D, E, and K.

CLIENT EDUCATION
• Discuss hereditary nature in German shepherd dogs.
• Discuss expense of pancreatic enzymes and need for lifelong therapy.
• Discuss the possibility of diabetes mellitus in patients with recurrent pancreatitis.

SURGICAL CONSIDERATIONS
N/A—mesenteric torsion reported in German shepherd dogs in Scandinavia but not North America.

MEDICATIONS

DRUGS OF CHOICE
• Powdered, non–enteric-coated pancreatic enzyme concentrates—therapy of choice
• Initially—mix enzyme powder in food at a dosage of 1 teaspoon with each meal per 10 kg body weight; feed two meals daily to promote weight gain.
• Preincubation of enzymes with food does *not* improve the effectiveness of oral enzyme therapy.
• Administration of bicarbonate or histamine blockers (famotidine, ranitidine, cimetidine) does *not* improve the effectiveness of enzyme therapy.

• Most dogs respond to therapy within 5–7 days; then the amount of daily pancreatic supplement may be gradually reduced to a dose that prevents return of clinical signs.
• Oral antibiotic therapy (metronidazole, 10–15 mg/kg PO q12h, oxytetracycline 20 mg/kg PO q12h) may be required for 5–7 days in dogs with concurrent SIBO.

CONTRAINDICATIONS
Avoid enteric-coated tablets; dissolution of their protective coating is unpredictable, and poor responses may be seen.

PRECAUTIONS
• Avoid tetracycline antibiotics in very young animals.
• Tetracycline antibiotics may cause fever, abdominal pain, hair loss, and depression in cats.

POSSIBLE INTERACTIONS
N/A

ALTERNATIVE DRUGS
N/A

FOLLOW-UP

PATIENT MONITORING
• Weekly for first month of therapy
• Diarrhea improves markedly—fecal consistency typically normalizes within 1 week.
• Gain in body weight
• Dogs that fail to respond after 1 week of enzyme therapy—place on antibiotics for SIBO.
• Once body weight and conditioning normalize, gradually reduce the daily dosage of enzyme supplements to a level that maintains normal body weight.

PREVENTION/AVOIDANCE
Do not breed affected animals.

POSSIBLE COMPLICATIONS
• 20% of dogs fail to respond to pancreatic enzymes.
• SIBO

EXPECTED COURSE AND PROGNOSIS
• Most causes are irreversible, and lifelong therapy will be required.
• Dogs with EPI alone—prognosis good with appropriate enzyme therapy and dietary management
• Prognosis is more guarded in patients with EPI and diabetes mellitus due to chronic pancreatitis.

MISCELLANEOUS

ASSOCIATED CONDITIONS
• SIBO
• Diabetes mellitus
• Associated vitamin K-responsive coagulopathy has been reported in a cat.

AGE-RELATED FACTORS
Consider EPI in young adult dogs with chronic diarrhea.

ZOONOTIC POTENTIAL
N/A

PREGNANCY
• Do not breed animals with EPI from pancreatic acinar atrophy.
• Do not use tetracycline antibiotics and metronidazole in pregnant animals.

SYNONYMS
• Juvenile pancreatic atrophy
• Pancreatic acinar atrophy

SEE ALSO
• Trypsin-like Immunoreactivity
• Cobalamin and Folate
• Diarrhea, Chronic—Dogs and Diarrhea, Chronic—Cats
• Small Intestinal Bacterial Overgrowth
• Pancreatitis

ABBREVIATIONS
• EPI = exocrine pancreatic insufficiency
• SIBO = small intestinal bacterial overgrowth
• TLI = trypsin-like immunoreactivity

Suggested Reading

Williams DA. New tests of pancreatic and small intestinal function. Compend Contin Educ Pract Vet 1987;9:1167–1174.
Williams DA. Sensitivity and specificity of serum trypsin-like immunoreactivity for the diagnosis of canine exocrine pancreatic insufficiency. J Am Vet Med Assoc 1988;192;195–201.
Williams DA. Exocrine pancreatic disease. In: Ettinger SJ, Feldman EC, eds. Textbook of veterinary internal medicine. 5th ed. Philadelphia: Saunders, 2000:1345–1367.
Author Albert E. Jergens
Consulting Editors Mitchell A. Crystal and Brett M. Feder

DISEASES

EYELASH DISORDERS (TRICHIASIS/DISTICHIASIS/ECTOPIC CILIA)

BASICS

OVERVIEW
• Trichiasis—when hair arising from normal sites contacts the corneal or conjunctival surfaces
• Distichiasis—when cilia emerge from or near the meibomian gland orifices on the lid margin and may or may not contact the cornea.
• Ectopic cilia—single or multiple hairs that arise from the palpebral conjunctival surface several millimeters from the lid margin, most commonly near the middle of the superior lid

SIGNALMENT
• Common in dogs; rare in cats
• Most common in young dogs
• Any breed may be affected
• Facial-fold trichiasis—breeds with prominent facial folds (e.g., Pekingese, pugs, and bulldogs)
• Distichiasis—found in some degree in most cocker spaniels
• Ectopic cilia—more common than average in dachshunds, lhasa apsos, and Shetland sheepdogs

SIGNS

Facial-Fold Trichiasis
• Nasal corneal vascularization and pigmentation
• Blepharospasm
• Epiphora

Distichiasis
• Usually asymptomatic
• Stiff, stout cilia contacting the cornea—may note blepharospasm, epiphora, corneal vascularization, pigmentation, and ulceration

Ectopic Cilia
• Ocular pain
• Severe blepharospasm
• Epiphora
• Superficial corneal ulcers with a linear appearance (corresponding to lid movement) on the superior cornea—common; resistant to healing until the underlying problem is diagnosed and corrected

CAUSES & RISK FACTORS
Usually related to facial conformation or breed predisposition or is idiopathic

DIAGNOSIS

DIFFERENTIAL DIAGNOSIS
• Other adnexal abnormalities—entropion)
• Keratoconjunctivitis sicca
• Conjunctival foreign body
• Infectious conjunctivitis
• Diagnosis based on direct observation of abnormal cilia

CBC/BIOCHEMISTRY/URINALYSIS
N/A

OTHER LABORATORY TESTS
N/A

IMAGING
N/A

DIAGNOSTIC PROCEDURES
N/A

TREATMENT

TRICHIASIS
• May be managed conservatively in some patients
• Keeping the periocular hair short may help; however, clipping the hair on facial folds may make it stiffer and more irritating.
• Surgical correction of adnexal abnormalities—indicated; entropion correction
• May resect facial folds
• Medial canthal closure—often a better procedure; also eliminates lagophthalmos and medial entropion

DISTICHIASIS
• Usually asymptomatic and requires no treatment
• Symptomatic—may treat surgically by cryotherapy, electrocautery or electroepilation, or resection from the conjunctival surface
• Lid splitting techniques—avoid; postoperative scarring may predispose patient to cicatricial entropion and impaired lid function.

ECTOPIC CILIA
• May be treated surgically—en-bloc resection of the cilia and associated meibomian gland
• Cryotherapy—may be used as the sole treatment or as an adjunct after surgical resection
• Warn client that patient is at risk for developing ectopic cilia at other locations.
• Advise client to have patient rechecked if clinical signs recur.

EYELASH DISORDERS (TRICHIASIS/DISTICHIASIS/ECTOPIC CILIA)

 MEDICATIONS

DRUGS
• Rarely indicated
• Lubricant ointments—sometimes valuable to soften cilia and lessen irritation before surgical correction
• Topical antibiotics—perioperative; recommended for patients undergoing surgery to minimize conjunctival flora in the surgical sites

CONTRAINDICATIONS/POSSIBLE INTERACTIONS
N/A

 FOLLOW-UP

Distichia—regrowth common because destructive procedures (cryotherapy and electroepilation) must be done conservatively to minimize lid damage.

✓ **MISCELLANEOUS**

Suggested Reading
Gelatt KN. Veterinary ophthalmology. 2nd ed. Philadelphia: Lea & Febiger, 1991.
Author Erin S. Champagne
Consulting Editor Paul E. Miller

DISEASES

FACIAL NERVE PARESIS/PARALYSIS

BASICS

DEFINITION
Dysfunction of the facial nerve (seventh cranial nerve), causing paralysis or weakness of the muscles of the ears, eyelids, lips, and nostrils

PATHOPHYSIOLOGY
Weakness or paralysis caused by impairment of the facial nerve or the neuromuscular junction peripherally or the facial nucleus in the brainstem

SYSTEMS AFFECTED
• Nervous—facial nerve peripherally or its nucleus in the brainstem
• Ophthalmic—if parasympathetic preganglionic neurons that supply the lacrimal glands and course with the facial nerve are involved, keratoconjunctivitis sicca develops because of lack of tear secretion.

GENETICS
N/A

INCIDENCE/PREVALENCE
More common in dogs than cats

GEOGRAPHIC DISTRIBUTION
N/A

SIGNALMENT

Species
Dogs and cats

Breed Predilections
Idiopathic paralysis—cocker spaniels, Pembroke Welsh corgis, boxers, English setters, and domestic longhair cats

Mean Age and Range
Adults

Predominant Sex
N/A

SIGNS

General Comments
• Assess strength of the palpebral closure; there should be full eyelid closure when a finger is gently passed over both eyelids simultaneously.
• Paresis—unilateral and idiopathic in most animals; not infrequently, unaffected facial nerve becomes affected within a few weeks to months; idiopathic paresis may rarely occur bilaterally.
• Most patients with bilateral nerve involvement have a systemic disease.
• Unilateral paresis or paralysis—may accompany other clinical signs; may indicate focal or systemic disease

Historical Findings
• Messy eating; food left around mouth
• Excessive drooling
• Facial asymmetry
• Eye—inability to close; rubbing; discharge; cloudy

Physical Examination Findings
• Ipsilateral ear and lip drooping
• Excessive drooling
• Food falling from the side of mouth
• Collapse of the nostril
• Inability to close the eyelids
• Wide palpebral fissure
• Decreased or absent menace response
• Palpebral reflex
• Chronic—patient may have deviation of the face toward the affected side.
• Mucopurulent discharge from the affected eye and exposure conjunctivitis or keratitis—may be noted
• When secondary to brainstem disease—altered mentation (e.g., depression or stupor); other cranial nerve and gait abnormalities may be noted.

CAUSES

Unilateral Peripheral
• Idiopathic*
• Metabolic—hypothyroidism*
• Inflammatory—otitis media or interna* (dogs and cats); nasopharyngeal polyps (cats)*
• Neoplasia
• Trauma—fracture of the petrous temporal bone; injury to the facial nerve external to the stylomastoid foramen or secondary to surgical ablation of external ear canal

Bilateral Peripheral
• Idiopathic—rare
• Inflammatory and immune-mediated—polyradiculoneuritis, including coonhound paralysis;* polyneuropathies;* myasthenia gravis*
• Metabolic—paraneoplastic polyneuropathy (e.g., insulinoma)
• Toxic—botulism
• Pituitary neoplasm—unknown cause

CNS
• Most unilateral
• Inflammatory—infectious (e.g., viral, bacterial, fungal, rickettsial, protozoal) and noninfectious (e.g., granulomatous meningoencephalomyelitis)
• Neoplastic—primary brain tumor; metastatic tumor

RISK FACTORS
Chronic ear disease

DIAGNOSIS

DIFFERENTIAL DIAGNOSIS
• Differentiate unilateral from bilateral.
• Look for other neurologic deficits.
• Idiopathic—likely if patient has no historical or physical signs of ear disease and no other neurologic deficits
• Hypothyroidism—with clinical evidence (e.g., lethargy and poor hair coat)
• Middle or inner ear disease—with head tilt or Horner syndrome
• CNS disease—suspect if the patient is depressed and displays neurologic signs related to the brainstem

CBC/BIOCHEMISTRY/URINALYSIS
•*Usually normal in idiopathic facial paralysis
• Hypercholesterolemia or nonregenerative anemia—may be seen with hypothyroidism-associated facial paralysis
• Hypoglycemia—with insulinoma

OTHER LABORATORY TESTS
• Mainly indicated for patients with bilateral weakness
• Amended insulin:glucose ratio—detect insulinoma
• Acetylcholine receptor antibodies—detect myasthenia gravis
• ELISA—detect coonhound paralysis
• Hypothyroidism tests

FACIAL NERVE PARESIS/PARALYSIS

IMAGING
• Radiographs—bullae (i.e., oblique, open mouthed); define middle ear disease and fractures
• CT and MRI—define ear or brainstem disease

DIAGNOSTIC PROCEDURES
• Schirmer tear test—evaluate tear production
• Electromyography and evaluation of motor nerve conduction velocity—detect polyradiculoneuritis and polyneuropathy
• CSF examination—detect brainstem disease

PATHOLOGIC FINDINGS
• Idiopathic—may see degeneration of large and small myelinated fibers without evidence of inflammation

 TREATMENT

APPROPRIATE HEALTH CARE
• Outpatient—idiopathic facial paralysis
• Inpatient—initial medical work up and management of systemic or CNS disease

NURSING CARE
N/A

ACTIVITY
N/A

DIET
No change required

CLIENT EDUCATION
• Advise client that the clinical signs are usually permanent, but as muscle fibrosis develops, there is a natural "tuck up" that reduces asymmetry; drooling usually stops within 2–4 weeks.
• Inform client that the other side can become affected.
• Discuss eye care: the cornea on the affected side may need lubrication; extra care may be needed if the animal is a breed with natural exophthalmos; client must regularly check for corneal ulcers.
• Inform client that most animals tolerate this nerve deficit well.

SURGICAL CONSIDERATIONS
Bulla osteotomy—may be useful in patients with disorders of the middle ear

 MEDICATIONS

DRUGS OF CHOICE
• Treat specific disease if possible
• Idiopathic disease—none specific; efficacy of steroids unknown
• Tear replacement—if Schirmer tear test value low; with ectropion or exophthalmic globes

CONTRAINDICATIONS
N/A

PRECAUTIONS
N/A

POSSIBLE INTERACTIONS
N/A

ALTERNATIVE DRUGS
N/A

 FOLLOW-UP

PATIENT MONITORING
• Re-evaluate early for evidence of corneal ulcers.
• Assess monthly for menace responses, palpebral reflexes, and lip and ear movements to evaluate return of function and condition of affected eye, although damage is usually permanent.

PREVENTION AVOIDANCE
N/A

POSSIBLE COMPLICATIONS
• Keratoconjunctivitis sicca
• Corneal ulcers
• Severe contracture on side of lesion

EXPECTED COURSE AND PROGNOSIS
• Depend on cause
• Inpatient with idiopathic disease—prognosis guarded for recovery
• Improvement may take weeks or months or may never occur.
• Lip contracture sometimes develops

 MISCELLANEOUS

ASSOCIATED CONDITIONS
N/A

AGE-RELATED FACTORS
N/A

ZOONOTIC POTENTIAL
N/A

PREGNANCY
N/A

SYNONYMS
Idiopathic facial paresis and paralysis

SEE ALSO
• Hypothyroidism
• Keratitis, Ulcerative
• Keratoconjunctivitis Sicca (KCS)
• Otitis Media and Interna

ABBREVIATIONS
• CSF = cerebrospinal fluid
• ELISA = enzyme-linked immunosorbent assay

Suggested Reading
Braund KG, Luttgen PJ, Sorjonen DC, et al. Idiopathic facial paralysis in the dog. Vet Rec 1979;105:297–299.
de Lahunta A. Veterinary neuroanatomy and clinical neurology. 2nd ed. Philadelphia: Saunders, 1983.
Kern TJ, Hollis NE. Facial neuropathy in dogs and cats: 95 cases (1975–1985). J Am Vet Med Assoc 1987191:1604–1609.
Author T. Mark Neer
Consulting Editor Joane M. Parent

DISEASES

FALSE PREGNANCY

BASICS

DEFINITION
Display of maternal behavior and physical signs of pregnancy in middle to late diestrus by a nonpregnant bitch

PATHOPHYSIOLOGY
• Underlying endocrinologic mechanism—poorly understood; all bitches that ovulate produce functional corpora lutea and remain under progesterone influence for 2–3 months.
• Serum progesterone concentrations—similar in pregnant, nonpregnant, and false pregnant animals, except for a sharp decline 1–2 days before parturition
• Thought that the falling serum progesterone concentration causes an increase in the serum prolactin concentration, which may be responsible for initiating the changes seen in false pregnant animals.
• Mating during the preceding estrus—no influence on occurrence
• Future fertility not affected

SYSTEMS AFFECTED
Reproductive

GENETICS
N/A

INCIDENCE/PREVALENCE
Unknown

GEOGRAPHIC DISTRIBUTION
N/A

SIGNALMENT
Nonpregnant females that were in estrus 2–3 months earlier and that are experiencing a decline in serum progesterone concentration

Species
• Common in dogs
• Rare in cats

Breed Predilections
None

Mean Age and Range
Any age

Predominant Sex
Female

SIGNS

General Comments
Severity variable among individuals and from one occurrence to the next within the same individual

Historical Findings
• Behavior changes—nesting, mothering activity, restlessness, and self-nursing
• Abdominal distention and mammary gland enlargement
• Vomiting, depression, and anorexia
• Signs of labor (rare)

Physical Examination Findings
Large mammary glands that secrete a brownish serous fluid or milk

CAUSES
• Progesterone and prolactin—inverse relationship; drop in progesterone concentration in late diestrus causes prolactin concentration to rise.
• Treatment with progestin for conditions not related to false pregnancy—may develop signs after drug withdrawal
• Oophorectomy or ovariohysterectomy during diestrus (when progesterone is high)—may develop signs postsurgery
• Hypothyroidism with high TSH concentration (stimulates prolactin secretion)—may note some associated clinical signs

RISK FACTORS
• Not thought to be influenced by previous pregnancy
• Does not cause predisposition to other reproductive diseases

DIAGNOSIS

DIFFERENTIAL DIAGNOSIS
• Diagnosis—made by a history of estrus within the preceding 2–3 months and clinical signs
• Other causes of mammary gland enlargement—neoplasia; mastitis
• Other causes of abdominal enlargement—ascites; organomegaly
• Closed pyometra—usually associated with more severe systemic signs than false pregnancy
• Pregnancy

CBC/BIOCHEMISTRY/URINALYSIS
Usually normal; if not, suspect other reproductive tract or systemic disease.

OTHER LABORATORY TESTS
N/A

IMAGING
Radiography or ultrasonography—recommended to rule out pyometra and normal pregnancy

DIAGNOSTIC PROCEDURES
N/A

PATHOLOGIC FINDINGS
N/A

TREATMENT

APPROPRIATE HEALTH CARE
• May discharge immediately if medical treatment is tried
• Inpatient—planned surgery
• Treatment usually unnecessary—all pregnant, nonpregnant, and false pregnant, ovulating dogs go through a similar diestrus stage.
• Progestins and androgens—suppress prolactin secretion.
• Ovariohysterectomy during anestrus—prevents recurrence

NURSING CARE
• Mammary glands—minimize stimuli that promote lactation (e.g., cold and warm packs)
• Elizabethan collar—prevent self-nursing or licking; but even rubbing of the collar on the mammary glands may be sufficient to prolong lactation.

ACTIVITY
N/A

DIET
Reduction of food over 3–4 days—may reduce lactation

CLIENT EDUCATION
• Inform client that false pregnancy is a normal phenomenon in ovulatory bitches.
• Assure client that there is no association between false pregnancy and reproductive abnormalities.
• Encourage client to attempt pregnancy during the next estrous cycle if bitch is to be bred.

SURGICAL CONSIDERATIONS
Ovariohysterectomy—fertility not an issue; recommend during the next anestrus; do not perform while patient has clinical signs, because surgery will not alleviate signs and medical treatment may be required.

 MEDICATIONS

DRUG
Bromocriptine—10 µg/kg PO q12h for 5 days; not approved for veterinary use in U.S. and Canada; will reduce lactation

CONTRAINDICATIONS
Bromocriptine—induces abortion in pregnant animals

PRECAUTIONS
Bromocriptine—with vomiting, give half the dosage for the next two doses; then give the full dosage again.

POSSIBLE INTERACTIONS
Concomitant use of erythromycin may increase bromocriptine plasma concentration.

ALTERNATIVE DRUGS
• Testosterone—1 mg/kg IM once; may cause virilizing effects (e.g., clitoral hypertrophy); contraindicated with hepatic or nephritic conditions; causes masculinization of female fetuses if given in pregnancy
• Mibolerone—Cheque, 40 µg/kg PO q24h for 5 days; same side effects as testosterone
• Megestrol acetate—Ovaban, 1–2 mg/kg PO q24h for 8 days; may cause mammary hyperplasia, pyometra, diabetes mellitus, increased appetite, weight gain, and atrophy of the adrenal cortex; signs may recur after discontinuation.
• Mild tranquilizers may reduce behavioral signs; do not use phenothiazines, which may increase prolactin concentration

 FOLLOW-UP

PATIENT MONITORING
N/A

PREVENTION/AVOIDANCE
Ovariohysterectomy during anestrus—prevents recurrence

POSSIBLE COMPLICATIONS
N/A

EXPECTED COURSE AND PROGNOSIS
• Usually resolves in 2–3 weeks without treatment
• Bromocriptine—may resolve condition in 1 week
• May develop during subsequent estrous cycles

 MISCELLANEOUS

ASSOCIATED CONDITIONS
N/A

AGE-RELATED FACTORS
N/A

ZOONOTIC POTENTIAL
N/A

PREGNANCY
Do not treat pregnant animals.

SYNONYMS
• Pseudopregnancy
• Pseudocyesis
• Phantom pregnancy

ABBREVIATION
• TSH = thyroid-stimulating hormone

Suggested Reading
Allen WE. Pseudopregnancy in the bitch: the current view on aetiology and treatment. J Small Anim Pract 1986;27:419–424.
Arbeiter K, Brass W, Ballabio R, et al. Treatment of pseudopregnancy in the bitch with cabergoline, an ergoline derivative. J Small Anim Pract 1988;29:781–788.
Johnson CA. False pregnancy, disorders of pregnancy, parturition. In: Nelson RW, Couto CG, eds., Essentials of small animal internal medicine. St. Louis: Mosby, 1992;669–683.
Johnston SD. Pseudopregnancy in the bitch. In: Morrow DA, ed. Current therapy in theriogenology 2. Philadelphia: Saunders, 1986;490–491.
Author Klass Post
Consulting Editor Sara K. Lyle

FANCONI'S SYNDROME

BASICS

OVERVIEW
A collection of abnormalities arising from defective renal tubular transport of water, sodium, potassium, glucose, phosphate, bicarbonate, and amino acids; impaired tubular reabsorption causes excessive urinary excretion of these solutes.

SIGNALMENT
• Documented in several breeds of dogs; not in cats
• Approximately 75% of the reported cases have occurred in the Basenji breed; estimates of the prevalence within the Basenji breed in North America range from 10 to 30%; it is presumed to be inherited in this breed, but the mode of inheritance is unknown.

Breed Predilections
• No sex predilection

Mean Age and Range
• Age at diagnosis ranges from 10 weeks to 11 years; most develop clinical signs from 2–4 years.

SIGNS
General Comments
• Vary depending on the severity of specific solute losses and whether renal failure has developed

• Loss of amino acids and glucose—usually not associated with clinical signs other than polyuria and polydipsia

Historical Findings
• Polyuria
• Polydipsia
• Weight loss
• ± Lethargy
• ± Reduced appetite

Physical Examination Findings
• Poor body condition
• Reduced and/or abnormal growth (rickets) in young, growing animals

CAUSES & RISK FACTORS
• Inherited (or idiopathic) in most cases; particularly in Basenjis, Norwegian elkhounds, Shetland sheepdogs, and schnauzer breeds
• Acquired Fanconi's syndrome—reported in dogs treated with gentamicin, streptozotocin, and amoxicillin; also reported secondary to primary hypoparathyroidism

DIAGNOSIS

DIFFERENTIAL DIAGNOSIS
Primary renal glucosuria—both cause glucosuria in the absence of hyperglycemia; documentation of aminoaciduria, mild proteinuria, or a normal anion gap metabolic acidosis (indicating bicarbonate loss) suggests Fanconi's syndrome

CBC/BIOCHEMISTRY/URINALYSIS
• CBC usually normal
• Hypokalemia in about one-third
• Azotemia if patient has renal failure
• Hypophosphatemia and hypocalcemia may occur in young, growing animals.
• Urine specific gravity usually low (1.005–1.018); mild proteinuria common
• Glucosuria in the absence of hyper-glycemia—found frequently; often the first suggestion of Fanconi's syndrome

OTHER LABORATORY TESTS
Blood gas analysis may reveal normal anion gap metabolic acidosis, which develops because of urinary bicarbonate loss (referred to as proximal renal tubular acidosis); urine remains acidic, and bicarbonate does not appear in the urine unless a bicarbonate load is administered.

IMAGING
Young, growing dogs may exhibit radiographic findings consistent with rickets (decreased bone density, wide irregular growth plates) and angular limb deformities; adult patients may exhibit decreased bone density.

DIAGNOSTIC PROCEDURES
Urinary clearance studies to document excessive excretion of solutes such as amino acids may be needed for confirmation.

PATHOLOGIC FINDINGS
Renal papillary necrosis in many patients

TREATMENT

• Discontinue any drug that may cause Fanconi's syndrome or treat for a specific intoxication.
• No treatment will reverse the transport defects in dogs with inherited or idiopathic disease.
• Because the number and severity of transport defects vary markedly between animals, treatments for hypokalemia, metabolic acidosis, renal failure, or rickets must be individualized. Treatments for hypokalemia, renal failure, and rickets are discussed elsewhere in this publication.
• Institute treatment for metabolic acidosis if blood bicarbonate concentration is <12 mEq/L; large doses of bicarbonate may be required because reduced tubular resorptive capacity results in marked urinary bicarbonate loss; the goal of bicarbonate therapy is to maintain blood bicarbonate concentration from 12 to 18 mEq/L.
• Young, growing dogs may require vitamin D and/or calcium and phosphorous supplementation.

MEDICATIONS

DRUGS
Sodium bicarbonate (10–50 mg/kg q8–12h) or potassium citrate (40–75 mg/kg q12h) as required (based on blood gas and electrolyte measurements) in patients with metabolic acidosis.

CONTRAINDICATIONS/POSSIBLE INTERACTIONS
Avoid drugs that are nephrotoxic or have the potential to cause Fanconi's syndrome (see Causes and Risk Factors).

FOLLOW-UP

• Monitor serum biochemistry at 10- to 14-day intervals to assess the effect of treatment and any change in parameters (especially BUN, creatinine, and potassium concentration); because bicarbonate therapy may aggravate renal potassium loss, monitor serum potassium concentration regularly; once stable, monitor serum chemistry at 2- to 4-month intervals. • Clinical course— varies; some dogs remain stable for years; others develop rapidly progressive renal failure over a few months; the cause of death is usually acute renal failure, often associated with severe metabolic acidosis.

MISCELLANEOUS

SEE ALSO
• Potassium, Hypokalemia
• Renal Failure, Chronic—Dogs
• Renal Failure, Acute—Dogs

Suggested Reading
Brown SA. Fanconi's syndrome. In: Kirk RW, ed. Current veterinary therapy X. Philadelphia: Saunders, 1989:1163–1165.
Author Darcy H. Shaw
Consulting Editors Larry G. Adams and Carl A. Osborne

FELINE IDIOPATHIC LOWER URINARY TRACT DISEASES

BASICS

DEFINITION
The terms *feline urologic syndrome* and *FUS* are used commonly by the veterinary profession as diagnostic terms to describe disorders of domestic cats characterized by hematuria, dysuria, pollakiuria, periuria, and partial or complete urethral obstruction, because varying combinations of these signs may be associated with any cause of feline lower urinary tract disease. The similarity of clinical signs with diverse causes is not surprising since the feline urinary tract responds to various diseases in a limited and predictable fashion. When used, the term *FUS* should be redefined as feline urologic *signs;* in this context, FUS is no more a diagnosis than are vomiting or pruritus. Idiopathic feline urinary tract disease is an exclusion diagnosis established only after known causes have been eliminated.

PATHOPHYSIOLOGY
• Refer to specific chapters describing diseases listed in section on differential diagnosis.
• Experimental and clinical studies have implicated calicivirus, feline syncytia-forming virus, and a gamma herpesvirus (bovine herpesvirus 4) as potential etiologic agents in some cats.
• Initial episodes of idiopathic lower urinary tract diseases usually occur in the absence of significant numbers of detectable bacteria and pyuria. Prospective diagnostic studies of male and female obstructed and nonobstructed cats identified bacterial urinary tract infections in <3% of patients.
• Some cats with lower urinary tract diseases exhibit findings similar to those observed in humans with interstitial cystitis, an idiopathic inflammatory disorder—decreased urine concentrations of glycosaminoglycans, increased urinary bladder permeability, and similar gross and light microscopic changes. These similarities prompted the hypothesis that some lower urinary tract diseases are analogous to human interstitial cystitis; further studies are essential to prove or disprove this hypothesis.

SYSTEMS AFFECTED
• Renal/Urologic—lower urinary tract
• Persistent urethral outflow obstruction results in postrenal azotemia.

GENETICS
N/A

INCIDENCE PREVALENCE
The incidence of hematuria, dysuria, and/or urethral obstruction in domestic cats in the United States and Great Britain was previously reported to be approximately 0.5–1.0% per year.

GEOGRAPHIC DISTRIBUTION
N/A

SIGNALMENT

Species
Cats

Breed Predilections
None

Mean Age and Range
• May occur at any age, but are most commonly recognized in young to middle-aged adults (mean age, 3.5 years).
• Uncommon in cats <1 year old and >10 years old

Predominant Sex
N/A

SIGNS

Historical Findings
• Dysuria
• Hematuria
• Pollakiuria
• Periuria—urinating in inappropriate locations
• Outflow obstruction

Physical Examination Findings
• Thickened, firm, contracted bladder wall
• May detect urethral plugs or uroliths by examination of the distal penis and penile urethra

CAUSES
• See Pathophysiology
• Noninfectious diseases including interstitial cystitis
• Viruses implicated

RISK FACTORS
Stress—may play a role in precipitating or exacerbating signs; an unlikely primary cause

DIAGNOSIS

DIFFERENTIAL DIAGNOSIS
• Metabolic disorders including various types of uroliths and urethral plugs
• Infectious agents including bacteria, mycoplasma/ureaplasma, fungal agents, and parasites
• Trauma
• Neurogenic disorders including reflex dyssynergia, urethral spasm, and hypotonic or atonic bladder (primary or secondary)
• Iatrogenic disease including reverse flushing solutions, urethral catheters, indwelling urethral catheters (especially open systems), postsurgical urethral catheters, and urethrostomy complications

• Anatomic abnormalities including urachal anomalies and acquired urethral strictures
• Neoplasia (benign and malignant)
• Clinical signs may be confused with constipation, which can be ruled out by abdominal palpation.

CBC/BIOCHEMISTRY/URINALYSIS
• Hematuria and proteinuria—usually present
• If urethral obstruction persists, serum chemistry profiles reveal azotemia, hyperphosphatemia, hyperkalemia, and reduced TCO_2.

OTHER LABORATORY TESTS
• Absence of bacteriuria—verify by quantitative urine culture; collect urine specimens by cystocentesis to avoid contamination with organisms that normally inhabit the distal urinary tract.
• Indirect fluorescent antibody test may reveal serum antibodies against bovine herpesvirus type 4 in some cats.
• Transmission electron microscopy may reveal calicivirus-like particles in some urethral plugs.

IMAGING
• Survey radiography—may exclude uroliths or urethral plugs
• Positive-contrast retrograde urethrocystography or antegrade cystography—may exclude urethral strictures, vesicourachal diverticula, and neoplasia
• Double-contrast cystography—may exclude small or radiolucent uroliths, blood clots, and thickening of the bladder wall due to inflammation or neoplasia
• Ultrasonography—may exclude uroliths

DIAGNOSTIC PROCEDURES
• Cystoscopy—may exclude uroliths and diverticula
• Biopsies obtained with urinary catheters, cystoscopes, or via surgery—may permit morphologic characterization of inflammatory or neoplastic lesions; not routinely needed

PATHOLOGIC FINDINGS
• Cystoscopy may reveal petechial hemorrhages (also called glomerulations) of the mucosal surface of the urinary bladder.
• Mucosal ulceration, congestion, submucosal edema, hemorrhage, and fibrosis; inflammatory cells may not be prominent, unless secondary bacterial urinary tract infections have resulted from catheterization or perineal urethrostomy.

TREATMENT

APPROPRIATE HEALTH CARE
• Patients with nonobstructive lower urinary tract diseases—typically managed as out-

FELINE IDIOPATHIC LOWER URINARY TRACT DISEASES

patients; diagnostic evaluation may require brief hospitalization.
• Patients with obstructive lower urinary tract diseases—usually hospitalized for diagnosis and management

NURSING CARE
N/A

ACTIVITY
N/A

DIET
• Management recommended for persistent crystalluria associated with matrix-crystalline urethral plugs
• Empirical observations suggest that recurrence of signs may be minimized by feeding moist rather than dry foods.

CLIENT EDUCATION
• Hematuria, dysuria, and pollakiuria—often self-limiting; subside within 4–7 days, but signs often recur unpredictably
• Lack of controlled studies that demonstrate efficacy of most drugs used to treat symptomatically
• Males should be monitored for signs of urethral obstruction.
• Reduce environmental stress by minimizing changes in the home, maintaining a constant diet, and providing safe places to hide.
• Provide proper litter box hygiene.

SURGICAL CONSIDERATIONS
• We do not recommend cystotomy to lavage and debride the bladder mucosa as a form of treatment.
• Do not perform perineal urethrostomies to minimize recurrent urethral obstruction without localizing obstructive disease to the penile urethra by contrast urethrography.

MEDICATIONS

DRUGS OF CHOICE
• Propantheline may be considered an anticholinergic to minimize hyperactivity of the bladder detrusor muscle and urge incontinence; because the smallest available tablet is 7.5 mg, suggested empirical dose is 0.25–0.5 mg/kg PO q12–24h.
• Amitriptyline, a tricyclic antidepressant and anxiolytic drug (with anticholinergic, antihistaminic, anti-α-adrenergic, antiinflammatory, and analgesic properties)—empirically advocated to treat cats with persistent signs; suggested empirical dosage is 5–10 mg/cat q24h given at night.
• Butorphanol—empirically recommended to reduce pain associated with lower urinary tract inflammation; suggested dosage is 1 mg/cat PO q12h.

• Phenoxybenzamine—may be used to minimize reflex dyssynergia and functional urethral outflow obstruction; suggested empirical dosage is 0.5 mg/kg PO q12h.
• Pentosan polysulfate sodium, a semisynthetic glycosaminoglycan—empirically recommended to help repair the glycosaminoglycan coating of the mucosa of the urinary tract; a controlled clinical trial is in progress, but results are not yet available.
• Corticosteroids—no detectable effect on remission of clinical signs demonstrated; predispose to bacterial urinary tract infections, especially in cats with indwelling transurethral catheters
• Dimethylsulfoxide (DMSO)—no detectable effect on remission of clinical signs demonstrated
• Antibiotics and methenamine—no detectable effect on remission of clinical signs in cats demonstrated

CONTRAINDICATIONS
• Phenazopyridine—a urinary tract analgesic used alone or in combination with sulfa drugs; may result in methemoglobinemia and irreversible oxidative changes in hemoglobin resulting in formation of Heinz bodies and anemia
• Methylene blue—a weak antiseptic agent; may cause Heinz bodies and severe anemia
• Bethanacol—a cholinergic drug used to manage hypotonic urinary bladders; do not use in patients with urethral obstruction.

PRECAUTIONS
• Cats with urethral obstruction and postrenal azotemia are at increased risk for adverse drug events, especially with drugs and anesthetics that depend on renal elimination or metabolism.
• Indwelling transurethral catheters, especially when associated with fluid-induced diuresis, predispose patients to bacterial urinary tract infections.

POSSIBLE INTERACTIONS
N/A

ALTERNATIVE DRUGS
N/A

FOLLOW-UP

PATIENT MONITORING
Monitor hematuria by urinalysis; cystocentesis may cause iatrogenic hematuria, so naturally voided samples are preferred.

PREVENTION/AVOIDANCE
• Empirical observations suggest that recurrence of signs may be minimized by feeding moist rather than dry foods.
• Reduce environmental stress.

POSSIBLE COMPLICATIONS
• Indwelling transurethral catheters—often cause trauma; predispose to ascending bacterial urinary tract infections
• Perineal urethrostomies—may predispose to bacterial urinary tract infections and urethral strictures

EXPECTED COURSE AND PROGNOSIS
Hematuria, dysuria, and pollakiuria often are self-limiting in patients with most idiopathic lower urinary tract diseases, subsiding within 4 to 7 days. These signs often recur unpredictably; the frequency of recurrence appears to decline with advancing age.

MISCELLANEOUS

ASSOCIATED CONDITIONS
N/A

AGE-RELATED FACTORS
Frequency of recurrence appears to decline with advancing age.

ZOONOTIC POTENTIAL
N/A

PREGNANCY
N/A

SYNONYMS
FUS (see section on definition), feline urological disease, feline urinary tract inflammation, feline interstitial cystitis, feline idiopathic cystitis

SEE ALSO
• Urolithiasis, Struvite—Cats
• Dysuria and Pollakiuria
• Lower Urinary Tract Infection
• Hematuria

ABBREVIATIONS
.None

Suggested Reading

Osborne CA, Kruger JM, Lulich JP, eds. Disorders of the feline lower urinary tract I. Etiology and pathophysiology. Vet Clin North Am 1996;26:169–421.

Osborne CA, Kruger JM, Lulich JP, eds. Disorders of the feline lower urinary tract II. Etiology and pathophysiology. Vet Clin North Am 1996;26:423–665.

Osborne, CA, Kruger, JM, Lulich JP, et al. Feline lower urinary tract diseases. In: Ettinger SJ, Feldman EC, eds. Textbook of veterinary internal medicine. 5th ed. Philadelphia: Saunders, 2000:1710–1747.

Authors Carl A. Osborne, John M. Kruger, Jody P. Lulich, and David J. Polzin
Consulting Editors Larry G. Adams and Carl A. Osborne

FELINE IMMUNODEFICIENCY VIRUS (FIV)

BASICS

DEFINITION
A retrovirus that causes an immunodeficiency disease in domestic cats; same subfamily (lentiviruses) as HIV, the causative agent of AIDS in humans

PATHOPHYSIOLOGY
• Infection disrupts immune system function; feline lymphocytes and macrophages serve as the main target cells for virus replication
• Acute infection—virus spreads from the site of entry to the lymph tissues and thymus, first infecting T lymphocytes then macrophages.
• CD4+ and CD8+ cells—both can be infected lytically in culture; virus selectively and progressively decreases CD4+ (T helper) cells; inversion of the CD4+:CD8+ ratio (from ~ 2:1 to < 1:1) develops slowly; an absolute decrease of CD4+ T cells is seen after several months of infection; patients are clinically asymptotic until cell-mediated immunity is disrupted.
• Humoral immune function—perturbed in advanced stages of infection
• Macrophages—main reservoir of virus in affected cats; transport virus to tissues throughout the body; defects in function (e.g., increased production of TNF)
• Astrocyte and microglial cells in the brain and megakaryocytes and mononuclear bone marrow cells may be infected.
• Co-infection with FeLV may increase the expression of FIV in many tissues, including kidney, brain, and liver.

SYSTEMS AFFECTED
• Hemic/Lymphatic/Immune—initially owing to loss of CD4+ T cells
• Nervous—alterations in sleep patterns and changes in visual, auditory, and spinal-evoked potentials; peripheral neuropathies
• Behavioral—repetitive movements, anxiety, or increased aggression may be seen.
• Other body systems—result of immuno-suppression and secondary infections

GENETICS
• No predisposition for infection
• May play a role in progression and severity

INCIDENCE/PREVALENCE
U.S. and Canada—1.5–3% in the healthy cat population; 9–15% in cats with signs of clinical illness

GEOGRAPHIC DISTRIBUTION
Worldwide; seroprevalence rates vary greatly

SIGNALMENT

Species
Cats

Breed Predilections
None

Mean Age and Range
• Prevalence of infection increases with age
• Mean age—5 years at time of diagnosis

Predominant Sex
Male—more aggressive; roaming

SIGNS

General Comments
• Diverse owing to immunosuppressive nature of infection
• Associated disease cannot be clinically distinguished from FeLV-associated immunodeficiencies.

Historical Findings
Recurrent minor illnesses, especially with upper respiratory and gastrointestinal signs

Physical Examination Findings
• Depend on occurrence of opportunistic infections
• Lymphadenomegaly—mild to moderate
• Gingivitis, stomatitis, periodontitis—25–50% of cases
• Upper respiratory tract—rhinitis; conjunctivitis; keratitis (~ 30% of cases); often associated with feline herpesvirus and calicivirus infections
• Persistent diarrhea—10–20% of cases; bacterial or fungal overgrowth parasite-induced inflammation; direct effect of FIV infection on the gastrointestinal epithelium
• Chronic, nonresponsive, or recurrent infections of the external ear and skin—from bacterial infections or dermatophytosis
• Fever and wasting—especially in later stage; possibly from high levels of TNF
• Ocular disease—anterior uveitis; pars planitis; glaucoma
• Lymphosarcoma or other neoplasia
• Neurologic abnormalities—disruption of normal sleep patterns; behavioral changes (pacing and aggression); peripheral neuropathies

CAUSES
• Cat-to-cat transmission; usually by bite wounds
• Occasional perinatal transmission

RISK FACTORS
• Male
• Free-roaming

DIAGNOSIS

DIFFERENTIAL DIAGNOSIS
• Primary bacterial, parasitic, viral, or fungal infections
• Toxoplasmosis—neurologic and ocular manifestations may be the result of *Toxoplasma* infection, FIV infection, or both
• Nonviral neoplastic diseases

CBC/BIOCHEMISTRY/URINALYSIS
• Hemogram may be normal.
• Anemia, lymphopenia, or neutropenia—may be seen; neutrophilia may occur in response to secondary infections.
• Urinalysis and serum chemistry profile—high serum protein from hypergamma-globulinemia; otherwise usually normal with no secondary infections

OTHER LABORATORY TESTS

Serologic Testing
• Detects antibodies to FIV
• ELISA—routine screening test; kits for in-house use to microtiter plates for diagnostic laboratory use; confirm positive results with additional testing, especially in healthy, low-risk cats or when diagnosis would result in euthanasia.
• Western blot (immunoblot)—confirmatory testing of ELISA-positive samples
• Kittens—when < 6 months old may test positive owing to passive transfer of anti-bodies from an FIV-positive queen; a positive test does not indicate infection; retest at 8–12 months to determine infection.

Others
• Virus isolation or detection—other methods occasionally available on an experimental basis; detection procedures usually not sensitive enough for diagnostic purposes
• CD4+:CD8+ evaluation—helps determine extent of immunosuppression

IMAGING
N/A

DIAGNOSTIC PROCEDURES
N/A

PATHOLOGIC FINDINGS
• Lymphadenopathy—associated with follicular hyperplasia and massive paracortical infiltration of plasmacytes; later, may see a mixture of follicular hyperplasia and follicular depletion or involution; in terminal stages, lymphoid depletion is predominant finding.
• Lymphocytic and plasmacytic infiltrates—gingiva, lymph nodes and other lymphoid tissues, spleen, kidney, liver, and brain
• Perivascular cuffing, gliosis, neuronal loss, white matter vacuolization, and occasional giant cells in the brain
• Intestinal lesions similar to those seen with feline parvovirus infection (feline panleukopenia-like syndrome)

TREATMENT

APPROPRIATE HEALTH CARE
• Outpatient sufficient for most patients
• Inpatient—with severe secondary infections until condition is stable

FELINE IMMUNODEFICIENCY VIRUS (FIV)

NURSING CARE
• Primary consideration—manage secondary and opportunistic infections
• Supportive therapy—parenteral fluids and nutritional supplements, as required

ACTIVITY
Normal

DIET
• Normal
• Diarrhea, kidney disease, or chronic wasting—special food, as needed

CLIENT EDUCATION
• Inform client that the infection is slowly progressive and healthy antibody-positive cats may remain healthy for years.
• Advise client that cats with clinical signs will have recurrent or chronic health problems that require medical attention.
• Discuss the importance of keeping cats indoors to protect them from exposure to secondary pathogens and to prevent spread of FIV.

SURGICAL CONSIDERATIONS
• Oral treatment or surgery—frequently required; dental cleaning, tooth extraction, gingival biopsy
• Biopsy or removal of tumors

MEDICATIONS

DRUGS OF CHOICE
• Immunomodulatory drugs—alleviate some clinical signs; hrα-interferon (Roferon) diluted in saline at 30 units/day PO for 7 days every other week; may increase survival rates and improve clinical status; also try propionibacterium acnes (Immunoregulin) at 0.5 mL/cat IV, once or twice weekly, or acemannan (Carrisyn) at 100 mg/cat PO daily
• Gingivitis and stomatitis—may be refractory to treatment
• Antibacterial or antimycotic drugs—useful for overgrowth of bacteria or fungi; prolonged therapy or high dosages may be required; for anaerobic bacterial infections use metronidazole (Flagyl) at 7–15 mg/kg PO q8h or q12h or clindamycin (Antirobe) at 11 mg/kg PO q12h.
• Corticosteroids or gold salts—judicious but aggressive use may help control immune-mediated inflammation.
• Anorexia—short-term appetite stimulation: diazepam (Valium) at 0.2 mg/kg IV or oral oxazepam (Serax) at 2.5 mg/cat IV; more prolonged appetite stimulation and reversal of cachexia: anabolic steroids or megestrol acetate; efficacy in FIV-positive cats unknown

• Topical corticosteroids—for anterior uveitis; long-term response may be incomplete or poor; pars planitis often regresses spontaneously and may recur.
• Glaucoma—standard treatment
• Yearly vaccination for respiratory and enteric viruses with inactivated vaccines is recommended.

CONTRAINDICATIONS
• Griseofulvin—avoid or use with extreme caution in FIV-positive cats; may induce severe neutropenia; neutropenia is reversible if the drug is withdrawn early enough but secondary infections associated with the condition can be life-threatening.
• MLV vaccines—may cause disease in immunosuppressed cats

PRECAUTIONS
Systemic corticosteroids—use with caution; may lead to further immunosuppression

POSSIBLE INTERACTIONS
See Contraindications

ALTERNATIVE DRUGS
N/A

FOLLOW-UP

PATIENT MONITORING
Varies according to secondary infections and other manifestations of disease

PREVENTION/AVOIDANCE
• Prevent contact with FIV-positive cats.
• Quarantine and test incoming cats before introducing into multicat households.
• Vaccines—efficacious vaccines not available; experimental vaccines have shown some promise; most not uniformly active against all strains of the virus

POSSIBLE COMPLICATIONS
N/A

EXPECTED COURSE AND PROGNOSIS
• Within the first 2 years after diagnosis or 4.5–6 years after the estimated time of infection, about 20% of cats die but > 50% remain asymptomatic.
• In late stages of disease (wasting and frequent or severe opportunistic infections), life expectancy is ≤ 1 year.

MISCELLANEOUS

ASSOCIATED CONDITIONS
• Secondary bacterial, viral, fungal, and parasitic disease
• Lymphoid tumors
• Immune-mediated disease

AGE-RELATED FACTORS
Kittens may test positive because of passive antibody transfer.

ZOONOTIC POTENTIAL
• None known; evidence against FIV transmission to humans is compelling but cannot be considered conclusive owing to the relatively short time the virus has been studied.
• Potential transmission of secondary pathogens (e.g., *Toxoplasma gondii*) to immunocompromised humans

PREGNANCY
FIV-positive queens—reported abortions and stillbirths; transmission to kittens is infrequent if the queen is antibody-positive before conception.

SYNONYMS
Feline immunodeficiency syndrome

SEE ALSO
Individual topics on secondary infectious diseases, ocular disease, gingivitis, and stomatitis

ABBREVIATIONS
• ELISA = enzyme-linked immunosorbent assay
• FeLV = feline leukemia virus
• HIV = human immunodeficiency virus
• hrα-interferon = human recombinant α-interferon
• MLV = modified live virus
• TNF = tumor necrosis factor

Suggested Reading

Barr MC, Olsen CW, Scott FW. Feline viral diseases. In: Ettinger SJ, Feldman EC, eds., Textbook of veterinary internal medicine. 4th ed. Philadelphia: Saunders, 1994:409–439.

English RV, Nelson P, Johnson CM, et al. Development of clinical disease in cats experimentally infected with feline immunodeficiency virus. J Infect Dis 1994;170:543–552.

Ishida T, Taniguchi A, Matsumura S, et al. Long-term clinical observations on feline immunodeficiency virus infected asymptomatic carriers. Vet Immunol Immunopathol 1992;35:15–22.

Sparger EE: Current thoughts on feline immunodeficiency virus infection. Vet Clin North Am Small Anim Pract 1993;23:173–191.

Author Margaret C. Barr
Consulting Editor Stephen C. Barr

DISEASE

FELINE INFECTIOUS PERITONITIS (FIP)

BASICS

DEFINITION
A systemic, viral disease characterized by insidious onset, persistent nonresponsive fever, pyogranulomatous tissue reaction, accumulation of exudative effusions in body cavities, and high mortality

PATHOPHYSIOLOGY
• FIP virus replicates locally in epithelial cells of the upper respiratory tract or oropharynx.
• Antiviral antibodies are produced, and the virus is taken up by macrophages.
• The virus is transported within monocytes/macrophages throughout the body; localizes at various vein wall and perivascular sites
• Local perivascular viral replication and subsequent pyogranulomatous tissue reaction produce the classic lesion.

SYSTEMS AFFECTED
• Multisystemic—pyogranulomatous or granulomatous lesions in the omentum, on the serosal surface of abdominal organs (e.g., liver, kidney, and intestines), within abdominal lymph nodes, and in the submucosa of the intestinal tract
• Respiratory—lesions on lung surfaces; pleural effusion in the wet form
• Nervous—vascular lesions can occur throughout the CNS, especially in the meninges.
• Ophthalmic—lesions may include uveitis and chorioretinitis.

GENETICS
N/A

INCIDENCE/PREVALENCE
• Prevalence of antibodies against FCoV—high in most populations, especially in multicat facilities
• Incidence of clinical disease—low in most populations, especially in single-cat households
• Because of the difficulty in diagnosis, control, and prevention, outbreaks within breeding catteries may be catastrophic; in endemic catteries, the risk of a FCoV antibody-positive cat eventually developing FIP is usually < 10%.

GEOGRAPHIC DISTRIBUTION
Worldwide

SIGNALMENT

Species
Cats—domestic and exotic

Breed Predilections
Some families or lines of cats appear more susceptible.

Mean Age and Range
• Highest incidence—in kittens 3 months to 3 years of age
• Incidence decreases sharply after cats reach 3 years of age

Predominant Sex
N/A

SIGNS

General Comments
• A wide range, depending on the virulence of the strain, effectiveness of the host immune response, and organ system affected
• Two classic forms—wet or effusive form, targets the body cavities; dry or noneffusive form, targets a variety of organs

Historical Findings
• Insidious onset
• Gradual weight loss and decrease in appetite
• Stunting in kittens
• Gradual increase in the size of the abdomen, giving a potbellied appearance
• Persistent fever—fluctuating; antibiotic unresponsive

Physical Examination Findings
• Depression
• Poor condition
• Stunted growth
• Weight loss
• Dull, rough hair coat
• Icterus
• Abdominal and/or pleural effusion
• Palpation of the abdomen—abdominal masses (granulomas or pyogranulomas) within the omentum, on the surface of viscera (especially the kidney), and within the intestinal wall; mesenteric lymph nodes may be enlarged.
• Ocular—anterior uveitis; keratic precipitates; color change to the iris; and irregularly shaped pupil
• Neurologic—brainstem, cerebrocortical, or spinal cord

CAUSES
• Two genomic types of FCoV—FCoV-1 (causes perhaps 85% of infections) and FCoV-2
• Distinguishing between forms—there has been great effort to distinguish between the low virulent or avirulent enteric strains (FECV) and the virulent strains; but FECV and FIP virus occur in both type 1 and type 2 forms; within each type is a spectrum from avirulent viruses that produce asymptomatic infections to those that produce fatal FIP.

RISK FACTORS
• Contact with a FCoV antibody-positive cat
• Breeding catteries or multicat facilities
• Less than 3 years of age
• FeLV infection

DIAGNOSIS
• Wet form—relatively easy to diagnose clinically
• Dry form—difficult to diagnose accurately
• No single diagnostic laboratory test

DIFFERENTIAL DIAGNOSIS
• Fever of unknown origin—when other causes of fever are ruled out
• Cardiac disease causing pleural effusion—effusion has low specific gravity and cell count
• Lesions of lymphoma, especially in the kidney, on palpation
• CNS tumors—most cats test positive for FeLV; for FeLV-negative cats, biopsy the lesion (if accessible) for histopathology and immunohistochemistry for FCoV
• Respiratory disease—FCV, FHV, chlamydiosis, or various bacteria
• Pansteatitis (yellow fat disease)—classic feel and appearance of fat within the abdominal cavity; pain on abdominal palpation; often a fish-only diet
• Panleukopenia producing enteritis—leukopenia; positive fecal canine parvovirus antigen assay

CBC/BIOCHEMISTRY/URINALYSIS
• Leukopenia—common early in the infection; later leukocytosis with neutrophilia and lymphopenia
• Mild to moderate anemia may occur.
• High total plasma globulin common
• Often hyperbilirubinemia and hyperbilirubinuria

OTHER LABORATORY TESTS
• Serum antibody tests—immunoassays, viral neutralization assays; detect antibodies against FCoV; positive tests not diagnostic, indicate only previous infection; correlation between height of titer and eventual confirmation of infection not high
• PCR assays—detect viral antigen; accuracy of positive tests correlating with clinical disease is still being evaluated.
• Immunohistochemistry (immunoperoxidase) assays detect FCoV within specific cells of biopsy samples or histopathologic sections of tissues from cats with fatal diseases; excellent for confirming cause of specific lesions, especially inflammatory abdominal disease, which is often is not diagnosed as FIP

IMAGING
• Generally not required
• May confirm abdominal and pleural effusions
• May detect granulomatous lesions

DIAGNOSTIC PROCEDURES
• Fluid obtained via thoracocentesis and abdominocentesis—pale to straw colored; viscous; flecks of white fibrin often seen; will clot upon standing; specific gravity usually high (1.030–1.040)
• Laparoscopy—to observe specific lesions of the peritoneal cavity; to obtain a biopsy sample for histopathology or immunohistochemistry confirmation

FELINE INFECTIOUS PERITONITIS (FIP)

- Exploratory laparotomy—may be indicated for difficult-to-diagnose patients if laparoscopy is not available

PATHOLOGIC FINDINGS

Gross
- Vary depending on the organs or tissues involved
- Patient will be emaciated, with a rough hair coat.

Wet Form
- Abdomen and/or thoracic cavity—may contain a thick, viscous exudate
- White, rough, pyogranulomatous plaques—may be on serosal surface of abdominal organs and the omentum
- Granulomatous lumps—may protrude from the surface of the kidney
- Granulomas—may be in the intestinal wall
- Fibrous strands—may extend between organs
- Liver—may have focal, pale lesions
- Iris—may be discolored
- Cornea—may see keratic precipitates
- Neurologic signs—may see lesions in the brain and/or the spinal cord

Histopathologic
- Granulomatous or pyogranulomatous in any affected tissue
- Lesions—start around veins; increase in size, involving large portions of tissue; microscopic appearance suggests the diagnosis.

TREATMENT

APPROPRIATE HEALTH CARE
Inpatient or outpatient, depending on stage and severity of disease and owner's willingness and ability to provide good supportive care

NURSING CARE
- Therapeutic paracentesis—to relieve pressure from excessive ascites or pleural effusions
- Important to encourage the affected cat to eat

ACTIVITY
Restrict to prevent exposure of other cats, although greatest degree of virus shed occurs before the patient shows signs

DIET
Any food that will entice the patient to eat

CLIENT EDUCATION
- Discuss the various aspects of disease, including the grave prognosis.
- Inform client of the high prevalence of FCoV infection but low incidence of actual clinical disease; > 10% of FCoV-positive cats < 3 years of age eventually develop clinical disease.

SURGICAL CONSIDERATIONS
- Generally none
- Rarely, inflammatory abdominal disease from FCoV may present with intestinal obstruction; abdominal surgery may be required.

MEDICATIONS

DRUGS OF CHOICE
- No treatment routinely effective
- Patients with generalized and typical signs almost invariably die
- Most FCoV-positive cats have subclinical infection or mild, localized granulomatous disease that is not diagnosed as FIP
- Immunosuppressive drugs (e.g., prednisolone and cyclophosphamide)—limited success
- Corticosteroids (subconjunctival injection)—may help ocular involvement
- Interferons—effective in vitro; limited success; a recombinant interferon reported to have some success in Japan
- Antibiotics—ineffective because generally not associated with secondary bacterial infections

CONTRAINDICATIONS
N/A

PRECAUTIONS
N/A

POSSIBLE INTERACTIONS
N/A

ALTERNATIVE DRUGS
No antiviral drugs proven to be efficacious

FOLLOW-UP

PATIENT MONITORING
Monitor for development of large quantities of pleural effusion.

PREVENTION/AVOIDANCE
- MLV intranasal vaccine—available against FIP virus; efficacy low; cannot rely on vaccination alone for control; may produce antibody-positive cats, complicating monitoring in catteries or colonies
- Mother/offspring—main method of transmission appears to be from asymptomatic carrier queens to their kittens at 5–7 weeks of age, after maternally derived immunity wanes; break cycle of transmission by early weaning at 4–5 weeks of age and isolating litter from direct contact with other cats, including the queen
- Routine disinfection—premise, cages, and water/food dishes; readily inactivates virus; reduces transmission
- Introduce only FCoV-negative cats to catteries or colonies that are free of virus

- Restrict household cats to indoor environments.

POSSIBLE COMPLICATIONS
- Pleural effusion may require thoracocentesis.
- Intestinal obstruction from inflammatory abdominal disease
- Neurologic disease from CNS lesions

EXPECTED COURSE AND PROGNOSIS
- Clinical course—a few days to several months
- Prognosis grave once typical signs occur; mortality nearly 100%

MISCELLANEOUS

ASSOCIATED CONDITIONS
- FeLV-positive cats—more prone to develop clinical disease

AGE-RELATED FACTORS
N/A

ZOONOTIC POTENTIAL
None

PREGNANCY
FIP virus can infect fetuses, resulting in fetal death or neonatal disease.

SYNONYMS
Feline coronavirus infection

ABBREVIATIONS
- FCoV = feline coronavirus
- FCV = feline calicivirus
- FECV = feline enteric coronavirus
- FeLV = feline leukemia virus
- FHV = feline herpes virus
- MLV = modified live virus
- PCR = polymerase chain reaction

Suggested Reading
Barr MC, Olsen CW, Scott FW. Feline viral diseases. In: Ettinger SJ, Feldman EC, eds. Veterinary internal medicine. 4th ed. Philadelphia: Saunders, 1995:409–439.

Report from the International FIP/FECV Workshop. Feline Pract 1995;23:2–111.

Sparkes AH, Gruffydd-Jones TJ, Harbour DA. An appraisal of the value of laboratory tests in the diagnosis of feline infectious peritonitis. J Am Anim Hosp Assoc 1994;30:345–350.

Author Fred W. Scott
Consulting Editor Stephen C. Barr

DISEASES

FELINE LEUKEMIA VIRUS (FeLV)

BASICS

DEFINITION
A retrovirus (oncovirus subfamily) that causes immunodeficiency and neoplastic disease in domestic cats

PATHOPHYSIOLOGY
• Early infection consists of five stages—(1) viral replication in tonsils and pharyngeal lymph nodes; (2) infection of a few circulating B lymphocytes and macrophages that disseminate the virus; (3) replication in lymphoid tissues, intestinal crypt epithelial cells, and bone marrow precursor cells; (4) release of infected neutrophils and platelets from the bone marrow into the circulatory system; and (5) infection of epithelial and glandular tissues, with subsequent shedding of virus into the saliva and urine
• An adequate immune response stops progression at stage 2 or 3 (4–8 weeks after exposure) and forces the virus into latency.
• Persistent viremia (stages 4 and 5) usually develops 4–6 weeks after infection, but may take 12 weeks.
Tumor Induction
• Occurs when the DNA provirus integrates into cat chromosomal DNA in critical regions (oncogenes)
• Virus integration near the cellular gene c-*myc* or near genes influencing the expression of c-*myc*—often results in thymic lymphosarcoma
• Changes in the virus's *env* gene—owing to mutations or recombinations with endogenous retroviral *env* sequences
• Feline sarcoma viruses—mutants of FeLV; arise by recombination between the genes of FeLV and host; virus–host fusion proteins are responsible for the efficient induction of fibrosarcomas.

SYSTEMS AFFECTED
• Hemic/Lymphatic/Immune—anemia; blood cell dyscrasias; neoplasias originating in the bone marrow; immunosuppression, possibly resulting from neuroendocrine dysfunction; absolute decrease in CD4+ and CD8+ subsets of T cells; decreased CD4+:CD8+ ratio
• All other body systems—immunosuppression with secondary infections or development of neoplastic disease

GENETICS
No genetic predisposition

INCIDENCE/PREVALENCE
Prevalence in U.S.—2–3% in the healthy cat population; three to four times greater in cats exhibiting signs of clinical illness

GEOGRAPHIC DISTRIBUTION
Worldwide

SIGNALMENT
Species
Cats

Breed Predilections
None

Mean Age and Range
• Prevalence highest between 1 and 6 years of age
• Mean—3 years

Predominant Sex
Male:female ratio—1.7:1

SIGNS
General Comments
• Onset of FeLV-associated disease—usually occurs over a period of months to years after infection
• Associated diseases—nonneoplastic or neoplastic; most of the nonneoplastic or degenerative diseases result from immunosuppression.
• Clinical signs of FeLV-induced immunodeficiency cannot be distinguished from those of FIV-induced immunodeficiency.

Historical Findings
• Patient allowed outdoors
• Member of a multicat household

Physical Examination Findings
• Depend on the type of disease (neoplastic or nonneoplastic) and occurrence of secondary infections
• Lymphadenomegaly—mild to severe
• Upper respiratory tract—rhinitis, conjunctivitis, and keratitis
• Persistent diarrhea—bacterial or fungal overgrowth; parasite-induced inflammation; direct effect of infection on crypt cells
• Gingivitis; stomatitis; periodontitis
• Chronic, nonresponsive or recurrent infections of the external ear and skin
• Fever and wasting
• Lymphoma (lymphosarcoma)—most common associated neoplastic disease; thymic and multicentric lymphomas highly associated; miscellaneous lymphomas (extranodal origin) most frequently involve the eye and nervous system
• Erythroid and myelomonocytic leukemias—predominant nonlymphoid leukemias
• Fibrosarcomas—in patients co-infected with mutated sarcoma virus; most frequently in young cats
• Peripheral neuropathies

CAUSES
• Cat-to-cat transmission—bites; close casual contact (grooming); shared dishes or litter pans
• Perinatal transmission—fetal and neonatal death of kittens from 80% of affected queens; transplacental and transmammary transmission in at least 20% of surviving kittens from infected queens

RISK FACTORS
• Male—result of behavior
• Free roaming
• Multicat household

DIAGNOSIS

DIFFERENTIAL DIAGNOSIS
• FIV
• Other infections—bacterial, parasitic, viral, or fungal
• Nonviral neoplastic diseases

CBC/BIOCHEMISTRY/URINALYSIS
• Anemia—often severe
• Lymphopenia
• Neutropenia—may be in response to secondary infections
• Thrombocytopenia and immune-mediated hemolytic anemia—may occur secondary to immune complexes
• Urinalysis and serum chemistry profile findings—depend on system affected and type of disease

OTHER LABORATORY TESTS
• IFA—identify FeLV p27 antigen in leukocytes and platelets in fixed smears of whole blood or buffy coat preparations; positive result indicates a productive infection in bone marrow cells; 97% IFA-positive cats remain persistently infected and viremic for life; p27 antigen can usually be detected by 4 weeks after infection, but may take up to 12 weeks to develop a positive test; for leukopenic cats, use buffy coat smears rather than whole blood smears.
• ELISA—detect soluble FeLV p27 antigen in whole blood, serum, plasma, saliva, or tears; more sensitive than IFA at detecting early or transient infections; a single positive test cannot predict which cats will be persistently viremic; retest in 12 weeks (many veterinarians test with IFA at this point); false-positive results more common when whole blood rather than serum or plasma is used; positive tests with saliva or tears should be checked with whole blood (IFA) or serum (ELISA).
• A few cats are persistently ELISA-positive and IFA-negative; recently, FeLV proviral genetic material has been detected in circulating blood cells from some of these cats; demonstrates infection despite no detectable viremia.
• Neither test detects FeLV-vaccinated cats, because the vaccine induces antibodies against gp70 antigen, not p27 antigen.

IMAGING
Thymic atrophy (fading kittens)

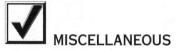

DIAGNOSTIC PROCEDURES

Bone marrow aspiration or biopsy—with erythroblastopenia (nonregenerative anemia), bone marrow often hypercellular owing to an arrest in differentiation of erythroid cells; true aplastic anemia with hypocellular bone marrow may be seen; some cases of anemia result from myeloproliferative disease.

PATHOLOGIC FINDINGS

• Lesions—depend on type of disease; bone marrow hypercellularity often accompanies neoplastic disease.
• Lymphocytic and plasmacytic infiltrates of the gingiva, lymph nodes, other lymphoid tissues, spleen, kidney, and liver
• Intestinal lesions similar to those seen with feline parvovirus infection (feline panleukopenia-like syndrome)

 TREATMENT

APPROPRIATE HEALTH CARE

• Outpatient for most cats
• Inpatient—may be required with severe secondary infections, anemia, or cachexia until condition stable
• Blood transfusions—emergency support; multiple transfusions may be necessary; passive antibody transfer reduces level of FeLV antigenemia in some cats; thus immunization of blood donor cats with FeLV vaccines is useful.

NURSING CARE

• Management of secondary and opportunistic infections—primary consideration
• Supportive therapy (e.g., parenteral fluids and nutritional supplements) may be useful.

ACTIVITY

Normal

DIET

• Normal
• Diarrhea, kidney disease, or chronic wasting—may require special diet

CLIENT EDUCATION

Discuss importance of keeping cats indoors and separated from FeLV-negative cats, to protect them from exposure to secondary pathogens and to prevent spread of FeLV

SURGICAL CONSIDERATIONS

• Biopsy or removal of tumors
• Oral treatment or surgery—dental cleaning, tooth extraction, gingival biopsy

 MEDICATIONS

DRUGS OF CHOICE

• Immunomodulatory drugs—may alleviate some clinical signs; hrα-interferon (Roferon, diluted in saline, 30 U/day PO for 7 days every

other week) may increase survival rates and improve clinical status; propionibacterium acnes (Immunoregulin, 0.5 mL/cat IV once or twice weekly); acemannan (Carrasyn, 100 mg/cat/day PO)
• *Haemobartonella* infection—suspect in all cats with regenerative hemolytic anemias; oxytetracycline (Terramycin, 15 mg/kg PO q8h or Liquamycin 7 mg/kg IM or IV q12h) or doxycycline (5 mg/kg PO q12h) for 3 weeks; short-term use of oral glucocorticoids in severe cases
• Lymphosarcoma—managed successfully with standard combination chemotherapy protocols; periods of remission average 3–4 months; some cats may remain in remission for much longer
• Myeloproliferative disease and leukemias—more refractory to treatment
• Yearly vaccination for respiratory and enteric viruses with inactivated vaccines recommended

CONTRAINDICATIONS

Modified live vaccines may cause disease in immunosuppressed cats.

PRECAUTIONS

Systemic corticosteroids—use with caution because of the potential for further immunosuppression.

POSSIBLE INTERACTIONS

N/A

ALTERNATIVE DRUGS

N/A

 FOLLOW-UP

PATIENT MONITORING

Varies according to the secondary infections and other manifestations of disease

PREVENTION/AVOIDANCE

• Prevent contact with FeLV-positive cats.
• Quarantine and test incoming cats before introduction into multiple cat households.
• Vaccines—most commercial vaccines induce virus-neutralizing antibodies specific for gp70; reported efficacy range from < 20% to almost 100%, depending on the trial and challenge system; test cats for FeLV before initial vaccination; if pre-vaccination testing is not done, clients should be aware that the cat may already be infected.

POSSIBLE COMPLICATIONS

N/A

EXPECTED COURSE AND PROGNOSIS

Persistently viremic cats—> 50% succumb to related diseases within 2–3 years after infection

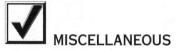 MISCELLANEOUS

ASSOCIATED CONDITIONS

• Secondary bacterial, viral, fungal, and parasitic disease
• Lymphoid tumors
• Fibrosarcomas
• Immune-mediated disease

AGE-RELATED FACTORS

• Neonatal kittens—most susceptible to persistent infection (70–100%)
• Older kittens—< 30% susceptible by 16 weeks of age

ZOONOTIC POTENTIAL

Probably low, but controversial—studies report conflicting results of antibodies to FeLV in humans and of correlation between certain human leukemias and exposure to cats.

PREGNANCY

• Abortions, stillbirths, and fetal resorptions common in FeLV-positive queens
• Transmission from queen to kittens—in at least 20% of live births

SYNONYMS

FeLV-AIDS—a mutated FeLV that causes immunodeficiency disease to develop rapidly

SEE ALSO

Individual topics on neoplasia, secondary infectious diseases, ocular disease, and gingivitis/stomatitis

ABBREVIATIONS

• ELISA = enzyme-linked immunosorbent assay
• FIV = feline immunodeficiency virus
• hrα-interferon = human recombinant interferon
• IFA = immunofluorescent antibody

Suggested Reading

Barr MC, Olsen CW, Scott FW. Feline viral diseases. In: Ettinger SJ, Feldman EC, eds. Textbook of veterinary internal medicine. 4th ed. Philadelphia: Saunders, 1994:409–439.
Loar AS. Feline leukemia virus: immunization and prevention. Vet Clin North Am Small Anim Pract 1993; 23:193–211.
Rojko JL, Hardy WD Jr. Feline leukemia virus and other retroviruses. In: Sherding RG, ed. The cat: diseases and clinical management. 2nd ed. New York: Churchill Livingston, 1994:263–432.
Author Margaret C. Barr
Consulting Editor Stephen C. Barr

DISEASES

FELINE PANLEUKOPENIA

BASICS

DEFINITION
An acute, enteric, vital infection of cats characterized by sudden onset, depression, vomiting and diarrhea, severe dehydration, and a high mortality

PATHOPHYSIOLOGY
The causative virus, FPV, infects only mitotic cells, causing acute cell cytolysis of rapidly dividing cells.

SYSTEMS AFFECTED
• Hemic/Lymphatic/Immune—severe panleukopenia; atrophy of the thymus
• Gastrointestinal—intestinal crypt cells of the jejunum and ileum destroyed; acute enteritis with vomiting and diarrhea; shortened, blunt villi with poor absorption of nutrients, dehydration, and secondary bacteremia
• Reproductive—in utero infection leading to fetal death, fetal resorption, abortion, stillbirth, or fetal mummification
• Nervous and Ophthalmic—in neonatal kittens, rapidly dividing granular cells of the cerebellum and retinal cells of the eye destroyed; cerebellar hypoplasia with ataxia and retinal dysplasia

GENETICS
N/A

INCIDENCE/PREVALENCE
• Unvaccinated populations—the most severe and important feline infectious disease
• Routine vaccination—almost total control of the disease
• Extremely contagious
• The virus is extremely stable, surviving for years on contaminated premises.

GEOGRAPHIC DISTRIBUTION
Worldwide in unvaccinated populations

SIGNALMENT

Species
• Felidae—all; domestic and exotic
• Canidae—susceptible to the closely related canine parvovirus; some exotic canids may be susceptible to FPV infection.
• Mustilidae—especially mink; may be susceptible
• Procyonidae—raccoon and coatimundi; susceptible

Breed Predilections
None

Mean Age and Range
• Unvaccinated and previously unexposed cats of any age can become infected once passively transferred maternal immunity has been lost.
• Kittens 2–6 months of age—most susceptible to develop severe disease
• Adults—often mild or subclinical infection

Predominant Sex
N/A

SIGNS

Historical Findings
• History of recent exposure (e.g., adoption shelter)
• Newly acquired kitten
• Kitten 2–4 months old from a premise with a history of the disease
• No vaccination history or last vaccinated when < 12 weeks of age
• Sudden onset, with vomiting, diarrhea, depression, and complete anorexia
• Owner may suspect poisoning.
• Cat may have disappeared or hid for 1 day or more before being found.
• Cat hangs head over water bowl or food dish but does not eat or drink.

Physical Examination Findings
• Depression—mild to severe
• Typical "panleukopenia posture"—sternum and chin resting on floor, feet tucked under body, and top of scapulae elevated above the back
• Dehydration—appears rapidly; may be severe
• Vomiting and diarrhea may occur.
• Body temperature—usually mild to moderate fever in the early stages; becomes severely subnormal as affected cat becomes moribund
• Abdominal pain—may be elicited on palpation
• Small intestine—either turgid and hose-like or flaccid
• Subclinical or mild infections with few or no clinical signs common, especially in adults
• Ataxia from cerebellar hypoplasia—kittens infected in utero or neonatally; signs evident at 10–14 days of age and persist for life; hypermetria; dysmetria; incoordination with a base-wide stance and an elevated "rudder" tail; alert, afebrile, and otherwise normal; retinal dysplasia sometimes seen

CAUSES

FPV
• Small, single-stranded DNA virus
• Single antigenic serotype
• Considerable antigenic cross-reactivity with canine parvovirus type 2 and mink enteritis virus
• Extremely stable against environmental factors, temperature, and most disinfectants
• Requires a mitotic cell for replication

RISK FACTORS
• Anything that increases the mitotic activity of the small intestinal crypt cells—intestinal parasites; pathogenic bacteria

• Secondary or co-infections—viral upper respiratory infections
• Age—kittens 2–6 months of age tend to be more severely affected.

DIAGNOSIS

DIFFERENTIAL DIAGNOSIS
• Panleukopenia-like syndrome of FeLV infection—chronic infection; chronic enteritis; chronic panleukopenia; often anemia; patient positive for FeLV antigen in the blood and/or saliva
• Salmonellosis—usually subclinical infection; severe gastroenteritis; total WBC counts usually high
• Acute poisoning—similar to acute or fulminating disease; severe depression; subnormal temperature; total WBC count not severely depressed
• Many diseases of cats can cause mild clinical signs that are hard to differentiate from mild panleukopenia; total WBC count is always low during the acute infection, even in subclinical cases.

CBC/BIOCHEMISTRY/URINALYSIS
• Panleukopenia—most consistent finding; leukocyte counts usually 500–3000 cells/dL with acute disease
• Biochemical findings usually nonspecific

OTHER LABORATORY TESTS
• Canine parvovirus antigen fecal immunoassay (CITE Canine Parvovirus Test Kit, IDEXX Labs)—not licensed for feline panleukopenia; will detect FPV antigen in feces
• Serologic testing—paired serum samples (acute and convalescent); detects rising antibody titer

IMAGING
N/A

DIAGNOSTIC PROCEDURES
• Viral isolation from feces or affected tissues (e.g., thymus, small intestine, spleen)
• Electron microscopy of feces—detect FPV particles

PATHOLOGIC FINDINGS

Gross
• Rough hair coat
• Severe dehydration
• Evidence of vomiting and diarrhea
• Edematous and turgid small intestine
• Petechial or ecchymotic hemorrhages on the serosal and/or mucosal surfaces of the jejunum and ilium
• Thymic atrophy
• Gelatinous or liquid bone marrow
• In utero infection—gross hypoplasia of the cerebellum

Microscopic
- Dilated small intestinal crypts with sloughing of epithelial cells
- Shortened and blunt intestinal villi
- Absence of lymphocytic infiltrates in all tissues
- Lymphocytic depletion of follicles of lymph nodes, Peyer's patches, and spleen
- Neonatal and fetal infection—disorientation and depletion of the granular and Purkinje's cells of the cerebellum
- Eosinophilic intranuclear inclusions in affected tissues during early stages of infection; not usually observed on routine histopathologic examination of formalin-fixed tissues

 TREATMENT

APPROPRIATE HEALTH CARE
- Main principles of treatment—rehydration; re-establishment of electrolyte balance; supportive care until the patient's immune system produces antiviral antibodies that neutralize the virus
- Inpatient—severe cases; hydration and replacement electrolyte therapy
- Outpatient—mild cases

NURSING CARE
- Fluid therapy—essential in severe cases; with electrolyte replacement and intravenous nutrient support may make the difference between survival and death
- Whole blood transfusions—if plasma protein falls < 4 g/dL or if total WBC counts fall < 2000 cells/dL

ACTIVITY
Keep patient indoors during acute disease—prevent contamination of the environment; prevent the cat from going into hiding

DIET
Temporarily withhold food until the acute gastroenteritis is controlled.

CLIENT EDUCATION
- Inform client that all current and future cats in the household must be vaccinated against FPV before exposure.
- Inform client that the virus remains infectious on the premises for years unless environment can be adequately disinfected with household bleach.

SURGICAL CONSIDERATIONS
None

 MEDICATIONS

DRUGS OF CHOICE
Broad-spectrum antibiotics—counter secondary bacteremia from intestinal bacteria

CONTRAINDICATIONS
Oral medications until gastroenteritis has been controlled

PRECAUTIONS
N/A

POSSIBLE INTERACTIONS
None known

ALTERNATIVE DRUGS
None

 FOLLOW-UP

PATIENT MONITORING
- Monitor hydration and electrolyte balance closely.
- Monitor CBC daily or at least every 2 days until recovery.
- Recovered cats are immune against FPV infection for life and do not require further vaccination.

PREVENTION/AVOIDANCE
- Contaminated environments (e.g., cages, floors, food and water dishes) should be disinfected with a 1:32 dilution of household bleach.
- FPV resistant to most commercial disinfectants

Vaccines
- Completely preventable by routine vaccination of kittens with either MLV or inactivated vaccines
- Immunity—long duration, perhaps even for life
- Kittens—vaccinate at 8–10 weeks of age; then after 12 weeks of age, when maternally derived immunity has waned
- Boosters—after 1 year; repeat every 3 years to provide excellent immunity.

POSSIBLE COMPLICATIONS
- Chronic enteritis—fungal or other cause
- Teratogenic effects (cerebellar hypoplasia resulting in ataxia for life)—virus infection of fetus
- Shock and other complications—severe dehydration and electrolyte imbalance

EXPECTED COURSE AND PROGNOSIS
- Most cases acute; lasting only 5–7 days
- If death does not occur during acute disease, recovery is usually rapid and uncomplicated; it may take several weeks for the patient to regain weight and body condition.
- Prognosis is guarded during acute disease, especially if the total WBC count is < 2000 cells/dL.

 MISCELLANEOUS

ASSOCIATED CONDITIONS
Viral upper respiratory diseases, including feline viral rhinotracheitis and feline calicivirus infection

AGE-RELATED FACTORS
- Clinical—generally a disease of kittens
- Subclinical—usually adults

ZOONOTIC POTENTIAL
None

PREGNANCY
- Unvaccinated pregnant cats are at great risk of infection.
- Fetuses almost always become infected with fatal or teratogenic effects, even when the dam has a subclinical infection.
- Fetal resorption, abortion, fetal mummification, stillbirth, or birth of weak, fading kittens
- Kittens may show ataxia from cerebellar hypoplasia when they become ambulatory.

SYNONYMS
- Feline distemper
- Feline viral enteritis
- Feline parvovirus infection

ABBREVIATIONS
- FeLV = feline leukemia virus
- FPV = feline parvovirus
- MLV = modified live virus

Suggested Reading
Barr MC, Olsen CW, Scott FW. Feline viral diseases. In: Ettinger SJ, Feldman EC, eds. Veterinary internal medicine. Philadelphia: Saunders, 1995:409–439.
Elston T, Rodan I, Flemming D, et al. 1998 report of the American Association of Feline Practitioners and Academy of Feline Medicine Advisory Panel on feline vaccines. J Am Vet Med Assoc 1998;212:227–241.
Greene CE. Feline panleukopenia. In: Greene CE, ed. Infectious diseases of the dog and cat. 2nd ed. Philadelphia: Saunders, 1998:52–57.
Pollock RVH, Postorino NC. Feline panleukopenia and other enteric viral diseases. In: Sherding RG, ed. The cat: diseases and clinical management. New York: Churchill Livingstone, 1994:479–487.
Author Fred W. Scott
Consulting Editor Stephen C. Barr

DISEASES

FELINE PARANEOPLASTIC SYNDROME

BASICS

OVERVIEW
• Rare—only seven reported cases
• Characterized by cutaneous lesions, which serve as markers of internal neoplasia

PATHOPHYSIOLOGY
• Most affected cats have had pancreatic adenocarcinomas with metastases to liver, lungs, pleura and/or peritoneum; one report of bile duct carcinoma.
• The link between internal malignancies and cutaneous lesions is unknown; may involve cytokines producing atrophy of the hair follicles.

SYSTEMS AFFECTED
• Skin/Exocrine—alopecia
• Gastrointestinal—weight loss, anorexia
• Other systems—result of metastasis of the pancreatic or biliary tumor (e.g., liver, lungs, pleura and/or peritoneal cavity)

SIGNALMENT
• All affected animals were mixed-breed or domestic shorthair cats.
• Mean age 12.5 years; range of 9–16 years
• Six cases were male.

SIGNS

Historical Findings
• Decrease in appetite followed by rapid weight loss and excessive shedding
• Pruritus—variable; sometimes with excessive grooming
• Hair loss—rapidly progressive
• Some affected cats may be reluctant to walk, owing to painful fissuring of the footpads.

Physical Examination Findings
• Hairs epilate easily
• Severe alopecia—ventral neck, abdomen and medial thighs
• The stratum corneum may "peel," leading to a glistening appearance to the skin.
• Gray lentigines may develop in alopecic areas.
• Footpads may be fissured and/or scaly.

CAUSES & RISK FACTORS
• The majority of cases are associated with an underlying pancreatic adenocarcinoma.
• Other internal carcinomas, such as bile duct carcinomas, may be involved.

DIAGNOSIS

DIFFERENTIAL DIAGNOSIS
• Hyperadrenocorticism—polyuria, polydipsia, and skin fragility
• Hyperthyroidism—polyphagia
• Hypothyroidism—spontaneous condition rare in cats; not associated with glistening skin
• Feline symmetrical alopecia—hair loss self-induced; not associated with easy epilation
• Demodicosis—mites are not associated with paraneoplastic alopecia.
• Dermatophytosis—hair loss often associated with breakage, not spontaneous shedding; inappetence and weight loss rare
• Alopecia areata—rarely involves the entire ventral surface; inappetence and weight loss rare
• Telogen effluvium—not associated with miniaturization of hair follicles
• Skin fragility syndrome—fragile skin not associated with paraneoplastic alopecia
• Superficial necrolytic dermatitis—not associated with marked exfoliation and miniaturization of hair follicles

CBC/BIOCHEMISTRY/URINALYSIS
Results usually unremarkable

OTHER LABORATORY TESTS
• Endocrine (thyroid profiles and a dexamethasone suppression test)—rule out endocrine disease
• Skin scrapings—rule out demodicosis
• KOH examination of hairs and/or fungal culture—rule out dermatophytosis

IMAGING
• Ultrasonography—pancreatic mass and/or nodular lesions in the liver or peritoneal cavity; failure to demonstrate nodules does not exclude the diagnosis, because they may be too small for detection.
• Thoracic radiographs—metastatic lesions in the lungs or pleural cavity

DIAGNOSTIC PROCEDURES
• Skin biopsies
• Laparoscopy or exploratory laparotomy—identify primary and metastatic tumors.

PATHOLOGIC FINDINGS
• Histopathologic examination of the skin—nonscarring alopecia; severe atrophy of hair follicles and adnexa; miniaturization of hair bulbs; mild acanthosis; variable absence of stratum corneum; variable mixed superficial perivascular infiltrates of neutrophils, eosinophils, and mononuclear cells
• Primary tumor—usually pancreatic adenocarcinoma, one case with a primary bile duct carcinoma
• Metastatic nodules—common in the liver, lungs, pleura, and peritoneum

TREATMENT
• Chemotherapy or other—no reported response; all cases have had metastatic disease at the time of diagnosis.
• Affected animals rapidly deteriorate; euthanasia should be suggested as a humane intervention.
• Supportive care—only if owners refuse to consider euthanasia; feed highly palatable, nutrient-dense foods and/or tube feed.

MEDICATIONS

DRUG(S)
N/A

CONTRAINDICATIONS/POSSIBLE INTERACTIONS
N/A

FOLLOW-UP
• Progressive deterioration
• Supportive care—ultrasonography and thoracic radiographs may demonstrate progression of metastatic disease.
• Expect death to occur within 2–8 weeks after onset of skin lesions.

MISCELLANEOUS

SYNONYMS
• Pancreatic paraneoplastic alopecia
• Paraneoplastic alopecia associated with internal malignancies
• Paraneoplastic alopecia associated with visceral neoplasia

SEE ALSO
Adenocarcinoma, Pancreas

Suggested Reading
Brooks DG, Campbell KL, Dennis JS, et al. Pancreatic paraneoplastic alopecia in three cats. J Am Anim Hosp Assoc 1994;30: 557–562.
Pascal-Tenorio A, Olivry T, Gross TL, et al. Paraneoplastic alopecia associated with internal malignancies in the cat. Vet Dermatol 1997;8:47–52.
Author Karen L. Campbell
Consulting Editor Karen Helton Rhodes

FELINE RHINOTRACHEITIS VIRUS

 BASICS

DEFINITION
Causes an acute disease in domestic and exotic cats, which is characterized by sneezing, fever, rhinitis, conjunctivitis, and ulcerative keratitis

PATHOPHYSIOLOGY
FHV-1—causes an acute cytolytic infection of respiratory or ocular epithelium after oral, intranasal, or conjunctival exposure

SYSTEMS AFFECTED
• Respiratory—rhinitis with sneezing and serous to purulent nasal discharge; tracheitis may occur; chronic sinusitis may be a sequela.
• Ophthalmic—often conjunctivitis with serous or purulent ocular discharge; ulcerative keratitis or panophthalmitis can occur
• Reproductive—in utero infection owing to infection of pregnant queens may result in severe herpetic infections in neonates.

GENETICS
N/A

INCIDENCE/PREVALENCE
• Common, especially in multicat households or facilities
• Perpetuated by latent carriers that harbor the virus in nerve ganglia, especially in the trigeminal ganglion

GEOGRAPHIC DISTRIBUTION
Found worldwide

SIGNALMENT
Species
Affects all domestic and many exotic felines
Breed Predilections
None
Mean Age and Range
• Cats of all ages
• Kittens most susceptible
Predominant Sex
N/A

SIGNS
Historical Findings
• Acute onset of paroxysmal sneezing
• Blepharospasm and ocular discharge
• Anorexia—from high fever, general malaise, or inability to smell
• Recurrent signs—carriers
• Abortion

Physical Examination Findings
• Fever—up to 106°F (41°C)
• Rhinitis—serous, mucopurulent, or purulent nasal discharge
• Conjunctivitis—serous, mucopurulent, or purulent nasal discharge
• Chronic rhinitis/sinusitis—chronic purulent nasal discharge
• Keratitis—ulceration, descemetocele, or panophthalmitis

CAUSES
FHV-1, of which there is only one serotype

RISK FACTORS
• Lack of vaccination for FHV-1
• Multiple cat facilities with overcrowding, poor ventilation, poor sanitation, poor nutrition, or physical or psychological stress
• Pregnancy and lactation
• Concomitant disease, especially owing to immunosuppressive organisms or other respiratory organisms
• Kittens born to carrier queens—infected about 5 weeks of age

 DIAGNOSIS

DIFFERENTIAL DIAGNOSES
• Feline calicivirus infection—less sneezing, conjunctivitis, ulcerative keratitis; may cause ulcerative stomatitis, pneumonia
• Feline chlamydiosis—more chronic conjunctivitis, which may be unilateral; pneumonitis; intracytoplasmic inclusions in conjunctival scrapings; responds to tetracyclines or chloramphenicol
• Bacterial infection (*Bordetella, haemophilus,* or *Pasteurella*)—less nasal and ocular involvement; often respond to antibiotics

CBC/BIOCHEMISTRY/URINALYSIS
• Not diagnostic
• Transient leukopenia followed by leukocytosis may occur.

OTHER LABORATORY TESTS
• Immunofluorescent assay—nasal or conjunctival scrapings; viral detection
• Viral isolation—pharyngeal swab sample
• Stained conjunctival smears—detect intranuclear inclusion bodies

IMAGING
Radiography—open mouth and skyline views of the skull reveal presence of chronic disease in the nasal cavity and frontal sinuses; infection cannot be reliably distinguished from neoplasia and inflammatory polyps; no abnormal radiographic findings with acute disease

DIAGNOSTIC PROCEDURES
N/A

PATHOLOGIC FINDINGS
• Gross—ocular and nasal discharge; mucosal edema of upper airway epithelium; tracheitis; sinusitis; ulcerative keratitis; and panophthalmitis
• Microscopic—submucosal edema; inflammatory cell infiltrates of upper respiratory and conjunctival tissues; chronic sinusitis; and intranuclear inclusion bodies in epithelial cells

 TREATMENT

APPROPRIATE HEALTH CARE
Inpatient—nutritional and fluid support to anorectic cats; prevent contagion

NURSING CARE
• Outpatient—keep patient indoors to prevent environmentally induced stress, which may lengthen the course of the disease.
• Fluids—intravenous or subcutaneous; to correct and prevent dehydration; to keep nasal secretions thin

ACTIVITY
Isolate affected cats during the acute phase, because they are contagious.

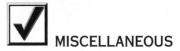

DIET
• Outpatient—entice food consumption to avoid anorexia, which induces a cascade of negative consequences; offer foods with appealing tastes and smells.
• Inpatients—forced enteral feeding for anorectic cats; remove nasal secretions (so nasal breathing can occur) before starting orogastric tube feeding; avoid nasoesophageal tubes because of rhinitis.

CLIENT EDUCATION
• Inform client of the contagious nature of the disease.
• Discuss proper vaccination protocols and early vaccination to cats in multicat facilities and households.
• Inform client that early weaning and isolation from all other cats except litter mates may prevent infections.

SURGICAL CONSIDERATIONS
Surgically implanted feeding tubes (esophagostomy tube, gastrostomy tube) may be needed when prolonged anorexia occurs.

MEDICATIONS

DRUGS OF CHOICE
• Broad-spectrum antibiotics—amoxicillin (22 mg/kg PO q12h) for secondary bacterial infections
• Antibiotic combinations—amoxicillin and enrofloxacin (2.5–5.0 mg/kg PO q12h) for secondary bacterial infections
• Ophthalmic antibiotics—for keratitis
• Ophthalmic antivirals—Herplex, Vira-A; for herpetic ulcers; must be instilled every 2 hours for significant effect
• Conjunctival vaccination with an intranasal FHV-1 vaccine—may help chronic keratitis

CONTRAINDICATIONS
• Systemic corticosteroids—may induce relapse in chronically infected cats
• Ophthalmic corticosteroids—may predispose to ulcerative keratitis
• Nasal decongestant drops—0.25% oxymetazoline HCl; decrease nasal discharge; contraindicated because some cats object and some experience rebound rhinorrhea

PRECAUTIONS
Death is usually the result of inadequate nutritional and fluid support.

POSSIBLE INTERACTIONS
None

ALTERNATIVE DRUGS
α-Interferon—Roferon; 30 units PO q24h; some efficacy in controlling the viral aspect of chronic infectious nasal discharge; for kittens: 2 units PO q24 when 3–8 weeks old to help prevent the effects of early exposure to FHV-1

FOLLOW-UP

PATIENT MONITORING
Monitor appetite closely; hospitalize for forced enteral feeding if anorexia develops.

PREVENTION/AVOIDANCE
Vaccines
• Routine vaccination with an MLV or inactivated virus vaccine—prevents development of severe disease; does not prevent infection and local viral replication with virus shedding
• Vaccinate at 8–10 weeks of age; at 12–14 weeks of age; and with annual boosters
• Endemic multicat facilities or households—vaccinate kittens with a dose of an intranasal vaccine at 10–14 days of age; then parenterally at 6, 10, and 14 weeks of age; isolate the litter from *all* other cats at 3–5 weeks of age; then use kitten vaccination protocol to prevent early infections

POSSIBLE COMPLICATIONS
• Chronic rhinosinusitis with lifetime sneezing and nasal discharge
• Herpetic ulcerative keratitis
• Permanent closure of the nasolacrimal duct with chronic ocular discharge

EXPECTED COURSE AND PROGNOSIS
• Usually 7–10 days before spontaneous remission, if secondary bacterial infections do not occur
• Prognosis generally good, if fluid and nutritional therapy are adequate

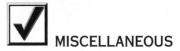

MISCELLANEOUS

ASSOCIATED CONDITIONS
Simultaneous viral or bacterial respiratory diseases

AGE-RELATED FACTORS
Primarily a disease of young kittens

ZOONOTIC POTENTIAL
None

PREGNANCY
Pregnant cats that develop disease may transmit FHV-1 to kittens in utero, resulting in abortion or neonatal disease

SYNONYMS
• Feline herpesvirus infection
• Rhino
• Coryza

SEE ALSO
• Bordetellosis—Cats
• Calicivirus—Cats

ABBREVIATIONS
• FHV-1 = feline herpesvirus type 1
• MLV = modified live virus

Suggested Reading
Barr MC, Olsen CW, Scott FW. Feline viral diseases. In: Ettinger SJ, Feldman EC, eds. Veterinary internal medicine. Philadelphia: Saunders, 1995:409–439.
Ford RB, Levy JK. Infectious diseases of the respiratory tract. In: Sherding RG, ed. The cat: diseases and clinical management. New York: Churchill Livingstone, 1994:489–500.
Ford RB. Role of infectious agents in respiratory disease. Vet Clin North Am Small Anim Pract 1993:23;17–35.
Gaskell R, Dawson S. Feline respiratory disease. In: Greene CE, ed. Infectious diseases of the dog and cat. Philadelphia: Saunders, 1998:97–106.
Author Gary D. Norsworthy
Consulting Editor Stephen C. Barr

DISEASES

FELINE SKIN FRAGILITY SYNDROME

BASICS

OVERVIEW
• A disorder of multifactorial causes characterized by extremely fragile skin
• Tends to occur in old cats that may have concurrent hyperadrenocorticism, diabetes mellitus, or excessive use of megestrol acetate or other progestational compounds
• A small number of cats have had no biochemical alterations.

SIGNALMENT
• Naturally occurring disease tends to be recognized in old cats.
• Iatrogenic cases have no age predilection.
• No breed or sex predilection

SIGNS
Historical findings
• Gradual onset of clinical signs
• Progressive alopecia (not always present)
• Often associated with weight loss, lusterless coat, poor appetite, and lack of energy

Physical Examination Findings
• The skin becomes markedly thin and tears with normal handling.
• The skin rarely bleeds upon tearing.
• Multiple lacerations (both old and new) may be noted on close examination
• Partial to complete alopecia of the truncal region may be noted
• Sometimes associated with rat tail, pinnal folding, pot-belly appearance

CAUSES & RISK FACTORS
• Hyperadrenocorticism—pituitary or adrenal dependent
• Iatrogenic—secondary to excessive corticosteroid or progestational drug use
• Diabetes mellitus—rare, unless associated with hyperadrenocorticism
• Possibly idiopathic

DIAGNOSIS

DIFFERENTIAL DIAGNOSIS
• Cutaneous asthenia
• Feline paraneoplastic syndrome—pancreatic neoplasia, hepatic lipidosis, cholangiocarcinoma
• Progestogen administration

CBC/BIOCHEMISTRY/URINALYSIS
• Of little diagnostic significance in most cases
• Approximately 80% of cats with hyperadrenocorticism have concurrent diabetes mellitus (hyperglycemia, glucosuria).

OTHER LABORATORY TESTS
• ACTH-stimulation test—70% of cats with hyperadrenocorticism have an exaggerated response.
• LDDST—15%–20% of normal cats may fail to decrease cortisol levels; typically unsuppressed with hyperadrenocorticism and nonadrenal illness
• HDDST—normal cats show decreases in cortisol concentrations; typically decreased with nonadrenal illnesses; considered by many clinicians to be the best screening test for hyperadrenocorticism; unreliable for discriminating between adrenal tumors and pituitary-dependent causes of hyperadrenocorticism, because both conditions fail to show suppression
• Endogenous ACTH levels—normal range for most labs is 20–100 pg/mL.

IMAGING
• Abdominal ultrasonography—adrenal masses are often small until end-stage disease.
• CT and MRI—small pituitary tumors may be difficult to visualize; MRI may be more successful.

DIAGNOSTIC PROCEDURES
N/A

PATHOLOGIC FINDINGS
Histopathology—suggestive, not diagnostic; epidermis and dermis are thin; attenuated collagen fibers are evident.

TREATMENT
• Underlying metabolic disease should be ruled out.
• Many patients are debilitated and require supportive care.
• Surgical correction of the lacerations—not helpful because the tissue cannot withstand any pressure from the sutures
• Hyperadrenocorticism—adrenalectomy is the preferred treatment.
• Cobalt 60 radiation therapy—variable success in the treatment of pituitary tumors

MEDICATIONS

DRUGS
• Medical management—may be useful for preparing patient for surgery and for minimizing postoperative complications (e.g., infections and poor wound healing)
• No known effective medical therapy for feline hyperadrenocorticism
• o,p′-DDD (mitotane)—12.5–50 mg/kg PO q12h; response has been equivocal; side effects include anorexia, vomiting, and diarrhea.
• Ketoconazole (nizoral)—10–15 mg/kg PO q12h; variable response
• Metyrapone—65 mg/kg PO q12h; clinical improvement noted more often with this drug than the others

CONTRAINDICATIONS/POSSIBLE INTERACTIONS
Hyperadrenocorticism—closely monitor diabetic cat; adjust insulin to prevent hypoglycemia when the cortisol levels fall.

FOLLOW-UP
Patients are often quite debilitated, making any form of treatment risky; close monitoring is required in all cases.

MISCELLANEOUS

ABBREVIATIONS
• HDDST = high-dose dexamethasone-suppression test
• LDDST = low-dose dexamethasone-suppression test
• o,p′-DDD = 1,1-(o,p′-dichlorodiphenyl)-2,2-dichloroethane

Suggested Reading
Gross TL, Ihrke PJ, Walder EJ. Veterinary dermatopathology. Philadelphia: Mosby, 1992.
Helton Rhodes, K. Cutaneous manifestations of hyperadrenocorticism. In: August JR, ed. Consultations in feline internal medicine. Philadelphia: Saunders, 1997:191–198.

Author Karen Helton Rhodes
Contributing Editor Karen Helton Rhodes

FELINE SYMMETRICAL ALOPECIA

 BASICS

OVERVIEW
• Alopecia in a symmetrical pattern with no gross changes in the skin
• Common clinical presentation in cats
• Manifestation of several underlying disorders

SIGNALMENT
No age, breed, or sex predilection

SIGNS
• Total to partial hair loss; most often symmetrical but can occur in a patchy distribution
• Areas of the trunk most commonly affected are the ventrum, caudal dorsum, and lateral and caudal thighs.
• Sometimes patchy areas of hair loss (unsymmetrical) on the distal extremities or trunk

CAUSES & RISK FACTORS
• Hypersensitivity reactions—fleas, food, atopy
• Parasites—fleas, *Cheyletiella*
• Infections—dermatophytosis
• Neurologic/behavioral—psychogenic
• Stress/metabolic—telogen effluvium
• Neoplasia—pancreatic neoplasia (paraneoplastic alopecia)
• Hyperadrenocorticism
• Alopecia areata
• Hyperthyroid (early sign)

 DIAGNOSIS

DIFFERENTIAL DIAGNOSIS
See Causes & Risk Factors

CBC/BIOCHEMISTRY/URINALYSIS
Eosinophilia in some allergic cats

OTHER LABORATORY TESTS
T_4-hyperthyroid

IMAGING
N/A

DIAGNOSTIC PROCEDURES
• Flea combing—identify fleas, flea excrement, or both
• Microscopic examination of hair—self-induced hair loss results in broken ends, whereas endogenous hair loss results in tapered ends.
• Fecal examination—excess hair, mites and ova (*Cheyletiella*), tapeworm, or fleas
• Food elimination diet trial—see Food Reactions (Dermatologic)
• Intradermal skin test—see Atopy
• Histopathologic examination—see below

PATHOLOGIC FINDINGS
• Biopsies—help confirm underlying cause (e.g., allergic dermatitis, psychogenic, or rarely, systemic disease)
• Histopathologic findings—vary depending on the cause
• Feline psychogenic alopecia—hair follicles and skin normal
• High numbers of mast cells, eosinophils, lymphocytes, or macrophages suggest allergic dermatitis.
• Alopecia areata—lymphocytic inflammation that encircles the bulb portions of the hair follicles; rare

 TREATMENT

• Effective management of the underlying causes is important.
• Inform the owner of the diagnostic plan and the time it could take to see a response (e.g., fleas, 4–6 weeks; diet, 3–12 weeks).

 MEDICATIONS

DRUGS
• Antihistamines—e.g., chlorpheniramine, 0.5 mg/kg PO q8h
• Glucocorticoids—0.5 mg/kg PO, alternate-day therapy
• Amitriptyline—1–2 mg/kg PO daily

CONTRAINDICATIONS/POSSIBLE INTERACTIONS
• Glucocorticoids—can cause alopecia, diabetes mellitus, polydipsia, polyuria, polyphagia, and weight gain; can suppress pruritus, making it difficult to determine the underlying cause
• Withdraw antipruritic medications (including glucocorticoids) as the diagnostic tests near completion (e.g., food hypersensitivity reactions)

 FOLLOW-UP

• Frequent examinations are essential in confirming the differential diagnoses.
• Successful identification of the underlying cause offers the best prognosis, if the cause can be controlled (e.g., flea bites or food hypersensitivity).

 MISCELLANEOUS

Suggested Reading
O'Dair HA, Foster AP. Focal and generalized alopecia. Vet Clin North Am Small Anim Pract 1995;25:851–870.
Author David Duclos
Consulting Editor Karen Helton Rhodes

FELINE SYNCYTIUM-FORMING VIRUS (FeSFV)

 BASICS

OVERVIEW
• A retrovirus in the Spumavirus subfamily that infects cats, apparently with little or no pathogenic effect
• Found worldwide; estimated prevalences, 10-70% or greater
• Infection linked statistically with chronic progressive polyarthritis; disease has not been reproduced by experimental infection.
• Research—disease potential low; nuisance when using feline-origin tissue culture cells; test cats and remove from study if FeSFV-positive

SIGNALMENT
• Cats
• The prevalence of virus—low in kittens; increases with age
• Males—more likely than females to be infected; chronic progressive polyarthritis occurs predominantly in males aged 1.5–5 years.

SIGNS
• Most affected cats healthy
• Co-infections with FIV and FeLV—fairly common, probably because of shared transmission modes and risk factors
• Statistical links with myeloproliferative disease and chronic progressive polyarthritis—may actually reflect co-infection with FIV
• Chronic progressive polyarthritis—swollen joints; abnormal gait; and lymphadenopathy

CAUSES & RISK FACTORS
• Transmission—primarily by biting; free-roaming cats at greater risk of infection
• Transmitted efficiently from infected queens to their offspring, probably in utero
• The high prevalence of infection in some cat populations suggests casual contact may play a role in transmission; this has not been demonstrated experimentally.

 DIAGNOSIS

DIFFERENTIAL DIAGNOSIS
Signs of chronic progressive polyarthritis—test for FIV, FeLV, and septic joint disease

CBC/BIOCHEMISTRY/URINALYSIS
Usually normal

OTHER LABORATORY TESTS
Serologic testing—for FeSFV antibodies and virus isolation; not readily available; not particularly useful because correlation between FeSFV infection and disease is so tenuous.

IMAGING
N/A

DIAGNOSTIC PROCEDURES
Joint fluid cytology—with chronic progressive polyarthritis; may reveal high numbers of neutrophils and large mononuclear cells

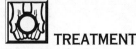 TREATMENT

None, except for chronic progressive polyarthritis

FELINE SYNCYTIUM-FORMING VIRUS (FeSFV)

 ## MEDICATIONS

DRUGS

Chronic progressive polyarthritis—immunosuppressive doses of prednisolone (10–15 mg/cat/day) and cyclophosphamide (7.5 mg/cat/day for 4 days each week)

CONTRAINDICATIONS/POSSIBLE INTERACTIONS

Immunosuppressive drugs—take care when using in patients co-infected with FIV or FeLV.

 ## FOLLOW-UP

EXPECTED COURSE AND PROGNOSIS

• Infection with FeSFV alone—adverse consequences unlikely
• Chronic progressive polyarthritis—often difficult to control; poor prognosis for long-term recovery

 ## MISCELLANEOUS

ASSOCIATED CONDITIONS

• Chronic progressive polyarthritis
• Co-infections with FIV and FeLV

SYNONYMS

• Feline syncytial virus
• Feline foamy virus

SEE ALSO

• Polyarthritis, Erosive Immune-mediated
• Polyarthritis, Nonerosive Immune-mediated

ABBREVIATIONS

• FeLV = feline leukemia virus
• FIV = feline immunodeficiency virus

Suggested Reading

Greene CE. Syncytium-forming virus infection. In: Greene CE, ed. Infectious diseases of the dog and cat. Philadelphia: Saunders, 1998:106–107.

Author Margaret C. Barr
Consulting Editor Stephen C. Barr

FIBROCARTILAGINOUS EMBOLIC MYELOPATHY

BASICS

DEFINITION
Acute ischemic necrosis of the spinal cord caused by fibrocartilaginous emboli

PATHOPHYSIOLOGY
• Emboli—found in spinal cord arteries, veins, or both; source is possibly intervertebral disk material.
• Exact mechanism of entry into the spinal vasculature unknown

SYSTEMS AFFECTED
Nervous

GENETICS
N/A

INCIDENCE/PREVALENCE
• Common cause of spinal cord disease in nonchondrodystophic breeds of dogs
• Not reported in chondrodystrophic breeds
• Rare in cats

GEOGRAPHIC DISTRIBUTION
N/A

SIGNALMENT
Species
Dogs and cats

Breed Predilections
• Giant- and large-breed dogs—highest prevalence
• Miniature schnauzers and Shetland sheepdogs—over-represented; hyperlipo-proteinemia and resultant hyperviscosity common in these breeds suspected causes of spinal cord infarction without contribution of fibrocartilaginous emboli

Mean Age and Range
• Most patients 3–5 years old
• Range 16 weeks to 10 years

Predominant Sex
Slight male predominance

SIGNS

Historical Findings
• Mild trauma or vigorous exercise at the onset of signs common
• Sudden onset
• Affected dog typically cries in pain; pain subsides in minutes to hours (at most).
• Signs of paresis or paralysis develop over a matter of seconds, minutes, or hours.
• Condition stabilizes within 12–24 hr.

Physical Examination Findings
N/A

Neurologic Examination Findings
• Deficits—usually lateralized; unaffected side usually mildly affected or normal; symmetrically distributed in a few patients
• Pain—at onset of signs and then generally absent; usually subsided by the time the patient is being examined; may be felt for a few hours in severely affected patients
• Any level of the spinal cord can be affected, depending on the distribution of the embolic material.
• Mild ataxia to paralysis
• Upper or lower motor neuron deficits
• Spinal cord injury—unilateral; or only the dorsal or ventral aspect of the spinal cord, causing an ipsilateral limb with sensory loss but muscle tone and motor function preserved (or vice versa); or other odd combinations are possible in patients with focal quadrant injuries.
• If signs progress beyond 24 hr, consider other diseases that cause ascending and descending myelomalacia.

CAUSES
Unknown

RISK FACTORS
• Vigorous exercise may trigger the incident.
• Hyperlipoproteinemia

DIAGNOSIS

DIFFERENTIAL DIAGNOSIS
• Acute nonprogressive, asymmetric, and nonpainful—characteristic; greatly helps in the diagnosis
• Back and neck pain with symmetrical signs—intervertebral disk disease; diskospondylitis; vertebral tumor; fracture and luxation; survey radiography and myelography help confirm the diagnosis.
• Parenchymal spinal cord hemorrhage secondary to a bleeding diathesis (e.g., caused by anticoagulant rodenticide ingestion, thrombocytopenia, or DIC)—rule out by carefully examining for evidence of hemorrhage, performing a platelet count, and determining blood clotting times.
• Focal myelitis—differentiate by progressive history and CSF analysis

CBC/BIOCHEMISTRY/URINALYSIS
Usually normal

OTHER LABORATORY TESTS
N/A

IMAGING
• Survey spinal radiograph—usually normal
• Myelography—in acute stage often demon-strates focal intramedullary swelling at the embolic site; later often normal or shows an area of cord atrophy

MRI of the Spine
• Most diagnostic technique in both acute and chronic stages
• Degenerative disk that was the source of the emboli—decreased signal intensity on T2 images
• Area of spinal cord infarction—increased signal intensity on T2 images

DIAGNOSTIC PROCEDURES
CSF Analysis
• Results depend on the location (e.g., lumbar vs. cerebellomedullary) and the time fluid was collected in relation to the onset of clinical signs.
• Acute stage—high RBC count and mildly high neutrophil count may be seen; a few days later, may see only mildly high protein
• Sometimes results are normal.

FIBROCARTILAGINOUS EMBOLIC MYELOPATHY

PATHOLOGIC FINDINGS
• Gross—focal spinal cord swelling with hemorrhage
• Microscopic—emboli of fibrocartilage in arteries and veins of the spinal cord and meninges; hemorrhagic necrosis and malacia in gray and white matter

TREATMENT

APPROPRIATE HEALTH CARE
Inpatient—for immediate medical treatment and diagnostic procedures.

NURSING CARE
• Keep recumbent patients on a padded surface; turn frequently to prevent pressure sores.
• Assist and encourage patients to ambulate as soon as possible.

ACTIVITY
Restrict until diagnosis is made.

DIET
Normal

CLIENT EDUCATION
• Inform client that recovery from paresis or paralysis is slow and gradual, when it occurs.
• Inform client that most patients need considerable supportive care at home during recovery.

SURGICAL CONSIDERATIONS
N/A

MEDICATIONS

DRUGS OF CHOICE
Methylprednisolone sodium succinate—may be beneficial if given within the first 8 hr after the onset of signs according to studies of acute spinal cord injury caused by spinal cord impact; 30 mg/kg IV as first treatment; then 15 mg/kg at 2 and 6 hr and every 6 hr thereafter for a total treatment period of 24–48 hr; give each dose slowly over 10–15 min; too rapid of an injection can cause vomiting.

CONTRAINDICATIONS
Nonsteroidal analgesics—do not administer with methylprednisolone sodium succinate; increases probability of gastrointestinal ulceration

PRECAUTIONS
• Methylprednisolone sodium succinate—no benefit with treatment for longer than 24–48 hr and dramatically increases adverse effects (e.g., gastrointestinal ulceration)
• High fiber diet during and after steroid treatment reduces gastrointestinal ulceration.

POSSIBLE INTERACTIONS
N/A

ALTERNATIVE DRUGS
N/A

FOLLOW-UP

PATIENT MONITORING
• Sequential neurologic evaluations—during the first 12–24 hr after examination
• Neurologic status—2, 3, and 4 weeks after onset of clinical signs
• Urinary incontinence—urinalysis and bacterial culture and sensitivity to detect urinary tract infection.

PREVENTION/AVOIDANCE
• Recurrence highly unlikely
• No known method of prevention

POSSIBLE COMPLICATIONS
• Fecal and urinary incontinence
• Urinary tract infection
• Urine scalding and pressure sores

EXPECTED COURSE AND PROGNOSIS
• Pain perception and upper motor neuron signs—prognosis for marked improvement generally good
• Loss of pain perception—prognosis poor
• Areflexia of limbs or sphincters—almost no chance of recovery; reduced purposeful movements and reflexes—functional recovery common; some degree of permanent deficit likely
• Progression of clinical signs from upper to lower motor neuron and an enlarging area of sensory loss indicate ascending or descending myelomalacia and a hopeless prognosis; consider euthanasia.
• Neurologic status—little change in the first 14 days after onset; most improvement occurs between days 21 and 42; remyelination is complete in most patients within 6–12 weeks after onset; if no improvement after 21–30 days, recovery is highly unlikely

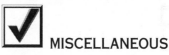

MISCELLANEOUS

ASSOCIATED CONDITIONS
Disorders that lead to a compromise in circulatory function may predispose or mimic fibrocartilaginous embolic myelopathy—hyperadrenocorticism; hypothyroidism; high systemic blood pressure; hyperviscosity syndrome; hyperlipidemia; bleeding diathesis; bacterial endocarditis

AGE-RELATED FACTORS
N/A

ZOONOTIC POTENTIAL
N/A

PREGNANCY
High-dose corticosteroid administration—may cause premature delivery

ABBREVIATIONS
• CSF = cerebrospinal fluid
• DIC = disseminated intravascular coagulation

Suggested Reading
Braughler JM, Hall ED. Current application of "high-dose" steroid therapy for CNS injury: a pharmacological perspective. J Neurosurg 1985;62:806–810.
Cauzinille L. Fibrocartilaginous embolism of the spinal cord. Paper presented at the 11th annual forum of the American College of Veterinary Internal Medicine, Washington, DC, 1993.
Cook JR. Fibrocartilaginous embolism. Vet Clin North Am Small Anim Pract 1988;18:581–592.
Summers BA, Cummings JF, de Lahunta A. Veterinary neuropathology. St. Louis: Mosby, 1995:246–249.
Author Allen Sisson
Consulting Editor Joane M. Parent

DISEASES

FIBROSARCOMA, BONE

 BASICS

OVERVIEW
• Usually develop in the axial skeleton
• Characterized histologically by well-to-poorly differentiated spindle-shaped cells
• Tends to be locally invasive but late to metastasize
• Metastasizes to lymph nodes, heart, pericardium, skin, and other bones
• Primary tumor uncommon in cats

SIGNALMENT
• Dogs and cats
• Breed predilections not reported
• More common in mature male dogs

SIGNS

Historical Findings
• Lameness
• Palpable mass

Physical Examination Findings
• Long bone tumor—monostotic swelling at a metaphyseal site
• Pain on palpation of tumor site
• Pathologic fracture
• Axial tumor—palpable mass

CAUSES & RISK FACTORS
Unknown

 DIAGNOSIS

DIFFERENTIAL DIAGNOSIS
• Other primary bone neoplasms—osteosarcoma; hemangiosarcoma; chondrosarcoma
• Metastatic neoplasia from another primary site
• Osteomyelitis—fungal or bacterial

CBC/BIOCHEMISTRY/URINALYSIS
Usually normal

OTHER LABORATORY TESTS
N/A

IMAGING
• Radiography—impossible to differentiate primary lesion from other primary bone tumors; lesions typically in metaphyseal sites of long bones and can be lytic, productive, or both (see Osteosarcoma)
• Thoracic radiography—detect metastasis
• CT—determine extent of local disease in patients with an axial tumor

DIAGNOSTIC PROCEDURES
Biopsy and histopathology of tumor—as described for osteosarcoma; take care to differentiate between fibrosarcoma and fibroblastic osteosarcoma.

 TREATMENT

• Aggressive surgical resection—amputation; limb salvage; hemipelvectomy; maxillectomy; mandibulectomy
• Radiotherapy—as an adjuvant to surgery

 MEDICATIONS

DRUGS
Chemotherapy—investigate, because late metastasis can be a problem

CONTRAINDICATIONS/POSSIBLE INTERACTIONS
N/A

 FOLLOW-UP

• Thoracic radiography—monthly for 3 months; then every 3rd month
• Believed to be less aggressive than osteosarcoma

 MISCELLANEOUS

Suggested Reading
Waters DJ, Cooley DM. Skeletal neoplasms. In: Morrison WB, ed. Cancer in dogs and cats: medical and surgical management. Philadelphia: Williams & Wilkins, 1998:639–654.

Author Terrance A. Hamilton
Consulting Editor Wallace B. Morrison

BASICS

OVERVIEW
• Slowly progressive (months) and locally invasive mesenchymal malignancy in the oral cavity of dogs and cats
• Third most common oral malignancy in dogs; second most common oral malignancy in cats
• Gingiva most commonly involved site
• Highly invasive to surrounding bone
• Metastasis—uncommon
• Death usually secondary to local recurrence, dysphagia, and cachexia
• A subset of histologically low-grade, yet biologically high-grade fibrosarcomas has been described.

SIGNALMENT
• Dogs and cats
• Breed predilections—none known; medium to large breeds more commonly affected; golden retrievers may be predisposed.
• Mean age—7.6 years (range, 0.5–15 years)
• Slight male predilection

SIGNS

Historical Findings
• Excessive salivation
• Halitosis
• Dysphagia
• Bloody oral discharge
• Weight loss

Physical Examination Findings
• Oral mass
• Loose teeth
• Facial deformity
• Occasional cervical lymphadenomegaly

CAUSES & RISK FACTORS
None identified

DIAGNOSIS

DIFFERENTIAL DIAGNOSIS
• Other oral malignancy
• Epulis
• Abscess
• Benign polyp

CBC/BIOCHEMISTRY/URINALYSIS
Usually normal

OTHER LABORATORY TESTS
Cytologic evaluation—rarely diagnostic

IMAGING
• Skull radiography—evaluate for bone involvement deep to the mass
• Thoracic radiography—evaluate lungs for metastasis

DIAGNOSTIC PROCEDURES
• Large, deep-tissue biopsy (down to the bone)—required to sufficiently differentiate from other oral malignancies
• Carefully palpate regional lymph nodes (mandibular and retropharyngeal).

TREATMENT

• Radical excision—required (e.g., hemi-mandibulectomy); well tolerated by most patients; at least 2-cm margins necessary
• Cryosurgery—indicated for small lesions minimally adherent to bone
• Inpatient radiotherapy—offers considerable long-term control if the tumor is deemed inoperable
• Most radiotherapy plans attempt 40–60 Gy over 3–6 weeks.
• Soft foods—may recommend to prevent tumor ulceration and after radical oral excision

MEDICATIONS

DRUGS
• Chemotherapy—good option for some patients; doxorubicin (adriamycin, 25–30 mg/m^2 IV once every 2 weeks for 5 treatments); median survival (dogs), 18 weeks; may provide marked palliation of clinical signs
• Cisplatin—intralesionally administered; local control (palliation) reported

CONTRAINDICATIONS/POSSIBLE INTERACTIONS
Chemotherapy may be toxic; seek advice before initiating treatment if you are unfamiliar with cytotoxic drugs.

FOLLOW-UP

EXPECTED COURSE AND PROGNOSIS
• Survival after excision—1-year, 25%–45%; 2-year, 20%–35%; median (dogs), 7–11 months; improves when excisional margins are free of neoplastic cells
• Survival after radiotherapy treatment—0–27 months; median, 7 months
• Survival after doxorubicin (dogs)—median, 18 weeks
• Cause of death—related to local recurrence and secondary anorexia and cachexia

MISCELLANEOUS

Suggested Reading
Ciekot PA, Powers BE, Withrow SJ, et al. Histologically low-grade, yet biologically high-grade, fibrosarcomas of the mandible and maxilla in dogs: 25 cases (1982–1991). J Am Vet Med Assoc 1994;204:610–615.
Oakes MG, Lewis DD, Hedlund CS, Hosgood G. Canine oral neoplasia. Compend Contin Educ Small Anim Pract 1993;15:15–31.

Author Kevin A. Hahn
Consulting Editor Wallace B. Morrison

DISEASES

FIBROSARCOMA, NASAL AND PARANASAL SINUS

BASICS

OVERVIEW
• Slow, progressive invasion of neoplastic mesenchymal cells within the nasal and paranasal sinuses
• Usually begins unilateral but progresses slowly to bilateral by the time the patient is examined
• Second most common nonepithelial histologic tumor type in dogs; prevalence of nonepithelial nasal neoplasia (dogs and cats), 0.3–4.7% of all tumors

SIGNALMENT
• More common in dogs than cats
• Median age (dogs and cats)—9–12 years (range, 1–16 years)
• Male predilection (2:1)

SIGNS

Historical Findings
• Intermittent and progressive history of unilateral to bilateral epistaxis (median duration, 3 months)
• Epiphora
• Sneezing
• Halitosis
• Anorexia
• Seizures secondary to brain invasion

Physical Examination Findings
• Noninfectious nasal discharge
• Facial deformity or exophthalmia
• Pain on examination of nasal or paranasal sinuses

CAUSES & RISK FACTORS
N/A

DIAGNOSIS

DIFFERENTIAL DIAGNOSIS
• Bacterial sinusitis—uncommon
• Viral infection (cats)
• Aspergillosis
• Cryptococcosis (cats)
• Foreign body
• Trauma
• Tooth root abscess
• Oronasal fistula
• Coagulopathy

CBC/BIOCHEMISTRY/URINALYSIS
Usually normal

OTHER LABORATORY TESTS
Cytologic and bacterial examination—rarely helpful

IMAGING
• Survey radiography (skull)—shows typical pattern of asymmetrical destruction of caudal turbinates with superimposition of a soft tissue mass; may find fluid density in the frontal sinuses secondary to outflow obstruction
• Thoracic radiography—detect lung metastasis (uncommon)
• CT or MRI—best method to observe integrity of cribriform plate or orbital invasion

DIAGNOSTIC PROCEDURES
• Rhinoscopy (visual observation is poor)—(firm, fleshy masses; avoid progressing caudally into the cribriform plate
• Tissue biopsy—necessary for definitive diagnosis
• Bacterial culture—often positive

TREATMENT
• Surgery alone—ineffective; turbinectomy may be done before external (teletherapy) or internal (brachytherapy) irradiation.
• Inpatient radiotherapy (with or without surgery)—60–80 Gy; provides the best clinical control in dogs

MEDICATIONS

DRUGS
Chemotherapy—good option for some patients; doxorubicin (30 mg/m^2 IV once every 2 weeks for 5 treatments in dogs weighing > 10 kg; 1 mg/kg for dogs < 10 kg and for cats); median survival (dogs) 18 weeks; may provide marked palliation of clinical signs

CONTRAINDICATIONS/POSSIBLE INTERACTIONS
Chemotherapy may be toxic; seek advice before initiating treatment if you are unfamiliar with cytotoxic drugs.

 FOLLOW-UP

PATIENT MONITORING
Survey radiography and/or CT or MRI (skull)—may be performed when clinical signs recur

EXPECTED COURSE AND PROGNOSIS
• Median survival if left untreated—3–5 months
• Median disease-free interval after radiotherapy—dogs, 8–25 months; cats, 1–36 months
• Survival rates with radiotherapy (dogs and cats)—1-year survival, 38%–57%; 2-year survival, 30%–48%; reports of shorter survival times with nonepithelial nasal tumors (8–16 months)
• Median survival after doxorubicin (dogs)—18 weeks
• Brain involvement—poor prognostic sign

 MISCELLANEOUS

Suggested Reading

Evans SM, Goldschmidt M, McKee LJ, Harvey CE. Prognostic factors and survival after radiotherapy for intranasal neoplasms in dogs: 70 cases (1974–1985). J Am Vet Med Assoc 1989;194:1460–1463.

Patnaik AK. Canine sinonasal neoplasms: soft tissue tumors. J Am Anim Hosp Assoc 1989;25:491–497.

Author Kevin A. Hahn

Consulting Editor Wallace B. Morrison

FLEAS AND FLEA CONTROL

BASICS

DEFINITION
• Flea allergy dermatitis—hypersensitivity reaction to antigens in flea saliva with or without evidence of fleas and flea dirt
• Flea infestation—large number of fleas and a large amount of flea dirt with or without a flea allergy dermatitis

PATHOPHYSIOLOGY
• Flea bite hypersensitivity (FBH)—caused by a low molecular weight hapten and two high molecular weight allergens that help initiate the allergic reaction
• High molecular weight allergens—increased binding to dermal collagen; when bound, form a complete antigen necessary for eliciting FBH
• Flea saliva—contains histamine-like compounds that irritate skin
• Intermittent exposure favors FBH; continuous exposure is less likely to result in hypersensitivity.
• Both IgE and IgG antiflea antibodies have been noted.
• Immediate and delayed hypersensitivity reactions have been noted.
• Late-phase IgE-mediated response—part of FBH reaction; occurs 3–6 hr after exposure
• Cutaneous basophil hypersensitivity—part of FBH reaction; an infiltration of basophils into the dermis; mediated either by IgE or IgG; subsequent exposures cause the basophils to degranulate; manifests as immediate and delayed hypersensitivity

SYSTEMS AFFECTED
Skin/Exocrine

GENETICS
FBH—unknown inheritance pattern; more common in atopic breeds

INCIDENCE/PREVALENCE
Varies with climatic conditions and flea population

GEOGRAPHIC DISTRIBUTION
• FBH—may occur anywhere; nonseasonal only in climates that are warm and humid year round and in animals housed indoors

SIGNALMENT
Species
Dogs and cats

Breed Predilection
FBH—any breed; most common in atopic breeds

Mean Age and Range
FBH—rare < 6 months of age; average age range, 3–6 years, but may be seen at any age

Predominant Sex
N/A

SIGNS
Historical Findings
• Compulsive biting
• Chewing (corncob nibbling)
• Licking, primarily in the back half of the body but may include the antebrachial regions
• Cats—scratching around the head and neck
• Signs of fleas and flea dirt

Physical Examination Findings
• Depends somewhat on the severity of the reaction and the degree of exposure to fleas (i.e., seasonal vs. year-round)
• Finding fleas and flea dirt is beneficial, although not essential, for the diagnosis of FBH; sensitive animals require a low exposure and tend to overgroom, making identification of the parasites difficult.
• Dogs—lesions concentrated in a triangular area of the caudal-dorsal-lumbosacral region; caudal aspect of the thighs, lower abdomen, inguinal region, and cranial forearms usually involved; primary lesions are papules; secondary lesions (e.g., hyperpigmentation, lichenification, alopecia, and scaling) common in uncontrolled FBH; secondary folliculitis and furunculosis may be seen.
• Cats—several patterns are seen; most common is a miliary crusting dermatitis in a wedge-shaped pattern over the caudal dorsal lumbosacral region and often around the head and neck; other presentations are alopecia of the inguinal region with or without inflammation or eosinophilic plaques and other forms of eosinophilic granuloma complex.
• Exposure to other animals and previous flea treatment should be ascertained.

CAUSES
See Pathophysiology

RISK FACTORS
FBH—intermittent exposure to fleas increases the likelihood of development; commonly seen in conjunction with atopy

DIAGNOSIS

DIFFERENTIAL DIAGNOSIS
• Food allergy
• Atopy
• Sarcoptic mange
• Cheyletiellosis
• Primary keratinization defects
• Diagnosis is best based on the history and laboratory tests.

CBC/BIOCHEMISTRY/URINALYSIS
• Usually normal
• Cats—hypereosinophilia may be detected

OTHER LABORATORY TESTS
• Skin scrapings—negative
• Flea combings—fleas or flea dirt, but often nothing is found
• RAST and ELISA—variable accuracy; both false-positive and false-negative results reported

IMAGING
N/A

DIAGNOSTIC PROCEDURES
• Diagnosis usually based on historical information and distribution of lesions
• Fleas or flea dirt is supportive but is often quite difficult to find, especially in cats.
• Identification of *Dipylidium caninum* segments is supportive.
• Intradermal allergy testing with flea antigen—reveals positive immediate reactions in 90% of flea-allergic animals; delayed reactions (24–48 hr) may sometimes be observed in allergic animals that show no immediate reaction.
• The most accurate test may be response to appropriate treatment.

PATHOLOGIC FINDINGS
• Superficial perivascular dermatitis
• Eosinophilic intraepidermal micro-abscesses—strongly suggest FBH
• Eosinophils as a major cellular component of the dermis—supportive of FBH
• Histopathologic evaluation—cannot accurately differentiate FBH from atopy, food allergy, or other hypersensitivities

TREATMENT

APPROPRIATE HEALTH CARE
Outpatient therapy

NURSING CARE
N/A

ACTIVITY
N/A

DIET
N/A

CLIENT EDUCATION
• Inform owners that there is no cure for FBH.
• Advise owners that flea-allergic animals often become more sensitive to flea bites as they age.
• Inform owners that controlling exposure to fleas is currently the only means of therapy; hyposensitization has not worked satisfactorily.

SURGICAL CONSIDERATIONS
N/A

MEDICATIONS

DRUGS OF CHOICE
- Corticosteroids—anti-inflammatory dosages for symptomatic relief while the fleas are being controlled
- Antihistamines—symptomatic relief
- Fipronil (GABA antagonist)—monthly spot treatment for cats and dogs and spray treatment for dogs; activity against fleas and ticks; resistant to removal with water; excellent safety and efficacy profile
- Imidacloprid—monthly spot treatment for cats and dogs; excellent safety and efficacy profile
- Systemic treatments—limited benefit because they require a flea bite that has already initiated FBH; may help animals with flea infestation; primarily licensed for use in only dogs; lufenuron, a chitin inhibitor, available as an oral formulation for cats and dogs and as an injection for cats; permethrin available as a spot treatment and reputed to have some repellent activity; imidacloprid (flea adulticide) available as a spot treatment for cats and dogs.
- Sprays—usually contain pyrethrins and pyrethroids (synthetic pyrethrins) with an insect growth regulator or synergist; generally effective < 48–72 hr; advantages are low toxicity and repellent activity; disadvantages are frequent applications and expense.
- Indoor treatment—fogs and premises sprays; usually contain organophosphates, pyrethrins, and/or insect growth regulators; apply according to manufacturer's directions; treat all areas of the house; can be applied by the owner; advantages are weak chemicals and generally inexpensive; disadvantage is labor intensity; premises sprays concentrate the chemicals in areas that most need treatment.
- Professional exterminators—advantages are less labor-intensive; relatively few applications; sometimes guaranteed; disadvantages are strength of chemicals and cost; specific recommendations and guidelines must be followed.
- Inert substances—boric acid, diatomaceous earth, and silica aerogel; treat every 6–12 months; follow manufacturer's recommendations; very safe and effective if applied properly
- Outdoor treatment—concentrated in shaded areas; sprays usually contain pyrethroids or organophosphates and an insect growth regulator; powders are usually organophosphates; product containing nematodes (*Steinerma carpocapsae*) is very safe and chemical-free.

CONTRAINDICATIONS
N/A

PRECAUTIONS
- Insecticidal sprays and dips should not be used on dogs and cats ≤ 3 months, unless otherwise specified on the label.
- Pyrethrin/pyrethroid-type flea products—adverse reactions include depression, hypersalivation, muscle tremors, vomiting, ataxia, dyspnea, and anorexia.
- Organophosphates—adverse reactions include hypersalivation, lacrimation, urination, defecation, vomiting, diarrhea, miosis, fever, muscle tremors, seizures, coma, and death.
- All pesticides must be applied according to label directions.
- Toxicity—if any signs are noted, the animal should be bathed thoroughly to remove any remaining chemicals and treated appropriately.
- Rodents and fish are very sensitive to pyrethrins.

POSSIBLE INTERACTIONS
- Organophosphate treatments—do not use more than one form at a time.
- Topical organophosphates—avoid in cats, very young animals (< 3months of age), and sick or debilitated animals.
- Straight permethrin sprays or spot-ons—do not use in cats.
- Cythioate—contraindicated in heartworm-positive dogs and greyhounds
- Piperonyl butoxide—do not use in concentrations > 1% in cats.

ALTERNATIVE DRUGS
- Powders—usually contain organophosphates or carbamates; advantage is high residual effectiveness; disadvantages are dry skin and toxicity; organophosphates and carbamates should be avoided in cats.
- Dips, sprays, powders, and foams—dips usually contain organophosphates and synthetic pyrethrins and should not be used more than once per week; follow manufacturer's instructions for safest and best results; after repeated use, these agents can be drying or irritating; newer, safer spot treatments have essentially replaced these products.

FOLLOW-UP

PATIENT MONITORING
- Pruritus—a decrease means the FBH is being controlled.
- Fleas and flea dirt—absence is not always a reliable indicator of successful treatment in very sensitive animals.

PREVENTION/AVOIDANCE
- See Medications
- Year-round warm climates—year-round flea control
- Seasonally warm climates—begin flea control in May or June

POSSIBLE COMPLICATIONS
- Secondary bacterial infections
- Acute moist dermatitis
- Acral lick dermatitis

EXPECTED COURSE AND PROGNOSIS
Prognosis is good, if strict flea control is instituted.

MISCELLANEOUS

ASSOCIATED CONDITIONS
Approximately 80% of atopic dogs are also allergic to flea bites.

AGE-RELATED FACTORS
Organophosphates—use with utmost caution in old animals; not recommended for use in very young animals (< 3 months).

ZOONOTIC POTENTIAL
In areas of moderate to severe flea infestation, people can be bitten by fleas; usually papular lesions are located on the wrists and ankles.

PREGNANCY
- Corticosteroids and organophosphates—do not use in pregnant bitches and queens.
- Carefully follow the label directions of each individual product to determine its safety.

SYNONYMS
- Flea bite allergy
- Flea bite hypersensitivity

ABBREVIATIONS
- ELISA = enzyme-linked immunosorbent assay
- GABA = γ-aminobutyric acid
- RAST = radioallergosorbent test

Suggested Reading
Bevier-Tournay DE. Fleas and flea control. In: Kirk RW, Bonagura JD, eds. Current veterinary therapy X. Philadelphia: Saunders, 1989:586–591.
Griffin CE, Kwochka KW, MacDonald JM. Current veterinary dermatology. St. Louis: Mosby, 1993.

Authors Karen A. Kuhl and Jean S. Greek
Consulting Editor Karen Helton Rhodes

DISEASES

FLUKES, LIVER

BASICS

OVERVIEW
• *Platynosum concinnum* infection • Occurs in cats in Florida, Hawaii, and many other tropical areas • Infestation acquired from ingestion of an infected intermediate host, usually a lizard or frog

SIGNALMENT
• Outdoor and outdoor/indoor cats in tropical areas • Reported 15%–85% of cats infected; few exhibit signs • Feral cats—higher prevalence of infection • Typical patient—young (6–24 months) feral cat that feeds on local fauna (e.g., lizards and frogs)

SIGNS
• Depend on severity of infection • Most affected cats have no clinical signs. • Jaundice • Emaciation • Anorexia • Mucoid diarrhea • Hepatomegaly • Abdominal distension • Vomiting • Malaise

CAUSES & RISK FACTORS
• *P. concinnum*—adults normally reside in the bile ducts and gallbladder; life cycle requires two intermediate hosts and tropical to semitropical climate • Embryonated eggs—passed in the cat's feces; ingested by first intermediate host, a land snail • Miracidia—hatch from eggs in the snail; penetrate host tissues; change into sporocysts • Mature daughter sporocysts—emerge from the snail; ingested by the second intermediate host, usually an anole lizard (but also skunks, geckos, frogs, and toads); enter bile ducts and reside there until host is ingested by the cat • Cercariae—released in the upper digestive tract of cat; migrate to the bile ducts; mature and shed eggs in about 8 weeks • Risk factors for infection—tropical or subtropical climate; existence of intermediate hosts; an outdoor or indoor/outdoor environment; successful hunting skills; consumption of infected intermediate host

DIAGNOSIS

DIFFERENTIAL DIAGNOSIS
• Other liver diseases of cats—cholangiohepatitis; hepatic lipidosis; hepatocellular carcinoma; bile duct carcinoma; hepatic lymphoma • Any disorder causing major bile duct occlusion • Differentiated by examination of cytologic specimens from hepatic or bile aspirates; most definitively from histopathology of biopsied liver tissue

CBC/BIOCHEMISTRY/URINALYSIS
• Various
• Usually circulating eosinophilia beginning 3 weeks after infection; persists for months
• Liver enzyme activities—increased, particularly ALT and AST; ALP may be normal or only slightly high
• Bilirubin—increased (up to 20 mg/dL) in advanced and severe disease
• Urinalysis—almost always discloses bilirubinuria
• Fasting bile acids—usually high

OTHER LABORATORY TESTS
• Fecal examination—definitive diagnosis; identification of *P. concinnum* eggs
• Technique—sedimentation most successful; Formalin-ether or-sodium acetate most reliable (demonstrate 8 times more eggs than will direct fecal examination); detects infection in only 25% of cats
• Patients with few parasites (one to five flukes)—may shed only 2–10 eggs/g of feces; may not discover eggs
• Serial examinations—may be necessary
• Routine examination—with jaundice in endemic areas; patients that have been in tropical or subtropical areas

IMAGING
• Survey abdominal radiographs—not helpful for diagnosis; provide only general information about liver size (mild hepatomegaly)
• Ultrasonography—helps differentiate biliary obstruction from hepatocellular disease; shows one or more of the following: (1) biliary obstruction: dilated gallbladder, common bile duct (> 2 mm), and intrahepatic ducts; (2) gallbladder sediment with flukes (oval hypoechoic structures with an echoic center): mildly thickened gallbladder wall with a double-layered appearance; (3) cholangiohepatitis: overall hypoechoic parenchyma with increased prominence of hyperechoic portal areas

DIAGNOSTIC PROCEDURES
Hepatic biopsy—reveal signs of infection

PATHOLOGIC FINDINGS
• Gross—may note enlarged, yellow, and thickened liver owing to dilated bile ducts and bile duct hyperplasia; may see flukes in the bile ducts or gallbladder; increased size and tortuosity of bile ducts on cut sections
• Histologic—depend on the number of flukes and duration of infection; early (4–6 weeks): enlarged bile ducts; periductal areas become infiltrated with inflammatory cells, especially eosinophils; middle (by 4 months): severe adenomatous hyperplasia of bile duct epithelium; coincident periductal inflammation; late (by 6 months): extensive peribiliary fibrous connective tissue that may cause bile duct stricture

TREATMENT

• Outpatient vs. inpatient—depends on severity of illness • Balanced electrolyte solution with supplemental potassium chloride—20–40 mEq/L; as appropriate; based on serum electrolytes • Diet—moderate- to high-protein canned food; restrict protein with liver failure severe enough to cause encephalopathic signs

MEDICATIONS

DRUGS

• Praziquantel—20 mg/kg SC q24h for 3–5 days; treatment of choice; eggs may be passed in feces for up to 2 months after treatment.
• Prednisolone—initial dose with an eosinophilia: 2.0 mg/kg/day for 2–4 weeks; then taper in 50% decrements every 2 weeks; long-term therapy required for severe changes
• Ursodeoxycholic acid—10–15 mg/kg PO q24h; once bile duct patency ensured
• Broad-spectrum antibiotic (e.g., enrofloxacin)—usually given

CONTRAINDICATIONS/POSSIBLE INTERACTIONS

N/A

FOLLOW UP

• Monitor clinical signs, appetite, body weight, liver enzymes, and fecal sedimentation (for fluke eggs). • Death—from liver failure; untreated symptomatic disease
• Uncomplicated recovery in most patients treated • Praziquantel prophylaxis—every 3 months; may be required for outdoor cats in endemic tropical climates

✓ MISCELLANEOUS

Pregnancy—use caution with drug use.

SEE ALSO

Cholangitis/Cholangiohepatitis

ABBREVIATIONS

• ALP = alkaline phosphatase • ALT = alanine aminotransferase • AST = aspartate aminotransferase

Suggested Reading

Tams TR. Hepatobiliary parasites. In: Sherding RG, ed. The cat: diseases and management. Philadelphia: Saunders, 1994:607–611.

Author Colin F. Burrows
Consulting Editor Sharon A. Center

DISEASES

FOOD REACTIONS (DERMATOLOGIC)

BASICS

DEFINITION
Pruritic, nonseasonal reactions associated with ingestion of one or more substances in the animal's food

PATHOPHYSIOLOGY
• Pathogenesis not completely understood
• Immediate and delayed reactions to specific ingredients—documented in the veterinary literature; immediate reactions presumed to be type I hypersensitivity reactions; delayed owing to type III or IV
• Food intolerance—nonimmunologic, idiosyncratic reaction; involves metabolic, toxic, or pharmacologic effects of offending ingredients
• Food hypersensitivity is the most common term used, because it is not easy to distinguish between immunologic and idiosyncratic reactions.

SYSTEMS AFFECTED
• Skin/Exocrine—pruritus in any location on the body; otitis externa
• Gastrointestinal—vomiting; diarrhea; more frequent bowel movements
• Nervous—very rare; seizures have been documented with food hypersensitivity/intolerance

GENETICS
N/A

INCIDENCE/PREVALENCE
• Approximately 5% of all skin diseases and 10–15% of all allergic skin diseases in dogs and cats are the result of food hypersensitivity
• Third-most-common pruritic skin disease in the dog; second-most-common in the cat
• Percentages vary greatly with clinicians and geographical location.

GEOGRAPHIC DISTRIBUTION
N/A

SIGNALMENT

Species
Dogs and cats

Breed Predilections
None

Mean Age and Range
Any age

Predominant Sex
None

SIGNS

General Comments
A wide range of signs that can mimic any of the other hypersensitivity reactions

Historical Findings
• Nonseasonal pruritus of any body location
• Poor response to anti-inflammatory doses of glucocorticoids suggests a food hypersensitivity.
• Vomiting
• Diarrhea
• Excessive borborygmus, flatulence, and frequent bowel movements

Physical Examination Findings
• *Malassezia* dermatitis, pyoderma, and otitis externa
• Plaques
• Pustules
• Erythema
• Crusts
• Scale
• Self-induced alopecia
• Excoriation
• Lichenification
• Hyperpigmentation
• Urticaria
• Angioedema
• Pyotraumatic dermatitis

CAUSES
• Immune-mediated reactions—result of the ingestion and subsequent presentation of one or more glycoproteins (allergens) either before or after digestion; sensitization may occur at the gastrointestinal mucosa, after the substance is absorbed, or both.
• Nonimmune (food intolerance) reactions—result of ingestion of foods with high levels of histamine or substances that induce histamine either directly or through histamine-releasing factors

RISK FACTORS
• Unknown
• It is speculated that in juvenile animals intestinal parasites or intestinal infections may cause damage to the intestinal mucosa, resulting in the abnormal absorption of allergens and subsequent sensitization.

DIAGNOSIS

DIFFERENTIAL DIAGNOSIS
• Flea bite hypersensitivity—usually confined to the caudal half of the body; often seasonal
• Atopy—associated with pruritus on the face, ventrum, and feet; often seasonal; if pruritus first occurs at < 6 months or > 6 years of age, then food hypersensitivity may be more likely than inhalant allergy.
• Drug reactions—history of drug administration before the development of signs and improvement after withdrawal of the suspected drug confirms the diagnosis.
• Scabies—pruritus often very specific in the location (ears, elbows and hocks); mites in skin scrapings and response to specific therapy confirm the diagnosis.

CBC/BIOCHEMISTRY/URINALYSIS
No important changes

OTHER LABORATORY TESTS
N/A

IMAGING
N/A

DIAGNOSTIC PROCEDURES

Food Elimination Diet
• Definitive test for food hypersensitivity
• Tailored to the individual patient
• The diet must be restricted to one protein and one carbohydrate to which the animal has had limited or no previous exposure.
• It may take up to 13 weeks for maximum improvement of the clinical signs.
• If the patient is sensitive to one or more foods, noticeable improvement will be seen by the 4th week of the diet.

Challenge and Provocation Diet Trials
• Used if the patient improves on the elimination diet
• Challenge—feed the patient with the original diet; a return of the signs confirms that something in the diet is causing the signs; the challenge period should last until the signs return but no longer than 10 days.

FOOD REACTIONS (DERMATOLOGIC)

• Provoke (provocation diet trial)—if the challenge confirmed the presence of a food hypersensitivity, add single ingredients to the elimination diet; test ingredients include a full range of meats (beef, chicken, fish, pork, lamb), a full range of grains (corn, wheat, soybean, rice), eggs, and dairy products; the provocation period for each ingredient should last up to 10 days or less if signs develop sooner (dogs usually develop signs within 1–2 days); results guide the selection of commercial foods that do not contain the offending substance(s).

PATHOLOGIC FINDINGS
• Skin biopsies—not diagnostic; help confirm other differentials
• Histopathologic findings—variable; common findings suggest hypersensitivity; a secondary pyoderma or *Malassezia* infection may be seen.

TREATMENT

APPROPRIATE HEALTH CARE
Outpatient management

NURSING CARE
N/A

ACTIVITY
No change

DIET
Avoid any food substances that caused the clinical signs to return during the provocation phase of the diagnosis.

CLIENT EDUCATION
• Make sure the client understands the principles involved in each phase of the diagnostic test diets.
• Inform client to eliminate treats, chewable toys, vitamins, and other chewable medications (e.g., heartworm preventative), which may contain ingredients from the patient's previous diet.
• Outdoor pets must be confined to prevent foraging and hunting, which might alter the test diet.
• Provide handouts for clients to take home.
• Advise client that all family members must be aware of the test protocol and must help keep the test diet clean and free of any other food sources.

SURGICAL CONSIDERATIONS
N/A

MEDICATIONS

DRUGS OF CHOICE
• Systemic antipruritic drugs—may be useful during the first 2–3 weeks of diet trial to control self-mutilation
• Antibiotics or antifungal medications—useful for secondary pyodermas or *Malassezia* infections

CONTRAINDICATIONS
• Antibiotics that are known to have anti-inflammatory effects (e.g., tetracycline, erythromycin, and trimethoprim-potentiated sulfas)
• Glucocorticoids and antihistamines must be discontinued for at least 10–14 days while on the diet trial to allow correct assessment of the animal's response.

PRECAUTIONS
N/A

POSSIBLE INTERACTIONS
Chewable vitamins and heartworm medications may contain offending food substances.

ALTERNATIVE DRUGS
None

FOLLOW-UP

PATIENT MONITORING
Examine patient and evaluate and document the pruritus and clinical signs every 3–4 weeks.

PREVENTION/AVOIDANCE
• Avoid intake of any of the proteins included in the previous diet.
• Treats and chewable toys should be limited to known safe substances (e.g., apples, vegetables).

POSSIBLE COMPLICATIONS
Other causes of pruritus (e.g., flea bite hypersensitivity; atopy; and external parasites such as sarcoptic, *Notoedres,* and *Cheyletiella* mites can mask the response to the food elimination diet trial.

EXPECTED COURSE AND PROGNOSIS
• Prognosis is good, if food ingredients are the only cause of the pruritus and offending ingredients are avoided.
• Rarely a dog or cat may develop hypersensitivity to new substances, which may require a new elimination diet trial.
• Any other hypersensitivities (flea or atopy) must also be treated.

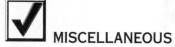

MISCELLANEOUS

ASSOCIATED CONDITIONS
• Superficial pyoderma
• *Malassezia* dermatitis
• Otitis externa

AGE-RELATED FACTORS
Animals who develop pruritus for the first time at < 6 months or > 6 years of age are more likely to have food hypersensitivity than atopy.

ZOONOTIC POTENTIAL
None

PREGNANCY
N/A

SYNONYMS
• Food allergy
• Food intolerance

SEE ALSO
• Atopy
• Contact Dermatitis
• Flea and Flea Control
• Malassezia Dermatitis
• Otitis Externa and Media
• Pyoderma

Suggested Reading
Jeffers JG, Shanley KJ. Diagnostic testing of dogs for food hypersensitivity. J Am Vet Med Assoc 1991;198:245–250.
MacDonald JM. Food allergy. In: Griffin CE, Kwochka KW, MacDonald JM, eds. Current veterinary dermatology. St. Louis Mosby, 1993:121.
Rosser EJ. Diagnosis of food allergy in dogs. J Am Vet Med Assoc 1993:203:259.
White SD. Food hypersensitivity in 30 dogs. J Am Vet Med Assoc 1986:188:695–698.
Author David Duclos
Consulting editor Karen Helton Rhodes

GASTRIC DILATION AND VOLVULUS SYNDROME (GDV)

BASICS

DEFINITION
A syndrome of dogs in which the stomach dilates and twists around its central axis, which results in complex local and systemic pathologic and physiologic changes

PATHOPHYSIOLOGY
• Fluid or ingesta accumulates in the stomach in conjunction with a mechanical or functional obstruction of the gastroesophageal and pyloric orifices. • Dilation of the stomach may progress, adding to functional obstruction and potentiating volvulus. • Twisting of the stomach may occur without dilation. • When viewing the dog in dorsal recumbency from caudal to cranial, the stomach may twist in a clockwise or counterclockwise direction. • The most common presentation is clockwise, with the duodenum passing ventrally from right to left; the rotation is around the long axis from the cardia to the pylorus; rotation varies from 90° to 360°. • Direct gastric damage and multiple systemic abnormalities occur secondary to ischemia and reperfusion injury. Ischemia results from rising intragastric pressures, decreased cardiac return as the stomach compresses the portal vein and caudal vena cava, direct outflow obstruction of gastric and splanchnic vessels due to twisting, infarction of the gastric mucosa due to neutrophil accumulation and margination, and edema due to multiple cell damage and inflammatory mediator release. • These changes account for the acute clinical signs, which include hypovolemic shock and cardiovascular failure. • Reperfusion injury is a complex entity involving the formation of oxygen free radicals and multiple inflammatory mediators.

SYSTEMS AFFECTED
• Gastrointestinal—fundus of the stomach is most severely compromised by occlusion of its blood supply during torsion • Cardiovascular—low venous return to the right side of the heart results in severe hypoxia to other organ systems and hypovolemic shock; arrhythmias occur secondary to the effects of hypoxia, inflammatory mediators, and other cardiogenic factors. • Respiratory—direct impedance of volume expansion caused by gastric distension and decreased cardiac output to the lungs • Hemic/Lymphatic/Immune—splenic infarction • Hepatobiliary—multiple factors including inflammatory mediators, hypoxia, endotoxemia, and potentially reperfusion injury of the liver

GENETICS
No direct genetic predisposition confirmed

INCIDENCE/PREVALENCE
• Vary • Metropolitan emergency clinics see these cases frequently.

GEOGRAPHIC DISTRIBUTION
N/A

SIGNALMENT

Species
Dog

Breed Predilections
• German shepherds • Great Danes • Saint Bernards • Rottweilers • Labrador retrievers • Alaskan malamutes • Any large, deep-chested breed • Rarely reported in dachshunds and Pekingese

Mean Age And Range
Any age; most commonly in middle-aged to older dogs

Predominant Sex
N/A

SIGNS

Historical Findings
• Nonproductive retching • Ptyalism • Progressive abdominal distension • Weakness or collapse • Depression • Frequent belching

Physical Examination Findings
• Tympanic cranial abdomen • Tachycardia • Tachypnea • Rectal body temperature may vary widely. • Signs of hypovolemic shock (e.g., pale mucous membranes, decreased capillary refill time, weak pulses)

CAUSES
Theories of interest include pyloric outflow obstruction, gastric myoelectric abnormalities, dynamic movement of the stomach following ingestion of food or water, and aerophagia.

RISK FACTORS
• Activity following ingestion of large quantities of food or water • Any intense activity or stress (including hospitalization and surgery)

DIAGNOSIS

DIFFERENTIAL DIAGNOSIS
• Gastric dilation without torsion—due to overdistension, usually from ingesting excessive quantities of food • Other diseases that cause acute abdominal distension (e.g., intestinal volvulus, splenic torsion, abdominal effusion or hemorrhage) • Differentiate non-GDV conditions via examination and imaging.

CBC/BIOCHEMISTRY/URINALYSIS
• Expect hemogram abnormalities consistent with acute inflammation and hemoconcentration/shock • Electrolyte abnormalities and acid–base alterations are common. • Urinalysis generally reflects hypovolemia—high urine specific gravity due to prerenal azotemia

OTHER LABORATORY TESTS
N/A

IMAGING
• Abdominal radiography—a right lateral abdominal radiograph is the imaging modality of choice; a "double bubble" compartmentalized stomach is considered pathognomonic; the pylorus is air filled on this view; a left lateral radiograph may help to determine if a volvulus is present; the pylorus is fluid-filled on this view. • Dorsoventral view—the pylorus may be shifted toward, or located in, the left cranial abdomen. • Stabilization may be necessary prior to imaging procedures.

DIAGNOSTIC PROCEDURES
Abdominocentesis and cytology may help determine if perforation has occurred.

PATHOLOGIC FINDINGS
• Gastric distension with resultant gastric edema, hyperemia, congestion, infarction, and necrosis, depending on the duration of the condition • Splenic torsion may also be present with similar changes.

TREATMENT

APPROPRIATE HEALTH CARE
• Emergency inpatient medical and surgical management • Patients require immediate medical therapy with special attention to establishing improved cardiovascular function and then gastric decompression. • Shock/fluid therapy should precede gastric decompression; give isotonic fluids at the rate of 90 mL/kg within the first 30–60 min, the general treatment of choice for hypovolemic (shock) patients; delivery of this volume may require placing two large-gauge intravenous catheters. • Supportive fluids on the basis of hydration status are recommended for animals not in shock. • Postoperative fluid support is needed until the patient is stable and able to eat and drink. • Use of colloid solutions has been advocated to restore cardiorespiratory function. • First try gastric decompression by orogastric intubation; light sedation with narcotics may facilitate this process. • Decompression by other techniques such as trocarization and indwelling catheters is described. • Maintain gastric decompression either by a pharyngo-gastric tube or an indwelling catheter until definitive treatment or surgical derotation and gastropexy. • Surgery is indicated in all cases of GDV, though the time interval from presentation to surgery may vary depending on response or lack of response to treatment. • Immediate surgery is indicated in patients unresponsive to cardiorespiratory stabilization and in all patients following successful stabilization.

NURSING CARE
• Maintain blood pressure with ample fluid support following volume replacement/shock therapy. • Electrolyte and acid–base management indicated; often potassium supplementation is necessary. • Monitor patients closely for reoccurrence of dilation or cardiorespira-

GASTRIC DILATION AND VOLVULUS SYNDROME (GDV)

tory decompensation.

ACTIVITY
Severely restrict activity prior to surgery and for a minimum of 10–14 days postsurgery

DIET
• Begin oral alimentation as soon as appropriate on the basis of gastric integrity at surgery. • Placing a jejunostomy feeding tube at the time of surgery when prolonged gastric healing is expected may allow early enteral supplementation. • Small multiple feedings of a high-quality, easily digested, easily assimilated diet is recommended during surgical recovery to prevent gastric distension. • Soaking dry food in water for 15–20 min prior to feeding helps prevent rapid expansion of food in the stomach. • Institute dietary changes on a permanent basis to prevent future dilatory episodes.

CLIENT EDUCATION
• Discuss potential risks of surgery and the potential for recurrence of the dilation. • Explain signs of recurrence of gastric dilation, so the client may detect the condition early.

SURGICAL CONSIDERATIONS
• Definitive treatment—exploratory celiotomy with gastric derotation and permanent right-sided gastropexy • Timing of surgery—controversial; based on the patient's cardiovascular condition, gastric decompression, and other physical parameters • Prolonged delay may result in death of the patient. • Derotation without gastropexy results in an 80% recurrence rate. • Multiple techniques for gastropexy are appropriate and are described in detail in surgical texts. • Partial gastrectomy may be required on the basis of gastric wall integrity, especially in the fundic region. • Thromboses of short gastric vessels, blue-to-black persistent serosal discoloration after derotation, and lack of hemorrhage from cut surfaces indicate nonviable tissue and necessitate excision. • Supplemental alimentation may be indicated with partial gastrectomies, depending on the remaining gastric integrity; a jejunostomy tube may be placed at the time of surgery for postoperative enteral support. • Splenic vasculature infarction is an indication for splenectomy. • Surgical exploration should be thorough and yet efficient to minimize surgical time. • Decreased survival time is associated with prolonged surgery and anesthesia in a hemodynamically unstable patient.

MEDICATIONS

DRUGS OF CHOICE
• Corticosteroids such as dexamethasone sodium phosphate (5 mg/kg slow IV) or prednisolone sodium succinate (22 mg/kg slow IV)—used to stabilize membranes, aid in cardiovascular support, and potentially help with treatment and prevention of reperfusion

injury • Antibiotics effective against gastrointestinal flora are often recommended because of the potential for endotoxemia associated with shock, gastric compromise, and potential abdominal contamination at the time of surgery. • Effective antibiotic choices include cefazolin sodium (20–35 mg/kg IV q8h or every 2 h interoperatively) or cefoxitin sodium (30 mg/kg IV q6–8h). • Additional antibiotics may be necessary, depending on cultures of abdominal contents at the time of surgery. • H_2-receptor antagonists may ameliorate or prevent gastric ulceration (e.g., famotidine 0.5 mg/kg IV or PO q12–24h; ranitidine 1.0 mg/kg IV or PO q12h).

CONTRAINDICATIONS
• Avoid drugs that may exacerbate hypovolemia (e.g., acetylpromazine). • Avoid drugs that may lead to renal compromise, until shock and hypovolemia are corrected (e.g., aminoglycosides). • Reserve drugs for correction of acid–base abnormalities until the patient is stabilized.

PRECAUTIONS
• Choose anesthetic agents for their cardiovascular supportive effects. • Pay special attention to maintaining the mean arterial pressure at or above 60 mm Hg. • Rapid administration of prednisolone sodium succinate may cause vomiting.

POSSIBLE INTERACTIONS
N/A

ALTERNATIVE DRUGS
• Hypertonic saline (7% NaCl solution) in 6% Dextran 70—5 mL/kg given over 5 min and followed with lactated Ringer's solution at 20 mL/kg/h • Colloids (e.g. hydroxylethyl starch [Hetastarch], 10–20 mL/kg IV administered slowly to effect; 6% dextran 70 in 0.9% sodium chloride [Dextran 70], 10–20 mL/kg IV administered slowly to effect; polymerized bovine hemoglobin glutamer-200 [Oxyglobin] 30 mL/kg IV given at 10 mL/kg/h) followed by lactated Ringer's solution at 20 mL/kg/h

FOLLOW-UP

PATIENT MONITORING
• Cardiorespiratory function for at least 24 h after surgery; blood pressure and perfusion • Electrocardiographic monitoring • Splenectomy frequently results in multifocal intermittent-to-continuous premature ventricular contractions. • Administer antiarrhythmics only when necessary. • Institute general supportive care with special attention to electrolyte and acid–base status. • Base treatment on serial laboratory analyses.

PREVENTION/AVOIDANCE
• Avoid ingestion of excessive amounts of food or fluids. • Feed small meals multiple times daily. • Avoid postprandial exercise.

POSSIBLE COMPLICATIONS
• Postoperative gastric ulceration may occur within 5–7 days if severe mucosal defects remain. • Rupture of gastric ulcers may result in septic peritonitis and its sequelae. • Other complications reported following gastropexy include belching and intermittent vomiting. • Gastric dilation may recur.

EXPECTED COURSE AND PROGNOSIS
• Based on surgical assessment and postoperative recovery • Patients recovering well after 7 days appear to have a good prognosis for complete recovery. • Gastropexy appears to be the most significant factor preventing recurrence; reoccurrence rates are as high as 80% without gastropexy and 3–5% with various gastropexy procedures.

MISCELLANEOUS

ASSOCIATED CONDITIONS
N/A

AGE-RELATED FACTORS
N/A

ZOONOTIC POTENTIAL
N/A

PREGNANCY
• No specific considerations aside from hemodynamic support • Associated hypoxia may be detrimental to the fetuses.

SYNONYMS
• Bloat • Gastric dilation—volvulus • Gastric torsion

SEE ALSO
• Shock • Sepsis and Bacteremia

ABBREVIATION
GDV = gastric dilation and volvulus syndrome

Suggested Reading
Guilford WG. Gastric dilatation, gastric dilatation-volvulus, and chronic gastric volvulus. In: Guilford WG, Center SA, Stombeck, et al., eds. Strombeck's small animal gastroenterology. 3rd ed. Philadelphia: Saunders, 1996:303–317.

Matthiesen DT. Gastric dilation-volvulus syndrome. In: Slatter D, ed. Textbook of small animal surgery. 2nd ed. Philadelphia: Lea & Febiger, 1993:580–593.

Matthiesen DT. Pathophysiology of gastric dilatation volvulus. In: Bojrab MJ, ed. Disease mechanisms in small animal surgery. 2nd ed. Philadelphia: Lea & Febiger, 1993: 220–231.

Schertel ER, Allen DA, Muir WW, et al. Evaluation of a hypertonic saline-dextran solution for treatment of dogs with shock induced by gastric dilatation-volvulus. J Am Vet Med Assoc 1997;210:226–230.

Author Michelle Joy Waschak
Consulting Editors Mitchell A. Crystal and Brett M. Feder

DISEASES

GASTRIC MOTILITY DISORDERS

BASICS

DEFINITION
Disorders resulting from conditions that directly or indirectly disrupt normal gastric emptying, which may then cause gastric distension and subsequent gastric signs

PATHOPHYSIOLOGY
• The stomach has two distinct motor regions.
• The proximal region relaxes to accommodate food and regulates expulsion of liquids; intrinsic slow contractions of this region push liquids through the pylorus.
• The distal stomach mechanically breaks down and expels solids through strong peristaltic contractions.
• Distal gastric motility and emptying is regulated by a gastric pacemaker, which is an area of intrinsic electrical activity found in the greater curvature.
• Gastric electrical activity, dietary composition, and extrinsic factors influence emptying.
• During fasting, nondigestible solids are expelled from the stomach by migrating myoelectric complexes that produce strong contractions that sweep through the stomach and intestine every 2 h in the fasted state; this motility is regulated by the hormone, motilin.
• Dysrhythmias in normal gastric electrical activity may be fundamental in the pathophysiology of disorders affecting gastric motility.

SYSTEMS AFFECTED
Gastrointestinal

GENETICS
N/A

INCIDENCE/PREVALENCE
• Unknown
• Many factors can affect gastric emptying, with or without resulting clinical disease.

GEOGRAPHICAL DISTRIBUTION
N/A

SIGNALMENT

Species
Dogs and cats

Breed Predilections
Unknown

Mean Age and Range
Symptoms can occur at any age, but primary motility disorders are uncommon in young animals.

Predominant Sex
N/A

SIGNS

General Comments
Often secondary to the primary cause of the disorder

Historical Findings
• Major clinical sign is chronic postprandial vomiting of food.
• The stomach in dogs should be empty 6–8 h after eating an average-size meal (4–6 h in cats).
• Vomiting undigested food >10 h after eating suggests a gastric motility disorder or outflow obstruction.
• Vomiting can occur anytime following eating.
• Other signs include gastric distension, nausea, anorexia, belching, pica, and weight loss.

Physical Examination Findings
• Normal or findings associated with the underlying cause of the disorder
• Palpation of a large, distended stomach
• Decreased gastric sounds on abdominal auscultation

CAUSES
• Primary idiopathic gastric motility disorders may arise from defects in normal myoelectric activity.
• Most motility disorders are secondary to other conditions.
• Metabolic disorders include hypokalemia, uremia, hepatic encephalopathy, and hypothyroidism.
• Nervous inhibition from stress, fear, pain, or trauma
• Drugs (e.g., anticholinergics, β-adrenergic agonists, and narcotics)
• Primary gastric disease (e.g., gastric outflow obstructions, gastritis, gastric ulcers, parvovirus) and gastric surgery
• GDV syndrome is suspected to result from a primary motility disorder of abnormal myoelectric and mechanical activity.
• Following surgical gastropexy, dogs may continue to have signs of gastric hypomotility.
• Gastroesophageal reflux and enterogastric reflux (see Bilious Vomiting Syndrome) may result from gastric hypomotility.
• Dysautonomia syndromes have gastric hypomotility as part of a generalized disease.

RISK FACTORS
Any potential gastric disease may result in secondary hypomotility.

DIAGNOSIS

DIFFERENTIAL DIAGNOSIS
• Extensive; include any condition causing vomiting
• Always rule out gastric outflow obstructions.

CBC/BIOCHEMISTRY/URINALYSIS
• Perform routine hemogram, serum chemistry profile, urinalysis, and fecal flotation to rule out the potential cause of gastric hypomotility.
• Continued vomiting may result in dehydration, electrolyte abnormalities, or acid–base imbalance.
• Hypokalemia is a common electrolyte abnormality associated with abnormal gastrointestinal motility.

OTHER LABORATORY TESTS
Specialized testing may be required to determine a specific cause; individualize for each patient.

IMAGING

Abdominal Radiography
Survey radiographs may reveal a gas-, fluid-, or ingesta-distended stomach.

Liquid Barium Contrast Radiography
• May be evidence of delayed gastric emptying and decreased gastric contractions if evaluated by fluoroscopy
• Some patients may have normal emptying of liquids but abnormal emptying of solids.

Food Barium Contrast Radiography
• Barium mixed with a standard meal may demonstrate delayed gastric emptying of solids.
• Normal animals should empty their stomachs by 6–8 h.
• Abnormal gastric retention is associated with longer gastric emptying times.

Food-Marker Contrast Radiography
Barium-impregnated small markers or other radiopaque markers mixed with a standard meal have delayed passage similar to that in the food barium contrast study.

Radionuclide Emission Imaging
Radionuclide markers mixed with a meal give the most clinically accurate measurement of emptying; gastric emptying times (time for a standard meal to leave the stomach) range from 4 to 8 h.

DIAGNOSTIC PROCEDURES

Endoscopy
• Findings are frequently normal in idiopathic conditions.

• Food may be found in the stomach when it should be empty after an 8- to 12-h preendoscopic fasting period.
• Endoscopy detects obstructive or inflammatory diseases of the stomach.

PATHOLOGIC FINDINGS
• Idiopathic conditions have normal gastric mucosa.
• Histology may identify inflammatory or neoplastic causes of gastric hypomotility.

TREATMENT

APPROPRIATE HEALTH CARE
• Most are outpatients.
• Severe vomiting or dehydration and electrolyte imbalance require hospitalization and specific therapy.

NURSING CARE
Dehydration with fluid and electrolyte imbalance requires appropriate fluid replacement.

ACTIVITY
Restrictions based on the underlying disease

DIET
• Manipulation is important in managing primary gastric motility disorders.
• Liquid or semiliquid and low in fat and fiber content
• Give small volumes with frequent feedings.
• Often dietary manipulation alone successfully manages patients with delayed gastric emptying from a motility disorder.

CLIENT EDUCATION
Discuss possible underlying causes of altered gastric motility and that response to therapy varies with individual case.

SURGICAL CONSIDERATIONS
• Dogs with chronic GDV syndrome and gastric retention—surgical gastropexy
• Following any gastric surgery it may take as long as 14 days for motility to return to normal.
• Gastric outflow obstructions require surgical correction.

MEDICATIONS

DRUGS OF CHOICE
Gastric Prokinetic Agents
• Metoclopramide—increases the amplitude of antral contractions; inhibits fundic receptive relaxation; coordinates duodenal and gastric

motility; also has antiemetic effects blocking the chemoreceptor trigger zone in the brainstem in dogs but not cats; oral dosage is 0.2–0.4 mg/kg q6–8h given 30 min before meals (use lower dose in cats).
• Cisapride—works directly by cholinergic neurotransmission of gastrointestinal smooth muscle stimulating motility; increases lower esophageal sphincter pressure; improves gastric emptying; promotes increased motility of both the small and large intestine; suggested dose is 0.1 mg/kg PO q8–12h given before meals; reportedly is more effective than metoclopramide in the dog and cat.
• Erythromycin—at low (submicrobiological) doses has a motilin hormone-like effect promoting gastric emptying; suggested dosage of erythromycin for specific motility effects is 1–5 mg/kg PO q8–12h, given 30 min before meals; appears to be more effective than metoclopramide

CONTRAINDICATIONS
• Do not administer gastric prokinetic agents to patients with a gastric outflow obstruction.
• Do not give metoclopramide with concurrent phenothiazine and narcotic administration or to patients with epilepsy.

PRECAUTIONS
• Metoclopramide may cause nervousness, anxiety, or depression.
• Cisapride may cause depression, vomiting, diarrhea, or abdominal cramping.
• Erythromycin may cause vomiting.

POSSIBLE INTERACTIONS
N/A

ALTERNATIVE DRUGS
N/A

FOLLOW-UP

PATIENT MONITORING
• Response to therapy depends on the underlying cause.
• Failure to respond medically necessitates further investigation for mechanical obstruction.

PREVENTION/AVOIDANCE
N/A

POSSIBLE COMPLICATIONS
N/A

EXPECTED COURSE AND PROGNOSIS
• Length of treatment depends on ability to resolve the underlying disorder and the clinical response.

• It may take parvovirus patients 10–14 days to regain normal gastric function following clinical recovery.
• Generalized dysautonomia has a grave prognosis.

MISCELLANEOUS

ASSOCIATED CONDITIONS
Both reflux esophagitis and reflux gastritis (bilious vomiting syndrome)

AGE-RELATED FACTORS
N/A

ZOONOTIC POTENTIAL
N/A

PREGNANCY
Avoid gastric prokinetic agents.

SYNONYMS
• Gastric hypomotility
• Gastric atony

SEE ALSO
• Gastroesophageal Reflux
• Gastric Dilatation Volvulus Syndrome
• Gastritis
• Bilious Vomiting Syndrome

ABBREVIATION
GDV = gastric dilatation volvulus syndrome

Suggested Reading
Hall JA, Burrows CF, Twedt DC. Gastric motility in dogs. Part 1. Normal gastric function. Compend Sm Anim 1988;10: 1282–1291.
Hall JA, Twedt DC, Burrows CF. Gastric motility in dogs. Part 2. Disorders of gastric motility. Compend Sm Anim 1990;12: 1373–1390.
Twedt DC. Diseases of the stomach. The cat diseases and clinical management. 2nd ed. New York: Churchill Livingstone, 1994: 1181–1210.
Willard MD. Diseases of the stomach. In: Ettinger SJ, Feldman EC, eds. Textbook of veterinary internal medicine. 4th ed. Philadelphia: Saunders, 1995:1143–1168.
Wise LA, Lappin MR. Canine dysautonomia. Semin Vet Med Surg (Sm Anim) 1990;5:72.
Author David C. Twedt
Consulting Editors Brett M. Feder and Mitchell A. Crystal

DISEASES

GASTRITIS, ATROPHIC

BASICS

OVERVIEW
A class of chronic gastritis characterized histologically by a focal or diffuse reduction in size and depth of gastric glands

SIGNALMENT
• Probably highly variable
• Not reported in cats
• A high prevalence reported in the Norwegian lundehunde

SIGNS
• Vomiting—usually intermittent
• Anorexia, lethargy, pica, weight loss

CAUSES & RISK FACTORS
• Unknown
• May reflect chronic gastritis due to any cause
• Immunization of dogs with their own gastric juice can induce chronic gastritis.
• *Helicobacter* spp. may be important in the development of canine and feline gastritis
• May be a genetic predisposition in the Norwegian lundehunde.

DIAGNOSIS

DIFFERENTIAL DIAGNOSIS
Other forms of chronic gastritis and chronic enteritis

CBC/BIOCHEMISTRY/URINALYSIS
Generally unremarkable

OTHER LABORATORY TESTS
N/A

IMAGING
Survey radiographs, contrast radiography, and ultrasonography are only useful to rule out other causes of chronic vomiting.

DIAGNOSTIC PROCEDURES
• Definitive diagnosis via gastroscopy and biopsy
• Gastroscopy may reveal prominent mucosal blood vessels caused by mucosal thinning.

PATHOLOGIC FINDINGS
• Histologic examination of gastric biopsy specimens reveals glandular atrophy.
• Urease activity in gastric biopsy specimens indicates infection with *Helicobacter* spp.

TREATMENT

• Typically, outpatient medical treatment
• Dietary elimination studies—warranted if underlying dietary sensitivity is suspected

MEDICATIONS

DRUGS

• Histamine type-2 receptor antagonists (e.g., famotidine 0.5 mg/kg PO qd to b.i.d.) or proton pump inhibitors (e.g., omeprazole 0.7 mg/kg PO qd) to inhibit gastric acid secretion
• Antibiotic treatment (e.g., amoxicillin at 10–20 mg/kg PO b.i.d. for 3 weeks) if infection with *Helicobacter* spp. is confirmed.
• If vomiting persists, prokinetic agents such as metoclopramide (0.2–0.5 mg/kg PO t.i.d.) or cisapride (0.1–0.5 mg/kg PO b.i.d. to t.i.d.) may be indicated.

CONTRAINDICATIONS/POSSIBLE INTERACTIONS

Be cautious with medications known to exacerbate gastritis, such as corticosteroids and nonsteroidal antiinflammatory drugs.

 FOLLOW-UP

• Long-term intermittent antacid therapy may be required.
• Associated with a high prevalence of gastric carcinoma in the Norwegian lundehunde.

 MISCELLANEOUS

With severe atrophy, gastric acid secretion may be impaired; this will likely be a subclinical abnormality.

ASSOCIATED CONDITIONS

Chronic enteritis

SEE ALSO

• Gastritis, chronic
• Vomiting, chronic

Suggested Reading

Twedt DC. Vomiting. In: Anderson NV, ed. Veterinary gastroenterology. Philadelphia: Lea & Febiger, 1992:336–367.

Williams DA, Melgarejo T. Gastroenteropathy in Norwegian Lundehunds in the USA. J Vet Int Med 1997;11:114–114.

Author David A. Williams

Consulting Editors Brett M. Feder and Mitchell A. Crystal

DISEASES

GASTRITIS, CHRONIC

BASICS

DEFINITION
• Intermittent vomiting of >1–2 weeks duration secondary to gastric inflammation
• Presence of gastric erosions and ulcers depends on the inciting cause and duration.

PATHOPHYSIOLOGY
• Chronic irritation of the gastric mucosa by chemical irritants, drugs, or infectious agents, resulting in an inflammatory response in the mucosal surface that may extend to involve submucosal layers
• Chronic allergen exposure or immune-mediated disease may also produce chronic inflammation.

SYSTEMS AFFECTED
• Gastrointestinal—esophagitis may result from chronic vomiting or gastroesophageal reflux.
• Respiratory—aspiration pneumonia is infrequently seen secondary to chronic vomiting; it is more likely if concurrent esophageal disease exists or patient is debilitated.

GENETICS
N/A

INCIDENCE/PREVALENCE
Relatively common

GEOGRAPHIC DISTRIBUTION
N/A

SIGNALMENT
Species
Dogs and cats
Breed Predilections
• Old, small-breed dogs (i.e., Lhasa apso, shih tzu, miniature poodle) are more commonly affected with antral mucosal hyperplasia and hypertrophy.
• Basenjis and the Drentse patrijshond breed can develop chronic hypertrophic gastritis.
Mean Age and Range
Varies with underlying cause
Predominant Sex
Varies with underlying cause

SIGNS
Historical Findings
• Vomit is frequently bile stained and may contain undigested food, flecks of blood, or digested blood ("coffee grounds").
• Frequency varies from daily to every few weeks and increases as gastritis progresses.
• Vomiting may be stimulated by eating or drinking.

• Early morning vomiting before eating may indicate bilious vomiting syndrome.
• May see weight loss with chronic anorexia
• May see melena with ulceration
• Diarrhea

Physical Examination Findings
• Often normal
• May be thin with persistent anorexia
• May have pale mucous membranes with anemia from chronic blood loss

CAUSES
• Inflammatory—immune-mediated, dietary allergy or intolerance, idiopathic
• Dietary indiscretion—plant material, foreign objects, chemical irritants
• Toxins—fertilizers, herbicides, cleaning agents, heavy metals
• Metabolic/endocrine disease—uremia, chronic liver disease, hypoadrenocorticism
• Parasitism—*Ollulanus tricuspis* and *Gnathostoma* spp. (cats); *Physaloptera* spp. (dogs)
• Drugs—NSAIDs, glucocorticoids
• Infectious—*Helicobacter* spp., viral (distemper in dogs, feline leukemias virus [FeLV] in cats),
• Miscellaneous—duodenogastric reflux (bilious vomiting syndrome), stress, achlorhydria

RISK FACTORS
• Medications—NSAIDs, glucocorticoids
• Environmental—unsupervised/free-roaming pets are more likely to ingest inappropriate foods or materials, intentionally or unintentionally.
• Ingestion of a dietary antigen to which an allergy or intolerance has been acquired

DIAGNOSIS

DIFFERENTIAL DIAGNOSIS
• Must differentiate chronic vomiting from chronic regurgitation
• All the causes listed above are included in the differential diagnosis of chronic gastritis; commonly no identifiable cause exists for the gastric inflammation.
• Idiopathic gastritis—diagnosis of exclusion; often characterized by a predominantly lymphoplasmacytic infiltrate (superficial or diffuse)
• Eosinophilic gastritis, hypertrophic gastritis, granulomatous/histiocytic gastritis, and atrophic gastritis are less common; often overlap of histologic changes exists in the types of inflammatory infiltrates.
• Atrophic gastritis differs on endoscopic

examination—visualization of the submucosal vessels secondary to thinning of the gastric mucosa
• Hypertrophic gastritis—prominent mucosal folds that do not flatten with gastric insufflation.

CBC/BIOCHEMISTRY/URINALYSIS
• Hemogram usually unremarkable unless systemic disease present
• Hemoconcentration if severe dehydration
• Anemia with ulceration—microcytic, hypochromic associated with iron deficiency if prolonged, severe blood loss
• May see eosinophilia with eosinophilic gastroenteritis
• Azotemia with low urine specific gravity in uremic gastritis
• Increased serum hepatic enzyme activities, total bilirubin or hypoalbuminemia with chronic hepatic disease
• Hyperkalemia and hyponatremia suggest Addison's disease.
• Hyponatremia, hypokalemia, hypochloremia, and an elevated bicarbonate level with an acidotic urine suggest a gastric outflow obstruction (hypochloremic metabolic alkalosis)

OTHER LABORATORY TESTS
Elevated serum gastrin level without azotemia suggests a gastrinoma.

IMAGING
• Survey abdominal radiographs—usually normal, but may reveal radiodense foreign objects, a thickened gastric wall, or gastric outlet obstruction with persistent gastric distension
• Contrast radiography—may detect foreign objects, outlet obstruction, delayed gastric emptying, or gastric wall defects
• Ultrasonography—may detect gastric wall thickening and gastric foreign objects

DIAGNOSTIC PROCEDURES
• Gastroscopy—usually adequate for visualization of the gastric mucosa and for biopsy
• Gastric biopsy and histopathology is required for diagnosis; should biopsy, even if gastric mucosa appears normal
• Foreign objects can be identified and retrieved via endoscopy.
• Do an exploratory celiotomy if a submucosal lesion of the gastric wall is suspected and a full-thickness biopsy is required.
• Fecal flotation may reveal intestinal parasites

PATHOLOGIC FINDINGS
• Idiopathic gastritis—inflammatory infiltrates vary; can be lymphocytes, plasma cells, neutrophils, eosinophils, and/or histiocytes
• Mucosal changes can be degenerative, hyperplastic, or atrophic.

• May be varying levels of edema and fibrous tissue; may be *Helicobacter* spp.; special stains can be requested for fungal hyphae.

TREATMENT

APPROPRIATE HEALTH CARE
• Most patients are stable at presentation unless vomiting is severe enough to cause dehydration.
• Can typically manage as outpatient, pending diagnostic testing or undergoing clinical trials of special diets or medications
• If patient is dehydrated or vomiting becomes severe, hospitalize and institute appropriate intravenous crystalloid fluid therapy (see Acute Vomiting).

NURSING CARE
N/A

ACTIVITY
N/A

DIET
• NPO for 12–24 h if vomiting frequently
• Soft, low-fat foods with a single carbo-hydrate and protein source
• Non-fat cottage cheese or tofu as a protein source, and rice, pasta, or potato as a carbo-hydrate source, in a ratio of 1:3
• Frequent, small meals
• Can use novel protein source if dietary allergy is suspected
• Feed diets for a minimum of 3 weeks to assess adequacy of response.

CLIENT EDUCATION
• Gastritis has numerous causes.
• Diagnostic workup—may be extensive; usually requires a biopsy for a definitive diagnosis

SURGICAL CONSIDERATIONS
• Surgical management if a granulomatous mass or hypertrophy is causing a gastric outflow obstruction
• Gastrotomy for removal of foreign objects if endoscopic retrieval is unsuccessful or is not available

MEDICATIONS

DRUGS OF CHOICE
• Treat any gastric erosions and ulcers (see Gastroduodenal Ulcer Disease).

• Give glucocorticoids (prednisone 1–2 mg/kg PO q12h; taper every 2–3 weeks over 2–3 months) for chronic gastritis secondary to suspected immune-mediated mechanisms if no clinical response to dietary management.
• Antiemetics for fluid and electrolyte disorders caused by frequent or profuse vomiting (see Acute Vomiting)
• Metoclopramide (0.4 mg/kg PO q6–8h or cisapride (0.5–1 mg/kg PO q8h) to increase gastric emptying and normalize intestinal motility gastric emptying is delayed or duodenogastric reflux is present

CONTRAINDICATIONS
• Do not use prokinetics, metoclopramide or cisapride, if gastric outlet obstruction is present.
• Antacids are not indicated with atrophic gastritis and achlorhydria.

PRECAUTIONS
N/A

POSSIBLE INTERACTIONS
N/A

ALTERNATIVE DRUGS
• Synthetic prostaglandin E (misoprostol 1–3 μg/kg PO q6–8h) to prevent gastric mucosal ulcers with NSAID toxicity
• Immunosuppressive drugs such as azathio-prine (50 mg/M^2 PO q24 h, tapering to every other day after 2–3 weeks) if an immune-mediated mechanism is suspected and response to dietary management and glucocorticoid administration is inadequate.

FOLLOW-UP

PATIENT MONITORING
• Resolution of clinical signs indicates a positive response.
• Electrolytes and acid–base status if initially abnormal
• Complete blood count for patients on myelosuppressive drugs (i.e., azathioprine)
• Repeat biopsy if signs decrease but do not resolve.

PREVENTION/AVOIDANCE
• Avoid medications (e.g., corticosteroids, NSAIDs) and foods that cause gastric irritation or allergic response in the patient.
• Prevent free roaming and potential for dietary indiscretion.

POSSIBLE COMPLICATIONS
• Progression of gastritis from superficial to atrophic gastritis
• Gastric erosions and ulcers with progressive mucosal damage
• Aspiration pneumonia
• Electrolyte or acid–base imbalances

EXPECTED COURSE AND PROGNOSIS
Varies with underlying cause

MISCELLANEOUS

ASSOCIATED CONDITIONS
N/A

AGE-RELATED FACTORS
Young animals are more likely to ingest foreign objects.

ZOONOTIC POTENTIAL
N/A

PREGNANCY
Do not administer misoprostol to pregnant animals.

SYNONYMS
N/A

SEE ALSO
• Vomiting, Chronic
• Gastroenteritis, Lymphocytic Plasmacytic
• Gastroenteritis, Eosinophilic
• Gastritis, Atrophic
• Gastroduodenal Ulcer Disease
• Physaloptera
• Chronic Hypertrophic Pyloric Gastropathy

ABBREVIATIONS
• FeLV = feline leukemia virus
• NPO = nothing per os
• NSAIDs = nonsteroidal antiinflammatory drugs

Suggested Reading
Guilford WG, Strombeck DR. Chronic gas-tric diseases. In: Guilford WG, Center SA, Strombeck DR, et al., eds. Small animal gastroenterology. Philadelphia: Saunders, 1996:275–302.
Willard MD. Diseases of the stomach. In: Et-tinger SJ, Feldman EC, eds. Textbook of veterinary internal medicine. Philadelphia: Saunders, 1995:1143–1168.
Author John Richard Hart, Jr.
Consulting Editors Brett M. Feder and Mitchell A. Crystal

DISEASES

GASTRODUODENAL ULCER DISEASE

 BASICS

DEFINITION
Erosive lesions that extend through the mucosa and into the muscularis mucosa

PATHOPHYSIOLOGY
• Gastroduodenal ulcers result from single or multiple factors altering, damaging, or overwhelming the normal defense and repair mechanisms of the "gastric mucosal barrier." • Factors that make up the "gastric mucosal barrier" and protect the stomach from ulcer formation include the mucus-bicarbonate layer over the epithelial cells, the gastric epithelial cells, gastric mucosal blood flow, epithelial cell restitution and repair, and prostaglandins produced by the gastrointestinal tract. • Factors that cause mucosal barrier damage and predispose to gastroduodenal ulcer formation include inhibiting the epithelial cell's ability to repair, decreasing the mucosal blood supply, and/or increasing gastric acid secretion. • The risk of gastroduodenal ulcer formation increases with the number of insults to the "gastric mucosal barrier."

SYSTEMS AFFECTED
• Gastrointestinal—gastric fundus and antrum are the most common sites of ulceration; gastrinomas (rare) usually cause ulcer formation in the proximal duodenum. • Cardiovascular/hemic—acute hemorrhage may result in anemia with subsequent tachycardia, systolic heart murmur, and/or hypotension. • Respiratory—tachypnea may be present with anemia; aspiration pneumonia rarely occurs secondary to vomiting.

GENETICS
N/A

INCIDENCE/PREVALENCE
True incidence unknown; probably more common than clinically recognized

GEOGRAPHIC DISTRIBUTION
Pythium spp.–induced ulcers have a regional distribution—states that border the Gulf of Mexico

SIGNALMENT

Species
Dogs; less commonly, cats

Breed Predilection
N/A

Mean Age and Range
All ages

Predominant Sex
Male dogs have increased incidence of gastric carcinoma.

SIGNS

General Comments
Some animals may be asymptomatic with significant gastroduodenal ulcer disease.

Historical Findings
• Vomiting—most common clinical sign • Hematemesis—fresh or digested (appear like coffee grounds) blood may or may not be present. • Melena may be present. • Cranial abdominal pain—patient may stand hunched in the back or assume the "praying position" (up in hind, down in front). • Anorexia • Weakness, pallor, and collapse if severe anemia or perforation/peritonitis develops

Physical Examination Findings
• Pale mucous membranes and weakness—if significant anemia • Systolic heart murmur—if anemia is acute and severe • Tachycardia, hypotension and prolonged capillary refill time if hypovolemic shock or perforation/septic peritonitis; hyperthermia and abdominal fluid distension may also be seen with perforation/septic peritonitis. • Edema—from blood/plasma loss causing hypoproteinemia • Weight loss and cachexia—if disease is chronic • May be a large cutaneous or subcutaneous mass, splenomegaly and/or hepatomegaly—if mast cell disease is the cause of the ulceration • May be icterus—if liver disease is cause of ulceration • May be oral ulceration and uremic breath—if ulceration is from renal failure

CAUSES
• Drugs—NSAIDs • Metabolic disease—hepatic disease, renal failure, hypoadrenocorticism, acute pancreatitis, hyperadrenocorticism • Stress/major medical illness—shock, severe illness, hypotension, trauma, major surgery, burns, heat stroke, sepsis, DIC • Gastric foreign bodies • Gastric neoplasia • Gastritis—lymphocytic/plasmacytic gastroenteritis, eosinophilic gastroenteritis • Mast cell tumor • Gastrinoma • Infectious agents—*Helicobacter* spp. (importance in dogs/cats unknown), pythiosis, *Ollulanus tricuspis* (in cats) • Neurologic disease—head trauma, intervertebral disk disease • Correction of chronic diaphragmatic hernia • Lead poisoning

RISK FACTORS
• Administration of ulcerogenic drugs (NSAIDs) • Concurrent administration of NSAIDS and glucocorticoids • Critically ill patients • Hypovolemic or septic shock

 DIAGNOSIS

DIFFERENTIAL DIAGNOSIS
• Esophageal disease (neoplasia, esophagitis, foreign body)—differentiate by contrast radiography and/or endoscopy • Thrombocytopenia (immune-mediated, paraneoplastic, infectious)—identified on CBC • Coagulopathies (DIC, anticoagulant rodenticide poisoning)—detected by coagulation panel

• Nasal disease (neoplasia, fungal infection)—blood may be swallowed, and hematemesis and melena can occur; may differentiate on clinical signs and physical examination findings alone or by skull radiographs and fiber-optic evaluation of nasopharyngeal area and nasal cavities • Oropharyngeal disease (neoplasia, foreign body)—distinguish by thorough oropharyngeal examination, often under sedation. • Pulmonary and airway disease (neoplasia, severe pneumonia, fungal infections, foreign body, headworm disease)—blood may be coughed up and/or swallowed and hematemesis/melena may occur; differentiate by thoracic radiographs, heartworm testing. • Administration of oral iron may stain vomitus; Pepto-Bismol may cause black, tarry stools.

CBC/BIOCHEMISTRY/URINALYSIS
• May be anemia—if acute (3–5 days) blood loss, nonregenerative anemia (normocytic, normochromic, minimal reticulocytosis); if blood loss >5 days duration, regenerative anemia (macrocytic, hyperchromic, reticulocytosis); if chronic blood loss, iron deficiency anemia (microcytic, hypochromic, poor reticulocytosis, ± thrombocytosis) • Panhypoproteinemia—may be present due to alimentary hemorrhage • May be mature neutrophilia, left-shift neutrophilia with sepsis and gastroduodenal ulcer perforation • BUN:creatinine ratio may be elevated with gastrointestinal hemorrhage. • May see elevated BUN, creatinine, hyperphosphatemia and isosthenuria—if ulcers are due to renal disease • May see elevated liver enzymes, hyperbilirubinemia and/or hypoalbuminemia—if ulcers are due to liver disease • May see hyperkalemia, hyponatremia, and azotemia—if ulcers are due to hypoadrenocorticism (atypical hypoadrenocorticism will not have electrolyte abnormalities) • Lipase and amylase may be elevated if ulcers are due to pancreatitis.

OTHER LABORATORY TESTS
• Fecal occult blood test may be positive—test is accurate if dog is eating dry food diet. • Fecal flotation—to screen for gastrointestinal parasitism • ACTH stimulation if suspect hypoadrenocorticism • Bile acids if suspect hepatic insufficiency • Buffy coat if suspect systemic mast cell disease • Gastrin levels if more common causes are ruled out

IMAGING
• Abdominal radiography usually unremarkable. • Contrast radiography (preferably double-contrast gastrogram) may identify a gastroduodenal ulcer or neoplastic disease. • Abdominal ultrasonography usually will not detect a gastroduodenal ulcer; it may identify a gastric or duodenal mass, gastric or duodenal wall thickening, and/or abdominal lymphadenopathy.

GASTRODUODENAL ULCER DISEASE

DIAGNOSTIC PROCEDURES
• Endoscopy—most definitive method for diagnosing; allows removal of foreign bodies; and collection of biopsy specimens from the gastric and/ or duodenal ulcerations • Urease testing of gastric biopsy specimens may confirm *Helicobacter* organisms. • If abdominal ultrasound shows a gastric or duodenal mass or gastroduodenal wall-thickening, perform an abdominal ultrasound-guided biopsy; occasionally ultrasound-guided gastroduodenal biopsy specimens will be diagnostic and the endoscopic biopsy specimens will not.
• Pythiosis-induced ulceration requires deep biopsies (ultrasound-guided or surgical); submit unrefrigerated samples in saline for culture and in formalin for histopathology with special staining. • Perform fine-needle aspiration or biopsies of cutaneous or intraabdominal masses to identify mast cell tumors. • May use abdominocentesis to identify septic peritonitis/gastroduodenal ulcer perforation

PATHOLOGIC FINDINGS
• Gastroduodenal inflammation and hemorrhage; may be necrosis, microthrombi, hemorrhage, and deep penetration • May identify *Helicobacter* spp. in gastric biopsy specimens (silver stains help identify *Helicobacter*) • May need special stains to detect pythiosis

TREATMENT

APPROPRIATE HEALTH CARE
• Treat any underlying causes. • Can treat on an outpatient basis if the cause is identified and removed, vomiting is not excessive, and gastroduodenal bleeding is minimal
• Inpatients—those with severe gastroduodenal bleeding and/or ulcer perforation, excessive vomiting, and/or undetermined cause • May need emergency management of hemorrhage or septic peritonitis

NURSING CARE
• Intravenous fluids to maintain hydration
• May need transfusions (whole blood or packed red blood cells) or oxygen-carrying hemoglobin solution infusions (Oxyglobin) in patients with severe gastroduodenal hemorrhage

ACTIVITY
Restricted

DIET
• Discontinue oral intake if vomiting. • When feeding is resumed, feed small amounts in multiple feedings; primarily an easily digestible diet.

CLIENT EDUCATION
Discuss potential causes

SURGICAL CONSIDERATIONS
Surgical treatment is indicated if medical treatment fails after 5–7 days, hemorrhage is uncontrolled and severe, gastroduodenal ulcer perforates, and/or potentially resectable tumor is identified.

MEDICATIONS

DRUG(S) OF CHOICE
• Histamine H_2-receptor antagonists competitively inhibit gastric acid secretion and are the initial drug of choice (famotidine 0.5 mg/kg PO, IV q12–24h, ranitidine 1–4 mg/kg SC, PO , IV q8–12h, cimetidine 5–10 mg/kg PO, SC, IV q8h); treat for at least 6–8 weeks; may couple with sucralfate • Sucralfate suspension (0.5–1 g PO q8h) protects ulcerated tissue (cytoprotection) by binding to ulcer sites.
• Administer antibiotic(s) with activity against enteric gram-negatives and anaerobes parenterally if a suspected break in the gastrointestinal mucosal barrier or aspiration pneumonia • Administer antiemetics (chlorpromazine 0.5–4 mg/kg q6–8h SC, IM, IV, prochlorperazine 0.1–0.5 mg/kg q6–8h SC, IM, IV, PO) if vomiting occurs frequently or causes significant fluid loss. • Omeprazole (0.7 mg/kg PO q24h)—the most potent inhibitor of gastric acid secretion; treatment of choice for ulcers nonresponsive to H_2 blockers and sucralfate and for gastrinomas with evidence of metastasis or nonresectable disease • If *Helicobacter* infection, institute appropriate therapy

CONTRAINDICATIONS
Do not administer phenothiazine derivatives to hypovolemic patients or those at risk for hypotension.

PRECAUTIONS N/A

POSSIBLE INTERACTIONS
• Cimetidine binds to hepatic cytochrome P450 enzyme and may interfere with metabolism of other drugs. • H_2-blockers prevent uptake of omeprazole by oxyntic cells. • Sucralfate may alter absorption of other drugs. • Patients taking H_2-blockers or in renal failure have elevated gastrin levels.

ALTERNATIVE DRUGS
Misoprostol, a synthetic prostaglandin analogue (2–5 μg/kg PO q6–12h), prevents or decreases the severity of NSAID-induced ulcers.

FOLLOW-UP

PATIENT MONITORING
• Assess improvement in clinical signs • Can check PCV, TP, BUN until they return to normal; test fecal samples intermittently for occult blood. • Repeat endoscopic evaluation is recommended for advanced cases to help determine duration of therapy.

PREVENTION/AVOIDANCE
• Avoid gastric irritants (e.g., NSAIDs, corticosteroids). • Concurrent use of misoprostol with NSAIDS • Administer NSAIDs with food.

POSSIBLE COMPLICATIONS
• Gastroduodenal ulcer perforation and possible sepsis • Severe blood loss requiring transfusion • Aspiration pneumonia—rare
• Death—sepsis, hemorrhage

EXPECTED COURSE AND PROGNOSIS
• Varies with underlying cause • Patients with malignant gastric neoplasia, renal failure, liver failure, pythiosis, systemic mastocytosis and sepsis, and gastric perforation—poor
• Gastroduodenal ulcers secondary to NSAID administration, *Helicobacter* infection, inflammatory bowel disease, or hypoadrenocorticism—may be good to excellent, depending on severity

MISCELLANEOUS

ASSOCIATED CONDITIONS N/A

AGE-RELATED FACTORS
Neoplasia more common in older animals

ZOONOTIC POTENTIAL
Further investigation needed to determine/evaluate a possible zoonotic potential for *Helicobacter* spp.

PREGNANCY
Synthetic prostaglandins (e.g., misoprostol) can cause abortion.

SYNONYMS N/A

SEE ALSO
• Acute Vomiting • Chronic Gastritis • Chronic Vomiting • *Helicobacter* • Hematemesis • Inflammatory Bowel Disease • Melena • Pythiosis • Pancreatitis

ABBREVIATIONS
• DIC = disseminated intravascular coagulation • NSAIDs = nonsteroidal antiinflammatory drugs

Suggested Readings

Guilford WO, Strombeck DR. Strombeck's small animal gastroenterology. 3rd ed. Philadelphia: Saunders, 1996.

Meddings JB, Kirk D, Olson M. Noninvasive detection of nonsteroidal anti-inflammatory drug-induced gastropathy in dogs. Am J Vet Res 1995;56:977–981.

Willard M. Diseases of the stomach. In: Ettinger SJ, Feldman EC, eds. Textbook of veterinary internal medicine. Philadelphia: Saunders, 1994:1143–1168.

Author Jocelyn Mott
Consulting Editors Mitchell A. Crystal and Brett M. Feder

DISEASES

GASTROENTERITIS, EOSINOPHILIC

BASICS

DEFINITION
An inflammatory disease of the stomach and intestine, characterized by an infiltration of eosinophils, usually into the lamina propria, but occasionally involving the submucosa and muscularis

PATHOPHYSIOLOGY
• Antigens bind to IgE on the surface of mast cells, resulting in mast cell degranulation.
• Some of the products released are potent eosinophil chemotactants.
• Eosinophils contain granules with substances that directly damage the surrounding tissues.
• Eosinophils also can activate mast cells directly, setting up a vicious cycle of degranulation and tissue destruction.

SYSTEMS AFFECTED
• Gastrointestinal—the large intestine may also be affected.
• In the cat, hypereosinophilic syndrome can involve the gastrointestinal tract, liver, spleen, kidney, adrenal glands, and heart.

GENETICS
N/A

INCIDENCE/PREVALENCE
• Eosinophilic gastroenteritis is reportedly more common in dogs than in cats.
• It is much less common than lymphocytic-plasmacytic gastroenteritis; occasionally, a mixed cellular infiltrate is present.

GEOGRAPHIC DISTRIBUTION
N/A

SIGNALMENT

Species
Dog and cat

Breed Predilections
German shepherd, rottweiler, and shar pei may be predisposed.

Mean Age and Range
• Dogs—most common in animals <5 years of age, although any age may be affected.
• Cats—median age, 8 years; range, 1.5–11 years reported

Predominant Sex
None reported

SIGNS

Historical Findings
• Intermittent vomiting, small bowel diarrhea, anorexia, and weight loss are the most common client complaints.
• One report states that 50% of cats with eosinophilic gastritis/enteritis had hematochezia or melena.

Physical Examination Findings
• Cats—thickened bowel loops may be palpated.
• May be evidence of weight loss
• If hypereosinophilic syndrome is the cause of the gastrointestinal disease, enlarged peripheral lymph nodes, mesenteric lymphadenopathy, hepatomegaly, and splenomegaly may be noted.

CAUSES
• Idiopathic eosinophilic gastroenteritis
• Parasitic
• Immune-mediated—food allergy; adverse drug reaction; associated with other forms of inflammatory bowel disease
• Systemic mastocytosis
• Hypereosinophilic syndrome
• Eosinophilic granuloma

RISK FACTORS
N/A

DIAGNOSIS

DIFFERENTIAL DIAGNOSIS
• All of the above-listed causes are included in the differential diagnosis of eosinophilic infiltrates in the stomach and small bowel.
• Idiopathic eosinophilic gastroenteritis is a diagnosis of exclusion.
• Multiple fecal flotations and direct smears are imperative to rule in or out intestinal parasitism.
• Intestinal biopsy differentiates the other causes of inflammatory bowel disease from eosinophilic gastroenteritis.
• Dietary trial will rule in or out food allergy or hypersensitivity.

CBC/BIOCHEMISTRY/URINALYSIS
• Hemogram may reveal a peripheral eosinophilia—more common in cats than dogs
• Panhypoproteinemia or hypoalbuminemia may be present if a protein-losing enteropathy is also present.
• Urinalysis is usually normal.

OTHER LABORATORY TESTS
Use a buffy-coat smear to rule out systemic mastocytosis.

IMAGING
• Plain abdominal radiographs provide little information.
• Barium contrast radiography may demonstrate thick intestinal walls and mucosal irregularities but does not provide any information about etiology or the nature of the thickening.
• Ultrasonography—may be used to measure stomach and intestinal wall thickness, and to rule out other diseases; can be used to examine the liver, spleen, and mesenteric lymph nodes in cats with hypereosinophilic syndrome

DIAGNOSTIC PROCEDURES
• Definitive diagnosis requires biopsy and histopathology, usually obtained via endoscopy.
• Bone marrow aspirates are recommended if systemic mastocytosis is suspected.
• Exploratory laparotomy may be indicated when portions of the gastrointestinal tract, unapproachable by endoscopy, are involved or abdominal organomegaly is present.

PATHOLOGIC FINDINGS
• Thickened rugal folds, erosions, ulcers, and increased mucosal friability may be present in the stomach, although grossly it can appear normal.
• Ulcerations and erosions may also be seen in the intestine.
• Eosinophilic infiltrates can be patchy in the intestine; multiple biopsies may be necessary to obtain a diagnostic sample.
• Histopathology reveals a diffuse infiltrate of eosinophils into the lamina propria; the submucosa and muscularis can also be involved (reportedly more common in cats with this disease).

TREATMENT

APPROPRIATE HEALTH CARE
• Most can be successfully treated on an outpatient basis.
• Patients with systemic mastocytosis, protein-losing enteropathies, or other concurrent illnesses may require hospitalization until they are stabilized.

NURSING CARE

• If the patient is dehydrated or must be NPO because of vomiting, any balanced fluid such as lactated Ringer's solution is adequate (for a patient without other concurrent disease); otherwise, select fluids on the basis of secondary diseases.
• If severe hypoalbuminemia from protein-losing enteropathy, consider colloids such as dextrans or hetastarch

ACTIVITY

No need to restrict unless severely debilitated.

DIET

• Manipulation—usually a critical component of therapy; may take several forms
• In patients with severe intestinal involvement and protein-losing enteropathy, total parenteral nutrition may be indicated until remission is obtained.
• Monomeric diets (e.g., elemental diet)—have nonallergenic components; can be used in patients who are not vomiting but have moderate-to-severe gastrointestinal inflammation; useful if a food allergy is suspected
• Highly digestible diets with limited nutrient sources—extremely useful for eliciting remission; can be used as maintenance diets once the patient is stabilized
• Dog—examples include Hill's prescription diets d/d and i/d, Iams chunks and Eukanuba Low Residue Diet, Canine Response Formula FP or KO, ANF, Hill's Science diets Maximum Stress and Canine Growth, or homemade diets.
• Cat—examples include Iams feline and Eukanuba Low Residue Diet, Tender Vittles, Hill's prescription diets i/d and d/d.
• Once the patient is stabilized, may institute an elimination diet trial if food allergy or intolerance is the suspected cause.

CLIENT EDUCATION

Explain the waxing and waning nature of the disease, the necessity for lifelong vigilance regarding inciting factors, and the potential for long-term therapy.

SURGICAL CONSIDERATIONS

N/A

MEDICATIONS

DRUGS OF CHOICE

• Corticosteroids—mainstay of treatment; prednisone used most frequently (1–2 mg/kg PO q12h in dogs; 2–3 mg/kg PO q12h in cats)

• Gradually taper corticosteroids; relapses are more common in patients that are taken off corticosteroids too quickly.
• Budesonide, a new oral glucocorticoid, has been used successfully to treat cats and dogs with inflammatory bowel disease; it is not yet approved in the United States but is available at some referral institutions.
• Occasionally other immunosuppressive drugs can be used to allow a reduction in corticosteroid dose and avoid some of the adverse effects of steroid therapy.
• Azathioprine (1–1.5 mg/kg q24h PO in dogs; 0.3 mg/kg q48h in cats) is the most common adjunctive immunosuppressive therapy.

CONTRAINDICATIONS

If secondary problems are present, avoid therapeutic agents that might be contraindicated for those conditions.

PRECAUTIONS

• Azathioprine rarely causes bone marrow suppression, usually more of a problem in cats than dogs.
• All patients on azathioprine—perform a complete blood count 10–14 days after the start of treatment, with rechecks monthly and then bimonthly thereafter; usually the condition is reversible when the drug is discontinued.
• Pancreatitis, hepatic damage, and anorexia are other potential side effects of this drug.

POSSIBLE INTERACTIONS

N/A

ALTERNATIVE DRUGS

N/A

FOLLOW-UP

PATIENT MONITORING

• Initially frequent for some more severely affected patients; peripheral eosinophil counts can be helpful; the corticosteroid dosage is usually adjusted during these visits.
• Patients with less severe disease—may be checked 2–5 weeks after the initial evaluation; monthly to bimonthly thereafter until corticosteroid therapy is completed.
• Patients receiving azathioprine—monitor as mentioned above; patients usually do not require long-term follow-up unless the problem recurs.

PREVENTION/AVOIDANCE

If a food intolerance or allergy is suspected or documented, avoid that particular item and adhere strictly to dietary changes.

POSSIBLE COMPLICATIONS

• Weight loss, debilitation in refractory cases
• Adverse effects of prednisone therapy
• Bone marrow suppression, pancreatitis, hepatitis, or anorexia caused by azathioprine

EXPECTED COURSE AND PROGNOSIS

• The vast majority of dogs with eosinophilic gastroenteritis respond to a combination of dietary manipulation and steroid therapy.
• Cats often have a more severe form of the disease, with a poorer prognosis than in dogs.
• Cats often require higher doses of corticosteroids for longer periods of time to elicit remission.

MISCELLANEOUS

ASSOCIATED CONDITIONS

N/A

AGE-RELATED FACTORS

N/A

ZOONOTIC POTENTIAL

A consideration only when eosinophilic infiltrates are secondary to parasites (e.g., *Ancylostoma, Giardia* and ascarids).

PREGNANCY

• Prednisone has been used safely in pregnant women; corticosteroids have been associated with increased incidence of congenital defects, abortion, and fetal death.
• Azathioprine has been used safely in pregnant women and may be a good substitute for corticosteroids in pregnant animals.

SYNONYMS

N/A

SEE ALSO

• Gastroenteritis, Lymphocytic-Plasmacytic
• Inflammatory Bowel Disease
• Mast Cell Tumors
• Gastrointestinal Parasites

ABBREVIATIONS

• IgE = immunoglobulin E
• NPO = nothing per os

Suggested Reading

Strombeck DR, Guilford WG. Idiopathic inflammatory bowel diseases. In: Guilford WG, Center SA, Strombeck DR, et al., eds. Strombeck's small animal gastroenterology. 3rd ed. Philadelphia: Saunders, 1996.
Tarris TR. Feline inflammatory bowel disease. Vet Clin North Am, 1993;23:569–586.

Author Kelly J. Diehl
Consulting Editors Brett M. Feder and Mitchell A. Crystal

DISEASES

GASTROENTERITIS, HEMORRHAGIC

BASICS

DEFINITION
A peracute hemorrhagic enteritis of dogs, characterized by a sudden onset of severe bloody diarrhea (often explosive), vomiting, and hypovolemia from dramatic loss of water and electrolytes into the intestinal lumen

PATHOPHYSIOLOGY
• Many conditions result in hemorrhagic diarrhea, but the HGE syndrome of dogs appears to have unique clinical features that distinguish it as an entity separate from other causes.
• HGE—a peracute loss of intestinal mucosal integrity, with rapid movement of blood, fluid, and electrolytes into the gut lumen
• Dehydration and hypovolemic shock occur quickly.
• Translocation of bacteria or toxins through the damaged intestinal mucosa may result in septic or endotoxic shock.

SYSTEMS AFFECTED
• Gastrointestinal
• Cardiovascular

GENETICS
Unknown; appears to be more common in certain breeds

INCIDENCE/PREVALENCE
Common clinical condition

GEOGRAPHIC DISTRIBUTION
Appears to occur more commonly in urban environments

SIGNALMENT

Species
Dogs

Breed Predilections
• All breeds can be affected; incidence is greater in small-breed dogs.
• Breeds most represented include miniature schnauzer, dachshund, Yorkshire terrier, and miniature poodle.

Mean Age and Range
• Usually occurs in adult dogs with a mean age of 5 years.

Predominant Sex
N/A

SIGNS

General Comments
• Clinical findings vary with both course and severity of the disease.
• Usually peracute and associated with concurrent hypovolemic shock
• Most patients have been healthy, with no historical environmental changes.

Historical Findings
• Signs usually begin with acute vomiting, anorexia, and depression, followed by severe bloody diarrhea.
• Signs—progress rapidly; become severe within hours (usually 8–12 h); result from hypovolemic shock and hemoconcentration

Physical Examination Findings
• Patient is generally depressed and weak, with prolonged capillary refill time and weak pulses.
• Skin turgor as a reflection of dehydration is normal because of the peracute nature of the disease and the lag time in fluid compartmental shifts.
• Abdominal palpation may be painful and reveal fluid-filled bowels.
• Rectal examination reveals bloody diarrhea; later in the course of disease a "raspberry jam" stool develops.
• Occasionally fever is present, but often the temperature is normal or even subnormal.

CAUSES
• Etiology unknown
• Endotoxic or anaphylactic shock, immune-mediated mechanisms directed against host enteric mucosa, or infectious etiologies have been proposed.
• Cultures from some dogs with HGE yield mostly pure cultures of *Clostridium perfringens,* but the significance is unknown.
• Searches for toxigenic *Escherichia coli* strains have been unrewarding.

RISK FACTORS
• Unknown
• Most dogs are previously healthy with no major concurrent illness.

DIAGNOSIS

DIFFERENTIAL DIAGNOSIS
• Parvovirus
• Bacterial enteritis (e.g., salmonellosis)
• Conditions resulting in endotoxic or hypovolemic shock
• Intestinal obstruction or intussusception
• Hypoadrenocorticism
• Pancreatitis
• Coagulopathy

CBC/BIOCHEMISTRY/URINALYSIS
• Hemoconcentration; PCV generally >60% and as high as 75%; often a stress leukogram
• Biochemistry profile may reveal secondary hepatic enzyme elevations and high BUN due to prerenal azotemia.

OTHER LABORATORY TESTS

Fecal Tests
• Stool—negative for parasites
• ELISA for parvovirus—negative
• Fecal cytology—shows many RBCs, occasional WBCs and possibly *C. perfringens* spores
• *Clostridium* may be cultured in high concentration, but cultures are negative for other enteric pathogens.

Coagulation Profile
Usually normal; occasionally secondary DIC is a complication.

IMAGING
Abdominal radiographs show fluid- and gas-filled small and large intestine.

DIAGNOSTIC PROCEDURES

Electrocardiogram
May note cardiac arrhythmias such as ventricular premature contractions and ventricular tachycardia

Endoscopy
Not indicated or helpful in the diagnosis; may show diffuse mucosal hemorrhage, ulceration, and hyperemia

PATHOLOGIC FINDINGS
Changes in the intestine include gross congestion and microscopic evidence of autolysis devoid of marked inflammation.

TREATMENT

APPROPRIATE HEALTH CARE
Hospitalize patients suspected of having HGE and treat aggressively; clinical deterioration is often rapid and can be fatal.

NURSING CARE
• Rapid fluid volume replacement for all patients
• Give balanced electrolyte solutions up to the rate of 40–60 mL/kg/h IV until the PCV is <50%.
• Give maintenance fluids to maintain circulatory function and correct any potassium or other electrolyte deficits during the recovery period.

ACTIVITY
Restrict

DIET
• NPO during acute disease
• During recovery period feed a bland, low-fat, low-fiber diet for several days before returning to the normal diet.

CLIENT EDUCATION
• Discuss the need for immediate, aggressive medical management.
• With appropriate therapy, mortality is usually low.
• Reoccurrence in about 10% of patients

SURGICAL CONSIDERATIONS
N/A

MEDICATIONS

DRUGS OF CHOICE
• Parenteral antibiotics are given because of the potential for septicemia and possible

implications of *C. perfringens;* ampicillin (10–20 mg/kg IV q6–8h) is recommended.
• Alternative choices include trimethoprim-sulfa or cephalosporins.
• Septicemia—ampicillin in combination with an aminoglycoside (e.g., gentamicin, 6–10 mg/kg IV q24h) or a fluoroquinolone (e.g., enrofloxacin, 5–10 mg/kg q24h) is suggested.
• Give short-acting glucocorticoids to dogs in shock (e.g., dexamethasone sodium phosphate 0.5–1.0 mg/kg IV).
• Excessive blood loss may require a blood transfusion (rare).

CONTRAINDICATIONS
N/A

PRECAUTIONS
Use aminoglycoside antibiotics with great care; do not give to patients with dehydration or renal compromise, because of the potential for nephrotoxicity.

POSSIBLE INTERACTIONS

Alternative Drugs
• Oral antibiotics and intestinal protectants—of little benefit and generally not administered
• Rectal administration of mucosal protectants—questionable value
• May give antiemetics to control severe vomiting; intestinal motility modifiers are not considered necessary or not recommended.

FOLLOW-UP

PATIENT MONITORING
• PCV and total solids frequently—at least every 4–6 h
• Modify the fluid replacement on the basis of PCV, continued GI fluid losses, and circulatory function.
• If no clinical improvement in 24–48 h, reevaluate the patient; other causes of hemorrhagic diarrhea are probable.

PREVENTION/AVOIDANCE
N/A

POSSIBLE COMPLICATIONS
• Occasionally DIC may develop; neurologic

signs or even seizures secondary to the hemoconcentration may occur.
• Cardiac arrhythmias occur from suspected myocardial reperfusion injury.

EXPECTED COURSE AND PROGNOSIS
• Course is generally short, 24–72 h.
• Prognosis is good; most patients recover with no complications.
• Sudden death is uncommon.

MISCELLANEOUS

ASSOCIATED CONDITIONS
N/A

AGE-RELATED FACTORS
N/A

ZOONOTIC POTENTIAL
Unknown

PREGNANCY
N/A

SYNONYMS
Acute hemorrhagic enterocolitis

SEE ALSO
• Diarrhea, Acute
• Vomiting, Acute

ABBREVIATIONS
• ELISA = enzyme-linked immunosorbent assay
• HGE = hemorrhagic gastroenteritis
• PCV = packed cell volume
• DIC = Disseminated intravascular coagulation

Suggested Reading
Burrows CF. Canine hemorrhagic gastroenteritis. JAAHA. 1977;13:451–458.
Spielman BL, Garvey MS. Hemorrhagic gastroenteritis in dogs. JAAHA. 1993;29:341–344.
Strombeck DR, Guilford WG. In: Guilford WG, Center SA, Strombeck DR, et al., eds. Strombeck's small animal gastroenterology. Philadelphia: Saunders, 1996:433–435.
Author David C. Twedt
Consulting Editors Brett M. Feder and Mitchell A. Crystal

GASTROENTERITIS, LYMPHOCYTIC-PLASMACYTIC

BASICS

DEFINITION
• A form of inflammatory bowel disease characterized by lymphocyte and/or plasma cell infiltration into the lamina propria of the stomach and intestine • Less commonly the infiltrates may extend into the submucosa and muscularis.

PATHOPHYSIOLOGY
• An abnormal immune response to environmental stimuli is most likely responsible for initiating gastrointestinal inflammation. • Continued exposure to antigen, coupled with self-perpetuating inflammation results in disease. • The exact mechanisms, antigens, and patient factors involved in initiation and progression remain unknown.

SYSTEMS AFFECTED
• Gastrointestinal—seldom is the stomach affected alone; the large bowel can also be affected. • Hemic/Lymphatic/Immune, Ophthalmic, Skin/Exocrine—other immune-mediated diseases frequently affect the hematopoietic system (autoimmune hemolytic anemia [AIHA], coagulopathies), eyes, and integument in humans with IBDs; animals may also develop these complications, although to date they are not as well characterized

GENETICS
Basenjis and lundehunds have particular familial forms of IBD.

INCIDENCE/PREVALENCE
A common problem in both cats and dogs; represents most of the cases of IBD.

GEOGRAPHIC DISTRIBUTION
N/A

SIGNALMENT

Species
Dogs and cats

Breed Predilections
• Lundehunds and basenjis have particular forms of IBD; gluten-sensitive enteropathy affects Irish setters. • German shepherds and shar peis are reportedly predisposed to lymphocytic-plasmacytic gastroenteritis. • No breed predilection reported in cats

Mean Age And Range
• Most common in middle-aged to old animals • Dogs as young as 8 months and cats as young as 5 months of age with IBD have been reported.

Predominant Sex
None reported

SIGNS

Historical Findings
• Signs associated with lymphocytic-plasmacytic gastritis with or without enteritis can vary greatly in type, severity, and frequency. • Generally have an intermittent, chronic course, but increase in frequency over time. • Cats—intermittent, chronic vomiting is the most common; chronic small bowel diarrhea is second. • Dogs—chronic small bowel diarrhea is the most common; if only the stomach is involved, vomiting is the most common. • Dogs and cats—anorexia (sometimes alternating with periods of ravenous appetite) and chronic weight loss are common; hematochezia, hematemesis, and melena are occasionally noted.

Physical Examination Findings
• Can vary from perfectly normal animal to a dehydrated, cachectic, and depressed patient • If only the stomach is involved, may be no discernible abnormalities

CAUSES
• Pathogenesis is most likely multifactorial. • Several causative factors have been identified.

Infectious Agents
Giardia, Salmonella, Campylobacter, and normal resident gastrointestinal flora have been implicated but not documented.

Dietary Agents
Meat proteins, food additives, artificial coloring, preservatives, milk proteins, and gluten (wheat) have all been proposed.

Genetic Factors
• Certain forms of IBD are more common in some breeds of dogs (see above). • Certain major histocompatibility genes, which are important components of normal immune responses, may render an individual susceptible to development of IBD.

RISK FACTORS
See Causes

DIAGNOSIS

DIFFERENTIAL DIAGNOSIS
• Other infiltrative inflammatory bowel conditions (e.g., eosinophilic gastroenteritis, granulomatous IBD) • Neoplastic conditions • Infectious diseases (e.g., histoplasmosis, giardiasis, salmonellosis, *Campylobacter* enteritis, and bacterial overgrowth) • Miscellaneous diseases (e.g., lymphangiectasia, gastrointestinal motility disorders, and exocrine pancreatic insufficiency) • In the cat, consider hyperthyroidism and systemic viral infection (e.g., FeLV, FIV, FIP).

CBC/BIOCHEMISTRY/URINALYSIS
• Often normal • Mild nonregenerative anemia and mild leukocytosis without a left shift—sometimes seen in cats • Neutrophilic leukocytosis, often with a left shift—frequently seen in dogs • Hypoproteinemia is more common in dogs than cats with IBD

OTHER LABORATORY TESTS
• Useful to eliminate other differentials • Dogs—tests include fasting serum TLI to evaluate exocrine pancreatic function, and fasting serum cobalamin and folate assays to evaluate for small intestinal function and bacterial overgrowth • Cats—T_4 and FeLV/FIV serology are recommended; fasting serum TLI (if exocrine pancreatic insufficiency suspected)

IMAGING
• Survey abdominal radiographs—usually normal. • Barium contrast studies—occasionally reveal mucosal abnormalities and thickened bowel loops; generally not helpful in establishing a definitive diagnosis; can be normal even in individuals with severe disease

DIAGNOSTIC PROCEDURES
• May first initiate a hypoallergenic diet trial to rule in or rule out dietary allergy or intolerance • Occasionally, certain forms of IBD respond to dietary manipulations alone. • If signs resolve completely, a diagnosis of dietary allergy or intolerance is likely, and no further workup is necessary. • Always perform fecal examination for parasites. • Definitive diagnosis requires biopsy and histopathology, usually obtained via endoscopy. • Duodenal aspirates for *Giardia* spp. may be collected during endoscopy. • Intestinal fluid obtained during endoscopy can also be submitted for quantitative culture if bacterial overgrowth is suspected. • Exploratory laparotomy may be indicated when portions of the gastrointestinal tract, unapproachable by endoscopy, are involved or if abdominal organomegaly is present.

PATHOLOGIC FINDINGS
• Grossly, stomach and intestinal appearance can range from normal to edematous, thickened, and ulcerated. • The hallmark histopathologic finding is an infiltrate of lymphocytes and plasma cells in the lamina propria. • The distribution may be patchy, so take several biopsy specimens.

TREATMENT

APPROPRIATE HEALTH CARE
Outpatient, unless the patient is debilitated from dehydration, hypoproteinemia, or cachexia

NURSING CARE
• If the patient is dehydrated or must be NPO because of vomiting, any balanced fluid such as lactated Ringer solution is adequate (for a patient without other concurrent disease); otherwise, select fluids on the basis of secondary diseases. • If severe hypoalbu-

minemia from protein-losing enteropathy, consider colloids (e.g., dextrans or hetastarch).

ACTIVITY
No restrictions

DIET
• Dietary therapy is an essential component of patient management. • Patients with severe intestinal involvement and protein-losing enteropathy may require total parenteral nutrition until remission. • Can feed monomeric diets such as elemental diets with nonallergenic components to patients that are not vomiting but have moderate-to-severe gastrointestinal inflammation; useful if a food allergy is suspected • Highly digestible diets with limited nutrient sources are extremely useful in eliciting remission and, after the patient is stabilized, can be used as maintenance diets. • Dog—examples include Hill's prescription diets d/d and i/d, Iams chunks and Eukanuba Low Residue Diet, Canine Response Formula FP or KO, ANF, Hill's Science diets Maximum Stress and Canine Growth, or homemade diets. • Cat—examples include Iams feline and Eukanuba Low Residue Diet, Tender Vittles, and Hill's prescription diets i/d and d/d. • Once the patient is stabilized, an elimination diet or food trial may be instituted if food allergy or intolerance is the suspected cause.

CLIENT EDUCATION
• IBD is not necessarily cured as much as controlled. • Relapses are common. • Patience is required during the various food and medication trials that are often necessary.

SURGICAL CONSIDERATIONS
N/A

MEDICATIONS

DRUGS OF CHOICE
• Corticosteroids—the mainstay of treatment for idiopathic lymphocytic-plasmacytic enteritis; prednisone used most frequently (1–2 mg/kg PO q12h in dogs; 2–3 mg/kg PO q12h in cats); cats may require a higher dose to control their disease; when signs resolve, gradually taper the corticosteroid dose; a new oral glucocorticoid, budesonide, has been used successfully to treat cats and dogs with IBD; the drug is not approved yet in the United States, but is available at some referral institutions; relapses are more common in individuals who are taken off corticosteroids too quickly. • Azathioprine (1–1.5 mg/kg q24h PO in dogs; 0.3 mg/kg q48h PO in cats)—an immunosuppressive drug that can be used to allow a reduction in corticosteroid dose and avoid some of the adverse effects of chronic steroid therapy • Metronidazole—has antibacterial and antiprotozoal properties; some evidence that it also has immune-modulating effects; the dosage for IBD in dogs and cats is 10 mg/kg PO q8–12h.

CONTRAINDICATIONS
If secondary problems are present, avoid therapeutic agents that might be contraindicated for those conditions.

PRECAUTIONS
• Azathioprine—causes bone marrow suppression rarely; usually more of a problem in cats than dogs • Perform a CBC on all individuals placed on azathioprine, 10–14 days after the start of treatment; recheck monthly and then bimonthly thereafter; usually the condition is reversible when the drug is discontinued. • Pancreatitis, hepatic damage, and anorexia are other potential adverse effects of this drug. • Metronidazole—can cause reversible neurotoxicity at high dosages; carcinogenic and mutagenic in laboratory animals; discontinuing the drug usually reverses the neurologic signs. • Cyclophosphamide—adverse effects include bone marrow suppression in dogs and cats and hemorrhagic cystitis (especially in dogs); a CBC every 2 weeks is recommended because adverse effects can occur months after initiating therapy; metabolized by the liver, so normal hepatic function should be established prior to use • Cyclosporine—can cause gastrointestinal irritation, gingival hyperplasia, and papillomatosis

POSSIBLE INTERACTIONS
• Cyclosporine can interfere with the metabolism of phenobarbital and phenytoin. • Ketoconazole, erythromycin, and cimetidine can decrease hepatic metabolism of cyclosporine. • Any drugs that are potentially nephrotoxic should be used with caution in conjunction with cyclosporine.

ALTERNATIVE DRUGS
• Cyclophosphamide and cyclosporine can be used in place of azathioprine. • Cyclophosphamide dosage for cats and dogs is 50 mg/m² PO q24h for four consecutive days in a cycle; cycles can be repeated weekly to every 3 weeks; caution clients to wear gloves when administering, because some people have contact dermal sensitivity. • Cyclosporine—currently undergoing evaluation for the treatment of IBD in humans; may be useful in the therapy of refractory cases of lymphocytic-plasmacytic gastroenteritis; a wide dose range, 0.5–8.5 mg/kg PO q12h, has been reported; initiate therapy at a high dose and taper as signs resolve; cost prohibits routine use of this drug.

FOLLOW-UP

PATIENT MONITORING
• For resolution of clinical signs • Severely affected patients require frequent monitoring; adjust medications during these visits. • Check patients with less severe disease 2–3 weeks after their initial evaluation and then monthly to bimonthly until immunosuppressive therapy is

discontinued. • Monitor patients receiving azathioprine or cyclophosphamide as mentioned above.

PREVENTION/AVOIDANCE
When a food intolerance or allergy is suspected or documented, avoid that particular item and adhere strictly to dietary changes.

POSSIBLE COMPLICATIONS
• Weight loss, debilitation in refractory cases • Side effects of prednisone therapy • Bone marrow suppression, pancreatitis, hepatitis, or anorexia caused by azathioprine

EXPECTED COURSE AND PROGNOSIS
• Dogs and cats with mild inflammation—good-to-excellent prognosis for full recovery • Patients with severe infiltrates, particularly if other portions of the GI tract are involved—more-guarded prognosis • Often the initial response to therapy sets the tone for a given individual's ability to recover.

MISCELLANEOUS

ASSOCIATED CONDITIONS
N/A

AGE-RELATED FACTORS
N/A

ZOONOTIC POTENTIAL
N/A

PREGNANCY
• Corticosteroids have been associated with increased incidence of congenital defects, abortion, and fetal death. • Azathioprine has been used safely in pregnant women, and may be a good substitute for corticosteroids in pregnant animals. • Metronidazole is mutagenic in laboratory animals; avoid

SYNONYMS
N/A

SEE ALSO
• Gastroenteritis, Eosinophilic • Inflammatory Bowel Disease

ABBREVIATIONS
• AIHA = autoimmune hemolytic anemia • FeLV = feline leukemia virus • FIP = feline infectious peritonitis • FIV = feline immunodeficiency virus • IBD = inflammatory bowel disease • NPO = nothing per os • TLI = trypsin-like immunoreactivity

Suggested Reading
Strombeck DR, Guilford WG. Idiopathic inflammatory bowel diseases. In: Guilford WG, Center SA, Strombeck DR, et al., eds. Strombeck's small animal gastroenterology. 3rd ed. Philadelphia: Saunders, 1996: 451–486.
Author Kelly J. Diehl
Consulting Editors Brett M. Feder and Mitchell A. Crystal

GASTROESOPHAGEAL REFLUX

BASICS

OVERVIEW
• Reflux of gastric or intestinal juice into the esophageal lumen
• Incidence unknown; probably more common than clinically recognized
• Transient relaxation of the gastroesophageal sphincter or chronic vomiting may permit reflux of gastrointestinal juices into the esophageal lumen.
• Gastric acid, pepsin, trypsin, and bile salts are all injurious to the esophageal mucosa.
• Esophagitis resulting from reflux may vary from mild inflammation of the superficial mucosa to severe ulceration involving the submucosa and muscularis.

SIGNALMENT
• Dogs and cats, male or female
• No breed predilections reported
• Can be associated with congenital hiatal hernia seen in Chinese shar-pei
• Occurs at any age; younger animals may be at increased risk because of developmental immaturity of the gastroesophageal sphincter.
• Young animals with congenital hiatal hernia may also be at increased risk.

SIGNS

Historical Findings
• Regurgitation
• Salivation
• Dysphagia
• Howling/crying during swallowing—odynophagia
• Anorexia
• Weight loss

Physical Examination Findings
• Often unremarkable
• Fever and ptyalism if severe ulcerative esophagitis

CAUSES & RISK FACTORS
• Anesthesia
• Failure to fast an animal prior to anesthesia
• Poor patient positioning during anesthesia
• Hiatal hernia
• Chronic vomiting
• Young age

DIAGNOSIS

DIFFERENTIAL DIAGNOSIS
• Oral or pharyngeal disease
• Ingestion of a caustic agent
• Esophageal foreign body
• Esophageal tumor
• Megaesophagus—idiopathic, myasthenia gravis, vascular ring anomaly
• Hiatal hernia
• Gastroesophageal intussusception

CBC/BIOCHEMISTRY/URINALYSIS
Usually normal

OTHER LABORATORY TESTS
N/A

IMAGING
• Survey thoracic radiographs are usually unremarkable.
• May be air in the distal esophagus
• Barium contrast radiography reveals gastro-esophageal reflux in some, but not all, animals.
• Barium paste may be more useful than liquid barium for evaluating esophageal function.

DIAGNOSTIC PROCEDURES
• Endoscopy and biopsy—probably the best means of documenting mucosal changes consistent with reflux esophagitis; patients may have an irregular mucosal surface with hyperemia or active bleeding in the distal esophagus.
• Esophageal manometry and pH-metry may help document this disorder in veterinary referral centers.

TREATMENT

• Generally managed as outpatients; it is not necessary to restrict activity; may withhold food for 1–2 days in moderate-to-severe cases
• Thereafter, feed low-fat, low-protein meals in small, frequent feedings; dietary fat decreases gastroesophageal sphincter pressure and delays gastric emptying; protein stimulates gastric acid secretion.

MEDICATIONS

DRUGS
Specific therapy may include
• Oral sucralfate suspensions (0.5–1.0 g PO q8h)
• Gastric acid anti-secretory agents—cimetidine 5–10 mg/kg PO q8h; ranitidine 0.5–2.0 mg/kg PO q12h; famotidine 0.5–1.0 mg/kg PO q12h; omeprazole 0.7 mg/kg PO q24h
• Prokinetic agents—cisapride 0.1–0.5 mg/kg PO q12h

CONTRAINDICATIONS/POSSIBLE INTERACTIONS
Sucralfate suspensions may interfere with the absorption of other drugs (e.g. cimetidine, ranitidine, omeprazole, cisapride,

FOLLOW-UP

• Patients do not necessarily require follow-up endoscopy.
• It may be appropriate in many patients to simply monitor clinical signs.
• Consider endoscopy for patients that do not respond to medical therapies.
• Clients should avoid feeding high-fat foods; they might exacerbate reflux.
• The most important complications are esophagitis and stricture formation.

MISCELLANEOUS

ASSOCIATED CONDITIONS
Hiatal hernia

AGE-RELATED FACTORS
N/A

ZOONOTIC POTENTIAL
N/A

PREGNANCY
N/A

SEE ALSO
N/A

ABBREVIATIONS
N/A

Suggested Reading

Evander A, Little AG, Riddell RH, et al. Composition of the reflux material determines the degree of reflux esophagitis in the dog. Gastroenterology 1987;93:280–286.
Callan MB, Washabau RJ, Saunders LPM, et al. Congenital esophageal hiatal hernia in the Chinese shar-pei dog. J Vet Int Med 1993;7:210–215.
Authors Robert J. Washabau and Nathaniel C. Myers III
Consulting Editors Brett M. Feder and Mitchell A. Crystal

DISEASES

GASTROINTESTINAL OBSTRUCTION

 BASICS

DEFINITION
• Partial or complete physical impedance to the flow of ingesta and/or secretions in an aboral direction through the pylorus into the duodenum (gastric outlet obstruction) or through the small intestine • Obstructions in the pharynx, esophagus, large intestine, or rectum, and motility disorders are addressed in separate chapters.

PATHOPHYSIOLOGY
Gastric Outflow Obstruction
• Ingesta and fluids accumulate in the stomach. • Vomiting often results in loss of fluids rich in hydrochloric acid (from gastric secretions) with subsequent hypochloremic metabolic alkalosis. • Varying degrees of dehydration, tissue compromise, malaise, and weight loss occur, depending on underlying cause, severity, and chronicity.

Small Intestinal Obstruction
• Ingesta and fluids accumulate proximal to the obstruction. • Vomiting often results in significant dehydration and electrolyte imbalances (particularly hypokalemia), depending on location (proximal vs. distal), partial or complete obstruction, and chronicity. • Mucosal damage and bowel ischemia can result in endotoxemia and sepsis.

SYSTEMS AFFECTED
• Behavioral—associated with abdominal discomfort or pain; praying position, change in temperament • Cardiovascular—hypovolemic shock • Gastrointestinal—anorexia, vomiting, diarrhea, malaise • Respiratory—aspiration pneumonia

GENETICS
Unknown (see Breed Predilections)

INCIDENCE/PREVALENCE
Common

GEOGRAPHIC DISTRIBUTION
N/A

SIGNALMENT
Species
• Dogs and cats • Foreign bodies more common in dogs because of indiscriminate ingestion.

Breed Predilections
• Congenital pyloric stenosis—more common in brachycephalic breeds (e.g., Boxer, Boston terrier) and Siamese cats • Acquired CHPG—more common in Lhasa apso, shih tzu, Pekingese, and Poodle breeds,. • Gastric dilation and volvulus—more common in large-breed dogs (e.g., German shepherd, Great Dane)

Mean Age and Range
• Foreign bodies are more common in young animals, but can occur at any age. • Pyloric stenosis occurs most often in young animals; CHPG occurs more commonly in middle-aged and old animals. • Intussusceptions occur most commonly in young animals.

Predominant Sex
None

SIGNS
Historical Findings
• The hallmark sign is vomiting. • Differentiate vomiting (forceful abdominal contractions) from regurgitation (passive). • Vomiting may occur soon after eating, especially with gastric outlet obstruction. • Vomiting food more than 8 h after ingestion is consistent with delayed gastric emptying. • Vomiting is usually more severe with gastric and proximal small intestinal obstructions; it may be characterized as projectile. • Other variable clinical signs include anorexia, lethargy, malaise, ptyalism, diarrhea, melena, and weight loss. • Continuing to have bowel movements does not rule out intestinal obstruction. • Ask clients about access to potential foreign bodies and tendency of the patient to ingest them.

Physical Examination Findings
• Can vary from normal to life-threatening crisis • May find dehydration, shock, presence of a foreign body, abdominal discomfort or pain, and abdominal mass (intussusception or tumor) • The physical examination is often the most useful diagnostic procedure for intestinal obstruction. • Do a careful sublingual examination to detect linear foreign bodies. • Although more common in cats, linear foreign bodies do occur in dogs also. • Sedation or anesthesia for oral examination and abdominal palpation often facilitates diagnosis.

CAUSES
Gastric Outflow Obstruction
• Foreign bodies • Pyloric stenosis • CHPG • Neoplasia • Gastric dilation and volvulus (GDV) • Granulomatous gastritis/gastroenteritis (e.g., pythiosis)

Small Intestinal Obstruction
• Foreign bodies • Intussusception • Hernias (with incarceration) • Mesenteric torsion/volvulus • Neoplasia • Granulomatous enteritis • Stricture

RISK FACTORS
• Exposure to foreign bodies • Tendency to ingest foreign bodies • Intussusceptions have been associated with intestinal parasitism and viral enteritis.

 DIAGNOSIS

DIFFERENTIAL DIAGNOSIS
• Metabolic disease (e.g., renal failure, hepatic disease, ketoacidotic diabetes mellitus, hypoadrenocorticism) • Infectious gastroenteritis—viral, bacterial, parasitic • Pancreatitis • Peritonitis • Toxicity • Gastroduodenal ulcer disease • Nonspecific gastroenteritis • CNS disease

CBC/BIOCHEMISTRY/URINALYSIS
• Useful to rule out other causes (e.g., renal failure, pancreatitis, liver disease, hypoadrenocorticism, and diabetic ketoacidosis) and to evaluate overall status of the patient • The hemogram may reveal anemia from gastrointestinal blood loss, stress leukocytosis, or possibly a degenerative left-shifted leukocytosis or leukopenia with severe mucosal injury or intestinal perforation and subsequent septic peritonitis. • The chemistry profile and blood gases often reveal a hypochloremic metabolic alkalosis with gastric outlet obstruction. • Hypokalemia and prerenal azotemia are variable findings.

OTHER LABORATORY TESTS
N/A

IMAGING
Survey Abdominal Radiography
• May reveal a foreign body in the stomach or intestine, severe gastric distension, or obstructed loops of intestine with dilation due to fluid and/or gas • Must differentiate adynamic ileus (usually diffuse) from obstruction (usually segmental) • Interpret radiographs within the context of the history, physical examination, and other laboratory data, to avoid misdiagnosis and unnecessary surgery.

Contrast Radiography
• Positive-contrast studies may reveal delayed gastric emptying (more than 4 h with liquid contrast and more than 8–10 h with liquid contrast mixed with food), foreign bodies, complete obstruction, and masses. • Can also use barium-impregnated spheres (BIPS) for radiographic evaluation of gastrointestinal obstruction • Barium enemas may be useful when ileocolic intussusception is suspected.

Abdominal Ultrasonography
May be useful in detecting foreign bodies and obstructions (especially intestinal intussusception)

DIAGNOSTIC PROCEDURES
Endoscopy
Can be useful for confirming gastric and proximal intestinal obstruction and for biopsy of masses; particularly useful with foreign bodies when retrieval may be possible

Abdominal Paracentesis and Cytology/Fluid Analysis
• More sensitive than physical examination and radiography—can detect small amounts of abdominal effusion • May reveal nonseptic inflammation associated with intestinal vascular compromise (prior to perforation) or septic peritonitis; can be an additional indication for exploratory laparotomy

PATHOLOGIC FINDINGS
Histopathology of gastrointestinal masses causing obstruction can reveal granulomatous inflammation, fungal infection (e.g., pythiosis), and neoplasia

TREATMENT

APPROPRIATE HEALTH CARE
• Manage these patients as inpatients for diagnosis, initial supportive medical care, and relief of the obstruction (usually with surgery). • Acute intestinal obstructions are emergencies; perform surgery as soon as possible after immediate supportive medical care; the intestines do not tolerate vascular compromise well. • Not uncommonly an intestinal resection and anastomosis procedure is required (with associated increased morbidity and potential complications) when an enterotomy might have succeeded with earlier diagnosis. • Even worse, a delayed diagnosis can result in intestinal necrosis, perforation, and septic peritonitis.

NURSING CARE
• Intravenous crystalloid fluids—necessary for rehydration, circulatory support, and correcting acid–base and electrolyte abnormalities • Severe circulatory compromise (shock)—administer isotonic crystalloid fluids (dogs, 90 mL/kg; cats, 70 mL/kg) over 1–2 h • Colloids (dextrans or hetastarch) may also be beneficial. • Evaluate hydration and electrolytes frequently—with treatment adjustments as necessary • Gastric outlet obstruction causing hypochloremic metabolic alkalosis—fluid of choice is 0.9% saline; otherwise, lactated Ringer's solution or another balanced electrolyte solution is adequate. • Appropriate potassium supplementation is important.

ACTIVITY
Restrict

DIET
Patients should be NPO until obstruction is relieved and vomiting resolved; then give a bland diet 1–2 days, with gradual return to normal diet.

CLIENT EDUCATION
• Warn clients that animals that tend to ingest foreign bodies are often repeat offenders. • Make all reasonable efforts to prevent access to foreign bodies.

SURGICAL CONSIDERATIONS
Gastric Outflow Obstruction
• Pyloroplasty or pyloromyotomy for pyloric stenosis or CHPG • Gastrotomy for foreign bodies that cannot be removed with endoscopy • Resection for granulomatous or neoplastic masses—Billroth I gastroduodenostomy and Billroth II gastrojejunostomy • Gastropexy—GDV

Intestinal Obstruction
• Enterotomy • Resection and anastomosis—bowel ischemia and necrosis • Open peritoneal lavage—with perforation and septic peritonitis • Prophylactic enteropexy—with intussusception

MEDICATIONS

DRUGS OF CHOICE
• Broad-spectrum parenteral antibiotics when significant mucosal injury or sepsis • Recommendations include ampicillin (10–20 mg/kg IV q8h) and an aminoglycoside (gentamicin 6.6 mg/kg IV q24h) or a fluoroquinolone (enrofloxacin 5–10 mg/kg IV or IM q24h). • For shock, give short-acting soluble glucocorticoids (dexamethasone sodium phosphate 0.5–1.0 mg/kg IV or prednisolone sodium succinate 5 mg/kg IV). • After the obstruction has been relieved, may give antiemetics (e.g., metoclopramide 0.2–0.5 mg/kg SC or IV q6–8h or 1–2 mg/kg/24 h as a CRI) • Mucosal ulceration—can use H_2-receptor antagonists (e.g., ranitidine 1–2 mg/kg PO, SC, IV q12h) and/or the gastric mucosal protectant, sucralfate (250 mg/cat PO q8–12h, 250–1000 mg/dog PO q8–12h)

CONTRAINDICATIONS
Prokinetic agents (e.g., metoclopramide and cisapride)

PRECAUTIONS
Do not use aminoglycoside antibiotics with shock, dehydration, or renal compromise, because of their potential nephrotoxicity.

POSSIBLE INTERACTIONS
N/A

ALTERNATIVE DRUGS
N/A

FOLLOW-UP

PATIENT MONITORING
Check hydration, PCV/TS, and electrolyte status closely, and adjust fluid therapy accordingly; postoperatively check for signs of peritonitis.

PREVENTION/AVOIDANCE
• Caution clients that some pets that tend to ingest foreign bodies may do so repeatedly. • Try to prevent ingestion of foreign bodies.

POSSIBLE COMPLICATIONS
• Aspiration pneumonia • Septic peritonitis—intestinal necrosis and perforation, dehiscence • Adynamic ileus and/or gastroparesis

EXPECTED COURSE AND PROGNOSIS
• Uncomplicated cases—good to excellent • Intestinal perforation and septic peritonitis—guarded, initially • Obstructive granulomatous gastroenteritis—guarded to poor, especially with pythiosis • Mesenteric torsion/volvulus—poor to grave; most patients die despite surgery.

MISCELLANEOUS

ASSOCIATED CONDITIONS
N/A

AGE-RELATED FACTORS
N/A

ZOONOTIC POTENTIAL
N/A

PREGNANCY
N/A

SYNONYMS
N/A

SEE ALSO
• Acute Abdomen • Constipation and Obstipation • Dysphagia • Esophageal Foreign Bodies • Esophageal Stricture • Gastric Dilation and Volvulus Syndrome (GDV) • Gastric Motility Disorders • Hiatal Hernia • Hypertrophic Pyloric Gastropathy, Chronic (CHPG) • Intussusception • Megacolon • Megaesophagus • Phycomycosis (Pythiosis) • Rectal Strictures • Regurgitation • Vomiting, Acute • Vomiting, Chronic

ABBREVIATIONS
• CHPG = chronic hypertrophic pyloric gastropathy • CRI = constant-rate infusion • GDV = gastric dilation and volvulus syndrome • PCV/TS = packed cell volume/total solids

Suggested Reading
Bjorling DE. Acute abdomen syndrome. In: Morgan RV, ed. Handbook of small animal practice. New York, Churchill Livingstone, 1992:483–487.

Slatter D. Textbook of small animal surgery. 2nd ed. Philadelphia: Saunders, 1993.

Strombeck DR, Guilford WG. Small animal gastroenterology. 2nd ed. Davis, CA: Stonegate Publishing, 1990:219–223, 391–401.

Tams TR. Small animal endoscopy. St. Louis, MO: CV Mosby, 1990.

Author Brett M. Feder

Consulting Editors Brett M. Feder and Mitchell A. Crystal

DISEASES

GIARDIASIS

 BASICS

OVERVIEW
• Enteric infection of dogs with *Giardia canis,* a protozoan parasite; occasionally cats
• Water-borne transmission of cysts
• Motile (flagellated) organisms attach to surface of enterocytes in small intestine, especially duodenum through jejunum.
• Malabsorption syndrome with soft voluminous stools
• Importance as a reservoir for human infections not known

SIGNALMENT
• Dogs—up to 50% for pups, up to 100% in kennels
• Cats—up to 11%

SIGNS
• May be acute, intermittent, or chronic
• Soft, frothy diarrhea, usually with rancid odor
• Persistence may lead to chronic debilitation.

CAUSES & RISK FACTORS
Giardia canis transmitted by oral ingestion of cysts, usually from water supplies.

 DIAGNOSIS

DIFFERENTIAL DIAGNOSIS
Other causes of maldigestion and malabsorption (e.g., pancreatic exocrine insufficiency, inflammatory bowel disease)

CBC/BIOCHEMISTRY/URINALYSIS
Usually normal

OTHER LABORATORY TESTS
N/A

IMAGING
N/A

DIAGNOSTIC PROCEDURES
• Motile organisms, tear-drop–shaped, 15 × 8 µm; "falling leaf" appearance in fresh fecal smear
• Cysts—seen as crescent shapes with fecal flotation; 12 µm
• Zinc sulfate flotation best
• Fecal ELISA not superior to zinc sulfate flotation
• Duodenal aspirates obtained via endoscopy

 TREATMENT

Treat as outpatients unless debilitated or dehydrated.

MEDICATIONS

DRUGS
• Albendazole 25 mg/kg PO q12h for 2 days 90% effective; 50× more effective than metronidazole; second 5-day course may be necessary.
• Fenbendazole 50 mg/kg PO q24h for 3 days effective; second 5-day course may be necessary.
• Metronidazole 25 mg/kg q12h for 5 days in dogs; 12–25 mg/kg PO for 5 days in cats
• Quinacrine hydrochloride 6.6 mg/kg q12h for 5 days

CONTRAINDICATIONS/POSSIBLE INTERACTIONS
• Metronidazole only 67% effective in dogs; bitter taste; anorexia; vomiting
• Quinacrine HCl may cause lethargy, fever; do not use in pregnant dogs or cats.

 FOLLOW-UP
• Serial fecal examinations to confirm efficacy of treatment
• May lead to chronic debilitation

 MISCELLANEOUS

ZOONOTIC POTENTIAL
• *Giardia* is the most common intestinal parasite in humans residing in North America.
• *Giardia* spp. may not be highly host-specific; no conclusive evidence indicates that cysts shed by dogs and cats are infective for humans.

PREGNANCY
Do not use quinacrine HCl in pregnant dogs or cats.

Suggested Reading
Barr SC, Bowman DD. Giardiasis in dogs and cats. Compend Cont Educ Pract Vet 16(5); 1994:603–614.
Author Robert M. Corwin
Consulting Editors Brett M. Feder and Mitchell A. Crystal

GLAUCOMA

 BASICS

DEFINITION
• High IOP that causes characteristic degenerative changes in the optic nerve and retina with subsequent loss of vision
• Diagnosis—IOP > 25–30 mm Hg (dogs) or > 31 mm Hg (cats) as determined via applanation tonometry or Schiotz tonometry (using the 1955 Friedenwald human conversion chart that accompanies the instrument) with changes in vision or the appearance of the optic nerve or retina

PATHOPHYSIOLOGY
• Develops when the normal outflow of aqueous humor is impaired
• May be result of primary eye disease (narrow or closed filtration angles and goniodysgenesis, which have a genetic predisposition)
• May be secondary to other eye diseases (primary lens luxation, anterior uveitis, intraocular tumor or hyphema)

SYSTEMS AFFECTED
Ophthalmic

GENETICS
Dogs—predisposing anomalous configuration of the filtration angles is thought to be inherited; mode of inheritance uncertain

INCIDENCE/PREVALENCE
Dogs—more common in some breeds; overall incidence is 0.5% of all hospital admissions to the veterinary teaching hospitals of the colleges of veterinary medicine of North America.

GEOGRAPHIC DISTRIBUTION
N/A

SIGNALMENT
Species
• Dogs—primary and secondary
• Cats—primary rare; secondary seen in patients with signs of long-standing uveitis or with lens luxation.

Breed Predilections
• Goniodysgenesis—Arctic circle breeds (e.g., Norwegian elkhounds, Siberian huskies, malamutes, akitas, Samoyeds); Bouvier des Flanders; basset hounds; chow chows; shar peis; spaniels (e.g., American and English cockers, English and Welsh springers)
• Narrow filtration angles—spaniels; chow chows; shar peis; toy breeds (e.g., poodles, Maltese, and shih tzus)
• Secondary to lens luxations—terriers (e.g., Boston, cairns, Manchesters, dandie dinmonts, Norfolks, Norwich, Scottish, Sealyhams, West Highland whites, and fox)

Mean Age and Range
• Primary (dogs)—any age; predominantly affects middle-aged (4–9 years of age)
• Secondary to lens luxations (dogs)—usually affects young (2–6 years of age)
• Secondary with chronic uveitis (cats)—usually affects older cats (> 6 yrs)

Predominant Sex
N/A

SIGNS
General Comments
• Cannot be accurately diagnosed without instrument tonometry
• All well-equipped small animal hospitals should have at least a Schiotz tonometer.

Historical Findings
• Acute angle closure—apparent pain (blepharospasm, tenderness about the head, serous to seromucoid discharge); may note a cloudy or red eye; unless bilateral, vision loss usually not noticed.
• Secondary—depend on primary disease
• Uveitis—may note pain (for many days), scleral injection, and corneal edema
• Anterior lens luxation—may note acute pain, scleral injection, and corneal edema; may see lens in the anterior chamber (if corneal edema is not severe)
• Chronic uveitis (cats)—may note no signs of pain; enlarged, seemingly painless eye or a dilated pupil common
• Globe enlargement—may be noticed first by owners

Physical Examination Findings
Acute Primary
• High IOP
• Blepharospasm
• Enophthalmos
• Episcleral injection
• Corneal edema
• Dilated pupil
• Vision loss—may be detected by lack of a menace or dazzle response and/or lack of a direct or consensual pupillary light reflex
•.Optic nerve may be depressed or cupped.

Chronic (End Stage)
• Globe enlargement (buphthalmos)
• Descemet streaks
• Subluxated lens with an aphakic crescent
• Optic nerve head atrophy
• Retinal necrosis—detected by peripapillary tapetal hyperreflectivity

Uveitis-induced
• Elevated IOP
• Episcleral injection
• Corneal edema
• Inflammatory debris in the anterior chamber
• Miotic pupil
• Posterior synechia
• Iris bombé

CAUSES
• Primary—filtration angle anomalies
• Secondary—impediment to aqueous humor outflow (e.g., uveitis: inflammatory cells or debris; lens luxation: lens or attached vitreous; hyphema: RBCs; ocular tumors: neoplastic cells)

RISK FACTORS
• Anterior uveitis
• Lens luxation
• Hyphema
• Intraocular neoplasia
• Topically applied mydriatics—may precipitate acute glaucoma in predisposed animals
• Primary (dogs)—consider all cases to be bilateral, even if one eye is normotensive; evaluation of the unaffected eye by a veterinary ophthalmologist for filtration angle anomalies is indicated to determine the risk for future glaucoma in that eye.

 DIAGNOSIS

DIFFERENTIAL DIAGNOSIS
• See Red Eye.
• Conjunctivitis—IOP not high; pupil not dilated; conjunctival hyperemia a more diffuse, red discoloration instead of episcleral vessel engorgement
• Uveitis—initially IOP is subnormal or hypotensive; usually results in a miotic pupil
• Tonometry—usually differentiates other causes of a red eye

CBC/BIOCHEMISTRY/URINALYSIS
• Primary—typically normal
• Secondary—abnormalities consistent with the primary systemic disease (e.g., thrombocytopenia with hyphema)

OTHER LABORATORY TESTS
Serologic testing for infectious diseases—may help diagnose cause of uveitis

IMAGING
• Radiography or ultrasonography—may demonstrate lesions consistent with fungal or neoplastic dissemination to the eye
• Ocular ultrasound (secondary disease)—may facilitate evaluation of the eye if the ocular media is opaque

DIAGNOSTIC PROCEDURES
• Instrument tonometry—essential
• Acute disease—refer to a veterinary ophthalmologist for a detailed ocular examination of both eyes, including evaluation of the filtration angles (gonioscopy).
• ERG—may help determine if affected eye is capable of vision restoration with medical and/or surgical treatment; normal tracing does not necessarily indicate that the eye will be visual; decreased amplitude or flat tracing guarantees that vision will not return.

PATHOLOGIC FINDINGS
• Collapse of the filtration apparatus
• Loss of retinal ganglion cells
• Photoreceptor disruption
• Gliosis of the optic nerve head

TREATMENT

APPROPRIATE HEALTH CARE
• Acute (dogs)—inpatient
• After discharge—reevaluate every 1–2 days for 1 week to monitor for return of increased IOP.

NURSING CARE
N/A

ACTIVITY
N/A

DIET
N/A

CLIENT EDUCATION
• Warn client that primary glaucoma is a bilateral disease; 50% develop glaucoma in the other eye in 8 months without prophylactic therapy.
• Warn client that 40% or more of dogs will be blind in the affected eye within the first year no matter what is done medically or surgically.

SURGICAL CONSIDERATION
• Most forms are best treated surgically.
• Primary (dogs)—< 10% of patients undergoing medical treatment alone will be visual at the end of the first year.
• Procedures—enhance aqueous humor outflow (filtration devices); decrease production of aqueous humor (e.g., Nd:YAG or diode laser surgery; cyclocryosurgery to cause ciliary body ablation); equally effective in maintaining normal IOP and vision
• Blind, painful eyes—enucleated, evisceration and intraocular prosthesis implantation (with no intraocular infection or neoplasia), or procedure to minimize long-term medical therapy

 MEDICATIONS

DRUGS OF CHOICE
• Use multiple agents to lower IOP into the normal range as quickly as possible in an attempt to salvage vision.

Acute Primary (Dogs)
• Emergency medical treatment includes the following:
• Topical miotic—2% pilocarpine solution (q6–12h) or 0.125% demecarium bromide (Humorsol; q12h); enhance aqueous outflow.
• Topically β-adrenergic antagonist—(0.5% timolol maleate (Timoptic; q8–12h); reduce aqueous humor production.
• Oral carbonic anhydrase inhibitor diuretic—dichlorphenamide (Daranide; 2–4 mg/kg q8–12h) or methazolamide (Neptazane; 2–4 mg/kg q8–12h); reduce production of aqueous

humor.
• Hyperosmotic agent—mannitol (1–2 g/kg IV over 20 min) or glycerin (1–2 mL/kg PO q8–12h); dehydrate the vitreous humor.

Uveitis-induced (Dogs)
• Treated like primary disease
• Miotic agents—do not use.
• Topical corticosteroids—used to reduce primary disease

Chronic Smoldering Uveitis (Cats)
• Topical corticosteroids
• Topical β-blockers
• Carbonic anhydrase inhibitor diuretics

CONTRAINDICATIONS
• Topical atropine—do not use.
• Miotic agents—do not use with primary anterior lens luxation or uveitis.

PRECAUTIONS
• Topical pilocarpine—irritating; may cause conjunctivitis and painful brow ache; may worsen uveitis
• Systemic absorption of topical β-adrenergic antagonists—may cause bronchoconstriction and bradycardia in small dogs and cats and in patients with compromised cardiovascular-pulmonary function
• Carbonic anhydrase inhibitor diuretics—cause metabolic acidosis and electrolyte imbalances seen clinically as panting or heavy breathing, weakness, disorientation, and/or behavioral change
• Osmotic diuretics—may initiate acute pulmonary edema in patients with compromised cardiovascular-pulmonary disease
• Glycerin—do not use with diabetes; causes hyperglycemia

POSSIBLE INTERACTIONS
Demecarium bromide—cholinesterase inhibitor; may lead to organophosphate poisoning if used in conjunction with organophosphate flea-repellent products

ALTERNATIVE DRUGS
• Other diuretics (furosemide, thiazides, etc.)—will not reduce IOP (as do the carbonic anhydrase inhibitor diuretics); worthless in the treatment of glaucoma
• Latanoprost 0.005%—SID at bedtime; may help improve outflow
• Dorzolamide 2%—BID or TID; topical carbonic anhydrase inhibitor

 FOLLOW-UP

PATIENT MONITORING
• IOP—monitored often and regularly after starting initial therapy; if a hypotensive level

is maintained for many weeks; *slowly* taper drug therapy.
• Monitor for drug reactions.

PREVENTION/AVOIDANCE
• Primary—bilateral disease; recommend that a veterinary ophthalmologist examine the unaffected eye to determine its risk of developing glaucoma.
• Prophylactic therapy for the predisposed, unaffected eye—0.125% demecarium bromide (1 drop SID at bedtime); delays onset of acute angle closure glaucoma so median time to an attack is 32 months.

POSSIBLE COMPLICATIONS
• Blindness
• Chronic ocular pain

EXPECTED COURSE AND PROGNOSIS
• Chronic disease that requires constant medical treatment
• With medical treatment only—most patients ultimately go blind.
• Surgical treatment—better chance of retaining vision longer; most patients do not remain visual for more than 2 years after initial diagnosis.
• Secondary to lens luxation—may carry a fair prognosis with successful removal of the luxated lens

 MISCELLANEOUS

ASSOCIATED CONDITIONS
N/A

AGE-RELATED FACTORS
N/A

PREGNANCY
• All listed drugs may affect pregnancy
• Primary—inherited; do not breed affected animals.

SEE ALSO
• Anterior Uveitis—Cats
• Anterior Uveitis—Dogs
• Red Eye

ABBREVIATIONS
• ERG = electroretinography
• IOP = intraocular pressure

Suggested Reading
Miller PE. Glaucoma. In: Bonagura JD, ed. Kirk's current veterinary therapy XII. Philadelphia: Saunders, 1995:1265–1272.
Author J. Phillip Pickett
Consulting Editor Paul E. Miller

DISEASES

GLOMERULONEPHRITIS

 BASICS

DEFINITION
Pathology associated with the presence of intraglomerular immune complexes even though inflammatory cells are not always present.

PATHOPHYSIOLOGY
Soluble, circulating antigen–antibody complexes may be deposited or trapped in the glomerulus. Alternatively, immune complexes can be formed in situ within the glomerular capillary wall when circulating antibodies react with "planted" antigens there. Following the formation or deposition of glomerular immune complexes, several factors, including activation of the complement system, infiltration of neutrophils and macrophages, platelet aggregation, activation of the coagulation system, and fibrin deposition, can contribute to glomerular damage. The glomerulus responds to these various insults by cellular proliferation (proliferative glomerulonephritis), thickening of the glomerular basement membrane (membranous glomerulonephritis), and, if the injury persists, hyalinization and sclerosis that can lead to chronic renal insufficiency and failure.

SYSTEMS AFFECTED
• Renal/Urologic—proteinuria initially; often the disease is progressive, resulting in irreversible glomerular damage, nephron loss, azotemia, and chronic renal failure. • Cardiovascular (with severe proteinuria)—hypoalbuminemia and sodium retention (edema and ascites), hypercholesterolemia, hypertension, hypercoagulability, and thromboembolic disease

GENETICS
Familial glomerular disease has been reported in Bernese mountain dogs, samoyeds, dobermans, cocker spaniels, rottweilers, greyhounds, soft-coated wheaten terriers, and cats.

INCIDENCE/PREVALENCE
• In some studies, 90% of random-source dogs have histologic evidence of disease. • Thought to be a leading cause of chronic renal failure in dogs

GEOGRAPHIC DISTRIBUTION
N/A

SIGNALMENT
Species
Dogs; less commonly, cats

Breed Predilections
• See Genetics above. • In some studies golden retrievers, miniature schnauzers, and long-haired dachshunds, in addition to those breeds listed above, appear to be overrepresented. • Labrador and golden retrievers appear to be predisposed to developing glomerulonephritis,

acute tubular necrosis, and interstitial inflammation associated with *Borrelia burgdorferi* infection.

Mean Age and Range
• Dogs—mean age 6.5–7.0 years; range, 0.8–17 years • Cats—mean age at presentation, 4.0 years

Predominant Sex
• Dogs—N/A • Cats—75% are males

SIGNS
General Comments
• Presenting complaint depends on the severity and duration of the proteinuria • Abnormal proteinuria is often discovered on yearly health screens or while working up other problems. • Occasionally, signs associated with an underlying infectious, inflammatory, or neoplastic disease may be why owners seek veterinary care.

Historical and Physical Examination Findings
• If protein loss is mild to moderate—nonspecific signs including weight loss and lethargy • If protein loss is severe (serum albumin concentration < 1.5–1.0 g/dL)—often edema and/or ascites • If disease leads to renal failure—polyuria–polydipsia, anorexia, nausea, and vomiting may occur. • Acute dyspnea or severe panting in dogs caused by a pulmonary thromboembolism (rare) • Acute blindness due to retinal hemorrhage or detachment (rare)

CAUSES
• True autoimmune or primary glomerulonephritis has not been documented in dogs or cats. • Several infectious and inflammatory diseases have been associated with glomerular deposition or in situ formation of immune complexes. In many cases no antigen source or underlying disease process is identified, and the disease is referred to as idiopathic. The following diseases have been associated with glomerulonephritis. • Dogs—infectious (e.g., infectious canine hepatitis, bacterial endocarditis, brucellosis, dirofilariasis, ehrlichiosis, leishmaniasis, pyometra, borreliosis, chronic bacterial infection, Rocky Mountain spotted fever, trypanosomiasis, and septicemia), neoplastic, inflammatory (e.g., pancreatitis, systemic lupus erythematosus, polyarthritis, and prostatitis), idiopathic, familial, endocrine (e.g., hyperadrenocorticism and diabetes mellitus and long-term administration of corticosteroids) • Cats—infectious (e.g., FeLV, FIP, and mycoplasma polyarthritis), neoplastic, inflammatory (e.g., pancreatitis, systemic lupus erythematosus, other immune-mediated diseases, and chronic skin disease), idiopathic, familial, and possibly endocrine (e.g., diabetes mellitus)

RISK FACTORS
See diseases/conditions listed above.

 DIAGNOSIS

DIFFERENTIAL DIAGNOSIS
• Proteinuria—most common cause is inflammation of the urinary tract (e.g., bacterial cystitis/pyelonephritis, urolithiasis, and neoplasia); urinary tract inflammation is usually associated with active urine sediment (i.e., increased numbers of RBC, WBC, epithelial cells, and bacteria/hpf). Like glomerulonephritis, renal amyloidosis often causes severe proteinuria with inactive urine sediment (hyaline casts may be present). Renal biopsy is the only accurate way to distinguish amyloidosis from glomerulonephritis. • Hypoalbuminemia—can be associated with decreased albumin production (severe liver disease) and increased albumin loss (protein-losing enteropathies and protein-losing nephropathies)

CBC/BIOCHEMISTRY/URINALYSIS
• Hypoalbuminemia and hypercholesterolemia are common. • Persistent, significant proteinuria with an inactive urine sediment (hyaline casts may be observed)

OTHER LABORATORY TESTS
Urine Protein:Creatinine Ratio
• Used to confirm and quantify abnormal proteinuria • Magnitude of proteinuria roughly correlates with the severity of glomerular lesions, making the urine protein:creatinine ratio a useful parameter to assess response to therapy or progression of disease.

Protein Electrophoresis
• Urine and serum protein electrophoresis may help identify the source of the proteinuria and establish a prognosis. • Proteinuria associated with hemorrhage into the urinary tract may have an electrophoretic pattern similar to that of the serum. • Early glomerular damage usually results principally in albuminuria; with disease progression an increasing amount of globulin may be lost as well. • Marked decreases in serum albumin and increased concentrations of larger-molecular-weight proteins, such as IgM, in the serum suggest severe glomerular proteinuria and the nephrotic syndrome. As the glomerular disease progresses and causes loss of three-quarters of the nephrons, the decreased glomerular filtration usually results in decreased proteinuria.

IMAGING
• No specific changes on abdominal radiographs or renal ultrasound, but these tests are useful in ruling out other concurrent conditions. • Can use ultrasonography to guide percutaneous renal biopsy

DIAGNOSTIC PROCEDURES
• Renal biopsy—if significant and persistent proteinuria with inactive urine sediment; histopathologic evaluation of renal tissue will

establish a diagnosis (e.g., glomerulonephritis vs. amyloidosis) and aid in formulation of a prognosis; consider only after performing less invasive tests (e.g., CBC, serum biochemistry profile, urinalysis, quantitation of proteinuria) and assessing blood clotting ability • Contraindications to renal biopsy—a solitary kidney, thrombocytopenia or other coagulopathy, and renal lesions associated with fluid accumulation (e.g., hydronephrosis and renal cysts and abscesses); renal biopsy should not be attempted by inexperienced clinicians or in patients that are not adequately restrained.

PATHOLOGIC FINDINGS

• Usually classified by histologic findings because the underlying cause is often unknown: glomerular basement membrane thickening—referred to as membranous glomerulonephritis; increased cellularity—referred to as proliferative glomerulonephritis; a combination of membrane-thickening and increased cellularity—referred to as membranoproliferative glomerulonephritis; glomerular scarring associated with increases in mesangial matrix—referred to as glomerulosclerosis • Whenever possible, use immunofluorescent and/or immunoperoxidase staining and electron microscopy to maximize the information gained from the biopsy specimen. • Request a Congo red stain in addition to routine stains since small amyloid deposits can be missed. Amyloid deposits appear green and birefringent when stained with Congo red and viewed under a polarized light source.

TREATMENT

APPROPRIATE HEALTH CARE

Most patients can be treated as outpatients; exceptions include severely azotemic and/or hypertensive patients and patients with thromboembolic disease.

NURSING CARE

NA

ACTIVITY

Restrict because of the possibility of thromboembolic disease

DIET

Sodium-reduced, high-quality, low-quantity protein diets

CLIENT EDUCATION

If the underlying cause cannot be identified and corrected, the disease is often progressive, resulting in chronic renal failure.

SURGICAL CONSIDERATIONS

N/A

MEDICATIONS

DRUGS OF CHOICE

• Since most glomerulonephritis is mediated by immunopathogenic mechanisms, the most specific and perhaps the most effective therapy is elimination of the source of antigenic stimulation. Unfortunately, this is often difficult because the disease process or antigen source is not identified or is impossible to eliminate (e.g., neoplasia). • Immunosuppressive drugs are often used in dogs and cats as a second line of treatment. Corticosteroids, azathioprine, chlorambucil, cyclophosphamide, and cyclosporine have been used clinically or experimentally to prevent immunoglobulin production by B cells or to alter the function of T helper or T suppressor cells. Despite widespread use of immunosuppressive agents, no controlled clinical trials in veterinary medicine have demonstrated their efficacy. • The third type of treatment is aimed at reducing glomerular inflammation. Thromboxane is a major cause of glomerular inflammation associated with immune complexes; thus low-dose aspirin has been recommended to decrease thromboxane production. Aspirin also decreases platelet aggregation and resultant thromboembolic disease. Low-dose aspirin (5–10 mg/kg PO q 24–48h) reportedly decreases platelet aggregation in dogs more effectively than 10 mg/kg once daily and may have less effect on the production of beneficial prostaglandins. • Enalapril (0.5 mg/kg q12–24h), an angiotensin-converting enzyme inhibitor, was recommended in dogs for both its antihypertensive and antiproteinuric effects. There are no controlled clinical trials that demonstrate the efficacy of this treatment.

CONTRAINDICATIONS

Do not use corticosteroids in azotemic patients.

PRECAUTIONS

• Exercise caution with the use of immunosuppressive drugs. • Dosages of highly protein bound drugs (e.g., aspirin) may need to be adjusted; serum albumin concentrations change with treatment or progression of disease. • Use enalapril cautiously in azotemic patients.

POSSIBLE INTERACTIONS

See Precautions above.

ALTERNATIVE DRUGS

N/A

FOLLOW-UP

PATIENT MONITORING

• Follow the urine protein:creatinine ratio closely. Immunosuppressive therapy may worsen proteinuria; if this happens, discontinue immunosuppressive therapy. • Also follow serum urea nitrogen, creatinine, albumin, and electrolyte concentrations, blood pressure, and body weight. • Ideally, reexamine 1, 3, 6, 9, and 12 months after initiation of treatment.

PREVENTION/AVOIDANCE

Do not breed affected animals of breeds with suspected familial

POSSIBLE COMPLICATIONS

• Nephrotic syndrome • Chronic renal insufficiency or failure

EXPECTED COURSE AND PROGNOSIS

• Long-term prognosis is guarded. • Often progresses to chronic renal insufficiency or failure despite treatment

MISCELLANEOUS

ASSOCIATED CONDITIONS

See associated diseases/conditions, nephrotic syndrome, and possible complications.

AGE-RELATED FACTORS

N/A

ZOONOTIC POTENTIAL

N/A

PREGNANCY

High risk for patients with severe hypoalbuminemia and/or hypertension

SYNONYMS

• Glomerular disease • Glomerulopathy • Protein-losing nephropathy

SEE ALSO

• Nephrotic Syndrome • Amyloidosis • Proteinuria

ABBREVIATIONS

• FeLP = feline leukemia virus
• FIP = feline infectious peritonitis
• GN = glomerulonephritis

Suggested Reading

Center SA, Smith CA, Wilkinson E, et al. Clinicopathologic, renal immunofluorescent, and light microscopic features of glomerulonephritis in the dog: 41 cases (1975–1985). J Am Vet Med Assoc 1987;190:81–90.

Cook AK, Cowgill LD. Clinical and pathologic features of protein-losing glomerular disease in the dog. A review of 137 cases (1985–1992). J Am Anim Hosp Assoc 1996;32:313–322.

Dambach DM, Smith CA, Lewis RM, Van Winkle TJ. Morphologic, immunohistochemical, and ultrastructural characterization of a distinctive renal lesion in dogs putatively associated with *Borrelia burgdorferi* infection: 49 cases (1987–1992). Vet Pathol 1997;34:85–96.

Grauer GF. Glomerulonephritis. Semin Vet Med Surg (Small Animal) 1992;7:187–197.

Author Gregory F. Grauer

Consulting Editors Larry G. Adams and Carl A. Osborne

DISEASES

GLUTEN ENTEROPATHY IN IRISH SETTERS

 BASICS

OVERVIEW
A rare inherited disease in which there is a predisposition to develop a sensitivity to dietary gluten present in wheat and other grains

SIGNALMENT
• Only reported in the Irish setter breed in the United Kingdom
• Mode of inheritance not known
• Signs develop in young to middle-aged dogs.

SIGNS
• Poor weight gain (or weight loss)
• Mild diarrhea

CAUSES & RISK FACTORS
The enteropathy and clinical signs are exacerbated by gluten-containing diet.

 DIAGNOSIS

DIFFERENTIAL DIAGNOSIS
Other chronic small intestinal diseases

CBC/BIOCHEMISTRY/URINALYSIS
Unremarkable

OTHER LABORATORY TESTS
• Serum folate concentrations are subnormal in some patients, reflecting chronic malabsorption.
• Serum trypsin-like immunoreactivity and cobalamin concentrations are usually normal.

IMAGING
Not useful

DIAGNOSTIC PROCEDURES
Intestinal biopsy specimens (jejunal) obtained via endoscopy or laparotomy

PATHOLOGIC FINDINGS
• Histologic examination of jejunal biopsy specimens from affected dogs reared on a wheat-containing diet reveals partial villus atrophy and accumulation of intraepithelial lymphocytes.
• Jejunal abnormalities improve following gluten withdrawal but recur with gluten challenge.

 TREATMENT

Avoid diets containing gluten.

 MEDICATIONS

DRUGS
Folate (0.5–2.0 mg PO q24 h for 2–4 weeks) if serum folate concentration is markedly subnormal (<4 µg/L)

CONTRAINDICATIONS/POSSIBLE INTERACTIONS
N/A

 FOLLOW-UP

Consider periodic assay of serum folate (q6–12 months)

 MISCELLANEOUS

SEE ALSO
Serum Cobalamin and Folate

Suggested Reading
Hall EJ, Batt RM. Dietary modulation of gluten sensitivity in a naturally occurring enteropathy of Irish setter dogs. Gut 1992;33:198–205.
Author David A. Williams
Consulting Editors Brett M. Feder and Mitchell A. Crystal

GROWTH HORMONE-RESPONSIVE DERMATOSES

BASICS

OVERVIEW
• Uncommon dermatoses resulting from a growth hormone deficiency or dermatoses responding to growth hormone therapy
• Pituitary dwarfism—the result of a primary growth hormone deficiency
• Adult-onset growth hormone–responsive dermatosis—a clinical syndrome that responds to growth hormone therapy; patients may be strictly growth hormone–deficient; may have one or more of a plethora of hormonal abnormalities, including possible imbalances of adrenal sex hormones

SIGNALMENT
• Pituitary dwarfism—most commonly seen in German shepherds; also reported in spitzes, toy pinschers, and Carnelian bear dogs; noted at 2–3 months of age • Adult-onset—reported in the chow chows, Pomeranians, poodles, keeshonds, Samoyeds, and American water spaniels; generally noted at 1–2 years of age; primarily affects males, although seen in both sexes (neutered and intact) and at all ages

SIGNS

Pituitary Dwarfism
• Patients appear normal at birth; by 2–3 months bilaterally symmetrical alopecia begins to be apparent; trunk, neck, and caudal thighs severely affected • Primary hair growth only over face and distal extremities only; retained puppy coat is easily epilated. • Skin—thin, hypotonic, scaly, and hyperpigmented; comedones noted

Adult-Onset Growth Hormone–Responsive Dermatosis
• Alopecia—bilaterally symmetrical; involves trunk, neck, caudomedial thighs, tail, ventral abdomen, perineum, and pinnae; the head and legs are spared. • Primary hairs are lost first; then loss of secondary hairs in the affected areas; hair readily epilates; tufts of regrowth at trauma or biopsy sites • Skin—thin and hyperpigmented; secondary seborrhea and pyoderma uncommon

CAUSES & RISK FACTORS
• Pituitary dwarfism—mediated by an autosomal recessive trait, which results in a developmental abnormality of the pituitary and lack of growth hormone production
• Adult-onset—unknown; breed predisposition suggests a hereditary influence; pituitary neoplasia has been suggested. • Although an absolute growth hormone deficiency may be noted, other causes may lead to a similar clinical syndrome that responds to growth hormone supplementation (e.g., castration-responsive dermatosis, congenital adrenal hyperplasia-like syndrome).

DIAGNOSIS

DIFFERENTIAL DIAGNOSIS
• Pituitary dwarfism—hypothyroidism, malnutrition, and metabolic disorders • Adult-onset—hypothyroidism, hyperadrenocorticism, castration-responsive dermatosis, cyclic flank alopecia, estrogen/testosterone-responsive dermatosis, follicular dysplasia, and congenital adrenal hyperplasia-like syndrome

CBC/BIOCHEMISTRY/URINALYSIS
Results usually unremarkable.

OTHER LABORATORY TESTS
• Growth hormone–stimulation test—dubious value; not currently available • Somatomedin C (insulin-like growth factor 1)—growth hormone dependent; concentrations parallel body size; release may be impaired by glucocorticoids and estrogens; an indirect assay of growth hormone levels; expected to be low in growth hormone–deficient states (performed at Michigan State University Animal Health Diagnostic Laboratory, Lansing, MI) • Pituitary dwarfism—low thyroid-stimulating hormone, ACTH, gonadotropin-releasing hormone, and human chorionic gonadotropin response test results
• Insulin response test—may aid diagnosis; causes severe hypoglycemia • Adrenal reproductive hormone testing—ACTH-stimulation test with evaluation of adrenocortical hormones and their precursors (performed at the University of Tennessee College of Veterinary Medicine Endocrinology Laboratory, Nashville, TN).

IMAGING N/A

DIAGNOSTIC PROCEDURES
• Skin biopsy—general endocrinopathy; orthokeratotic hyperkeratosis; epidermal atrophy; follicular keratosis, dilation, and atrophy; telogenization of hair follicles; atrophy of sebaceous glands; amounts and sizes of dermal elastin fibers are small • Castration-responsive or growth hormone–responsive dermatoses (dogs)—hypereosinophilic tricholemmal keratinization of hair follicles ("flame follicles")

TREATMENT
Outpatients

MEDICATIONS

DRUGS
• L-Thyroxine—0.02 mg/kg PO q12h for a 6-week trial; recommended if the baseline total T_4 is low or low normal • o,p′-DDD (Lysodren)—15–25 mg/kg PO q24h for 2–7 days; an ACTH-stimulation test to evaluate the response should demonstrate suppression of the baseline cortisol to a low-normal range; poststimulation range is 30–50 ng/mL (3.0–5.0 μg/dL); conduct ACTH-stimulation testing quarterly. • Methyltestosterone—1 mg/kg (maximum dose, 30 mg/dog) PO q48h for a maximum of 3 months; after hair regrowth, maintain at 1 mg/kg (maximum dose, 30 mg/dog) PO every 4–7 days. • Bovine, porcine, or synthetic human growth hormone—0.15 IU/kg SC twice weekly for 6 weeks; may repeat if no response within 3 months.

CONTRAINDICATIONS/POSSIBLE INTERACTIONS
Intact male dogs—neuter to rule out castration-responsive dermatosis.

FOLLOW-UP

PATIENT MONITORING
• Growth hormones—monitor blood glucose before each treatment; growth hormone is diabetogenic • Methyltestosterone—cholangiohepatitis, seborrhea, and behavioral changes; monitor liver enzymes and clinical status • If post-ACTH stimulation blood cortisols are too low, evaluate serum electrolytes to determine the need for mineralocorticoid treatment.

PREVENTION/AVOIDANCE N/A

POSSIBLE COMPLICATIONS
Growth hormone therapy—anaphylaxis with repeated dosing; diabetes mellitus (transient or permanent)

EXPECTED COURSE AND PROGNOSIS
• Pituitary dwarfism—hair regrowth will begin within 4–8 weeks of beginning therapy and lasts 6 months to 2 years; retreatment is usually necessary. • Adult-onset—hair regrowth is usually observed in 2–12 weeks after therapy and lasts 6 months to 3 years; retreatment is often necessary. • o,p′-DDD—gives a good prognosis for hair regrowth if imbalance of adrenal sex hormone concentrations is suspected; may be a transient increase in epilation, but hair regrowth may be noted 4–12 weeks after beginning therapy • Signs are confined to the skin, so treatment is not mandatory; owners may decline therapy because of the possible side effects.

MISCELLANEOUS

ABBREVIATION
o,p′-DDD = 1,1-(o,p′-dichlorodiphenyl)-2,2-dichloroethane

Suggested Reading
Schmeitzel LP. Sex hormone–related and growth hormone-related alopecias. Vet Clin North Am Small Anim Pract 1990;20:1579–1601.

Author Margaret S. Swartout
Consulting Editor Karen Helton Rhodes

DISEASES

HAEMOBARTONELLOSIS

BASICS

OVERVIEW
RBC destruction and anemia caused by parasite attachment to the external surface of RBCs and immune response by the host

SIGNALMENT
• Dogs and cats
• Most common in adults
• In cats, more common in males
• No sex prevalence in dogs

SIGNS

Cats
• Variable disease severity ranging from inapparent infection to marked depression and death
• Intermittent fever (50%) during the acute phase, depression, weakness, anorexia, pale mucous membranes, splenomegaly and (occasionally) icterus

Dogs
Mild or inapparent signs (e.g., pale mucous membranes and listlessness), except when dogs have been splenectomized

CAUSES & RISK FACTORS
• *Haemobartonella felis* (cats) and *Haemobartonella canis* (dogs)—currently classified as rickettsial organisms, but recent genetic studies indicate that *H. felis* is a mycoplasma
• Cats—anemia more severe if FeLV-infected
• Dogs—likelihood of severe anemia greatly increased if splenectomized or with pathologic changes in the spleen

DIAGNOSIS

DIFFERENTIAL DIAGNOSIS
• Other causes of hemolytic anemia, including AIHA, babesiosis (not in cats in the U.S.), cytauxzoonosis (cats only), Heinz body hemolytic anemia, microangiopathic hemolytic anemia, pyruvate kinase deficiency, and phosphofructokinase deficiency (dogs only)
• Differentiated from AIHA only by recognition of parasites in the blood; both disorders may be Coombs', test positive
• *Babesia* and *Cytauxzoon* species are protozoal organisms that differ in morphology from *Haemobartonella*.
• New methylene blue stain used to identify Heinz bodies
• Enzyme assays or specialized DNA tests used to diagnose pyruvate kinase and phosphofructokinase deficiencies

CBC/BIOCHEMISTRY/URINALYSIS
• Anemia, with reticulocytosis in most animals with clinically important hemobartonellosis—may appear poorly regenerative if a precipitous decrease in PCV has occurred early in the disease, or if patient has concurrent disorders (e.g., FeLV or FIV infection in cats)
• Autoagglutination may be seen in feline blood samples after they cool to below body temperature.
• Variable total and differential leukocyte counts of little diagnostic value
• Slight hemoglobinemia rarely observed; no hemoglobinuria reported
• Hyperbilirubinemia may be measured at times but is seldom severe.
• Substantial bilirubinuria seen in some dogs
• Abnormalities related to anemic hypoxia may be shown by biochemical analysis, but profile can be normal.
• Hypoglycemia possible in moribund cats
• Plasma protein concentration usually normal but may be high

OTHER LABORATORY TESTS
• Routine blood stains (e.g., Wright-Giemsa) to identify organisms in blood films, which must be examined for organisms before treatment is begun
• Reticulocyte stains cannot be used, because punctate reticulocytes in cats appear similar to the parasites.
• Organisms must be differentiated from precipitated stain, refractile drying or fixation artifacts, poorly staining Howell-Jolly bodies, and basophilic stippling.
• *H. felis*—small, blue-staining cocci, rings, or rods on RBCs
• *H. canis*—commonly forms chains of organisms that appear as filamentous structures on the surface of RBCs
• Parasitemia is cyclic and thus organisms not always identifiable in blood (especially in cats).
• In cats, a PCR-based assay can detect parasites in blood below the number required to make a diagnosis by a stained blood film.
• Direct Coombs test may be positive.

IMAGING
N/A

DIAGNOSTIC PROCEDURES
In patients with nonregenerative anemia, bone marrow biopsy should be performed to detect other disorders (e.g., myeloproliferative disorders).

TREATMENT
• Without treatment, mortality may reach 30% in cats.
• Outpatient treatment unless severely anemic or moribund
• Blood transfusions required when the anemia is considered life-threatening
• IV administration of glucose-containing fluid recommended in moribund animals

MEDICATIONS

DRUGS OF CHOICE
• Doxycycline (5 mg/kg PO q12h), tetracycline (20 mg/kg PO q8h), or oxytetracycline (20 mg/kg PO q8h) antibiotics should be given for 3 weeks.
• Glucocorticoids, such as prednisolone (1–2 mg/kg PO q12h), may be given to severely anemic animals; gradually decrease dosage as the PCV increases.

CONTRAINDICATIONS/POSSIBLE INTERACTIONS
• Tetracycline may cause fever or evidence of gastrointestinal disease in cats; use a low dosage, different tetracycline product, or discontinue drug altogether.
• Chloramphenicol should not be used to treat cats, because it causes dose-dependent erythroid hypoplasia.

FOLLOW-UP
• Examine animal after 1 week of treatment to confirm that PCV has risen.
• Alert owners that cats remain carriers even after completion of treatment but seldom relapse with clinical disease once the PCV returns to normal.

MISCELLANEOUS

ASSOCIATED CONDITIONS
FeLV

ABBREVIATIONS
• AIHA = autoimmune hemolytic anemia
• FeLV = feline leukemia virus
• FIV = feline immunodeficiency virus
• PCR = polymerase chain reaction
• PCV = packed cell volume

Suggested Reading
Harvey JW. Haemobartonellosis. In: Greene CE, ed., Infectious diseases of the dog and cat. 2nd ed. Philadelphia: Saunders, 1997: 166–171.

Messick JB, Berent LM, Cooper SK. Development and evaluation of a PCR-based assay for the detection of *Haemobartonella felis* infection in cats and differentiation of H. felis from related bacteria by restriction fragment length polymorphism analysis. J Clin Microbiol 1998 36(2):462–466.

Author John W. Harvey
Consulting Editor Susan M. Cotter

HAIR FOLLICLE TUMORS

BASICS

OVERVIEW
• Two main types—trichoepithelioma, which arises from keratinocytes in the outer root sheath of the hair follicle or from both the sheath and the hair matrix; pilomatricoma, which arises from the hair matrix
• Both types—generally benign; a few published reports of malignant pilomatricoma

SIGNALMENT
• Age—usually > 5 years
• No sex predisposition
• Trichoepithelioma—common in dogs; rare in cats; cocker spaniels and basset hounds may be predisposed; no breed predisposition in cats
• Pilomatricoma—uncommon in dogs and cats; Kerry blue terriers and poodles may be predisposed; no known breed predisposition in cats

SIGNS
• Usually a solitary mass
• Trichoepithelioma—common on the back and head (cats)
• Pilomatricoma—common on the back, shoulders, flanks, and limbs
• Firm, round, elevated, well-circumscribed, hairless, or ulcerated dermoepithelial masses; cut surface gray (trichoepithelioma) or lobulated with white chalky areas (pilomatricoma)

CAUSES & RISK FACTORS
Unknown

DIAGNOSIS

DIFFERENTIAL DIAGNOSIS
Histopathologic examination—distinguish from basal cell tumor and squamous cell carcinoma

CBC/BIOCHEMISTRY/URINALYSIS
Usually normal

OTHER LABORATORY TESTS
N/A

IMAGING
N/A

DIAGNOSTIC PROCEDURES
Tissue biopsy

PATHOLOGIC FINDINGS
• Trichoepithelioma—varies in degree of differentiation and site of origin (root sheath or hair matrix); horn cysts, lack of desmosomes, and differentiation toward hair follicle-like structures and formation of hair common
• Pilomatricoma—characterized by a variable proliferation of basophilic cells resembling hair matrix cells and fully keratinized, faintly eosinophilic cells with a central unstained nucleus (shadow cells); calcification common

TREATMENT
Complete excision—curative

MEDICATIONS

DRUGS
N/A

CONTRAINDICATIONS/POSSIBLE INTERACTIONS
N/A

FOLLOW-UP
• Monitor for local recurrence.
• Prognosis usually excellent

MISCELLANEOUS

Suggested Reading

Muller GH, Kirk RW, Scott DW. Neoplastic diseases. In: Muller GH, Kirk RW, Scott DW, eds. Small animal dermatology. 4th ed. Philadelphia: Saunders, 1989:858–866.
Thomas RC, Fox LE. Tumors of the skin and subcutis. In: Morrison WB, ed. Cancer in dogs and cats: medical and surgical management. Philadelphia: Williams & Wilkins 1998:489–510.

Author Joanne C. Graham
Consulting Editor Wallace B. Morrison

HEARTWORM DISEASE—CATS

 BASICS

OVERVIEW
- Disease caused by infection with *Dirofilaria immitis*
- Microfilaremia uncommon (< 20%)
- Prevalence one-tenth that of unprotected dogs
- Low average worm burden
- Worms are physically smaller and have a shorter life span in cats.

SIGNALMENT
- Cats
- No age or breed predisposition
- Males more commonly infected

SIGNS

Historical Findings
- Coughing
- Dyspnea
- Vomiting
- PTE frequently results in acute respiratory failure and death.
- Vomiting and respiratory signs predominate in chronic disease.

Physical Examination Findings
- Usually normal
- Increased bronchovesicular sounds
- Murmur or gallop rhythm should increase suspicion of primary cardiac disease.

CAUSES & RISK FACTORS
- Outdoor cats at increased risk (2:1)
- FeLV infection is not a predisposing factor.

 DIAGNOSIS

DIFFERENTIAL DIAGNOSIS
- Asthma
- Cardiomyopathy
- Chylothorax
- *Aelurostrongylus abstrusus* infection
- *Paragonimus kellicotti* infection

CBC/BIOCHEMISTRY/URINALYSIS
- Mild nonregenerative anemia
- Eosinophilia inconsistent
- Basophilia should increase suspicion.
- Hyperglobulinemia

OTHER LABORATORY TESTS

Heartworm Concentration Tests
Low sensitivity, high specificity

Heartworm Antigen Tests
- ELISA or immunochromatographic tests
- Tests that detect circulating HWAg are more specific than antibody tests; a positive antigen test result is strong evidence of heartworm disease.
- Low worm burdens (fewer than 5 worms) and single-sex infections commonly result in false negative results.
- Negative result does not rule out heartworm disease; more than 40% of cats with adult infection are antigen-negative.

Heartworm Antibody Tests
- ELISA or immunochromatographic tests
- Tests that detect circulating antibodies to immature and adult heartworm antigen are the most sensitive tests for feline heartworm disease.
- A positive result simply documents exposure to heartworms.
- The more intense the antibody response (higher titer or antibody unit [ABU] level), the more likely is an adult infection.

IMAGING

Radiography/Angiography
- Enlarged (>pulmonary vein, >1.6 times the width of the 9th rib), blunted, tortuous pulmonary arteries
- Patchy perivascular pulmonary infiltrates
- Pulmonary arterial obstruction and linear filling defects seen on nonselective angiography

Echocardiography
- Dilated main pulmonary artery
- Identification of worms in heart or main pulmonary artery; most commonly seen in the right pulmonary artery
- Excludes or confirms other primary cardiac diseases (cardiomyopathy)

DIAGNOSTIC TESTS
N/A

 TREATMENT
- Asymptomatic cats should not receive adulticide therapy; perhaps no cats should.
- Symptomatic cats should be stabilized.
- Spontaneous "cure" is probably much more common in cats than dogs (shorter heartworm life span).

MEDICATIONS

DRUGS

Initial Stabilization
- Supplemental oxygen
- Theophylline (Theo-Dur) 25 mg/kg PO q24h in the evening
- Prednisolone 1–2 mg/kg PO q24h for 10–14 days; then reduce gradually
- Cautious balanced fluid therapy if indicated

Adulticide/Thromboembolism
- Thiacetarsamide: 2.2 mg/kg IV q12h for 2 days
- 30% mortality should be expected from adulticide therapy and subsequent PTE
- Supportive care for PTE the same as initial stabilization
- PTE complications most severe 5–10 days after adulticide therapy; commonly fatal

CONTRAINDICATIONS /POSSIBLE INTERACTIONS
- Aspirin therapy—no documented benefit
- Current information does not support the use of melarsomine (Immiticide) in cats.

 FOLLOW-UP

PATIENT MONITORING
Serial evaluation of clinical response, thoracic radiographs, and heartworm antigen and antibody tests are most informative.

PREVENTION/AVOIDANCE
- Ivermectin (Heartgard for Cats)—24 μg/kg PO every 30 days
- Milbemycin oxime—0.5–0.1 mg/kg PO every 30 days (not currently approved for use in cats)

 MISCELLANEOUS

ABBREVIATIONS
- ABU = antibody unit
- HWAg = adult heartworm antiagent
- PTE = pulmonary thromboembolism

Suggested Reading
Miller MW. Feline dirofilariasis. Clin Tech Small Anim Pract 1998;13(2):99–108.
Author Matthew W. Miller
Consulting Editors Larry P. Tilley and Francis W. K. Smith, Jr.

HEARTWORM DISEASE—DOGS

BASICS

DEFINITION
Disease caused by infection with *Dirofilaria immitis*

PATHOPHYSIOLOGY
Disease is directly related to the number of worms, duration of infection, and host response. Endothelial damage leads to myo-intimal proliferation. Lobar arterial enlargement, tortuosity, and obstruction cause impaired compliance, loss of collateral recruitment, pulmonary hypertension, and thrombosis. Pulmonary damage exacerbated after the death of adult worms.

SYSTEMS AFFECTED
• Cardiovascular—high right ventricular afterload causes myocardial hypertrophy and, in some animals, congestive heart failure (CHF)
• Respiratory—pulmonary hypertension, embolization, allergic pneumonitis, eosino-philic and granulomatous
• Renal/urologic—immune complex glomerulopathy

GENETICS
None

INCIDENCE/PREVALENCE
• Varies with geographic location
• Virtually 100% in unprotected dogs living in highly endemic regions

GEOGRAPHIC DISTRIBUTION
• Most common in tropical and semitropical zones
• Common along the Atlantic and Gulf coasts and Ohio and Mississippi River basins
• Gradually extending across the United States
• Numerous pockets of infection in otherwise low prevalence regions

SIGNALMENT

Species
Dogs

Breed Predilection
• Medium- to large-breed dogs that spend a lot of time outdoors
• All unprotected dogs at risk in endemic regions

Mean Age and Range
Infection can occur at any age; most affected animals are 3–8 years old.

Predominant Sex
None

SIGNS

Historial Findings
• Animals often asymptomatic or exhibit minimal signs such as occasional coughing (Class I)

• Coughing and exercise intolerance associated with moderate pulmonary damage
• Cachexia, exercise intolerance, syncope, and ascites (right-sided CHF [R-CHF]) in severely affected dogs (Class III)

Physical Examination Findings
• No abnormalities—animals with mild infection (Class I) and some with moderately severe infection (Class II)
• Labored breathing or crackles—dogs with severe pulmonary hypertension (Class III) or pulmonary thromboembolic complications
• Tachycardia, ascites, and hepatomegaly indicate R-CHF (Class III).
• Hemoptysis—occasionally occurs; indicates severe pulmonary thromboembolic complications

CAUSE
Infection with *D. immitis*

RISK FACTORS
• Residence in endemic regions
• Outside habitus
• Lack of prophylaxis

DIAGNOSIS

DIFFERENTIAL DIAGNOSIS
• Other causes of pulmonary hypertension and thrombosis (e.g., hyperadrenocorticism)
• Allergic lung disease
• Other causes of ascites (e.g., dilated cardiomyopathy)

CBC/BIOCHEMISTRY/URINALYSIS
• Anemia—absent, mild, or moderate depending on chronicity and severity of disease and thromboembolic complications
• Eosinophilia and basophilia—vary
• Inflammatory leukogram and thrombocyto-penia associated with thromboembolism
• Hyperglobulinemia—inconsistent finding
• Proteinuria—common in animals with severe and chronic infection; may be caused by immune-complex glomerulonephritis or amyloidosis

OTHER LABORATORY TESTS
• Highly specific, sensitive serologic tests that identify adult *D. immitis* antigen are widely available.
• Microfilaria identification tests include the modified Knott's test, filter tests, and direct smear.

IMAGING

Radiographic Findings
• Main pulmonary artery segment enlargement and lobar arterial enlargement and tortuosity vary from absent (Class I) to severe (Class III).
• Parenchymal lung infiltrates of variable severity—surround lobar arteries; may extend

into most or all of one or multiple lung lobes when thromboembolism occurs
• Diffuse, symmetrical, alveolar, and interstitial infiltrates occasionally occur because of an allergic reaction to microfilaria.

Echocardiographic Findings
• Often unremarkable; may reflect right ventricular dilation and wall hypertrophy
• Parallel, linear echodensities produced by heartworms may be detected in the right ventricle, right atrium, and pulmonary arteries.

Angiography
Little practical clinical importance

DIAGNOSTIC PROCEDURES

Electrocardiographic Findings
• Usually normal
• May reflect right ventricular hypertrophy in dogs with severe (Class III) infection
• Heart rhythm disturbances—occasionally seen (atrial fibrillation most common) in severe infection

PATHOLOGIC FINDINGS
• Large right heart
• Pulmonary arterial myointimal proliferation
• Pulmonary thromboembolism
• Pulmonary hemorrhage
• Hepatomegaly and congestion in animals with R-CHF

TREATMENT

APPROPRIATE HEALTH CARE
• Most patients hospitalized during adulticide administration
• Appropriate patients should be given microfilaricide in the morning and discharged in the evening.
• Hospitalization recommended for dogs experiencing thromboembolic complications

ACTIVITY
• Severe restriction of activity required for 4–6 weeks after adulticide administration
• Cage confinement recommended for 3 weeks after adulticide administration for severe (Class III) disease
• Cage confinement for 7 days recommended for dogs experiencing pulmonary thromboembolic complications

DIET
Restricted sodium diet recommended for dogs with CHF

CLIENT EDUCATION
• Good prognosis for animals with mild-to-moderate infection
• Postadulticide pulmonary complications likely in patients with moderate-to-severe infection
• Reinfection can occur unless appropriate prophylaxis administered

SURGICAL CONSIDERATIONS
• Treatment of choice for vena cava syndrome
• Worm removal from right heart and pulmonary artery via jugular vein by use of fluoroscopy and a long, flexible, alligator forceps is highly effective for treating high worm burden when employed by an experienced operator.

MEDICATIONS

DRUGS OF CHOICE
• Stabilize animals with R-CHF with diuretics, cage rest, and sodium restriction before adulticide treatment.
• Stabilize pulmonary failure with anti-thrombotic agents (e.g., aspirin or heparin) or antiinflammatory dosages of corticosteroid, depending on the clinical and radiographic findings.
• Melarsomine dihydrochloride (Immiticide, 2.5 mg/kg IM)—an adulticide drug with the advantage of IM administration and less hepatotoxicity, and better efficacy against both sexes of adult worms of all ages than thiacetarsamide sodium
• Class I and II infections—two injections 24 h apart are given into the epaxial muscles (first on one side, then on the opposite side, using 22-gauge needles); apply pressure over the injection site during and after needle withdrawal. A positive antigen test result 4 months later usually indicates repeat treatment; with a weakly positive antigen test result, repeat test in 1–2 months before deciding to repeat adulticide treatment.
• Class III infections—one injection administered; 1 month later; two injections 24 h apart are recommended
• Microfilaricide administration indicated for most dogs with circulating microfilariae, 4–6 weeks after adulticide. Ivermectin (50 µg/kg) or interceptor is administered in the morning, and the patient observed for the day and discharged in the evening.

CONTRAINDICATIONS
• Adulticide treatment with icterus or hepatic failure
• Diethylcarbamazine in microfilaremic dogs

PRECAUTIONS
• Adulticide treatment—not indicated in patients with renal failure, hepatic failure, or nephrotic syndrome
• Standard adulticide therapy in dogs with severe infection is associated with high mortality due to subsequent pulmonary thromboembolism

POSSIBLE INTERACTIONS
None

ALTERNATIVE DRUGS
• Heparin (75 units/kg SQ q8h) or aspirin (5–7 mg/kg PO q24h) for 1–3 weeks before and during, and for 3 weeks after, adulticide administration is a controversial recommendation for the most severe cases of Class III disease; therapy is combined with strict, extended cage confinement.
• Heparin (75 units/kg SQ q8h) is recommended for dogs with pulmonary thrombosis, thrombocytopenia, or hemoglobinuria.

FOLLOW-UP

PATIENT MONITORING
• Perform a microfilaria concentration test in appropriate patients 3–4 weeks after microfilaricide administration; if positive, repeat the microfilaricide protocol immediately. Give another microfilaria test 3–4 weeks later; if positive, adulticide failure should be suspected. Institute heartworm prophylaxis when microfilaremia is eradicated or immediately in patients with occult infection.
• Give an antigen test—4 months after adulticide treatment; if positive, must decide whether or not to repeat the adulticide treatment. If a weakly positive test result; repeat in 1–3 months. Some dogs with persistent adult infection may not require retreatment—determined by age, severity of infection, degree of improvement since the first treatment, strength of the positive antigen test result, and concomitant disease.

PREVENTION/AVOIDANCE
Heartworm prophylaxis should be provided for all dogs at risk:
• Ivermectin (Heartgard)—a highly effective, monthly preventative that, when combined with pyrantel pamoate (Heartgard Plus), also controls hookworm and roundworm infection; can be given safely to microfilaremic dogs
• Milbemycin oxime (Interceptor)—a highly effective, monthly prophylaxis that also controls hookworms, roundworms, and whipworms; the preventative dosage is microfilaricidal; acute reactions may occur when given to microfilaremic dogs.
• Moxidectin (ProHeart)—a monthly prophylactic drug that can be given to microfilaremic dogs.
All of the monthly prophylactic drugs can be administered safely to collies at the appropriate dosages
• Diethylcarbamazine—a safe and effective prophylactic drug that should be administered daily; marketed as tablets and chewable tablets; in combination with pyrantel pamoate (Filaribits Plus) it also controls roundworms and hookworms; do not use in microfilaremic dogs.

POSSIBLE COMPLICATIONS
• Postadulticide pulmonary thromboembolic complications—may occur up to 4–6 weeks after treatment; usually more severe in dogs with severe heartworm infection (Class III) and those not properly confined
• Thrombocytopenia, disseminated intravascular coagulation
• Melarsomine adverse effects—pulmonary thromboembolism (usually 7–30 days after therapy); anorexia (13% incidence); injection site reaction (myositis) 32% incidence but mild and only lasts 1–2 days; lethargy or depression (15% incidence); causes elevations of hepatic enzymes

EXPECTED COURSE AND PROGNOSIS
• Usually uneventful with excellent prognosis in asymptomatic and mildly symptomatic animals (Class I)
• Guarded prognosis with higher risk of complications in dogs with severe infection (Class III)

MISCELLANEOUS

ASSOCIATED CONDITIONS
N/A

AGE-RELATED FACTORS
Old dogs may not require treatment, since heartworm infection may not be the life-limiting factor.

ZOONOTIC POTENTIAL
N/A

PREGNANCY
• Adulticide treatment should be delayed.
• Transplacental infection by microfilaria can occur.

SYNONYMS
N/A

SEE ALSO
• Congestive Heart Failure, Right-sided
• Disseminated Intravascular Coagulation
• Hepatotoxins
• Nephrotic Syndrome
• Pulmonary Hypertension
• Pulmonary Thromboembolism

ABBREVIATIONS
CHF = congestive heart failure

Suggested Reading

Dillon R, Dirofilariosis in dogs & cats. In: Ettinger SJ, Feldman EC, eds. Textbook of canine and feline veterinary internal medicine. Philadelphia: Saunders, 2000.

Authors Clay A. Calvert and Clarence A. Rawlings

Consulting Editors Larry P. Tilley and Francis W. K. Smith, Jr.

HEAT STROKE AND HYPERTHERMIA

BASICS

DEFINITION
• Hyperthermia—elevation in body temperature above the normal range (101–102° F); can be differentiated into pyrogenic hyperthermia (pyrexia or fever) and nonpyrogenic hyperthermia
• Heat stroke—a form of nonpyrogenic hyperthermia that occurs when heat-dissipating mechanisms of the body cannot accommodate excessive heat; can lead to multisystemic organ dysfunction. Temperatures of 106°F or above without signs of inflammation suggest nonpyrogenic hyperthermia.
• Malignant hyperthermia—an uncommon, familial, nonpyrogenic hyperthermia that occurs secondary to some anesthetic agents
• Other causes of nonpyrogenic hyperthermia include excessive exercise, thyrotoxicosis, and hypothalamic lesions.

PATHOPHYSIOLOGY
• Hypothalamic set point—changed with true fever, most likely mediated by the endogenous pyrogen, interleukin 1
• Nonpyrogenic hyperthermia does not change the hypothalamic set point.
• The critical temperature leading to multiple organ dysfunction is 109°F.
• The primary pathophysiologic processes of heat stroke are related to thermal damage that can lead to cellular necrosis, hypoxemia, and protein denaturalization.

SYSTEMS AFFECTED
• Nervous—neuronal damage, parenchymal hemorrhage, and cerebral edema
• Cardiovascular—hypovolemia, cardiac arrhythmias, myocardial ischemia, and necrosis
• Gastrointestinal—mucosal ischemia and ulceration, bacterial translocation, and endotoxemia
• Hepatobiliary—hepatocellular necrosis
• Renal/Urologic—acute renal failure
• Hemic/Lymph/Immune—hemoconcentration, thrombocytopenia, disseminated intravascular coagulopathy (DIC)
• Musculoskeletal—rhabdomyolysis

GENETICS
N/A

GEOGRAPHIC DISTRIBUTION
May be seen in any climate but more common in warm and or humid environments

SIGNALMENT

Species
Dogs or cats

Breed Predilection
• May occur in any breed
• Long-haired animals
• Brachycephalic breeds

Mean Age and Range
All ages; often age extremes

Predominant Sex
None

SIGNS

Historical Findings
• Identifiable underlying cause—hot day, locked in car, grooming accident, excessive exercise
• Predisposing underlying disease—laryngeal paralysis, cardiovascular disease, neuromuscular disease, previous history of heat-related disease

Physical Examination Findings
• Panting
• Hypersalivation
• Hyperthermia
• Hyperemic mucous membranes
• Tachycardia
• Cardiac arrhythmias
• Shock
• Respiratory distress
• Hematemesis
• Hematochezia
• Melena
• Petechiation
• Seizures
• Muscle tremors
• Coma
• Oliguria/anuria
• Respiratory arrest
• Cardiopulmonary arrest

CAUSES
• Excessive environmental heat and humidity*—may be due to weather conditions or accidents such as enclosed in unventilated room, car, or grooming dryer cages
• Upper airway disease
• Exercise
• Toxicosis—strychnine and metaldehyde cause hyperthermia secondary to seizure activity.
• Anesthesia (malignant hyperthermia)

RISK FACTORS
• Previous history of heat-related disease
• Age extremes
• Heat intolerance due to poor acclimatization
• Obesity
• Poor cardiopulmonary conditioning
• Hyperthyroidism
• Underlying cardiopulmonary disease
• Brachycephalic breeds
• Thick hair coat
• Dehydration

DIAGNOSIS

DIFFERENTIAL DIAGNOSIS
• If temperatures exceed 106°F without evidence of inflammation, consider heat stroke.
• Panting and hypersalivation may not be seen with true fever, as hypothalamic set point has been raised.

CBC/BIOCHEMISTRY/URINALYSIS
• May help identify underlying disease process
• May help identify sequelae to hyperthermia
• CBC abnormalities may include stress leukogram, anemia, thrombocytopenia, or hemoconcentration
• Biochemistry profile may show azotemia, hyperalbuminemia, high ALT, high AST, high CK, hypernatremia, hyperchloremia, hyperglycemia, hyperphosphatemia, hyperkalemia, hypokalemia
• Urinalysis may show hypersthenuria, proteinuria, cylindruria, hemoglobinuria, myoglobinuria.

OTHER LABORATORY TESTS
• Blood gas analysis may show mixed acid/base disorder, respiratory alkalosis, or metabolic acidosis.
• Coagulation profile may indicate prolonged activated clotting time (ACT), prothrombin time (PT), or partial thromboplastin time (PTT); may be fibrin degradation products (FDP); may be DIC if PT and PTT are prolonged along with FDPs and thrombocytopenia

IMAGING
• Thoracic radiographs may help identify underlying cardiopulmonary disease or predisposing factors.
• Abdominal radiographs may help identify underlying disease process.
• Computed tomography may help identify hypothalamic lesion.

DIAGNOSTIC PROCEDURES
Continuous temperature monitoring

HEAT STROKE AND HYPERTHERMIA

TREATMENT

APPROPRIATE HEALTH CARE
• Hospitalize patients until temperature is stabilized.
• Most patients need intensive care for several days.

NURSING CARE
• Immediate correction of hyperthermia:
Spray with water or immerse in water before transporting to veterinary facility
Convection cool with fans
Evaporative cool (e.g., alcohol on foot pads, axilla, and groin)
• Stop cooling procedures when temperature reaches 103°F, to avoid hypothermia.
• Supplement oxygen via oxygen cage, mask, or nasal catheter.
• Give ventilatory support if required.
• Give fluid support with shock doses of crystalloids.
• Treat complications such as DIC, renal failure, cerebral edema.
• Treat underlying disease or correct predisposing factors.

ACTIVITY
Restricted

DIET
Nothing per os until animal is stable

CLIENT EDUCATION
• Be aware of clinical signs.
• Know how to cool animals.
• An episode of heatstroke may predispose pets to additional episodes.

SURGICAL CONSIDERATIONS
Tracheostomy may be required if upper airway obstruction is underlying cause.

MEDICATIONS

DRUGS OF CHOICE
• No specific drugs are required for hyperthermia or heat stroke; therapy depends on clinical presentation.
• Acute renal failure—dopamine continuous-rate intravenous infusion (2–5 μg/kg/min), furosemide intravenously (2–4 mg/kg prn)
• Cerebral edema—mannitol (1 g/kg IV over 15–30 min), furosemide (1 mg/kg IV) 30 min after mannitol infusion; corticosteroids (dexamethasone sodium phosphate, (1–2 mg/kg IV), prednisone sodium succinate (10–20 mg/kg IV), or methyl prednisolone (15 mg/kg IV))

• Ventricular arrhythmia—lidocaine bolus (2 mg/kg IV) followed by continuous-rate intravenous infusion (25–75 μg/kg/min) or procainamide (6–8 mg/kg IV)
• Metabolic acidosis—sodium bicarbonate (0.3 × BW(kg) × BE); give 1/2 as bolus IV
• DIC—plasma (20 mL/kg); heparin (50–100 U/kg SC q6–8h); first dose of heparin can be put in unit of plasma
• Hemorrhagic vomiting diarrhea—broad-spectrum antibiotics
• Seizures—diazepam (0.5–1 mg/kg IV); phenobarbital (6 mg/kg IV as needed)

CONTRAINDICATIONS
• Nonsteroidal antiinflammatory agents not indicated in nonpyrogenic hyperthermia because the hypothalamic set point is not altered
• Cooling with ice—may lead to peripheral vasoconstriction and poor heat dissipation

PRECAUTIONS
Refer to manufacturers' recommendations.

POSSIBLE INTERACTIONS
Refer to manufacturers' recommendations.

ALTERNATIVE DRUGS
N/A

FOLLOW-UP

PATIENT MONITORING
Closely during cooling-down period and for a minimum of 24 h postepisode; most need several days, depending on clinical presentation and sequelae; thorough physical examination daily; also consider
• Body temperature
• Body weight
• Blood pressure
• Central venous pressure
• Activated clotting time
• ECG
• Thoracic auscultation
• Urinalysis and urine output
• PCV, TP
• CBC, biochemical profile

PREVENTION/AVOIDANCE
Avoid risk factors.

POSSIBLE COMPLICATIONS
• Cardiac arrhythmias
• Organ failure
• Coma
• Seizures
• Acute renal failure
• DIC
• Pulmonary edema—acute respiratory distress

• Rhabdomyolysis
• Hepatocellular necrosis
• Respiratory arrest
• Cardiopulmonary arrest

EXPECTED COURSE AND PROGNOSIS
• Depends on underlying cause or disease process
• Guarded—depending on complications and duration of episode
• May predispose to further episodes because of damage to thermoregulatory center

MISCELLANEOUS

ASSOCIATED CONDITIONS
N/A

AGE-RELATED FACTORS
N/A

ZOONOTIC POTENTIAL
N/A

PREGNANCY
N/A

SYNONYMS
• Heat stroke
• Heat exhaustion
• Heat prostration
• Heat-related disease

SEE ALSO
Fever

Suggested Reading

Haskins SC. Thermoregulation, hypothermia, hyperthermia. In: Ettinger SJ, Feldman EC, eds., Textbook of veterinary internal medicine. Philadelphia: Saunders, 1995:26–30.

Lee-Parritz DE, Pavletic MM. Physical and chemical injuries: heatstroke, hypothermia, burns, and frostbite. In: Murtaugh RJ, Kaplan PM, eds. Veterinary emergency and critical care medicine. St. Louis: Mosby Year Book, 1992:194–196.

Rushlander D. Heat stroke. In: Kirk RW, Bonagura JD, eds. Current veterinary therapy. 11th ed. Philadelphia: Saunders, 1992:143–146.

Author Steven L. Marks

Consulting Editors Larry P. Tilley and Francis W. K. Smith, Jr.

HELICOBACTER INFECTION

BASICS

DEFINITION
Helicobacter spp. are microaerophilic Gram-negative urease-positive bacteria ranging from coccoid to curved to spiral.

PATHOPHYSIOLOGY

Gastric Helicobacter
• The discovery of the association of *Helicobacter pylori* with gastritis, peptic ulcers, and gastric neoplasia has fundamentally changed the understanding of gastric disease in humans. • Investigation of the relationship of gastric disease to HLOs in other species has resulted in the discovery of *H. mustelae* in ferrets with gastritis and peptic ulcers, *H. acinonyx* in cheetahs with severe gastritis, and *H. heilmannii* in pigs with gastric ulcers. • The relationship of *Helicobacter* spp. to gastric inflammation in cats and dogs is unresolved; inflammation or glandular degeneration accompanies infection in some but not all subjects. • The presence of multiple species complicates the investigation of pathogenicity. • Experiments to determine the pathogenicity of *H. pylori* in SPF cats and *H. pylori* and *H. felis* in gnotobiotic dogs demonstrated gastritis, lymphoid follicle proliferation, and humoral immune responses after infection.

Intestinal and Hepatic Helicobacter
• The role of *Helicobacter* spp. in intestinal and hepatic disease in dogs and cats is unclear. • *H. canis* has been isolated from healthy dogs and dogs with diarrhea. • No clear association of the organism with diarrhea • *H. canis* has also been isolated from the liver of a dog with active, multifocal hepatitis. • *H. fennelliae* has been isolated from dogs and *H. cinaedi* from dogs and cats; neither has been associated with clinical signs.

SYSTEMS AFFECTED
• Gastrointestinal—stomach: gastric *Helicobacter* spp. may be related to gastritis; intestines: diarrhea observed in some dogs with *H. canis* infection • Hepatobiliary—acute hepatitis has been associated with *H. canis* infection.

GENETICS
N/A

INCIDENCE/ PREVALENCE

Gastric Helicobacter spp.
• Gastric HLOs are highly prevalent in dogs and cats—86% of random-source cats, 90% of clinically healthy pet cats, 67–86% of clinically healthy pet dogs, and almost 100% of laboratory beagles and shelter dogs infected • HLOs demonstrated in gastric biopsy specimens from 57–76% of cats and 61–82% of dogs presented for investigation of recurrent vomiting. • Recent polymerase chain reaction (PCR)-based studies of the prevalence of individual *Helico-*

bacter spp. identified *H. heilmannii* in 38 of 49 (78%) Swiss cats and *H. felis* in 20 of 24 (83%) American dogs. • Coinfection of dogs with HLOs consistent with *H. felis* and *H. heilmannii/bizzozeronii* was common in two electron-microscopic studies. • To date *H. pylori* has only been identified in a colony of laboratory cats.

Intestinal and Hepatic Helicobacter spp.
• *H. canis* was isolated from 4% of 1000 dogs. • Only one case of *H. canis*–associated hepatitis has been reported. • The prevalence of *H. fennelliae* and *H. cinaedi* is undetermined.

GEOGRAPHIC DISTRIBUTION
• *Helicobacter* infection in humans has a higher prevalence rate in less-developed countries. • Crowded and/or less sanitary conditions may result in higher infection rates.

SIGNALMENT

Species
Dogs and cats

Breed Predilections
N/A

Mean Age and Range
• Infection with gastric *Helicobacter* spp. appears to be acquired at a young age. • The dog with *H. canis*–associated hepatitis was 2 months old.

Predominant Sex
N/A

SIGNS

Historical Findings
• Vomiting, anorexia, abdominal pain, weight loss, and/or borborygmus in dogs and cats with gastric *Helicobacter* spp. • Diarrhea in dogs may be associated with *H. canis* infection. • Vomiting, weakness, and sudden death in a dog with hepatic *H. canis* • Asymptomatic *Helicobacter* infection is common

Physical Examination Findings
• Usually unremarkable • May have signs of dehydration from fluid and electrolyte loss due to vomiting or diarrhea

CAUSES

Gastric Helicobacter spp.
• *H. felis, H. pylori, H. heilmannii* have been found in cats. • *H. felis, H. heilmannii, H. bizzozeronii, H. salomonis, H. bilis,* and *Flexispira rappini* have been identified in dogs. • *H. pylori* has not been isolated from pet cats.

Intestinal and Hepatic Helicobacter spp.
• *H. fennelliae*—dog (significance unknown) • *H. cinaedi*—dogs and a cat (significance unknown) • *H. canis*—normal and diarrheic dogs; one dog with acute hepatitis

RISK FACTORS
Potentially poor sanitary conditions and overcrowding may facilitate the spread of infection.

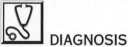

DIAGNOSIS

DIFFERENTIAL DIAGNOSIS

General Comments
High *Helicobacter* spp. prevalence rates exist in dogs and cats, so both exclusion of other diagnoses and positive *Helicobacter* testing are necessary to support clinical disease due to *Helicobacter* infection.

Gastric Helicobacteriosis
Distinguish from other causes of vomiting (both gastrointestinal and nongastrointestinal).

Intestinal Helicobacteriosis
Distinguish from other causes of diarrhea (both gastrointestinal and nongastrointestinal).

Hepatic Helicobacteriosis
Distinguish from other causes of hepatobiliary disease.

CBC/BIOCHEMISTRY/URINALYSIS
• May reflect fluid and electrolyte abnormalities secondary to vomiting and/or diarrhea
• May reflect changes consistent with hepatic disease in *H. canis*–associated hepatitis

OTHER LABORATORY TESTS
• Culture—*H. canis, H. fennelliae, H. cinaedi* (feces), and gastric HLOs (gastric biopsies) require specialized isolation techniques and media; success rates are low.
• Urease testing—see Diagnostic Procedures
• No reliable, noninvasive serologic test available at this time

IMAGING
Radiography and ultrasonography—usually normal

DIAGNOSTIC PROCEDURES

Gastric Helicobacteriosis
• Endoscopy and gastric biopsy with histopathology enable definitive diagnosis of gastric *Helicobacter* infection.
• Endoscopy may reveal superficial pockmarks that suggest lymphoid follicle hyperplasia.
• Other endoscopic reported findings include diffuse gastric rugal thickening, mucosal flattening, punctate hemorrhages, and erosions.
• Urease test (also known as CLO test or *Campylobacter*-like organism test) of gastric biopsy specimens—identify HLOs; commercial tests are available for in-house use that typically yield results within minutes.
• Examination of impression smears

Hepatobiliary Helicobacteriosis
Hepatic biopsy/histopathology (Warthin-Starry staining) and culture

PATHOLOGICAL FINDINGS

• Requires histopathology of gastric (gastric HLOs) or hepatic (hepatobiliary HLOs) biopsy specimens along with special staining of tissue samples with Warthin-Starry or modified-Steiner stain; routine H&E staining may reveal larger *Helicobacter* organisms, smaller organisms are often missed.
• Stomach—gastric spiral organisms on silver-stained sections; lymphocytic plasmacytic gastritis and lymphoid follicle hyperplasia; rarely neutrophil involvement; no ulcers reported in dogs and cats
• *H. canis*–associated hepatitis—hepatocellular necrosis, mononuclear cells, and neutrophils; spiral to curved bacteria predominantly in bile canaliculi

 TREATMENT

APPROPRIATE HEALTH CARE

• The pathogenicity of *Helicobacter* spp. in dogs and cast is still under debate, so it is premature to give clear-cut indications for treatment.
• No indication at present for treating asymptomatic animals with *Helicobacter* infection.
• The author attempts to eradicate gastric *Helicobacter* in infected dogs and cats with vomiting and idiopathic gastritis prior to initiating immunosuppressive therapy.

NURSING CARE

Fluid therapy for dehydration from vomiting

ACTIVITY

N/A

DIET

Diets to facilitate gastric emptying—easily assimilated, high in digestible carbohydrate

CLIENT EDUCATION

Explain the difficulty of establishing a diagnosis, the high prevalence rates in normal dogs and cats, the potential for recurrence, and the zoonotic aspects of the disease.

SURGICAL CONSIDERATIONS

N/A

 MEDICATIONS

GENERAL COMMENTS

• A combination of two antibiotics and one antisecretory drug is effective in people with *H. pylori* infection—cure rates approach/exceed 90%.
• Combination therapy may eliminate *Helicobacter* in dogs and cats less effectively than in humans.
• Treat for 2–3 weeks.

DRUGS OF CHOICE

Antibiotics (Two with One Antisecretory Agent)

• Amoxicillin (20 mg/kg PO q12h)
• Azithromycin (5 mg/kg PO q24h)
• Bismuth subsalicylate (17–20 mg/kg PO q12h or 1 mL/kg of regular strength preparation [262 mg/15 mL] PO q12h)
• Clarithromycin (5 mg/kg PO q12h)
• Metronidazole (dogs, 15–20 mg/kg PO q12h; cats, 12.5 mg/kg PO q12h)
• Tetracycline (20 mg/kg PO q8h)

Antisecretory Agents (One with Two Antibiotics)

• Famotidine (0.5 mg/kg PO q12–24h)
• Omeprazole (0.7 mg/kg PO q24h)
• Ranitidine (1.0 mg/kg PO q12h)
• Cimetidine (10 mg/kg PO q8h)

Intestinal and Hepatic Helicobacter spp. in Dogs

The combination of amoxicillin and metronidazole may be effective.

CONTRAINDICATIONS

N/A

PRECAUTIONS

N/A

POSSIBLE INTERACTIONS

N/A

 FOLLOW-UP

PATIENT MONITORING

• No noninvasive tests are currently available to confirm eradication of gastric HLOs. • If vomiting persists or recurs after cessation of combination therapy, do a repeat endoscopic biopsy to determine whether the infection has been eradicated.

PREVENTION/AVOIDANCE

Overcrowding and unsanitary conditions

POSSIBLE COMPLICATIONS

• Recurrence • Zoonotic potential

EXPECTED COURSE AND PROGNOSIS

• The efficacy of present therapy for eradicating *Helicobacter* is questionable. • Patients with *Helicobacter* and gastritis that do not respond to antibiotic therapy usually are given immunosuppressive therapy (prednisolone, other) for inflammatory bowel disease. • Metronidazole (20 mg/kg PO q12h), amoxicillin (20 mg/kg PO q12h), and famotidine (0.5 mg/kg PO q12h) for 14 days effectively eradicated *Helicobacter* in 6 of 8 dogs evaluated 3 days posttreatment, but all dogs were recolonized 28 days after infection. • Clarithromycin (30 mg/cat PO q12h), metronidazole (30 mg/cat PO q12h), ranitidine (20 mg/cat PO q12h), and bismuth (40 mg PO q12h) for 4 days effectively eradicate *H. heilmannii* in 11 of 11

cats by 10 days, but 2 cats were reinfected 42 days after treatment. • Amoxicillin (20 mg/kg PO q8h), metronidazole (20 mg/kg PO q8h), and omeprazole (0.7 mg/kg PO q24h) for 21 days transiently eradicated *H. pylori* in 6 cats, but all were reinfected 6 weeks posttreatment (*Note*: this dose of metronidazole has the potential for toxicity). • Unclear if recurrent infection following therapy is due to reinfection or recrudescence of infection

 MISCELLANEOUS

ASSOCIATED CONDITIONS

Gastrointestinal erosions

AGE-RELATED FACTORS

Gastric HLO appears to be acquired at a young age.

ZOONOTIC POTENTIAL

• The high prevalence of *Helicobacter* spp. in dogs and cats raises the possibility that household pets may serve as a reservoir for the transmission of *Helicobacter* spp. to people.
• *H. pylori, H. heilmannii,* and *H. felis* have been isolated from humans with gastritis.
• *H. fennelliae* and *H. cinaedi* have been isolated from immunocompromised people with proctitis and colitis. • *H. cinaedi* has also been associated with septicemia in people.
• *H. canis* has also been isolated from people.

PREGNANCY

Avoid metronidazole and tetracycline in pregnant animals.

SYNONYMS

• Gastric spiral bacterial • Gastrospirillum

SEE ALSO

• Gastritis, Chronic • Gastroduodenal Ulcer Disease • Inflammatory Bowel Disease
• Vomiting, Chronic

ABBREVIATIONS

• HLO = Helicobacter-like organism
• PCR = polymerase chain reaction

Suggested Reading

Crystal MA. Helicobacter. In: Norsworthy GD, Crystal MA, Fooshee SK, eds. The feline patient. Essentials of diagnosis and treatment. Baltimore: Williams & Wilkins, 1998:243–247.
Fox JG. *Helicobacter*-associated gastric disease in ferrets, dogs and cats. In: Bonagura JD, ed. Kirk's current veterinary therapy XII small animal practice. Philadelphia: Saunders, 1995:720–723.
Fox JG, Lee A. The role of *Helicobacter* species in newly recognized gastrointestinal tract disease of animals. Lab Anim Sci 1997;47:222–255.
Author Kenneth W. Simpson
Consulting Editors Mitchell A. Crystal and Brett M. Feder

HEMANGIOPERICYTOMA

BASICS

OVERVIEW
• A soft tissue sarcoma arising from pericytes, which are cells surrounding capillaries in subcutaneous tissue
• Locally invasive, often extending far beyond visible margins
• Metastasizes in up to 20% of patients
• Local growth can interfere with limb function.

SIGNALMENT
• More common in large-breed than in small-breed dogs
• Rare in cats

SIGNS

Historical Findings
• Typically, slow-growing mass (weeks to months)
• Rapid growth uncommon unless high-grade variant

Physical Examination Findings
• Soft tissue mass, usually located on extremity; less commonly found on trunk
• Soft, fluctuant, or firm
• Generally adhered to underlying tissue
• Regional lymph node metastasis uncommon

CAUSES & RISK FACTORS
Unknown

DIAGNOSIS

DIFFERENTIAL DIAGNOSIS
• Other soft tissue sarcomas—nerve sheath tumor; fibrosarcoma
• Lipoma and other tumors—benign and malignant
• Biopsy—essential to confirm diagnosis

CBC/BIOCHEMISTRY/URINALYSIS
N/A

OTHER LABORATORY TESTS
N/A

IMAGING
• Thoracic radiographs—recommended before treatment, although metastasis uncommon
• CT or MRI—may be required to determine extent of disease and to optimize surgical treatment

DIAGNOSTIC PROCEDURES
• Biopsy—essential to confirm diagnosis and determine grade of the tumor
• Regional lymph node evaluation—appropriate for high-grade tumors

TREATMENT

• Early, aggressive surgical excision—treatment of choice
• Local recurrence, metastasis, and overall survival time—greatly affected by surgical margin width as determined by a pathologist
• Radiotherapy—good option when complete surgical excision is not possible

Surgical Technique
• Microscopically, cancer cells extend far beyond gross tumor borders.
• Pseudocapsule composed of cancer cells common
• Excise tumor en bloc; if it is peeled out, a healthy bed of cancer cells is left behind.
• Submit the entire sample to a pathologist for surgical margin evaluation; mark two edges of the tissue with suture material to orient the pathologist and allow for proper margin evaluation.
• Toe or limb amputation may be necessary.
• Rib resection or abdominal wall resection—may be required for tumors of the trunk

MEDICATIONS

DRUGS
Chemotherapy—not consistently reported as beneficial; recommended after excision of a high-grade (grade III) tumor; doxorubicin is drug of choice.

CONTRAINDICATIONS/POSSIBLE INTERACTIONS
N/A

FOLLOW-UP

PATIENT MONITORING
Incomplete surgical excision—perform a second surgery or start radiotherapy as soon as possible.

EXPECTED COURSE AND PROGNOSIS
• Cure—possible when surgery is aggressive and surgical margins are tumor free
• Recurrence—inevitable if treatment is not aggressive; increased risk for metastatic disease
• Long-term tumor control—radiotherapy after surgically debulking the tumor gives 1- to 5-year control rates of 60%–85%.

MISCELLANEOUS

Suggested Reading

Kuntz CA, Dernell WS, Powers BE, et al. Prognostic factors for surgical treatment of soft tissue sarcomas in dogs: 75 cases (1986–1996). J Am Vet Med Assoc 1997;211:1147–1151.

Postorino NC, Berg RJ, Powers BE, et al. Prognostic variables for canine hemangiopericytoma: 50 cases (1979–1984). J Am Anim Hosp Assoc 1988;24:501–509.

Salisbury SK. Aggressive cancer surgery and aftercare. In: Morrison WB, ed. Cancer in dogs and cats: medical and surgical management. Baltimore: Williams & Wilkins 1998:265–321.

Author Robyn Elmslie
Consulting Editor Wallace B. Morrison

BASICS

OVERVIEW
• A highly metastatic malignant tumor of vascular endothelial cells
• Primary disease rare
• Incidence rates—3%–8% of all bone tumors
• May be difficult to distinguish primary from metastatic lesions

SIGNALMENT
• Mean age—dogs, 6 years; cats, 17–18 years
• Boxers, Great Danes, and German shepherds predisposed
• Male dogs have higher incidence

SIGNS

Historical Findings
• Tumor on limb—lameness; swelling; pathologic fracture
• Tumor on rib—thoracic wall swelling; dyspnea if patient has pleural effusion

Physical Examination Findings
• Soft tissue swelling at tumor site
• Palpable fracture
• Quiet or absent ventral lung sounds (if pleural effusion present)
• Pale mucous membranes

CAUSES & RISK FACTORS
Unknown

DIAGNOSIS

DIFFERENTIAL DIAGNOSIS
• Other primary or metastatic bone tumors
• Osteomyelitis (bacterial or fungal)

CBC/BIOCHEMISTRY/URINALYSIS
• Regenerative anemia
• Nucleated RBC
• Poikilocytosis—acanthocytes; schistocytes; spherocytes
• Anisocytosis
• Thrombocytopenia
• Leukocytosis
• Hypoproteinemia

OTHER LABORATORY TESTS
High fibrin degradation products, PT, PTT, and low fibrinogen concentration—may indicate DIC

IMAGING
• Radiology of bone—reveals poorly marginated osteolytic lesion with minimal periosteal reaction; pathologic fractures possible
• Thoracic radiography—evaluate lungs for metastasis
• Abdominal and cardiac ultrasound—look for primary tumor or metastasis
• CT scan—may help determine extent of bone tumor before surgery

DIAGNOSTIC PROCEDURES
Biopsy—incisional may be helpful, but because of the vascular nature of the tumor, blood contamination of specimen may preclude a diagnosis; excisional may be preferred.

PATHOLOGIC FINDINGS
• Dark, friable mass within the medullary cavity of the bone
• Histopathologic—vascular spaces and clefts filled with RBCs, thrombi, and necrotic debris; spaces lined by pleomorphic tumor cells with round, ovoid, or pleomorphic nuclei

TREATMENT
• Aggressive surgical excision of tumor sites
• Amputation—required if limbs affected
• Axial tumors—may be more difficult to remove
• Adjunctive chemotherapy—indicated in all cases

MEDICATIONS

DRUGS
Doxorubicin—30 mg/m^2 dogs > 10 kg; 1 mg/kg dogs < 10 kg and cats every 3 weeks for 4–6 treatments; treatment of choice after surgical resection

CONTRAINDICATIONS/ POSSIBLE INTERACTIONS
Doxorubicin—cardiotoxic; do not use with pre-existing heart disease

FOLLOW-UP

PATIENT MONITORING
• Thoracic radiography, cardiac and abdominal ultrasound, and physical examination—1, 3, 6, 9, 12, 18, and 24 months after treatment
• Creatinine—monitor in small dogs and cats receiving doxorubicin because of potential nephrotoxicity.

POSSIBLE COMPLICATIONS
• Pathologic fractures
• Tumors and metastatic lesions may rupture causing serious acute blood loss.

EXPECTED COURSE AND PROGNOSIS
• Mean survival—unknown
• Median survival (all locations) after surgery and chemotherapy—180 days

MISCELLANEOUS

ASSOCIATED CONDITIONS
High incidence of DIC

ABBREVIATIONS
• DIC = disseminated intravascular coagulation
• PT = prothrombin time
• PTT = partial thromboplastin time

Suggested Reading
Straw RC. Tumors of the skeletal system. In: Withrow SJ, MacEwen EG, eds. Small animal clinical oncology. 2nd ed. Philadelphia: Saunders, 1996:287–315.
Waters DJ, Cooley DM. Skeletal neoplasms. In: Morrison WB, ed. Cancer in dogs and cats: medical and surgical management. Baltimore: Williams & Wilkins, 1998: 639–654.
Author Joanne C. Graham
Consulting Editor Wallace B. Morrison

HEMANGIOSARCOMA, HEART

 ## BASICS

OVERVIEW
- The most common cardiac tumor in dogs
- The heart can be a primary or metastatic site in dogs and cats.
- Most tumors involve the right atrium or right auricular appendage, or both.
- Rarely involves the right ventricular wall or heart valve

SIGNALMENT
- Dogs and rarely cats
- Most commonly reported in German shepherds and golden retrievers

SIGNS

General Comments
Most relate to the development of pericardial effusion and right-sided congestive heart failure rather than to the tumor itself.

Physical Examination Findings
- Abdominal effusion
- Quiet or absent ventral lung sounds—with pleural effusion
- Dyspnea
- Weight loss
- Muffled heart sounds with pericardial effusion
- Syncope
- Arrhythmia
- Pulse deficits
- Pulsus paradoxus
- Exercise intolerance
- Hepatomegaly
- Jugular distension

CAUSES & RISK FACTORS
Unknown

 ## DIAGNOSIS

DIFFERENTIAL DIAGNOSIS
- Other causes of right heart failure—heart worm disease
- Other cardiac neoplasia
- Idiopathic hemorrhagic pericardial effusion

CBC/BIOCHEMISTRY/URINALYSIS
- May find anemia and nucleated RBCs
- Prerenal azotemia with congestive heart failure

OTHER LABORATORY TESTS
N/A

IMAGING
- Radiographs—often reveal evidence of pericardial and/or pleural effusion; rarely detect cardiac mass
- Ultrasound (heart)—useful for identifying cardiac location of tumor

DIAGNOSTIC PROCEDURES
Biopsy of mass—required for definitive diagnosis

 ## TREATMENT

- Surgery and chemotherapy—primary choices
- Periodic centesis of pericardial and pleural effusion—may provide symptomatic relief

 ## MEDICATIONS

DRUGS
Chemotherapy—doxorubicin; may be effective in providing palliation for varying periods of time

CONTRAINDICATIONS/POSSIBLE INTERACTIONS
N/A

 ## FOLLOW-UP

PATIENT MONITORING
Physical examination, thoracic radiographs, and cardiac ultrasound—monthly intervals

PREVENTION/AVOIDANCE
N/A

POSSIBLE COMPLICATIONS
Relate to centesis of pericardial and pleural space (e.g., arrhythmia, pneumothorax, and infection) or from primary treatment by surgery and/or chemotherapy

EXPECTED COURSE AND PROGNOSIS
Prognosis—guarded to poor

 ## MISCELLANEOUS

ASSOCIATED CONDITIONS
- Concurrent hemangiosarcoma at other sites (e.g., liver and spleen)
- Clinical signs of congestive heart failure secondary to pericardial effusion

Suggested Reading
Morrison WB. Nonpulmonary intrathoracic cancer. In: Morrison WB, ed. Cancer in dogs and cats: medical and surgical management. Baltimore: Williams & Wilkins 1998:537–550.

Author Wallace B. Morrison
Consulting Editor Wallace B. Morrison

BASICS

OVERVIEW
• Malignant tumor arising from endothelial cells
• Primary tumor develops within dermal or subcutaneous tissues.
• Accounts for 14% of all hemangiosarcoma in dogs
• Prevalence (dogs)—0.3%-2.0%

SIGNALMENT
• Dogs and rarely cats
• Pit bulls, boxers, and German shepherds—affected more commonly than other breeds
• Multicentric dermal hemangiosarcoma—whippet dogs and related breeds
• Median age, 9 year; range, 4.5–15 years

SIGNS
• Usually solitary mass; may see multiple masses
• Dermal—firm, raised, dark nodules primarily on the limbs, prepuce, and ventral abdomen
• Subcutaneous—firm or soft, fluctuant masses with or without associated bruising; masses may appear to change size quickly because of intratumoral bleeding; typically larger than dermal; often found on the pelvic limbs, but may arise in any location

CAUSES & RISK FACTORS
• Vascular stasis, radiotherapy, trauma, and sun exposure—predisposing factors in humans; may be risk factors in dogs
• Pit bulls, boxers, and German shepherds—may have genetic predisposition
• Whippets—may be genetically predisposed to multicentric dermal hemangiosarcoma

 DIAGNOSIS

DIFFERENTIAL DIAGNOSIS
• Trauma—subcutaneous hematoma
• Other benign or malignant tumors

CBC/BIOCHEMISTRY/URINALYSIS
• Usually normal
• May see laboratory abnormalities compatible with DIC—prolonged bleeding times, thrombocytopenia, low fibrinogen, and high fibrin split products

OTHER LABORATORY TESTS
N/A

IMAGING
• Thoracic radiographs—detect pulmonary metastasis
• CT or MRI—delineate extent of disease; often required to determine feasibility of surgery

DIAGNOSTIC PROCEDURES
Skin biopsy—required to confirm diagnosis; differentiate between dermal and subcutaneous

PATHOLOGIC FINDINGS
• Dermal—well circumscribed; confined to the dermis
• Subcutaneous—poorly circumscribed; very invasive

 TREATMENT

• Aggressive surgical excision—treatment of choice; complete surgical excision of subcutaneous tumor difficult
• DIC and bleeding—important intraoperative and postoperative concerns

 MEDICATIONS

DRUGS
• Chemotherapy (subcutaneous tumor)—recommended after excision; may be administered to patients before surgery to cytoreduce tumor and increase the likelihood of successful surgical outcome; treatment with doxorubicin, cyclophosphamide, and vincristine shown to improve survival time in dogs
• Multicentric dermal—etretinate (0.75–1 mg/kg q24h) and vitamin E (400 IU PO q12h); author successfully induced partial remission in whippets with nonresectable disease

CONTRAINDICATIONS/POSSIBLE INTERACTIONS
Aspirin and other NSAIDs—avoid because of associated increased potential for bleeding

 FOLLOW-UP

EXPECTED COURSE AND PROGNOSIS
• Dermal—median survival, 780 days
• Subcutaneous—median survival, > 6 months; depends on the degree of invasion
• Metastasis—may occur

 MISCELLANEOUS

ABBREVIATIONS
DIC = disseminated intravascular coagulation
NSAIDs = non-steroidal antiinflammatory drugs

Suggested Reading
Ward H, Fox LE, Calderwood-Mays MB, et al. Cutaneous hemangiosarcoma in 25 dogs: a retrospective study. J Vet Intern Med 1994:8:345–348.
Author Robyn Elmslie
Consulting Editor Wallace B. Morrison

HEMANGIOSARCOMA, SPLEEN AND LIVER

 BASICS

DEFINITION
Highly metastatic malignant vascular neoplasm arising from endothelial cells

PATHOPHYSIOLOGY
• A large mass develops in the liver or spleen.
• Metastasis—rapidly via hematogenous routes; most frequently to the liver (from the spleen) and lungs (from the spleen and liver)
• Can rupture, leading to acute hemorrhage, collapse, and sudden death

SYSTEMS AFFECTED
• Hepatobiliary
• Hemic/Lymphatic/Immune—spleen
• Possible metastasis—lungs; kidneys; muscle; peritoneum; omentum; lymph nodes; mesentery; adrenal glands; spinal cord; brain; subcutaneous tissue; diaphragm

GENETICS
N/A

INCIDENCE/PREVALENCE
• Dogs—0.3%–2.0% of recorded necropsies; 7% of all malignancies; about 50% hemangiosarcomas splenic and 5% hepatic
• Cats—18 affected cats out of 3145 necropsies; liver most common site

GEOGRAPHIC DISTRIBUTION
N/A

SIGNALMENT
Species
Dogs and cats

Breed Predilections
• Dogs—German shepherds, boxers, Great Danes, English setters, golden retrievers, pointers
• Cats—domestic shorthair

Mean Age and Range
• Dogs—mean age, 8–10 years; can be seen < 1 year old
• Cats—mean age, 10 years

Predominant Sex
• Dogs—possible male predilection
• Cats—none

SIGNS
General Comments
• Related to the organs involved
• Also caused by bleeding secondary to rupture of the mass or DIC

Historical Findings
• Sudden death because of acute blood loss
• Weight loss
• Weakness
• Intermittent collapse
• Ataxia
• Lameness
• Seizures
• Dementia
• Paresis

Physical Examination Findings
• Pale mucous membranes
• Tachycardia
• Peritoneal fluid
• Palpable cranial abdominal mass

CAUSES
• Dogs and cats—unknown
• Humans—arsenicals; vinyl chloride; thorium dioxide
• Minks—methyl nitrosamine

RISK FACTORS
N/A

 DIAGNOSIS

DIFFERENTIAL DIAGNOSIS
• Other causes of splenic and hepatic masses—lymphosarcoma; leiomyosarcoma; liposarcoma; hematoma; hemangioma; splenic cyst; hepatoma; hepatocellular carcinoma; hepatic cyst
• One study reported 43 of 100 splenic masses as hemangiosarcoma.

CBC/BIOCHEMISTRY/URINALYSIS
• Regenerative anemia with polychromasia, reticulocytosis, anisocytosis, and nucleated RBCs
• Leukocytosis—caused by mature neutrophilia
• Thrombocytopenia
• High liver enzyme activity—with liver involvement

OTHER LABORATORY TESTS
• High PT, PTT, and fibrin degradation products—with DIC
• Evaluate clotting cascade—evidence of spontaneous hemorrhage; considering surgery

IMAGING
Radiography
• Abdominal—reveals cranial abdominal mass; possible evidence of abdominal fluid
• Thoracic radiography—detects metastasis
• Area of any lameness—pain from metastasis to bone possible; bone lysis with little to no proliferation common

Ultrasonography
• Reveals splenic masses with multiple cavitations
• Hepatic involvement—usually appears as multiple hypoechoic nodules

Echocardiography
• Perform in patients with evidence of pericardial effusion.
• May detect cardiac masses—primary cardiac (often right atrial location) or metastasis

DIAGNOSTIC PROCEDURES
Peritoneocentesis—with evidence of abdominal effusion; usually obtain serosanguinous fluid or frank blood that does not clot; may see spindle-shaped neoplastic cells

PATHOLOGIC FINDINGS
• Spleen—a large hemorrhagic, friable mass; usually some degree of abdominal hemorrhage
• Liver—multiple, variable-sized, hemorrhagic nodules in many patients
• Spleen and liver—widespread abdominal metastasis in many patients
• Histopathologic examination—necessary for definitive diagnosis; three patterns predominate: large blood spaces lined by endothelial cells, numerous small capillary structures, and solid areas of endothelial cells without apparent vascular structure

TREATMENT

APPROPRIATE HEALTH CARE
Inpatient—initial medical and surgical management

NURSING CARE
• Balanced isotonic electrolyte solutions—correct dehydration
• Fresh whole blood transfusion—with severe anemia
• Manage DIC as necessary.

ACTIVITY
Restricted until after initial surgical management; spontaneous hemorrhage may occur.

DIET
No change

CLIENT EDUCATION
• Inform client that emergency surgery may be indicated.
• Warn client that sudden death is possible.
• Discuss the importance of follow-up chemotherapy.

SURGICAL CONSIDERATIONS
Initial treatment of choice

MEDICATIONS

DRUGS OF CHOICE

Chemotherapy Cycle
• Day 1—doxorubicin (30 mg/m² IV for dogs > 10 kg; 1 mg/kg for dogs and cats < 10 kg) and cyclophosphamide (100–150 mg/m² IV); diphenhydramine (2.2 mg/kg IM) 20 min before the doxorubicin to prevent anaphylactoid reaction
• Days 8 and 15—vincristine (0.75 mg/m² IV)
• Repeat every 21 days; generally, four cycles are given after surgery.

CONTRAINDICATIONS
• Doxorubicin—do not use with arrhythmias or reduced fractional shortening of the heart.
• Chemotherapy may cause gastrointestinal, bone marrow, and cardiac toxicity; seek advice before treatment if unfamiliar with cytotoxic drugs.

PRECAUTIONS
• Monitor WBC count—delay chemotherapy if neutrophil count < 2,000/μL
• Monitor platelets—delay chemotherapy if platelets < 100,000/μL

POSSIBLE INTERACTIONS
None

ALTERNATIVE DRUGS
None

FOLLOW-UP

PATIENT MONITORING
Thoracic and abdominal radiography and abdominal ultrasound—every 3 months after treatment; monitor for recurrence or metastasis.

PREVENTION/AVOIDANCE
N/A

POSSIBLE COMPLICATIONS
• Sepsis—because of neutropenia
• Doxorubicin-induced cardiomyopathy
• Skin sloughs—caused by extravasation of doxorubicin or vincristine
• Vomiting and diarrhea

EXPECTED COURSE AND PROGNOSIS
• Mean time to recurrence (cats)—4–5 months
• Median survival time with surgery alone (dogs)—19–65 days
• Median survival time with surgery plus chemotherapy (dogs)—145 days (mean survival, 271 days)

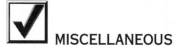

MISCELLANEOUS

ASSOCIATED CONDITIONS
DIC

AGE-RELATED FACTORS
None

ZOONOTIC POTENTIAL
None

PREGNANCY
Do not use chemotherapy in pregnant animals.

SYNONYMS
• Malignant hemangioendothelioma
• Angiosarcoma

SEE ALSO
• Hemangiosarcoma, bone
• Hemangiosarcoma, heart
• Hemangiosarcoma, skin

ABBREVIATIONS
• DIC = disseminated intravascular coagulation
• PT = prothrombin time
• PTT = partial thromboplastin time

Suggested Reading

Hammer AS, Couto G, Filppi J, et al. Efficacy and toxicity of VAC chemotherapy (vincristine, doxorubicin, and cyclophosphamide) in dogs with hemangiosarcoma. J Vet Intern Med 1991;5:160–166.

Johnson KA, Powers BE, Withrow SJ, et al. Splenomegaly in dogs: predictors of neoplasia and survival after splenectomy. J Vet Intern Med 1989;3:160–166.

Morrison WB. Blood vascular, lymphatic, and splenic cancer. In: Morrison WB, ed. Cancer in dogs and cats: medical and surgical management. Baltimore: Williams & Wilkins, 1998:705–715.

Prymals C, McKee LJ, Goldschmidt MH, et al. Epidemiologic, clinical, pathologic, and prognostic characteristics of splenic hemangiosarcoma and splenic hematoma in dogs: 217 cases (1985). J Am Vet Med Assoc 1988;193:706–712.

Scavelli TD, Patnaik AK, Melhaff CJ, et al. Hemangiosarcoma in the cat: retrospective evaluation of 31 surgical cases. J Am Vet Med Assoc 1985;187:817–819.

Author Terrance A. Hamilton
Consulting Editor Wallace B. Morrison

DISEASES

HEMOTHORAX

BASICS

OVERVIEW
• Collection of blood in the pleural space
• May range from peracute to chronic
• Cardiovascular and respiratory systems commonly affected

SIGNALMENT
Any age, breed, or sex of dogs and cats

SIGNS
• Peracute to acute onset—hypovolemic signs usually occur before sufficient blood volume accumulates in the pleural space to impair respiration.
• Respiratory distress
• Pale membranes
• Weakness and collapse
• Weak, rapid pulse
• Ventral thoracic dullness; dorsal hyperresonance if concurrent pneumothorax
• Associated with causative factor—trauma or coagulopathy

CAUSES & RISK FACTORS
• Trauma—bleeding from any artery or vein of the thoracic wall, mediastinum, or thoracic spine; damaged heart, lungs, thymus, and diaphragm; herniated abdominal viscera (liver or spleen)
• Neoplasia—involving any structure adjacent to the pleural cavity
• Coagulopathies—congenital or acquired; rodenticide ingestion common
• Lung lobe torsion
• Acute thymic hemorrhage in young animals

DIAGNOSIS

DIFFERENTIAL DIAGNOSIS
• Pulmonary contusion
• Pneumothorax
• Diaphragmatic hernia
• Flail chest
• Nonhemorrhagic pleural effusions—chylothorax; pyothorax; modified transudates; transudates

CBC/BIOCHEMISTRY/URINALYSIS
PCV and hemoglobin—reflect blood loss after initial fluid compartment shifts have occurred

OTHER LABORATORY TESTS
Fluid Analysis
• Hemorrhage-produced effusion—PCV and protein content similar to that of the peripheral blood; platelets common
• Inflammation- or vascular congestion–produced effusion—PCV < 8%
• Cytologic examination—often fails to identify malignant causes

COAGULATION TESTS
• ACT and blood smear evaluation—may provide rapid diagnostic information
• PT, APTT, and platelet count—may be mildly to moderately abnormal with DIC
• Specific tests—may diagnose congenital defect or acquired coagulopathy

IMAGING
• Radiology—reveals pleural effusion varying from a diffuse increase in radiopacity to ventral leafing, interlobar fissures, and localized pleural densities; may see associated lesions (e.g., rib fractures, pneumothorax, pulmonary contusions, diaphragmatic lesions, and masses)
• Ultrasound—confirm pleural effusion; look for masses, lung lobe torsion, and herniation of liver, gallbladder, spleen, or bowel

DIAGNOSTIC PROCEDURES
• Thoracentesis
• Surgical exploration—may be necessary to establish a diagnosis; if imaging does not suggest the appropriate side to enter, the left side is recommended.

TREATMENT
• Acute—fluids to treat hypovolemia
• Coexisting pneumothorax—generally requires needle thoracentesis or tube thoracostomy
• Pulmonary contusion—may require ventilator support
• Drain large volumes of hemorrhage to relieve dyspnea; may leave small volumes of blood unassociated with contamination or extensive tissue devitalization
• Severe or recurrent thoracic hemorrhage—may require surgical exploration in conjunction with appropriate medications
• Oxygen therapy
• Maintenance of body heat
• Blood transfusion—may be needed for RBC or clotting factors

MEDICATIONS

DRUGS
• Hypovolemia—see Shock, Hemorrhagic
• Vitamin K or specific factor replacement—if indicated
• Analgesics—systemically or as nerve blocks
• Broad-spectrum antibiotics—when indicated

CONTRAINDICATIONS/POSSIBLE INTERACTIONS
Avoid aspirin and other NSAIDs.

FOLLOW-UP

PATIENT MONITORING
• Clinical signs
• Temperature
• Urine production
• Relief from pain
• Follow-up radiographs at 48-hr intervals

POSSIBLE COMPLICATIONS
• Pyothorax
• Sepsis
• Entrapment and constriction of lungs by scar tissue and fibrosis

MISCELLANEOUS

ASSOCIATED CONDITIONS
• Peritonitis—with penetrating wounds (e.g., gunshot) into the abdomen
• Esophageal perforation

SEE ALSO
• Disseminated Intravascular Coagulation (DIC)
• Lung Lobe Torsion
• Pleural Effusion
• Pulmonary Contusions
• Rodenticide Anticoagulant Poisoning

ABBREVIATIONS
• ACT = activated clotting time
• APTT = activated partial thromboplastin time
• DIC = disseminated intravascular coagulation
• PCV = packed cell volume
• PT = prothrombin time

Suggested Reading
Glaus TM, Rawlings CA, Mahaffey EA, Mahaffey MB. Acute thymic hemorrhage and hemothorax in a dog. J Am Anim Hosp Assoc 1993;29:481–491.
Author Bradley L. Moses
Consulting Editor Eleanor C. Hawkins

BASICS

OVERVIEW
• Amyloidoses—disorders that share the common feature of pathologic deposition of an extracellular insoluble fibrillar proteinaceous matrix • Amyloid—accumulates secondary to inflammatory or lymphoproliferative disorders or as a familial tendency • Dogs and cats—usually reactive or secondary amyloidosis; underlying primary inflammatory disorder common • Associated familial disorders—certain kindreds of dogs and cats • Multiple organs commonly involved; clinical signs usually owing to renal or liver involvement • Liver involvement—may be insidious; may lead to high liver enzymes, severe hepatomegaly, coagulopathy, liver rupture leading to hemoabdomen, and/or liver failure

SIGNALMENT
• Dogs—some Chinese shar peis with cyclic fevers (shar pei fever syndrome), akitas with cyclic fever and polyarthropathy, and collies with gray collie syndrome predisposed; usually develop renal signs; may develop signs of liver failure or rupture • Cats—Asian shorthair and Siamese cats predisposed; usually < 5 years of age (hepatic signs predominant); familial disorder in Abyssinians (renal signs)

SIGNS
Historical Findings
• Shar peis—episodic fever; swollen hocks • Akitas—episodic polyarthropathy; pain; signs of meningitis • Acute lethargy • Anorexia • Polyuria and polydipsia • Vomiting

Physical Examination Findings
• Pallor • Abdominal effusion—hemorrhage or ascites • Jaundice • Hepatomegaly • Edema • Joint pain • Nonlocalized pain

CAUSES & RISK FACTORS
• Familial immunoregulatory disorders—kindreds of predisposed dogs and cats • Chronic infection—coccidioidomycosis; blastomycosis • Cyclic neutropenia—gray collie syndrome • Bacterial endocarditis • Chronic inflammation—SLE • Neoplasia

 DIAGNOSIS

DIFFERENTIAL DIAGNOSIS
• Chronic hepatic inflammation • Hepatic neoplasia • Primary coagulopathy • Glomerulonephritis • Pyelonephritis • SLE • Abdominal trauma

CBC/BIOCHEMISTRY/URINALYSIS
• Anemia secondary to hepatic hemorrhage or rupture • Chronic inflammation • Leukocytosis with a left shift during febrile episodes—shar peis and akitas • Normal to high liver enzymes, total bilirubin, and serum bile acids • Azotemia • Proteinuria • Dilute urine—with renal involvement or failure

OTHER LABORATORY TESTS
• Coagulation tests—normal to prolonged • Synovial fluid—with joint swelling or pain shows suppurative, nonseptic inflammation • CSF—with meningeal pain demonstrates increased protein and neutrophilic inflammation

IMAGING
• Abdominal radiography—hepatomegaly; renomegaly, or normal kidney size; effusion • Abdominal ultrasonography—hepatomegaly; hypoechoic parenchyma with diffuse amyloid; enlarged or normal kidney; normal or equivocally hypoechoic parenchyma; may note mesenteric lymphadenopathy and thickened gut wall owing to amyloid deposition; abdominal effusion

DIAGNOSTIC PROCEDURES
• Liver or kidney biopsy • Abdominocentesis—may reveal hemorrhagic effusion or transudate

PATHOLOGIC FINDINGS
Gross
• Liver—normal to pale color; large, firm to friable; hemorrhages (subcapsular hematomas, capsular tears) or obvious fractures in parenchyma • Kidneys—large, normal, or small with renal amyloidosis; surface smooth to finely irregular; glomeruli usually primarily involved in dogs with renal amyloidosis (stain positively with Lugol iodine); renal deposition in shar peis similar to Abyssinian cats (medullary involvement)

Microscopic
• Liver—acellular amorphous material diffusely deposited in the space of Disse associated with hepatic cord atrophy; may note primarily involved blood vessels in the portal triad (often observed in Abyssinian cats); may note amyloid in both intrahepatic locations with severe disease • Kidney—amorphous material in glomeruli (dogs) or renal medulla (cats, shar peis); birefringent and apple green amyloid when stained with Congo red and viewed with polarized light

 TREATMENT

• Dictated by the severity of clinical signs • No curative treatment; manage underlying disease when identified. • Fluids—for dehydration • Blood transfusion—for acute blood loss • Diet—individually tailored to the patient • Liver failure—consider measures appropriate for hepatic encephalopathy.

• Pathologic proteinuria—see Nephrotic Syndrome • Warn client that this syndrome is difficult to treat and has a guarded to poor prognosis. • Surgical considerations—hepatic lobe resection as an emergency measure for catastrophic hemorrhage

 MEDICATIONS

DRUGS
• Colchicine—dogs, 0.03 mg/kg PO q24h; may block formation of amyloid in the early phases; side effects include vomiting, diarrhea (bloody), and bone marrow suppression. • DMSO—dogs, 80–125 mg/kg PO q12h or as an 18% solution in sterile water SC given three times a week; may promote dissolution of amyloid fibrils or provide a unique anti-inflammatory or anti-amyloid effect; side-effects include garlic smell and objectionable taste.

CONTRAINDICATIONS/POSSIBLE INTERACTIONS
Colchicine combined with probenecid may cause vomiting.

 FOLLOW-UP

• Shar peis—may live > 2years; will have episodes of fever and cholestasis • Akitas with cyclic clinical signs—grave prognosis • Cats that survive liver hemorrhage eventually succumb to renal failure.

 MISCELLANEOUS

SEE ALSO
Amyloidosis

ABBREVIATIONS
• CSF = cerebrospinal fluid • DMSO = dimethyl sulfoxide • SLE = systemic lupus erythematosus

Suggested Reading
Center SA. Hepatic lipidosis, glucocorticoid hepatopathy, vacuolar hepatopathy, storage disorders, amyloidosis, and iron toxicity. In: Guilford WG, Center SA, Strombeck DR, et al., eds. Strombeck's small animal gastroenterology. 3rd ed. Philadelphia: Saunders, 1996:766–801.
Loevan KO. Hepatic amyloidosis in two Chinese shar pei dogs. J Am Vet Med Assoc 1994;204:1212–1216.
Author Susan E. Johnson
Consulting Editor Sharon A. Center

DISEASES

HEPATIC ENCEPHALOPATHY

 BASICS

DEFINITION
A metabolic disorder affecting the CNS and developing secondary to advanced hepatic disease

PATHOPHYSIOLOGY
• Complex pathophysiologic state with a multifactorial origin • Gut-derived substances of bacterial and protein metabolism—important in the pathogenesis; dietary protein modification or therapeutic agents that reduce gut bacterial flora often improve neurologic function without altering the underlying liver disease. • Current theories concerning pathogenesis—ammonia as the putative neurotoxin with or without other synergistic toxins; alteration in monoamine or catecholamine neurotransmitters as a result of perturbed aromatic amino acid metabolism; alteration in amino acid neurotransmitters, GABA, and/or glutamate; increased cerebral levels of an endogenous benzodiazepine-like substance

SYSTEMS AFFECTED
• Nervous—generally a decrease in neuronal function; seizures occur, particularly in cats • Gastrointestinal—presumably as a result of liver dysfunction; vomiting, diarrhea, and anorexia • Renal/Urologic—formation of ammonium biurate crystals owing to increased ammonia excretion; renal pelvic and cystic calculi

Genetics
Congenital PSVA—inherited in a polygenic manner in certain breeds

Incidence/Prevalence
Uncommon in small animal practice

Geographic Distribution
N/A

SIGNALMENT
Species
Dogs and cats

Breed Predilections
PSVA—usually in purebred dogs; apparent increased occurrence in some breeds in different geographic locations (e.g., Yorkshire terriers, Australian cattle dogs, Maltese terriers, and Irish wolfhounds)

Mean Age and Range
• PSVA—usually young dogs • Acquired liver disease resulting in acquired portosystemic shunting—dogs and cats of any age

Predominant Sex
None

SIGNS
General Comments
• Neurologic—may be related to meal ingestion • Dramatic temporary resolution—may occur after initiating antibiotic therapy • Prolonged recovery from sedation or anaesthesia • Cats and dogs similar; important differences noted below

Historical Findings
• Episodic abnormalities • Lethargy • Anorexia • Vomiting • Disorientation—aimless wandering; compulsive pacing; head pressing • Polyuria or polydipsia • Amaurotic blindness • Seizures • Coma • More frequent in cats than in dogs—ptyalism; seizures; aggression; disorientation; ataxia; stupor • More frequent in dogs than in cats—compulsive behavior (head pressing, circling, aimless wandering); vomiting; diarrhea; polyuria or polydipsia

Physical Examination Findings
• PSVA—stunted growth (less common in cats); copper-colored eyes (cats) • Ptyalism (cats) • Depression • Disorientation • Palpable urolith

CAUSES
• PSVA (dogs)—usually single large intrahepatic or extrahepatic vessels (see Portosystemic Shunt) • Acquired portosystemic shunting—occurs with diseases that induce portal hypertension (cirrhosis; intrahepatic arteriovenous fistula; fibrosis; see Hypertension, Portal) • Acute hepatic failure—induced by drugs, toxins, or infection (see Hepatic Failure, Acute)

RISK FACTORS
• Alkalosis • Hypokalemia • Certain anesthetics and sedatives • Gastrointestinal bleeding—most common precipitating cause • Transfusion of stored blood products containing high concentrations of ammonia • Infections • Constipation • Methionine

 DIAGNOSIS

DIFFERENTIAL DIAGNOSIS
• Lead toxicity • Urinary tract infection—cystic calculi • Intestinal parasitism • Primary gastrointestinal disease • Hypoglycemia • Toxoplasmosis • Congenital CNS disease or malformation—hydrocephalus; storage diseases • Acute ethylene glycol toxicity • Rabies • CNS neoplasia • Canine distemper • Thiamine deficiency—Wernicke encephalopathy • Drug intoxication

CBC/BIOCHEMISTRY/URINALYSIS
CBC
• Acquired portosystemic shunting and PSVA—RBC microcytosis • Poikilocytosis—common, especially in cats • Leukogram—reflects specific liver disease or causal conditions

Biochemistry
• Hypoalbuminemia—with hepatic synthetic failure, negative acute phase response, or other disorder causing extracorporeal albumin loss • ALT and ALP—high; may be normal or only slightly high with PSVA or end-stage cirrhosis • BUN—low; reflects hepatic urea cycle dysfunction, protein-restricted diet, polyuria or polydipsia associated with increased GFR • Creatinine—low; reflects reduced muscle mass, hepatic synthetic failure, and polyuria or polydipsia causing increased GFR • Hypoglycemia—especially in young dogs with PSVA; fulminant hepatic failure; end-stage cirrhosis

Urinalysis
Ammonium biurate crystalluria

OTHER LABORATORY TESTS
• Ammonia—high fasting ammonemia common; condition may occur without hyperammonemia owing to its multifactorial complex pathophysiology; normal or high blood values cannot alone be used for diagnosis (see Ammonia) • Intolerance to oral or rectal ammonium chloride (all patients)—more reliable for confirmation of hepatic insufficiency or acquired portosystemic shunting • High-serum bile acids—confirm hepatic insufficiency

IMAGING
• Abdominal radiography—reveal a small liver in dogs; less reliable in cats • Abdominal ultrasonography—may identify PSVA, acquired portosystemic shunting, intrahepatic arteriovenous fistula, or echogenic patterns consistent with acquired liver disorders may note a relatively hypovascular liver in dogs with microvascular hepatoportal dysplasia • Portovenography—confirms PSVA or acquired portosystemic shunting; does not reveal arteriovenous fistula; shows associated acquired portosystemic shunting • Celiac artery/hepatic artery angiography—required for confirmation of intrahepatic arteriovenous fistula • Colorectal scintigraphy—rectal instillation of technetium pertechnetate and gamma camera imaging of circulatory distribution to

the liver and heart; detect portosystemic shunting via calculation of a shunt fraction

DIAGNOSTIC PROCEDURES

Hepatic biopsy—confirm underlying liver disorder

PATHOLOGIC FINDINGS

• Gross—none specific; brain herniation may develop with acute disease.
• Microscopic—CNS: mild vacuolation of glial cells and cerebral edema with severe disease (usually acute); hepatic: depends on the primary hepatic condition

TREATMENT

APPROPRIATE HEALTH CARE
• Depends on underlying condition
• PSVA—surgical correction

NURSING CARE
• Depends on underlying condition
• Avoid risk factors.
• Fluids—0.9% saline or Ringer with 2.5%–5.0% dextrose and 20–30 mEq of potassium chloride/L; do not use lactate with fulminant hepatic failure (rare); use sodium-restricted fluids with acquired liver disease with acquired portosystemic shunting and ascites.
• Colloids—may be essential with low albumin (< 1.5 g/dL); use fresh-frozen plasma rather than synthetic colloids.
• Minimize exposure to drugs that require hepatic biotransformation or elimination.

ACTIVITY
Keep patient quiet, warm, and adequately hydrated.

DIET
• Adequate calories—avoid catabolism
• Dietary protein restriction—cornerstone of medical management for chronic disease; only as needed to ameliorate signs; dairy and vegetable proteins best tolerated
• Good-quality vitamin supplement (without methionine)—vitamin metabolism often perturbed with liver dysfunction
• Ensure thiamine repletion—avoid Wernicke encephalopathy

CLIENT EDUCATION
• Inform client that surgical treatment is potentially curative for PSVA.
• Inform client that medical management may be attempted if surgical correction is not feasible.
• Warn client that treatment is otherwise palliative and provides temporary alleviation of signs.
• Advise client that high vigilance is required to avoid precipitating circumstances or conditions.

SURGICAL CONSIDERATIONS
• See Portosystemic Shunt
• Acquired portosystemic shunting—do not ligate.

MEDICATIONS

DRUGS OF CHOICE
• Medications that increase dietary protein tolerance alter gastroenteric flora or enteric conditions, reducing production or availability of substances that precipitate the disease.
• Antibiotics—spectrum against intestinal flora (aerobic and anaerobic); nonabsorbable (neomycin, 10–20 mg/kg PO q8–12h); local and systemic (metronidazole, 7.5–10 mg/kg q12h); used in combination with lactulose
• Nonabsorbable-fermented carbohydrates—lactulose, lactitol, or lactose (if lactase deficient); decrease production or absorption of ammonia; increase rate of stool transit; lactulose most commonly used (starting dose, 0.5–1 mL/kg given two or three times daily); therapeutic goal is passage of two to three soft stools per day; may also be administered as an enema for acute hepatic coma
• Enemas—cleansing (warmed polyionic fluids) mechanically clean the colon (10–15 mL/kg); retention directly deliver fermentable substrates or directly alter colonic pH; lactulose, lactitol, or lactose diluted 1:2 in water; neomycin in water (do not exceed oral dose); diluted Betadine (1:10, rinse well after 15 min); diluted vinegar (diluted 1:10 in water)

CONTRAINDICATIONS
Avoid drugs metabolized by the liver.

PRECAUTIONS
• Use anesthetics, sedatives, tranquillizers, potassium-wasting diuretics, and analgesics cautiously.
• If possible, avoid drugs that rely on hepatic metabolism, biotransformation, or excretion.
• Consider altered pharmacokinetics owing to hypoalbuminemia and reduced protein binding of certain drugs.

POSSIBLE INTERACTIONS
Drugs that affect or depend on hepatic metabolism—cimetidine; chloramphenicol; barbiturates

ALTERNATIVE DRUGS
N/A

FOLLOW-UP

PATIENT MONITORING
• Albumin—monitor in patients with nonsurgically correctable disease. • Blood

glucose concentration—monitor to avoid neuroglycopenia (exacerbates or worsens the disease) • Electrolytes, especially potassium—monitor to avoid hypokalemia (aggravates hyperammonemia)

PREVENTION/AVOIDANCE
Avoid dehydration, azotemia, hemolysis, constipation, hypokalemia, gastrointestinal bleeding, infusion of stored blood, ammonium challenge, urinary tract infections (especially with urease-producing organisms), hypokalemia, hypomagnesemia, and alkalemia.

POSSIBLE COMPLICATIONS
Permanent neurologic damage—rare

EXPECTED COURSE AND PROGNOSIS
• Depend on underlying disease • With acute or chronic hepatic failure—usually fully reversible with the amelioration of the underlying liver disease

MISCELLANEOUS

ASSOCIATED CONDITIONS
N/A

AGE-RELATED FACTORS
N/A

ZOONOTIC POTENTIAL
N/A

PREGNANCY
N/A

SYNONYMS
• Hepatic coma • Portosystemic encephalopathy

SEE ALSO
• Ammonia • Hepatic Failure, Acute • Portosystemic Shunt

ABBREVIATIONS
• ALP = alkaline phosphatase
• ALT = alanine aminotransferase
• GABA = gamma aminobutyric acid
• GFR = glomerular filtration rate
• PSVA = portosystemic vascular anomaly

Suggested Reading
Maddison JE. Current concepts of hepatic encephalopathy. J Vet Intern Med 1992;6:341–353.
Maddison JE. Medical management of chronic hepatic encephalopathy. In: Kirk RW, Bonagura J, eds. Current veterinary therapy XII. Philadelphia: Saunders, 1995:1153–1158.
Author Jill E. Maddison
Consulting editor Sharon A. Center

HEPATIC FAILURE, ACUTE

BASICS

DEFINITION
• Sudden loss of > 75% functional hepatic mass, occurring primarily because of acute, massive hepatic necrosis
• Causes—vary; include drugs, environmental toxins, infectious agents, thermal injury, and severe hypoxia

PATHOPHYSIOLOGY
• Necrosis—occurs when the liver undergoes an insult secondary to poor perfusion, hypoxia, hepatotoxic drugs or chemicals, heat excess, or infectious agents; consequences to hepatic function depend on insult type and its preferred distribution within the lobule; accompanied by enzyme leakage and impairment in multiple hepatic functions, resulting in failure
• Events that decrease perfusion or cause hypoxia—commonly affect zone 3 of the hepatic acinus, corresponding to the peri-central region
• Ingested toxins—affect the more meta-bolically active zone 1 of the acinus, located periportally;
• Failure—associated with myriad metabolic derangements in glucose homeostasis, protein synthesis (procoagulant and anticoagulant factors), and detoxification; may result in death

SYSTEMS AFFECTED
• Hepatobiliary—hepatocellular necrosis; hepatic failure
• Nervous—hepatic encephalopathy
• Gastrointestinal—vomiting; diarrhea; melena; hematochezia
• Hemic/Lymphatic/Immune—procoagulant and anticoagulant factor imbalances; DIC

Genetics
N/A

Incidence/Prevalence
• Mild to moderate necrosis—common in association with many primary and secondary hepatobiliary diseases
• Severe necrosis resulting in acute failure—less common; prevalence difficult to assess (several causes)

Geographic Distribution
N/A

SIGNALMENT

Species
Dogs more common than cats

Breed Predilections
N/A

Mean Age and Range
N/A

Predominant Sex
N/A

SIGNS
• Acute onset
• Vomiting
• Jaundice
• Small intestinal diarrhea—may be bloody
• Hepatic encephalopathy
• Seizures
• Bleeding
• Tender hepatomegaly

CAUSES
See also Hepatotoxins

Drugs
• Antimicrobials
• Chemotherapy agents
• Anthelminthics
• Analgesics
• Diazepam—oral preparation (cats)
• Anesthetics

Biologic Toxins
• *Amanita phylloides* mushrooms
• Cycads
• Aflatoxins

Infectious Agents
• Canine infectious hepatitis virus
• Leptospirosis

Other
• Heatstroke
• Post-whole body hyperthermia treatment for cancer
• Thromboembolic disease
• Shock
• DIC
• Acute circulatory failure from any cause

RISK FACTORS
• Administration of any potentially hepato-toxic drug
• Exposure to environmental toxins—*Amanita phylloides* mushroom

DIAGNOSIS

DIFFERENTIAL DIAGNOSIS
• Severe acute pancreatitis or gastroenteritis—differentiated via laboratory data
• Acute decompensation of chronic hepato-biliary disease—distinguished by abdominal ultrasonography and liver biopsy

CBC/BIOCHEMISTRY/URINALYSIS
• Anemia and panhypoproteinemia—associated with bleeding
• Thrombocytopenia
• Liver enzyme activity—dramatically high ALT and AST; less strikingly abnormal ALP

• Hypoglycemia
• Normal to low BUN concentration
• High serum and urine bilirubin concentrations

OTHER LABORATORY TESTS
• Serum bile acids—high values confirm hepatic dysfunction.
• Plasma ammonia—high values confirm hepatic dysfunction.
• Coagulation tests—identifies coagulation factor deficiencies and DIC

IMAGING
• Abdominal radiography—may identify a normal to slightly enlarged liver
• Abdominal ultrasonography—disclose evidence of nonhepatic disease (e.g., pancreatitis) and severe chronic hepatobiliary disease (e.g., heterogeneous liver texture, multiple nodules, hepatopetal portal blood flow); rule out biliary obstruction

DIAGNOSTIC PROCEDURES
Liver biopsy—required to confirm necrosis

PATHOLOGIC FINDINGS
• Gross—may note slightly enlarged and mottled liver
• Microscopic—reveals necrosis; identifying the most affected zone helps determine specific cause; hypoxic changes commonly pericentral; toxic changes commonly periportal

TREATMENT

APPROPRIATE HEALTH CARE
Inpatient—intensive care required

NURSING CARE
• Fluids—non-lactate-containing; initially at a resuscitation rate
• Low oncotic pressure from bleeding and protein loss—provide colloidal fluid; plasma preferred; may use dextran 70, hetastarch, or a plasma extender
• Potassium and glucose—supplemented as appropriate
• Fluid regimen—changed to maintenance composition and rate after normovolemia is achieved
• Phosphate—supplemented if clinically significant hypophosphatemia is discovered

ACTIVITY
Restricted—promote healing and regeneration of the liver

DIET
• Vomiting—withhold food until stops
• Small, easily digestible meals

• Protein—moderate restriction is initially recommended; gradually increase, as tolerated, to ensure positive nitrogen balance necessary for hepatic regeneration
• Energy intake—increase over several days until caloric requirements are met for maintenance and stress
• Enteral route optimal; if food must be withheld for > 5 days, institute TPN.
• Branched-chain amino acid solutions (intravenous)—controversial; advocated by some clinicians
• Supplemental vitamins essential—water-soluble (twofold normal); K_1 (0.5–1.5 IU/kg for three doses; then once weekly); E as antioxidant (see Drugs of Choice)

CLIENT EDUCATION
• Inform client that acute hepatic failure is a serious condition.
• Warn client that some patients die even with optimal treatment.
• Inform client that an underlying cause for the necrosis (e.g., exposure to a drug or toxin) should be investigated.

SURGICAL CONSIDERATIONS
N/A

MEDICATIONS

DRUGS OF CHOICE
Vomiting
• Metoclopramide—1–2 mg/kg/day continuous IV infusion; for mild or infrequent vomiting; contraindicated if spironolactone is used for ascites mobilization
• Chlorpromazine (dogs)—0.5 mg/kg SC, IM q8–24h; for severe vomiting
• Cimetidine (5 mg/kg IV q8h) or famotidine (0.5 mg/kg IM, SC q12–24h)—for gastrointestinal bleeding; cimetidine may inhibit formation of injurious metabolites of some toxins.

Hepatic Encephalopathy
• Lactulose—0.5 mL/kg PO q8h
• Metronidazole—7.5 mg/kg PO q12h
• Abnormal mentation and impaired swallowing—administer drugs per rectum
• Mannitol—1g/kg over 10–20 min via a blood filter; if no brisk diuresis noted within 1 hr, check plasma osmolality (measured) and blood pressure for excessive volume expansion; for cerebral edema
• Furosemide—0.5–1.0 mg/kg IV q8–24h; for increasing free water excretion and reducing CSF production; monitor hydration and serum potassium to avoid dehydration and hypokalemia.

Coagulopathy
Fresh whole blood or frozen plasma—for clinically significant bleeding

Free-Radical Scavengers
• For ongoing damage attributable to membrane damage and reperfusion injury and hypoxia
• Vitamin E—10–100 IU/kg PO q24h
• Vitamin C—100–500 IU per day
• N-acetylcysteine—140 mg/kg PO, IV loading dose; then 70 mg/kg PO, IV, q6h for five to seven treatments
• s-adenosylmethionine—10 mg/kg PO q12h

CONTRAINDICATIONS
Avoid drugs that are biotransformed primarily by the liver and/or that alter liver blood flow or metabolic enzyme activity—may be impractical, because metabolism of many drugs involves the liver in some way

PRECAUTIONS
Administration of stored whole blood or packed RBCs may precipitate or exacerbate hepatic encephalopathy.

POSSIBLE INTERACTIONS
N/A

ALTERNATIVE DRUGS
N/A

FOLLOW-UP

PATIENT MONITORING
• Temperature, pulse, respiration, and mental status—every 1–2 hr for the first 24 hr
• High vigilance for signs of infection, especially iatrogenic catheter-associated nosocomial organisms
• Body weight—twice a day; to guide fluid therapy
• Acid–base balance, electrolyte balance (especially potassium and phosphate), and glucose—every 12–24 hr for the first 72 hr
• Liver enzyme activities and serum bilirubin concentration—every 2–3 days until marked improvement observed

PREVENTION/AVOIDANCE
• Dogs—vaccination against infectious canine hepatitis virus
• Avoid drugs and toxins associated with hepatotoxicity.

POSSIBLE COMPLICATIONS
• Hypoglycemia
• DIC
• Uncontrolled gastrointestinal bleeding
• Hepatic encephalopathy
• Chronic hepatic insufficiency
• Hepatic cirrhosis and fibrosis
• Death

EXPECTED COURSE AND PROGNOSIS
• Prognosis—depends on quantity of liver mass destroyed
• Adequate support may permit hepatic regeneration and recovery.

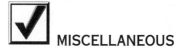

MISCELLANEOUS

ASSOCIATED CONDITIONS
• Pancreatitis
• Sepsis
• Shock
• Intestinal bleeding
• DIC

AGE-RELATED FACTORS
N/A

ZOONOTIC POTENTIAL
N/A

PREGNANCY
N/A

SYNONYMS
• Acute hepatic necrosis
• Fulminant hepatic failure

SEE ALSO
• Alanine Aminotransferase (ALT)/Aspartate Aminotransferase (AST)
• Alkaline Phosphatase (ALP)/γ-Glutamyl transferase (GGT)
• Ammonia
• Bilirubin, High
• Coagulopathy of Liver Disease
• Hepatic Encephalopathy
• Hepatitis, Infectious Canine
• Hepatotoxins

ABBREVIATIONS
• ALP = alkaline phosphatase
• ALT = alanine aminotransferase
• AST = aspartate aminotransferase
• CSF = cerebrospinal fluid
• DIC = disseminated intravascular coagulation

Suggested Reading
Center SA, Elston TH, Rowland PH, et al. Fulminant hepatic failure associated with oral administration of diazepam in 11 cats. J Am Vet Med Assoc 1996;209:618–625.
Center SA. Acute hepatic injury: hepatic necrosis and fulminant hepatic failure. In: Guilford GW, Center SA, Strombeck DR, et al., eds. Small animal gastroenterology. Philadelphia: Saunders, 1996:654–704.
Holloway SA. Heatstroke in dogs. Compend Contin Educ Pract Vet 1992;14: 1598–1604.
Hughes D, King LG. The diagnosis and management of acute liver failure in dogs and cats. Vet Clin North Am Small Anim Pract 1995;25:437–460.
Rudloff E, Kirby R. The critical need for colloids: selecting the right colloid. Compend Contin Educ Pract Vet 1997;19:811–825.
Author Susan E. Bunch
Consulting Editor Sharon A. Center

DISEASES

HEPATIC LIPIDOSIS

BASICS

DEFINITION
• Feline hepatic lipidosis syndrome—occurs when > 50% of hepatocytes accumulate excessive triglycerides, resulting in severe cholestasis and liver dysfunction • Untreated—progressive metabolic dysregulation and death • May be a secondary or idiopathic condition • Most patients have an underlying disease causing anorexia.

PATHOPHYSIOLOGY
• Cats have an unusual propensity for accumulation of lipid vacuoles in the liver. • Energy and protein deprivation—excess accumulation of hepatic triglycerides; protein deficiency may play a leading role, limiting formation of apoproteins essential for mobilization of triglycerides from the liver. • Causal factors—increased peripheral mobilization of fat; increased de novo hepatic triglyceride synthesis; impaired B-oxidation of fatty acids; reduced hepatocellular exportation of triglyceride-bearing lipoproteins • Triglyceride vacuoles accumulation—hepatocellular swelling; displacement of organelles; organelle dysfunction; canalicular compression • Hepatic failure with severe disease

SYSTEMS AFFECTED
• Hepatobiliary—severe intrahepatic cholestasis; hepatic dysfunction or failure • Gastrointestinal—anorexia; vomiting • Musculoskeletal—peripheral tissue wasting • Nervous—hepatic encephalopathy • Hemic/Lymphatic/Immune—abnormal erythrocyte shapes (poikilocytes)

GENETICS
N/A

INCIDENCE/PREVALENCE
Most common severe feline hepatopathy in North America causing jaundice

GEOGRAPHIC DISTRIBUTION
Worldwide

SIGNALMENT

Species
Cats and rarely dogs (reported in puppies)

Breed Predilection
None

Mean Age and Range
• Mean—8 years • Range—1–16 years • Primarily middle-aged adults

Predominant Sex
Inconsistent predilection for obese female cats

SIGNS

Historical Findings
• Anorexia • Weight loss • Jaundice • Lethargy • Vomiting • Diarrhea or constipation • Weakness • Ptyalism • Hepatic encephalopathy • Collapse • Abnormalities caused by an unrelated underlying disease

Physical Examination Findings
• Jaundice • Hepatomegaly • Dehydration • Weakness, neck ventriflexion, recumbency • Ptyalism • Obtunded mentation • Depend on underlying or primary disease

CAUSES
Idiopathic—common; no underlying disease

Secondary
• Primary liver disease—portosystemic vascular anomaly; cholangitis/cholangiohepatitis syndrome; extrahepatic bile duct occlusion; cholelithiasis; neoplasia • Diabetes mellitus • Small intestinal disease—obstruction; neoplasia; inflammatory bowel disease • Pancreatitis • Urogenital disease—chronic interstitial nephritis; renal failure (acute or chronic); feline lower urinary tract disease • Neurologic conditions • Infectious diseases—toxoplasmosis; FIP; FeLV-related • Hyperthyroidism • B$_{12}$ deficiency • Other systemic conditions, including toxins

RISK FACTORS
• Obesity • Anorexia • Negative nitrogen balance—catabolism • Severe rapid weight loss

DIAGNOSIS

DIFFERENTIAL DIAGNOSIS
• Primary underlying liver diseases—cholangitis/cholangiohepatitis syndrome, cholelithiasis, extrahepatic bile duct occlusion, and neoplasia; most important differentials; differentiated by abdominal ultrasonography, liver aspirate, and definitively by liver biopsy • Congenital portosystemic vascular anomalies—rarely confused; differentiated by ultrasonography or colorectal scintigraphy • Hepatic toxoplasmosis or FIP—differentiated via liver biopsy • Pancreatitis—differentiated by abdominal ultrasonography, serum tests (high trypsin-like immunoactive substances, high amylase, high lipase; amylase and lipase not reliable), and/or direct inspection and biopsy • Gastrointestinal disease—inflammatory bowel disease (differentiate by endoscopic or full-thickness bowel biopsy), obstruction (differentiate by survey radiographs, barium contrast study, ultrasonography) • Toxicities—suspected on the basis of history (e.g., administration of oral diazepam or acetaminophen); hyperthyroidism differentiated via a serum thyroid panel

CBC/BIOCHEMISTRY/URINALYSIS
• Hematology—poikilocytosis common; mild nonregenerative anemia; hemolytic anemia with severe hypophosphatemia; leukogram reflects underlying disorder. • Biochemistry—hyperbilirubinemia; high ALP, ALT, and AST; normal or mildly high GGT; low BUN; normal creatinine; variable glucose (hypoglycemia rare); variable cholesterol and albumin; globulins usually normal (may note hyperglobulinemia with underlying inflammatory conditions); hypokalemia (associated with failure to survive); may note severe hypophosphatemia (< 2 mg/dL) during initial 72 hr of hospitalization (associated with hemolytic anemia) • Urinalysis—lipiduria common

OTHER LABORATORY TESTS
• Prolonged coagulation times—PT, APTT, and ACT; 50% of patients • Fibrinogen—usually normal • Hyperammonemia—may occur; ammonium urate crystalluria is extremely rare. • Serum bile acids—increase before bilirubin; determination redundant after jaundice is established

IMAGING

Survey Abdominal Radiography
• Hepatomegaly • May note other features that indicate primary or underlying disease

Abdominal Ultrasonography
• Diffuse hepatic parenchymal hyperechogenicity—reflects abnormal hepatic lipid content; renal tubule lipid vacuolation complicates comparison to kidney; comparison to falciform fat recommended • Cannot differentiate idiopathic from secondary, unless an underlying disease causes overt lesions

DIAGNOSTIC PROCEDURES
• Fine-needle aspirate—liver tissue; confirm hepatocellular vacuolation; > 50% of hepatocytes should contain overt cytosolic vacuoles • Aspiration cytology—based on historical and clinical features, high ALP, normal or slightly high GGT, and diffuse hepatic parenchymal hyperechogenicity; cannot rule out underlying primary hepatic disorders or causal diseases in other organ systems • Biopsy—liver; provides a definitive diagnosis for primary liver disorders • Give vitamin K$_1$ (0.5–1.5 mg/kg IM) at least 12 hr before aspiration or biopsy.

PATHOLOGIC FINDINGS
• Gross—diffuse hepatomegaly with a smooth surface contour; friable, greasy, and yellow golden tissue that may have a reticulated appearance; biopsy specimens float in formalin. • Microscopic—diffuse severe vacuolation of hepatocytes; few and large (macrovesicular) or numerous and small (microvesicular) vacuoles; neutral fat (triglycerides) content of vacuoles confirmed by staining non–paraffin-embedded tissue with oil red O or Sudan black

TREATMENT

APPROPRIATE HEALTH CARE
• Inpatient—supportive care for severe disease; discharge home after stabilization and

institution of a feeding route. • Frequent re-evaluations are imperative. • Outpatient—reduces the influence of stress, which can complicate recovery

NURSING CARE
• Balanced polyionic fluids—initial management; use caution with lactated Ringer (patients may develop impaired lactate metabolism); potassium chloride supplementation provided according to the sliding scale (see Potassium, Hypokalemia). • Dextrose—supplementation contraindicated unless hypoglycemia noted; may augment hepatic triglyceride accumulation • Vomiting, nausea, and gastroparesis—may treat with metoclopramide (0.2–0.5 mg/kg SC q8h 30 min before feeding or as a continuous IV drip at 0.01–0.02 mg/kg/hr, or 1–2 mg/kg/day)

Hypophosphatemia
• Serum phosphate < 2.0 mg/dL • Treat at an initial dose of 0.01–0.03 mmol/kg/hr IV (commercial parenteral phosphate solutions contain 3 mmol/mL phosphate or 93 mg/mL elemental phosphorus); monitor serum phosphate concentration every 3–6 hr; discontinue when concentration reaches > 2 mg/dL. • Too much phosphate—hypocalcemia; soft tissue mineralization • Phosphate infusion—lowers ionized calcium if the calcium-phosphorus product is > 58 mg/dL • Affect on potassium chloride supplementation—use of potassium phosphate may lead to iatrogenic hyperkalemia if this source of potassium is not considered.

ACTIVITY
• Most patients initially limit their own activity. • Mobilization—may augment gastric motility when gastroparesis complicates feeding tube utility

DIET
Nutritional support—cornerstone of recovery

Tube Feeding
• Forced alimentation is usually required; forced oral feeding may lead to food aversion. • Recommended by nasogastric, esophageal, or gastrostomy intubation • Initially place a nasogastric tube; establish a more substantial route later. • May place gastrostomy tube blindly, via endoscopy, or exploratory laparotomy • Best outcomes—when patient is not subjected to exploratory surgery • Offered oral food daily—appraise patient's interest in eating

Food Content
• High-protein, high-calorie food • Calories—gradually increase over 72 hr; attain intake of 60–90 kcal/kg/day • Supplementations—controversial; seem to accelerate recovery in author's experience; not challenged by rigorous, controlled studies; L-carnitine (250 mg/day); taurine (250–500 mg/day); thiamine (50–100 mg/day); water-soluble vitamins (twice normal dose); vitamin E (100–400 IU/day); potassium gluconate (with

hypokalemia); zinc (7–8 mg/day); fish oil (2000 mg/day) • Human stress formula—if used must supplement with protein and arginine • Vitamin K_1—0.5–1.5 mg/kg; may initially require two to three doses at 12-hr intervals; avoid overdosage (induction of erythrocyte oxidant injury).

CLIENT EDUCATION
• Instruct client to perform the tube feeding regimen. • Warn client that the gastrostomy tubes may be retained for 4–6 months. • Inform client that recurrence is unlikely.

SURGICAL CONSIDERATIONS
• Exploratory laparotomy—if indicated, also perform liver biopsy; careful inspection for an underlying disorder, and biopsy of pancreas, stomach, and intestines, as indicated. • Avoid surgical interventions until the patient is stable or has improved.

MEDICATIONS

DRUGS OF CHOICE
• Lactulose (0.5–1 mL/kg PO q8–12h; titrate to achieve two to three soft stools daily); metronidazole (7.5 mg/kg PO q8–12h); and/or neomycin (22 mg/kg PO q12h) • Antibiotics—as needed for concurrent infections

CONTRAINDICATIONS
• Avoid medications that rely on hepatic biotransformation or excretion. • Avoid medications that react at the GABA-benzodiazepine receptor (e.g., barbiturates, diazepam). • Appetite stimulants (e.g., diazepam, oxazepam, and cyproheptadine)—do not provide dependable energy intake; may produce sedation • Ursodeoxycholic acid—no evidence for use in affected cats

PRECAUTIONS N/A

POSSIBLE INTERACTIONS N/A

ALTERNATIVE DRUGS N/A

FOLLOW-UP

PATIENT MONITORING
• Body weight and hydration status—judicious adjustments in energy intake and fluid therapy important • Serum bilirubin concentrations—improve after 5–7 days of adequate dietary intake and supplement administration • Liver enzyme activity—slow to normalize • Discharge for home care—when vomiting is controlled, gastroparesis resolves, total bilirubin values decline, patient is ambulatory, and tube-feeding apparatus is problem-free • Tube feeding—discontinue only after patient demonstrates the ability and willingness to eat normally for 1 week.

PREVENTION/AVOIDANCE
• Obesity—prevent; weight reduction must not exceed 1.5% loss per week. • Caution owner to observe food intake of obese patients during periods of environmental stress (moving, newly introduced persons or pets, home construction).

POSSIBLE COMPLICATIONS
• Feeding tube malfunction—obstruction of gastrostomy tube relieved by papaya juice; cola soft drink, or pancreatic enzyme digestion of food debris • Peritubal infection • Worsening hepatic encephalopathy after dietary support introduced • Disseminated intravascular coagulation (rare) • Hepatic failure leading to death

EXPECTED COURSE/PROGNOSIS
• Optimal response to tube feeding and nutritional supplements—recovery of strength and vigor within 1 week • Complete recovery—14–21 days; sometimes longer • Therapy described here—80% of patients recover. • Secondary disease—recovery depends on the nature and management of the condition initiating the anorexia. • Rarely recurs

MISCELLANEOUS

ASSOCIATED CONDITIONS
• Primary liver disorders • Pancreatitis • Diabetes mellitus • Neoplasia—hepatic and systemic • Hepatic encephalopathy • Any systemic illness that limits nutritional intake

SYNONYMS
• Fatty liver syndrome • Hepatosteatosis • Feline hepatic vacuolation • Vacuolar hepatopathy • Vacuolar degeneration

SEE ALSO
• Cholangitis/Cholangiohepatitis • Hepatic Encephalopathy

ABBREVIATIONS
• ACT = activated clotting time • APTT = activated partial thromboplastin time • FeLV = feline leukemia virus • FIP = feline infectious peritonitis • GABA = γ-aminobutyric acid • PT = prothrombin time

Suggested Reading
Center SA. Hepatic lipidosis, glucocorticoid hepatopathy, vacuolar hepatopathy, storage disorders, amyloidosis, and iron toxicity. In: Guilford WG, Center SA, Strombeck DR, et al., eds., Strombeck's small animal gastroenterology. 3rd ed. Philadelphia: Saunders, 1996:766–801.
Author Sharon A. Center
Consulting Editor Sharon A. Center

HEPATITIS, CHRONIC ACTIVE

 BASICS

DEFINITION
Chronic ongoing hepatic inflammation resulting in accumulation of inflammatory cells and fibrosis in the liver; a syndrome, with many causes, found in dogs

PATHOPHYSIOLOGY
• Caused by any event that alters normal hepatic architecture or activates cell-mediated immunity in the liver • Infectious agents and toxins—inciting agents • Inflammatory cells (predominantly lymphocytes and plasma cells)—initially accumulate in the periportal area; eventually bridge across hepatic lobules as fibrosis ensues • Released cytokines—cause areas of hepatocyte necrosis; eventually bridge across hepatic lobules as fibrosis ensues • Cirrhosis and hepatic failure—late-stage disease

SYSTEMS AFFECTED
• Hepatobiliary—inflammation; necrosis; cholestasis; fibrosis • Nervous—hepatic encephalopathy • Gastrointestinal—vomiting; diarrhea; anorexia • Urinary—polydipsia; polyuria • Hemic/Lymph/Immune—coagulopathies

Genetics
• Inheritable copper hepatotoxicity—Bedlington terriers; possibly West Highland white terriers; perhaps other breeds (see Copper Hepatopathy) • May play a role—Doberman pinschers; cocker spaniels; Labrador retrievers

Incidence/Prevalence
Relatively uncommon in dogs; extremely rare in cats

Geographic Distribution
N/A

SIGNALMENT
Species
Dogs

Breed Predilections
• Bedlington terriers • Doberman pinschers • Cocker spaniels • Labrador retrievers • Skye terriers • Standard poodles • West Highland white terriers

Mean Age and Range
Mean—6 years (range, 2–10 years)

Predominant Sex
• Many breeds—females may be at risk
• Cocker spaniels—males more common

SIGNS
Historical Findings
• Anorexia • Lethargy • Weight loss • Vomiting • Diarrhea • Polyuria or polydipsia • Ascites • Jaundice

Physical Examination Findings
• Depression or lethargy • Weight loss • Jaundice • Ascites • Hepatic encephalopathy

CAUSES
• Infectious—canine hepatitis virus (adenovirus 1); leptospirosis; canine acidophil cell hepatitis (controversial)
• Immune-mediated
• Toxic—copper storage disease; drugs (e.g., anticonvulsants, diethylcarbamazine-oxibendazole, dimethylnitrosamine)

RISK FACTORS
• Breed
• Age
• Gender
• Drug exposure—anticonvulsants

 DIAGNOSIS

DIFFERENTIAL DIAGNOSIS
• Acute hepatitis—history; biopsy
• Portosystemic shunting (congenital or late onset)—contrast angiography; biopsy
• Hepatic neoplasia—radiographic or ultrasonographic imaging; biopsy
• Other causes of ascites—hypoalbuminemia (gastrointestinal or renal loss); right heart failure; carcinomatosis
• Other causes of portal hypertension—see Hypertension, Portal)
• Other causes of jaundice—EHBDO; hemolysis.

CBC/BIOCHEMISTRY/URINALYSIS
• CBC—nonregenerative anemia; RBC microcytosis with acquired shunting; variable thrombocytopenia; low total protein
• Biochemistry—high liver enzymes (ALT, AST, ASP, GGT); variable total bilirubin, albumin, BUN, glucose, and cholesterol; hepatic failure suggested by low albumin, BUN, glucose, and cholesterol, in the absence of other explanations
• Urinalysis—variable urine concentration; bilirubinuria; ammonium biurate crystalluria with hyperammonemia

OTHER LABORATORY TESTS
• High fasting and postprandial total serum bile acids
• Ammonia intolerance
• Prolonged coagulation times—PT, APTT, ACT, and PIVKA; sometimes high fibrin degradation products

IMAGING
• Abdominal radiography—microhepatia in late-stage disease; image obscured by ascites
• Abdominal ultrasonography—normal to small liver; hyperechoic parenchyma; nodules and lumpy margin (cirrhosis); rule out EHBDO

DIAGNOSTIC PROCEDURES
• Liver biopsy—definitive diagnosis and prognosis
• Samples—obtained via laparotomy, laparoscopy, ultrasound guided-needle; submitted for biopsy, culture and sensitivity, and cytology

PATHOLOGIC FINDINGS
• Gross—microhepatia; fine or coarse nodules; visible extrahepatic portosystemic shunting; normal biliary tree
• Microscopic—accumulation of inflammatory cells in periportal regions (lymphocytes, plasma cells, neutrophils); piecemeal and/or bridging necrosis; erosion of limiting plate; with cirrhosis periportal fibrosis, bile duct hyperplasia, and nodular regeneration
• Special stains—consider copper, iron, and leptospires; save a sample saved for quantitative copper analysis if copper stains are positive; increased iron likely reflects inflammation and may be noxious.

 TREATMENT

APPROPRIATE HEALTH CARE
• Inpatient—most affected dogs for diagnostics and initiation of medical management
• Outpatient—once stable and accepting medications

NURSING CARE
• Fluid therapy—Ringer solution supplemented with potassium and dextrose (if needed); ideal for initial management in patients without ascites; 0.45% saline plus 2.5% dextrose or another sodium-restricted polyionic fluid combined with dextrose recommended with ascites
• Potassium chloride—judicious use avoids hypokalemia; supplementation according to the conventional sliding scale; 20 mEq/L fluid for maintenance
• Paracentesis—for ascites; therapeutic (large-volume) used initially only with respiratory distress owing to ventilatory compromise or patient discomfort owing to tense abdominal distention; perform with strict attention to aseptic procedure.

ACTIVITY
Moderate restriction—initial management; may promote hepatic regeneration, euglycemia, and ascites mobilization

DIET
• Calories—adequate intake essential
• Nitrogen—maintenance of positive balance
• Protein—restrict with hepatic encephalopathy; avoid meat, fish, and egg proteins; preferentially use vegetable (soy, wheat germ) and/or dairy proteins.

• Small frequent meals—3–5 per day; optimize nutritional benefit; avoid hypoglycemia
• Sodium—restriction is essential (fluids and food) with ascites.

CLIENT EDUCATION
• Warn client that medication is required for life.
• Inform client that many dogs may be managed for years, but few are cured.
• Warn client that although some patients achieve full remission, the disease recrudesces without chronic medication

SURGICAL CONSIDERATIONS
N/A

 MEDICATIONS

DRUGS OF CHOICE
• Diuretics—combination furosemide (1–2 mg/kg IV, SC, PO q12h) and spironolactone (1–2 mg/kg PO q12h) to carefully mobilize ascites
• Vitamins—water-soluble at twice the normal dosage; with abnormal coagulation tests, vitamin K_1 (0.5–1.5 mg/kg SC or PO; two to three doses at 12-hr intervals; then every 7–21 days, depending on response of PIVKA, PT, or APTT)
• Lactulose, metronidazole, and possibly neomycin—for hepatic encephalopathy; modify diet (see Hepatic Encephalopathy)
• Antioxidants—vitamin E (10–100 IU/kg PO q24h); S-adenosylmethionine (20 mg/kg PO divided q12h)
• Zinc acetate—elemental zinc 25–100 mg PO per day (20–30-kg dog); adjust dosage to maintain plasma zinc concentrations of 200–400 mg/dL (see Copper Hepatopathy).
• Copper chelation—when copper concentration is > 3000 ppm dry liver, administer D-penicillamine, followed by chronic zinc acetate (see Copper Hepatopathy).

Immunomodulation
• Prednisone—for immune-mediated disease; 1–2 mg/kg PO q12h
• Azathioprine—adjunctive therapy for immune-mediated disease; 0.5–1.0 mg/kg PO q24h for 1 week; then every other day
• After 4–6 weeks of therapy, titrate to lowest effective dose—depending on biochemical evidence of response (e.g., declining total bilirubin and liver enzyme levels and rarely normal serum bile acids)
• These drugs cannot be discontinued.
• Glucocorticoid with mineralocorticoid effects—avoid with ascites; worsen sodium and water retention; use dexamethasone at an appropriate dose reduction (give every 3 days).
• Ursodeoxycholic acid (Actigall)—immunomodulatory, antifibrotic,

hepatoprotectant, and choleretic effects; 10–15 mg/kg PO q24h or divided q12h

CONTRAINDICATIONS
• Avoid drugs that are primarily metabolized or eliminated by the liver and drugs that alter liver blood flow or metabolism.
• Avoid choleretic agents (e.g., ursodeoxycholic acid or dehydrocholic acid) with EHBDO.

PRECAUTIONS
• Corticosteroids—may precipitate hepatic encephalopathy, gastrointestinal bleeding, and ascites
• Azathioprine—may suppress bone marrow, cause gastrointestinal toxicity, and pancreatitis
• Furosemide—may promote electrolyte disturbances, dehydration, and hepatic encephalopathy
• Zinc—overdose may cause hemolytic anemia.

POSSIBLE INTERACTIONS
Important to avoid drugs that impair cytochrome P450 microsomal enzymes—cimetidine; fluoroquinolones; quinidine; chloramphenicol

ALTERNATIVE DRUGS
Colchicine—0.03 mg/kg/day PO; used occasionally to manage hepatic fibrosis in dogs (anecdotal clinical reports)

 FOLLOW-UP

PATIENT MONITORING
• Serum biochemistry—every 1–2 weeks initially in seriously ill dogs to assess biochemical improvement or deterioration • Serum electrolytes—every 2–4 weeks (more often in patients on diuretics) until ascites mobilized and electrolyte balance evident • CBC—monthly for 6 months (patients on azathioprine); then four times a year • Serum zinc concentration—avoid hemolytic crisis (patients on zinc acetate) • Serum biochemistry and total bile acid values—every 6–8 weeks (stable or improving patients) • Liver biopsies—ideally, at 6 months and 1 year after initiating treatment

PREVENTION/AVOIDANCE
Susceptible breeds—biochemical analyses every 6 months; early detection; initiate therapy in presymptomatic stages

POSSIBLE COMPLICATIONS
• Sepsis secondary to immunosuppression
• Worsening hepatic encephalopathy • Disseminated intravascular coagulation • Gastrointestinal ulceration • Hepatic failure and death

EXPECTED COURSE AND PROGNOSIS
• Underlying cause can be corrected (e.g., remove toxic drugs, chelate copper)—fair

prognosis • Involved immune-mediated disease—survival is quite variable (several months to years after diagnosis) • Ascites and cirrhosis noted at diagnosis—survival usually short; some patients have lived several years.

 MISCELLANEOUS

ASSOCIATED CONDITIONS
N/A

AGE-RELATED FACTORS
N/A

ZOONOTIC POTENTIAL
Suspected leptospirosis—inform client of possible exposure; inspect titers from other household pets.

PREGNANCY
N/A

SYNONYMS
• Doberman hepatitis • Cocker spaniel hepatitis

SEE ALSO
• Cirrhosis/Fibrosis of the Liver • Copper Hepatopathy • Hepatic Encephalopathy • Hypertension, Portal

ABBREVIATIONS
• ACT = activated clotting time • ALP = alkaline phosphatase • ALT = alanine aminotransferase • APTT = activated partial thromboplastin time • AST = aspartate aminotransferase • EHBDO = extrahepatic bile duct obstruction • GGT = gamma-glutamyltransferase • PIVKA = proteins invoked by vitamin K absence or antagonism • PT = prothrombin time

Suggested Reading
Center SA. Chronic liver disease. In: Guilford WG, Center SA, Strombeck DR, et al., eds. Strombeck's small animal gastroenterology. 3rd ed. Philadelphia: Saunders, 1996:705–765.
Dill-Macky E. Chronic hepatitis in dogs. Vet Clin North Am Small Anim Pract 1995;25:387–398.
Franklin JE, Saunders GK. Chronic active hepatitis in Doberman pinschers. Compend Contin Educ Pract Vet 1988;10:1247–1254.
Leveille-Webster CR, Center SA. Chronic hepatitis: therapeutic considerations. In: Bonagura JD, ed. Kirk's current veterinary therapy XII. Philadelphia: Saunders, 1995:749–756.
Sevelius E. Diagnosis and prognosis of chronic hepatitis and cirrhosis in dogs. J Small Anim Pract 1995;36:521–528.
Author Robert M. Hardy
Consulting Editor Sharon A. Center

HEPATITIS, GRANULOMATOUS

BASICS

OVERVIEW
• Occurs secondary to infection by specific bacterial, viral, parasitic, protozoal, or fungal organism, resulting in granuloma formation or mononuclear phagocyte infiltration and inflammation of the liver • May be localized to the liver or may be part of a multisystemic disease, which may mask the underlying hepatic disease • Rarely reflects an immuno-regulatory disorder (immune-mediated disease) or reticuloendothelial neoplasia

SIGNALMENT
• Dogs and cats • No breed, sex, or age pre-dilection • No known genetic basis • Suspicion that immunoregulatory or reticuloendothelial neoplasia causing granulomatous hepatitis may be more common in golden retrievers

SIGNS
General Comments
Depend on cause
Historical Findings
• Anorexia • Lethargy • Weight loss • Vomiting • Diarrhea • Polyuria or polydipsia
Physical Examination Findings
• Severe hepatomegaly • Abdominal pain • Jaundice • Ascites • Fever • Tachypnea

CAUSES & RISK FACTORS
• Systemic fungal infection—most common; histoplasmosis; blastomycosis; coccidioido-mycosis • Bacterial infection—brucellosis; mycobacterial disease • Parasitism—visceral larval migrans; liver flukes; dirofilariasis • Viral—FIP • Protozoal disease—toxo-plasmosis • Miscellaneous—intestinal lymph-angiectasia; neoplasia; immune-mediated disorders; idiopathic disease

DIAGNOSIS

DIFFERENTIAL DIAGNOSIS
Degree of suspicion needed to make the diagnosis, because of the disease's multisystemic nature

CBC/BIOCHEMISTRY/URINALYSIS
• CBC—inflammatory or stress leukogram; nonregenerative anemia (chronic inflam-mation) • Biochemistry—high liver enzymes; hyperbilirubinemia; hypoglycemia; hypo-albuminemia; low BUN; high or low total serum proteins; hypergammaglobulinemia; may note electrolyte abnormalities with fluid and acid–base disturbances • Urinalysis- may be normal; may note nonspecific abnormalities, proteinuria, RBC, WBC, cellular casts, other casts, and bilirubinuria

OTHER LABORATORY TESTS
• High serum bile acid concentrations • Co-agulation assays—normal, except with end-stage liver failure • Serologic tests—high fungal titer (fungal disease); must evaluate with caution and procure convalescent titers; increased IgM titers to toxoplasmosis support active infection • Antinuclear antibody titer—positive with SLE

IMAGING
• Abdominal radiography—hepatomegaly; abdominal mass; loss of detail owing to ascites • Abdominal ultrasonography—assess liver size and parenchymal distribution of disease (diffuse vs. focal); define mass lesions in liver, other viscera, and mesenteric lymphadenopathy

DIAGNOSTIC PROCEDURES
• Abdominocentesis—bacterial culture and sensitivity tests; cytology may be useful. • Liver biopsy—definitive diagnosis • Blood, liver aspirates, and liver biopsy—fungal stain; gram stain; culture and sensitivity

PATHOLOGIC FINDINGS
• Gross—hepatomegaly; normal appearance; firm texture; blunted margins; finely irregular surface • Microscopic—pyogranulomatous reaction with no consistent orientation; may observe Kupffer cell hemophagocytic activity (immune-mediated hemolytic anemia); lesions depend on inciting cause

TREATMENT
• Inpatient vs. outpatient—dictated by severity of clinical signs • Fluid therapy—with balanced polyionic solution (e.g., lactated Ringer solution) for dehydration; may require dextrose (2.5%–5%) and potassium • Nutritional support (enteral or parenteral)—may be required if patient is unwilling or unable to eat; positive nitrogen balance essential; do not use a protein-restricted diet without evidence of hepatic encephalopathy • Inform client that the causes of the syndrome are often difficult to treat (e.g., systemic blastomycosis and FIP).

MEDICATIONS

DRUGS
• Depend on the initiating cause; see specific chapters • Idiopathic disease (no underlying cause or possibly markers of autoimmunity)—glucocorticoids combined with azathioprine proven successful; risky if undetected infectious condition exists • Vomiting—antiemetics (e.g., metoclopramide, 0.2–0.5 mg/kg PO or SC q6–8h) • Gastrointestinal bleeding—H_2-receptor antagonists (e.g., famotidine 0.2 mg/kg PO q24h or IV, SC q12h)

CONTRAINDICATIONS/POSSIBLE INTERACTIONS
• Important to consider possible drug interactions once a definitive diagnosis is made, because of the broad spectrum of possible causes. • May need to adjust dosages of medications that require hepatic activation, biotransformation, or elimination • Glucocorticoids and azathioprine—may worsen clinical signs when an underlying infectious agent exists

 ## FOLLOW-UP

PATIENT MONITORING
• Routine monitoring of fluids, acid–base balance, and general response to treatment • Repeat hematologic testing and ultrasound examination—may be useful

POSSIBLE COMPLICATIONS
• Chronic hepatitis • Cirrhosis • Hepatic failure

EXPECTED COURSE AND PROGNOSIS
• Depend on the primary cause • Prognosis is usually guarded at best, owing to the multisystemic nature of the syndrome.

 ## MISCELLANEOUS

ZOONOTIC POTENTIAL
• Brucellosis—main causal agent of concern. • Blastomycosis and coccidioidomycosis—not contagious; may be contracted when humans and pets share common environments

PREGNANCY
No special considerations; fetuses are likely to be affected (aborted or stillborn).

SEE ALSO
• Blastomycosis • Coccidioidomycosis • Feline Infectious Peritonitis (FIP) • Histoplasmosis • Lupus Erythematosus, Systemic (SLE)

ABBREVIATIONS
• FIP = feline infectious peritonitis • SLE = systemic lupus erythematosus • Toxoplasmosis

Suggested Reading
Center SA. Chronic liver disease. In: Guilford WG, Center SA, Strombeck DR, et al., eds. Strombeck's small animal gastroenterology. 3rd ed. Philadelphia: Saunders, 1996:705–765.

Author Robert M. Hardy
Consulting Editor Sharon A. Center

HEPATITIS, INFECTIOUS CANINE

 BASICS

OVERVIEW
• Viral disease of dogs and other Canidae caused by canine adenovirus 1 (CAV-1), which is serologically homogeneous and antigenically distinct from CAV-2, the respiratory virus • Infection—targets parenchymal organs (especially liver), eyes, and endothelium • Oro-nasal exposure—leads to tonsillar localization and viremia within 4–8 days; saliva and feces infectious during initial viremia • Virus—initially localizes in Kupffer cells and endothelium; replicates in Kupffer cells; release and damage of adjacent hepatocytes and massive viremia; with adequate antibody response, cleared from most organs within 10–14 days; persists in the renal tubules where it may be excreted in urine for 6–9 months • Chronic hepatitis—may develop with only a partial neutralizing antibody response • Cytotoxic ocular injury—leads to anterior uveitis and the classic hepatitis blue eye

SIGNALMENT
• Dogs • No breed or sex predilections • Un-vaccinated dogs susceptible • Usually occurs < 1 year of age

SIGNS
• Depend on the immunologic status of the host and degree of initial cytotoxic injury • Peracute—fever (39.4–41.1°C; 103–106°F); CNS signs; vascular collapse; DIC; death within hours • Acute—fever; anorexia; lethargy; vomiting; diarrhea; hepatomegaly; abdominal pain; abdominal effusion (serosanguinous or hemorrhagic); vasculitis (petechia, bruising); lymphadenopathy; active urine sediment; DIC; hepatic encephalopathy; rarely, a nonsuppurative encephalitis • Uncomplicated—lethargy; anorexia; transient fever; tonsillitis; vomiting; diarrhea; lymphadenopathy; hepatomegaly; abdominal pain • Late—20% of patients develop anterior uveitis and corneal edema 4–6 days after infection; usually recover within 21 days; may progress to glaucoma and corneal ulceration

 DIAGNOSIS

DIFFERENTIAL DIAGNOSIS
• Infectious hepatitis—bacterial; fungal; other • Leptospirosis • Granulomatous hepatitis • Toxic hepatopathy • Fulminant infectious disease—parvovirus; canine distemper

CBC/BIOCHEMISTRY/URINALYSIS
• Leukopenia (lymphopenia, neutropenia) during the acute viremic stage, followed by leukocytosis • Reactive lymphocytes and high numbers of nucleated RBCs after the acute viremic stage • Initially high ALT, AST, ALP, and GGT activities; begin to decrease within 14 days • Hypoglycemia and hypoalbuminemia—reflect fulminant hepatic failure, vasculitis, and secondary endotoxemia • Hyponatremia and hypokalemia—from vomiting and diarrhea • Proteinuria—acute glomerular injury • Predisposition to pyelonephritis • Cellular casts—WBC; epithelial • Bilirubinuria

OTHER LABORATORY TESTS
• Bile acids—mild to moderately high • Coagulation tests—during the viremic stage may see thrombocytopenia, prolonged PT, APTT, hypofibrinogenemia, and increased fibrin degradation products (with DIC); may note schistocytes on blood smears • Serologic testing—fourfold increase in IgM and IgG (not routinely performed); ELISA for CAV-1 antibodies recommended, but results may be confused with vaccine-induced antibodies. • Viral isolation—from anterior chamber of the eye, kidney, tonsils, and urine (chronically); difficult from parenchymal organs (especially liver) unless within the first week of infection

IMAGING
• Abdominal radiographs—may observe hepatomegaly or poor abdominal detail owing to ascites • Abdominal ultrasonography—may observe hepatomegaly, hypoechoic hepatic parenchyma (multifocal or diffuse), and abdominal effusion

DIAGNOSTIC PROCEDURES
Liver biopsy

PATHOLOGIC FINDINGS
Gross
• Acute—edema and hemorrhage of lymph nodes; abdominal effusion; surface serosal hemorrhages on viscera and peritoneum; large, dark, and mottled liver common; gallbladder may be thickened and discolored (blue or white); may note a fibrinous exudate on the liver, gallbladder, and other abdominal viscera; large spleen; may see infarcts on kidneys • Chronic—may note small fibrotic or cirrhotic liver

Microscopic
• Acute or peracute—associated with centrolobular to panlobular hepatic necrosis • Mild hepatic necrosis—may see sharply demarcated margins segregating normal from necrotic areas • Neutrophilic and mononuclear infiltrate—associated with resolving lesions • Intranuclear inclusions—found first in Kupffer cells and later in hepatocytes; may be noted in endothelial cells and histiocytes • Other tissues may demonstrate endothelial damage (vasculitis), causing edema and a neutrophilic–mononuclear inflammatory infiltrate.

 TREATMENT

• Usually inpatient • Fluid therapy—balanced polyionic fluids for maintenance and ongoing contemporary fluid support; carefully monitor fluid balance to avoid dehydration and over-hydration; overhydration may lead to pulmonary edema and anasarca owing to vasculitis. • With vasculitis, hypoalbuminemia, and DIC—include plasma or whole blood, colloids, and crystalloids in the intravenous fluid. • With fulminant hepatic failure—avoid lactate-rich fluids • Potassium supplementation—according to the conventionally used sliding scale to avoid hypokalemia. • Maintain euglycemia—frequent feeding of small meals or intravenous dextrose (2.5%) infusions in crystalloids • With DIC—use blood component therapy; use fresh whole blood transfusions to avoid hepatic encephalopathy; may use plasma for colloid support and clotting factors • Schistocytes or other evidence of DIC—consider low-dose heparin (50–75 U/kg). • Monitor patient for acute renal failure; intervene, as appropriate, with fluids, colloids, and mannitol, followed by furosemide combined with a dopamine infusion (see Renal Failure, Acute). • Activity—restricted to permit recovery and avoid virus dissemination to other animals • Diet—oral alimentation possible: feed a highly digestible diet and ensure a positive nitrogen balance; restrict dietary protein only with hepatic encephalopathy; oral alimentation not possible for > 48 hr: offer TPN. • Inform client of the importance of a vaccination program in young dogs; clarify the high efficacy of vaccines. • Warn client of the possibility of chronic liver or renal disease after recovery from acute disease.

MEDICATIONS

DRUGS
• Prophylactic antimicrobials—recommended because of danger of transmural migration of enteric flora and subsequent endotoxemia • Broad-spectrum antimicrobials (combinations)—cover for gut flora (gram-negative bacteria), including anaerobic bacteria; common agents: amoxicillin/ clavulanic acid, ticarcillin, cephalexin, and cefadroxil combined with either amikacin or gentamicin and clindamycin or metronidazole • Metoclopramide infusion—persistent vomiting • With hepatic encephalopathy—appropriate dietary modifications; colonic lavage; metronidazole (reduced dose to 7.5 mg/kg PO BID); lactulose (see Hepatic Encephalopathy)

CONTRAINDICATIONS/POSSIBLE INTERACTIONS
• Use caution when administering drugs that require hepatic metabolism for activity, detoxification, or elimination in patients with hepatic insufficiency. • Avoid diets rich in meat-, fish-, or egg-derived protein with hepatic encephalopathy. • Avoid lactated fluids with fulminant hepatic failure. • Future vaccinations for hepatitis are not indicated.

FOLLOW-UP

PATIENT MONITORING
• Routine monitoring of fluid; acid–base balance; physical assessment; body weight; serial electrolyte assessments • Central venous pressure—avoid jugular catheter with coagulopathy • Evaluate liver enzymes, serum albumin, and total bilirubin—indicators of continued hepatocellular damage, repair, and nitrogen balance • Monitor renal function—BUN; creatinine; urine volume; urine sediment

PREVENTION/AVOIDANCE
• MLV vaccination—6–8 weeks of age; two boosters 3–4 weeks apart until 16 weeks; booster at 1 year; annual vaccinations not proven to be essential and likely not necessary (highly efficacious vaccination) • MLV CAV-1 vaccines—long-lasting immunity with a single dose; viral shedding occurs; < 0.5% of dogs develop blue eye uveitis. • MLV CAV-2 vaccines—effective; do not cause urine shedding or anterior uveitis

POSSIBLE COMPLICATIONS
• Fulminant hepatic failure • Acute renal failure • DIC • Glaucoma • Chronic active hepatitis • Septicemia owing to hepatic failure • Hepatic encephalopathy • Pyelonephritis—increased susceptibility

EXPECTED COURSE AND PROGNOSIS
• Peracute—poor prognosis; death within hours of clinical signs • Acute—guarded to good prognosis • Poor antibody response (titer 1:16–1:50)—may develop chronic hepatitis • Good antibody response (> 1:500 IgG titer)—may undergo a complete recovery within 5–7 days • Recovered patients—may develop chronic liver or renal disease

MISCELLANEOUS

AGE-RELATED FACTORS
• Maternal antibody—may provide protection in some pups for the first 8 weeks of life; depends on antibody concentration in the bitch and its effective passive transfer • Vaccination of pups with high levels of passively acquired maternal antibodies—successful at 14–16 weeks of age

ZOONOTIC POTENTIAL
None

SYNONYMS
• Canine adenovirus 1 • Fulminant hepatic failure

SEE ALSO
• Hepatic Encephalopathy • Hepatic Failure, Acute • Renal Failure, Acute • Disseminated Intravascular Coagulation (DIC)

ABBREVIATIONS
• ALP = alkaline phosphatase
• ALT = alanine aminotransferase
• APTT = activated partial thromboplastin time
• AST = aspartate aminotransferase
• DIC = disseminated intravascular coagulation
• ELISA = enzyme-linked immunoadsorbent assay
• GGT = gamma-glutamyltransferase
• MLV = modified live virus
• PT = prothrombin time

Suggested Reading

Greene CE. Infectious canine hepatitis and canine acidophil cell hepatitis. In: Greene CE, ed. Infectious diseases of the dog and cat. 2nd ed. Philadelphia: Saunders, 1998:22–28.

Author Sharon A. Center
Consulting Editor Sharon A. Center

DISEASES

HEPATITIS, LEPTOSPIROSIS

 BASICS

OVERVIEW

• Bacterial disease caused by pathogenic leptospires • Serovars (dogs)—identified: *L. icterohaemorrhagiae, L. canicola, L. pomona, L. grippotyphosa, L. ballum, L. Bratislava, L. australis, L. tarassovi,* and *L. autumnalis;* most common: *L. grippotyphosa, L. pomona, L. icterohaemorrhagiae,* and *L. canicola*

• *L. canicola*—dogs are maintenance hosts (carriers). • Cats—uncommon and rarely associated with clinical disease; low prevalence of antibodies to leptospira; reports of organism isolation rare; reported antibodies: *L. bataviae, L. canicola, L. grippotyphosa,* and *L. pomona*

• Infection—via oronasal exposure; primarily from water contaminated by urine of infected animals; may note direct, venereal, placental, or indirect (fomites) transmission, including infected meat; may directly invade abraded skin and mucous membranes

• Organisms—can survive for weeks in a warm, moist environment; do not survive freezing

• Leptospiremia—peaks 4–12 days after infection; associated with a fever

• Primary site and clinical signs—depend on host and infecting serovar

• Peracute infection—death may be so rapid that it precludes development of signs of renal or liver disease or a positive antibody titer.

SIGNALMENT

• Dogs, rarely cats • Breed predilection—possibly German shepherds

• Sex—no clear predisposition; intact males may be over-represented.

• Season—more common in late summer and fall

• Age—may note severe disease in both young and adult animals

SIGNS

General Comments

• Dogs—depend on host and infecting serovar; may be acute, subacute, or chronic; subclinical infection common

• Cats—do not develop clinical signs, despite experimental infection and development of leptospiremia and leptospiruria; leptospires have been isolated from patients with clinical disease, but it is unclear if leptospirosis is a causal agent of chronic nephritis.

Historical Findings

• Anorexia
• Lethargy
• Polydipsia and polyuria
• Vomiting
• Weight Loss • Weakness
• Diarrhea
• Hematuria
• Cough
• Labored breathing
• Melena

Physical Examination Findings

• Abdominal pain
• Lethargy
• Oculonasal discharge
• Renomegaly
• Hepatomegaly
• Myalgia • High or low body temperature
• Uveitis
• Jaundice
• Cough
• Dyspnea
• Petechiae
• *L. icterohaemorrhagiae* (dogs)—associated with hepatic necrosis, azotemia, or acute hemorrhagic disease
• *L. canicola* (dogs)—associated with acute interstitial nephritis or a subclinical renal carrier state
• *L. pomona* and *L. grippotyphosa* (dogs)—associated with renal and hepatic injury
• *L. grippotyphosa* (dogs)—associated with chronic active hepatitis

CAUSES & RISK FACTORS

• *L. pomona* and *L. grippotyphosa* (dogs)—the most common serovars in the northeastern U.S.

• Widespread vaccination against *L. icterohaemorrhagiae* and *L. canicola*—may be responsible for the apparent decline in disease attributed to these serovars

• Exposure to wildlife, rodents, livestock, and contaminated stagnant or slow-moving water—important risk factors

 DIAGNOSIS

DIFFERENTIAL DIAGNOSIS

Any acute infectious disease or toxicity that causes anorexia, fever, myalgia, vomiting or diarrhea, acute renal failure, and/or high liver enzymes

CBC/BIOCHEMISTRY/URINALYSIS

• Depend on serovar, host, and severity of disease

• Mild nonregenerative anemia

• Leukocytosis—usually without a left shift

• Stress leukogram—lymphopenia, eosinopenia, and monocytosis

• Leukopenia—peracute disease

• Thrombocytopenia—owing to vasculitis, response to acute systemic infection, or DIC

• High BUN, creatinine, and phosphorus

• High liver enzymes, total bilirubin, and creatinine kinase • Electrolyte and acid–base abnormalities—may occur in association with metabolic acidosis with vomiting, diarrhea, or renal azotemia

• Isosthenuria or hyposthenuria, glucosuria, hematuria, proteinuria, bilirubinuria, granular casts, and pyuria

OTHER LABORATORY TESTS

MAT

• Most common and most definitive test; uses serovar-specific antigens; cross-reactions between serovars occur.

• Magnitude of titer—does not correlate with prognosis or development of carrier state; does not distinguish between classes of antigens; both IgM and IgG can cause agglutination of organisms.

• Peak titer—3–4 weeks postinfection; may remain positive for months or years; a single high, nonvaccinal titer or fourfold increase is diagnostic; serovar eliciting the highest titer usually considered the infecting organism

• Early antibiotic or corticosteroid therapy may inhibit convalescent titer development.

• Titers—negative: early infection or not infected; 1:100: residual infection, early response to infection, or vaccination; 1:100–300: significant for unvaccinated patient; > 1:300: suggests active infection for nonvaccinal serovar; > 1:1000: diagnostic unless measured within 2–3 months of vaccination and is against vaccinal serovar (*L. icterohaemorrhagiae* or *L. canicola*)

ELISA

• Greater sensitivity than MAT
• Paired IgM and IgG titers best
• Acute disease—may note a high antileptopiral IgM titer with a low or negative IgG titer
• IgG—may not detect until 2 weeks after infection; may persist for months to years
• Vaccinated dogs or dogs with previous infection—may note high IgG titers but low IgM titers

Detection of Organisms

• Bacterial culture—leptospires are aerobic, fastidious, slow-growing, and susceptible to environmental conditions; use blood (acute stages only), urine (4–10 days after onset of clinical illness), kidney, liver, or aqueous humor; best to obtain samples before initiating antibiotic therapy

• Darkfield microscopy—screening tool; rapid; low specificity and sensitivity owing to artifacts; limited use because of the large number of organisms required and their short survival in voided urine

• Fluorescent antibody test—detects leptospires in tissues, blood, or urine sediment; rapid; good sensitivity; may use frozen samples; not serovar-specific; best within 4–10 days of onset of clinical illness and before initiation of antibiotic therapy
• Furosemide—a single injection (if clinical condition of the patient permits) may flush leptospires into urine, creating a favorable environment (dilute urine) for organism detection by any method.

Coagulation
• Usually within normal limits
• With DIC—high fibrin degradation products; low fibrinogen; prolonged ACT, PT, and APTT

IMAGING
• Abdominal radiography—hepatomegaly; renomegaly; splenomegaly; reduced abdominal contrast (e.g., may note effusion or ascites)
• Thoracic radiography—may disclose interstitial and alveolar opacities with pulmonary hemorrhage
• Abdominal ultrasonography—may note hepatomegaly with hypoechoic parenchymal regions owing to hepatic necrosis; renomegaly or normal kidney volume; possible dilation of renal pelves; possible hyperechoic or mineralized renal cortices

DIAGNOSTIC PROCEDURES
• Liver and/or renal biopsy—specimen from aspiration, laparoscopy, or laparotomy
• Silver or immunohistochemical stains—visualize organisms; low sensitivity for detecting organisms

PATHOLOGIC FINDINGS
• Depend on infecting serovar
• Gross—discrete yellow to white hemorrhages on renal surfaces; generalized icterus; diffuse petechial hemorrhages in lungs and gastric mucosa
• Microscopic—lymphoplasmacytic and neutrophilic interstitial nephritis; mild to severe hepatic necrosis, which may lead to hepatic fibrosis; may note leptospires in renal or liver tissue (Warthin-Starry stain or fluorescent antibody test); consistent with uremic gastritis and pleuritis

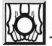 ## TREATMENT

• Supportive and symptomatic, depending on severity
• Peritoneal dialysis—with anuria due to acute renal failure
• Inpatient—fluid and parenteral antimicrobial therapy

• Fluids—balanced polyionic electrolyte solutions (e.g., lactated Ringer solution) with added potassium (10–20 mEq/L) administered intravenously
• Diuretics—osmotic, loop, or low-dose dopamine with oliguria or anuria owing to renal damage
• Diet—adequate energy and protein intake for rapid recovery; nutritional support with vomiting and diarrhea precludes adequate nutrient intake
• Inform client that the infectious agent was acquired in the local environment and recommend screening other pets in the household.
• Warn client of the zoonotic potential.

 ## MEDICATIONS

DRUGS
• Penicillin—effective (14-day course); ampicillin (10–20 mg/kg IV or 20–40 mg/kg PO q8h); procaine penicillin G (20,000–40,000 IU/kg IM q12h until oral therapy is possible); adjust dosages with azotemia; continue with oral therapy when feasible (amoxicillin-clavulanic acid, amoxicillin, ampicillin).
• Cefotaxime and enrofloxacin—alternatives to penicillin
• Doxycycline—following penicillin; 5 mg/kg PO q12h for 10–14 days; eliminate renal carrier state
• Minocycline and dihydrostreptomycin—alternatives to doxycycline; dihydrostreptomycin contraindicated with renal failure
• Gastroprotectants—famotidine or sucralfate for vomiting or uremia

CONTRAINDICATIONS/POSSIBLE INTERACTIONS
Use all drugs with caution because of reduced renal and hepatic elimination.

 ## FOLLOW-UP

PATIENT MONITORING
• Titers—assess diagnostic accuracy; may not decline for months to years • Renal and hepatic biochemistries—routine monitoring; assess progress and treatment

PREVENTION/AVOIDANCE
• Vaccination—effective only for the serovars that the vaccine contains (*L. canicola* and *L. icterohaemorrhagiae*); short duration of

immunity (6–12 months maximum); may revaccinate show animals, hunting dogs, and animals in high-risk areas more than once a year • Immunity to one serovar does not convey immunity to others. • Environmental control—important for prevention; control rodents; eliminate standing water; isolate all infected animals; elimination of carrier state unrealistic owing to wild animal reservoirs and subclinical infections, which are widespread

POSSIBLE COMPLICATIONS
• Chronic active hepatitis • Chronic renal dysfunction • Shedding

EXPECTED COURSE/PROGNOSIS
• Depend on serovar, severity of disease, and host immunity • Subacute infection treated with appropriate antibiotics—good prognosis for recovery • Acute infection—guarded prognosis

 ## MISCELLANEOUS

ZOONOTIC POTENTIAL
Contaminated urine is highly infectious to humans and animals.

PREGNANCY
• No special considerations • Fetuses are likely to be affected, aborted, or stillborn

ABBREVIATIONS
• ACT = activated coagulation time
• APTT = activated partial thromboplastin time
• DIC = disseminated intravascular coagulation
• ELISA = enzyme-linked immunoadsorbent assay
• MAT = microscopic agglutination test
• PT = prothrombin time

Suggested Reading
Birnbaum N, Barr SC, Center SA, et al. Natural infection with canine leptospirosis in 36 dogs: serological and clinicopathological features. J Small Anim Pract 1998;39.231–236.
Greene CE, Miller MA, Brown CA. Leptospirosis. In: Greene C, ed. Infectious diseases of the dog and cat. 2nd ed. Philadelphia: Saunders, 1998:273–281.
Author Nichole Birnbaum
Consulting Editor Sharon A. Center

DISEASES

HEPATITIS, SUPPURATIVE AND HEPATIC ABSCESS

 BASICS

OVERVIEW
Bacterial infections restricted to the hepato-biliary system—uncommon; consist of multi-focal microabscessation; diffuse cholangitis/cholangiohepatitis, cholecystitis, and chole-dochitis; or discrete unifocal suppurative, necrotic lesions; usually associated with pyogenic organisms

SIGNALMENT
• No breed or sex predilections • Hepatic abscess—most common in old dogs; may develop subsequent to omphalitis in neonates • Suppurative cholangitis or cholangio-hepatitis—most common in young to middle-aged male cats

SIGNS
Historical Findings
• Anorexia • Lethargy • Vomiting • Diarrhea • Trembling • Polyuria or polydipsia • Weight loss.

Physical Examination Findings
• Fever • Abdominal pain • Dehydration • Tachypnea • Hepatomegaly • Bleeding • Ab-dominal distention or fluid wave • Jaundice

CAUSES & RISK FACTORS
• Ascending biliary tract infection • Hema-togenous infection via the portal vein, hepatic artery, or umbilical vein • Penetrating wounds • Complication of hepatic biopsy • Diabetes mellitus • Glucocorticoid administration or hyperadrenocorticism • Immunosuppressive therapy for cancer or immune-mediated disease • Pre-existing disease of the liver, biliary tree, or pancreas—major bile duct occlusion; hepatocellular neoplasia; pancreatitis

 DIAGNOSIS

DIFFERENTIAL DIAGNOSIS
• Infectious or necroinflammatory disease—most patients are febrile. • Hepatic abscess—fever, abdominal pain, and/or hepatomegaly (especially with a risk factor) • Pancreatitis or pancreatic abscess • Hepatobiliary neoplasia • Gastrointestinal obstruction or perforation • Peritonitis or other intra-abdominal abscess

CBC/BIOCHEMISTRY/URINALYSIS
• CBC—neutrophilic leukocytosis with a left shift; toxic changes in WBCs; monocytosis;, thrombocytopenia; nonregenerative anemia • Chemistry—may note high ALP, ALT, and AST; hypoalbuminemia, hyperglobulinemia, inconsistent hyperbilirubinemia, and hypogly-cemia; may note features of endotoxemia owing to infection with gram-negative organisms • Urinalysis—usually normal; bilirubinuria; culture usually negative but may disclose hematogenously dispersed organisms

OTHER LABORATORY TESTS
• Preprandial and postprandial serum bile acid—may be high; depends on the degree of hepatic involvement or cholestasis • Coagu-lation assessments (PT, APTT, fibrinogen, platelet count) and red cell morphology (schistocytes)—may be consistent with DIC

IMAGING
Abdominal Radiography
• Hepatomegaly or hepatic mass effect (abscess) • Loss of abdominal detail (effusion) • Gas within the hepatic parenchyma or biliary tree (gas-producing organism)

Ultrasonography
• Abscess—most noninvasive method of detection (> 0.5 cm); solitary, variably echogenic, cavitated lesions • Dystrophic tissue mineralization or entrapped gas—may have an hyperechoic appearance • Multiple masses—occasionally have mixed echogenicity • Highly echogenic interface in a cavitated mass—may be gas; in combination with an abdominal effusion and highly echogenic perilesional fat supports an abscess • Miliary abscesses—cannot discern from other parenchymal hepatic disorders

DIAGNOSTIC PROCEDURES
Cytology
• Histologic specimens rarely reveal bacteria • Impression smears essential • Samples—abdominocentesis, ultrasound-guided abscess or hepatic parenchymal aspiration; cholecys-tocentesis • Stains—Wright-Giemsa; gram, if bacterial organisms are visualized • Look for bacterial organisms within WBCs and for signs of a more primary disease process

Culture and Sensitivity
• Specimens yielding a suppurative or pyogran-ulomatous reaction—culture for aerobic and anaerobic bacteria • Blood (aerobic and anaerobic cultures)—more likely to be positive in patients with multiple abscesses • Poly-microbial infections—common (40%) • Gram-negative bacteria—common; *E. coli* (most common); *Enterobacter* spp.; *Klebsiella* spp.; *Proteus* spp. • Gram-positive bacteria—*Staphylococcus* spp. • Anaerobic organisms—less common; suspected with polymicrobial population

 TREATMENT

• Inpatient—patients often critically • Intra-venous fluid and antibiotics—aggressive therapy essential • Fluid support—correct dehydration deficits; rectify acid–base and electrolyte disturbances; potassium chloride supplementation as appropriate • Abscess—drain via hepatic lobectomy during laparotomy or under ultrasound guidance; after drainage monitor body temperature and liver enzymes and repeat ultrasonographic assessment (look for generalized or loculated abdominal fluid); repeat drainage if required;

may use an indwelling catheter directly inserted into the area of suppuration for continued extra-corporeal drainage • Bile duct occlusion—biliary decompression essential; must administer antimicrobials intravenously before performing biliary tree manipulations to avoid septicemia

 MEDICATIONS

DRUGS
• Antibiotics—based on culture and sensitivity results; continued for a minimum of 3 months • Initial treatment—first-generation cephalo-sporins (cefazolin, 20 mg/kg IV q8h) combined with either metronidazole (15 mg/kg IV q12h) or clindamycin (10–16 mg/kg SC per day); or penicillins (ampicillin, 20 mg/kg IV q8h) combined with an aminoglycoside (gentamicin, 2–3 mg/kg IV q12–24h) or ehrofloxicin (2.5 mg/kg PO, IM, SC q12h)

CONTRAINDICATIONS/POSSIBLE INTERACTIONS
• Aminoglycosides—do not give until hydration status is normalized. • Metro-nidazole—reduce dose by 50% with severe hepatic dysfunction. • Avoid drugs metabolized or excreted by the liver or those known to be hepatotoxic.

 FOLLOW-UP

PATIENT MONITORING
• Assess vital signs and physical condition • Ultrasound examination—determine abscess reoccurrence

POSSIBLE COMPLICATIONS
• DIC • Septicemia • Fulminant hepatic failure • Septic peritonitis • Endotoxemia

EXPECTED COURSE AND PROGNOSIS
• Favorable prognosis—early detection and aggressive interventional management • Worse prognosis—concurrent diseases; required surgical intervention

 MISCELLANEOUS

ABBREVIATIONS
• APTT = activated partial thromboplastin time
• PT = prothrombin time

Suggested Reading
Center SA. Hepatobiliary infections. In: Greene, CE, ed. Infectious diseases of the dog and cat. 2nd ed. Philadelphia: Saun-ders, 1998:615–625.
Author Cynthia R. L. Webster
Consulting Editor Sharon A. Center

HEPATOCELLULAR ADENOMA (HEPATOMA)

 BASICS

OVERVIEW
• A benign tumor of epithelial origin • More common than primary malignant liver tumors

SIGNALMENT
• Rare in dogs and very rare in cats • Affected dogs commonly > 10 years of age • Breed predispositions unknown

SIGNS
• Usually clinically silent • Rupture may lead to hemoperitoneum, resulting in weakness. • Single or multiple, well-circumscribed liver masses that may be pedunculated • Occasionally, cranial abdominal pain, vomiting, and inappetence

CAUSES & RISK FACTORS
• Unknown • May be associated with chronic inflammation or hepatotoxicity

 DIAGNOSIS

DIFFERENTIAL DIAGNOSIS
• Hepatic adenocarcinoma • Hepatic abscess • Abdominal mass • Splenomegaly • Nodular hyperplasia

CBC/BIOCHEMISTRY/URINALYSIS

CBC
• Usually normal • Anemia—rarely unexplained; regenerative anemia if tumor is bleeding • Leukocytosis with a left shift—tumors with necrotic centers

Biochemistry
• Liver enzymes variable • ALP, ALT, AST—normal or mild to markedly high • Serum total bilirubin values—usually normal

Urinalysis
No significant abnormalities

OTHER LABORATORY TESTS
• Serum bile acids—normal unless tumor strategically impairs hepatic perfusion and bile flow in the porta hepatis • Coagulation—abnormalities consistent with DIC (rare) associated with necrotic tumors and bleeding

IMAGING

Radiography
• May demonstrate a single mass lesion or apparent asymmetry of hepatic silhouette • Rarely, gas in necrotic center of tumor

Abdominal Ultrasonography
• Discrete mass lesion with variable echogenicity, depending on intratumor necrosis, hemorrhage, gas, or cystic cavities • A mixed echogenic pattern—most common

DIAGNOSTIC PROCEDURES
• Hepatic aspiration cytology—use a 23- or 25-gauge 1–1.5-inch needle under ultrasonographic guidance; may find normal hepatocytes or cells with mild atypia, making differentiation from hepatocellular adenocarcinoma impossible • Hepatic biopsy—with needle biopsy, several core biopsies necessary to provide enough tissue for histopathologic characterization, so not recommended (insufficient tissue may impair accurate characterization); often confused with regenerative or hyperplastic nodules; histopathology of resected mass preferred method of diagnosis; wide resection recommended because mass may be hepatocellular carcinoma

PATHOLOGIC FINDINGS

Gross
• Usually well-circumscribed single nodules < 10 cm in diameter • May be yellow brown • Often soft, highly vascular, and friable • Occasionally multiple • Occasionally very large (> 20 cm)

Microscopic
• May be difficult to distinguish from nodular hyperplasia or normal liver tissue; misdiagnosis of hepatocellular carcinoma may occur • Usually well-defined trabecular pattern; not necessarily encapsulated • Compression of adjacent hepatic parenchyma common • Mitotic figures infrequent • Affected liver cells resemble normal hepatocytes but often are larger and have a clear cytosol. • Conspicuous absence of portal tracts • Normal reticulin pattern helps differentiate adenomas from regenerative nodules and hepatocellular carcinoma

 TREATMENT

• Symptomatic care to minimize discomfort • Outpatient—appropriate unless surgical intervention requires postoperative critical care • Bleeding tumor—requires blood transfusion; surgical excision advised • Activity—normal, unless massive liver lobe enlargement causes discomfort or hemorrhage; confine to cage if actively bleeding.

Surgery
• Excision recommended for large single mass lesions • Between 60% and 70% of the liver lobes can be resected if the patient is given appropriate critical care. • Biopsy local lymph nodes and normal liver for histologic evaluation.

 MEDICATIONS

DRUGS
N/A

CONTRAINDICATIONS/POSSIBLE INTERACTIONS
N/A

 FOLLOW-UP

PATIENT MONITORING
• Abdominal palpation—every 3–4 months; evaluate for recurrence (low-yield method of evaluation) • Liver enzymes—sequential evaluation; assess recurrence of mass-associated enzyme liberation • Abdominal ultrasonography—every 3–4 months for the first year; preferred method of reappraisal

POSSIBLE COMPLICATIONS
• Avoid making a definitive diagnosis on the basis of aspiration cytology; solid tissue biopsy best for accurate diagnosis; resection better than needle biopsy for definitive diagnosis • Risk of tumor necrosis and massive abdominal hemorrhage if unresected

EXPECTED COURSE AND PROGNOSIS
Usually good

 MISCELLANEOUS

SYNONYMS
Hepatoma—a confusing term that should be avoided; refers to hepatocellular carcinoma in human medicine although considered synonymous with hepatocellular adenoma in veterinary medicine

SEE ALSO
Hepatocellular Carcinoma (HCCA)

ABBREVIATIONS
• ALP = alkaline phosphatase • ALT = alanine aminotransferase • AST = aspartate aminotransferase • DIC = disseminated intravascular coagulation

Suggested Reading
Guilford WG, Strombeck DR. Hepatic neoplasms. In: Guilford WG, Center SA, Strombeck DR, et al., eds. Strombeck's small animal gastroenterology. 3rd ed. Philadelphia: 1996:847–859.
Morrison WB. Primary cancers and cancer-like lesions of the liver, biliary epithelium, and exocrine pancreas. In: Morrison WB, ed., Cancer in dogs and cats: medical and surgical management. Baltimore: Williams & Wilkins, 1998:559–568.
Authors Wallace B. Morrison
Consulting Editor Wallace B. Morrison

DISEASES

HEPATOCELLULAR CARCINOMA (HCCA)

 BASICS

OVERVIEW
• A malignant tumor of epithelial origin • Less common than benign liver tumors in dogs, but accounts for > 50% of malignant hepatic tumors

SIGNALMENT
• Rare in dogs and very rare in cats • Affected dogs commonly > 10 years of age • No breed predispositions

SIGNS
• Typically absent until disease is advanced • Lethargy • Weakness • Anorexia • Weight loss • Polydipsia • Diarrhea • Vomiting • Hepatomegaly (asymmetric)—consistent; precedes development of overt clinical signs • Abdominal hemorrhage

CAUSES & RISK FACTORS
• Unknown • May be associated with chronic inflammation or hepatotoxicity • Toxins—induce tumor in experimental animals (e.g., aflatoxins, dimethylnitrosamine, CCl_4) and in humans (e.g., chronic hepatitis viruses)

 DIAGNOSIS

DIFFERENTIAL DIAGNOSIS
• Hepatic adenoma • Hepatic abscess • Abdominal mass • Splenomegaly • Nodular hyperplasia • Biliary cystadenoma • Bile duct adenoma/carcinoma • Metastatic carcinoma • Polycystic liver disease—less common form; fibrous stroma hyperplasia with anaplastic duct cells; few cysts • Hepatic lymphosarcoma • Hepatic hemangiosarcoma • Hepatic carcinoids

CBC/BIOCHEMISTRY/URINALYSIS

CBC
• Usually normal • Anemia—rarely unexplained anemia; may develop a regenerative anemia if tumor is a bleeding tumor • Leukocytosis with a left shift—tumors with necrotic centers

Biochemistry
• Liver enzymes variable • ALT, AST, ALP, and GGT—usually very high; suggests a pathologic process more severe than indicated by the clinical signs • Serum total bilirubin values—usually normal • May note hypoalbuminemia, hyperglobulinemia, hypoglycemia, and hypercholesterolemia

OTHER LABORATORY TESTS
• Serum bile acids—normal unless tumor strategically impairs hepatic perfusion and bile flow in the porta hepatis • Coagulation—may see abnormalities consistent with DIC in patients with necrotic tumors and abdominal bleeding

IMAGING

Radiography
• May demonstrate a single mass lesion or apparent asymmetry of hepatic silhouette associated with a single lobe • Caudolateral displacement of stomach owing to marked hepatomegaly • Rarely, gas in necrotic center of tumor • Thoracic—may reveal pulmonary metastases

Abdominal Ultrasonography
• Discrete mass lesion with variable echogenicity, depending on the intratumor necrosis, hemorrhage, gas, or cystic cavities • Mixed echogenic pattern—most common • Target lesions may develop.

DIAGNOSTIC PROCEDURES
• Hepatic aspiration cytology—often reflect dysplasia and overt malignant features; occasionally only necrotic cells; discordant findings between cytology and histopathology; use histologic features to make a definitive diagnosis. • Hepatic biopsy—needle biopsy not recommended

PATHOLOGIC FINDINGS

Gross
• Usually a discrete mass; sometimes multiple nodules or infiltrative tumor into adjacent liver lobes • May be friable • Color varies from almost white to normal liver color • Necrotic core may be obvious • Diffusely infiltrated tumors may not be grossly apparent other than hepatomegaly (of involved lobes).

Microscopic
Varies from well differentiated and closely resembling the cell of origin to severely anaplastic

Hepatocellular Carcinoma (HCCA)

TREATMENT

Outpatient, unless surgical intervention requires postoperative critical care during recuperation or bleeding tumors require blood component or whole blood transfusion

Nutrition
• Consider strategies appropriate for neoplasia—frequent small meals; increased calorie intake; shift balance of energy intake to protein and fat rather than from carbohydrate (if fat assimilation normal) • Supplement with ω-3 fatty acids, water-soluble vitamins (twice normal), and vitamin E • Administer vitamin K_1—with EHBDO

Surgery
• Excision recommended • Between 60% and 70% of the liver lobes can be resected if the patient is given appropriate critical care. • Resect primary or metastatic focal lesions. • Biopsy local lymph nodes and normal-appearing liver.

MEDICATIONS

DRUGS
• Chemotherapy—none generally effective
• Mitoxantrone—one of four treated dogs had a complete remission for 65 days

CONTRAINDICATIONS/POSSIBLE INTERACTIONS
N/A

FOLLOW-UP

PATIENT MONITORING
• Abdominal palpation—every 2–4 months; evaluate recurrence (low-yield method of evaluation) • Abdominal ultrasonography—every 2–4 months for the first year; preferred method of reappraisal monitor liver enzymes

PREVENTION/AVOIDANCE
N/A

POSSIBLE COMPLICATIONS
• Risk of tumor necrosis and massive abdominal hemorrhage if unresected

EXPECTED COURSE AND PROGNOSIS
• Prognosis is variable histologic classification is not prognostic.
• Mean survival with surgical resection (lobectomy or partial hepatectomy)—> 300 days • Metastatic rate—61%; lungs, hepatic lymph nodes, and peritoneum common metastatic sites

MISCELLANEOUS

ASSOCIATED CONDITIONS
• Chronic hepatitis • Cholangiohepatitis • Polycystic liver disease • Chronic toxin ingestion

SEE ALSO
Hepatocellular Adenoma (Hepatoma)

ABBREVIATION
• EHBDO = extrahepatic bile duct obstruction

Suggested Reading
Hammer AS, Sikkema DA. Hepatic neoplasia in the dog and cat. Vet Clin North Am Small Anim Pract 1995;25:419–435.
Authors Wallace B. Morrison
Consulting Editor Wallace B. Morrison

HEPATOPORTAL MICROVASCULAR DYSPLASIA (MVD)

 BASICS

DEFINITION
• An intrahepatic vascular abnormality causing intrahepatic shunting between the portal and systemic circulation
• Clinicopathologic hallmark—increased concentration of TSBA
• Macroscopic portosystemic vascular anomalies—suspected association; coexists with irreversible disease in many small dogs; likely explains failure of TSBA to normalize after ligation

PATHOPHYSIOLOGY
• Vascular defect not precisely known; suspected abnormal microperfusion between intrahepatic portal and hepatic venules
• Hepatic encephalopathy—seen in a small number of dogs (rare)

SYSTEMS AFFECTED
• Nervous—hepatic encephalopathy; seizures; slow recovery from anesthesia
• Gastrointestinal—vomiting; diarrhea
• Behavioral—vague abnormalities
• Renal/Urologic—ammonium biurate urolithiasis

GENETICS
• Inherited in Cairn terriers
• Genetic basis likely in other breeds, especially Yorkshire terriers in which it is seemingly most prevalent
• Inheritance—complex; not recessive; not sex-linked, may be autosomal dominant with variable expression or polygenic with complex expression
• Unaffected parents may produce affected progeny.

INCIDENCE/PREVALENCE
• Estimates not available
• Clinical experience—common in certain small-breed dogs (Yorkshire terriers, Cairn terriers, Maltese terriers)

GEOGRAPHIC DISTRIBUTION
Worldwide

SIGNALMENT

Species
Dogs

Breed Predilections
• Usually small breeds
• Well-described in Cairn terriers
• Commonly affected—Yorkshire terriers; Maltese; Lhasa apsos; bichon frise
• Documented—dachshunds; miniature schnauzers; shih tzus; Pekinese; and miniature poodle breeds

Mean Age and Range
Congenital; patients detected as juveniles (by 4–6 months)

Predominant Sex
N/A

SIGNS

General Comments
• Two groups—asymptomatic (diagnosed in the course of routine screening or a diagnostic workup for an unrelated health problem) and symptomatic (manifest subtle or severe signs related to hepatic encephalopathy, gastro-intestinal problems, and renal/urologic problems)
• Take care to rule out other possible causes; concurrent illness may complicate interpretation of bile acid values

Historical Findings
• Asymptomatic dogs—usually unremarkable history; occasionally delayed anesthetic recovery or drug intolerance
• Symptomatic (no concurrent illness)—nonspecific complaints (anorexia, lethargy, vomiting, and diarrhea) complaints related to a specific body system (abnormal behavior, acute seizure activity, dysuria, or hematuria); may note slow recovery from anesthesia or sedation

Physical Examination Findings
• Usually unremarkable
• Hepatic encephalopathy—diffuse cerebral abnormalities (altered behavior, aggression, stupor), blindness, or seizures (see Hepatic Encephalopathy)

CAUSES
Congenital and likely inheritable disorder

RISK FACTORS
Pure-bred terrier heritage or lineage

 DIAGNOSIS

DIFFERENTIAL DIAGNOSIS
• Portosystemic vascular anomaly—any asymptomatic young dog with increased TSBA values or in any young dog with hepatic encephalopathy
• Symptomatic (> 2 years of age)—acquired portosystemic shunting owing to inflammatory, infiltrative, neoplastic, toxic, or cirrhotic hepatopathies; intrahepatic or extrahepatic cholestatic disease

CBC/BIOCHEMISTRY/URINALYSIS
• CBC—usually normal; no microcytosis or poikilocytosis
• Biochemistry—generally unremarkable; hepatic enzyme activities usually normal; may note increased ALP activity in young patients; mild hypoglobulinemia or hypoalbuminemia noted in approximately 50% of young patients
• Urinalysis—rarely may reveal ammonium biurate crystalluria; urine specific gravity usually normal

OTHER LABORATORY TESTS

TSBA
• Preprandial and postprandial measurement—recommended laboratory screening test; by definition, all affected have increased TSBA.
• Shunting pattern—commonly observed (postprandial concentrations severalfold higher than preprandial); also seen with portosystemic vascular anomaly (see Bile Acids)
• Generally, magnitude of elevation lower than with portosystemic vascular anomaly; occasionally see marked elevations (in the range normally associated with portosystemic vascular anomaly); impossible to distinguish between MVD and portosystemic vascular anomaly on this basis

Clearance Studies
• Affected Cairn terriers—impaired clearance; increased 30-min retention of indocyanine green, an organic anion used to assess liver perfusion and function
• Complements TSBA measurements but does not add additional useful clinical information

IMAGING
• Abdominal radiography—usually normal; microhepatia and renomegaly not noted (occur with portosystemic vascular anomaly)
• Abdominal ultrasonography—cannot identify abnormal shunting vessels; liver size usually normal; experienced ultrasonographer may suspect a hypovascular liver (reduced portal venous arborization); the cross section of the caudal vena cava compared to that of the aorta at the same level (usually 1:1 in normal dogs) is significantly larger in Cairn terriers with MVD or portosystemic vascular anomaly (diagnostic utility of this finding uncertain).
• Mesenteric portography—routine techniques reveal normal findings in affected dogs; rapid film change technique shows blunted terminal portal venules and a prolonged parenchymal blush phase in affected dogs; rule out portosystemic vascular anomaly.

HEPATOPORTAL MICROVASCULAR DYSPLASIA (MVD)

• Colorectal scintigraphy—normal or slightly increased shunt fractions in affected dogs; rule out portosystemic vascular anomaly

DIAGNOSTIC PROCEDURES

• Liver biopsy
• Microscopic examination of liver tissue—required for definitive diagnosis and to rule out other liver disorders that cause increased TSBA
• Needle biopsies—often inadequate
• Wedge or laparoscopically retrieved large-pinch biopsies—reliably diagnostic
• Obtain samples from multiple liver lobes—histologic abnormalities may be subtle and asymmetrically distributed within and between liver lobes.
• Cannot discriminated between MVD and portosystemic vascular anomaly; similar histologic lesions; must consider histologic changes in light of history, clinical and laboratory findings, and results of diagnostic imaging
• Severely affected liver lobes—may identify visible portal venules (absent with portosystemic vascular anomaly)

PATHOLOGIC FINDINGS

Liver—grossly normal; normal size

Microscopic

• Abnormalities restricted to the hepatic vasculature, except occasional multifocal lipogranulomas
• Lesions—nearly identical to those typical of portosystemic vascular anomaly but less pronounced; no hepatic atrophy; apparent apposition of hepatic venules and portal veins without intercalated hepatic parenchyma (unique)
• Characteristics—hepatic arteriolar proliferation in portal triads; juvenile-appearing portal structures; increased number of ill-defined vascular spaces (develop between sinusoids and adjacent arterioles and portal veins)

TREATMENT

APPROPRIATE HEALTH CARE

• Asymptomatic—no specific medical care recommended
• Hepatic encephalopathy and protracted vomiting or diarrhea—hospitalize for supportive care and diagnostic evaluation
• Mild hepatic encephalopathy—controlled with a protein-restricted diet
• With a progressive decline in hepatic function that may ultimately result in hepatic failure—manage like any dog with hepatic failure.

NURSING CARE
N/A

ACTIVITY
N/A

DIET

• Hepatic encephalopathy—low-protein diet; sole therapy for control of signs
• Asymptomatic—no modification

CLIENT EDUCATION

• Counsel breeder that the MVD trait cannot be culled from a kindred.
• Warn breeder that proven nonaffected males and females have produced affected progeny.
• Inform client that the value of the TSBA test to detect disease is to identify susceptible dogs and that test results will not obfuscate future health care issues.

SURGICAL CONSIDERATIONS
N/A

MEDICATIONS

DRUG(S) OF CHOICE
N/A

CONTRAINDICATIONS
N/A

PRECAUTIONS
N/A

POSSIBLE INTERACTIONS
N/A

ALTERNATIVE DRUGS
N/A

FOLLOW-UP

PATIENT MONITORING

• No specific recommendations—long-term prognosis unknown
• Asymptomatic—limited follow-up demonstrated that some patients experience a progressive increase in TSBA.

PREVENTION/AVOIDANCE

• Specific recommendations to eliminate disease from a particular genetic line or breed are not possible—mode of inheritance and long-term prognosis remain unclear.
• Cairn terriers—seems unlikely that simply breeding unaffected dogs will eliminate the condition from a kindred.
• Other breeds—extending observations in Cairn terriers to include all breeds speculative; probable that it will be equally difficult to eliminate the disease

POSSIBLE COMPLICATIONS
N/A

EXPECTED COURSE AND PROGNOSIS

• Most affected dogs remain asymptomatic for life.
• Progressive elevation of TSBA values with age—documented in some asymptomatic patients
• Affected Yorkshire terriers, Maltese, and bichon frises—may develop a progressive hepatopathy characterized by worsening clinical signs, portal hypertension, acquired portosystemic shunting, and ascites
• A few patients developed a hepatopathy concurrent with inflammatory bowel disease that was complicated by portal thromboembolism.

MISCELLANEOUS

ASSOCIATED CONDITIONS

• Breeds most frequently diagnosed with portosystemic vascular anomaly are also most frequently affected with MVD.

AGE-RELATED FACTORS

• TSBA screening of young Cairn terriers—majority of patients diagnosed by 4 months of age
• A few puppies with normal TSBA at 4 months of age had abnormally elevated TSBA by 9 months, suggesting a developmental component.

ZOONOTIC POTENTIAL
N/A

PREGNANCY
N/A

SYNONYMS

• Hepatic microvascular dysplasia
• Microscopic portovascular dysplasia

SEE ALSO

• Hepatic Encephalopathy
• Portosystemic Shunt

ABBREVIATIONS

• ALP = alkaline phosphatase
• TSBA = total serum bile acids

Suggested Reading

Phillips L, Tappe J, Lyman R, et al. Hepatic microvascular dysplasia in dogs. Prog Vet Neurol 1996;7:88–96.
Schermerhorn T, Center SA, Dykes NL, et al. Characterization of hepatoportal microvascular dysplasia in a kindred of Cairn terriers. J Vet Intern Med 1996;10:219–230.
Author Thomas Schermerhorn
Consulting Editor Sharon A. Center

HEPATORENAL SYNDROME

 BASICS

OVERVIEW
• Signifies the development of acute functional renal failure as a consequence of severe liver dysfunction
• A marked reduction in renal blood flow and GFR; no morphologic lesions
• Increased renal vascular resistance reduces cortical perfusion and precedes onset of renal failure.
• Renal function improves if liver disease improves.
• Pathogenesis—controversial; appears to involve complex interrelationships between homeostatic mechanisms and locally acting vasomodulatory factors
• Causal mechanisms—may involve the renin-angiotensin-aldosterone axis, sympathetic nervous system, atrial natriuretic peptide, nitric oxide, endothelin, prostaglandins, and the renal kallikrein-kinin system
• Prevalence—some disagreement; rarely recognized in veterinary patients

SIGNALMENT
Cats and dogs of any age

SIGNS
Urine output—initially high; then precipitously declines, resulting in oliguria

CAUSES & RISK FACTORS
• Acquired hepatic insufficiency
• Jaundice
• Hypoalbuminemia
• Portal hypertension
• Ascites
• Diuretic administration
• Therapeutic abdominocentesis
• Iatrogenic hypovolemia

 DIAGNOSIS

DIFFERENTIAL DIAGNOSIS
• Acute nephrosis, prerenal azotemia, and concurrent chronic renal failure and liver disease—may be difficult to differentiate if pre-existing or if pretreatment laboratory values are not available
• May be associated with the polyuria; characterized by renal azotemia; occasionally seen in dogs with acute liver disease
• Essential diagnostic criteria (humans)—spontaneously acquired acute decline in GFR; low urine sodium concentration (< 10 mEq/L); urine:plasma creatinine ratio > 30:1; urine osmolality greater than plasma osmolality; no other cause of renal failure

CBC/BIOCHEMISTRY/URINALYSIS
• Hypoalbuminemia
• Hyperbilirubinemia
• Creatinine—high; may rise rapidly or increase gradually over several weeks
• Hyposthenuria—more common than isosthenuria

OTHER LABORATORY TESTS
• Depend on nature of the liver disease
• Leptospirosis—must rule out

IMAGING
• Survey abdominal radiography—difficult to interpret because of ascitic effusion
• Arteriography of renal circulation—disclose vasoconstriction in humans
• Ultrasonography—unable to discern changes in renal blood flow; kidney size within normal limits

DIAGNOSTIC PROCEDURES
• Imperative to conduct a diligent search for an underlying cause of the declining GFR
• Ultrasound-guided percutaneous renal biopsy—may be performed at the time of hepatic biopsy
• Biopsy—will not disclose morphologic lesions that can alter the course of therapy

 TREATMENT

• Inpatient—for impaired renal function
• Mainstay (humans)—judiciously limit sodium and water intake
• Fluid and oncotic pressure imbalances—correct with appropriate replacement fluids
• Electrolyte abnormalities and metabolic alkalosis—particularly hypokalemia, hyponatremia, or hypernatremia; correct
• Blood volume—expand with plasma, if possible; may use hetastarch or gelatins if adequate quantities of fresh-frozen plasma are unavailable
• Commercial colloids—may provoke bleeding tendencies
• Limit activity—in an attempt to improve renal perfusion
• Inform client of the grave prognosis and predisposing variables.

Diet
• Maintain positive nitrogen balance and adequate caloric intake.
• Azotemic—restrict protein during therapeutic attempts at diuresis.
• Hepatic encephalopathy—protein-restricted diet; avoid meat, fish, and egg proteins; vegetable (soy, wheat germ) and/or dairy protein preferred
• Small frequent meals (3–5 per day)—optimize nutritional benefit; avoid hypoglycemia

MEDICATIONS

DRUGS
• Underlying hepatic disease—treat with appropriate medications.
• Vasomotor drugs, peritoneovenous shunts, aggressive paracentesis, thromboxane inhibitors, dialysis, and orthotopic liver transplantation—objects of recent attention in human treatment

CONTRAINDICATIONS/ POSSIBLE INTERACTIONS
Avoid aminoglycosides (nephrotoxic), furosemide (promotes dehydration, augments aminoglycoside toxicity), hypotensive agents (e.g., acepromazine), and NSAIDs (cause papillary tubular necrosis).

 FOLLOW-UP

PATIENT MONITORING
• Monitor urine output, total plasma protein, body weight, peripheral blood pressure, plasma osmolality, and oncotic pressure—help guide fluid (crystalloids) and colloid administration
• Determination of central venous pressure—may be hazardous owing to bleeding tendencies and risks of catheter insertion
• Creatinine and BUN—unreliable in patients with severe hepatic insufficiency (cirrhosis, portosystemic shunting)

PREVENTION/AVOIDANCE
• Consider possibility of diagnosis in patients undergoing diuresis and therapeutic abdominocentesis.
• Provide oncotic support and monitor renal function proactively in patients fitting the pathologic profile.
• Diuretic dosages—adjust to avoid hypovolemia and vasopressor stimulation.

POSSIBLE COMPLICATIONS
Expect progressive decline in renal function.

EXPECTED COURSE AND PROGNOSIS
Grave prognosis

 MISCELLANEOUS

ASSOCIATED CONDITIONS
• Severe liver disease
• Ascites
• Diuretic therapy
• Therapeutic abdominocentesis

SEE ALSO
Renal Failure, Acute

ABBREVIATION
GFR = glomerular filtration rate

Suggested Reading

Epstein M. Hepatorenal syndrome: emerging perspectives of pathophysiology and therapy. J Am Soc Nephrol 1994;4:1735–1753.
Author Mark E. Hitt
Consulting Editor Sharon A. Center

HEPATOTOXINS

BASICS

DEFINITION
• Endogenous or exogenous substances that cause dysfunction, clinical or overt pathologic changes in the liver
• Direct—causes predictable injury
• Idiosyncratic—unpredictable

PATHOPHYSIOLOGY
• May cause cytopathic (necrosis, marked hepatocellular injury), cholestatic, or mixed histopathologic patterns of injury
• The liver is targeted by a wide array of substances because of its location and central role in metabolic and detoxification pathways.
• Susceptibility and severity of injury—affected by age, species, nutrition, concurrent drug administration, co-existent disease, hereditary factors, and current or prior exposure to the same or similar compounds

SYSTEMS AFFECTED
• Hepatobiliary—injury depends on factors listed above, toxin concentration, and duration and intermittence of exposure; effects range from high serum enzyme activity and absence of clinical signs to fulminant hepatic failure.
• Nervous—hepatic encephalopathy
• Renal—hepatorenal syndrome (rare)

GENETICS
N/A

INCIDENCE/PREVALENCE
• Not uncommon
• Cats appear to be more susceptible than dogs owing to their lower endogenous detoxification abilities (lower hepatic concentration of glucuronides, lower acetylation, and sulfation).

GEOGRAPHIC DISTRIBUTION
N/A

SIGNALMENT
Species
Dogs and cats

Breed Predilections
• Siamese cats—some kindreds suspected to have higher risk because of lower concentrations of glucuronides
• Dogs at greater risk for certain drug toxicities—Doberman pinschers and Samoyeds for trimethoprim sulfa; Doberman pinschers for oxibendazole; Labrador retrievers for Caprofen

Mean Age and Range
Young (< 16 weeks of age)—immature hepatic drug and toxin metabolism and excretion

Predominant Sex
N/A

SIGNS
General Comments
• Depend on chronic long-term exposure or single acute exposure
• Detailed history—important; include environment, drug, and past medical history

HISTORICAL FINDINGS
• Severe malaise
• Anorexia
• Vomiting
• Diarrhea
• Jaundice

Physical Examination Findings
• Variable fever
• Icterus—may develop later (e.g., 48–96 hr postexposure)
• Ascites—rare; grave sign
• Severe hepatic failure—hepatic encephalopathy or coma
• DIC secondary to hemorrhagic liver necrosis—hemorrhage; petechia; ecchymosis

CAUSES
Most Commonly Reported Drugs
• Caprofen (dogs)
• Diazepam (cats)
• Danocrine (dogs)
• Acetaminophen (dogs)
• Diethylcarbamazine—*Dirofilaria immitis* microfilaria positive (dogs)
• Diethylcarbamazine-oxibendazole (dogs)
• Galactosamine
• Glucocorticoids (dogs)
• Griseofulvin (cats)
• Halothane (dogs)
• Mebendazole (dogs)
• Methimazole (cats)
• Methoxyflurane (dogs)
• Phenytoin (dogs)
• Primidone (dogs)
• Phenobarbital (dogs)
• Tetracycline
• Thiacetarsemide (dogs)
• Trimethoprim-sulfadiazine (dogs)

Chemicals
• Amanita mushrooms
• Aflatoxins or mycotoxins
• Chlorinated compounds
• Dimethylnitrosamine
• Dinitrophenol
• Heavy metals
• Phenols

Endotoxins
• Enteric organisms—*Clostridium perfringens; C. difficile*
• Food poisoning

RISK FACTORS
• Medications influencing hepatic metabolism—phenobarbital; chloramphenicol; halothane; cimetidine
• Primary liver disease

DIAGNOSIS

DIFFERENTIAL DIAGNOSIS
• Must distinguish from other disorders affecting the liver.
• Infectious canine hepatitis
• FIP
• Toxoplasmosis
• Suppurative cholangitis
• DIC
• Rocky Mountain spotted fever
• Acute hemorrhagic necrotizing pancreatitis
• Leptospirosis
• Any drug is a potential idiosyncratic hepatotoxin.

CBC/BIOCHEMISTRY/URINALYSIS
• PCV and total solids—normal or high in acute hepatotoxicoses (shock or dehydration)
• Schistocytes—predict DIC
• Serum ALT and AST—extremely high without trauma; proportionately higher than serum ALP activity; monitor for peak values (often in the thousands) that quickly decline within 7–14 days (many hepatotoxins associated with acute exposure); no prognostic importance to a single high value; markedly high values may reflect myonecrosis
• Creatinine kinase—must determine; high activity associated with myonecrosis
• Hyperbilirubinemia—may be marked
• Albumin, BUN, and glucose—variable
• Loss of hepatic function—variable

OTHER LABORATORY TESTS
• Coagulation profile—PT, APTT, FDP, and platelets; assess DIC
• Nonicteric—serum bile acids to assess hepatic function
• Drug assays—costly; results often delayed

IMAGING
• Radiography—acute toxicity: normal to large liver; chronic injury: small, normal, or large liver
• Ultrasonography—variable echogenicity and hepatic margins (from normal to overtly abnormal)

DIAGNOSTIC PROCEDURES
Needle biopsy (liver)—confirms or supports the diagnosis; assess severity

PATHOLOGIC FINDINGS
• Findings variable
• Marked periportal changes—suggest portal delivery of toxin

TREATMENT

APPROPRIATE HEALTH CARE
Inpatient—critical care setting required

NURSING CARE
• Prevent or correct shock.
• Fluid therapy—maintain hepatic microvascular perfusion and improve oxygen delivery and waste removal; administer 1.5-fold maintenance; pay attention to oncotic pressure and overhydration; administer colloid if albumin < 1.5 g/dL.
• Monitor urine output.
• Hypoglycemia—administer dextrose containing solutions to achieve euglycemia.

ACTIVITY
Quiet and rest

DIET
• Protein—normal, unless overt hepatic encephalopathy noted
• Calories—must be accurately calculated
• Water-soluble vitamins—administered at twofold normal recommendations
• Vitamin K_1—0.5–1.5 mg/kg per day for 3 days; then weekly
• TPN—may be necessary

CLIENT EDUCATION
• Discuss the potential for 3–10 days in intensive care.
• Warn client that fibrosis or cirrhosis may develop if the patient has experienced chronic, recurrent injury.

SURGICAL CONSIDERATIONS
N/A

MEDICATIONS

DRUGS OF CHOICE
• Short-acting glucocorticoids—may give for shock; prednisolone sodium succinate
• Penicillin or ampicillin (intravenous)—for infection derived from transmural migration of enteric flora (aerobic and anaerobic bacteria); with parenteral aminoglycoside or enrofloxacin

• Free-radical scavengers (vitamin E at 10–20 IU/kg per day; vitamin C at 100–1000 mg/day), s-adenosylmethionine (20 mg/kg), or N-acetylcysteine (as for acetaminophen toxicity)—may improve recovery for a variety of toxic injuries
• Choleretic agents—usually not justified except for chronic liver injury; if necessary, ursodeoxycholic acid (10–15 mg/kg q24h PO) recommended

CONTRAINDICATIONS
Avoid or assess risk for drugs known to lead to hepatotoxicosis or that require or inhibit hepatic metabolism.

PRECAUTIONS
• Drugs listed as hepatotoxins—use with caution.
• Catheterizing large vessels—use caution with coagulopathy.

POSSIBLE INTERACTIONS
N/A

ALTERNATIVE DRUGS
N/A

FOLLOW-UP

PATIENT MONITORING
• Prevent hypothermia.
• Blood glucose, electrolytes, and PCV—daily; fluctuations may occur rapidly.
• Serum biochemical analysis—every 48 hr

PREVENTION/AVOIDANCE
Close scrutiny of the environment and future medications

POSSIBLE COMPLICATIONS
• DIC
• Hepatic encephalopathy
• Progressive hepatic failure

EXPECTED COURSE AND PROGNOSIS
• Usually 3–5 days are needed to estimate prognosis.
• Progressive worsening of status, intractable emesis and hematemesis, intolerance to supportive treatments, oliguria, DIC, and hepatic encephalopathy—negative indicators
• Postnecrotic cirrhosis—possible

✓ MISCELLANEOUS

ASSOCIATED CONDITIONS
• Hepatitis
• Fibrosis
• Hepatic encephalopathy
• Hepatic lipidosis in cats
• Icterus

AGE-RELATED FACTORS
• Young—may have greater exposure to and ingestion of toxic substances
• Old—may have diseases requiring drugs that increase risk

ZOONOTIC POTENTIAL
N/A

PREGNANCY
N/A

SEE ALSO
• Cirrhosis/Fibrosis of the Liver
• Hepatic Encephalopathy
• Hepatic Failure, Acute
• Hepatorenal Syndrome
• Poisoning (Intoxication)

ABBREVIATIONS
• ALP = alkaline phosphatase
• ALT = alanine aminotransferase
• APTT = activated partial thromboplastin time
• AST = aspartate aminotransferase
• DIC = disseminated intravascular coagulation
• FDP = fibrin degradation products
• FIP = feline infectious peritonitis
• PCV = packed cell volume
• PT = prothrombin time
• TPN = total parental nutrition

Suggested Reading
Center SA. Acute hepatic injury: hepatic necrosis and fulminant hepatic failure. In: Guilford WG, Center SA, Strombeck DR, et al., eds. Strombeck's small animal gastroenterology. 3rd ed. Philadelphia: Saunders, 1996:654–704.
George CF, George RH. The liver and response to drugs. In: Wright R, ed. Liver and biliary disease. Philadelphia: Saunders, 1985:415–452.
Author Mark E. Hitt
Consulting Editor Sharon A. Center

DISEASES

HEPATOZOONOSIS

 ## BASICS

OVERVIEW
- Systemic infection with the protozoan *Hepatozoon canis*
- May involve bone, liver, spleen, muscles, capillaries of the myocardium, and small intestinal epithelium
- Dogs—more common in the southern and southwestern U.S.
- Cats—uncommon the U.S.; one reported case from Hawaii

SIGNALMENT
- Dogs and rarely cats
- No age, breed, or sex predilections

SIGNS
- Usually subclinical infection
- May be intermittent and recurrent
- Severe clinical disease—fever; inappetence; weight loss; bloody diarrhea; neurologic (hyperesthesia over the paralumbar regions)

CAUSE & RISK FACTORS
Rhipicephalus sanguineus—tick; bite or ingestion

 ## DIAGNOSIS

DIFFERENTIAL DIAGNOSIS
- Neoplasia
- Endocarditis
- Immune-mediated polyarthritis or polymyositis
- Chagas disease
- Leishmaniasis
- Babesiosis
- Ehrlichiosis
- Diskospondylitis

CBC/BIOCHEMISTRY/URINALYSIS
- Neutrophilic leukocytosis, sometimes with a left shift
- Anemia—mild to moderate
- High serum ALP activity

OTHER LABORATORY TESTS
Blood films—identify organisms in circulating neutrophils and monocytes

IMAGING
Radiographs—pelvis, lumbar vertebrae, and long bones; reveal periosteal proliferation

DIAGNOSTIC PROCEDURES
Muscle biopsy

PATHOLOGIC FINDINGS
- Cachexia
- Muscle atrophy
- Enlarged liver and spleen—may contain schizont stages on histopathology
- Periosteal proliferation of bone

 ## TREATMENT
- Inpatient—for severe pain; provide symptomatic relief.
- Pain management—as for any musculoskeletal disease
- General activity level and appetite—depend on pain level
- Not possible to predict responsiveness to drug therapy (except pain management) because data are limited

 ## MEDICATIONS

DRUGS
- Mostly palliative
- Glucocorticoids—may give temporary relief
- NSAIDs
- Primaquine phosphate—0.5 mg/kg SC once
- Diminazene aceturate—3.5 mg/kg IM once
- Imidocarb dipropionate—5 mg/kg SC once
- Imidocarb dipropionate (5 mg/kg SC once every 14 days) combined with tetracycline (22 mg/kg PO q8h for 14 days)
- Clarithromycin—5–10 mg/kg PO q12h for 14–21 days

CONTRAINDICATIONS/POSSIBLE INTERACTIONS
None

 ## FOLLOW-UP

PATIENT MONITORING
- Difficult to monitor organisms in chronically infected dogs
- Best to monitor for improvement

PREVENTION/AVOIDANCE
Control ticks within the household or kennel

POSSIBLE COMPLICATIONS
- Glucocorticoids—may exacerbate clinical disease
- Radiographic changes may never occur.

EXPECTED COURSE AND PROGNOSIS
- Infection often asymptomatic
- Long-term quality of life may not be satisfactory, even with good therapeutic results.

 ## MISCELLANEOUS

ZOONOTIC POTENTIAL
No reported risk to humans

ABBREVIATION
ALP = alkaline phosphatase

Suggested Reading
Craig TM. Hepatozoonosis. In: Greene CE, ed., Infectious diseases of the dog and cat. Philadelphia: Saunders, 1990:786–791.
Author Johnny D. Hoskins
Consulting Editor Stephen C. Barr

BASICS

OVERVIEW
• A systemic, usually fatal disease in young pups caused by CHV • CHV—common in the worldwide dog population but disease is infrequent; remains latent in several tissues after primary infection; latent in the trigeminal nerve ganglia; may be excreted in nasal secretions at unpredictable intervals; recrudescence can be provoked by stress or corticosteroid treatment; isolated from dogs with respiratory illness, but no causal link demonstrated • Litter mortality high; poor regulation of body temperature and immature immune response mechanisms believed responsible for the exceptional susceptibility of pups < 2–3 weeks of age • All organ systems are affected. • Clinical disease rare in dogs older than 3–4 weeks of age • Mature nonpregnant animals usually have inapparent, localized infections in the nasopharynx or external genitalia. • Transplacental infections during the last 3–4 weeks of gestation—fetal deaths, often with mummification; abortions; birth of dead or dying pups • Localized genital infections have been reported in both sexes.

SIGNALMENT
• Only members of the canine family (dogs, coyotes, and wolves) are susceptible. • Death usually occurs between 9 and 14 days after birth; range is from 1 day (prenatal infection) to about 1 month (neonatal infection). • Most commonly reported in purebred dogs, although there is no breed predilection.

SIGNS
• Dyspnea • Serous to mucopurulent nasal discharge • Anorexia • Grayish yellow or green, soft, odorless stool • Persistent, agonizing crying • Encephalitic signs • Severe gasping before death • Petechial hemorrhages on the mucous membranes occasionally seen • The incubation period in neonatal pups 4–6 days • Onset sudden; death occurs 12–36 hr later. • Some pups are found dead without premonitory signs. • Occasionally, pups with mild signs survive but often later develop ataxia, persistent vestibular signs, ataxia, or blindness. • Mature females may have lymphofollicular or hemorrhagic lesions in the vagina. • Conjunctivitis—observed on rare occasions • CHV keratitis—reported but not confirmed

CAUSES & RISK FACTORS
• CHV—typical herpesvirus; only one serotype described; an atypical virus was isolated in Great Britain from dog-pox–like lesions on the genital tract that was associated with male genital lesions, abortions, and stillbirths.

• Young, susceptible females and their newborn pups at greatest risk
• Closed breeding kennels—CHV endemic; infection is less common and most adults are immune; newly introduced susceptible breeding bitches at high risk
• Abortion storms with massive pup losses have occurred when pregnant bitches maintained in private homes were assembled for whelping.

DIAGNOSIS

DIFFERENTIAL DIAGNOSIS
• Bacteria (brucellosis, coliform bacteria, or streptococci), toxoplasmosis, toxic substances—no typical gross lesions of CHV
• MVC (canine parvovirus type 1)—causes enteric or respiratory disease; no characteristic CHV lesions
• Distemper and canine adenovirus type 1 (canine hepatitis)—uncommon; no characteristic CHV renal lesions

CBC/BIOCHEMISTRY/URINALYSIS
Thrombocytopenia may occur.

OTHER LABORATORY TESTS
Serologic testing of little value

IMAGING
N/A

DIAGNOSTIC PROCEDURES
• Frozen tissue sections—immuno-fluorescence or immunoperoxidase staining; reveal viral antigen in most organs, especially in the lesion areas
• Cell cultures—viral isolation readily accomplished from several tissues, especially lung and kidney; refrigerate, do not freeze, samples.

PATHOLOGIC FINDINGS
Gross
• Characteristic lesions—disseminated focal necrosis; hemorrhages in several organs
• Kidneys—diffuse hemorrhagic areas, necrotic foci, and hemorrhagic infarcts pathognomonic
• Lungs, liver, adrenal glands—diffuse foci of hemorrhage and necrosis
• Small intestine variably affected
• Lymph nodes and spleen—generalized enlargement; consistent finding

Histopathologic
• Foci of perivascular necrosis—with or without mild cellular infiltration; kidney, lung, liver, spleen, small intestine, and brain
• Lesions in the CNS of recovered pups—nonsuppurative ganglioneuritis; meningoencephalitis; necrotic changes in the cerebellum and retina; acidophilic intranuclear inclusions may be observed but are not abundant.

• Necrotizing lesions—may be seen in fetal placentas

TREATMENT
• Not recommended
• Antiviral drug therapy—generally unsuccessful
• Immune sera from recovered bitches—beneficial in reducing pup deaths when antiserum is given before onset of illness

MEDICATIONS
DRUG(S) N/A

CONTRADINDICATIONS/POSSIBLE INTERACTIONS N/A

FOLLOW UP
• Normal litters can be expected from bitches that have suffered pup losses or abortions.
• Currently, no vaccine licensed in the U.S.
• Isolate pregnant dams, especially young bitches, when introduced into a kennel; adults commonly shed latent CHV in nasal secretions for 1–2 weeks after encountering newly introduced dogs. • Surviving pups may suffer deafness, blindness, encephalopathy, or renal damage.

MISCELLANEOUS
AGE-RELATED FACTORS
• Dogs of all ages susceptible • Fatal illness occurs only in pups infected during the neonatal period (1–10 days after birth).

ZOONOTIC POTENTIAL
None

PREGNANCY
Infection of dams during last 3 weeks of gestation—fetal infections with death and mummification, or ill pups that die shortly after birth

ABBREVIATIONS
• CHV = canine herpesvirus
• MVC = minute virus of canines

Suggested Reading
Carmichael LE, Greene CE. Canine herpesvirus infection. In: Greene CE, ed. Infectious diseases of the dog and cat. Philadelphia: Saunders, 1998:28–32.
Author Leland Carmichael
Consulting Editor Stephen C. Barr

DISEASES

HIATAL HERNIA

BASICS

OVERVIEW
• Protrusion of abdominal contents into the thoracic cavity through the esophageal hiatus of the diaphragm; can be intermittent or persistent
• Three basic types—(1) sliding (axial or bell): gastroesophageal junction moves cranially to the diaphragm (most common); (2) paraesophageal: gastroesophageal junction remains in the normal position but the gastric fundus moves cranial to the diaphragm (rare); (3) combination of sliding and paraesophageal

SIGNALMENT
• Dogs and cats
• Congenital in most patients (<1 year old), but can be acquired from trauma
• Possible predilection for males
• Chinese shar-pei breed may be over-represented.

SIGNS
• Vomiting
• Regurgitation
• Hypersalivation—ptyalism
• Hematemesis
• Dyspnea

CAUSES & RISK FACTORS
• Congenital
• Traumatic
• May be concurrent gastroesophageal reflux and subsequent esophagitis—depends on the amount of functional intraabdominal esophagus remaining

DIAGNOSIS

DIFFERENTIAL DIAGNOSIS
• Megaesophagus
• Esophageal obstruction
• Gastroesophageal intussusception—characterized by a highly fatal acute onset of severe vomiting, hematemesis, abdominal pain, and dyspnea in young, large-breed dogs with concurrent esophageal disease (usually megaesophagus); German shepherd breed appears to be over represented; rare

CBC/BIOCHEMISTRY/URINALYSIS
Generally within normal limits

OTHER LABORATORY TESTS
N/A

IMAGING

Thoracic Radiography
May show a dilated esophagus, soft tissue density in the caudal thorax dorsal to the vena cava, absence of the right crus of the diaphragm, or an alveolar pattern indicating aspiration pneumonia; because of the dynamic nature, false-negative results are often obtained.

Contrast Esophagram
Evaluates esophageal size and gastric fundus location

Contrast Fluoroscopy
Best way to evaluate gastric motility and intermittent herniation

DIAGNOSTIC PROCEDURES
Esophagoscopy may reveal evidence of inflammation consistent with reflux esophagitis in the distal esophagus.

TREATMENT
• Best initial approach is conservative medical treatment to control esophagitis and clinical signs.
• A low-fat diet and elevated feedings
• Lack of response warrants surgical intervention.
• Untreated animals are predisposed to developing chronic esophagitis with mucosal ulceration, aspiration pneumonia, strictures, and strangulation of abdominal organs.
• Surgical intervention consists of anatomic replacement of herniated organs, reduction in size of the esophageal hiatus, phrenicoesophageal pexy, and a left-sided fundic gastropexy.
• Use of an antireflux surgical procedure (fundoplication) is controversial and is indicated for patients with documented primary incompetence of the lower esophageal sphincter (rare).
• Client education should include the importance of dietary management and the potential for aspiration pneumonia.
• Parenteral fluids and aggressive nursing care are needed if concurrent aspiration pneumonia exists.

MEDICATIONS

DRUGS OF CHOICE

• Histamine H_2-antagonist (e.g., cimetidine 10 mg/kg PO q6–8h or ranitidine 2 mg/kg PO q12h) to reduce gastric acid production and treat gastroesophageal reflux; an alternative antisecretory drug is the proton pump inhibitor, omeprazole (0.7 mg/kg PO q24h).
• Prokinetic agent (e.g., metoclopramide 0.2–0.5 mg/kg PO q8h) to increase lower esophageal sphincter pressure
• Appropriate antibiotics on the basis of culture and sensitivity results as needed to treat concurrent aspiration pneumonia

CONTRAINDICATIONS/POSSIBLE INTERACTIONS

Avoid anticholinergic agents because of their negative effects on gastric motility.

 FOLLOW-UP

• Postoperative megaesophagus has been reported.
• Aspiration pneumonia—common secondary complication
• Prognosis guarded; postsurgical complications include recurrent herniation, gastric dilatation (without volvulus), and gastroesophageal reflux.

 MISCELLANEOUS

Suggested Reading

Ellison G, Lewis D, Phillips L, et al. Esophageal hiatal hernia in small animals: literature review and a modified surgical technique. J Am Anim Hosp Assoc 1987;23:391–399.

Prymak C, Saunders M, Washabau R. Hiatal hernia repair by restoration and stabilization of normal anatomy. Vet Surg 1989;18(5):386–391.

Waldron D, Leib M. Hiatal hernia. In: Bojrab MJ, ed. Disease mechanisms in small animal surgery. 2nd ed. Philadelphia: Lea & Febiger, 1993:210–213.

Author James E. Williams, Jr.
Consulting Editors Brett M. Feder and Mitchell A. Crystal

DISEASES

BASICS

DEFINITION
The malformation and degeneration of the coxofemoral joints

PATHOPHYSIOLOGY
• Developmental defect initiated by a genetic predisposition to subluxation of the immature hip joint
• Poor congruence between the femoral head and acetabulum—creates abnormal forces across the joint; interferes with normal development (leading to irregularly shaped acetabula and femoral heads); overloads the articular cartilage (causing microfractures and DJD)

SYSTEMS AFFECTED
Musculoskeletal

GENETICS
• Complicated, polygenetic transmission
• Expression—determined by an interaction of genetic and environmental factors
• Heritability index—depends on breed

INCIDENCE/PREVALENCE
• One of the most common skeletal diseases encountered clinically in dogs
• Actual incidence—unknown; depends on breed

GEOGRAPHIC DISTRIBUTION
N/A

SIGNALMENT
Species
Dogs

Breed Predilections
• Large breeds—St. Bernards; German shepherds; Labrador retrievers; golden retrievers; rottweilers
• Smaller breeds—may be affected; less likely to demonstrate clinical signs

Mean Age and Range
• Begins in the immature dog
• Clinical signs—may develop after 4 months of age; may develop later with DJD

Predominant Sex
None

SIGNS
General Comments
• Depend on the degree of joint laxity, degree of DJD, and chronicity of the disease
• Early—related to joint laxity
• Later—related to joint degeneration

Historical Findings
• Decreased activity
• Difficulty rising
• Reluctance to run, jump, or climb stairs
• Intermittent or persistent hind limb lameness—often worse after exercise
• Bunny hopping or swaying gait
• Narrow stance in the hind limbs

Physical Examination Findings
• Pain
• Joint laxity (positive Ortolani sign)—characteristic of early disease; may not be seen in chronic cases owing to periarticular fibrosis
• Crepitus
• Decreased range of motion in the hip joints
• Atrophy of thigh muscles
• Hypertrophy of shoulder muscles

CAUSES
• Genetic predisposition for hip laxity
• Rapid weight gain, nutrition level, and pelvic muscle mass—influence expression and progression

RISK FACTORS
N/A

DIAGNOSIS

DIFFERENTIAL DIAGNOSIS
• Degenerative myelopathy
• Lumbosacral instability
• Bilateral stifle disease
• Panosteitis
• Polyarthropathies

CBC/BIOCHEMISTRY/URINALYSIS
N/A

OTHER LABORATORY TESTS
N/A

IMAGING
• Ventrodorsal hip-extended radiographs—commonly used for diagnosis; may need sedation or general anesthesia for accurate positioning
• Early radiographic signs—subluxation of the hip joint with poor congruence between the femoral head and acetabulum; initially normally shaped acetabulum and femoral head; with disease progression, shallow acetabulum and flattened femoral head
• Radiographic evidence of DJD—flattening of the femoral head; shallow acetabulum; periarticular osteophyte production; thickening of the femoral neck; sclerosis of the subchondral bone; periarticular soft tissue fibrosis
• Distraction radiographs—quantify joint laxity; may accentuate the laxity for more accurate diagnosis
• Dorsal acetabular rim view radiographs—evaluate acetabular rim; assess dorsal coverage of the femoral head

DIAGNOSTIC PROCEDURES
N/A

PATHOLOGIC FINDINGS
• Early—normal femoral head and acetabulum; may note joint laxity and excess synovial fluid
• With progression—malformed acetabulum and femoral head; synovitis; articular cartilage degeneration
• Chronic—may note full-thickness cartilage erosion

TREATMENT

APPROPRIATE HEALTH CARE
• May treat with conservative medical therapy or surgery
• Outpatient unless surgery is performed
• Depends on the patient's size, age, and intended function; severity of joint laxity; degree of DJD; clinician's preference; and financial considerations of the owner

NURSING CARE
• Physiotherapy (passive joint motion)—decreases joint stiffness; helps maintain muscle integrity
• Swimming (hydrotherapy)—excellent nonconcussive form of physical therapy; encourages joint and muscle activity without exacerbating joint injury

ACTIVITY
• As tolerated
• Swimming—recommended to maintain joint mobility while minimizing weight-bearing activities

DIET
• Weight control—important; decrease the load applied to the painful joint; minimize weight gain associated with reduced exercise

CLIENT EDUCATION
• Discuss the heritability of the disease.
• Explain that medical therapy is palliative, because the joint instability is not corrected.
• Warn the client that joint degeneration often progresses unless a corrective osteotomy procedure is performed early in the disease.
• Explain that surgical procedures can salvage joint function once severe joint degeneration occurs.

SURGICAL CONSIDERATIONS

Triple Pelvic Osteotomy
• Corrective procedure; designed to re-establish congruity between the femoral head and the acetabulum
• Immature patient (6–12 months of age)
• Rotate acetabulum—improve dorsal coverage of the femoral head; correct the forces acting on the joint; minimize the progression of DJD; may allow development of a more normal joint if performed early (before severe degeneration develops)

Total Hip Replacement
• Indicated to salvage function in mature dogs with severe degenerative disease that is unresponsive to medical therapy
• Pain-free joint function—reported as >90% of cases
• Unilateral joint replacement—provides acceptable function in ~80% of cases
• Complications—luxation; sciatic neuropraxia; infection

Excision Arthroplasty
• Removal of the femoral head and neck to eliminate joint pain
• Primarily a salvage procedure—for significant DJD; when pain cannot be controlled medically; when total hip replacement is cost-prohibitive
• Best results—small, light dogs (< 20 kg); patients with good hip musculature
• A slightly abnormal gait often persists.
• Postoperative muscle atrophy—common, particularly in large dogs

MEDICATIONS

DRUGS OF CHOICE
• Analgesics and anti-inflammatory drugs—minimize joint pain (and thus stiffness and muscle atrophy caused by limited usage); decrease synovitis
• Medical therapy—does not correct biomechanical abnormality; degenerative process likely to progress; often provides only temporary relief of signs

• Agents—aspirin (10–25 mg/kg q8–12h); meclofenamic acid (1.1 mg/kg divided q12h for 1 week, then maintenance); piroxicam (10–20 mg q24h, then taper to maintenance); carprofen (2.2 mg/kg q12h); etodolac (10–15 mg/kg, q24h)

CONTRAINDICATIONS
Avoid corticosteroids—potential side effects; articular cartilage damage associated with long-term use.

PRECAUTIONS
• NSAIDs—gastrointestinal upset may preclude use in some patients.
• Carprofen—reported to cause acute hepatotoxicity in some dogs

POSSIBLE INTERACTIONS
N/A

ALTERNATIVE DRUGS
Polysulfated glycosaminoglycans, glucosamine, and chondroitin sulfate—may have a chondroprotective effect in DJD; not fully evaluated for treatment of hip dysplasia

FOLLOW-UP

PATIENT MONITORING
• Clinical and radiographic monitoring—assess progression
• Medical treatment—clinical deterioration suggests an alternate dosage or medication or surgical intervention.
• Triple pelvic osteotomy—monitored radiographically; assess healing, implant stability, joint congruence, and progression of DJD
• Hip replacement—monitored radiographically; assess implant stability

PREVENTION/AVOIDANCE
• Best prevented by not breeding affected dogs
• Pelvic radiographs—may help identify phenotypically abnormal dogs; may not identify all dogs carrying the disease
• Do not repeat dam–sire breedings that result in affected offspring.
• Special diets designed for rapidly growing large-breed dogs—may decrease the severity

POSSIBLE COMPLICATIONS
N/A

EXPECTED COURSE AND PROGNOSIS
Joint degeneration usually progresses—most patients lead normal lives with proper medical or surgical management.

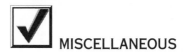

MISCELLANEOUS

ASSOCIATED CONDITIONS
N/A

AGE-RELATED FACTORS
N/A

ZOONOTIC POTENTIAL
N/A

PREGNANCY
Do not breed affected dogs; added weight owing to pregnancy may exacerbate clinical signs.

ABBREVIATION
DJD = degenerative joint disease

Suggested Reading
Manley PA. The hip joint. In: Slatter D, ed. Textbook of small animal surgery. 2nd ed. Philadelphia: Saunders, 1993:1786–1804.
McLaughlin RM, Tomlinson J. Alternative surgical treatments for canine hip dysplasia. Vet Med 1996;91:137–143.
McLaughlin RM, Tomlinson J. Radiographic diagnosis of canine hip dysplasia. Vet Med 1996;91:36–47.
McLaughlin RM, Tomlinson J. Treating canine hip dysplasia with triple pelvic osteotomy. Vet Med 1996;91:126–136.
Rettenmaier JL, Constantinescu GM. Canine hip dysplasia. Compend Contin Educ Pract Vet 1991;13:643–653.
Tomlinson J, McLaughlin RM. Canine hip dysplasia: developmental factors, clinical signs and initial examination steps. Vet Med 1996;91:26–33.
Tomlinson J, McLaughlin RM. Medically managing canine hip dysplasia. Vet Med 1996;91:48–53.
Tomlinson J, McLaughlin RM. Total hip replacement. Vet Med 1996;91:118–124.
Wallace LJ. Canine hip dysplasia: past and present. Semin Vet Med Surg 1987;2:92–106.
Author Ron M. McLaughlin
Consulting Editor Peter D. Schwarz

DISEASES

HISTIOCYTOMA

 BASICS

OVERVIEW
Benign skin tumor arising from Langerhans cells (e.g., histiocytes) of the skin

SIGNALMENT
• Common in dogs but extremely rare in cats
• More than 50% of patients are dogs < 2 years old.
• Boxers, dachshunds, cocker spaniels, Great Danes, and Shetland sheepdogs—may be predisposed
• No breed predilection in cats
• No sex predilection in cats or dogs

SIGNS
• Small, firm, dome- or button-shaped, dermoepithelial mass that may be ulcerated
• Fast growing, nonpainful, usually solitary
• Common sites—head, ear pinna, and limbs
• Occasionally multiple cutaneous nodules or plaques

CAUSES & RISK FACTORS
Unknown

 DIAGNOSIS

DIFFERENTIAL DIAGNOSIS
Histopathologic examination and immuno-histochemical stains—distinguish from focal granulomatous inflammation, transmissible venereal tumor, lymphosarcoma, and mast cell tumor (latter stains positive with tolui-dine blue; histiocytoma does not)

CBC/BIOCHEMISTRY/URINALYSIS
Usually normal

OTHER LABORATORY TESTS
N/A

IMAGING
N/A

OTHER DIAGNOSTIC PROCEDURES
• Cytologic examination—fine-needle aspirate; reveals pleomorphic round cells, 12–24 μm in diameter; variable-sized and -shaped nuclei; variable amounts of pale blue cytoplasm that resemble monocytes
• Mitotic index usually high
• May see substantial lymphocyte, plasma cell, and neutrophil infiltration

PATHOLOGIC FINDINGS
• Histopathologic—characterized by uniform sheets of histiocytes that penetrate the dermis and subcutis; cells may be densely packed in deeper layers of the dermis.
• Collagen fibers and skin adnexa—may be displaced
• Immunophenotyping—confirm cell origin

 TREATMENT

• May spontaneously regress within 3 months
• Surgical excision or cryosurgery—generally curative
• Important to differentiate histiocytoma from malignant tumor if client elects the wait-and-see approach

MEDICATIONS

DRUG(S)
N/A

CONTRAINDICATIONS/POSSIBLE INTERACTIONS
N/A

 FOLLOW-UP

PATIENT MONITORING
Surgical excision—recommended if mass has not spontaneously regressed within 3 months

EXPECTED COURSE AND PROGNOSIS
• Prognosis—excellent with surgical removal
• Spontaneous regression possible within 3 months

 MISCELLANEOUS

Suggested Reading
Thomas RC, Fox LE. Tumors of the skin and subcutis. In: Morrison WB, ed. Cancer in dogs and cats: medical and surgical management. Baltimore: Williams & Wilkins 1998:489–510.

Author Joanne C. Graham
Consulting Editor Wallace B. Morrison

HISTIOCYTOSIS—DOGS

BASICS

OVERVIEW
• Rare disorder resulting from proliferation of cells from the monocyte-macrophage lineage
• Many authors attempt to differentiate systemic from malignant disorders based on cytologic appearance of the histiocytes and tissue distribution.
• Organ systems affected include skin, hemic/lymphatic, nervous, ophthalmic, and respiratory.

SIGNALMENT
Systemic
• Young to middle-aged dogs (mean age at onset, 4 years)
• Usually male
• Usually Bernese mountain dogs

Malignant
• Old male dogs (mean age at onset, 7 years)
• Most commonly reported in Bernese mountain dogs
• Has been documented in cats

SIGNS
Historical Findings
• Lethargy
• Anorexia
• Weight loss
• Respiratory stertor
• Coughing
• Dyspnea
• Dogs with systemic disorder may not have signs of systemic illness.

Physical Examination Findings
Systemic histiocytosis
• Marked predilection for skin and lymph nodes
• Cutaneous masses—multiple; nodular; well-circumscribed; and often ulcerated, crusted, or alopecic; occur commonly on the muzzle, nasal planum, eyelids, flank, and scrotum.
• Moderate to severe peripheral lymphadenomegaly often present

• Ocular manifestations—conjunctivitis, chemosis, scleritis, episcleritis, episcleral nodules, corneal edema, anterior and posterior uveitis, retinal detachment, glaucoma, and exophthalmos
• Abnormal respiratory sounds and/or nasal mucosa infiltration
• Organomegaly occurs with systemic involvement.
Malignant histiocytosis
• Pallor, weakness, dyspnea with abnormal lung sounds, and neurologic signs (e.g., seizures, central disturbances, and posterior paresis) common
• Moderate to severe lymphadenomegaly and hepatosplenomegaly
• Occasionally masses are palpated in the liver and/or spleen.
• Eyes and skin are rarely affected.

CAUSES & RISK FACTORS
• Systemic—nonneoplastic disease
• Malignant—neoplastic disorder
• Both disorders—may represent variable manifestations of a common underlying defect; may represent stages in a range of histiocytic proliferative disorders, although intermediate stages have not been identified.
• Familial disease of Bernese mountain dogs—polygenic mode of inheritance; heritability of 0.298; accounts for up to 25% of all tumors in this breed

DIAGNOSIS

DIFFERENTIAL DIAGNOSIS
• Histiocytic lymphoma—differentiation and definitive diagnosis often require special staining for immunohistochemical markers.
• Lymphomatoid granulomatosis—extensive pulmonary infiltrate of lymphocytes, plasma cells, histiocytes, and atypical lymphoreticular cells; affects young to middle-aged dogs, with respiratory disease as the chief complaint; lack of lymph node, organ, or bone marrow involvement

• Cutaneous histiocytosis—benign histiocytic proliferative disorder in young dogs of any breed; characterized by multiple dermal and subcutaneous nodules or plaques; no ocular involvement; fluctuating clinical course over months to years regardless of treatment
• Periadnexal multinodular granulomatous dermatitis—benign, well-demarcated cutaneous nodules, commonly on the muzzle and may affect the eye; histologically distinct granulomas and variable numbers of inflammatory cells; may be indistinguishable from cutaneous histiocytosis
• Cutaneous histiocytoma—common benign skin tumor of young dogs; solitary, alopecic, frequently ulcerated lesions; may regress without treatment
• Granulomatous diseases—dogs with infectious diseases (e.g., nocardiosis, actinomycosis, and mycotic diseases) may have nodular pulmonary opacities
• Malignant fibrous histiocytoma—locally aggressive soft tissue sarcoma composed of histiocytes and fibroblasts; no breed predilection; distant metastases rare
• Fibrous histiocytoma—lesion involving the eye(s), generally appearing as a raised limbal mass; involvement of the cornea, conjunctiva, nictitans, eyelid, and periocular areas possible
• Hemophagocytic syndrome (histiocytosis)—benign histiocytic proliferation secondary to infectious, neoplastic, or metabolic disease; can affect bone marrow, lymph nodes, liver, and spleen; causes cytopenia of at least two cell lines
• Anaplastic carcinoma or sarcoma—histopathologic findings in dogs with histiocytosis may indicate a poorly differentiated tumor; immunostaining for tissue-specific markers will differentiate

CBC/BIOCHEMISTRY/URINALYSIS
• Mild to severe anemia (regenerative or nonregenerative) and thrombocytopenia common
• Biochemistry results reflect the degree of organ involvement.

OTHER LABORATORY TESTS
Serum ferritin—may be a tumor marker for malignant histiocytosis; one affected dog had very high serum ferritin concentration, suggesting secretion by neoplastic mononuclear phagocytes.

IMAGING
• Thoracic radiographs—well-defined, nodular pulmonary opacities (single or multiple), pleural effusion, lung lobe consolidation, diffuse interstitial infiltrates, mediastinal masses, and sternal and bronchial lymphadenomegaly
• Abdominal radiographs—hepatomegaly, splenomegaly, abdominal effusion

DIAGNOSTIC PROCEDURES
• Biopsy of affected organs and/or lymph nodes
• Cytologic examination of bone marrow aspirate or biopsy may show histiocytic infiltration.
• Immunohistochemistry—diagnosis of histiocytosis may be difficult because results of cytologic/histologic examinations not always definitive; cytochemical staining may be useful in determining the histiocytic origin of the cells.

PATHOLGIC FINDINGS
Gross Findings
• Skin masses
• Lymphadenomegaly
• Ill-defined white foci in the spleen, lung, kidney, testes, liver, pancreas, skeletal muscles of the head
• Splenomegaly or hepatomegaly with possible mass lesions

Histopathologic Findings
Systemic
• Histiocytic infiltrates fail to demonstrate the bizarre cytologic characteristics of the mononuclear cells typical of malignant disorder.
• Histiocytes appear to target small blood vessels.
• Multinucleated giant cells rarely seen

• Immunohistochemistry—special stains for histiocytic markers such as lysozyme or α-1-antitrypsin may be required for a definitive diagnosis.

Malignant
• Cytologic atypia is the hallmark characteristic in affected dogs.
• Histiocytes are large and pleomorphic with foamy cytoplasm.
• The mitotic index is generally high and abnormal mitotic figures may be present.
• Multinucleated giant cells often seen
• Classically, erythrophagocytosis by neoplastic histiocytes is evident.
• Occasionally, leukophagocytosis and thrombophagocytosis are evident.

TREATMENT
Fluid therapy or blood transfusions may be required depending on clinical findings.

MEDICATIONS
DRUGS
• No definitive treatment
• Immunotherapy with a human leukemic T cell line being investigated

Systemic
• Palliative responses to corticosteroids, lasting from 4 to 18 months, reported
• Anecdotal responses to bovine thymic extract reported

Malignant
Responses to corticosteroids, cyclophosphamide, vincristine, and doxorubicin-based protocols reported; optimal choice of drugs is unknown.

CONTRAINDICATIONS/POSSIBLE INTERACTIONS
N/A

FOLLOW-UP
• Effectiveness of treatment is determined by repeated physical examinations, CBC and biochemistry profiles, and diagnostic imaging.
• Patients with systemic disorder have a fluctuating debilitating disease that can be characterized by multiple clinical episodes and asymptomatic periods.
• Prognosis for malignant disorder extremely poor; death usually occurs within a few months of diagnosis.

MISCELLANEOUS
Suggested Reading
Padgett GA, Madewell BR, Keller ET, et al. Inheritance of histiocytosis in Bernese mountain dogs. J Small Anim Pract 1995:36; 93–98.
Author Kenneth M. Rassnick
Consulting Editor Susan M. Cotter

HISTOPLASMOSIS

 BASICS

DEFINITION
A systemic fungal infection cause by *Histoplasma capsulatum*

PATHOPHYSIOLOGY
• Mycelial form grows in bird manure or organically enriched soil.
• Mycelium—produces infectious spores (microconidia); inhaled into the terminal airways
• Spores—germinate in the lungs; develop into yeasts, which are phagocytized by macrophages
• Macrophages—distribute the organisms throughout the body
• Ingested organisms may directly infect the intestinal tract.
• Immune response—determines whether disease develops; affected animals often develop transient, asymptomatic infection.

SYSTEMS AFFECTED
• Cats—respiratory tract main site of infection; bone, bone marrow, liver, spleen, skin, and lymph nodes also affected; intestinal tract, eyes, kidneys, adrenals, and brain less frequently involved
• Dogs—intestinal tract most frequently involved site; liver, lung, spleen, and lymph nodes often involved; bones, bone marrow, kidneys, adrenals, oral cavity, tongue, eyes, and testes less frequently affected

GENETICS
N/A

INCIDENCE/PREVALENCE
Prevalence of clinically relevant histoplasmosis relatively low in cats and dogs; an active practice, even in endemic areas, would see 3–4 cases a year.

GEOGRAPHIC DISTRIBUTION
• Endemic areas—Ohio, Missouri, Mississippi, Tennessee, and St. Lawrence River basins
• Also seen in Texas, the southeastern U.S., and the Great Lakes region

SIGNALMENT
Species
Cats and dogs

Breed Predilection
N/A

Mean Age and Range
• Cats—predominantly young; many < 1 year of age; all ages can be infected.
• Dogs—most often middle-aged; all ages can be infected.

Predominant Sex
N/A

SIGNS
Historical Findings
Cats
• Insidious onset over days to weeks
• Anorexia, weight loss, and dyspnea—most common
• Coughing
• Lameness
• Ocular discharges
• Diarrhea
Dogs
• Weight loss, depression, and diarrhea—most common
• Coughing
• Dyspnea
• Exercise intolerance
• Lymphadenopathy
• Lameness and eye and skin changes—less common

Physical Examination Findings
Cats
• Fever to 40°C (104.0°F)
• Increased respiratory effort and harsh lung sounds
• Mucous membranes pale
• Enlarged lymph nodes
• Lameness and ocular changes may be found.
Dogs
• Thin to emaciated
• Fever to 40°C (104.0°F)
• Hepatosplenomegaly
• Mucous membranes often pale
• Icterus occasionally seen
• Coughing and dyspnea associated with harsh lung sounds

CAUSES
H. capsulatum

RISK FACTORS
• Bird roosts where the soil is enriched with bird droppings are high-risk environments; old chicken coops have been implicated.
• Exposure to airborne dust contaminated with fungal spores coming from sites of fungal growth (especially cats)
• Tissue samples from nearly half of stray dogs and cats from an endemic area were positive for *Histoplasma,* supporting the theory that many people and animals are infected but few develop clinically significant disease.

 DIAGNOSIS

DIFFERENTIAL DIAGNOSIS
Cats
• Dyspnea from fungal pneumonia—differentiate from heart failure, feline asthma, lymphosarcoma, pneumonia, pyothorax, and other fungal pneumonias.
• Lameness—differentiate from trauma.
• Ocular changes—differentiate from lymphosarcoma, toxoplasmosis, and feline infectious peritonitis.

Dogs
• Severe chronic diarrhea and weight loss—consider lymphocytic plasmacytic enteritis, eosinophilic enteritis, lymphosarcoma, chronic parasitism, and pancreatic exocrine insufficiency.
• Diarrhea and anemia—consider severe hookworm infection.
• Hepatosplenomegaly and peripheral lymphadenopathy—consistent with lymphosarcoma
• Respiratory signs—distemper, bacterial pneumonia, and heart disease

CBC/BIOCHEMISTRY/URINALYSIS
• Moderate to severe nonregenerative anemia common
• Leukocyte counts—usually normal; some patients have a leukocytosis; patients with bone marrow involvement may be leukopenic.
• *Histoplasma* organisms—may be found in circulating neutrophils and monocytes
• Severe liver involvement—may see hyperbilirubinemia and high ALT activity
• Dogs with severe intestinal histoplasmosis often have low total protein.

OTHER LABORATORY TESTS
• AGID test—for antibodies; supports diagnosis; positive results indicate active disease; previous infections may produce false-positive results; many animals with active disease are negative on serology.
• Coombs test—may be positive because antibodies to *Histoplasma* may cross-react with RBCs; steroid therapy contraindicated

IMAGING
Thoracic Radiography
• Dogs—diffuse interstitial to nodular pneumonia; enlarged tracheobronchial lymph nodes compressing the tracheal bifurcation; old lung lesions may be calcified, coin-like opacities that suggest metastatic tumors.
• Cats—usually a diffuse interstitial pattern of lung involvement; calcification and tracheobronchial lymphadenopathy uncommon

Abdominal and Bone Radiography
• Dogs—splenic, mesenteric lymph node, and hepatic enlargement
• Cats and less often dogs—bone lesions predominantly osteolytic and usually occur distal to the elbows and stifles

DIAGNOSTIC PROCURES
• Identification of organisms on cytology, histopathology, or culture—definitive diagnosis
• Tissue samples—enlarged lymph nodes, liver, and spleen are good sites; rectal scrapings may be rich in organisms; bone

marrow; lung aspirates (when less-invasive procedures are not diagnostic); tracheal washes inconsistent

PATHOLOGIC FINDINGS

• Multifocal, granulomatous lesions in organs rich in reticuloendothelial cells (e.g., spleen, liver, lymph nodes, lungs, and bone marrow)
• Dogs—gut prime site of involvement; tracheobronchial lymph node enlargement common
• Cats—predominantly respiratory involvement

 TREATMENT

APPROPRIATE HEALTH CARE

• Usually outpatient with oral itraconazole
• Inpatient with intravenous amphotericin B—dogs with severe intestinal disease and malabsorption

NURSING CARE

• Dogs on amphotericin B therapy—keep well hydrated with a balanced electrolyte solution to decrease potential for renal toxicity.
• Emaciated animals with malabsorption—give total parenteral nutrition to reverse wasting until the intestinal disease is resolved enough for adequate food absorption.
• Animals with severe dyspnea—oxygen supplementation

ACTIVITY

Dogs with dyspnea—reduce

DIET

Good-quality, easily absorbed, palatable food required

CLIENT EDUCATION

• Discuss possible areas of exposure in the home environment.
• Inform client that both pets and family members may have been exposed to the same source and that the animal is not a hazard to the family.

SURGICAL CONSIDERATIONS

N/A

 MEDICATIONS

DRUGS OF CHOICE

Itraconazole
• Drug of choice if adequate intestinal function for drug absorption exists.
• Dogs and cats—5mg/kg PO q12h; give with a high-fat meal.
• Duration depends on the clinical response; minimum treatment is 90 days.

Intravenous Amphotericin B
Dogs
• With severe inflammatory bowel disease and malabsorption—use until patient begins to gain weight; then start on itraconazole.
• Patient must be well hydrated before starting treatment; avoid electrolyte solutions that may precipitate the drug.
• BUN—check before each dose; discontinue if level approaches 50 mg/dL and maintain hydration; resume when level < 30 mg/dL
• Usual dose—0.5 mg/kg IV q48h
• Reconstitute in 5% dextrose and dilute for administration
• Normal renal function—dilute in 60–120 mL 5% dextrose and give over 15 min.
• Some renal compromise—dilute in 0.5–1 L 5% dextrose and give over 3–4 hr to reduce renal toxicity.
Cats
• Use cautiously
• Usual dose—0.25 mg/kg IV in 5% dextrose over 3–4 hr
• More sensitive to the drug than are dogs

Fluconazole
• Use for dogs that cannot be given amphotericin B.
• Usual dose (intravenous form)—5 mg/kg IV q12h until intestinal absorption allows oral itraconazole treatment

CONTRAINDICATIONS

Amphotericin B—renal failure precludes use

PRECAUTIONS

• Steroids—use with caution; will allow proliferation of *Histoplasma;* life-threatening respiratory distress justifies use of short-acting corticosteroids, but treatment time with antifungal drugs is likely to be increased.
• Itraconazole and fluconazole—hepatic toxicity; temporarily discontinue if patient becomes anorexic or if serum ALT activity > 300 U/L; restart at half dose after appetite improves.

POSSIBLE INTERACTIONS

Itraconazole—contraindicated with terfenadine and cisapride in humans

ALTERNATIVE DRUGS

None

 FOLLOW-UP

PATIENT MONITORING

• Serum ALT—with itraconazole treatment; check monthly or if the patient becomes anorexic.
• Chest radiographs—with pulmonary involvement; check after 60 days of treatment to assess improvement; repeat at 30-day intervals and stop treatment when infiltrates are clear or remaining lung lesions fail to improve; may be difficult to differentiate

between residual fibrotic lesions and active disease; continue treatment for at least 1 month after all signs of active disease have resolved.

PREVENTION/AVOIDANCE

• Avoid suspected areas of exposure (e.g., bird roosts).
• Recovered dogs are probably immune.

POSSIBLE COMPLICATIONS

Recurrence possible; requires a second course of treatment

EXPECTED COURSE AND PROGNOSIS

• Treatment—duration is usually about 4 months; drugs are expensive, especially for large dogs.
• Prognosis—good for stable patients without severe dyspnea; influenced by severity of lung involvement and debility of patient

 MISCELLANEOUS

ASSOCIATED CONDITIONS

• No apparent predisposing conditions

AGE-RELATED FACTORS

N/A

ZOONOTIC POTENTIAL

• Not spread from animals to people
• Care must be taken to avoid needlesticks when collecting aspirates.
• Infection can occur from cuts when doing necropsies on infected animals.

PREGNANCY

Itraconazole—no teratogenic effects in rats and mice at therapeutic doses; embryotoxicity found at high doses; no dog or cat studies; one dog given the drug halfway through her pregnancy delivered a normal litter.

ABBREVIATIONS

• AGID = agar gel immunodiffusion
• ALT = alanine aminotransferase

Suggested Reading

Clinkenbeard KD, Cowell RL, Tyler RD. Disseminated histoplasmosis in cats: 12 cases. J Am Vet Med Assoc 1987;190:1445–1448.
Hodges RD, Legendre AM, Adams LG, et al. Itraconazole for the treatment of histoplasmosis in cats. J Vet Intern Med 1994;8:409–413.
Wolf AM. Histoplasmosis. In: Greene CE, ed. Infectious diseases of the dog and cat. Philadelphia: Saunders, 1998:378–383.
Author Alfred M. Legendre
Consulting Editor Stephen C. Barr

DISEASES

HOOKWORMS (ANCYLOSTOMIASIS)

BASICS

OVERVIEW
• Nematode parasites of the species *Ancylostoma caninum* in the small intestine of dogs, *A. tubaeforme* of cats, and *A. braziliense* and *Uncinaria stenocephala* in both dogs and cats
• *A. braziliense* is found in southern states; the others are in the temperate zone as well.
• Voracious blood-sucking adults and fourth-stage larvae of *A. caninum* and *A. tubaeforme* cause blood-loss anemia and enteritis; active worms leave bite sites with continuing seepage of blood. • Of special concern is infection in neonates with acute to peracute disease; infections may be acute to chronic compensatory at weaning or chronic noncompensatory in those immunosuppressed or debilitated.
• *Uncinaria* is of little clinical concern.
• *A. braziliense* is the major cause of CLM.
• Coughing may result from larval migration following skin penetration.
• *A. caninum* is transmitted via colostrum to pups; all species are transmitted by ingestion of infective larvae or by skin penetration.

SIGNALMENT
Acute disease in young; chronic disease in mature dogs and cats.

SIGNS
Historical Findings
• Pale mucous membranes
• Dark, tarry stools (melena); diarrhea; constipation
• Loss of condition
• Poor appetite
• Dry cough
• Sudden death

Physical Examination Findings
• Poor condition
• Pale mucous membranes

CAUSES & RISK FACTORS
• Infected bitch or queen
• Contaminated environment
• Concurrent enteric infections
• Other compromising conditions (e.g., pregnancy)

DIAGNOSIS

DIFFERENTIAL DIAGNOSIS
• Toxocariasis—large roundworm infection
• Coccidiosis
• Strongyloidosis
• *Uncinaria* eggs, 70 μm; *A. caninum*, 60 μm

CBC/BIOCHEMISTRY/URINALYSIS
• Eosinophilia
• Anemia—may be microcytic, hypochromic due to chronic iron deficiency

OTHER LABORATORY TESTS
N/A

IMAGING
N/A

DIAGNOSTIC PROCEDURES
• Fecal flotation; fecal egg examination—*A. caninum, A. tubaeforme* at 60 × 40 μm
• Necropsy of sibling pups, kittens that have died following appearance of similar clinical signs

PATHOLOGIC FINDINGS
Eosinophilic enteritis due to larval activity in wall of small intestine

TREATMENT
• Pups in an environment with a history of hookworm infections—routine treat at 2-week intervals to weaning
• Acute, severe cases—inpatients for fluid therapy and blood transfusion (as indicated by severity of anemia and clinical signs)
• Alert owner to potential for sudden death.
• Chronic compensatory cases, including breeding females—deworming program to eliminate intestinal and somatic infections

MEDICATIONS

DRUGS
A/L Anthelmintic Activity
• Fenbendazole—50 mg/kg PO q24h for 3 consecutive days
• Milbemycin oxime—0.5 mg/kg PO q30d

Adulticide Activity
• Pyrantel pamoate—15 mg/kg PO in dogs; 20–30 mg/kg PO in cats
• Praziquantel/pyrantel pamoate/febantel

tablets for dogs; praziquantel/pyrantel pamoate tablets for cats
• Ivermectin—6 μg/kg PO (with pyrantel pamoate)
• Dichlorvos packets/tablets biweekly

Adulticide Activity—Dogs
• A/L dewormer (fenbendazole) during third trimester of pregnancy to kill migrating larvae in somatic tissue and adults
• A/L dewormer on daily or monthly basis for pups and mature dogs
• Treat pup biweekly until weaning if at risk

Adulticide Activity—Cats
• A/L dewormer for queen prior to breeding and after littering
• Adulticide dewormer by 4 weeks for kitten

CONTRAINDICATIONS/POSSIBLE INTERACTIONS
• Do not give organophosphates to heartworm-positive dogs or cats.
• Do not give dichlorvos concurrently with other organophosphates such as insecticides

FOLLOW-UP
• Monitor fecal egg counts posttreatment.
• Hematocrit if infection resulted in blood loss

MISCELLANEOUS

AGE-RELATED FACTORS
Disease more acute in young animals and chronic in adults

ZOONOTIC POTENTIAL
CLM, especially with *A. braziliense;* infective larvae penetrate skin

SYNONYMS
Ancylostomiasis

ABBREVIATIONS
• A/L = adulticide/larvicide
• CLM = cutaneous larva migrans

Suggested Reading
Bowman DD. Hookworm parasites of dogs and cats. Comp Contin Educ Pract Vet 1992;14(5):585–595.
Author Robert M. Corwin
Consulting Editors Brett M. Feder and Mitchell A. Crystal

BASICS

OVERVIEW
• Sympathetic denervation of the eye
• Anatomical pathway very important
Hypothalamus
↓
brainstem/cervical cord
T1-T3 spinal cord segments
and nerve roots
↓
vagosympathetic trunk
↓
cranial cervical ganglion
↓
middle ear
↓
ophthalmic branch (cranial nerve V)
↓
long ciliary nerve
↓
iris dilator muscle
↓
other fibers: smooth muscle in periorbita
upper and third eyelid
• Affects the ophthalmic and nervous systems

SIGNALMENT
• Idiopathic—one study suggests male golden retrievers 4–13 years of age.• Idiopathic—dogs, 50–93%; cats, 45% • Other causes—N/A

SIGNS
• Miosis • Protruding third eyelid • Ptosis (drooping) of upper eyelid • Enophthalmia • See Table 1 • Otitis—possible • Other neurologic abnormalities—possible

CAUSES & RISK FACTORS
See Table 1

DIAGNOSIS

DIFFERENTIAL DIAGNOSIS
Anterior uveitis—IOP abnormal; aqueous flare

CBC/BIOCHEMISTRY/URINANLYSIS
N/A

OTHER LABORATORY TESTS
N/A

IMAGING
• See Table 1 • Spinal radiographs and myelogram—may reveal spinal cord lesion • Thoracic radiographs—may reveal cause of injury to the sympathetic trunk (e.g., trauma and mediastinal tumor) • Skull radiographs—may reveal middle ear problem • CT and MRI—may help identify brainstem lesion, retrobulbar mass, or middle ear problem • Ultrasonography—orbit; may reveal retrobulbar mass

DIAGNOSTIC PROCEDURES
• See Table 1 • CSF tap—investigate brain and spinal cord disease • Electromyography—look for brachial plexus avulsion • Pharmacologic testing—see Anisocoria

TREATMENT
• Treat underlying disease

MEDICATIONS

DRUGS
• Depend on underlying disease • Idiopathic—none

CONTRAINDICATIONS/POSSIBLE INTERACTIONS
N/A

FOLLOW-UP
• Depends on severity of underlying disease
• Idiopathic—may take up to 4 months for a partial or complete recovery

MISCELLANEOUS

ABBREVIATIONS
• CSF = cerebrospinal fluid • FCE = fibrocartilaginous embolism • LMN = lower motor neuron • UMN = upper motor neuron

Suggested Reading
Scagliotti RH. Comparative neuro-opthalmology. In: Gelatt KN, ed. Veterinary opthalmology 3rd ed. Philadelphia: Lippincott Williams & Wilkins; 1999:1307–1400.
Author David Lipsitz
Consulting Editor Paul E. Miller

Table 1.

Summary of Lesions Resulting in Horner Syndrome			
Location	*Causes*	*Associated Neurologic Signs*	*Diagnostic Plan*
brainstem	trauma; neoplasm; infectious; inflammatory	altered mental status; ipsilateral motor defects; ipsilateral cranial nerve deficits	CT or MRI; CSF analysis
cervical spinal cord	trauma; disk; neoplasm; FCE	ipsilateral hemiparesis/paralysis; tetraparesis/paralysis; UMN; thoracic/pelvic limbs	spinal films; CSF analysis; myelogram
T1-T3 spinal cord	trauma; disk; neoplasm; FCE	LMN: thoracic limb(s); UMN: pelvic limb(s)	spinal films; CSF analysis; myelogram
T1-T3 ventral roots	brachial plexus avulsion	ipsilateral brachial plexus injury; ipsilateral loss of panniculus reflex	Neurologic examination; EMG
sympathetic trunk, cranial cervical ganglion	trauma; mediastinal neoplasm; iatrogenic-surgical trauma	unilateral: none; bilateral: laryngeal/pharyngeal dysfunction	chest radiographs
middle ear	trauma; neoplasm; otitis media/interna; nasopharyngeal polyp (cat)	ipsilateral peripheral vestibular disease; ipsilateral facial nerve paralysis	otic examination; bullae radiographs or CT; myringotomy
retrobulbar	trauma; neoplasm; abscess	variable: none or involvement of cranial nerves II, III, IV, VI	CT or MRI; ultrasound orbit

HYDROCEPHALUS

 BASICS

DEFINITION
• Abnormal dilation of the ventricular system from an increased volume of CSF
• May be symmetrical or asymmetrical
• May involve the entire ventricular system or only elements proximal to a site of ventricular system obstruction

PATHOPHYSIOLOGY
• Two types—compensatory and obstructive
• Compensatory—CSF fills the space where the nervous parenchyma was destroyed and/or failed to develop; intracranial pressure normal; ventricular dilation incidental to the primary disease
• Obstructive—CSF accumulates in front of an obstruction along the normal CSF circulatory pattern (noncommunicating) or at its resorption site by the meningeal arachnoid villi (communicating); intracranial pressure high or normal; clinical signs may be noted when intracranial pressure is normal.
• Congenital obstruction—primary obstructive hydrocephalus; most common site is at the level of the mesencephalic aqueduct; prenatal infections (especially parainfluenza virus) may cause aqueductal stenosis with subsequent hydrocephalus; may result in considerable disruption of the architecture of the brain
• Acquired obstruction—secondary obstructive hydrocephalus; caused by tumors, abscesses, and inflammatory diseases (including inflammation resulting from hemorrhage caused by traumatic injuries or other causes of bleeding); sites include the interventricular foramina, mesencephalic aqueduct, or lateral apertures of the fourth ventricle.
• Overproduction of CSF—rare; caused, for example, by a choroid plexus tumor

SYSTEMS AFFECTED
Nervous

GENETICS
Siamese cats—autosomal recessive

INCIDENCE/PREVALENCE
Unknown

GEOGRAPHIC DISTRIBUTION
N/A

SIGNALMENT
Species
Dogs and cats

Breed Predilections
• Congenital—small and brachycephalic dogs: bulldogs, Chihuahuas, Maltese, Pomeranians, toy poodles, Yorkshire terriers, Lhasa apsos, cairn terriers, Boston terriers, pugs, and Pekingese
• Inherited—Siamese cats
• Acquired—any breed of cat or dog

Mean Age and Range
• Congenital—usually becomes apparent at a few weeks up to 1 year of age
• Acquired—any age

Predominant Sex
None

SIGNS
General Comments
• Congenital—may occur without clinical signs, especially in dogs of toy breeds; other malformations or anomalies of the CNS may be noted (e.g., malformations of the cerebellum or syringomyelia), which may further contribute to the constellation of signs.
• Acquired—signs attributable to the underlying disease may be as or more prominent than the signs attributable to the hydrocephalus.
• Severity of the clinical signs may not correspond to the degree of ventricular enlargement.

Historical Findings
• Behavioral—decreased consciousness; lack of or loss of training ability (including house-training); excessive sleepiness; vocalization; sometimes hyperexcitability
• Blindness
• Seizures—may be noted

Physical Examination Findings
Head—may appear large and dome-shaped with an exaggerated "stop"; open sutures and/or fontanelles

Neurologic Examination Findings
• Cerebral disease—abnormal behavior (especially dullness and sleepiness), cortical blindness (loss of vision with normal eyes and pupillary light reflexes), inappropriate vocalization, sometimes hyperexcitable
• Gait abnormalities—incoordination, ataxia, and decreased postural reactions
• Seizures—may occur

• Congenital form—malformation of the orbit during growth may result in a ventrolateral strabismus with normal oculocephalic eye movements.
• Severely increased intracranial pressure—stupor or coma, pinpoint or dilated fixed pupils, abnormal respiratory patterns, and decerebrate posture; may lead to fatal tentorial herniation

CAUSES
• Congenital—unclear
• Acquired—intracranial inflammatory diseases or mass lesions

RISK FACTORS
Animals with compensated hydrocephalus may decompensate in the face of an insult such as infection or trauma.

 DIAGNOSIS

DIFFERENTIAL DIAGNOSIS
• Other congenital brain anomalies
• Metabolic or toxic diseases resulting in cerebral dysfunction
• Brain mass lesions or infectious diseases resulting in high intracranial pressure (hydrocephalus may coexist)
• Traumatic injury to the brain (hydrocephalus may coexist)

CBC/BIOCHEMISTRY/URINALYSIS
• Usually normal

OTHER LABORATORY TESTS
N/A

IMAGING
• Skull radiography (congenital)—reveal an enlarged domed cranium with sutures and fontanelles open past their normal closure time; cranial vault may have a ground-glass appearance.
• CT and MRI—provide definite diagnosis
• Ultrasound scan through open fontanelle may reveal enlarged ventricles.

DIAGNOSTIC PROCEDURES
• CSF analysis—use caution when collecting sample if patient has high intracranial pressure (may lead to fatal brain herniation through the foramen magnum and/or beneath the tentorium cerebelli); composition normal if no other intracranial disease (e.g., neoplasia, inflammation), otherwise protein may be high and/or abnormal cells may be noted

• EEG—congential: usually characteristic, including hypersynchrony, high amplitude (25–300 μV), and low frequency (1–7 Hz); acquired: varies

PATHOLOGIC FINDINGS
• Brain—may be large with loss of the normal pattern of sulci and gyri; may see distortion of the parenchyma, including thinning of the cerebral cortex, rupture of the septum pellucidum, and atrophy of other adjacent structures; with severe disease, brain herniation may occur, either of the cerebrum and midbrain under the tentorium cerebelli or of the cerebellum and caudal medulla oblongata through the foramen magnum.
• Ventricular system—mildly to severely distended (either entirely or only the part rostral to the obstructive lesion); with noncommunicating form, narrowing or blockage of the ventricular system owing to inflammation or mass lesions

 TREATMENT

APPROPRIATE HEALTH CARE
• Inpatient—intensive care for patients with severe signs or when undergoing surgical therapy
• Outpatient—patients with mild to moderate signs that can be treated medically

NURSING CARE
Prevent secondary complications of recumbency for stuporous or comatose patients—avoid pressure sores; drying eyes; and hypostatic lung congestion

ACTIVITY
N/A

DIET
N/A

CLIENT EDUCATION
Advise client to observe for deterioration in mental alertness, vision, and behavior, which may signal worsening of the problem.

SURGICAL CONSIDERATIONS
• Surgical shunting of the CSF from the ventricles to the peritoneal cavity—definitive treatment

• Complications—infection and shunt blockage common; shunt revision commonly needed
• Clinical signs may not resolve completely; residual signs usually indicate irreversible brain damage.
• Surgery for a brain tumor or other mass lesion—consider if it is the underlying cause.

 MEDICATIONS

DRUGS OF CHOICE
• Reduce CSF production—corticosteroids: prednisone (0.25–0.5 mg/kg PO q12h) or dexamethasone (0.25 mg/kg PO q12h, tapered to an alternate-day regimen); or carbonic anhydrase inhibitors: acetazolamide (10 mg/kg PO q6h)
• Reduce intracranial pressure—osmotic diuretics: mannitol (1 g/kg slow IV infusion over 20 min; may repeat twice at 6-hr intervals); and/or loop diuretics: furosemide (dogs, 2–8 mg/kg IV, IM, SC q12h; cats, 1–2 mg/kg IV, IM, SC q12h)
• Treat underlying cause—administer specific drugs when possible (e.g., antibiotics for bacterial infection).

CONTRAINDICATIONS
Fluid therapy—use with caution with severe disease; do not overhydrate.

PRECAUTIONS
• Corticosteroids—long-term treatment may cause iatrogenic hyperadrenocorticism or hypoadrenocorticism if drug is suddenly withdrawn.
• Diuretics—may cause shock or electrolyte imbalances, especially hypokalemia with furosemide administration

POSSIBLE INTERACTIONS
N/A

ALTERNATIVE DRUGS
N/A

 FOLLOW-UP

PATIENT MONITORING
• Monitor for exacerbation of the hydrocephalus and for signs attributable to an underlying cause (e.g., intracranial neoplasia).

PREVENTION/AVOIDANCE
N/A

POSSIBLE COMPLICATIONS
• Brain herniation and death
• Infection and blockage when ventriculoperitoneal shunting is carried out; shunt revision and specific treatment for bacterial infection are then indicated.

EXPECTED COURSE AND PROGNOSIS
• Depend on cause and severity
• Mild congenital form—good prognosis; may require only occasional medical treatment

 MISCELLANEOUS

ASSOCIATED CONDITIONS
Cerebellar hypoplasia in kittens congenitally infected with feline panleukopenia virus

AGE-RELATED FACTORS
Congenital—usually seen in animals < 1 year old

ZOONOTIC POTENTIAL
N/A

PREGNANCY
N/A

SYNONYMS
N/A

SEE ALSO
Stupor and Coma

ABBREVIATION
CSF = cerebrospinal fluid

Suggested Readings

Harrington ML, Bagley RS, Moore MP. Hydrocephalus. Vet Clin North Am Small Anim Pract 1996;26:4:843–856.
Oliver JE, Lorenz MD, Kornegay JN. Handbook of veterinary neurology. 3rd. ed. Philadelphia: Saunders, 1997.
Summers BA, Cummings JF, de Lahunta A. Veterinary neuropathology. St. Louis: Mosby, 1995.
Author Mary O. Smith
Consulting Editor Joane M. Parent

DISEASES

HYDRONEPHROSIS

BASICS

OVERVIEW
• Causes progressive distension of the renal pelvis and diverticula, with atrophy of the renal parenchyma secondary to obstruction in most patients; the disease is usually unilateral and occurs secondary to complete or partial obstruction of the kidney or ureter by uroliths, neoplasia, retroperitoneal disease, trauma, radiotherapy, and accidental ligation of the ureter during ovariohysterectomy and after ectopic ureter surgery.
• Bilateral hydronephrosis—rare; usually secondary to trigonal, prostatic, or urethral disease

SIGNALMENT
Dogs affected more often than cats

SIGNS

Historical Findings
• None in some animals
• Anorexia
• Restlessness
• Polydipsia and polyuria
• Hematuria
• Signs of uremia in patients with bilateral hydronephrosis or if the contralateral kidney has compromised function
• May be referable to the cause of the obstruction

Physical Examination Findings
• Normal in some patients
• Renomegaly
• Renal, abdominal, or lumbar pain
• Abdominal mass—bladder or prostate
• Trigonal, prostatic, vaginal, or urethral mass palpable on rectal examination

CAUSES & RISK FACTORS
Any cause of ureteral obstruction including uroliths, ureteral stenosis, atresia, fibrosis (cats), or neoplasia; trigonal mass; prostatic disease; vaginal mass; retroperitoneal abscess, cysts, hematoma, or other mass; inadvertent ureteral ligation during ovariohysterectomy; postoperative complication from ectopic ureter surgery; perineal hernia

DIAGNOSIS

DIFFERENTIAL DIAGNOSIS
• Other causes of renomegaly—e.g., amyloidosis, neoplasia, granuloma, cysts, and perinephric pseudocysts (cats)
• Other causes of abdominal pain—e.g., pancreatitis and peritonitis
• Intervertebral disk disease leading to lumbar pain
• Pyelonephritis without obstruction

CBC/BIOCHEMISTRY/URINALYSIS
• Normal in some patients
• Loss of urine-concentrating ability (first abnormality detected), hematuria, pyuria

• Azotemia, hyperphosphatemia, hyperkalemia, and acidemia in patients with severe, bilateral hydronephrosis resulting in renal failure

OTHER LABORATORY TESTS
N/A

IMAGING
• Abdominal radiographs may be normal or show renomegaly, prostatomegaly, uroliths, reduced retroperitoneal contrast, or urinary bladder distension.
• Excretory urography, cystography, or injection of radiographic contrast by nephropyelocentesis may be required to determine the location and cause of obstruction.
• Ultrasonography reveals dilation of the renal pelvis and diverticula, with thinning of the renal parenchyma; dilation of one or both ureters is detected in some animals.

DIAGNOSTIC PROCEDURES
Transurethral urethocystoscopy or vaginoscopy may help determine the cause and location of some obstructions.

TREATMENT
• Treat as an inpatient and start supportive care (e.g., fluids ± antibiotics) while performing diagnostic tests. Correct fluid and electrolyte deficits with intravenous fluid therapy (0.9% NaCl or lactated Ringer solution) over 4–6 hr, followed by maintenance fluids as needed. Some patients may be extremely polyuric, necessitating higher maintenance fluid rates.

• Relieve lower urinary tract obstruction as soon as possible by catheterization, serial cystocentesis, or tube cystostomy, pending surgical correction.
• Discuss renal disease versus failure and possible need for surgery with the owner.
• Specific treatment (usually surgical) depends on the cause and whether there is concurrent renal failure or other disease process (e.g., metastatic neoplasia).
• Emergency surgery rarely required; treat metabolic and electrolyte abnormalities prior to surgery.
• Kidney removal may not be necessary unless infected or neoplastic.
• If mild disease is secondary to nephroliths or ureteroliths, extracorporeal shock wave lithotripsy may be used as an alternative to surgery.

MEDICATIONS

DRUGS
• Administer sodium bicarbonate to treat severe metabolic acidemia. For a measured acid deficit, give one-quarter of the calculated dose (weight in kg × 0.3 × base deficit) of bicarbonate as a slow intravenous bolus and the remainder with intravenous fluids. If the base deficit is not known, give bicarbonate at a dosage of 2–4 mEq/kg, depending on the severity of signs.

• Hyperkalemia (mild to moderate) often resolves with fluid replacement and/or bicarbonate administration. Severe, symptomatic hyperkalemia requires more-aggressive medical management such as regular insulin (0.5 u/kg IV) and 50% dextrose (2.0 g/kg IV). Some veterinary literature implies that potassium-containing solutions (e.g., lactated Ringer solution) should be avoided in hyperkalemic patients, but current data do not support this.
• See chapters on acute or chronic renal failure for additional treatment principles for patients with bilateral hydronephrosis.

CONTRAINDICATIONS/POSSIBLE INTERACTIONS
• Do not add or mix sodium bicarbonate with calcium-containing fluids.
• Many contraindications and potential complications are associated with the use of sodium bicarbonate; consider them before administering bicarbonate.
• Do not give radiographic contrast material intravenously until the patient is rehydrated.

FOLLOW-UP

PATIENT MONITORING
• Ultrasonography—can repeat at 2- to 4-week intervals after relief of obstruction, to assess improvement; often some signs of resolution appear by 3 months after relief of obstruction.

• BUN, creatinine, and electrolytes
• After relief of obstruction—polyuria and postobstructive diuresis leading to hypokalemia, weight loss, dehydration, and possibly renal failure

POSSIBLE COMPLICATIONS
Rupture of the excretory system and irreversible renal damage

EXPECTED COURSE AND PROGNOSIS
Depends on the cause, duration of obstruction, and presence or absence of concurrent infection. Irreversible damage to the kidney usually begins 15–45 days after obstruction. If the obstruction is relieved within 1 week, renal damage is reversible; some function may be regained with relief of obstruction present for as long as 4 weeks. Concurrent infection accelerates the severity of renal damage.

MISCELLANEOUS

Suggested Reading
Christie BA, Bjorling DE. Kidneys. In: Slatter D, ed. Textbook of small animal surgery. 2nd ed. Philadelphia: Saunders, 1993: 1428–1442.
Author Marc G. Bercovitch
Consulting Editors Larry G. Adams and Carl A. Osborne

HYPERADRENOCORTICISM (CUSHING DISEASE)

BASICS

DEFINITION
• Spontaneous hyperadrenocorticism (HAC) is a disorder caused by excessive production of cortisol by the adrenal cortex. • Iatrogenic HAC results from excessive exogenous administration of glucocorticoids. • In either instance, clinical signs are due to the deleterious effects of the elevated circulating cortisol concentrations on multiple organ systems.

PATHOPHYSIOLOGY
• Some 85–90% of cases of naturally occurring HAC are due to bilateral adrenocortical hyperplasia resulting from pituitary corticotroph tumors or hyperplasia oversecreting ACTH • In the remaining 10–15% of cases, cortisol-secreting adrenocortical neoplasia is present; approximately one-half of these are malignant. • Iatrogenic HAC results from excessive exogenous administration of glucocorticoids.

SYSTEMS AFFECTED
• HAC is a multisystemic disorder. • The degree to which each system is involved varies considerably; in some patients signs referable to one system may predominate; others have several systems involved to a comparable degree. • Signs referable to the urinary tract or skin often predominate.

GENETICS
N/A

INCIDENCE/PREVALENCE
• No exact figures available • Considered one of the most common endocrine disorders in dogs; rare in cats

GEOGRAPHIC DISTRIBUTION
N/A

SIGNALMENT
Dogs and cats

Breed Predilections
• Dogs—poodles, dachshunds, Boston terriers, boxers, and beagles are reportedly at increased risk • Cats—no apparent predilection

Predominant Sex
• No predilection for pituitary-dependent hyperadrenocorticism (PDH) in dogs; two-thirds to three-quarters of those a renal tumor are female • No apparent predilection in cats

Mean Age and Range
HAC is generally a disorder of middle-aged to old animals; PDH can be seen in dogs as young as 1 year.

SIGNS

General Comments
• Severity may vary greatly, depending on the duration and severity of cortisol excess. • In some cases, the physical presence of the neoplastic process (pituitary or adrenal) contributes.

Historical and Physical Examination Findings
Polyuria and polydipsia, polyphagia, pendulous abdomen, hepatomegaly, hair loss, lethargy, muscle weakness, anestrus, obesity, muscle atrophy, comedones, increased panting, testicular atrophy, hyperpigmentation, calcinosis cutis, facial nerve palsy

CAUSES
• Pituitary dependent—adenoma or hyperplasia of corticotrophs • Adrenal tumor—adenoma or carcinoma • Iatrogenic—due to glucocorticoid administration

RISK FACTORS
N/A

DIAGNOSIS

DIFFERENTIAL DIAGNOSIS
• Depends on the clinical and laboratory abnormalities displayed • Includes hypothyroidism, sex hormone dermatoses, acromegaly, diabetes mellitus, hepatopathies, renal disease, and other causes of polyuria/polydipsia

CBC/BIOCHEMISTRY/URINALYSIS
• Hemogram may show eosinopenia, lymphopenia, leukocytosis and erythrocytosis. • Serum chemistry may show elevated alkaline phosphatase, liver enzymes, cholesterol, glucose, and total CO_2. • Urinalysis may reveal decreased specific gravity, proteinuria, hematuria, pyuria, or bacteruria.

OTHER LABORATORY TESTS
• Diagnosing HAC—ACTH response test, low-dose dexamethasone suppression test (0.015 mg/kg dexamethasone [Azium] in dogs; 0.1 mg/kg in cats); urinary cortisol:creatinine ratio (negative result virtually excludes HAC; a positive result must be confirmed with blood test); be cognizant of the effects of nonadrenal illness on these tests (false positive results). • Differentiating PDH from AT—high-dose dexamethasone suppression (Current Veterinary Therapy Isone, Azium), plasma ACTH level, CRH response test.

IMAGING
• Abdominal radiographs may differentiate PDH from AT, demonstrating mineralization in one-third of AT; chest radiographs are indicated in AT to check for metastases. • Ultrasonography, CT, and MR—useful for differentiating PDH from AT and for staging AT • CT and MR—often useful for demonstrating macroadenomas

DIAGNOSTIC PROCEDURES
N/A

PATHOLOGIC FINDINGS
• PDH—gross examination reveals normal-sized pituitary to pituitary macroadenoma and bilateral adrenocortical enlargement • Microscopically, see pituitary adenoma or corticotroph hyperplasia of pars distalis or pars intermedia and adrenocortical hyperplasia • AT—gross examination reveals variable-sized adrenal mass, atrophy of contralateral gland (rarely bilateral tumors), and metastasis in some patients with adrenal carcinoma • Microscopically, see adrenocortical adenoma or carcinoma

TREATMENT

APPROPRIATE HEALTH CARE
Dictated by the severity of clinical signs, the patient's overall condition, and any complicating factors (e.g., diabetes mellitus, pulmonary embolism)

NURSING CARE
N/A

ACTIVITY
No alteration of activity necessary.

DIET
Usually no need to alter; appropriate reducing or high-fiber diet if concurrent diabetes mellitus

CLIENT EDUCATION
• Lifelong therapy required • If adverse reaction to mitotane—discontinue drug, give prednisone, and reevaluate in next few days; if no response to prednisone in a few hours, evaluate immediately

SURGICAL CONSIDERATIONS
• Hypophysectomy—described, but generally not recommended for treatment of PDH in dogs or cats because of the difficulty of the procedure and the need for intensive monitoring and lifelong hormonal supplementation. • Bilateral adrenalectomy, likewise, is a demanding procedure not generally used for the treatment of PDH in dogs; cats seem to tolerate the surgery somewhat better than dogs; given the appropriate personnel and facilities, it is one of the treatments of choice for feline PDH. • Surgery is probably the treatment of choice for adrenocortical adenomas and small carcinomas unless the patient is a poor surgical risk or the client refuses surgery. • Medical control of adrenal-dependent hyperadrenocorticism with ketoconazole is recommended prior to surgery, if possible.

MEDICATIONS

DRUGS OF CHOICE
• Mitotane (*o,p'*-DDD) remains the drug of choice for medical management of both PDH and AT in the dogs • PDH—give an initial loading dose of 40–50 mg/kg/day until both

basal and post-ACTH cortisol levels are in the normal resting range (1–5 μg/dL); then 50 mg/kg/week divided; dosage adjustments are based on ACTH response testing (maintain basal and post-ACTH cortisol levels between 1 and 5 μg/dL); if relapse occurs, as indicated by cortisol levels outside the normal resting range, reload for 5–7 days and increase weekly maintenance dose by approximately 50%; give prednisone (0.2 mg/kg/day) during initial and subsequent loading periods • AT—use mitotane (goal is low-to-undetectable basal and post-ACTH cortisol levels) or administer mitotane at highest tolerated dosage; give prednisone at 0.2 mg/kg/day • *l*-Deprenyl (selegiline hydrochloride; Anipryl, Deprenyl Animal Health, Inc., Topeka, KN)—may be used as an alternative treatment for PDH; decreases pituitary ACTH secretion by increasing dopaminergic tone to the hypothalamic-pituitary axis, thus decreasing serum cortisol concentrations; indicated only for the treatment of uncomplicated PDH; not recommended for treatment of PDH in dogs with concurrent illnesses such as diabetes mellitus; cannot be used to treat cortisol-secreting adrenocortical neoplasia; initiate therapy with 1 mg/kg daily and increase to 2 mg/kg/day after 2 months if the response is inadequate; if this dose is also ineffective, give alternative therapy • The multicenter trial performed by Deprenyl Animal Health, Inc., reported that 75–80% of dogs had a good response to therapy as assessed by resolution of clinical signs and monthly low dose dexamethasone suppression testing; other investigators reported lower efficacy rates (50% or less in some studies); further independent clinical trials are necessary to assess the efficacy of this medication in controlling PDH; adverse effects such as anorexia, lethargy, vomiting and diarrhea are uncommon (<5% of dogs) and usually mild; disadvantages include the need for lifelong daily administration and the expense of the medication • Ketoconazole (10 mg/kg BID initially; up 20 mg/kg BID in some dogs)—indicated for dogs unable to tolerate mitotane at doses necessary to control HAC and preoperative control of HAC in dogs with AT scheduled for adrenalectomy; may be useful for palliation of clinical signs of HAC in dogs with AT; over one-third of dogs reportedly fail to respond adequately to the drug; adverse effects include anorexia, vomiting, diarrhea, lethargy, and an idiosyncratic hepatopathy • Feline HAC—the drug of choice for medical management is controversial; further studies are needed; mitotane (50 mg/kg/day then 50 mg/ kg/week divided, dosage adjustments based on ACTH response testing) or metyrapone (65 mg/kg BID to TID, dosage adjustments based on ACTH response testing) should be considered; *l*-deprenyl is a newly described alternative for therapy of canine PDH, but its use has not been described in cats with HAC; a short-term

safety study in normal cats revealed no significant adverse effects

CONTRAINDICATIONS
N/A

PRECAUTIONS
• Side effects of mitotane—not uncommon; mild in most dogs; include lethargy, weakness, anorexia, vomiting, diarrhea, ataxia, and iatrogenic hypoadrenocorticism • Side effects are more common in dogs with AT given high doses of mitotane. • Side effects of ketoconazole—seem to be less common; include anorexia, vomiting, diarrhea, and transient liver enzyme elevation • Side effects of *l*-deprenyl are uncommon.

POSSIBLE INTERACTIONS
N/A

ALTERNATIVE DRUGS
• Consider radiation therapy for animals with pituitary macroadenomas. • ACTH levels may take several months to decrease; control HAC with above drugs in the interim.

 FOLLOW-UP

PATIENT MONITORING
• Response to therapy—use periodic ACTH response testing (see references); test after the initial 7–10 days of mitotane or ketoconazole therapy to ensure adequate response, then at 1, 3, and 6 months of maintenance mitotane therapy and every 6–12 months thereafter; adequacy of any necessary mitotane reloading period is checked with an ACTH response test before higher maintenance mitotane dose initiated; depending on the problem, clinical signs resolve within several days to months of appropriate therapy; current label recommendations are to evaluate the efficacy of *l*-deprenyl therapy solely on the basis of resolution of clinical signs of HAC; the ACTH stimulation test is not indicated for assessing the response to treatment • Some clinicians choose to do low-dose dexamethasone suppression tests every 4–6 weeks to evaluate for normalization (or improvement) of the pituitary-adrenal axis.

PREVENTION/AVOIDANCE
N/A

POSSIBLE COMPLICATIONS
N/A

EXPECTED COURSE/PROGNOSIS
• Untreated HAC—generally a progressive disorder with a poor prognosis • Treated PDH—usually a good prognosis; the average survival time for a dog with PDH treated with mitotane is 2 years; at least 10% survive 4 years; dogs living longer than 6 months tend to die of causes unrelated to their HAC • Macroadenomas and neurologic signs—poor to grave prognosis • Adrenal adenomas—usually a good to excellent prognosis; small carcinomas (not metastasized) have a fair to good prognosis

• Large carcinomas and AT with widespread metastasis—generally a poor to fair prognosis, but impressive responses to high doses of mitotane are occasionally seen.

 MISCELLANEOUS

ASSOCIATED CONDITIONS
Neurologic signs in dogs with large pituitary tumors; glucose intolerance or concurrent diabetes mellitus; pulmonary thromboembolism; increased incidence of urinary tract and skin infections; hypertension; proteinuria/glomerulopathy

AGE-RELATED FACTORS
N/A

ZOONOTIC POTENTIAL
N/A

PREGNANCY
N/A

SYNONYMS
Cushing's disease.

SEE ALSO
N/A

ABBREVIATIONS
• AT = adrenal tumor
• CRH = corticotropin releasing hormone
• HAC = hyperadrenocorticism
• PDH = pituitary-dependent hyperadrenocorticism

Suggested Reading

Bruyette DS, Ruehl WW, Entrikent, et al: Management of canine hyperadrenocorticism with l-deprenyl (Anipryl). Vet Clin North Am 1997;27(2):273–286.

Duesberg C, Peterson ME. Adrenal disorders in cats. Vet Clin North Am 1997; 27(2): 321–348.

Guptill L, Scott-Moncrieff JC, Widmer WR. Diagnosis of canine hyperadrenocorticism. Vet Clin North Am 1997; 27(2):215–236.

Kintzer PP, Peterson ME. Mitotane treatment of cortisol secreting adrenocortical neoplasia: 32 cases (1980–1992). J Am Vet Med Assoc 1994;205:54–61.

Kintzer PP, Peterson ME. Mitotane therapy of canine hyperadrenocorticism. In: Kirk RW, Bonagura JD, eds. Current veterinary therapy XII. Philadelphia: Saunders, 1995:.

Kintzer PP, Peterson ME. Diagnosis and management of canine cortisol-secreting adrenal tumors. Vet Clin North Am 1997; 27(2):299–308.

Peterson ME. Hyperadrenocorticism. In: Kirk RW, ed. Current veterinary therapy IX. Philadelphia: Saunders, 1986; 27(2):255– 272.

Peterson ME, Kintzer PP. Medical therapy of pituitary-dependent hyperadrenocorticism: mitotane. Vet Clin North Am 1997;27(2): 255–272.

Author Peter P. Kintzer
Consulting Editor Deborah Greco

DISEASES

HYPERANDROGENISM

 BASICS

OVERVIEW
• High absolute or relative concentrations of masculinizing sex hormones such as testosterone and its derivatives
• Androgens are produced by testicular interstitial (i.e., Leydig) cells, ovaries, the adrenal cortex, and peripheral conversion of weak androgens to more potent androgens.
• Hyperandrogenism can cause behavioral changes, abnormalities of the reproductive tract, and dermatologic problems.

SIGNALMENT
• Dogs and cats
• Pomeranians at higher risk than other breeds

SIGNS

Historical Findings
• Aggression
• High libido
• Virilization in females—lifting the leg to urinate, excessive mounting behavior, irregular estrous cycles
• Stunted growth may be caused by early closure of epiphyseal growth plates.

Physical Examination Findings
• Clitoral hypertrophy
• Gynecomastia can be caused by aromatization of excess androgens to estrogens.
• Priapism
• Alopecia or hirsutism
• Hyperpigmentation of the skin
• Seborrhea oleosa
• Perianal adenoma
• Prostatomegaly
• Tail gland hyperplasia

CAUSES & RISK FACTORS
• Exogenous administration of androgens and anabolic steroids
• High endogenous secretion of testosterone by gonadal tissue
• Testicular tumor
• Exposure of female fetuses to androgens
• High concentrations of gonadotrophin-releasing hormone and luteinizing hormone

 DIAGNOSIS

DIFFERENTIAL DIAGNOSIS
• Hyperadrenocorticism and hypothyroidism are ruled out by endocrine testing.
• Consider behavioral problems and CNS disease in overly aggressive animals.
• Immune-mediated skin diseases can be differentiated by skin biopsies and direct immunofluorescent studies.
• Rule out parasitic skin diseases (e.g., mange) by examining multiple skin scrapings.
• Rule out intersex abnormalities (e.g., hermaphrodites and pseudohermaphrodites) by physical examination or karyotyping.

CBC/BIOCHEMISTRY/URINALYSIS
Usually normal

OTHER LABORATORY TESTS
Repeated serum testing, gonadotropin-releasing hormone response test, and luteinizing hormone response tests are superior to single serum testing to detect high concentrations of testosterone (see Appendix for test protocols).

IMAGING
Abdominal radiography, abdominal ultrasound, and exploratory laparotomy may be useful to detect intraabdominal gonadal tissue or testosterone-secreting neoplasms.

DIAGNOSTIC PROCEDURES
Skin biopsies are consistent with other endocrinopathies.

 TREATMENT
• Neuter intact animals.
• Surgical excision of testosterone-secreting tumors

 MEDICATIONS

DRUGS
• Megestrol acetate (Ovaban) and finasteride (Proscar) inhibit 5-α-reductase in the prostate.
• Dogs—finasteride, 1–5 mg/kg/day; not approved for use in dogs

• Megestrol acetate, 1.1–2.2 mg/kg PO once daily for 7 days, then 0.5–1.1 mg/kg once daily for 2 weeks; use in conjunction with behavior modification.
• Mitotane (Lysodren) in dogs with increased adrenal androgens
• Dogs—see Hyperadrenocorticism for dosages.

CONTRAINDICATIONS/POSSIBLE INTERACTIONS
None

 FOLLOW-UP
• Repeat serum testosterone concentration after neutering.
• Serum testosterone levels may not decrease after finasteride and thus cannot be used to determine drug efficacy.
• Aggressive behavior, dermatologic abnormalities, and gynecomastia resolve after castration in some animals.
• Virilization of females may be prevented by avoiding in utero exposure to androgens and by avoiding exogenous administration of androgens and anabolic steroids postnatally.

☑ MISCELLANEOUS

ASSOCIATED CONDITIONS
• High concentrations of adrenal androgens are associated with growth hormone–responsive dermatosis in the Pomeranian.
• Hyperandrogenism in male dogs enhances perianal gland adenomas and benign prostatic hyperplasia.

SEE ALSO
• Dermatoses, Growth Hormone Responsive
• Dermatoses, Sex Hormone Responsive
• Benign Prostatic Hyperplasia

ABBREVIATIONS
N/A

Suggested Reading
Schmeitzel LP. Growth hormone-responsive alopecia and sex hormone-associated dermatoses. In: Birchard SJ, Sherding RG, eds., Saunders manual of small animal practice. Philadelphia: Saunders, 1994:326–329.
Author Margaret R. Kern
Consulting Editor Deborah S. Greco

BASICS

OVERVIEW
• An imbalance between coagulation factors and inhibitors that shifts the balance toward clot formation, resulting in a (comparatively) high risk of thrombosis.
• Mechanisms include congenital or acquired deficiency of coagulation inhibitors or dysfibrinogenemia.
• Most common mechanism is loss of antithrombin III and perhaps other factors because of protein-losing nephropathy
• Effects of thrombosis vary according to thrombus location; pulmonary arteries a common site

SIGNALMENT
• Dogs and cats (uncommon)
• No breed or sex predilection

SIGNS
• None, before onset of thrombosis
• Patients with pulmonary thromboembolism have acute respiratory distress, hepatomegaly, cyanosis, weakness, and jugular distention on examination.
• Patients with aortic thromboembolism have acute paresis or paralysis, limb pain, absent or weak femoral pulses, cold limbs, cyanotic nailbeds, and peripheral neuropathy on examination.

CAUSES & RISK FACTORS
• Protein-losing nephropathy
• DIC
• Congenital deficiencies in factors related to clotting

DIAGNOSIS

DIFFERENTIAL DIAGNOSIS
• Vascular damage secondary to septicemia or trauma; use CBC, history, and results of physical examination to differentiate.
• Stasis of blood flow as in cardiomyopathy of cats and polycythemia (rare in dogs and cats)

CBC/BIOCHEMISTRY/URINALYSIS
• Hypoalbuminemia, proteinuria, and possibly hypercholesterolemia if hypercoagulability is secondary to protein-losing nephropathy
• Thrombocytopenia and schistocytosis in some animals with DIC

OTHER LABORATORY TESTS
• APTT, PT, fibrinogen, and fibrin degradation products—abnormal in some animals with DIC
• Thrombin time—rules out dysfibrinogenemia
• Specific assays of coagulation factors and inhibitors—necessary to identify deficiencies
• Urine protein:creatinine ratio, if protein-losing nephropathy suspected

IMAGING
Angiography may be necessary to localize thrombus.

DIAGNOSTIC PROCEDURES
None

TREATMENT
• Treat animals with protein-losing nephropathy as inpatients only if thrombosis has resulted in dysfunction of important organs.
• Restrict activity that may lead to trauma, and warn owner of dangers of thrombosis.
• Treat animals with DIC as inpatients by severely restricting activity.
• Administer fluids if necessary to avoid dehydration

MEDICATIONS

DRUGS

Protein-losing Nephropathy
• Administer heparin, then warfarin, to inhibit coagulation; use aspirin as an alternative to warfarin.
• Provide fresh-frozen plasma or whole plasma to replace inhibitors, especially antithrombin III.
• Consider thrombolytic therapy with streptokinase or urokinase if thrombosis has occurred.

DIC
See Disseminated Intravascular Coagulation (DIC)

CONTRAINDICATIONS/POSSIBLE INTERACTIONS
Do not treat with warfarin initially or exclusively; its effect on anticoagulant proteins C and S and on vitamin K–dependent factors leads to initial hypercoagulability.

FOLLOW-UP
• PT—monitor every 3 days to titrate the dose of warfarin to 1.5–2 times the baseline prothrombin value; monitor weekly after a stable dosage has been achieved (typically no sooner than 2 weeks).
• Use international normalization ratios to minimize the effects of test kit variability on measurement of PT.

MISCELLANEOUS

SEE ALSO
• Amyloidosis
• Aortic Thromboembolism
• Disseminated Intravascular Coagulation (DIC)
• Glomerulonephritis
• Nephrotic Syndrome
• Pulmonary Thromboembolism

ABBREVIATIONS
• DIC = disseminated intravascular coagulation
• PT = prothrombin time
• APTT = activated partial thromboplastin time

Suggested Reading
Bick RL, Pegram M. Syndromes of hypercoagulability and thrombosis: a review. Semin Thromb Hemost 1994;20:109–132.
Author G. Daniel Boon
Consulting Editor Susan M. Cotter

HYPEREOSINOPHILIC SYNDROME

BASICS

OVERVIEW
• Idiopathic persistent eosinophilia caused by sustained overproduction of eosinophils in the bone marrow
• Hypothesized to be caused by severe reaction to an undefined antigen or dysregulation of immunologic control of eosinophil production
• Multisystemic syndrome with invasion of tissues by eosinophils and subsequent organ damage and dysfunction, leading to death
• Organ damage caused by effects of eosinophil granule products and eosinophil-derived cytokines that are released in the tissues from activated or necrotic cells
• Probably includes a heterogeneous group of disorders
• Common sites of infiltration—gastrointestinal tract (especially intestine and liver), spleen, and lymph nodes (especially mesenteric nodes)
• Less common sites of infiltration—skin, kidney, heart, thyroid, lung, adrenal glands, and pancreas

SIGNALMENT
• Cats—may occur more frequently in female, middle-aged, domestic shorthair animals than others
• Dogs—rare and incompletely described

SIGNS
Historical Findings
• Lethargy
• Anorexia
• Intermittent vomiting and diarrhea
• Weight loss
• Less frequently—fever, pruritus, and seizures

PHYSICAL EXAMINATION FINDINGS
• Fever
• Emaciation
• Hepatosplenomegaly
• Thickened (diffuse or segmental) intestine that is nonpainful
• Mesenteric, and possible peripheral, lymphadenopathy
• Mass lesions caused by eosinophilic granulomatous inflammation involving lymph nodes or organs
• Pruritic erythroderma

CAUSES & RISK FACTORS
• Unknown, but believed to be a severe reaction to an underlying, but unidentifiable, antigenic stimulus
• Cats—eosinophilic enteritis may be an early form.

DIAGNOSIS

DIFFERENTIAL DIAGNOSIS
• Identifiable causes of eosinophilia—parasitism, hypersensitivity disorder, infectious disease, immune-mediated disease, and neoplasia; with these conditions, eosinophilia is usually limited in degree and remains confined to a specific organ, such as the lungs in feline asthma.
• Eosinophilic leukemia—distinction is controversial; differentiating criteria of this leukemia: (1) immature eosinophils seen in higher numbers in the circulation and constitute a higher percentage of the leukocyte differential; (2) anemia more common; (3) myeloid:erythroid ratio in bone marrow is higher (> 10:1) and blast forms are more numerous; (4) tissue infiltrates consist of immature eosinophils and may show a sinusoidal pattern in the liver without fibrosis; (5) in cats, chloroma-like masses in the kidneys reported.

CBC/BIOCHEMISTRY/URINALYSIS
• Leukocytosis with eosinophilia (usually marked), possibly with a left shift in the eosinophil series; eosinophil count range: 3,200–130,000 cells/μL
• Basophilia
• Anemia in some animals
• In animals with organ dysfunction, biochemical abnormalities may be seen.

OTHER LABORATORY TESTS
Rule out identifiable causes of eosinophilia—fecal flotation, heartworm test, fungal culture, and biopsy to detect neoplasm

IMAGING
Intestinal mucosal irregularities and thickened intestine seen on radiographic contrast studies

DIAGNOSTIC PROCEDURES
• Bone marrow—hypercellularity, eosinophilic hyperplasia (up to 40% of nucleated cells consist of eosinophils), lack of morphologic abnormalities, and high myeloid:erythroid ratio (mean 7.27:1)
• Biopsy of affected organ or mass

PATHOLOGIC FINDINGS
- Spleen—eosinophilic infiltrate in red pulp, sometimes in white pulp
- Gastrointestinal tract—mucosal and submucosal eosinophilic infiltrates in small intestine, sometimes in colon and stomach
- Lymph nodes—reactive hyperplasia and infiltration of cords and sinuses with eosinophils
- Heart—eosinophilic infiltrates in the myocardium and endocardium; fibrosis and thrombus formation
- Less frequently—eosinophilic infiltrates in the skin, liver, lung, pancreas, kidney, adrenal, and thyroid gland

TREATMENT
- Use long-term maintenance therapy to control or reduce the eosinophilia and organ damage.
- Massive tissue infiltration impedes treatment and usually lends a poor prognosis.
- High serum IgE concentration portends a good response to treatment with prednisone and a better prognosis.

MEDICATIONS

DRUGS
- Corticosteroids—prednisolone, 1–3 mg/kg/day initially; then taper to alternate-day administration if eosinophilia is suppressed; if eosinophilia returns, resume higher daily dose.
- Chemotherapeutic agents—try if eosinophilia is steroid resistant, but the paucity of case reports describing these therapies precludes recommending their use
- Hydroxyurea (inhibits DNA synthesis)—administer to reduce the eosinophil count if not normal or near normal after 7–14 days of treatment with steroids; most likely would be used long-term if effective in conjunction with steroids
- Cyclosporin A—suppresses production of eosinophilopoietic factors by T cells
- Vincristine and alkylating agents, such as chlorambucil, effective in humans
- Reduce dosage or discontinue drug if bone marrow suppression or thrombocytopenia develops.

CONTRAINDICATIONS/POSSIBLE INTERACTIONS
Aggressive cytotoxic therapy has been deleterious in some human patients.

FOLLOW-UP
- Monitor eosinophil count (not always indicative of tissue infiltrates) and myelosuppression if chemotherapeutic drugs are used.
- Monitor clinical signs (e.g., anorexia, lethargy, vomiting, and diarrhea) and any physical abnormalities.

MISCELLANEOUS

SEE ALSO
Eosinophilia and Basophilia

Suggested Reading
Huibregtse BA, Turner JL. Hypereosinophilic syndrome and eosinophilic leukemia: a comparison of 22 hypereosinophilic cats. J Anim Hosp Assoc 1994;30:591–599.
Author Karen M. Young
Consulting Editor Susan M. Cotter

HYPERESTROGENISM

 BASICS

OVERVIEW
• High absolute or relative concentrations of feminizing sex hormones such as estradiol, estriol, and estrone
• Estrogens are produced by the ovary, testes, adrenal cortex, and by peripheral conversion of precursor hormones.
• The main organs affected are skin, urogenital tract, and hematopoietic system.

SIGNALMENT
• Dogs and cats
• Endogenous hyperestrogenism is more common in middle-aged to old dogs.

SIGNS

Historical Findings
• Low libido in males
• Infertility
• Males attracting other males
• Failure of male dogs to lift their leg to urinate
• Hematuria
• Abnormal estrous cycles; prolonged proestrus or estrus
• Nymphomania, excessive mounting of other females
• Failure of hair to grow after clipping

Physical Examination Findings
• Testicular mass or enlarged testicles in animals with endogenous hyperestrogenism
• Bilateral testicular atrophy in animals with exogenous hyperestrogenism
• Cryptorchidism
• Pale mucous membranes are manifestations of anemia and bone marrow suppression in dogs.
• Petechiation or other signs of hemorrhage
• Large clitoris and vulva
• Vaginal hyperplasia and prolapse
• Pendulous prepuce
• Gynecomastia
• Galactorrhea
• Bilateral, symmetrical alopecia beginning at the flank and perineum
• Cutaneous hyperpigmentation
• Prostatomegaly
• Prostatic cyst or abscess
• Fever, depression, and pyometra may be caused by neutropenia associated with bone marrow suppression

CAUSES & RISK FACTORS
• Cystic ovaries
• Functional ovarian tumors (e.g., granulosa-theca cell)
• A functional testicular tumor is usually a Sertoli cell tumor, but it can be a seminoma or interstitial cell tumor.
• Exogenous estrogen administration

 DIAGNOSIS

DIFFERENTIAL DIAGNOSIS
• Rule out hyperadrenocorticism and hypothyroidism initially.
• Intersex abnormalities (e.g., hermaphroditism and pseudohermaphrodism)
• Allergic skin disease
• Autoimmune skin disease
• Demodicosis and dermatophytosis

CBC/BIOCHEMISTRY/URINALYSIS
• Nonregenerative anemia, thrombocytopenia, and leukocytosis initially, followed by leukopenia
• Hematuria

OTHER LABORATORY TESTS
• High serum estrogen (estradiol) concentration to help confirm a suspected diagnosis
• Separate serum from RBCs, refrigerate, and ship on ice; lipemia may interfere with the radioimmunoassay.
• Examination of prepucial or vaginal cytology may reveal numerous cornified cells with pyknotic nuclei or anuclear cells.
• Gonadotropin-releasing (GnRH) response test to detect suspected ovarian tissue after ovariohysterectomy

IMAGING
Radiography and ultrasonography to detect cryptorchid testicles or intraabdominal mass

DIAGNOSTIC PROCEDURES

• Examination of bone marrow aspirate or biopsy specimen may reveal hypoplasia, aplasia, or fatty infiltration.
• Laparoscopy or laparotomy to detect cryptorchid testicles or intraabdominal mass
• Skin biopsy findings may be consistent with those of other endocrinopathies—orthokeratotic hyperkeratosis, epidermal thinning, follicular keratosis, dilation and atrophy, increased telogen hair follicles, sebaceous gland atrophy

 TREATMENT

• Neutering is the treatment of choice for endogenous hyperestrogenism.
• Castration of dogs with testicular neoplasia may result in permanent resolution of clinical signs.
• Ovariohysterectomy for functional ovarian tumor and cystic ovaries
• Discontinue exogenous drug administration.

 MEDICATIONS

DRUGS

• Supportive and symptomatic therapy as indicated
• Severe bone marrow suppression may require whole blood transfusions or blood component therapy.
• Administer antibiotics to treat secondary infection.

• May try androgens, lithium, G-CSF, GM-CSF, and IL-3 to stimulate hypoplastic marrow
• May use GnRH to treat persistent estrus and vaginal hyperplasia caused by follicular cysts

CONTRAINDICATIONS/POSSIBLE INTERACTIONS

• Do not use myelosuppressive chemotherapeutic agents in patients with bone marrow suppression.
• Estrogens may increase serum concentrations of thyroxine (T_4) and triiodothyronine (T_3).

 FOLLOW-UP

• Repeat CBC to monitor effectiveness of therapy or disease progression.
• Male feminization signs usually have resolved by 2–6 weeks after castration without metastatic disease.
• Serum estrogen concentrations should return to normal after surgical removal of functional tumors.
• Bone marrow aplasia usually does not respond to castration.
• Bone marrow suppression may be a permanent sequela.
• Measure serum progesterone after GnRH administration for cystic ovaries; if ovulation occurred, serum progesterone should be >1 ng/mL, and the bitch should be bred at the next estrus.

 MISCELLANEOUS

ASSOCIATED CONDITIONS

• Canine male-feminizing syndrome, usually caused by a Sertoli cell tumor
• Prostatic neoplasia
• Ovarian imbalance type I dermatosis
• Discontinue exogenous estrogen in dogs with acute pancreatitis.
• Exogenous estrogen administration is potentially hepatotoxic.

ABBREVIATIONS

• GnRH = gonadotropin-releasing hormone
• G-CSF = granulocyte colony-stimulating factor
• GM-CSF = granulocyte-macrophage colony-stimulating factor
• IL-3 = interleukin-3

Suggested Reading

Schmeitzel LP. Growth hormone-responsive alopecia and sex hormone-associated dermatoses. In: Birchard SJ, Sherding RG, eds. Saunders manual of small animal practice. Philadelphia: Saunders, 1994:326–329.
Author Margaret R. Kern
Consulting Editor Deborah S. Greco

HYPERPARATHYROIDISM

BASICS

DEFINITION
A pathologic, sustained, high, circulating concentration of parathyroid hormone (PTH)

PATHOPHYSIOLOGY
• PTH—secreted by the parathyroid glands in response to changes in the concentration of ionized calcium in the serum; raises the serum calcium concentration through its effects on bone and renal tubular calcium resorption and vitamin D–dependent intestinal calcium absorption
• Can develop as a primary condition or be secondary to a disorder of calcium homeostasis; primary hyperparathyroidism is associated with benign (usually) adenoma of the parathyroid gland(s); secondary hyperparathyroidism can be caused by a deficiency of calcium and vitamin D associated with malnutrition or chronic renal disease

SYSTEMS AFFECTED
• Renal/urologic
• Gastrointestinal
• Neuromuscular
• Cardiovascular

GENETICS
• None known for primary hyperparathyroidism, but its association with certain breeds suggests a possible hereditary basis in some cases.
• Secondary hyperparathyroidism can develop in association with hereditary nephropathy, but is not inherited per se.

INCIDENCE/PREVALENCE
• Prevalence of primary form is unknown.
• More commonly diagnosed in dogs than in cats.
• Fairly common among causes of hypercalcemia, but much less common than hypercalcemia of malignancy (at least in dogs)
• Nutritional secondary hyperparathyroidism is decreasing in prevalence as the public becomes more educated in pet nutrition.
• Chronic renal failure with secondary hyperparathyroidism is extremely common, more so in cats than in dogs.

GEOGRAPHIC DISTRIBUTION
N/A

SIGNALMENT

Species
Cats and dogs

Breed Predilections
• Keeshond
• Siamese cat

Mean Age and Range
• Cats—mean age, 13 years; range 8–15 years
• Dogs—mean age, 10 years; range 5–15 years

Predominant Sex
None

SIGNS

General Comments
• Most dogs and cats with primary hyperparathyroidism do not appear ill.
• Signs are usually mild and are due solely to the effects of hypercalcemia.
• Signs become apparent when hypercalcemia is severe and chronic.

Historical Findings
• Polyuria
• Polydipsia
• Anorexia
• Lethargy
• Vomiting
• Weakness
• Urolithiasis
• Stupor and coma

Physical Examination Findings
• Often unremarkable.
• Parathyroid adenoma is not palpable in dogs but often is in cats.
• Nutritional secondary disease is sometimes associated with pathologic bone fractures and general poor body condition.

CAUSES
• Primary hyperparathyroidism—PTH-secreting adenoma of the parathyroid gland
• Renal secondary hyperparathyroidism—renal calcium loss and reduced gut absorption of calcium due to deficiency in calcitriol production by the renal tubular cells
• Nutritional secondary hyperparathyroidism—a nutritional deficiency of calcium and vitamin D

RISK FACTORS
• Primary hyperparathyroidism—unknown
• Secondary hyperparathyroidism—coexisting renal tubular disease or calcium/vitamin D malnutrition

DIAGNOSIS

DIFFERENTIAL DIAGNOSIS
The differential list includes causes of hypercalcemia.
• Lymphosarcoma—common in dogs, rare in cats
• Anal sac apocrine gland adenocarcinoma—dogs
• Other miscellaneous carcinomas—dogs and cats
• Myeloproliferative disease—cats
• Fibrosarcoma—cats
• Chronic renal failure
• Hypoadrenocorticism
• Vitamin D rodenticide intoxication—no such products are currently marketed in the U.S.

CBC/BIOCHEMISTRY/URINALYSIS
• High serum calcium concentration
• Low or low-normal serum phosphorus concentration in primary hyperparathyroidism
• Hyperphosphatemia in secondary hyperparathyroidism or hypervitaminosis D
• BUN and creatinine concentrations are usually normal in patients with primary hyperparathyroidism, except those with hypercalcemia-induced renal failure.

OTHER LABORATORY TESTS
• Serum ionized calcium determination is often normal in patients with chronic renal failure and high in patients with primary hyperparathyroidism or hypercalcemia associated with malignancy.
• High serum PTH concentration is diagnostic for primary hyperparathyroidism in the absence of azotemia; assays that measure the intact PTH molecule are most useful.

IMAGING
• Radiography can be useful to assess urolithiasis, renal morphology, and bone density and to identify occult neoplasia.
• Ultrasonography of the ventral cervical area sometimes reveals a parathyroid gland adenoma
• Ultrasound of the abdomen can reveal lymphadenopathy, urolithiasis, or renal morphologic abnormalities.

DIAGNOSTIC PROCEDURES
Surgical exploration of the ventral cervical area

PATHOLOGIC FINDINGS
• Parathyroid adenoma is usually a solitary, small (=1 cm), round, light brown or reddish mass located in the proximity of the thyroid gland.
• Occasionally multiple adenomas are found.
• The histologic distinctions between adenomas, hyperplasia, and carcinomas of the parathyroid gland are often unclear.

 TREATMENT

APPROPRIATE HEALTH CARE
• Primary hyperparathyroidism generally requires inpatient care and surgery.
• Nutritional or renal secondary hyperparathyroidism in noncritical patients can be managed on an outpatient basis.

NURSING CARE
N/A

ACTIVITY
No alterations recommended

DIET
Calcium supplementation for secondary forms

CLIENT EDUCATION
Explain signs referable to changes in calcium status, since hypocalcemia is a potential complication of parathyroidectomy.

SURGICAL CONSIDERATIONS
Surgery is the treatment of choice for primary hyperparathyroidism and is often important in establishing the diagnosis.

 MEDICATIONS

DRUGS OF CHOICE
• Normal saline is the fluid of choice for treatment of hypercalcemia
• Diuretics (furosemide) and corticosteroids can be useful in treating hypercalcemia.
• No medical treatment exists for primary hyperparathyroidism per se.

CONTRAINDICATIONS
• Do not use glucocorticoids until the diagnosis of lymphoma has been excluded; they can obfuscate the diagnosis.
• Avoid calcium-containing fluids.

PRECAUTIONS
• Use furosemide only in patients with adequate hydration.
• Mithramycin has been used in patients with severe hypercalcemic crises; avoid if possible, because of associated nephrotoxicity and hepatotoxicity.

POSSIBLE INTERACTIONS
N/A

ALTERNATIVE DRUGS
None

 FOLLOW-UP

PATIENT MONITORING
• Postoperative hypocalcemia is relatively common after treatment of primary hyperparathyroidism in patients with a presurgery serum calcium concentration >14 mg/dL; check serum calcium once or twice daily for 1 week after surgery.
• In patients with renal impairment, check serum concentrations of urea nitrogen and creatinine.

PREVENTION/AVOIDANCE
• No strategies exist for prevention of primary hyperparathyroidism.
• Nutritional secondary hyperparathyroidism is prevented by proper nutrition.

POSSIBLE COMPLICATIONS
Irreversible renal failure secondary to hypercalcemia

EXPECTED COURSE AND PROGNOSIS
• Untreated disease usually progresses to end-stage kidney or neurologic disease.
• Prognosis for treatment of parathyroid adenoma is excellent.
• Recurrence is seen in a small percentage of cases

 MISCELLANEOUS

ASSOCIATED CONDITIONS
Calcium-containing urolithiasis

AGE-RELATED FACTORS
N/A

ZOONOTIC POTENTIAL
N/A

PREGNANCY
N/A

SYNONYMS
None

SEE ALSO
• Calcium, Hypercalcemia
• Renal Failure, Chronic
• Hyperparathyroidism, Renal Secondary

ABBREVIATIONS
PTH = parathyroid hormone

Suggested Reading
Chew DJ, Nagode LA, Carothers M. Disorders of calcium: hypercalcemia and hypocalcemia. In: DiBartola SP. Fluid therapy in small animal practice. Philadelphia: WB Saunders, 1992:116–176.
Feldman EC. Disorders of the parathyroid glands. In: Ettinger SJ, Feldman ED, eds. Textbook of veterinary internal medicine. 4th ed. Philadelphia: WB Saunders, 1994:1437–1464
Richter KP, Kallet AJ, Feldman EC, Primary hyperparathyroidism in the cat. In: Kirk RW, Bonagura JD, eds. Current veterinary therapy XI. Philadelphia: WB Saunders, 1992.

Author Thomas K. Graves
Consulting Editor Deborah S. Greco

HYPERPARATHYROIDISM, RENAL SECONDARY

BASICS

OVERVIEW
• Clinical syndrome characterized by a high concentration of biologically active PTH secondary to chronic renal failure; major cause is the absolute or relative lack of calcitriol synthesis, though low concentrations of ionized calcium also contribute.
• Hyperphosphatemia secondary to declining renal function reduces the activity of 1α-hydroxylase in the kidney, which in turn reduces production of calcitriol (1,25-dihydroxycholecalciferol). Reduced renal tubular mass also contributes to reduced calcitriol synthesis. Normal calcitriol concentrations exert a negative effect on PTH synthesis within the parathyroid gland nucleus. Low calcitriol and serum ionized calcium concentrations result in increased PTH production and parathyroid gland hyperplasia. High PTH production increases serum calcitriol and calcium concentrations at the expense of chronically high PTH concentration.
• Calcitrol synthesis is impaired in patients with severe chronic renal failure and low numbers of renal tubules regardless of the level of PTH compensation. PTH may act as a uremic toxin and may promote nephrocalcinosis and progression of chronic renal failure.

SIGNALMENT
Dogs and cats; see Chronic Renal Failure for age and breed predilections

SIGNS
• Those associated with underlying chronic renal failure are the usual reason for examination.
• Severe renal osteodystrophy or "rubber jaw" occurs in some patients, most commonly young dogs with severe renal secondary hyperparathyroidism.

CAUSES & RISK FACTORS
Any disease that causes chronic renal failure

DIAGNOSIS

DIFFERENTIAL DIAGNOSIS
• Hypercalcemic nephropathy—renal disease (or failure) caused by ionized hypercalcemia; can be difficult to differentiate from long-standing renal secondary hyperparathyroidism in which the parathyroid glands lose their negative feedback responsiveness to high levels of ionized calcium (tertiary hyperparathyroidism)
• The total serum calcium concentration is usually higher in patients with hypercalcemic nephropathy than in those with renal secondary hyperparathyroidism; the ionized serum calcium concentration is usually low or normal with renal secondary hyperparathyroidism and high with hypercalcemic nephropathy.
• Serum PTH concentration is low in animals with hypercalcemia of malignancy; may detect underlying causes of hypercalcemia such as lymphoma or apocrine gland adenocarcinoma of the anal sac
• Primary hyperparathyroidism—initially characterized by hypercalcemia (ionized and total), normal or low serum phosphorus concentration, and high PTH concentration; renal function is initially normal but may become compromised later in the course of disease.

CBC/BIOCHEMISTRY/URINALYSIS
• Azotemia
• Hyperphosphatemia
• Urine specific gravity < 1.030 in dogs and < 1.035 in cats
• Possible hypocalcemia (ionized calcium); the total serum calcium concentration may be low, normal, or slightly high; see Chronic Renal Failure.

OTHER LABORATORY TESTS
• Definitive diagnosis and therapeutic monitoring of renal secondary hyperparathroidism require measurement of high serum PTH concentration; an immunoassay for PTH directed against the amino-terminal or intact PTH molecule and validated for dogs or cats is preferred.
• A low ionized serum calcium concentration is useful to differentiate renal secondary hyperparathyroidism from other causes of hypercalcemia.

IMAGING
Radiographs may reveal low bone density, loss of the lamina dura around the teeth, and soft-tissue mineralization of the gastric mucosa or other tissues.

DIAGNOSTIC PROCEDURES
N/A

TREATMENT
• See Chronic Renal Failure for general treatment principles.
• Patients with renal secondary hyperparathyroidism—feed a diet low in phosphorus content and give free access to fresh water.

MEDICATIONS

DRUGS

Intestinal Phosphate Binders

• Prescribe if dietary management does not return phosphorous concentration to normal.
• Aluminum hydroxide (30–90 mg/kg/day PO with meals), calcium carbonate (90–150 mg/kg/day PO with meals), or calcium acetate (60–90 mg/kg/day PO with meals)
• Hypercalcemia may uncommonly develop when a calcium-containing phosphate binder is combined with calcitriol. Aluminum- and calcium-containing phosphate binders can be used in combination to reduce the dosage of each and minimize the risk of hypercalcemia.

Calcitriol

• Low-dose calcitriol (1.5–3.5 ng/kg PO q24 h)—may use after initiation of dietary phosphorus restriction and oral phosphate binders; note that this dose is in ng/kg rather than mg/kg; a pharmacy that specializes in reformulation into low doses is needed to provide this prescription.
• Maintain serum phosphorus concentration within the normal range before and during calcitriol therapy.

CONTRAINDICATIONS/POSSIBLE INTERACTIONS

• Calcitriol administration may result in hypercalcemia, especially if combined with a calcium-containing intestinal phosphate binder. Hypercalcemia sometimes develops in patients with long-standing chronic renal failure but is not related to calcitriol treatment. In these instances, ionized calcium concentration is normal or low and hypercalcemia does not resolve when calcitriol treatment is discontinued.
• Do not use calcium-containing intestinal phosphate binders in patients with hyperphosphatemia or with a calcium × phosphorus product > 70. Use aluminum-containing intestinal phosphate binders initially to correct hyperphosphatemia, followed by calcium-containing intestinal phosphate binders once the serum phosphorus concentration is normal.

FOLLOW-UP

PATIENT MONITORING

• Serum concentrations of calcium, phosphorus, creatinine, and urea nitrogen—weekly to monthly depending on therapy and the severity of chronic renal failure
• Patients receiving calcitriol—weekly for 4 weeks, then monthly for hypercalcemia and hyperphosphatemia
• Serial evaluations of PTH concentration—most dogs and cats treated with low doses of calcitriol achieve near-normal levels of PTH within 3 months; it may be necessary to increase the dose in those with severe parathyroid gland hyperplasia.

PREVENTION/AVOIDANCE

Dietary phosphorus restriction in patients with chronic renal failure may delay the onset of renal secondary hyperparathyroidism.

POSSIBLE COMPLICATIONS

Renal osteodystrophy and pathologic fractures (rare)

EXPECTED COURSE AND PROGNOSIS

• Progression of the underlying chronic renal failure may be slowed by treatment of renal secondary hyperparathyroidism.
• Long-term prognosis is guarded to poor for patients with chronic renal failure and renal secondary hyperparathyroidism.
• Short-term prognosis depends on severity of chronic renal failure.

MISCELLANEOUS

AGE-RELATED FACTORS

Young animals can develop severe renal osteodystrophy and may benefit from treatment with calcitriol and calcium carbonate.

ABBREVIATION

PTH = Parathyroid hormone

Suggested Reading

Chew DJ, Nagode LA. Calcitriol in the treatment of chronic renal failure. In: Kirk RW, Bonagura JD, eds. Current veterinary therapy. XI Philadelphia: Saunders, 1992: 857–860.

Authors Larry G. Adams and Dennis J. Chew
Consulting Editors Larry G. Adams and Carl A. Osborne

HYPERSENSITIVITY REACTION (ANAPHYLAXIS)

 BASICS

DEFINITION
• Acute manifestation of a type I hypersensitivity reaction mediated through the rapid introduction of an antigen into a host having antigen-specific antibodies of the IgE subclass
• The binding of antigen to mast cells sensitized with IgE results in the release of preformed and newly synthesized chemical mediators.
• Anaphylactic reactions may be localized (atopy) or systemic (anaphylactic shock).
• Anaphylaxis not mediated by IgE is designated an anaphylactoid reaction and will not be discussed.

PATHOPHYSIOLOGY
• First exposure of the patient to a particular antigen (allergen) causes a humoral response and results in production of IgE, which binds to the surface of mast cells; the patient is then considered to be sensitized to that antigen.
• Second exposure to the antigen results in cross-linking of two or more IgE molecules on the cell surface, resulting in mast cell degranulation and activation; release of mast cell granules initiates an anaphylactic reaction.
• Major mast cell–derived mediators include histamine, eosinophilic chemotactic factor, arachidonic acid, metabolites (e.g., prostaglandins, leukotrienes, and thromboxanes), platelet-activating factor, and proteases, which cause an inflammatory response of increased vascular permeability, smooth muscle contraction, inflammatory cell influx, and tissue damage.
• Clinical manifestations depend on the route of antigen exposure, the dose of antigen, and the level of the IgE response.

SYSTEMS AFFECTED
• Skin/Exocrine—pruritus, urticaria, and edema
• Respiratory (cats)—dyspnea and cyanosis
• Gastrointestinal—salivation, vomiting, and diarrhea
• Hepatobiliary (dogs)—because of portal hypertension and vasoconstriction

GENETICS
Familial basis reported for type I hypersensitivity reaction in dogs

INCIDENCE/PREVALENCE
• Localized type I hypersensitivity reactions not uncommon
• Systemic type I hypersensitivity reactions rare

GEOGRAPHIC DISTRIBUTION
None

SIGNALMENT

Species
Dogs and cats

Breed Predilections
• Dogs—numerous breeds documented as having a predilection for developing atopy.
• Cats—no breeds documented as having predilection for atopy

Mean Age and Range
• Dogs–age of clinical onset ranges from 3 months to several years of age; most affected animals 1–3 years old
• Cats–age of clinical onset ranges from 6 months to 2 years.

Predominant Sex
• Dogs–atopy more common in females
• Cats–no reported sex predilection

SIGNS

General Comments
• Initial clinical signs vary depending on the route of exposure to the inciting antigen (allergen).
• Shock—end result of a severe anaphylactic reaction
• Shock organ—dogs, liver; cats, respiratory and gastrointestinal systems
• May be localized to the site of exposure, but may progress to a systemic reaction

Historical Findings
• Onset of signs immediate (within minutes)
• Dogs—pruritus, urticaria, vomiting, defecation, and urination
• Cats—intense pruritus about the head, dyspnea, salivation, and vomiting

Physical Examination Findings
• Localized cutaneous edema at the site of exposure
• Hepatomegaly in some dogs
• Hyperexcitability possible in early stages
• Depression and collapse terminally

CAUSES
Virtually any agent; those commonly reported include venoms, blood-based products, vaccines, foods, and drugs.

RISK FACTORS
Previous exposure (sensitization) increases the chance of the animal developing a reaction.

 DIAGNOSIS

DIFFERENTIAL DIAGNOSIS
• Other types of shock
• Trauma
• Depends on the major organ system involved or if reaction is localized; diagnosis can be made largely on the basis of history and clinical signs.

CBC/BIOCHEMISTRY/URINALYSIS
Because of the acute onset of disease, no tests available that reliably predict individual susceptibility

OTHER LABORATORY TESTS
• Intradermal skin testing to identify allergens
• Radioallergosorbent test to quantify the concentration of serum IgE specific for a particular antigen

IMAGING
N/A

DIAGNOSTIC PROCEDURES
Limited because a severely allergic animal can develop an anaphylactic reaction when exposed to even small quantities of antigen

PATHOLOGIC FINDINGS
• Lesions vary, depending on severity of reaction, from localized cutaneous edema to severe pulmonary edema (in cats) and visceral pooling of blood (in dogs).
• Other nonspecific findings vary and are characteristic of shock.
• Nonspecific characteristics of localized reactions include edema, vasculitis, and thromboembolism.

HYPERSENSITIVITY REACTION (ANAPHYLAXIS)

 TREATMENT

APPROPRIATE HEALTH CARE
In an acutely affected animal, the reaction is considered a medical emergency requiring hospitalization.

NURSING CARE
Elimination of inciting antigen, if possible

Systemic Anaphylaxis
• Goal—emergency life support through the maintenance of an open airway, preventing circulatory collapse, and re-establishing physiologic parameters
• Administer fluids intravenously at shock dosages to counteract hypotension.

Localized Anaphylaxis
Goal—limit the reaction and prevent progression to a systemic reaction.

ACTIVITY
N/A

DIET
If a food-based allergen is suspected (uncommon), avoid foods associated with hypersensitivity reaction.

CLIENT EDUCATION
• Discuss the unpredictable nature of the disease.
• Discuss the need to recognize that the animal has an allergic condition that may require immediate medical care.

SURGICAL CONSIDERATIONS
None

 MEDICATIONS

DRUGS OF CHOICE

Systemic Anaphylaxis
• Epinephrine hydrochloride parenterally (1:1000; 0.01 mL/kg) for shock
• Corticosteroids for shock—prednisolone sodium succinate (10–30 mg/kg IV q8h) or dexamethasone sodium phosphate (6–15 mg/kg IV q12h)
• Atropine sulfate (0.04 mg/kg IM) to counteract bradycardia and hypotension
• Aminophylline (10 mg/kg IM or slowly IV) in severely dyspneic patients

Localized Anaphylaxis
• Diphenhydramine hydrochloride (1–2 mg/kg IV or IM)
• Prednisolone (2 mg/kg PO)
• Epinephrine hydrochloride (0.15 ml SC at site of initiation)
• If shock develops, initiate treatment for a systemic anaphylaxis.

CONTRAINDICATIONS
None

PRECAUTIONS
Localized reaction can develop into systemic reaction.

POSSIBLE INTERACTIONS
N/A

ALTERNATIVE DRUGS
N/A

 FOLLOW-UP

PATIENT MONITORING
Closely monitor hospitalized patients for 24–48 hr.

PREVENTION/AVOIDANCE
If inciting antigen (allergen) can be identified, eliminate or reduce exposure.

POSSIBLE COMPLICATIONS
None

EXPECTED COURSE AND PROGNOSIS
• If localized reaction is treated early, prognosis is good.
• If the animal is in shock on examination, prognosis guarded to poor

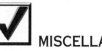 MISCELLANEOUS

ASSOCIATED CONDITIONS
None

AGE-RELATED FACTORS
None

ZOONOTIC POTENTIAL
None

PREGNANCY
N/A

SYNONYMS
None

SEE ALSO
• Atopy
• Shock, Cardiogenic

Suggested Reading
Mueller DL, Noxon JO. Anaphylaxis: pathophysiology and treatment. Compend Contin Ed Pract Vet 1990;12:157–170.
Author Paul W. Snyder
Consulting Editor Susan M. Cotter

HYPERTENSION, PORTAL

BASICS

DEFINITION
Portal pressure > 13 cm H_2O

PATHOPHYSIOLOGY
• Caused by an increase in portal blood flow, an increase in resistance to portal blood flow, or a combination • Increased resistance—most common cause; owing to disease; anatomic site used to classify the mechanism: prehepatic (abdominal portion of the portal vein), hepatic (within the liver), or posthepatic (hepatic veins, caudal vena cava, and heart) • Consequences—development of multiple acquired portosystemic shunts with subsequent hepatic encephalopathy; alterations in abdominal lymph production • Acquired portosystemic shunts—usually connect the abdominal portal system and the caudal vena cava; may develop with any cause of portal hypertension; occur within 1–2 months of onset of hypertension • Ascitic fluid (secondary to posthepatic disorders)—modified transudate (protein > 2.5 g/dL); represents increased production of protein-rich hepatic and mesenteric lymph • Ascitic effusion (secondary to severe liver disease)—typically a pure transudate (protein < 2.5 g/dL and acellular) • Ascites (prehepatic causes)—often short-lived; low protein content, which reflects splanchnic lymph; more likely to develop when portal hypertension coexists with symptomatic hypoalbuminemia (albumin < 1.5 g/dL)

SYSTEMS AFFECTED
• Hepatobiliary—obstruction of blood flow causes distention of the venous bed behind the obstruction; passive congestion of the spleen causes splenomegaly; passive congestion of the liver caused by posthepatic disorders only results in hepatomegaly. • Nervous—hepatic encephalopathy • Cardiovascular—multiple portosystemic shunts and ascites • Gastrointestinal—splanchnic tissue edema; increased gut wall permeability; endotoxemia; predisposition to ulceration; malnutrition owing to reduced nutrient assimilation

GENETICS
Increased occurrence in some breeds and kindreds—hepatic vascular anomalies; idiopathic hepatic fibrosis; copper storage hepatopathy; some chronic hepatopathies

INCIDENCE/PREVALENCE
N/A

GEOGRAPHIC DISTRIBUTION
N/A

SIGNALMENT
Species
• Dogs and cats • More common in dogs

BREED PREDILECTIONS
Familial hepatic vascular disorders reported—Dobermans (noncirrhotic portal hypertension); St. Bernards (arteriovenous fistula), black standard poodles (idiopathic hepatobiliary fibrosis), German shepherds (idiopathic hepatobiliary fibrosis)

Mean Age and Range
• Juveniles—familial or inherited disorders; congenital vena cava and cardiac malformations • Young dogs (< 2 years of age)—idiopathic hepatic fibrosis • Young dogs (< 6 months of age)—onset of signs associated with congenital vascular malformations

Predominant Sex
N/A

SIGNS
General Comments
• Depend on the site, degree, and rate of development and on the underlying cause • Most underlying disorders are chronic.

Historical Findings
• Abdominal distention • Ascites • Hepatic encephalopathy—may be secondary to acquired portosystemic shunts • Cardiac disorder—cough; exercise intolerance; dyspnea • Portal thromboembolism—bloody diarrhea; ileus; abdominal pain

Physical Examination Findings
• Abdominal effusion • Splenomegaly • Hepatomegaly—posthepatic causes only • Jugular vein distention—cardiogenic causes • Hepatojugular reflex • Muffled heart sounds—pericardial disease; concurrent pleural effusion • Cardiac arrhythmias or murmur—cardiac disease • Pulmonary crackles (edema)—cardiogenic causes • Hepatic encephalopathy • Jaundice • Hepatic bruit—(arteriovenous fistula) • Changes noted after ligation of PSVA (see Portosystemic Shunt)

CAUSES
Prehepatic
• Portal vein thrombosis, stenosis, or neoplasia • Congenital portal vein hypoplasia • Portal vein compression—large lymph node; neoplasm; granuloma; abscess • Postoperative complication of congenital portosystemic shunt ligation

Intrahepatic
• Cirrhosis or fibrosis of the liver • Chronic hepatitis or cholangiohepatitis • Chronic extrahepatic bile duct obstruction • Idiopathic hepatic fibrosis • Hepatic neoplasia—porta hepatis location • Liver entrapment in diaphragmatic hernia • Veno-occlusive disease • Noncirrhotic portal hypertension • Portal vein hypoplasia • Hepatic arteriovenous fistula

Posthepatic
• Right-sided congestive heart failure • Heartworm disease • Pericardial tamponade • Pericarditis—restrictive or constrictive • Cardiac neoplasia • Cor triatriatum dexter • Thrombosis of supradiaphragmatic caudal vena cava • Kinked caudal vena cava • Diaphragmatic hernia with vascular entrapment

RISK FACTORS
Depend on underlying cause

DIAGNOSIS

DIFFERENTIAL DIAGNOSIS
• Physicochemical analysis of abdominal effusion—helps narrow diagnosis • Pure transudate—hypoalbuminemia secondary to PLE; PLN; liver failure • Modified transudate with normal or low albumin—PLE; PLN; liver failure (chronic effusion); neoplasia; abdominal thromboembolism; visceral entrapment in diaphragmatic hernia • Modified transudate with large liver, jugular distention, and hepatojugular reflex—cardiac abnormalities; pericardial abnormalities; heartworms • Modified transudate with large liver and without jugular distention, muffled heart, and pulmonary edema—kinked vena cava; Budd-Chiari syndrome • Hepatic encephalopathy—liver fibrosis; cirrhosis; juvenile liver disorders; intrahepatic arteriovenous fistula • Jaundice—liver disease • Bloody diarrhea, abdominal pain, ileus, signs of endotoxemia—acute abdominal portal venous thromboembolism

CBC/BIOCHEMISTRY/URINALYSIS
• CBC—schistocytes with thromboembolism; RBC microcytosis with acquired portosystemic shunt or PSVA; jaundiced plasma with liver disease • Biochemistry—liver disease associated variably with high liver enzymes, low BUN, creatinine, cholesterol, glucose, hyperbilirubinemia, and coagulation abnormalities; posthepatic disorders associated with high liver enzymes, sometimes azotemia, and anicteric plasma • Urinalysis—ammonium biurate crystalluria and low urine specific gravity with acquired portosystemic shunt; may note granular casts with thromboembolism; may note proteinuria with heartworm disease

OTHER LABORATORY TESTS
• Serum bile acids—shunting pattern with acquired portosystemic shunts • Blood ammonia—hyperammonemia associated with underlying liver disease and acquired portosystemic shunts • Physicochemical characterization of abdominal effusion

IMAGING
Radiography
• Thoracic—reveals abnormalities attributable to posthepatic disorders (e.g., kinked vena

cava, pericardial tamponade, pulmonary edema, pleural effusion, diaphragmatic hernia) • Abdominal—may reveal ascites, splenomegaly, liver size (large in congestion, arteriovenous fistula; small in PSVA and most disorders causing acquired portosystemic shunts)

Abdominal Ultrasonography
• Inspect portal perfusion dynamics and vessel distention • Detect acquired portosystemic shunts or PSVA • Appraise visceral parenchyma and lymph nodes (neoplasia, other disorders) • Identify portal hypoplasia, stricture, and occlusion in porta hepatis • Estimate hepatic venous distention—intrahepatic and supradiaphragmatic • Echocardiography—detect congenital disorders, neoplasia, thrombi, heartworms, pleural effusion, malformed or thrombosed vena cava, and diaphragmatic hernia

Angiography and Nuclear Imaging
• Colorectal scintigraphy—confirm portosystemic shunting • Angiography—demonstrate celiac trunk or proper hepatic artery for arteriovenous fistula • Nonselective or selective studies—congenital cardiac and thromboembolic disorders • Portovenogram—veno-occlusive or Budd-Chiari syndromes

DIAGNOSTIC PROCEDURES
• Electrocardiography and central venous pressure—with cardiac disease • Liver biopsy—required with hepatic disorders • Portal pressure—may measure during laparotomy; unreliable in deducing underlying causes; somewhat blunted with acquired portosystemic shunts

 TREATMENT

APPROPRIATE HEALTH CARE
Inpatient—severe signs of hepatic encephalopathy

NURSING CARE
• Fluid therapy—with all causes; restrict sodium concentration (avoid 0.9% NaCl) because of the high likelihood of total body sodium loading • Monitor body weight, girth circumference, plasma proteins, and PCV—assess hydration status and tolerance of fluid infusion • Low oncotic pressure—colloid or albumin indicated; avoid dextran with hepatic dysfunction; plasma preferred for liver patients (or use hetastarch at 20 mL/kg/day) • Glucose supplementation–with hepatic dysfunction and hypoglycemic; 2.5% dextrose with half-strength polyionic fluids initially; titrate dextrose concentration to achieve euglycemia and avoid hyperglycemia. • Therapeutic abdominocentesis—only if abdominal distention is causing discomfort or impairing ventilatory

effort or when medical efforts at ascites mobilization have failed; repeated large-volume procedure may cause dehydration, hypoproteinemia, electrolyte depletions, and introduce infection.

ACTIVITY
Depends on cause

DIET
• Ascites—restricted sodium • Hepatic encephalopathy—restricted protein

CLIENT EDUCATION
• Inform client that definitive diagnosis requires a logical progressive diagnostic strategy. • Inform client that there can be no prediction for cure or chronic amelioration until a definitive diagnosis is ascertained.

SURGICAL CONSIDERATIONS
• Ligation of acquired portosystemic shunts—contraindicated; may result in fatal portal hypertension; if acute symptomatic portal, hypertension develops after the procedure; the ligature must be removed. • Embolectomy of thrombi—not recommended; streptokinase or tissue-plasminogen activator • Correction of chronic diaphragmatic hernia—high-risk procedure • Surgical correction and cure of cor triatriatum dexter and kinked vena cava—possible • Pericardectomy—pericardial restriction or tamponade • Remove tumor or fibrous adhesions causing veno-occlusion.

 MEDICATIONS

DRUGS OF CHOICE
• Diuretics—spironolactone (1–2 mg/kg PO q12h) combined with furosemide (1–2 mg/kg PO q12h) with liver disease; furosemide and enalapril with cardiac dysfunction
• See also Hepatic Encephalopathy

CONTRAINDICATIONS
N/A

PRECAUTIONS
N/A

POSSIBLE INTERACTIONS
• Avoid drugs that rely on first-pass hepatic extraction, biotransformation, or hepatic elimination, if possible; if not possible, reduce the dosage.
• Reduce dose of highly protein-bound drugs with hypoalbuminemia.

ALTERNATIVE DRUGS
N/A

 FOLLOW-UP

PATIENT MONITORING
• Body weight and girth—sequentially • Hydration • Electrolytes • Acid–base status

• Central venous pressure • Blood pressure • Albumin—with hypoalbuminemia • Glucose—with liver disease • Lung sounds, pulse oximetry, ventilatory effort, and central venous pressure—with cardiovascular and/or pulmonary disorder; guard against iatrogenic pulmonary edema during fluid therapy (especially with hypoalbuminemia)

PREVENTION/AVOIDANCE
N/A

POSSIBLE COMPLICATIONS
• Thrombosis • Endotoxemia • Hypotension

EXPECTED COURSE AND PROGNOSIS
Depend on cause

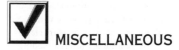 MISCELLANEOUS

ASSOCIATED CONDITIONS
• Chronic liver disease • Disorders causing prehepatic or posthepatic venous occlusion

AGE-RELATED FACTORS
N/A

ZOONOTIC POTENTIAL
N/A

PREGNANCY
Complicates uterine perfusion and likely leads to abortion or stillbirth

SEE ALSO
• Ascites (Abdominal Effusion) • Cirrhosis/Fibrosis of the Liver • Congestive Heart Failure, Right-sided • Hepatic Encephalopathy • Pericarditis • Portosystemic Shunt

ABBREVIATIONS
• PCV = packed cell volume • PLE = protein-losing enteropathy • PLN = protein-losing nephropathy • PSVA = portosystemic venous anomaly

Suggested Reading
Center SA. Pathophysiology of liver disease: normal and abnormal function. In: Guilford WG, Center SA, Strombeck DR, et al., eds. Strombeck's small animal gastroenterology. 3rd ed. Philadelphia: Saunders, 1996:553–632.
Johnson S. Portal hypertension. Part I. Pathophysiology and clinical consequences. Compend Contin Educ Pract Vet 1987;741–750.
Johnson S. Portal hypertension. Part II. Clinical assessment and treatment. Compend Contin Educ Pract Vet 1987;9:7917–930.
Author Susan E. Johnson
Consulting Editor Sharon A. Center

DISEASES

HYPERTENSION, PULMONARY

BASICS

DEFINITION
Elevation in systolic pulmonary artery pressure > 30 mm Hg or mean pulmonary arterial pressure > 20 mm Hg

PATHOPHYSIOLOGY
• Several events can lead to elevations in pulmonary artery pressure. Primary pulmonary hypertension, a congenital abnormality in the pulmonary vasculature, has not been identified in cats or dogs. Secondary pulmonary hypertension can be caused by pulmonary artery or capillary vasoconstriction, pulmonary artery obstruction, high left atrial pressure with resultant pulmonary capillary pressure elevation, or excessive pulmonary arterial blood flow. Hypoxia and associated acidemia commonly result in pulmonary vasoconstriction. • As pressures in the pulmonary capillaries and pulmonary artery rise, the right ventricle hypertrophies to maintain pulmonary blood flow. Pulmonary hypertension leads to abnormalities in pulmonary blood flow and filling of the left ventricle, which can cause dyspnea, weakness, exercise intolerance, and cyanosis. High right heart pressures can cause venous congestion, tricuspid regurgitation, and right-sided congestive heart failure (R-CHF).
• Secondary causes of pulmonary hypertension include severe pulmonary disease (vasoconstriction and obstruction), heartworm disease (vasoconstriction and obstruction), severe left heart disease (high left atrial pressure), pulmonary thromboembolism (obstruction and vasoconstriction), and congenital heart disease with left-to-right shunting (excessive pulmonary blood flow). Extrapulmonary causes of chronic hypoxia such as hypoventilation and high altitude disease can also lead to pulmonary hypertension.

SYSTEMS AFFECTED
• Cardiovascular—pulmonary artery hypertrophy and dilation, right ventricular hypertrophy and dilation (cor pulmonale), right atrial dilation, possible secondary tricuspid regurgitation, possible R-CHF • Respiratory—pulmonary abnormalities may cause pulmonary hypertension

GENETICS
No genetic basis found; pulmonary hypertension can be secondary to several congenital heart defects that may have a genetic basis.

INCIDENCE/PREVALENCE
• Unknown • No cases of idiopathic primary pulmonary hypertension documented in the veterinary literature

GEOGRAPHIC DISTRIBUTION
Unknown; may be a relatively higher prevalence in heartworm endemic areas and at high altitudes

SIGNALMENT

Species
Dogs and cats

Breed Predilections
May be based on underlying cause of pulmonary hypertension (e.g. congenital heart disease)

Mean Age and Range
N/A

Predominant Sex
N/A

SIGNS

General Comments
May be due to pulmonary hypertension or the underlying primary disease

Historical Findings
• Exercise intolerance • Dyspnea • Coughing/hemoptysis • Syncope • Abdominal distention • Weight loss

Physical Examination Findings
• Dyspnea • Coughing • Hemoptysis • Loud or split second heart sound • Abnormal lung sounds • Cyanosis • Heart murmur • Abdominal distention • Jugular distention • Weight loss

CAUSES

Pulmonary Parenchymal Disease (Vasoconstriction from Chronic Hypoxia and Acidemia)
• Vascular obstruction from pulmonary fibrosis, vascular hypertrophy, and infiltrative disease • Chronic bronchitis • Eosinophilic bronchitis • Disseminated neoplasia • Adult respiratory distress syndrome

Pulmonary Thromboembolism (Vascular Obstruction and Secondary Vasoconstriction)
• Hyperadrenocorticism • Protein-losing nephropathy • Sepsis • Heartworm disease • Immune-mediated hemolytic anemia • Neoplasia • Pancreatitis • Endocarditis • Disseminated intravascular coagulation • Cardiac disease

Congenital Heart Disease with Left-to-Right Shunting (Excessive Pulmonary Blood Flow and Reactive Vasoconstriction)
• Patent ductus arteriosus • Ventricular septal defect • Atrial septal defect • Probably a rare cause of pulmonary hypertension

Heartworm Disease (Vascular Obstruction Secondary to Vascular Hypertrophy and Thromboembolism—Reactive Vasoconstriction)

Left Heart Disease (High Left Atrial Pressure)
• Mitral regurgitation • Dilated cardiomyopathy • Hypertrophic cardiomyopathy • Restrictive cardiomyopathy • Mitral stenosis • Left atrial tumors

Extrapulmonary Causes of Chronic Hypoxia (Vasoconstriction from Hypoxia and Acidemia)
• Hypoventilation (Pickwickian syndrome, neuromuscular disorders) • High altitude disease • Idiopathic primary pulmonary hypertension • Not documented in dogs or cats

RISK FACTORS
• Cardiac and pulmonary disease • Heartworm disease • Diseases associated with pulmonary thromboembolism • Obesity • High altitude

DIAGNOSIS

DIFFERENTIAL DIAGNOSIS
• L-CHF without pulmonary hypertension • Collapsing trachea • Primary right-sided heart disease • Significant pulmonary disease without pulmonary hypertension • Heartworm disease • Pneumothorax • Pyothorax • Hemothorax • Laryngeal paralysis

CBC/BIOCHEMISTRY/URINALYSIS
• Findings vary with underlying cause. • No consistent findings associated with pulmonary hypertension • Polycythemia can be seen if marked hypoxia

OTHER LABORATORY TESTS
• Arterial blood gases (hypoxemia) • Occult heartworm test • Workup for causes of pulmonary thromboembolism (urine protein: creatinine ratio, antithrombin III level, coagulation profile, ACTH stimulation test, low-dose dexamethasone suppression test) • Fluid analysis of pleural or abdominal effusions

IMAGING

Radiography
• Large pulmonary artery • Large right ventricle • Dilated caudal vena cava • Pleural effusion • Hepatomegaly • Ascites • Other findings vary with cause, but might include evidence of primary pulmonary disease, pulmonary embolism, and heartworm disease.

Echocardiography
• Right ventricular hypertrophy • Right ventricular dilation • Right atrial dilation • Pulmonary artery dilation • Pleural effusion • Mild pericardial effusion • If tricuspid valve insufficiency, systolic pressure gradients can be estimated with Doppler (>30 mm Hg) • Evidence of left heart disease, heartworm disease, congenital heart disease, or pulmonary thromboembolism, depending on cause of pulmonary hypertension

DIAGNOSTIC PROCEDURES
Transtracheal wash or bronchoalveolar lavage

Electrocardiography
• Right mean electrical axis deviation • Deep S waves in leads I, II, III, and aVF • Widening of QRS complex • Tall P waves (i.e., P pulmonale) • ST segment depression may occur with significant hypoxia.

Cardiac Catheterization and Pulmonary Angiography
• May be required to confirm pulmonary hypertension • May demonstrate abnormalities such as heartworms, pulmonary thromboembolism, or vascular changes supporting the underlying cause of pulmonary hypertension

PATHOLOGIC FINDINGS
• Consistent with underlying disease • Pulmonary artery thrombus • Dilated pulmonary artery • Right heart enlargement • Heartworms • Pleural effusion • Ascites • Medial hypertrophy of pulmonary vasculature • Intimal proliferation and sclerosis of pulmonary vasculature • Necrotizing arteritis

TREATMENT

APPROPRIATE HEALTH CARE
• Hospitalize patients in severe respiratory distress until stable. • Administer oxygen therapy, bronchodilators, diuretics, and antibiotics on an emergency basis in accordance with underlying disease.

NURSING CARE
• Monitor hydration and body temperature closely. • Administer fluid therapy judiciously on basis of hydration status and presence of right-sided cardiac disease; right-sided cardiac disease may contraindicate fluid therapy. • Maintain low-stress environment.

ACTIVITY
Restricted

DIET
Specific guidelines based on underlying disease; if heart failure, restricted sodium diet may have benefit

CLIENT EDUCATION
• Diagnosis often presumptive without catheterization or Doppler echocardiography • Prognosis varies with reversibility of the underlying disease, but is very guarded in most cases. • Avoid environments that may predispose to respiratory distress—excessively cold or dry air, excessive heat, second-hand smoke, high altitudes

SURGICAL CONSIDERATIONS
N/A

MEDICATIONS

DRUGS OF CHOICE
• Medical management is controversial; direct treatment at the primary underlying disease process. • The ideal therapeutic agent should reduce pulmonary vascular resistance and hypertension without affecting the systemic circulation; oxygen can accomplish this, but long-term oxygen administration is not feasible in these patients; short-term or intermittent use of oxygen may be beneficial.

Vasodilators
• Ideally, base selection on pulmonary and systemic blood pressure response during cardiac catheterization. • Choices include ACE inhibitors (e.g., enalapril, benazepril), hydralazine, and calcium channel blockers. • Often not useful due to development of systemic hypertension.

Bronchodilators
• May benefit treatment of hypoxia-mediated pulmonary hypertension (i.e. pulmonary disease) • Choices include sympathomimetics (e.g., terbutaline) and methylxanthines (e.g., theophylline, aminophylline). • Bronchodilators may have additional positive inotropic effects.

Positive Inotropes (Digoxin, Dobutamine)
• Not a primary treatment of pulmonary hypertension • May improve right heart function and resolve CHF • Monitor closely for digoxin-related arrhythmias.

Anticoagulant Therapy
• Indicated if thromboembolic disease diagnosed • Questionable efficacy • Choices include heparin, warfarin, and aspirin.

CONTRAINDICATIONS
• Drugs or situations that worsen pulmonary hypoxia (e.g., respiratory depressants) • Drugs that depress cardiac function (e.g., β-blockers) • Drugs that cause vasoconstriction

PRECAUTIONS
• Excessive administration of vasodilators can cause systemic hypotension. • Excessive use of bronchodilators can lead to detrimental tachycardia and hyperexcitability. • Monitor coagulation profiles closely during anticoagulation.

POSSIBLE INTERACTIONS
N/A

ALTERNATIVE DRUGS
N/A

FOLLOW-UP

PATIENT MONITORING
• Physical examination with careful cardiac and pulmonary auscultation • Clinical signs, closely • Thoracic radiography • Arterial blood gases • Echocardiography • Electrocardiography

PREVENTION/AVOIDANCE
Give client complete understanding of conditions that predispose to pulmonary hypertension.

POSSIBLE COMPLICATIONS
• Right-sided heart failure • Syncope • Cardiac arrhythmias • Sudden death

EXPECTED COURSE AND PROGNOSIS
• Based on ability to reverse underlying disease • When changes are irreversible, treatment is palliative. • In general very guarded

MISCELLANEOUS

ASSOCIATED CONDITIONS
See causes

AGE-RELATED FACTORS
N/A

ZOONOTIC POTENTIAL
None

PREGNANCY
High risk

SYNONYMS
N/A

SEE ALSO
Diseases causing pulmonary hypertension

ABBREVIATIONS
ACE = angiotensin-converting enzyme

Suggested Reading
Hawkins EC. Disease of the lower respiratory tract. In: Ettinger SJ, Feldman EC, eds. Textbook of veterinary internal medicine. 4th ed. Philadelphia: Saunders, 1995.

Johnson LR, Hamlin RL. Recognition and treatment of pulmonary hypertension. In: Bonagura, JD, ed. Current veterinary therapy XII. Philadelphia: Saunders, 1995.

Perry LA, Dillon AR, Bowers TL. Pulmonary hypertension. Compend Cont Ed Pract Vet 1991;13:226.

Rich S, Braunwald E, Grossman W. Pulmonary hypertension. In: Braunwald E, ed. Heart disease. 5th ed. Philadelphia: Saunders, 1997.

Wiedmann HP, Matthay RA. Cor Pulmonale. In: Braunwald E, ed. Heart disease. 5th ed. Philadelphia: Saunders, 1997.

Author Donald P. Schrope

Consulting Editors Larry P. Tilley and Francis W. K. Smith, Jr.

HYPERTENSION, SYSTEMIC

 BASICS

DEFINITION
Sustained elevation in systolic or diastolic (or both) arterial blood pressure

PATHOPHYSIOLOGY
• Blood pressure is determined by cardiac output and systemic vascular resistance; cardiac output determined by heart rate and stroke volume; systemic arterial blood pressure regulation depends on integration of complex mechanisms within the central and peripheral nervous systems, renal and cardiac tissues, and humoral factors, which synergistically affect cardiac output and peripheral vascular resistance.
• Baroreceptors in the carotid sinus and aortic arch respond to changes in blood pressure; a fall in blood pressure increases sympathetic discharge, causing vasoconstriction and increased cardiac contractility and heart rate to return blood pressure to normal, humoral substances that modulate blood pressure include catecholamines, vasopressin, kinins, renin, angiotensin, aldosterone, prostaglandins, and atrial natriuretic peptide; the renin-angiotensin-aldosterone system is probably the most important component. • Hypertension—primary (e.g., essential or idiopathic) or secondary to an underlying disease process; secondary hypertension is more common in veterinary medicine; cause of primary hypertension is not fully understood but some has a hereditary component.

SYSTEMS AFFECTED
• Cardiovascular • Renal/Urologic • Ocular • Nervous

GENETICS
Colonies of hypertensive dogs have been produced by mating dogs with essential hypertension; mode of inheritance not known

INCIDENCE/PREVALENCE
Unknown; diagnosed more frequently now that more veterinarians are monitoring blood pressure. One study found that 65% of cats with chronic renal failure and 87% of cats with hyperthyroidism had mild hypertension. A study of clinically normal dogs documented hypertension in 10% (blood pressure more than 2 standard deviations above the mean).

SIGNALMENT

Species
Dogs and cats

Breed Predilection
None

Mean Age and Range
• Dogs—mean age 8.9 ± 3.6 years; range 2–14 years • Cats—mean age 15.1 ± 3.8 years; range 4–20 years

SIGNS
• Acute blindness • Ocular hemorrhage • Dilated pupils • Retinal detachment • Swollen or shrunken kidneys • Hematuria • Epistaxis • Seizures, disorientation, ataxia, circling, hemiparesis, paraparesis, nystagmus • Cardiac murmurs and gallops; less commonly, CHF • Palpable thyroid gland (when hyperthyroid)

CAUSES

Primary or Essential
Not known

Secondary
• Renal disease—end-stage renal disease, glomerulonephritis, amyloidosis, renal artery stenosis • Hyperadrenocorticism • Hyperthyroidism • Diabetes mellitus—uncommon • Pheochromocytoma—rare condition • Hyperaldosteronism—rare condition • Central nervous system disease

 DIAGNOSIS

DIFFERENTIAL DIAGNOSIS
• Cardiovascular—hypertrophic cardiomyopathy, hyperthyroid heart disease, aortic stenosis, arterial thromboembolic disease • Ophthalmic—ocular trauma, systemic infections (bacterial, fungal, viral), coagulopathies, vasculopathy • Neurologic—primary brain, spinal cord, or peripheral nerve disease • Physical examination and results of biochemistry tests and urinalysis important for establishing the underlying cause for secondary hypertension

CBC/BIOCHEMISTRY/URINALYSIS
• CBC usually normal • Biochemistry may reveal azotemia and hyperphosphatemia (renal insufficiency), hyperglycemia (diabetes mellitus), high serum alkaline phosphatase (hyperadrenocorticism), or electrolyte imbalances. • Urinalysis may reveal proteinuria and hematuria (glomerulonephritis and amyloidosis), poor concentration ability (renal insufficiency, hyperadrenocorticism), or glucosuria (diabetes mellitus).

OTHER LABORATORY TESTS
• Glomerulonephropathy—high urine protein:urine creatinine ratio, low creatinine clearance • Renal dysfunction—low creatinine clearance • Hyperadrenocorticism—exaggerated ACTH response test, failure to suppress with dexamethasone, high urine cortisol:creatinine ratio • Hyperthyroidism (cats)—high T_4, inadequate suppression with a T_3 suppression test • Hypothyroidism (dogs)—low T_3, T_4, free T_3, free T_4; possibly high T_3 and T_4 autoantibodies, high endogenous TSH, and depressed TSH stimulation test result • Pheochromocytoma—high urinary vanillylmandelic acid • Hyperaldosteronism—24-h urine aldosterone and plasma aldosterone concentrations high

IMAGING
• Thoracic radiograph to evaluate secondary cardiac changes (mild cardiomegaly) • Abdominal radiographs to evaluate liver, adrenals, and kidneys • Echocardiogram to evaluate hypertensive heart disease (left ventricular free wall and/or interventricular septal hypertrophy and mild left atrial dilation) • Abdominal ultrasound to evaluate kidneys and adrenal glands • CT or MRI scan if brain tumor or hyperadrenocorticism suspected • Thyroid scintigraphy to evaluate hyperthyroidism

DIAGNOSTIC PROCEDURES
Definitive diagnosis of hypertension requires documentation of high arterial blood pressure via direct or indirect methods.

Direct (Invasive)
Measurement using arterial catheterization or puncture and pressure transducer (PDS Monitor, Baxter) is considered the gold standard; equipment is expensive and the technique can cause animal discomfort and is seldom performed in clinical practice.

Indirect (Noninvasive)
Performed correctly, indirect blood pressure measurements correlate well with direct blood pressure measurements. Indirect blood pressure measurements obtained with oscillometric or Doppler techniques; require an inflatable cuff (width of the cuff should be approximately 40% of the circumference of the limb at the site of placement) wrapped around a distal limb or tail

Oscillometric Technique
• Oscillometric technique (Dinamap, Critikon) detects pulse pressure oscillations beneath the cuff bladder that result from changes in arterial diameter; proper cuff size critical for accurate measurement • Place animal in lateral or sternal recumbency or allow to stand in a calm environment. Place artery arrow marker on the cuff on the palmar aspect of the metacarpal region (or proximal to the carpus with arrow pointed medially), over the craniomedial metatarsal region (or proximal to the tarsus) or on the ventral aspect of the tail in a snug position. Cuff inflates and deflates automatically with blood pressure (systolic, diastolic, and mean); heart rate is automatically calculated and digitally displayed.

Doppler Technique
• Ultrasonic Doppler flow detector (Parks Medical Electronics; Silogic; SDI) • Uses ultrasound waves to detect and audibilize blood flow in an artery distal to the blood pressure cuff • Apply pneumatic cuff in snug position. Distal to the cuff, place the transducer probe crystal over moistened skin, just proximal to the large carpal pad (common digital branch of the radial artery), in a bed of ultrasound gel, and tape or hold in place. Inflate cuff bladder to suprasystemic pressure

until the audible signal is cut off. Deflate cuff at approximately 3 mm Hg/sec). Return of the Doppler signal determines systolic blood pressure. Mark diastolic pressure (not as easy to detect) when Doppler signal pitch changes abruptly or disappears. Doppler technique also detects blood pressure on the ventral aspect of the proximal tail and over the craniomedial aspect of the tarsus.

Blood Pressure Guidelines for Dogs and Cats

Hypertension is currently defined by most investigators as the following:
• Dog: Systolic > 180 mm Hg; diastolic > 100 mm Hg • Cat: Systolic > 170–180 mm Hg; diastolic > 120 mm Hg
Average a series of 3–5 measurements for the most reliable measurement. Interpret all results in light of the animal's excitement level during the procedure and repeat if results are questionable.

PATHOLOGIC FINDINGS

• Arteriolar hypertrophy, tunica media vasorum hyperplasia, and destruction of the internal elastic lamina layer; vascular damage in the eye, kidney, and cardiovascular and nervous system tissues leads to hemorrhage, thrombosis, edema, and necrosis. • Ventricular hypertrophy develops in response to an increased workload.

 TREATMENT

APPROPRIATE HEALTH CARE

Hospitalization may be stressful to the patient; make every attempt to manage them as outpatients. Inpatient care may be necessary depending upon the underlying condition (e.g., fluid therapy in a cat with renal failure) or serious complications related to hypertension (e.g., neurologic signs).

DIET

Influenced by underlying cause; sodium restriction generally advised, although unlikely to lower blood pressure when used alone

CLIENT EDUCATION

• Unless underlying cause is curable (e.g., hyperthyroidism) or controllable (e.g., hyperadrenocorticism), patient is likely to be on antihypertensive medication indefinitely.
• Alert owners to end-organ effects of uncontrolled hypertension (e.g., retinal hemorrhage, retinal detachment, progressive renal impairment, cardiac disease, neurological signs).

SURGICAL CONSIDERATIONS

Dictated by underlying cause; may be indicated for hyperthyroidism, pheochromocytoma, some forms of hyperadrenocorticism

 MEDICATIONS

DRUGS OF CHOICE

Preferred Therapy

• Treat underlying cause. • Cats—calcium channel blocker (i.e., amlodipine) or ACE inhibitor (i.e., benazepril) and sodium-restricted diet • Dogs—calcium channel blocker (i.e., amlodipine) or ACE inhibitor (e.g., enalapril or benazepril) and sodium-restricted diet • β-Blocker or α-adrenergic blocker if no response to ACE inhibitor or calcium channel blocker

ACE Inhibitors

• Lower peripheral vascular resistance and stroke volume by blocking the conversion of angiotensin I to angiotensin II. • Enalapril—dogs, 0.5 mg/kg PO q12–24h; cats, 0.25–0.5 mg/kg PO q24–48h • Benazepril—dogs and cats, 0.25–0.5 mg/kg PO q24h

Calcium Channel Blockers

• Lower peripheral vascular resistance by vasodilation; some lower cardiac output through negative chronotropic and inotropic effects. • Amlodipine—dogs, 0.15–0.25 mg/kg q24h (anecdotal); cats, 0.18 mg/kg PO q24h • Diltiazem: dogs, 0.5–1.5 mg/kg PO q8h; cats, 1.5–2.5 mg/kg PO q8h; diltiazem-CD: cats 10 mg/kg PO q24h

CONTRAINDICATIONS

• β-Blockers might worsen bronchiolar disease, CHF; do not use in patients with second- and third-degree AV blocks.
• Diltiazem—use with caution in patients with CHF and do not use in patients with second- or third-degree AV block.

PRECAUTIONS

Diuretics might induce hypokalemia and metabolic alkalosis; arterial vasodilators can cause reflex tachycardia; any treatment can cause hypotension.

POSSIBLE INTERACTIONS

Combinations of drugs may increase risk of hypotension.

ALTERNATIVE DRUGS

• Diuretics • Lower blood volume and cardiac output • Of little use as a single agent

β-Adrenergic Blockers

• Lower heart rate and cardiac output and suppress renin secretion • Propranolol—dogs, 0.2–1.0 mg/kg PO q8h; cats, 2.5–5 mg/cat PO q8h • Atenolol—dogs, 0.25–1 mg/kg PO q12–24h PO; cats, 6.25–12.5 mg/cat PO q12–24h

Vasodilators

• Lower peripheral vascular resistance by direct action on arteriole smooth muscle. • Hydralazine HCl-dogs, 0.5–2 mg/kg PO q12h; cats, 0.5–0.8 mg/kg PO q12h

 FOLLOW-UP

PATIENT MONITORING

• Blood pressure and hypertensive complications (especially retinopathy) weekly until blood pressure is controlled • Laboratory tests to measure clinical disease response and side effects of medications (e.g., proteinuria, hematuria, anemia, thrombocytopenia, potassium balance, sodium balance, azotemia, albumin)

POSSIBLE COMPLICATIONS

• CHF • Glomerulonephropathy (proteinuria, hematuria) • Renal failure • Retinopathy (hemorrhage, detached retina)
• Cerebral vascular accident (various central nervous system signs)

EXPECTED COURSE AND PROGNOSIS

Dictated by underlying cause; in most patients can be controlled with appropriate therapy

 MISCELLANEOUS

AGE-RELATED FACTORS

Renal failure and hyperthyroidism—more common in older animals

SYNONYM

High blood pressure

SEE ALSO

• Diabetes Mellitus, Uncomplicated
• Glomerulonephritis • Hyperadrenocorticism
• Hyperthyroidism • Pheochromocytoma
• Renal Failure, Acute • Renal Failure, Chronic

ABBREVIATION

• ACE = angiotensin-converting enzyme
• CHF = congestive heart failure

Suggested Reading

Kobayashi DL, Peterson ME, Graves TK, et al. Hypertension in cats with chronic renal failure or hyperthyroidism. J Vet Int Med 1990;4:58–62.
Littman MP. Spontaneous systemic hypertension in 24 cats. J Vet Int Med 1994;8:79–86.
Snyder PS. Amlodipine: a randomized, blinded clinical trial in 9 cats with systemic hypertension. J Vet Intern Med 1998;12(3):157–162.
Snyder PS. Canine hypertensive disease. Compend Cont Ed Pract Vet 1991;13:1785–1793.
Author Patti S. Snyder and Jerry A. Thornhill
Consulting Editors Larry P. Tilley and Francis W. K. Smith, Jr.

DISEASES

HYPERTHYROIDISM

 BASICS

DEFINITION
A pathologic, sustained, high overall metabolism caused by high circulating concentrations of thyroid hormones

PATHOPHYSIOLOGY
• Hyperthyroidism in cats is most often caused by autonomously hyperfunctioning nodules of the thyroid gland that secrete T_4 and T_3, uncontrolled by normal physiologic influences (e.g., TSH secretion); one or both lobes of the thyroid gland can be affected.
• Rare cases of feline hyperthyroidism (1–2%) are caused by hyperfunctioning thyroid carcinoma.
• Extremely uncommon in dogs, it has been seen in some dogs with thyroid carcinoma (most dogs with thyroid gland neoplasia are euthyroid) and in dogs with oversupplementation of exogenous thyroid hormone.

SYSTEMS AFFECTED
• Musculoskeletal—cachexia
• Cardiovascular—myocardial hypertrophy and hypertension
• Gastrointestinal—chronic cellular malnutrition, decreased gastrointestinal transit time, malabsorption, and hepatocellular damage
• Renal/urologic—high GFR may mask underlying chronic renal failure, possible hyperfiltration injury, and decreased urine-concentrating ability
• Nervous
• Behavioral

GENETICS
No known genetic predisposition

INCIDENCE/PREVALENCE
• Most common endocrine disease of cats; one of the most common diseases in late middle-aged and old cats; true incidence is unknown, but diagnosis of the disease is increasing.
• Rare in dogs

GEOGRAPHIC DISTRIBUTION
N/A

SIGNALMENT
Species
Cats and (rarely) dogs
Breed Predilections
None
Mean Age and Range
Mean age in cats, approximately 13 years; range 4–22 years
Predominant Sex
None

SIGNS
General Comments
• Multisystemic; reflect the overall increase in metabolism
• Less than 10% of patients are referred to as "apathetic"; these patients exhibit atypical signs (e.g. poor appetite, anorexia, depression, and weakness).

Historical Findings
• Weight loss
• Polyphagia
• Vomiting
• Diarrhea
• Polydipsia
• Tachypnea
• Hyperactivity
• Dyspnea
• Aggression

Physical Examination Findings
• Large thyroid gland—70% of patients are affected bilaterally
• Poor body condition
• Heart murmur
• Tachycardia
• Gallop rhythm
• Unkempt appearance
• Thickened nails

CAUSES
• Cats—Autonomously hyperfunctioning nodules; rarely, thyroid carcinoma
• Dogs—T_4 or T_3 secretion by a thyroid carcinoma

RISK FACTORS
Unknown

 DIAGNOSIS

DIFFERENTIAL DIAGNOSIS
The clinical signs of feline hyperthyroidism can overlap with those of chronic renal failure, chronic hepatic disease, and neoplasia (especially intestinal lymphoma); they can be excluded on the basis of routine laboratory findings and thyroid function tests.

CBC/BIOCHEMISTRY/URINALYSIS
• Erythrocytosis (mild) and, less commonly, leukocytosis, lymphopenia, and eosinopenia—stress response associated with high T_3 and T_4
• High ALT activity—common
• High ALP, LDH, AST, BUN, creatinine, glucose, phosphorus, and bilirubin—less common; caused by more severe complications of hyperthyroidism

OTHER LABORATORY TESTS
• Serum total T4 concentration (TT_4)—measures for protein-bound and free (unbound) T_4; high resting concentration confirms the diagnosis of hyperthyroidism
• Serum total T_3 concentration—high concentration less reliable than serum TT_4
• Free T_4 (FT_4) by equilibrium dialysis—useful to diagnose mild or early hyperthyroidism in cats; which may have normal resting serum TT_4 concentrations
• In theory, FT_4 more accurately reflects true thyroid gland secretory status, but some cats with nonthyroidal illness exhibit unexplained elevations in FT_4; do not use FT_4 alone as a first-line screening test.
• T_3 suppression test—useful to diagnose mild hyperthyroidism (see Appendix for protocol and interpretation)
• TRH stimulation test—useful to diagnose mild hyperthyroidism (see Appendix for protocol and interpretation)

IMAGING
• Thoracic radiography and echocardiography may be useful in assessing the severity of myocardial disease.
• Dogs—do thoracic radiography to detect pulmonary metastasis.
• Cats—abdominal ultrasound may be useful to explore underlying renal disease.

DIAGNOSTIC PROCEDURES
• Treatment of hyperthyroidism can significantly decrease renal function; pursue any abnormal value revealed by CBC, serum biochemical testing, or urinalysis by bacterial culture of the urine, abdominal radiography, and ultrasonography of the urinary tract.
• Can measure GFR by plasma disappearance of iohexol or appropriate radiopharmaceuticals (if available) in cats with suspected underlying renal disease
• Noninvasive blood pressure measurement may be useful in complete pretreatment assessment and monitoring or therapy.

PATHOLOGIC FINDINGS
• Adenomatous hyperplasia of one or both lobes of the thyroid gland
• Carcinoma in dogs and 1–2% of cats

 TREATMENT

APPROPRIATE HEALTH CARE
• Outpatient management usually suffices for cats, if antithyroid drugs are used.
• Radioiodine treatment and surgical thyroidectomy require inpatient treatment and monitoring.
• Rare cases of overt congestive heart failure require emergency inpatient intensive care.

NURSING CARE
N/A

ACTIVITY
No alterations recommended

DIET

- Resolution of thyrotoxicosis obviates the need for modifications.
- Poor absorption of many nutrients and high metabolism suggest the need for a highly digestible diet with high bioavailability of protein in untreated hyperthyroidism.

CLIENT EDUCATION
- Inform clients of adverse effects of antithyroid drugs (see below) and surgical complications.
- Clients should be aware of possible (rare) recurrence after treatment.

SURGICAL CONSIDERATIONS
- Surgical thyroidectomy is one recommended treatment for hyperthyroidism in cats.
- Surgical treatment of thyroid carcinoma (dogs and cats) is usually not curative, but can be palliative.

MEDICATIONS

DRUGS OF CHOICE
- Methimazole (Tapazole) is most often recommended (10–15 mg/day divided q8–12h).
- β-Adrenergic blocking drugs—sometimes used to treat some of the cardiovascular and neurologic effects of excess thyroid hormone; can be used in combination with methimazole; mainly used to prepare the patient for surgical thyroidectomy or radioiodine therapy
- Radioiodine is a safe and effective treatment; availability of veterinary facilities offering this treatment is limited but increasing.

CONTRAINDICATIONS
N/A

PRECAUTIONS
- Antithyroid drugs have several side effects.
- Anorexia and vomiting are common side effects of methimazole; rare side effects include self-induced excoriation of the face, thrombocytopenia, bleeding diathesis, agranulocytosis, serum antinuclear antibodies, and hepatopathy.
- Side effects usually develop within the first 3 months of treatment and may or may not necessitate drug cessation and alternative treatment (depending on severity).
- Bleeding, jaundice, and agranulocytosis necessitate immediate withdrawal of the drug.

POSSIBLE INTERACTIONS
N/A

ALTERNATIVE DRUGS
- Carbimazole—another useful antithyroid drug; not available in the United States.
- Propylthiouracil—can be useful if methimazole is unavailable; adverse effects may be more common and more severe than with methimazole.
- Ipodate—a radiographic contrast agent; can be used to treat some cases of mild hyperthyroidism, but not effective in most hyperthyroid patients; long-term effectiveness has not been established.

FOLLOW-UP

PATIENT MONITORING
- Methimazole—physical examination, CBC (with platelet count), serum biochemical analysis, and serum T_4 determination every 2–3 weeks for the initial 3 months of treatment; adjust the dosage to maintain serum T_4 concentration in the low-normal range.
- Surgical thyroidectomy—watch for development of hypocalcemia and/or laryngeal paralysis during the initial postoperative period; measure serum T_4 concentrations in the first week of surgery and every 3–6 months thereafter to check for recurrence.
- Radioiodine—measure serum T_4 concentrations 2 weeks after treatment and every 3–6 months subsequently.
- Renal function—GFR declines following treatment in most patients; therefore, perform a physical examination, serum biochemistry, and urinalysis 1 month after treatment and then as indicated by the clinical history.

PREVENTION/AVOIDANCE
N/A

POSSIBLE COMPLICATIONS
- Untreated disease can lead to congestive heart failure, intractable diarrhea, renal damage, retinal detachment (as a result of hypertension), and death.
- Complications of surgical treatment include hypoparathyroidism, hypothyroidism, and laryngeal paralysis.
- Hypothyroidism is rare following radioiodine therapy.

EXPECTED COURSE AND PROGNOSIS
- Uncomplicated disease—prognosis is excellent; recurrence is possible and is most commonly associated with poor owner compliance with medical management; regrowth of hyperthyroid tissue is possible but uncommon after surgical thyroidectomy or radioiodine treatment.
- Dogs or cats with thyroid carcinoma—prognosis is poor; treatment with radioiodine, surgery, or both is usually followed by recurrence of disease; adjuvant chemotherapy is of questionable benefit.

MISCELLANEOUS

ASSOCIATED CONDITIONS
- In cats with underlying renal disease (either secondary to chronic hypertension or unrelated to thyroid disease), the prognosis is less favorable.
- Renal insufficiency may not become apparent until euthyroidism has been established; for this reason, a reversible form of treatment (i.e., antithyroid drugs) is recommended if renal disease is suspected in a cat with hyperthyroidism.
- In some patients, hyperthyroidism might best be left untreated.

AGE-RELATED FACTORS
N/A

ZOONOTIC POTENTIAL
N/A

PREGNANCY
N/A

SYNONYMS
- Thyrotoxicosis
- Multinodular toxic goiter
- Plummer's disease

SEE ALSO
- Hypoparathyroidism
- Cardiomyopathy, Hypertrophic—Cats
- Congestive Heart Failure, Left-sided
- Hypertension, Systemic

ABBREVIATIONS
- ALP = alkaline phosphatase
- FT_4 = free thyroxine
- GFR = glomerular filtration rate
- TT_4 = total thyroxine
- T_4 = thyroxine
- T_3 = triiodothyronine
- TSH = thyrotropin
- TRH = thyrotropin-releasing hormone

Suggested Reading

Graves TK, Peterson ME. Occult hyperthyroidism in cats. In: Kirk RW, Bonagura JD, eds. Current veterinary therapy XI. Philadelphia: Saunders, 1992:334–337

Graves TK. Complications of treatment and concurrent illness associated with feline hyperthyroidism. In: Kirk RW, Bonagura JD, eds. Current veterinary therapy XII. Philadelphia: Saunders, 1995:

Graves TK. Hyperthyroidism and the kidney. In August JR, ed. Consultations in feline internal medicine 3, Philadelphia: Saunders, 1997:

Peterson ME. Hyperthyroid diseases. In: Ettinger SJ, Feldman EC, eds. Textbook of veterinary internal medicine. 4th ed. Philadelphia: Saunders, 1994:

Author Thomas K. Graves
Consulting Editor Deborah S. Greco

HYPERTROPHIC OSTEODYSTROPHY

BASICS

DEFINITION
An inflammatory disease of bone that affects rapidly growing puppies

PATHOPHYSIOLOGY
• Characterized by nonseptic suppurative inflammation within metaphyseal trabeculae of long bones
• Rapidly growing bones more severely affected
• Metaphyses—widened owing to perimetaphyseal swelling and bone deposition
• Trabecular microfracture and metaphyseal separation—occur adjacent and parallel to the physis
• Bone formation defective
• Ossifying periostitis—may be extensive

SYSTEMS AFFECTED
• Musculoskeletal—symmetrical distribution; distal forelimbs most severely affected; may note soft tissue mineralization in other organs; widened costochondral junctions
• Respiratory—interstitial pneumonia
• Gastrointestinal—diarrhea

GENETICS
No basis

INCIDENCE/PREVALENCE
Low

GEOGRAPHIC DISTRIBUTION
N/A

SIGNALMENT

Species
Dogs

Breed Predilections
• Large, rapidly growing breeds
• Great Danes—most common
• Reported—Irish wolfhounds; St. Bernards; kuvasz; Irish setters; Weimaraners; Doberman pinschers; German shepherds; Labrador retrievers; many others

Mean Age and Range
• Affects only growing puppies
• Mean—3–4 months
• Range of onset—2–8 months

Predominant Sex
Males more than females

SIGNS

General Comments
Lameness—may be episodic; degree varies from mild to non–weight-bearing; initial episode may resolve without relapse.

Historical Findings
• Depend on severity of the episode
• Owners often describe a depressed puppy that is reluctant to move.
• Inappetence—common

Physical Examination Findings
• Lameness—symmetrical, more severe in forelimbs
• Metaphyses—painful; warm; swollen
• Pyrexia—as high as 41.1°C (106°F)
• Inappetence
• Depression
• Weight loss
• Dehydration
• Diarrhea
• Cachexia
• Debilitation
• Manifestations of systemic illness—respiratory or gastrointestinal

CAUSES
Unknown; the following hypotheses have been proposed.

Metabolic
• Hypovitaminosis C—discounted; many patients have normal ascorbic acid values; supplementation does not resolve disease or prevent relapses; dogs synthesize their own vitamin C; histologic changes differ from those of disease.
• Hypocuprosis—produces histologic changes in rats similar to those seen in affected puppies; does not cause similar changes in dogs

Nutritional
• Overnutrition and oversupplementation—association is inconsistent at best.
• Only one or two affected puppies within a litter; however, all receive the same diet and supplementation.
• Has occurred in puppies that were not over-fed or oversupplemented
• Correcting diet does not alter the course of the disease or eliminate relapses.

Infectious
• Bacterial or fungal organisms—not identified histopathologically in tissues from affected puppies
• Unable to transmit the disease hematogenously from affected to unaffected puppies
• Canine distemper virus RNA—detected in bone cells of patients; unaffected dogs injected with blood from patients developed distemper (3 of 7 dogs) but not hypertrophic osteodystrophy.
• Secondary development may depend on the timing of the neonate's exposure.

RISK FACTORS
None proven

DIAGNOSIS

DIFFERENTIAL DIAGNOSIS
• Juvenile bone and joint disorders
• Panosteitis—no metaphyseal swelling; cottony intramedullary densities in long bones on radiographs
• Elbow dysplasia—no metaphyseal swelling; no fever; pain localized to the elbow(s); typical radiographic signs
• Osteochondritis dissecans—no metaphyseal swelling or fever; pain localized to shoulder or elbow; subchondral defects on radiographs
• Septic polyarthritis—swelling more localized to joint capsule; soft tissue swelling localized to the joint on radiographs; septic suppurative inflammation on arthrocentesis; culture
• Nonseptic polyarthritis—nonseptic suppurative inflammation on arthrocentesis; direct diagnostics toward other causes (e.g., *Ehrlichia canis*).
• Septic metaphysitis—radiographs of the extremities not typical of hypertrophic osteo-dystrophy; asymmetrical; may note septic suppurative inflammation on needle aspiration of metaphyseal lesions; hematologic findings implicate bacterial infection (neutrophilia with accompanying left shift).
• Retained cartilage cores—young large and giant breeds; valgus deformity of the distal forelimbs caused by retained cartilage core in the distal ulnar physes; retained cartilage on radiographs; afebrile; less perimetaphyseal swelling; less or no pain with manipulation
• Canine osteochondrodysplasias—developmental disorders; various breeds; cartilage abnormalities and abnormal bone growth result in limb shortening and bowing deformities of the distal limbs; afebrile; nonpainful; heritable

CBC/BIOCHEMISTRY/URINALYSIS
• Do not contribute to diagnosis
• Stress leukogram
• Normal serum parameters
• Hypocalcemia uncommon

OTHER LABORATORY TESTS
N/A

IMAGING
• Distal extremity radiographs—irregular radiolucent zones within metaphyses, parallel and adjacent to physes; flared metaphyses; extraperiosteal new bone extending up the diaphyses; mineralization of perimetaphyseal soft tissues; asynchronous growth in paired bones; cranial bowing; valgus deformity

• Vertebrae and mandible—rarely affected
• Thoracic radiographs—may reveal interstitial infiltrates

DIAGNOSTIC PROCEDURES
N/A

PATHOLOGIC FINDINGS
• Distal metaphyses of the radius and ulna—most severe changes; similar abnormalities in all long bones
• Gross—wide metaphyses; peripheral mineralization; soft tissue swelling

Histologic
• Nonseptic suppurative inflammation of the metaphysis (osteochondritis), especially adjacent to growth plates
• Necrosis and probable secondary failure of osseous tissue deposition onto the calcified cartilage lattice of the primary spongiosa
• Trabecular microfractures and impaction
• Metaphyseal infraction
• Defective bone formation—thought to be secondary to osteochondral complex inflammation
• Mineralization of perimetaphyseal soft tissues and soft tissues in other regions of the body
• Interstitial pneumonia

TREATMENT

APPROPRIATE HEALTH CARE
• None specific
• Supportive—from none to intensive care for severely affected puppies
• Depends on the severity of the episode, pyrexia, and the patient's ability to maintain normal hydration and willingness to eat

NURSING CARE
• Some patients will not stand or move—prone to develop pressure sores; turn every 2–4 hr to prevent sores and hypostatic congestion of the dependent lung
• Intravenous fluid therapy—for dehydration; maintenance fluid thereafter

ACTIVITY
• Restricted—running and jumping may exacerbate metaphyseal injury and result in further inflammation.
• Confine to a small well-padded area—recommended
• Leash walking only

DIET
• Normal commercial puppy ration
• Avoid supplements

CLIENT EDUCATION
• Warn the client of the disease's relapsing nature.
• Inform client that bony deformities will remodel to some degree with time but that bowing and valgus deformations are permanent.
• Warn client that the more severe the disease, the more severe the bowing deformity.

SURGICAL CONSIDERATIONS
• Generally none
• Consider surgical methods of alimentation (pharyngostomy tube, esophagostomy tube, gastrostomy tube)—debilitated puppies that will not eat or drink and have frequently relapsing episodes of acute clinical signs

MEDICATIONS

DRUGS OF CHOICE
• Anti-inflammatory drugs—for pain and antipyretic effects; may try aspirin (10 mg/kg PO q12h), carprofen (1–2 mg/kg IM or PO q12h), or etodalac (10–15 mg/kg PO q24h)
• Prednisone—0.5–1.0 mg/kg PO q24h); only when there is no response to NSAIDs

CONTRAINDICATIONS
Vitamin C—may be contraindicated; may accelerate dystrophic calcification and decrease bone remodeling

PRECAUTIONS
• Avoid immunosuppressive drugs if an infectious cause is proven or if secondary infection is seen.
• NSAIDs—may cause gastric ulceration; watch for hematemesis or melena.

POSSIBLE INTERACTIONS
None

ALTERNATIVE DRUGS
None

FOLLOW-UP

PATIENT MONITORING
Signs of improvement—less metaphyseal sensitivity; patient gets up; appetite improves; pyrexia resolves.

PREVENTION/AVOIDANCE
N/A

POSSIBLE COMPLICATIONS
• Cachexia
• Permanent bowing deformities
• Secondary bacterial infection

• Pressure sores
• Muscle fasciculations, seizure—with hypocalcemia
• May see secondary septicemia

EXPECTED COURSE AND PROGNOSIS
• Course—days to weeks
• Most patients—one or two episodes and recover
• Some patients—seem to have intractable relapsing episodes of pain and pyrexia; rarely die or are euthanized
• Prognosis—usually good; guarded with multiple relapses or complicating secondary problems
• Persistent bowing deformity—eliminates many purebred puppies from the show ring

MISCELLANEOUS

ASSOCIATED CONDITIONS
Craniomandibular osteopathy—may be associated with mineralization of soft tissues (ossifying periostitis) around long bones; similar to hypertrophic osteodystrophy; may result in lameness

AGE-RELATED FACTORS
None

ZOONOTIC POTENTIAL
None

PREGNANCY
Occurs only in juveniles

SYNONYMS
Metaphyseal osteopathy

SEE ALSO
• Elbow Dysplasia
• Osteochondrosis
• Panosteitis

Suggested Reading
Bellah JR. Hypertrophic osteodystrophy. In: Bojrab MJ, ed. Disease mechanisms in small animal surgery. 2nd ed. Philadelphia: Lea & Febiger, 1993:858–864.
Lenehan TM, Fetter AW. Hypertrophic osteodystrophy. In: Newton CD, Nunamaker DM, eds. Textbook of small animal orthopedics. Philadelphia: Lippincott, 1985:597–601.
Mee AP, Gordon MT, May C, et al. Canine virus transcripts detected in the bone cells of dogs with metaphyseal osteopathy. Bone 1993;14:59–67.
Author Jamie R. Bellah
Consulting Editor Peter D. Schwarz

HYPERTROPHIC OSTEOPATHY

BASICS

OVERVIEW
• Results in increased peripheral blood flow and periosteal new bone proliferation along the diaphyseal region of long bones, often beginning in the distal phalanges, metacarpals, and metatarsals
• Pathogenesis—speculative; theories: chronic anoxia, obscure toxins, hyperestrogenism, and autonomic neurovascular reflex mechanisms mediated by afferent branches of the vagus or intercostal nerves
• Considered a manifestation of a primary disease process
• Affects the musculoskeletal system

SIGNALMENT
• More common in dogs than cats
• Age of highest frequency—8 years; coincides with the peak incidence of pulmonary neoplasms
• Mean age—5.6 years for dogs with nonneoplastic lung lesions
• Large-breed dogs—12 years of age with embryonal rhabdomyosarcoma

SIGNS

Historical Findings
• Listlessness
• Reluctance to move
• Enlargement of the distal portion of the extremities

Physical Examination Findings
• Lame, sore, and painful limbs
• Extremities—enlarged and firm to the touch; not edematous
• Swelling—predominantly below level of elbow and stifle joints, extending distally to toes

CAUSES & RISK FACTORS
• Primary and metastatic lung tumors
• Nonneoplastic thoracic conditions—pneumonia; heartworm disease; congenital or acquired heart disease; bronchial foreign bodies; *Spirocerca lupi* infestation of esophagus; focal lung atelectasis
• Esophageal sarcoma
• Embryonal rhabdomyosarcoma of the urinary bladder
• Adenocarcinoma of the liver or prostate gland
• Thoracic and abdominal mesotheliomas

DIAGNOSIS

DIFFERENTIAL DIAGNOSIS
• Osteomyelitis—not symmetrical and generally edematous; lysis; history of penetrating trauma or systemic infection
• Metastatic neoplasia—not symmetrical

CBC/BIOCHEMISTRY/URINALYSIS
• Depend on the underlying cause
• Serum ALP—may be elevated

OTHER LABORATORY TESTS
Ultrasound—help identify and differentiate primary lesions

IMAGING
• Radiographs of affected long bones—bilaterally symmetric extensive, rough, PNB formation on diaphyseal regions; buds project outward from the cortex and perpendicular to the long axis; PNB forms around the entire circumference of the bone; joints not affected
• Radiographs of the thoracic and abdominal cavities—indicated; identify underlying cause

DIAGNOSTIC PROCEDURES
Bone biopsy and culture (bacterial and fungal)—necessary only in atypical cases; rule out neoplasia and osteomyelitis

TREATMENT

• Directed at underlying primary cause
• Options in selected cases—unilateral vagotomy on the side of a lung lesion; incising through parietal pleura; subperiosteal rib resection; bilateral cervical vagotomy

 MEDICATIONS

DRUGS

• Depend on underlying cause
• Glucocorticoids (e.g., prednisone)—may be used to improve clinical signs and reduce the extent of swelling
• Analgesics—as needed

CONTRAINDICATIONS/POSSIBLE INTERACTIONS

N/A

 FOLLOW-UP

PATIENT MONITORING

• Condition indicates other disease processes—important to recognize need for further diagnostic tests to identify the primary cause
• Removal of the inciting cause—may bring about regression of clinical signs

EXPECTED COURSE AND PROGNOSIS

• Bony changes—may take several months to regress
• Prognosis—guarded to poor owing to the common occurrence of neoplastic causes

 MISCELLANEOUS

SYNONYMS

• Hypertrophic pulmonary osteopathy (HPO)
• Hypertrophic pulmonary osteoarthropathy (HPOA)
• Hypertrophic osteoarthropathy (HOA)

ABBREVIATIONS

PNB = periosteal new bone

Suggested Reading

Halliwell WH. Tumorlike lesions of bone. In: Bojrab MJ, ed. Disease mechanisms in small animal surgery. Philadelphia: Lea & Febiger, 1993:933–934.

Author Peter D. Schwarz
Consulting Editor Peter D. Schwarz

HYPERTROPHIC PYLORIC GASTROPATHY, CHRONIC

BASICS

DEFINITION
Pyloric stenosis or chronic hypertrophic pyloric gastropathy is an obstructive narrowing of the pyloric canal resulting from varying degrees of muscular hypertrophy or mucosal hyperplasia.

PATHOPHYSIOLOGY
• Can result from a congenital lesion composed primarily of hypertrophy of the smooth muscle or be one of three types of acquired form—primarily circular muscle hypertrophy (type 1), a combination of muscular hypertrophy and mucosal hyperplasia (type 2), or primarily mucosal hyperplasia (type 3)
• The cause is unknown; proposed factors include increased gastrin levels (which have a trophic effect on the muscle and mucosa) or changes in the myenteric plexus that lead to chronic antral distension and its associated effects.

SYSTEMS AFFECTED
• Gastrointestinal—chronic intermittent vomiting
• Musculoskeletal—weight loss
• Respiratory—possible aspiration pneumonia

GENETICS
Inheritance pattern unknown

INCIDENCE/PREVALENCE
Uncommon

GEOGRAPHIC DISTRIBUTION
N/A

SIGNALMENT

Species
• More common in dogs
• Rare in cats

Breed Predilections
• Congenital—brachycephalic breeds (boxer, Boston terrier, bulldog); Siamese cats
• Acquired—Lhasa apso, shih tzu, Pekingese, poodle

Mean Age And Range
• Congenital—shortly after weaning and up to 1 year of age
• Acquired—9.8 years of age

Predominant Sex
Twice as many males as females

SIGNS

General Comments
• Clinical signs are related to the degree of pyloric narrowing.
• Projectile vomiting is generally not a presenting complaint.

Historical Findings
• Chronic intermittent vomiting of undigested or partially digested food (rarely containing bile) within a few hours of eating
• Congenital lesions begin to produce clinical signs shortly after weaning.
• Frequency of vomiting increases with time.
• Weight loss
• Lack of response to antiemetics or motility agents
• Anorexia

Physical Examination Findings
• Most dogs are generally in good physical condition.
• Some may present with weight loss or abdominal distension.

CAUSES
• Congenital or acquired
• May be influenced by infiltrative mural diseases
• Chronic elevations in gastrin levels
• Neuroendocrine factors may play a role.

RISK FACTORS
Chronic stress, inflammatory disorders, chronic gastritis, gastric ulcers, and genetic predispositions influence the disease process in humans and may play a role in small animals.

DIAGNOSIS

DIFFERENTIAL DIAGNOSIS
• Gastric neoplasia—most common
• Foreign body
• Granulomatous fungal disease (e.g., pythiosis)
• Eosinophilic granuloma
• Motility disorders
• Cranial abdominal mass—pancreatic or duodenal

CBC/BIOCHEMISTRY/URINALYSIS
• Findings vary, depending on the degree and chronicity of obstruction.
• Hypochloremia metabolic alkalosis (characteristic of pyloric outflow obstruction) or metabolic acidosis (or mixed acid–base imbalance)
• Hypokalemia
• Anemia—if concurrent gastrointestinal (GI) ulceration
• Prerenal azotemia—if dehydration present

OTHER LABORATORY TESTS
N/A

IMAGING

Abdominal Radiographs
Normal to markedly distended stomach

Upper GI Barium Contrast Study
• May display a "beak" sign created by pyloric narrowing, allowing minimal barium to pass into the pyloric antrum
• Retention of most of the barium in the stomach after 6 h indicates delayed gastric emptying
• Intraluminal filling defects or pyloric wall thickening

Fluoroscopy
• Normal gastric contractility
• Delayed passage of barium through the pylorus

Abdominal Ultrasound
Measurable thickening of the wall of the pylorus and antrum

HYPERTROPHIC PYLORIC GASTROPATHY, CHRONIC

DIAGNOSTIC PROCEDURES

Endoscopy—allows evaluation of the mucosa for ulceration, hyperplasia, and mass lesions; samples can be obtained for histopathological evaluation.

PATHOLOGIC FINDINGS

• Include focal to multifocal mucosal polyps, diffuse mucosal thickening, and pyloric wall-thickening, with variable degree of pyloric narrowing
• Changes range from hypertrophy of the circular smooth muscle to hyperplasia of the mucosa and associated glandular structures; a wide spectrum of inflammatory cell infiltration exists.

TREATMENT

APPROPRIATE HEALTH CARE

• Depends on severity of clinical signs
• Patients should be evaluated and surgery scheduled at the earliest convenience.

NURSING CARE

• Appropriate parenteral fluids to correct any electrolyte imbalances and metabolic alkalosis or acidosis
• Isotonic saline (with potassium supplementation) is the fluid of choice for hypochloremic metabolic alkalosis.
• Consideration of postoperative nutritional support is important.
• In severe cases treated with gastroduodenostomy or gastrojejunostomy, surgical placement of a jejunostomy tube for enteral nutrition may be advantageous.

ACTIVITY

Restrict

DIET

Highly digestible, low-fat—until surgical intervention is feasible

CLIENT EDUCATION

• Surgical treatment is highly successful.
• If clinical signs recur postoperatively, more-aggressive surgical procedures may be indicated.

SURGICAL CONSIDERATIONS

• Surgical intervention is the treatment of choice.
• Goals involve establishing a diagnosis with histopathological samples, excising abnormal tissue, and restoring GI function with the least-invasive procedure.
• Surgical procedures depend on the extent of obstruction—pyloromyotomy (Fredet-Ramstedt), pyloroplasty (Heineke-Mikulicz or antral advancement flap), gastroduodenostomy (Bilroth 1), gastrojejunostomy (Bilroth 2)

MEDICATIONS

DRUGS OF CHOICE

Antiemetics and motility modifiers are generally ineffective.

CONTRAINDICATIONS

• Evidence of complete pyloric obstruction precludes metoclopramide use.
• Avoid anticholinergic agents because of their effects on GI motility.

PRECAUTIONS

N/A

POSSIBLE INTERACTIONS

N/A

ALTERNATIVE DRUGS

N/A

FOLLOW-UP

PATIENT MONITORING

Postoperatively for recurrence of clinical signs because of poor choice of surgical procedure.

PREVENTION/AVOIDANCE

N/A

POSSIBLE COMPLICATIONS

Postoperative surgical complications include recurrence of clinical signs, gastric ulceration, pancreatitis, bile duct obstruction, and incisional dehiscence with peritonitis.

EXPECTED COURSE AND PROGNOSIS

• 85% of dogs show good-to-excellent results with resolution of clinical signs upon proper surgical intervention.
• Poor prognosis if gastric neoplasia (especially adenocarcinoma) is an underlying cause

MISCELLANEOUS

ASSOCIATED CONDITIONS

Gastric ulceration

AGE-RELATED FACTORS

• Intermittent vomiting in young brachycephalic breeds upon weaning indicates congenital stenosis.
• Chronic intermittent vomiting in adult (8–10 years old) small breed dogs supports a diagnosis of an acquired obstruction.

ZOONOTIC POTENTIAL

None

PREGNANCY

High gastrin levels in pregnant females may predispose to development of the syndrome.

SYNONYMS

• Chronic hypertrophic antral gastropathy
• Hypertrophic gastritis
• Acquired antral pyloric hypertrophy
• Congenital pyloric stenosis

SEE ALSO

N/A

Suggested Reading

DeNovo R. Antral pyloric hypertrophy syndrome In: Kirk R, ed. Current veterinary therapy X. Philadelphia: Saunders, 1989: 918–921.

Matthiesen D. Chronic gastric outflow obstruction. In: Slatter D, ed. Textbook of small animal surgery. 2nd ed. Philadelphia: Saunders, 1993:561–571.

Stanton M. Gastric outlet obstruction. In: Bojrab MJ, ed. Disease mechanisms in small animal surgery. 2nd ed. Philadelphia: Lea & Febiger, 1993:235–236.

Author James E. Williams, Jr.
Consulting Editors Brett M. Feder and Mitchell A. Crystal

DISEASES

HYPERVISCOSITY SYNDROME

BASICS

OVERVIEW
• An assortment of clinical signs caused by high blood viscosity
• Typically results from markedly high concentration of plasma proteins, although can result (rarely) from extremely high erythrocyte count
• Most frequently seen as a paraneoplastic syndrome, often associated with multiple myeloma and other lymphoid tumors or leukemia
• Total plasma protein may exceed 10 g/dL, with serum protein electrophoresis showing monoclonal gammopathy.
• Clinical signs caused by reduced blood flow through smaller vessels, high plasma volume, and associated coagulopathy
• Systems affected include hemic/lymphatic/immune, ophthalmic, and nervous.

SIGNALMENT
• Dogs more frequently affected than cats
• No sex or breed predilections
• More common in older animals

SIGNS

Historical Findings
• No consistent signs
• Anorexia
• Lethargy
• Depression
• Polyuria and polydipsia
• Blindness, ataxia, and seizures
• Bleeding tendencies

Physical Examination Findings
• Neurologic deficits, including seizures and disorientation
• Tachycardia and tachypnea if congestive heart failure present owing to volume overload
• Epistaxis or other mucosal bleeding
• Hepatomegaly/splenomegaly/lymphadenopathy
• Visual deficits associated with engorged retinal vessels, retinal hemorrhage or detachment, and papilledema

CAUSES & RISK FACTORS
• Multiple myeloma and plasma cell tumors (IgM > IgA > IgG)
• Lymphocytic leukemia or lymphoma
• Marked polycythemia (PCV > 65%)
• Chronic atypical inflammation with monoclonal gammopathy (e.g., ehrlichiosis in dogs)
• Chronic autoimmune disease (e.g., systemic lupus erythematosus and rheumatoid arthritis)

DIAGNOSIS

DIFFERENTIAL DIAGNOSIS
• Other unexplained neurologic disease or bleeding disorders
• Appropriate polycythemia (e.g., right to left cardiac shunt)
• Hyperviscosity is a syndrome, not a final diagnosis.

CBC/BIOCHEMISTRY/URINALYSIS
• Nonregenerative anemia (in patients without polycythemia as a cause of hyperviscosity), thrombocytopenia, or leukopenia
• Hyperproteinemia (total plasma protein > 9.0 g/dL) and hyperglobulinemia (> 5.0 g/dL)
• Azotemia and hypercalcemia if hyperviscosity caused by a paraneoplastic syndrome
• Isosthenuria and marked proteinuria

OTHER LABORATORY TESTS
• High concentration of IgG, IgA, or IgM, as detected by radial immunodiffusion
• High plasma or serum viscosity (> 3 relative to water)
• Prolonged prothrombin time or activated partial thromboplastin time

IMAGING
Hepatosplenomegaly, cardiomegaly, and osteolytic lesions (in association with multiple myeloma) are possible.

DIAGNOSTIC PROCEDURES
• Plasma cell or lymphoid infiltrate revealed by bone marrow biopsy
• Bence-Jones proteinuria in patients with multiple myeloma

 TREATMENT

APPROPRIATE HEALTH CARE
• Generally treat as inpatient
• Treat underlying disease
• Phlebotomy (15–20 mL/kg) with crystalloid fluid volume replacement
• Plasmapheresis (10–15 mL/kg), if available

NURSING CARE
As dictated by underlying disease

 MEDICATIONS

DRUGS
• Provide treatment for underlying neoplastic or inflammatory condition
• See other topics for drug therapy for the underlying cause (e.g., plasma cell tumor, lymphocytic leukemia, lymphoma, ehrlichiosis, and polycythemia).

CONTRAINDICATIONS/POSSIBLE INTERACTIONS
• Avoid use of medications that might increase vascular volume, including synthetic colloids (e.g., hetastarch and dextran)
• Avoid medications that alter platelet function (e.g., NSAIDs).

 FOLLOW-UP

• Monitor serum or plasma proteins frequently as a marker of treatment efficacy.
• CBC, biochemistry panel, and urinalysis to monitor other laboratory abnormalities

 MISCELLANEOUS

SEE ALSO
• Ehrlichiosis
• Leukemia, Chronic Lymphocytic
• Lymphosarcoma (Lymphoma)—Cats
• Lymphosarcoma (Lymphoma)—Dogs
• Multiple Myeloma
• Plasmacytoma, Mucocutaneous
• Polycythemia

ABBREVIATION
PVC = packed cell volume

Suggested Reading
Hohenhaus AE. Syndromes of hyperglobulinemia: diagnosis and therapy. In: Kirk RW, ed. Current veterinary therapy. Vol. 12. Philadelphia: Saunders, 1995:523–530.
Author Elizabeth Rozanski
Consulting Editor Susan M. Cotter

HYPHEMA

 BASICS

DEFINITION
Blood in the anterior chamber

PATHOPHYSIOLOGY
• Results from any condition that causes intraocular vessel damage sufficient to allow egress of erythrocytes
• Bleeding vessels—resident or acquired vessels (neovascularization); may be in the retina, vitreous (hyaloid artery or primary vitreous), choroid, ciliary body, or iris; resident: bleed as a result of trauma, inflammation, defects in hemostasis, or neoplastic infiltration; new: inherently leaky and prone to bleed spontaneously
• Most common causes of iris neovascularization—chronic retinal detachment, chronic uveitis, and intraocular neoplasia, especially lymphosarcoma
• May be the presenting sign of systemic hypertension, especially in old cats—occurs as a result of precapillary, arteriole ischemia secondary to the eye's attempt to autoregulate blood flow to maintain normal perfusion of ocular tissue
• Usually does not in itself cause any adverse secondary effects
• Secondary glaucoma—persistent bleeding; referred to as ghost cell glaucoma; occurs because the plasma membranes of aged erythrocytes lose their plasticity, predisposing the patient to plugging of the trabecular spaces

SYSTEMS AFFECTED
Ophthalmic

GENETICS
N/A

INCIDENCE/PREVALENCE
May be a presenting sign of many ocular and systemic diseases

GEOGRAPHIC DISTRIBUTION
N/A

SIGNALMENT
Species
Dogs and cats

Breed Predilections
N/A

Mean age and Range
Any

Predominant Sex
N/A

SIGNS
General Comments
Depend on how much bleeding has occurred, whether vision is impaired, and whether there is an associated systemic disease

Historical Findings
• Extremely diverse, reflecting the multitude of causes
• History of vision loss uncommon
• Rarely bilateral and complete

Physical Examination Findings
• Blood seen within the anterior chamber of the eye; if severe, cannot see other intraocular structures
• Corneal edema—common
• Lymphosarcoma—blood often mixed with WBCs
• Secondary to trauma—often see eyelid, conjunctival, or corneal lesions
• IOP—may be elevated with long-standing duration of condition

CAUSES
• Trauma
• Chronic retinal detachment
• Uveal neoplasia—especially lymphosarcoma, hemangiosarcoma, and primary uveal melanoma
• Uveitis—especially if caused by FIP (cats) and rickettsial disease (dogs)
• Coagulopathies
• Vasculitis—immune-mediated or secondary to rickettsial diseases (e.g., Rocky mountain spotted fever, ehrlichiosis)
• Systemic hypertension—primary or secondary to renal disease; hyperthyroidism
• Parasite migration—ophthalmomyiasis interna
• Secondary to congenital ocular defects—collie eye anomaly; persistent primary vitreous; severe retinal dysplasia

RISK FACTORS
• Uveitis
• Metastatic neoplasia
• Chronic retinal detachment
• Any disease causing vasculitis or vascular fragility
• Chronic renal disease
• Coagulopathies
• Congenital ocular defects

 DIAGNOSIS

DIFFERENTIAL DIAGNOSIS
• Bilateral condition—indicates systemic disease
• Unilateral condition in old dogs—suspect retinal detachment
• No conjunctival or episcleral vascular injection—suspect coagulopathy
• With retinal hemorrhage or detachment in old cats—strongly suspect systemic hypertension
• With chronic uveitis or recurrent condition—rule out intraocular neoplasia

CBC/BIOCHEMISTRY/URINALYSIS
• Usually normal with localized ocular disease
• Anemia or thrombocytopenia—may be noted with a systemic bleeding disorder

OTHER LABORATORY TESTS
• Suspected coagulopathy—special laboratory tests to assess hemostasis indicated; intrinsic coagulation (ACT and PTT); extrinsic coagulation (one-stage PT); thrombocyte and reticulocyte counts; thrombin time; fibrinogen levels; fibrinogen degradation products
• Secondary to chronic uveitis—uveitis workup indicated (see Anterior Uveitis—Dogs and Anterior Uveitis—Cats)

IMAGING
• Ocular ultrasonography—indicated when condition is severe enough to obstruct view of the intraocular structures; easily identify retinal detachment and intraocular tumors
• Thoracic radiographs and possibly abdominal ultrasound—may help rule out disseminated neoplasia

DIAGNOSTIC PROCEDURES
• Suspected bleeding disorders—bone marrow examination; buccal bleeding time
• Blood pressure measurement—indicated when condition cannot be attributed to ocular disease
• Lymph node aspiration and biopsy—indicated for suspected lymphosarcoma

PATHOLOGIC FINDINGS
Gross—anterior chamber partially or completely filled with blood

Histologic
- Erythrocytes—in a matrix of proteinaceous fluid
- RBCs—in the iridocorneal angle and trabecular spaces
- Vitreal hemorrhage
- Posterior synechia and inflammatory cells in the anterior uvea—common with primary uveitis
- Pre-iridal fibrovascular membranes—common with primary retinal detachment or chronic uveitis

TREATMENT

APPROPRIATE HEALTH CARE
Usually outpatient

NURSING CARE
N/A

ACTIVITY
Restricted only if caused by a clotting disorder

DIET
N/A

CLIENT EDUCATION
- Explain that hyphema is a clinical sign and not a specific disease.
- Inform client that no specific treatments for hyphema exist and that treatment is directed at eliminating the underlying cause.

SURGICAL CONSIDERATIONS
- Trauma—surgical intervention indicated to repair accompanying adnexal or corneal defects
- Secondary glaucoma caused by chronic condition—surgical procedure indicated to remove (e.g., enucleation) or possibly salvage the globe (e.g., evisceration and intrascleral prosthesis; gentamicin injection)
- Irreversibly lost vision—consider enucleation or possibly a globe salvage procedure.
- Surgical evacuation of blood from the anterior chamber—rarely indicated

MEDICATIONS

DRUGS OF CHOICE
- None specific
- Topical antibiotics—not indicated unless associated with conjunctival or corneal epithelial defects (trauma)

- Topical corticosteroids—q6h; 1% prednisolone acetate or 0.1% dexamethasone; often empirically used to control uveal inflammation
- Systemic corticosteroids—usually indicated only when caused by a corticosteroid-responsive systemic disease (e.g., lymphosarcoma) or posterior segment inflammation
- Systemic hypotensive therapy—indicated if caused by hypertension
- Topical 1% atropine solution—given to effect; indicated to prevent synechia formation unless secondary glaucoma has occurred
- Dichlorphenamide—2–4 mg/kg PO q8–12h; for secondary glaucoma; may help lower IOP
- Topical 0.5% timolol (q12 h) or dipivefrin HCl (q8–12h)—may be used in place of epinephrine
- Formed clots—may be dissolved if tissue-plasminogen activator (0.1–0.2 mL, 250 µg/mL) is injected into the anterior chamber within 5–7 days of hemorrhage

CONTRAINDICATIONS
Do not treat with tissue plasminogen activator if a clot has not formed and if the cause of the bleeding has not been eliminated, because rebleeding is likely.

PRECAUTIONS
Pilocarpine—may exacerbate breakdown of the blood–aqueous barrier; may cause further bleeding

POSSIBLE INTERACTIONS
N/A

ALTERNATIVE DRUGS
N/A

FOLLOW-UP

PATIENT MONITORING
- Severe disease—IOP monitored daily
- Less severe disease—examined every 2–3 days until resolution

PREVENTION/AVOIDANCE
Restricted activity if caused by a clotting disorder

POSSIBLE COMPLICATIONS
- Glaucoma
- Vision loss

EXPECTED COURSE AND PROGNOSIS
- Trauma—prognosis generally good unless irrevocable damage has occurred to the lens, ciliary body, or retina
- Secondary to retinal detachment and anterior segment neovascularization—

typically will not resolve; secondary glaucoma eventually results, necessitating some type of surgical intervention to relieve pain (e.g., enucleation; evisceration with prosthesis).

MISCELLANEOUS

ASSOCIATED CONDITIONS
- Clotting disorders
- Systemic hypertension
- Uveitis
- Metastatic neoplasia—lymphosarcoma; hemangiosarcoma
- Retinal detachment
- Von Willebrand disease

AGE-RELATED FACTORS
Systemic hypertension—more common in elderly patients

ZOONOTIC POTENTIAL
N/A

PREGNANCY
N/A

SEE ALSO
- Anterior Uveitis—Cats
- Anterior Uveitis—Dogs
- Clotting Factor Deficiencies
- Hypertension, Systemic
- Red Eye

ABBREVIATIONS
- ACT = activated clotting time
- FIP = feline infectious peritonitis
- IOP = intraocular pressure
- PT = prothrombin time
- PTT = partial thromboplastin time

Suggested Reading
Collins BK, Moore CP. Diseases and surgery of the canine anterior uvea. In: Gelatt KN, ed., Veterinary ophthalmology. 3rd ed. Philadelphia: Lippincott Williams & Wilkins, 1997:775–795.
Littman MP. Spontaneous systemic hypertension in 24 cats. J Vet Intern Med 1994;8:79–86.
Morgan RV. Systemic hypertension in 4 cats: ocular and medical findings. J Am Anim Hosp Assoc 1986;22;615–621.
Nelms S, Nasisse MP, Davidson MG, Kirschner S. Hyphema associated with retinal disease in dogs: 17 cases. J Am Vet Med Assoc 1993;202:1289–1292.
Author Mark P. Nasisse
Consulting Editor Paul E. Miller

DISEASES

HYPOADRENOCORTICISM

 BASICS

DEFINITION
An endocrine disorder resulting from deficient production of glucocorticoids and/or mineralocorticoids

PATHOPHYSIOLOGY
• Mineralocorticoid (aldosterone) deficiency results in an inability to excrete potassium and retain sodium; sodium deficiency leads to diminished effective circulating volume that in turn contributes to prerenal azotemia, hypotension, dehydration, weakness, and depression.
• Hyperkalemia (along with other metabolic derangements) may result in myocardial toxicity.
• Glucocorticoid (cortisol) deficiency contributes to anorexia, vomiting, melena, lethargy, and weight loss, predisposes to hypoglycemia, and results in impaired excretion of water free of sodium.

SYSTEMS AFFECTED
Multiple organ systems involved; extent of involvement varies from case to case.

GENETICS
N/A

INCIDENCE/PREVALENCE
No exact figures available; considered uncommon to rare in dogs and very rare in cats

GEOGRAPHIC DISTRIBUTION
N/A

SIGNALMENT
Species
Dogs and cats

Breed Predilections
• Great Danes, rottweilers, Portuguese water dogs, standard poodles, West Highland white terriers, and wheaten terriers have increased relative risk.
• No predilection in cats

Mean Age and Range
• Dogs—range, <1 to >12 years; median, 4 years
• Cats—range, 1–9 years; most are middle-aged

Predominant Sex
Female dogs are at an increased relative risk; no predilection in cats

SIGNS
General Comments
Vary from mild and few in some patients with chronic hypoadrenocorticism to severe and life-threatening in an acute addisonian crisis

Historical Findings
• Dogs—lethargy, anorexia, vomiting, weight loss, waxing/waning course, diarrhea, previous response to therapy, shaking, PU/PD
• Cats—lethargy, anorexia, vomiting, PU/PD, weight loss

Physical Examination Findings
• Dogs—depression, weakness, dehydration, collapse, hypothermia, slow CRT, melena, weak pulse, bradycardia, painful abdomen, hair loss
• Cats—dehydration, weakness, slow CRT, weak pulse, bradycardia

CAUSES
• Primary hypoadrenocorticism—idiopathic (immune-mediated), mitotane overdose, granulomatous disease, metastatic tumors
• Secondary hypoadrenocorticism—iatrogenic following withdrawal of long-term glucocorticoid administration, isolated ACTH deficiency, panhypopituitarism, nonfunctional pituitary tumor

RISK FACTORS
N/A

 DIAGNOSIS

DIFFERENTIAL DIAGNOSIS
• Signs are nonspecific and are seen in other, more common medical disorders, particularly gastrointestinal and renal diseases.
• Although no signs are pathognomonic, a waxing and waning course and previous response to nonspecific medical intervention ("fluids and steroids") should alert the clinician to consider the diagnosis.

CBC/BIOCHEMISTRY/URINALYSIS
• Hematologic abnormalities may include anemia, eosinophilia, and lymphocytosis.
• Serum biochemical findings may include hyperkalemia, azotemia, hyponatremia, hypochloremia, decreased total CO_2, hypercalcemia, increased liver enzymes, increased serum alkaline phosphatase, and hypoglycemia.
• Urinalysis often reveals impaired urine-concentrating ability.
• Some patients with hypoadrenocorticism exhibit normal electrolyte levels.

OTHER LABORATORY TESTS
• Definitive diagnosis is by demonstration of undetectable-to-low serum cortisol concentrations that fail to increase after administration of either ACTH gel IM (20 U in dogs, 10 U in cats) or synthetic ACTH IV (0.25 mg in dogs, 0.125 mg in cats).
• In hypovolemic dehydrated animals, use synthetic ACTH IV or delay testing until after initial fluid administration is completed.
• Determine the plasma ACTH concentration in patients with normal electrolyte levels, to differentiate primary from secondary hypoadrenocorticism; must collect sample before administering glucocorticoids

IMAGING
Radiographs may reveal microcardia, narrowed vena cava or descending aorta, hypoperfused lung fields, and very rarely megaesophagus.

DIAGNOSTIC PROCEDURES
N/A

PATHOLOGIC FINDINGS
• Gross examination—atrophy of the adrenal glands
• Microscopically—lymphocytic-plasmacytic adrenalitis and/or adrenocortical atrophy

 TREATMENT

APPROPRIATE HEALTH CARE
• An acute addisonian crisis is a medical emergency requiring intensive therapy.
• Treatment of chronic hypoadrenocorticism depends on severity of clinical signs; usually initial stabilization and therapy are conducted on an inpatient basis.

NURSING CARE
Treat acute addisonian crisis with rapid correction of hypovolemia using isotonic fluids (preferably 0.9% NaCl).

ACTIVITY
No alteration necessary

DIET
No need to alter

CLIENT EDUCATION
• Lifelong glucocorticoid and/or mineralocorticoid replacement therapy is required.
• Increased dosages of replacement glucocorticoid are required during periods of stress such as travel, hospitalization, and surgery.

SURGICAL CONSIDERATIONS
N/A

 MEDICATIONS

DRUGS OF CHOICE
• Chronic primary hypoadrenocorticism—treat with glucocorticoid replacement (prednisone, 0.2 mg/kg/day) and mineralocorticoid replacement (fludrocortisone acetate, 10–20 μg/kg/day divided, adjusted by 0.05- to 0.1-mg increments on the basis of serial serum electrolyte determinations or DOCP, 2 mg/kg IM or SC every 21–30 days adjusted if needed on the basis of serum electrolyte determinations)
• Parenteral administration of a rapidly acting glucocorticoid such as dexamethasone sodium phosphate or prednisolone sodium succinate; dexamethasone sodium phosphate is preferred because prednisolone cross-reacts with cortisol assays
• Patients with confirmed secondary hypoadrenocorticism require only glucocorticoid supplementation (prednisone, 0.2 mg/kg/day).

CONTRAINDICATIONS
N/A

PRECAUTIONS
N/A

POSSIBLE INTERACTIONS
N/A

ALTERNATIVE DRUGS
N/A

 FOLLOW-UP

PATIENT MONITORING
• Adjust the daily dose of fludrocortisone by 0.05- to 0.1-mg increments as needed, based on serial serum electrolyte determinations; following initiation of therapy, check serum electrolyte levels weekly until they stabilize in the normal range; thereafter, check serum electrolyte concentrations and BUN or creatinine monthly for the first 3–6 months and then every 3–12 months
• In many dogs given fludrocortisone, the daily dose required to control the disorder increases incrementally, usually during the first 6–24 months of therapy; in most dogs, the final fludrocortisone dosage needed is 20–30 μg/kg /day; very few can be controlled on 10 μg/kg/day or less.
• After the first 2 injections of DOCP, ideally measure serum electrolyte levels at 2, 3, and 4 weeks to determine the duration of effect; thereafter, check electrolyte levels at the time of injection for the next 6 months (and adjust the dosage of DOCP if necessary) and then every 6–12 months
• DOCP is usually required at 3- to 4-week intervals, but a few patients need injections every 2 weeks; alternatively, to maintain monthly injections, the dosage of DOCP can be incrementally increased; almost all hypoadrenocorticism will be well controlled on a maintenance DOCP dose of 2 mg/kg/injection.

PREVENTION/AVOIDANCE
• Continue hormonal replacement therapy for the lifetime of the patient.
• Increase the dosage of replacement glucocorticoid during periods of stress such as travel, hospitalization, and surgery.

POSSIBLE COMPLICATIONS
• PU/PD may occur from prednisone administration, necessitating decreasing or discontinuing the drug.
• PU/PD may occur from fludrocortisone administration, necessitating a change to DOCP therapy.

EXPECTED COURSE AND PROGNOSIS
Except for patients with primary hypoadrenocorticism caused by granulomatous or metastatic disease and secondary hypoadrenocorticism caused by a pituitary mass, the vast majority of patients carry a good to excellent prognosis following proper stabilization and treatment.

✓ MISCELLANEOUS

ASSOCIATED CONDITIONS
Concurrent endocrine gland failure occurs in up to 5% of dogs—hypothyroidism, diabetes mellitus and/or hypoparathyroidism

AGE-RELATED FACTORS
N/A

ZOONOTIC POTENTIAL
N/A

PREGNANCY
N/A

SYNONYMS
Addison's disease (primary hypoadrenocorticism)

SEE ALSO
• Hyperkalemia
• Hyponatremia

ABBREVIATION
PD/PU = polydipsia, polyuria

Suggested Reading
Greco DS, Peterson ME. Feline hypoadrenocorticism. In: Kirk RW, ed. Current veterinary therapy X. 1989:1042–1045.

Kintzer PP, Peterson ME. Canine hypoadrenocorticism. In: Kirk, RW, Bonagura JD, eds. Current veterinary therapy XII. 1995:

Kintzer PP, Peterson ME. Primary and secondary hypoadrenocorticism. Vet Clin N Am 1997;27(2):349–358.

Peterson ME, Kintzer PP, Kass PH. Pretreatment clinical and laboratory findings in dogs with hypoadrenocorticism: 225 cases (1979–1993). J Am Vet Med Assoc 1996;208:85–91.

Author Peter P. Kintzer
Consulting Editor Deborah S. Greco

DISEASES

HYPOANDROGENISM

BASICS

DEFINITION
Relative or absolute deficiency of masculinizing sex hormones such as testosterone and its derivatives

PATHOPHYSIOLOGY
• Androgens—have both masculinizing and anabolic effects; are produced by the adrenal cortex, ovaries, and testes; interstitial (Leydig) cells of the testes primarily produce testosterone along with small amounts of DHT, dehydroepiandrosterone, and androstenedione; weak androgens may be converted peripherally to more powerful androgens.
• Hypoandrogenism develops because of inadequate production of androgens, an androgen receptor defect, or an enzymatic defect.
• Androgen-responsive tissues (e.g., testes, penis, prepuce, prostate gland, and perineum) become less sensitive to the effects of androgens as a result of receptor-mediated problems.
• Enzymatic defects include deficiency of 5α-reductase, which results in failure to convert testosterone to DHT.
• Castration, testicular agenesis, and testicular hypoplasia, as well as inadequate synthesis of adrenocortical androgens, result in low androgen production.
• Patients usually have male phenotypes with XY chromosomes.

SYSTEMS AFFECTED
• Renal/Urologic—anatomic and functional abnormalities
• Reproductive—anatomic and functional abnormalities
• Skin—alopecia and seborrheic dermatosis

GENETICS
• Androgen resistance associated with testicular feminization is thought to be X-linked recessive.
• Hypospadias in the Boston terrier breed are considered familial; the mode of inheritance is unknown.

INCIDENCE/PREVALENCE
Uncommon

GEOGRAPHIC DISTRIBUTION
N/A

SIGNALMENT
Species
Dogs and cats

Breed Predilections
• Boston terriers—hypospadias
• Calico and tortoiseshell cats—Klinefelter's syndrome (39 XXY)

Mean Age and Range
• Congenital—behavioral problems are usually recognized around puberty.
• Anatomic abnormalities may be detected sooner.

Predominant Sex
Male

SIGNS
Historical Findings
• Postpuberty—infertility and low libido
• Prepuberty—failure of male dogs to lift their legs to urinate; absence of urine spraying in tom cats

Physical Examination Findings
• Clinical signs vary.
• Subnormal development of male secondary sex characteristics
• Smaller than expected stature for breed and age
• Small, underdeveloped, or hypoplastic testes, penis, prepuce, and scrotum; soft consistency to testes
• Poor semen quality
• Hypospadia
• Absence of penile spines in male cats
• Gynecomastia possible in male dogs
• Bilaterally symmetrical alopecia and seborrhea sicca that usually begins in the perineum
• Hyperpigmentation and pruritus usually not seen
• Urinary incontinence

CAUSES
• Castration
• Gonadotropin deficiencies caused by hypothalamic and pituitary problems result in low GnRH, LH, and FSH concentrations, which cause low testosterone secretion and secondary hypogonadism.
• Pituitary tumor may cause low LH and FSH.
• Hypothalamic tumor may cause low GnRH.
• Primary hypogonadism and reduced testicular size and function cause gonadotropin hyperactivity with high GnRH, LH, and FSH concentrations.
• Cryptorchidism
• Hyperprolactinemia inhibits LH and testosterone secretion.
• Reduced sensitivity of androgen-responsive tissues

RISK FACTORS
• Drugs—ketoconazole, megestrol acetate, cimetidine, spironolactone, and some antineoplastic agents (busulfan, chlorambucil, cisplatin, cyclophosphamide, methotrexate, vincristine) decrease testosterone in humans; megestrol acetate and finasteride inhibit DHT production within the prostate.
• Exogenous administration of steroid compounds that act via negative feedback on the pituitary gland; anabolic steroids, estrogens, progestogens, and glucocorticoids inhibit LH and, thus, testosterone secretion.

DIAGNOSIS

DIFFERENTIAL DIAGNOSIS
• Can confirm hypothyroidism by a TSH stimulation test, determination of TSH concentration, or equilibrium dialysis assay for free T_4
• Intersex abnormalities (e.g., male pseudo-hermaphrodite and XX male syndrome) have distinct anatomic or histologic abnormalities and karyotype.

CBC/BIOCHEMISTRY/URINALYSIS
Results usually normal

OTHER LABORATORY TESTS
• Serum testosterone concentration—testosterone secretion is episodic, so repetitive testing or a stimulation test is more diagnostic than a single serum test for testosterone.
• GnRH stimulation test or HCG stimulation test (see Appendix for protocol)—serum testosterone concentration should not increase in response to GnRH or HCG in patients with primary gonadal problems and hypoplastic testes.
• Karyotyping
• Neutrophils in buccal smears may contain sex-chromatin (Barr bodies) in phenotypic males.

- Gonadotropin assay
- Prolactin assay
- Low sperm count or high numbers of abnormal sperm

IMAGING
CT and MRI to detect a brain tumor

DIAGNOSTIC PROCEDURES
- Testicular biopsy may be indicated in patients with small testicles, abnormally shaped testicles, or testicles with abnormal consistency
- Skin biopsy in patients with alopecia and seborrhea sicca

PATHOLOGIC FINDINGS
- Hypospadia
- Testicular hypoplasia or atrophy
- Persistent müllerian duct in male pseudo-hermaphrodites

TREATMENT

APPROPRIATE HEALTH CARE
- May attempt hormone replacement on an outpatient basis
- Hospitalization is required for surgical procedures.

NURSING CARE
N/A

ACTIVITY
N/A

DIET
N/A

CLIENT EDUCATION
Do not breed affected animals.

SURGICAL CONSIDERATIONS
Neuter animals with abnormal karyotypes and anatomic defects such as hypospadias and cryptorchidism.

MEDICATIONS

DRUGS OF CHOICE
- Discontinue drugs that may be contributing to hypogonadism (see Causes).
- May try replacement therapy with GnRH (Cystorelin) and gonadotropins (e.g., LH, FSH) to increase libido in male dogs

- Can administer testosterone (oral methyltestosterone or injectable repositol testosterone) to castrated male dogs with testosterone-responsive alopecia and urinary incontinence

CONTRAINDICATIONS
Drugs that predispose to hypoandrogenism

PRECAUTIONS
- Testosterone can cause aggression and cholestatic liver disease and aggravate chronic prostatitis and perianal adenomas.
- Chronic administration of GnRH can cause infertility by negative inhibition of the hypothalamic-pituitary-testis axis.
- Exogenous testosterone decreases testicular size and sperm counts.

POSSIBLE INTERACTIONS
N/A

ALTERNATIVE DRUGS
N/A

FOLLOW-UP

PATIENT MONITORING
Reassess libido, sperm count, and serum testosterone concentration after initiating replacement therapy.

PREVENTION/AVOIDANCE
Avoid drugs known to cause hypoandrogenism in breeding animals.

POSSIBLE COMPLICATIONS
Permanent infertility and hypogonadism are possible.

EXPECTED COURSE AND PROGNOSIS
Hypoandrogenism can be intermittent, transient, or permanent, depending on the cause.

MISCELLANEOUS

ASSOCIATED CONDITIONS
- Cryptorchidism is commonly associated with hypospadias.
- Hypoandrogenism is associated with benign prostatic hyperplasia and squamous metaplasia because of low androgen secretion and high estrogen associated with advanced age.

- Hypoandrogenism is theorized to be the cause of testosterone responsive dermatosis and testosterone-responsive urinary incontinence.
- Idiopathic male-feminizing syndrome
- Intersex abnormalities—XX male syndrome

AGE-RELATED FACTORS
Testosterone secretion normally diminishes in older males.

ZOONOTIC POTENTIAL
N/A

PREGNANCY
Low adrenal androgen production by the fetus is thought to cause hypospadias.

SYNONYMS
N/A

SEE ALSO
- Infertility, Male dogs
- Sexual Development Disorders
- Dermatoses, Sex Hormone Responsive
- Incontinence, Urinary

ABBREVIATIONS
- GnRH = gonadotropin-releasing hormone
- FSH = follicle-stimulating hormone
- HCG = human chorionic gonadotropin
- DHT = dihydrotestosterone
- LH = luteinizing hormone

Suggested Reading

Feldman EC, Nelson RW. Disorders of the male reproductive tract. In: Feldman EC, Nelson RW, eds. Canine and feline endocrinology and reproduction. Philadelphia: Saunders, 1987:481–524.

Meyers-Wallen VN, Patterson DF. Disorders of sexual development in dogs and cats. In: Kirk RW, ed. Current veterinary therapy X: small animal practice. Philadelphia: Saunders, 1989:1261–1269.

Purswell BJ. Pharmaceuticals used in canine reproduction. Semin Vet Med Surg (Sm Anim) 1994;9:54–60.

Schmeitzel LP. Sex hormone-related and growth hormone-related alopecias. Vet Clin North Am (Sm Anim Pract) 1990;20: 1579–1601.

Shille VM, Olson PN. Dynamic testing in reproductive endocrinology. In: Kirk RW, ed. Current veterinary therapy X: small animal practice. Philadelphia: Saunders, 1989: 1282–1288.

Author Margaret R. Kern
Consulting Editor Deborah S. Greco

DISEASES

HYPOMYELINATION—CENTRAL AND PERIPHERAL NERVOUS SYSTEM

BASICS

DEFINITION
• Congenital condition caused by insufficient myelin production
• All axons > 1–2 mm in diameter are invested with a covering of myelin that arises from oligodendrocytes in the CNS and Schwann cells in the PNS.
• Myelin insulates axons and facilitates propagation of action potentials.

SIGNALMENT
CNS
• Dogs
• Welsh springer spaniels, Samoyeds, chow chows, Weimaraners, Bernese mountain dogs, Dalmatians, and lurchers (an English cross-breed)—reported
• Clinical signs appear within days of birth.
• Predominant sex—springer spaniels and Samoyed male puppies clinically affected, whereas females remain largely asymptomatic carriers; no sex differences reported in other breeds

PNS
• Dogs
• Golden retrievers—reported in both sexes
• Clinical signs appear at 5–7 weeks of age.

SIGNS
CNS
• Generalized body tremors that worsen with exercise and subside during rest
• Improve by 1 year of age, except for springer spaniels and Samoyeds, which are affected for life

PNS
• Generalized weakness, pelvic limb ataxia, muscle wasting, and hyporeflexia
• Do not resolve with age

CAUSES & RISK FACTORS
• Genetic—sex-linked recessive condition proven for CNS disease in springer spaniels; speculative for other breeds
• Viral or toxic—possible in chow chows, Weimaraners, Bernese mountain dogs, Dalmatians, and lurchers, because clinical signs of CNS disease improve or resolve.
• PNS—undetermined; possibly genetic

DIAGNOSIS

DIFFERENTIAL DIAGNOSIS
CNS
• Cerebellar hypoplasia or abiotrophy—tremors in neonates; but ataxia and intention tremors more prominent
• Storage diseases—associated with tremors; neonates are normal.
• Idiopathic tremors in white dogs—do not develop before 8 months of age

PNS
• Muscular dystrophy
• Congenital myasthenia gravis
• Other polyneuropathies or myopathies

CBC/BIOCHEMISTRY/URINALYSIS
Usually normal

OTHER LABORATORY TESTS
N/A

IMAGING
MRI—detect CNS form

DIAGNOSTIC PROCEDURES
CNS
• Diagnosis based on clinical signs
• Brain biopsy
• Necropsy

PNS
• Electromyography—usually normal to mild diffuse spontaneous activity
• Motor nerve conduction velocity—small or no evoked potentials and slowed conduction
• Nerve biopsy—insufficient myelin surrounding peripheral axons

HYPOMYELINATION—CENTRAL AND PERIPHERAL NERVOUS SYSTEM

 TREATMENT
• None effective for either form

MEDICATIONS

DRUG(S) OF CHOICE
N/A

CONTRAINDICATIONS/POSSIBLE INTERACTIONS
N/A

 FOLLOW-UP

PREVENTION/AVOIDANCE
Avoid breeding animals in which a genetic cause is suspected.

EXPECTED COURSE AND PROGNOSIS
• CNS—springer spaniels and Samoyeds affected for life; other breeds improve by 1 year of age.
• PNS—signs do not resolve with age.

 MISCELLANEOUS

ABBREVIATION
PNS = peripheral nervous system

Suggested Reading

Duncan ID. Abnormalities of myelination of the central nervous system associated with congenital tremor. J Vet Intern Med 1987;1:10–23.

Matz ME, Shell L, Braund K. Peripheral hypomyelinization in two golden retriever litter mates. J Am Vet Med Assoc 1990;197:228–230.

Author Karen Dyer Inzana
Consulting Editor Joane M. Parent

HYPOPARATHYROIDISM

BASICS

DEFINITION
Absolute or relative deficiency of parathyroid hormone secretion leading to hypocalcemia

PATHOPHYSIOLOGY
• Dogs—most commonly idiopathic immune-mediated parathyroiditis • Cats—most commonly iatrogenic secondary to damaged or removed parathyroid glands during thyroidectomy for hyperthyroidism; idiopathic atrophy and immune-mediated parathyroiditis also seen (uncommon)

SYSTEMS AFFECTED
• Nervous/neuromuscular—seizures, tetany, ataxia, and weakness caused by increased neuromuscular activity resulting from diminished neuronal membrane stability • Cardiovascular—ECG changes and bradycardia caused by altered neuromuscular activity • Gastrointestinal—anorexia and vomiting (especially cats) of unknown cause, possibly changes in gastrointestinal muscular activity • Ophthalmic—posterior lenticular cataracts of unknown cause • Respiratory—panting caused by neuromuscular weakness and anxiety associated with neurologic and neuromuscular changes • Renal/urologic—polyuria and polydipsia (PU/PD) of unknown cause

INCIDENCE/PREVALENCE
• Dogs—uncommon; exact prevalence not reported • Cats—common in thyroidectomized cats (10–82% of patients, depending on surgical technique and surgical skill); spontaneous occurrence rare (6 cases reported)

SIGNALMENT

Species
Dogs and cats

Breed Predilections
Toy poodle, miniature schnauzer, German shepherd, Labrador retriever, and Scottish terrier; mixed-breed cats

Mean Age and Range
• Dogs—mean age, 6 years; range, 6 weeks to 12 years • Cats—secondary to thyroidectomy: mean age 12–13 years, range 4–22 years; spontaneous: mean age 2.25 years, range 6 months to 6.7 years

Predominant Sex
• Dogs—female • Cats—none

SIGNS

Dogs
• Seizures (54–73%) • Muscle trembling, twitching, and fasciculations (54%) • Tense, splinted abdomen (50%) • Ataxia/stiff gait (43%) • Fever (30–40%) • Panting (35%) • Posterior lenticular cataracts (15–20%) • Weakness • PU/PD • Facial rubbing • Vomiting • Anorexia • Up to 20% may have nor-

mal physical examination results

Cats (based on 6 reported cases)
• Lethargy, anorexia, and depression (100%) • Seizures (50%) • Muscle trembling, twitching, and fasciculations (83%) • Panting (33%) • Posterior lenticular cataracts (33%) • Bradycardia (17%) • Fever (17%) • Hypothermia (17%)

RISK FACTORS
• Dogs—N/A • Cats—thyroidectomy for hyperthyroidism

DIAGNOSIS

DIFFERENTIAL DIAGNOSIS
The main problems associated with hypoparathyroidism, which must be differentiated from other disease processes, are seizures, weakness, and muscle trembling, twitching, and fasciculations.

Seizures
• Cardiovascular—syncope • Metabolic—hepatoencephalopathy and hypoglycemia • Neurologic—epilepsy, neoplasia, toxin, and inflammatory disease

Weakness
• Cardiovascular—congenital anatomic defects, arrhythmias, heart failure, and pericardial effusion • Metabolic—hypoadrenocorticism, hypoglycemia, anemia, hypokalemia (especially cats), and hypothyroidism • Neurologic/neuromuscular—myasthenia gravis, polymyositis, polyradiculoneuropathy, and spinal cord disease • Toxic—tick paralysis, botulism, chronic organophosphate exposure, and lead poisoning

Muscle Trembling, Twitching, and Fasciculations
• Metabolic—hypercalcemia, hyperadrenocorticism, and puerperal tetany (i.e., eclampsia) • Toxic—tetanus and strychnine poisoning

CBC/BIOCHEMISTRY/URINALYSIS
• Results of hemogram and urinalysis usually normal; these tests are performed to rule out other differential diagnoses • Hypocalcemia (usually <6.5 mg/dL) and normal or mild to moderate hyperphosphatemia • Evaluate serum albumin carefully in all patients with hypocalcemia; hypoalbuminemia is the most common cause of hypocalcemia; in dogs with hypoalbuminemia, one of the following formulas should be used to correct the serum calcium:

$$\text{Corrected Ca} = \text{Ca (mg/dL)} - \text{albumin (g/dL)} + 3.5$$

or

$$\text{Corrected Ca} = \text{Ca (mg/dL)} - [0.4 \times \text{total protein (g/dL)}] + 3.3$$

• Hypocalcemia caused by hypoalbuminemia in cats cannot be corrected by these formulas, although hypoalbuminemia causes reduced serum calcium in cats. • The only other disease process that reduces serum calcium and raises serum phosphorus is renal failure, which is easily distinguished from hypoparathyroidism by the presence of azotemia.

OTHER LABORATORY TESTS
Serum PTH determination—demonstrates undetectable or very low concentration of PTH; patients with other processes causing hypocalcemia (e.g., renal failure) have a normal-to-high concentration of PTH.

IMAGING
Radiography and ultrasonography are normal

DIAGNOSTIC PROCEDURES
• ECG changes seen in patients with hypocalcemia include prolongation of the ST and Q-T segments; sinus bradycardia and wide T waves or T wave alternans is occasionally seen. • Cervical exploration reveals absence or atrophy of the parathyroid glands.

PATHOLOGIC FINDINGS
• Dogs—normal tissue with mature lymphocytes, plasma cells, and fibrous connective tissue along with chief cell degeneration • Cats—parathyroid gland atrophy is more common, although histopathologic findings similar to those in dogs were found in one cat

TREATMENT

APPROPRIATE HEALTH CARE
• Hospitalize for medical management of hypocalcemia until clinical signs of hypocalcemia are controlled and serum calcium concentration is >7.0 mg/dL. • See Calcium, Hypocalcemia for emergency inpatient management and appropriate fluid therapy.

MEDICATIONS

DRUGS OF CHOICE

Emergency/Acute Therapy
See Calcium, Hypocalcemia.

Short-term Post-tetany Therapy
See Calcium, Hypocalcemia.

Long-term Therapy
• Vitamin D administration is needed indefinitely; The dosage should be increased or tapered on the basis of serum calcium concentration (see Table 1). • Shorter-acting prep-

arations of vitamin D are preferred so that overdosage (hypercalcemia) can be quickly corrected (see Table 1). • A more economical approach to treatment is to maximize oral administration of calcium and reduce oral administration of vitamin D; calcium is usually less expensive than vitamin D.

PRECAUTIONS
All calcium preparations given orally can cause gastrointestinal disturbances; calcium carbonate may be less irritating because of its high calcium availability and lower dosage requirement.

POSSIBLE INTERACTIONS
• Injectable calcium solutions are reportedly incompatible with tetracycline drugs, cephalothin, methylprednisolone sodium succinate, dobutamine, metoclopramide, and amphotericin B. • Thiazide diuretics used in conjunction with large doses of calcium may cause hypercalcemia. • Patients on digitalis are more likely to develop arrhythmias if calcium is administered intravenously. • Calcium administration may antagonize effects of calcium channel blocking agents (e.g., diltiazem, verapamil, nifedipine, and amlodipine).

FOLLOW-UP

PATIENT MONITORING
• Hypocalcemia and hypercalcemia are both concerns with long-term management. • Serum calcium concentration monthly for the first 6 months then every 2–4 months; goal is to maintain serum calcium between 8 and 10 mg/dL. • Inform clients about clinical signs of hypo- and hypercalcemia.

POSSIBLE COMPLICATIONS
• Hypocalcemia • Hypercalcemia, which can lead to renal failure (see Hypercalcemia)

EXPECTED COURSE AND PROGNOSIS
• With close monitoring of serum calcium and client dedication, the prognosis for long-term survival is excellent. • Adjustments in vitamin D and oral calcium administration can be expected during the course of management, especially during the initial 2–6 months. • Cats with hypoparathyroidism secondary to thyroidectomy usually require only transient treatment because they typically regain normal parathyroid function within 4–6 months, often within 2–3 weeks.

MISCELLANEOUS

ASSOCIATED CONDITIONS
Excess muscular activity can lead to hyperthermia, which may necessitate treatment.

PREGNANCY
Hypocalcemia can lead to weakness and dystocia.

SEE ALSO
• Calcium, Hypercalcemia • Calcium, Hypocalcemia • Hyperthyroidism

ABBREVIATIONS
• Ca = calcium • ECG = electrocardiography • PTH = parathyroid hormone • PU/

PD = polyuria and polydipsia

Suggested Reading

Bruyette DS, Feldman EC. Primary hypoparathyroidism in the dog. Report of 15 cases and review of 13 previously reported cases. J Vet Int Med 1988;2:7–14.

Feldman EC, Nelson RW. Hypocalcemia and primary hypoparathyroidism. In: Feldman EC, Nelson RW, eds. Canine and feline endocrinology and reproduction. Philadelphia: WB Saunders, 1996:497–516.

Peterson ME, James KM, Wallace M, et al. Idiopathic hypoparathyroidism in five cats. J Vet Int Med 1991;5:47–51.

Waters CB, Scott-Moncrieff JCR. Hypocalcemia in cats. Compend Contin Educ Pract Vet 1992;14:497–507.

Author Mitchell A. Crystal
Consulting Editor Deborah S. Greco

Table 1

Calcium Preparations			
Preparation	*Dose*	*Available Calcium*	*Size Available*
Calcium carbonate	Canine: 1–4 g/day Feline: 0.5–1 g/day	40%	350–1500 mg tablets
Calcium gluconate	Canine: 1–4 g/day Feline: 0.5–1 g/day	10%	1000 mg tablets
Calcium lactate	Canine: 1–4 g/day Feline: 0.5–1 g/day	13%	

Table 2

Vitamin D Preparations			
Preparation	*Dose*	*Maximal Effect*	*Size*
1,25 Dihydroxycholecalciferol (active vitamin D_3, calcitriol)	0.003–0.006 µg/kg/day	1–4 days	0.25 and 0.5 µg capsules
Dihydrotachysterol	Initial: 0.02–0.03 mg/kg/day Maint: 0.01–0.02 mg/kg/24–48 h	1–7 days	0.125, 0.2, 0.4 mg capsules and 0.25 mg/mL syrup
Ergocalciferol (vitamin D_2)	Initial: 4000–6000 U/kg/day Maint: 1000–2000 U/kg/day-week	5–21 days	25,000 and 50,000 U capsules and 8,000 U/mL syrup

DISEASES

HYPOPYON AND LIPID FLARE

BASICS

OVERVIEW
- White anterior chamber opacities
- Hypopyon—more common than lipid flare; an accumulation of WBCs in the anterior chamber that develops in animals with an extreme breakdown of the blood–aqueous barrier; cellular components typically settle homogeneously in the ventral anterior chamber, forming a horizontal line.
- Lipid flare—lipid-laden aqueous humor in the anterior chamber, giving the entire aqueous humor a milky white color; aqueous humor becomes laden with lipids with a breakdown of the blood–aqueous barrier and concurrent hyperlipidemia.

SIGNALMENT
- Hypopyon—dogs and cats of any age, breed, or sex that have severe anterior uveitis from any cause
- Lipid flare—hyperlipidemic miniature schnauzers are prone, rare in cats

SIGNS
- Turbidity of aqueous humor—diffuse with lipid flare; ventral with hypopyon
- Anterior uveitis of some degree

CAUSES & RISK FACTORS
Any cause of anterior uveitis may lead to hypopyon or lipid flare (see Anterior Uveitis—Dogs; Anterior Uveitis—Cats).

Hypopyon
- May be composed of inflammatory cells with severe keratitis and anterior uveitis
- May be composed of neoplastic cells with intraocular neoplasia (e.g., lymphosarcoma)

Lipid Flare
- Primary hyperlipidemia—idiopathic hyperlipidemia in miniature schnauzers; lipoprotein lipase deficiency in cats
- Secondary hyperlipidemia—diabetes mellitus; pancreatitis; hypothyroidism; cholestatic liver disease; hyperadrenocorticism; nephrotic syndrome

DIAGNOSIS

DIFFERENTIAL DIAGNOSIS
Aqueous flare solely as a result of a high anterior chamber protein concentration—not milky white; will not obscure one's ability to see the iris

CBC/BIOCHEMISTRY/URINALYSIS

Hypopyon
Dogs—typically normal unless secondary to a systemic disease

Lipid Flare
- High serum cholesterol or triglyceride concentration—common
- High cholesterol—mild, < 500 mg/dL; moderate, 500–750 mg/dL; marked, > 750 mg/dL
- High triglyceride—mild, < 400 mg/dL; moderate, 400–1000 mg/dL; marked, > 1000 mg/dL
- Cats—lower cutoff points are appropriate.

OTHER LABORATORY TESTS
- Standing plasma test—determine if lipemia is caused by chylomicrons, very low density lipoproteins, or both; chylomicrons form a cream layer on top of the sample; very low density lipoprotein particles remain suspended.
- Lipoprotein electrophoresis
- Measurement of lipoprotein lipase activity—detects low activity

IMAGING
N/A

DIAGNOSTIC PROCEDURES
- Workup for ulcerative keratitis or anterior uveitis may be indicated.
- Anterior chamber paracentesis—seldom worthwhile unless globe perforation has occurred and bacterial endophthalmitis is suspected; or if lymphosarcoma is suspected

TREATMENT
- Hypopyon—inpatient for aggressive medical therapy; warn client of the potential for blindness.
- Primary hyperlipidemia; secondary hyperlipidemia not responding to treatment of primary disease—outpatient; provide a low-fat, low-calorie diet.

MEDICATIONS

DRUGS
- Hypopyon—usually sterile, unless globe perforation has occurred; if secondary to corneal ulceration, cornea may be infected and aggressive antibiotic therapy indicated (see Keratitis, Ulcerative)
- Topical 1% prednisolone acetate or 0.1% dexamethasone—q1–2h initially, then q4–8h for severe hypopyon; q6–8h for lipid flare; if the cornea is not ulcerated
- Subconjunctival steroids—triamcinolone acetonide (4–8 mg/eye); adjunct to topical treatment in severe cases.
- Systemic corticosteroids—1.0–2.0 mg/kg/day for 7 days, then gradually decrease dosage
- Topical 1% atropine—q4–6h initially, then q6–12h; for severe disease

CONTRAINDICATIONS/POSSIBLE INTERACTIONS
- Topical or subconjunctival corticosteroids—avoid if the cornea is ulcerated.
- Topical NSAIDs—flurbiprofen or suprofen (q6h) for severe hypopyon when topically applied corticosteroids are contraindicated; safety in cats undetermined
- Atropine—use with caution or not at all with high IOP

FOLLOW-UP
- Check with frequent (initially daily) ocular examinations, including tonometry to rule out secondary glaucoma.
- Hypopyon—guarded prognosis; depends on the response to treatment
- Lipid flare—usually resolves quickly with topical agents and treatment of the primary disease

MISCELLANEOUS

PREGNANCY
Avoid systemic steroids in pregnant animals.

SEE ALSO
- Anterior Uveitis—Cats
- Anterior Uveitis—Dogs
- Keratitis, Ulcerative

ABBREVIATION
IOP = intraocular pressure

Suggested Reading
Collins BK, Moore CP. Diseases and surgery of the canine anterior uvea. In: Gelatt KN, ed., Veterinary ophthalmology. 3rd ed. Philadelphia: Lippincott Williams & Wilkins, 1999:755–795.

Author Michael J. Ringle
Consulting Editor Paul E. Miller

BASICS

OVERVIEW
• A condition resulting from destruction of the pituitary gland by a neoplastic, degenerative, or anomalous process
• Associated with low production of pituitary hormones including thyroid-stimulating hormone (TSH), adrenocorticotropin hormone (ACTH), luteinizing hormone, follicle-stimulating hormone, and growth hormone (GH)

SIGNALMENT
• Age: 2–6 months
• Breeds—German shepherd dog, Carnelian bear dog, spitz, toy pinscher, and Weimaraner
• Simple autosomal recessive in German shepherd dog and Carnelian bear dog

SIGNS

Historical Findings
• Mental retardation manifested as difficulty in house-breaking
• Slow growth noticed in first 2–3 months of life
• Proportionate dwarfism

Physical Examination Findings
• Retained puppy haircoat
• Thin, hypotonic skin
• Shrill bark
• Truncal alopecia
• Cutaneous hyperpigmentation
• Infantile genitalia
• Delayed dental eruption

CAUSES & RISK FACTORS

Congenital
• Cystic Rathke's pouch
• Isolated GH deficiency

Acquired
• Pituitary tumor
• Trauma
• Radiotherapy

 DIAGNOSIS

DIFFERENTIAL DIAGNOSIS
• Hypothyroid dwarfism; breed predilection and disproportionate dwarfism observed in patients with hypothyroidism.
• Other causes of stunted growth—portosystemic shunt, diabetes mellitus, hyperadrenocorticism, malnutrition, parasitism

CBC/BIOCHEMISTRY/URINALYSIS
• Eosinophilia
• Lymphocytosis
• Hypophosphatemia
• Hypoglycemia

OTHER LABORATORY TESTS
• Corticotropin and TSH response tests
• Subnormal response to TSH and ACTH
• Growth hormone and insulin-like growth factor assays
• Growth hormone assay not currently available in the U.S.; recommend measurement of IGF-1, which is low

IMAGING
Radiography may reveal epiphyseal dysgenesis and abnormal retention of physeal growth plates.

DIAGNOSIS
N/A

 TREATMENT
N/A

 MEDICATIONS

DRUGS OF CHOICE
• Growth hormone—human, porcine, or bovine, if available; 0.1 IU/kg SC 3 times weekly for 4–6 weeks; repeat if necessary
• Treat hypothyroidism with levothyroxine (22 µg/kg PO q24h)
• Glucocorticoid (e.g., prednisone, 0.2 mg/kg PO q24h) if ACTH response test results are subnormal; higher dosage of steroids needed during periods of stress.

CONTRAINDICATIONS/POSSIBLE INTERACTIONS
Hypersensitivity reactions and carbohydrate intolerance may develop with growth hormone supplementation.

 FOLLOW-UP

PATIENT MONITORING
• Blood and urinary glucose concentration
• Stop growth hormone supplementation if glucosuria develops or blood glucose is >150 mg/dL

POSSIBLE COMPLICATIONS
Neurologic complications of expansion of Rathke's pouch

EXPECTED COURSE AND PROGNOSIS
• Skin and haircoat improve within 6–8 weeks of initiating growth hormone and thyroid supplementation.
• Generally no increase in stature, because growth plates have usually closed by the time of diagnosis
• Dogs often die at a young age (3–4 years) because of neurologic complications.
• Poor long-term prognosis

 MISCELLANEOUS

SEE ALSO
• Hypothyroidism
• Hypoadrenocorticism (Addison's disease)

ABBREVIATIONS
• TSH = thyroid-stimulating hormone
• ACTH = adrenocorticotropin
• GH = growth hormone

Suggested Reading
Campbell KL. Growth hormone-related disorders in dogs. Compend Cont Educ Pract Vet 1988;10:477–482.
Author Deborah S. Greco
Consulting Editor Deborah S. Greco

DISEASES

HYPOTHYROIDISM

 BASICS

DEFINITION
• Clinical condition that results from inadequate production and release of tetraiodothyronine (levothyroxine, T_4) and triiodothyronine (liothyronine, T_3) by the thyroid gland
• Characterized by a generalized decrease in cellular metabolic activity

PATHOPHYSIOLOGY

Acquired Hypothyroidism
• In dogs, primary acquired hypothyroidism is the most common (>95% of cases) type.
• Caused by lymphocytic thyroiditis (50%) or idiopathic thyroid atrophy (50%) • Lymphocytic thyroiditis is thought to be immune mediated (cellular and humoral).
• Circulating autoantibodies to thyroglobulin, T_3, or T_4 are usually present, but these autoantibodies can also be found in a variable percentage (13–40%) of normal, euthyroid dogs.
• Rarely, primary hypothyroidism is caused by neoplastic (primary or metastatic) destruction of the thyroid gland or dietary iodine deficiency.
• Rare in cats and is most commonly seen following bilateral thyroidectomy or radioactive iodine therapy; it is often transitory and frequently does not require therapy.
• Accessory thyroid tissue in the neck or thoracic cavity usually undergoes hyperplasia and produces physiologic amounts of thyroid hormones.
• Acquired secondary hypothyroidism is very uncommon in dogs and cats; it is caused by pituitary dysfunction or destruction leading to decreased thyrotropin (thyroid-stimulating hormone, TSH) production.
• Thyrotropin is the pituitary hormone responsible for stimulating thyroid hormone synthesis and secretion.
• Increased circulating levels of glucocorticoids (endogenous or exogenous) can transitorily suppress TSH secretion by anterior pituitary thyrotropes; this leads to decreased blood levels of T_4 and free T_4.
• Thyrotrope secretion of TSH normalizes when blood glucocorticosteroid levels return to normal.
• Tertiary hypothyroidism caused by decreased thyrotropin-releasing hormone (TRH) production by the hypothalamus has not been documented in dogs or cats.

Congenital Hypothyroidism
• Congenital hypothyroidism is very rare in both dogs and cats.
• Reported causes of primary congenital hypothyroidism in dogs and cats include thyroid agenesis or dysgenesis, dyshormonogenesis, and iodine deficiency.
• Secondary congenital hypothyroidism is most commonly observed in German shepherd dogs with a panhypopituitarism caused by a cystic Rathke's pouch.
• A congenital deficiency in pituitary TSH production was reported in a family of giant schnauzers.

SYSTEMS AFFECTED
• Endocrine/metabolic
• Skin/exocrine
• Behavioral
• Neuromuscular
• Reproductive
• Gastrointestinal
• Ophthalmic
• Cardiovascular
• Nervous

GENETICS
• No known genetic basis for the inheritance of primary hypothyroidism in canines.
• Familial lymphocytic thyroiditis has been reported in individual colonies of borzois, beagles, and great Danes.

INCIDENCE/PREVALENCE
• Primary hypothyroidism is the most common endocrinopathy of dogs; the reported prevalence of hypothyroidism in dogs 1:156–1:500.
• Hypothyroidism is rare in cats.

GEOGRAPHIC DISTRIBUTION
N/A

SIGNALMENT

Species
Dogs and rarely cats

Breed Predilections
• Primary acquired hypothyroidism is more common in medium to large-sized dogs.
• Breeds reported to be predisposed to developing primary acquired hypothyroidism include the golden retriever, Doberman pinscher, Irish setter, great Dane, airedale terrier, old English sheepdog, dachshund, miniature schnauzer, cocker spaniel, poodle and boxer.

Mean Age And Range
Most common in middle-aged dogs (4–10 years)

Predominant Sex
No definitive sex predilection has been identified; however, castrated male dogs and spayed female dogs appear to be at increased risk.

SIGNS

Historical Findings
• Most common—lethargy, inactivity, mental dullness, weight gain, hair loss or excessive shedding, lack of hair regrowth following clipping, dry or lusterless haircoat, excessive scaling, hyperpigmentation, recurrent skin infections, and cold intolerance
• Uncommon—generalized weakness, incoordination, head tilt, facial paralysis, seizures and infertility
• Clinical signs develop slowly and are progressive.

Physical Examination Findings
Dermatologic abnormalities—very common
• Bilaterally symmetric truncal alopecia that spares the head and extremities—common
• Alopecia is usually nonpruritic unless a secondary pyoderma or other pruritic dermatitis is also present.
• Hairs epilate easily; the haircoat is often dry and lusterless.
• Alopecia often initially involves the flank area, base of the ears, tail (rat tail) and friction areas (axillae, ventrum of thorax, abdomen and neck, and under the collar).
• Early in the disease course, alopecia may be multifocal and asymmetric; alopecic lesion may have irregular margins.
• Hyperpigmentation and increased thickness of the epidermis are common, particularly in friction areas.
• Seborrhea—common; can be generalized, multifocal, or localized
• A secondary superficial pyoderma occurs frequently; deep pyoderma is less common.
• Dermal accumulation of mucopolysaccharides can lead to nonpitting edema (myxedema), particularly in the facial area; this produces the classic "tragic" expression associated with hypothyroidism.
General/metabolic—very common
• Lethargy, mental dullness
• Weight gain
• Mild hypothermia Reproductive
• Infertility and prolonged anestrus in females
• Inappropriate galactorrhea in sexually intact bitches

Neuromuscular—uncommon
• A peripheral neuropathy (localized or generalized) involving lower motor neurons occasionally occurs in hypothyroid dogs.
• Generalized weakness is the most common clinical sign; dogs may have a stiff, stilted gait. Other neurologic findings may include proprioceptive deficits, hyporeflexia, head tilt, facial paralysis/paresis, and ataxia.
• A secondary myopathy characterized by denervation atrophy is usually present in dogs with hypothyroid polyneuropathy.
• Some hypothyroid dogs develop a generalized myopathy without concurrent neurologic involvement; these dogs present for generalized weakness.
• Seizures secondary to marked cerebral atherosclerosis have been rarely reported in hypothyroid dogs with marked hyperlipidemia.
• Laryngeal paralysis, megaesophagus, and Homer's syndrome have been associated with hypothyroidism, but definitive proof of a causal relationship is lacking.
Ophthalmic
• Corneal lipid deposits • Lipemia retinalis
Felines—rare
• Unkempt appearance, matting of hair, nonpruritic seborrhea sicca, pinnal alopecia
• Lethargy
• Obesity
Congenital hypothyroidism—cretinism
• Mental dullness/retardation, lethargy, inactivity
• Disproportionate dwarfism (large, broad head with short neck and limbs), shortened mandible, protruding tongue, delayed dental eruption
• Constipation/obstipation—particularly in cats
• Hypothermia
• Retention of puppy coat, progressive truncal alopecia (dogs)

CAUSES
Lymphocytic thyroiditis, idiopathic thyroid atrophy, congenital disease, pituitary disease, dietary iodine deficiency, neoplasia and iatrogenic.

RISK FACTORS
• Neutering may slightly increase risk of developing primary hypothyroidism.
• Bilateral thyroidectomy may result in hypothyroidism.

 DIAGNOSIS

DIFFERENTIAL DIAGNOSIS
• Dermatologic abnormalities are frequently the predominant clinical abnormality in dogs with hypothyroidism.
• Consider endocrine causes of alopecia (e.g., hyperadrenocorticism, sex hormone–related dermatopathies, growth hormone–responsive dermatosis, and adrenal sex hormone abnormalities).
• If fasting hyperlipidemia (the most common laboratory abnormality in hypothyroid dogs) must rule out diabetes mellitus, hyperadrenocorticism, nephrotic syndrome, acute pancreatitis, bilary obstruction, and primary lipid metabolism abnormalities.

CBC/BIOCHEMISTRY/URINALYSIS
• Hypercholesterolemia—observed in up to 80% of hypothyroid dogs
• Hypertriglyceridemia and gross lipemia—less common
• Mild, normochromic, normocytic, nonregenerative anemia—up to 50% of hypothyroid dogs
• Mildly elevated serum creatine kinase levels are intermittently identified.

OTHER LABORATORY TESTS
• Do endocrine testing in dogs with clinical signs or laboratory abnormalities suggesting hypothyroidism.
• Routine endocrine testing of sick dogs for hypothyroidism is unnecessary if they do not show signs consistent with hypothyroidism.
• Please see Appendix for table of endocrine test protocols.

Basal Serum Thyroid Hormone Concentrations
• Basal serum T_4 levels in the midnormal to high-normal range rule out a diagnosis of hypothyroidism; further endocrine testing is not indicated.

• A subnormal T_4 concentration is compatible with, but not diagnostic for, hypothyroidism.
• Subnormal T_4 levels can be seen in healthy, euthyroid dogs.
• Serum T_4 levels often drop below normal in dogs with nonthyroidal illness (sick euthyroid syndrome); these animals are not hypothyroid and do not require thyroid hormone supplementation.
• Basal serum T_3 levels are not an accurate means for evaluating thyroid function; one study found normal serum T_3 levels in 74% of hypothyroid dogs; serum T_3 levels can be subnormal in healthy, euthyroid dogs and in euthyroid dogs with nonthyroidal illness.
• Markedly elevated T_4 or T_3 levels in dogs indicate the presence of thyroid hormone autoantibodies; these autoantibodies can cause false elevations or, much less commonly, false decreases in T_4 or T_3 concentrations determined by radioimmunoassay.
• Determination of serum free T_4 (FT_4) levels by equilibrium dialysis is a sensitive and specific way to evaluate a patient for hypothyroidism.
• Low FT_4 concentrations in a patient with compatible clinical signs and low total 14 levels strongly indicate hypothyroidism; however, FT_4 levels are low in up to 25% of euthyroid dogs with hyperadrenocorticism.
• Severe nonthyroidal illness may suppress FT_4 levels in some euthyroid dogs.
• Determination of serum FT_3 levels is noncontributory to diagnosing hypothyroidism.

Endogenous Thyrotropin (TSH) Concentrations
• Thyrotropin concentrations are increased in most dogs with primary hypothyroidism, but 18–38% of dogs with confirmed hypothyroidism have normal serum ISH levels.
• Elevated TSH levels have been reported in up to 14% of euthyroid dogs with nonthyroidal illness.
• High TSH levels combined with low T_4 or FT_4 concentrations strongly indicate hypothyroidism.

HYPOTHYROIDISM

Autoantibodies to Thyroid Hormones and Thyroglobulin (Tg)

• Autoantibodies to Tg and to a lesser extent T_3 and T_4 occur frequently in dogs with hypothyroidism and are consistent with a diagnosis of lymphocytic thyroiditis; these autoantibodies can also occur in healthy, euthyroid dogs.

• Autoantibodies to Tg were found in up to 43% of dogs with nonthyroidal endocrine diseases.

• Healthy dogs with normal T_4 concentrations and autoantibodies to Tg, T_3, or T_4 may be at increased risk for developing hypothyroidism, but this is not proven.

TSH Stimulation Test

• Considered the gold standard for diagnosing clinical hypothyroidism • Administer exogenous TSH to the patient and determine pre- and poststimulation serum T_4 concentrations

• In hypothyroid dogs, the T_4 concentration following TSH administration does not rise into the normal reference range and frequently does not exceed the pre–TSH stimulation T_4 concentration.

• T_4 levels increase beyond the upper limit of the normal reference range following TSH stimulation of healthy, euthyroid dogs.

• Dogs with moderate or severe nonthyroidal illness, early primary hypothyroidism, or early secondary or tertiary hypothyroidism may show a muted response to TSH administration.

• T_4 concentrations increase but frequently not above the normal reference range.

• Reevaluate these animals in 3–4 months or following resolution of their nonthyroidal disease, if they still have clinical signs compatible with hypothyroidism.

• Because of the difficulty and expense of obtaining ISH, TSH stimulation testing is not commonly done in private practice; similar diagnostic information can be obtained by evaluating baseline serum T_4, FT_4, and endogenous TSH concentrations.

TRH Stimulation Testing

• Exogenous TRH is administered IV; pre- and poststimulation T_4 or TSH concentrations are measured.

• In euthyroid dogs, both T_4 and TSH concentrations increase above baseline values.

• In hypothyroid dogs, T_4 concentration does not increase significantly over the baseline T_4 value.

• Changes in T_4 concentration in healthy, euthyroid dogs are small and variable, making it difficult to differentiate normal dogs from hypothyroid dogs.

• Thyrotropin levels also increase in dogs with primary hypothyroidism, but the percentage increase over baseline concentrations is less than in euthyroid dogs.

• TRH stimulation testing is not recommended for diagnosing hypothyroidism; better tests are available; evaluating TSH concentrations following TRH administration can differentiate primary hypothyroidism from central hypothyroidism.

IMAGING

Radiography

• Epiphyseal dysgenesis, delayed epiphyseal ossification, and shortened vertebral bodies are present in patients with congenital hypothyroidism; these patients frequently develop radiographic signs of degenerative joint disease as adults.

• Megacolon is a common radiographic finding in cats with congenital hypothyroidism.

Echocardiography

Indices of left ventricular systolic function are commonly abnormal; these changes are usually not clinically significant unless the dog has concurrent primary heart disease.

DIAGNOSTIC PROCEDURES

Electrocardiography—low-amplitude R-waves are commonly observed, bradycardia less frequently

PATHOLOGIC FINDINGS

• Lymphocytic thyroiditis is characterized by a diffuse infiltration of lymphocytes and plasma cells into the thyroid parenchyma with eventual destruction of the gland.

• Idiopathic thyroid atrophy is characterized by parenchymal atrophy and replacement with adipose and connective tissue.

• Epidermal and dermal abnormalities are common.

• Dermatohistopathologic abnormalities commonly seen with hypothyroidism include orthokeratotic hyperkeratosis, sebaceous gland atrophy, epidermal hyperplasia, follicular atrophy, myxedema, and vacuolation of the arrector pili muscles.

 TREATMENT

APPROPRIATE HEALTH CARE
Outpatient

NURSING CARE
N/A

ACTIVITY
N/A

DIET
Reduced-fat diet until body weight is satisfactory and T_4 concentrations are normal

CLIENT EDUCATION

• Dogs with primary hypothyroidism respond well to treatment with oral synthetic levothyroxine (L-thyroxine).

• The appropriate dosage for L-thyroxine varies between individuals because of differences in gastrointestinal (GI) absorption and hormone metabolism; possible after patient has responded to therapy and T_4 levels have normalized.

• Treatment is lifelong.

• Most clinical and laboratory abnormalities resolve over a few weeks to a few months.

• Occasionally, dermatologic abnormalities worsen transiently during the first month of therapy.

SURGICAL CONSIDERATIONS
N/A

MEDICATIONS

DRUGS OF CHOICE
• Levothyroxine is the treatment of choice.
• The starting dosage is 0.02–0.04 mg/kg/day or 0.5 mg/m²/day divided BID. •
 Adjust dosage on the basis of on serum T_4 concentration and clinical response to therapy; initially, use a veterinary name brand product.
• If the patient responds to therapy, once-daily therapy can be tried; however, some patients require continued BID therapy.
• Different brands of L-thyroxine frequently have different GI absorption kinetics; the dosage may change if the brand is changed.

CONTRAINDICATIONS
None

PRECAUTIONS
• The initial dosage of L-thyroxine may need to be decreased in animals with concurrent heart failure, diabetes mellitus, renal failure, liver disease, or hypoadrenocorticism.
• The initial dosage of L-thyroxine is 25% of the standard daily dosage.
• Slowly increase the dosage over 2–4 months until the appropriate dosage is obtained; this allows the patient to adjust slowly to the increased basal metabolic rate.
• Start glucocorticoid replacement therapy prior to L-thyroxine therapy in hypothyroid animals with concurrent hypoadrenocorticism.

POSSIBLE INTERACTIONS
• Glucocorticoids, phenytoin, salicylates, androgens, and furosemide may enhance the metabolism of L-thyroxine by inhibiting serum protein binding.
• Sucralfate and aluminum hydroxide can inhibit GI absorption.

ALTERNATIVE DRUGS
• Therapy with synthetic liothyronine (T_3) is not indicated or recommended in the vast majority of hypothyroid dogs.
• Liothyronine therapy is only indicated if a dog fails to achieve a normal serum T_4 concentration following appropriate therapy with at least two different brands of L-thyroxine.
• This probably indicates a lack of intestinal absorption; liothyronine is almost completely absorbed from the gut.

• The initial dosage is 4–6 mg/kg PO TID; final dosage is based on clinical response and on serum T_3 levels in the normal range; some patients can be maintained on BID therapy.

FOLLOW-UP

PATIENT MONITORING
• Mental alertness and activity levels usually increase within 1–2 weeks after initiation of therapy.
• Dermatologic abnormalities slowly resolve over 1–4 months, as do neurologic deficits that are secondary to hypothyroidism.
• Reproductive abnormalities resolve more slowly.
• If significant clinical improvement does not occur within 3 months of initiation of therapy, with serum T_4 levels in the normal range, the diagnosis of hypothyroidism may be incorrect.
• Check serum T_4 levels after 1 month of therapy.
• Determine peak serum T_4 concentrations 4–8 h after L-thyroxine administration.
• Serum T_4 concentrations should be in the normal range or mildly increased.
• Patients on once-daily therapy that do not respond to therapy and have a normal or high peak T_4 concentration should have their prepill T_4 concentration (trough T_4) assessed; if the trough T_4 concentration is low, twice-daily therapy is indicated.
• Following initial normalization of serum T_4 values, check them yearly, or sooner if clinical signs of hypothyroidism or thyrotoxicosis develop.
• Recheck serum T_4 concentrations 1 month after any change in dosage or brand of L-thyroxine being administered.

PREVENTION/AVOIDANCE
Proper treatment prevents disease recurrence.

POSSIBLE COMPLICATIONS
• Prolonged administration of an inappropriately high dosage of L-thyroxine can cause iatrogenic hyperthyroidism.
• Clinical signs of thyrotoxicosis include panting, polyphagia, weight loss, polyuria/polydipsia, anxiety, and diarrhea.
• Keep peak serum T_4 concentrations at or below 7.5 mg/dL.

EXPECTED COURSE AND PROGNOSIS
• Dogs treated for acquired primary hypothyroidism have an excellent prognosis; life expectancy is normal.
• Patients with acquired central hypothyroidism may have a poor prognosis if condition is secondary to a tumor or destructive process affecting the pituitary or hypothalamus.

MISCELLANEOUS

ASSOCIATED CONDITIONS
Primary hypothyroidism has been reported to occur concurrently with primary hypoadrenocorticism, and/or insulin dependent diabetes mellitus in a small number of animals.

AGE-RELATED FACTORS
None

ZOONOTIC POTENTIAL
None

PREGNANCY
N/A

SYNONYMS
None

SEE ALSO
Myxedema and Myxedema Coma

ABBREVIATIONS
• T_4 = L-thyroxine, tetraiodothyronine
• T_3 = liothyronine, triiodothyronine
• FT_4 = free T_4
• FT_3 = free T_3
• TSH = thyroid-stimulating hormone, thyrotropin
• TRH = thyrotropin-releasing hormone

Suggested Readings

Chastain CB, Panciera DL. Hypothyroid diseases. In: Ettinger SJ, Feldman EC, eds. Textbook of veterinary internal medicine. 4th ed. Philadelphia: WB Saunders, 1995: 1487–1501.

Panciera DL. Hypothyroidism in dogs: 66 cases (1987–1992). J Am Vet Med Assoc 1994;204:761–767.

Peterson ME, Melian C, Nichols R. Measurement of serum total thyroxine, triiodothyronine, free thyroxine and thyrotropin concentrations for diagnosis of hypothyroidism in dog. J Am Vet Med Assoc 1997;211:1396–1402.

Author John W. Tyler
Consulting Editor Deborah S. Greco

DISEASES

IMMUNODEFICIENCY DISORDERS, PRIMARY

BASICS

DEFINITION
• Diminished ability to mount an effective immune response
• Caused by heritable defects in the immune system (secondary disease—diminished immune response acquired as a consequence of some other primary disease)

PATHOPHYSIOLOGY
• The identification of a specific defect in the immune response requires an adequate understanding of the cellular and genetic basis of the immune system.
• The types and causes are diverse; defects in the cell-mediated, humoral, complement, and phagocytic systems have all been described in the veterinary literature.
• Defects involving the humoral immune response—associated with a high susceptibility to bacterial infection
• Defects involving the cell-mediated immune response—associated with a high susceptibility to viral, fungal, and protozoal infections
• Defects in the phagocytic or complement system—associated with disseminated infection.

SYSTEMS AFFECTED
• Hemic/Lymph/Immune—defect in a specific cell population in lymphoid tissue
• Skin/Exocrine, Respiratory, Gastrointestinal—chronic or recurrent infections
• Musculoskeletal—failure to thrive
• Other organ systems—dissemination of infection

GENETICS
Typically breed-specific with variable modes of inheritance

INCIDENCE/PREVALENCE
Rare

GEOGRAPHIC DISTRIBUTION
None

SIGNALMENT

Species
Dogs and cats

Breed Predilections
• X-linked severe combined immuno-deficiency—Bassett hounds
• IgA deficiency—beagles, German shepherds, and Chinese shar-peis
• IgM deficiency—Doberman pinschers
• Thymic hypoplasia—dwarfed Weimaraners
• Cyclic hematopoiesis—gray collies
• Chediak-Higashi syndrome—Persian cats
• Leukocyte adhesion deficiency—Irish setters
• Complement deficiency—Brittany spaniels
• Bactericidal defect—Doberman pinschers
• Transient hypogammaglobulinemia—Samoyeds

Mean Age and Range
Primary immunodeficiency diseases typically expressed in the first year of life

Predominant Sex
X-linked recessive severe combined immuno-deficiency disease of Bassett hounds–males affected and females carriers for the defect

SIGNS

General Comments
Depend on the level at which the immune response is defective; range from chronic respiratory and gastrointestinal signs and skin infections to life-threatening conditions

Historical Findings
• High susceptibility to infection and failure to respond to appropriate, conventional antibiotic therapy
• Lethargy
• Anorexia
• Skin infection
• Failure to thrive
• Signs often appear when maternal antibody concentrations decline.
• Vaccine-induced disease by modified live virus preparation

Physical Examination Findings
• Hallmark—failure to thrive
• Clinical signs attributable to infections

CAUSES
Congenital

RISK FACTORS
None

DIAGNOSIS

DIFFERENTIAL DIAGNOSIS
• Patients must be rigorously evaluated for underlying disease process that may cause secondary (acquired) immunodeficient state (e.g., hyperadrenocorticism, FeLV, and FIV).
• Patients are typically young with recurrent infection that fails to respond to conventional treatment

CBC/BIOCHEMISTRY/URINALYSIS
CBC may indicate deficiencies in specifically affected cell lines or a chronic inflammatory process.

OTHER LABORATORY TESTS
• Serum protein electrophoresis—demonstrate gross deficiency in immunoglobulin concentration
• Serum immunoglobulin quantitation—evaluate humoral immune system, identify selective immunoglobulin deficiency, support diagnosis of agammaglobulinemia
• The lymphocyte transformation test—evaluate the cell-mediated immune system and identify animals with T lymphocyte deficiency.
• Bactericidal assays—evaluate neutrophil function.
• Serum concentration of complement components—diagnose complement deficiency.
• Enumeration of lymphocyte subsets by immunofluorescence with monoclonal antibodies—identify deficiency of specific cell lines.
• Other more specific tests to evaluate immune function in veterinary species are available, but to get reliable results generally requires access to research laboratories that perform these tests.

IMAGING
N/A

DIAGNOSTIC PROCEDURES
In some patients, bone marrow and lymph node biopsy aids in classifying the type of immune deficiency.

X

IMMUNODEFICIENCY DISORDERS, PRIMARY

PATHOLOGIC FINDINGS
• Lesions vary; depend on the specific defect; most the result of recurrent or opportunistic infection involving the skin, ear canal, and respiratory and gastrointestinal systems
• Lesions of septicemia common in animals with severe defects
• T lymphocyte defects—hypoplastic or dysplastic lesions of the thymus and T lymphocyte–dependent areas of secondary lymphoid tissues
• B lymphocyte defects—hypoplastic or dysplastic lesions of the bone marrow or B lymphocyte–dependent areas of secondary lymphoid tissues
• Lymphoid hypoplasia or hyperplasia may be seen, depending on the overall defect and the occurrence of infection.

 TREATMENT

APPROPRIATE HEALTH CARE
• Hospitalization may be necessary to control life-threatening infection.
• Outpatient management possible for some patients

NURSING CARE
Supportive care appropriate to the nature of the infection

ACTIVITY
Determined largely by the severity of the defect and the occurrence of infection

DIET
• Dietary management may be required to ensure that the patient is maintained at an adequate level of nutrition.
• Potential sources of infectious agents such as raw meat must be avoided.

CLIENT EDUCATION
• Inform client that the animal cannot be cured.
• Discuss why the patient has high susceptibility to infection.
• Discuss and advise as to the heritability of the disease.
• Discuss the possibility of other litter mates being affected.
• Avoid exposure to ill animals.

SURGICAL CONSIDERATIONS
N/A

 MEDICATIONS

DRUGS OF CHOICE
• Antibiotics to control infections
• γ-Globulin or plasma preparations can be used in conjunction with antibiotics to control infection in patients with humoral defect.
• Symptomatic treatment for secondary disease states

CONTRAINDICATIONS
γ-Globulin or plasma preparations should not be administered to patients with selective IgA deficiency, because many affected patients have high concentrations of anti-IgA antibodies and may develop an anaphylactic reaction.

PRECAUTIONS
Modified live virus vaccines should not be administered to patients with suspected T lymphocyte deficiencies, because it may induce disease in these patients.

POSSIBLE INTERACTIONS
None

ALTERNATIVE DRUGS
None

 FOLLOW-UP

PATIENT MONITORING
• For clinical signs of secondary infection
• Routine physical examination to assess efficacy of antibiotic therapy in control of secondary infection

PREVENTION/AVOIDANCE
• Affected animals should not be bred.
• Pedigree analysis to determine the mode of inheritance and prevent propagating the defect

POSSIBLE COMPLICATIONS
Infection

EXPECTED COURSE AND PROGNOSIS
• The severity of the defect determines the course of disease and prognosis.
• Patients with minor defects can be successfully managed.

 MISCELLANEOUS

ASSOCIATED CONDITIONS
None

AGE-RELATED FACTORS
Usually expressed early in life

ZOONOTIC POTENTIAL
None

PREGNANCY
N/A

SYNONYMS
None

SEE ALSO
Neutropenia

ABBREVIATIONS
• FeLV = feline leukemia virus
• FIV = feline immunodeficiency virus

Suggested Readings
Guliford WG. Primary immunodeficiency diseases of dogs and cats. Compend Cont Ed Pract Vet 1987;9:641–648.
Lewis RM, Picut CA. Veterinary clinical immunology. Philadelphia: Lea & Febiger, 1989.
Author Paul W. Snyder
Consulting Editor Susan M. Cotter

DISEASES

IMMUNOPROLIFERATIVE ENTEROPATHY OF BASENJIS

BASICS

OVERVIEW
• An immunologically mediated disease characterized by chronic intermittent diarrhea, anorexia, and weight loss associated with lymphoplasmacytic enteritis, protein-losing enteropathy, malabsorption, maldigestion, and hypergammaglobulinemia due to increased concentrations of serum IgA
• Pathogenesis unclear but related to abnormal immune responses
• Systems affected include GI, immune, skin, renal, endocrine, and hepatobiliary

SIGNALMENT
• Young to middle-aged Basenjis—usually <3 years of age
• Related dogs often affected

SIGNS
• Chronic intermittent diarrhea
• Severe progressive weight loss
• Anorexia often precedes diarrhea
• Bilaterally symmetric alopecia
• Scaling and ulceration of ear margins
• Attitude—usually bright and alert
• Vomiting occasionally noted

CAUSES & RISK FACTORS
• Cause unknown
• Immune, genetic, and environmental factors are likely.
• Episodes of diarrhea are associated with stressful events—boarding, estrus, transport, vaccination, etc.

DIAGNOSIS

DIFFERENTIAL DIAGNOSIS
• Lymphangiectasia, lymphoplasmacytic enteritis, eosinophilic enteritis, histoplasmosis, EPI, intestinal lymphoma, metabolic disorders, intestinal parasitism
• Signalment, age of onset, fecal, CBC, chemistry profile, urinalysis, serum (TLI)/B$_{12}$/folate, serum IgA levels, and GI histology are used to differentiate.

CBC/BIOCHEMISTRY/URINALYSIS
• Hypoproteinemia
• Severe hypoalbuminemia
• Hyperglobulinemia
• Mature neutrophilia is often present.
• Poorly regenerative anemia—advanced disease
• Moderately increased hepatic enzymes—advanced disease

OTHER LABORATORY TESTS
• Hypergammaglobulinemia due to increased serum IgA
• Depression xylose absorption curve correlates with severity of clinical disease
• SIBO may cause functional EPI, but TLI depression is normal.
• May be hypergastrinemia and hyperchlorhydria

IMAGING
Abdominal ultrasound may demonstrate diffuse small bowel thickening, normal GI wall layering, and lack of other visceral abnormalities.

OTHER DIAGNOSTIC PROCEDURES
Endoscopic appearance of the small bowel typically is abnormal.

PATHOLOGIC FINDINGS
• Consistent pathologic lesions include uniform thickening of the small bowel, generalized infiltration of the intestinal lamina propria with lymphocytes and plasma cells, and blunting and fusion of villous tips.
• May be gastric mucosal hypertrophy, lymphocytic gastritis, parietal and chief cell hyperplasia, and gastric ulceration
• Presence and severity of gastric lesions do not correlate with severity of intestinal lesions.
• Other associated lesions include thyroid parafollicular cell atrophy, gastric acinar atrophy, and glomerulonephritis.

IMMUNOPROLIFERATIVE ENTEROPATHY OF BASENJIS

TREATMENT

• Outpatient medical management unless dehydration or other severe complications exist
• Advise owners not to breed affected dogs or their littermates.
• Minimize stressful episodes.
• Use dietary trials to determine what diet is best tolerated.

MEDICATIONS

DRUGS

Antibiotics
• Used for SIBO
• Metronidazole (10–20 mg/kg PO q12–24h)
• Tylosin (10 mg/kg PO q12h)
• Oxytetracycline (10–20 mg/kg PO q8h)

Corticosteroids
• Used for immunosuppression and anti-inflammation
• Prednisone (1 mg/kg PO q 12h for 2–4 weeks then slowly taper over 4–6 months to achieve 0.5–1 mg/kg PO q48h)

CONTRAINDICATIONS

Anticholinergics

FOLLOW-UP

• Diarrhea and weight loss usually show initial improvement with antibiotic or corticosteroid therapy.
• Recurrence of signs is common.
• Long-term prognosis poor

MISCELLANEOUS

ABBREVIATIONS

• EPI = exocrine pancreatic insufficiency
• GI = gastrointestinal
• SIBO = small intestinal bacterial overgrowth
• TLI = trypsin-like immunoreactivity

Suggested Reading

Breitschwerdt EB. Immuno-proliferative enteropathy of Basenjis. Semin Vet Med Surg (Sm Anim) 1992;7:153–161.

Author Amy M. Grooters
Consulting Editors Mitchell A. Crystal and Brett M Feder

INFLAMMATORY BOWEL DISEASE (IBD)

BASICS

DEFINITION
A group of gastrointestinal diseases characterized by inflammatory cellular infiltrates in the lamina propria of the small or large intestine, with associated clinical signs

PATHOPHYSIOLOGY
• An abnormal mucosal immune response to certain causative factors that results in the recruitment of inflammatory cells to the intestine.
• Damage results from the elaboration of cytokines, release of proteolytic and lysosomal enzymes, complement activation secondary to immune complex deposition, and generation of oxygen free radicals.
• Certain environmental agents and hereditary factors may also influence the development of IBD.

SYSTEMS AFFECTED
• Gastrointestinal
• Hepatobiliary
• Hemic/Lymphatic/Immune—rarely
• Musculoskeletal—rarely
• Ophthalmic—rarely
• Respiratory—rarely
• Skin/Exocrine—rarely

GENETICS
N/A

INCIDENCE/PREVALENCE
Common

GEOGRAPHIC DISTRIBUTION
N/A

SIGNALMENT

Species
Dogs and cats

Breed Predilections
Breed predisposition with some forms of the disease (e.g., immunoproliferative enteropathy of basenjis and lundehunds, histiocytic colitis of French bulldogs and boxers, and gluten-sensitive enteropathy in Irish setters)

Mean Age and Range
More common in animals >2 years of age, although younger animals can be affected.

Predominant Sex
N/A

SIGNS

Historical Findings
• Dogs—chronic intermittent vomiting, diarrhea, and weight loss are common.
• Cats—vomiting is most common, followed by diarrhea.
• Borborygmus, flatulence, anorexia or ravenous appetite, hematochezia, abdominal pain, and mucoid stools are less commonly reported.

Physical Examination Findings
• Vary from an apparently healthy animal to a thin, depressed one
• Poor haircoat is frequently noted.
• Abdominal palpation may reveal pain, thickened bowel loops, and mesenteric lymphadenopathy (especially in cats).

CAUSES
• Pathogenesis is most likely multifactorial.
• Several causative factors have been identified.

Infectious Agents
• No convincing link definitively established between one microbial agent and IBD
• *Giardia, Salmonella, Campylobacter,* and normal resident gastrointestinal flora have been implicated.

Dietary Agents
Meat proteins, food additives, artificial coloring, preservatives, milk proteins, gluten (wheat) are all proposed causative agents.

Genetic Factors
• Certain forms of IBD are more common in some breeds of dogs (see above).
• Association of inherited chromosome fragility with IBD suggested in humans
• Certain major histocompatibility genes, which are important components of normal immune responses, may render an individual susceptible to the development of IBD.

RISK FACTORS
See Causes.

DIAGNOSIS

DIFFERENTIAL DIAGNOSIS
• Cats—hyperthyroidism, intestinal neoplasia (especially infiltrative lymphosarcoma or mast cell tumor), dietary intolerance/hypersensitivity, granulomatous FIP, other viral infections (e.g., FeLV and FIV), exocrine pancreatic insufficiency, intestinal parasitism, and bacterial overgrowth are primary differentials.
• Dogs—intestinal neoplasia, motility disorders, dietary intolerance/hypersensitivity, lymphangiectasia, exocrine pancreatic insufficiency, intestinal parasitism, and bacterial overgrowth are primary differentials.

CBC/BIOCHEMISTRY/URINALYSIS
• Results often normal; these tests help rule in or out some other differential diagnoses.
• Occasionally a mild, nonregenerative anemia and mild leukocytosis without a left shift occur in cats.
• Dogs with IBD frequently have a neutrophilic leukocytosis with a left shift.
• Hypoproteinemia tends to be more common in dogs with IBD than cats.

OTHER LABORATORY TESTS
• Useful to eliminate other differentials
• Dogs—tests include fasting serum TLI to evaluate exocrine pancreatic function and fasting serum cobalamin and folate assays to evaluate small intestinal function and bacterial overgrowth.
• Cats—T_4 and FeLV/FIV serology are recommended; fasting serum TLI (if exocrine pancreatic insufficiency is suspected)

IMAGING
• Survey abdominal radiographs—usually normal
• Barium contrast studies—occasionally reveal mucosal abnormalities and thickened bowel loops, but are generally not helpful in establishing a definitive diagnosis; can be normal in individuals with even severe disease
• Ultrasonography—may use to measure stomach and intestinal wall thickness and to rule out other diseases

DIAGNOSTIC PROCEDURES
• May initiate a hypoallergenic diet trial first to rule in or rule out dietary allergy or intolerance
• Occasionally, certain forms of IBD respond to dietary manipulations alone; if signs resolve completely, a diagnosis of dietary allergy or intolerance is likely and no further workup is necessary.
• Always perform fecal examination for parasites.

INFLAMMATORY BOWEL DISEASE (IBD)

• Definitive diagnosis requires biopsy and histopathology, usually obtained via endoscopy.
• May collect duodenal aspirates for *Giardia* spp. detection during endoscopy
• Intestinal fluid obtained during endoscopy can also be submitted for quantitative culture if bacterial overgrowth is suspected.
• Exploratory laparotomy may be indicated if involved portions of the gastrointestinal tract are unapproachable by endoscopy or if abdominal organomegaly is present.

PATHOLOGIC FINDINGS
Infiltration of intestines with inflammatory cells

TREATMENT

APPROPRIATE HEALTH CARE
Outpatient, unless the patient is debilitated from dehydration, hypoproteinemia, or cachexia

NURSING CARE
• If the patient is dehydrated or must be NPO because of vomiting, any balanced fluid such as lactated Ringer solution is adequate (for a patient without other concurrent disease); otherwise, select fluids on the basis of secondary diseases.
• If severe hypoalbuminemia from protein-losing enteropathy, consider colloids such as dextrans or hetastarch.

ACTIVITY
No restrictions

DIET
• Manipulation is important.
• For detailed description of possible regimens, see specific diseases.

CLIENT EDUCATION
• Emphasize to the client that IBD is not necessarily cured as much as controlled.
• Relapses are common; the client must be prepared to be patient during the various food and medication trials that are often necessary to get the disease under control.
• A severely debilitated patient may need hospitalization and parenteral nutrition.

SURGICAL CONSIDERATIONS
Unlike the situation with human beings, no surgical procedures are available for relief of IBD in veterinary patients.

MEDICATIONS

DRUGS OF CHOICE
See discussion under specific diseases.

CONTRAINDICATIONS
If secondary problems are present, avoid therapeutic agents that might be contraindicated for those conditions.

PRECAUTIONS
See discussion under specific diseases.

POSSIBLE INTERACTIONS
See discussion under specific diseases.

ALTERNATIVE DRUGS
See discussion under specific diseases.

FOLLOW-UP

PATIENT MONITORING
• Periodic reevaluation may be necessary until the patient's condition stabilizes.
• No other follow-up may be required except yearly physical examinations and assessment during relapse.

PREVENTION/AVOIDANCE
N/A

POSSIBLE COMPLICATIONS
Dehydration, malnutrition, adverse drug reactions, hypoproteinemia, anemia, and diseases secondary to therapy or resulting from the above mentioned problems

EXPECTED COURSE AND PROGNOSIS
• Varies with specific type of IBD
• See discussion under specific diseases.

MISCELLANEOUS

ASSOCIATED CONDITIONS
See discussion under specific diseases.

AGE-RELATED FACTORS
• See discussion of specific diseases.
• The workup and differentials are essentially the same, regardless of age.
• Some differentials are more likely in younger individuals (i.e., intestinal parasitism versus neoplasia).
• Younger individuals with confirmed IBD may have other immune system defects.
• Counsel clients about breeding and monitoring for the appearance of other diseases.

ZOONOTIC POTENTIAL
N/A

PREGANANCY
See discussion under specific diseases.

SYNONYMS
N/A

SEE ALSO
• Gastroenteritis, Lymphocytic-Plasmacytic
• Gastroenteritis, Eosinophilic
• Colitis and Proctitis

ABBREVIATIONS
• FeLV = feline leukemia virus
• FIP = feline infectious peritonits
• FIV = feline immunodeficiency virus
• IBD = inflammatory bowel disease
• TLI = trypsin-like immunoreactivity

Suggested Reading
Strombeck DR, Guilford WG. Idiopathic inflammatory bowel diseases. In: Guilford WG, Center SA, Strombeck DR, et al., eds. Strombeck's small animal gastroenterology. 3rd ed. Philadelphia: Saunders, 1996: 451–486.
Tams TR. Feline inflammatory bowel disease. Vet Clin North Am 1993;23.
Author Kelly J. Diehl
Consulting Editors Brett M. Feder and Mitchell A. Crystal

DISEASES

INSULINOMA

 BASICS

DEFINITION
Pancreatic islet β-cell neoplasm that secretes an excess quantity of insulin

PATHOPHYSIOLOGY
Excessive insulin secretion leads to excessive glucose uptake and use by insulin-sensitive tissues and reduced hepatic production of glucose; this causes hypoglycemia and its associated clinical signs.

SYSTEMS AFFECTED
• Nervous—seizures, disorientation, abnormal behavior, collapse, posterior paresis, and ataxia
• Musculoskeletal—weakness and muscle fasciculations
• Gastrointestinal—polyphagia and weight gain

GENETICS
N/A

INCIDENCE/PREVALENCE
• Dogs—uncommon
• Cats—rare (4 reports)

GEOGRAPHIC DISTRIBUTION
N/A

SIGNALMENT
Species
Dogs and cats
Breed Predilections
• Dogs—standard poodle, boxer, fox terrier, Irish setter, German shepherd, golden retriever, and collie
• Cats—none; possibly Siamese
Mean Age and Range
• Dogs—middle-aged to old; mean, 10.5 years; range, 3–14 years (rare in dogs <6 years old)
• Cats—(4 cases) mean, 14.75 years; range, 12–17
Predominant Sex
None

SIGNS
General Comments
• Episodic
• May or may not be related to fasting, excitement, exercise, and eating
• Dogs usually demonstrate more than one clinical sign, and they progress with time.

Historical Findings
• Dogs—seizures (generalized and focal) most common; also, posterior paresis, weakness, collapse, muscle fasciculations, abnormal behavior, lethargy and depression, ataxia, polyphagia, weight gain, polyuria and polydipsia, and exercise intolerance
• Cats—seizures, ataxia, muscle fasciculations, weakness, lethargy and depression, anorexia, weight loss, and polydipsia

Physical Examination Findings
• Usually within normal limits
• Obesity in some dogs
• Rarely, polyneuropathy in dogs

CAUSES
Most patients have malignant, insulin-producing carcinoma or adenocarcinoma of the pancreas; tumors considered benign according to histopathologic findings usually metastasize later.

RISK FACTORS
Fasting, excitement, exercise, and eating may increase the risk of hypoglycemic episodes.

 DIAGNOSIS

DIFFERENTIAL DIAGNOSIS
• Extrapancreatic tumor hypoglycemia—paraneoplastic hypoglycemia has been documented in dogs with hepatocellular carcinoma, metastatic mammary carcinoma, primary pulmonary carcinoma, and others; these tumors secrete insulin or insulin-like factors
• Differentiate from Beta-cell pancreatic tumor by a complete hypoglycemic workup, including imaging.
• Seizures and collapse—must consider cardiovascular (e.g., syncope), metabolic (e.g., hepatoencephalopathy, hypocalcemia, anemia, and hypoadrenocorticism) and neurologic (e.g., epilepsy, neoplasia, toxin, and inflammatory disease) causes
• Posterior paresis and weakness—consider cardiovascular (e.g., congenital anatomic defect, arrhythmias, heart failure, and pericardial effusion), metabolic (e.g., hypoadrenocorticism, hypocalcemia, anemia, hypokalemia, and hypothyroidism), neurologic and neuromuscular (e.g., spinal cord disease, myasthenia gravis, polymyositis, and polyradiculoneuropathy), and toxic (e.g., tick paralysis, botulism, chronic organophosphate exposure, and lead poisoning) causes

• Muscle fasciculations—consider metabolic (e.g., hypercalcemia, hypocalcemia, and hyperadrenocorticism) and toxic (e.g., tetanus and strychnine poisoning) causes

CBC/BIOCHEMISTRY/URINALYSIS
• Results usually normal, except hypoglycemia (< 70 mg/dL in > 90% of patients)
• Normoglycemia in some patients, due to counterregulatory hormone production (epinephrine, glucocorticoids, etc.)

OTHER LABORATORY TESTS
• Simultaneous fasting glucose and insulin determination—on initiating fasting, collect blood samples hourly or bihourly for serum glucose determination and serum storage; when the serum glucose drops below 60 mg/dL (usually within 8–10 h in dogs, at presentation in cats), submit that sample for serum insulin determination; interpretation: high insulin, insulinoma likely; normal insulin, insulinoma possible; low insulin, insulinoma unlikely
• Amended insulin:glucose ratio (AIGR)—this test is intended to diagnose insulinoma when the insulin concentration is within the normal range but inappropriately high for the degree of hypoglycemia.

$$AIGR = \frac{[\text{plasma insulin } (\mu U/mL) \times 100]}{[\text{plasma glucose } (mg/dL) - 30]}$$

use 1 as denominator if glucose is < 30; AIGR > 30 suggests insulinoma, AIGR = 19–30, gray zone, repeat test; AIGR < 19, insulinoma unlikely
• **Note:** False-positive results are possible, especially when serum glucose is < 40 mg/dL.

IMAGING
Thoracic and abdominal radiography and abdominal ultrasonography are usually normal but help evaluate for extrapancreatic tumor–induced hypoglycemia as well as some other differential diagnoses.

DIAGNOSTIC PROCEDURES
N/A

PATHOLOGIC FINDINGS
• Insulinoma is usually a small, solitary nodule, but multiple nodules or diffuse infiltration can be seen.
• Most insulinomas can be identified grossly at surgery, occasionally gentle palpation is required for detection, and very rarely no tumor can be identified.
• Metastasis is seen in 40% of patients at surgery; common areas include the regional

lymph nodes and liver; other areas include the duodenum, mesentery, omentum, and spleen.
• Histopathologically they appear as either carcinoma or adenoma, but both behave malignantly.

TREATMENT

APPROPRIATE HEALTH CARE
• Hospitalize for workup, surgery, and (if clinically hypoglycemic) treatment.
• Treat as outpatient if the owner declines surgery and the patient is not clinically hypoglycemic.

NURSING CARE
• Administer 50% dextrose, 1 mL/kg IV slow bolus (1–3 min) to control seizures/severe hypoglycemic signs.
• Fluid therapy with 2.5% dextrose (increase to 5% if needed to control clinical signs) should follow dextrose bolus; alternatively, if the patient can eat, frequent feedings of an appropriate diet (see Diet) may replace dextrose-containing fluids in some patients.

ACTIVITY
Restricted

DIET
• The first and most important aspect of management (with or without surgery)
• Feed 4–6 small meals a day.
• Should be high in protein, fat, and complex carbohydrates and low in simple sugars; avoid semimoist food.

CLIENT EDUCATION
Owner should be aware of signs of hypoglycemia and seek immediate attention if they occur.

SURGICAL CONSIDERATIONS
Confirms diagnosis, improves survival time, can potentially provide prolonged remission, and improves response to medical treatment

MEDICATIONS

DRUGS OF CHOICE
Emergency/Acute Therapy
See Nursing Care above.

Long-term Therapy
• Glucocorticoids (prednisone at an initial dosage of 0.25 mg/kg PO q12h; increased to 2–3 mg/kg PO q12h if needed)—initial

medical treatment if diet alone is ineffective; begin with the low dosage and gradually increase as signs of hypoglycemia recur.
• Diazoxide (Proglycem, 5 mg/kg PO q12h; gradually increased to 30 mg/kg PO q12h if needed)—added after diet and glucocorticoids have proven ineffective
• Sandostatin (Ocreotide, 10–20 µg SC q8–12h)—a synthetic somatostatin analogue; prevents hypoglycemia in some dogs refractory to conventional treatment; can be used with diet, steroids, and diazoxide; expensive

CONTRAINDICATIONS
Insulin

PRECAUTIONS
• Dextrose bolus—suitable for acute hypoglycemic crisis if followed by continuous dextrose-containing fluids or appropriate feeding; may precipitate further hypoglycemic crises if given alone
• Glucocorticoids used at high dosages for prolonged periods can cause iatrogenic hyperadrenocorticism.
• Diazoxide—can cause gastrointestinal irritation; causes bone marrow suppression, cataract formation, aplastic anemia, tachycardia, and thrombocytopenia in humans

POSSIBLE INTERACTIONS
N/A

ALTERNATIVE DRUGS
N/A

FOLLOW-UP

PATIENT MONITORING
• At home for return or progression of clinical signs of hypoglycemia
• In-hospital serum glucose determinations—single, intermittent serum glucose determinations may not truly reflect the glycemic status of the patient because insulinomas occasionally respond to normal feedback mechanisms and because of production of counterregulatory hormones.
• Adjust medication on the basis of clinical signs and serum glucose levels.

PREVENTION/AVOIDANCE
N/A

POSSIBLE COMPLICATIONS
Recurrent or progressive episodes of hypoglycemia

EXPECTED COURSE AND PROGNOSIS
• Likelihood of malignancy is high; metastasis is seen in 40% of patients at the time of surgery.
• Dogs—mean survival time, about 16–19 months; range, 2–60 months; surgery improves survival time.
• Cats—mean survival time, about 6.5 months; range, 0–18 months

MISCELLANEOUS

ASSOCIATED CONDITIONS
Obesity

AGE-RELATED FACTORS
Younger dogs have shorter survival times.

ZOONOTIC POTENTIAL
N/A

PREGNANCY
N/A

SYNONYMS
• Insulin-secreting tumor
• B-cell tumor
• Hyperinsulinism
• Islet cell tumor
• Islet cell adenocarcinoma
• Insulin-producing pancreatic tumor

SEE ALSO
Glucose, Hypoglycemia

ABBREVIATION
AIGR = amended insulin:glucose ratio

Suggested Reading
Feldman EC, Nelson RW. Feldman beta-cell neoplasia: insulinoma. In: Feldman EC, Nelson RW, eds. Canine and feline endocrinology and reproduction. 2nd ed. Philadelphia: Saunders, 1996:422–441.
Hawks D, Peterson ME, Hawkins KL, Rosebury WS. Insulin-secreting pancreatic (islet cell) carcinoma in a cat. J Vet Int Med 1992;6:193–196.
Peterson ME. Islet cell tumors secreting insulin, pancreatic polypeptide, gastrin, or glucagon. In: Kirk RW, Bonagura JD, eds. Current veterinary therapy XI. Philadelphia: WB Saunders, 1992:368–375.
Author Mitchell A. Crystal
Consulting Editor Deborah S. Greco

DISEASES

INTERDIGITAL DERMATITIS

 BASICS

OVERVIEW
- Disease of the feet of dogs
- Also known as pododermatitis, interdigital pyoderma, pedal folliculitis, and furunculosis

SIGNALMENT
- Dogs of any age, sex, or breed
- Short-coated male dogs (e.g., English bull dogs, Great Danes, basset hounds, mastiffs, bull terriers, boxers, dachshunds, Dalmatians, German short-haired pointers, and weimaraners) may be predisposed.
- Some long-coated breeds (e.g., German shepherds, Labrador retrievers, golden retrievers, Irish setters, and Pekingese) are possibly predisposed.

SIGNS
- May affect one foot and one interdigital space or multiple interdigital spaces and feet
- Diseased tissue—usually erythematous and swollen; has either intact bullae, ruptured draining tracts, or both
- Sometimes mild to severe swelling of the affected feet
- Mild to severe lameness may be seen.

CAUSES & RISK FACTORS

One Affected Foot
- Foreign bodies (e.g., grass awns, wood slivers, suture material)
- Osteomyelitis
- Neoplasia
- Infection

More Than One Affected Foot
- Hypersensitivity reaction—food, atopy, contact dermatitis
- Infection—bacterial, fungal, yeast
- Trauma—clipper burns, cuts
- Chemical—contact irritant dermatitis
- Metabolic—hypothyroidism, hyperadrenocorticism
- Parasitic—demodicosis often complicated by the presence of furunculosis and draining tracts; heartworm, hookworm, and pelodera result in erythema, pruritus, and patchy alopecia of the feet; pelodera affects the limbs and the ventral abdomen.
- Idiopathic
- Recurrent pododermatitis—clinically important footpad involvement with the interdigital dermatitis
- Immune mediated—pemphigus, pemphigoid, systemic lupus erythematosus
- Zinc deficiency or zinc responsive
- Superficial necrolytic dermatitis

 DIAGNOSIS

DIFFERENTIAL DIAGNOSIS
Adult onset demodicosis—underlying hypothyroidism, hyperadrenocorticism, allergic disease, neoplasia, or idiopathic

CBC/BIOCHEMISTRY/URINALYSIS
- Usually normal
- Superficial necrolytic dermatitis—may have high liver and pancreatic enzyme activities

OTHER LABORATORY TESTS
- Blood tests—heartworm microfilaria
- Thyroid hormone tests—hypothyroidism
- Adrenal response tests (low-dose dexamethasone-suppression test, urine cortisol: creatinine ratio, ACTH stimulation)—hyperadrenocorticism

IMAGING
Radiographs—underlying osteomyelitis

DIAGNOSTIC PROCEDURES
- Biopsies—foreign bodies, demodicosis, neoplasia, infectious agents (fungi, bacteria) or other parasites (heartworm and, rarely, hookworm)
- Skin scrapings—identify parasites (demodicosis), pelodera, or fungi (dermatophytosis)
- Fecal flotation—identify hookworm ova
- Cytologic examination of the exudate with Wright-Giemsa stain—identify yeast, bacteria, and (rarely) parasites; evaluate the type of inflammatory response (e.g., eosinophils may suggest parasites or hypersensitivity)

PATHOLOGIC FINDINGS
Other than causal findings listed above (e.g., parasites and bacteria), the reaction pattern is a folliculitis, perifolliculitis, and pyogranulomatous dermatitis if the follicles have ruptured.

 TREATMENT

- Treatments directed at underlying cause, if known.
- Antibiotics—if bacteria are present; must be used until the deep tissues have healed; selection of appropriate drug depends on culture and sensitivity; begin as soon as possible with the correct drug, because treatment usually lasts several months.
- Draining lesions—twice-daily foot soaks (10 min each) until draining stops
- May be beneficial to restrict activity or protect feet
- Severe refractory cases—surgical débridement and removal of the interdigital tissue and joining the digits together (fusion podoplasty)

 MEDICATIONS

DRUGS
- Broad-spectrum antibiotic—for the deep bacterial infection (furunculosis); use one that is effective against the staphylococcal organisms based on culture and sensitivity; try amoxicillin with clavulanate, fluoroquinolones, or cephalosporin; 6–8 weeks of therapy needed
- Rifampin—use with caution for short periods (30–60 days) at 5–10 mg/kg q24h; penetrates deep lesions well, owing to its lipid solubility; must be accompanied by a good antibiotic, because bacteria rapidly develop resistance

CONTRAINDICATIONS/POSSIBLE INTERACTIONS

Rifampin
- Monitor liver enzymes and CBC every 2 weeks.
- Do not use with liver disease.
- Stimulates liver enzymes involved in drug metabolism and thus can influence the metabolism of concurrently administered drugs; concentrations of anticoagulants, digitoxin, corticosteroids, and other drugs become subtherapeutic.
- When rifampin and ketoconazole are administered concurrently, both drugs are subtherapeutic.
- Use caution when concurrently administering other drugs.

 FOLLOW-UP

- Monitor closely to detect the underlying cause, if not previously determined; determining the cause can be tedious and frustrating but is essential for complete resolution and healing.
- Continue medication for bacterial infection for 2 weeks after all palpable dermal lesions are resolved.

 MISCELLANEOUS

Suggested Reading
Scott DW. Canine pododermatitis. In: Kirk RW, ed. Current veterinary therapy, small animal practice VII. Philadelphia: Saunders, 1980:467–469
Author David Duclos
Consulting Editor Karen Helton Rhodes

INTERSTITIAL CELL TUMOR, TESTICLE

BASICS

OVERVIEW
Benign tumor of the testicle that arises from interstitial (e.g., Leydig) cells

SIGNALMENT
• Common in dogs and rare in cats
• Usually old male dogs

SIGNS
• Usually none unless associated with estrogen secretion, causing feminization and bone marrow hypoplasia (see Sertoli Cell Tumor)
• Single or multiple discrete tumor masses (usually 1 to 2 cm) within a single testis

CAUSES & RISK FACTORS
• Generally unknown
• Cryptorchidism—may predispose

DIAGNOSIS

DIFFERENTIAL DIAGNOSIS
• Sertoli cell tumor
• Seminoma
• Hyperadrenocorticism—with feminization
• Hypothyroidism—with feminization

CBC/BIOCHEMISTRY/URINALYSIS
• Usually normal, unless estrogen excess causes bone marrow hypoplasia
• Various cytopenias—with estrogen excess

OTHER LABORATORY TESTS
• High serum estradiol concentration
• Low serum testosterone concentration

IMAGING
Ultrasonography—tumors < 3 cm in diameter tend to be hypoechoic; tumors > 5 cm tend to have mixed echogenic patterns.

DIAGNOSTIC PROCEDURES
N/A

TREATMENT
Castration and histopathologic examination of appropriate tissue

MEDICATIONS

DRUGS
• None, unless bone marrow hypoplasia
• Recombinant hematopoietic colony-stimulating factors—may be useful in treating bone marrow hypoplasia

CONTRAINDICATIONS/POSSIBLE INTERACTIONS
N/A

FOLLOW-UP

PATIENT MONITORING
None required, unless bone marrow hypoplasia

POSSIBLE COMPLICATIONS
Cytopenias caused by estrogen excess

EXPECTED COURSE AND PROGNOSIS
Usually excellent

MISCELLANEOUS

ASSOCIATED CONDITIONS
• Prostate disease—with testicular tumor
• Reported as a functional ectopic tumor in one cat

Suggested Reading
Morrison WB. Cancers of the reproductive tract. In: Morrison WB, ed., Cancer in dogs and cats: medical and surgical management. Baltimore: Williams & Wilkins 1998.
Suess RP, Barr SC, Sacre BJ, et al. Bone marrow hypoplasia in a feminized dog with an interstitial cell tumor. J Am Vet Med Assoc 1992;200:1346–1348.
Author Wallace B. Morrison
Consulting Editor Wallace B. Morrison

DISEASES

INTERVERTEBRAL DISK DISEASE, CERVICAL

BASICS

DEFINITION
Age-related change in the cervical intervertebral disks, which may result in disk protrusion or extrusion into the spinal canal with consequent trauma to and/or compression of the meninges, spinal cord, and nerve roots

PATHOPHYSIOLOGY
• Classified as Hansen type I or type II disease • Type I—rupture of the annulus fibrosus of the intervertebral disk with extrusion of nucleus pulposus into the spinal canal; usually associated with chondroid degeneration of the disk, disk mineralization, and acute extrusion • Type II—insidious bulging of the dorsal annulus fibrosus and its protrusion into the vertebral canal; usually associated with gradual fibroid metaplasia of the disk • Disk extrusion or protrusion into the spinal canal—results in compression of the spinal cord and focal myelopathy • Pathological consequences of spinal cord compression—include ischemia and demyelination • Lateral or ventral extrusion or protrusion of the disk—less common than dorsal extrusion or protrusion; usually not associated with clinical signs • Vertebral anomalies (e.g., fusions of vertebrae)—may increase mechanical stresses on adjacent intervertebral disk; may predispose disks to protrusion or extrusion

SYSTEMS AFFECTED
Nervous—focal, compressive myelopathy

GENETICS
• No known basis • Chondrodystrophic breeds (dachshunds, beagles, and Pekingese)—predisposed to type I disease • Large breeds (especially Doberman pinschers)—predisposed to type II disease

INCIDENCE/PREVALENCE
• Unknown • Cervical lesions—account for 14–16% of intervertebral disk disease cases in dogs

GEOGRAPHIC DISTRIBUTION:
N/A

SIGNALMENT
Species
Dogs

Breed Predilections
• Type I—beagles; toy poodles; dachshunds; all chondrodystrophic breeds • Type II—Doberman pinschers

Mean Age and Range
• Type I—3–6 years • Type II—8–10 years

Predominant Sex
None recognized

SIGNS
General Comments
Severity of signs and nervous tissue pathology depend on the rate and force of disk extrusion or protrusion, the volume of the compressive mass, and the diameter of the spinal canal relative to the diameter of the spinal cord at the site.

Historical Findings
• Neck pain—most prominent complaint; may be exacerbated by picking up the patient or manipulating its neck • Unwillingness to extend the neck or to flex it either ventrally or laterally—common • Paresis and postural reaction deficits of all four limbs—may be worse on one side; may occur with sufficient damage to long motor and sensory tracts in the spinal cord • Disk extrusion impinging on a nerve root in the lower cervical region—patient may appear lame in one forelimb and may hold the limb off the ground (root signature). • Compression of spinal cord or ventral nerve roots in the lower cervical spine—may result in focal atrophy of shoulder or forelimb muscles • Paralysis of all four limbs—uncommon

Physical Examination Findings
• Neck pain—most common; elicited by flexing and extending the neck or turning the neck side to side; elicited on deep palpation of the cervical muscles • Root signature sign—approximately 50% of patients • May note paresis with postural reaction deficits involving both limbs on one side or all four limbs; may be more severe on one side • Paralysis—rare • Hindlimb paresis—may be more pronounced than forelimb paresis • Hindlimb spinal reflexes—normal to exaggerated • Forelimb reflexes—may be normal or exaggerated when lesion affects the C1 to C6 region; may be normal to decreased when lesion affects the C6 to T2 region

CAUSES
Age-related chondroid degeneration or fibroid metaplasia of the cervical intervertebral disks

RISK FACTORS
Obesity

DIAGNOSIS

DIFFERENTIAL DIAGNOSIS
• Type I—trauma; fibrocartilaginous embolism; meningitis; neoplasia; diskospondylitis
• Type II—lower cervical vertebral instability (Wobbler syndrome); neoplasia; diskospondylitis; meningitis

CBC/BIOCHEMISTRY/URINALYSIS
N/A

OTHER LABORATORY TESTS
CSF analysis—performed routinely when myelography is to be carried out or when the diagnosis is in doubt; usually reveals mildly to moderately elevated total protein levels (<100 mg/dL) with mild to moderate mixed pleocytosis; more abnormal in acute severe disease than in mild or chronic disease

IMAGING
Cervical Spinal Radiography
• Often reveals a narrowed, wedged-shaped disk space, small intervertebral foramen, and collapsed articular facets; may be less prominent with type II disease
• Type I—may see mineralized disk material within the spinal canal or intervertebral foramen
• Dorsolateral view—may reveal a round button-shaped density overlying the disk space

Myelography
• Sometimes recommended only when the diagnosis or exact location of the lesion remains uncertain after plain radiography
• Recommended for all surgical patients—plain radiography may be misleading
• Cisternal injection of contrast material—may be used for cervical lesions
• Injection of contrast into the lumbar subarachnoid space (between L5 and L6 or L4 and L5)—generally produces the best results
• Lateral view—usually reveals dorsal deviation of the ventral contrast column at the location of disk extrusion
• Dorsoventral view—may reveal contrast column deviated to one side; may show widened right to left columns at the site of disk extrusion

DIAGNOSTIC PROCEDURES
N/A

PATHOLOGIC FINDINGS
Gross
• Type I—white to yellow extruded disk material that is granular in consistency; with chronic disease, material may be hardened and difficult to remove.
• Type II—firm, grayish white protruded disk material that is adherent to the floor of the spinal canal
• Spinal cord—may be swollen and discolored with acute severe disease; may be narrowed and atrophied with chronic disease; often normal

Histopathologic
• Decreased water and proteoglycans in degenerate disks
• Increased collagen
• Type I—granular and calcified nucleus pulposus
• Type II—cartilaginous disk

• Pathological changes in the spinal cord—vary considerably with the type and severity of the disk extrusion or protrusion; chronic, mild disease: usually demyelination and gliosis; acute, severe disease: predominately hemorrhage, edema, and tissue necrosis

TREATMENT

APPROPRIATE HEALTH CARE
• Outpatient—patients with a first time episode of neck pain
• Inpatient—patients with repeated episodes of neck pain; patients with neck pain plus neurologic deficits; aggressively treated with myelography and surgery

NURSING CARE
• Handling—take great care to protect the neck; important to minimize cervical spine manipulation when withdrawing blood and using restraint measures.
• Transporting patient under general anesthesia—protect the neck; support the body on a flat surface (e.g., board or gurney).
• Mild neurologic deficits treated with medical therapy alone—observe for worsening signs.
• Urination—monitor all patients for appropriate and complete emptying of the bladder; may need to manually express, use intermittent urinary catheterization, or place an indwelling urinary catheter.
• Defecation—may need to manually evacuate bowel or use enemas.
• Recumbent patient—keep on padded bedding; turn every 4 hr to prevent formation of decubital ulcers.
• Physical therapy, including hydrotherapy—appropriate for patients with neurologic deficits

ACTIVITY
• Reduced for all patients
• Use harnesses, not collars, for leash walking.
• Discourage any form of jumping.
• Patient with an initial episode of neck pain only—cage confinement for 2–4 weeks may alleviate signs and should be tried before surgical treatment.

DIET
• Reducing—for all obese patients

CLIENT EDUCATION
• Discuss the signs of spinal cord compression.
• Emphasize the importance of cage rest for a patient being treated conservatively.

SURGICAL CONSIDERATIONS
• Indicated for most patients with repeated episodes of neck pain and all patients with neurologic deficits
• Disk material extruding into spinal canal and lying ventral to the spinal cord—ventral slot procedure indicated; may perform ventral fenestration of adjacent disks prophylactically
• Disk material lying lateral to the spinal cord or within the intervertebral foramen—may achieve decompression through a dorsal laminectomy, with or without facetectomy
• Hemilaminectomy—can be performed in the cervical region; technically demanding owing to the complex arrangement of the cervical musculature and the passage of the vertebral artery through foramina in the lateral aspect of the spine throughout most of the cervical region
• Patients with neck pain alone—myelography usually reveals disk material within the spinal canal; fenestration without decompression may not resolve clinical signs; ventral slot indicated
• More than one herniated disk—may perform multiple ventral slots; carries a higher risk of complications (e.g., instability of the spine), particularly when the affected disks are directly adjacent to one another

MEDICATIONS

DRUGS OF CHOICE
• Glucocorticoids (e.g., prednisone)—low doses may decrease pain in patient treated conservatively
• Glucocorticoids without concurrent cage confinement—may decrease pain and encourage excessive activity, resulting in further disk extrusion; important to impose cage rest if conservative treatment is attempted
• Methylprednisolone sodium succinate—30 mg/kg IV within 8 hr of onset of clinical signs or at the time of surgery for acute spinal cord compression; for severe cases, may repeat at half the dose 2 hr after the first dose, then q6h for 24 hr
• Prednisone or prednisolone—0.25mg/kg PO twice daily for 3–4 days, then tapering over 2–3 weeks for conservative treatment; always combine with strict cage rest and close observation for exacerbation of clinical signs.

CONTRAINDICATIONS
Avoid concomitant use of glucocorticoids and NSAIDs—combined negative effects on the gastrointestinal tract

PRECAUTIONS
• NSAIDs—may result in life-threatening gastrointestinal hemorrhage; avoid, particularly when glucocorticoids are being administered.

POSSIBLE INTERACTIONS
NSAIDs in combination with glucocorticoids—increased risk of life-threatening gastrointestinal hemorrhage; avoid combination in all patients.

ALTERNATIVE DRUGS
Vitamin E—beneficial in cats with spinal cord injury; no data available for dogs; may be a useful adjunctive therapy

FOLLOW-UP

PATIENT MONITORING
Re-evaluate weekly until clinical signs have resolved.

PREVENTION/AVOIDANCE
• Unavoidable in certain breeds • May slow or avoid exacerbation of clinical signs by keeping the patient lean and having it avoid strenuous exercise and jumping

POSSIBLE COMPLICATIONS
• Recurrence of neck pain with or without neurologic deficits possible • Patients treated surgically—may be less likely to have recurrences • Catastrophic spinal cord compression—almost never occurs

EXPECTED COURSE AND PROGNOSIS
• Many patients treated conservatively have recurrence and ultimately require surgery.
• Most patients treated surgically do not have recurrent episodes.

MISCELLANEOUS

ASSOCIATED CONDITIONS
Predisposed breeds are also predisposed to thoracolumbar disk disease.

AGE-RELATED FACTORS
N/A

ZOONOTIC POTENTIAL
N/A

PREGNANCY
N/A

SEE ALSO
Intervertebral Disk Disease, Thoracolumbar

ABBREVIATION
CSF = cerebrospinal fluid

Suggested Reading
Braund KG. Canine intervertebral disk disease. In: Bojrab MJ, ed. Disease mechanisms in small animal surgery. Philadelphia: Saunders, 1993:960–969.
Oliver JE, Lorenz MD, Kornegay JN. Handbook of veterinary neurology. 3rd ed. Philadelphia: Saunders, 1997:174–187.
Toombs JP. Cervical intervertebral disk disease in dogs. Compend Contin Educ Pract Vet 1992;14:1477–1487.
Author Mary O. Smith
Consulting Editor Peter D. Schwarz

DISEASES

INTERVERTEBRAL DISK DISEASE, THORACOLUMBAR

 BASICS

DEFINITION
Caused by age-related changes within the intervertebral disks; may result in disk protrusion or extrusion

PATHOPHYSIOLOGY
• Classified as Hansen type I or II disease • Type I—involves rupture of the annulus fibrosus of the intervertebral disk, with extrusion of nucleus pulposus into the spinal canal; associated with chondroid degeneration of the disk, disk mineralization, and acute extrusion • Type II—involves an insidious bulging of the dorsal annulus fibrosus and its protrusion into the vertebral canal; usually is associated with gradual fibroid metaplasia of the disk • Disk extrusion or protrusion into the spinal canal—leads to compression of the spinal cord and focal myelopathy • Spinal cord compression—ischemia; demyelination • Lateral or ventral extrusion or protrusion of the disk—less common than dorsal extrusion or protrusion; usually not associated with clinical signs

SYSTEMS AFFECTED
Nervous—focal compressive myelopathy

GENETICS
• No known basis • Chondrodystrophic breeds (e.g., dachshunds, beagles, and Pekingese)—predisposed to Hansen type I disease • Large breeds—predisposed to Hansen type II disease

INCIDENCE/PREVALENCE
• Unknown • Thoracolumbar disk disease—approximately 85% of disk disease in dogs

GEOGRAPHIC DISTRIBUTION
N/A

SIGNALMENT

Species
Dogs

Breed Predilections
• Type I—dachshunds; shih tzus; Pekingese; Welsh corgis; beagles; all chondrodystrophic breeds • Type II—large breeds

Mean Age and Range
• Type I—3–6 years of age • Type II—8–10 years of age

Predominant Sex
None recognized

SIGNS

General Comments
Depend on the type of disk disease and the severity of spinal cord contusion and compression

Historical Findings
• Range from back pain without neurologic deficits to paraplegia, depending on the severity of disk extrusion and spinal cord injury; typically, back pain and some degree of paraparesis • Onset—sometimes follows jumping or vigorous activity; small-breed dogs (type I disease) usually acute; large-breed dogs (type II disease) usually insidious • Usually no history of trauma • May remain static, show some resolution, or (usually) worsen after initial onset

Physical Examination Findings
• Thoracolumbar pain—common; usually elicited by palpation of the dorsal spinous processes of the vertebrae and/or the epaxial musculature of the thoracolumbar region; may be evident by the patient's hunched posture and reluctance to ambulate; commonly mistaken for abdominal pain (palpation of the cranial abdomen also may elicit signs of pain in such cases) • May note some degree of paraparesis • May note decreased to absent proprioception in the hindlimbs • Spinal reflexes in the hindlimbs—normal to exaggerated: lesion affects the spinal cord between segments T3 and L3; decreased: lesion affects spinal cord segments caudal to L3. • Superficial and deep pain perception in the hindlimbs—may be diminished or absent; loss of all pain perception indicates a grave prognosis. • Forelimb neurologic function—normal; Schiff-Sherrington phenomenon may cause increased extensor tone in the forelimbs. • May note urinary incontinence or retention—owing to involvement of motor and sensory pathways within the spinal cord that convey information between the urinary bladder and appropriate centers in the CNS

CAUSES
Age-related chondroid degeneration or fibroid metaplasia of the thoracolumbar intervertebral disks

RISK FACTORS
Type I—chondrodystrophic breeds

 DIAGNOSIS

DIFFERENTIAL DIAGNOSIS
• Type I—trauma, neoplasia, and fibrocartilaginous embolism; differentiated by history and radiography (myelography) • Type II—degenerative myelopathy, neoplasia, and diskospondylitis; differentiated by history and radiography (myelography) • Discitis without spondylitis—relatively rare; differentiated via MRI and blood and urine cultures

CBC/BIOCHEMISTRY/URINALYSIS
Urinary incontinence or retention—patient at risk for lower urinary tract infections; urinalysis reveals leukocytes, proteinuria, and (possibly) bacteria.

OTHER LABORATORY TESTS
CSF analysis—routinely performed for myelography and when diagnosis is in doubt; may be normal, typically shows mildly to moderately increased protein concentration, with or without mild to moderate mixed pleocytosis; more abnormal in acute severe disease than in mild or chronic disease

IMAGING
• Thoracolumbar spinal radiography—often reveals a narrowed, wedge-shaped disk space, small intervertebral foramen, and collapsed articular facets at sites of intervertebral disk extrusion; more common with Hansen type I than type II disease; may see mineralized disk material within the spinal canal or intervertebral foramen with type I disease • Myelography—indicated in all patients with planned surgical therapy; injections of contrast usually made at the L5–6 intervertebral space (L4–5 space may be preferable in large-breed dogs); usually reveals an extradural mass lesion overlying or adjacent to the affected disk; shows extradural mass ventral, lateral, or (rarely) dorsal to the spinal cord; may note swelling of the spinal cord • CT or MRI—when results of myelography are not definitive

DIAGNOSTIC PROCEDURES
• Usually none • CSF analysis—see above

PATHOLOGIC FINDINGS

Gross
• Extruded disk material (type I disease)—white to yellow and granular in consistency; if chronic, may be hardened and difficult to remove from the spinal canal • Protruded disk material (type II disease)—usually firm, grayish white, and adherent to the floor of the spinal canal; may note swollen and discolored spinal cord in acute severe disease; may note narrowed cord owing to atrophy in chronic disease; cord may appear normal

Histopathologic
• Degenerate disks—water and proteoglycans decreased; collagen increased • Type II—disk becomes more cartilaginous. • Type I—nucleus pulposus becomes granular and calcified. • Spinal cord—depends on type and severity of the disk extrusion or protrusion; chronic, mild disease: demyelination and gliosis; acute, severe disease: hemorrhage, edema, and tissue necrosis

 TREATMENT

APPROPRIATE HEALTH CARE
• Four categories of patients—(1) first-time episode of back pain only; (2) repeated episodes of back pain; (3) some degree of paraparesis with deep pain perception; (4) complete paraparesis and loss of deep pain perception

INTERVERTEBRAL DISK DISEASE, THORACOLUMBAR

• Medical therapy—category 1 patients only
• Surgical therapy—categories 1–4

NURSING CARE
• Take great care to protect the spine when handling these patients
• Minimize thoracolumbar spine manipulation when withdrawing blood and performing restraint measures
• Protect the back and support the body on a flat surface (board or gurney) when transporting patients that are under general anesthesia
• Category 1 patients—watch for worsening signs
• Ensure that all patients are able to urinate appropriately and that they can empty the urinary bladder completely; may require manual expression, or intermittent urinary catheterization, or an in-dwelling urinary catheter
• Recumbent patients—kept on padded bedding and turned every 4 hr to prevent formation of decubital ulcers
• Inability to defecate—manual evacuation of the bowel, or enemas
• Physical therapy (including hydrotherapy)—appropriate for neurologic deficits

ACTIVITY
• Restricted—all patients
• Cage confinement for 2–4 weeks—category 1 patients; may alleviate signs; attempt before surgical treatment

DIET
Weight reduction—obese patients

CLIENT EDUCATION
• Discuss the signs of spinal cord compression.
• Inform client that patients with worsening clinical signs should be re-evaluated immediately.
• Emphasize the importance of cage rest when treating the patient with medical therapy alone and when the patient is recovering from surgery

SURGICAL CONSIDERATIONS
• Indicated for category 2–4 patients
• Directed toward relieving spinal cord compression via hemilaminectomy, dorsal laminectomy, or (less common) pediculectomy
• Back pain without concurrent neurologic deficits—disk material usually within the spinal canal; benefits from decompressive surgery rather than disk fenestration alone
• Concurrent prophylactic fenestration—controversial
• Acute loss of deep pain perception—may benefit from emergency decompressive surgery

 MEDICATIONS

DRUGS OF CHOICE
• Methylprednisolone sodium succinate—30 mg/kg IV, within 8 hr of onset or at time of surgery for acute spinal cord compression; may repeat 2 hr after first dose and then q6h for 24 hr for severe acute disease
• Prednisone or prednisolone—0.25mg/kg PO twice daily for 3–4 days, then taper over 2–3 weeks; for patients not undergoing surgery; always combined with strict cage rest and close observation for exacerbation of clinical signs

CONTRAINDICATIONS
Avoid concomitant use of glucocorticoids and NSAIDs—owing to combined negative effects on the gastrointestinal tract

PRECAUTIONS
• Glucocorticoids without concurrent cage confinement—may lessen pain, encouraging excessive activity and leading to further disk extrusion or protrusion; used particularly in combination with surgical therapy may predispose patient to gastrointestinal hemorrhage; generally safe when course is short and dose is low; prolonged or high dosage may result in life-threatening hemorrhage or even gut perforation.
• Avoid NSAIDs—may result in life-threatening gastrointestinal hemorrhage

POSSIBLE INTERACTIONS
Avoid combination of NSAIDs and glucocorticoids in all patients—increases risk of life-threatening gastrointestinal hemorrhage

ALTERNATIVE DRUGS
• Vitamin E (cats)—suggested as beneficial for spinal cord injury; no data available for dogs; may be a useful adjunctive therapy
• NSAIDs alone—not shown to be efficacious; pose severe risks of complications

 FOLLOW-UP

PATIENT MONITORING
• Patients treated medically—re-evaluated twice daily for worsening neurologic signs for the first few days after onset; if stable, re-evaluated weekly until clinical signs have resolved • Patients treated surgically—evaluated twice daily for neurologic function until improvement is evident; monitor urinary bladder and bowel function closely (see Nursing Care).

PREVENTION/AVOIDANCE
• May be unavoidable in some breeds • Avoid or slow exacerbation of clinical signs—keeping patient lean; and avoiding strenuous exercise and jumping

POSSIBLE COMPLICATIONS
Recurrence of signs; less likely with surgical treatment

EXPECTED COURSE AND PROGNOSIS
• Conservative treatment—may note recurrence; may ultimately require surgery • Surgical treatment—no recurrent episodes
• Patients that have lost all pain perception in the hindlimbs—guarded to poor prognosis; recoveries occasionally occur

 MISCELLANEOUS

ASSOCIATED CONDITIONS
Predisposed breeds are also predisposed to cervical disk disease.

AGE-RELATED FACTORS
N/A

ZOONOTIC POTENTIAL
N/A

PREGNANCY
N/A

SEE ALSO
• Intervertebral Disk Disease, Cervical
• Schiff-Sherrington Phenomenon

ABBREVIATION
CSF = cerebrospinal fluid

Suggested Reading
Braund KG. Canine intervertebral disk disease. In: Bojrab MJ, ed. Disease mechanisms in small dog surgery. Philadelphia: Lea & Febiger, 1993:960–969.
Levine SH, Caywood DD. Recurrence of neurological deficits in dogs treated for thoracolumbar disk disease. J Am Anim Hosp Assoc 1984;20:889–894.
Oliver JE, Lorenz MD, Kornegay J. Handbook of veterinary neurology. 3rd ed. Philadelphia: Saunders, 1997.
Prata RG. Neurosurgical treatment of thoracolumbar disks: the rationale and value of laminectomy with concomitant disk removal. J Am Anim Hosp Assoc 1981;17:17–26.
Toombs JT, Bauer MB. Intervertebral disk disease. In: Slatter DH, ed. Textbook of small dog surgery. 2nd ed. Philadelphia: Saunders, 1993:1070–1086.
Author Mary O. Smith
Consulting Editor Peter D. Schwarz

DISEASES

INTUSSUSCEPTION

BASICS

DEFINITION
• Prolapse or invagination of one portion of the GI tract into the lumen of an adjoining segment
• The invaginated segment is the *intussusceptum* and the ensheathing segment is the *intussuscipiens.*
• Classified according to location within the alimentary tract—enterocolic (ileocolic; most common location), cecocolic, enteroenteric, duodenogastric, gastroesophageal
• High intussusceptions may be defined as those proximal to the jejunum; low intussusceptions are those distal to the duodenum.

PATHOPHYSIOLOGY
• Exact physical and mechanical events that lead to intussusception are unknown.
• Uncoordinated peristalsis is probably involved; vigorous contraction of a bowel segment causes invagination of that segment into an adjacent flaccid segment.
• Regions of the GI tract that undergo abrupt change in anatomic diameter (e.g. ileocolic, or gastroesophageal junctions) are at high risk.
• Results in partial or complete GI obstruction leading to hypovolemia and dehydration
• Vascular compromise is common, especially to the intussusceptum, ranging from venous and lymphatic obstruction to arterial obstruction with full-thickness necrosis.
• Disruption of the mucosal barrier may allow absorption of bacteria and/or endotoxin, and shock.

SYSTEMS AFFECTED
• Gastrointestinal
• Cardiovascular—hypovolemic or septic shock
• May be multiple organ failure in severe, untreated cases

GENETICS
Heritability unproven, although gastroesophageal intussusception (GEI) has been reported in multiple littermates.

INCIDENCE/PREVALENCE
Unknown

GEOGRAPHIC DISTRIBUTION
N/A

SIGNALMENT
Species
• Dogs and cats
• GEI reported only in dogs.

Breed Predilections
• German shepherd dogs and Siamese cats
• German shepherd dogs have an especially high prevalence of GEI (64%).

Mean Age and Range
• Higher incidence in puppies and kittens: ~ 80% are <1 year of age; for GEI, 80% of dogs are >3 months of age).
• Reported range—5 days to 9 years

Predominant Sex
• None for intussusception in general
• Male:female ratio approximately 2:1 for GEI

SIGNS
General Comments
• Clinical signs and disease progression vary markedly depending upon location, degree of vascular compromise, and completeness of obstruction.
• In general, high intussusceptions have a more acute onset of signs and a more rapid clinical deterioration with higher mortality than low intussusceptions.

Historical Findings
• High intussusceptions—frequent vomiting, regurgitation, hematemesis, dyspnea, abdominal discomfort, and collapse
• Low intussusceptions—may include bloody mucoid diarrhea, tenesmus, intermittent vomiting, and weight loss

Physical Examination Findings
• Intermittent vomiting, bloody mucoid stools, and/or palpation of a sausage-shaped abdominal mass—mass is often caudal since ileocolic intussusception is most common.
• Most patients are mildly to severely dehydrated.
• May be signs of shock
• Abdominal pain—variable; may make palpation of the mass more difficult
• Ileocolic intussusception may present with the intussusceptum protruding through the anus.

CAUSES
• Idiopathic
• Enteritis—viral, bacterial
• Intestinal parasites
• Foreign bodies
• Previous abdominal surgery
• Intestinal mass
• Megaesophagus associated with GEI

RISK FACTORS
Any condition leading to altered GI motility

DIAGNOSIS

DIFFERENTIAL DIAGNOSIS
• Many of the disease conditions that may mimic intussusception are also predisposing factors for development of intussusception; thorough examination and close patient monitoring are of utmost importance.

• Viral enteritis—usually can diagnose on the basis of typical changes in CBC (leukopenia/neutropenia) and commercial fecal antigen test kits
• Foreign bodies—may be radiopaque or may cause plication of intestinal loops (linear foreign bodies); contrast studies can usually differentiate a foreign body from an intussusception, although the distinction is often made at the time of exploratory celiotomy.
• Mesenteric volvulus—can exhibit signs similar to those of intussusception; plain radiographic distinction may be difficult; mesenteric volvulus tends to have a more rapidly fatal course, and emergency celiotomy is indicated to differentiate the two conditions.
• Intestinal parasites—diagnosed by fecal examination and response to an anthelmintic
• HGE can be differentiated by a lack of radiographic sign of obstruction.
• Ileocolic intussusception with the intussusceptum protruding through the anus is differentiated from rectal prolapse by passing a blunt probe between the prolapsed segment and the anus; if the probe passes into the pelvic canal, the protrusion is due to an intussusception.
• GEI has inappropriately been confused with hiatal hernia.

CBC/BIOCHEMISTRY/URINALYSIS
• Leukogram—variable; ranges from leukopenia (underlying viral enteritis) to leukocytosis (with bowel necrosis or peritonitis)
• Hematocrit—may be low if significant GI hemorrhage; high with dehydration
• Electrolyte abnormalities—hyponatremia, hypochloremia, and hypokalemia tend to be more profound with high intussusceptions.
• Prerenal azotemia with dehydration
• Urinalysis—usually normal or nonspecific

OTHER LABORATORY TESTS
• Blood gas evaluation usually reveals a metabolic acidosis.
• High intussusception—metabolic alkalosis may prevail from loss of gastric acid in the vomitus (hypochloremia with metabolic alkalosis strongly supports pyloric outflow obstruction).

IMAGING
• Definitive diagnosis from plain films may be difficult.
• Usually radiographic signs of obstruction—bowel loops distended with gas and fluid; more pronounced with complete obstruction
• A tissue-dense tubular mass strongly supports a diagnosis of intussusception
• In GEI, thoracic radiographs show dilation of the esophagus with a tissue-dense mass in the caudal esophagus; the normal gastric air bubble may be absent in the cranial abdomen.

• Abdominal ultrasound—can be used to identify the intussusception; a cylindrical intestinal mass with excessive wall layering is highly specific for intussusception.
• Contrast studies (upper GI, barium enema)—can be used to outline an intussusception, but often with unnecessary delays in definitive treatment

DIAGNOSTIC PROCEDURES
• Esophagoscopy can identify a soft tissue mass (stomach) within the lumen of the esophagus in patients with GEI.
• Colonoscopy may help identify enterocolic or cecocolic intussusceptions.

PATHOLOGIC FINDINGS
• The basic lesion is grossly obvious.
• Histopathologic changes in the affected bowel range from areas of mucosal erosion and hemorrhages to full-thickness mural necrosis.

TREATMENT

APPROPRIATE HEALTH CARE
• Inpatient medical and surgical management; surgical emergency once patient is stabilized
• Life-threatening condition

NURSING CARE
• Aggressive intravenous fluid support to correct dehydration and replace ongoing GI losses
• A balanced electrolyte solution (e.g., lactated Ringer solution; use NaCl if profound
• Profound hyponatremia and hypochloremia indicates 0.9% NaCl.
• Potassium supplementation—base on measured serum levels, but usually required; use 20 mEq of KCl/L of IV fluid if serum potassium concentration is unknown; do not exceed an administration rate of 0.5 mEq/kg/h.

ACTIVITY
Restrict during treatment and postoperative periods (~ 7–10 days).

DIET
• Maintain vomiting patients NPO.
• Can usually initiate oral intake of fluid and food 12–24 h following surgical correction
• Early oral alimentation with small, frequent meals promotes normal peristalsis and avoids further ileus.

CLIENT EDUCATION
• A poor-to-grave prognosis is associated with nonoperative treatment of intussusception.
• GEI is associated with a high mortality in all cases.
• Correction of the intussusception may not address the underlying GI disorder.

SURGICAL CONSIDERATIONS
• A surgical emergency
• Celiotomy and correction should follow initial patient stabilization.
• Attempt manual reduction of the intussusception by gently "milking" the invaginated segment.
• Assess bowel viability by color, pulsation, intestinal contraction, and Wood's lamp fluorescence following IV fluorescein injection.
• If the intussusception is nonreducible or nonviable, resection and anastomosis are indicated.
• Can minimize risk of postoperative recurrence by enteroplication of the small intestines
• GEI recurrence is prevented by a left-sided gastropexy of the fundus.

MEDICATIONS

DRUGS OF CHOICE
• Administer broad-spectrum antibiotics or combinations with efficacy against coliforms and anaerobes, intravenously prior to surgery.
• Histamine blockers (e.g., famotidine, ranitidine) and/or protectants (e.g., sucralfate) may be indicated if GI ulceration is suspected.

CONTRAINDICATIONS
• Motility-enhancing antiemetics (e.g., metoclopramide, cisapride)
• Antiemetics mask signs of GI obstruction.

PRECAUTIONS
Anticholinergics exacerbate postoperative ileus and are not recommended.

POSSIBLE INTERACTIONS
N/A

ALTERNATE DRUGS
N/A

FOLLOW-UP

PATIENT MONITORING
• Watch closely for recurrence or worsening of signs for the first 3–5 days following surgery, when serious complications are most likely to occur.
• Recurrence is common (20–30%) in patients that do not receive enteroplication and usually occurs within 3 days.
• Suspect anastomotic dehiscence or leakage with a deterioration of clinical signs; diagnostic peritoneal lavage is the most sensitive method for detecting dehiscence.

PREVENTION/AVOIDANCE
Routine veterinary care of puppies and kittens (e.g., vaccinations and treatment of intestinal parasites) will eliminate many predisposing factors.

POSSIBLE COMPLICATIONS
• Recurrence
• Persistence of underlying GI problem if undiagnosed or untreated
• Peritonitis
• Short bowel syndrome may occur with resection of large segments of intestine.

EXPECTED COURSE AND PROGNOSIS
• Presence and severity of underlying condition will affect prognosis.
• Low intussusceptions: <20% mortality with proper treatment
• GEI: ~ 95% mortality

MISCELLANEOUS

ASSOCIATED CONDITIONS
May accompany other GI abnormalities

AGE-RELATED FACTORS
In old animals may be more commonly associated with mural mass lesions; routinely submit resected bowel segments in old patients for histopathology.

ZOONOTIC POTENTIAL
N/A

PREGNANCY
The stress of the metabolic and hemodynamic derangements, coupled with anesthesia and surgery, may result in pregnancy termination.

SYNONYMS
Cecocolic intussusception is commonly termed *cecal inversion*.

SEE ALSO
• Shock • Peritonitis • Gastrointestinal Obstruction

ABBREVIATIONS
• GEI = gastroesophageal intussusception
• GI = gastrointestinal
• HGE = hemorrhagic gastroenteritis

Suggested Reading
Leib MS, Blass CE. Gastroesophageal intussusception in the dog: a review of the literature and a case report. JAAHA 984;20:783–790.
Lewis DD. Intussusception in dogs and cats. Compend Contin Educ Pract Vet 1987;9:523–533.
Oaks MG, Lewis DD, Hosgood G, et al. Enteroplication for the prevention of intussusception recurrence in dogs: 31 cases. JAVMA 1994;205:72–75.
Orsher RJ, Rosin E. Small intestine. In: Slatter D, ed. Textbook of small animal surgery. 2nd ed. Philadelphia: Saunders, 1993: 593–612.
Author Bradford C. Dixon
Consulting Editors Mitchell A. Crystal and Brett M. Feder

DISEASES

IRIS ATROPHY

BASICS

OVERVIEW
- Degeneration of the pupillary margin or stroma (or both portions) of the iris, resulting in an iris that is thin or has areas of full-thickness tissue loss
- May be a senile or secondary change
- Secondary—may be a potential sequela of chronic inflammation (uveitis) or high IOP (glaucoma)
- Iris sphincter muscle—frequently affected, resulting in incomplete pupillary constriction
- Margin may remain unaffected; loss of stroma and iris dilator muscle causes large holes in the iris that resemble multiple pupillary openings
- Vision unaffected

SIGNALMENT
- Dogs—common aging change; all breeds, but affects small breeds (e.g., miniature and toy poodles, miniature schnauzers, and Chihuahuas) more commonly
- Cats—uncommon; most common with blue irides
- Secondary—any breed of dog or cat

SIGNS

Historical Findings
- Photophobia
- Previous episodes of uveitis or glaucoma

PHYSICAL EXAMINATION FINDINGS
- Incomplete pupillary light reflex, accompanied by a normal menace response
- Unilateral—may note anisocoria
- Irregular, scalloped edge to the pupillary margin
- Thin or absent areas of the iris on transillumination
- Strands of iris occasionally remain, spanning across portions of the pupil.
- Holes within the iris stroma—may resemble additional pupils
- Secondary—may be accompanied by any sign associated with chronic glaucoma or uveitis (e.g., conjunctival or episcleral injection, corneal edema, posterior synechiae, high IOP, and buphthalmia)

CAUSES & RISK FACTORS
- Normal aging
- Uveitis
- Glaucoma

DIAGNOSIS

DIFFERENTIAL DIAGNOSIS
- Must differentiate from congenital iris anomalies
- Iris aplasia—rare in dog and cats
- Iris hypoplasia
- Iris coloboma—a complete, full-thickness area of lack of development of all layers of the iris; frequently associated with the merle condition; may also see associated lack of lens zonules and an indentation of the lens deep to the colobomatous area
- Polycoria—more than one pupil, each with the ability to constrict
- Persistent pupillary membranes—arise from the collarette (midportion) of the iris, not from the free pupillary margin

CBC/BIOCHEMISTRY/URINALYSIS
N/A

OTHER LABORATORY TESTS
N/A

IMAGING
N/A

DIAGNOSTIC PROCEDURES
Tonometry—high IOP if secondary to glaucoma; possibly low IOP if secondary to uveitis

TREATMENT
- Nonreversible
- Secondary to uveitis or glaucoma—aimed at controlling the underlying disease
- May halt progression of the condition
- Patient may exhibit photophobia because of inability to constrict the pupil; provide adequate shade.

MEDICATIONS

DRUGS
- Senile—none
- Secondary—depend on underlying disease

CONTRAINDICATIONS/POSSIBLE INTERACTIONS
Topical atropine—exacerbates photophobia and pupillary dilation

FOLLOW-UP
- Senile—may continue to progress with age
- Secondary—usually does not progress once the primary disease is controlled

✓ MISCELLANEOUS

SEE ALSO
- Anterior Uveitis—Cats
- Anterior Uveitis—Dogs
- Glaucoma

ABBREVIATION
IOP = intraocular pressure

Suggested Reading
Collins BK, Moore CP. Diseases and surgery of canine anterior uvea. In: Gelatt, KN, ed., Veterinary ophthalmology. 3rd ed. Philadelphia: Lippincott Williams & Wilkins, 1999: 755–795.

Author Stephanie L. Smedes
Consulting Editor Paul E. Miller

BASICS

OVERVIEW
• Iron—essential element for living organisms; may be lethal when ingested in large quantities
• Sources of large concentrations of readily ionizable iron—multivitamins; dietary mineral supplements; human pregnancy supplements
• Overdose—loss of the normal mucosal limitations of iron absorption; corrosive to the gastrointestinal mucosa • Circulating iron in excess of the TIBC—very reactive; causes oxidative damage to any cell type • Damage to mitochondria—loss of oxidative metabolism
• Affected primary systems—gastrointestinal; hepatic; cardiovascular; nervous

SIGNALMENT
Dogs; possible in other species

SIGNS

General Comments
• History—generally indicates pill ingestion
• Unlikely to develop in patients that remain asymptomatic for 6–8 hr • Occur in four stages

Stage I (0–6 hr)
• Vomiting • Diarrhea • Depression • Gastrointestinal hemorrhage • Abdominal pain

Stage II (6–24 hr)
Apparent recovery

Stage III (12–96 hr)
• Vomiting • Diarrhea • Depression • Gastrointestinal hemorrhage • Shock • Tremors
• Abdominal pain

Stage IV (2–6 weeks)
Gastrointestinal obstruction

CAUSES & RISK FACTORS
• Generally associated with ingestion of iron-fortified pills
• Dogs—likely to ingest a large number of pills, owing to relatively indiscriminate eating behavior
• Toxic dose (dogs)—> 20 mg/kg of elemental iron
• Metallic iron and iron oxide (rust)—not readily ionizable; not associated with toxicoses
• Take care when calculating iron ingestion; iron salts in supplements and medications vary in elemental iron content (between 12% and 63%).

ELEMENTAL IRON IN IRON SALTS

Salt Form	Elemental Iron (%)
Ferric ammonium citrate	15%
Ferric chloride	34%
Ferric hydroxide	63%
Ferric phosphate	37%
Ferrous fumarate	33%
Ferrous carbonate	48%
Ferrous gluconate	12%
Ferrous lactate	24%
Ferrous sulfate	20%
Peptonized iron	16%

DIAGNOSIS

DIFFERENTIAL DIAGNOSIS
Other causes of gastroenteritis

CBC/BIOCHEMISTRY/URINALYSIS
• Leukocytosis
• Hyperglycemia
• Normal to high AST, ALT, ALP, and serum bilirubin

OTHER LABORATORY TESTS
Metabolic acidosis

Serum Analysis for Total Iron and TIBC
• Normal binding capacity—3–4 times the serum iron
• Serum iron in excess of TIBC—indicates poisoning; treatment required; monitor at 2–3 hr and at 5–6 hr postingestion and in asymptomatic patients (absorption rates vary with tablet dissolution and serum iron concentrations change rapidly).

IMAGING
Radiography—intact iron-containing pills are radiodense; able to visualize pill bezoars or pills adhered to the esophageal mucosa

DIAGNOSTIC PROCEDURES
• Postmortem analysis for iron in tissues—often ineffective, because of the reactive nature of free iron and the systemic distribution of reactive binding
• Analysis of gastrointestinal or stomach contents—may aid in documenting high iron exposures

PATHOLOGIC FINDINGS
Primary gross lesions—hemorrhage in the gastrointestinal tract and liver; hepatomegaly

TREATMENT
• Correct hypovolemic shock—intravenous fluids
• Correct acidosis—bicarbonate added to intravenous fluids

DECONTAMINATION AND PROTECTION
• Prevent further gastrointestinal and systemic damage—removal of unabsorbed iron from the stomach; lessens duration and severity of signs
• Treat gastrointestinal damage—gastric demulcents or sucralfate for severe gastrointestinal damage
• Emesis—induced for asymptomatic patient
• Gastric or enterogastric lavage—lessens absorption; performed when emesis is contraindicated or when pill bezoars are identified
• Emergency gastrotomy—indicated if lavage fails to remove adherent pills or bezoars

CHELATION
• Chelate excess systemic iron.
• Deferoxamine mesylate—iron chelator
• Duration of therapy—until TIBC is greater than serum iron

MEDICATIONS

DRUGS
• Deferoxamine mesylate—15 mg/kg/hr IV infusion or 40 mg/kg IM q4–6h or 40 mg/kg slow IV q4–6h; for chelation; indicated when serum iron exceeds TIBC
• Sucralfate—0.5–1 g PO q8–12h; for gastrointestinal protection

CONTRAINDICATIONS/POSSIBLE INTERACTIONS
• Activated charcoal—does not bind iron
• Gastric lavage—contraindicated with hematemesis, owing to increased risk of perforation
• Intravenous deferoxamine—must be given slowly or may precipitate cardiac arrhythmias
• Deferoxamine—teratogenic; use in pregnant patients only if the benefit outweighs the risks.

FOLLOW-UP
• Liver enzymes—monitored up to 24 hr after excess circulating iron is controlled
• Instruct client to watch for evidence of gastrointestinal obstruction for 4–6 weeks after poisoning.

MISCELLANEOUS

SEE ALSO
Poisoning (Intoxication)

ABBREVIATIONS
• ALP = alkaline phosphatase • ALT = alanine aminotransferase • AST = aspartate aminotransferase • TIBC = total iron binding capacity

Suggested Reading
Greentree WF, Hall JO. Iron toxicosis. In: Bonagura JD, ed. Kirk's current veterinary therapy XII. Philadelphia: Saunders, 1983:240–242.
Author Jeffery O. Hall
Consulting Editor Gary D. Osweiler

IRRITABLE BOWEL SYNDROME

BASICS

DEFINITION
A condition characterized by chronic intermittent signs of colonic dysfunction in the absence of structural gastrointestinal pathology

PATHOPHYSIOLOGY
• Unknown causes
• Potential causes include abnormal colonic myoelectrical activity and motility, dietary fiber deficiency, dietary intolerances, stress, and changes in neural or neurochemical regulation of colonic function.

SYSTEMS AFFECTED
Gastrointestinal

GENETICS
N/A

INCIDENCE/PREVALENCE
• An estimated 10–15% of dogs with chronic large bowel diarrhea have IBS.
• This disorder is poorly characterized and the diagnosis is based on exclusion of other causes, so accurate assessment of its prevalence is difficult.

GEOGRAPHICAL DISTRIBUTION
N/A

SIGNALMENT
Species
Dogs

Breed Predilections
Any breed; especially working dogs

Mean Age And Range
N/A

Predominant Sex
N/A

SIGNS
Historical Findings
• Chronic, intermittent signs of large bowel diarrhea, including frequent passage of small amounts of feces and mucus, and dyschezia
• Hematochezia is uncommon.
• Abdominal pain, bloating, vomiting, and nausea may also occur.

Physical Examination Findings
• Often unremarkable
• May be evident abdominal pain
• Rectal examination is normal aside from large bowel diarrhea.

CAUSES
Unknown

RISK FACTORS
• Stress (e.g., changes in the household or being left alone for extended periods) may be associated with episodes of diarrhea.
• In many dogs, stress appears to play no role.

DIAGNOSIS
• Based on the exclusion of all other potential causes of large bowel diarrhea
• Reserve for patients that have undergone a thorough diagnostic evaluation, therapeutic deworming, and bland diet trials without resolution of signs.

DIFFERENTIAL DIAGNOSIS
Causes of Large Bowel Diarrhea
• Whipworms
• Inflammatory colitis
• *Clostridium perfringens*
• Fiber-responsive large bowel diarrhea
• Dietary indiscretion or intolerance
• *Giardia*
• Histoplasmosis
• Pythiosis
• Colonic neoplasia
• Cecal inversion

Diseases with Similar Signs
• Dysuria/stranguria—exclude with observation, urinalysis, and imaging
• Prostatic disease—exclude with rectal examination and imaging

CBC/BIOCHEMISTRY/URINALYSIS
Normal

OTHER LABORATORY TESTS
Direct fecal examination, fecal flotation, and fecal/rectal scraping cytology—normal

IMAGING
• Survey and contrast radiographic studies of the abdomen—normal
• Abdominal ultrasonography—normal

DIAGNOSTIC PROCEDURES
• Colonoscopy generally normal; colonic spasm, excessive intraluminal mucus, and hypermotility are occasionally present.
• Mucosal biopsy specimens from multiple areas in the colon are histologically normal.

PATHOLOGIC FINDINGS
Normal

TREATMENT

APPROPRIATE HEALTH CARE
Outpatient medical management

ACTIVITY
N/A

DIET
A highly digestible diet with added soluble fiber (Metamucil, 1–3 tbs per day) often improve the diarrhea, but rarely completely resolves clinical signs.

CLIENT EDUCATION
• Inform clients that response to treatment varies and affected dogs may have long-term intermittent clinical signs.
• Eliminate any stressful factors in the dog's environment if possible.

SURGICAL CONSIDERATIONS
N/A

 ## MEDICATIONS

DRUGS OF CHOICE
Drug therapy for several days up to 1 to 2 weeks during episodes

Motility Modifiers
• Opiate antidiarrheals improve signs by increasing rhythmic segmentation.
• Loperamide (Imodium), 0.1–0.2 mg/kg PO q8–12h
• Diphenoxylate (Lomotil), 0.05–0.2 mg/kg PO q8–12h

Antispasmodic–Tranquilizer Combinations
• Used to relieve abdominal cramping, bloating, and distress
• Chlordiazepoxide and clidinium bromide (Librax), 0.1–0.25 mg of clidinium/kg PO q8–12h
• Isopropamide and prochlorperazine (Darbazine), 0.14–0.22 mg/kg SC q12h; oral: see package insert.

Parenteral Antiemetics
• If nausea and vomiting preclude the use of oral medication, administer antiemetics

parenterally for 1–2 days.
• Chlorpromazine (Thorazine), 0.2–0.5 mg/kg q6–24h SC or IM

CONTRAINDICATIONS
• Opiates—respiratory dysfunction, hepatic encephalopathy and/or severe debilitation
• Anticholinergics—cardiac disease, hepatobiliary disease, renal disease, hypertension, and/or hyperthyroidism

PRECAUTIONS
N/A

POSSIBLE INTERACTIONS
N/A

ALTERNATIVE DRUGS
Sulfasalazine (Azulfidine), 22–30 mg/kg PO q8h—reported to improve signs in some dogs with significant dyschezia

 ## FOLLOW-UP

PATIENT MONITORING
Have owner monitor stool consistency and watch for signs of dyschezia and abdominal discomfort.

PREVENTION/AVOIDANCE
Minimize any stressful factors in the patient's environment that might precipitate an episode.

POSSIBLE COMPLICATIONS
N/A

EXPECTED COURSE AND PROGNOSIS
• Should see improved stools, decreased mucus, and relief of dyschezia and abdominal distress within 1–2 days of starting medication
• In some dogs, signs completely resolve following treatment and dietary alterations; others have long-term episodic signs.

 ## MISCELLANEOUS

ASSOCIATED CONDITIONS
N/A

AGE RELATED FACTORS
N/A

ZOONOTIC POTENTIAL
N/A

PREGNANCY
N/A

SYNONYMS
• Spastic colon
• Nervous colon
• Spastic colitis
• Mucous colitis

SEE ALSO
• Diarrhea, Chronic—Dogs
• Colitis and Proctitis
• Dyschezia and Hematochezia

ABBREVIATION
• IBS = irritable bowel syndrome

Suggested Reading
Leib MS, Monroe WE, Codner EC. Management of chronic large bowel diarrhea in dogs. Vet Med 1991;86:922–929.
Strombeck DR, Guilford WG. Strombeck's small animal gastroenterology. 3rd ed. Philadelphia: Saunders, 1996.
Tams TR. Irritable bowel syndrome. In: Kirk RW, Bonagura JD, eds. Current veterinary therapy XI. Philadelphia: Saunders, 1992:604–608.
Author Amy M. Grooters
Consulting Editors Mitchell A. Crystal and Brett M. Feder

DISEASES

IVERMECTIN TOXICITY

 BASICS

OVERVIEW
• Toxicity—dogs given large extra-label dosages (≥ 10–15 times recommended dosage)
• Ivermectin—potentiates the release and binding of the neuroinhibitory substance GABA at certain synapses in the CNS; metabolized and excreted by the liver
• Sensitivity—some dogs unusually sensitive; differences may relate to a defect in the blood–brain barrier, higher than normal amounts of unbound ivermectin in the plasma, or an ivermectin-specific blood–brain transport mechanism.

SIGNALMENT
• Collies—most commonly affected; not all are sensitive.
• Australian shepherds—common
• May be a genetic component in sensitive animals
• No age or sex predilections

SIGNS
• Mydriasis
• Depression
• Drooling
• Vomiting
• Ataxia
• Tremors
• Disorientation
• Weakness, recumbency
• Nonresponsiveness
• Blindness
• Bradycardia
• Hypoventilation
• Coma
• Death

CAUSES & RISK FACTORS
• Extra-label use at high dosage
• Breed sensitivity—collies; Australian shepherds

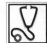 **DIAGNOSIS**

• Based on history and clinical signs
• No specific tests useful in confirming the diagnosis

DIFFERENTIAL DIAGNOSIS
• Overdoses of other avermectin compounds—milbemycin oxime
• Other toxicants or diseases affecting CNS

CBC/BIOCHEMISTRY/URINALYSIS
N/A

OTHER LABORATORY TESTS
Arterial blood gases—may reveal high $PaCO_2$ and low PaO_2 caused by respiratory depression and hypoventilation

IMAGING
N/A

DIAGNOSTIC PROCEDURES
Physostigmine—1 mg IV; temporary (30–40-min) return to consciousness or resumed alertness and muscle activity after the administration supports but does not confirm diagnosis; does not speed recovery; not indicated for treatment; glycopyrrolate administered first may prevent severe bradycardia

 TREATMENT

• Mainstay—supportive and symptomatic care
• Proper fluid therapy, maintenance of electrolyte balance, nutritional support, and prevention of secondary complications—important goals
• Nutritional support—institute early, preferably within 2–3 days of exposure; severe CNS depression or coma may last for weeks.
• Frequent turning of patient, appropriate bedding, physical therapy, attentive nursing care, and other standard treatment measures for a recumbent patient important
• Apply ocular lubricants.

• Mechanical ventilation—may be required with respiratory depression

 MEDICATIONS

DRUG(S)
• No known reversal agent
• Atropine or glycopyrrolate—may be administered as needed to treat bradycardia

CONTRAINDICATIONS/POSSIBLE INTERACTIONS
Avoid other drugs that stimulate the GABA receptor—benzodiazepine tranquilizers

 FOLLOW-UP

• Prognosis and eventual outcome—depend on individual and breed sensitivity, amount of drug ingested or injected, how rapidly clinical signs develop, response to supportive treatment, and overall health of patient
• Convalescence may be prolonged (several weeks); good supportive care in many seemingly hopeless cases has resulted in complete recovery.

 MISCELLANEOUS

SEE ALSO
• Heartworm Disease—Dogs
• Poisoning (Intoxication)

ABBREVIATION
GABA = γ-aminobutyric acid

Suggested Reading
Paul AJ, Tranquilli WJ. Ivermectin. In: Kirk RW, ed. Current veterinary therapy X. Philadelphia: Saunders, 1989:140–142.
Author Allan J. Paul
Consulting Editor Gary D. Osweiler

JUVENILE POLYARTERITIS (BEAGLE PAIN SYNDROME)

BASICS

OVERVIEW
A systemic necrotizing vasculitis most commonly reported in young beagles

SIGNALMENT
• Age at onset—4–10 months old
• Males and females equally affected
• Most reported cases from colonies of beagles bred for research; pet beagles may also be affected.

SIGNS
• Cervical pain
• Fever—40–41.5°C (104–107°F)
• Lethargy
• Anorexia
• Hunched stance
• Unwillingness to move the head and neck
• General hyperesthesia

CAUSES & RISK FACTORS
• Hereditary predisposition in some colonies
• Suspected to be immune-mediated

DIAGNOSIS

DIFFERENTIAL DIAGNOSIS
• Bacterial meningitis—signs are persistent and progressive rather than relapsing and remitting; rule out by CSF analysis and culture
• Cervical disk disease—cervical pain; affected dogs usually older; no fever, leucocytosis, or CSF pleocytosis
• Diskospondylitis—cervical pain and fever; CSF usually normal
• Granulomatous and infectious meningo-encephalomyelitis—differentiated by signalment, CSF analysis, and appropriate serologic testing and culture
• Aseptic meningitis—similar; differentiated on the basis of breed (large breed dogs); concurrent in some akitas with juvenile polyarthritis syndrome
• Polyarthritis—cervical pain; other joints usually affected; CSF normal; some beagles may have both conditions
• Protozoal infection—toxoplasmosis, *Neospora* caninum, or hepatozoonosis; may cause fever and muscle pain; differentiated by serology and muscle biopsy

CBC/BIOCHEMISTRY/URINALYSIS
• Leucocytosis with neutrophilia—neutrophil count 21–76 × 10³/μL)
• Nonregenerative anemia—hematocrit 21–32%
• Hypoalbuminemia—1.7–2.9 g/dL
• Urinalysis—usually normal; occasionally mild increase in protein:creatinine ratio

OTHER LABORATORY TESTS
• Serum electrophoresis—hypoalbuminemia with high a alpha₂-globulin fraction
• Antinuclear antibody test, Coombs test, and rheumatoid factor test—negative

IMAGING
• Thoracic, abdominal, and cervical radiographs—normal

DIAGNOSTIC PROCEDURES
• CSF analysis—neutrophilic pleocytosis normal results do not rule out the diagnosis.
• Synovial fluid analysis—may show neutrophilic inflammation
• Bacterial cultures (CSF, blood, and urine)—negative
• Serology for other infectious diseases—negative

PATHOLOGIC FINDINGS
• Severe necrotizing vasculitis, perivasculitis, and thrombosis of small to medium vessels in the leptomeninges of the cervical spinal cord, cranial mediastinum, and coronary arteries
• Other affected organs—thyroid, thymus, lymph nodes, testes, small intestine, diaphragm, esophagus, and urinary bladder
• Minimal vascular lesions—in clinically asymptomatic dogs
• Amyloidosis—identified occasionally in severely affected patients

TREATMENT
• Restrict activity.
• Fluid therapy—may be necessary with severe clinical signs if patient is unwilling to eat or drink

MEDICATIONS

DRUGS
Prednisone—1 mg/kg q12h; clinical signs should resolve in 12–48 hr; taper to minimum dose that will control signs (usually 0.25–0.5 mg/kg q48h); usually can be discontinued after 2–6 months of treatment

CONTRAINDICATIONS/POSSIBLE INTERACTIONS
N/A

FOLLOW-UP

PATIENT MONITORING
• Monitor for neck pain and gastrointestinal hemorrhage.
• Monitor CBC and biochemical panel for inflammation or organ dysfunction.
• Some patients may relapse despite treatment.
• Often will spontaneously resolve when patient is 12–18 months old

PREVENTION/AVOIDANCE
N/A

POSSIBLE COMPLICATIONS
N/A

EXPECTED COURSE AND PROGNOSIS
• Episodic—signs usually persist 2–7 days and then resolve; most patients experience multiple episodes but some have only 1–2 episodes before apparently becoming normal.
• Some patients may have persistent clinical signs.
• Clinical signs appear to resolve in all but the most severely affected patients by 12–18 months of age.

MISCELLANEOUS

ASSOCIATED CONDITIONS
Polyarthritis

AGE-RELATED FACTORS
N/A

ZOONOTIC POTENTIAL
N/A

PREGNANCY
N/A

SEE ALSO
• Steroid-responsive Meningitis—arteritis dogs
• Arteritis—Dogs
• Neck and Back Pain

ABBREVIATION
CSF = cerebrospinal fluid

Suggested Reading
Scott-Moncrieff JCR, Snyder PW, Glickman LT, et al. Systemic necrotizing vasculitis in nine young beagles. J Am Vet Med Assoc 1992:201;1553–1558.
Author Andrea Tipold
Consulting Editor Joane M. Parent

DISEASES

KERATITIS, NONULCERATIVE

BASICS

DEFINITION
• Any inflammation of the cornea that does not retain fluorescein stain

PATHOPHYSIOLOGY
• Alteration of corneal clarity indicates a pathologic response—edema; neovascularization; inflammatory cell infiltration; pigmentation; lipid or calcium deposition; enzymatic destruction; scarring • Neovascularization—superficial vessels: dendritic or tree branching, usually indicate superficial or external eye disease; deep vessels: shorter and straighter indicate deep corneal or intraocular disease

GENETICS
• No proven genetic basis in dogs or cats • Chronic superficial keratitis (pannus) in German shepherds—may be recessive • Environmental factors (e.g., altitude and solar radiation

INCIDENCE/PREVALENCE
Common cause of eye disease in dogs and, to a lesser extent, in cats

SIGNALMENT

Species
• Dogs—chronic superficial (pannus); nodular granulomatous episclerokeratitis; pigmentary (or corneal pigmentation); KCS • Cats—herpetic (stromal form); eosinophilic; corneal sequestration; KCS uncommon and usually secondary to chronic herpesvirus infection

Breed Predilections
Dogs: • Chronic superficial—may occur in any breed; high prevalence in German shepherds and Belgian tervurens • Nodular granulomatous episclerokeratitis—occurs primarily in collies; also noted in Shetland sheepdogs and border collies • Corneal pigmentation—brachycephalic breeds with nasal folds, nasal trichiasis, and exposure keratopathy; notably pugs, Pekingese, Lhasa apsos, and shih tzus • KCS—brachycephalic breeds; notably English bulldogs, cocker spaniels, Cavalier King Charles spaniels, Lhasa apsos, shih tzus, pugs, Pekingese, and West Highland white terriers *Cats:* • Eosinophilic and herpetic—none known • Corneal sequestration—most prevalent in Persians, Siamese, Burmese, and Himalayans

Mean Age and Range
Dogs: • Chronic superficial—may occur at any age; higher risk at 4–7 years of age • Nodular granulomatous episclerokeratitis—young to middle-aged collies; mean age 3.8 years • KCS—usually middle-age or old *Cats:* • Herpetic—all ages • Eosinophilic and corneal sequestration—all ages except neonates

SIGNS

Historical Findings
• May cause variable corneal discoloration and ocular discomfort

Physical Examination Findings
Associated with or secondary to chronic uveitis or glaucoma—may be unilateral or bilateral; often characterized by diffuse and marked corneal edema (bluish white), circumcorneal and deep vascularization, and evidence of ocular discomfort

Dogs: Chronic Superficial
• Usually bilateral • Often symmetrical pinkish white lesions with variable pigmentation (e.g., granulation tissue) that begin at the lateral or ventrolateral cornea • The lateral, medial, ventral, and dorsal corneal quadrants are usually affected in that order. • May note white lipid deposits in adjacent corneal stroma • Advanced condition—may lead to blindness • Third eyelids—may be affected; may appear thickened or depigmented • Nodular granulomatous

Nodular Granulomatous Episclerokeratitis
• Usually bilateral, raised, pink, vascular, and often symmetrical lesions of the lateral cornea • Lesions—may be slowly or rapidly progressive • White lipid deposits may occur in adjacent corneal stroma • Third eyelids may be affected; may appear thickened

Pigmentary
• Appears as focal to diffuse brown or black discoloration of the cornea, often in association with corneal neovascularization or scarring • May be unilateral or bilateral

KCS
• Variable findings • May be unilateral or bilateral • Early—mucoid or mucopurulent ocular discharge and conjunctival hyperemia • Chronic or severe—corneal neovascularization; pigmentation (brown); variable scarring

Cats: Herpetic Nonulcerative (Stromal)
• May be unilateral or bilateral • Often occurs with ulceration • Causes stromal edema (bluish white), scarring, and vascularization • Stromal scarring—may threaten vision

Eosinophilic
• Usually unilateral • Usually affects the lateral or medial cornea; but may affect any quadrant • Appears as a white, pinkish white, or gray corneal plaque, usually with a roughened or cobblestone surface • Corneal epithelium—usually intact; some fluorescein stain retention is possible. • Vascularization variable

Corneal Sequestration
• Usually unilateral • Appears as an amber, brown, or black, oval-to-circular plaque of the central or paracentral cornea • Affected cornea—usually ulcerated; retains fluorescein stain only at the periphery of the lesion • Corneal vascularization variable • Edges of the plaque—usually slightly elevated because of edema, thickened epithelium, or granulation tissue

CAUSES
Dogs: • Chronic superficial—presumed to be immune-mediated; influenced by environmental factors, notably altitude and solar radiation; has a breed predilection • Nodular granulomatous episclerokeratitis—presumed to be immune-mediated; has a breed predilection • Pigmentary—secondary condition; look for the primary cause; usually associated with exposure keratopathy, nasal trichiasis, nasal folds, KCS, or chronic superficial keratitis; congenital predisposition in some breeds (e.g., Pekingese and pugs) • KCS—usually caused by immune-mediated dacryoadenitis (see Keratoconjunctivitis Sicca) *Cats:* • Herpetic stromal—believed to be an immune-mediated, T-cell lymphocyte reaction to herpesvirus antigen rather than a cytopathic effect of the virus • Eosinophilic—unknown; some patients are concurrently infected with feline herpesvirus. • Corneal sequestration—unknown; patients have some evidence of previous corneal trauma or irritation; suggested relationship with previous herpesvirus keratitis

RISK FACTORS
Dogs: • Chronic superficial—more likely to occur at high altitudes with intense sunlight • Nodular granulomatous episclerokeratitis, pigmentary, and KCS *Cats:* • Herpesvirus infection—may be a risk factor for • Corneal sequestration—see Breed Predilections.

DIAGNOSIS

DIFFERENTIAL DIAGNOSIS
Dogs: • Infectious keratitis—usually ulcerative and painful • Noninfectious and nonulcerative keratitis • Nodular granulomatous episclerokeratitis—distinguished from neoplasia by age of onset, breed predilection, bilateral nature, and therapeutic response to antiinflammatory therapy *Cats:* • Herpetic stromal—may be associated with corneal ulceration or respiratory disease • Eosinophilic—relatively distinct in appearance; differentiate from fungal keratitis, acid-fast granuloma, neoplasia, and granulation tissue of other causes • Corneal sequestration—unique in appearance; distinguish from melanoma; sequestration usually affects the central or paracentral cornea, whereas melanoma affects the limbal cornea and sclera.

CBC/BIOCHEMISTRY/URINALYSIS
Usually normal

OTHER LABORATORY TESTS
• Serologic test for herpesvirus (cats)—may be positive with herpetic, corneal sequestration, or KCS; consider titers >1:100 significant. • Viral culture or IFA for herpesvirus (cats)—conjunctival scrapings; may be positive with herpatic, eosinophilic, corneal sequestration, or KCS (see Diagnostic Procedures)

DIAGNOSTIC PROCEDURES
Dogs: • Cytologic evaluation of corneal or conjunctival scrapings (chronic superficial)—reveals a preponderance of lymphocytes and plasma cells • Schirmer tear test (pigmentary, suspected KCS, any corneal disease of undetermined cause)—values > 15 mm/min, normal; values < 10 mm/min, consistent with KCS; values between 10 and 15 suggest KCS but

should be interpreted with consideration of the breed and concurrent ocular findings.

Cats: • IFA (herpetic)—cellular material obtained by conjunctival or corneal scrapings; place on a glass slide, air dry, and submit for testing (Virology Laboratory, College of Veterinary Medicine, University of Tennessee, 615-974-5643). • Histopathologic examination of affected cornea (eosinophilic or corneal sequestration)—obtain by superficial keratectomy; diagnostic (but diagnosis is usually possible by clinical signs alone)

PATHOLOGIC FINDINGS

Dogs: • Histopathologic examination of affected cornea (chronic superficial)—fibrovascular infiltrate of the superficial stroma accompanied by lymphocytes, plasma cells, and variable pigmentation • Histopathologic testing (ocular granulomatous episclerokeratitis)—increased vascularization of the limbal cornea with variable numbers of lymphocytes, plasma cells, and histiocytes; may note reticulin fibers; fibrosis is not a prominent feature; intact corneal and conjunctival epithelium

Cats: • Histopathologic examination of affected cornea (eosinophilic)—usually reveals granulomatous inflammation of the superficial stroma with eosinophils, lymphocytes, plasma cells, and histiocytes; may note mast cells; epithelium may be intact, thin, or ulcerated. • Corneal sequestration—coagulation necrosis of the corneal stroma with ulceration or necrosis of the epithelium; vascularization and variable numbers of polymorphonuclear and mononuclear inflammatory cells

TREATMENT

APPROPRIATE HISTOLOGY CARE

• Outpatient—initially • Inpatient—inadequate therapeutic response or continued ocular discomfort; may warrant surgery

CLIENT EDUCATION

Dogs: • Chronic superficial—warn client that this disease is controlled rather than cured • Nodular granulomatous episclerokeratitis • Pigmentary keratitis—inform client that the primary cause must be sought and corrected to prevent progression. • KCS—warn client that this disease requires lifelong treatment and sometimes surgery. ***Cats:*** • Herpetic keratitis—warn client that ocular discomfort and corneal opacity are often recurrent. • Eosinophilic—warn client that this disease is controlled rather than cured. • Corneal sequestrum—inform client that the sequestrum may slough spontaneously, but that it requires months or even years and that the clinical course is prolonged without surgery; warn client that removal of the sequestrum by keratectomy may be incomplete and that sequestration may recur postoperatively.

SURGICAL CONSIDERATIONS

Dogs

Chronic Superficial: • Superficial keratectomy—may be performed for severe disease; usually unnecessary; still requires indefinite medical treatment to prevent recurrence • β-irradiation with a Strontium-90 probe—noninvasive; may be preferred because lym-phocytes, plasma cells, and melanocytes are sensitive to effects of irradiation

Nodular Granulomatous Episclerokeratitis: • Superficial keratectomy—diagnostic; usually unnecessary; only temporarily resolves clinical signs • Medical treatment preferred

Pigmentary: • Superficial keratectomy—may be per-formed; should be done only after the initial problem is corrected; is indicated only if severe enough to threaten vision • β-irradiation and cryotherapy—have been used to resolve condition

KCS: Parotid duct transposition surgery or partial permanent tarsorrhaphy—may be indicated

Cats

Eosinophilic
• Superficial keratectomy—diagnostic; usually unnecessary; only temporarily resolves clinical signs • Medical treatment preferred

Corneal Sequestration: • Keratectomy—may be curative; recurrence possible • Primary indication for surgery—ocular discomfort

MEDICATIONS

DRUGS OF CHOICE

Dogs

Chronic superficial: • Topical corticosteroids—q6–12h; cause regression of corneal blood vessels; may try prednisolone, dexamethasone, flumethasone, or betamethasone • Sub-conjunctival corticosteroid injection—for severe disease; adjunct to topical therapy; may try triamcinolone acetonide (Vetalog; 4–8 mg), methylprednisolone acetate (Depo-Medrol; 4–8 mg), or betamethasone phosphate/acetate (Betasone; 0.75–1.5 mg) • Topical 1% or 2% cyclosporine solution—q8–12h; may use alone or in combination with topical corticosteroids; combination may be synergistic.

Granulomatous Episclerokeratitis: • Cortico-steroids—topical or subconjunctival as described above • Systemic azathioprine—2 mg/kg/day initially, then gradually reduce; effective when used alone or in combination with topical corticosteroids; may be treatment of choice

Pigmentary: • Topical treatment—directed at primary cause • Topical corticosteroids—if primary condition is inflammatory • Lubri-cants or cyclosporine—if primary condition is exposure keratopathy or KCS

KCS: Topical 1% or 2% cyclosporine—treatment of choice; see Keratoconjunctivitis Sicca (KCS). ***Cats:*** • Topical antiviral agents—trifluridine (Viroptic) or idoxuridine (Herplex);

q4–6h • Stromal—topical corticosteroids concurrent with antiviral agents; use judiciously because of possible viral recrudescence. • Eosinophilic—usually responds well to topical corticosteroids (q6–12h), causing remission (as in dogs); megastrol acetate (Ovaban; 5 mg PO q24h for 5 days, then 5 mg PO q48h for 1 week, then 5 mg PO weekly for maintenance) for difficult-to-manage cases • Corneal sequestration—treat initial problem if possible; usually requires topical (triple) antibiotics (q6–12h); may also use antiviral drugs for suspected herpesvirus infection; topical 1% atropine ointment (q12h, then reduce to q24h or q48h) to relieve discomfort associated with concurrent uveitis

CONTRAINDICATIONS

• Topical corticosteroids—contraindicated with corneal ulcers • Megestrol acetate—contraindi-cated in sexually intact female cat or cats with marginal liver function • Topical atropine—contraindicated with glaucoma and lens luxation

PRECAUTIONS

• Azathioprine—may cause gastrointestinal signs, hepatotoxicity, and myelosuppression • Megestrol acetate—not FDA approved for use in cats; possible side effects: polyphagia, transient diabetes mellitus, mammary hyper-plasia, mammary neoplasia, and pyometra

FOLLOW-UP

PATIENT MONITORING

• Periodic ocular examination—recommended to evaluate efficacy of topical and systemic medications • Examine at 1–2-week intervals, gradually lengthening the interval with remission or resolution of signs.

POSSIBLE COMPLICATIONS

• Advanced chronic superficial, nodular granu-lomatous episclerokeratitis, pigmentary, KCS, eosinophilic, or herpetic keratitis—may lead to visual deficit or blindness • Herpetic or corneal sequestration—may cause continued ocular discomfort

MISCELLANEOUS

Suggested Reading

Chavkin MJ, Roberts SM, Salman MD, et al. Risk factors for development of chronic su-perficial keratitis in dogs. J Am Vet Med As-soc 1994;204:1630–1634.

Author B. Keith Collins

Consulting Editors Paul E. Miller

DISEASES

KERATITIS, ULCERATIVE

BASICS

DEFINITION
• Inflammation of the cornea associated with loss of the corneal epithelium (corneal erosion) and, possibly, variable amounts of underlying corneal stroma (corneal ulcer)

PATHOPHYSIOLOGY
• May be caused by any condition (traumatic or nontraumatic) that disrupts the corneal epithelium or stroma • Ulcers—classified as superficial or deep, uncomplicated or complicated • Superficial—involves only the epithelium and possibly the superficial stroma • Deep—involves a greater thickness of stroma and may extend to Descemet's membrane, which may cause the globe to rupture • Complicated—occur with persistence of the inciting cause, microbial infection, or production of degradative enzymes • Epithelial wound healing—adjacent epithelial cells loosen and begin to migrate over the defect within a few hours; mitosis occurs within a few days; normal epithelial thickness is restored; the healing process is complete in 5–7 days. • Stromal wound healing—slower, more complex; may occur in an avascular or vascular manner; for relatively shallow wounds, epithelial migration and mitosis may be sufficient to fill the defect; epithelium may cover some ulcers, even when epithelial and stromal regeneration are insufficient to restore normal corneal thickness (the nonulcerated, crater-like defect is called a facet); usually heal by fibrovascular infiltration, which may require several weeks • Stromal ulcers—commonly complicated by microbial infection or enzymatic destruction initiated by corneal epithelial or stromal cells, host inflammatory cells, or microbial organisms • EBMD—may delay healing of superficial ulcers; interferes with attachment of the regenerating epithelium to the underlying stroma; results in a protracted clinical course; referred to as a refractory ulcer • Excessive enzymatic destruction—may result in a tenacious or gelatinous appearance of the corneal stroma—a melting or collagenase ulcer

GENETICS
• No proven basis, although breed predilections are seen • May occur secondary to other corneal diseases that have breed predispositions and, presumably, a genetic basis—corneal epithelial dystrophy in the Shetland sheepdogs; corneal endothelial dystrophy in Boston terriers

SIGNALMENT

Species
Dogs and cats

Breed Predilections
• Dogs—brachycephalic breeds; refractory ulcers most common in boxers, may occur in any breed • Cats—Persian, Himalayan, Siamese, and Burmese predisposed to feline corneal sequestration (see Keratitis, Nonulcerative)

Mean Age and Range
• Age of onset—highly variable; determined by cause • Refractory ulcers—tend to affect middle-aged and old dogs

SIGNS

General Comments
May be acute or chronic

Historical Findings
• Tearing, squinting, and rubbing at the eyes • Appearance of a film over the eye—corneal edema and prolapsed third eyelid • Sometimes a history of trauma • Herpetic ulcers (cats)—may have a history of respiratory disease

Physical Examination Findings
• Nonspecific—serous to mucopurulent ocular discharge; blepharospasm; photophobia; nictitans prolapse; conjunctival hyperemia (red eye) • May note one or more circumscribed, linear, or geographic (map-like) defects in the cornea • Deep stromal ulcer or descemetocele—may appear as a crater-like defect • Depending on size, cause, and duration—neovascularization; pigmentation; edema; scarring; mineral or lipid deposition; inflammatory cell infiltrate; collagenolytic activity (or melting) of the corneal stroma; may note focal to diffuse areas of corneal opacity • Refractory ulcers—loose or redundant epithelial edges; may demonstrate undermining of fluorescein stain in areas with seemingly intact epithelium • Usually stimulates tear production, possibly resulting in overflow of tears onto the face (epiphora); absence of obvious lacrimation suggests concurrent dry eye component or KCS. • Reflex anterior uveitis—mild or severe; secondary to ulceration • Visible anterior chamber exudates—most common with ulcers caused by penetrating corneal wounds or concurrent bacterial infection.

CAUSES
• Trauma—blunt; penetrating; perforating • Adnexal disease—distichiasis; ectopic cilia; entropion; ectropion; trichiasis; eyelid mass • Tear-film abnormality—quantitative tear deficiency (e.g., KCS); qualitative tear deficiency caused by conjunctival goblet cell (or mucin) deficiency or some other unidentified tear abnormality • Infection—primary corneal infection most common in cats; caused by herpesvirus • Lagophthalmos (inability to close the eyelids completely)—results in exposure keratitis and drying; may be breed-related in brachycephalic dogs and, to a lesser extent, in some cat breeds; may be caused by exophthalmos, buphthalmos, or neuroparalytic from idiopathic facial nerve paralysis (especially in cocker spaniels) • Innate corneal disease—EBMD; endothelial dystrophy; other endothelial disease • Miscellaneous—foreign body; chemical burns; neurotrophic keratitis (loss of trigeminal sensation); immune-mediated disease

RISK FACTORS
• Trauma • KCS from any cause • Feline herpesvirus infection

DIAGNOSIS

DIFFERENTIAL DIAGNOSIS
• Fluorescein dye retention—diagnostic • Other causes of a red and painful eye—conjunctivitis; KCS; uveitis; glaucoma (see Red Eye) • May develop concurrently with other causes of a red eye (e.g., secondary to KCS)

OTHER LABORATORY TESTS
• Serologic test for feline herpesvirus (cats)—may confirm the cause; however, a negative test result does not rule out herpesvirus infection; titer > 1:100 considered consistent with infection

DIAGNOSTIC PROCEDURES

Flourescein Staining
• Three patterns recognized • Homogenous green—superficial or stromal ulcer; may be circular, irregular, linear, or any combination thereof; interpretation of depth subjective • Crater-like defect that retains stain at the periphery and is clear at the center—des-cemetocele; may see Descemet's membrane bulging anteriorly • Crater-like defect that pools stain transiently but from which stain is rinsed easily—previous stromal ulcer that has re-epithelialized (facet); must be distinguished from a descemetocele

Other
• Rose bengal stain to the eye (cats)—may facilitate diagnosis of superficial linear ulcers (dendritic ulcers), which are considered pathognomonic for herpesvirus infection • Microbial culture and susceptibility testing—aerobic bacteria and fungi; indicated with rapidly progressive or deep corneal ulcers • Schirmer tear test—identify KCS-associated ulceration • Cytologic evaluation (cells obtained by corneal scraping) and gram, giemsa, or Wright staining—may reveal microbial organisms; may direct initial antimicrobial therapy

TREATMENT

APPROPRIATE HEALTH CARE
• Inpatient—deep or rapidly progressive ulcers; may require surgery and/or frequent medical treatments

ACTIVITY
• Restrict with deep stromal ulcer or descemetocele; may rupture • Self-trauma to the eye—prevented with an Elizabethan collar

CLIENT EDUCATION

• If more than one ophthalmic solution is prescribed, instruct client to allow at least 5 min between the applications of different drugs to prevent chemical incompatibility or dilution. • Advise client to contact the veterinarian if the patient appears more painful or if the ulcer appears to be deteriorating.

SURGICAL CONSIDERATIONS

• Superficial ulcers—do not usually require surgery if the inciting cause has been eliminated • Refractory ulcers—debrided with a dry, sterile, cotton-tipped swab to remove loose epithelial edges after topical anesthesia is applied • Ulcer that extends to one-half or greater corneal thickness and particularly to Descemet's membrane—may benefit from surgery • Descemetocele—considered a surgical emergency • Full-thickness corneal lacerations—repair immediately

Procedures

• Creating a nictitans flap; keratotomy; superficial keratectomy; conjunctival flap surgery • Punctate or grid keratotomy—performed easily; recommended as the first surgical procedure after corneal debridement • Rotational pedicle conjunctival flap—most versatile and amenable to use by the clinical practitioner

MEDICATIONS

DRUGS OF CHOICE

Antibiotics

• Topical agents—indicated for all patients • Frequency of application—determined by severity and the preparation used; ointments have a relatively long contact time and are applied q6–12h; solutions require more frequent application and are applied 4, 6, or even 8 times daily, particularly in the initial treatment of complicated ulcers. • Commonly used agents—chloramphenicol; oxytetracycline/polymyxin B (Terramycin); erythromycin; triple antibiotic; gentamicin; tobramycin (Tobrex) • Combination of neomycin, polymyxin B, and bacitracin (i.e., triple antibiotic)—excellent first choice; broad-spectrum of antimicrobial activity • Gentamicin and tobramycin—good choices for rapidly progressive ulcers with suspected *Pseudomonas* spp. or another gram-negative organism • Fluoroquinolone solution (Ciloxan)—topical; for aminoglycoside-resistant *Pseudomonas* spp.

Atropine

• 1% ointment or solution • Indicated for reflex anterior uveitis that occurs with corneal ulcers • Used frequently enough to cause mydriasis (usually q8–24h)

Antiviral Agents

• Indicated for herpetic ulcers in cats • Trifluridine (Viroptic) or idoxuridine (Herplex) solutions—q4–6h until clinical response is

observed; then reduce for 1–2 weeks after clinical signs have subsided

Acetylcysteine (Mucomyst)

• Anticollagenolytic agents • Most commonly used for treatment of melting ulcers; efficacy is controversial • May dilute 20% stock solution to 5%-10% with artificial tears and applied q2–4h • May be mixed with antibiotics—5 mL 20% acetylcysteine, 2 mL gentamicin injection (50 mg/mL), and 8 mL artificial tear solution for a concentration of 0.6% gentamicin and 6.6% acetylcysteine

NSAIDs

• May be indicated for their antiinflammatory and analgesic properties • Aspirin—dogs: 10–15 mg/kg PO q12h; cats: use judiciously, 10 mg/kg PO q48h

Contact Lenses

• Therapeutic—act as a bandage to reduce both frictional irritation from the eyelids and pain • Available from The Cutting Edge, Ltd (800-468-2275) • May also provide sustained drug release • Additional advantages—easy application with only topical anesthesia; continued visualization of the eye • Refractory ulcers—offer greatest benefit; may be used as an alternative to or in conjunction with surgery • Disadvantages—include relatively high cost ($13–15/lens); may be displaced by the third eyelid • Available in different diameters (13.5–17.0 mm) and base curvatures (8.5–9.0 mm) for use in different breeds; short radius of curvature (i.e., more curved) may provide a better fit for small-breed dogs.

CONTRAINDICATIONS

• Topical corticosteroids—contraindicated with a corneal erosion or ulcer • Topical NSAIDs—contraindicated with herpetic ulcers • Topical atropine—contraindicated with glaucoma and lens luxation; relatively contraindicated with KCS • Topical cyclosporine—contraindicated with distemper and herpesvirus-associated ulcers

PRECAUTIONS

• Atropine—use judiciously (if at all) with KCS; further compromises tear production; perform Schirmer tear tests for suspected KCS; extended use may require periodic tear tests • Topical NSAIDs (e.g., flurbiprofen and diclofenac)—may delay corneal healing; do not potentiate enzymatic corneal destruction as do corticosteroids • Topical cyclosporine (primarily used to treat KCS)—may be used safely unless the ulcer is related to canine distemper or feline herpesvirus infection

ALTERNATIVE DRUGS

Autologous plasma (collected in EDTA)—used by some ophthalmologists in place of acetylcysteine as an anticollagenolytic agent; keep refrigerated; avoid contamination; discard after 48 hr.

FOLLOW-UP

PATIENT MONITORING

• Fluorescein staining—periodically to assess healing; restain superficial ulcers in 3–5 days. • Superficial ulcer that persists for 7 days or longer—either inciting cause has not been eliminated or the patient has EBMD (which is treated as a refractory ulcer) • Deep stromal or rapidly progressive ulcers—assessed every 1–2 days initially (outpatient) until improvement is seen or the ulcer has stabilized; many of these patients are hospitalized or undergo surgery.

PREVENTION/AVOIDANCE

• Brachycephalic dogs—lubricant ointment administration (e.g., Lacrilube), permanent partial tarsorrhaphy surgery, or both may help prevent recurrent ulceration. • KCS-related ulcers (dogs)—require continued medical treatment of the KCS or parotid duct transposition surgery to prevent continued ulceration • Herpesvirus (cats)—chronic or intermittent antiviral therapy may be necessary to prevent recurrent ulceration.

POSSIBLE COMPLICATIONS

• Progressive corneal ulceration—rupture of the globe; endophthalmitis; secondary glaucoma; phthisis bulbi; blindness • Blind and painful eye—may require enucleation

EXPECTED COURSE AND PROGNOSIS

• Uncomplicated superficial ulcer—usually heals in 5–7 days, about 1 mm/day • Refractory ulcer—may persist for weeks or months despite medical therapy; will often heal within 2 weeks after punctate or grid keratotomy • Deep corneal ulcer treated only medically—may require several weeks for the fibrovascular infiltrate to reach the defect; does not always granulate satisfactorily; continued deterioration of the ulcer and globe rupture are possible. • Deep ulcer treated with a conjunctival flap—frequently results in more comfort within a few days after surgery; often removed in 4–6 weeks if healing is uneventful

MISCELLANEOUS

Suggested Reading

Collins BK. Diseases of the globe: cornea and sclera. In: Bojrab MJ, ed. Disease mechanisms in small animal surgery. 2nd ed. Philadelphia: Lea & Febiger, 1993;130–138.

Kirschner SE. Persistent corneal ulcers: what to do when ulcers won't heal. Vet Clin North Am Small Anim Pract 1990;20:627–642.

Author B. Keith Collins
Consulting Editor Paul E. Miller

KERATOCONJUNCTIVITIS SICCA (KCS)

BASICS

OVERVIEW
A deficiency of aqueous tear film, resulting in drying and inflammation of the cornea and conjunctiva

SIGNALMENT
- Very common in dogs; much rarer in cats
- Predisposed dog breeds—include cocker spaniels, bulldogs, West Highland white terriers, lhaso apsos, and shih tzus
- Inheritance—undefined
- Age of onset—depends on inciting cause
- Some studies report females are predisposed.

SIGNS
- Cats tend to be less symptomatic than dogs.
- Blepharospasm
- Conjunctival hyperemia
- Chemosis
- Prominent nictitans
- Mucoid to mucopurulent ocular discharge
- Corneal changes (chronic disease)—superficial vascularization; pigmentation; ulceration
- Severe disease—impaired or loss of vision

CAUSES & RISK FACTORS
- Immunologic—immune-mediated adenitis most common and often associated with other immune-mediated diseases (e.g., atopy)
- Congenital—pugs; Yorkshire terriers; sporadically in other breeds
- Neurogenic—occasionally seen after traumatic proptosis or neurologic disease that interrupts innervation of the lacrimal gland, often has a dry nose on same side as dry eyes.
- Drug-induced—general anesthesia and atropine cause transient KCS.
- Drug toxicity—some sulfa-containing drugs (e.g., trimethoprim-sulfamethoxazole) may cause transient or permanent condition
- Iatrogenic—removal of the nictitans gland may predispose, especially in at-risk breeds.
- Radiotherapy— when periocular area is in or near the primary beam
- Systemic disease—canine distemper virus; any debilitating disease
- Chronic conjunctivitis (cats)—chronic herpes or chlamydia conjunctivitis
- Chronic blepharoconjunctivitis (dogs)
- Breed-related predisposition

DIAGNOSIS

DIFFERENTIAL DIAGNOSIS
Often confused with bacterial conjunctivitis; most dogs with chronic KCS have secondary bacterial overgrowth; differentiated by use of the Schirmer tear test

CBC/BIOCHEMISTRY/URINALYSIS
N/A

OTHER LABORATORY TESTS
N/A

IMAGING
N/A

DIAGNOSTIC PROCEDURES
- Schirmer tear test—decreased results diagnostic; normal value (dogs): at least 15 mm/min of wetting; symptomatic patients: usually < 10 mm/min of wetting
- Fluorescein staining—corneal ulcers
- Aerobic bacterial culture and sensitivity if initial treatment is unsuccessful; not routinely recommended because bacterial overgrowth common with chronic disease
- Conjunctival cytology—may indicate the nature and degree of bacterial overgrowth

TREATMENT
- Outpatient—unless secondary disease (e.g., ulcerative keratitis) identified
- Clean eyes before instilling medication.
- Instruct owners to keep the eyes and adnera clean and free of dried discharge.
- Advise owners to call at once if ocular pain increases because patients are predisposed to severe corneal ulceration.
- Parotid duct transposition—surgical procedure that reroutes the parotid duct to deliver saliva to the inferior cul-de-sac; performed much less frequently since cyclosporine was introduced; saliva can be irritating to the cornea; some patients are uncomfortable after surgery and require ongoing medical therapy.

MEDICATIONS

DRUGS
- Cyclosporine A (dogs)—drug of choice; may be used as a 0.2% ointment; most effective for immune-mediated disease; shown to be effective in promoting lacrimation in 80% of patients; for unresponsive disease, some ophthalmologists advocate use of a 1% or 2% solution in corn oil (q12h initially, then q12–24h thereafter, depending on response).
- Pilocarpine—0.25% topically q12h; alternatively may use 1 drop of 2% pilocarpine/10 kg body weight q12h on food and slowly increase by 1 drop increments until increased tearing or systemic side effects noted (anorexia, salivation, vomiting, diarrhea, bradycardia). Most effective in neurogenic KCS.

- Artificial tears and lubricant ointments—help moisten the cornea; must be used frequently; only transiently relieve drying; preparations vary greatly in their composition; thicker agents (Hylashield) may be soothing for very dry eyes in patients that fail to respond to cyclosporine therapy.
- Broad-spectrum antibiotics—topical (solutions or ointments); frequently indicated for secondary bacterial overgrowth; rarely indicated once the bacterial overgrowth is controlled and tear production improves
- Corticosteroids—topical; frequently used before cyclosporine was introduced; minimize inflammation; effective in reducing corneal vascularization and pigmentation; now not commonly used
- Mucolytic agents (e.g., acetylcysteine)—occasionally used to help break up tenacious mucous discharge; add significantly to the cost of treatment; rarely indicated once tear production has improved

CONTRAINDICATIONS/POSSIBLE INTERACTIONS
- Topical cyclosporine—occasionally irritating
- Topical pilocarpine—initially irritating
- Topical corticosteroids—avoided with ulcerative keratitis

FOLLOW-UP
- Recheck at regular intervals—monitor response and progress.
- Schirmer tear test—performed 4–6 weeks after initiating cyclosporine; evaluate response (patient should have received the drug the day of the visit).
- Immune-mediated disease—usually requires life-long treatment
- Other types of disease—may be transient (e.g. atropine therapy); require treatment only until tear production returns.

MISCELLANEOUS

Suggested Reading
Moore CP. Diseases and surgery of the lacrimal system. In: Gelatt KN ed., Philadelphia: Lippincott Williams & Wilkins 1999: 583–607.
Author Erin S. Champagne
Consulting Editor Paul E. Miller

L-FORM BACTERIAL INFECTIONS

 BASICS

OVERVIEW
Caused by bacteria variants with defective or absent cell walls

L-Form Bacteria
- Isolated from humans, animals, and plants
- Named for Lister Institute (London), where discovered in 1935
- Differ from the mycoplasma by lack of sterols in their membranes (similar to bacteria)
- Soft, fragile, pleomorphic, spherical, and osmotically fragile; structurally equivalent to protoplasts and spheroplasts, which cannot divide
- Can grow and replicate by cell fission in an irregular manner, yielding daughter cells that differ in size, nucleic acid content, and amount of cytoplasm
- Formed as spontaneous variant of bacteria or when cell wall synthesis is inhibited or impaired by antibiotics (e.g., penicillin), specific immunoglobulins, or lysosomal enzymes that degrade cell walls
- Can be induced from virtually all gram-positive and -negative bacteria under suitable conditions
- May revert to normal cell wall strain in a suitable host or favorable medium
- Usually no pathogenicity

SIGNALMENT
- Sporadic in cats and dogs
- Most common in free-roaming cats of all ages

SIGNS
- Dogs—arthritis
- Cats—penetrating wound (usually cat bite); infected surgical site; cellulitis; fever; arthritis; synovitis

CAUSES & RISK FACTORS
- Bites, scratches, or trauma may allow organism to enter skin and subcutaneous tissue.
- Environmental reservoir unknown
- Formation encouraged by antibiotic treatment of host, resistance of host, suitability of in vivo site for establishment of infective locus, and relatively low to moderate virulence of the infecting bacterium
- Greatly reduced infectivity but may revert and display the pathogenic properties of the original bacterium

 DIAGNOSIS

DIFFERENTIAL DIAGNOSIS
- Mycoplasma—differentiate by phase microscopy, by electron microscopy, or by measuring penicillin-binding proteins
- Suppurative skin infections caused by mycobacteria, yeast, or fungi
- Arthritis caused by immune-mediated disease, bacteria, spirochetes, mycoplasma, rickettsia, chlamydia, viruses, or fungus

CBC/BIOCHEMISTRY/URINALYSIS
- Neutrophilia with left shift
- Monocytosis
- Lymphocytosis
- Eosinophilia
- Mild normochromic, normocytic anemia
- High serum total protein

OTHER LABORATORY TESTS
- Cytology—exudate from draining lesions contains macrophages and neutrophils.
- Joint fluid—high neutrophil count
- Culture—difficult; requires special media (Hayflick); "Fried-egg" appearance of colonies on solid agar (center portion embedded in agar; thin vacuolated growth on agar surface)
- Light microscopy—difficult to demonstrate
- Electron microscopy—may show characteristic pleomorphic, cell wall–deficient organisms in phagocytes
- Precise characterization and speciation—the organism must revert to the parental cell-walled state (may take years)

IMAGING
Radiographs—periarticular soft tissue swelling; periosteal proliferation

DIAGNOSTIC PROCEDURES
N/A

PATHOLOGIC FINDINGS
- Biopsy—pyogenic cellulitis; panniculitis; chronic pyogranulomatous arthritis; tenosynovitis
- Stains—neither conventional (H&E) nor specialized (gram, acid-fast, silver, PAS) reveal organisms

 TREATMENT

- Gentle cleaning degrades fragile organisms.
- Allow open wounds to heal by secondary intention

 MEDICATIONS

DRUGS
- Variable antibiotic sensitivity
- Tetracycline—22 mg/kg PO q8h for at least 1 week after signs disappear
- Fever usually breaks within 24–48 hr.
- β-lactam antibiotics—inhibit cell wall synthesis; not effective

CONTRAINDICATIONS/POSSIBLE INTERACTIONS
N/A

 FOLLOW-UP

Arthritic changes persistent

 MISCELLANEOUS

- Public health significance unknown
- Ubiquitous; therefore, role in disease questioned

ABBREVIATIONS
- H&E = hematoxylin and eosin
- PAS = periodic acid–Schiff

Suggested Reading
Carro T. L-forms and mycoplasmal infections. In: August JR, ed., Consultations in feline internal medicine. 2nd ed. Philadelphia: Saunders, 1994:13–20.
Author J. Paul Woods
Consulting Editor Stephen C. Barr

LARYNGEAL DISEASE

 BASICS

DEFINITION

Suggests a disease process that alters normal structure and, usually, function of the larynx

PATHOPHYSIOLOGY

- Signs depend on the cause and severity of the resulting dysfunction.
- With severe obstruction to laryngeal airflow—hyperpyrexia and heat prostration possible
- Air hunger syndrome (e.g., hypoventilation, hypoxemia)—may note retching, vomiting, aspiration pneumonia, and even respiratory or cardiac arrest

SYSTEMS AFFECTED

- Respiratory—interference with air–oxygen delivery to the alveoli (hypoventilation); aspiration pneumonia; pulmonary edema possible in dogs
- Gastrointestinal—retching and vomiting secondary to severe hypoxemia
- Cardiovascular and nervous—hyperpyrexia and heat prostration

GENETICS

- Paralysis (dogs)—Bouvier des Flandres (autosomal dominant trait); Siberian huskies and husky mixed breeds (mode of inheritance under study)
- Cats—no studies reported

INCIDENCE/PREVALENCE

- Paralysis—hereditary forms: high incidence; acquired (idiopathic) form: fairly high prevalence, undefined incidence; rare in cats
- Trauma—rare in dogs and cats
- Tumors (primary and as part of a generalized neoplastic process)—rare in dogs; more common in domestic cats but incidence poorly defined

GEOGRAPHIC DISTRIBUTION

N/A

SIGNALMENT

Species

Dogs and cats

Breed Predilections

Paralysis (Dogs)
- Hereditary—Bouvier des Flandres, Siberian huskies, and husky mixed breeds
- Part of generalized polyneuropathy syndrome—Dalmatians
- Acquired—over represented in giant breeds (St. Bernards, Newfoundlands) and large breeds (Irish setters, Labradors, golden retrievers)

Mean Age and Range

Paralysis
- Hereditary—onset of signs at 4–8 months of age
- Acquired—1–12 years of age; reported mean, 9–12 years
- Cats—usually old

Neoplasia
- Middle-aged to old dogs and cats

Predominant Sex

Paralysis—hereditary: reported 3:1 male predominance; acquired: reported small to moderate male predominance

SIGNS

General Comments

Directly related to the degree of impairment of laryngeal airflow

Historical Findings

- Change in character of the bark or meow
- Occasional coughing
- Reduced activity
- Exercise intolerance
- Abnormal breathing sounds with exertion or stress
- Associated with exertion, stress, or heat—severely difficult breathing; gagging and retching; vomiting; weakness and lethargy; collapse; even sudden death

Physical Examination Findings

- Noisy respiration and a high-pitched inspiratory sound (stridor)—most common
- Cats—inspiratory stridor less characteristic than in dogs
- Upper airway sounds—referred over the trachea and to hilar lung fields, bilaterally
- With aspiration—focal or bilateral rales may be ausculted
- Rectal temperature—usually high

CAUSES

Paralysis

- Congenital
- Acquired—suggested hormonal deficiencies (e.g., hypothyroidism), central or peripheral vagal nerve abnormality, cervical trauma, abnormality involving the recurrent laryngeal nerves, disease in the anterior thorax, generalized peripheral neuropathy, myopathy, and other immune-mediated disorders
- Thyroid adenocarcinoma—may impinge or invade recurrent laryngeal nerves

Trauma

- Penetrating (e.g., bite wounds) or blunt neck
- Injury secondary to ingested foreign materials—bones; sticks; needles; pins

Neoplasia

- Dogs—squamous cell adenocarcinoma (most common); leiomyoma; rhabdomyosarcoma; osteosarcoma; hemangiosarcoma; mast-cell tumors; lymphosarcoma
- Cats—quite rare; squamous cell adenocarcinoma; lymphosarcoma

RISK FACTORS

- Systemic disorders—See Causes
- Concomitant pulmonary abnormalities

 DIAGNOSIS

DIFFERENTIAL DIAGNOSIS

- Laryngeal collapse—potential complication of long-standing brachycephalic airway syndrome and (rarely) laryngeal paralysis; noisy, obstructed breathing pattern with no inspiratory stridor; more likely than paralysis in brachycephalic dog; complete laryngeal examination under heavy sedation needed to confirm the diagnosis.
- Chronic proliferative, pyogranulomatous laryngitis—may cause a mass lesion requiring surgical removal; histopathologic examination; tapered administration of corticosteroids
- Obstructing processes involving the trachea and the tracheobronchial junction—may mimic laryngeal disease on physical examination; causes include tracheal collapse (e.g., tracheomalacia) and intraluminal and peritracheal masses.

CBC/BIOCHEMISTRY/URINALYSIS

- Usually normal
- With aspiration pneumonia—high WBC count with a left shift possible

OTHER LABORATORY TESTS

- Arterial blood gas analysis—detect hypoxemia and respiratory acidosis
- Thyroid testing—routinely performed because hypothyroidism is a suggested cause for idiopathic paralysis; < 10% of affected dogs test positive; hormone replacement in a few dogs did not result in improved laryngeal function.

IMAGING

- Routine imaging procedures—little benefit as primary diagnostic procedures
- Radiography, fluoroscopy, and bronchoscopy—help rule out the differential diagnoses; detect aspiration pneumonia
- Barium swallow with or without fluoroscopy (dogs)—perform in every patient in which occasional vomiting is reported; a low incidence (< 10%) of esophageal motor dysfunction found with idiopathic paralysis

DIAGNOSTIC PROCEDURES

Electromyography—define partial or complete denervation potentials (e.g., fibrillation and/or positive waves) with or without pseudomyotonia

Laryngoscope

• Visual inspection with the patient under heavy sedation or anesthesia required for proper evaluation
• Paralysis—dogs: even light barbiturate anesthesia makes evaluation difficult; recommend acepromazine (0.033 mg/kg IM, SC); cats: ketamine HCl (6–10 mg/kg IV) alone or ketamine HCl (3–5 mg/kg) with diazepam (0.1–0.2 mg/kg), or Telesol (9–12 mg/kg IM, SC) provides sedation without interfering with laryngeal function
• Abduction of laryngeal cartilages—normally observed during deep inspiration; with paralysis may note passive opening of the larynx during expiration

PATHOLOGIC FINDINGS

• Gross—redness and swelling of the mucosa over the arytenoid cartilages and the vocal folds
• Histopathologic—inflammation and edema of the perilaryngeal mucous membranes; denervation atrophy of the laryngeal muscles

 TREATMENT

APPROPRIATE HEALTH CARE

• Outpatient—while awaiting surgery if stable
• Emergency—marked respiratory distress; oxygen therapy combined with sedation and corticosteroids (dexamethasone sodium phosphate at 1–2 mg/kg IV; then 0.5–1.0 mg/kg SC q12h for 24 hr; then 0.2 mg/kg SC q12h in tapering doses) or emergency tracheotomy

NURSING CARE
N/A

ACTIVITY

Severe restriction—patients pending surgery; when owner refuses surgery

DIET
N/A

CLIENT EDUCATION

Paralysis

• Discuss potential complications of heat prostration and asphyxia if surgery is not pursued.
• Discuss the improved quality of life and normal life expectancy with successful surgery.
• Discuss the heritability of the congenital forms of laryngeal paralysis.
• Discuss the increased risk for aspiration pneumonia after surgery.

SURGICAL CONSIDERATIONS

• Paralysis—surgical management treatment of choice; variety of procedures reported; efficacy of any one procedure depends on the surgeon's experience and expertise and perhaps other minor factors.
• Trauma—temporary tracheotomy may be life-saving and curative.
• Neoplasia—tumor excision with or without modified surgery to enlarge the laryngeal airway may be curative in dogs; for squamous cell adenocarcinoma, surgical excision coupled with radiotherapy management of choice; permanent tracheostomy may improve quality of life.

 MEDICATIONS

DRUGS OF CHOICE

• Acquired paralysis (dogs) when surgery is declined—may benefit from mild sedatives (acepromazine, promazine, or diazepam) and corticosteroids (prednisone at 2.2 mg/kg divided q12h initially; then gradually reduce to alternate-day administration)
• Tonsillar lymphosarcoma—responds to chemotherapy

CONTRAINDICATIONS
N/A

PRECAUTIONS

• Heavy sedation without a tracheotomy in a hot environment may predispose the patient to heat prostration.
• Corticosteroids—chronic use may predispose the patient to gastric ulcerations and, if susceptible, to diabetes mellitus and systemic or focal infection

POSSIBLE INTERACTIONS
N/A

ALTERNATIVE DRUGS
N/A

 FOLLOW-UP

PATIENT MONITORING

• Re-examination of larynx—recommended 3–4 weeks after surgery
• Arterial blood gases—should normalize after surgery
• Improvement in activity and exercise tolerance—reported by owners after surgery

PREVENTION/AVOIDANCE

Dogs with inheritable laryngeal paralysis should not be used for breeding.

POSSIBLE COMPLICATIONS

• Recurrence of clinical signs—with tumor regrowth; with inadequate surgery to treat paralysis

• Laryngeal web formation (dogs)—after bilateral vocal cord resection; transect and treat with tapered corticosteroids
• Increased risk of aspiration pneumonia—after any laryngeal surgical protocol
• Risk of aspiration—particularly high if evidence of aspiration noted before surgical treatment of paralysis

EXPECTED COURSE AND PROGNOSIS

• Paralysis—long-term prognosis good to excellent with successful surgery; with unsatisfactory initial surgery, additional surgery may improve prognosis.
• Trauma—progress usually satisfactory with conservative management, even after emergency tracheotomy
• Neoplasia—squamous cell adenocarcinoma (dogs and cats): prognosis poor, even with radiotherapy; lymphosarcoma (cats): prognosis depends on chemotherapy used and patient response.

 MISCELLANEOUS

ASSOCIATED CONDITIONS

• Cervical masses, notably thyroid adenocarcinoma, occasionally
• Generalized esophageal motor dysfunction—low incidence in dogs with acquired paralysis, suggesting polyneuropathy

AGE-RELATED FACTORS

Hereditary paralysis—onset of clinical signs within the first year of life

ZOONOTIC POTENTIAL
N/A

PREGNANCY

Increased risk in patients with clinical signs of laryngeal dysfunction

SEE ALSO

• Brachycephalic Airway Syndrome
• Lymphosarcoma—Cats
• Stertor and Stridor
• Tracheal Collapse—Dogs

Suggested Reading

Harvey CE. The larynx. In: Bojrab MJ, ed. Pathophysiology in small animal surgery. Philadelphia: Lea & Febiger, 1981: 350–358.
Venker-van Haagen AJ. Diseases of the larynx. Vet Clin North Am Small Anim Pract 1992;22:1155–1172.
Venker-van Haagen AJ. Laryngeal disease of dogs and cats. In: Kirk RW, ed. Current veterinary therapy IX. Philadelphia: Saunders, 1986:265–269.
Author Neil K. Harpster
Consulting Editor Eleanor C. Hawkins

LEAD POISONING

BASICS

DEFINITION
Intoxication (blood lead > 0.4 ppm) owing to acute or chronic exposure to some form of lead

PATHOPHYSIOLOGY
- Lead—interacts with sulfhydryl groups; interferes with numerous enzymes, including those involved in heme synthesis; causes fragility and decreased survival of RBCs
- Release of reticulocytes and nucleated RBCs from bone marrow
- Inhibition of 5′-pyrimidine nucleotidase—retention of RNA degradation products; aggregation of ribosomes (e.g., basophilic stippling)
- Damage to CNS capillaries—may account for brain lesions
- Young patients—weaker blood–brain barrier may permit more lead to reach the brain.

SYSTEMS AFFECTED
- Hemic/Lymph/Immune—interference with hemoglobin synthesis
- Gastrointestinal—unknown mechanism
- Nervous—capillary damage; possible direct toxic affect
- Renal/Urologic—damage to proximal tubule cells

GENETICS
N/A

INCIDENCE/PREVALENCE
- Incidence unknown
- Less prevalent in dogs—owing to elimination of sources
- More prevalent in cats—increased awareness and diagnosis
- Higher number of cases during warmer months

GEOGRAPHIC DISTRIBUTION
Low socioeconomic status of pet-owning family associated with high blood lead concentration in pets

SIGNALMENT

Species
Dogs more commonly than cats

Breed Predilections
N/A

Mean Age and Range
Mainly dogs < 1 year of age

Predominant Sex
N/A

SIGNS

General Comments
- Primarily gastrointestinal and neurologic
- Gastrointestinal—often precede CNS signs; predominant with chronic, low-level exposure
- CNS—occur more often with acute exposure
- History of renovation of older house or ingestion of lead objects

Physical Examination Findings
- Vomiting
- Diarrhea
- Anorexia
- Abdominal pain
- Lethargy
- Hysteria
- Seizures
- Blindness

CAUSES
- Ingestion of some form of lead—paint and paint residues or dust from sanding; car batteries; linoleum; solder; plumbing materials and supplies; lubricating compounds; putty; tar paper; lead foil; golf balls; lead object (e.g., shot, fishing sinkers, drapery weights)
- Use of improperly glazed ceramic food or water bowl

RISK FACTORS
- Age < 1 year
- Living in economically depressed areas
- Living in old house or building that is being renovated

DIAGNOSIS

DIFFERENTIAL DIAGNOSIS

Dogs
- Canine distemper
- Infectious encephalitides
- Bromethalin or methylxanthine toxicosis
- NSAID toxicosis
- Heat stroke
- Intestinal parasitism
- Intussusception
- Pancreatitis
- Infectious canine hepatitis

Cats
- Degenerative or storage diseases
- Hepatic encephalopathy
- Infectious encephalitides
- Organophosphate toxicosis

CBC/BIOCHEMISTRY/URINALYSIS
- Between 5 and 40 nucleated RBCs/100 WBCs without anemia
- Absence of nucleated RBC changes does not rule out the diagnosis.
- Anisocytosis, polychromasia, poikilocytosis, target cells, hypochromasia
- Basophilic stippling of RBCs
- Neutrophilic leukocytosis
- Urinalysis—mild, nonspecific renal damage

OTHER LABORATORY TESTS

Lead Concentration
- Toxic—antemortem whole blood: > 0.4 ppm (40 μg/dL); postmortem liver and/or kidney: > 5 ppm (wet weight)
- Lower values—must be interpreted in conjunction with history and clinical signs
- Blood levels—do not correlate with occurrence or severity of clinical signs
- $CaNa_2EDTA$ mobilization test—collect one 24-hr urine sample; administer $CaNa_2EDTA$ (75 mg/kg IM); collect a second 24-hr urine sample; with toxicosis, urine lead increases 10–60-fold post-EDTA.

IMAGING
May note radiopaque material in gastro-intestinal tract; not diagnostic

DIAGNOSTIC PROCEDURES
N/A

PATHOLOGIC FINDINGS
- Gross—may note paint chips or lead objects in gastrointestinal tract
- Intranuclear inclusion bodies—may note in hepatocytes or renal tubule epithelial cells; intracellular storage form of lead; considered pathognomonic

TREATMENT

APPROPRIATE HEALTH CARE
- Inpatient—first course of chelation, depending on severity of clinical signs
- Outpatient—orally administered chelators

NURSING CARE
• Balanced electrolyte fluids—Ringer solution; replacement of hydration deficit
• Gastric or enterogastric lavage—may be indicated

ACTIVITY
N/A

DIET
N/A

CLIENT EDUCATION
• Inform client of the potential of adverse human health effects of lead.
• Notify public health officials.
• Determine the source of the lead.

SURGICAL CONSIDERATIONS
Removal of lead objects from the gastrointestinal tract

MEDICATIONS

DRUGS OF CHOICE
• Evacuation of gastrointestinal tract—saline cathartics; sodium or magnesium sulfate (dogs, 2–25 g; cats, 2–5 g PO as 20% solution or less)
• Control of seizures—diazepam (0.5 mg/kg IV; repeat if necessary) or phenobarbital (intravenous dose to effect)
• Alleviation of CNS signs—mannitol (0.25–2 g/kg IV, slow infusion over 30–60 min) and dexamethasone (2.2–4.4 mg/kg IV)
• Reduction of lead body burden—CaNa$_2$EDTA (dogs and cats, 25 mg/kg SC, IM, IV q6h for 2–5 days); dilute to a 1% solution with D$_5$W before administration; may need multiple treatments if blood lead concentration is $\geq$ 1 ppm; allow a 5-day rest period between treatments.

CONTRAINDICATIONS
• EDTA—do not administer to patients with renal impairment or anuria; establish urine flow before administration.
• D-Penicillamine—do not give if there is lead in the gastrointestinal tract (increases absorption)
• Succimer—does not increase gastrointestinal absorption

PRECAUTIONS
CaNa$_2$EDTA—safety in pregnancy not established

POSSIBLE INTERACTIONS
Depletion of zinc, iron, and manganese—concern with long-term chelation therapy

ALTERNATIVE DRUGS
• Alternatives to CaNa$_2$EDTA
• D-Penicillamine—alternative to EDTA; 10–15 mg/kg PO q12h for 7–14 days; allow a 7-day rest period between treatments.
• Succimer—alternative to EDTA; new orally administered chelating agent; may become the future drug of choice; 10 mg/kg PO q8h for 5 days, followed by 10 mg/kg PO q12h for 2 weeks; allow a 2-week rest period between treatments; may administer per rectum if clinical signs preclude oral administration

FOLLOW-UP

PATIENT MONITORING
Blood lead—should be < 0.4 ppm; assess 10–14 days after cessation of chelation therapy.

PREVENTION/AVOIDANCE
Determine source of lead and remove it from the patient's environment.

POSSIBLE COMPLICATIONS
Permanent neurologic signs (e.g., blindness) occasionally

EXPECTED COURSE AND PROGNOSIS
• Signs should dramatically improve within 24–48 hr after initiating chelation therapy.
• Prognosis—favorable with treatment
• Uncontrolled seizures—guarded prognosis

MISCELLANEOUS

ASSOCIATED CONDITIONS
N/A

AGE-RELATED FACTORS
Dogs < 1 year of age—more likely to be affected

ZOONOTIC POTENTIAL
None; however, humans in the same environment may be at risk for exposure.

PREGNANCY
• Transplacental passage—may cause neonatal poisoning
• Lactation—lead mobilized from bones unlikely to poison nursing animals

SYNONYMS
Plumbism

SEE ALSO
Poisoning (Intoxication)

Suggested Reading
Braton, R, Kowalczyk, D. Lead poisoning. In: Kirk R, ed. Current veterinary therapy X. Philadelphia: Saunders, 1989:152–159.

Morgan RV, Moore FM, Pearce LK, et al. Clinical and laboratory findings in small companion animals with lead poisoning: 347 cases (1977–1986). J Am Vet Med Assoc 1991;199:93–97.

Morgan RV, Pearce LK, Moore FM, et al. Demographic data and treatment of small companion animals with lead poisoning: 347 cases (1977–1986). J Am Vet Med Assoc 1991;199:98–102.

Morgan RV. Lead poisoning in small companion animals: an update (1987–1992). Vet Hum Toxicol 1994;36:18–22.

Ramsey DT, Casteel SW, Fagella AM, et al. Use of orally administered succimer (meso-2,3-dimercaptosuccinic acid) for treatment of lead poisoning in dogs. J Am Vet Med Assoc 1996;208:371–375.

VanAlstine WG, Wickliffe LW, Everson RJ, et al. Acute lead toxicosis in a household of cats. J Vet Diagn Invest 1993;5:496–498.

Author Robert H. Poppenga
Consulting Editor Gary D. Osweiler

DISEASES

LEGG-CALVÉ-PERTHES DISEASE

BASICS

DEFINITION
A spontaneous degeneration of the femoral head and neck leading to collapse of the coxofemoral joint and osteoarthritis

PATHOPHYSIOLOGY
• Precise cause unknown; a specific vascular lesion not identified
• Histologic evidence—points to infarction of vessels serving the proximal femur
• Necrosis of subchondral bone—leading to collapse and deformation of the femoral head during normal loading
• Articular cartilage—becomes thickened; cleft development; fraying of superficial layers
• Simultaneous osseous degeneration and repair—characteristic of ischemia and revascularization of bone

SYSTEMS AFFECTED
Musculoskeletal—causes a hind leg lameness; insidious in onset

GENETICS
• Manchester terriers—multifactorial inheritance pattern with a high degree of heritability
• Hereditary predisposition likely

INCIDENCE/PREVALENCE
• Common among miniature, toy, and small dog breeds
• No accurate estimates available

GEOGRAPHIC DISTRIBUTION
N/A

SIGNALMENT

Species
Dogs

Breed Predilections
• Toy breeds and terriers—most susceptible
• Manchester terriers, miniature pinschers, toy poodles, Lakeland terriers, west Highland white terriers, and cairn terriers—higher than expected incidence

Mean Age and Range
• Most patients are 5–8 months of age.
• Range—3–13 months

Predominant Sex
None

SIGNS

General Comments
Usually unilateral; only 12%–16% of cases are bilateral.

Historical Findings
Lameness—usually gradual onset over 2–3 months; weight-bearing; occasionally leg is carried.

Physical Examination Findings
• Pain on manipulation of the hip—most common
• Crepitation of the joint—inconsistent
• Atrophy of the thigh muscles—nearly always noted
• Patient otherwise normal

CAUSES
• Unknown
• Tamponade of the intracapsular subsynovial vessels serving the femoral head—suggested cause of ischemia leading to the pathologic changes

RISK FACTORS
• Small, toy, and miniature breeds—increased risk
• Trauma to the hip region

DIAGNOSIS

DIFFERENTIAL DIAGNOSIS
• Medial patellar luxation—may occur independently; primary differential in young dogs
• Rupture of the cranial cruciate ligament—primary differential in old dogs

CBC/BIOCHEMISTRY/URINALYSIS
N/A

OTHER LABORATORY TESTS
N/A

IMAGING
• Early radiographic changes—widening of the joint space; decreased bone density of the epiphysis; sclerosis and thickening of the femoral neck
• Later radiographic changes—lucent areas within the femoral head
• End-stage radiographic changes—flattening and extreme deformation of the femoral head; severe osteoarthrosis

DIAGNOSTIC PROCEDURES
N/A

PATHOLOGIC FINDINGS
• Femoral head—removed during FHNE; usually deformed with a thickened irregular articular surface
• Early disease—histologically characterized by loss of lacunar osteocytes and necrosis of marrow elements; trabeculae surrounded by granulation tissue
• Later disease—thickened metaphyseal trabeculae; mixture of necrosis and repair tissue typical of revascularization of bone
• Advanced disease—osteoclastic activity; new bone formation

TREATMENT

APPROPRIATE HEALTH CARE
• Rest and analgesics—reportedly successful in alleviating lameness in a minority of patients
• Ehmer sling—successful in one patient; maintained for 10 weeks
• Insidious onset often prevents early recognition and possibility of conservative treatment.
• FHNE with early and vigorous exercise after surgery—treatment of choice

NURSING CARE

Postsurgery
• Physical therapy—extremely important for rehabilitating the affected limb
• Analgesics, anti-inflammatory drugs, and cold packing—3–5 days; important
• Range-of-motion exercises—extension and flexion; initiated immediately
• Small lead weights—attached as ankle bracelets above the hock joint; encourage early use of the treated limb

ACTIVITY
• Postsurgery—early activity encouraged to improve leg use
• Conservative therapy—restricted activity recommended

DIET
Avoid obesity.

LEGG-CALVÉ-PERTHES DISEASE

CLIENT EDUCATION
• Warn owners of Manchester terriers of the genetic basis of the disease; discourage breeding affected dogs.
• Warn client that recovery after FHNE may take 3–6 months.

SURGICAL CONSIDERATIONS
FHNE—treatment of choice

MEDICATIONS

DRUGS OF CHOICE
NSAIDs—preoperative or postoperatively; minimize joint pain; reduce synovitis; may try buffered or enteric-coated aspirin (10–25 mg/kg PO q8h or q12h), caroprofen (2.2 mg/kg PO q12h), etodolac (10–15 mg/kg PO q24h), phenylbutazone (3–7 mg/kg PO q8h, total dose < 800 mg/day), meclofenemic acid (0.5 mg/kg PO q12h), or piroxicam (0.3 mg/kg PO q24h for 3 days, then q48h)

CONTRAINDICATIONS
NSAIDs—gastrointestinal upset may preclude use in some patients.

PRECAUTIONS
• NSAIDs—inhibition of platelet activity may increase hemorrhage at surgery; discontinue aspirin for at least 1 week before surgery, if possible; usually cause some degree of gastric ulceration
• Acetaminophen—unsuitable; potential for toxicity

POSSIBLE INTERACTIONS
NSAIDs—do not use in conjunction with glucocorticoids; risk of gastrointestinal tract ulceration

ALTERNATIVE DRUGS
Chondroprotective drugs (e.g., polysulfated glycosaminoglycans, glucosamine, and chondroitin sulfate)—little in advanced disease; no evidence to suggest that these drugs prevent the disease.

FOLLOW-UP

PATIENT MONITORING
• Postsurgical progress checks—2-week intervals; necessary to ensure compliance with exercise recommendations
• Conservative therapy—re-evaluated (physical examination, radiographs) to determine if surgery is needed

PREVENTION/AVOIDANCE
• Discourage breeding of affected animals.
• Do not repeat dam–sire breedings that result in affected offspring.

POSSIBLE COMPLICATIONS
Limiting postoperative exercise may result in less than optimal limb use.

EXPECTED COURSE AND PROGNOSIS
• FHNE—good to excellent prognosis for full recovery (84%–100% success rate)
• Conservative therapy—reported to alleviate lameness after 2–3 months in about 25% of patients

MISCELLANEOUS

ASSOCIATED CONDITIONS
N/A

AGE-RELATED FACTORS
Usually affects juvenile small-breed dogs, but maturer dogs may be affected by chronic disease.

ZOONOTIC POTENTIAL
N/A

PREGNANCY
N/A

SYNONYMS
• Perthes disease
• Coxa plana
• Coxa magna
• Avascular necrosis of the femoral head
• Aseptic necrosis of the femoral head
• Osteochondritis juvenilis

SEE ALSO
• Cruciate Disease, Cranial
• Hip Dysplasia—Dogs
• Patella Luxation

ABBREVIATION
FHNE = femoral head and neck excision

Suggested Reading

Brinker WO, Piermattei DL, Flo GL, eds. Diagnosis and treatment of orthopedic conditions of the hindlimb. In: Handbook of small animal orthopedics and fracture treatment. 3rd ed. Philadelphia: Saunders 1997:465–466.

Gambardella PC. Legg-Calvé-Perthes disease in dogs. In: Bojrab MJ, ed. Disease mechanisms in small animal surgery. 2nd ed. Philadelphia: Saunders, 1993:804–807.

Gibson KL, Lewis DD, Perchman RD. Use of external coaptation for the treatment of avascular necrosis of the femoral head in a dog. J Am Vet Med Assoc 1990;197:868–869.

Piek, CJ, Hazewinkel HAW, Wolvekamp WTC, et al. Long term follow-up of avascular necrosis of the femoral head in the dog. J Small Anim Pract 1996;37:12–18.

Smith MM. Perthes' disease. In: Slatter DH, ed. Textbook of small animal surgery. 2nd ed. Philadelphia: Saunders, 1993:1981–1984.

Author Larry Carpenter
Consulting Editor Peter D. Schwarz

DISEASES

LEIOMYOMA, STOMACH, SMALL AND LARGE INTESTINE

 BASICS

OVERVIEW
Uncommon benign tumor arising from the smooth muscle of the stomach and intestinal tract

SIGNALMENT
• Middle-aged to old (> 6 years) dogs and cats
• Dogs more commonly affected than are cats
• No breed predisposition

SIGNS

Historical Findings
• Usually nonspecific; owners report poor quality of life
• Stomach—vomiting
• Small intestine—vomiting; weight loss; borborygmus; flatulence
• Large intestine and rectum—tenesmus; sometimes rectal prolapse

Physical Examination Findings
• Stomach—no specific abnormalities
• Small intestine—midabdominal mass; occasionally distended, painful loops of small bowel
• Large intestine and rectum—palpable mass per rectum

CAUSES & RISK FACTORS
Unknown

 DIAGNOSIS

DIFFERENTIAL DIAGNOSIS
• Gastric foreign body
• Gastrointestinal adenocarcinoma
• Leiomyosarcoma
• Malignant lymphoma
• Pancreatitis

CBC/BIOCHEMISTRY/URINALYSIS
• Usually normal
• Hypoglycemia—occasionally

OTHER LABORATORY TESTS
N/A

IMAGING
• Abdominal ultrasound—may reveal a thickened wall of stomach or bowel; gastric leiomyoma most common at esophageal–gastric junction
• Contrast radiography (stomach and small intestine—may reveal a space-occupying mass
• Double-contrast radiography (large intestine and rectum)—reveals a space-occupying mass

DIAGNOSTIC PROCEDURES

Upper Gastrointestinal Tract
Perform upper gastrointestinal tract endoscopy and mucosal biopsy but frequently nondiagnostic because tumors are deep to the mucosal surface; surgical biopsy often required to confirm the diagnosis

Large Intestine and Rectum
Colonoscopy may reveal a mass; mucosal biopsy may be nondiagnostic because of normal mucosal covering of the tumor; perform deep surgical biopsy if possible

 TREATMENT

Surgical resection—treatment of choice; curative if tumor is resectable

 MEDICATIONS

DRUG(S)
N/A

CONTRAINDICATIONS/POSSIBLE INTERACTIONS
N/A

 FOLLOW-UP

• Complete resection—normal postoperative care; no additional follow-up necessary
• Some affected dogs have clinical signs of hypoglycemia (e.g., weakness and seizures).

 MISCELLANEOUS

ASSOCIATED CONDITIONS
Hypoglycemia—recently recognized as an associated paraneoplastic syndrome

Suggested Reading
Morrison WB. Nonlymphomatous cancers of the esophagus, stomach, and intestines. In: Morrison WB, ed., Cancer in dogs and cats: medical and surgical management. Baltimore: Williams & Wilkins, 1998:551–558.
Takiguci M, Yasuda J, Hashimoto A, et al. Esophageal/gastric adenocarcinoma in a dog. J Am Anim Hosp Assoc 1997;33:42–44.
Author Ralph C. Richardson
Consulting Editor Wallace B. Morrison

LEIOMYOSARCOMA, STOMACH, SMALL, AND LARGE INTESTINE

BASICS

OVERVIEW
• Uncommon malignant tumor arising from the smooth muscle of the stomach and intestinal tract
• Tends to be locally invasive (remaining confined to the intestinal tract) and slow to metastasize
• Early diagnosis and complete resection may be curative.
• Prognosis guarded

SIGNALMENT
• Mostly middle-aged to old (> 6 years) dogs and cats
• Dogs more commonly affected than are cats
• No breed predisposition

SIGNS
Historical Findings
• Usually vague and nonspecific
• Stomach—abdominal discomfort; weight loss; vomiting
• Small intestine—vomiting; weight loss; borborygmus; flatulence
• Large intestine and rectum—tenesmus, may lead to rectal prolapse

Physical Examination Findings
• Stomach—nonspecific
• Small intestine—midabdominal mass; sometimes distended, painful loops of small bowel on abdominal palpation
• Large intestine and rectum—palpable mass per rectum

CAUSES & RISK FACTORS
Unknown

DIAGNOSIS

DIFFERENTIAL DIAGNOSIS
• Gastric foreign body
• Gastrointestinal adenocarcinoma
• Leiomyoma
• Malignant lymphoma of the intestines
• Pancreatitis

CBC/BIOCHEMISTRY/URINALYSIS
• Usually normal
• Hypoglycemia—reported as a paraneoplastic syndrome

OTHER LABORATORY TESTS
N/A

IMAGING
• Abdominal ultrasonography—may reveal a thickened wall of the stomach or bowel
• Positive contrast radiography (stomach and small intestine)—reveals a space-occupying mass
• Double-contrast radiography (large intestine and rectum)—reveals a space-occupying mass

DIAGNOSTIC PROCEDURES
Upper Gastrointestinal Tract
• Endoscopy and mucosal biopsy—perform, but results frequently nondiagnostic because tumors deep to the mucosal surface
• Surgical biopsy—often required to confirm diagnosis

Large Intestine and Rectum
• Colonoscopy—may allow a mass to be seen; mucosal biopsy may be nondiagnostic because of the normal mucosal covering of the tumor
• Deep biopsy—perform if possible.

TREATMENT
• Surgical resection—treatment of choice; curative because usually confined to the gastrointestinal tract and slow to metastasize
• Carefully evaluate for metastasis before extensive surgery (e.g., mesenteric lymph nodes, liver, and lungs).

MEDICATIONS

DRUG(S)
None reported

CONTRAINDICATIONS/POSSIBLE INTERACTIONS
N/A

FOLLOW-UP
• Complete resection—routine physical examination and abdominal and thoracic radiography at 1, 3, 6, 9, and 12 months after surgery
• Incomplete resection—symptomatic support to relieve clinical signs

✓ MISCELLANEOUS

ASSOCIATED CONDITIONS
Hypoglycemia—reported as a paraneoplastic syndrome

Suggested Reading
Morrison WB. Nonlymphomatous cancers of the esophagus, stomach, and intestines. In: Morrison WB, ed. Cancer in dogs and cats: medical and surgical management. Baltimore: Williams & Wilkins, 1998:551–558.
Author Ralph C. Richardson
Consulting Editor Wallace B. Morrison

DISEASES

BASICS

OVERVIEW
- Protozoan—genus *Leishmania;* causes two types of disease: cutaneous and visceral
- Organ systems affected—cutaneous: skin, hepatobiliary, spleen, kidneys, eyes, and joints; visceral: hemorrhagic diathesis
- Affected dogs in the U.S. invariably acquired infection in another country.
- *L. donovani infantum*—Mediterranean basin, Portugal, and Spain; sporadic cases in Switzerland, northern France, and the Netherlands
- *L. donovani* complex or *L. braziliensis*—endemic areas of South and Central American and southern Mexico
- Endemic cases in dogs (Oklahoma and Ohio) and cats (Texas) have been reported in the U.S., although the disease is not considered endemic here.
- Sandfly vectors—transmit flagellated parasites into the skin of a host
- Cats—often localizes in skin
- Dogs—invariably spreads throughout the body to most organs; renal failure is the most common cause of death.
- Incubation period—1 month to several years

SIGNALMENT
- Dogs—virtually all develop visceral, or systemic, disease; 90% also have cutaneous involvement; no sex or breed predilection
- Cats—cutaneous disease (rare); no sex or breed predilection

SIGNS
Visceral
- Exercise intolerance
- Severe weight loss and anorexia
- Diarrhea, vomiting, epistaxis, and melena—less common
- Dogs—lymphadenopathy; cutaneous lesions; emaciation; signs of renal failure (polyuria, polydipsia, vomiting) possible; neuralgia, polyarthritis, polymyositis, osteolytic lesions, and proliferative periostitis rare; about one-third of patients have fever and splenomegaly.

Cutaneous
- Hyperkeratosis—most prominent finding; excessive epidermal scale with thickening, depigmentation, and chapping of the muzzle and footpads
- Hair coat—dry; brittle; hair loss
- Dogs—intradermal nodules and ulcers may be seen; abnormally long or brittle nails are a specific finding in some patients.
- Cats—cutaneous nodules usually develop.

CAUSES & RISK FACTORS
- Travel to endemic regions (usually the Mediterranean), where dogs are exposed to infected sandflies
- Transfusion from infected animals can occur.

DIAGNOSIS

DIFFERENTIAL DIAGNOSIS
- Visceral—mycoses (blastomycosis, histoplasmosis); systemic lupus erythematosus; metastatic neoplasia; distemper; vasculitis
- Cutaneous—other causes of hyperkeratosis: primary idiopathic seborrhea and nutritional dermatoses (vitamin A responsive, zinc responsive); idiopathic nasodigital hyperkeratosis, lichenoid-psoriasiform dermatosis, epidermal dysplasia, and Schnauzer comedo syndrome are rare and breed-specific
- Skin biopsy—hyperkeratotic and nodular lesions; existence of organisms confirms diagnosis
- Hyperglobulinemia—differentiate from chronic ehrlichiosis and multiple myeloma

CBC/BIOCHEMISTRY/URINALYSIS
- Hyperproteinemia with hyperglobulinemia—100% of cases
- Hypoalbuminemia—95% of cases •
Proteinuria—85% of cases
- High liver enzyme activity—55% of cases
- Thrombocytopenia—50% of cases
- Azotemia—45% of cases
- Leukopenia with lymphopenia—20% of cases

OTHER LABORATORY TESTS
- Coombs, antinuclear antibody, and lupus erythematosus cell tests—sometimes positive
- Serologic diagnosis available

IMAGING
N/A

DIAGNOSTIC PROCEDURES
- Cultures—skin, spleen, bone marrow, or lymph node biopsies or aspirates; by the Center for Disease Control and Prevention
- Cytology and histopathology—identify intracellular organisms in biopsies or aspirate specimens (listed above)

PATHOLOGIC FINDINGS
- Cell infiltration (mainly histiocytes and macrophages) and characteristic intracellular amastigote forms—identified in many tissues: skin, lymph nodes, liver, spleen, and kidney
- Mucosal ulcerations—stomach, intestine, and colon, occasionally found

TREATMENT
- Outpatient
- Emaciated, chronically infected animals—consider euthanasia; prognosis very poor
- Diet—high-quality protein; special for renal insufficiency, if necessary
- Cats—single dermal nodule lesions are best surgically removed.
- Advise client of potential zoonotic transmission of organisms in lesions to humans.
- Inform client that organisms will never be eliminated, and relapse, requiring treatment, is inevitable.

MEDICATIONS

DRUGS
- Sodium stibogluconate—available from the Center for Disease Control and Prevention; 30–50 mg/kg IV or SC q24h for 3–4 weeks
- Meglumine antimonate—100 mg/kg IV or SC q24h for 3–4 weeks
- Allopurinol—very efficacious in treating one dog; 7 mg/kg PO q8h for 3 months
- γ-interferon given with antimonials—good success in humans

CONTRAINDICATIONS/POSSIBLE INTERACTIONS
- Seriously ill dogs—start antimonial drugs at lower doses
- Renal insufficiency—treat before giving antimonial drugs; prognosis depends on renal function at the onset of treatment

FOLLOW-UP
- Treatment efficacy—monitor by clinical improvement and identification of organisms in repeat biopsies
- Relapses—a few months to a year after therapy; recheck at least every 2 months after completion of treatment.
- Prognosis for a cure—very guarded; antimonial therapy gives dogs some quality of life.

MISCELLANEOUS

Suggested Reading

Slappendel RJ, Ferner L. Leishmaniasis. In: Greene CE, ed. Infectious diseases of the dog and cat. Philadelphia: Saunders, 1998:450–458.

Author Stephen C. Barr
Consulting Editor Stephen C. Barr

LENS LUXATION

BASICS

OVERVIEW
• Lens displacement into the anterior chamber or posterior segment/vitreous
• Occurs when the lens capsule separates 360° from the zonules, that hold the lens in place
• Subluxation—partial separation of the lens from its zonular attachments; the lens remains in a normal or near-normal position in the pupil.
• Primary luxation—result of an inherited tendency for the zonules to weaken and break or, rarely, a congenital malformation of the zonular attachments
• Congenital luxation—often associated with microphakia
• Secondary luxation—most common form in cats; results from zonular rupture caused by buphthalmia, chronic intraocular inflammation, or intraocular neoplasia

SIGNALMENT
• Dogs—primary usually seen in adults; most commonly affected breeds: poodle, shar pei, whippet, Norwegian elkhound, and terrier
• Dogs and cats—secondary; any age/breed.

SIGNS
• Acute or chronically painful eye with episcleral injection and diffuse corneal edema, especially if glaucoma also present
• Central corneal edema—may be caused by the lens touching the endothelium, resulting in mechanical disruption of endothelial cells
• Abnormally shallow or deep anterior chamber
• Iridodonesis (iris trembling)
• Aphakic crescent (an area of pupil devoid of the lens)
• Malpositioned clear lens—sometimes observed in an otherwise asymptomatic eye

CAUSES & RISK FACTORS
• Primary—inheritance pattern uncertain
• Primary luxation and primary glaucoma—may occur simultaneously in some breeds (e.g., Jack Russell terriers and shar peis)
• Uveitis, especially chronic lens-induced uveitis
• Intraocular neoplasia—may physically luxate the lens
• Trauma—rarely causes a normal lens to luxate without signs of severe uveitis or hyphema

DIAGNOSIS

DIFFERENTIAL DIAGNOSIS
• Uveitis and glaucoma—also cause painful, red eyes with corneal edema and may be concurrent

• Buphthalmia may cause lens luxation; usually differentiated from primary lens luxation by history
• Corneal endothelial dystrophy—may also cause corneal edema, making it difficult to see the intraocular structures; usually differentiated from primary lens luxation by history.
• Diagnosis usually made by careful ophthalmic examination and history.

CBC/BIOCHEMISTRY/URINALYSIS
Normal, unless sequela of a systemic disease that causes uveitis or dissemination of neoplasia

OTHER LABORATORY TESTS
N/A

IMAGING
• Thoracic radiographs and abdominal ultrasonography—may be indicated if secondary to intraocular neoplasia
• Ocular ultrasonography—useful if corneal edema or cloudy ocular media preclude examination and history.

DIAGNOSTIC PROCEDURES
Complete ophthalmic examination, including tonometry

TREATMENT
• Potentially visual eyes—best treated by removing the lens
• Occasionally topical miotic therapy can keep a posteriorly luxated lens behind the pupil and surgery can be avoided.
• Irreversibly blind eyes or secondary to intraocular neoplasia—often best treated by enucleation or, if appropriate, one of the globe-salvage procedures (e.g., cyclocryosurgery, evisceration, intrascleral prosthesis)

MEDICATIONS

DRUGS
• Initiate the following medications, and if the eye has the potential for vision, refer the patient to a veterinary ophthalmologist immediately for intracapsular lens extraction.
• Topical miotic—0.125% demecarium bromide (q12–24h); indicated with normal IOP, primary luxation, and lens is in the posterior segment; potentially lessens the chance of anterior lens luxation and secondary glaucoma
• Mannitol—1 g/kg IV over 20 min; indicated for high IOP (> 40 mm Hg)
• Carbonic anhydrase inhibitors—dichlorphenamide (2–4 mg/kg PO q12h); initiated to reduce aqueous production
• Topical antiinflammatory—0.1% dexamethasone sodium phosphate (q6h)

CONTRAINDICATIONS/POSSIBLE INTERACTIONS
• Topical miotics—contraindicated if the lens is in the anterior chamber. • Owner must verify location of lens prior to applying a miotic

FOLLOW-UP
• Medically treated primary posterior luxation—IOP rechecked 24 hr after starting treatment and frequently thereafter; once IOP is stable, reexamine patient at least quarterly.
• Monitor for secondary glaucoma and retinal detachment
• If only one lens is involved at the time of examination, the other lens may eventually become involved.

MISCELLANEOUS

ABBREVIATION
IOP = intraocular pressure

Suggested Reading

Davidson MG, Nelms SR. Diseases of the lens and cataract formation. In: Gelatt KN ed., Veterinary Opthamology, 3rd ed. Philadelphia: Lippincott Williams & Wilkins 1999; 797–825.
Author Denise M. Lindley
Consulting Editor Paul E. Miller

DISEASES

LEPTOSPIROSIS

BASICS

DEFINITION
• Caused by pathogenic members of the genus *Leptospira* • Acute and chronic diseases of dogs (mainly nephritis and hepatitis) and other animals, including, although rarely, cats • Dogs—most disease caused by the serovars *L. grippotyphosa* and *L. pomona* • Vaccine (dogs)—contains the serovars *L. canicola* and *L. icterohaemorrhagiae;* promotes immunity to homologous serovars and protection from overt clinical disease; may not prevent colonization of the kidneys, resulting in a chronic carrier state; serovar specific; does not promote protection against other serovars present in nature

PATHOPHYSIOLOGY
• *Leptospira*—penetrate intact or cut skin or mucous membranes; rapidly invade bloodstream (4–7 days); spread to all parts of the body (2–4 days) • Invasion leads to fever, leukocytosis, transitory anemia (hemolysis), mild hemoglobinuria, and albuminuria. • Fever and bacteremia soon resolve. • Capillary and endothelial cell damage; occasionally results in petechial hemorrhages • Liver—hepatic necrosis and jaundice • Kidney—leptospiruria; *Leptospira* may localize in damaged renal tubules; organism replicates readily in tubular epithelial cells. • Early serum antibodies appear • Death—usually a result of interstitial nephritis, vascular damage, and renal failure; may result from acute septicemia or DIC

SYSTEMS AFFECTED
Subacute to Acute/Severe Disease
• Renal/Urologic—focal interstitial nephritis; hemoglobinuric nephrosis; tubular damage/failure • Hepatobiliary—hepatitis; dysfunction; necrosis • Respiratory—vasculitis; interstitial pneumonia • Cardiovascular—endothelial cell damage; hemorrhage • Nervous—meningitis
Chronic Disease
• Renal/Urologic—chronic renal failure • Reproductive—abortion; weak puppies • Ophthalmic—anterior uveitis

GENETICS N/A

INCIDENCE/PREVALENCE
• Usually one or more serovars account for endemic disease in a geographic area. • *L. canicola* and *L. icterohaemorrhagiae*—usual serovars; clinical disease in dogs; *L. canicola* most common worldwide; *L. icterohaemorrhagiae* most common in Australia • *L. grippotyphosa* and *L. pomona*—becoming more prominent • Reported incidence (dogs)—falsely low; most infections are inapparent and remain undiagnosed. • Prevalence (dogs)—city, 37.8%; suburban, 18.7%

GEOGRAPHIC DISTRIBUTION
• Worldwide, especially in warm, wet climates or seasons • Standing water and neutral or slightly alkaline soil promotes presence in environment.

SIGNALMENT

Species
Dogs and rarely cats

Breed Predilections N/A

Mean Age and Range
• Young dogs without passive maternal antibody—more likely to exhibit severe disease • Old dogs with adequate antibody titer levels—seldom exhibit clinical disease unless exposed to a serovar not in the vaccine

Predominant Sex
Traditionally, male dogs more commonly affected; disputed by recent reports

SIGNS

General Comments
• Vary with the age and immune status, environmental factors that affect leptospira survival, and virulence of the infecting serovar • Primary reservoir host—may spread particular serovar via urine shedding; may have no clinical signs or less severe disease (acute diffuse to chronic interstitial nephritis, e.g., *L. canicola* in dogs with relatively weak antibody response) • Incidental (accidental) host—acute severe disease (e.g., *L. icterohaemorrhagiae* in dogs with severe antibody response)

Historical Findings
Peracute to Subacute Disease
• Fever • Sore muscles • Stiffness • Shivering • Weakness • Anorexia • Depression • Vomiting • Rapid dehydration • Diarrhea—with or without blood • Icterus • Spontaneous cough • Difficulty breathing • PD-PU progressing to anuria • Bloody vaginal discharge • Death—without clinical signs
Chronic Disease
• No apparent illness • Fever of unknown origin • PD-PU—chronic renal failure

Physical Examination Findings
Peracute to Acute Disease
• Tachypnea • Rapid irregular pulse • Poor capillary perfusion • Hematemesis • Hematochezia • Melena • Epistaxis • Injected mucous membranes • Widespread petechial and ecchymotic hemorrhages • Reluctance to move, paraspinal hyperesthesia, stiff gait • Conjunctivitis • Rhinitis • Hematuria • Mild lymphadenopathy

CAUSES
• Dogs—*L. canicola, L. icterohaemorrhagiae, L. pomona,* * *L. grippotyphosa,* * *L. Bratislava, copenhagenii, L. australis, L. autumnalis, L. ballum,* and *L. bataviae* • Cats—*L. canicola, L. grippotyphosa, L. pomona,* and *L. bataviae*

RISK FACTORS

Transmission
• Direct—host-to-host contact via infected urine, postabortion discharge, infected fetus/discharge, and sexual contact (semen) • Indirect—exposure (via urine) to a contaminated environment (vegetation, soil, food, water, bedding) under conditions in which *Leptospira*

can survive • Disease agent—*Leptospira* serovar, each with its own virulence factors, infectious dose, and route of exposure

Host Factors
• Vaccine—protection is serovar-specific; prevents clinical disease as a result of homologous serovar; may not prevent kidney colonization and urine shedding; nonvaccine serovars may infect and cause disease in vaccinated hosts. • Outdoor animals or hunting dogs—exposure of mucous membranes to water; exposure of abraded or water-softened skin increases risk of infection.

Environmental Factors
• Warm and moist environment; wet season (high rainfall areas) of temperate regions; low-lying areas (marshy, muddy, irrigated); warm humid climates of tropical and subtropical regions • Temperature range—7–10°C (44.6–50°F) to 34–36°C (93–96°F) • Water—organism survives better in stagnant than in flowing water; neutral or slightly alkaline pH • Organism survives 180 days in wet soil and longer in standing water. • Dense animal population—kennels and urban settings; increases chances of urine exposure • Exposure to rodents and other wildlife

DIAGNOSIS

DIFFERENTIAL DIAGNOSIS
Subclinical infections and chronic carrier states generally go undetected

Subacute to Acute Disease
• Dogs—heartworm disease; immune-mediated hemolytic anemia; bacteremia/septicemia (bite wound, prostatitis, endocarditis, dental disease); infectious canine hepatitis virus; canine herpesvirus; hepatic neoplasia; trauma; lupus; Rocky Mountain spotted fever; ehrlichiosis; toxoplasmosis; renal neoplasia; renal calculi • Cats—hemobartonellosis; drugs (acetaminophen); bacteremia/septicemia; FIV- and FeLV-associated diseases; cholangitis; toxoplasmosis; FIP; hepatic neoplasia, autoimmune disease (e.g., systemic lupus erythematosus); trauma; renal calculi; renal neoplasia

Reproductive/Neonatal Disease
• Dogs—brucellosis; distemper; herpes • Cats—FIP; FeLV; panleukopenia; herpesvirus; toxoplasmosis; salmonellosis

CBC/BIOCHEMISTRY/URINALYSIS
• PCV and total plasma solids—high owing to dehydration; rarely PCV low (hemolysis) • Leukocytosis with left shift—leukopenia initially during leptospiremic phase • Thrombocytopenia • Increased fibrin degradation products • BUN—high • Creatinine—high; mainly renal; depends on degree of renal failure • Electrolyte alterations—depend on degree of renal and gastrointestinal dysfunction • Hyponatremia • Hypochloremia • Hypokalemia—hyperkalemia with kidney failure • Hyperphos-

phatemia • Hypoalbuminemia • Acidosis—serum bicarbonate low • Alanine aminotransferase, aspartate aminotransferase, lactate dehydrogenase, and alkaline phosphatase—high • Proteinuria • Isosthenuria—acute renal failure

OTHER LABORATORY TESTS

Serology (Microscopic Agglutination Test)
• Test in acute stage and 3–4 weeks later (conva-lescent serum). • Unvaccinated patients—titers may be low initially (1:100–1:200); may be higher in the convalescent serum (1:800– 1:1600 or higher) if a homologous *Leptospira* serovar is tested • Vaccinated patients—expect low (usually not higher than 1:400) titers for the vaccine serovars *L. canicola* and *L. icterohaemorrhagiae;* titers for other serovars are the same as for unvaccinated patients; run all serum samples at the same time, if possible.

Dark Field Microscopy of Urine
• Often inconclusive • Difficult to read • Requires fresh urine

Fluorescent Antibody Test of Urine
• More conclusive • *Leptospira* does not need to be viable; submit urine to laboratory on ice by overnight courier • Pretreat with furosemide 15 min before urine collection to increase success rate. • Correlate results with clinical history.

IMAGING N/A

DIAGNOSTIC PROCEDURES
• Culture of body fluids antemortem (urine, blood, aqueous humor) and tissues postmortem (kidney, liver, fetus, placenta)—usually not practical because of the fastidiousness of *Leptospiras;* contact laboratory for the proper transport medium • Fluorescent Antibody Test—done on all tissues submitted for postmortem workup, especially kidney and liver • Special stains (Warthin-Starry silver stain)—attempt immunohistochemistry with monoclonal antibodies on formalin-fixed sections of kidney, liver, and fetal/placental tissues. • Polymerase chain reaction—some laboratories have developed protocols for both urine and tissue specimens.

PATHOLOGIC FINDINGS
• Degree of kidney and liver disease depends on the serovar and the host's immunity • Cats—generally less severe lesions • Dogs (acute disease)—lungs may be edematous; kidneys pale and enlarged; liver enlarged and may be friable with multifocal necrosis and hemorrhage; gastrointestinal tract may hemorrhage • Histopathology—hepatocellular degeneration and necrosis possible with some serovars; kidney lesions vary from minor inflammation to interstitial necrosis and renal fibrosis.

TREATMENT

APPROPRIATE HEALTH CARE
Acute severe disease—inpatient; extent of

supportive therapy depends on severity; renal failure requires closely monitored diuresis.

NURSING CARE
• Depends on severity • Dehydration and shock—parenteral, balanced, polyionic, isotonic intravenous solution (lactated Ringer's) • Severe hemorrhage—blood transfusion may be needed in association with treatment for DIC. • Oliguria or anuria—initially rehydrate; then give intravenous osmotic diuretics or tubular diuretics; peritoneal dialysis may be necessary.

ACTIVITY
Acutely ill and bacteremic/septicemic patients—restricted activity; cage rest; monitoring; and warmth

DIET
Severely ill patients—often anorexic, in shock, and lethargic; parental nutrition for prolonged anorexia

CLIENT EDUCATION
Inform client of zoonotic potential from contaminated urine of affected dogs and their environment.

SURGICAL CONSIDERATIONS N/A

MEDICATIONS

DRUGS OF CHOICE
• Procaine penicillin G—40,000–80,000 U/kg IM q24h or divided q12h until kidney function returns to normal • Dihydrostreptomycin—10–15 mg/kg IM q12h for 2 weeks to eliminate organism from kidney interstitial tissues; try streptomycin if no renal failure • Doxycycline—5 mg/kg PO or IV q12h for 2 weeks; use alone to clear both leptospiremia and leptospiruria

CONTRAINDICATIONS N/A

PRECAUTIONS
• Aminoglycoside—monitor patients with renal insufficiency carefully. • Penicillins (dogs)—adjust doses with renal insufficiency.

POSSIBLE INTERACTIONS N/A

ALTERNATIVE DRUGS
• Ampicillin or amoxicillin—instead of penicillin • Erythromycin

FOLLOW-UP

PATIENT MONITORING
• Monitor kidney function, liver function, and electrolytes. • Monitor BUN, serum creatinine, and urine specific gravity in dogs with renal failure for indication of prognosis.

PREVENTION/AVOIDANCE
• Vaccines—vaccinate dogs per current label recommendations; bacteria-induced immunity lasts only 6–8 months and is serovar specific (no cross-protection outside of the serogroup);

revaccination at least yearly; vaccinate dogs at risk (hunter, show dogs, dogs with access to water/ponds) every 4–6 months, especially in endemic areas. • Kennels—strict sanitation to avoid contact with infected urine; control rodents; monitor and remove carrier dogs until treated; isolate affected animals during treatment. • Activity—limit access to marshy/muddy areas, ponds, low-lying areas with stagnant surface water, heavily irrigated pastures, and access to wildlife.

POSSIBLE COMPLICATIONS
• DIC • Liver and kidney dysfunction may be permanent. • Uveitis and abortion sequelae

EXPECTED COURSE AND PROGNOSIS
• Most infections subclinical or chronic • Prognosis guarded for acute severe disease

MISCELLANEOUS

AGE-RELATED FACTORS
Severe clinical disease in young dogs (nonvaccinated or lacking maternal antibody)

ZOONOTIC POTENTIAL
• High; organisms spread in urine of infected animals • Strict kennel hygiene and disinfection of premises (iodine-based disinfectant or stabilized bleach solutions) • Acutely infected and carrier animals must be treated.

PREGNANCY
• Possible abortion sequelae • Antimicrobial therapy—consider effect of drug on developing fetus.

SYNONYMS
In humans—Weil disease; swineherd disease; rice field disease; water-fever disease; cane-fever disease

ABBREVIATIONS
• DIC = disseminated intravascular coagulation • FeLV = feline leukemia virus • FIP = feline infectious peritonitis • FIV = feline immunodeficiency virus
• PCV = packed cell volume
• PD-PU = polydipsia and polyuria

Suggested Reading
Baldwin CJ, Atkins CE. Leptospirosis in dogs. Compend Contin Educ Pract Vet 1987;9:499–508.
Birnbaum N, Barr SC, Center SA, et al. Naturally acquired leptospirosis in 36 dogs: serological and clinicopathological features. J Small Anim Pract 1998;39:231–236.
Greene CE, Miller MA, Brown CA. Leptospirosis. In: Greene CE, ed. Infectious diseases of the dog and cat. Philadelphia: Saunders, 1998:273–281.
Heath SE, Johnson R. Leptospirosis. J Am Vet Med Assoc 1994;205:1518–1523.
Author Patrick L. McDonough
Consulting Editor Stephen C. Barr

LEUKEMIA, ACUTE LYMPHOBLASTIC

BASICS

OVERVIEW
• Lymphoproliferative disorder defined as the presence of circulating neoplastic prolymphocytes and lymphoblasts in the blood
• Patients have impaired humoral and cellular immunity.
• Characterized by bone marrow infiltration (and extramedullary sites) and displacement of normal hematopoietic stem cells
• May infiltrate other organs

SIGNALMENT
• Dogs—male to female ratio, 3:2; mean age, 6.2 years (range, 1–12 years)
• Rare in cats

SIGNS
• Often nonspecific
• Large liver and spleen
• Lymphadenomegaly
• Petechial or ecchymotic hemorrhages
• Other—reflect specific organ infiltration

CAUSES & RISK FACTORS
• Dogs—ionizing radiation; oncogenic viruses; chemical agents suspected but unproved
• Cats—FeLV infection

DIAGNOSIS

DIFFERENTIAL DIAGNOSIS
• Acute or chronic infection—toxoplasmosis; canine distemper; ehrlichiosis
• Aplastic anemia
• Metastatic neoplasia
• Multicentric lymphosarcoma—with acute lymphoblastic leukemia, only moderately large peripheral lymph nodes, marked splenomegaly, and signs of systemic illness with relatively acute onset
• Other leukemias and myeloproliferative disorders

CBC/BIOCHEMISTRY/URINALYSIS
• CBC—normocytic, normochromic, nonregenerative anemia; thrombocytopenia; lymphoblastosis; leukocytosis or leukopenia
• Serum chemistry profile—high liver enzyme activities

OTHER LABORATORY TESTS
• Cytologic examination (bone marrow or core biopsies)—lymphoblastic infiltration with low numbers of myeloid and erythroid precursors and low numbers of megakaryocytes
• Immunohistochemical or enzymatic biochemical studies—may be needed to differentiate from other leukemic cells

IMAGING
Plain film radiography and ultrasound—often reveal hepatomegaly and splenomegaly

DIAGNOSTIC PROCEDURES
Bone marrow biopsy

TREATMENT
• Usually outpatient, unless supportive care required
• Patients are immunocompromised and should not be exposed to infectious disease.
• Transfusions—as indicated, to restore RBCs, platelets, or coagulation factors

MEDICATIONS

DRUGS
Combination chemotherapy—prednisone (20 mg/m² PO q12h) and vincristine (0.7 mg/m² IV weekly); may result in partial or short-lived complete remission

CONTRAINDICATIONS/POSSIBLE INTERACTIONS
Chemotherapy may have toxic side effects; seek advice before starting treatment if you are unfamiliar with cytotoxic drugs.

FOLLOW-UP
• Monitor peripheral blood count and bone marrow—judge success and toxicity of treatment
• Hemorrhage from thrombocytopenia—major cause of death in dogs
• Prognosis grave

MISCELLANEOUS

PREGNANCY
Chemotherapy—contraindicated in pregnant animals

ABBREVIATION
FeLV = feline leukemia virus

Suggested Reading
Hamilton TA. The leukemias. In: Morrison WB, ed. Cancer in dogs and cats: medical and surgical management. Baltimore: Williams & Wilkins, 1998:721–729.
Reagan WJ, DeNicola DB. Myeloproliferative and lymphoproliverative disorders. In: Morrison WB, ed. Cancer in dogs and cats: medical and surgical management. Baltimore: Williams & Wilkins, 1998:95–122.
Author Linda S. Fineman
Consulting Editor Wallace B. Morrison

LEUKEMIA, CHRONIC LYMPHOCYTIC

 BASICS

OVERVIEW
• Rare, lymphoproliferative disorder
• Circulating neoplastic lymphocytes that are mature and well differentiated
• May note impaired humoral and cellular immunity
• Systems affected—hematopoietic, lymphatic, and integument

SIGNALMENT
• Dogs and cats
• Dogs—mean age, 9.4 years (range, 3–15 years); male to female ratio, 2:1

SIGNS
• Nonspecific
• Polydipsia and polyuria
• Lymphadenmegaly
• Lameness
• Fever
• Bruising

CAUSES & RISK FACTORS
Ionizing radiation, oncogenic viruses, and chemical agents—suspected but unproved

 DIAGNOSIS

DIFFERENTIAL DIAGNOSIS
• Lymphosarcoma—may have a leukemic phase
• Immune-mediated hematologic diseases

CBC/BIOCHEMISTRY/URINALYSIS
• Mild to moderate normocytic, normochromic anemia
• Normal to low platelet count
• Lymphocytosis—range, 5,000>100,000 cells/μL
• Normal to mildly high serum globulins
• May see high ALP

OTHER LABORATORY TESTS
• Cytologic examination (bone marrow or core biopsy)—shows high numbers of mature lymphocytes; crowding out of normal cell lines in advanced stages
• Serum protein electrophoresis—detects monoclonal spikes (usually IgM) in about 50% of patients
• Bence Jones proteinuria—about 50% of patients
• Direct Coombs test—may be positive with secondary immune-mediated hemolytic anemia

IMAGING
Radiography and ultrasonography—may reveal cranial organomegaly or internal lymphadenomegaly

DIAGNOSTIC PROCEDURES
Bone marrow biopsy

 TREATMENT

• Usually outpatients
• Splenectomy—indicated with secondary, immune-mediated hemolytic anemia or thrombocytopenia or if hypersplenism cannot be controlled medically
• Treatment advised only when patient is symptomatic.

 MEDICATIONS

DRUGS
• Chlorambucil—0.2 mg/kg PO q24h for 7 days; then 0.1 mg/kg q24h to effect
• Prednisone—20 mg/m^2 PO q12h; in combination with chlorambucil

CONTRAINDICATIONS/POSSIBLE INTERACTIONS
• Chemotherapy—myelosuppression; may need to alter dosage, depending on neutrophil and platelet counts

 FOLLOW-UP

• Periodic cytologic examination of bone marrow—response to treatment and disease progression
• Weekly examination of CBC—response to treatment and disease progression
• Variable course, but progressive
• Severe hemolytic anemia and pneumonia may cause death.

 MISCELLANEOUS

PREGNANCY
Chemotherapy contraindicated in pregnant animals.

ABBREVIATION
ALP = alkaline phosphatase

Suggested Reading

Hamilton TA. The leukemias. In: Morrison WB, ed. Cancer in dogs and cats: medical and surgical management. Baltimore: Williams & Wilkins, 1998:721–729.
Reagan WJ, DeNicola DB. Myeloproliferative and lymphoproliverative disorders. In: Morrison WB, ed. Cancer in dogs and cats: medical and surgical management. Baltimore: Williams & Wilkins, 1998:95–122.
Author Linda S. Fineman
Consulting Editor Wallace B. Morrison

DISEASES

LEUKOENCEPHALOMYELOPATHY IN ROTTWEILERS

 BASICS

OVERVIEW
• A progressive, degenerative, demyelinating disease primarily affecting the cervical spinal cord in rottweilers
• Occurs worldwide
• Probably inherited

SIGNALMENT
• Dogs
• Rottweilers—either sex; 1.5–3.5 years old at onset

SIGNS
• No history of injury or illness
• Owners do not report discomfort.
• Insidious, progressive onset
• Proprioceptive ataxia and upper motor neuron weakness involving all four limbs; proprioceptive positioning disappears as the disease progresses.
• Spinal reflexes normal to exaggerated
• Crossed extensor reflexes in all four limbs in later stages

CAUSES & RISK FACTORS
Unknown; possibly a myelinolytic disease

 DIAGNOSIS

DIFFERENTIAL DIAGNOSIS
• Neuroaxonal dystrophy and distal sensorimotor polyneuropathy—neurologic disorders in rottweilers; differentiated on the basis of neurologic deficits; neuroaxonal dystrophy: deficits relate to the cerebellum; distal sensorimotor polyneuropathy: tetraparesis associated with lower motor neuron signs
• Diskospondylitis, fracture or luxation, and intervertebral disk disease—neck pain; disk disease rarely seen in large-breed dogs at a young age
• Cervical vertebral instability (wobbler)—differentiate on the basis of spinal survey and myelographic studies; stenosis of the vertebral canal
• Canine distemper virus or other inflammatory cause of myelitis—progresses faster; CSF analysis abnormal
• Spinal cord tumors—old dogs; myelography reveals spinal cord compression.

CBC/BIOCHEMISTRY/URINALYSIS
Normal

OTHER LABORATORY TESTS
N/A

IMAGING
Spinal cervical survey radiographs normal

DIAGNOSTIC PROCEDURES
• CSF analysis normal
• Myelography normal

 TREATMENT

• Outpatient, unless the severity of neurologic deficits precludes nursing care at home
• Activity—whatever can be tolerated
• Diet—ensure proper intake of food; patient may have difficulty reaching the feeding area.
• Neurologic status—slowly and progressively deteriorates; eventually, the patient is unable to walk or get up.

 MEDICATIONS

DRUGS
None available

CONTRAINDICATIONS/POSSIBLE INTERACTIONS
N/A

 FOLLOW-UP

• Neurologic examination—monitor monthly to assess progression
• Avoid bed sores and urine and fecal scalding by keeping the patient on a clean, dry, and cushioned pad (e.g., synthetic sheepskin).
• Severe tetraparesis—within 6–12 months after onset of clinical signs
• Euthanasia—because of severe debility

 MISCELLANEOUS

ABBREVIATION
CSF = cerebrospinal fluid

Suggested Reading
Wouda W, van Nes JJ. Progressive ataxia due to central demyelination in rottweiler dogs. Vet Q 1986;8:89–97.
Author Joane M. Parent
Consulting Editor Joane M. Parent

BASICS

OVERVIEW
• Plants in the *Lilium* and *Hemerocallis* genera—widely used ornamental plants; very toxic to cats; Easter lilies, tiger lilies, Japanese show lilies, rubrum lilies, numerous *Lilium* hybrids, and day lilies
• Ingestion of leaves or flowers—results in a severe nephrotoxic syndrome; as little as 2–3 leaves reported to be lethal
• Toxic principle(s) not elucidated

SIGNALMENT
• Cats—systemic poisoning
• Dogs—only mild gastrointestinal upset, even after ingestion of large quantities of plant material
• No age or breed predilections noted

SIGNS
• Sudden onset of vomiting—gradually subsides within 2–4 hr
• Depression and anorexia—onset about the same time as vomiting; persist throughout the syndrome
• Polyuria and dehydration—by 12–24 hr; lead to anuric renal failure
• Vomiting—reoccurs by 36 hr; accompanied by progressive weakness
• Recumbency—by 3–4 days
• Death—by 4–7 days postingestion

CAUSES & RISK FACTORS
• Plants—Easter lilies; tiger lilies; Asiatic hybrid lilies; Japanese show lilies; *Lilium* hybrids; day lilies; primarily when used in cut-flower arrangement or as household potted plants
• All ingestions by cats of plant material from the *Lilium* and *Hemerocallis* genera should be considered potentially toxic.
• Indoor cats—exclusively predisposed to ingestion of newly introduced plants

DIAGNOSIS

DIFFERENTIAL DIAGNOSES

Nephrotoxins
• Aspirin and other NSAIDs
• Zinc
• Boric acid
• Ethylene glycol
• Mercury
• Nephrotoxic antibacterials—aminoglycosides

Systemic Diseases
• Acute chronic renal failure
• Urinary obstruction
• Immune-mediated renal disease
• Leptospirosis
• Pyelonephritis
• Lymphosarcoma

CBC/BIOCHEMISTRY/URINALYSIS
• Stress leukogram
• Moderate to severely high BUN, phosphate, and potassium
• Creatinine—severe increase common; usually 15–29 mg/dl; may be into the 40s
• Increased AST, ALT, and ALP late in disease
• Severe proteinuria, glucosuria, low specific gravity, and numerous tubular epithelial casts
• Crystalluria—not caused by ingestion of these plants

OTHER LABORATORY TESTS
N/A

IMAGING
N/A

DIAGNOSTIC PROCEDURES
If possible, examine plant to verify that it has been chewed.

PATHOLOGIC FINDINGS
• Gross—swollen kidneys; empty gastrointestinal tract; moderate to severe perirenal edema
• Histologic—severe acute renal tubular necrosis with intact basement membranes; mild to severe interstitial edema; severe cast formation in the collecting ducts; may note evidence of mitotic figures in the remaining tubular epithelium

TREATMENT
• Early decontamination—lessens duration and severity of signs
• Fluid therapy—initiation within 24 hr of ingestion prevents anuric renal failure; intravenous normal saline at two to three times maintenance for 24 hr
• Anuric renal failure—peritoneal dialysis only treatment; 7 days of therapy has returned renal function.

MEDICATIONS

DRUGS
• Decontamination—activated charcoal (2 g/kg)
• Cathartic—sorbitol (2.1 g/kg) or magnesium sulfate (0.5 g/kg)

CONTRAINDICATIONS/POSSIBLE INTERACTIONS
• Avoid fluids containing potassium.
• Avoid drugs eliminated by renal clearance.
• Diuretics (mannitol, hypertonic fluids, furosemide, thiazides)—not effective at initiating urine production

FOLLOW-UP
• Successful prevention of anuric renal failure or after peritoneal dialysis—periodically follow serum chemistries to ensure normal renal function.

EXPECTED COURSE & PROGNOSIS
• Dehydration—from polyuric renal failure; required for the disease to progress to anuria

MISCELLANEOUS

SEE ALSO
• Poisoning (Intoxication)
• Renal Failure, Acute

ABBREVIATIONS
• ALP = alkaline phosphatase
• ALT = alanine aminotransferase
• AST = aspartate aminotransferase

Suggested Reading
Groff RM, Miller JM, Stair EL, et al. Toxicoses and toxins. In: Norsworthy GD, ed., Feline practice. Philadelphia: Lippincott, 1993:551–569.
Author Jeffery O. Hall
Consulting Editor Gary D. Osweiller

DISEASES

LIPOMA, INFILTRATIVE

BASICS

OVERVIEW
• Invasive, nonencapsulated, lipoma variant that does not metastasize
• A benign neoplasm that infiltrates soft tissues, particularly muscles, and including fasciae, tendons, nerves, blood vessels, salivary glands, lymph nodes, and joint capsules, and occasionally bones
• Muscle infiltration typically extensive
• Surgical cures difficult to obtain
• Occurs much less frequently than does lipoma

SIGNALMENT
• Usually middle-aged dogs
• Cats—one report; extremely rare
• Labrador retrievers—possibly over-represented
• No breed predilection definitively demonstrated
• About 3–4 times more common in females than in males

SIGNS
• Large, diffuse, soft tissue mass
• Clinically appears as localized muscle swelling
• Infiltration of pelvic, thigh, shoulder, sternum, and lateral cervical musculature—most common; recent evidence suggests no clear site prediction.

CAUSES & RISK FACTORS
Unknown

DIAGNOSIS

DIFFERENTIAL DIAGNOSIS
• Rhabdomyoma or rhabdomyosarcoma
• Lipoma or liposarcoma
• Mast cell neoplasia
• Fibrosarcoma
• Hemangiopericytoma

CBC/BIOCHEMISTRY/URINALYSIS
Normal

OTHER LABORATORY TESTS
N/A

IMAGING
Radiography—reveals fat dense tissue between soft tissue dense structures

DIAGNOSTIC PROCEDURES
Cytologic examination of aspirate—reveals mature adipocytes

PATHOLOGIC FINDINGS
• Histologic examination—well-differentiated adipocytes; may be indistinguishable from normal adipose tissue
• Distinctive feature—tumor infiltration into and between muscle bundles

TREATMENT

Surgery
• Characteristic invasiveness makes excision extremely difficult; difficult to distinguish between tumor and normal adipose tissue
• Poorly defined tumor margins—may contribute to the observed high recurrence rate after surgical excision
• Inform client that at least 50% of patients have recurrence within 3–16 months, except with limb amputation for appendicular tumor.
• Amputation of an affected limb—recommended only when the quality of life is affected; tumor causes little inconvenience unless it interferes with movement, causes pressure-related pain, or develops in a vitally important anatomic site

External Beam Radiotherapy
• Had been used; efficacy remains unknown

• Unlikely to kill mitotically inactive mature adipocytes but may inhibit progressive infiltration by damaging tumor microcirculation

MEDICATIONS

DRUG(S)
Chemotherapy—unlikely to be beneficial; partial response observed after doxorubicin administration in one dog

CONTRAINDICATIONS/POSSIBLE INTERACTIONS
N/A

FOLLOW-UP
• Focus—whether and when to recommend surgery
• Re-evaluations—schedule as dictated by tumor growth and other characteristics

MISCELLANEOUS

SYNONYMS
• Lipomatosis
• Well-differentiated liposarcoma

Suggested Reading
Bergman PJ, Withrow SJ, Straw RC, et al. Infiltrative lipoma in dogs: 16 cases (1981–1992). J Am Vet Med Assoc 1994;205:322–324.
Author James P. Thompson
Consulting Editor Wallace B. Morrison

BASICS

OVERVIEW
• Poisonous lizards—found only in the U.S. Southwest and Mexico; *Heloderma suspectum* (Gila monster) and *H. horridum* (Mexican beaded lizard); tenacious bite; deliver venom from glands on the lower jaw by aggressive chewing action over grooved teeth; non-aggressive; animal envenomations rare
• Venom components—less well-characterized than other venoms; no evidence of altered coagulation in the victim

SIGNALMENT
Dogs and cats

SIGNS

Historical Findings
• Sudden outset of pain
• Bite—usually on the face, especially the lower lip; lizard may still be attached to patient (pathognomonic).

Physical Examination Findings
• Bleeding from bite site
• May note hypotension
• Extremely painful bite site
• Localized swelling
• Ptyalism—excessive salivation
• Excessive lacrimation
• Frequent urination and defecation
• May note aphonia in cats

CAUSES & RISK FACTORS
Outdoor activities

DIAGNOSIS

DIFFERENTIAL DIAGNOSIS
• Trauma
• Venomous snake bite—usually fewer punctures; depression and clotting abnormalities more prominent

CBC/BIOCHEMISTRY/URINALYSIS
N/A

OTHER LABORATORY TESTS
N/A

IMAGING
N/A

DIAGNOSTIC PROCEDURES
Electrocardiography—may detect arrhythmias

TREATMENT
• Remove lizard—place a prying instrument between the jaws; push into the back of the mouth; a flame held underneath the jaw often releases grip.
• Inpatient—monitor and treat hypotension, as necessary, with crystalloid fluid therapy
• Bite site—flush with lidocaine; probe to identify and remove fragments of lizard teeth (if not removed, they will become sequestra and abscess); soak with Burow solution or similar solution every 8 hr.

MEDICATIONS

DRUGS
• Control pain—Rimadyl (dogs) or narcotics (if severe)
• Broad-spectrum antibiotics indicated

CONTRAINDICATIONS/POSSIBLE INTERACTIONS
• Corticosteroids—not generally used by the author, unless marked hypotension; authorities differ on the value of corticosteroids
• Antihistamines—not useful

FOLLOW-UP
• ECG—monitor for arrhythmias.
• Bite site—monitor for infection.

MISCELLANEOUS

Suggested Reading
Peterson ME, Meerdink G. Bites and stings of venomous animals. In: Kirk RW, ed. Current veterinary therapy X. Philadelphia: Saunders, 1989:177–186.
Author Michael E. Peterson
Consulting Editor Gary D. Osweiler

DISEASES

LOWER URINARY TRACT INFECTION

BASICS

DEFINITION
Result of microbial colonization of the urinary bladder and/or proximal portion of the urethra

PATHOPHYSIOLOGY
Microbes, usually aerobic bacteria, ascend the urinary tract under conditions that permit them to persist in the urine or adhere to the epithelium and subsequently multiply. Urinary tract colonization requires at least transient impairment of the mechanisms that normally defend against infection. Inflammation of infected tissues results in the clinical signs and laboratory test abnormalities exhibited by patients.

SYSTEMS AFFECTED
Renal/Urologic—lower urinary tract

GENETICS
N/A

INCIDENCE/PREVALENCE
Common in female dogs; less common in male dogs; uncommon in cats

GEOGRAPHIC DISTRIBUTION
N/A

SIGNALMENT
Species
More common in dogs than in cats

Breed Predilections
None

Mean Age and Range
All ages affected, but occurrence increases with age because of a greater frequency of other urinary lesions (e.g., uroliths, prostate disease, and tumors) that predispose to secondary urinary tract infection.

Predominant Sex
More in female than male dogs; occurrence in male and female cats is similar.

SIGNS
Historical Findings
• None in some patients
• Pollakiuria—frequent voiding of small volumes
• Dysuria
• Urgency (or an apparent loss of ability to control urination during periods of confinement)
• Urinating in places that are not customary
• Hematuria and cloudy or malodorous urine in some patients

Physical Examination Findings
• No abnormalities in some animals
• Acute infection—bladder or urethra may seem tender on palpation
• Palpation of the bladder may stimulate urination.

• Chronic infection—wall of the bladder or urethra may be palpably thickened or abnormally firm.
• Secondary infection—findings referable to the underlying problem

CAUSES
• Aerobic bacteria—most common
• Most common—*Escherichia, Staphylococcus,* and *Proteus* spp. (more than half of all cases)
• Common—*Streptococcus, Klebsiella, Enterobacter, Pseudomonas,* and *Corynebacterium* spp.
• Rare—a few other bacterial and fungal agents

RISK FACTORS
• Conditions that cause urine stasis or incomplete emptying of the bladder
• Conditions that disrupt mucosal defense properties
• Conditions that reduce or bypass anatomic and functional barriers to microbial ascent of the urinary tract (e.g., loss of muscle tone or length of the urethra and the vesicoureteral junctions)
• Conditions that compromise the antibacterial properties of urine (e.g., changes in urine pH or osmolality and low concentrations of urea and certain organic acids)

DIAGNOSIS

DIFFERENTIAL DIAGNOSIS
• Any other disease of the bladder or urethra
• Conditions commonly confused with, or complicated by, urinary tract infection include urolithiasis and neoplasia. In cats, idiopathic hemorrhagic cystitis is also a common problem that must be distinguished.
• Lower urinary tract disease can become complicated by secondary urinary tract infection; this is termed *complicated urinary tract infection* and requires different therapeutic strategies than are used for uncomplicated (i.e., simple) episodes of urinary tract infection.
• Frequent reinfection (more than one episode of newly acquired urinary tract infection within a year) usually indicates impaired host defense mechanisms. Seek an underlying cause. If the no underlying cause can be identified and corrected, consider prophylactic antibacterial drug therapy.

CBC/BIOCHEMISTRY/URINALYSIS
• Results of CBC and serum biochemistry normal
• Pyuria is most commonly associated with urinary tract infection, but noninfectious urinary lesions can also cause pyuria. Hematuria and proteinuria are also common. Bacteria may or may not be detected by microscopic examination of urinary sediment. Bacteriuria is sometimes reported in animals that do not have urinary tract infection.

OTHER LABORATORY TESTS
Urine Culture and Sensitivity Testing
• Urine culture is necessary for definitive diagnosis.
• Correct interpretation of urine culture results requires obtaining the specimen in a manner that minimizes contamination, handling and storing the specimen so that numbers of viable bacteria do not change in vitro, and using a quantitative culture method. Keep the specimen in a sealed sterile container; if the culture is not started right away, the urine can be refrigerated up to 8 h without important change in the results.
• Cystocentesis is the preferred technique for obtaining urine for culture.
• Cutoff values for significant bacteriuria in urine of dogs—obtained by cystocentesis, >1,000/mL; obtained by catheterization, > 10,000/mL; voided urine specimen, >100,000/mL
• Cutoff values for significant bacteriuria in urine of cats—obtained by cystocentesis or catheterization, >1,000/mL; voided urine specimen, >10,000/mL
• Values that approach but do not exceed these cutoffs (i.e., less than one order of magnitude below) are suspicious, and retesting is indicated. Urine cultures that produce values more than one order of magnitude below these cutoffs are negative.
• In vitro susceptibility testing that determines the minimum inhibitory concentration (MIC) of each drug against the isolated organism is preferred for urinary pathogens. Drugs commonly used to treat urinary tract infection are highly concentrated in the urine, and any drug with an MIC value of one fourth or less of the average urine concentration of the drug during treatment is likely to be effective.

IMAGING
Survey and contrast radiographic studies as well as ultrasound of the bladder or urethra may detect an underlying urinary tract lesion (i.e., complicated urinary tract infection).

DIAGNOSTIC PROCEDURES
N/A

PATHOLOGIC FINDINGS
N/A

TREATMENT

APPROPRIATE HEALTH CARE
Treat as outpatient unless another urinary abnormality (e.g., obstruction) requires inpatient treatment

NURSING CARE
N/A

ACTIVITY
• Unrestricted
• Regulating the patient's urination to coordinate with antibacterial drug treatments may improve therapeutic efficacy.

DIET
Restrictions not necessary but may be indicated for other concurrent urinary diseases (e.g., urolithiasis)

CLIENT EDUCATION
Prognosis for cure of simple urinary tract infection is excellent; prognosis for complicated urinary tract infection depends on the underlying abnormality. Compliance with recommendations for treatment and follow-up evaluations is crucial for optimum results.

SURGICAL CONSIDERATIONS
Except when a concomitant disorder requires surgical intervention, management does not involve surgery.

MEDICATIONS

DRUGS OF CHOICE
• An appropriate antibiotic can be selected on the basis of the genus of the infecting bacteria—penicillin (e.g., ampicillin, 25 mg/kg PO q8h) for *Staphylococcus, Streptococcus,* or *Proteus* spp; trimethoprim-sulfadiazine (15 mg/kg combined PO q12h) for *Escherichia coli;* cephalexin (30 mg/kg PO q8h) for *Klebsiella* spp.; tetracycline (20 mg/kg PO q8h) for *Pseudomonas* spp.
• For an organism whose predictable susceptibility to a specific drug is not known or that does not respond as expected to the first drug, base choice of drug on results of sensitivity test.
• Antibacterial drugs are usually most effective when given q8h; however, fluoroquinolones and trimethoprim-sulfa products are effective when given q12h.
• For acute, uncomplicated infection, treat with antimicrobial drugs for 7–10 days. Chronic bacterial cystitis may need treatment for up to 4–6 weeks. Appropriate duration of treatment for complicated lower urinary tract infection depends on the underlying problem.
• Low-dose, bedtime antibacterial therapy can be used to prevent infections in animals that have frequent reinfections. Start such prophylactic treatment immediately after cure of the most recent episode of urinary tract infection by conventional treatment. Administer an appropriate antibacterial drug, usually ampicillin or nitrofurantoin, once daily for 4–6 months or longer. Dosage should be about one third of the conventional daily dose for the chosen drug, and the drug should be given after the animal has urinated for the last time each evening.

CONTRAINDICATIONS
Allergic reaction to a drug

PRECAUTIONS
• Long-term or repeated use of antimicrobial drugs is associated with adverse effects (e.g., allergic reaction) in some animals.
• Keratoconjunctivitis sicca is associated with administration of trimethoprim-sulfa products.
• Because of potential nephrotoxicity with long-term administration, use aminoglycosides only when there are no alternatives.

POSSIBLE INTERACTIONS
Patients with impaired renal function may have reduced urinary excretion of drugs used to treat urinary tract infection. Besides leading to unintended drug accumulation in such patients, impaired urinary excretion might reduce the drug's effectiveness.

ALTERNATIVE DRUGS
• Enrofloxacin and nitrofurantoin
• Ceftiofur, gentamicin, or amikacin, which must be given by injection

FOLLOW-UP

PATIENT MONITORING
• When antibacterial drug efficacy is in doubt, culture the urine 2–3 days after starting treatment. If the drug is effective, the culture will be negative. • Continue treating at least 1 week after resolution of hematuria, pyuria, and proteinuria. Failure of urinalysis findings to return to normal while an episode of urinary tract infection is being treated with an effective antibiotic (i.e., as indicated by negative urine culture) generally indicates some other urinary tract abnormality (e.g., urolith, tumor). Rapid recrudescence of signs when treatment is stopped generally indicates either a concurrent urinary tract abnormality or that the infection extends into some deep-seated site (e.g., prostatic or renal parenchyma). • Successful cure of an episode of urinary tract infection is best demonstrated by performing a urine culture 7–10 days after completing antimicrobial therapy. • Animals being given low-dose bedtime antibacterial prophylactic treatment for frequent reinfection should have a urine culture performed via cystocentesis every 1–2 months.

PREVENTION/AVOIDANCE
• Avoid indiscriminate use of urinary catheters • Animals with frequent reinfection can be given bedtime therapy to augment host defenses and prevent reinfection.

POSSIBLE COMPLICATIONS
Failure to detect or treat effectively may lead to pyelonephritis or formation of struvite uroliths.

EXPECTED COURSE AND PROGNOSIS
• If not treated, expect infection to persist indefinitely. Associated health risks include development of urolithiasis and extension of infection to other portions of the urinary tract (e.g., the kidneys) or beyond (e.g., septicemia, diskospondylitis, and bacterial endocarditis). • Generally, the prognosis for animals with uncomplicated lower urinary tract infection is good-to-excellent. Patients that have frequent reinfection are candidates for low-dose bedtime prophylactic therapy, as described, but even these patients usually do well. The prognosis for animals with complicated infection is determined by the prognosis for the other urinary abnormality.

MISCELLANEOUS

ASSOCIATED CONDITIONS
• Struvite urolithiasis • Diabetes mellitus or hyperadrenocorticism

AGE-RELATED FACTORS
Complicated infection is more common in middle-aged to old than in young animals.

ZOONOTIC POTENTIAL
N/A

PREGNANCY
Depending on the stage of pregnancy, intensity of signs, and presence or absence of concomitant abnormalities, consider deferring treatment. Avoid using tetracycline, nitrofurantoin, or enrofloxacin.

SYNONYMS
Bacterial cystitis, urethrocystitis, and urethritis

SEE ALSO
• Pyelonephritis • Urolithiasis, Struvite—Dogs and Cats

ABBREVIATION
MIC = minimum inhibitory concentration

Suggested Reading

Grauer GF. Urinary tract infections. In: Nelson RW, Couto CG, eds. Essentials of small animal internal medicine. St Louis: Mosby-Year Book, 1992:494–500.

Lees GE, Rogers KS. Treatment of urinary tract infections in dogs and cats. J Am Vet Med Assoc 1986;189:648–652.

Lulich JP, Osborne CA. Bacterial infections of the urinary tract. In: Ettinger SJ, Feldman EC, eds. Textbook of veterinary internal medicine. 4th ed. Philadelphia: Saunders, 1995:1775–1788.

Author George E. Lees

Consulting Editors Larry G. Adams and Carl A. Osborne

DISEASES

LUMBOSACRAL STENOSIS (CAUDA EQUINA SYNDROME)

BASICS

DEFINITION
• Caused by dorsoventral narrowing of the lumbosacral vertebral canal with compression of the L7, sacral, or caudal nerve roots
• Syndrome refers to the clinical signs related to injury of these nerve roots.

PATHOPHYSIOLOGY
• Congenital—abnormal development of the dorsal arch of the L7-S1 vertebrae causes narrowing of the lumbosacral spinal canal; chronic biomechanical stress may contribute to degenerative changes that reduce the canal diameter and cause compression of the spinal nerve roots; the smaller the canal, the less stenosis required before clinical signs appear.
• Acquired—caused by bony and soft tissue degenerative changes that lead to a gradual but progressive reduction in the lumbosacral spinal canal

SYSTEMS AFFECTED
Nervous—specifically nerve roots, from L7 caudally

GENETICS
No known genetic basis

INCIDENCE/PREVALENCE
Unknown

GEOGRAPHIC DISTRIBUTION
N/A

SIGNALMENT
Species
• Common in dogs
• Rare in cats

Breed Predilections
• Congenital—small to medium dogs; border collies
• Acquired—large-breed dogs; German shepherds

Mean Age and Range
• Congenital—3–8 years
• Acquired—average age at onset 6–7 years

Predominant Sex
• Congenital—none
• Acquired—male

SIGNS
• Relate to varying degrees of compression of the L7, sacral, and caudal nerve roots
• Lumbosacral pain—salient clinical feature; may be the only sign
• Sciatic nerve dysfunction—may initially manifest as a lameness; may progress to pelvic limb weakness, muscle wasting, and postural reaction deficits
• Pudendal nerve root involvement—urinary and/or fecal incontinence
• Caudal nerve root involvement—weakness to paralysis of the tail
• Both meninges and nerve root compression—sensory disturbances that vary from unpleasant sensations to obvious low lumbar pain
• Congenital—self-inflicted lesions common
• Patients with both forms—extension of the pelvic limbs or dorsiflexion of the tail over the back reduces the lumbosacral canal diameter and usually elicits a painful response.

CAUSES
• Congenital vertebral malformation
• Type II disk protrusion
• Hypertrophy or hyperplasia of the inter-arcuate ligament
• Proliferation of the articular facets
• Subluxation or instability of the lumbosacral junction

RISK FACTORS
N/A

DIAGNOSIS

DIFFERENTIAL DIAGNOSIS
• Hip dysplasia or other orthopedic injury—low lumbar pain; distinguish via thorough orthopedic examination
• Chronic diskospondylitis, osteomyelitis, and primary or metastatic vertebral tumors—cannot be differentiated by clinical signs alone
• Vertebral fractures and subluxations—acute; characterized by more bilateral signs
• Localized myelitis or radiculoneuritis—usually more diffuse pain

CBC/BIOCHEMISTRY/URINALYSIS
• Usually normal
• Urinalysis—may reveal lower urinary tract infection secondary to urinary incontinence

OTHER LABORATORY TESTS
N/A

IMAGING
• Radiology—spondylosis at the lumbosacral junction; narrowing of the L7-S1 disk space; ventral displacement of the sacrum relative to the lumbar vertebrae; interpret with caution because all can be seen in clinically normal animals.
• Myelography—rarely of benefit because the subarachnoid space rarely extends beyond vertebra L6 in large-breed dogs; indicated to rule out lesions rostral to the lumbosacral junction
• Epidurography—may outline a space-occupying mass over the lumbosacral disk space
• Discography of the L7-S1 space—may help highlight elevation of the dorsal annulus fibrosis
• Intraosseous venography—technically difficult; least reliable diagnostic procedure
• CT and MRI—enhance the ability to recognize the condition

DIAGNOSTIC PROCEDURES
Electromyography—diagnostic and prognostic; denervation may be detected in the muscles innervated by the nerve roots L7 to caudal; denervation confirms the localization of the lesion and implies permanent deficits.

PATHOLOGIC FINDINGS
• May see one or more of the following features
• Hypertrophy of the ligamentum flavum
• Type II disk disease
• Hypertrophy of the interarcuate ligament
• Spondylosis causing stenosis of the intervertebral foramen with ensuing compression of nerve roots
• Ventral displacement of the sacrum in relation to lumbar vertebrae
• Proliferation of articular facets
• Congenital malformation consisting of shortened pedicles
• Thickened and sclerotic lamina and articular processes

LUMBOSACRAL STENOSIS (CAUDA EQUINA SYNDROME)

TREATMENT

APPROPRIATE HEALTH CARE
• Urinary continence—outpatient pending surgery
• Urinary incontinence—inpatient for initial medical management

NURSING CARE
Urinary incontinence—catheterize the bladder until adequate voluntary control returns; monitor closely for urinary tract infection and administer appropriate antibiotics if necessary.

ACTIVITY
• After surgical decompression—restrict for 4 weeks; then gradually return to athletic function
• Nonsurgical treatment—confinement and restricted leash walks, alone or combined with corticosteroids, frequently alleviate pain; clinical signs often return with increasing levels of exercise.

DIET
Avoid obesity; excess weight increases biomechanical stress on the spine.

CLIENT EDUCATION
• Inform client that without treatment there will be progressive neurologic impairment of the pelvic limbs, urinary and fecal incontinence, and paralysis of the tail.
• Inform client that pelvic limb lameness and self-inflicted lesions result from pain associated with nerve root irritation and compression.
• Discuss surgical treatment, noting that it stops the progression and removes the source of pain, that some neurologic deficits may remain, and that medical management alone is usually unsatisfactory.

SURGICAL CONSIDERATIONS
• Surgical decompression—preferred treatment
• Dorsal laminectomy of the L7-S1 vertebrae—effectively relieves compression in most patients; may combine with facetectomy or foraminotomy if nerve roots are compressed by spondylitic bone
• Fusion of the lumbosacral joint—consider if the lumbosacral junction appears unstable (on radiographs or during surgery); through a dorsal approach by fixation of the L7-S1 articular process to the wing of the ilium or through a ventral approach with an ileal graft placed in a ventral slot

MEDICATIONS

DRUGS OF CHOICE
NSAIDs or corticosteroids—usually unsatisfactory

CONTRAINDICATIONS
N/A

PRECAUTIONS
N/A

POSSIBLE INTERACTIONS
N/A

ALTERNATIVE DRUGS
N/A

FOLLOW-UP

PATIENT MONITORING
N/A

PREVENTION/AVOIDANCE
N/A

POSSIBLE COMPLICATIONS
• Seroma formation—frequent sequel to surgery; can be effectively managed by cage rest and surgical drainage
• Excessive fibrous tissue formation (laminectomy membrane) in the surgical area—infrequent cause of recurrence of clinical signs; minimize by proper surgical technique; surgical removal is difficult and has a lower success rate than the initial dorsal laminectomy.

EXPECTED COURSE AND PROGNOSIS
• Vary with the degree of neurologic injury
• Low lumbar pain and mild neurologic deficits (dogs)—good prognosis after surgery; most fully recover within a few months.
• Fecal and urinary incontinence (dogs)—guarded prognosis

MISCELLANEOUS

ASSOCIATED CONDITIONS
Lower urinary tract infections frequently accompany urinary incontinence.

AGE-RELATED FACTORS
German shepherds—concurrent coxofemoral osteoarthritis and/or degenerative myelopathy

ZOONOTIC POTENTIAL
N/A

PREGNANCY
N/A

SYNONYMS
• Lumbosacral malarticulation or malformation
• Lumbosacral instability
• Lumbosacral spondylopathy
• Lumbosacral spondylolisthesis

SEE ALSO
• Diskospondylitis
• Intervertebral Disk Disease—Thoracolumbar

ABBREVIATIONS
N/A

Suggested Reading

Morgan JP, Bailey CS. Cauda equina syndrome in the dog: radiographic evaluation. J Small Anim Pract 1990;31:69–77.
Ness MG. Degenerative lumbosacral stenosis in the dog: a review of 30 cases. J Small Anim Pract 1994;35:185–190.
Oliver JE Jr, Selcer RR, Simpson S. Cauda equina compression from lumbosacral malarticulation and malformation in the dog. J Am Vet Med Assoc 1978;173: 207–214.
Sisson AF, LeCouteur RA, Ingram JT, et al. Diagnosis of cauda equina abnormalities by using electromyography, discography, and epidurography in dogs. J Vet Intern Med 1992;6: 253–263.
Tarvin G, Prada RG. Lumbosacral stenosis in dogs. J Am Vet Med Assoc 1980;177: 154–159.

Author Karen Dyer Inzana
Consulting Editor Joane M. Parent

DISEASES

LUNG LOBE TORSION

BASICS

OVERVIEW
• Twisting of lung lobe(s) at the hilus with occlusion of the bronchus, lymphatics, vein, and (finally) arteries
• Affected lobes—right middle lobe most commonly affected; other lobes may twist singly or in pairs.
• Initially, the lobe becomes engorged with blood, which causes it to enlarge; infarction and necrosis may follow; hemorrhagic pleural effusion typically develops.
• Chronic survivors—may note shrinkage and fibrosis of the lobe

SIGNALMENT
• Most common in large, deep-chested dogs
• Less common in cats

SIGNS
• Fever
• Weakness
• Collapse
• Dyspnea
• Orthopnea
• Cough
• Hemoptysis
• Ventral thoracic dullness
• Tachycardia
• Cyanosis
• Shock

CAUSES & RISK FACTORS
• Lobar torsion—usually associated with pre-existing condition that causes pleural effusion (e.g., trauma, neoplasia, and chylothorax)
• Thoracic or diaphragmatic surgery
• Spontaneous or idiopathic

DIAGNOSIS

DIFFERENTIAL DIAGNOSIS
• Pulmonary contusion
• Diaphragmatic hernia
• Pulmonary abscess or infarction
• Neoplasia—lymphomatoid granulomatosis
• Coagulopathy
• Pneumonia, embolization, or thrombosis
• Uncomplicated pleural effusion and compression atelectasis
• Fungal or foreign body granuloma
• Lobar consolidation or bronchial obstruction from a foreign body

CBC/BIOCHEMISTRY/URINALYSIS
N/A

OTHER LABORATORY TESTS
N/A

IMAGING

Radiography
• Initially may reveal air bronchograms with disorientation of the torsed bronchus
• Pleural effusion—suggested by ventral leafing and interlobar fissures
• Consolidation and swelling of the torsed lobe with possible displacement of the heart and mediastinum
• May see lack of expansion of other lobes
• Thoracentesis may improve visualization and provide therapeutic benefits.

Ultrasound
• May allow further characterization
• Fine-needle aspiration contraindicated

DIAGNOSTIC PROCEDURES
• Pleural effusion—typically hemorrhagic; PCV and WBC count similar to that of the peripheral blood; no platelets; chronicity or pre-existing effusions (e.g., chyle) may alter observations
• Bronchoscopy—may reveal occlusion of the associated bronchus
• Surgical exploration—definitive diagnosis and treatment

TREATMENT

• Thoracentesis or chest tube placement
• Re-expansion pulmonary edema—may be a serious problem (especially in cats) if large volumes of pleural fluid are withdrawn quickly or if chronically compressed lungs are acutely inflated at surgery.
• Intravenous fluid administration
• Administer oxygen and treat for shock—when indicated
• Anesthesia—requires adequate ventilatory support; carefully monitor patient.
• Surgical removal of the involved lobe(s)—only effective treatment; do not salvage (may lead to recurrence or necrosis); in situ ligation of the vessels or clamping with noncrushing forceps has been advocated; closely inspect remaining thoracic structures for any abnormalities.
• Postsurgery—monitoring; supportive care; tube drainage

MEDICATIONS

DRUGS
• Antibiotics—perioperatively
• Treatment for shock—when indicated

CONTRAINDICATIONS/POSSIBLE INTERACTIONS
N/A

FOLLOW-UP

• Observe for recurrence of pleural effusion.
• Thoracic radiographs—before discharge; as needed thereafter
• Prognosis—good if no underlying abnormality remains

MISCELLANEOUS

ABBREVIATION
PCV = packed cell volume

Suggested Reading

Nelson AW. Lower respiratory system. In: Slatter DH, ed. Textbook of small animal surgery. Vol 1. 2nd ed. Philadelphia: Saunders, 1993:797–804.

Author Bradley L. Moses

Consulting Editor Eleanor C. Hawkins

LUPUS ERYTHEMATOSUS, SYSTEMIC (SLE)

BASICS

DEFINITION
A multisystem autoimmune disease characterized by the formation of autoantibodies against a wide array of self-antigens and circulating immune complexes

PATHOPHYSIOLOGY
• Cause unknown
• An immunoregulatory defect causes the production of autoantibodies to non-organ-specific nuclear and cytoplasmic antigens and to organ-specific antigens.
• Immune complexes are formed and deposited in the glomerular basement membrane, synovial membrane, skin, blood vessels, and other sites.
• Tissue injury—caused by activation of complement by immune complexes and infiltration of inflammatory cells and by a direct cytotoxic effect of autoantibodies against membrane-bound antigens
• Clinical manifestations depend on the localization of the immune complexes and the specificity of the autoantibodies.

SYSTEMS AFFECTED
• Musculoskeletal—deposition of immune complexes in the synovial membranes
• Skin/Exocrine—deposition of immune complexes in the skin
• Renal/Urologic—deposition of immune complexes in the glomeruli
• Hemic/Lymph/Immune—autoantibodies against RBCs, leukocytes, or platelets
• Other organ systems—if there is deposition of immune complexes or autoantibodies

GENETICS
• Hereditary in a colony of German shepherds
• Linked to the major histocompatibility complex allele DLA-A7

INCIDENCE/PREVALENCE
Rare, but probably underdiagnosed

GEOGRAPHIC DISTRIBUTION
None

SIGNALMENT

Species
Dogs and cats

Breed Predilection
None

Mean Age and Range
Mean age 6 years, but can occur at any age

Predominant Sex
None

SIGNS

Historical Findings
• The onset can be acute or insidious.
• Depend on the site of immune complex deposition and specificity of the autoantibodies
• Waxing and waning course with clinical manifestations often changing over time
• Lethargy
• Anorexia
• Shifting leg lameness
• Skin lesions
• Altered behavior

Physical Examination Findings
• Joints may be swollen and painful.
• Symmetric or focal cutaneous lesions—characterized by erythema, scaling, ulceration, and alopecia; mucocutaneous and oral lesions common
• Fever
• Lymphadenopathy and hepatosplenomegaly
• Arrhythmias, heart murmurs, and pleural frictions rubs (i.e., associated with myocarditis, pericarditis, or pleuritis)
• Muscle wasting

CAUSES
• Definitive causes unidentified
• Exposure to drugs and viral infection suspected

RISK FACTORS
Exposure to UV light may exacerbate the disease.

DIAGNOSIS

• Definitive diagnosis—positive ANA or LE cell test (or both) and two major signs or one major and two minor signs
• Probable diagnosis—positive ANA or LE cell test (or both) and one major or two minor signs
• Major signs—polyarthritis, proteinuria, dermatitis, hemolytic anemia, leukopenia, thrombocytopenia, and polymyositis
• Minor signs—fever of unknown origin, oral ulcers, peripheral lymphadenopathy, pleuritis, pericarditis, myocarditis, depression, and seizures

DIFFERENTIAL DIAGNOSIS
• Neoplastic disease—may be associated with circulating immune complexes; patient may have similar signs as SLE.
• Important to rule out infectious disease, because SLE is treated with immunosuppressive drugs

CBC/BIOCHEMISTRY/URINALYSIS
• CBC—anemia, leukopenia, and thrombocytopenia; leukocytosis (i.e., monocytosis and neutrophilia) resulting from chronic inflammation
• Anemia—moderate and nonregenerative (e.g., anemia of chronic disease) or severe and regenerative (e.g., hemolytic)
• Biochemical analysis—results vary widely, depending on the organ(s) affected.
• High urine protein:urine creatinine ratio (> 1) indicates true proteinuria that may be caused by glomerulonephritis.
• Patients with hemolytic anemia may have bilirubinuria.

OTHER LABORATORY TESTS
• Serum electrophoresis—usually shows high concentration of β- and γ-globulins
• ANA test—a sensitive assay; positive results support diagnosis of SLE; false-positive results associated with some infectious diseases (e.g., leishmaniasis and subacute bacterial endocarditis in dogs; FeLV, cholangiohepatitis, and treatment with propylthiouracil in cats)
• LE test—positive result supports diagnosis of SLE; less sensitive than the ANA test and cumbersome to perform
• Direct antiglobulin test (Coombs test)—positive in patients with immune-mediated hemolytic anemia

LUPUS ERYTHEMATOSUS, SYSTEMIC (SLE)

IMAGING

Radiography of affected joints reveals nonerosive arthritis, unlike the erosive lesions of rheumatoid arthritis.

DIAGNOSTIC PROCEDURES

• Arthrocentesis in patients with lameness or swollen joints; high cell count, with nondegenerate neutrophils and monocytes and low viscosity is a characteristic finding.
• Bacterial culture of synovial fluid is negative.
• Skin biopsy in patients with skin lesions; save specimen in 10% buffered formalin (for histopathologic examination) and Michel's solution (for immunofluorescence testing).
• Bone marrow biopsy in patients with nonregenerative anemia reveals excess iron deposition (anemia of chronic disease).

PATHOLOGIC FINDINGS

• Nonerosive polyarthritis with infiltration of synovial membrane by neutrophils and lymphocytes; no pannus formation
• Membranous or membranoproliferative glomerulonephritis
• Mononuclear interface dermatitis with hydropic degeneration of keratinocytes and eosinophilic round bodies representing apoptotic basal keratinocytes
• Vasculitis of dermal blood vessels and panniculitis in some patients
• Immunofluorescence—deposition of immune complexes along the basement membrane of the dermal-epidermal junction
• Vasculitis may be seen in any organ, especially myocardium, pericardium, and meninges.
• Reactive lymphoid hyperplasia in the lymph nodes and spleen

TREATMENT

APPROPRIATE HEALTH CARE

Hospitalization may be necessary for initial management (e.g., in a patient with hemolytic crisis); outpatient management is usually possible.

NURSING CARE

Supportive care varies with systems affected.

ACTIVITY

During episodes of acute polyarthritis, enforced rest is indicated.

DIET

Dietary protein restriction recommended in animals with severe renal disease caused by glomerulonephritis

CLIENT EDUCATION

• Discuss the progressive and unpredictable course of the disease.
• Discuss the need for long-term, immunosuppressive therapy and its side effects.
• Discuss heritability of the disease.

SURGICAL CONSIDERATIONS

None

MEDICATIONS

DRUGS OF CHOICE

• Goal of treatment—to control the abnormal immune response and to reduce the inflammation
• Corticosteroids—target both objectives; basis of treatment (prednisone, 1–2 mg/kg PO q12h)
• Cytotoxic immunosuppressive drug—add when prednisone fails to improve the condition or when the patient is steroid intolerant; reduce prednisone to 0.5–1 mg/kg PO q12h; use azathioprine (dogs, 2 mg/kg PO q24h), cyclophosphamide (dogs; 50 mg/m² PO for 4 consecutive days, then 3 days off, repeat weekly), or chlorambucil (dogs, 2–3 mg/m² PO; cats,1.5 mg/m² PO).
• Reduce immunosuppressant drug dosage to lowest possible once remission is achieved.
• For painful joints—aspirin (dogs, 10–25 mg/kg PO q12h; cats, 10–40 mg/kg PO q72h) or carprofen (dogs, 2.2 mg/kg PO q12h)

CONTRAINDICATIONS

Aspirin should not be give to patients with thrombocytopenia or gastrointestinal ulcers.

PRECAUTIONS

• Cats are susceptible to azathioprine toxicity; this drug should be used with caution, if at all (dosage, 1 mg/cat PO q48h).
• Cyclophosphamide can induce hemorrhagic cystitis and bone marrow suppression.
• Treatment with immunosuppressive drugs increases the risk of severe infection.

POSSIBLE INTERACTIONS

Concurrent use of aspirin and prednisone increases the risk of gastrointestinal ulceration.

ALTERNATE DRUGS

Cyclosporin A (5–10 mg/kg PO q12h) may be tried in refractory patients; use with caution and withdraw if side effects occur (e.g., gastritis, lymphocytoid dermatitis, papillomatosis, and gingival hyperplasia).

FOLLOW-UP

PATIENT MONITORING

• Weekly physical examination
• CBC and biochemical analysis to monitor side effects of the immunosuppressive drugs, initially weekly
• ANA remains high during remission and is not useful for monitoring the disease.

PREVENTION/AVOIDANCE

Do not breed affected animals.

POSSIBLE COMPLICATIONS

Renal failure and nephrotic syndrome secondary to glomerulonephritis

EXPECTED COURSE AND PROGNOSIS

• Prognosis guarded to poor
• The presence of hemolytic anemia and glomerulonephritis and the development of bacterial infection warrant a poor prognosis.

MISCELLANEOUS

ASSOCIATED CONDITIONS

None

AGE-RELATED FACTORS

None

ZOONOTIC POTENTIAL

None

PREGNANCY

The use of cytotoxic immunosuppressive drugs in pregnant animals is contraindicated.

SYNONYMS

None

SEE ALSO

• Anemia, Immune-Mediated
• Thrombocytopenia, Primary Immune-Mediated
• Glomerulonephritis
• Polyarthritis, Nonerosive Immune-Mediated

ABBREVIATIONS

• ANA = antinuclear antibody
• FeLV = feline leukemia virus
• LE = lupus erythematosus

Suggested Reading

Lewis RM, Picut CA. Veterinary clinical immunology. Philadelphia: Lea & Febiger, 1989.

Halliwell REW, Gorman NT. Veterinary clinical immunology. Philadelphia: Saunders, 1989.

Pedersen NC, Barlough JE. Systemic lupus erythematosus in the cat. Feline Pract 1991;19:5–13.

Author Harm HogenEsch
Consulting Editor Susan M. Cotter

DISEASES

LUPUS ERYTHEMATOSUS, CUTANEOUS (DISCOID)

 BASICS

OVERVIEW
- Considered to be a benign variant of SLE
- Its comparative nature to the human form is controversial.
- One of the most common immune-mediated skin diseases
- Predominantly involves the planum nasale, face, ears, and mucous membranes; rarely other areas

SIGNALMENT
- Predominantly in dogs; rarely in cats
- Predominant breeds—collies, German shepherds, Siberian huskies, Shetland sheepdogs, Alaskan malamutes, chow chows, and their crosses
- No age predilection

SIGNS
- Usually starts with depigmentation of planum nasale and/or lips
- Depigmentation progresses to erosions and ulcerations.
- Tissue loss and scarring can occur.
- May also involve pinnae and periocular region; rarely feet and genitalia

CAUSES & RISK FACTORS
- Exact mechanism undetermined
- Genetic predisposition likely
- Suspected causes—drug reactions, viral initiation, and UV light exposure
- Seasonal exacerbations—associated with increased photoperiod and UV radiation
- UV exposure is a major concern.

 DIAGNOSIS

DIFFERENTIAL DIAGNOSIS
Major Considerations
- Other immune-mediated diseases—pemphigus foliaceus, pemphigus erythematosus, SLE, and uveodermatologic syndrome
- Drug reactions, erythema multiforme, and toxic epidermal necrolysis—nasal and facial lesions
- Dermatomyositis—affects some of the same predisposed breeds (collies and Shetland sheepdogs)
- Nasal pyoderma and nasal dermatophytosis—infectious conditions; can mimic discoid lupus erythematosus
- Insect hypersensitivity—one form creates a nasal inflammatory disease.

Other (Rare) Considerations
- Contact allergy
- Zinc-responsive dermatosis
- Metabolic epidermal necrosis
- T cell epidermotropic lymphoma—may start on the planum and rostral aspect of the muzzle and lips
- Squamous cell carcinoma—may affect the planum; may occur at a slightly higher incidence in chronic discoid lupus lesions
- Idiopathic leukoderma leukotrichia (vitiligo)—may cause depigmentation of the tissue and hair without concurrent inflammation

CBC/BIOCHEMISTRY/URINALYSIS
Usually normal

OTHER LABORATORY TESTS
ANA, LE preparation, and Coombs tests—usually normal or negative

IMAGING
N/A

OTHER DIAGNOSTIC PROCEDURES
Biopsies of nonulcerated, slate gray depigmented lesions—often characterized by interface lichenoid dermatitis with pigment incontinence and variable degrees of dermal mucin

PATHOLOGIC FINDINGS
Immunopathologic examination of nonulcerated samples preserved in Michel's solution—may reveal positive basal laminal fluorescence

 TREATMENT

- Not life-threatening
- May be disfiguring
- May create a source of trauma-induced bleeding
- Avoid direct solar exposure and use waterproof sunblocks with an SPF > 15.

LUPUS ERYTHEMATOSUS, CUTANEOUS (DISCOID)

 MEDICATIONS

DRUGS
• Tetracycline and niacinamide—250 mg each PO q8h for dogs < 10 kg; 500 mg PO q8h for larger dogs
• Vitamin E—10–20 IU/kg PO q12h; may help reduce inflammation
• Topical corticosteroids—initially, a potent fluorinated product (e.g., 0.1% amcinonide) q24h for 14 days; then q48–72h for 28 days; if in remission switch to less-potent product (e.g., 0.5% or 2.5% hydrocortisone)
• Prednisone—consider for severe or nonresponsive cases; 2–3 mg/kg daily either solely or in combination with azathioprine 2 mg/kg PO on alternate days; taper prednisone to 0.5–1 mg/kg PO q48h for long-term maintenance

CONTRAINDICATIONS/POSSIBLE INTERACTIONS
N/A

 FOLLOW-UP

PATIENT MONITORING
• Recheck 14 days after initiating treatment for clinical response.
• CBC and biochemistry—every 3–6 months if using topical or oral corticosteroids for control
• CBC and platelet counts—every 2 weeks for the first 3–4 months; then every 3–6 months while on azathioprine

PREVENTION/AVOIDANCE
• Avoid using affected animals for breeding.
• Prone animals should avoid sunlight.

POSSIBLE COMPLICATIONS
• Scarring
• Secondary pyoderma
• Bleeding
• Disfigurement

EXPECTED COURSE AND PROGNOSIS
• Progressive but not usually life-threatening if left untreated
• With proper treatment, expect remission in majority of cases.
• The need for chronic immunosuppressive therapy suggests a more guarded prognosis, but remissions are common with more aggressive therapy.

 MISCELLANEOUS

ABBREVIATIONS
• ANA = antinuclear antibody
• LE = lupus erythematosus
• SLE = systemic lupus erythematosus

Suggested Reading
Rosenkrantz WS. Discoid lupus erythematosus: current veterinary dermatology. St. Loius: Mosby, 1993.
Author Wayne S. Rosenkrantz
Consulting Editor Karen Helton Rhodes

DISEASES

LYME DISEASE

BASICS

DEFINITION
• One of the most common tick-transmitted zoonotic diseases in the world
• Caused by the spirochete *Borrelia burgdorferi*
• Dominant clinical feature (dogs)—recurrent acute arthritis with lameness, sometimes with anorexia and depression; may develop cardiac, neurologic, or renal diseases
• Reported in horses, cattle, and cats

PATHOPHYSIOLOGY
• Arthritis—pathogenesis unclear; caused directly by migrating spirochetes
• Local skin infestation after a tick bite is followed by a generalized infection of predominantly connective tissues, joint capsules, muscle, and lymph nodes.
• The incubation period in experimental dogs is 2–5 months.

SYSTEMS AFFECTED
• Persistent *B. burgdorferi*—found in skin, muscle, connective tissues, joints, and lymph nodes; rarely in body fluids (blood, CSF, and synovial fluid)
• Pathologic changes—with few exceptions restricted to joints, local lymph nodes, skin at the tick bite site; in specific cases, glomeruli of the kidney

GENETICS
Genetic basis known for mice; not established for dogs

INCIDENCE/PREVALENCE
• Percentage of seropositive dogs within a population varies greatly with exposure to infected ticks in endemic areas; reported range 5%–80%.
• About 5% of seropositive dogs in endemic areas develop Lyme disease.

GEOGRAPHIC DISTRIBUTION
• Worldwide distribution
• Variation in distribution of endemic areas
• U.S.—northwest > 90% of cases; also upper Mississippi region, California, and some southern states

SIGNALMENT

Species
Dogs and rarely cats

Breed Predilections
None

Mean Age and Range
Young dogs appear to be more susceptible than old dogs.

Sex Predispositions
None

SIGNS
• Recurrent acute arthritis with lameness—characteristic
• Lameness—lasts for only 3–4 days; responds well to antibiotic treatment; when acute, one or more joints may be swollen and warm; a pain response is elicited by palpation.
• Affected dogs may walk stiffly with an arched back and may be sensitive to touch.
• Fever, anorexia, and depression may accompany arthritis.
• Superficial cervical and/or popliteal lymph nodes may be swollen.
• Cardiac—reported but rare; include complete heart block and neurologic complications
• Kidneys—reported glomerulonephritis with immune complex deposition in the glomeruli leading to fatal renal disease; patients may present with renal failure (vomiting, diarrhea, anorexia, weight loss, polyuria/polydipsia, peripheral edema or ascites).

CAUSES
• *B. burgdorferi* or related *Borrelia* sp.—transmitted by the small, hard-shell deer tick *Ixodes scapularis* or related *Ixodes* tick
• Infection—only after tick (nymphal stage in spring or adult female in fall) is partially engorged; 24–48 hr after the initial infestation

Ixodes ticks
• Have a 2-year life cycle
• Larvae—hatch in spring; become infected by feeding on white-footed mice (*Peromyscus leucopus*), which are persistently infected
• Nymphs—larvae molt into nymphs in the spring of the following year; stay infected or become infected by feeding on mice
• Adults—nymphs molt into adults in late fall of the second year; females engorge after mating on deer or other mammals, fall off, and hide under leaves until the following spring, when they each lay about 2000 eggs; males tend to stay on the deer.

RISK FACTORS
• Roaming tick-infested environment in Lyme-endemic area
• Speculated that urine from infected dogs and vectors other than ticks may be sources of infection; little supporting evidence

DIAGNOSIS

DIFFERENTIAL DIAGNOSIS
• Lyme arthritis—differentiate from other inflammatory arthritides
• Infectious agents—Rocky Mountain spotted fever; ehrlichiosis
• Fungal agents—histoplasma; cryptococcus; blastomycosis
• Protozoa—leishmania
• Bacteria—streptococcus; staphylococcus; others
• Immune-mediated diseases—idiopathic, lupus erythematosus, rheumatoid arthritis
• Specific breed diseases—akita arthritis, sharpei fever
• Culture of the joint fluid, serological assays, and immune testing (antinuclear antibodies; lupus erythematosus preparations)—rule out other disorders

CBC/BIOCHEMISTRY/URINALYSIS
• Arthritis only—unremarkable
• With protein-loosing glomerulopathy—uremia, proteinuria, hypercholesterolemia, hyperphosphatemia, and hypoalbuminemia usually occur.

OTHER LABORATORY TESTS
• Fluid from affected joints—high WBC counts
• Positive serology by ELISA and Western blot—indicates previous exposure to *B. burgdorferi;* may indicate disease; ELISA cannot differentiate between sera from vaccinated and from naturally infected dogs but Western blot can; cross-reactions with antibody responses to *Leptospira* spp. minimal

IMAGING
Radiographs—help identify effusions in the joint; may help distinguish erosive from nonerosive joint disease

DIAGNOSTIC PROCEDURES
PCR from skin biopsy specimens—*B. burgdorferi* frequently isolated or demonstrated; time-consuming and expensive (not practical)

PATHOLOGIC FINDINGS

Gross
• Swollen joints with excess synovial fluid
• Sometimes enlarged lymph nodes

Histophatholgy
• Acute arthritis—fibrinopurulent synovitis
• Other joints—may have mild synovitis with infiltration of lymphocytes and plasma cells
• Lymph nodes—may show cortical hyperplasia with multiple enlarged follicles and expanded parafollicular areas

• Skin near tick bite site—may be perivascular infiltrates of plasma cells, lymphocytes, and some mast cells in the superficial dermis
• Renal lesions—glomerulonephritis, diffuse tubular necrosis with regeneration, and interstitial inflammation

TREATMENT

APPROPRIATE HEALTH CARE
Outpatient

NURSING CARE
Keep patient warm and dry.

ACTIVITY
Reduced activity advisable until clinical signs improve

DIET
No change needed

CLIENT EDUCATION
Inform client of importance of regular application of antibiotics as prescribed.

SURGICAL CONSIDERATIONS
Aspiration of synovial fluid—consider for diagnostic purposes

MEDICATIONS

DRUGS OF CHOICE
• Most commonly used antibiotics—doxycycline (10 mg/kg PO q12h) or amoxicillin (20 mg/kg PO q8–12h)
• Antibiotics—do not eliminate persistent infection; significantly improve clinical signs and pathology
• Recommended treatment period—4 weeks

CONTRAINDICATIONS
N/A

PRECAUTIONS
Do not treat young and growing animals with tetracyclines (doxycycline).

POSSIBLE INTERACTIONS
Jarisch-Herxheimer reaction—rare occurrence within the first 3 days of antibiotic treatment reported in humans; not known in animals; toxic byproducts from killed spirochetes may intensify symptoms.

ALTERNATIVE DRUGS
• Corticosteroids—may initially ameliorate signs; mask effects of antibiotics for diagnostic purposes; enhance clinical signs later by immunosuppression
• Pain medications (nonsteroidal)—use judiciously to avoid masking signs

FOLLOW-UP

PATIENT MONITORING
• Improvement—seen within 3 days of antibiotic treatment
• If no improvement—consider a differential diagnosis.

PREVENTION/AVOIDANCE
• Prevent tick engorgement—repellents containing DEET or permethrin; tick collars; groom dogs daily
• Controlling tick population in the environment—restricted to small areas; limited results from reducing deer and/or rodent population
• Vaccine—two commercially available bacterins consisting of killed *B. burgdorferi* in adjuvant; one was shown to reduce the incidence of disease from 4.7% of seropositive dogs to about 1%; value still debated; single protein vaccine (OspA) protects dogs from infection and disease.

POSSIBLE COMPLICATIONS
• Heart block
• CNS disorders
• Fatal renal failure

EXPECTED COURSE AND PROGNOSIS
• Recovery from initial lameness expected 2–3 days after initiation of antibiotic treatment
• Disease may be recurrent with intervals of weeks to months; responds again to antibiotic treatment
• The nonresponsive chronic arthritis seen in humans is not known in dogs.

MISCELLANEOUS

AGE-RELATED FACTORS
• Young pups appear to be more susceptible than old dogs.
• Disease can occur in dogs of all ages; there is no difference in treatment.

ZOONOTIC POTENTIAL
• Occurs in humans; source of infection is ticks.
• Speculated that *B. burgdorferi* in the saliva or urine of affected dogs might be transmissible to humans—experiments have failed to prove this.
• Speculated that dogs can transport ticks home that then become attached to humans—*Ixodid* are not intermittent feeders and attach quickly; once tick starts feeding on a dog, it feeds to repletion and does not change hosts.

PREGNANCY
• Although possible, there is no convincing evidence that *B. burgdorferi* infection is transmitted in utero in dogs.
• Pregnant animals tolerate antibiotic treatment; do not use tetracyclines.

SYNONYMS
• Lyme borreliosis
• Lyme arthritis

ABBREVIATIONS
• CSF = cerebrospinal fluid
• ELISA = enzyme-linked immunosorbent assay
• PCR = polymerase chain reaction

Suggested Reading
Appel MJG, Allan S, Jacobson RH, et al. Experimental Lyme disease in dogs produces arthritis and persistent infection. J Infect Dis 1993;167:651–664.
Dambach DM, Smith CA, Lewis RM, et al. Morphological, immunohistochemical, and ultrastructural characterization of a distinctive renal lesion in dogs putatively associated with *Borrelia burgdorferi* infection: 49 cases (1987–1992). Vet Pathol 1997;34:85–170.
Greene CE, Appel MJG, Straubinger RK. Lyme borreliosis. In: Greene CE, ed. Infectious diseases of the dog and cat. Philadelphia: Saunders, 1998:282–293.
Levy SA, Barthold SW, Daubach DM, et al. Canine Lyme borreliosis. Compend Contin Educ Pract Vet 1993;15:833–848.
Straubinger RK, Summers BA, Chang Y-F, et al. Persistence of *Borrelia burgdorferi* in experimentally infected dogs after antibiotic treatment. J Clin Microbiol 1997;35:111–116.

Author Max J. G. Appel
Consulting Editor Stephen C. Barr

LYMPHADENITIS

 BASICS

DEFINITION
• Inflammation of one or more lymph nodes characterized by active migration of neutrophils, macrophages, or eosinophils into the node
• Lymphoid hyperplasia is not a form of lymphadenitis.

PATHOPHYSIOLOGY
• Usually the result of an infectious agent gaining access to a lymph node and establishing infection; because of the filtration functions of lymph nodes, they are likely to be exposed to infectious agents.
• Many organisms can cause inflammation; but agents such as fungi and mycobacteria that reside within macrophages and elicit a granulomatous inflammatory response are especially prone to establish infection within lymph nodes.
• Noninfectious—occurs infrequently; an example is eosinophilic lymphadenitis that occurs as an occasional component of eosinophilic inflammatory diseases.

SYSTEMS AFFECTED
• Hemic/Lymphatic/Immune
• May be a component of a more widespread infectious disease

GENETICS
• No known genetic basis
• Exception—rare cases of immunodeficiency; e.g., the familial susceptibility of certain basset hounds to mycobacteriosis, of which lymphadenitis is a frequent manifestation

INCIDENCE/PREVALENCE
• Frequent manifestation of a number of infectious diseases
• Precise incidence is unknown.

GEOGRAPHIC DISTRIBUTION
Same as for systemic fungal infections such as histoplasmosis (central U.S.) and blastomycosis (central and eastern U.S.) and, less commonly, leishmaniasis (southern and southwestern U.S.)

SIGNALMENT
Species
Dogs and cats
Breed Predilection
None

Mean Age and Range
Because of their susceptibility to infection, neonates may have a higher rate of occurrence than older animals.
Predominant Sex
None

SIGNS
General Comments
• Complications of infection in another organ—usually relate to that organ rather than to the inflamed lymph node
• Component of systemic infection—associated with systemic inflammatory disease: fever, malaise, and anorexia

Historical Findings
• Seldom causes lymph node enlargement that is severe enough to be observed by owners
• Systemic signs of inflammatory disease or organ dysfunction

Physical Examination Findings
• Inflamed lymph nodes are typically large and firm and may be painful.
• Bacterial—animal may develop abscesses within the nodes that may open to the exterior and present as draining tracts.
• Animals may also have fever and other systemic signs of infection.

CAUSES
Bacteria
• Most pathogenic aerobic and anaerobic species have occasionally been reported.
• More likely agents—*Pasteurella, Bacteroides,* and *Fusobacterium* spp.
• A few, such as *Yersinia pestis* (bubonic plague) and *Francisella tularensis* (tularemia), have a particular affinity for lymph nodes and are especially likely to be manifest as lymphadenitis, especially in cats.

Fungi
• Infections commonly include lymphadenitis as one manifestation of systemic disease.
• Likely organisms include *Blastomyces, Cryptococcus, Histoplasma, Coccidiodes,* and *Sporothrix.*
• Many other mycotic agents have occasionally been reported.

Viruses
• Many viral infections implicated because of lymphoid hyperplasia
• Coronavirus FIP
• Mesenteric lymph nodes are most commonly affected.

Other
• Protozoa—animals with toxoplasmosis and leishmaniasis frequently have lymphadenitis, although it is unlikely to be the most obvious clinical finding.
• Algae—lymphadenitis is often one manifestation of canine prototothecosis.
• Noninfectious (e.g., associated with pulmonary or systemic eosinophilic disease)—usually unknown

RISK FACTORS
• Animals with compromised immune function are susceptible to infection and, therefore, to lymphadenitis.
• FeLV and FIV are among the more common causes of immune compromise in veterinary patients.

 DIAGNOSIS

DIFFERENTIAL DIAGNOSIS
• Must ascertain that a palpable or visible mass is actually a lymph node and not a neoplastic mass or inflammatory process such as sialoadenitis
• Frequently cannot be distinguished on the basis of clinical findings from other causes of lymphadenomegaly, such as lymphoid hyperplasia, lymphoma, and metastatic neoplasia
• Fever and painful lymph nodes are likely to be associated with lymphadenitis.
• Lymphoma and lymphoid hyperplasia are more common causes of generalized lymph node enlargement than is lymphadenitis.

CBC/BIOCHEMISTRY/URINALYSIS
• Although affected animals may have an inflammatory leukogram, the absence of such changes does not exclude the diagnosis.
• Some animals with systemic causes of lymphadenitis (e.g., fungal infections, leishmaniasis) may have marked hyperglobulinemia.
• Circulating eosinophilia, often severe, is a relatively consistent finding in animals with eosinophilic diseases that are extensive and severe enough to cause lymphadenitis.
• Biochemistry results may reflect the degree of organ involvement from the underlying disease process.

OTHER LABORATORY TESTS
Serologic tests for the various systemic fungal diseases can be useful for identification, although these tests are best used only when attempts to demonstrate the organisms fail.

IMAGING
Radiography and ultrasonography—involvement of internal nodes, such as those in the thoracic and abdominal cavities, in patients with systemic inflammatory disease; valuable in assessing involvement of other organs, e.g., pneumonia in a patient with blastomycosis or histoplasmosis

DIAGNOSTIC PROCEDURES
• Fine-needle aspiration cytology is sufficient to diagnose most cases; a simple differential stain (e.g., Diff-Quik) is usually suitable.
• Gram staining can be performed in patients suspected of bacterial infection.
• Cytologic findings—high proportion of neutrophils, macrophages, eosinophils, or some combination of those cell types, which are only rarely seen in normal lymph nodes
• Bacteria, fungal agents, protozoa, and algae—often present in fine-needle aspirates of lymph nodes from animals with those infections; cytologic examination frequently is the most efficient means of detecting and identifying specific infectious agents in animals with either lymphadenitis of an isolated node or systemic infection.
• Eosinophilic lymphadenitis should not be diagnosed by cytologic examination of specimens, unless the proportion of eosinophils is markedly high, because mild eosinophilic infiltrates occur commonly in peripheral nodes of animals with allergic or parasitic skin disease.
• When a diagnosis is not made by cytologic examination, a lymph node biopsy may be indicated; specimens can be used for both histopathologic evaluation and culture.

PATHOLOGIC FINDINGS
• Although affected lymph nodes may be grossly normal, they are more frequently large and firm; the extent of enlargement varies widely and often distorts the shape of the node.
• Severe lymphadenitis may extend through the capsule of the node into adjacent tissues.
• On cut surface, affected nodes are often hyperemic and may have poorly defined nodules; in extreme examples of purulent lymphadenitis, abscesses may develop.
• Histologic lesions of purulent lymphadenitis include diffuse or multifocal infiltration of the affected node by neutrophils; the normal cortical-medullary architecture of the node may be disrupted.
• Granulomatous lymphadenitis—accumulations of activated macrophages involving the parenchyma of the node
• Eosinophilic lymphadenitis—large numbers of eosinophils both within sinuses and in the cortical parenchyma
• Necrosis common in all forms

 TREATMENT

APPROPRIATE HEALTH CARE
• Because lymphadenitis is a lesion rather than a specific disease, no single set of therapeutic recommendations is appropriate.
• The characteristics of the inflammation and the causative agent dictate appropriate treatment.

NURSING CARE
N/A

ACTIVITY
N/A

DIET
N/A

CLIENT EDUCATION
N/A

SURGICAL CONSIDERATIONS
N/A

 MEDICATIONS

DRUGS OF CHOICE
• Effective drug therapy requires identification of the causative agent.
• Purulent lymphadenitis of a single lymph node is likely to be of bacterial cause and can be treated with broad-spectrum systemic antibiotics if no organism is detected on initial cytologic evaluation.

CONTRAINDICATIONS
N/A

PRECAUTIONS
N/A

POSSIBLE INTERACTIONS
N/A

ALTERNATIVE DRUGS
N/A

 FOLLOW-UP

PATIENT MONITORING
N/A

PREVENTION/AVOIDANCE
N/A

POSSIBLE COMPLICATIONS
N/A

EXPECTED COURSE AND PROGNOSIS
N/A

 MISCELLANEOUS

ASSOCIATED CONDITIONS
• Multiple affected lymph nodes—frequently a manifestation of systemic infection that also affects many other organs
• Detection of fungi, protozoa, or algae in any inflamed node should alert one to the possibility of systemic infection by that agent.

AGE-RELATED FACTORS
None

ZOONOTIC POTENTIAL
• Bubonic plague, tularemia, and mycotic organisms present some risk of human infection.
• Specimens from affected animals should be handled cautiously.

PREGNANCY
N/A

SYNONYMS
None

SEE ALSO
See Causes.

ABBREVIATIONS
• FeLV = feline leukemia virus
• FIP = feline infectious peritonitis
• FIV = feline immunodeficiency virus

Suggested Reading
Duncan JR The lymph nodes. In: RL Cowell, RD Tyler, eds. Diagnostic cytology of the dog and cat. Goleta, CA: American Veterinary, 1989:93–98.
Rogers KS, Barton CL, Landis M. Canine and feline lymph nodes. II. Diagnostic evaluation of lymphadenopathy. Compend Contin Ed Pract Vet 15:1493–1503.
Author Kenneth M. Rassnick
Consulting Editor Susan M. Cotter

DISEASES

LYMPHANGIECTASIA

 BASICS

DEFINITION
An obstructive disorder involving the lymphatic system of the gastrointestinal tract, resulting in protein-losing enteropathy

PATHOPHYSIOLOGY
• Lymphatic obstruction results in dilation and rupture of intestinal lacteals with subsequent loss of lymphatic contents (plasma proteins, lymphocytes, and chylomicrons) into the intestinal lumen.
• Although the proteins may be digested and reabsorbed, excessive enteric loss results in hypoproteinemia.
• Hypoproteinemia causes decreased plasma oncotic pressure, leading to edema formation, ascites, and pleural effusion.

SYSTEMS AFFECTED
• Gastrointestinal—diarrhea, ascites
• Respiratory—pleural effusion
• Skin/Exocrine—subcutaneous edema

GENETICS
• Familial tendency for protein-losing enteropathy reported in soft-coated wheaten terriers, basenjis, and lundehunds.
• Mode of inheritance unknown

INCIDENCE/PREVALENCE
Uncommon

GEOGRAPHIC DISTRIBUTION
N/A

SIGNALMENT
Species
Dogs

Breed Predilections
Increased incidence reported in soft-coated Wheaten terriers, Basenjis, Lundehunds, and Yorkshire terriers.

Mean Age and Range
Mean age, 4.9 ± 1.9 years; age range, 2–9 years

Predominant Sex
Increased incidence seen in female soft-coated Wheaten terriers

SIGNS
• Clinical signs are variable.
• Diarrhea—chronic, intermittent, with watery to semisolid consistency
• Ascites
• Subcutaneous edema
• Dyspnea from pleural effusion
• Weight loss
• Flatulence
• Vomiting

CAUSES
Primary or Congenital Lymphangiectasia
• Focal—intestinal lymphatics only
• Diffuse lymphatic abnormalities (e.g., chylothorax, lymphedema, chyloabdomen, thoracic duct obstruction)

Secondary Lymphangiectasia
• Right-sided congestive heart failure
• Constrictive pericarditis
• Budd-Chiari syndrome
• Neoplasia (lymphosarcoma)

RISK FACTORS
N/A

 DIAGNOSIS

DIFFERENTIAL DIAGNOSIS
• Must differentiate from other causes of hypoproteinemia
• Hypoalbuminemia can be caused by decreased hepatic synthesis due to severe hepatic disease.
• Globulins often normal or increased
• Hypoalbuminemia can be caused by glomerulonephritis or amyloidosis; urinalysis should detect proteinuria.
• Acute or chronic blood loss can cause hypoproteinemia.
• A rare cause of hypoproteinemia is inadequate protein intake (i.e., starvation).

CBC/BIOCHEMISTRY/URINALYSIS
• Usually lymphopenia
• Hypoalbuminemia and hypoglobulinemia (panhypoproteinemia)
• Hypocholesterolemia
• Hypocalcemia

OTHER LABORATORY TESTS
• Serum protein electrophoresis—quantitate and identify protein loss
• Gastrointestinal protein loss is characterized by loss of albumin and globulins.
• Liver disease is characterized by low levels of albumin with normal or high globulins; renal disease characteristically causes hypoalbuminemia with normal serum globulins.
• Urine protein:creatinine ratio—rule out proteinuria.
• Serum bile acids (pre- and postprandial)—assess hepatic function.
• Fluid analysis of body cavity effusions—the effusion associated with lymphangiectasia is usually a transudate, but chyloabdomen and chylothorax are occasionally present.

IMAGING
• Survey thoracic and abdominal radiographs—rule out cardiac disease and neoplasia.
• Radiographs—detect or confirm ascites or pleural effusion.
• Cardiac ultrasound—rule out right-sided congestive heart failure.

DIAGNOSTIC PROCEDURES
• An ECG can aid in evaluating the heart and ruling out right-sided congestive heart failure.
• Endoscopy allows mucosal visualization and biopsy.
• Laparotomy allows visualization of dilated intestinal lymphatics and biopsies of intestines (full-thickness) and lymph nodes.

PATHOLOGIC FINDINGS
• Gross findings at laparotomy may include dilated lymphatics that are visible as a weblike network throughout the mesentery and serosal surface.

• May see small yellow-white nodules and foamy granular deposits adjacent to lymphatics
• Histopathology findings include ballooning distortion of villi, caused by markedly dilated lacteals.
• Villi can be edematous; some have a blunted appearance.
• Usually mucosal edema; diffuse or multifocal accumulations of lymphocytes and plasma cells can be identified in the lamina propria.

TREATMENT

APPROPRIATE HEALTH CARE
• Most treated as outpatients
• May need hospitalization for plasma transfusion

NURSING CARE
N/A

ACTIVITY
Normal

DIET
• Long-chain triglycerides stimulate intestinal lymph flow and subsequent protein loss.
• Therapy involves feeding a low-fat diet with ample high-quality protein such as Prescription Diet r/d or w/d (Hill's Pet Products, Topeka, KS) or Eukanuba Restricted-Calorie (The Iams Company, Dayton, OH).
• Feed MCTs to supplement fat and increase the calories.
• Commercial sources of MCTs—MCT oil or Portagen (Mead Johnson, Evansville, IN)
• Supplement with fat-soluble vitamins—A, D, E, and K

CLIENT EDUCATION
Discuss unpredictable nature of prognosis and response to therapy.

SURGICAL CONSIDERATIONS
• When intestinal lymphangiectasia is secondary to an identifiable lymphatic obstruction, consider surgery to relieve the obstruction.
• Pericardiectomy is indicated in cases of constrictive pericarditis.

MEDICATIONS

DRUGS OF CHOICE
• Can use corticosteroids if dietary therapy is unsuccessful
• Oral prednisone is administered at a dose of 1–2 mg/kg q12h; after remission of the disease, adjust the dosage to a lower maintenance level.
• Can administer antibiotics to control secondary bacterial overgrowth
• Tylosin (10–20 mg/kg PO q12h) and metronidazole (10–20 mg/kg PO q12h) have been used.

CONTRAINDICATIONS
N/A

PRECAUTIONS
N/A

POSSIBLE INTERACTIONS
N/A

ALTERNATIVE DRUGS
N/A

FOLLOW-UP

PATIENT MONITORING
Body weight, serum protein concentration, and evidence of recurrent clinical signs (pleural effusion, ascites, and/or edema) every 7–14 days

PREVENTION/AVOIDANCE
N/A

POSSIBLE COMPLICATIONS
• Respiratory difficulty from pleural effusion
• Severe protein-calorie depletion
• Intractable diarrhea

EXPECTED COURSE AND PROGNOSIS
• Prognosis guarded
• Some animals fail to respond to treatment.
• Remissions of several months to more than 2 years can be maintained in some patients.

MISCELLANEOUS

ASSOCIATED CONDITIONS
Soft-coated Wheaten terriers may also have protein-losing nephropathy.

AGE-RELATED FACTORS
N/A

ZOONOTIC POTENTIAL
N/A

PREGNANCY
N/A

SYNONYMS
N/A

SEE ALSO
Protein-losing Enteropathy

ABBREVIATION
MCTs = medium-chain triglycerides

Suggested Reading
Davies C, Leib MS. Endoscopy case of the month. Vet Med 1996;91:422–434.
Fossum TW. Protein-losing enteropathy. Semin Vet Med Surg (Sm Anim) 1989;4:219–225.
Fossum TW, Sherding RG, Zack PM, et al. Intestinal lymphangiectasia associated with chylothorax in two dogs. J Am Vet Med Assoc 1987;190:61–64.
Suter MM, Palmer DG, Schenk H. Primary intestinal lymphangiectasia in three dogs: a morphological and immunopathological investigation. Vet Pathol 1985;22:123–130.
Tams TR, Twedt DC. Canine protein-losing gastroenteropathy syndrome. Compend Contin Educ Pract Vet 1981;3:105–114.
Author Mollyann Holland
Consulting Editors Brett M. Feder and Mitchell A. Crystal

LYMPHEDEMA

BASICS

OVERVIEW
• Abnormal accumulation of protein-rich lymph fluid into interstitial spaces, especially subcutaneous fat
• Chronic lymphedema causes tissue fibrosis.
• May be congenital or acquired

SIGNALMENT
• More common in dogs than cats
• Congenital in bulldogs and hereditary/congenital in a family of poodles; possible breed predilection in Labrador retrievers and Old English sheepdogs

SIGNS

Historical Findings
• Primary/congenital—usually peripheral limb swelling at birth or develops in first several months
• Typically starts at distal extremity and slowly advances proximally

Physical Examination Findings
• Most common in limbs, especially pelvic limbs; may be unilateral or bilateral
• Less common in ventral thorax, abdomen, ears, and tail
• Pitting, nonpainful; temperature of affected area is normal.
• Pitting quality lost with chronicity as fibrosis occurs
• Lameness and pain uncommon unless cellulitis develops

CAUSES & RISK FACTORS
• Hereditary/congenital malformation of the lymphatic system—aplasia, valvular incompetence, and lymph node fibrosis
• Excessive interstitial fluid production secondary to venous hypertension (associated with congestive heart failure and obstruction of venous drainage) or increased vascular permeability (associated with infection, trauma, heat, and irradiation)
• Secondary damage to lymphatic vessels or lymph nodes—associated with trauma, infection, and neoplasia

DIAGNOSIS

DIFFERENTIAL DIAGNOSIS
• Edema caused by venous stasis (e.g., congestive heart failure and cirrhosis); look for varices, hyperpigmentation, and ulceration
• Arteriovenous fistulae—listen for machinery murmur; feel for pulsatile vessels; confirm with angiogram
• Edema caused by hypoproteinemia—protein-losing nephropathy or enteropathy, hepatic failure, serum loss from burns or hemorrhage; check serum protein concentration
• Trauma—review history; look for bruising and lacerations
• Neoplasia—if swelling firm, obtain aspirate for cytologic examination
• Cellulitis—look for fever, pain, and warm swelling

CBC/BIOCHEMSITRY/URINALYSIS
Results normal

OTHER LABORATORY TESTS N/A

IMAGING
Lymphography useful in documenting abnormalities within the lymphatic system; best results obtained with an injection of water-based contrast media directly into a lymphatic vessel. See references for detailed description of the technique.

DIAGNOSTIC PROCEDURES
N/A

TREATMENT

• No curative therapy—a number of surgical and medical treatments may be tried.
• Rest and massage of the affected limbs—does not help
• Conservative care—long-term use of pressure wraps, coupled with skin care and use of antibiotics to treat cellulitis and lymphangitis; may be successful in some patients
• Surgical procedures—can be attempted when conservative care and medications fail; lymphangioplasty, bridging techniques, lymphaticovenous shunts, superficial and deep lymphatic anastomosis, and excisional procedures; none is consistently beneficial, and only excisional procedures reported in dogs
• In humans—microwave heating of affected areas appears beneficial and adds to the effect of benzopyrones (see Drugs)
• Diets severely restricted in long-chain triglycerides are being investigated in humans.

MEDICATIONS

DRUGS
• Benzopyrones reduce high-protein edema by stimulating macrophages to release proteases; beneficial effects recorded in experimental studies in dogs. Rutin 50 mg/kg PO q8h may benefit. A recent study in humans showed combined usage of oral and topical benzopyrones to be more effective than either alone.
• Diuretics, steroids, anticoagulants, and fibrinolytic agents have been used, but no confirmed benefit

CONTRAINDICATIONS/POSSIBLE INTERACTIONS
Diuretics—initially reduce swelling but increase protein content of interstitial fluid, resulting in further tissue damage and fibrosis.

FOLLOW-UP

• Puppies with severe lymphedema may die.
• Resolution seen in some puppies with pelvic limb involvement only

MISCELLANEOUS

Suggested Reading
Fossum TW, King LA, Miller MW, et al. Lymphedema: clinical signs, diagnosis, and treatment. J Vet Int Med 1992;6:312–319.
Fossum TW, Miller MW. Lymphedema: etiopathogenesis. J Vet Int Med 1992;6:283–293.
Author Francis W. K. Smith, Jr.
Consulting Editors Larry P. Tilley and Francis W. K. Smith, Jr.

BASICS

OVERVIEW
• Rare pulmonary disease of dogs characterized by angiocentric and angiodestructive infiltration by atypical lymphoid cells
• Not a granulomatous disease as previously reported

SIGNALMENT
• Dogs
• Median age—5.75 years (range, 1.5–14 years)
• No breed predilection, but more common in large breeds and pure breeds

SIGNS
• Progressive respiratory signs including cough and dyspnea
• Exercise intolerance
• Weight loss
• Anorexia
• Fever in 50% of patients
• Duration—days to weeks

CAUSES & RISK FACTORS
Unknown

DIAGNOSIS

DIFFERENTIAL DIAGNOSIS
• Mycotic, bacterial, or aspiration pneumonia
• Primary or metastatic pulmonary neoplasia

CBC/BIOCHEMISTRY/URINALYSIS
• Neutrophilic leukocytosis common
• Eosinophilia common
• Basophilia common

OTHER LABORATORY TESTS
N/A

IMAGING
• Radiography—reveals lobar pulmonary consolidation (e.g., mass lesions), hilar lymphadenomegaly, and pleural effusion
• Lesions—unilateral or bilateral

DIAGNOSTIC PROCEDURES
Biopsy—for definitive diagnosis

PATHOLOGIC FINDINGS
• Histologic—characterized by pleomorphic, angioinvasive mononuclear cells that often cause vascular obliteration
• Cytologic—may appear as sterile eosinophilic and neutrophilic inflammation with reactive macrophages

TREATMENT
Cytotoxic drugs combined with surgical excision when appropriate

MEDICATIONS

DRUGS
Combination protocol—COP suitable for lymphosarcoma

CONTRAINDICATIONS/POSSIBLE INTERACTIONS
• Myelosuppression—caused by cytotoxic drugs
• Hemorrhagic cystitis—caused by cyclophosphamide

FOLLOW-UP

PATIENT MONITORING
Same as for lymphosarcoma treated by chemotherapy

POSSIBLE COMPLICATIONS
• Dyspnea as disease progresses
• Depression
• Anorexia
• Myelosuppression caused by chemotherapy

EXPECTED COURSE AND PROGNOSIS
Median survival with COP chemotherapy—12.5 months (range, days to 4 years)

MISCELLANEOUS

ASSOCIATED CONDITIONS
May progress to lymphosarcoma

SYNONYMS
• Eosinophilic pulmonary granulomatosis
• Lymphoid granulomatosis
• Lymphoproliferative angiitis
• Granulomatosis

ABBREVIATION
COP = cyclophosphamide, vincristine (Oncovin), and prednisone

Suggested Reading
Berry CR, Moore PF, Thomas WP, et al. Pulmonary lymphomatoid granulomatosis in seven dogs (1976–1987). J Vet Intern Med 1990;4:157–166.
Morrison WB. Tumors of uncertain origin. In: Morrison WB, ed. Cancer in dogs and cats: medical and surgical management. Baltimore: Williams & Wilkins, 1998: 779–784.
Author Wallace B. Morrison
Consulting Editor Wallace B. Morrison

LYMPHOSARCOMA—CATS

BASICS

DEFINITION
Malignant transformation of lymphocytes that reside mainly in lymphoid tissues

PATHOPHYSIOLOGY
Depends on the organs involved

SYSTEMS AFFECTED
• Hemic/Lymphatic/Immune
• Gastrointestinal
• Renal/Urologic
• Ophthalmic
• Nervous
• Skin/Exocrine

GENETICS
N/A

INCIDENCE/PREVALENCE
• About 90% of hematopoietic tumors and 33% of all tumors in cats
• Prevalence—41.6–200 per 100,000 cats

GEOGRAPHIC DISTRIBUTION
• On the East Coast (U.S.)—mediastinal lymphosarcoma most common (40%–52% of all patients)
• On the West Coast (U.S.)—alimentary lymphosarcoma most common (36% of all patients)

SIGNALMENT

Species
Cats

Breed Predilections
None

Mean Age and Range
• Mean age of FeLV-positive cats—3 years
• Mean age of FeLV-negative cats—7 years
• Median age of cats with localized extranodal lymphosarcoma—13 years

Predominant Sex
None

SIGNS

General Comments
• Depend on anatomic form

Historical Findings
• Mediastinal form—open-mouthed breathing; coughing; regurgitation; anorexia; weight loss
• Alimentary form—anorexia; weight loss; lethargy; vomiting; constipation; diarrhea; melena; frank blood in the stool
• Renal form—consistent with renal failure (e.g., vomiting, anorexia, polydipsia, polyuria, and lethargy)
• Multicentric form—possibly none in early stages; anorexia, weight loss, and depression with progression of disease
• Solitary form—depends on location; nasal lymphosarcoma: usually sneezing, nasal discharge, and occasionally facial deformity; spinal cord lymphosarcoma: quickly progressing posterior paresis may be seen; cutaneous lymphosarcoma: pruritic, hemorrhagic, or alopecic dermal masses may be seen

Physical Examination Findings
• Mediastinal form—noncompressible cranial thorax
• Alimentary form—thickened intestines or abdominal masses
• Renal form—large, irregular kidneys
• Multicentric form—generalized lymphadenomegaly
• All forms—fever; dehydration; depression; cachexia in some patients

CAUSES
FeLV—cause; patients inconsistently test positive during illness (e.g., 85% with mediastinal, 45% with renal, 20% with multicentric, and 15% with alimentary)

RISK FACTORS
FeLV exposure

DIAGNOSIS

DIFFERENTIAL DIAGNOSIS
• Mediastinal form—congestive heart failure; cardiomyopathy; chylothorax; pyothorax; hemothorax; pneumothorax; diaphragmatic hernia; allergic lung disease; thymoma; ectopic thyroid carcinoma; pleural carcinomatosis; acetaminophen toxicity
• Alimentary form—foreign body ingestion; intestinal ulceration; intestinal fungal infection; inflammatory bowel disease; intussusception; lymphangiectasia; other gastrointestinal tumor
• Renal form—pyelonephritis; amyloidosis; glomerulonephritis; chronic renal failure
• Multicentric form—systemic mycotic infection; immune-mediated disease; toxoplasmosis; lymphoid hyperplasia; hypersensitivity reaction

CBC/BIOCHEMISTRY/URINALYSIS
• May see anemia, leukocytosis, and lymphoblastosis
• May find high creatinine, high serum urea nitrogen, high hepatic enzyme activity, hypercalcemia (rare), and monoclonal gammopathy
• May see isosthenuria, bilirubinuria, and proteinuria

OTHER LABORATORY TESTS
FeLV testing

IMAGING
• Thoracic radiography—evaluate for a mediastinal mass, pleural effusion, abnormal pulmonary parenchymal patterns (rare), and perihilar or retrosternal lymphadenomegaly
• Abdominal radiography—detect masses, hepatomegaly, splenomegaly, mesenteric or ileac (sublumbar) lymphadenomegaly, and unilateral or bilateral renomegaly
• Abdominal ultrasonography—reveal diffuse echotexture changes in the liver, spleen, and kidneys and focal thickening of the intestines

DIAGNOSTIC PROCEDURES
• Examination of bone marrow aspirate or core biopsy—evaluate bone marrow reserves
• Cytologic examination of a mass or lymph node
• Biopsy of a mass or lymph node

PATHOLOGIC FINDINGS
• Gross—likely to be white to gray in color with areas of hemorrhage and necrosis
• Cytologic—monomorphic population of pleomorphic lymphoid cells, sometimes with prominent, multiple nucleoli and coarse nuclear chromatin
• Histopathologic—vary; several morphologic classification schemes in use

TREATMENT

APPROPRIATE HEALTH CARE
Outpatient whenever possible

NURSING CARE
N/A

ACTIVITY
Normal

DIET
No change

CLIENT EDUCATION
• Warn client that a cure is possible but not likely.
• Inform client that the goal is to induce remission and achieve a good quality of life for patients for as long as possible.

SURGICAL CONSIDERATIONS
• To relieve intestinal obstructions and remove solitary masses
• To obtain specimens for histopathologic examination

 MEDICATIONS

DRUGS OF CHOICE
• Chemotherapy—used in a combination or sequential protocol; some protocols have induction and maintenance periods.
• Induction for combination chemotherapy—vincristine (0.5 mg/m^2 IV once weekly), cyclophosphamide (50 mg/m^2 PO q48h), cytosine arabinoside (100 mg/m^2 SC days 1 and 2), and prednisone (40 mg/m^2 q24h for 1 week; then 20 mg/m^2 PO q48h); use for 6 weeks.
• Maintenance for combination chemotherapy—methotrexate (2.5 mg/m^2 PO 3 times a week), chlorambucil (20 mg/m^2 PO every 2 weeks), prednisone (20 mg/m^2 PO q48h), and vincristine (0.5 mg/m^2 IV every 4 weeks)
• Relapsing lymphoma—doxorubicin, vinblastine, actinomycin-D, mitoxantrone, nitrogen mustard, and procarbazine
• Radiotherapy—may be used for localized lymphoma; relapses outside the radiation field are not uncommon.

CONTRAINDICATIONS
None

PRECAUTIONS
• Myelosuppression secondary to chemotherapy—more common than average in FeLV-positive cats
• Seek advice before initiating treatment if you are unfamiliar with cytotoxic drugs.

POSSIBLE INTERACTIONS
None

ALTERNATIVE DRUGS
• Sequential chemotherapy—week 1: vincristine (0.025 mg/kg IV), L-asparaginase (400 IU/kg IM), and prednisone (2 mg/kg PO divided twice a day); week 2: cyclophosphamide (10 mg/kg IV); week 3: vincristine (0.025 mg/kg IV); week 4: methotrexate (0.8 mg/kg IV); then repeat the cycle; maintenance: lengthen the time between each treatment.
• Prednisone alone—temporary palliation

 FOLLOW-UP

PATIENT MONITORING
• Physical examination, CBC, and platelet count—before each weekly cycle
• Radiography—as necessary

PREVENTION/AVOIDANCE
Avoid exposure to or breeding FeLV-positive cats.

POSSIBLE COMPLICATIONS
• Leukopenia
• Sepsis

EXPECTED COURSE AND PROGNOSIS
• Depends on initial response to chemotherapy, anatomic type, FeLV status, and tumor burden
• Mean survival with complete remission—7 months
• Median survival with partial remission—2.5 months
• Median survival with no response to treatment—1.5 months
• Mediastinal—about 10% of patients with live > 2 years
• Median survival with alimentary form—8 months
• Median survival with peripheral multicentric form—23.5 months
• Median survival with renal form—FeLV-negative, 11.5 months; FeLV-positive, 6.5
• Median survival with lymphosarcoma—FeLV-negative, 7 months; FeLV-positive, 3.5 months
• Median survival with a low tumor burden—FeLV-negative, 17.5 months; FeLV-positive, 4 months
• Treated with prednisone alone—patients live 1.5–2 months.
• Median duration of complete remission from localized lymphosarcoma—114 weeks

 MISCELLANEOUS

ASSOCIATED CONDITIONS
• Hypoglycemia (rare)
• Monoclonal gammopathy (rare)
• Hypercalcemia (rare)

AGE-RELATED FACTORS
• Young cats with lymphosarcoma are generally FeLV-positive.

ZOONOTIC POTENTIAL
None

PREGNANCY
Do not use chemotherapy in pregnant animals.

SYNONYMS
• Lymphoma
• Malignant lymphoma

ABBREVIATION
FeLV = feline leukemia virus

Suggested Reading

Elmslie RE, Ogilive GK, Gillette EL, et al. Radiotherapy with and without chemotherapy for localized lymphoma in 10 cats. Vet Radiol 1991;32:277–280.

Jeglum KA, Whereat A, Young KA. Chemotherapy of lymphoma in 75 cats. J Am Vet Med Assoc 1987;190:174–178.

Mooney SC, Hayes AA, MacEwen EG, et al. Treatment and prognostic factors in lymphoma in cats: 103 cases (1977–1981). J Am Vet Med Assoc 1989;194:696–699.

Mooney SC, Hayes AA, Matus RE, et al. Renal lymphoma in cats: 28 cases (1977–1984). J Am Vet Med Assoc 1987;191:1473–1477.

Vonderhaar MA, Morrison WB. Lymphosarcoma. In: Morrison WB, ed. Cancer in dogs and cats: medical and surgical management. Baltimore: Williams & Wilkins, 1998:667–695.

Author Terrance A. Hamilton
Consulting Editor Wallace B. Morrison

DISEASES

LYMPHOSARCOMA—DOGS

 BASICS

DEFINITION
Clonal proliferation of neoplastic lymphocytes in solid tissues, primarily in lymph nodes, bone marrow, and visceral organs

PATHOPHYSIOLOGY
• Usually unifocal in origin with follicle-associated B lymphocytes that retain growth characteristics and the ability to migrate
• Ease of migration may account for spread of clinical disease.
• T lymphocyte lymphosarcoma—usually epitheliotropic (cutaneous) or mediastinal
• Clonal proliferation and high growth fraction may account for sudden onset of clinical signs.

SYSTEMS AFFECTED
• Hemic/Lymphatic/Immune—generalized, often peripheral, lymphadenomegaly with or without splenic, hepatic, and or bone marrow involvement and circulating malignant lymphocytes
• Gastrointestinal—infiltration of stomach, intestines, and associated lymph nodes
• Respiratory—proliferation of neoplastic lymphocytes in mediastinal lymph nodes, thymus, or lung parenchyma
• Miscellaneous (extranodal)—proliferation of or invasion by neoplastic lymphocytes in the bone marrow and ocular, cutaneous, mucocutaneous, neural, renal, cardiac, and other tissues

GENETICS
No consistent documentation of genetic basis

INCIDENCE/PREVALENCE
Reported as 6–30 per 100,000 dogs per year

GEOGRAPHIC DISTRIBUTION
N/A

SIGNALMENT

Species
Dogs

Breed Predilections
• Boxers, basset hounds, golden retrievers, Saint Bernards, Scottish terriers, Airedale terriers, and bulldogs—reported high-risk breeds
• Dachshunds and Pomeranians—reported low-risk breeds

Mean Age and Range
Patients usually 5–10 years old

Predominant Sex
None

SIGNS

General Comments
Depend on anatomic form and stage of disease

Historical Findings
• All forms of malignant lymphoma—nonspecific; anorexia; lethargy; weight loss
• Multicentric—generalized, painless lymphadenomegaly most common; may note distended abdomen secondary to hepatomegaly, splenomegaly, or ascites
• Gastrointestinal—vomiting; diarrhea; anorexia; abdominal discomfort
• Mediastinal—coughing; difficulty swallowing; anorexia; drooling; labored breathing; exercise intolerance secondary to mass(es) and/or effusion
• Extranodal—vary with the anatomic site; ocular: photophobia and conjunctivitis; CNS: seizures; cutaneous: plaque-like lesion; renal: lumbar pain; cardiac: exercise intolerance or syncope

Physical Examination Findings
• Multicentric—generalized, painless, irregular, movable, large lymph node(s) with or without hepatosplenomegaly
• Gastrointestinal—marked weight loss or palpable abdominal mass; thickened gut loops; rectal mucosal irregularities
• Mediastinal—dyspnea; tachypnea; muffled heart sounds secondary to pleural effusion
• Extranodal—ocular: anterior uveitis, retinal hemorrhages, and hyphema; cutaneous: raised plaque; neural: dementia, seizures, and paralysis; renal: renomegaly and renal failure; cardiac: arrhythmias

CAUSES
No specific cause proven

RISK FACTORS
N/A

 DIAGNOSIS

DIFFERENTIAL DIAGNOSIS
• Infectious, neoplastic, immune-mediated, and inflammatory disease
• Cytologic and histologic evaluation and complete staging—differentiate from other diseases

CBC/BIOCHEMISTRY/URINALYSIS
• Anemia, lymphocytosis, lymphopenia, neutrophilia, monocytosis, circulating blasts, and thrombocytopenia common
• High ALT or ALP activity and hypercalcemia common
• Urinalysis usually normal

OTHER LABORATORY TESTS
N/A

IMAGING
• Thoracic radiography—may reveal sternal or tracheobronchial lymphadenomegaly, widened mediastinum, pulmonary densities, and pleural effusion
• Abdominal radiography—may reveal sublumbar or mesenteric lymphadenomegaly, intestinal mass, abdominal effusions, and hepato(spleno)megaly
• Ultrasonography—lymphadenomegaly (obscured by effusion on radiographs) or nodules in visceral organs
• ECHO—evaluate cardiac contractility before doxorubicin administration

DIAGNOSTIC PROCEDURES
• Examine bone marrow aspirate and core biopsy—identify the extent of disease, which affects the chemotherapy choices
• CSF tap—if patient has CNS signs
• ECG—identify arrhythmias before doxorubicin administration

PATHOLOGIC FINDINGS
• Cut section—homogenous, white masses with areas of necrosis
• Monomorphic population of discrete round neoplastic cells that efface and replace parenchyma of lymph nodes and visceral organs or bone marrow

 TREATMENT

APPROPRIATE HEALTH CARE
• Inpatient—intravenous chemotherapy
• Outpatient—after remission, some protocols allow owner to administer drugs orally at home; instruct owner to wear latex gloves when administering these drugs.
• Radiotherapy—may be used to treat refractory lymph nodes, large mediastinal involvement, and solitary cutaneous areas

NURSING CARE
• Fluid therapy—may benefit patients with advanced disease; may benefit clinically ill and dehydrated patients
• Thoracocentesis or abdominocentesis—recommended with marked pleural or abdominal effusion

ACTIVITY
Restrict in patients with low WBC or platelet count

DIET
N/A

CLIENT EDUCATION
• Warn client that chemotherapy is rarely curative and relapse usually occurs.
• Inform client that the side effects of chemotherapy drugs depend on the type used but are usually associated with the gastrointestinal tract and bone marrow.
• Advise client that most dogs have leukopenia by day 7–10.
• Inform client that there is a 70%–80% response rate to most chemotherapy protocols.
• Note that the quality of life is good while the patient is receiving chemotherapy and

while it is in remission; add that some protocols are associated with serious morbidity, whereas others have little morbidity.

SURGICAL CONSIDERATIONS
Rarely successful unless limited to one accessible site

MEDICATIONS

DRUGS OF CHOICE
• Combination chemotherapy—many protocols exist with similar remission and survival times
• Single-agent therapy (doxorubicin)—associated with remission and survival times that are similar to those for combination chemotherapy
• Corticosteroids alone—effective in the short term (1–2 months)
• Retinoids—may be used for cutaneous lymphosarcoma (3–4 mg/kg isotretinoin PO q24h)

Doxorubicin Protocol
Administer 30 mg/m² IV every 21 days (1 mg/kg for dog < 10 kg) for 3–5 treatments past complete remission (4–6 total treatments)

Combination Chemotherapy Protocol I
Induction
• Vincristine—0.5 mg/m² IV; day 1
• Cyclophosphamide—50 mg/m² PO; days 4–7
• Prednisone—20 mg/m² PO q12h
• Repeat weekly for 6 weeks; then begin maintenance
Maintenance
• Methotrexate—5.0 mg/m² PO; days 1 and 5
• Cyclophosphamide—100 mg/m² PO; day 3
• Prednisone—20 mg/m² q48h
• Continue for 6 weeks; then administer 1 week of induction; then 6 weeks of maintenance
• Continue for 1 year or until relapse

Combination Chemotherapy Protocol II (COPLA)
Induction
• L-asparaginase—10,000 units/m² SC; day 1 of weeks 1 and 2
• Vincristine—0.5–0.7 mg/m² IV; day 1 of weeks 1–8
• Cyclophosphamide—50 mg/m² PO q48h
• Prednisone—20 mg/m² PO q24h for 7 days; then q48h for 2–5 weeks; then 10 mg/m² PO q48h for 6 weeks; then stop
• Doxorubicin—30 mg/m² IV (1 mg/kg for dog < 10 kg); day 1 of weeks 6, 9, and 12
Maintenance
• Vincristine—0.5–0.7 mg/m² IV; day 1 every other week for 2 times; then day 1 every third week for 3 times; then day 1 every

fourth week for 4 times; then day 1 every sixth week for 1 year
• Chlorambucil—4 mg/m² PO q48h for up to 2 years, starting on day 1 of week 1 and continuing for up to 2 years if remission is maintained

CONTRAINDICATIONS
N/A

PRECAUTIONS
• Doxorubicin—use cautiously or not at all with poor cardiac contractility or arrhythmias; use cautiously in patients with > 80% of bone marrow replaced by cancer cells.
• L-asparaginase or doxorubicin—pretreat with diphenhydramine (1 mg/kg SC) 20 min before administration
• Always use a catheter when administering intravenous drugs.

POSSIBLE INTERACTIONS
All chemotherapy drugs must be given according to published protocols, because many have overlapping side effects.

ALTERNATIVE DRUGS
• Many alternative treatment protocols exist
• Lomustine (CCNU) or dacarbazine (DTIC)—may use for refractory cases

FOLLOW-UP

PATIENT MONITORING
• Physical examination and cytologic or histologic evaluation—all nonresponsive lymph nodes
• CBC and platelet count—(1) on day 10 after first treatment; if severe leukopenia or neutropenia (WBC < 2000 cells/mm³; neutrophils < 1000 cells/mm³) is noted, reduce dosage (15%–25%) or add colony-stimulating factors to the protocol; (2) before each anthracycline chemotherapy or weekly (on day 1) with combination chemotherapy; if moderate or severe leukopenia (WBC < 4000 cells/mm³) is noted, delay treatment until cell counts return to normal (usually 1 week).
• After 2–3 courses of chemotherapy treatments, repeat tests with abnormal results before administering next treatment to confirm response.
• Echocardiography and ECG—periodically during and after doxorubicin administration to identify development of cardiotoxicity

PREVENTION/AVOIDANCE
N/A

POSSIBLE COMPLICATIONS
• Leukopenia and neutropenia
• Vomiting and diarrhea
• Anorexia
• Cardiotoxicity—owing to doxorubicin; usually after total cumulative dose of 180–240 mg/m²

• Alopecia
• Pancreatitis
• Sepsis
• Tissue sloughing—with extravasated dose

EXPECTED COURSE AND PROGNOSIS
• Median duration of first remission with combination chemotherapy or doxorubicin—6 months (range, 45–334 days); 58%–90% of patients achieve complete remission.
• Median survival time with combination chemotherapy or doxorubicin—6–12 months (range, 112–365 days)
• Mediastinal form and/or hypercalcemia—poorer prognosis
• Primary CNS, diffuse gastrointestinal, and multisite cutaneous forms—associated with poor response to treatment

MISCELLANEOUS

ASSOCIATED CONDITIONS
None

AGE-RELATED FACTORS
None

ZOONOTIC POTENTIAL
None

PREGNANCY
Treatment of pregnant dogs is contraindicated.

SYNONYMS
• Lymphoma • Malignant lymphoma

SEE ALSO
• Leukemia, Chronic Lymphocytic • Leukemia, Acute Lymphoblastic • Calcium, Hypercalcemia

ABBREVIATIONS
• ALP = alkaline phosphatase • ALT = alanine aminotransferase • CCNU = chloroethylcyclohexylnitrosourea • COPLA = cyclophosphamide, vincristine (Oncovin), prednisone, and L-asparaginase • DTIC = (dimethyltriazeno)imidazole carboxamide • CSF = cerebrospinal fluid

Suggested Reading
Keller E, MacEwen E, Rosenthal R, et al. Evaluation of prognostic factors and sequential combination chemotherapy for canine lymphoma. J Vet Intern Med 1993;7;289–295.

Teske E. Canine malignant lymphosarcoma: a review and comparison with human non-Hodgkin's lymphosarcoma. Vet Q 1994;4:209–219.

Vonderhaar MA, Morrison WB. Lymphosarcoma. In: Morrison WB, ed. Cancer in dogs and cats: medical and surgical management. Baltimore: Williams & Wilkins, 1998: 667–695.

Author Mary Ann Vonderhaar
Consulting Editor Wallace B. Morrison

DISEASES

LYMPHOSARCOMA (LYMPHOMA), EPIDERMOTROPIC

 BASICS

OVERVIEW
- A subset of cutaneous T cell lymphosarcoma
- An uncommon malignant neoplasia affecting many species, including dogs and cats
- Mycosis fungoides and Sézary syndrome (mycosis fungoides with associated leukemia)—most common forms of cutaneous T cell lymphosarcoma
- Pagetoid reticulosis—rare; the lymphoid infiltrate is generally confined to the epidermis in the early stages of the disease.

SIGNALMENT
- More common in dogs than in cats
- Affects old dogs and cats; mean age 9–12 years
- No apparent breed or sex predilection

SIGNS

Historical Findings
- Chronic skin disease—months to years before diagnosis
- Erythema
- Depigmentation
- Scaling
- Alopecia
- Sometimes pruritus

Physical Examination Findings
- Erythema
- Scaling
- Depigmentation
- Alopecia
- Infiltrative plaques
- Ulceration
- Crusting
- Multiple nodules or mass formation
- Pruritus
- Lesions—throughout the skin; marked tendency for involvement of mucocutaneous junctions (lip, eyelids, nasal planum, anorectal junction, or vulva) or the oral cavity (gingiva, palate, or tongue)
- Usually three principal phases—patch, plaque, and tumor; progression to the tumor stage is very rapid in dogs (compared to humans); may also occur in tumor stage from the onset (tumor d'emblee form)

CAUSES & RISK FACTORS
None identified

 DIAGNOSIS

DIFFERENTIAL DIAGNOSIS
- Dermatophytosis, demodicosis—alopecia, erythema, scaling
- Allergies, scabies—generalized pruritus, erythema, scaling
- Cutaneous lupus erythematosus, erythema multiforme, other immune-mediated diseases—mucocutaneous depigmentation/ulceration
- Nonneoplastic chronic stomatitis—infiltrative and ulcerative oral mucosal disease
- Histiocytoma, cutaneous histiocytosis, mast cell tumor, or any other cutaneous neoplasia—nodule or mass formation

CBC/BIOCHEMISTRY/URINALYSIS
- Laboratory abnormalities—vary, depending on the stage and form of cutaneous T cell lymphosarcoma (mycosis fungoides vs. Sézary syndrome)
- Generally not helpful in the early stages

OTHER LABORATORY TESTS
N/A

IMAGING
Radiographs and ultrasound—not commonly used in the early stages; imaging is eventually necessary to confirm system disease and/or for tumor staging.

DIAGNOSTIC PROCEDURES
- Skin scrapings and fungal culture—rule out demodicosis and dermatophytosis, if applicable.
- Skin biopsy—definitive diagnosis

PATHOLOGIC FINDINGS
- Lymphoid infiltrate—into epidermis and epithelium of hair follicles and adnexal structures; distributed diffusely or as discrete Pautrier microaggregates within the epithelium
- Dermal infiltrate—polymorphous; also consists of malignant lymphocytes that obscure the dermoepidermal junction; in the patch and plaque stages, limited to the superficial dermis; in the tumor stage, extends to the deep dermis and subcutis
- Lymphocyte epitheliotropism—usually remains prominent throughout all stages

 TREATMENT

- Inform the client that a cure is extremely unlikely.
- The goal is to maintain a good quality of life for as long as possible.
- Therapy is usually of little benefit; rarely, solitary nodules can be surgically excised, resulting in long-term remissions or "cures."

LYMPHOSARCOMA (LYMPHOMA), EPIDERMOTROPIC

MEDICATIONS

DRUGS
• Chemotherapy—several protocols used with limited to no success, including various combinations of prednisolone, chlorambucil, vincristine, cyclophosphamide, doxorubicin, and methotrexate
• Topical chemotherapy—mechlorethamine (nitrogen mustard) has resulted in some success in managing early lesions; it has not been shown to alter the fatal course of the disease.
• α-Interferon, retinoids, extracorporeal photophoresis, and anti–T cell monoclonal antibodies—recently investigated in therapeutic trials with variable results

CONTRAINDICATIONS/POSSIBLE INTERACTIONS
• Depend on the chemotherapeutic or treatment protocol
• Seek advice from a veterinary oncologist or dermatologist before initiating therapy if you are unfamiliar with cytotoxic drugs and/or to learn about the most recent treatment protocols.

FOLLOW-UP
• Prognosis grave
• Average survival time for dogs, from the onset of skin lesions to death, is 5–10 months
• Death is usually the result of euthanasia.
• Rarely, dogs and cats may live for longer than 2 years after the diagnosis is made.

MISCELLANEOUS

Suggested Reading

Moore PF, Olivry T. Cutaneous lymphomas in companion animals. Clin Dermatol 1994;12:499–505.
Scott DW, Miller WH, Griffin CE. Muller & Kirk's small animal dermatology. 5th ed. Philadelphia: Saunders, 1995.
Author K. Marcia Murphy
Consulting Editor Karen Helton Rhodes

DISEASES

MALASSEZIA DERMATITIS

 BASICS

OVERVIEW
• *Malassezia pachydermatis* (syn. *Pityrosporum canis*)—yeast; normal commensal of the skin, ears, and mucocutaneous areas; can overgrow and cause dermatitis, cheilitis, and otitis in dogs
• Yeast numbers in diseased areas are usually excessive, although this is a variable finding.
• The causes of the transformation from harmless commensal to pathogen are poorly understood but seem related to allergy, seborrheic conditions, and possibly congenital and hormonal factors.
• *Malassezia* dermatitis and *Malassezia*-associated seborrheic dermatitis—common in all geographic regions of the world
• Cats—similar disease, but rare

SIGNALMENT
• Any dog breed; however, west Highland white terriers, poodles, basset hounds, cocker spaniels and dachshunds are predisposed.
• No gender predilection

SIGNS
• Pruritus—with varying degrees of erythema, alopecia, scale. and greasy malodorous exudation; affects lips, ears, feet, axilla, inguinal area, and ventral neck
• Hyperpigmentation and lichenification—chronic cases
• Concurrent black waxy to seborrheic otitis—frequent
• Frenzied facial pruritus—uncommon but characteristic
• Often a history of suspected allergy that worsens and seems to develop resistance to or is resistant to glucocorticoid treatment
• Concurrent pyoderma, hypersensitivities, endocrine, and keratinization disorders

CAUSES & RISK FACTORS
• High humidity and temperature—may increase the frequency
• Concurrent hypersensitivity disease (particularly atopy, flea allergy, and some food allergy/intolerances) may be a predisposing factor.
• Defects of cornification and seborrheas (especially in young dogs) in predisposed breeds
• Endocrinopathies (especially in old dogs)—suspected to be associated predisposing factors
• Genetic factors—suspected for young onset in predisposed breeds
• Concurrent increase in cutaneous *Staphylococcus intermedius* population and resultant pyoderma—confirmed finding; canine seborrheic dermatitis is proposed, in selected cases, to be a result of this combination pathogen overgrowth; treatment of one alone does not result in resolution of all signs, but just unmasks the other; antiyeast treatment alone resolves all signs of *Malassezia* dermatitis.
• Idiopathic

 DIAGNOSIS

DIFFERENTIAL DIAGNOSIS
• Allergic dermatitis, including flea allergy, atopy, and food allergy
• Superficial pyoderma
• Primary and secondary seborrheas
• All associated diseases mentioned above

CBC/BIOCHEMICAL/URINALYSIS
Changes reflect predisposing conditions (e.g., hypothyroidism, hyperadrenocorticism) rather than yeast infection.

OTHER LABORATORY TESTS
• Fungal culture—use contact plates (small agar plates made from bottle lids and filled with Sabouraud agar or preferably modified Dixon agar); press plates onto the affected skin surface; then incubate at 32–37°C for 3–7 days; count the distinctive yellow or buff, round, domed colonies (1–1.5 mm); provides semiqualitative data
• Nonquantitative culture methods—no value, because *Malassezia* is a normal commensal

IMAGING
N/A

DIAGNOSTIC PROCEDURES
Skin cytology—touch, cotton swab, or cellophane tape preparation stained with Diff-Quick; apply stain as a drop directly onto the slide (yeast may wash off during staining); pass a flame under the slide to improve stain penetration and visualization.

PATHOLOGICAL FINDINGS

• Histopathology—valuable if the skin reaction pattern (spongiotic, hyperplastic, superficial, perivascular) is recognized and yeast is seen in the superficial scale; yeast is often lost during collection or processing.
• Surface cytology—more reliable; simple, inexpensive, and rapid

 TREATMENT

• Goals—confirm diagnosis by associating elimination of signs with reduction in yeast and bacterial numbers
• Identify and treat any predisposing factors or diseases.
• Topical therapy—yeast is principally located in the stratum corneum.
• Shampoo treatment—remove scale, exudation, and malodor.
• Topical therapies with trial data— (miconazole, selenium sulfides); twice-weekly treatments effective
• Other topical antifungal and antibacterial shampoo treatments may also be of value if given with suitable systemic drugs.
• Alternative combinations—topical keratolytic shampoo treatment with systemic antiyeast and antibacterial drugs.

 MEDICATIONS

DRUGS

• Localized cases—may respond to creams and lotions containing imidazole compounds
• Ketoconazole—10 mg/kg q24h for 2–4 weeks; widespread or chronic lichenified cases
• Chronic lichenified cases—ketoconazole at 5–10 mg/kg q24h as a short diagnostic for 5–7 days with effective topical antimycotic shampoo treatment; quick response confirms the diagnosis; response can be slow in chronic cases when yeasts are buried deep in epidermal folds.
• Topical antimicrobial shampoo—to maintain remission in chronic cases

CONTRAINDICATIONS/POSSIBLE INTERACTIONS

Ketaconazole—rarely may cause hepatic reaction; will mask the signs of hyper-adrenocorticism and interfere with adrenal function tests

 FOLLOW-UP

• Physical examinations and skin cytology findings after 2–4 weeks to monitor therapy
• Treat until only rare organisms can be demonstrated or 7 days after a complete response is achieved.
• Pruritus and odor—usually noticeably improved within 1 week
• Recurrences—common when underlying dermatoses are not well controlled; regular bathing with antifungal-antibacterial shampoo combinations (miconazole plus chlorhexidine) help decrease recurrence.

 MISCELLANEOUS

PREGNANCY

Ketoconazole contraindicated

Suggested Reading

Scott DW, Miller WH, Griffin CE. Muller & Kirk's small animal dermatology. 5th ed. Philadelphia: Saunders, 1995.
Author K. V. Mason
Consulting Editor Karen Helton Rhodes

DISEASES

MALFORMATIONS—CONGENITAL, CENTRAL NERVOUS SYSTEM

BASICS

DEFINITION
Morphologic abnormalities of the brain and/or spinal cord that are present at birth

PATHOPHYSIOLOGY
May be inherited or induced in utero by infectious agents or other teratogens; some agents and teratogens affect specific sites in the CNS, whereas others produce diffuse abnormalities.

SYSTEM AFFECTED
Nervous—affected secondarily by malformations of the spinal column (e.g., spinal cord compression by hemivertebrae)

GENETICS
• Encephalocele—Burmese cats; autosomal dominant
• Congenital hydrocephalus—Siamese cats; autosomal recessive
• Hypomyelination—springer spaniels; X-linked recessive
• Myelodysplasia—weimaraners; codominant lethal gene with variable penetrance
• Sacrocaudal dysgenesis—Manx cats; autosomal dominant with incomplete penetrance

INCIDENCE/PREVALANCE
Unknown

GEOGRAPHIC DISTRIBUTION
N/A

SIGNALMENT

Species
Dogs and cats

Breed Predilections
• Congenital hydrocephalus—dogs: Boston terriers, bulldogs, cairn terriers, Chihuahuas, Lhasa apsos, Maltese, Pekingese, Pomeranians, pugs, toy poodles, Yorkshire terriers; cats: Siamese
• Hypomyelination—Bernese mountain dogs, chow chows, Dalmatians, lurchers, Samoyeds, weimaraners
• Lissencephaly—Lhasa apsos
• Optic nerve hypoplasia—miniature poodles
• Optic chiasm malformation—Belgian sheepdogs

• Intracranial intra-arachnoid cyst—possibly small-breed, brachycephalic dogs
• Spina bifida, meningomyelocele, and myelodysplasia—bulldogs

Mean Age and Range
By definition, present at birth; clinical signs may not be apparent until the malformed portion of the nervous system is used by the patient or secondary signs (e.g., seizures) appear.

Predominant Sex
Hypomyelination in Samoyeds and springer spaniels—males

SIGNS

General Comments
Reflect the location of the neural lesion

Historical Findings
Maternal—illness or exposure to teratogens

Physical Examination
• Malformation of overlying structures—may be evident
• Congenital hydrocephalus—enlarged cranium; open fontanelles; bilateral divergent strabismus of the eyes
• Encephalocele (Burmese cats)—craniofacial and ophthalmic malformations

CAUSES

Inherited (Dogs)
• Hypomyelination—springer spaniels
• Myelodysplasia—Weimaraners

Noninherited (Dogs)
• Usually unknown
• Viral infections suspected

Inherited (Cats)
• Encephalocele—Burmese
• Hydrocephalus—Siamese
• Sacrocaudal dysgenesis—Manx

Noninherited (Cats)
• Griseofulvin—craniofacial malformation; microphthalmia; optic nerve hypoplasia
• Panleukopenia virus (maternal infection or vaccination with MLV)—cerebellar hypoplasia

RISK FACTORS
• Breeding affected animals
• Maternal illness or exposure to teratogens during pregnancy

DIAGNOSIS

DIFFERENTIAL DIAGNOSIS
• Suggested by nonprogressive neurologic deficits that are present at or shortly after birth
• Other causes of neurologic deficits in the neonate—metabolic disease; neoplasia (rare); inflammatory disease; trauma; toxins

CBC/BIOCHEMISTRY/URINALYSIS
Usually normal

IMAGING
• MRI—most accurate, least invasive method of detection
• Myelography—may reveal spinal malformations
• Radiography or CT—examination of associated skeletal elements

DIAGNOSTIC PROCEDURES
CSF analysis—rule out other causes (particularly inflammatory)

PATHOLOGIC FINDINGS
• Characteristic for the specific defects
• Hypoplasia—after destruction of progenitor cells by the inciting agent
• Atrophy—destructive effect on already differentiated growing tissues

TREATMENT

APPROPRIATE HEALTH CARE
• Usually outpatient
• Surgical intervention—may be indicated to correct or prevent neurologic problems

NURSING CARE
Paretic or paralyzed animals—maintenance of effective elimination of urine and feces; prevention of pressure sores; maintenance of skin cleanliness; physical therapy

ACTIVITY
Watch—prevent injuries as patient moves about

MALFORMATIONS—CONGENITAL, CENTRAL NERVOUS SYSTEM

DIET
N/A

CLIENT EDUCATION
• Discuss the care of paretic or paralyzed patients, including maintaining effective elimination of urine and feces, preventing pressure sores, maintaining skin cleanliness, and conducting physical therapy.
• Discuss the management of seizures, if they occur.

SURGICAL CONSIDERATIONS
• Congenital hydrocephalus—ventriculo-peritoneal shunt
• Intracranial intra-arachnoid cysts—fenestration, shunt
• Meningeal malformations that communicate with the skin—surgical ablation or closure of communication

MEDICATIONS

DRUGS OF CHOICE
• None for most malformations.
• Hydrocephalus—reduce CSF production and/or reduce intracranial pressure (see Hydrocephalus)
• Antibiotics—meningeal malformations that communicate with the skin

CONTRAINDICATIONS
N/A

PRECAUTIONS
N/A

POSSIBLE INTERACTIONS
N/A

ALTERNATIVE DRUGS
N/A

FOLLOW-UP

PATIENT MONITORING
• Monitor for any secondary physical problems.
• Watch for worsening of any neurologic signs.
• Monitor for later developing signs (e.g., seizures).

PREVENTION/AVOIDANCE
• Inherited—do not breed affected carrier animals; pedigree analysis or test breeding for determining genetic basis
• Noninherited—maintain health of the dam.

POSSIBLE COMPLICATIONS
• Cavitary malformations (intra-arachnoid cysts, spinal arachnoid cysts, hydrocephalus, hydromyelia/syringomyelia)—additional or progressive neurologic signs may occur if CSF continues to accumulate within the lesion.
• Sacrocaudal dysgenesis (Manx cats)—uterine inertia

EXPECTED COURSE AND PROGNOSIS
• Usually stable
• Hypomyelination—Bernese mountain dogs, chow chows, Dalmatians, and Weimaraners; may improve to near normal
• Cavitary malformations—may cause progressive signs; prognosis uncertain

MISCELLANEOUS

ASSOCIATED CONDITIONS
• Labrador retriever axonopathy—aplasia or hypoplasia of the corpus callosum
• Dandy-Walker syndrome—dysgenesis of the cerebellar vermis; hydrocephalus; dilated 4th ventricle; stenosis of the mesencephalic aqueduct; agenesis of the corpus callosum; syringomyelia
• Intracranial intra-arachnoid cysts—hydrocephalus
• Occipital dysplasia—hydrocephalus
• Hypoplasia (feline panleukopenia virus)—hydrocephalus or hydranencephaly
• Hydrocephalus (lateral aperture obstruction)—hydromyelia; syringomyelia
• Hydrocephalus—intraventricular hematoma
• Spina bifida—meningocele or myelomeningocele

AGE-RELATED FACTORS
• Neurologic deficits are usually evident at birth or within the first few weeks of life.
• Abnormal musculoskeletal morphology may be evident at birth.

ZOONOTIC POTENTIAL
• N/A

PREGNANCY
• N/A

SYNONYMS
• N/A

SEE ALSO
• Cerebellar Hypoplasia
• Dysraphism, Spinal
• Hydrocephalus
• Hypomyelination—Central and Peripheral Nervous System

ABREVIATIONS
• CSF = cerebrospinal fluid
• MLV = modified live virus

Suggested Reading

Braund KG. Clinical syndromes in veterinary neurology. 2nd ed. St. Louis: Mosby, 1994.

Oliver JE, Lorenz MD, Kornegay JN. Handbook of veterinary neurology. 3rd ed. Philadelphia: Saunders, 1997.

Summers BA, Cummings JF, de Lahunta A. Veterinary neuropathology. St. Louis: Mosby, 1995.

Vernau KM, Kortz GD, Koblik PD, et al. Magnetic resonance imaging and computed tomography characteristics of intracranial intra-arachnoid cysts in 6 dogs. Vet Radiol Ultrasound 1997;38:171–176.

Author Cleta Sue Bailey
Consulting Editor Joane M. Parent

DISEASES

MALIGNANT FIBROUS HISTIOCYTOMA (GIANT CELL TUMOR)

BASICS

OVERVIEW
- Name based on histologic features of fibroblast- and histiocyte-like cells
- Mesenchymal neoplasm, but definitive cellular origin unknown; likely possibilities include fibroblasts, histiocytes, and primitive mesenchymal cells
- Several histologic variants
- Storiform-pleomorphic and giant-cell—two major variants; both locally invasive; firm, subcutaneous or visceral masses on examination
- Despite previous reports to the contrary, metastatic potential in dogs appears to be high.

SIGNALMENT
- More commonly reported in cats than in dogs
- Mean age—cats: 9 years (range, 2–12 years); dogs: 8 years (range, < 1–10 years); reported in a 4-month-old, mixed-breed, male puppy
- No breed or sex predilection

SIGNS

Historical Findings
- Anorexia, weight loss, and lethargy may occur.
- Depend on site of involvement

Physical Examination Findings
- Firm, invasive tumor arising in subcutaneous tissue
- May exhibit deep extension into underlying skeletal muscle
- May develop adjacent to bone and induce bone destruction and proliferation
- Most common sites—dorsal thoracic and scapular area, limbs, and pelvic region
- Distant metastasis—common

CAUSES & RISK FACTORS
- Unknown
- Can be induced with carcinogens in laboratory animal species

DIAGNOSIS

DIFFERENTIAL DIAGNOSIS
- Fibrosarcoma
- Chondrosarcoma
- Osteosarcoma
- Mast cell neoplasia
- Rhabdomyoma or rhabdomyosarcoma
- Liposarcoma

CBC/BIOCHEMISTRY/URINALYSIS
- CBC—may vary; may be normal; may see regenerative or nonregenerative anemia
- Biochemistry—variably abnormal
- Urinalysis—usually normal

OTHER LABORATORY TESTS
Cytologic examination of aspirate—may reveal histiocyte- and fibroblast-like cells

IMAGING
Radiography—reveals soft tissue dense mass; may note bone proliferation or destruction

DIAGNOSTIC PROCEDURES
Histologic examination of biopsy specimen—necessary for definitive diagnosis

PATHOLOGIC FINDINGS
Classification—considerable debate exists among pathologists, which may account for the apparent differences in behavior reported in the literature

TREATMENT
- Surgical excision—difficult owing to local invasive nature; recurrence rate is high.
- Amputation of an affected limb—may be appropriate; thoracic and abdominal radiographs and abdominal ultrasound critical for evaluating for detectable metastasis before amputation
- Radiotherapy—may be helpful as adjuvant treatment for localized tumor not amenable to surgical resection

MEDICATIONS

DRUGS
Chemotherapy—may be helpful; doxorubicin (patient > 10 kg, 30 mg/m^2 IV every 3 weeks; patients < 10 kg, 1 mg/kg IV every 3 weeks); preliminary results suggest a survival time of 1–12 months.

CONTRAINDICATIONS/POSSIBLE INTERACTIONS
N/A

FOLLOW-UP
Re-examination—according to growth of tumor

MISCELLANEOUS

Suggested Reading
Waters CB, Morrison WB, DeNicola DB, et al. Giant cell variant of malignant fibrous histiocytoma in dogs: 10 cases (1986–1993). J Am Vet Med Assoc 1994;205:1420–1424.

Author James P. Thompson
Consulting Editor Wallace B. Morrison

MAMMARY GLAND HYPERPLASIA—CATS

BASICS

OVERVIEW
A progesterone-dependent enlargement of one or more mammary glands

SIGNALMENT
• Young, intact, cycling, or pregnant queens
• Cats of either gender that are receiving exogenous progestogen (e.g., megestrol acetate)

SIGNS
• Localized or diffuse enlargement of one or more mammary glands
• Firm and nonpainful masses
• No concurrent signs of systemic illness

CAUSES & RISK FACTORS
• Secondary to a progesterone influence
• High progesterone—false pregnancy in queen induced to ovulate but nonpregnant for 40–50 days after ovulation induction; throughout gestation; with exogenous progestogens

DIAGNOSIS

DIFFERENTIAL DIAGNOSIS
• Mastitis—lactating queen; mammary glands erythematous and painful; systemic illness with fever and immature neutrophilia; inflammatory cells and bacteria in fluid expressed from the affected gland(s)

• Mammary neoplasia—old queens (> 6 years of age); gross appearance may be indistinguishable; differentiated by biopsy of affected tissue

CBC/BIOCHEMISTRY/URINALYSIS
Normal

OTHER LABORATORY TESTS
N/A

IMAGING
N/A

DIAGNOSTIC PROCEDURES
• Cytologic examination of fluid expressed from affected glands—noninflammatory
• Excision biopsy—benign fibroglandular proliferation with no inflammation or necrosis

TREATMENT

• Hypertrophy—owing to high endogenous progesterone; regresses when progesterone falls at the end of false pregnancy or gestation
• Consider ovariohysterectomy if fertility is not an issue.
• Hypertrophy—owing to exogenous progestogens; regresses when medication is withdrawn

MEDICATIONS

DRUGS
• Bromocriptine mesylate—0.25 mg PO q24h for 5–7 days; not approved for use in cats; may cause nausea

• Nausea—metoclopramide (0.2 mg/kg PO q6–8h) or divided bromocriptine dose (give twice daily)
• Milbolerone (Cheque) and megestrol acetate (Ovaban)—reported success equivocal

CONTRAINDICATIONS/POSSIBLE INTERACTIONS
N/A

FOLLOW-UP

• Likelihood of recurrence in cats left intact—unknown
• Correlation with other abnormal conditions of the reproductive tract—unknown

MISCELLANEOUS

SYNONYMS
• Benign mammary hypertrophy
• Mammary fibroadenomatosis
• Fibroglandular mammary hypertrophy

Suggested Reading
Hayden DW, Johnston SD, Krang DT, et al. Feline mammary hypertrophy/fibroadenoma complex: clinical and hormonal aspects. Am J Vet Res 1981;42:1699–1703.
Author Margaret V. Root
Consulting Editor Sara K. Lyle

DISEASES

MAMMARY GLAND TUMORS—CATS

 BASICS

DEFINITION
Malignant and benign tumors of the mammary glands in cats

PATHOPHYSIOLOGY
• Hormonal influences—may be involved
• Between 80% and 90% are malignant.

SYSTEMS AFFECTED
• Reproductive—mammary glands and metastatic sites
• Metastases at the time of euthanasia—> 80% of patients; one or more of the following sites: lymph nodes, lungs, pleura, liver, diaphragm, adrenal gland, and kidneys

GENETICS
• Unknown
• Siamese cats—may have twice the risk of other breeds

INCIDENCE/PREVALENCE
• Third most common neoplasia in cats (after hematopoietic and skin tumors)
• Accounts for 17% of neoplasms in female cats

GEOGRAPHIC DISTRIBUTION
N/A

SIGNALMENT

Species
Cats

Breed Predilections
• Domestic shorthair and Siamese cats—higher reported incidence rates than other breeds

Mean Age and Range
• Mean—10–12 years
• Range—9 months to 23 years

Predominant Sex
Most (99%) develop in intact females

SIGNS

Historical Findings
• Many patients have advanced disease on examination—average of 5 months after the tumors are first noticed

Physical Examination Findings
• Firm, nodular mass which may adhere to the skin but not to underlying abdominal wall
• Approximately 60% of patients have multiple gland involvement; one third have simultaneous involvement of both right and left mammary gland chains.
• Any or all glands may be involved; slightly higher incidence observed for the two cranial glands
• Nipples—often red and swollen; may exude tan or yellow fluid
• Ulceration—noted in one quarter of patients
• Infiltrated lymphatic vessels—may appear as subcutaneous, linear, beaded chains
• Pelvic limbs—may be edematous and uncomfortable; temperature may be abnormal owing to tumor thrombi or impaired vascular return

CAUSES
• Unknown
• Strong association with prior use of progesterone-like drugs
• Only 10% of tumors are positive for estrogen receptors.

RISK FACTORS
• Intact females have a sevenfold higher risk than do spayed females.
• Genetic—Siamese breed
• Administration of progesterone-like drugs (e.g., megestrol acetate)—associated with development of benign and malignant masses
• Early ovariohysterectomy—protective effect not as clearly defined as in dogs

 DIAGNOSIS

DIFFERENTIAL DIAGNOSIS
• Lobular hyperplasia
• Fibroepithelial hyperplasia
• Papillary cystic hyperplasia
• Mastitis
• Cysts

CBC/BIOCHEMISTRY/URINALYSIS
Anemia and leukocytosis—may occur

OTHER LABORATORY TESTS
Coagulation profile—with large, ulcerated tumors; rule out DIC

IMAGING
• Thoracic radiographs—detect lung metastases or pleural effusion; metastatic patterns may vary from discreet nodules to a diffuse interstitial pattern.
• Abdominal radiographs or ultrasound of sublumbar lymph nodes or ascites

DIAGNOSTIC PROCEDURES
• Preliminary biopsy—not recommended because of the high frequency of malignancy, unless results will change owner's willingness to treat; tissue for histopathologic examination obtained at the time of mastectomy
• Cytologic examination—mass(es): may rule out nonmammary malignancies; lymph nodes: with suspected metastasis; pleural fluid (if noted)

PATHOLOGICAL FINDINGS
• Gross—adherence to overlying skin and ulceration common
• Histopathology—> 80% of tumors are adenocarcinomas: tubular, papillary, and solid most common; most are a combination of tumor types; often contain extensive areas of necrosis with lymphocytic and plasma-cell infiltration
• Metastasis to regional lymph nodes—50% of patients

 TREATMENT

APPROPRIATE HEALTH CARE
Discharge after surgery if stable.

NURSING CARE
Provide supportive fluids and appropriate antibiotics as needed.

ACTIVITY
N/A

DIET
N/A

CLIENT EDUCATION
- Stress the importance of early detection and removal.
- Stress the potential benefits of early ovariohysterectomy.

SURGICAL CONSIDERATIONS
- Radical mastectomy—patients without radiographic evidence of metastasis regardless of tumor size; removal of all four glands of the affected chain; significantly reduces the chance of local recurrence; include the ipsilateral axillary (if large or cytologically suspect) and inguinal lymph nodes.
- Tumors in both mammary chains—perform two radical mastectomies, usually 2–4 weeks apart.
- Concurrent ovariohysterectomy—may address coexisting ovarian and uterine disease

 MEDICATIONS

DRUGS OF CHOICE
Combination chemotherapy—doxorubicin (1 mg/kg IV q 3 weeks) and cyclophosphamide (50 mg/m² PO on days 3, 4, 5, and 6); repeat every 3–4 weeks; shown to induce short-term partial and complete responses in about half of patients with metastatic or nonresectable local disease

CONTRAINDICATIONS
- Renal disease
- Compromised myocardial function
- Severe myelosuppression

PRECAUTIONS
- Doxorubicin—do not exceed a cumulative dose of 200 mg/m².
- Chemotherapy may be toxic; seek advice before initiating treatment if you are unfamiliar with cytotoxic drugs.
- Hepatic disease
- Renal disease

POSSIBLE INTERACTIONS
Verapamil—may potentiate doxorubicin-induced cardiomyopathy; avoid concurrent use.

ALTERNATIVE DRUGS
- Mitoxantrone—may substitute for doxorubicin
- No available biological response modifier has shown efficacy.

 FOLLOW-UP

PATIENT MONITORING
- Complete physical examination—bi-monthly; emphasis on palpation of previous incision line(s), remaining mammary glands, and axillary and inguinal lymph node regions
- Thoracic radiographs—every 1–3 months

PREVENTION/AVOIDANCE
Ovariohysterectomy—0.6% the risk of intact cats; optimum age for it to be sparing unknown

POSSIBLE COMPLICATIONS
- Tumor—anemia; osteoporosis; hypercalcemia; DIC; ascites; pleural effusion
- Chemotherapy—dilated cardiomyopathy; myelosuppression; anorexia; gastrointestinal toxicity; renal insufficiency; hepatopathy; agents may be carcinogenic and mutagenic.

EXPECTED COURSE AND PROGNOSIS
- High incidence of recurrence (66% with conservative surgery) and metastasis
- Time to recurrence—related to the type of surgery; radical mastectomy disease-free interval, 575 days (survival, 800 days); conservative surgery disease-free interval, 325 days (survival, 500 days)
- Single most important prognostic factor—tumor size; median survival with diameter > 3 cm, 6 months after surgery; median survival with diameter < 2 cm, approximately 3 years

 MISCELLANEOUS

ASSOCIATED CONDITIONS
- Cystic ovaries
- Mastitis
- Uterine disease
- Other unrelated tumors

AGE-RELATED FACTORS
- Middle-aged cats most commonly affected
- Siamese cats—develop tumors at a younger age; incidence reaches a plateau at approximately 9 years.

ZOONOTIC POTENTIAL
None

PREGNANCY
Do not use chemotherapy in pregnant animals.

ABBREVIATION
DIC = disseminated intravascular coagulation

Suggested Reading

Jeglum KA, DeGuzman E, Young KM. Chemotherapy of advanced mammary adenocarcinoma in 14 cats. J Am Vet Med Assoc 1985;187:157–160.

MacEwen EG, Withrow SJ. Tumors of the mammary gland. In: Withrow SJ, MacEwen EG, eds. Small animal clinical oncology. 2nd ed. Philadelphia: Saunders, 1996;365–372.

Morrison WB. Canine and feline mammary gland tumors. In: Morrison WB, ed. Cancer in dogs and cats: medical and surgical management. Baltimore: Williams & Wilkins, 1998:591–598.

Author Sue Downing
Consulting Editor Wallace B. Morrison

DISEASES

BASICS

DEFINITION
Benign or malignant tumors of the mammary glands in dogs

PATHOPHYSIOLOGY
• Malignancy—about 50%
• About 50% of patients have multiple tumors.
• Lymphatic connections—exist between right and left series of glands; generally, cranial glands drain to axillary lymph nodes, caudal glands drain to inguinal lymph nodes, and in-between glands drain variably to either or both types of nodes; plexiform connections help explain occurrence of lymphatic metastasis against predicted lymph flow.
• Hormonal influence—suggested by lower incidence in dogs spayed at an early age (see Prevention/Avoidance)

SYSTEMS AFFECTED
• Reproductive
• Metastasis—respiratory, nervous, and other systems

GENETICS
N/A

INCIDENCE/PREVALENCE
Females—198.8 per 100,000

GEOGRAPHIC DISTRIBUTION
Similar worldwide

SIGNALMENT

Species
Dogs

Breed Predilection
None

Mean Age and Range
• Median age—about 10.5 years (range, 1–15 years)
• Uncommon in dogs < 5 years

Predominant Sex
Female; extremely rare in males

SIGNS

Historical Findings
Usually slow-growing single or multiple masses

Physical Examination Findings
• Single or multiple masses—about 50% of patients have multiple tumors.
• May be ulcerated
• May be freely movable—implies benign behavior
• May be fixed to skin or body wall—implies malignant behavior

CAUSES
Unknown; likely hormonal

RISK FACTORS
Circumstantial evidence—incriminates treatment with progestins and estrogen in combination, prolactin, and growth hormone

DIAGNOSIS

DIFFERENTIAL DIAGNOSIS
• Lipoma
• Mast cell tumor
• Mammary hyperplasia
• Mastitis

CBC/BIOCHEMISTRY/URINALYSIS
• Usually normal
• Hypercalcemia and hypoglycemia—occasionally reported

OTHER LABORATORY TESTS
N/A

IMAGING
• Thoracic radiography—may detect metastasis
• Abdominal radiography—may detect metastasis to iliac (sublumbar) lymph nodes
• Radionuclide bone scanning—rarely positive in dogs

DIAGNOSTIC PROCEDURES
• Examination of cytologic preparations—often misleading; inflammation may mimic criteria of malignancy.
• Excisional biopsy—definitive diagnosis

PATHOLOGIC FINDINGS
• Gross—associated with considerable inflammation; may find ulceration
• Histopathologic—50% benign; 42% adenocarcinoma; 4% inflammatory carcinoma; 4% sarcoma

TREATMENT

APPROPRIATE HEALTH CARE
• Surgery—primary mode of treatment
• Chemotherapy—may be effective; infrequently reported

NURSING CARE
N/A

ACTIVITY
N/A

DIET
N/A

CLIENT EDUCATION
• Advise client that a mammary lump should never be left in place and observed.
• Inform client that early surgical intervention is best.
• Advise spaying before first estrus.

SURGICAL CONSIDERATIONS
Local excision (e.g., simple, regional , or unilateral mastectomy) with wide and deep margins (at least 2 cm in all directions)—may be as effective in terms of disease-free interval as radical bilateral mastectomy

MEDICATIONS

DRUGS OF CHOICE
Doxorubicin—30 mg/m^2 IV every 21days; reported to have induced partial remission in two dogs for 12 and 16 months, respectively

CONTRAINDICATIONS
Myocardial failure

PRECAUTIONS
Chemotherapy may be toxic; seek advice before treatment if you are unfamiliar with cytotoxic drugs.

POSSIBLE INTERACTIONS
Doxorubicin—side effects include myelotoxicity, vomiting and diarrhea, pancreatitis, and cardiac damage.

ALTERNATIVE DRUGS
Tamoxifen—helpful in some humans with breast cancer; ineffective in dogs and has serious side effects; do not use in dogs and cats.

FOLLOW-UP

PATIENT MONITORING
Physical examination and thoracic radiographs—1, 3, 6, 9, and 12 months after treatment

PREVENTION/AVOIDANCE
• Spayed before first estrous cycle—0.5% risk compared to intact bitch
• Spayed before second estrous cycle—8.0% risk compared to intact bitch
• Spayed after second estrus—26% risk compared to intact bitch
• Spayed after 2.5 years of age—no sparing effect on risk

POSSIBLE COMPLICATIONS
N/A

EXPECTED COURSE AND PROGNOSIS
• Median survival after mastectomy with tubular adenocarcinoma—24.6 months
• Median survival after mastectomy with solid carcinoma—6.5 months
• Benign tumor—excellent prognosis after mastectomy
• Carcinoma < 5 cm in diameter—usually a good prognosis

MISCELLANEOUS

Inflammatory carcinoma—very aggressive subtype; characterized by rapid growth, firmness, diffuse involvement, erythema, limb edema, color change, and pain; patient may be anemic, have leukocytosis, and develop DIC; tumor may be mistaken for mastitis, abscess, or dermatitis; prognosis poor

ASSOCIATED CONDITIONS
• Hypertrophic osteopathy
• Metastasis to lungs and CNS

AGE-RELATED FACTORS
N/A

ZOONOTIC POTENTIAL
N/A

PREGNANCY
N/A

ABBREVIATION
DIC = disseminated intravascular coagulation

Suggested Reading

Allen SW, Mahaffey EA. Canine mammary neoplasia: prognostic indicators and response to surgical therapy. J Am Anim Hosp Assoc 1989;25:540–546.

Hahn KA, Richardson RC, Knapp DW. Canine malignant mammary neoplasia: biological behavior, diagnosis, and treatment alternatives. J Am Anim Hosp Assoc 1992;28:251–256.

Morris JS, Dobson JM, Bostock DE. Use of tamoxifen in control of canine mammary neoplasia. Vet Rec 1993;133:539–542.

Morrison WB. Canine and feline mammary tumors. In: Morrison WB, ed. Cancer in dogs and cats: medical and surgical management. Baltimore: Williams & Wilkins, 1998:591–598.

Authors Wallace B. Morrison and Kevin A. Hahn
Consulting Editor Wallace B. Morrison

MAST CELL TUMORS

BASICS

DEFINITION
Neoplasia arising from mast cells

PATHOPHYSIOLOGY
• Histamine and other vasoactive substances released from mast cell tumors—may cause erythema and edema; histamine may cause gastric and duodenal ulcers. • Heparin release—increases likelihood of bleeding

SYSTEMS AFFECTED
• Skin/Exocrine—skin and subcutaneous tissue most common tumor sites in dogs and cats • Hemic/Lymphatic/Immune—spleen: common primary location in cats and uncommon primary location in dogs; common location for metastasis from the skin or subcutaneous sites • Gastrointestinal—intestinal mast cell tumor uncommon in cats and rare in dogs; gastric and duodenal ulcers possible

GENETICS
N/A

INCIDENCE/PREVALENCE
• Compose 20–25% of all skin and subcutaneous tumors in dogs • Fourth most common skin tumor in cats

GEOGRAPHIC DISTRIBUTION
N/A

SIGNALMENT

Species
Dogs and cats

Breed Predilections
• Boxers and Boston terriers • Siamese cats—predisposed to histiocytic cutaneous mast cell tumors

Mean Age and Range
• Dogs—mean age, 8 years • Cats—mean age, 10 years • Reported in animals < 1 year old and in cats as old as 18 years

Predominant Sex
None

SIGNS

General Comments
Depend on the location and grade of the tumor

Historical Findings
Dogs
• Patient may have had skin or subcutaneous tumor for days to months at the time of examination. • May have appeared to fluctuate in size • Recent rapid growth after months of quiescence common • Recent onset of erythema and edema most common with high-grade skin and subcutaneous tumors

Cats
• Anorexia—most common complaint with splenic tumor • Vomiting—may occur secondary to both splenic and gastrointestinal tumors

Physical Examination Findings
Dogs
• Extremely variable; may resemble any other type of skin or subcutaneous tumor (benign and malignant); may resemble an insect bite or allergic reaction • Primarily a solitary skin or subcutaneous mass; but may be multifocal • Approximately 50% located on the trunk and perineum; 40% on extremities; 10% on the head and neck region • Regional lymphadenopathy—may develop when a high-grade tumor metastasizes to draining lymph nodes • Hepatomegaly and splenomegaly—features of disseminated mast cell neoplasia
Cats
• Cutaneous—primarily found in the subcutaneous tissue or dermis; may be papular or nodular, solitary or multiple, and hairy or alopecic or have an ulcerated surface; slight predilection for the head and neck regions • Splenic—splenomegaly is only consistent finding • Intestinal—firm, segmental thickenings of the small intestinal wall; measure 1–7 cm in diameter; metastases to the mesenteric lymph nodes, spleen, liver and (rarely) lungs

CAUSES
Unknown

RISK FACTORS
• Hereditary • Previous inflammation

DIAGNOSIS

DIFFERENTIAL DIAGNOSIS
• Any other skin or subcutaneous tumor, benign or malignant, including lipoma • Insect bite or allergic reaction • Splenic—most common cause of splenomegaly in cats; must differentiate from lymphoma • Intestinal (cats)—may resemble any primary gastrointestinal disorder (e.g., inflammatory and neoplasia)

CBC/BIOCHEMISTRY/URINALYSIS
Anemia and mastocythemia—may find in cats with splenic tumor and dogs with systemic mastocytosis

OTHER LABORATORY TESTS
N/A

IMAGING
• Abdominal radiography—may reveal splenomegaly in cats with splenic tumor and dogs with systemic mastocytosis • Ultrasonography—helpful for evaluating visceral (liver, spleen) metastasis in dogs with high-grade tumors

DIAGNOSTIC PROCEDURES
• Cytologic examination of fine-needle aspirate—most important preliminary diagnostic test; reveals round cells with basophilic cytoplasmic granules that do not form sheets or clumps; if malignant mast cells are agranular, occurrence large eosinophilic infiltrate may suggest mast cell tumor. • Tissue biopsy—necessary for definitive diagnosis and grading • Staging—to determine the extent of disease and appropriate treatment • Additional tests to achieve complete staging—cytologic examination or biopsy of local draining lymph node; cytologic examination of bone marrow aspirate; and thoracic radiography and abdominal ultrasonography with cytologic evaluation of hepatic and splenic aspirates

PATHOLOGIC FINDINGS
• Histopathologic examination (dogs)—grading of tumor to predict biologic behavior; graded I–III (III is the most aggressive type) • Cats—grading system; no correlation between histopathologic appearance of cutaneous tumor and prognosis

TREATMENT

APPROPRIATE HEALTH CARE

Dogs
• Aggressive surgical excision—treatment of choice • Histopathologic evaluation of the entire surgically excised tissue—essential to determine completeness of excision and predict the biological behavior; if tumor cells extend close to the surgical margins, perform a second aggressive surgery as soon as possible. • Lymph node involvement but no systemic involvement—aggressive excision of the affected lymph node(s) and the primary tumor required; follow-up chemotherapy useful to prevent further metastasis • Primary tumor and/or affected lymph node cannot be excised to microscopic disease—chemotherapy has minimal benefit. • Systemic metastasis—excision of primary tumor and affected lymph nodes and follow-up chemotherapy have minimal effect on survival time. • Radiotherapy—good treatment option for cutaneous tumor in a location that does not allow aggressive surgical excision; if possible, perform surgery before radiotherapy to reduce the tumor to a microscopic volume; tumors on an extremity respond better than do tumors located on the trunk.
Cats
• Surgery—treatment of choice for cutaneous tumors • Splenectomy—treatment of choice for splenic tumor • Splenectomy and chemotherapy—recommended when mastocythemia accompanies splenic tumor

NURSING CARE
N/A

ACTIVITY
N/A

DIET
N/A

CLIENT EDUCATION
• Warn client that a patient that has had more than one cutaneous tumor is predisposed to developing new mast cell tumors. • Advise client that fine needle aspiration and cytologic examination should be performed as soon as possible on any new mass. • Inform client that appropriate surgical excision should be done as soon as possible.

SURGICAL CONSIDERATIONS
• Complete surgical excision with 2 cm margins in all planes—vital • Excisional biopsy rather than incisional biopsy—necessary • Biopsy of lymph nodes and other suspicious visceral organs—appropriate

 MEDICATIONS

DRUGS OF CHOICE
• Prednisone—has been mainstay; recent evidence suggests that, used alone, achieves only short-term remission • Other drugs (e.g., vinblastine and cyclophosphamide)—add to lengthen the remission of prednisone-sensitive tumors • Cutaneous tumor not controlled by surgery or radiotherapy—medical treatment appropriate; in author's experience, prednisone and chemotherapy not beneficial for aggressive tumors in cats • Prednisone-resistant tumor—chemotherapy does not appear to be beneficial. • Intestinal tumor and systemic mastocytosis after splenectomy (cats)—prednisone and chemotherapy indicated • Measurable tumor (dogs)—vincristine alone induced partial remission in 21% of patients.

Combination Chemotherapy
• Author's preferred treatment • Prednisone—1 mg/kg PO q24h; taper slowly after 4 months; discontinue after 7 months • Vinblastine—2–3 mg/m^2 IV; administer on day 1 of each 21-day cycle; initiate at a dosage of 2 mg/m^2; increase by 10%–30% with each subsequent cycle, depending on tolerance and response (e.g., check CBC 1 week after ad-

ministration); perform CBC before each administration; continue for 6 months • Cyclophosphamide—250–300 mg/m^2 PO divided over 4 days; administer on days 8, 9, 10, and 11 of each 21-day cycle; initiate at 250 mg/m^2 for two cycles; increase to 300 mg/m^2 for cycle three if well tolerated; continue for 6 months

CONTRAINDICATIONS
N/A

PRECAUTIONS
N/A

POSSIBLE INTERACTIONS
N/A

ALTERNATIVE DRUGS
Histamine-blocking agents (e.g., cimetidine)—helpful, particularly for systemic mastocytosis or when massive histamine release is a concern

 FOLLOW-UP

PATIENT MONITORING
• Evaluate any new masses cytologically or histologically. • Evaluate regional lymph nodes at regular intervals to detect metastasis of grade II to III tumor.

PREVENTION/AVOIDANCE
N/A

POSSIBLE COMPLICATIONS
• Bleeding • Hemorrhagic gastroenteritis

EXPECTED COURSE AND PROGNOSIS
Dogs
• Tumors in the inguinal region—tend to be more aggressive than similarly graded tumors in other locations; always consider to have the potential to metastasize • Survival times 6 months after surgery (Bostock)—grade I, 77% alive; grade II, 45% alive; grade III, 13% alive • Lymph node metastasis—survival may be prolonged if prednisone and chemotherapy are given after the primary tumor and affected lymph node(s) are aggressively excised. • Prednisone alone—effectively induced remission and prolonged survival time in 20% of patients with grade II or III tumors; only one of the five responding patients had documented lymph node metastasis when prednisone was initiated.

Cats
• Solitary cutaneous tumor—prognosis excellent; rate of recurrence low (16%–36%) despite incomplete excision; < 20% of patients develop metastasis • Survival after splenectomy for splenic tumor—reports of > 1 year • Concurrent development of mastocythemia—prognosis poor; prednisone and chemotherapy may achieve short-term remission. • Intestinal tumor—prognosis poor; survival times rarely > 4 months after surgery

 MISCELLANEOUS

ASSOCIATED CONDITIONS
N/A

AGE-RELATED FACTORS
N/A

ZOONOTIC POTENTIAL
N/A

PREGNANCY
N/A

Suggested Reading

Liska WD, MacEwen EG, Zaki FA, et al. Feline systemic mastocytosis: a review and results of splenectomy in seven cases. J Am Anim Hosp Assoc 1979;15:589–597.

McCaw DL, Miller MA, Ogilvie GK, et al. Response of canine mast cell tumors to treatment with oral prednisone. J Vet Intern Med 1994;8:406–408.

Molander-McCray H, Henry CJ, Potter K, et al. Cutaneous mast cell tumors in cats: 32 cases (1991–1994). J Am Anim Hosp Assoc 1998;34:281–284.

Patnaik AK, Ehler WN, MacEwen EG. Canine cutaneous mast cell tumors: morphologic grading and survival time in 83 dogs. Vet Pathol 1984;21:469–474.

Author Robyn E. Elmslie
Consulting Editor Wallace B. Morrison

DISEASES

MASTITIS

BASICS

OVERVIEW
• Bacterial infection of one or more lactating glands
• Result of ascending infection, trauma to the gland, or hematogenous spread
• *Escherichia coli, Staphylococci,* and B-hemolytic *Streptococci*—most commonly involved
• Potentially life-threatening infection; may lead to septic shock
• Sepsis—direct effect on mammary glands with systemic involvement

SIGNALMENT
Postpartum bitch and queen

SIGNS
Historical Findings
• Anorexia
• Lethargy
• Neglect of puppies or kittens
• Failure of puppies or kittens to thrive

Physical Examination Findings
• Firm, swollen, warm, and painful mammary gland(s) from which purulent or hemorrhagic fluid can be expressed
• Fever, dehydration, and septic shock—with systemic involvement
• Abscessation or gangrene of gland(s)

CAUSES & RISK FACTORS
• Trauma inflicted by puppy or kitten toenails and teeth
• Poor hygiene
• Systemic infection originating elsewhere (e.g., metritis)

DIAGNOSIS

DIFFERENTIAL DIAGNOSIS
• Galactostasis—no systemic illness; cytologic examination and culture of milk and culture help differentiation.
• Inflammatory mammary adenocarcinoma—affected gland does not produce milk; differentiated by biopsy

CBC/BIOCHEMISTRY/URINALYSIS
• Leukocytosis with left shift
• Leukopenia—with sepsis
• Mildly high PCV, total protein, and BUN—with dehydration

IMAGING
N/A

OTHER LABORATORY TESTS
N/A

DIAGNOSTIC PROCEDURES
Milk—normally slightly more acidic than serum; may become alkaline with infection; neutrophils, macrophages, and other mononuclear cells common; degenerative neutrophils with intracellular bacteria noted with septic disease; bacterial culture to identify the organism

TREATMENT
• Inpatient until stable
• Puppies and kittens—hand-raised or placed on healthy surrogate dam; for selected patients, neonates may be allowed to continue nursing (pay special attention to antibiotics used and weight gain of neonates).
• Dehydration or sepsis—intravenous fluid therapy
• Correct electrolyte imbalances and hypoglycemia.
• Treat shock, if indicated.
• Apply warm compress and milk out affected gland(s) several times daily.
• Abscessed or gangrenous glands—require surgical débridement

MEDICATIONS

DRUGS
• Acidic milk—weak bases; erythromycin (10 mg/kg PO q8h, dogs and cats) or lincomycin
• Alkaline milk—weak acids; amoxicillin or cephalosporin (20 mg/kg q8h, dogs and cats)
• Either alkaline or acidic milk—chloramphenicol and enrofloxacin (2.5 mg/kg q12h)

• May infuse affect gland(s) with 1% Betadine solution by lacrimal cannula

CONTRAINDICATIONS/POSSIBLE INTERACTIONS
Patient allowed to nurse—avoid tetracycline, enrofloxacin, and chloramphenicol; may use cephalosporins, amoxicillin, and amoxicillin with clavulanic acid

FOLLOW-UP

PATIENT MONITORING
Physical examination and CBC

PREVENTION/AVOIDANCE
• Clean environment
• Hair shaved from around mammary glands
• Toenails of puppies and kittens clipped

POSSIBLE COMPLICATIONS
• Abscessation or gangrene—may cause loss of gland(s)
• Hand-raising puppies and kittens—requires considerable commitment by the owner

EXPECTED COURSE AND PROGNOSIS
Prognosis—good with treatment

MISCELLANEOUS

ABBREVIATION
PCV = packed cell volume

Suggested Reading
Olson JD, Olson PN. Disorders of the canine mammary gland. In: Morrow DA, ed., Current therapy in theriogenology 2. Philadelphia: Saunders, 1986:506–509.
Author Joni L. Freshman
Consulting Editor Sara K. Lyle

BASICS

OVERVIEW
• An inflammatory process involving the mediastinal space, usually the result of an infectious process
• Acute disease—severe infection may be life-threatening and may spread to the pleural space; sepsis may develop
• Chronic—mediastinal granuloma or abscess may develop and may result in cranial vena cava syndrome.
• Systems affected—primarily cardiovascular system because of interference with venous return or respiratory system secondary to intrathoracic mass effect or pleural effusion; may also interfere with esophageal function

SIGNALMENT
Rare in dogs and cats

SIGNS
• Lethargy and weakness
• Dysphagia and regurgitation
• Edema of head, neck, and forelimbs
• Polypnea and dyspnea

CAUSES & RISK FACTORS
• Acute disease—usually result of esophageal perforation or tracheal tear; may be secondary to neck wounds (e.g., bite or gunshot), sepsis, pneumonia, pericarditis, or pyothorax; may be complicated by gram-negative bacteria
• Chronic disease—usually result of a bacterial (e.g., *Actinomyces* and *Nocardia* spp.) or fungal (e.g., *Coccidioides, Cryptococcus, Blastomyces,* and *Histoplasma* spp.) infection
• Predisposing factors—esophageal foreign body; cervical or thoracic trauma; immuno-suppressed state

DIAGNOSIS

DIFFERENTIAL DIAGNOSIS
• Isolated pericarditis, pyothorax, and pneumonia
• Cranial mediastinal mass—lymphosarcoma; thymoma, thyroid, or parathyroid tumor; neurogenic tumor; mesenchymal tumor (usually lipoma or other fat accumulation); mediastinal cyst
• Esophageal motor dysfunction or other esophageal abnormality
• Gastroesophageal disorder

CBC/BIOCHEMISTRY/URINALYSIS
• High WBC count with left shift
• PCV and total protein—may be high owing to volume depletion

OTHER LABORATORY TESTS
N/A

IMAGING
• Thoracic radiographs—reveal a wide mediastinum; may see pneumothorax or bilateral pleural effusion
• Esophageal contrast study—evaluate esophageal perforation or other abnormality; use a water-soluble contrast media with suspected perforation.
• Thoracic ultrasound—differentiate between mediastinal fluid accumulation (e.g., cyst and abscess), inflammatory reaction, and tumor
• Computed homograph and MRI—more definitive than ultrasound

DIAGNOSTIC PROCEDURES
• Cytology—thoracentesis of any pleural effusion; transthoracic fine-needle aspirate; cutting-needle biopsy of the mediastinal enlargement
• Submit all samples submitted for bacterial culture and sensitivity testing.

TREATMENT

• Inpatient with restricted activity until infection is controlled and condition is stable
• Pleural effusion of marked quantity or pyothorax of any degree—managed by tube thoracostomy
• Physiologically balanced electrolyte solutions—administer parenterally until oral alimentation is possible and water and food intake returns to normal or near normal.
• Esophageal perforation—surgical emergency; after surgical repair, enforce either parenteral alimentation or gastric tube feeding for 3–5 days.
• Chronic disease—best treated by surgical exploration when associated with an abscess or a granuloma
• Tube thoracostomy—maintain postsurgery by continuous water seal suction for 5–7 days or until negligible fluid is removed; follow a similar course with or without pleural cavity lavage when surgery is not performed.
• Warn client that this is a serious disease with a guarded prognosis.

MEDICATIONS

DRUGS
Broad-spectrum bactericidal antibiotic—choose on the basis of bacterial culture and sensitivity testing; parenterally for at least the first week of treatment, then orally

CONTRAINDICATIONS/POSSIBLE INTERACTIONS
Aminoglycoside antibiotics—avoid or accurately base dosage on creatinine clearance with azotemia

FOLLOW-UP

PATIENT MONITORING
• Daily temperature recording
• Hemogram—every 2–3 days during hospitalization (usually 7–10 days)
• Thoracic radiographs—at 7–10-day intervals (more often if drainage is needed)
• Antibiotics—generally continue for 1 week after hemogram and radiographs return to normal; with abscessation, continue an additional 4–6 weeks.

POSSIBLE COMPLICATIONS
• Pyothorax
• Sepsis
• Mediastinal fibrosis

EXPECTED COURSE AND PROGNOSIS
• With early diagnosis and aggressive treatment—prognosis fair to good
• With mediastinal fibrosis—long-term prognosis guarded to poor

MISCELLANEOUS

ABBREVIATION
PCV = packed cell volume

Suggested Reading

Bauer T. Mediastinal, pleural and extrapleural diseases. In: Ettinger SJ, ed. Textbook of veterinary internal medicine. 3rd ed. Philadelphia: Saunders, 1989:867–897.

Author Neil K. Harpster

Consulting Editor Eleanor C. Hawkins

MEGACOLON

 BASICS

DEFINITION
A condition of persistent increased large bowel diameter associated with chronic constipation/obstipation and low-to-absent colonic motility

PATHOPHYSIOLOGY
• Acquired megacolon results from chronic retention of fecal material that leads to colonic absorption of fecal water and solidified fecal concretions.
• Prolonged distension of the colon results in irreversible changes in colonic motility that leads to colonic inertia.
• Congenital absence of colonic ganglionic cells (Hirschsprung's disease) is not clearly documented in small animals.
• Recent work strongly suggests that the pathogenesis of idiopathic megacolon in cats involves a disturbance of colonic smooth muscle function.

SYSTEMS AFFECTED
Gastrointestinal

GENETICS
N/A

INCIDENCE/PREVALENCE
Unknown

GEOGRAPHIC DISTRIBUTION
N/A

SIGNALMENT
Species
• Idiopathic megacolon—cats
• Acquired megacolon—cats and dogs

Breed Predilections
Some evidence for increased risk in Manx cats

Mean Age and Range
• Idiopathic megacolon—middle-aged to old cats (mean age, 4.9 years; range, 1–15 years)
• Acquired megacolon—none

Predominant Sex
None

SIGNS
Historical Findings
• Idiopathic megacolon—typically a chronic/recurrent problem; signs often present for months to years.
• Acquired megacolon—signs may be acute or chronic.
• Constipation/obstipation
• Tenesmus with small or no fecal volume

• Hard, dry feces
• Infrequent defecation
• Small amount of diarrhea (often mucoid) may occur after prolonged tenesmus.
• Occasional vomiting, anorexia, and/or depression
• Weight loss

Physical Examination Findings
• Abdominal palpation reveals an enlarged colon with a hard fecal mass.
• Digital rectal examination may indicate an underlying (obstructive) cause and confirms fecal impaction.
• Dehydration
• Scruffy, unkempt haircoat

CAUSES
• Idiopathic—cats
• Mechanical obstruction—pelvic fracture malunion, foreign body or improper diet (especially bones), stricture, pseudocoprostasis, prostatic disease, perineal hernia, neoplasia, anal or rectal atresia
• Causes of dyschezia—anorectal disease (anal sacculitis, anal sac abscess, perianal fistula, proctitis), trauma (fractured pelvis, fractured limb, dislocated hip, perianal bite wound or laceration, perineal abscess)
• Metabolic disorders—hypokalemia, severe dehydration
• Drugs—vincristine, barium, antacids, sucralfate, anticholinergics
• Neurologic/neuromuscular disease—congenital abnormalities of the caudal spine (especially Manx cats), paraplegia, spinal cord disease, intervertebral disk disease, dysautonomia, sacral nerve disease, sacral nerve trauma (e.g., tail fracture/pull injury), trauma to colonic innervation

RISK FACTORS
• Conditions leading to inability to posture (limb and pelvic fractures, neuromuscular disease etc.) or rectoanal pain
• Prior pelvic fractures
• Possible association with low physical activity and obesity
• Perineal hernias

 DIAGNOSIS

DIFFERENTIAL DIAGNOSIS
• Other causes of palpable colonic masses (e.g. lymphoma, carcinoma, intussusception)—distinguish on the basis of texture, rectal examination, and imaging.

• Dysuria/stranguria—exclude by palpation of the bladder and colon, and by urinalysis.
• Tenesmus due to inflammation of the lower bowel (colitis)—exclude by palpation, rectal examination, and imaging.

CBC/BIOCHEMISTRY/URINALYSIS
• May show evidence of dehydration (elevated packed cell volume, total protein) and stress leukogram
• Electrolyte abnormalities may develop depending on duration of obstipation; may be prerenal azotemia with dehydration
• Urinalysis—no consistent changes; important to confirm normal renal function in dehydrated animals and to rule out lower urinary tract disease as a differential diagnosis

OTHER LABORATORY TESTS
N/A

IMAGING
• Abdominal/pelvic radiographs to identify any underlying causes
• Can easily see the enlarged, fecal-filled colon on plain abdominal radiographs
• Abdominal ultrasound may help to identify mural or obstructive masses.

DIAGNOSTIC PROCEDURES
May need colonoscopy to rule out mural or intraluminal obstructive lesions

PATHOLOGIC FINDINGS
• The most severe dilation typically occurs in the transverse and descending colon, although the entire length of the colon can be involved.
• The colon is usually histologically normal.

 TREATMENT

APPROPRIATE HEALTH CARE
• Inpatient medical management; surgery may be indicated if recurrent/severe problem
• Medical therapy—restore normal hydration, followed by anesthesia and manual evacuation of the colon using warm water enemas, water-soluble jelly, and gentle extraction of feces with a gloved finger or sponge forceps; do not traumatize the colonic mucosa excessively.
• Continue long-term therapy at home.

NURSING CARE
• Most patients require parenteral fluid support to correct dehydration.
• Intravenous administration of balanced electrolyte solutions is the preferred route.

MEGACOLON

ACTIVITY
• Encourage activity and exercise.
• Restriction indicated in the postoperative period if surgery is performed.

DIET
• Many patients require a low-residue-producing diet; bulk-forming fiber diets can worsen or lead to recurrence of colonic fecal distension.
• A high-fiber diet is occassionally helpful.
• A more palatable, maintenance-type diet can be supplemented with products such as Metamucil or pumpkin pie filler.

CLIENT EDUCATION
• In idiopathic disease or with severe colonic injury, medical therapy is often lifelong and can be frustrating.
• Recurrence is common.
• Surgery (subtotal colectomy) is indicated if medical therapy fails.

SURGICAL CONSIDERATIONS
• An underlying obstructive cause requires surgical correction.
• Avoid enema administration/colonic evacuation prior to subtotal colectomy.
• Subtotal colectomy with ileorectal or colo-rectal anastomosis—treatment of choice for idiopathic megacolon refractory to medical management
• Colectomy may also be required with obstructive megacolon caused by irreversible changes in colonic motility.

MEDICATIONS

DRUGS OF CHOICE
• Can improve colonic motility in less severe cases with cisapride, a prokinetic GI drug (dogs, 0.1–0.5 mg/kg PO q8–12h; cats, 2.5–10.0 mg/cat q8–12h)
• Stool softeners (e.g., lactulose, 1 mL/4.5 kg PO q8–12h to effect) are recommended in conjunction with cisapride and diet.
• Broad-spectrum prophylactic antibiotics are recommended prior to colon evacuation and during the perioperative period if surgery is elected.

CONTRAINDICATIONS
• Sodium phosphate retention enemas (e.g., Fleet; C.B. Fleet Co., Inc.)—because of their association with severe hypocalcemia
• Mineral oil and white petrolatum—because of danger of fatal lipoid aspiration pneumonia due to lack of taste

PRECAUTIONS
Common hairball laxatives (e.g., Laxatone, Cat-a-Lax) are typically ineffective.

POSSIBLE INTERACTIONS
N/A

ALTERNATIVE DRUGS
Docusate sodium can be used as a stool softener in place of lactulose.

FOLLOW-UP

PATIENT MONITORING
• Following colonic resection and anastomosis—for 3–5 days check for signs of dehiscence and peritonitis.
• Clinical deterioration warrants abdomino-centesis and/or peritoneal lavage to detect anastomotic leakage.
• Continue fluid support until the patient is willing to eat and drink.

PREVENTION/AVOIDANCE
• Repair pelvic fractures that narrow the pelvic canal.
• Avoid exposure to foreign bodies and feeding bones.

POSSIBLE COMPLICATIONS
• Recurrence or persistence—most common
• Potential surgical complications include peritonitis, persistent diarrhea, stricture formation, and recurrence of obstipation.
• Traumatic perforation of the colon is a serious complication of overzealous fecal evacuation.

EXPECTED COURSE AND PROGNOSIS
• Historically, medical management has been unrewarding.
• Cisapride appears to improve the prognosis with medical management in some patients, but may not suffice in severe or long-standing cases.
• Postoperative diarrhea—expected; typically resolves within 6 weeks (80% of cats with idiopathic megacolon undergoing subtotal colectomy) but can persist for several months; stools become more formed as the ileum adapts by increasing reservoir capacity and water absorption.
• Subtotal colectomy is well tolerated by cats; constipation recurrence rates are typically low.

✓ MISCELLANEOUS

ASSOCIATED CONDITIONS
Perineal hernia

AGE-RELATED FACTORS
Concurrent medical conditions (e.g., chronic renal insufficiency, hyperthyroidism) may occur with idiopathic megacolon, since many cats are old.

ZOONOTIC POTENTIAL
N/A

PREGNANCY
• The effect of cisapride on the fetus is unknown.
• Patients would be at increased risk for dystocia if they carried a pregnancy to term.

SYNONYMS
N/A

SEE ALSO
• Constipation and Obstipation
• Dyschezia and Hematochezia
• Perineal Hernia

ABBREVIATIONS
N/A

Suggested Reading

Bertoy RW. Megacolon. In: Bojrab MJ, ed. Disease mechanisms in small animal surgery. 2nd ed. Philadelphia: Lea & Febiger, 1993:262–265.

Holt D, Johnston DE. Idiopathic megacolon in cats. Compend Contin Educ Pract Vet 1991;13:1411–1416.

Rosin E. Megacolon in cats: the role of colectomy. In: Lieb MS, ed. Small animal practice. Philadelphia: Saunders, Vet Clin North Am 1993;23(3):587–594.

Tams TR. Cisapride: clinical experience with the newest GI prokinetic drug. (Abstract) Proceedings of the 12th Annual Veterinary Medical Forum-ACVIM. 1994:100–101.

Author Bradford C. Dixon
Consulting Editors Mitchell A. Crystal and Brett M. Feder

DISEASES

MEGAESOPHAGUS

 BASICS

DEFINITION
Rather than a single disease entity, megaesophagus refers to esophageal dilation and hypomotility, which may be a primary disorder or secondary to esophageal obstruction or neuromuscular dysfunction.

PATHOPHYSIOLOGY
• Esophageal motility is decreased or absent, resulting in accumulation and retention of food and liquid in the esophagus. • Reflex esophageal motility begins when food stimulates sensory afferents in the esophageal mucosa, which then sends afferent messages to the brainstem swallowing center via the vagus nerve. • Efferent messages from lower motor neurons in the nucleus ambiguus travel via the vagus to stimulate contraction of esophageal striated and smooth muscle. • Lesions anywhere along this pathway, including the myoneural junction, may result in esophageal hypomotility and distention. • Increased lower esophageal sphincter tone is not an important cause of megaesophagus in veterinary patients.

SYSTEMS AFFECTED
• Gastrointestinal—regurgitation, weight loss/cachexia • Neuromuscular—may be manifestation of neuromuscular disease • Respiratory—if aspiration pneumonia occurs

GENETICS
Congenital idiopathic megaesophagus is heritable in Wire-haired fox terriers (simple autosomal recessive) and Miniature schnauzers (simple autosomal dominant or 60% penetrance autosomal recessive).

INCIDENCE/PREVALENCE
Most common cause of regurgitation in dogs and cats

GEOGRAPHIC DISTRIBUTION
N/A

SIGNALMENT

Species
More common in dogs than cats

Breed Predilections
• Hereditary in wire-haired fox terriers and miniature schnauzers • Familial predispositions reported in the German shepherd, Newfoundland, Great dane, Irish setter, Sharpei, Pug, Greyhound, and Siamese cats.

Mean Age and Range
• Congenital megaesophagus—signs of regurgitation first appear at weaning • Acquired forms—reported most often in young adults to middle-aged animals.

Predominant Sex
N/A

SIGNS

Historical Findings
• May include regurgitation of food and water, weight loss or poor growth, hypersalivation and a gurgling sound with swallowing • History relating to the underlying cause of megaesophagus may include weakness, paresis or paralysis, ataxia, gagging, dysphagia, pain, or depression. • May see coughing, mucopurulent nasal discharge, and dyspnea with concurrent aspiration pneumonia

Physical Examination Findings
• Occasionally normal • Related to megaesophagus—regurgitation, weight loss, auscultation of retained fluid and food in the esophagus, halitosis, ptyalism, bulging of the esophagus at the thoracic inlet, and pain associated with palpation of the cervical esophagus • Related to the cause or sequelae of megaesophagus—respiratory crackles, tachypnea, pyrexia, myalgia, muscle weakness, muscle atrophy, hyporeflexia, proprioceptive and postural deficits, autonomic disorders (mydriasis with loss of pupillary light reflex, dry nasal and ocular mucous membranes, diarrhea, bradycardia), cranial nerve deficits (especially cranial nerves VI, IX, and X), paresis or paralysis, and mentation changes

CAUSES
• Congenital idiopathic megaesophagus • Esophageal obstruction—esophageal foreign body, stricture, neoplasia, granuloma, vascular ring anomalies (e.g., persistent right aortic arch), periesophageal compression • Neurologic and neuromuscular diseases—myasthenia gravis (focal or generalized), polymyositis (including systemic lupus erythematosus [SLE]), polyneuritis/polyradiculoneuritis, botulism, dysautonomia, central nervous system (CNS) disorders, degenerative, infectious/inflammatory, neoplasia, traumatic disorders of the brainstem and spinal cord, bilateral vagal damage. • Miscellaneous—esophagitis, hypothyroidism, hypoadrenocorticism, thymoma (with secondarily acquired myasthenia gravis), toxicosis (lead, thallium, acetylcholinesterase inhibitors)

RISK FACTORS
N/A

 DIAGNOSIS

DIFFERENTIAL DIAGNOSIS
• Other disorders causing regurgitation. • Obstructive pharyngeal disease (foreign bodies, inflammation, neoplasia, cricopharyngeal achalasia) and palate disorders may produce regurgitation with normal esophageal motility. • Pharyngeal pain and dysphagia often occur with obstructive pharyngeal disease. • Distinguish regurgitation from dysphagia and vomition. • Regurgitation is a passive process with no forceful abdominal contraction, anticipatory salivation, nausea, or retching. • Bile-stained ingesta suggests vomition. • The time relationship between eating and expulsion of food does not help to distinguish regurgitation and vomiting.

CBC/BIOCHEMISTRY/URINALYSIS
• No characteristic findings, but may aid in identifying the underlying cause • Hyponatremia and hyperkalemia suggest hypoadrenocorticism. • Hypercholesterolemia is usually present with hypothyroidism.

OTHER LABORATORY TESTS
• Acetylcholine receptor antibody titers to screen for acquired myasthenia gravis • Antinuclear antibody titers to evaluate for SLE • ACTH stimulation to evaluate adrenal function • Free T_4/TSH level to evaluate thyroid function • Blood lead and cholinesterase levels to evaluate for toxicity

IMAGING

Survey Thoracic Radiographs
• Esophagus dilated with gas, fluid, or ingesta • The trachea is often displaced ventrally by the distended esophagus.

Contrast Esophagram and Fluoroscopy
• An esophagram using either barium liquid or paste may demonstrate contrast pooling and abnormal esophageal motility. • Abnormal primary and secondary esophageal peristalsis can be visualized with fluoroscopy. • Contrast studies—not necessary for diagnosing most cases of megaesophagus; use with caution in animal patients with known megaesophagus, because of the risk of aspiration.

Nuclear Scintigraphy
Measures the rate of transport of radiolabeled food through the esophagus

DIAGNOSTIC PROCEDURES
• Endoscopy—can use to visualize a dilated esophagus, foreign bodies, neoplasia, and esophagitis; mucosal biopsy specimens and cytology samples may be obtained; esophageal foreign bodies may be removed. • EMG and NCV—fibrillation potentials, positive sharp waves, and complex repetitive discharges suggest neuromuscular disease; prolonged NCV suggests peripheral neuropathy. • Repetitive nerve stimulation and edrophonium challenge—muscular weakness following edrophonium chloride (0.1–0.2 mg/kg IV) and a decremental response of the compound action potential support the diagnosis of myasthenia gravis; false-positive and false-negative results can occur. • Muscle and nerve biopsies/histopathology—useful to confirm diagnosis of inflammatory and degenerative disorders of muscles and nerves • Cerebrospinal fluid analysis—pleocytosis and/or protein elevations suggest CNS disease • Autonomic nervous system testing—ocular

pharmacologic testing (e.g. 0.05–0.1% pilocarpine eyedrops to demonstrate postganglionic denervation of the iris constrictor muscle) and measurement of blood pressure (hypotension) support autonomic dysfunction. • Fecal examination for *Spirocerca lupi* ova

PATHOLOGIC FINDINGS
Gross and histopathologic findings vary, depending on the underlying disease.

 TREATMENT

APPROPRIATE HEALTH CARE
• Many can be diagnosed and treated as outpatients. • Hospitalize patients with aspiration pneumonia, obstructive megaesophagus, severe debilitation, or advanced neurologic disease.

NURSING CARE
Aspiration pneumonia and/or dehydration warrant appropriate antibiotic and fluid therapy.

ACTIVITY
No change necessary for megaesophagus alone; restriction may be necessary for associated neuromuscular disorders.

DIET
• Feed in upright position (45–90° angle to the floor) and maintain position for 10–15 min following feeding. • Feeding a gruel often produces the least regurgitation, although dietary consistency must be individualized for each patient; the consistency that produces the least regurgitation may change with time. • Patients with severe regurgitation may need parenteral feeding via gastrotomy tube.

CLIENT EDUCATION
Emphasize the danger of aspiration pneumonia and the importance of the special feeding requirements.

SURGICAL CONSIDERATIONS
• Surgery may be necessary to remove esophageal foreign bodies or neoplasia or correct vascular ring anomalies. • No surgical procedures improve esophageal motility. • The modified Heller's cardiomyotomy reduces lower esophageal tone and may improve gravity-facilitated movement of ingesta into the stomach. • Surgical treatment of megaesophagus has not been critically evaluated in dogs and cats and is not currently recommended.

 MEDICATIONS

DRUGS OF CHOICE
• No drugs are commonly used to treat megaesophagus alone; direct treatment at the underlying disease or associated conditions (e.g., aspiration pneumonia). • Sucralfate (0.5–1.0 g/dog PO q8h), H_2 blockers (e.g., famotidine 0.5 mg/kg PO q12–24h in dogs) or omeprazole (0.7 mg/kg PO q24h in dogs) can be used if reflux esophagitis is present. • Metoclopramide (0.2–0.5 mg/kg PO q6–8h in dogs) speeds gastric emptying, increases gastroesophageal sphincter tone, and is most useful when reflux esophagitis is a contributing or the primary cause; use of metoclopramide for other causes has had limited success. • Broad-spectrum antibiotics—necessary for patients with aspiration pneumonia; parenteral antibiotics or enteral administration via a gastrotomy tube may be required for patients with severe regurgitation. • Immunosuppressive agents (e.g., prednisone, cyclophosphamide, azathioprine) are required for immune-mediated diseases. • Prednisone and acetylcholinesterase inhibitors (pyridostigmine) are used to treat myasthenia gravis.

CONTRAINDICATIONS
N/A

PRECAUTIONS
• Corticosteroids may be necessary to treat conditions causing megaesophagus; use with caution in patients with aspiration pneumonia. • Cisapride (0.1–0.5 mg/kg PO q8–12h in dogs) has been used to treat megaesophagus, but its use is controversial; it decreases esophageal transit time and increases lower esophageal tone in normal dogs; both of these effects are undesirable when treating megaesophagus; despite this, regurgitation decreases in some patients receiving cisapride; if symptoms of megaesophagus worsen, discontinue cisapride.

POSSIBLE INTERACTIONS
N/A

ALTERNATIVE DRUGS
N/A

 FOLLOW-UP

PATIENT MONITORING
• Reexamine patients if signs of aspiration pneumonia develop—fever, cough, mucopurulent nasal discharge • May use repeat thoracic radiographs, esophagrams, and fluoroscopic and neurologic examinations to follow progression or resolution of megaesophagus.

PREVENTION/AVOIDANCE
Esophageal obstruction may be prevented if pets are not allowed access to bones, garbage, or other tempting items.

POSSIBLE COMPLICATIONS
Aspiration pneumonia

EXPECTED COURSE AND PROGNOSIS
• Poor, with or without treatment • Aspiration pneumonia, owner noncompliance, and malnutrition are leading causes of death. • Additional neurologic abnormalities may develop if the megaesophagus is caused by neuromuscular disease. • Megaesophagus caused by myasthenia gravis may improve with treatment. • Occasionally congenital idiopathic megaesophagus may resolve with age; probably much less frequently than previously reported.

 MISCELLANEOUS

ASSOCIATED CONDITIONS
Aspiration pneumonia

AGE-RELATED FACTORS
Regurgitation at weaning suggests congenital or obstructive megaesophagus.

ZOONOTIC POTENTIAL
Determine rabies vaccination status for all patients.

PREGNANCY
N/A

SYNONYMS
Do not use the term *achalasia,* which describes esophageal hypomotility and lower esophageal sphincter hypertonicity in humans, because megaesophagus in animals is rarely associated with lower esophageal sphincter hypertonicity.

SEE ALSO
• Dysphagia • Regurgitation • Esophageal Foreign Bodies • Myasthenia Gravis • Pneumonia, Bacterial

Suggested Reading
Boudrieau RJ. Megaesophagus in the dog: a review of 50 cases. JAAHA 1985;21:33–40.
Guilford WG. Megaesophagus in the dog and cat. Semin Vet Med Surg (Small Anim) 1990;5:37–45.
Leib MS. Megaesophagus. In: Bojrab MJ, ed. Disease mechanisms in small animal surgery. 2nd ed. Philadelphia: Lea & Febiger, 1993:205–209.
Washabau RJ, Hall JA. Diagnosis and management of gastrointestinal motility disorders in dogs and cats. Compend Cont Educ Pract Vet 1997;19:721–736.
Author Randall C. Longshore
Consulting Editors Brett M. Feder and Mitchell A. Crystal

DISEASES

MELANOCYTIC TUMORS, ORAL

 BASICS

OVERVIEW
• Tumors characterized by progressive local invasion of neoplastic melanocytic cells within the oral cavity of dogs or cats
• Arise from the gingival surface and grow rapidly
• Generally characterized by a nonencapsulated, raised, irregular, ulcerated, and/or necrotic surface; highly invasive to bone
• Melanoma—most common oral malignancy in dogs; third most common in cats
• Metastasis—common; spread to the lymph nodes more common than to the lungs
• Cause of death—secondary to local recurrence, dysphagia, and subsequent cachexia

SIGNALMENT
• Occurs more commonly in dogs and cats > 10 years in age
• No sex or breed predilection

SIGNS

Historical Findings
• Excessive salivation
• Halitosis
• Dysphagia
• Bloody oral discharge
• Weight loss

Physical Examination Findings
• Oral mass
• Loose teeth
• Facial deformity
• Occasionally, cervical lymphadenomegaly

CAUSES & RISK FACTORS
None identified

 DIAGNOSIS

DIFFERENTIAL DIAGNOSIS
• Other oral malignancy
• Epulis
• Abscess
• Benign polyp

CBC/BIOCHEMISTRY/URINALYSIS
Usually normal

OTHER LABORATORY TESTS
Cytologic evaluation of an impression smear—obtain from an incisional biopsy specimen (wedge); may yield a diagnosis

IMAGING
• Skull radiography—evaluate for bone involvement deep to the mass.
• Thoracic radiographs—evaluate lungs for metastasis.

DIAGNOSTIC PROCEDURES
• Large, deep tissue biopsy (down to bone)—required to sufficiently differentiate from other oral malignancies
• Carefully palpate regional lymph nodes (mandibular and retropharyngeal).

 TREATMENT

SURGERY
• Radical surgical excision—required (e.g., hemimaxillectomy); well tolerated by most patients; must have margins of at least 2 cm; improved survival when excisional margins are free of neoplastic cells
• Cryosurgery—not indicated because of extensive bony invasion
• Soft foods—may be recommended to prevent tumor ulceration or after radical oral excision

RADIATION
• Coarse fraction external beam radiotherapy (teletherapy)—may offer considerable long-term control if tumor is deemed inoperable
• Current radiotherapy plans—attempt 24 Gy given in three fractions at 0, 7, and 21 days
• Response in cats not reported
• Complications—common; include mucositis, anorexia, and dehydration requiring aggressive supportive care
• Combined with low-dose cisplatin—may improve overall survival
• Combined with hyperthermia—does not improve overall survival

MEDICATIONS

DRUGS
• No effective chemotherapeutic agents described for local or systemic control of oral melanoma in dogs or cats
• Local control (palliation) with intralesionally administered cisplatin reported

CONTRAINDICATIONS/POSSIBLE INTERACTIONS
• Chemotherapy can be toxic; seek advice before initiating treatment if you are unfamiliar with cytotoxic drugs.
• Cisplatin should not be used in cats.

FOLLOW-UP

EXPECTED COURSE AND PROGNOSIS
• Radical excision involving normal bone—best long-term control and survival
• Survival after complete surgical excision (dogs)—median, 340 days; mean, 567 days
• Survival after incomplete surgical excision (dogs)—median, 260 days; mean, 210 days
• Survival after any form of surgical excision (cats)—< 60 days
• Survival with radiotherapy treatment (dogs)—0–19 months
• Positive prognostic features at the time of diagnosis—location (e.g., rostral mandible and caudal maxilla), small tumor size, and low mitotic index
• Distant metastasis at examination—low (< 10%); but is most often the cause of death late in the course of the disease
• Overall prognosis in cats—poor; most tumors are locally invasive and diagnosed late in the course of the disease; cause of death is secondary to local recurrence, dysphagia, and subsequent cachexia.

MISCELLANEOUS

Suggested Reading

Bateman KE, Catton PA, Pennock PW, Kruth SA. 0-7-21 radiation therapy for the treatment of canine oral melanoma. J Vet Intern Med 1994;8:267–272.

Hahn KA, DeNicola DB, Richardson RC, Hahn EA. Canine oral malignant melanoma: prognostic utility of an alternative staging system. J Small Anim Pract 1994;35:251–256.

Patnaik AK, Mooney S. Feline melanoma: a comparative study of ocular, oral, and dermal neoplasms. Vet Pathol 1988;25:105–112.

Author Kevin A. Hahn
Consulting Editor Wallace B. Morrison

DISEASES

MELANOCYTIC TUMORS, SKIN AND DIGIT

BASICS

DEFINITION
Benign or malignant neoplasm arising from melanocytes and melanoblasts (melanin-producing cells)

PATHOPHYSIOLOGY
• Locally invasive
• Malignant—may invade bone and metastasize to regional lymph nodes

SYSTEMS AFFECTED
• Skin/Exocrine
• Metastatic sites—bone, lymph nodes, lung, and viscera

GENETICS
Unknown

INCIDENCE/PREVALENCE
• Dogs—4%–20% of all skin tumors
• Cats—0.8%–7% of all skin tumors

GEOGRAPHIC DISTRIBUTION
N/A

SIGNALMENT
Species
Dogs and cats

Breed Predilections
• Dogs—Scottish terriers, Boston terriers, Airedale terriers, cocker spaniels, boxers, springer spaniels, Irish setters, Irish terriers, chow chows, Chihuahuas, and Doberman pinschers
• Cats—none

Mean Age and Range
• Dogs—9 years
• Cats—8–14 years

Predominant Sex
• Dogs—males may be predisposed.
• Cats—none

SIGNS
Historical Findings
• Slow or rapidly growing mass
• Lameness if digit is involved

Physical Examination Findings
• Pigmented or nonpigmented (amelanotic) mass, usually solitary
• Develops anywhere but may be more common on face, trunk, feet, and scrotum in dogs and head and pinna in cats
• Regional lymph nodes—may be large
• Advanced disease—may have dyspnea or harsh lung sounds because of pulmonary metastasis

CAUSES
Unknown

RISK FACTORS
Unknown

DIAGNOSIS

DIFFERENTIAL DIAGNOSIS
Histopathologic examination and special stains—may distinguish amelanotic melanoma from poorly differentiated mast cell tumors, lymphosarcoma, and carcinoma

CBC/BIOCHEMISTRY/URINALYSIS
Usually normal

OTHER LABORATORY TESTS
Immunohistochemical stains—may help differentiate melanoma (especially amelanotic) from other tumors; melanoma stains positive with vimentin, S-100, neuron-specific enolase, and human melanosome–specific antigen.

IMAGING
• Thoracic radiography—detect metastasis
• Area radiography—determine if underlying bone is involved, especially with melanoma of the digit.

DIAGNOSTIC PROCEDURES
Cytologic examination of fine-needle aspirate—reveals brown, rod-like intracellular granules (melanin) in cells of various sizes and shapes; pigment may be absent in the case of amelanotic melanoma; may see macrophages (melanophages) containing phagocytosed melanin

PATHOLOGIC FINDINGS
Gross
• Masses—vary in color and appearance; may be ulcerated
• Benign—generally slow-growing; brown to black; varies from macules and plaques to firm, dome-shaped nodules, 0.5–2 cm in diameter
• Malignant—generally rapidly growing; amelanotic to dark brown, gray, or black
• Melanomas of the digit (dog) and eyelid (cat) tend to be malignant.

Histopathologic Findings
• Often difficult to distinguish benign from malignant lesions because both may have cells that vary in shape (e.g., epithelioid, fusiform, dendritic, and mixed), degree of pigmentation, and cytoplasmic morphology
• Malignant—generally high mitotic index; nuclear and nucleolar pleomorphism; invasive into surrounding tissues; amelanotic may pose a diagnostic challenge; special stains may be particularly useful.
• Benign and malignant—may note associated inflammation, predominantly lymphoplasmacytic

TREATMENT

APPROPRIATE HEALTH CARE
Inpatient if undergoing surgery

NURSING CARE
Fluid administration—indicated during surgery
• Melanoma of the digit—may require bandaging of the distal limb after surgery

ACTIVITY
• Depends on location of tumor
• Generally, restrict until sutures are removed.

DIET
Normal

MELANOCYTIC TUMORS, SKIN AND DIGIT

CLIENT EDUCATION
• Discuss the need for early surgical removal.
• Do not advise a wait-and-see approach.
• Warn client that malignant melanoma may metastasize early in the course of the disease; thus prognosis is guarded.

SURGICAL CONSIDERATIONS
• Wide surgical excision—treatment of choice
• Amputation of digit—nail bed or digit affected

MEDICATIONS

DRUGS OF CHOICE
• Adjunctive chemotherapy—recommended if surgical excision is incomplete or the mass is nonresectable
• Dacarbazine (DTIC), doxorubicin, and carboplatin—reported to induce partial and complete remission in a small number of animals; may be the drugs of choice

CONTRAINDICATIONS
Doxorubicin—cardiotoxic; contraindicated with heart disease

PRECAUTIONS
Veterinarians administering chemotherapeutics should follow published guidelines on the safe use of these drugs and should be familiar with potential side effects.

POSSIBLE INTERACTIONS
None reported

ALTERNATIVE DRUGS
Cimetidine—shown to be of some benefit in horses and humans with malignant melanoma; believed to act as a biologic response modifier by reversing suppressor T-cell–mediated immune suppression; has not been evaluated for this purpose in dogs and cats

FOLLOW-UP

PATIENT MONITORING
• Evaluate for evidence of recurrence and metastasis—1, 3, 6, 9, 12, 18, and 24 months after surgery; if the owner believes the mass is returning; if the patient is otherwise not normal
• Thoracic radiography—at the time of rechecks and periodically thereafter

PREVENTION/AVOIDANCE
N/A

POSSIBLE COMPLICATIONS
None

EXPECTED COURSE AND PROGNOSIS
• Dogs—25%–50% of melanomas reported to be malignant; melanomas on the digit and scrotum have a greater likelihood of being malignant.
• Survival with benign melanomas (dogs)—mean: skin, > 24 months; digit, 19.3 months; 2-year: skin, 94.3%; digit: 38%
• Survival with malignant melanoma (dogs)—skin: 8–13.5 months; digit: 16.9 months; 2-year: skin, 34.1%; digit: 22%–36%
• Cats—35%–50% of melanomas reported to be malignant
• Mean survival with melanoma of the skin or digit (cats)—not frequently reported; 4.5 months after surgery in one study of 57 cats

MISCELLANEOUS

ASSOCIATED CONDITIONS
None

AGE-RELATED FACTORS
None

ZOONOTIC POTENTIAL
None

PREGNANCY
N/A

SYNONYMS
• Benign—melanocytic nevus; melanocytoma
• Malignant—melanosarcoma (rarely used)

ABBREVIATION
DTIC = (dimethyltriazeno)imidazole carboxamide

Suggested Reading
Aronsohn MG, Carpenter JL. Distal extremity melanocytic nevi and malignant melanomas in dogs. J Am Anim Hosp Assoc 1990;26:605–612.

Bostock DE. Prognosis after surgical excision of canine melanomas. Vet Pathol 1979;16:32–40.

Miller WH, Scott DW, Anderson WI. Feline cutaneous melanocytic neoplasms: a retrospective analysis of 43 cases (1979–1991). Vet Dermatol 1993;4:19–26.

Pulley LT, Stannard AA. Tumors of the skin and soft tissues. In: Moulton JE, ed. Tumors in domestic animals. 3rd ed. Berkeley: University of California Press, 1990:75–82.

Thomas RC, Fox LE. Tumors of the skin and subcutis. In: Morrison WB, ed. Cancer in dogs and cats: medical and surgical management. Baltimore: Williams & Wilkins, 1998:489–510.

Author Joanne C. Graham
Consulting Editor Wallace B. Morrison

DISEASES

MENINGIOMA

 BASICS

OVERVIEW
• Tumors of the meninges most commonly found intracranially over the cerebrum
• Usually solitary masses; occasionally multiple
• May occur as plaque-like masses on the floor of the calvaria, paranasally, or (rarely) in a retrobulbar location in dogs more than cats; also develop along the spinal cord but less frequently and with an intradural, extramedullary predilection site
• Compress the adjacent tissue, causing vasogenic edema
• Dogs—tends to be more invasive into brain parenchyma or surrounding vasculature

SIGNALMENT
• Dogs and cats
• Dogs—no breed predilection; mesocephalic breeds may have a higher incidence of paranasal meningiomas; most > 7 years of age; range 11 weeks to 14 years; a spinal meningeal sarcoma was diagnosed in an 11-week-old rottweiler; slight predominance for females
• Cats—most > 9 years of age; range 1–24 years; slight predominance for males

SIGNS
• Vary with tumor location
• Typically chronic and insidiously progressive over weeks to months
• May be acute if vascular invasion results in focal ischemia or if edema develops rapidly
• Lateralizing deficits predominate.

Intracranial
• Cerebral disease—predominates; abnormal behavior and mentation; contralateral visual and proprioceptive deficits; seizures
• Dogs—late-onset seizures common, presenting signs without evidence of neurologic examination deficits (silent area disease)
• Cats—may suggest herniation (e.g., anisocoria and stupor)

Intraspinal
• Ataxia and motor dysfunction—vary with location of the tumor along the spinal column
• Neck and back pain

CAUSE & RISK FACTORS
• Uncertain
• Documentation in young cats with mucopolysaccharidosis type I suggests a causal relationship.

 DIAGNOSIS

DIFFERENTIAL DIAGNOSIS
• Other primary CNS (e.g., glioma) or secondary (e.g., extensional or metastatic) tumors—more rapid onset and progression of signs; differentiate by brain imaging
• Cryptococcus granuloma—reported to have same appearance on CT as a meningioma in a cat
• Granulomatous meningoencephalitis—may cause progressive focal deficits in dogs
• Silent area meningiomas—may mimic a metabolic encephalopathy
• Nerve sheath tumors, gliomas, and type II intervertebral disk disease—differentiate from a spinal cord syndrome

CBC/BIOCHEMISTRY/URINALYSIS
Usually normal

OTHER LABORATORY TESTS
CSF analysis—infrequently performed because of the characteristic results of diagnostic imaging; results normal or reveal high protein, sometimes with a suppurative inflammation if the tumor is necrotic

IMAGING
• CT and MRI scans of the head—preferred diagnostic techniques for intracranial disease; more commonly reveal a homogenous enhancement of well-circumscribed lesions than ring enhancement in postcontrast scans
• Skull radiography and CT—may reveal hyperostosis of the calvaria adjacent to the meningioma and increased tissue density if the tumor is calcified
• Myelography—typically reveals an intradural–extramedullary mass with spinal disease; golf tee appearance makes differentiation from a nerve sheath tumor difficult without biopsy.

DIAGNOSTIC PROCEDURES
Electroencephalography—reveals slow-wave, medium- to high-voltage activity indicating cortical depression; may show paroxysmal waveforms characteristic of seizure activity

TREATMENT

- Outpatient, if treated medically
- Inpatient—dehydration; anorexia; frequent seizures
- Surgical excision—necessary for definitive management; usually successful if the tumor is accessible; incomplete excision more common in dogs because of invasiveness
- Radiation therapy—after excision; may be associated with prolonged survival time
- Medical management—palliative only; expect patient to deteriorate.
- Fluids—avoid overzealous administration; may exacerbate cerebral edema and neurologic deficits

MEDICATIONS

DRUGS

Cerebral Edema

- Corticosteroids—improve neurologic deficits associated with vasogenic edema
- Stuporous, severely ataxic, or showing signs of herniation—methylprednisolone sodium succinate (30 mg/kg IV) or dexamethasone sodium phosphate (2–3 mg/kg IV)
- Continued deterioration or no improvement—20% mannitol solution (0.5–2.0 g/kg CRI over 20 min)

- Once stable—prednisone (0.5 mg/kg q12h) or dexamethasone (cat or small dog: 0.25 mg PO q8h; medium to large dog: 0.5 mg q8h; giant dog: 0.75mg q8h; then taper as needed)

Seizures

- Anticonvulsants—if seizures occur more frequently than one per 6–8 weeks
- Phenobarbital—2–3 mg/kg IV q12h
- Cluster seizures—consider a loading dose of phenobarbital (12–16 mg/kg IV) or diazepam (0.5mg/kg/hr CRI)

CONTRAINDICATIONS/POSSIBLE INTERACTIONS

Chloramphenicol and cimetidine—avoid with phenobarbital because they delay its metabolism.

FOLLOW-UP

- Serial neurologic examinations—detect marked improvement in deficits within 24–48 hr after initiation of corticosteroids

Cats

- Surgical excision—prognosis good in ~ 70% of patients that undergo surgical excision; tumor may grow; seizure activity may persist.
- Medical management—neurologic deficits become more severe, but may take many months because meningiomas tend to be slow growing; thoracolumbar disease progresses to paralysis and inability to control urination, causes urinary retention, and (possibly) bladder atony and cystitis.

MISCELLANEOUS

ABBREVIATIONS

- CRI = constant rate infusion
- CSF = cerebrospinal fluid

Suggested Reading

Braund KG, Ribas JL. Central nervous system meningiomas. Compend Contin Educ Pract Vet 1986;8:241–248.

Nafe LA. Meningiomas in cats: a retrospective clinical study of 36 cases. J Am Vet Med Assoc 1979;174:1224–1227.

Author Richard J. Joseph
Consulting Editor Joane M. Parent

DISEASES

MENINGITIS/MENINGOENCEPHALITIS/MENINGOMYELITIS, BACTERIAL

BASICS

DEFINITION
- Meningitis—inflammation of the meninges
- Meningoencephalitis—inflammation of the meninges and brain
- Meningomyelitis—inflammation of the meninges and spinal cord

PATHOPHYSIOLOGY
- Bacterial infection of the CNS by extension of an infected extraneural site or by hematogenous route
- Inflammation of the meninges can lead to secondary inflammation of the brain or spinal cord, resulting in neurologic deficits.

SYSTEMS AFFECTED
- Nervous—meninges, brain, or spinal cord
- Multisystemic signs—may develop because the infection usually originates in an extraneural site

GENETICS
N/A

INCIDENCE/PREVALENCE
Rare

GEOGRAPHIC DISTRIBUTION
N/A

SIGNALMENT

Species
Dogs and cats

Breed Predilections
N/A

Mean Age and Range
- Any age
- Neonates may have a relatively higher risk because of omphalophlebitis.

Predominant Sex
N/A

SIGNS

General Comments
- Patients are nearly always systemically ill.
- Depression, shock, hypotension, and DIC may be found.
- May be fulminating

Physical Examination Findings
- May find site of underlying infection
- Cervical rigidity
- Hyperesthesia
- Pyrexia
- Vomiting and bradycardia—may occur

- Neurologic deficits—reflect the location of the involved parenchyma; increased intracranial pressure (e.g., stupor or coma, anisocoria, or poor physiologic nystagmus) may be seen.

CAUSES
- Meningoencephalitis—usually secondary to local extension from infection of the ears, eyes, sinuses, nasal passages
- Meningomyelitis—secondary from diskospondylitis or osteomyelitis
- Hematogenous spread of bacterial infection less often occurs from extracranial foci in dogs with bacterial endocarditis, prostatitis, metritis, or diskospondylitis.
- The point of origin is not always found.

RISK FACTORS
- Untreated bacterial infection
- Immunocompromised state
- Injury involving the CNS or adjacent structures

DIAGNOSIS

DIFFERENTIAL DIAGNOSIS

Fungal Meningitis
- Affected extraneural sites (dogs)—common with CNS cryptococcus (e.g., nasal, skin, and bone), blastomycosis (e.g., lung, lymph nodes, eyes, skin, and bone), and coccidioidomycosis (e.g., lung, bones, and joints)
- Diagnosis often made by biopsy or cytologic examination of affected tissues
- Serologic testing available
- Organisms—sometimes observed in the CSF; may be cultured

Distemper Virus Meningoencephalitis
- Patients usually young and unvaccinated
- CNS signs may be preceded by mild gastrointestinal and respiratory signs.
- Chorioretinitis common
- Inclusion bodies—may be observed on cytologic examination
- Virus—may be detected in a conjunctival scraping or tracheal wash specimen by fluorescent antibody technique
- CSF analysis—typically reveals a high number of small lymphocytes and high protein concentration, primarily albumin; neutrophils not seen

FIP Virus Meningoencephalitis
- Often accompanied by uveitis and chorioretinitis
- Patients generally < 3 years old; may have a protracted history

Toxoplasma Meningoencephalitis
- May be accompanied by pneumonia, hepatitis, myositis, and uveitis, especially in cats
- Toxoplasmosis—usually seen in young dogs; frequently involves the nerve roots and muscles
- Serum toxoplasma titer—may rise with active infection
- Serum IgM—may be detected in the serum and CSF of affected dogs
- Biopsy of affected tissues—may reveal the organism

Aseptic (Immune-mediated) Meningitis
Observed mainly in young large-breed dogs that have cervical pain alone and are not systemically ill

Neoplasia of the CNS
- Signs—limited to the CNS
- Standard laboratory tests—normal
- The diagnosis is made by CT or MRI and CSF analysis.

Granulomatous Meningoencephalomyelitis
- Clinical signs—usually not systemic
- CSF analysis—lymphocytes, monocytes, occasional plasma cells, and aplastic mononuclear cells; sometimes mature nontoxic neutrophils
- CSF culture—negative

CBC/BIOCHEMISTRY/URINALYSIS
- Leukocytosis common; left shift or toxicity may be seen.
- Evidence of other organ involvement (e.g., liver and kidney) and hyperglobulinemia in response to chronic infection
- Pyuria and bacteriuria—with underlying urinary tract or prostatic infection; with hematogenous spread of bacteria

OTHER LABORATORY TESTS
- Positive serologic tests—differentiate fungal, protozoal, rickettsial, and viral from bacterial disease; cats: toxoplasma titer may be positive without clinical disease.
- Cytologic examination of infected tissues—skin, eyes, nasal discharge, and sputum; helps identify the organism, especially in patients with fungal disease
- Blood and urine culture—may be positive

MENINGITIS/MENINGOENCEPHALITIS/MENINGOMYELITIS, BACTERIAL

IMAGING
• Spinal radiography—diskospondylitis as a focus of infection
• Skull radiography—sinus, nasal cavity, or ear as initiating site
• Echocardiography—valvular endocarditis suspected

DIAGNOSTIC PROCEDURES
Biopsy—infected tissue; may help identify the organism

CSF Analysis
• Collection—contraindicated with signs that suggest high intracranial pressure, because it may precipitate brain herniation
• Analysis—neutrophilic pleocytosis with high protein concentration; sometimes the neutrophils appear toxic or degenerated and bacteria are seen; difficult to differentiate aseptic from bacterial meningitis by this alone
• Culture—aerobic or anaerobic; may be positive

PATHOLOGIC FINDINGS
• May note subdural empyema, herniation, or purulent material on the surface of the brain
• Diffuse suppurative leptomeningeal infiltration common

 TREATMENT

APPROPRIATE HEALTH CARE
Inpatient—treat aggressively; intensive care monitoring often necessary

NURSING CARE
Fluid therapy and supportive care—as indicated for shock

ACTIVITY
Restricted

DIET
N/A

CLIENT EDUCATION
Inform client that rapid and aggressive treatment is important.

SURGICAL CONSIDERATIONS
N/A

 MEDICATIONS

DRUGS OF CHOICE
Antibiotics
• Agents that penetrate the blood–brain barrier—chloramphenicol, trimethoprim, sulfonamides, metronidazole, moxalactam, and cefotaxime
• Cultures—CSF, blood, urine, primary site; determine drug sensitivity; if cultures cannot be obtained, choose a broad-spectrum agent that is effective against aerobes and anaerobes.
• Inflammation and suspected staphylococcal infection—use penicillin or ampicillin, which enter the CNS; use in combination with another antibiotic that enters the CNS.

Anticonvulsants
• Indicated for seizures
• Diazepam initially and then phenobarbital

CONTRAINDICATIONS
Aminoglycosides and first-generation cephalosporins—do not penetrate the blood–brain barrier even in the presence of inflamed meninges; do not use.

PRECAUTIONS
N/A

POSSIBLE INTERACTIONS
Chloramphenicol—do not use in combination with phenobarbital; inhibits the hepatic metabolism of phenobarbital, leading to a toxic concentration

ALTERNATIVE DRUGS
N/A

 FOLLOW-UP

PATIENT MONITORING
Nervous system signs, fever, leukocytosis, and systemic signs

PREVENTION/AVOIDANCE
Treat local infections adjacent to the CNS (e.g., infections of the eyes, ears, sinuses, nose, and spine) early and aggressively to prevent extension to the CNS.

POSSIBLE COMPLICATIONS
Damage caused by inflammation of the brain and spinal cord or associated thrombosis may be irreversible.

EXPECTED COURSE AND PROGNOSIS
• Response to antibiotics—variable; prognosis guarded
• Many patients die despite treatment.
• Some patients recover completely.
• Treatment for at least 4 weeks after resolution of all signs is recommended.

 MISCELLANEOUS

ASSOCIATED CONDITIONS
N/A

AGE-RELATED FACTORS
N/A

ZOONOTIC POTENTIAL
N/A

PREGNANCY
N/A

SYNONYMS
N/A

SEE ALSO
• Encephalitis
• Meningoencephalomyelitis, Granulomatous

ABBREVIATIONS
• DIC = disseminated intravascular coagulation
• CSF = cerebrospinal fluid
• FIP = feline infectious peritonitis

Suggested Reading
Dow SW, LeCouteur RA, Henik RA, et al. Central nervous system infection associated with anaerobic bacteria in two dogs and two cats. J Vet Intern Med 1988;2:171–176.
Fenner WR. Bacterial infections of the central nervous system. In: Greene CE, ed., Infectious diseases of the dog and cat. Philadelphia: Saunders, 1990:184–196.
Meric SM. Canine meningitis. J Vet Intern Med 1988;2:26–35.
Oliver JE, Lorenz MD, Kornegay JN. Handbook of veterinary neurology. Philadelphia: Saunders, 1997:383–385.
Thomas WB, Sorjonen DC, Steiss JE. A retrospective evaluation of 38 cases of canine distemper encephalomyelitis. J Am Anim Hosp Assoc 1993;29:129–133.
Author Susan M. Taylor
Consulting Editor Joane M. Parent

DISEASES

MENINGOENCEPHALOMYELITIS, EOSINOPHILIC

 BASICS

OVERVIEW
• Diffuse or multifocal meningoencephalomyelitis
• CSF analysis reveals eosinophilic pleocytosis.
• Eosinophils—in response to a parasite or an allergic reaction
• Underlying cause of the idiopathic syndrome unknown
• Meningeal involvement can be marked.

SIGNALMENT
• Dogs
• Golden retrievers may be predisposed.
• Age range—14 weeks to 5.5 years
• Occurs more commonly in males

SIGNS
• Vary in location and severity
• Neurologic abnormalities—often relate to the cerebrum; dementia, seizures, circling, and cortical blindness

CAUSES & RISK FACTORS
• Idiopathic or allergic—more common than other causes
• Neoplasia—reaction to foreign material
• Parasitic—cerebral cysticerci, *Neospora caninum, Toxoplasma gondii, Dirofilaria immitis*

 DIAGNOSIS

DIFFERENTIAL DIAGNOSIS
• Cannot be differentiated from the other encephalitides on the basis of clinical signs alone; CSF analysis must be done.
• After eosinophils are identified in the CSF—consider parasitic disease, allergic response, and tumor
• Parasitic disease—differentiate on the basis of systemic signs, laboratory data, and serologic test results.
• Allergic and idiopathic disease—predominance of cerebral signs; negative serologic test results; marked eosinophilic pleocytosis
• Brain tumor—old patient; relatively long history; clinical signs relate to a focal lesion; eosinophils may be found, but usually in low numbers; confirm by brain imaging and biopsy.

CBC/BIOCHEMISTRY/URINALYSIS
• Peripheral eosinophilia—not always a reliable indicator of brain disease; degree does not correlate with the number of eosinophils in the CSF.
• Biochemical analysis and urinalysis—usually normal with idiopathic and allergic disease; liver enzyme activity and creatine kinase may be high with parasitic disease.

OTHER LABORATORY TESTS
N/A

IMAGING
N/A

DIAGNOSTIC PROCEDURES

CSF Analysis
• Idiopathic and allergic disease—marked eosinophilic pleocytosis
• Parasitic disease—less pleocytosis; may see neutrophils
• Neoplasia—low WBC; small numbers of eosinophils

Serologic Testing
• If CSF analysis confirms existence of eosinophils, look thoroughly for parasitic disease.
• Always test for heartworm, *N. caninum,* and *T. gondii.*

 TREATMENT

• Usually inpatient, because of severity of clinical signs
• Activity—as tolerated
• Regular diet

MENINGOENCEPHALOMYELITIS, EOSINOPHILIC

 MEDICATIONS

DRUGS
• Idiopathic disease—steroid administration; dexamethasone (0.25 mg/kg q12h for 3 days; then q24h for 3 days); follow with prednisone (1 mg/kg q24h for 2 weeks; then q48h for 6–8 weeks); then slowly wean patient over 6 weeks
• Parasitic disease—clindamycin, sulfonamides, and pyrimethamine
• Heartworm—microfilarial migration to the CNS is rare; no available treatment other than supportive

CONTRAINDICATIONS/POSSIBLE INTERACTIONS
Steroids—contraindicated with parasitic disease

 FOLLOW-UP

PATIENT MONITORING
Repeat neurologic examination every 6 hr to monitor progress.

EXPECTED COURSE AND PROGNOSIS
• Idiopathic disease—good prognosis with early and aggressive treatment; improvement usually seen in the first 72 hr; full recovery in 6–8 weeks; may repeat CSF analysis to determine if treatment can be stopped
• Parasitic disease—poor to grave prognosis
• Larval migration (e.g., heartworm)—prognosis guarded to poor and depends on location of the lesion; signs may resolve, but larvae often continue to migrate and death may ensue.
• Degradation of eosinophils is toxic to nervous tissue; patient may have permanent deficits from not only the primary disease but also the eosinophils.

 MISCELLANEOUS

ABBREVIATION
CSF = cerebrospinal fluid

Suggested Reading
Smith-Maxie LL, Parent JM, Rand J, et al. Cerebrospinal fluid analysis and clinical outcome of eight dogs with eosinophilic meningoencephalomyelitis. J Vet Intern Med 1989;3:167–174.

Author Joane M. Parent
Consulting Editor Joane M. Parent

DISEASES

MENINGOENCEPHALOMYELITIS, GRANULOMATOUS

 BASICS

DEFINITION
Progressive, idiopathic, inflammatory disease that can affect the brain, spinal cord, or meninges in dogs

PATHOPHYSIOLOGY
• Immunologic basis supported by immunohistologic studies and the histologic resemblance to experimental allergic encephalomyelitis
• Host response to an infectious agent suggested by similarities to viral encephalomyelitis
• No infectious agents have been identified.
• Three forms—focal, disseminated, and ocular
• Focal—usually affects the brainstem, cerebral cortex, cerebellum, or cervical spinal cord
• Disseminated—usually affects the caudal brainstem (vestibular system), cervical cord, and meninges
• Ocular—primarily affects the optic nerves and optic chiasm; may occur alone or in combination with the CNS form, focal or disseminated

SYSTEMS AFFECTED
• Nervous
• Ophthalmic

GENETICS
No heritability demonstrated

INCIDENCE/PREVALENCE
The literature indicates sporadic occurrence, but field evidence suggests it may be one of the most common causes of progressive CNS dysfunction in adult dogs.

GEOGRAPHIC DISTRIBUTION
N/A

SIGNALMENT

Species
• Dogs
• Inflammatory CNS lesions without recognized infectious agents can occur in any species, including cats.

Breed Predilections
• Poodles and terriers—may be predisposed
• Other small breeds—commonly affected
• Large-breed dogs—may be affected, particularly with disseminated disease

MEAN AGE AND RANGE
• Mean—5 years
• Range—6 months to 10 years
• Old dogs occasionally affected
• Approximately 30% of affected dogs < 2 years old

Predominant Sex
Both sexes affected with a slightly higher prevalence in females

SIGNS

Historical Findings
• Focal—acts as a slowly enlarging, space-occupying mass; signs progressing over 3–6 months
• Disseminated—acute onset; rapid progression over 1–8 weeks; 25% die within 1 week.
• Ocular—acute blindness; often remains static; progression usually occurs when other forms coexist.

Physical Examination Findings
• Fever—in some patients with the disseminated form
• Neurologic abnormalities—reflect location of the lesion(s)
• Cerebral involvement—seizures, circling, head pressing, and central blindness
• Brainstem involvement—head tilt, nystagmus, and trigeminal or facial nerve paralysis
• Ocular form—acute blindness; bilaterally dilated, nonresponsive pupils.
• Meningeal and cervical spinal cord involvement—cervical pain with ataxia and tetraparesis common

CAUSES
Unknown

RISK FACTORS
Unknown

 DIAGNOSIS

DIFFERENTIAL DIAGNOSIS
• Cannot be differentiated from other causes of meningoencephalomyelitis by clinical signs alone
• Infectious causes—viral, fungal, rickettsial, and protozoal diseases; differentiate by signalment (e.g., rarely occurs in dogs < 2 years old, whereas canine distemper, toxoplasmosis, and neosporium meningoencephalomyelitis are most common in young dogs), systemic signs, and results of serologic testing and CSF culture.
• CSF analysis—typically not pathognomonic for a specific cause; the following generalizations have been reported; bacterial infections: severe polymorphonuclear pleocytosis and very high protein levels; distemper: mild mononuclear pleocytosis and mildly elevated protein levels; protozoal and fungal infections: mixed mononuclear and polymorphonuclear

pleocytosis and fungal organisms (especially cryptococcosis) may be noted; rickettsial infections: mild mononuclear pleocytosis with mildly high protein levels
• Aseptic meningitis—cervical pain without neurologic deficits; CSF analysis usually reveals neutrophilic pleocytosis.
• Brain tumors—differentiate from focal by CSF analysis combined with diagnostic imaging.
• Cervical intervertebral disk disease and atlantoaxial luxation—commonly seen in toy and brachycephalic breeds; can produce clinical signs similar to the focal form

CBC/BIOCHEMISTRY/URINALYSIS
• Usually normal
• Occasional leukocytosis may be seen

OTHER LABORATORY TESTS
• None required
• Serum titers help rule out infectious disease.

IMAGING
• CT (brain)—variably dense, nonenhancing intra-axial mass most common finding
• MRI (brain)—nonenhancing intra-axial mass with attendant edema

DIAGNOSTIC PROCEDURES

CSF Analysis
• Total WBC—varies widely; mean = 800 cells/mm³; range = 9–5400 cells/mm³
• Mononuclear pleocytosis with a high number of lymphocytes and monocytes and occasional plasma cells common
• Large, foamy mononuclear cells frequently seen
• Neutrophil population—1–20% in most patients
• Total protein—varies widely; range = 40–250 mg/dL
• Occasionally, proteins are high without pleocytosis or results are normal.

PATHOLOGIC FINDINGS
• Meninges may be thickened and cloudy.
• Brain sections—may have circumscribed areas that are soft and grayish
• Optic nerves—large with ocular form
• Dense perivascular aggregations of mononuclear cells (lymphocytes, monocytes and plasma cells) arranged in a whirling pattern—characteristic

MENINGOENCEPHALOMYELITIS, GRANULOMATOUS

TREATMENT

APPROPRIATE HEALTH CARE
• Inpatient—initial treatment for severe or progressive disease
• Antiepileptics—patients with seizures
• Diuretics—Lasix (1 mg/kg IV q6–8h) and/or mannitol (1 g/kg IV q6h); for patients with marked neurologic disabilities and/or evidence of edema on imaging
• Outpatient—stable patients can be discharged after the diagnosis has been made.

NURSING CARE
• Intravenous fluids—patients that are not drinking; maintenance fluid therapy indicated, unless the patient is dehydrated; avoid overhydration, which leads to cerebral edema.
• Seizures—monitor patient continuously; treat as needed.
• Patients unable to ambulate should be maintained on soft bedding, turned frequently, and checked for appropriate urinary and fecal function.

ACTIVITY
Restricted

DIET
• Adequate caloric intake is indicated.
• Special diet and caloric considerations—for patients undergoing stress, anorexia, or accelerated metabolism because of illness

CLIENT EDUCATION
• Inform client that this condition has an inexorable course, although some dogs respond to treatment for a short time (weeks to a few months).
• Discuss the importance of the initial diagnostic evaluation for differentiating the disease from more treatable disorders.

SURGICAL CONSIDERATIONS
• Histologic evaluation of affected CNS tissue—diagnostic gold standard
• Low-morbidity brain biopsy—for a confirmed focal mass to differentiate from other focal diseases

MEDICATIONS

DRUGS OF CHOICE
Corticosteroids
• Primary treatment
• Relatively benign clinical conditions—prednisolone (1 mg/kg PO q12h); continue treatment until the patient achieves a response zenith; then slowly decrease dose; recrudescence of signs prompts re-establishment of the lowest dose that maintains a clinically acceptable pet.
• Severe clinical conditions—high-dose (2–4 mg/kg IV) for the first 48–72 hr; after signs improve, initiate oral corticosteroids.
• Some patients do not respond to corticosteroid treatment.
• Most patients require continued treatment to prevent recrudescence of clinical signs.
• To prevent steroid-induced gastric ulceration—cimetidine (10 mg/kg PO q8h) and/or sucralfate (0.5–1.0 g PO q8–12h)

CONTRAINDICATIONS
It is important to eliminate infectious differentials before treating with corticosteroids.

PRECAUTIONS
Rapid reduction in corticosteroid dosage may precipitate a refractory recrudescence of clinical signs.

POSSIBLE INTERACTIONS
N/A

ALTERNATIVE DRUGS
• Azathioprine—2 mg/kg PO daily; add to the regimen when the side effects of prednisolone (e.g., polyuria and polyphagia) are too pronounced or when prednisolone has failed.
• Cyclophosphamide—50 mg/m² PO q48h; try when prednisolone is ineffective.
• Radiotherapy—may be beneficial

FOLLOW-UP

PATIENT MONITORING
• Nervous system signs
• Perform CBC and biochemical analysis regularly to monitor for toxicity if azathioprine or cyclophosphamide is administered.

PREVENTION/AVOIDANCE
N/A

POSSIBLE COMPLICATIONS
Disease may progress despite appropriate treatment.

EXPECTED COURSE AND PROGNOSIS
• Corticosteroids—may slow or reverse progress of signs; must be continued for life
• Disease progresses in most patients despite treatment.

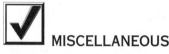

MISCELLANEOUS

ASSOCIATED CONDITIONS
N/A

AGE-RELATED FACTORS
N/A

ZOONOTIC POTENTIAL
N/A

PREGNANCY
Corticosteroid administration and the short life expectancy of affected dogs make successful gestation unlikely.

SYNONYMS
Reticulosis, inflammatory and neoplastic

SEE ALSO
• Encephalitis
• Meningitis/Meningoencephalitis/Meningomyelitis, Bacterial
• Meningoencephalomyelitis, Eosinophilic

ABBREVIATION
CSF = cerebrospinal fluid

Suggested Reading
Cook JR. Granulomatous meningoencephalitis. Applying what we know. Vet Med Rep 1989;1:321–327.
Oliver JE, Lorenz MO, Kornegay JN. Handbook of veterinary neurology. 3rd ed. Philadelphia: Saunders, 1997.
Sorjonen DC. Clinical and histopathological features of granulomatous meningoencephalomyelitis in dogs. J Am Anim Hosp Assoc 1990;26:141–147.
Summers BA, Cummings SF, de Lahunta A. Veterinary pathology. St. Louis: Mosby, 1994.
Author D. C. Sorjonen
Consulting Editor Joane M. Parent

DISEASES

MESOTHELIOMA

BASICS

OVERVIEW
• Rare tumor of the epithelial lining of body cavities
• Dogs—thoracic cavity, pericardial sac, abdominal cavity, and vaginal tunic of the scrotum
• Cats—thoracic cavity, pericardial sac, and abdominal cavity
• Highly effusive

SIGNALMENT
• Dogs and cats
• Sclerosing mesothelioma—primarily in male dogs
• German shepherds—most commonly affected breed

SIGNS
• Displacement of viscera
• Dyspnea
• Exercise intolerance
• Muffled heart and ventral lung sounds
• Vomiting
• Large scrotum
• Abdominal distension with ascites
• Low chest compliance owing to mediastinal mass and pleural effusion

CAUSES & RISK FACTORS
Exposure to asbestos

DIAGNOSIS

DIFFERENTIAL DIAGNOSIS
• Other causes of effusion—congestive heart failure; liver disease; hypoalbuminemia; pyothorax; lymphosarcoma; idiopathic pericardial effusion
• Other mediastinal masses—lymphosarcoma; thymoma; thyroid carcinoma; chemodectoma

CBC/BIOCHEMISTRY/URINALYSIS
No specific abnormalities

OTHER LABORATORY TESTS
N/A

IMAGING
• Radiography—shows body cavity effusion and/or masses
• Ultrasound—detects pericardial sac thickening and effusion

DIAGNOSTIC PROCEDURES
• Cytologic examination of fluid—interpret results cautiously because it can be difficult to distinguish mesothelioma from physiologic mesothelial proliferation.
• Exploratory surgery or laparoscopy—reveals nodules, plaques, or thickenings of the mesothelial lining of the body cavity
• Histologic evaluation—reveals morphologic characteristics of epithelial neoplasms and mesenchymal proliferation

TREATMENT

• Outpatient
• Activity—restrict with dyspnea
• Partial pericardectomy—relieve pericardial effusion
• Centesis or pleurodesis—palliative therapy for pleural effusion

MEDICATIONS

DRUGS
Cisplatin—has been successful; may be given intracavitary but penetrates the tumor only a few cells deep and is effective only when the mass is not large; administer according to established protocols that include adequate diuresis.

CONTRAINDICATIONS/POSSIBLE INTERACTIONS
Cisplatin—do not use in cats; do not use in dogs with renal disease.

FOLLOW-UP
• Thoracic radiography—every treatment and every 3 months after treatment
• Laboratory tests—assess renal status after cisplatin administration.
• Avoid exposure to asbestos.
• Survival after intracavitary cisplatin—3 dogs: 410 days, > 129 days, and 306 days

MISCELLANEOUS

Suggested Reading

Moore AS, Kirk C, Cardona A. Intracavitary cisplatin chemotherapy experience with six dogs. J Vet Intern Med 1991;5:227–231.

Morrison WB. Nonpulmonary intrathoracic cancer. In: Morrison WB, ed. Cancer in dogs and cats: medical and surgical management. Baltimore: Williams & Wilkins 1998:537–550.

Author Terrance A. Hamilton
Consulting Editor Wallace B. Morrison

DISEASES

METALDEHYDE POISONING

BASICS

DEFINITION
• Metaldehyde—polycyclic polymer of acetaldehyde; primarily affects the nervous system; an ingredient of slug and snail baits; used as solid fuel for some camp stoves
• Baits—liquid or dry; usually pellets mixed with feed material (e.g., soybeans, rice, oats, sorghum, and apples); may contain other toxicants (e.g., arsenate and insecticides)

PATHOPHYSIOLOGY
• Exact mechanism unknown
• May increase excitatory neurotransmitters or decrease inhibitory neurotransmitters

SYSTEMS AFFECTED
• Nervous
• Respiratory—death usually as a result of respiratory failure
• Hepatobiliary—even if patient survives the initial convulsive period, it may die of liver disease 2–3 days later.

GENETICS
N/A

INCIDENCE/PREVALENCE
Depend on geographic location

GEOGRAPHIC DISTRIBUTION
• More commonly found in coastal and low-lying areas, which have a higher prevalence of snails and slugs than other areas

SIGNALMENT

Species
Dogs and cats

Breed Predilections
N/A

Mean Age and Range
Any

Predominant Sex
N/A

SIGNS

General Comments
May occur immediately after ingestion or may be delayed for up to 3 hr

Historical Findings
• Bizarre behavior
• Ataxia
• Convulsions

Physical Examination Findings
• Convulsions—continuous or intermittent; not necessarily evoked by external stimuli
• Between convulsions—may note muscle tremors and anxiety; may be hyperesthetic
• Hyperthermia—temperature up to 42.2°C (108°F) common; probably caused by excessive muscle activity
• Tachycardia
• Nystagmus
• Mydriasis
• Hyperpnea
• Hypersalivation
• Ataxia
• Vomiting
• Cyanosis
• Diarrhea
• Dehydration
• Depression or narcosis—may occur late in the course
• Death—usually owing to respiratory failure, which occurs 4–24 hr after exposure; owing to liver disease, 2–3 days after exposure if patient survives initial convulsive period

CAUSES
Ingestion of metaldehyde

RISK FACTORS
Living in area with high prevalence of snails and slugs

DIAGNOSIS

DIFFERENTIAL DIAGNOSIS
• Strychnine toxicosis—causes intermittent seizures that can be evoked by external stimuli
• Penitrem A—mycotoxin usually found in moldy English walnuts or cream cheese; has been reported in other foodstuffs; causes a tremorogenic syndrome
• Roquefortine—mycotoxin found in moldy bleu cheese and other foodstuffs; causes a tremorogenic syndrome
• Lead toxicosis—may cause seizures, behavior changes, blindness, and gastrointestinal upset
• Organochlorine insecticides—cause seizures in most mammals
• Anticholinesterase insecticides—organophosphates and carbamates; may cause seizures; usually accompanied by excessive salivation, lacrimation, urination, and defecation
• Seizures—may be the result of a host of nontoxic conditions (e.g., neoplasia, trauma, infection, metabolic disorder, and congenital disorder)

CBC/BIOCHEMISTRY/URINALYSIS
Not diagnostic

OTHER LABORATORY TESTS

Metaldehyde testing—vomitus, stomach contents, or serum

IMAGING

N/A

DIAGNOSTIC PROCEDURES

N/A

PATHOLOGIC FINDINGS

• Hepatic, renal, and pulmonary congestion
• Petechial and ecchymotic hemorrhages
• Subendocardial and subepicardial hemorrhages

 TREATMENT

APPROPRIATE HEALTH CARE

Emergency inpatient intensive care management until convulsions cease

NURSING CARE

Fluids—may be necessary for dehydration or acidosis

ACTIVITY

Restricted

DIET

Do not feed patients that are vomiting, convulsing, or heavily sedated.

CLIENT EDUCATION

N/A

SURGICAL CONSIDERATIONS

N/A

 MEDICATIONS

DRUGS OF CHOICE

• No antidote available
• Prevent further absorption—emetics or gastric lavage followed by administration of activated charcoal
• Convulsions—tranquilize with diazepam or barbiturates

CONTRAINDICATIONS

Never induce vomiting in a convulsing patient.

PRECAUTIONS

• Do not use depressants in an already depressed patient
• Barbiturates—may lead to cardiac arrest

POSSIBLE INTERACTIONS

N/A

ALTERNATIVE DRUGS

N/A

 FOLLOW-UP

PATIENT MONITORING

Periodically allow tranquilizers to wear off to re-evaluate convulsive condition.

PREVENTION/AVOIDANCE

Do not apply metaldehyde in areas accessible to pets.

POSSIBLE COMPLICATIONS

Liver disease—if patient survives the initial convulsive phase

EXPECTED COURSE AND PROGNOSIS

• Reported sequelae—diarrhea; memory loss; temporary blindness
• Liver disease—may be a secondary problem
• Prognosis—principally depends on the amount ingested
• Without successful treatment—death 4–12 hr after exposure

 MISCELLANEOUS

ASSOCIATED CONDITIONS

Concurrent toxicoses from additional ingredients (arsenate and insecticides) in the molluscicide

AGE-RELATED FACTORS

N/A

ZOONOTIC POTENTIAL

N/A

PREGNANCY

Not known to be mutagenic, genotoxic, or immunotoxic

SYNONYMS

• Polyacetaldehyde
• Limovet
• Limax
• Antimilace
• Snail bait

SEE ALSO

Poisoning (Intoxication)

Suggested Reading

Andreasen JR. Metaldehyde toxicosis in ducklings. J Vet Diagn Invest 1993; 5:500–501.

Booze TF, Oehme FW. Metaldehyde toxicity: a review. Vet Hum Toxicol 1985;27:11–19.

Von Burg R, Stout T. Metaldehyde. J Appl Toxicol 1991;11:377–378.

Author Konstanze H. Plumlee
Consulting Editor Gary D. Osweiler

DISEASES

METRITIS

BASICS

OVERVIEW
• Bacterial uterine infection that develops in the immediate postpartum period (usually within the first week); occasionally develops after an abortion or non-sterile artificial insemination—rarely after breeding
• Bacteria—ascend through the open cervix to the uterus; a large, flaccid, postpartum uterus provides an ideal environment for growth; gram-negative (e.g., *Escherichia coli*) commonly isolated
• Potentially life-threatening infection; may lead to septic shock
• Directly affects uterus; systemic involvement as sepsis develops
• Can become chronic and lead to infertility

SIGNALMENT
• Postpartum bitch and queen
• No age or breed predilection

SIGNS

Historical Findings
• Malodorous, purulent, sanguinopurulent, or dark green vulvar discharge
• Depression
• Anorexia
• Neglect of puppies and kittens
• Reduced milk production

Physical Examination Findings
• Fever
• Large uterus on abdominal palpation
• Dehydration
• Injected mucous membranes
• Tachycardia—with sepsis

CAUSES & RISK FACTORS
• Dystocia
• Obstetric manipulation
• Retained fetuses or placenta
• Postabortion and postnatural or artificial insemination (rare)

DIAGNOSIS

DIFFERENTIAL DIAGNOSIS
• Subinvolution of placental sites—no sign of infection on cytologic examination of vagina
• Eclampsia—differentiated by serum calcium concentration
• Mastitis—differentiated by physical examination findings

CBC/BIOCHEMISTRY/URINALYSIS
• Neutrophilia with left shift
• Leukopenia—occasionally with endotoxic shock
• High PCV, total protein, creatinine, BUN, and urine specific gravity—secondary to dehydration
• High liver enzyme—with endotoxemia
• Low urine specific gravity—may see with endotoxemia

OTHER LABORATORY TESTS
N/A

IMAGING
• Radiography—reveals a large uterus and possibly retained fetuses.
• Ultrasonography—reveals intrauterine fluid accumulation, retained placenta, and retained fetuses; shows abdominal effusion secondary to uterine rupture

DIAGNOSTIC PROCEDURES
• Vaginal cytologic examination—detect degenerative neutrophils with intracellular and extracellular bacteria
• Guarded anterior vaginal culture—aerobes and anaerobes; identify organism

TREATMENT
• Inpatient until systemic signs resolve
• Dehydration—intravenous balanced electrolyte solution
• Treat shock
• Electrolyte imbalances and hypoglycemia—correct; identified by serum chemistry profile
• Ovariohysterectomy—treatment of choice for retained fetus or placenta, uterine rupture, or severe infection and if future breeding is not desired
• Chronically affected patient that does not respond to medical treatment—may perform hysterotomy and lavage as long as the uterus has no friable areas
• Friable uterus—pack off and handle gently at surgery.

MEDICATIONS

DRUGS
• Antibiotics—start with broad-spectrum agents (oral if patient is stable; intravenous if patient is in shock); choice confirmed by bacterial culture and sensitivity; continued at least 14 days
• Nursing planned—amoxicillin-clavulanic acid (dogs, 12.5 mg/kg PO q12h; cats, 62.5 mg/cat PO q12h) or oxacillin to start
• Nursing not planned—enrofloxacin (2.5 mg/kg PO q12h) to start
• Oxytocin—0.5–1.0 U/kg IM; then repeat in 1–2 hr; may note inadequate response if > 48 hr since parturition
• PGF$_{2\alpha}$—100–250 µg/kg SC q12h for 5–8 days; to evacuate uterus

CONTRAINDICATIONS/POSSIBLE INTERACTIONS
• Prostaglandin—may induce uterine rupture if the tissue is devitalized
• Oxytocin—may not be effective beyond 48 hr postpartum
• Uterine flushing—may cause rupture of devitalized wall

FOLLOW-UP

PATIENT MONITORING
• CBC, temperature, vaginal cytologic examination, and clinical signs
• Ultrasonography—monitor evacuation of uterine fluid

POSSIBLE COMPLICATIONS
• Ovariohysterectomy—necessary when medical treatment is ineffective
• Uterine rupture and peritonitis—may occur with medical treatment
• Owners may need to handraise puppies and kittens

EXPECTED COURSE AND PROGNOSIS
• Ovariohysterectomy—prognosis for recovery good; recommended for old patients
• Medical treatment—prognosis for recovery fair; may adversely affect future reproduction

MISCELLANEOUS

ABBREVIATION
PCV = packed cell volume

Suggested Reading
Magne ML. Acute metritis in the bitch. In: Morrow DA, ed. Current therapy in theriogenology 2. Philadelphia: Saunders, 1986:505–506.

Author Joni L. Freshman
Consulting Editor Sara K. Lyle

BASICS

OVERVIEW
• Form of cardiac dysfunction associated with an abnormal number of moderator bands spanning the ventricular cavity, interventricular septum, papillary muscles, or ventricular free walls
• Can cause systolic and diastolic dysfunction
• May be an incidental congenital anomaly in many instances

SIGNALMENT
• Primarily in cats
• All Ages affected

SIGNS
Historical Findings
• Lethargy
• Tachypnea and dyspnea
• Anorexia
• Weight loss
• Hind limb paresis or paralysis due to thromboembolic disease

Physical Examination Findings
• Gallop rhythm
• Systolic murmur
• Arrhythmias
• Hypothermia
• Left- or right-sided CHF

CAUSES & RISK FACTORS
• Congenital anomaly
• Secondary to acquired myocardial disease

DIAGNOSIS

DIFFERENTIAL DIAGNOSIS
• Restrictive cardiomyopathy
• Hypertrophic cardiomyopathy
• Dilated cardiomyopathy
• Hypertension
• Other congenital defects

CBC/BIOCHEMISTRY/URINALYSIS
No consistent findings

OTHER LABORATORY TESTS
Plasma taurine concentration useful in diagnosing taurine-responsive dilated cardiomyopathy

IMAGING
Thoracic Radiography
Radiographs may reveal one or more of the following:
• Generalized cardiomegaly
• Atrial enlargement
• Pulmonary edema
• Pleural effusion
• Ascites

Echocardiography
Two-dimensional echocardiography may confirm excessive moderator bands.

DIAGNOSTIC PROCEDURES
• ECG——detect arrhythmias; incidence of bradycardia and conduction disturbances may be higher in cats with increased moderator bands than in those with other myocardial diseases.
• Blood pressure determination

TREATMENT

• Treat as inpatient if patient has CHF.
• Minimize stress during initial treatment.
• Treatment strategy may vary——base on underlying pathophysiologic process
• Alert owner to possibility of animal developing thromboembolic disease.
• Sudden death is possible.

MEDICATIONS

DRUGS
CHF
• Furosemide—1 mg/kg IV initially, then switch to 1 mg/kg SC or PO q8–12h
• 2% nitroglycerin ointment—cats: apply 1/8–1/4 inch topically to hairless area q4–6h until congestive signs resolve (e.g., pulmonary edema)
• Manually remove pleural fluid.
• Administer oxygen

LONG-TERM MANAGEMENT (IN ADDITION TO DIURETIC ADMINISTRATION)
• Digoxin to increase myocardial contractility or treat supraventricular tachyarrhythmias—1/4 of a 0.125-mg tablet per cat PO q48–72h
• Diltiazem to improve myocardial relaxation or treat supraventricular tachyarrhythmias—1–2.5 mg/kg PO q8h
• Enalapril for balanced vasodilation—0.5 mg/kg PO q24–48h
• Treat any thromboembolic disease

CONTRAINDICATIONS/POSSIBLE INTERACTIONS
• Concurrent azotemia warrants judicious use of diuretics; azotemia is a relative contraindication for the use of enalapril and requires careful monitoring.
• Hypokalemia may predispose animal to digoxin toxicity.

FOLLOW-UP

• Monitor radiographs for resolution of congestive state.
• Monitor serial ECG for arrhythmias.
• Monitor serum biochemical analysis for azotemia and electrolyte imbalances.

MISCELLANEOUS

SEE ALSO
• Dilated Cardiomyopathy, Cats
• Hypertension, Systemic
• Hypertrophic Cardiomyopathy, Cats
• Restrictive Cardiomyopathy, Cats

ABBREVIATIONS
• CHF = congestive heart failure
• ECG = electrocardiogram

Suggested Reading
Fox RP. Feline cardiomyopathies. In: Fox PR, Sisson D, Moise NS, eds. Textbook of canine and feline cardiology. 2nd ed. Philadelphia: Saunders, 1999:621–678.
Author Michael B. Lesser
Consulting Editors Larry P. Tilley and Francis W. K. Smith, Jr.

DISEASES

MUCOPOLYSACCHARIDOSIS (MPS)

BASICS

OVERVIEW
• A group of heritable lysosomal storage disorders caused by deficiency of lysosomal enzymes needed for the stepwise degradation of GAGs (mucopolysaccharides)
• Undegraded GAGs are stored in lysosomes, resulting in progressive tissue and organ dysfunction.
• Features depend on the specific lysosomal enzyme deficiency, type of GAG stored, and the tissues in which storage occurs.

Types of MPSs Reported in Dogs and Cats
• MPS I—α-L-iduronidase deficiency; dermatan and heparan sulfate stored
• MPS II—iduronate sulfatase deficiency; dermatan and heparan sulfate stored
• MPS IIIA—heparan N-sulfatase deficiency; heparan sulfate stored
• MPS VI—arylsulfatase B deficiency; dermatan sulfate stored
• MPS VII—β-glucuronidase deficiency; dermatan, heparan, and chondroitin sulfate stored

SIGNALMENT
• Cats—MPS I and VII, domestic shorthair; MPS VI, Siamese and domestic shorthair
• Dogs—MPS I, Plott hounds; MPS II, Labrador retrievers; MPS IIIA, wire-haired dachshunds; MPS VI, miniature pinschers, miniature schnauzers, and Welsh corgis; MPS VII, mixed-breeds and German shepherds.
• Both sexes equally affected by MPS I, III, VI, and VII; primarily males affected by MPS II

SIGNS
• Dwarfism (except cats with MPS I)
• Severe bone disease (dysostosis multiplex)
• Degenerative joint disease, including hip subluxation
• Facial dysmorphia—more evident in Siamese cats, which normally have an elongated face, than in other cats
• Hepatomegaly (except cats with MPS VI)
• Corneal clouding—a result of fine granular opacities in the corneal stroma, first apparent at approximately 8 weeks of age
• Large tongue (dogs)
• Thickening of the heart valves
• Excess urinary excretion of GAG
• Metachromatic granules (Alder-Reilly bodies) in blood leukocytes
• Disease progresses; clinical signs apparent at 2–4 months of age
• Affected animals may live several years, but locomotor difficulty is progressive.
• Skeletal abnormalities more severe in cats with MPS VI than in those with MPS I; some MPS VI cats develop posterior paresis owing to spinal cord compression.
• Manipulation of the head or neck usually painful
• CNS disease not clinically apparent in dogs or cats with any type of MPS, although there is microscopic evidence of neuronal storage.

CAUSES & RISK FACTORS
• MPS transmission is autosomal recessive, except MPS II, which is X-linked recessive.
• In-breeding increases risk if the defective gene is present in the family.

DIAGNOSIS

DIFFERENTIAL DIAGNOSIS
• Metachromatic granules within neutrophils and lymphocytes—suggest MPS; also observed with GM$_2$ gangliosidosis, a lysosomal storage disease that, unlike MPS, is characterized by progressive neurologic disease and early death; also observed in neutrophils of some Burmese cats that have normal lymphocytes and have no clinical abnormalities; very rarely, toxic granulation of neutrophils can have a similar appearance.
• Corneal clouding—also observed with numerous other lysosomal storage diseases, including acid lipase deficiency, GM$_1$ and GM$_2$ gangliosidosis, and mannosidosis; lysosomal enzyme panels can be performed to definitely diagnose the type of storage disorder; corneal edema and corneal dystrophy may have a similar appearance.
• Whereas the radiographic appearance of MPS is characteristic, other disorders with similarities include congenital hypothyroidism, epiphyseal dysplasia, and hypervitaminosis A.

CBC/BIOCHEMISTRY/URINALYSIS
• Examination of Wright's-stained blood films reveals neutrophils and monocytes containing numerous distinctive metachromatic granules.
• Granules quite indistinct in animals with MPS I
• Granules usually not apparent when stained with Diff-Quik
• Occasional lymphocytes have vacuoles that contain metachromatic granules, particularly in animals with MPS VII.

OTHER LABORATORY TESTS
• Wright's-stained cytologic preparations of lymph node, liver, bone marrow, and joint fluid specimens reveal characteristic metachromatic granules within cells.
• Presence of excess GAG in urine usually indicates MPS.
• Definitive diagnosis made by measuring lysosomal enzyme activity in serum, leukocyte pellets, or frozen liver.

IMAGING
• Radiography—low bone density with thin cortices
• Epiphyseal abnormalities—vary from slight irregularities to large scalloped defects in subchondral bone
• Joint changes—acetabular flattening and periarticular osteophyte formation
• In some cats, proliferative bone is present around all articular facets of vertebrae, causing fusion of cervical vertebrae.

DIAGNOSTIC PROCEDURES
None

PATHOLOGIC FINDINGS
Distended lysosomes seen in cells of many tissues examined by light and electron microscopy

TREATMENT

DEFINITIVE TREATMENT
• BMT—the most successful treatment to date; after engraftment, donor-derived normal leukocytes provide missing enzyme to various tissues; when performed at a very early age, affected animals lead near-normal lives; not as helpful when performed after skeletal maturity; expensive, life-threatening, and a normal sibling is needed as a donor
• Enzyme-replacement therapy, using recombinant enzyme at birth, followed by BMT, has been quite effective in animal models of MPS.
• Both BMT and enzyme replacement are expensive and have been employed primarily in animal models to determine the potential success in children; very few privately owned animals have been treated.

NURSING CARE
• Fluid administration often required to correct dehydration.
• With increasing age, difficulty eating progresses; a diet of soft food may be helpful.

MEDICATIONS

DRUGS
Affected animals are susceptible to viral and bacterial respiratory infection; antibiotics may be indicated.

CONTRAINDICATIONS/POSSIBLE INTERACTIONS
None

FOLLOW-UP

PREVENTION/AVOIDANCE
• Avoid inbreeding in family with history of disease
• Enzyme assays should be performed to diagnose heterozygotes.

EXPECTED COURSE AND PROGNOSIS
• Prognosis reasonably good in animals treated with BMT
• Untreated animals usually develop severe skeletal and joint disease and may become nonambulatory at 3 to 5 years of age.

MISCELLANEOUS

ABBREVIATIONS
• BMT = bone marrow transplant
• GAG = glycosaminoglycan

Suggested ReadingReading
Haskins M, Giger U. Lysosomal storage diseases. In: Kaneko JJ, Harvey JW, Bruss ML, eds. Clinical biochemistry of domestic animals. 5th ed. San Diego: Academic Press, 1997:741–760.
Author Mary Anna Thrall
Section Editor Susan M. Cotter

DISEASES

MULTIPLE MYELOMA

BASICS

DEFINITION
• Rare malignant neoplasm of hematopoietic tissue derived from a clonal population of plasma cells, usually in the bone marrow
• Three of four defining features must be present for diagnosis: monoclonal gammopathy; neoplastic plasma cells or bone marrow plasmacytosis; lytic bone lesions; and Bence Jones (light-chain) proteinuria

PATHOPHYSIOLOGY
• Proliferation of a single clone of plasma cells that produces immunoglobulins (IgA or IgG) or subunits (heavy or light chains)
• Overproduction of IgM—Waldenstrom's macroglobulinemia
• Polymerized IgA or IgG—may increase serum viscosity (8–10 times normal)
• Bleeding diathesis—caused by effect of paraprotein coating of platelets, thrombocytopenia, increased viscosity of blood, and interference with normal coagulation factors
• Nephrotoxicity—secondary to protein deposition of amyloid or direct effect of the protein on renal tubular epithelial cells

SYSTEMS AFFECTED
• Musculoskeletal—multiple areas of active bone lysis in the skeleton including vertebral column (especially lumbar), pelvis, skull and, occasionally, appendicular bones
• Soft tissues—neoplastic plasma cells may be present in extraskeletal sites (e.g., liver, spleen, lymph nodes, kidney, pharynx, lung, muscle, and gastrointestinal tract)
• Nervous, cardiovascular, and respiratory—possible abnormalities secondary to hyperviscosity

GENETICS
N/A

INCIDENCE/PREVELANCE
• Dogs—reported prevalence < 1% of all malignant tumors; < 8% of hematopoietic malignant tumors
• Cats—reported prevalence < 1% of hematopoietic tumors

GEOGRAPHIC DISTRIBUTION
N/A

SIGNALMENT
Species
Dogs and cats

Breed Predilections
German shepherds and other purebred dogs

Mean Age and Range
Primarily middle-aged or old dogs and cats (6–13 years)

Predominant Sex
None

SIGNS
General Comments
Attributed to bone infiltration and lysis, effects of proteins produced by the tumor (e.g., hyperviscosity and nephrotoxicity), and infiltration of organ(s) by neoplastic cells

Historical Findings
• Depend on location and extent of disease
• Weakness
• Lameness
• Pain
• Paresis
• Urinary incontinence
• Epistaxis—unilateral or bilateral
• Blindness
• Dementia
• Malaise
• Labored breathing
• Polyuria
• Polydipsia
• Gastrointestinal bleeding

Physical Examination Findings
Dogs
• Bleeding—especially from the nose or mucous membranes (36%)
• Blindness, retinal hemorrhage, or dilated retinal vessels (35%)
• Lameness (47%), bone pain and weakness (60%)—with lytic bone lesions
• Dementia, malaise, (11%), and coma (rare)
• Polydipsia and polyuria (25%)—with hypercalcemia or renal dysfunction
• Pale mucous membranes
• Fever
• Lethargy
• Hepatosplenomegaly
Cats
• Anorexia
• Weight loss
• Malaise
• Polydipsia
• Polyuria
• Fever

CAUSES
Unknown

RISK FACTORS
N/A

DIAGNOSIS

DIFFERENTIAL DIAGNOSIS
• Infectious—bacterial, fungal, and parasitic disorders (e.g., ehrlichiosis)
• Neoplastic—metastatic (e.g., carcinoma, sarcoma, mast cell tumor, lymphosarcoma, and lymphoid leukemia)
• Immune-mediated—benign hypergammaglobulinemia; rheumatoid arthritis; plasmacytic gastroenterocolitis

CBC/BIOCHEMISTRY/URINALYSIS
• Hemogram—anemia (70% of dogs); neutropenia (25% of dogs); thrombocytopenia (30% of dogs); eosinophilia; plasma cell leukemia (very rare)
• High RBC Rouleaux formation, high serum viscosity, or high serum total protein with hypoalbuminemia (65% of dogs) and hyperglobulinemia
• Hypercalcemia (17% of dogs)
• High BUN, creatinine, ALP, or ALT
• Bence Jones proteins—undetectable on routine urinalysis (dip stick)
• Urine proteinuria, isosthenuria, cylindruria, pyuria, hematuria, or bacteriuria

OTHER LABORATORY TESTS
• Serum protein electrophoresis—identify monoclonal gammopathy (i.e., protein spike), even if globulin concentration is normal
• Serum immunoglobulin quantification
• Urine protein electrophoresis—identify Bence Jones proteins (immunoglobulin light chain); positive in 30%–40% of dogs
• Protein:creatinine ratio—assess the extent of urine protein loss
• Coagulation profile
• Serum viscosity—high
• Bleeding time or platelet function tests

IMAGING
• Radiography (dogs)—axial and appendicular skeleton; show multifocal, lytic (punched-out) lesions in 50%
• Radiography (cats)—bony lesions rare
• Extraskeletal sites may be identified by organomegaly.
• Ultrasonography—detect changes in echotexture of visceral organs (e.g., infiltration)

DIAGNOSTIC PROCEDURES
Cytologic examination of bone marrow and skeletal and extraskeletal lesions—determine if > 20%–25% of normal cell population are plasma cells

PATHOLOGIC FINDINGS
• Color—greenish in soft tissue; red-grey within bone marrow
• Sheets or isolated discrete round cells with eosinophilic cytoplasm, eccentric nuclei, perinuclear clear zone, and cartwheel appearance of the nuclear chromatin
• Neoplastic cells may grow between osseous trabeculae or cause erosion and lysis of bony trabeculae and cortex.

TREATMENT

APPROPRIATE HEALTH CARE
• Inpatient—azotemia, hypercalcemia, or clinically important bacterial infection
• Plasmapheresis—lowers protein burden; for symptomatic patient, withdraw a volume of

venous blood, centrifuge it, discard the plasma, and return the RBCs in intravenous fluids (crystalloid) to the patient; with signs of hyperviscosity, perform phlebotomy and replace intravenously with an equal volume of isotonic fluids
• Radiotherapy—may be used on isolated areas with curative or palliative intent

NURSING CARE
• Venipuncture—use aseptic technique.
• Bacterial infection—treat aggressively with appropriate antibiotics.
• Hypercalcemia and renal failure—treat appropriately.

ACTIVITY
Multiple myeloma—treat as immune compromised; take care to prevent bacterial infection (e.g., caused by puncture wounds from dog or cat fights).

DIET
N/A

CLIENT EDUCATION
• Inform client that chemotherapy is palliative but long remissions are possible.
• Warn client that relapse will occur.
• Discuss side effects, which depend on the drugs used.
• Inform client that most patients develop mild leukopenia with chemotherapy.

SURGICAL CONSIDERATIONS
Areas nonresponsive to chemotherapy or solitary lesions can be removed surgically.

 MEDICATIONS

DRUGS OF CHOICE
• Dogs—melphalan (0.1 mg/kg PO q24h for 10 days; then 0.05 mg/kg PO q24h) and prednisone (0.5 mg/kg PO q24h for 10 days; then 0.5 mg/kg q48h for 60 days, then stop); cyclophosphamide can be used in addition to or in place of melphalan (200–300 mg/m^2 IV once weekly or 50 mg/m^2 PO q24h for 4 days/week).
• Cats—melphalan (0.5 mg PO q24h for 10 days; then 0.5 mg PO q48h) and prednisone (2.5 mg PO q24h)

CONTRAINDICATIONS
N/A

PRECAUTIONS
• Melphalan—very bone marrow suppressive, especially to platelets
• Cyclophosphamide—may be beneficial to substitute for melphalan with thrombocytopenia
• Affected animals may have low numbers of neutrophils or nonfunctional lymphocytes; take care to minimize exposure to infectious agents (e.g., viral, bacterial, and fungal).

• Use septic or very clean technique when performing any invasive techniques, even drawing blood.
• Chemotherapy may be toxic; seek advice before initiating any treatment if you are not familiar with cytotoxic drugs.

POSSIBLE INTERACTIONS
N/A

ALTERNATIVE DRUGS
Dogs—more aggressive combination chemotherapy protocol; cyclophosphamide (200 mg/m^2 IV every 14 days), vincristine (0.7 mg/m^2 IV every 14 days), melphalan (0.10 mg/kg PO q24h for 10 days; then 0.05 mg/kg PO q24h), and prednisone (0.5 mg/kg PO q24h)

 FOLLOW-UP

PATIENT MONITORING
• CBC and platelet counts—weekly for at least 4 weeks; assess bone marrow response
• Tests with abnormal results—monthly 2 times; evaluate response to treatment
• Protein electrophoresis; monthly for several months, until normal levels obtained; monitor periodically for relapse.
• Abnormal skeletal radiographs—monthly 2 times; then every other month until normal; evaluate response to treatment

PREVENTION/AVOIDANCE
N/A

POSSIBLE COMPLICATIONS
• Bleeding
• Secondary infections
• Pathologic fractures
• Even with treatment, it may be several months before clinical signs resolve.
• Chemotherapy—may cause leukopenia or thrombocytopenia, anorexia, alopecia, hemorrhagic cystitis, or pancreatitis

EXPECTED COURSE AND PROGNOSIS
Continuous care must be taken to protect patients from secondary infection.

Dogs
• Median survival with alkylating agents and prednisone—18 months
• Median survival with prednisone—7 months
• Complete response in 43%; partial response in 49%
• Hypercalcemia, extensive bone lysis, or Bence Jones proteinuria—shorter survival times

Cats
Survival with alkylating agents and prednisone—2–9 months

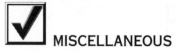 **MISCELLANEOUS**

ASSOCIATED CONDITIONS
None

AGE-RELATED FACTORS
None

ZOONOTIC POTENTIAL
None

PREGNANCY
Chemotherapy is contraindicated in pregnant animals.

SYNONYMS
• Plasma cell myeloma
• Plasmacytoma
• Myelocytoma
• Myelosarcoma
• Plasma cell leukemia
• Erythrocytoma
• Lymphocytoma

SEE ALSO
• Calcium, Hypercalcemia
• Renal Failure, Chronic

ABBREVIATIONS
• ALP = alkaline phosphatase
• ALT = alanine aminotransferase

Suggested Readings

Couto, CG. Oncology. In: Sherding RD, ed. The cat: diseases and clinical management. New York: Churchill Livingstone, 1989:589–647.

Hammer AS, Couto CG. Complications of multiple myeloma. J Am Anim Hosp Assoc 1994;30:9–14.

Matus RE, Leifer CE, MacEwan EG, Hurvitz AI. Prognostic factors for multiple myeloma in the dog. J Am Vet Med Assoc 1986;11:1288–1292.

Morrison WB. Plasma cell neoplasms. In: Morrison WB, ed. Cancer in dogs and cats: medical and surgical management. Baltimore: Williams & Wilkins, 1998:697–704.

Vail DM. Hematopoietic tumors: plasma cell neoplasms. In: Withrow SJ, MacEwan EG, eds., Clinical veterinary oncology. Philadelphia: Lippincott, 1996;509–520.

Author Mary Ann Vonderhaar
Consulting Editor Wallace B. Morrison

DISEASES

MUMPS

 BASICS

OVERVIEW
• Common illness in humans
• Dogs contract the disease from infected children.
• Incidence (dogs)—low

SIGNALMENT
• Dogs of all ages
• No sex or breed predilections

SIGNS
• Enlarged parotid salivary glands
• Fever
• Anorexia

CAUSES & RISK FACTORS
Mumps virus—family Paramyxoviridae; genus *Paramyxovirus*

 DIAGNOSIS

DIFFERENTIAL DIAGNOSIS
• Benign parotid salivary gland enlargement
• Neoplasia

CBC/BIOCHEMISTRY/URINALYSIS
No specific findings

OTHER LABORATORY TESTS
N/A

IMAGING
N/A

DIAGNOSTIC PROCEDURES
Serologic—mumps viral antibodies

 TREATMENT

Usually not required

 MEDICATIONS

DRUG(S)
None

CONTRAINDICATIONS/POSSIBLE INTERACTIONS
None

 FOLLOW-UP

PATIENT MONITORING
Monitor hydration, electrolytes, acid–base balance, and body temperature.

EXPECTED COURSE AND PROGNOSIS
Patients usually recover within 5–10 days of infection.

 MISCELLANEOUS

ZOONOTIC POTENTIAL
Mumps virus spreads only from acutely infected humans to susceptible dogs.

Suggested Reading

Greene CE. Mumps and influenza virus infections. In: Greene CE, ed. Infectious diseases of the dog and cat. 2nd ed. Philadelphia: Saunders, 1998:130.

Author Johnny D. Hoskins
Consulting Editor Stephen C. Barr

BASICS

OVERVIEW
• Toxic mushrooms—classified into four categories on the basis of clinical signs and their time of onset and into seven groups on the basis of the toxin; *Amanita* most important genus
• Onset of signs after ingestion of category B, C, or D mushrooms—20 min to 3 hr
• Systems affected—hepatobiliary (hepatic necrosis); renal/urologic (renal tubular necrosis); nervous (autonomic and central)

Category A
• Most toxic
• Cause of cellular destruction, most often of liver and kidneys
• Group I toxin—cyclopeptides; found in *Amanita* spp. and *Galerina* spp.
• Group II toxin—monomethylhydrazine; found in *Gyromitra* spp.; onset of signs > 6 hr after ingestion

Category B
• Affect the autonomic nervous system
• Group III toxin—coprine; found in *Coprinus* spp.
• Group IV toxin—muscarinic effects; found in *Clitocybe* spp. and *Inocybe* spp.

Category C
• Affect the CNS; cause delirium
• Groups V toxin—ibotenic acid-muscimol; found in *Amanita* spp.
• Group VI toxin—hallucinogens; *Psilocybe* spp. and *Panceobus* spp.

Category D
• Cause gastrointestinal irritation
• Group VII toxin—found in a variety of genera

SIGNALMENT
Primarily dogs; mostly puppies

SIGNS

General Comments
• Depend on the type of mushroom ingested
• Toxicity of a particular species—not consistent; depends on the local environment

Physical Examination Findings
• Vomiting
• Diarrhea
• Abdominal pain
• Lethargy
• Icterus
• Ataxia
• Seizures
• Coma

Group IV Toxins
• Ptyalism (excess salivation)
• Lacrimation
• Diarrhea

CAUSES & RISK FACTORS
Exposure to and ingestion of toxic mushroom

DIAGNOSIS

DIFFERENTIAL DIAGNOSIS
• Diagnosis usually relies on owner observation.
• Seasonal occurrence; primarily summer and fall

CBC/BIOCHEMISTRY/URINALYSIS
• High ALT, AST, total bilirubin, BUN, and creatinine; may be delayed 24–48 hr after ingestion
• Hypoglycemia
• Hypokalemia

OTHER LABORATORY TESTS
• Identification of mushroom (refrigerate) or spores in vomitus or stomach contents—submit to an experienced mycologist

IMAGING
N/A

DIAGNOSTIC PROCEDURES
N/A

PATHOLOGIC FINDINGS
Hepatocellular and renal tubular necrosis

TREATMENT
• Inpatient—monitor vital signs; supportive and symptomatic care
• NPO if vomiting
• Parental fluids—maintain hydration and induce diuresis
• Warn client that temporary improvement in gastrointestinal signs with group I toxicity is often followed by delayed onset of hepatic and renal failure.

MEDICATIONS

DRUGS
• Induce emesis—ipecac syrup (1–2 mL/kg PO up to 15 mL) or apomorphine (0.04 mg/kg IV)
• Activated charcoal—1–4 g/kg q3–6h for 24–36 hr; mix in water (1 g/5–10 mL water)
• Furosemide—2–4 mg/kg IV q8–12h; for oliguric or anuric renal failure in patents with normal hydration status
• Atropine—0.02–0.04 mg/kg half-dose IV, half-dose IM; block muscarinic signs; group IV toxins only
• Penicillin G—20,000 U/kg IM q12–24h
• Diazepam—0.25–0.5 mg/kg IV or IM; for seizures

CONTRAINDICATIONS/POSSIBLE INTERACTIONS
Atropine—contraindicated with group IV toxicosis

FOLLOW-UP
• Monitor hepatic and renal function for at least 48 hr.
• Group I toxicosis—temporary improvement in gastrointestinal signs often followed by delayed onset of hepatic and renal failure
• Prognosis—good, except for group I toxicosis

MISCELLANEOUS

SEE ALSO
Poisoning (Intoxication)

ABBREVIATIONS
• ALT = alanine aminotransferase
• AST = aspartate aminotransferase

Suggested Reading
Lincoft G, Mitchel DH. Toxic and hallucinogenic mushroom poisoning. New York: Van Nostrand Reinhold, 1977.

Author Ronald B. Wilson
Consulting Editor Gary D. Osweiler

MYASTHENIA GRAVIS

 BASICS

DEFINITION
A disorder of neuromuscular transmission characterized by muscular weakness and excessive fatigability

PATHOPHYSIOLOGY
Transmission failure at the neuromuscular junction—results from structural or functional abnormalities of the nicotinic AChRs (congenital form) and from autoantibody-mediated destruction of AChRs and post-synaptic membranes (acquired form)

SYSTEMS AFFECTED
• Neuromuscular—result of abnormalities or destruction of AChRs
• Respiratory—may find aspiration pneumonia secondary to megaesophagus

GENETICS
• Congenital familial forms—Jack Russell terriers, springer spaniels, smooth fox terriers; autosomal recessive mode of inheritance
• Acquired—as with other autoimmune diseases, requires appropriate genetic background for disease to occur; multifactorial, involving environmental, infectious, and hormonal influences

INCIDENCE/PREVALENCE
• Congenital—rare
• Acquired—not uncommon in dogs; rare in cats

GEOGRAPHIC DISTRIBUTION
Worldwide

SIGNALMENT

Species
Dogs and cats

Breed Predilections
• Congenital—Jack Russell terriers; springer spaniels; smooth fox terriers
• Acquired—several breeds: golden retrievers; German shepherds; Labrador retrievers; dachshunds; Scottish terriers

Mean Age and Range
• Congenital—6–8 weeks of age
• Acquired—bimodal age of onset; dogs: 1–4 years of age and 9–13 years of age

Predominant Sex
• Congenital—none
• Acquired—may be a slight predilection for females in the young age group; none in the old age group

SIGNS

General Comments
• Acquired—may have several clinical presentations ranging from focal involvement of the esophageal, pharyngeal, and extraocular muscles to acute generalized collapse
• Should be on the differential diagnosis of any dog with acquired megaesophagus or lower motor neuron weakness

Historical Findings
• Vomiting—common; important to differentiate between vomiting and regurgitation
• Voice change
• Exercise-related weakness
• Acute collapse

Physical Examination Findings
• Patient may look normal at rest.
• Excessive drooling, regurgitation, and repeated attempts at swallowing
• Muscle atrophy—usually not found
• Dyspnea—with aspiration pneumonia
• Fatigue or cramping—with mild exercise
• Careful neurologic examination—subtle findings: decreased or absent palpebral reflex (may be fatigable); may note a poor or absent gag reflex; spinal reflexes usually normal but fatigable (rarely absent and dog unable to support its weight)

CAUSES
• Congenital
• Immune-mediated
• Paraneoplastic

RISK FACTORS
• Appropriate genetic background
• Neoplasia—particularly thymoma
• Methimazole treatment (cats)—may result in reversible disease

 DIAGNOSIS

DIFFERENTIAL DIAGNOSIS
• Other disorders of neuromuscular transmission—tick paralysis; botulism; cholinesterase toxicity
• Acute or chronic polyneuropathies
• Polymyopathies—including polymyositis
• Diagnosis depends upon a careful history, thorough physical and neurologic examinations, and specialized laboratory testing.

CBC/BIOCHEMISTRY/URINALYSIS
• Normal
• Serum creatine kinase—usually normal; may be elevated with polymyositis associated with concurrent thymoma

OTHER LABORATORY TESTS
• Serum AChR antibody titer—diagnostic for acquired form
• Thyroid and adrenal function—may see abnormalities associated with acquired form

IMAGING
Thoracic radiographs—megaesophagus; cranial mediastinal mass

DIAGNOSTIC PROCEDURES
• Ultrasound-guided biopsy of cranial mediastinal mass—may support diagnosis of thymoma
• Dramatic increase in muscle strength after administration of edrophonium chloride (0.1 mg/kg IV)—may see false-negative and false-positive responses
• Decreased or absent palpebral reflex—may return after edrophonium chloride administration
• Electrophysiologic evaluation—necessity questionable with increased availability of AChR antibody testing; many patients with acquired form are poor anesthetic risks.
• Electrocardiogram—with bradycardia; third-degree heart block was recently documented in some patients with acquired disease.

PATHOLOGIC FINDINGS
Biopsy of a cranial mediastinal mass—may reveal thymoma or thymic hyperplasia

TREATMENT

APPROPRIATE HEALTH CARE
• Inpatient—until adequate dosages of anticholinesterase drugs are achieved
• Aspiration pneumonia—may require intensive care
• Gastrostomy tube—may be required if patient is unable to eat or drink without significant regurgitation

NURSING CARE
• Oxygen therapy, intensive antibiotic therapy, intravenous fluid therapy, and supportive care—generally required for aspiration pneumonia
• Nutritional maintenance with a gastrostomy tube—multiple feedings of a high-caloric diet; good hygiene care

ACTIVITY
• Self-limited owing to the severity of muscle weakness and extent of aspiration pneumonia

DIET
• Increased food and water
• May try different consistencies of food—gruel; hard food; soft food; evaluate what is best tolerated

CLIENT EDUCATION
• Warn client that, although the disease is treatable, most patients require months of special feeding and medication.
• Inform client that a dedicated owner is important to a favorable outcome for acquired myasthenia.

SURGICAL CONSIDERATIONS
• Cranial mediastinal mass—thymoma
• Before attempting surgical removal, stabilize patient with anticholinesterase drugs and treat aspiration pneumonia.
• Weakness may not be seen initially.
• Suspected thymoma—test all patients for acquired disease before surgery.

 MEDICATIONS

DRUGS OF CHOICE
• Anticholinesterase drugs—prolong the action of acetylcholine at the neuromuscular junction; pyridostigmine bromide syrup (Mestinon syrup) at 1–3 mg/kg PO q 8–12h diluted half and half in water
• Corticosteroids—0.5 mg/kg q24h; initiated if there is a poor response to pyridostigmine or if there is no response to the edrophonium chloride challenge
• Prednisone—immunosuppressive dosages; may initially worsen weakness

CONTRAINDICATIONS
Avoid drugs that may reduce the safety margin of neuromuscular transmission—aminoglycoside antibiotics; antiarrhythmic agents; phenothiazine's; anesthetics; narcotics; muscle relaxants; magnesium

PRECAUTIONS
• Avoid large volumes of barium for evaluating megaesophagus.
• Large air-filled esophagus seen on survey radiographs—barium study not indicated

POSSIBLE INTERACTIONS
N/A

ALTERNATIVE DRUGS
N/A

 FOLLOW-UP

PATIENT MONITORING
• Return of muscle strength should be evident.
• Thoracic radiographs—evaluated every 4–6 weeks for resolution of megaesophagus
• AChR antibody titers—evaluated every 6–8 weeks; decrease to the normal range with clinical remission

PREVENTION/AVOIDANCE
N/A

POSSIBLE COMPLICATIONS
• Aspiration pneumonia
• Respiratory arrest

EXPECTED COURSE AND PROGNOSIS
• No severe aspiration pneumonia or pharyngeal weakness—good prognosis for complete recovery; resolution usually within 4–6 months
• Thymoma present—guarded prognosis unless complete surgical removal and control of myasthenic symptoms are achieved

 MISCELLANEOUS

ASSOCIATED CONDITIONS
• Other autoimmune disorders—thyroiditis; skin disorders; hypoadrenocorticism
• Disorders of the thymus—thymoma; thymic hyperplasia
• Other neoplasias

AGE-RELATED FACTORS
• Bimodal age of onset—1–4 years of age and 9–13 years of age

ZOONOTIC POTENTIAL
N/A

PREGNANCY
• Humans—weakness may improve during pregnancy but worsens after delivery; some neonates of affected mothers have a temporary myasthenia gravis–like weakness that lasts several days to weeks owing to in utero transfer of autoantibodies from the mother.
• Documented in dogs after whelping

SEE ALSO
• Chapters covering autoimmune diseases
• Megaesophagus

ABBREVIATION
AChR = acetylcholine receptor

Suggested Reading
Drachma DB. Myasthenia gravis. N Engle J Med 1994;330:1797–1810.
Shelton GD. Canine myasthenia gravis. In: Kirk WR, Bangor JD, eds. Current veterinary Therapy XI. Philadelphia: Saunders, 1992:1039–1040.
Shelton GD. Megaesophagus secondary to myasthenia gravis. In: Kirk WR, Bonagura JD, eds. Current veterinary therapy XI. Philadelphia: Saunders, 1992:580–583.
Author G. Diane Shelton
Consulting Editor Peter D. Schwarz

DISEASES

MYCOBACTERIAL INFECTIONS

BASICS

OVERVIEW
• Mycobacteria—gram-positive, acid-fast, higher bacteria (genus *Mycobacterium*); obligate or sporadic pathogens in humans and animals • Tuberculosis—caused by *M. tuberculosis* (humans), *M. bovis* (cattle and some wild mammals), and *M. microti* (voles); dogs and cats exposed to infected primary hosts sporadically infected; disseminated or multi-organ disease caused by obligately parasitic organism; rare in dogs and cats in developed countries • Leprosy—*M. leprae* (human) and *M. lepraemurium* (murine); cats: well-localized skin infection associated with intracellular acid-fast organism that cannot be cultured by any standard microbiologic methods; causal organism debated • Subcutaneous or systemic infections (dogs and cats)—*M. abscessus, M. avium, M. chelonae, M. fortuitum, M. phlei, M. smegmatis, M. thermoresistable,* and *M. xenopi;* sporadic infections; usually as the result of traumatic tissue introduction of the organism • Atypical mycobacteriosis—systemic or localized infection with *Mycobacterium* species not otherwise classified as causing tuberculosis or leprosy; most organisms free-living saprophytes • Disseminated infection with *M. avium* (dogs and cats)—often classified as tuberculosis, but epidemiologically and therapeutically better classified as an atypical mycobacteriosis

SIGNALMENT
Tuberculosis
• Cats and dogs of any age • Bassett hounds and Siamese reported as most susceptible; evidence unclear (possible statistical aberration)

Feline Leprosy
• Adult free-roaming cats and kittens • Cases sporadically reported in northeastern USA

Atypical Mycobacteriosis
• Adult cats—subcutaneous • Adult dogs—occasional report of respiratory or systemic disease; rarely cutaneous

SIGNS
Tuberculosis
• Correlated with route of exposure • Major sites of involvement—oropharyngeal lymph nodes; cutaneous and subcutaneous tissues of the head and extremities; pulmonary system; gastrointestinal system • Dogs—respiratory, especially coughing; dyspnea uncommon • Cats—from contaminated milk: weight loss, chronic diarrhea, and thickened intestines; from predation: cutaneous nodules, ulcers, and draining tracts • Virtually all dogs and many cats—pharyngeal and cervical lymphadenopathy; retching, ptyalism, or tonsillar abscess; lymph nodes visible or pal-

pably firm, fixed, tender, may ulcerate and drain • Fever • Depression • Partial anorexia and weight loss • Hypertrophic osteopathy may occur. • Disseminated disease—body cavity effusion; visceral masses; bone or joint lesions; dermal and subcutaneous masses and ulcers; lymphadenopathy and/or abscesses; CNS signs; and sudden death

Feline Leprosy
• Cutaneous nodules and plaques—single or multiple; usually on head and extremities; may be covered with normal epithelium and hair; may be alopecic or ulcerated and crusted; nonpainful; not attached to underlying structures • Regional lymphadenopathy may be seen. • Systemic—none

Atypical Mycobacteriosis
• Cutaneous—traumatic lesion that fails to heal with appropriate therapy; spreads locally in the subcutaneous tissue (panniculitis); original lesion enlarges, forming a deep ulcer that drains greasy hemorrhagic exudate; surrounding tissue becomes firm; satellite pinpoint ulcers open and drain. • Cutaneous and subcutaneous—systemic signs rare • Pulmonary and systemic infections—same as for tuberculosis • *M. avium*—infection most often disseminated

CAUSES & RISK FACTORS
Tuberculosis
• Source of exposure—always an infected typical host • Dogs—usually exposed from an infected person in the household (*M. tuberculosis*); route is ingestion of expectorated infectious material; aerosol exposure possible; patients most often found in urban areas with Third World immigrants • Cats—classically exposed by drinking unpasteurized milk of infected cattle (*M. bovis*); much less common now than in the past; may be exposed by predation on infected small mammals (*M. bovis,* or undefined tuberculosis species)

Feline Leprosy
• Patients often located near seaports and other coastal locales • History of bite wound—possible • Exposure—thought to be by predation on infected rodents

Atypical Mycobacteriosis
• Natural habitat of saprophytic species of *Mycobacterium* is a moist environment. • Trauma and accidental inoculation of the subcutaneous fat may result in infection; history of bite wound possible (subcutaneous disease) • Fat animals may be more at risk than lean ones. • Exposure—routes for pulmonary and systemic diseases unknown

DIAGNOSIS

DIFFERENTIAL DIAGNOSIS
The mycobacterial infections have different prognoses, treatment recommendations, and

public health consequences but may initially have similar signs, especially cutaneous lesions.

Tuberculosis
• Other mycobacterial infections • Systemic mycoses • Lymphosarcoma • Disseminated mast cell tumor • Systemic histiocytosis • Plague • Disseminated nocardiosis

Feline Leprosy
• Other mycobacterial infections—especially cutaneous tuberculosis • Plague • L-form bacterial infection • *Rhodococcus equi* infection • Chronic bite wound abscess • Neoplasia • Mycetoma • Dermatophyte pseudomycetoma • Cytology and biopsy—if acid-fast organisms are identified, consider tuberculosis or cutaneous nocardiosis, both of which can be fastidious and slow growing in culture, leading to the suspicion of unculturable leprosy organism

Atypical Mycobacteriosis
• Foreign body • Bacterial abscess • L-form bacterial infection • Feline leprosy • Cutaneous tuberculosis • *Rhodococcus equi* infection • Nocardiosis • Sterile nodular panniculitis • Deep pyoderma and cellulitis • Leishmaniasis • Mast cell tumor • Sweat gland neoplasia

CBC/BIOCHEMISTRY/URINALYSIS
• Variable abnormalities, depending on extent of systemic disease • Tuberculosis—anemia common

OTHER LABORATORY TESTS
Tuberculosis (dogs)—intradermal skin testing with BCG may produce false-positive results.

IMAGING
Radiography
• Thoracic, abdominal, or skeletal lesions—suggest granulomatous infectious disease • No specific lesions for the mycobacterioses • Pulmonary tuberculosis lesions—may become calcified or cavitated

DIAGNOSTIC PROCEDURES
• Based on histopathologic and microbiologic evaluation of biopsy material from affected tissue • Biopsy specimens—should be uncontaminated by surface bacteria; must incorporate the center of a granulomatous focus • Smears from affected tissues—for detection with acid-fast bacilli; swabs or aspirations of draining cutaneous lesions or lymph nodes; transtracheal wash; endoscopic brushing; rectal cytology; impression taken at surgical biopsy • Culture—submit heat-fixed smears and tissue; special media and techniques required; identification of isolates may take several weeks.

PATHOLOGIC FINDINGS
Tuberculosis
• Granulomas—with prominent necrosis; often poorly demarcated; often surrounded and admixed with other inflammatory cells • Abundant epithelioid macrophages • Giant

cells uncommon • Acid-fast bacteria—low numbers detected with ZN acid-fast stain; within epithelioid macrophages
• Lymph nodes—generally obliterated by the pyogranulomatous inflammatory reaction

Feline Leprosy
• Lesions—chronic pyogranulomas; lack central necrosis characteristic of tuberculosis
• Organisms—identify by ZN acid-fast stain; usually numerous within epithelioid histiocytes; may be sparse in some chronic lesions

Atypical Mycobacteriosis
• Pyogranulomatous panniculitis
• Dermatitis
• Lesions—typically associated with fat necrosis and extracellular accumulations of lipid; surrounded by a cuff of neutrophils
• Organisms—within the fat vacuoles; identify by H&E stain or modified Fite-Faraco acid-fast stains; typical ZN acid-fast staining technique may wash out fat accumulations and organisms from specimens.
• Pulmonary and systemic disease—pyogranulomas; occasional areas of necrosis; no giant cells (as in tuberculosis); organisms usually numerous within macrophages

TREATMENT
• Feline leprosy—cured by surgical excision of lesions
• Subcutaneous atypical mycobacteriosis—may be aided by debulking surgery; benefit of surgery in conjunction with aggressive medical treatment undefined
• Humans—cutaneous lesions have been treated with controlled local heating.

MEDICATIONS

DRUGS

Tuberculosis
Primary
• Always use double- or triple-drug oral therapy; never attempt single-drug therapy for any organism.
• Current recommendation—fluoroquinolone (e.g., enrofloxacin), clarithromycin, and rifampin for 6–9 months
• Enrofloxacin, orbifloxacin, and ciprofloxacin—5–15 mg/kg PO q24h
• Rifampin—10–20 mg/kg PO q24h or divided q12h (maximum, 600 mg/day)
• Clarithromycin—5–10 mg/kg PO q24h
Alternatives
• Isoniazid and rifampin—combinations have been used; little is known about their use in cats; one recent report of treatment (cat) with isoniazid, rifampin, and dihydrostreptomycin

for 3 months noted weight loss but eventual successful outcome
• Isoniazid—10–20 mg/kg (up to 300 mg total) PO q24h
• Ethambutol—15 mg/kg PO q24h
• Pyrazinamide—instead of ethambutol; 15–40 mg/kg PO q24h
• Dihydrostreptomycin—15 mg/kg IM q24h

Feline Leprosy
• Dapsone—1 mg/kg up (to 50 mg/cat) PO q12h for 2–4 weeks
• Clofazimine—2–8 mg/kg PO q24h for 6 weeks; then every 3–4 days for 1–2 months
• Rifampin—10–20 mg/kg PO q24h or divided q12h

Atypical Mycobacteriosis
• Chemotherapy—may use in vitro sensitivity testing to choose drug
• Antibiotics—macrolides, sulfonamides, tetracyclines, aminoglycosides, and fluoroquinolones generally effective
• Fluoroquinolones and/or clarithromycin—good empirical treatment; same dosages as for tuberculosis; treat for 2–6 months; relapses during course of or after completion of treatment common
• Single-agent therapy has been typically recommended, but double-agent therapy may be warranted owing to poor response over the long term.
• M. avium—clofazimine at 2–8 mg/kg PO q24h for 6 weeks; then every 3–4 days for 1–2 months
• Subcutaneous disease (M. fortuitum)—topical treatment with a 1:1 solution of 2.27% enrofloxacin in 90% DMSO used successfully in cats; applied 1 mL q12h for a total of 5 mg/kg
• Humans (systemic disease)—ancillary therapy with γ-interferon resulted in resolution of a refractory case

CONTRAINDICATIONS/POSSIBLE INTERACTIONS
• Traditional antituberculosis drugs—be alert for any adverse reactions; experience limited, especially in cats
• Isoniazid—liver toxicity, seizures, neuritis, and drug eruption in humans
• Ethambutol—optic neuritis in humans
• Pyrazinamide—liver toxicity in humans
• Rifampin—anorexia, vomiting, and liver toxicity
• Dapsone—hemolytic anemia, other immune-mediated blood dyscrasias, and liver toxicity
• Clofazimine—orange discoloration of fat, diarrhea and/or weight loss, and hepatic enzyme elevation
• Dihydrostreptomycin—hearing loss and renal damage

FOLLOW-UP

PATIENT MONITORING
• Antituberculosis and antileprosy drugs—examine at least monthly; monitor for anorexia and weight loss. • Monitor liver enzymes monthly. • Instruct owners to report cutaneous lesions immediately.

PREVENTION/AVOIDANCE
Clinicians aware of a human tuberculosis case in a household with dogs or cats should counsel owners about the risk of reverse zoonosis.

EXPECTED COURSE AND PROGNOSIS
• Tuberculosis—guarded, but currently undefined because experience with modern drugs is limited • Feline leprosy—fair, especially if lesions are amenable to surgical excision • Subcutaneous atypical mycobacteriosis—good for survival but guarded for resolution; relapse after cessation of long-term antibiotic therapy occurs in > 40% of cats treated with single-agent therapy. • Pulmonary and disseminated atypical mycobacteriosis—guarded, but may be improved with modern agents and double-drug treatment

MISCELLANEOUS

ZOONOTIC POTENTIAL
• Tuberculosis—affected domestic pets are possible serious zoonotic threats to owners; public health authorities should be notified of any antemortem or postmortem diagnosis (may be required by law); do not attempt treatment without concurrence of public health authorities. • M. tuberculosis—greatest potential for zoonosis, especially with draining cutaneous lesions • Disease transmission from dogs and cats to humans—very rarely recorded; in recent outbreaks of tuberculosis in cats, no such case was documented.

ABBREVIATIONS
• BCG = Bacillus of Calmette-Guérin
• DMSO = dimethyl sulfoxide • H&E = hematoxylin and eosin • ZN = Ziehl-Neelson

Suggested Reading
Greene CE. Mycobacterial infections. In: Greene CE, ed. Infectious diseases of the dog and cat. Philadelphia: Saunders, 1998:313–325.

Author Carol Foil
Consulting Editor Stephen C. Barr

MYCOPLASMA

BASICS

DEFINITION
• Class Mollicutes (Latin, *mollis*, "soft"; *cutis*, "skin"); > 80 genera; three families: myco-plasmas, T-mycoplasmas or ureaplasmas, and acholeplasmas
• Smallest (0.2–0.3 μm) and simplest procaryotic cells capable of self-replication
• Fastidious, facultative anaerobic, gram-negative rods
• Lack a cell wall; thus plastic, highly pleo-morphic, and sensitive to lysis by osmotic shock, detergents, alcohols, and specific anti-body plus complement; enclosed by a trilayered cell membrane built of amphipathic lipids (phospholipids, glycolipids, lipoglycans, sterols) and proteins; most require sterols for growth.
• Different from wall-defective or wall-less L-form bacteria, which can revert to the normal cell wall strain
• Reproduce by binary fission; genome replication not necessarily synchronized with cell division, resulting in budding forms and chains of beads
• Ubiquitous in nature as parasites, commensals, or saprophytes in animals, plants, and insects; many are pathogens of humans, animals, plants, and insects.

PATHOPHYSIOLOGY
• Often part of the resident flora as commensals on mucous membranes of the upper respiratory, digestive, and genital tracts; pathogenicity and role in disease often controversial
• Species show considerable host specificity
• Mechanisms by which disease is caused are poorly understood.
• Some species attach to cells by specific receptors; small size and plastic nature enable them to adapt to the shape and contours of host cell surfaces.
• Intimate contact with host cells—necessary for assimilation of vital nutrients and growth factors (e.g., nucleic acid precursors), which organism cannot synthesize; along with the tendency of exogenous proteins to bind to mycoplasmal membrane may allow organism to evade the host's immune response; may incorporate host cell antigen onto myco-plasma membrane (capping) because lack of cell wall; conversely, mycoplasmal protein antigen may become incorporated onto surface of host cell, thereby involving host cell in deleterious immunologic reactions intended against the organism
• Products produced during growth—capsular carbohydrate, hemolysins, proteolytic enzymes, ammonia, and endonucleases; accumulation of mycoplasma metabolites (i.e., H_2O_2, NH_3) may contribute to cytopathic effects and tissue damage; cytotoxic

glycoproteins and proteins have been isolated from the membranes of several species.
• Immune response—predominantly humoral; as with bacterial infections, IgM and IgA are first antibodies to appear, followed by IgG.
• Fibrinous exudate accompanying infections—protects organism from antibodies and anti-microbial drugs; contributes to chronicity
• Secondary bacterial invaders—common (e.g., attachment respiratory tract cells results in destruction of cilia, which predisposes patient to secondary bacterial infection)

SYSTEMS AFFECTED
Dogs
• Respiratory—pneumonia and upper respiratory infections; caused by *M. cynos;* associated with *M. canis, M. spumans, M. edwardii, M. feliminutum, M. gateae,* and *M. bovigenitalium*
• Renal/Urologic—urinary and genital tract infections (e.g., balanoposthitis, urethritis, prostatitis, cystitis, nephritis, vaginitis, endometritis); caused by *M. canis* and *M. spumans*
• Reproductive—mycoplasma and ureaplasma; associated with infertility, early embryonic death, abortion, stillbirths or weak newborns, and neonatal mortality
• Musculoskeletal—arthritis; from *M. spumans*
• Gastrointestinal—associated with colitis
Cats
• Ophthalmic—conjunctivitis; associated with *M. felis* (5%–25%)
• Respiratory—pneumonia, associated with *M. gateae, M. feliminutum,* and *M. felis;* upper respiratory infections, associated with *M. felis*
• Musculoskeletal—chronic fibrinopurulent polyarthritis and tenosynovitis; associated with *M. gatea* and unspecified mycoplasmal organisms
• Renal/Urologic—urinary tract infections
• Reproductive—abortions and fetal deaths; associated with *M. gateae* and ureaplasmas
• Skin/Exocrine—chronic cutaneous abscesses

GENETICS
N/A

INCIDENCE/PREVALENCE
• Frequent inhabitants of mucosal membranes; *M. gatea* and/or *M. felis* found in oral cavity or urogenital tract of 70%–80% of healthy cats
• Rate of isolation in diseased dogs much higher than in normal dogs (e.g., lung, uterus, prepuce)

GEOGRAPHIC DISTRIBUTION
Ubiquitous

SIGNALMENT

Species
Dogs and cats

Breed Predilections
None

Mean Age and Range
All ages

Predominant Sex
None

SIGNS

General Comments
Pathogenic role controversial

Historical Findings
• Polyarthritis—chronic intermittent lameness; reluctance to move; joint pain
• Fever
• Malaise
• Conjunctivitis—unilateral or bilateral

Physical Examination Findings
• Polyarthritis—diffuse limb edema; joint swelling; pain
• Conjunctivitis—blepharospasm; chemosis; conjunctival hyperemia; epiphora; and serous or purulent ocular discharge
• Mild rhinitis—sneezing

CAUSES
• Mycoplasma flora of dogs—*M. canis, M. spumans, M. maculosum, M. edwardii, M. cynos, M. molare, M. opalescens, M. feliminutum, M. gateae, M. arginini, M. bovigenitalium, Acholeplasma laidlawii,* and ureaplasms
• Mycoplasma flora of cats—*M. felis, M. gateae, M. feliminutum, M. arginini, M. pulmonis, M. arthritidis, M. gallisepticum, Acholeplasma laidlawi,* and ureaplasms

RISK FACTORS
• Commensals—occasionally cause systemic infection associated with immunodeficiency, immunosuppression, or cancer
• Impaired resistance of the host—may allow organism to cross the mucosal barrier and disseminate
• Organism may be opportunistic—one factor in a multifactorial causal complex (e.g., impaired pulmonary clearance from viral infection may allow organism to establish infection in lungs as secondary opportunistic pathogen)
• Predisposing factors—stresses (e.g., reproductive problems associated with overcrowded operations) and other factors (e.g., urinary tumors and urinary calculi)
• Rate of isolation of organism in diseased dogs much higher than in normal dogs

DIAGNOSIS

DIFFERENTIAL DIAGNOSIS
• Upper respiratory infection (dogs and cats)—viruses (parainfluenza virus, canine distemper, herpesvirus, feline calicivirus, reovirus); *Chlamydia psittaci;* bacteria (*Bordetella bronchiseptica,* staphylococci, streptococci, coliforms)

• Urinary tract infection (dogs and cats)—bacteria (staphylococci, streptococci, coliforms); fungus (*Candida*); parasites
• Infertility, early embryonic death, abortion, stillbirths or weak newborns, and neonatal mortality (dogs)—bacteria (*Brucella, Salmonella, Campylobacter, E. coli,* streptococcus); viruses (canine herpesvirus, canine distemper, canine adenovirus); *Toxoplasma gondii,* endocrinopathies (progesterone deficiency, hypothyroidism)
• Prostatitis (dogs)—bacteria (*E. coli, Brucella canis*); fungi (*Blastomyces, Cryptococcus*)
• Arthritis (dogs and cats)—immune-mediated, bacteria (staphylococci, streptococci, coliforms, anaerobes); L-form bacteria; rickettsia (*Ehrlichia*); *Borrelia burgdorferi;* fungi (*Coccidioides, Cryptococcus, Blastomyces*); protozoa (*Leishmania*); viruses (feline calicivirus)
• Conjunctivitis (cats)—feline herpesvirus; feline calicivirus; feline reovirus; *Chlamydia psittaci;* bacteria

CBC/BIOCHEMISTRY/URINALYSIS

With Polyarthritis
• Mild anemia
• Neutrophilic leukocytosis
• Hypoalbuminemia
• Hypoglobulinemia
• Proteinuria, resulting from immune-complex glomerulonephritis

OTHER LABORATORY TESTS
• Serologic tests—complement fixation, agar gel immunodiffusion, ELISA; detect organism
• Difficult to demonstrate in and from tissues
• Extremely pleomorphic—in smears (e.g., conjunctival scrapings) seen as coccobacilli, coccal forms, ring forms, spirals, and filaments
• Stains—stain poorly (gram-negative); preferred: Giemsa or other Romanowsky stain
• Fluorescent antibody test—definitive diagnosis; isolate and identify or detect the organism in tissues; can submit cotton swabs placed in Hayflick broth medium or commercially available swabs; organisms fragile; refrigerate specimens and deliver to the laboratory within 48 hr; freeze to preserve longer

IMAGING
Polyarthritis—no radiographic changes

DIAGNOSTIC PROCEDURES
• Polyarthritis—high numbers of nondegenerative neutrophils in synovial fluid
• Prostatic fluid—inflammatory cells with negative bacterial culture

TREATMENT

APPROPRIATE HEALTH CARE
Outpatient

NURSING CARE
N/A

ACTIVITY
N/A

DIET
N/A

CLIENT EDUCATION
N/A

SURGICAL CONSIDERATIONS
N/A

MEDICATIONS

DRUGS OF CHOICE
• Sensitive to antibiotics that specifically inhibit synthesis in procaryotes
• Tetracyclines—22 mg/kg PO q8h
• Doxycycline—5mg/kg PO q12h
• Chloramphenicol—40–50 mg/kg IV, IM, SC, PO q8–12h
• No standardized procedure for in vitro antimicrobial susceptibility tests
• Topical antibiotic—conjunctivitis

CONTRAINDICATIONS
• Topical steroid ointments—improper use for conjunctivitis may prolong infection and predispose patient to corneal ulceration.
• Tetracyclines—avoid use in animals < 6 months of age.
• Tetracycline and chloramphenicol—avoid use in pregnant animals.

PRECAUTIONS
Sulfonamides and β-lactams—inhibit peptidoglycan synthesis; organism resistant because of lack of cell walls

POSSIBLE INTERACTIONS
N/A

ALTERNATIVE DRUGS
• Gentamicin
• Kanamycin
• Spectinomycin
• Spiramycin
• Tylosin
• Erythromycin
• Nitrofurans
• Fluoroquinolones

CONTRAINDICATIONS/POSSIBLE INTERACTIONS
N/A

FOLLOW-UP

PATIENT MONITORING
Treat for an extended period of time.

PREVENTION/AVOIDANCE
• No vaccines are available.
• Organism readily killed by drying, sunshine, and chemical disinfection.

POSSIBLE COMPLICATIONS
N/A

EXPECTED COURSE AND PROGNOSIS
Prognosis good in animals with competent immune systems and given appropriate antibiotic therapy

MISCELLANEOUS

ASSOCIATED CONDITIONS
M. pneumoniae—infects respiratory tracts in humans worldwide; causes mycoplasma pneumonia, bronchitis, or upper respiratory infection; usually self-limited; rarely fatal

AGE-RELATED FACTORS
Tetracyclines—avoid in animals < 6 months of age.

ZOONOTIC POTENTIAL
• Not generally considered zoonotic
• Reported development of suppurative mycoplasmal tenosynovitis in a veterinarian who was scratched by a cat being treated for colitis

PREGNANCY
Tetracycline and chloramphenicol—do not use in pregnant animals.

SYNONYMS
Pleuropneumonia-like organisms

ABBREVIATION
ELISA = enzyme-linked immunosorbent assay

Suggested Reading
Greene CE. Mycoplasmal, ureaplasmal, and L-form infections. In: Greene CE, ed. Infectious diseases of the dog and cat. Philadelphia: Saunders, 1998:174–178.
Author J. Paul Woods
Consulting Editor Stephen C. Barr

MYELODYSPLASTIC SYNDROMES

 BASICS

OVERVIEW
Characterized by alterations in the normal development and maturation of hematopoietic stem cells

SIGNALMENT
More common in cats than in dogs

SIGNS
- Pale mucous membranes
- Lethargy
- Weight loss
- Hepatosplenomegaly
- Peripheral lymphadenomegaly varies

CAUSES & RISK FACTORS
- Associated with FeLV infection in cats
- Bone marrow dysplasia—may be caused by ehrlichiosis and Rocky Mountain spotted fever
- Drugs (e.g., trimethoprim and sulfa combination, estrogen, Butazolidin, and cytotoxic anticancer agents)—may cause myelodysplasia

 DIAGNOSIS

DIFFERENTIAL DIAGNOSIS
Differentiate from infectious causes and drug toxicity (see Causes & Risk Factors)

CBC/BIOCHEMISTRY/URINALYSIS
- Cytopenias
- Megaloblastic anemia
- Circulating, nucleated RBC
- Large, bizarre platelets
- Immature granulocytes with abnormal morphologic characteristics
- Monocytosis

OTHER LABORATORY TESTS
Examination of bone marrow aspirate and core biopsy—reveals ineffective erythropoiesis and granulopoiesis within a specimen with normal cellularity

IMAGING
N/A

DIAGNOSTIC PROCEDURES
Bone marrow biopsy

 TREATMENT

- Nonspecific, unless a treatable cause is identified
- Intensive nursing care often necessary
- Supportive care—may require multiple blood transfusions and nutritional support

 MEDICATIONS

DRUGS
Antibiotics—for secondary bacterial infection, if necessary

CONTRAINDICATIONS/POSSIBLE INTERACTIONS
N/A

 FOLLOW-UP

- CBC and cytologic examination of bone marrow aspirate or biopsy—repeat to monitor progression of disease
- Transfuse as necessary.
- Possible complications—sepsis; hemorrhage; profound anemia
- Prognosis—guarded to poor

 MISCELLANEOUS

ABBREVIATON
FeLV = feline leukemia virus

Suggested Reading

Harvey JW. Myeloproliferative disorders in dogs and cats. Vet Clin North Am Small Anim Pract 1981;11:349–381.

Reagan WJ, DeNicola DB. Myeloproliferative and lymphoproliferative disorders. In: Morrison WB, ed. Cancer in dogs and cats: medical and surgical management. Baltimore: Williams & Wilkins, 1998:95–122.

Author Linda S. Fineman
Consulting Editor Wallace B. Morrison

Myelomalacia—Diffuse, Hemorrhagic (Hematomyelia)

BASICS

OVERVIEW
• Acute, progressive, ischemic necrosis of the spinal cord after acute spinal cord trauma
• First appears at the site of injury; then progresses both cranially and caudally
• Death may be caused by respiratory paralysis if the intercostal and phrenic nerves are affected.

SIGNALMENT
• Any age or breed
• Because of the close association between acute type I disk herniation and myelomalacia, breeds predisposed to the former are more commonly affected.

SIGNS
• Acute paralysis from spinal injury—initial clinical sign
• Thoracolumbar injury—paralysis with exaggerated spinal reflexes in the pelvic limbs
• Pain perception—usually absent caudal to the lesion
• Spinal cord malacia—progresses to involve the lumbosacral spinal segments within 72 hr, causing pelvic limb areflexia and atonia; dilated anus, and flaccid, easily expressed urinary bladder; thoracic and cervical spinal cord segments may be involved 7–10 days after the initial insult.
• Subarachnoid hemorrhage secondary to necrosis of the microvasculature in the spinal cord—may cause hyperthermia and extreme meningeal pain

CAUSES & RISK FACTORS
• Type I disk disease
• Vertebral or spinal cord trauma

DIAGNOSIS

DIFFERENTIAL DIAGNOSIS
• Cannot be differentiated from spinal trauma
• Diagnosis based on hind limb upper motor neuron paralysis that progresses to a lower motor neuron paralysis and a rostrally advancing line of analgesia.

CBC/BIOCHEMISTRY/URINALYSIS
• Usually normal, initially
• Road accident—nonspecific abnormalities related to other organ injury
• After condition has developed, degenerative left shift caused by massive spinal cord necrosis may occur.

OTHER LABORATORY TESTS
N/A

IMAGING
• Spinal survey radiography—evidence of herniated disk; vertebral fracture or luxation
• Myelogram—cord compression; edema

DIAGNOSTIC PROCEDURES
N/A

TREATMENT
• None to reverse spinal cord damage
• Agents useful for treating the secondary effects of spinal cord trauma (e.g., methylprednisolone sodium succinate and 21-aminosteroid compounds)—not evaluated for myelomalacia; may be useful in halting progression

MEDICATIONS

DRUGS OF CHOICE
• Methylprednisolone sodium succinate—30 mg/kg IV initially; follow with 15 mg/kg IV 2 and 6 hr after the initial dose; follow with 2.4 mg/kg/hr for 42 hr
• Histamine H_2-blocker (e.g., cimetidine), sucralfate, or misoprostol—protect against gastrointestinal ulcers in patients receiving corticosteroids

CONTRAINDICATIONS/POSSIBLE INTERACTIONS
Rise in incidence of infection associated with methylprednisolone administration in humans.

FOLLOW-UP
• In a few patients, condition progresses only caudally; paralysis is permanent, but respiratory compromise does not occur.
• Reported after decompressive laminectomy, suggesting that surgery does not prevent its occurrence.

MISCELLANEOUS

Suggested Reading
Griffiths IR. The extensive myelopathy of intervertebral disc protrusions in dogs (the ascending syndrome). J Small Anim Pract 1972;13:425–428.
Author Karen Dyer Inzana
Consulting editor Joane M. Parent

MYELOPATHY, DEGENERATIVE

BASICS

DEFINITION
Syndrome characterized by slow, progressive degeneration of axons and myelin in the spinal cord

Pathophysiology
Vitamin B_{12} deficiency, vitamin E deficiency, progressive increase in circulating suppressor T lymphocytes, an autoimmune response to a neural antigen, and dying-back neuropathy—examined as possible links; none is established as an important factor

Systems Affected
Nervous

Genetics
Suspected, but not proven, hereditary basis—German shepherds, German shepherd mixed breeds, and Siberian huskies

Incidence/Prevalence
• Data unavailable
• Most common cause of pelvic limb paresis in middle-aged, German shepherds and German shepherd mixed breeds
• Rare in other breeds of dogs and in cats

Geographic Distribution
N/A

SIGNALMENT

Species
Dogs and cats

Breed Predilections
• Most commonly affected—German shepherds and German shepherd mixed breeds
• Other large and medium breeds occasionally affected—collies and collie crosses, Labrador retrievers, Siberian huskies, Chesapeake Bay retrievers, Kerry blue terriers, and Welsh corgis (observed by author)

Mean Age and Range
• Mean age of onset—9.6 years
• Range—4–14 years
• German shepherds—two cases reported at 6 and 7 months old

Predominant Sex
Males

SIGNS

Historical Findings
• Insidious onset
• Bilateral but not necessarily symmetrical
• Initially—mild ataxia and paresis of the pelvic limbs; thoracic limbs not affected

• Owners often bring their dog in for examination several months after onset of clinical signs, suspecting arthritis.
• Knuckling and scuffing of the toes of the pelvic limbs—most common complaint
• Crossing over and swaying of the rear quarters—often occur when patient is turning
• Urination and defecation—voluntary control retained until extremely late in the disease
• Caudal paraspinal and pelvic limb muscles—often atrophy from disuse late in the disease
• Pain or discomfort—not evident

Neurologic Examination Findings
• Deficits limited to the pelvic limbs
• Ataxia and upper motor neuron paresis—localized to the T3-L3 spinal cord segments
• Proprioception deficits—worse than expected for the mild degree of paresis observed early in the disease; may be considerably asymmetric
• Withdrawal reflexes—normal to exaggerated; may see a crossed extensor reflex
• Anal sphincter tone, perineal reflex, and tail tone—normal
• Patellar reflexes—usually normal to exaggerated; sometimes impaired or absent unilaterally or bilaterally because of degeneration of the dorsal root ganglia or dorsal gray matter of the spinal cord; ventral motor roots not affected, so this is not a true lower motor neuron sign but indicates the disease
• Pain perception—preserved

CAUSES
Unknown

RISK FACTORS
N/A

DIAGNOSIS

DIFFERENTIAL DIAGNOSIS
• Hansen type II intervertebral disk protrusion and spinal neoplasia—most likely to resemble degenerative myelopathy; back pain at the lesion site is common but may not be observed; differentiated by survey radiography and myelography
• Myelitis—usually more acute and progressive; ruled out by CSF analysis at the time of myelography
• Diskospondylitis—differentiated by occurrence of back pain; survey radiography helpful

• Lumbosacral stenosis—generally causes pain; to rule out, may need electromyography and epidurography
• Vertebral spondylosis and dural ossification—common radiographic findings in old, large-breed dogs; almost never cause clinical signs

CBC/BIOCHEMISTRY/URINALYSIS
Usually normal

OTHER LABORATORY TESTS
Abnormal cell-mediated immune studies—depressed responses to concanavalin A, phytohemagglutinin P, and pokeweed mitogens in most affected dogs; tests are not readily available; diagnostic accuracy not confirmed by double-blind studies

IMAGING
• Thoracic and abdominal radiography—screen for metastatic disease; consider the age of the patient and the possibility of spinal neoplasia.
• Spinal survey radiography—generally normal; may reveal dural ossification or spondylosis; findings are generally of no clinical significance.
• Myelography—normal
• CT—normal
• MRI—normal

DIAGNOSTIC PROCEDURES
CSF analysis—collect from the lumbar subarachnoid space; usually contains a high protein concentration (40–100 mg/dL) with a normal WBC count; unfortunately, these findings are also seen with type II disk protrusion, the main differential.

PATHOLOGIC FINDINGS
• Gross necropsy findings—normal
• Histologic examination—demyelination, axonal degeneration, and astrocytosis of the white matter
• Lesions—most severe in the thoracic spinal cord in dorsolateral and ventromedial funiculi; bilateral but not necessarily symmetrical; lesions discontinuous
• May see marked degeneration in the lumbar dorsal nerve roots but not the ventral nerve roots

TREATMENT

APPROPRIATE HEALTH CARE
• Outpatient
• Inpatient—for diagnostic workup only

MYELOPATHY, DEGENERATIVE

NURSING CARE
• Dog should be encouraged to be active as long as possible to delay onset of a nonambulatory state.
• Nonambulatory patients—pay careful attention to prevent pressure sores; provide good bedding.
• A cart may be beneficial.

ACTIVITY
Encourage exercise to prevent muscle atrophy; the stronger and more active the patient is, the longer it will stay ambulatory as the paresis progresses.

DIET
Avoid excess weight.

CLIENT EDUCATION
• Inform client that this is a nontreatable disease that progresses slowly and steadily.
• Inform client that euthanasia is recommended once a nonambulatory state is reached.

SURGICAL CONSIDERATIONS
• No effective surgery available
• It is possible for a dog to have concurrent type II disk protrusion; unless the spinal cord compression caused is extreme, surgery should not be done until a therapeutic trial of corticosteroids is completed; if marked improvement is seen, then decompressive surgery is warranted; CAUTION: surgery to remove a type II disk protrusion in a patient with clinical signs that are actually the result of degenerative myelopathy often causes irreversible neurologic deterioration.

MEDICATIONS

DRUGS OF CHOICE
• No proven effective treatment available
• Proposed treatment—suggested by one author; combination of exercise, vitamin supplements, and epsilon aminocaproic acid (Amicar, Lederle, NY; 500 mg PO q8h mixed with a hematinic compound); apparently slows the progression in 50% of patients; 15%–20% of patients do not deteriorate further if treatment is maintained; no controlled trials have been done.

CONTRAINDICATIONS
• Corticosteroids—do not use; not beneficial in the treatment of this disease
• Steroid myopathy—may worsen muscle atrophy and pelvic limb weakness, hastening the onset of a nonambulatory state

PRECAUTIONS
N/A

POSSIBLE INTERACTIONS
N/A

ALTERNATIVE DRUGS
N/A

FOLLOW-UP

PATIENT MONITORING
• Epsilon aminocaproic acid administration—if effective, improvement should be seen within 8 weeks; preform a neurologic examination at that time to access therapeutic response; if patient has deteriorated, discontinue treatment because it is expensive.
• Re-evaluate patient on a regular basis to monitor progression and avoid complications.

PREVENTION/AVOIDANCE
N/A

POSSIBLE COMPLICATIONS
Pressure sores and urine scalding once a nonambulatory state is reached

EXPECTED COURSE AND PROGNOSIS
• Most affected dogs gradually lose function in the pelvic limbs, reaching a nonambulatory state within 6 months to 2 years after onset.
• Nonambulatory patients eventually lose thoracic limb function and may develop urinary and fecal incontinence.

MISCELLANEOUS

ASSOCIATED CONDITIONS
• Enteropathy—seen in some patients; leads to subnormal serum vitamin B_{12} and vitamin E concentrations; speculated cause is degenerative myelopathy that leads to autonomic nerve dysfunction, which, in turn, leads to impaired intestinal motility and intestinal bacterial overgrowth.
• Depressed cell-mediated immunity—seen in some patients; may be a response to the lesion or may indicate that the disease has an immunologic basis

AGE-RELATED FACTORS
• Clinical signs develop in dogs > 4 years old.
• A few cases of a similar nature have been reported in dogs < 1 year old.

ZOONOTIC POTENTIAL
N/A

PREGNANCY
Because the disease is slowly progressive, an ambulatory affected dog should reach term normally; important to discuss with the client the probable heritability of the disease.

SYNONYMS
Degenerative radiculomyelopathy of the aged German shepherd

SEE ALSO
Intervertebral Disk Disease, Thoracolumbar

ABBREVIATION
CSF = cerebrospinal fluid

Suggested Reading
Clemmons RM. Degenerative myelopathy. In: Kirk RW, ed. Current veterinary therapy X. Philadelphia: Saunders, 1989:830–833.
Kornegay JN. Congenital and degenerative diseases of the central nervous system: axonal and myelin lesions—degenerative myelopathy. In: Kornegay JN, ed. Neurologic disorders. New York: Churchill Livingstone, 1986:120–122.
LeCouteur RA, Child G. Diseases of the spinal cord: degenerative myelopathy of dogs. In: Ettinger SJ, ed. Textbook of veterinary internal medicine. 3rd ed. Philadelphia: Saunders, 1989:648–649.
Longhofer SL, Duncan ID, Messing A. A degenerative myelopathy in young German shepherd dogs. J Small Anim Pract 1990;31:199–203.
Oliver JE, Lorenz MD. Handbook of veterinary neurology. 3rd ed. Philadelphia: Saunders, 1997.
Author Allen Sisson
Consulting Editor Joane M. Parent

MYELOPROLIFERATIVE DISORDERS

 BASICS

OVERVIEW
• Neoplastic proliferation of nonlymphoid cell lines of bone marrow origin
• Believed to represent a spectrum of disorders in which the stem cell involved is a hematopoietic precursor capable of differentiating into all blood cell types except lymphocytes
• Leukemia (acute and chronic)—may develop from granulocytic, monocytic, erythrocytic, and megakaryocytic cell lines

SIGNALMENT
Dogs and cats

SIGNS
• Pale mucous membranes
• Lethargy
• Weight loss
• Hepatosplenomegaly
• Peripheral lymphadenomegaly—occasionally

CAUSES & RISK FACTORS
• Cats—most commonly associated with FeLV infection; when recovering from panleukopenia or hemobartonellosis, may be a relatively higher risk of developing a mutant cell line induced by FeLV
• Dogs—unknown

 DIAGNOSIS

DIFFERENTIAL DIAGNOSIS
• Acute lymphocytic leukemia—usually differentiated by special staining techniques
• Leukemoid response
• Other causes of eosinophilia—parasitism; allergic disease; eosinophilic gastroenteritis; differentiate from eosinophilic leukemia
• Severe hemolytic anemia must be differentiated from acute erythroleukemia.

CBC/BIOCHEMISTRY/URINALYSIS
• Severe, nonregenerative anemia
• Circulating nucleated RBCs
• Megaloblastic erythrocytes
• Leukocytosis or leukopenia
• Thrombocytopenia with abnormal platelet morphology

OTHER LABORATORY TESTS
• Examination of bone marrow aspirate or core biopsy—reveals hypercellular bone marrow with abnormal morphology in all cell lines; neoplastic proliferation or absence of one cell line
• Immunohistochemical or other special stain—may be necessary to determine cell type

IMAGING
Plain radiographs and ultrasound—hepatomegaly and splenomegaly common

DIAGNOSTIC PROCEDURES
Examination of one marrow aspirate or core biopsy

 TREATMENT

• Outpatient or inpatient
• Supportive care—blood transfusions and fluid administration to correct dehydration

 MEDICATIONS

DRUGS
• Little information available in the literature regarding treatment
• Cytosine arabinoside—may be used; 100 mg/m² SC divided q12h 4 days per week
• Hydroxyurea—30–45 mg/kg q24h for 7–10 days; then 30–45 mg/kg q48h; essentially, titrate dosage to patient response
• Antibiotics—may be indicated to combat secondary infection

CONTRAINDICATIONS/POSSIBLE INTERACTIONS
Chemotherapy can be toxic; seek advice before treatment if unfamiliar with cytotoxic drugs.

 FOLLOW-UP

• CBC and examination of bone marrow aspirate—determine response to treatment and progression of disease
• Prognosis—grave; usually rapid and fatal clinical course

 MISCELLANEOUS

PREGNANCY
Chemotherapy drugs are contraindicated in pregnant animals.

ABBREVIATION
FeLV = feline leukemia virus

Suggested Reading
Hamilton TA. The leukemias. In: Morrison WB, ed. Cancer in dogs and cats: medical and surgical management. Baltimore: Williams & Wilkins, 1998:721–729.
Reagan WJ, DeNicola DB. Myeloproliferative and lymphoproliferative disorders. In: Morrison WB, ed. Cancer in dogs and cats: medical and surgical management. Baltimore: Williams & Wilkins, 1998:95–122.
Author Linda S. Fineman
Consulting Editor Wallace B. Morrison

MYOCARDIAL INFARCTION

BASICS

OVERVIEW
• Rapid development of myocardial necrosis resulting from sustained, complete reduction of blood flow to a portion of the myocardium, caused by thrombus formation • Uncommon as a naturally occurring disease in dogs • Microscopic intramural myocardial infarctions and focal areas of myocardial fibrosis are common in dogs with acquired cardiovascular disease. • Consistent ECG characteristics of spontaneous myocardial infarction are not well characterized in dogs and cats.

SIGNALMENT
Rare in dogs and cats

SIGNS

Historical Findings
• Lethargy • Anorexia • Weakness • Dyspnea • Collapse • Vomiting • Obesity • Unexpected death

Physical Examination Findings
• Lameness • Tachycardia • Heart murmur • Cardiac rhythm disturbances • Low-grade fever

CAUSES AND RISK FACTORS
• Atherosclerosis and coronary artery disease • Nephrotic syndrome • Vasculitis • Hypothyroidism • Bacterial endocarditis • Neoplasia • Septicemia • Intramural coronary arteriosclerosis in old dogs • Subvalvular aortic stenosis

Cats
• Cardiomyopathy • Thromboembolism

DIAGNOSIS
Generally presumptive, based on acute onset of signs in a patient with predisposing factors and consistent ECG changes

DIFFERENTIAL DIAGNOSIS

Other Causes of S-T Segment Changes
• Normal variation • Myocardial ischemia/hypoxia • Hyper-, hypokalemia • Digitalis toxicity • Trauma to the heart • Pericarditis • Artifact—wandering baseline

Other Causes of Weakness and Collapse
• Trauma • Neurologic disease • Thromboembolism • Pericardial effusion • Arrhythmia

CBC/BIOCHEMISTRY/URINALYSIS
• Mild leukocytosis • High liver enzymes • Hyperlipidemia—if animal is hypothyroid • High amylase • High creatinine and cardiac isoenzymes • High LDH

OTHER LABORATORY TESTS
Low T4 and T3

IMAGING
• Echocardiography—2-D and M-mode echocardiography useful in evaluating wall motion abnormalities and overall left ventricular function • Angiocardiography—rarely, if ever, used in clinical veterinary cardiology

DIAGNOSTIC PROCEDURES

Electrocardiographic Findings
• Sudden deviation of the ST segment • Tall peaked T waves—first few hours • Sudden development of Q waves or a change in direction of the T wave • Axis shift of the frontal plane • Low-voltage QRS complexes • Sudden development of bundle branch block or heart block • Sudden onset of ventricular arrhythmias because of myocardial ischemia • Sloppy "R" wave descent may be associated with intramural myocardial infarction

TREATMENT
• Direct at the underlying disorder; likewise the symptomatic therapy (e.g., congestive heart failure [CHF]) • Must identify and immediately treat life-threatening arrhythmias • Restrict activity

MEDICATIONS

DRUGS
• Thrombolytic agents, IV—(e.g., streptokinase); cost prohibitive and lack of experience in veterinary medicine with dosage and use • Lidocaine for ventricular arrhythmias • β-Blockers—use cautiously with dilated cardiomyopathy because of possible development of low-output CHF • Propranolol—dogs, 0.2–1.0 mg/kg PO q8h; cats, 2.5–5 mg/cat PO q8–12h • Atenolol—dogs, 0.25–1.0 mg/kg PO q12–24h; cats, 6.25–12.5 mg PO q24h • Antithrombotic agents (e.g., warfarin, heparin, and aspirin)

CONTRAINDICATIONS/POSSIBLE INTERACTIONS
N/A

FOLLOW-UP
• Determined by clinical status and diagnosis of underlying disorder • Monitor anticoagulated patient; CBC and bleeding profiles, including fibrinogen

MISCELLANEOUS

SEE ALSO
• Ventricular Tachycardia • Atherosclerosis

Suggested Reading
Driehuys E, Van Winkle TJ, Sammarco CD, Drobatz KJ. Myocardial infarction in dogs and cats: 37 cases (1985–1994)
Liu SK, Fox PR. Cardiovascular pathology. In: Fox PR, Sisson D, Moise NS, eds. Canine and feline cardiology. 2nd ed. Philadelphia: Saunders, 1999:837–838.
Author Larry P. Tilley
Consulting Editors Larry P. Tilley and Francis W. K. Smith, Jr.

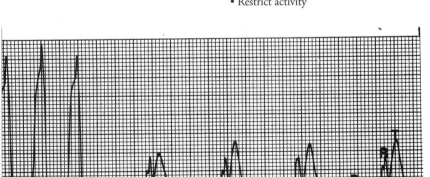

Transmural infarction of the left ventricle in a dog with arteriosclerosis and hypothyroidism. The first three rapid successive complexes represent ventricular tachycardia. The sinus rhythm that follows illustrates small complexes, marked elevation of the S-T segment, and first degree AV block (prolonged P-R interval). (From: Tilley LP. Essentials of canine and feline electrocardiography. 3rd ed. Baltimore: Williams & Wilkins, 1992, with permission).

MYOCARDIAL TUMORS

 BASICS

OVERVIEW
• Rare
• Reported types—hemangiosarcoma, hemangioma, fibrosarcoma, fibroma, lymphosarcoma, myxosarcoma, myxoma, rhabdomyoma, and neurofibroma

SIGNALMENT
• Dogs and cats
• More common in old animals

SIGNS
• Depend on location and infiltration
• May include—sudden collapse caused by cardiac arrhythmia or signs of heart failure caused by pericardial effusion, venous obstruction, myodynamic failure, or valvular obstruction

CAUSES & RISK FACTORS
Unknown

 DIAGNOSIS

DIFFERENTIAL DIAGNOSIS
• Idiopathic pericardial effusion
• Pericarditis
• Cardiomyopathy
• Congestive heart failure
• Valvular insufficiency
• Heart base tumor

CBC/BIOCHEMISTRY/URINALYSIS
Anemia in a few patients

OTHER LABORATORY TESTS
N/A

IMAGING
• Thoracic radiography—evaluate heart size and shape
• Echocardiography—assess myocardial texture

DIAGNOSTIC PROCEDURES
• Electrocardiography—determine presence of arrhythmia
• Surgical biopsy

 TREATMENT

• Inpatient—restrict activity until recovered from surgery
• Surgical excision—may be curative for benign tumors
• Pericardiectomy—may provide relief from cardiac tamponade
• Chemotherapy—probably most effective after surgical excision
• Alert the client to the potential for sudden death.

MEDICATIONS

DRUGS
• Lidocaine infusion (25–75 µg/kg/min) or procainamide (8–20 mg/kg PO q8h)—treat symptomatic ventricular premature contractions and ventricular tachycardia
• Atenolol (cats: 6.25–12.5 mg/cat PO q12h; dogs: 0.25–1.0 mg/kg PO q12–24h) or propranolol (dogs: 0.2–1 mg/kg PO q8h) or diltiazem (1–1.5 mg/kg PO q8h)—treat paroxysmal supraventricular tachycardia
• Combination chemotherapy—doxorubicin (30 mg/m² every 3 weeks), cyclophosphamide (100–150 mg/m² every 3 weeks), and vincristine (0.7 mg/m² weeks 2 and 3); used successfully to treat cardiac hemangiosarcoma

CONTRAINDICATIONS/POSSIBLE INTERACTIONS
Chemotherapy may have gastrointestinal, bone marrow, cardiac, and other toxicities; seek advice before treatment if you are unfamiliar with cytotoxic drugs.

 ## FOLLOW-UP

• Serial cardiac ultrasonography—monitor response to treatment and doxorubicin toxicity
• Thoracic radiography—monitor effusion and metastasis
• CBC and platelet count—monitor myelo-suppression caused by chemotherapy
• Prognosis—guarded to poor

 ## MISCELLANEOUS
Chemotherapy should not be used in pregnant animals.

Suggested Reading
deMadron NE, Helfand SC, Stebbins KE. Use of chemotherapy for treatment of cardiac hemangiosarcoma in a dog. J Am Vet Med Assoc 1987;190:887–891.

Morrison WB. Nonpulmonary intrathoracic cancer. In: Morrison WB, ed. Cancer in dogs and cats: medical and surgical management. Baltimore: Williams & Wilkins, 1998:537–550.

Author Terrance A. Hamilton
Consulting Editor Wallace B. Morrison

DISEASES

MYOCARDITIS

 BASICS

DEFINITION
• Inflammation of the heart muscle, often caused by infectious agents affecting the myocytes, interstitium, vascular elements, or pericardium.
• Viral, bacterial, rickettsial, fungal, and protozoal diseases are all associated with myocardial inflammation (i.e., myocarditis).
• Pharmacologic agents (e.g., doxorubicin) can also be causative.

PATHOPHYSIOLOGY
• Mechanisms—toxin production, direct invasion of myocardial tissue, and immune-mediated myocardial damage; vasculitis associated with systemic disease; allergic reactions and direct myocyte damage caused by pharmacologic agents. Protozoa (e.g., *Trypanosoma cruzi*) lead to granulomatous myocarditis; viral myocarditis is associated with cell-mediated immunologic reactions.
• Myocardial involvement may be focal or diffuse. Clinical manifestations depend on the extent of the lesions. Diffuse, severe involvement may lead to global myocardial damage and CHF; discrete lesions involving the conduction system may cause profound arrhythmias.

SYSTEMS AFFECTED
• Systemic organ involvement depends on the causative agent.
• Cardiovascular—myocardial failure or arrhythmias
• Respiratory—if pulmonary edema develops

GENETICS
N/A

INCIDENCE/PREVALENCE
• Viral myocarditis (e.g., parvovirus, distemper virus, and herpesvirus)—rare; very young puppies in their first months of life may be profoundly affected; in a second form (parvo-viral), dilated cardiomyopathy develops in dogs 5–6 months of age that were infected during their first weeks of life.
• Protozoal myocarditis associated with *T. cruzi* (i.e., Chagas' disease) reported in dogs < 2 years old from the southeastern United States. Males are more commonly affected than females. *Toxoplasma gondii* occasionally causes myocarditis. Immunosuppressed animals (e.g., cats with feline leukemia virus) are at high risk. *Hepatozoon canis* reported in dogs living in the Texas Gulf.
• Fungal myocarditis—primarily seen in association with systemic fungal infection; myocardial involvement varies with regional prevalence and prevalence of the systemic manifestation.

• Bacterial myocarditis—can be caused by generalized sepsis and bacteremia.
• Doxorubicin cardiotoxicity—reported in dogs receiving cumulative doses = 150–240 mg/M^2
• Spirochetal myocarditis associated with *Borrelia burgdorferi*—documented in 10% of humans with Lyme's disease; incidence and prevalence in dogs not well documented

GEOGRAPHIC DISTRIBUTION
Suspect myocarditis associated with infectious agents wherever these diseases are endemic (see above).

SIGNALMENT
Species
Dogs and cats
Breed Predilections
N/A
Mean Age and Range
Viral myocarditis—seen primarily in animals < 1 year of age
Predominant Sex
N/A

SIGNS
General Comments
• Related to the degree and location of myocardial involvement
• Range from those of arrhythmias to those of CHF
• Onset of cardiac dysfunction in association with systemic illness or the use of specific pharmacologic agents is often the hallmark of myocarditis.
Historical Findings
• Coughing, exercise intolerance, dyspnea—associated with CHF
• Syncope and weakness—associated with arrhythmias
• Concurrent systemic manifestations—often seen with infective myocarditis
• Use of antineoplastic or other pharmacologic agents—associated with the onset of cardiac dysfunction
Physical Examination Findings
• Gallop rhythm or murmur may be found—depends on the nature of the myocardial damage
• Arrhythmias—may be ausculted.
• Fever—common in patients with active infection associated with myocarditis

CAUSES
• Virus (e.g., parvovirus, distemper virus, herpesvirus)
• Protozoa (e.g., *T. cruzi, T. gondii,* and *H. canis*)
• Bacteria
• Fungus (e.g., *Cryptococcus neoformans, Coccidioides immitis,* and *Aspergillus terreus*)
• Algae (e.g., *Prototheca* spp.)
• Doxorubicin

RISK FACTORS
• Exposure to infectious agents
• Use of myocardiotoxic compounds
• Immunosuppression
• Debilitating diseases

 DIAGNOSIS

DIFFERENTIAL DIAGNOSIS
• Always consider preexisting heart disease, including congenital defects, cardiomyopathy, and acquired valvular disease.
• History of a heart murmur or the presence of arrhythmias before onset of systemic illness helps differentiate from other diseases.
• Extracardiac organ involvement and identification of infectious agents may aid in the diagnosis.

CBC/BIOCHEMISTRY/URINALYSIS
Abnormalities—vary, depending on organ involvement

OTHER LABORATORY TESTS
Serologic Tests to Help Identify an Infectious Agent
• Cytologic examination of pericardial, pleural, and peritoneal effusions to identify the infectious organism
• Blood culture to diagnose bacteremia

IMAGING
Thoracic Radiographic Findings
• Cardiac silhouette may appear large or normal depending on the extent of involvement.
• Pulmonary edema, congestion, or pleural effusion in patients with CHF
• Globoid heart in some animals with pericardial effusion
• Pulmonary granuloma may be found in animals with granulomatous myocardial infection.

Echocardiographic Findings
• Reflect the extent of myocardial damage; may be normal if lesions are small or primarily affect the conduction system
• Pericardial effusion in some patients; pericardium may appear thickened and hyperechoic, depending on the extent of pericardial involvement.
• Myocardium may appear mottled with patchy areas of hyperechogenicity caused by myocardial inflammation, fibrosis, or granulomas.
• Regional dyskinesis caused by focal involvement may be appreciated on 2-D echocardiography.

Angiography
• Because of the quality and noninvasive nature of echocardiography, cardiac catheterization is rarely indicated for the diagnosis.

• May use angiography to detect specific chamber involvement or pericardial effusion, if echocardiography is not available

DIAGNOSTIC PROCEDURES

Electrocardiographic Findings
• LV, LA, RV, or RA enlargement patterns in some patients—depending on the extent of chamber involvement.
• Arrhythmias—include both atrial and ventricular tachyarrhythmias
• Differentiate right and left bundle branch blocks and hemiblocks from ventricular enlargement patterns.
• Atrioventricular nodal conduction disturbances in some patients

Endomyocardial Biopsy
Useful for detection of infectious agents (e.g., protozoa, fungal elements) or inflammatory cell infiltrates

Pericardiocentesis
• Alleviates pericardial effusion
• Submit fluid for cytologic examination and possible bacterial culture.

Holter Monitor Study
• To detect arrhythmias, frequency and severity
• To monitor antiarrhythmic therapy

Pathologic Findings
• Dilated cardiac chambers with patchy areas of hyperemia, necrosis, or fibrosis
• Granulomas seen grossly in some patients
• Microscopic examination of the myocardium or pericardium may reveal inflammatory cells (e.g., lymphocytes, plasma cells, and macrophages), patchy fibrosis, or the infectious agents themselves.
• Myofiber dropout—seen in patients with doxorubicin toxicity.

TREATMENT

APPROPRIATE HEALTH CARE
• Hospitalize patients with CHF for initial medical management.
• Hospitalize patients with severe ventricular arrhythmias for initial antiarrhythmic therapy.
• Hospitalize patients with severe systemic manifestations for aggressive medical therapy.

NURSING CARE
N/A

ACTIVITY
Restricted

DIET
Sodium restriction if CHF

CLIENT EDUCATION
• Cardiac manifestations may persist even with resolution of systemic illness.
• Certain arrhythmias (i.e., ventricular tachyarrhythmias) may predispose to sudden death.
• Antemortem diagnosis may be difficult.
• Some infectious agents may pose a public health risk.

SURGICAL CONSIDERATIONS
Complete atrioventricular block may require pacemaker implantation.

MEDICATIONS

DRUGS OF CHOICE
• If a specific etiologic agent is identified, direct treatment against it
• Tailor antiarrhythmic therapy to the predominant arrhythmia.
• Treat CHF with furosemide (1–2 mg/kg PO q6–12h), enalapril (0.25–0.5 mg/kg PO q12–24h), and digoxin (0.22 mg/M² PO q12h)

CONTRAINDICATIONS
Public health considerations may preclude treatment of some infectious diseases (i.e., *T. cruzi*).

PRECAUTIONS
• All antiarrhythmic drugs have proarrhythmic properties and should be monitored closely.
• Systemic organ involvement (e.g., renal involvement) may necessitate modifying drug dosages or use of various cardiac drugs; monitor systemic function carefully.

POSSIBLE INTERACTIONS
N/A

ALTERNATIVE DRUGS
N/A

FOLLOW-UP

PATIENT MONITORING
• Antiarrhythmic therapy—frequent auscultation and ECG
• Serologic titers when appropriate
• Auscultation and follow-up radiographs—treatment of CHF
• Hemograms and serum biochemical analysis—systemic effects

PREVENTION/AVOIDANCE
• Avoid breeding animals with a poor vaccination history.
• Avoid endemic areas if possible.
• Monitor ECG and echocardiogram when using doxorubicin.

EXPECTED COURSE AND PROGNOSIS
• Depend on the extent and severity of myocardial involvement
• Many systemic fungal and protozoal diseases do not respond well to medical management.
• Patients with extensive myocardial inflammation, degeneration, and signs of CHF—very poor prognosis
• Patients with isolated, controllable arrhythmias—good prognosis if the underlying cause can be treated successfully

MISCELLANEOUS

ASSOCIATED CONDITIONS
Often accompanies systemic illness

AGE-RELATED FACTORS
Viral myocarditis—most often seen in animals , 1 year old

ZOONOTIC POTENTIAL
• Varies with infectious agent involved.
• May be high with protozoal and mycotic infections

PREGNANCY
Some viral diseases (e.g., canine herpesvirus and parvovirus) have been passed to the fetus during pregnancy.

SYNONYMS
N/A

SEE ALSO
• Infectious diseases listed under causes
• Ventricular premature complexes
• Ventricular tachycardia

ABBREVIATIONS
• CHF = congestive heart failure
• LA = left atrium
• RA = right atrium
• LV = left ventricle
• RV = right ventricle

Suggested Reading
Liu SK, Fox PR. Cardiovascular pathology. In: Fox PR, Sisson D, Moise NS, eds. Textbook of canine and feline cardiology. 2nd ed. Philadelphia: WB Saunders, 1999:817–844.
Wynne J, Braunwald E. The cardiomyopathies and myocardities In: Braunwald E, ed. Heart disease: a textbook of cardiovascular medicine. 5th ed. Philadelphia: Saunders, 1997:1404–1463.
Author Michael B. Lesser
Consulting Editors Larry P. Tilley and Francis W. K. Smith, Jr.

BASICS

DEFINITION
• Masticatory—focal inflammatory myopathy affecting the muscles of mastication (temporalis and masseter muscles) and sparing the limb muscles
• Extraocular—selectively affects the extraocular muscles, sparing limb and masticatory muscles

PATHOPHYSIOLOGY
• Masticatory—suspected immune-mediated cause owing to autoantibodies against type 2M fibers and a positive clinical response to immunosuppressive doses of corticosteroids
• Extraocular—suspected immune-mediated cause owing to positive clinical response to corticosteroids

SYSTEMS AFFECTED
Neuromuscular—muscles of mastication; extraocular muscles

GENETICS
• Unknown
• As with autoimmune diseases in general, the appropriate genetic background must exist.
• Extraocular—golden retrievers may have a genetic predisposition.

INCIDENCE/PREVALENCE
• Unknown
• Masticatory—not rare

GEOGRAPHIC DISTRIBUTION
Probably worldwide

SIGNALMENT
Species
Dogs

Breed Predilections
• Various
• Extraocular—golden retrievers

Mean Age and Range
• No obvious age predisposition

Predominant Sex
• None obvious

SIGNS
General Comments
Masticatory—usually related to abnormalities of jaw movement and jaw pain; not a "table-top" diagnosis; usually requires laboratory testing to confirm diagnosis

Historical Findings
• Masticatory—acute or chronic pain when opening the jaw; inability to pick up a ball or get food into the mouth; acutely swollen muscles; progressive muscle atrophy
• Extraocular—bilateral exophthalmos

Physical Examination Findings
• Masticatory—marked jaw pain with manipulation and/or trismus; acute muscle swelling with exophthalmos; muscle atrophy with enophthalmos; inability to open the jaw under anesthesia
• Extraocular—bilateral proptosis; impaired vision

CAUSES
Immune mediated

RISK FACTORS
• Appropriate genetic background
• Possible previous bacterial or viral infection

 DIAGNOSIS

DIFFERENTIAL DIAGNOSIS
• Retro-orbital abscess—probe behind last upper molar
• Temporomandibular joint disease—radiographically abnormal joint
• Polymyositis—markedly high serum creatine kinase; generalized EMG abnormalities; diagnostic muscle biopsies
• Neurogenic atrophy of temporalis muscles—determined by EMG and muscle biopsy
• Atrophy of masticatory muscles from corticosteroids—history of corticosteroid use; characteristic changes on muscle biopsy

CBC/BIOCHEMISTRY/URINALYSIS
• Serum creatine kinase—normal or mildly elevated

OTHER LABORATORY TESTS
• Muscle biopsy—diagnostic test of choice for masticatory disease
• Immunocytochemical assay—demonstrate autoantibodies against masticatory muscle type 2M fibers; negative in polymyositis and extraocular disease

IMAGING
• Radiography of the temporomandibular joints
• Orbital sonogram—for extraorbital disease; demonstrate swollen extraocular muscles

DIAGNOSTIC PROCEDURES
EMG—differentiate between extraocular disease and polymyositis; abnormal masticatory muscles in masticatory disease only; generalized abnormalities in polymyositis

PATHOLOGIC FINDINGS
Masticatory
• Swelling or atrophy of the masticatory muscles
• Biopsy specimen—may see myofiber necrosis, phagocytosis, mononuclear cell infiltration with a multifocal and perivascular distribution; may see myofiber atrophy and fibrosis with chronic condition; eosinophils rare

Extraocular
Mononuclear cell infiltration—restricted to extraocular muscles

 TREATMENT

APPROPRIATE HEALTH CARE
Outpatient

NURSING CARE
Gastrostomy tube—may be required with severe restrictions in jaw mobility; requires good hygiene and supportive care

ACTIVITY
N/A

MYOPATHY, FOCAL INFLAMMATORY—MASTICATORY MUSCLE MYOSITIS AND EXTRAOCULAR MYOSITIS

DIET
Masticatory—may require liquid food or gruel until jaw mobility is regained; may need a gastric feeding tube to facilitate fluid and caloric intake

CLIENT EDUCATION
• Warn client that long-term corticosteroid therapy may be required.
• Inform client that residual muscle atrophy may occur with chronic masticatory disease.

SURGICAL CONSIDERATIONS
• Not indicated

MEDICATIONS

DRUGS OF CHOICE
Coricosteroids—immunosuppressive dosages, tapered as jaw mobility, swelling, and serum creatine kinase return to normal; maintained at lowest alternate-day dosage that prevents restricted jaw mobility; treated for a minimum of 6 months

CONTRAINDICATIONS
N/A

PRECAUTIONS
• Corticosteroids—watch for infection and undesirable side effects.
• Clinical signs may reoccur if treatment is stopped too soon.

POSSIBLE INTERACTIONS
N/A

ALTERNATIVE DRUGS
Intolerable side effects of corticosteroids—institute a lower dose of corticosteroids and combine with another drug (e.g., azathioprine).

FOLLOW-UP

PATIENT MONITORING
• Masticatory—return of jaw mobility and decreased serum creatine kinase
• Extraocular—decreased swelling of extraocular muscles

PREVENTION/AVOIDANCE
N/A

POSSIBLE COMPLICATIONS
• Corticosteroids—undesirable side effects;
• Recurrence of clinical signs—treatment stopped too early
• Poor clinical response—inadequate dosages of corticosteroids

EXPECTED COURSE AND PROGNOSIS
• Masticatory—jaw mobility should return to normal unless the condition is chronic and severe fibrosis develops; good prognosis if treated early with adequate dosages of corticosteroids
• Extraocular—good response to corticosteroids; good prognosis

MISCELLANEOUS

ASSOCIATED CONDITIONS
Other concurrent autoimmune disorders

AGE-RELATED FACTORS
N/A

ZOONOTIC POTENTIAL
N/A

PREGNANCY
Unknown

SYNONYMS
• Eosinophilic myositis
• Atrophic myositis

SEE ALSO
• Myopathy, Generalized Inflammatory–Polymyositis and Dermatomyositis
• Myopathy, Noninflammatory–Endocrine

ABBREVIATION
EMG = electromyogram

Suggested Reading

Carpenter JL, Schmidt GM, Moore FM, et al. Canine bilateral extraocular polymyositis. Vet Pathol 1989;26:510–512.

Orvis JS, Cardinet GH III. Canine muscle fiber types and susceptibility of masticatory muscles to myositis. Muscle Nerve 1981;4:354–359.

Shelton GD, Cardinet GH III, Bandman E. Canine masticatory muscle disorders: a clinicopathological and immunochemical study of 29 cases. Muscle Nerve 1987;10:753–766.

Shelton GD. Canine masticatory muscle disorders. In Kirk RW, ed. Current veterinary therapy X. Philadelphia: Saunders, 1989;816–819.

Author G. Diane Shelton
Consulting Editor Peter D. Schwarz

MYOPATHY, GENERALIZED INFLAMMATORY—POLYMYOSITIS AND DERMATOMYOSITIS

BASICS

DEFINITION
• Polymyositis—a condition in which skeletal muscles are damaged by a nonsuppurative inflammatory process dominated by lymphocytic infiltration
• Dermatomyositis—polymyositis is associated with characteristic skin lesions

PATHOPHYSIOLOGY
• Inflammation of skeletal muscles—results in muscle weakness, myalgia, and atrophy
• Muscle inflammation—may be a result of immune-mediated, infectious, or paraneoplastic disorders; may be a sequela to certain drug therapies

SYSTEMS AFFECTED
• Neuromuscular—generalized muscle involvement including masticatory and limb muscles
• Gastrointestinal—particularly the pharyngeal and esophageal muscles, because they are composed predominantly of skeletal muscle in dogs
• Skin/Exocrine—particularly if related to a generalized immune-mediated connective tissue disorder

GENETICS
• Unknown
• As for autoimmune diseases in general, the appropriate genetic background must exist.
• Dermatomyositis—reported to have an autosomal dominant inheritance pattern in rough-coated collies and Shetland sheepdogs

INCIDENCE/PREVALENCE
• Unknown
• Generalized inflammatory myopathies—not common

GEOGRAPHIC DISTRIBUTION
Probably worldwide

SIGNALMENT
Species
Dogs and rarely cats

Breed Predilections
• Polymyositis—various breeds of dogs and cats may be affected
• Dermatomyositis—reported in rough-coated collies, Shetland sheepdogs, and Australian cattle dogs

Mean Age and Range
• Polymyositis—none obvious
• Dermatomyositis—3–5 months of age

Predominant Sex
None obvious

SIGNS
General Comments
• Polymyositis—usually associated with a stiff-stilted gait, muscle pain, and/or muscle weakness
• Elevated serum creatine kinase—supports but does not make the diagnosis of myositis
• Muscle biopsy—needed to confirm the diagnosis

Historical Findings
• Stiff-stilted gait—acute or chronic
• Muscle swelling and/or atrophy
• Generalized muscle pain
• Generalized muscle weakness and exercise intolerance
• Regurgitation of food or difficulty swallowing

Physical Examination Findings
• Pain upon palpation of muscle groups
• Generalized muscle atrophy, including the muscles of mastication
• Gait abnormalities, including a stiff-stilted gait
• Neurologic examination—not abnormal; may be a decreased gag reflex if the pharyngeal muscles are affected
• Dermatomyositis (dogs)—typical skin lesions

CAUSES
• Immune-mediated
• Infectious—*Toxoplasma gondii; Neospora canis; Hepatozoon canis; Ehrlichia canis;* bacterial infection uncommon
• Drug-induced
• Paraneoplastic syndrome

RISK FACTORS
• Appropriate genetic background
• Possibly previous bacterial or viral infection
• Neoplasia, possibly occult

DIAGNOSIS

DIFFERENTIAL DIAGNOSIS
• Polyarthritis—differentiated by physical examination and evaluation of joint fluid
• Noninflammatory muscle disorders—differentiated by muscle biopsy
• Polyneuropathy—differentiated by neurologic examination, electrophysiology, and muscle biopsy
• Chronic intervertebral disk disease—differentiated by physical examination and serum creatine kinase

CBC/BIOCHEMISTRY/URINALYSIS
Serum creatine kinase—markedly elevated

OTHER LABORATORY TESTS
• Serum antinuclear antibody titer—may be positive in connective tissue disorders
• May see concurrent hypothyroidism

IMAGING
• Regurgitation—evaluate thoracic radiography for esophageal dilatation.
• Pharyngeal weakness—perform a dynamic study for the evaluation of the swallowing process.

DIAGNOSTIC PROCEDURES
• Muscle biopsy—single most important test for diagnosing polymyositis; sample multiple

muscles, because condition may be missed if distribution is patchy
• Electromyographic evaluation—performed to determine the distribution of muscle involvement and the muscles to be biopsied; should help differentiate myopathic from neuropathic causes of muscle weakness

PATHOLOGIC FINDINGS
• Muscle swelling or atrophy
• Biopsy specimens—usually contain mononuclear cell infiltrates
• Rare neutrophils or eosinophils—may be noted
• Regenerating myofibers—may be observed
• Intramyofiber parasite cyst—rare
• Chronic condition—may see extensive myofiber atrophy and fibrosis

 TREATMENT

APPROPRIATE HEALTH CARE
Outpatient

NURSING CARE
Supportive care—may be required to prevent skin wounds and decubital ulcers in non-ambulatory severely affected patients

ACTIVITY
Should increase, along with muscle strength, as muscle inflammation decreases

DIET
• Megaesophagus—may require feeding from an elevation; try foods of different consistencies.
• Severe regurgitation—may need to place a gastric feeding tube to maintain hydration and nutrition

CLIENT EDUCATION
• Warn client that long-term immunosuppressive therapy may be required for an immune-mediated condition.
• Inform client that residual muscle atrophy may be occur with chronic disease and extensive fibrosis.
• Suggest genetic counseling for familial disorders.

SURGICAL CONSIDERATIONS
Only for concurrent neoplasia.

 MEDICATIONS

DRUGS OF CHOICE
• Corticosteroids—immunosuppressive dosages usually result in clinical improvement of immune-mediated condition; decrease to the lowest alternate-day dosage that maintains normal creatine kinase and improved muscle strength and mobility; may require long-term therapy
• Identified infectious agent—initiate specific therapy.

CONTRAINDICATIONS
N/A

PRECAUTIONS
Corticosteroids—observe for infection and undesirable side effects; remember that chronic therapy may lead to muscle atrophy.

POSSIBLE INTERACTIONS
N/A

ALTERNATIVE DRUGS
Intolerable side effects of corticosteroids—institute a lower dose of corticosteroids combined with another drug (e.g., azathioprine).

 FOLLOW-UP

PATIENT MONITORING
• Serum creatine kinase—periodic evaluation; if elevated, should decrease into the normal range
• Corticosteroids—side effects

PREVENTION/AVOIDANCE
N/A

POSSIBLE COMPLICATIONS
• Corticosteroids—undesirable side effects
• Recurrence of clinical signs—treatment stopped too early
• Poor clinical response—inadequate dosages of corticosteroids

EXPECTED COURSE AND PROGNOSIS
• Immune-mediated condition—good to fair prognosis
• Paraneoplastic disorder associated with occult neoplasia—guarded prognosis

 MISCELLANEOUS

ASSOCIATED CONDITIONS
• Other concurrent autoimmune disorders
• Neoplasia

AGE-RELATED FACTORS
N/A

ZOONOTIC POTENTIAL
N/A

PREGNANCY
Unknown

SEE ALSO
Myopathy, Noninflammatory–Endocrine

Suggested Reading
Hargis AM, Haupt KH, Prieur DJ, Moore MP. A skin disorder in three Shetland sheepdogs: comparison with familial canine dermatomyositis of collies. Compend Contin Educ Pract Vet 1985;7:306–318.
Kornegay JN, Gorgacz EJ, Dawe DL, et al. Polymyositis in dogs. J Am Vet Med Assoc 1980;176: 431–438.
Shelton GD, Cardinet GH III. Pathophysiologic basis of canine muscle disorders. J Vet Intern Med 1987;1:36–44.
Author G. Diane Shelton
Consulting Editor Peter D. Schwarz

MYOPATHY, NONINFLAMMATORY—ENDOCRINE

BASICS

DEFINITION
Myopathies associated with various endocrinopathies (including hypothyroidism, hyperthyroidism, hypoadrenocorticism, hyperadrenocorticism) and associated with exogenous corticosteroid use (steroid myopathy)

PATHOPHYSIOLOGY
With Adrenal Dysfunction
• Glucocorticoid excess—impaired muscle protein metabolism; may accelerate degradation of myofibrillar and soluble protein in skeletal muscle; impairment of carbohydrate metabolism owing to induction of an insulin-resistant state; may note elevated ACTH levels
• Adrenal insufficiency—circulatory insufficiency; fluid and electrolyte imbalance; impaired carbohydrate metabolism
With Thyroid Disease
• Hyperthyroidism—increased mitochondrial respiration; accelerated protein degradation and lipid oxidation; glycogen depletion; impaired glucose uptake
• Hypothyroidism—impaired muscle energy metabolism by reduced glycogen breakdown, gluconeogenesis, and oxidative and glycolytic capacity; impaired insulin-stimulated carbohydrate metabolism

SYSTEMS AFFECTED
• Neuromuscular—impaired energy metabolism
• Cardiovascular—impaired energy metabolism; circulatory disorders

GENETICS
N/A

INCIDENCE/PREVALENCE
• Exact incidence unknown
• Myopathies related to exogenous corticosteroids—common
• Myopathies associated with Cushing syndrome and hypothyroidism—not uncommon

GEOGRAPHIC DISTRIBUTION
Probably worldwide

SIGNALMENT
Species
• Dogs—steroid myopathy; weakness associated with hyperadrenocorticism and hypoadrenocorticism; hypothyroidism
• Cats—weakness associated with hyperthyroidism

Breed Predilections
Affects several breeds

MEAN AGE AND RANGE
• Steroid myopathy—dogs of any age
• Other disorders—see specific disease

Predominant Sex
None found

SIGNS
General Comments
Corticosteroid use in dogs—muscles very susceptible; muscle atrophy (particularly the masticatory muscles) is not uncommon with prolonged corticosteroid use

Historical Findings
• Muscle weakness, atrophy, and stiffness
• Regurgitation
• Dysphagia
• Dysphonia

Physical Examination Findings
• Muscle weakness, stiffness, cramping, and myalgia
• Muscle hypertrophy or atrophy
• May not note other clinical signs of an endocrine disorder

CAUSES
• Endocrine dysfunction
• Autoimmune
• Neoplastic

RISK FACTORS
N/A

DIAGNOSIS

DIFFERENTIAL DIAGNOSIS
• Inflammatory myopathies—distinguished by muscle biopsy
• Noninflammatory myopathies—distinguished by muscle biopsy

CBC/BIOCHEMISTRY/URINALYSIS
• Baseline testing—abnormalities consistent with endocrine disorder
• Serum creatine kinase—usually normal

OTHER LABORATORY TESTS
Thyroid and adrenal function—should be diagnostic

IMAGING
• Dynamic studies—evaluate pharyngeal and esophageal function; with regurgitation and dysphagia
• Cardiac evaluation—for cats with hyperthyroidism

DIAGNOSTIC PROCEDURES
• Muscle biopsy—fresh frozen sections
• Electromyography

PATHOLOGIC FINDINGS
• Hyperadrenocorticism and steroid myopathies—selective atrophy of type 2 muscle fibers; may see lobulated to ragged-red fibers with associated myotonia
• Hypoadrenocorticism—normal
• Hyperthyroidism (cats)—unknown if pathologic abnormalities occur within muscle
• Hypothyroidism—atrophy of type 2 fibers; may see an increase in type 1 fibers; may see PAS-positive deposits in type 2 fibers

MYOPATHY, NONINFLAMMATORY—ENDOCRINE

 TREATMENT

APPROPRIATE HEALTH CARE
Depends on specific endocrine disorder

NURSING CARE
Support bandaging, wound management (decubital ulcers), and physical therapy—with musculoskeletal manifestations

ACTIVITY
• Clinical corticosteroid myopathy (humans)—inactivity worsens condition; increased muscle activity may partially prevent atrophy.
• Physical therapy—may help prevent and treat muscle weakness and wasting in dogs receiving glucocorticoids

DIET
• Regurgitation and megaesophagus—feed from an elevation.
• Dysphagia and esophageal dilation—give food with the best-tolerated consistency.
• Gastric feeding tube—if oral feeding is not tolerated

CLIENT EDUCATION
Depends on specific endocrine disorder

SURGICAL CONSIDERATIONS
Removal of neoplasia

 MEDICATIONS

DRUGS OF CHOICE
• Depend on specific endocrine disorder
• Corticosteroid myopathy—decrease corticosteroid dosage to the lowest possible level; use a nonfluorinated corticosteroid and alternate-day dosing.
• Intramyofiber lipid storage with steroid myopathy—L-carnitine (50 mg/kg q12h) may improve muscle strength.

CONTRAINDICATIONS
N/A

PRECAUTIONS
Depend on specific endocrine disorder

POSSIBLE INTERACTIONS
N/A

ALTERNATIVE DRUGS
Fluorinated corticosteroids, triamcinolone, betamethasone, and dexamethasone—most likely to produce muscle weakness; use an equivalent dose of another corticosteroid.

 FOLLOW-UP

PATIENT MONITORING
• Depends on specific endocrine disorder
• Steroid myopathy—should note return of muscle strength and mass with decreased steroid use

PREVENTION/AVOIDANCE
N/A

POSSIBLE COMPLICATIONS
Depend on specific endocrine disorders

EXPECTED COURSE AND PROGNOSIS
• Myotonia associated with hyperadrenocorticism—poor prognosis for resolution
• Steroid myopathy—good prognosis for return of muscle strength and mass; recovery may take weeks
• Hypothyroid myopathy—improvement in muscle pain and stiffness common
• Hyperthyroidism (cats)—good prognosis for return of muscle strength and return to euthyroid state
• Hypoadrenocorticism—good prognosis for return of muscle strength
• Dysphagia and regurgitation—may resolve with adequate treatment

 MISCELLANEOUS

ASSOCIATED CONDITIONS
• May note multiple endocrinopathies
• Hypothyroidism (dogs)—concurrent myasthenia gravis

AGE-RELATED FACTORS
N/A

ZOONOTIC POTENTIAL
N/A

PREGNANCY
Unknown

Suggested Reading
Jaggy A, Oliver JE, Ferguson DC, et al. Neurological manifestations of hypothyroidism: a retrospective study of 29 cases. J Vet Intern Med 1994;8:328–330.
LeCouteur RA, Dow SW, Sisson AF. Metabolic and endocrine myopathies of dogs and cats. Semin Vet Med Surg Small Anim 1989;4:146–155.
Shelton GD, Cardinet GH III. Pathophysiologic basis of canine muscle disorders. J Vet Intern Med 1987;1:36–44.
Author G. Diane Shelton
Consulting Editor Peter D. Schwarz

DISEASES

MYOPATHY, NONINFLAMMATORY—HEREDITARY LABRADOR RETRIEVER

BASICS

OVERVIEW
- An inherited progressive and degenerative generalized myopathy of Labrador retrievers
- Simple autosomal recessive mode of inheritance
- Pathophysiologic mechanism(s) unknown
- Histologic examination of muscle—more typical of a neurogenic than a myopathic cause; no morphologic changes in the CNS or peripheral nerves identified

SIGNALMENT
- Occurs in black and yellow Labrador retrievers
- Age of onset—variable (6 weeks to 7 months); most common at 3–4 months
- Affects males and females

SIGNS
- Severity ranges from stilted gait to muscle weakness, bunny hopping pelvic limb gait, ventriflexion of the neck, arched back, and abnormal joint posture (cow-hocked stance, hyperextended carpi)
- Worsen with exercise, excitement, and cold weather
- Patient may collapse with forced exercise.
- Some improvement with rest
- Worsen with excitement and cold weather
- Generalized muscle atrophy—mild to severe
- Atrophy of proximal limb and masticatory muscles—often most prominent
- Tendon reflexes—normal, hypoactive, or absent
- Occasionally, patients become recumbent or develop megaesophagus.

CAUSE & RISK FACTORS
Autosomal recessive mode of inheritance

DIAGNOSIS

DIFFERENTIAL DIAGNOSIS
- With little muscle atrophy—exercise intolerance may mimic signs of myasthenia gravis or cardiac or orthopedic disease.
- With marked muscle atrophy—consider other myopathies (infectious, immune-mediated, metabolic, congenital) and generalized lower motor neuron disorders.

CBC/BIOCHEMISTRY/URINALYSIS
Creatine kinase—normal or mildly or moderately elevated

OTHER LABORATORY TESTS
N/A

IMAGING
N/A

DIAGNOSTIC PROCEDURES
- EMG—spontaneous activity, including complex repetitive discharges, especially in proximal limb and masticatory muscles; may reveal no abnormalities with mild disease
- Muscle histology—reveals variation in fiber size, angular atrophy of both type 1 and 2 myofibers, grouped atrophy, increase in central nuclei, muscle degeneration and regeneration, and fibrosis; may note deficiency or increase in type 2 myofibers

TREATMENT
- None specific
- Avoid cold, because it exacerbates clinical signs.
- Discourage breeding of affected animals.
- Do not repeat dam–sire breedings that result in affected offspring.

MEDICATIONS

DRUGS
Diazepam—may be beneficial

CONTRAINDICATIONS/POSSIBLE INTERACTIONS
None known

FOLLOW-UP
- Clinical signs generally stabilize.
- Mild disease—may be an acceptable pet; may show some improvement in exercise tolerance
- Aspiration pneumonia—a risk with megaesophagus

MISCELLANEOUS

ASSOCIATED CONDITIONS
N/A

AGE-RELATED FACTORS
N/A

ZOONOTIC POTENTIAL
N/A

PREGNANCY
N/A

ABBREVIATION
EMG = electromyography

Suggested Reading
McKerrell RE, Braud KG. Hereditary myopathy of Labrador retrievers. In: Kirk RW, Bonagura JD, eds. Current veterinary therapy X. Philadelphia: Saunders, 1989:820–821.

Author Georgina Child
Consulting Editor Peter D. Schwarz

MYOPATHY, NONINFLAMMATORY—HEREDITARY MYOTONIA

BASICS

OVERVIEW
• Myopathy characterized by persistent contraction of muscle fibers on initiation of movement or when stimulated to contract
• May affect all skeletal muscles
• Congenital or acquired
• Congenital—may be associated with abnormal chloride conductance of muscle membrane
• Affects neuromuscular system

SIGNALMENT
• Congenital—described in young chow chows; rarely seen in other dog breeds
• Acquired—all breeds potentially susceptible
• Not reported in cats

SIGNS
Historical Findings
• Difficulty rising
• Stiffness after rest
• May note dyspnea, dysphagia, and/or regurgitation
• May improve with exercise
• Exacerbated by cold

PHYSICAL EXAMINATION FINDINGS
• Hypertrophy of proximal limb muscles, neck muscles, and tongue
• Abduction of thoracic limbs
• Bunny-hopping pelvic limb gait
• Patient may fall and remain rigid in lateral recumbency for short periods.

CAUSES & RISK FACTORS
Chow chows—suspected autosomal recessive mode of inheritance

DIAGNOSIS

DIFFERENTIAL DIAGNOSIS
Other myopathies—distinguished by signalment and clinical and electromyographic findings

CBC/BIOCHEMISTRY/URINALYSIS
Creatinine kinase—may be slightly elevated

OTHER LABORATORY TESTS
N/A

IMAGING
N/A

DIAGNOSTIC PROCEDURES
• Percussion of muscles and tongue in conscious and anesthetized dogs—causes sustained dimpling
• Electromyography—reveals multifocal or generalized high-frequency discharges that wax and wane in amplitude and frequency (dive bomber–sounding potentials) and that are increased after muscle percussion

PATHOLOGIC FINDINGS
• Muscle histology—shows mild changes (e.g., some angular atrophy, central nuclei, variation in fiber size)

TREATMENT
• None specific
• Discourage activities that result in hyper-ventilation.
• Avoid cold.
• Anesthesia (induction and recovery)—possible risk of respiratory obstruction owing to adduction of vocal cords or regurgitation

MEDICATIONS

DRUGS
Membrane-stabilizing drugs—procainamide and quinidine; may decrease severity of clinical signs

CONTRAINDICATIONS/POSSIBLE INTERACTIONS
None

FOLLOW-UP

PREVENTION/AVOIDANCE
• Chow chows—inherited condition; advise owner regarding breeding.
• Discourage breeding of affected animals.
• Do not repeat dam–sire breedings that resulted in affected offspring.

POSSIBLE COMPLICATIONS
Respiratory obstruction and/or aspiration of regurgitated food—may be life-threatening; advise owners of the clinical symptoms and treatment.

EXPECTED COURSE AND PROGNOSIS
• Prognosis guarded

MISCELLANEOUS

ASSOCIATED CONDITIONS
N/A

AGE-RELATED FACTORS
• Aging—signs may stabilize or worsen.

ZOONOTIC POTENTIAL
N/A

PREGNANCY
N/A

Suggested Reading
Duncan ID, Griffiths IR. Myotonia in the dog. In: Kirk RW, ed. Current veterinary therapy Vlll. Philadelphia: Saunders, 1983:686–689.
Author Georgina Child
Consulting Editor Peter D. Schwarz

MYOPATHY, NONINFLAMMATORY—HEREDITARY SCOTTY CRAMP

 BASICS

OVERVIEW
• Inherited neurologic disorder in Scottish terriers characterized by episodic muscle hypertonicity or cramping
• Not associated with any morphologic changes in muscle, peripheral nerve, or the CNS
• Thought to be the result of a disorder in serotonin metabolism within the CNS
• Similar condition reported in young Dalmatians and Labrador retrievers—may be result of low numbers of neurotransmitter glycine receptors in the CNS
• Affects the neuromuscular system

SIGNALMENT
• Young Scottish terriers, typically < 1 year of age
• No known sex predilection

SIGNS
• Normal at rest and on initial exercise
• Further exercise or excitement—abduction of the thoracic limbs; arching of the lumbar spine; stiffening or overflexion of the pelvic limbs (goose-stepping gait)
• Patient may fall, with tail and pelvic limbs flexed tightly against the body
• Respiration—may cease for a short time
• Facial muscles—may be contracted
• No loss of consciousness
• Severity varies
• Episodes—may last up to 30 min

CAUSES & RISK FACTORS
Inherited condition with probable recessive mode of transmission

 DIAGNOSIS

DIFFERENTIAL DIAGNOSIS
Seizure disorder—distinguished on basis of family history, typical clinical signs with no loss of consciousness, and induction of signs with serotonin antagonists

CBC/BIOCHEMISTRY/URINALYSIS
Normal

OTHER LABORATORY TESTS
N/A

IMAGING
N/A

DIAGNOSTIC PROCEDURES
Clinical signs may be induced by giving the serotonin antagonist, methysergide.

 TREATMENT

Behavioral modification and/or environmental changes—eliminating triggering situations (excitement, stress); may be adequate

 MEDICATIONS

DRUGS
Acepromazine, diazepam, or vitamin E—may reduce the incidence and severity of episodes

CONTRAINDICATIONS/POSSIBLE INTERACTIONS
• Serotonin antagonists—increase severity of clinical signs
• Aspirin, indomethacin, phenylbutazone, Benamine, and penicillin—may exacerbate clinical signs

 FOLLOW-UP

PATIENT MONITORING
Nonprogressive

PREVENTION/AVOIDANCE
• Discourage breeding affected animals.
• Do not repeat dam–sire breedings that result in affected offspring.

EXPECTED COURSE AND PROGNOSIS
• Mild to moderate—fair to good long-term prognosis; usually acceptable disability to owners; nonprogressive
• Severe—guarded to poor prognosis

 MISCELLANEOUS

ASSOCIATED CONDITIONS
N/A

AGE-RELATED FACTORS
N/A

ZOONOTIC POTENTIAL
N/A

PREGNANCY
N/A

Suggested Reading
Meyers KM, Clemmons RM. Scotty cramp. In: Kirk RW, ed. Current veterinary therapy VIII. Philadelphia: Saunders, 1983:702–704.

Author Georgina Child
Consulting Editor Peter D. Schwarz

BASICS

OVERVIEW
- Inherited, progressive, and degenerative generalized myopathy with X-linked mode of inheritance
- Patients lack muscle membrane–associated protein dystrophin
- RNA processing defect—identified in golden retrievers, Irish terriers, Samoyeds, rottwielers, Belgian shepherds, and one miniature schnauzer
- Affects neuromuscular system

SIGNALMENT
- Seen primarily in neonate and young dogs
- Described in cats
- Primarily affects males
- Females—usually carriers of gene defect; homozygotes may be affected.

SIGNS
Dogs
- Golden retrievers—exercise intolerance; stilted gait; bunny-hopping pelvic limb gait; plantigrade stance; partial trismus; muscle atrophy (especially the truncal and temporalis muscles); hypertrophy of some muscles (especially the tongue); kyphosis; lordosis; drooling; dysphagia; aspiration pneumonia (owing to pharyngeal and/or esophageal involvement)
- Other breeds—similar; include vomiting and megaesophagus
- Vary in severity, onset, and progression; may be seen as early as 6 weeks; tend to stabilize by 6 months
- Stunting and ineffective suckling—may be evident in younger pups
- Cardiac failure—may occur owing to cardiomyopathy and severe muscle contractures
- Spinal reflexes—normal initially; may become hypoactive

Cats
- Dystrophin deficient—muscle hypertrophy; stiff gait; cervical rigidity; exercise intolerance; vomiting
- Not apparent in one cat until 21 months of age

CAUSES & RISK FACTORS
Inherited defect of the X chromosome

DIAGNOSIS

DIFFERENTIAL DIAGNOSIS
Other inherited, infectious (protozoal), immune-mediated, or metabolic myopathies; distinguished by muscle histology and demonstration of dystrophin deficiency

CBC/BIOCHEMISTRY/URINALYSIS
Normal except for marked elevation in serum creatine kinase (may be > 10,000 U/L; further increased after exercise)

OTHER LABORATORY TESTS
- Dystrophin deficiency—demonstrated immunocytochemically or by Western blot analysis; diagnostic
- Serologic testing—may be warranted to rule out infectious and immune-mediated causes

IMAGING
N/A

DIAGNOSTIC PROCEDURES
Electromyography—shows complex repetitive discharges

PATHOLOGIC FINDINGS
Histologic examination of muscle—muscle fiber necrosis and regeneration; myofiber mineralization (may be dramatic); myofiber hypertrophy (may be variation in myofiber size or fibrosis)

TREATMENT
None proven effective

MEDICATIONS

DRUGS
Glucocorticosteriods—may provide some improvement; reason unknown

CONTRAINDICATIONS/POSSIBLE INTERACTIONS
None

FOLLOW-UP

PATIENT MONITORING
Monitor periodically for aspiration pneumonia or cardiomyopathy.

PREVENTION/AVOIDANCE
- Discourage breeding of affected animals.
- Do not repeat dam–sire breedings that result in affected offspring.

POSSIBLE COMPLICATIONS
Aspiration pneumonia or cardiomyopathy may be life threatening.

EXPECTED COURSE AND PROGNOSIS
- Overall prognosis—guarded to poor owing to no effective palliative treatment
- Golden retrievers—signs tend to stabilize at 6 months.
- Other dog breeds and cats—progression variable

MISCELLANEOUS

ASSOCIATED CONDITIONS
N/A

AGE-RELATED FACTORS
N/A

ZOONOTIC POTENTIAL
N/A

PREGNANCY
N/A

Suggested Reading
Kornegay JN. The X-linked muscular dystrophies. In: Kirk RW, Bonagura JD, eds. Current veterinary therapy XI. Philadelphia: Saunders, 1992:1042–1047.
Author Georgina Child
Consulting Editor Peter D. Schwarz

MYOPATHY, NONINFLAMMATORY—METABOLIC

BASICS

DEFINITION
• Myopathy associated with disorders of glycogen metabolism, lipid metabolism, or oxidative phosphorylation and mitochondrial metabolism
• Currently poorly characterized in veterinary medicine

PATHOPHYSIOLOGY
• Usually associated with inherited or acquired enzyme defects involving major metabolic pathways
• May result in storage of the abnormal metabolic byproduct or morphologic abnormalities of mitochondria

SYSTEMS AFFECTED
• Neuromuscular—dependence on oxidative metabolism for energy
• Nervous—dependence on glycolytic and oxidative metabolism for energy
• Cardiovascular—dependence on oxidative metabolism for energy
• Hemic/Lymphatic/Immune—RBCs depend on glycolytic metabolism.
• Storage products in other organs—liver; spleen

GENETICS
Undetermined

INCIDENCE/PREVALENCE
Rare, except lipid-storage myopathies

GEOGRAPHIC DISTRIBUTION
Unknown; probably worldwide

SIGNALMENT
Species
Dogs and cats

Breed Predilections
• Inherited muscle phosphofructokinase deficiency—English springer spaniels
• Acid maltase deficiency—Laplands
• Debranching enzyme deficiency—German shepherds
• Suspected mitochondrial abnormalities—clumber spaniels, Sussex spaniels, Old English sheepdogs

Mean Age and Range
• Inherited metabolic defects—2–3 months
• Acquired metabolic defects—adults

Predominant Sex
None found

SIGNS
General Comments
Very few of these conditions have been adequately described.

Historical Findings
• Muscular weakness
• Exercise intolerance
• Cramping
• Collapse
• Regurgitation and/or dysphagia
• Esophageal and/or pharyngeal abnormalities
• Dark urine; myoglobinuria; hemoglobinuria
• Encephalopathy
• Vomiting

Physical Examination Findings
• Exercise-related weakness, stiffness, and/or cramping
• Abnormal neurologic examination—disorientation; stupor; coma
• Abdominal distention—storage product accumulation in liver
• May appear normal, with fluctuating clinical signs

CAUSES
• Inborn error of metabolism
• Acquired metabolic defect
• Viral infections
• Drug induced
• Environmental factors

RISK FACTORS
• Inherited disorders
• Appropriate genetic background
• Others unknown

DIAGNOSIS

DIFFERENTIAL DIAGNOSIS
• Inflammatory myopathies—differentiated by muscle biopsy
• Other noninflammatory myopathies—differentiated by muscle biopsy
• Other metabolic encephalopathies—differentiated by laboratory evaluation

CBC/BIOCHEMISTRY/URINALYSIS
• Plasma lactate levels—elevated resting or postexcercise with disorders of fatty acid oxidation or oxidative phosphorylation; no elevation with glycolytic disorders
• Serum creatine kinase levels—may be elevated with exercise and normal at rest; may be persistently elevated
• Hypoglycemia—may occur with some glycolytic and oxidative disorders
• Hyperammonemia—may occur with urea cycle defects

OTHER LABORATORY TESTS
• Quantitation of plasma and urine amino acids—abnormal accumulations
• Quantitation of urine organic acids—demonstrate abnormal organic acid production
• Quantitation of plasma, urine, and muscle carnitine—may be low with primary disorders of carnitine; low with primary organic acidurias
• Specific enzyme assays—depend on suspected metabolic defect
• Fibroblast cultures—study metabolic defect

IMAGING
MRI—evaluate the CNS; reveals abnormalities in humans

MYOPATHY, NONINFLAMMATORY—METABOLIC

DIAGNOSTIC PROCEDURES
• Light microscopy—fresh frozen muscle sections; demonstrates storage products (glycogen, lipid) or abnormal mitochondria
• Electron microscopy of muscle (fresh frozen sections)—reveals abnormal mitochondria, paracrystalline inclusions, and glycogen accumulation
• Cardiovascular system evaluation—may have concurrent cardiomyopathy
• Other organ biopsies—with organomegaly

PATHOLOGIC FINDINGS
• Triglyceride droplets in muscle—lipid storage myopathy
• Ragged-red fibers in muscle—mitochondrial myopathy
• Glycogen deposition in muscle—glycogen storage disorder

 TREATMENT

APPROPRIATE HEALTH CARE
• Inpatient—may required intensive care for severe encephalopathy, seizures, lactic acidemia, hypoglycemia, or hyperammonemia
• Outpatient—clinical signs related only to neuromuscular system

NURSING CARE
Depends on type and severity of disorder

ACTIVITY
• Exercise restriction—with muscle weakness, stiffness, or exercise-induced collapse

DIET
• Avoid prolonged periods of fasting.
• Restrictions—depend on underlying defect
• Vitamin and co-factor therapy—determined by underlying defect

CLIENT EDUCATION
• Warn client that most inherited metabolic defects cannot be cured, although some can be treated.
• Advise against breeding affected individuals.

SURGICAL CONSIDERATIONS
N/A

 MEDICATIONS

DRUGS OF CHOICE
• Depend on the abnormality and clinical signs
• Lipid storage myopathies—l-carnitine (50 mg/kg PO q12h); riboflavin (50–100 mg PO q24h); coenzyme Q (1 mg/kg PO q24h)
• Mitochondrial myopathies—may benefit from therapy similar to that listed for lipid storage myopathies

CONTRAINDICATIONS
None known

PRECAUTIONS
Avoid fasting and strenuous exercise if they precipitate clinical signs.

POSSIBLE INTERACTIONS
N/A

ALTERNATIVE DRUGS
N/A

 FOLLOW-UP

PATIENT MONITORING
• Lipid storage myopathies—return of muscle strength; elimination of muscle pain
• Elevated serum creatine kinase—should return to normal

PREVENTION/AVOIDANCE
N/A

POSSIBLE COMPLICATIONS
Severe neurologic impairment

EXPECTED COURSE AND PROGNOSIS
• Untreatable disorder—poor prognosis
• Lipid storage myopathies—good prognosis if no underlying organic acidemia

 MISCELLANEOUS

ASSOCIATED CONDITIONS
• Iatrogenic and naturally occurring Cushing syndrome
• Lipid storage myopathies—found in some dogs
• Hemolytic anemia—owing to underlying metabolic defect

AGE-RELATED FACTORS
• Inborn errors—usually found in young dogs
• Acquired defects—found in adult dogs

ZOONOTIC POTENTIAL
N/A

PREGNANCY
Unknown

SYNONYMS
• Lipid storage myopathies
• Mitochondrial myopathies
• Glycogen storage disorders
• Cori disease—glycogenosis type III
• Phosphofructokinase deficiency—glycogenosis type VII
• Acid maltase deficiency—glycogenosis type II)

Suggested Reading
LeCouteur RA, Dow SW, Sisson AF. Metabolic and endocrine myopathies of dogs and cats. Semin Vet Med Surg Small Anim 1989;4:146–155.
Shelton GD, Gardinet GH III. Pathophysiologic basis of canine muscle disorders. J Vet Intern Med 1987;1:36–44.
Shelton GD. Canine lipid storage myopathies. In: Bonagura JD, Kirk RW, eds. Current veterinary therapy XII. Philadelphia: Saunders, 1995;1161–1163.
Author G. Diane Shelton
Consulting Editor Peter D. Schwarz

MYXEDEMA AND MYXEDEMA COMA

BASICS

OVERVIEW
• Myxedema coma is a rare complication that can develop in dogs with severe hypothyroidism; in addition to the clinical signs usually seen with hypothyroidism, patients also develop hypothermia, extreme weakness, lethargy, and profound mental obtundation that can progress from marked depression to coma and death.
• Clinical signs develop secondary to a marked decrease in cellular oxidative metabolism, calorigenesis, and an overall decreased basal metabolic rate; myxedema refers to the nonpitting edema that frequently occurs in patients, most prominently in the skin of the facial region particularly above the eyes and in the jowls; myxedema develops because of increased dermal ground substance (mucopolysaccharides, hyaluronic acid, and water).
• Myxedema coma has a high mortality rate; successful treatment depends on appropriate and timely therapy, based on clinical recognition of the syndrome.

SIGNALMENT
• Dog • Myxedema coma is a rare syndrome; the great majority of reported cases have been in Doberman pinschers.
• Age range was 2.5– 5 years.
• No apparent sex predilection
• Myxedema coma not reported in felines

SIGNS

Historical Findings
• Dogs are usually presented for profound weakness, collapse, lethargy, and mental obtundation; these signs may develop acutely over a day or may exist for a few weeks before presentation.

• Rapid development of clinical signs has been most commonly observed in animals that were being boarded or were hospitalized.
• In addition, affected animals commonly have a history of alopecic skin disease or a poor haircoat; the owner may report other clinical signs of hypothyroidism.

Physical Examination
• Extreme weakness, depressed level of consciousness, and *hypothermia without shivering* have been present in all reported cases of myxedema coma.
• Other common abnormalities are bradycardia, bradypnea, alopecia, dry haircoat, and myxedema of the face and jowls.
• Mucous membranes may be slightly cyanotic secondary to poor peripheral perfusion and hypoxia; hypoxia can be caused by hypoventilation and/or pulmonary edema; 50% of reported patients have had hilar pulmonary edema and pleural effusion; heart and lung sounds may be diminished or crackles may be heard if pulmonary edema exists.
• A small percentage of patients have abdominal fluid detected by abdominal palpation.

CAUSES & RISK FACTORS
• Myxedema coma develops in canines secondary to severe primary hypothyroidism.
• Both lymphocytic thyroiditis and thyroid atrophy have been reported in affected dogs.
• Risk factors for development of myxedema coma include infectious diseases, respiratory disease, central nervous system or respiratory system depressants (anesthetics and tranquilizers), heart failure, and hypovolemia.
• Exposure to cold environmental temperatures can also precipitate myxedema coma.

DIAGNOSIS

DIFFERENTIAL DIAGNOSIS
• Consider diseases that cause cardiovascular, metabolic/endocrine, respiratory, neuromuscular, or central nervous system abnormalities when patients present with a primary complaint of weakness; however, metabolic/endocrine and central nervous system diseases are more likely to be associated with marked mental dullness.
• Hypothermia may be seen with shock, fulminant heart failure, hypothalamic and metabolic/endocrine disorders, or with exposure to cold temperatures.
• Dilative cardiomyopathy is a primary differential in Doberman pinschers.
• Specific metabolic/ endocrine diseases that should be ruled out include hypoadrenocorticism, hypoglycemia, diabetic ketoacidosis, and hepatoencephalopathy.
• Clinical abnormalities that help differentiate myxedema coma include hypothermia without shivering, myxedema, bradycardia, and epidermal abnormalities (nonpruritic alopecia and poor haircoat).

CBC/BIOCHEMISTRY/URINALYSIS
• Mild, nonregenerative anemia
• Inappropriately normal lymphocyte count
• Inflammatory leukogram—increased bands
• Hypercholesterolemia
• Hyponatremia
• Hypertriglyceridemia
• Hypoxia
• Hypercarbia
• Hypoglycemia

OTHER LABORATORY TESTS

Endocrine Testing
• A definitive diagnosis is made when subnormal baseline serum T_4 levels and either subnormal free T_4 or increased endogenous TSH levels are documented in a dog with compatible clinical signs.
• A TSH stimulation test is not recommended because it would delay definitive treatment for 6 h.

Cytology and Fluid Analysis
Pleural and peritoneal effusions are usually identified as high-protein transudates.

IMAGING
• Thoracic radiographs—50% of reported patients have had hilar pulmonary edema; pleural effusion also observed
• Abdominal radiographs—may be loss of abdominal serosal detail secondary to intraabdominal fluid
• Echocardiography—method of choice for ruling out dilative cardiomyopathy; dogs with hypothyroidism can have echocardiographic evidence of abnormal left ventricular systolic function (decreased fractional shortening, increased end-systolic diameter, increased preejection period, and decreased left ventricular free wall and interventricular septal wall thickness); these abnormalities are usually mild and not as severe as those seen in patients with dilative cardiomyopathy.

DIAGNOSTIC PROCEDURES
ECG—bradycardia, decreased P and R wave amplitude, and a prolonged PR interval may be seen.

PATHOLOGIC FINDINGS
• Thyroid gland—lymphocytic thyroiditis and/or atrophy
• Skin—may see increased dermal thickness, myxedema, orthokeratotic hyperkeratosis, follicular atrophy, and vacuolation of the arrector pilli muscles

TREATMENT
• Myxedema coma is a medical emergency.
• Successful treatment depends on early clinical recognition of the characteristic clinical signs and laboratory abnormalities.
• Treatment is initiated on the basis of a presumptive clinical diagnosis.

NURSING CARE
• Rewarm patients passively with blankets and place them in a warm environment.
• Avoid active attempts (e.g., warm fluids or heating pads) to warm patients; they could cause a precipitous increase in peripheral tissue perfusion and O_2 use.
• Cautious intravenous administration of sodium-containing isotonic fluids at maintenance rates (20 mL/lb/day) is indicated.
• Can add dextrose to the fluids if hypoglycemia is present
• Patients with marked hypoxia should receive oxygen therapy (oxygen cage, oxygen face mask, or oxygen nasal catheter); however, the profound hypoventilation that is causing the hypoxia may necessitate mechanical respiratory support in patients with severe hypoxia and hypercarbia.

MEDICATIONS

DRUGS
• Intravenous levothyroxine (0.02 mg/kg q12h for 1–2 doses as needed) is the definitive treatment.
• Can switch patients to oral levothyroxine therapy (0.01 mg/kg BID) after their condition has stabilized
• Treatment with glucocorticosteroids and broad-spectrum antibiotics is recommended.

CONTRAINDICATIONS/POSSIBLE INTERACTIONS
• Avoid active rewarming.
• Inappropriate intravenous fluid therapy can precipitate or aggravate pulmonary edema.
• Avoid the use of narcotics, tranquilizers, or anesthetics in most instances.

FOLLOW-UP
• The patient's mental alertness, temperature, pulse, and respiration should improve significantly within 6–8 h.
• Most reported patients have died within 12–24 h following initiation of therapy even though their vital signs have improved.
• Myxedema coma has a grave prognosis.

MISCELLANEOUS

SEE ALSO
Hypothyroidism

ABBREVIATIONS
• T_4 = levothyroxine

Suggested Readings
Chastain CB, Graham CL, Riley MG. Myxedema coma in two dogs. Canine Pract 1982;9:20–34.
Kelly MJ, Hill JR. Canine myxedema stupor and coma. Compend Contin Ed Pract Vet 1984;6:1049–1055.
Author John W. Tyler
Consulting Editor: Deborah S. Greco

DISEASES

NARCOLEPSY AND CATAPLEXY

BASICS

OVERVIEW
Sleep disorders

Narcolepsy

Excessive daytime sleepiness, lethargy, or brief periods of collapse and unconsciousness that resolve spontaneously

Cataplexy

• Brief episodes of muscle paralysis with loss of tendon reflexes that are completely and spontaneously reversible
• Patient stays alert and will follow with its eyes.

SIGNALMENT
• Dogs and rarely cats
• Multiple breeds of dogs
• Proven hereditary—Labrador retrievers, poodles, dachshunds, and Doberman pinschers
• Recessive inheritance with complete penetrance—Labradors and Dobermans
• Clinical signs usually appear < 6 months of age.

SIGNS
• Physical and neurologic examinations—normal except during an attack
• Onset—rapid (peracute) in both conditions
• Episodes—usually last only a few seconds to minutes, but can last up to 30 min; usually characterized by collapse into lateral or sternal recumbency with no movements and atonic muscles; commonly elicited during eating, excitement, playing, and sexual activity; may see multiple episodes in one day
• Eye movements, muscular twitching, and whining (as in REM sleep)—frequently observed during episodes
• Patients usually aroused by loud noises, petting, or other external stimuli.

CAUSES & RISK FACTORS
• Unknown
• Neurotransmitter disturbance
• Possible immune system involvement

DIAGNOSIS

DIFFERENTIAL DIAGNOSIS
• Seizure activity—urinary or fecal incontinence, excessive salivation, and muscle rigidity are not characteristic of sleep disorders.
• Cataplexy—myasthenia gravis; hypoglycemia; hypocalcemia; hypokalemia; adrenal insufficiency; polymyositis; syncope; nonconvulsive seizure (drop attacks)
• Narcolepsy—hypothyroidism; chronic hypoxia; obesity (Pickwickian syndrome); other metabolic illnesses

CBC/BIOCHEMISTRY/URINALYSIS
• Normal
• Perform to rule out differentials.

OTHER LABORATORY TESTS
N/A

IMAGING
N/A

DIAGNOSTIC PROCEDURES
• Observe an episode—if a consistent activity elicits attacks, attempt to simulate the activity; probably helpful only for severely affected animals
• Food-elicited cataplexy test—place 10 pieces of food in a row 12–24 in. apart; record the time required for the patient to eat all the pieces and the number, type, and duration of any attacks that occur; normal dogs eat all food in < 45 sec and have no attacks; affected dogs take > 2 min to eat the food and can have 2–20 attacks
• Yohimbine challenge (cataplexy)—administer 25–50 μg/kg IV bolus; positive: 90% reduction in the number or severity of episodes; response should occur within 20–30 min after administration and last for about 4 hr
• Physostigmine challenge (cataplexy)—administer 0.025 mg/kg IV; repeat the food-elicited test 5–15 min after the injection; increase dosage if necessary (0.05 mg/kg; 0.075 mg/kg; 0.10 mg/kg); produces signs in affected patients, causing up to a 300% increase in the number and duration of episodes; effects of each dose last 15–45 min.

TREATMENT

• Primary goal—reduce the severity and frequency of cataplectic attacks
• Inform client that cataplexy is not a fatal disease, choking on food and airway obstruction do not occur, and the pet is not suffering.
• Inform client that activities such as hunting, swimming, and unleashed exercise put the patient at risk.

MEDICATIONS

DRUGS
• Yohimbine—drug of choice; 50–100 μg/kg SC or PO q8–12h
• Imipramine—Tofranil; 0.5–1.0 mg/kg PO q8h
• Methylphenidate—Ritalin—5–10 mg PO q24h
• Dextroamphetamine—5–10 mg PO q24h

CONTRAINDICATIONS/POSSIBLE INTERACTIONS
• Many patients develop drug tolerance; change of drug may become necessary.
• Monamine oxidase inhibitors—contraindicated in dogs because of possible toxic cardiovascular side effects

FOLLOW-UP

• Avoiding inciting activities may reduce episodes so that medication is not needed.
• Patients with the inherited form may improve with age.
• Prognosis—varies because the disease is not curable; even with treatment, some patients remain symptomatic.

MISCELLANEOUS
REM = rapid eye movement

Suggested Reading

Fenner WR. Seizures, narcolepsy, and cataplexy. In: Birchard SJ, Sherding RG, eds. Saunders manual of small animal practice. Philadelphia: Saunders, 1994:1147–1156.

Author T. Mark Neer

Consulting Editor Joane M. Parent

NASAL AND NASOPHARYNGEAL POLYPS

 BASICS

OVERVIEW
• Protruding, pink, polypoid growths (benign) arising from the mucous membranes
• Nasal—originate from the nasal mucosa in dogs and cats
• Nasopharyngeal—originate from the base of the eustachian tube in cats; may extend into the external ear canal, middle, pharynx, and nasal cavity

SIGNALMENT
• Nasopharyngeal—kittens and young adult cats
• Nasal—dogs and cats

SIGNS
Nasal
• Nonresponsive to antibiotics, or recurrent
• Chronic mucopurulent nasal discharge
• Noisy breathing
• Nasal congestion
• Sneezing or epistaxis
• Unilaterally decreased nasal airflow

Nasopharyngeal
• Same as for nasal
• Inspiratory dyspnea and choking or gagging
• Dysphagia
• Chronic, nonresponsive otitis
• Head tilt
• Horner syndrome

CAUSES & RISK FACTORS
Unknown

 DIAGNOSIS

DIFFERENTIAL DIAGNOSIS
• Upper respiratory infection
• Upper airway obstruction
• Chronic otitis
• Neurologic disease
• Nasopharyngeal stenosis
• Foreign body
• Neoplasia

CBC/BIOCHEMISTRY/URINALYSIS
N/A

OTHER LABORATORY TESTS
N/A

IMAGING
• Radiographs of nasal cavity—may show a soft tissue structure within the nasal passages
• Radiographs of nasopharynx—may show a soft tissue mass
• Closely evaluate radiographs for involvement of the tympanic bullae.

DIAGNOSTIC PROCEDURES
• Rhinoscopy (rigid or flexible cystoscope or arthroscope)—allows visualization and biopsy of the mass
• Dental mirror or flexible cystoscope or bronchoscope of the nasopharynx—palpation and visual examination; often reveals polyp
• Deep otoscopic examination

 TREATMENT
• Surgery—treatment of choice; excision via the oral cavity or rhinotomy with nasal polyps; complete excision of root and base mandatory to prevent recurrence
• Concurrent bulla osteotomy—may prevent recurrence of nasopharyngeal polyps

 MEDICATIONS

DRUGS
Postsurgery—appropriate agent for secondary bacterial or yeast infection of the nasal or otic cavity; choose on the basis of culture and sensitivity testing

CONTRAINDICATIONS/POSSIBLE INTERACTIONS
N/A

 FOLLOW-UP
• Incomplete removal of polyp and stalk—may result in recurrence
• Horner syndrome or facial paralysis—may develop after bulla osteotomy; generally transient

 MISCELLANEOUS

Suggested Reading
Bedford PGC. Diseases of the nose. In: Ettinger SJ, Feldman EC, eds. Textbook of veterinary internal medicine. 4th ed. Philadelphia: Saunders, 1995:551–567.
Author James C. Prueter
Consulting Editor Eleanor C. Hawkins

NASOPHARYNGEAL STENOSIS

 BASICS

OVERVIEW
• Formation of a thin but tough membrane at the internal nasal meatus, resulting in the narrowing of the orifice from a 5–6-mm oval opening to a 1–2-mm opening.
• Chronic inflammation and fibrosis on histologic examination suggest an infectious or allergic cause.

SIGNALMENT
• Cats of any breed or sex
• Age—range, 8 months to 10 years; any age as long as ample time has passed since exposure to the inciting cause

SIGNS
• Evidence of upper respiratory obstruction
• Whistling or snoring noise
• Minimal nasal discharge
• Duration of at least several months
• Aggravation of signs during eating
• Failure to respond to antibiotics or corticosteroids

CAUSES & RISK FACTORS
• Viral upper respiratory or chlamydial infection
• Foreign body or irritant contacting affected area

 DIAGNOSIS

DIFFERENTIAL DIAGNOSIS
• Nasopharyngeal polyps—seen during oral examination or by radiography or endoscopy
• Chronic rhinitis or sinusitis—moderate to severe nasal discharge and sneezing; obvious radiographic changes commonly seen
• Foreign body—unilateral mucopurulent nasal discharge; radiographic abnormalities
• Intranasal neoplasia—unilateral obstruction; nasal discharge often bloody; radiographic changes
• Mycotic rhinitis—moderate to severe nasal discharge, often hemorrhagic; radiographic changes
• Laryngeal disease—no improvement with open-mouth breathing; lack of snorting and nasal discharge; abnormalities on oral examination

CBC/BIOCHEMISTRY/URINALYSIS
N/A

OTHER LABORATORY TESTS
N/A

IMAGING
Near-normal radiographic findings

DIAGNOSTIC PROCEDURES
• Inability to pass a 3.5 French catheter through the ventral meatus into the pharynx
• Visualization of the membrane by use of a retroflexed pediatric bronchoscope or a dental mirror

 TREATMENT

Surgery—under general anesthesia; patient in dorsal recumbency with the mouth wide open; incise soft palate; resect membrane; suture soft palate.

 MEDICATIONS

DRUGS
Antibiotics after surgery

CONTRAINDICATIONS/POSSIBLE INTERACTIONS
N/A

 FOLLOW-UP

• Warn client that recurrence is possible.
• Consider high levels of corticosteroids if a second surgery is necessary.

 MISCELLANEOUS

Suggested Reading
Mitten RW. Acquired nasopharyngeal stenosis in cats. In: Kirk RW, Bonagura JD, eds. Current veterinary therapy XI. Philadelphia: Saunders, 1992:801–803.
Author Justin H. Straus
Consulting Editor Eleanor C. Hawkins

NECROTIZING ENCEPHALITIS OF YORKSHIRE TERRIERS

BASICS

OVERVIEW
• One of the breed-restricted encephalitides defined by highly characteristic morphologic features.
• First described in 1993 in Switzerland; occurs in several other European countries and in North America
• CNS only organ system affected
• A genetic basis probable

SIGNALMENT
• Dogs
• Yorkshire terriers
• Occasionally in other small breeds—Chihuahuas; shi-tzus
• Usually affects young adults (1–5 years of age); may affect older animals

SIGNS
• Initially variable
• Acute in onset; uniformly progressive
• Seizures—may occur; not always observed (unlike the breed-specific encephalitides of Maltese and pug dogs)
• Brainstem symptoms with central vestibular signs—predominate
• Rarely, cortical involvement

CAUSES & RISK FACTORS
• Unknown
• An infectious agent might be suspected.

DIAGNOSIS

DIFFERENTIAL DIAGNOSIS
• Rule out other inflammatory or infectious diseases of the CNS
• Neoplasia

CBC/BIOCHEMISTRY/URINALYSIS
Usually normal

OTHER LABORATORY TESTS
N/A

IMAGING
• CT and MRI (brain)—nonspecific changes; may support the clinical diagnosis considering breed, age, multifocal lesions, and course of the disease
• Neurosonography, CT, and MRI (brain)—nonspecific moderate hydrocephalus

DIAGNOSTIC PROCEDURES
CSF analysis—moderate pleocytosis (12–76 leukocytes/mm³) with mononuclear cells; mild to marked elevation of protein

PATHOLOGIC FINDINGS
Lesions
• In the CNS—multifocal; predominantly in the brainstem and cerebral white matter
• Active—large malacic gliotic center surrounded by a wall of extremely severe mononuclear inflammation
• Old—rarefied or cystic areas surrounded by intense astroglial sclerosis

TREATMENT
• Outpatient
• No specific treatment known
• Supportive only—prevent seizures

MEDICATIONS

DRUGS
• None specific
• Steroids—may suppress the clinical signs to a considerable degree; prednisolone or prednisone (1–2 mg/kg PO q24h for the first 1–2 weeks; then taper dosage slowly).
• Phenobarbital—to reduce seizures; 2–8 mg/kg PO q12h; monitor serum concentration

CONTRAINDICATIONS/POSSIBLE INTERACTIONS
N/A

FOLLOW-UP

PATIENT MONITORING
• Monitor serum concentration of phenobarbital.
• Perform regular clinical and neurologic examinations.

PREVENTION/AVOIDANCE
N/A

POSSIBLE COMPLICATIONS
N/A

EXPECTED COURSE AND PROGNOSIS
• Chronic for months or even years
• In every described case, the neurologic signs were progressive.
• Prognosis—guarded

MISCELLANEOUS

SEE ALSO
• Necrotizing Meningoencephalitis of Maltese Dogs
• Pug Encephalitis (Meningoencephalitis)
• Seizures (Convulsions, Status Epilepticus)—Dogs

ABBREVIATION
CSF = cerebrospinal fluid

Suggested Reading
Tipold A, Fatzer R, Jaggy A, et al. Necrotizing encephalitis in Yorkshire terriers. J Small Anim Pract 1993;34:623–628.
Author Andrea Tipold
Consulting Editor Joane M. Parent

NECROTIZING MENINGOENCEPHALITIS OF MALTESE DOGS

BASICS

OVERVIEW
• One of the breed-restricted encephalitides that are defined by highly characteristic morphologic features
• Rare; found only in North America
• CNS only organ system affected

SIGNALMENT
• Maltese dogs between 9 months and 4 years of age
• A genetic basis probable

SIGNS
• Acute and progressive
• Mostly mild to severe symptoms consistent with a forebrain lesion
• Seizures—observed in all described patients

CAUSES & RISK FACTORS
• Unknown
• An infectious agent might be suspected.

DIAGNOSIS

DIFFERENTIAL DIAGNOSIS
Rule out neoplasia and other inflammatory or infectious CNS diseases.

CBC/BIOCHEMISTRY/URINALYSIS
Usually normal

OTHER LABORATORY TESTS
N/A

IMAGING
CT and MRI (brain)—nonspecific changes

DIAGNOSTIC PROCEDURES
• CSF analysis—moderate pleocytosis (50–247 leucocytes/mm^3); mononuclear cells or mixed cell population in the differential cell count; mild protein elevation
• Brain biopsy—helps the diagnosis in vivo

PATHOLOGIC FINDINGS
Necrosis and nonsuppurative inflammation of the cerebral gray and white matter

TREATMENT
• Inpatient or outpatient
• No specific treatment known
• Supportive only—prevent seizures

MEDICATIONS

DRUGS
• None specific
• Seizures—phenobarbital (2–8 mg/kg PO q12h); monitor serum concentrations
• Inflammatory response—corticosteroids; prednisolone or prednisone (1–2 mg/kg PO q24h for the first 1–2 weeks; then taper dosage slowly)

CONTRAINDICATIONS/POSSIBLE INTERACTIONS
N/A

FOLLOW-UP

PATIENT MONITORING
• Monitor serum concentration of phenobarbital.
• Perform regular clinical and neurologic examinations.

EXPECTED COURSE AND PROGNOSIS
• Outcome not known exactly because only a few cases have been described.
• Prognosis—regarded as poor; because pug dogs with a similar disease may survive a few years, a prolonged course of the disease may be expected in Maltese dogs too.

MISCELLANEOUS

SEE ALSO
• Necrotizing Encephalitis in Yorkshire Terriers
• Pug Encephalitis (Meningoencephalitis)
• Seizures (Convulsions, Status Epilepticus)—Dogs

ABBREVIATION
CSF = cerebrospinal fluid

Suggested Reading
Stalis IH, Chadwick B, Dayrell-Hart B, et al. Necrotizing meningoencephalitis of Maltese dogs. Vet Pathol 1995;32:230–235.
Author Andrea Tipold
Consulting Editor Joane M. Parent

BASICS

OVERVIEW
• *Neospora caninum*—recently recognized coccidian protozoon previously confused with *Toxoplasma gondii;* tachyzoites and tissue cysts resemble *T. gondii* under light microscopy.
• Complete life cycle unknown.
• Disease caused by necrosis associated with tissue damage from cyst rupture and tachyzoite invasion
• Only known natural mode of transmission—transplacental, resulting in congenital infection

SIGNALMENT
• Dogs—natural infections (mainly puppies); hunting dogs overrepresented
• Cats—experimentally infected

SIGNS
• Similar to those of toxoplasmosis, except neurologic and muscular abnormalities predominate and are often more severe
• Young dogs (< 6 months)—ascending paralysis more common; distinguished from other forms of paralysis by gradual muscle atrophy; stiffness of pelvic limbs more affected than thoracic limbs; progresses to rigid contracture of limbs
• Cervical weakness and dysphagia—gradually develop, eventually leading to death
• Ataxia secondary to atrophy of the cerebellum
• Old dogs—usually CNS involvement (seizures, tremors), polymyositis, myocarditis, and dermatitis; as in toxoplasmosis, virtually any organ may be affected.

CAUSES & RISK FACTORS
N. caninum

DIAGNOSIS

DIFFERENTIAL DIAGNOSIS
• Young dogs—other causes of peripheral multifocal neurologic signs, mainly including infectious diseases (toxoplasmosis, distemper);

progressive polyradiculomyositis; other causes of diffuse lower motor neuron muscular diseases rare
• Old dogs with CNS disease—other infectious diseases (fungal, rabies, pseudorabies); toxicity (lead, organophosphorous, carbamate, chlorinated hydrocarbon, strychnine); nonsuppurative encephalitis; meningitis; granulomatous meningoencephalitis; metabolic disease (hypoglycemia, hepatic encephalopathy)

CBC/BIOCHEMISTRY/URINALYSIS
• Depending on the organ system involved
• Muscle involvement—creatine phosphokinase and AST activities may be high.

OTHER LABORATORY TESTS
• Serologic testing (IFA)—CSF or serum
• Antibodies do not cross-react with *T. gondii.*

IMAGING
N/A

DIAGNOSTIC PROCEDURES
CSF—slight increase in protein and nucleated cell number; cells mainly mononuclear; neutrophils may be seen

PATHOLOGIC FINDINGS
• Nonsuppurative encephalomyelitis
• Myositis
• Myofibrosis
• Polyradiculoneuritis
• Pneumonia, cerebella atrophy, multifocal necrotizing myocarditis, and nodular dermatitis—described
• *N. caninum* seems to induce more inflammation than does *T. gondii.*
• Histology—differentiation by location in host cell cytoplasm (not within a parasitophorous vacuole as *T. gondii*)
• Tissue cysts—those of *N. caninum* have thicker walls; differentiated from *T. gondii* by immunohistochemical staining
• Electronmicroscopy—rhoptries of *N. caninum* tachyzoites electron dense; those of *T. gondii* honeycomb

TREATMENT
• Once muscle contracture or ascending paralysis has occurred, the prognosis for clinical improvement is poor.
• Progression of clinical disease might be arrested by treatment.

MEDICATIONS

DRUGS
• See Toxoplasmosis
• Clindamycin—25–50 mg/kg PO or IM per day, divided into 2 doses; continue for at least 2 weeks after clinical signs cleared

CONTRAINDICATIONS/POSSIBLE INTERACTIONS
N/A

FOLLOW-UP
Treat for an extended period of time.

MISCELLANEOUS

ZOONOTIC POTENTIAL
None identified (unlike *T. gondii*)

ABBREVIATIONS
• AST = aspartate aminotransferase
• CSF = cerebrospinal fluid
• IFA = immuno fluorescent antibody

Suggested Reading
Dubey JP. Neosporosis. Paper presented at the 11th annual meeting of the American College of Veterinary Internal Medicine, Washington, DC, May 1993.
Author Stephen C. Barr
Consulting Editor Stephen C. Barr

DISEASES

NEPHROLITHIASIS

BASICS

DEFINITION
• Nephroliths—uroliths (i.e., polycrystalline concretions or calculi) located in the renal pelvis or collecting diverticula of the kidney • Nephroliths or nephrolith fragments may pass into the ureters (ureteroliths). • Nephroliths that are not infected, not causing obstruction or clinical signs, and not progressively enlarging are termed *inactive*.

PATHOPHYSIOLOGY
Nephroliths can obstruct the renal pelvis or ureter, predispose to pyelonephritis, and result in compressive injury of the renal parenchyma leading to renal failure; see chapters on the different urolith types for pathophysiology of urolithiasis; in cats, nephroliths composed of blood clots mineralized with calcium phosphate can form secondarily to chronic renal hematuria.

SYSTEMS AFFECTED
• Renal/Urologic—affects the urinary tract, with potential for obstruction, recurrent urinary tract infections, or renal failure • Obstruction of the renal pelvis or ureter in an animal with pyelonephritis may result in septicemia (urosepsis) and thus affect any body system.

GENETICS
N/A

INCIDENCE/PREVALENCE
• Nephroliths compose ~1.3–2.8% of uroliths in dogs and cats submitted to stone centers for analysis; the true incidence of nephroliths is likely much higher because many animals with nephroliths are asymptomatic. • Most common mineral compositions of canine nephroliths submitted for analysis, in descending frequency—calcium oxalate, struvite, ammonium urate, mixed, and calcium phosphate • Most common mineral compositions of nephroliths in cats submitted for analysis, in descending frequency—calcium oxalate, matrix, calcium phosphate, mixed, and struvite

GEOGRAPHIC DISTRIBUTION
N/A

SIGNALMENT
Species
Dogs and cats

Breed Predilections
Canine
• Calcium oxalate nephroliths—miniature schnauzer, Lhasa apso, Yorkshire terrier, miniature poodle, and shih tzu • Struvite nephroliths—miniature schnauzer, bichon frise, shih tzu, Yorkshire terrier, Lhasa apso, cocker spaniel, and miniature poodle • Urate nephroliths—dalmatian, Yorkshire terrier, and English bulldog

Feline
• Domestic shorthair (33%), domestic longhair (17%), Persian (8%), Siamese (6%), unknown breed (19%)

Mean Age and Range
• Dogs—mean age of affected animals, 9 years (range, 4 months to 14 years) • Cats—mean age of affected animals, 8 years (range, 2 months to 18 years)

Predominant Sex
• Overall, nephroliths in dogs are slightly more common in females (55%) than males (41%), with 4% unspecified; for struvite nephroliths, females > males; for calcium oxalate, cystine, and urate nephroliths males > females • In cats, nephroliths are slightly more common in females (55%) than males (45%).

SIGNS
General Comments
Many patients are asymptomatic, and the nephroliths are diagnosed during workup of other problems.

Historical Findings
• None or hematuria, vomiting, and recurrent urinary tract infection; dysuria and pollakiuria in animals with urinary tract infection • Signs attributable to uremia in animals with bilateral obstruction or renal failure • Signs referable to lower urinary tract urolithiasis if uroliths are present in the upper and lower urinary tract • So-called renal colic with acute abdominal/lumbar pain and vomiting is uncommon.

Physical Examination Findings
Abdominal or lumbar pain upon palpation or no significant findings

CAUSES
• For an extensive listing of causes, see chapters on each urolith type. Oversaturation of the urine with calculogenic minerals may contribute to urolithiasis. • Calcium oxalate urolithiasis—hypercalciuria, hypercalcemia, hypocitraturia, hyperoxaluria, primary hyperparathyroidism, excessive dietary calcium intake • Calcium phosphate urolithiasis—chronic renal bleeding (cats), hypercalcemia, hyperparathyroidism, excessive dietary calcium and phosphorus, renal tubular acidosis • Cystine urolithiasis—cystinuria • Struvite urolithiasis—urinary tract infection with urease-producing microbes, diets that produce alkaline urine pH • Urate urolithiasis—genetic defect in conversion of uric acid to allantoin (dalmatians), portosystemic shunt • Xanthine urolithiasis—allopurinol administration and high dietary purine intake in dogs predisposed to urate urolithiasis

RISK FACTORS
• Alkaline urine—struvite and calcium phosphate uroliths • Acid urine—calcium oxalate, cystine, urate, and xanthine uroliths • Urine retention and formation of highly concentrated urine • Lower urinary tract infection—ascending infection and

pyelonephritis • Conditions that predispose to urinary tract infection (e.g., perineal urethrostomy, ectopic ureters, hyperadrenocorticism, vesicoureteral reflux, and exogenous steroid administration or hyperadrenocorticism (calcium oxalate uroliths)

DIAGNOSIS

DIFFERENTIAL DIAGNOSIS
Consider nephroliths in any patient with renal failure, recurrent urinary tract infection, acute vomiting (acute pancreatitis, acute gastroenteritis, intestinal or gastric obstruction, etc.), or abdominal or lumbar pain (e.g., intervertebral disk protrusion, peritonitis); nephroliths are usually confirmed by radiographs or ultrasonography; differentiate mineralization of the renal pelvis or collecting diverticula from true nephrolithiasis.

CBC/BIOCHEMISTRY/URINALYSIS
• CBC results—usually normal unless the patient has pyelonephritis; patients with pyelonephritis may have leukocytosis and neutrophilia with a left shift. • Serum biochemistry analysis—usually normal unless bilateral obstruction, pyelonephritis, or compressive renal injury leads to renal failure (azotemia with an inappropriate urine specific gravity, hyperphosphatemia); hypercalcemia may contribute to formation of calcium oxalate or calcium phosphate nephroliths. • Urinalysis—may reveal hematuria and crystalluria; crystal type may indicate mineral composition; pyuria, proteinuria, and bacteriuria may also be seen in animals with urinary tract infection.

OTHER LABORATORY TESTS
• Submit all retrieved nephroliths or nephrolith fragments for quantitative analysis to allow implementation of appropriate preventative strategies. Although definitive identification of nephrolith type requires quantitative analysis, composition can frequently be predicted on the basis of signalment, radiographic appearance, and urinalysis findings. • Results of bacterial culture of urine may confirm urinary tract infection in animals with concurrent pyelonephritis.

IMAGING
• Can detect radiopaque nephroliths (e.g., calcium phosphate, calcium oxalate, struvite) by survey radiography; cystine, urate, and xanthine are radiolucent to slightly radiopaque. • May use ultrasonography or excretory urography to confirm the presence, size, and number of nephroliths or ureteroliths regardless of radiographic density

DIAGNOSTIC PROCEDURES
After ESWL, nephrolith fragments can be retrieved for quantitative analysis by voiding, catheter-assisted retrieval, or voiding

urohydropropulsion.

PATHOLOGIC FINDINGS

Histopathology required only to confirm the presence of secondary renal lesions.

TREATMENT

APPROPRIATE HEALTH CARE

Manage patients with inactive nephroliths as outpatients. Medical dissolution protocols can be administered to outpatients. Removal of nephroliths by surgery or ESWL requires hospitalization.

NURSING CARE

N/A

ACTIVITY

Unlimited

DIET

Medical dissolution of nephroliths requires a diet appropriate to the specific nephrolith type. See Medications section.

CLIENT EDUCATION

• Inactive nephroliths—may not require removal but should be monitored periodically by urinalysis, urine culture, and radiography; can potentially cause obstruction at any time, which can result in hydronephrosis without clinical signs, so conservative management and monitoring carries a slight risk of undetected and potentially irreversible renal damage, which must be weighed against the potential renal damage from nephrotomy • Nephroliths (especially metabolic uroliths) tend to recur after removal; monitor the patient periodically.

SURGICAL CONSIDERATIONS

• Indications for removal of nephroliths—obstruction, recurrent infection, symptomatic nephroliths, progressive nephrolith enlargement, and a nonfunctional contralateral kidney • Treatment options for nephroliths—medical dissolution, surgery, and ESWL. Calcium oxalate nephroliths , the most common mineral composition in dogs and cats, are not amenable to medical dissolution. Ureteroliths or nephroliths causing complete obstruction are also not amenable to medical dissolution. • Surgical options—nephrotomy or pyelolithotomy. Because the nephroliths are surrounded by renal tissue, nephrotomy is required in most dogs and cats. Experimental nephrolith removal by percutaneous nephrolithotomy has been reported in dogs. • ESWL—safe and effective method of treating canine nephroliths and ureteroliths; nephrolith fragments pass down the ureter into the bladder and are voided in the urine. • ESWL—not effective for treatment of nephroliths and ureteroliths in cats

MEDICATIONS

DRUGS OF CHOICE

• Antibiotics on the basis of urine culture and sensitivity testing as needed; periprocedural antibiotics are recommended when infected nephroliths are treated by ESWL or surgically removed. • Medical dissolution protocols are limited to struvite, urate, and cystine uroliths. • Medical dissolution protocols for *struvite* nephroliths include a calculolytic diet (Prescription Diet s/d, Hill's) and appropriate antibiotic therapy (i.e., if patient has a urinary tract infection) for the duration of treatment. • Medical dissolution of canine *urate* nephrolithiasis can be attempted by a protein- and purine-restricted, alkalinizing diet (Prescription diet Canine u/d, Hill's), allopurinol (15 mg/kg PO q12h), and supplemental potassium citrate as needed to maintain urine pH ~7.0. • Medical dissolution of canine *cystine* nephrolithiasis can be attempted using a protein-restricted, alkalinizing diet (Prescription diet Canine u/d, Hill's), 2-MPG (Thiola, 15 mg/kg PO q12h), and supplemental potassium citrate as needed to maintain urine pH ~7.5.

CONTRAINDICATIONS

• Do not use allopurinol without dietary purine restriction—it may cause xanthine nephrolithiasis in dogs predisposed to urate urolithiasis. • Do not give acidifying diets to azotemic patients unless blood pH and total CO_2 are monitored for development of metabolic acidosis.

PRECAUTIONS

N/A

POSSIBLE INTERACTIONS

N/A

ALTERNATIVE DRUGS

N/A

FOLLOW-UP

PATIENT MONITORING

Abdominal radiographs (ultrasonography for radiolucent uroliths), urinalysis, and urine culture every 3 to 6 months to detect nephrolith recurrence. Dogs treated with ESWL—check every 2 to 4 weeks by radiographs and ultrasonography until nephrolith fragments have passed through the excretory system.

PREVENTION/AVOIDANCE

Eliminate factors predisposing to individual urolith type, augment urine volume, and correct factors contributing to urine retention.

POSSIBLE COMPLICATIONS

Hydronephrosis, renal failure, recurrent urinary tract infection, and pyelonephritis

EXPECTED COURSE AND PROGNOSIS

• Highly variable; depends on nephrolith type, location, and size, and the presence of secondary complications (e.g., obstruction, infection, renal failure) • Inactive nephroliths may remain inactive for years resulting in an excellent prognosis. • We have had excellent results using ESWL to treat dogs with nephroliths—return to normal health and an excellent prognosis • The prognosis for patients with renal failure caused by nephrolithiasis depends on the severity and rate of progression of renal failure.

MISCELLANEOUS

ASSOCIATED CONDITIONS

Hyperadrenocorticism and chronic glucocorticoid administration are associated with calcium oxalate uroliths and with urinary tract infection resulting in struvite urolithiasis.

AGE-RELATED FACTORS

Geriatric dogs that are poor surgical candidates may be treated with ESWL.

ZOONOTIC POTENTIAL

N/A

PREGNANCY

Contraindication to ESWL

SYNONYMS

Kidney stones, renal calculi, renoliths, kidney calculi

SEE ALSO

• Renal Failure, Chronic • Hydronephrosis • Pyelonephritis • Urinary Tract Obstruction • Urolithiasis, Calcium Oxalate • Urolithiasis, Calcium Phosphate • Urolithiasis, Cystine • Urolithiasis, Struvite—Cats • Urolithiasis, Struvite—Dogs • Urolithiasis, Urate • Urolithiasis, Xanthine

ABBREVIATIONS

ESWL = extracorporeal shock wave lithotripsy

Suggested Reading

Block G, Adams LG, Widmer WR, et al. The use of extracorporeal shock wave lithotripsy for treatment of spontaneous nephrolithiasis and ureterolithiasis in dogs. J Am Vet Med Assoc 1996;208:531–536.

Ling GV. Nephrolithiasis: prevalence of mineral type. In: Kirk RW, Bonagura JD, eds. Current Veterinary Therapy. XII Philadelphia: Saunders, 1995:980.

Osborne CA, Unger LK, Lulich JP. Canine and feline nephroliths. In: Kirk RW, Bonagura JD, eds. Current Veterinary Therapy. XII. Philadelphia: Saunders, 1995:981–985.

Stone EA. Canine nephrotomy. Compend Contin Educ Pract Vet 1987;9:883–888.

Author Larry G. Adams

Consulting Editors Larry G. Adams and Carl A. Osborne

NEPHROTOXICITY, DRUG-INDUCED

BASICS

DEFINITION
Renal injury caused by a pharmacologic agent used to diagnose or treat a medical disorder

PATHOPHYSIOLOGY
• Drugs can cause nephrotoxicosis by interfering with renal blood flow, glomerular function, or tubular function.
• Many drugs are nephrotoxic because they are excreted primarily by the kidneys.
• Most nephrotoxic drugs cause proximal renal tubular necrosis.
• If renal injury is severe, acute renal failure develops.

SYSTEMS AFFECTED
• Renal/Urologic
• Gastrointestinal—inappetence, vomiting, diarrhea, or melena due to gastrointestinal irritation or ulceration in patients with uremia
• Endocrine/Metabolic—metabolic acidosis due to decreased elimination of acid by kidneys and inability to resorb bicarbonate
• Hemic/Lymphatic/Immune—anemia due to blood loss or decreased red blood cell survival in patients with uremia; increased susceptibility to infections because of immune dysfunction in patients with uremia
• Nervous—depression, lethargy associated with effect of uremic toxins on central nervous system
• Respiratory—tachypnea or dyspnea due to uremic pneumonitis or compensatory response for metabolic acidosis

GENETICS
N/A

INCIDENCE/PREVALENCE
N/A

GEOGRAPHIC DISTRIBUTION
N/A

SIGNALMENT
Species
More common in dogs than cats
Breed Predilections
N/A
Mean Age and Range
Any age; old patients are more susceptible.
Predominant Sex
N/A

SIGNS
Historical Findings
• Polyuria and polydipsia
• Inappetence
• Depression
• Vomiting
• Diarrhea

Physical Examination Findings
• Dehydration
• Oral ulcers
• Foul-smelling breath

CAUSES
Antimicrobial Drugs*
• Aminoglycosides—all drugs in this class are potentially nephrotoxic, including neomycin, gentamicin, amikacin, kanamycin, and streptomycin. Nephrotoxicosis due to treatment with gentamicin occurs most often, probably because it is the most frequently used aminoglycoside.
• Tetracyclines—outdated products can cause acquired Fanconi-like syndrome characterized by glucosuria, proteinuria, and renal tubular acidosis; IV administration to dogs at high dosages (>30 mg/kg) can cause acute renal failure.
• Administration of sulfa drugs (e.g., trimethoprim-sulfadiazine) has been associated with acute renal failure in dogs, but no causal relationship has been proven.

Antifungal Drugs
Amphotericin B—only one that causes clinically important nephrotoxicosis

Antineoplastic Drugs
• Cisplatin—only antineoplastic agent that causes clinically important nephrotoxicosis in dogs
• Doxorubicin—may be associated with nephrotoxicosis in cats; rarely of clinical importance

NSAIDS
• Aspirin, ibuprofen, naproxen, piroxicam, and flunixin meglumine may cause nephrotoxicosis.
• Most likely to cause renal injury in patients with preexisting renal disease or those with concomitant dehydration or other causes of hypovolemia.

ACE Inhibitors
• Include captopril, enalapril, and lisinopril
• Most likely to cause acute renal failure in patients with hyponatremia, dehydration, or congestive heart failure.

Antiparasitic Drugs
Thiacestarsamide is the only antiparasitic drug that causes clinically important nephrotoxicosis.

Radiographic Contrast Agents
Intravenous administration of radiographic contrast agents can cause acute renal failure, especially in patients with dehydration, hypovolemia, or hypotension associated with inhalational anesthesia.

RISK FACTORS
• Dehydration
• Advanced age, probably because older patients have preexisting renal disease
• Renal disease, inactive or active
• Renal hypoperfusion; potential causes include any disorder associated with hypovolemia (e.g., vomiting, hemorrhage, hypoadrenocorticism), low cardiac output (e.g., congestive heart failure, pericardial disease, cardiac arrhythmias, inhalational anesthesia), or renal vasocontriction (e.g., NSAID administration)
• Electrolyte and acid–base abnormalities including hypokalemia, hyponatremia, hypocalcemia, and metabolic acidosis
• Concurrent drug therapy—adminstration of furosemide increases nephrotoxicosis of aminoglycosides; treatment with cytotoxic drugs (e.g., cyclophosphamide) may increase nephrotoxic potential of drugs
• Fever
• Sepsis

DIAGNOSIS

DIFFERENTIAL DIAGNOSIS
• Must differentiate from other causes of acute renal failure including causes of acute tubular necrosis such as ethylene glycol toxicosis and renal ischemia, and causes of nephritis such as leptospirosis and bacterial urinary tract infection
• Most patients have a history of recent treatment (i.e., within the previous 2 weeks) with a potentially nephrotoxic drug; acute renal failure may occur several days after discontinuation of an aminoglycoside.
• Determine all drugs that have been administered to the patient, including over-the-counter preparations (e.g., aspirin, ibuprofen, and naproxen) and medications prescribed for human use (e.g., NSAID or ACE inhibitor).

CBC/BIOCHEMISTRY/URINALYSIS
• Hemogram—usually normal unless concomitant problems exist (e.g., gastrointestinal hemorrhage associated with administration of NSAIDs)
• Biochemical analysis—normal in early stages of drug-induced nephrotoxicosis or reveals signs consistent with acute renal failure including azotemia, hyperphosphatemia, and metabolic acidosis
• Urinalysis—may reveal low urinary specific gravity (often < 1.025) proteinuria, glucosuria, or cylindruria

OTHER LABORATORY TESTS
Measuring serum aminoglycoside concentration may help prevent nephrotoxicosis in patients receiving these drugs, especially those with risk factors.

IMAGING
N/A

DIAGNOSTIC PROCEDURES
Renal biopsy may be indicated to determine cause of acute renal failure and potential for reversibility, especially in patients that do not respond to treatment as expected.

PATHOLOGIC FINDINGS
Most nephrotoxic drugs cause proximal renal tubular necrosis.

TREATMENT

APPROPRIATE HEALTH CARE
• Manage patients with acute renal failure as inpatients.
• Manage patients without azotemia that can eat and drink enough to maintain hydration as outpatients.

NURSING CARE
• Administer 0.9% saline intravenously in patients with renal failure; lactated Ringer solution can be used but it contains a small amount of potassium, which may not be ideal in patients with acute renal failure and hyperkalemia.
• Correct hydration deficits rapidly (i.e., over 6–8 h) to minimize further renal injury. Calculate volume of fluid to administer using the formula volume (mL) = body weight (kg) × % dehydration × 1000 mL.
• In addition to correcting hydration deficits, administer maintenance requirements (66 mL/kg/day) and replace any ongoing losses caused by vomiting and diarrhea. As a minimum, assume that patients with acute renal failure are losing 3–5% of their body weight because of ongoing losses.

ACTIVITY
Reduce

DIET
• Outpatients can be fed their regular diet.
• Modify for patients with acute renal failure; avoid oral feeding until vomiting is controlled.
• When oral feeding is initiated, a moderately protein-restricted diet such as canine k/d (Hill's Pet Products, Topeka) can help control signs of uremia.

CLIENT EDUCATION
• Avoid unnecessary stress (e.g., boarding and elective surgery); provide unlimited access to clean, fresh water at all times.
• If any signs of illness such as inappetence, vomiting, or diarrhea develop, return the patient immediately for veterinary care to minimize worsening of renal function.

SURGICAL CONSIDERATIONS
• Avoid elective surgery until renal disease is resolved.
• If surgery is necessary, administer fluids (5–20 mL/kg/h) during anesthesia to maintain adequate mean arterial blood pressure (>60 mm Hg) and renal perfusion. Monitor urine output and adjust rate fluid administration to maintain urine production of 1–2 mL/kg/h.

MEDICATIONS

DRUGS OF CHOICE
None

CONTRAINDICATIONS
Do not use furosemide to promote diuresis in patients with aminoglycoside nephrotoxicosis.

PRECAUTIONS
Avoid drugs that may worsen renal injury in patients with nephrotoxicosis, including NSAIDs, vasodilators, and ACE inhibitors.

POSSIBLE INTERACTIONS
N/A

ALTERNATIVE DRUGS
N/A

FOLLOW-UP

PATIENT MONITORING
• Weigh hospitalized patients several times daily to detect changes in fluid balance and adjust fluid therapy accordingly.
• Biochemical analysis and electrolytes every 1–2 days to evaluate severity of azotemia and detect electrolyte and acid/base abnormalities
• Patients receiving aminoglycosides—urinalysis every 1–2 days to detect early signs of nephrotoxicosis such as glucosuria, increased proteinuria, and cylindruria; discontinue aminoglycoside if any of these signs are observed
• Urine output to determine if patient is polyuric or oliguric; adjust fluid therapy on basis of these findings and determine need for additional treatment to stimulate urine production

PREVENTION/AVOIDANCE
• Avoid or correct risk factors that predispose to development of drug-induced nephrotoxicosis.
• Administer saline diuresis to all dogs receiving cisplatin.
• Avoid using nephrotoxic drugs unless they are necessary (e.g., use aminoglycosides only if patient has overwhelming sepsis and culture results indicate aminoglycosides are the only effective antimicrobial).
• Monitor serum aminoglycoside concentration and perform frequent urinalyses while administering an aminoglycoside. Monitoring urinary GGT:creatinine ratio may detect renal injury early in aminoglycoside toxicity.
• Do not administer furosemide with an aminoglycoside.

POSSIBLE COMPLICATIONS
Acute renal failure

EXPECTED COURSE AND PROGNOSIS
• Patients without azotemia may develop acute renal failure within several days, especially with aminoglycosides.
• Renal injury caused by nephrotoxic drugs may lead to development of chronic renal failure months to years later.

MISCELLANEOUS

ASSOCIATED CONDITIONS
N/A

AGE-RELATED FACTORS
N/A

ZOONOTIC POTENTIAL
N/A

PREGNANCY
N/A

SYNONYMS
N/A

SEE ALSO
Renal failure, acute

ABBREVIATIONS
• ACE = angiotensin-converting enzyme
• NSAID = nonsteroidal antiinflammatory drug

Suggested Reading

Behrend EN, Grauer GF, Mani I, et al. Hospital-acquired acute renal failure in dogs: 29 cases (1983–1992). J Am Vet Med Assoc 1996;208:537–541.

Brown SA, Barsanti JA. Gentamicin nephrotoxicosis in the dog. In: Kirk RW, ed. Current veterinary therapy IX. Philadelphia: Saunders, 1986:1146–1150.

Brown SA, Barsanti JA, Crowell WA. Gentamicin-associated acute renal failure in the dog. J Am Vet Med Assoc 1985;186:686–690.

Rubin SI. Nonsteroidal antiinflammatory drugs, prostaglandins, and the kidney. J Am Vet Med Assoc 1986;188:1065–1068.

Vaden SL, Levine J, Breitschewerdt EB. A retrospective case-control of acute renal failure in 99 dogs. J Vet Intern Med 1997;11:58–64.

Author S. Dru Forrester
Consulting Editors Larry G. Adams and Carl A. Osborne

NEUROAXONAL DYSTROPHY

 BASICS

OVERVIEW
• Inherited abiotrophies of neurons in diverse regions of the CNS, particularly the cerebellum and associated pathways
• Axonal spheroids—present throughout the CNS gray matter, except the cerebral cortex
• Inheritance—usually thought to be autosomal recessive

SIGNALMENT
• Dogs and cats
• Dogs—rottweilers, collies, Chihuahuas, German shepherds, and boxers
• Age at onset—breed-specific, ranging from 5 weeks (cats) to 1–2 years (rottweilers)

SIGNS
• Cerebellar ataxia—progressive dysmetria and hypermetria of the limbs (rarely hypometria) with patellar hyperreflexia
• Strength and proprioception normal
• Loss of menace responses despite normal vision and facial nerve function
• Mild intention tremor or head and neck dysmetria in some patients

CAUSES & RISK FACTORS
• Specific cause unknown
• Believed to be neuronal abiotrophy with autosomal recessive inheritance
• Breed predisposition

 DIAGNOSIS

DIFFERENTIAL DIAGNOSIS
• Distemper encephalitis—differentiated on the basis of systemic signs preceding or accompanying the neurologic deficits and on results of CSF analysis (normal with neuroaxonal dystrophy)
• Cerebellar hypoplasia—apparent by 3–6 weeks of age; nonprogressive
• Infectious encephalitides—fungal, rickettsial, and protozoal; differentiated on the basis of multisystemic signs, serologic testing, and CSF analysis
• Cervical spinal cord disease—proprioceptive deficits and tetraparesis
• Diagnosis is by exclusion; it may not be possible to reach an antemortem diagnosis.

CBC/BIOCHEMISTRY/URINALYSIS
Normal

OTHER LABORATORY TESTS
N/A

IMAGING
N/A

DIAGNOSTIC PROCEDURES
All antemortem diagnostic tests are normal.

 TREATMENT

• None available that will alter the course of the disease
• Outpatient, unless severe deficits preclude nursing care at home
• Activity—restrict activity to areas where a fall can be avoided (avoid stairs, swimming pools, etc.).

 MEDICATIONS

DRUGS
N/A

CONTRAINDICATIONS/POSSIBLE INTERACTIONS
N/A

 FOLLOW-UP

• Rottweilers—worsen over 1–5 years; develop clonic patellar reflexes and crossed extensor reflexes
• Not fatal but severely incapacitating

 MISCELLANEOUS

ABBREVIATION
CSF = cerebrospinal fluid

Suggested Reading
De Lahunta A. Abiotrophy in domestic animals: a review. Can J Vet Res 1990;54:65–76.
Author Mary O. Smith
Consulting Editor Joane M. Parent

BASICS

OVERVIEW
• An uncommon infection of dogs and cats
• Organism—soil saprophyte; enters body through contamination of wounds or by respiratory inhalation
• A compromised immune system enhances the likelihood of infection.
• Systems affected—respiratory, skin/exocrine, lymphatic, musculoskeletal, nervous

SIGNALMENT
Dogs and cats of any breed

SIGNS
• Depends on the site of infection
• Pleural—pyothorax, resulting in dyspnea, emaciation, and fever
• Cutaneous—chronic, nonhealing wounds; often accompanied by fistulous tracts; if extended, may result in lymphadenopathy, draining lymph nodes, and osteomyelitis
• Disseminated—most common in young dogs; usually begins in the respiratory tract; lethargy, fever, and weight loss; cyclic fever may be characteristic; CNS may be affected; pleural and/or abdominal effusion may occur.

CAUSES & RISK FACTORS
• *Nocardia asteroides** (dogs and cats)
• *N. brasiliensis* (cats only)
• *Proactinomyces* spp. (rare)

DIAGNOSIS

DIFFERENTIAL DIAGNOSES

Cutaneous
• Actinomycosis
• Atypical mycobacteriosis
• Leprosy
• Bite wound abscesses
• Draining tracts resulting from foreign bodies

Pleural
• Bacterial pyothorax
• Thoracic neoplasia
• Chronic diaphragmatic hernia

Disseminated
• Systemic fungal infections
• Feline infectious peritonitis

CBC/BIOCHEMISTRY/URINALYSIS
• Neutrophilic leukocytosis
• Nonregenerative anemia—with long-standing infections (anemia of chronic disease)
• Chemistries—usually normal; hypergamma-globulinemia may be seen with long-standing infections.

OTHER LABORATORY TESTS
N/A

IMAGING
Radiographs—may reveal pleural or peritoneal effusion, pleuropneumonia, or osteomyelitis

DIAGNOSTIC PROCEDURES
• Cytology—thoracentesis or abdomino-centesis for samples; stain these or other exudates with Romanowsky, gram, and modified acid-fast stains for rapid diagnosis; may reveal gram-positive branching fila-mentous rods and cocci; cannot be distin-guished from *Actinomyces* spp.
• Culture—diagnostic; aerobic culturing on Sabouraud medium

PATHOLOGIC FINDINGS
• *N. asteroides*—more suppurative pyogranulomatous reaction than with *Actinomyces* spp.
• *N. brasiliensis*—granulomatous reaction with extensive fibrosis
• Although the organism is usually present, it cannot be distinguished histopathologically from *Actinomyces* spp.

TREATMENT
• Pleural or peritoneal effusions and disseminated form—inpatient until clinically stable and effusion removed; fluid therapy for rehydration and maintenance often needed
• Long-term antibiotic therapy and draining fistulous tracts—outpatient
• Diet—encourage consumption by offering foods with appealing tastes and smells; forced enteral feeding for anorectic inpatients essential; orogastric tube feeding preferred
• Surgery—when feasible, surgical drainage should accompany medical therapy; impor-tant to place a thoracostomy tube for pleural effusion; attempt surgical drainage and débridement of draining tracts and lymph nodes; take care to identify foreign bodies.

MEDICATIONS

DRUGS
• Cultured organism—antibiotic sensitivity testing
• No culture or results pending—good first-choice drugs: sulfonamides (e.g., sulfadiazine at 100 mg/kg IV, PO as a loading dose followed by 50 mg/kg IV, PO q12h) and sulfonamide-trimethoprim combinations (30 mg/kg PO q24h)
• Aminoglycosides—gentamicin (3 mg/kg IV, IM, SC q8h); amikacin (6.5 mg/kg IV, IM, SC q8h)
• Tetracyclines—doxycycline (10 mg/kg PO q24h); tetracycline hydrochloride (15–20 mg/kg PO q8h); minocycline (5–12.5 mg/kg PO q12h)
• Erythromycin—10–20 mg/kg PO q8h; or combined with ampicillin (20–40 mg/kg PO q8h) or amoxicillin (6–20 mg/kg PO q8–12h)
• Amoxicillin plus an aminoglycoside—synergistic combination; consider in any serious infection when culturing is not possible or is pending
• Average treatment period is 6 weeks; however, medical treatment should extend several weeks past apparent remission of the disease.

CONTRAINDICATIONS/POSSIBLE INTERACTIONS
Tetracyclines (cats)—may cause fever up to 41.5°C (107°F); discontinue and replace if fever increases during therapy.

FOLLOW-UP
Monitor carefully for fever, weight loss, seizures, dyspnea, and lameness the first year after apparently successful therapy because of the potential for bone and CNS involvement.

MISCELLANEOUS

Suggested Reading

Edwards DF. Actinomycosis and nocardiosis. In: Greene CE, ed. Infectious diseases of the dog and cat. Philadelphia: Saunders, 1998:303–313.
Author Gary D. Norsworthy
Consulting Editor Stephen C. Barr

DISEASES

NONSTEROIDAL ANTI-INFLAMMATORY DRUGS (NSAID) TOXICITY

 BASICS

DEFINITION
• Toxicity secondary to the acute or chronic ingestion of an NSAID
• NSAIDs—classified as carboxylic acids (aspirin, indomethacin, and sulindac; ibuprofen, naproxen, and carprofen; meclofenamic acid and flunixin meglumine) or enolic acids (phenylbutazone, dipyrone, piroxicam)

PATHOPHYSIOLOGY
• Action—analgesic, antipyretic, and anti-inflammatory owing to the inhibition of cyclooxygenase; decreases production of prostaglandins that act as mediators of inflammation
• Well absorbed orally
• Clearance—varies greatly among species; eliminated slowly in dogs and cats
• Metabolized in the liver to active or inactive metabolites
• Excreted in the kidney via glomerular filtration and tubular secretion

SYSTEMS AFFECTED
• Gastrointestinal—erosions and ulcers
• Renal/Urologic—acute renal failure; acute interstitial nephritis
• Hemic/Lymphatic/Immune—may note bleeding disorders secondary to decreased platelet aggregation
• Hepatobiliary—idiosyncratic hepatocellular damage

GENETICS
Species differences in absorption, excretion, and metabolism of different agents are dramatic; avoid extrapolation of data from other species or dosages.

INCIDENCE/PREVALENCE
Among the 10 most common toxicoses reported to the National Animal Poison Control Center

GEOGRAPHIC DISTRIBUTION
N/A

SIGNALMENT
• Dogs and cats
• No breed, age or sex predilections

SIGNS

General Comments
• Gastrointestinal irritation—usually develops within a few hours
• Renal involvement or gastrointestinal ulceration—may be delayed several days

Historical Findings
• Evidence of accidental consumption of owner's medication
• Lethargy
• Anorexia
• Vomiting—with or without blood
• Diarrhea
• Icterus
• Melena
• Collapse and sudden death—may occur secondary to a perforated gastric ulcer
• Polyuria, polydipsia, and oliguria
• Ataxia, seizures, coma—may occur with large ingestions

Physical Examination Findings
• Depression
• Pale mucous membranes
• Painful abdomen
• Dehydration
• Fever
• Tachycardia
• Icterus

CAUSES
Accidental exposure or inappropriate administration

RISK FACTORS
Animals predisposed to renal disease—old age; pre-existing renal, hepatic, or cardio-vascular disease; hypotension; other concurrent illness and/or medications; previous history of gastrointestinal ulcer or bleeding

 DIAGNOSIS

DIFFERENTIAL DIAGNOSIS
Other conditions (medical or toxicologic) that cause gastrointestinal and renal effects; diagnosis based on history of exposure and compatible clinical signs

CBC/BIOCHEMISTRY/URINALYSIS
• Anemia—regenerative or nonregenerative, depending on duration of bleeding
• Leukocytosis—associated with perforated gastric ulcer and accompanying peritonitis
• BUN and creatinine—may be high secondary to prerenal azotemia or primary renal insult
• High liver enzymes—occasionally
• May note hematuria, pyuria, proteinuria, and isosthenuria

OTHER LABORATORY TESTS
N/A

IMAGING
N/A

DIAGNOSTIC PROCEDURES
Endoscopy—verify gastrointestinal ulceration

PATHOLOGIC FINDINGS
• Gastrointestinal irritation, ulceration, or hemorrhage with possible gastric perforation and peritonitis
• Renal tubular or papillary necrosis or interstitial nephritis

 TREATMENT

APPROPRIATE HEALTH CARE
• Outpatient—mild clinical signs; managed at home with appropriate medication, dietary, and symptomatic measures
• Inpatient—high ingested dose; potential for renal toxicosis; relatively serious clinical signs (frequent vomiting, bloody vomitus, melena, anemia, or evidence of renal involvement); aggressive treatment to avoid life-threatening complications

NURSING CARE
• Fluid therapy—restore hydration when moderate to severe vomiting; administration of at least twice maintenance rates with known or potential renal involvement (see Renal Failure, Acute)
• If severely anemic, a blood transfusion may be indicated.

ACTIVITY
N/A

NONSTEROIDAL ANTI-INFLAMMATORY DRUGS (NSAID) TOXICITY

DIET
- Vomiting—NPO
- Vomiting resolved—begin with a bland, low-protein diet

CLIENT EDUCATION
- Stress the importance of contacting a veterinarian or the National Animal Poison Control Center whenever an animal is exposed to a nonprescribed NSAID.
- Inform client that dogs and particularly cats have a low tolerance to NSAIDs.
- With a prescribed NSAID, instruct client to look for adverse or idiosyncratic effects and to stop the drug and contact the clinic if they occur.

SURGICAL CONSIDERATIONS
Surgical intervention may be required for a perforated gastric ulcer.

MEDICATIONS

DRUGS OF CHOICE

Recent Ingestion
- Ingestion within a few hours and no vomiting—induce emesis (apomorphine or hydrogen peroxide) unless patient has seizures or marked CNS depression.
- After emesis—activated charcoal (1–2 g/kg PO) and a cathartic (magnesium or sodium sulfate at 0.25 tsp/5 kg or 70% sorbitol at 3 mL/kg) if no diarrhea
- Repeat activated charcoal—one-half the original dose

H_2-Receptor Antagonists
- For gastrointestinal upset or ulceration
- Cimetidine—5–10 mg/kg PO, IV, IM q6–8h; primarily effective for treating ulcers from acute overdose or from chronic administration after the drug withdrawn
- Ranitidine—alternative; dogs, 2 mg/kg PO, IV q8h; cats, 2.5 mg/kg IV q12h or 3.5 mg/kg PO q12h; may be a better choice because cimetidine may inhibit liver microsomal enzymes

Other
- Sucralfate—dogs, 0.5–1 g PO q8–12h; cats, 0.25 g PO q8h; binds to proteins in the ulcer base; stimulates mucus and bicarbonate secretion

- Misoprostol—1–3 μg/kg PO q8h; PGE_2 analogue; prevents gastrointestinal bleeding and ulceration; promotes healing during chronic use in humans and dogs treated with aspirin
- Omeprazole—patients > 20 kg, 1 capsule (20 mg) daily; patients < 20 kg one-half capsule; patients < 5 kg, one-quarter capsule; potent inhibitor of gastric acid secretion; blocks the final step of hydrochloric acid production
- Dopamine—may be indicated for acute renal failure
- Standard anticonvulsant therapy—diazepam, pentobarbital, phenobarbital, if needed
- Duration of treatment—depends on the half-life of the particular agent ingested

CONTRAINDICATIONS
Avoid concomitant use of corticosteroids or multiple NSAIDs together; contraindicated in pregnancy (abortifacient effect)

PRECAUTIONS
Patients using other nephroactive or nephro-toxic drugs (e.g., aminoglycosides and ACE inhibitors)—at higher risk for developing NSAID nephropathy

POSSIBLE INTERACTIONS
NSAIDs—highly protein bound; may be affected by concurrent use of other highly protein bound drugs

ALTERNATIVE DRUGS
N/A

FOLLOW-UP

PATIENT MONITORING
- Urine output—monitor carefully for oliguria; examine for casts, protein, and glucose
- Stool and vomitus—check for gastrointestinal bleeding (may not develop for several days)
- BUN and creatinine—twice daily for several days (full extent of renal damage may not be immediately evident)

PREVENTION/AVOIDANCE
- Store medications out of the reach of pets.
- Discourage owners from medicating pet without supervision of a veterinarian.
- Pretest high-risk patients with appropriate laboratory tests before beginning therapy.

POSSIBLE COMPLICATIONS
- Perforation of a gastric ulcer and peritonitis
- Irreversible acute and chronic renal failure

EXPECTED COURSE AND PROGNOSIS
- Gastric upset or ulceration—usually complete recovery with appropriate treatment
- Renal effects—generally reversible with early and aggressive treatment
- Acute hepatopathies—generally resolve after discontinuation of drug

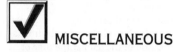

MISCELLANEOUS

ASSOCIATED CONDITIONS
N/A

ZOONOTIC POTENTIAL
N/A

PREGNANCY
- Exposure during pregnancy—risk for fetal cardiopulmonary and renal effects
- May prolong pregnancy, especially if administered during the third trimester and before the onset of labor

SEE ALSO
- Aspirin Toxicity
- Poisoning (Intoxication)
- Renal Failure, Acute

ABBREVIATION
ACE = angiotensin-converting enzyme

Suggested Reading
Johnston SA, Budsburg SC. Nonsteroidal anti-inflammatory drugs and corticosteroids in the management of canine osteoarthritis. Vet Clin North Am Small Anim Pract 1997;27:841–862.
Kore AC. Toxicology of nonsteroidal anti-inflammatory drugs. Vet Clin North Am Small Anim Pract 1990;20:419–431.
Author Judy Holding
Consulting Editor Gary D. Osweiler

OPHTHALMIA NEONATORUM

BASICS

OVERVIEW
• Infection of the conjunctiva or cornea before, or just after, the separation of the eyelids in the neonate
• Occurs in puppies and kittens
• Associated with *Staphylococcus* spp. or *Streptococcus* spp. in dogs and cats, and with Herpesvirus in cats
• Potentially vision-threatening
• Source of infection—believed to be from a vaginal infection of the dam at the time of birth or from a nonhygenic environment

SIGNALMENT
• Affects all breeds of cats and dogs
• Neonates before the time that they open their eyelids (10–14 days postpartum)

SIGNS
• Upper and lower eyelids are still adherent (physiologic ankyloblepharon) and bulge outward because of the accumulation of debris and discharge within the conjunctival fornices and between the cornea and lids
• May note a mucoid to mucopurulent discharge extruding through the medial canthus
• Cornea and conjunctiva—may be ulcerated
• May note adhesions (symblepharon) of the conjunctiva to the cornea or to other areas of the conjunctiva (including that of the nictitans)
• Perforation of the cornea with iris prolapse and collapse of the globe—occasionally seen

CAUSES & RISK FACTORS
• Vaginal infections in the dam near the time of birth
• Unclean environment for the neonates

DIAGNOSIS

DIFFERENTIAL DIAGNOSIS
Neonates with entropion in which the eyelids have already separated—may have mucoid to mucopurulent discharge; view of the cornea may be obscured; may have appearance of ankyloblepharon; differentiated by age

(patients older than 10–14 days) and no ankyloblepharon when eyelids are everted

CBC/BIOCHEMISTRY/URINALYSIS
Normal unless there is a concurrent systemic infection

OTHER LABORATORY TESTS
• Immunofluorescent antibody or polymerase-chain reaction tests (cats)—feline herpesvirus
• Cultures of neonate's ocular discharge and/or dam's vaginal discharge—may help diagnose bacterial infection
• Cytology of the affected tissues—may help determine presence of bacteria

IMAGING
N/A

DIAGNOSTIC PROCEDURES
• Full physical examination of the dam and neonate
• Fluorescein staining—corneal or conjunctival ulceration

TREATMENT

• Separation of the eyelids—cornerstone of treatment; can be accomplished by manual traction beginning at the medial canthus or introduction into the medial canthus of a small blunt scissor blade or the blunt, butt end of a scalpel blade and gently separating (not cutting) the eyelids.
• Conjunctival sacs and cornea—lavaged with warm saline to remove the discharge
• Warm compresses—may aid in separation of the eyelids and in preventing readherence
• Systemic support—as needed

MEDICATIONS

DRUGS
• Broad spectrum, topical antibiotics—neomycin, bacitracin, or polymyxin B; applied four times daily for at least 1 week; antibiotic chosen on basis of bacterial culture and sensitivity, if available

CONTRAINDICATIONS/POSSIBLE INTERACTIONS
• Tetracycline—do not use in neonates because of the risks of affecting bone or teeth; topical chloramphenicol or ciprofloxacin is drug of choice for *Chlamydia*
• Topical corticosteroids—contraindicated

FOLLOW-UP

PATIENT MONITORING
• Warm compresses—may be necessary for a few days to keep the eyelids from re-adhering
• Topical antibiotics—continued for a minimum of 7 days
• Observe littermates that are not initially affected
• Treat vaginal infections in the dam with appropriate medications.

PREVENTION/AVOIDANCE
• Keep the external environment and the dam's nipples clean.
• Treat vaginal infection in the dam before delivery, if possible.

POSSIBLE COMPLICATIONS
• Severe keratitis with scarring and symblepharon
• Rupture of the cornea with secondary phthisis; blindness may be irreversible.

MISCELLANEOUS

Suggested Reading
Williams MM. Neonatal ophthalmic disorders. In: Kirk RW, ed. Current veterinary therapy X. Philadelphia: Saunders, 1989: 658–673.
Author Stephanie L. Smedes
Consulting Editor Paul E. Miller

OPTIC NEURITIS

 BASICS

OVERVIEW
• Inflammation of one or both optic nerves, resulting in reduction of visual function
• May be a primary disease or secondary to systemic CNS disease because the optic nerve communicates with the subarachnoid space
• Affects the ophthalmic and nervous systems

SIGNALMENT
• Dogs and cats
• Primary—uncommon; usually affects dogs > 3 years of age
• Secondary—N/A

SIGNS
Historical Findings
• Acute onset blindness
• Partial visual deficits—often overlooked

Physical Examination Findings
• Blind or reduced vision in one or both eyes
• Pupils fixed and dilated—may have intact but diminished pupillary light reflex
• Funduscopic examination—optic disk swelling; focal hemorrhage; active or inactive chorioretinitis
• Often normal fundus with retrobulbar or intracranial optic nerve disease

CAUSES & RISK FACTORS
• Idiopathic*
• Systemic mycoses*
• Canine distemper
• FIP
• Neoplasm—primary or metastatic
• Toxoplasmosis
• Neosporum caninum
• Granulomatous meningoencephalomyelitis
• Toxicity—lead

 DIAGNOSIS

DIFFERENTIAL DIAGNOSIS
• Cortical blindness—normal pupillary light reflex; normal fundus examination; possibly other neurologic deficits
• SARDS (dogs)—minimal to absent pupillary light reflex; normal fundus (early in course); flat electroretinogram

CBC/BIOCHEMISTRY/URINALYSIS
No specific abnormalities

OTHER LABORATORY TESTS
Specific viral, protozoal, or fungal serologic tests on serum

IMAGING
Neuroimaging—CT and/or MRI

DIAGNOSTIC PROCEDURES
• CSF analysis
• Electroretinogram—investigate retinal function; normal in optic neuritis, flat in SARDS
• Visual evoked potentials—investigate optic nerve function

 TREATMENT

• Based on underlying disease

 MEDICATIONS

DRUGS
• Depend on primary disease process when identifiable
• Idiopathic–Prednisone—2 mg/kg q12h for 14 days; then 1 mg/kg q12h for 14 days; then gradual reduction to maintenance dosage

CONTRAINDICATIONS/POSSIBLE INTERACTIONS
N/A

 FOLLOW-UP

• Monitor clinical signs or visual evoked potentials, if available.
• Prognosis—depends on underlying disease
• Blindness may be permanent with idiopathic optic neuritis
• Clinical course—unpredictable
• Flare ups—may occur if medication is inadequate

✓ MISCELLANEOUS

ABBREVIATIONS
• CSF = cerebrospinal fluid
• FIP = feline infectious peritonitis
• SARDS= sudden acquired retinal degeneration syndrome

Suggested Reading
Braund KG. Clinical syndromes in veterinary neurology. 2nd ed. St. Louis: Mosby, 1994.
Author David Lipsitz
Consulting Editor Paul E. Miller

DISEASES

ORAL CAVITY TUMORS, UNDIFFERENTIATED MALIGNANT TUMORS

 BASICS

OVERVIEW
• Highly aggressive, rapidly growing masses in the area of the hard palate, upper molar teeth, or maxilla and orbit.
• Most are highly invasive to the bone and are nonencapsulated with a smooth to slightly nodular surface (mistaken as benign); may become ulcerated
• Biopsy—reveals undifferentiated malignancy of undetermined histogenesis
• Highly metastatic
• Cervical lymphadenopathy common

SIGNALMENT
• All dogs < 2 years old; range, 6–22 months
• Primarily a disease of large breeds
• No sex predilection

SIGNS

Historical Findings
• Excessive salivation
• Halitosis
• Dysphagia
• Bloody oral discharge
• Weight loss

Physical Examination Findings
• Oral mass
• Loose teeth
• Facial deformity
• Cervical lymphadenopathy—occasionally

CAUSES & RISK FACTORS
None identified

 DIAGNOSIS

DIFFERENTIAL DIAGNOSIS
• Other oral malignancy
• Epulis
• Abscess
• Benign polyp

CBC/BIOCHEMISTRY/URINALYSIS
May be normal

OTHER LABORATORY TESTS
Cytologic evaluation of an impression smear obtained from an incisional biopsy specimen (wedge)—may yield diagnosis

IMAGING
• Skull radiography—detect bone invasion deep to the mass
• Thoracic radiography—detect lung metastasis

DIAGNOSTIC PROCEDURES
• Carefully palpate regional lymph nodes (mandibular and retropharyngeal).
• Large, deep tissue biopsy (down to bone)—required to differentiate from other oral malignancies

 TREATMENT

• Surgical excision—usually ineffective because of extensive local disease or metastasis on examination; if attempted, radical recommended (e.g., hemimaxillectomy) with margins of at least 2 cm into normal bone and soft tissues
• Inpatient radiotherapy—efficacy unreported; most undifferentiated tumors are poorly responsive.
• Soft foods—may be recommended to prevent tumor ulceration or after radical oral excision

ORAL CAVITY TUMORS, UNDIFFERENTIATED MALIGNANT TUMORS

MEDICATIONS

DRUGS
• Chemotherapy—efficacy unreported; most undifferentiated tumors are poorly responsive.
• Local control (palliation) with intralesionally administered cisplatin—reported

CONTRAINDICATIONS/POSSIBLE INTERACTIONS
Chemotherapy can be toxic; seek advice before initiating treatment if you are unfamiliar with cytotoxic drugs.

FOLLOW-UP
Dogs—most have lymph node metastasis on examination; usually euthanatized within 30 days of diagnosis because tumor growth is progressive and uncontrolled, resulting in dysphagia and cachexia.

MISCELLANEOUS

Suggested Reading

Frazier DL, Hahn KA. Cancer chemotherapeutics. In: Hahn KA, Richardson RC, eds. Cancer chemotherapy, a veterinary handbook. Baltimore: Williams & Wilkins, 1995:77–150.

Patnaik AL, Lieberman PH, Erlandson RA, et al. A clinicopathologic and ultrastructural study of undifferentiated malignant tumors of the oral cavity in dogs. Vet Pathol 1986;23:170–175.

Author Kevin A. Hahn
Consulting Editor Wallace B. Morrison

ORAL MASSES

 BASICS

DEFINITION
Oral cavity growth

PATHOPHYSIOLOGY
N/A

SYSTEMS AFFECTED
N/A

GENETICS
N/A

INCIDENCE/PREVALENCE
• Males are more commonly affected with oral melanomas and fibrosarcomas than females.
• Breed predilection—golden retriever, German shorthaired pointer, Weimaraner, St. Bernard, and cocker spaniels more prone to oral tumors; dachshunds and beagles less prone to oral tumors; boxer, gingival hyperplasia

GEOGRAPHIC DISTRIBUTION
N/A

SIGNALMENT

Cat
• Squamous cell carcinoma—age range, 3–21 years (mean, 12.5); most common site, the sublingual area; two forms are tonsillar and nontonsillar; common presenting signs include excessive drooling and/or bleeding from the mouth; frequently invades bone, loosening teeth; morbidity and mortality result from local disease rather than distant metastasis.
• Fibrosarcomas—age range, 1–21 years (mean, 10.3); no particular predilection site; all associated with local tissue destruction; muscle and bone invasion are occasionally seen.

Dog
• Epulides are the most common benign oral tumor; three types occur.
• Fibromatous epulis—common in dogs (and cats); age range 1–17 (mean, 7.5); both pedunculated and sessile forms; they usually have a smooth, pink surface.
• Peripheral odontogenic fibroma (ossifying epulis)—similar to fibromatous, but has an osteoid matrix
• Peripheral ameloblastoma (acanthomatous

epulis)—classified as benign but tends to invade adjacent bone
• Malignant melanoma—the most common oral malignant tumor in the dog; cocker spaniels, German shepherds, chow chows, and dogs with heavily pigmented mucous membranes are predisposed; males more frequently affected than females
• Melanoma—many places in the oral cavity (gingiva, buccal mucosa, hard or soft palate, and tongue); locally invasive and metastasize to lungs and regional lymph nodes; presenting complaint is commonly oral bleeding, ptyalism, or halitosis; tumor size on presentation is important to patient survival; in the dog, melanomas <2 cm carry a better survival rate (median 511 days) than those >2 cm (164 days); tumors located rostrally have better prognosis than those located distally.
• Squamous cell carcinoma—the next most common oral malignancy; originates from the gingival epithelium; red, ulcerated, and may have cauliflower projections; large-breed dogs are predisposed; prognosis depends on location in the oral cavity; those located rostrally carry a better prognosis than those at the base of the tongue or occurring in the tonsils, which tend to metastasize and are the most aggressive.
• Papillary squamous cell carcinoma—a rapidly growing tumor of young dogs (<1 year); in the papillary gingiva; locally aggressive but does not metastasize; treatment of choice is excision.
• Fibrosarcomas—the third most common oral malignancy in dogs (and the second most common in the cat); fibrosarcomas have a predilection for the maxilla of large, male, older dogs; the gingiva is commonly affected, especially around the maxillary fourth premolar, followed by the hard palate and oral mucosa; invasive but rarely metastasize
• Tumors of dental laminar epithelium—originate from epithelial cells of the dental lamina; form from dental epithelium during development or may originate from nests of epithelial cells that maintain the ability to function as dental lamina
• Ameloblastoma—the most common tumor of dental laminar epithelium in dogs; behave as slowly expansible tumors occurring deep within bone; may be cystic or solid

• Other tumor types include undifferentiated carcinomas, osteosarcomas, lymphosarcomas, mast cell tumors, giant cell tumors, neurofibromas, and myxofibrosarcomas.

SIGNS
May include halitosis, oral hemorrhage, and reluctance to chew; often are none

CAUSES
N/A

RISK FACTORS
• Tonsillar squamous cell carcinoma occurs ten times more commonly in dogs from urban settings than in rural dogs.
• Squamous cell carcinoma—more prevalent in white dogs in one study

 DIAGNOSIS

DIFFERENTIAL DIAGNOSIS
Infection—viral/bacterial/fungal

CBC/BIOCHEMISTRY/URINALYSIS
N/A

OTHER LABORATORY TESTS
N/A

IMAGING
Take radiographs of the affected jaw for bony invasion, lungs for metastases.

DIAGNOSTIC PROCEDURES
Aspirate enlarged regional lymph nodes for cytology or biopsy to evaluate metastasis.

PATHOLOGIC FINDINGS
• Must biopsy; sample deep tissue surrounding the mass; use excision, wedge, or needle-punch techniques.
• Cytology may also be helpful but is not as definitive as histopathology.

 TREATMENT

• Depends on the tumor type
• Benign tumors are treatable with long-term success via surgery.
• Malignant tumors are treated surgically with varying success depending on tumor type, location, and metastasis at presentation.
• In advanced circumstances, combined

therapy (surgery, chemotherapy, and radiation) may provide the best care.
• Dogs with tumors caudal to the first premolar had a three times greater risk of dying from the disease than those with tumors rostral to the first premolar.

SURGICAL CONSIDERATIONS
• Fibromatous epulis—marginal excision is the treatment of choice; cryotherapy and radiation treatment also give long-term success.
• Peripheral odontogenic fibromas (ossifying epulis)—treat the same as fibromatous epulis.
• Acanthomatous epulis—excision with at least 1-cm margins is usually curative; radiation has also been used successfully; the combination of surgery and radiation may be most effective (requiring less aggressive surgery), but if radiation is not readily available, surgery may be the only option; surgery must be aggressive; the best chance to resolve the problem surgically is the first time; extract any teeth that may impede incisional healing.
• Multiple (10) injections of bleomycin (5 mg) injected at the tumor site has been effective in a small number of reported cases.
• Melanoma—prognosis improves if the tumor is small and located in the rostral mandible; if surgery is chosen for therapy, it should be aggressive; typically mandibulectomy or maxillectomy; median survival times average 8 months; combination of surgery, radiation, and chemotherapy (low-dose cisplatin) yielded a median survival of 14 months in one study; pigmentation does not affect the prognosis; relatively radioresistant; one study showed a median survival time of 14 months after radiation only; the problem with melanoma is not local disease management but metastasis.
• Squamous cell carcinoma—better long-term prognosis than malignant melanoma or fibrosarcoma in the dog; may be widely surgically excised or irradiated in the dog, especially if the lesion is rostral (better prognosis than those located caudally); perform a maxillectomy or mandibulectomy with a 2-cm clean surgical margin as a goal; in dogs, radiation alone delivers a median survival rate of 15–17 months; in dogs, prognosis for survival following treatment of lingual involvement is poor; dogs tolerate partial glossotomy involving 40–60% of the tongue; for tumors larger

than 2-cm or those with incomplete resections; surgery, radiation, and chemotherapy (mitoxantrone) may be the best options.
• Fibrosarcoma—surgical excision with at least 2-cm margins usually results in a 12-month median survival rate; usually require a maxillectomy or mandibulectomy; palatine fibrosarcomas carry the poorest prognosis because of the inability to surgically resect adequately.

APPROPRIATE HEALTH CARE
N/A

NURSING CARE
N/A

ACTIVITY
N/A

DIET
N/A

CLIENT EDUCATION
N/A

MEDICATIONS

DRUGS OF CHOICE
N/A

CONTRAINDICATIONS
N/A

PRECAUTIONS
N/A

POSSIBLE INTERACTIONS
N/A

ALTERNATIVE DRUGS
N/A

FOLLOW-UP

PATIENT MONITORING
N/A

PREVENTION/AVOIDANCE
N/A

POSSIBLE COMPLICATIONS
• Surgical removal of part of the tongue may result in avascular necrosis if the tongue is transected just caudal to the origin of dorsal branches of the lingual arteries.

• Postoperative complications of mandibulectomy include wound dehiscence, prehension dysfunction, tongue lag, medial drift, excessive drooling, palatal ulceration secondary to malocclusion, and pressure necrosis.
• Feline mandibulectomies can be performed, but they result in greater complications (tongue swelling, ranula formation) than in the canine patient.

EXPECTED COURSE AND PROGNOSIS
• Dogs with inadequate tumor-free surgical margins were two-and-a-half times more likely to die of the tumor than those with complete histologic excision; some surgical patients need gastrostomy tubes to facilitate nutritional supplementation during the treatment period.
• Dogs with tumors located caudal to the first premolar had three times greater risk of dying from the disease than those with tumors located rostral to the first premolar.

MISCELLANEOUS

ASSOCIATED CONDITIONS
N/A

AGE-RELATED FACTORS
N/A

ZOONOTIC POTENTIAL
N/A

PREGNANCY
N/A

SYNONYMS
N/A

SEE ALSO
N/A

ABBREVIATIONS
N/A

Suggested Reading

Harvey CE, Emily PP. Small animal dentistry. Philadelphia: Mosby, 1993.
Wiggs RB, Lobprise HB. Veterinary dentistry: principles and practice. Philadelphia: Lippincott-Raven, 1997.
Author James Anthony
Consulting Editor Jan Bellows

ORGANOPHOSPHATE AND CARBAMATE TOXICITY

BASICS

DEFINITION
• Results from exposure to organophosphorous compounds or carbamate, which are common active ingredients in household and agricultural insecticide products
• Animal products—organophosphate: chlorpyrifos, coumaphos, cythioate, diazinon, famphur, fenthion, phosmet, and tetrachlorvinphos; carbamate: carbaryl and propoxur
• Agricultural, lawn, and garden products—organophosphate: acephate, chlorpyrifos, diazinon, disulfoton, malathion, parathion, terbufos, and others; carbamate: carbofuran and methomyl

PATHOPHYSIOLOGY
• Cause nervous system effects by inhibiting cholinesterase, which includes acetylcholinesterase, pseudocholinesterase, and other esterases
• Acetylcholinesterase—normally hydrolyzes the neurotransmitter acetylcholine in nervous tissue, RBCs, and muscle, resulting in termination of nervous transmission
• Pseudocholinesterase—found in plasma, liver, pancreas, and nervous tissue, mainly in cats
• Cholinesterase inhibition—allows acetylcholine accumulation at the postsynaptic receptor; causes stimulation of effector organs; spontaneous reactivation after organophosphorous compound binding is very slow and once aging occurs is virtually nonexistent; reversible after carbamate binding

SYSTEMS AFFECTED
Nervous—result from overriding stimulation of parasympathetic pathways; may also result from sympathetic stimulation; acetylcholine stimulates nicotinic receptors of the somatic nervous system (skeletal muscle), parasympathetic preganglionic nicotinic and postganglionic muscarinic receptors (cardiac muscle, pupil, blood vessels, smooth muscles in lung and gastrointestinal tract, exocrine glands), and sympathetic preganglionic nicotinic receptors (adrenal and indirectly cardiac muscle, pupil, blood vessels, smooth muscles in lung and gastrointestinal tract, exocrine glands).

GENETICS
• Animals with inherently low cholinesterase activity—more susceptible to cholinesterase depression
• Cholinesterase activity—more easily inhibited in cats than in dogs

INCIDENCE/PREVALENCE
Common in small animals

GEOGRAPHIC DISTRIBUTION
• More common in areas of high flea prevalence and intense agricultural activity

SIGNALMENT

Species
Cats and small or exceptionally lean dogs—most susceptible

Breed Predilections
Lean dogs (e.g., sight hounds and racing breeds) and lean longhair cats—more susceptible to cholinesterase inhibition because of lack of fat; many organophosphorous compounds and metabolites are stored in fat and slowly released into circulation.
• Organophosphate-containing dips labeled for dogs only—inappropriately applied to cats

Mean Age and Range
Young animals—more likely intoxicated due to lower detoxification capability

Predominant Sex
Intact males more susceptible to some organophosphates

SIGNS

General Comments
• Parasympathetic stimulation—usually predominates
• Sympathetic stimulation—may result in lack of specific expected signs; may note opposite signs from those expected

Historical Findings
• Medical history—often discloses heavy or repeated applications of flea and tick insecticides; evidence of exposure to an agricultural product
• Carbamate insecticides (methomyl and carbofuran)—may cause rapid onset of seizures and respiratory failure; treat aggressively without delay.
• Organophosphate insecticides (cats)—chronic anorexia, muscle weakness, and muscle twitching, with or without episodes of acute toxicosis, which may last for days to weeks

Physical Examination Findings
• Hypersalivation
• Vomiting
• Diarrhea
• Miosis
• Bradycardia
• Depression
• Ataxia
• Muscle tremors
• Seizures
• Hyperthermia

• Dyspnea
• Respiratory failure
• Death
• Patient may not exhibit all signs
• Sympathetic stimulation—signs reversed

CAUSES
• Overuse, misuse, or use of multiple cholinesterase-inhibiting insecticides
• Misuse of organophosphate insecticides in cats
• Intentional dermal application of house or yard insecticides

RISK FACTORS
• Concurrent exposure to multiple organophosphate- and/or carbamate-containing products
• Exposure to floors that are damp with organophosphorous premise products
• Incorrect dilution of insecticides

DIAGNOSIS

DIFFERENTIAL DIAGNOSIS
• History of exposure, amount of exposure, and clinical signs—should be consistent with toxicosis
• Exposure to other insecticidal products—pyrethrin/pyrethroids (flea and tick); D-limonene (citrus flea and tick); fipronil (flea and tick); imidacloprid (flea)
• Other pesticides—strychnine; fluoroacetate (1080); 4-aminopyridine (avicide); metaldehyde (snail bait); zinc/aluminum phosphide (rodenticide); bromethalin (rodenticide)
• Other toxicants—chocolate; caffeine; cocaine; amphetamine

CBC/BIOCHEMISTRY/URINALYSIS
N/A

OTHER LABORATORY TESTS

Cholinesterase Activity
• Reduced to < 25% of normal in whole blood, retina, or brain—suggests exposure to a cholinesterase-inhibiting compound
• Test results—must be interpreted in context of the amount of exposure and the clinical signs and the time of their onset
• Use laboratories experienced in handling animal samples.
• Chlorpyrifos—experimentally exposed animals may remain clinically normal with no detectable cholinesterase activity.
• Carbamate inhibition—reactivation may can occur during sample transport and testing, giving false-negative results.

ORGANOPHOSPHATE AND CARBAMATE TOXICITY

IMAGING
N/A

DIAGNOSTIC PROCEDURES
• Detection of insecticides—tissue (e.g., brain, liver, kidney, and fat); stomach contents; gastrointestinal tract; fur or hair; negative results do not rule out toxicosis.
• May find pieces of chewed containers in the gastrointestinal tract.

PATHOLOGIC FINDINGS
• Histopathologic lesions—rare
• Delayed neuropathy—not usually associated with commercially available organophosphorous compounds

 TREATMENT

APPROPRIATE HEALTH CARE
• Outpatient—mild signs from exposure to flea and tick collars and powders; treated by simply removing the collar or brushing excess powder from the coat
• Inpatient—continued salivation, tremors, or dyspnea

NURSING CARE
• Basis—stabilization; decontamination; antidotal treatment with atropine (and pralidoxime chloride for organophosphate toxicosis); supportive care
• Oxygen—if necessary, until respiration returns to normal
• Fluid therapy—may be needed in anorexic cats
• Bathing (dermal exposure)—use hand dishwashing detergent; rinse with copious amounts of water.

ACTIVITY
N/A

DIET
Chronically anorexic cats—maintain nutritional and fluid requirements.

CLIENT EDUCATION
• Stress the importance of following insecticide label directions.
• Caution client that cats with chronic anorexia and weakness may need days to weeks of supportive care for full recovery.

SURGICAL CONSIDERATIONS
N/A

 MEDICATIONS

DRUGS OF CHOICE
• Diazepam (0.05–1.0 mg/kg IV) or phenobarbital (3.0–30 mg/kg IV to effect, low dosage in cats)—controls seizures
• Atropine sulfate—0.2 mg/kg one-quarter IV, remaining SC, as needed; administered immediately; repeated only as needed to control life-threatening clinical signs from muscarinic stimulation
• Pralidoxime chloride (Protopam)—10–15 mg/kg IM, SC q8–12h until recovery; discontinue after three doses if no response; reduces muscle fasciculations; most beneficial against organophosphorous insecticides when started within 24 hr of exposure; even several days after dermal exposure may stimulate anorexic cats (with or without tremors) to resume eating; if refrigerated and wrapped in foil, reconstituted bottles may be successfully used for up to 2 weeks.
• Ingestion of liquid insecticidal solution—avoid inducing emesis; risk of aspiration because many solutions contain hydrocarbon solvents
• No clinical signs, liquid solvent not ingested, and very recent ingestion—3% hydrogen peroxide (2.2 mL/kg PO to a maximum of 45 mL) after feeding a moist meal
• Evacuation of the stomach for patient with clinical signs—gastric lavage with the patient intubated, under anesthesia, with a large-bore stomach tube; then administration of activated charcoal (2.0 g/kg PO) containing sorbitol as a cathartic in a water slurry
• Diarrhea—do not administer sorbitol-containing product.

CONTRAINDICATIONS
Phenothiazine tranquilizers may potentiate organophosphate toxicosis.

PRECAUTIONS
Atropine—avoid overuse; may cause tachycardia, CNS stimulation, seizures, disorientation, drowsiness, and respiratory depression

POSSIBLE INTERACTIONS
N/A

ALTERNATIVE DRUGS
N/A

 FOLLOW-UP

PATIENT MONITORING
Monitor heart rate, respiration, and fluid and caloric intake.

PREVENTION/AVOIDANCE
• Closely follow directions on insecticidal labels.
• Avoid use on sick or debilitated animals.
• Avoid simultaneous use of organophosphate and carbamate products.

POSSIBLE COMPLICATIONS
N/A

EXPECTED COURSE AND PROGNOSIS
• Chronic organophosphate insecticide–induced weakness and anorexia (cats)—may last 2–4 weeks; most patients fully recover with aggressive nursing care.
• Acute toxicosis treated promptly—good prognosis

 MISCELLANEOUS

ASSOCIATED CONDITIONS
N/A

AGE-RELATED FACTORS
N/A

ZOONOTIC POTENTIAL
N/A

PREGNANCY
N/A

SEE ALSO
Poisoning (Intoxication)

Suggested Reading
Fikes JD. Feline chlorpyrifos toxicosis. In: Kirk RW, Bonagura JD eds. Current veterinary therapy XI. Philadelphia: Saunders, 1992:188–191.
Fikes JD. Organophosphate and carbamate insecticides. Vet Clin North Am Small Anim Pract 1990;20:353–367.
Authors Steven R. Hansen and Elizabeth A. Curry-Galvin
Consulting Editor Gary D. Osweiler

DISEASES

ORONASAL FISTULA

 BASICS

OVERVIEW
- A hole between the oral and nasal cavity
- Communication between the mouth and nasal cavity can occur from pathology of any of the maxillary teeth; defects are vertical.

SIGNALMENT
Dog—dolichocephalic head types are affected most often, especially dachshunds.

SIGNS
- Chronic rhinitis—with or without blood
- Sneezing—also common, especially when the maxillary canines are digitally palpated

CAUSES AND RISK FACTORS
- Can be caused by trauma, penetration of a foreign body, bite wounds, traumatic tooth extraction, electrical shock, or oral cancer
- Usually associated with a periapical abscess of the maxillary canine tooth caused by end-stage periodontitis leading to lysis of the bone separating the nasal and oral cavities
- Fistula width is related to the size of the dog; fistula depth to the chronicity of the periodontal infection.
- Dogs with uncorrected base-narrow canines and those with prognathic (overbite) mal-occlusions causing the mandibular canines to penetrate the hard palate are predisposed.

 DIAGNOSIS

- Maxillary canines are most commonly affected.
- The palatal root of the maxillary fourth premolar is next most common.
- Inserting a periodontal probe into the pocket along the palatine surface of the maxillary canine tooth often causes hemorrhage from the ipsilateral nostril, confirming an oronasal fistula.

DIFFERENTIAL DIAGNOSIS
- Periodontal disease
- Oral cancer
- Trauma
- Foreign body penetration

CBC/BIOCHEMISTRY/URINALYSIS
N/A

IMAGING
- Radiographs rarely diagnose oronasal fistula because the lesions are generally isolated to the medial surface.
- Radiographs may show foreign body entrapment, or lysis consistent with neoplasia.

DIAGNOSTIC PROCEDURES
Periodontal probing—if probing leads to epistaxis; an oronasal fistula exists

 TREATMENT

- Repair to prevent foreign material and infection from passing from the mouth into the nose causing rhinitis, sinusitis, and possibly, pneumonia
- Extract the tooth and close the defect; after extraction, the goal of surgical closure is to place an epithelial layer in both the oral and nasal cavities.
- When the palatal root of the maxillary fourth premolar causes the oronasal fistula, perform conventional or surgical endodontics on the mesial and distal roots, and amputate the palatal root.
- Full-thickness flap—after tooth extraction, a mucoperiosteal pedical flap may be elevated from the dorsal aspect of the fistula, advanced to cover the defect, and sutured in place; a successful full-thickness flap requires some attached gingiva above the defect, sutures at the edge of the defect (not over the void), and no tension on the suture line.
- Double reposition flap—used for large fistulas or repair failures where no attached gingiva remains or where periosteal tissue cannot be included; after extraction, the first flap is harvested from the hard palate and inverted so that the oral epithelium is toward the nasal passage; the second flap is muco-buccal and harvested from the alveolar mucosa and underside of the lip rostral to the fistula; it is sutured over the first flap and donor site.

- Guided tissue regeneration of the maxillary canine—may be used for reconstruction and elimination of the fistula despite marked support compromise of the canine tooth; a palatal flap is elevated to approach the infrabony defect; soft tissue and calculus is removed from the defect with a curette.
- Bone grafts such as PerioGlas, synthetic and natural hydroxyapatite, autogenous and heterologous bone, polylactic acid, and plaster of Paris have been used to exclude regrowth of gingival connective tissue and epithelium, promoting regeneration of bone and periodontal ligament.
- Can surgically repair oronasal fistulas located in the central portion of the hard palate with a transposition flap of the hard palate mucoperiosteum from tissue adjacent to the defect

 MEDICATIONS
N/A

DRUGS
N/A

CONTRAINDICATIONS/POSSIBLE INTERACTIONS
N/A

 FOLLOW-UP
Normal postoperative monitoring

 MISCELLANEOUS

Suggested Readings
Harvey CE, Emily PP. Small animal dentistry. St. Louis: Mosby, 1993.
Wiggs RB, Lobprise HB. Veterinary dentistry: principles and practice. Philadelphia: Lippincott-Raven, 1997.
Author Jan Bellows
Consulting Editor Jan Bellows

BASICS

OVERVIEW
• A growth and developmental abnormality of cartilage and bone; encompasses many disorders involving bone growth
• Results from delayed endochondral ossification
• Skeletal defects—usually involve the appendicular skeleton; specifically the metaphyseal growth plates
• Achondroplasia—failure of cartilage growth; characterized by a proportionate short-limbed dysplasia; evident soon after birth
• Hypochondrodysplasia—less severe form of achondrodysplasia
• Characteristic breeds—result of selection of certain desirable traits
• Affects musculoskeletal and ophthalmic systems

SIGNALMENT
• Achondroplastic breeds—bulldogs; Boston terriers; pugs; Pekingese; Japanese spaniels; shih tzus
• Hypochondroplastic breeds—dachshunds; basset hounds; beagles; Welsh corgis; dandie Dinmont terriers; Scottish terriers; Skye terriers
• Reported nonselected chondrodysplastic abnormalities—Alaskan malamutes; Samoyeds; Labrador retrievers; English pointers; Norwegian elkhounds; Great Pyrenees; cocker spaniels; Scottish terriers; Scottish deerhounds
• Ocular-skeletal dysplasia—diagnosed in Labrador retrievers and Samoyeds

SIGNS
Historical Findings
• Obvious skeletal deformities
• Retarded growth

Physical Examination Findings
• Usually affects the appendicular skeleton; may affect axial skeleton
• Long bones—appear shorter than normal; often bowed
• Major joints (elbow, stifle, carpus, tarsus)—appear enlarged
• Radius and ulna—often severely affected owing to asynchronous growth
• Lateral bowing of the forelimbs
• Enlarged carpal joints
• Valgus deformity of the paws

• Shortened maxilla—relative mandibular prognathism
• Spinal deviations—owing to hemivertebrae
• Retina—dysplasia; partial to complete detachment

CAUSES & RISK FACTORS
• Achondrodysplastic and hypochondrodysplastic breeds—autosomal dominant trait
• Nonselected chondrodysplastic breeds—simple autosomal recessive or polygenic trait
• Littermates often affected

DIAGNOSIS

DIFFERENTIAL DIAGNOSIS
Premature closure of the ulnar or radial physes—history of trauma; no other bones affected; unilateral or bilateral abnormalities

CBC/BIOCHEMISTRY/URINALYSIS
N/A

OTHER LABORATORY TESTS
Bone biopsy of growth plate—definitive diagnosis

IMAGING
• Radiography of affected limbs—irregular flattening of the metaphysis; widening of the physeal line; retained endochondral cores; irregularities in ossification of the affected long bone; degenerative joint disease and joint laxity owing to abnormal stress and weight bearing on the limbs
• Radiography of the spine—hemivertebrae; wedge-shaped vertebrae

PATHOLOGIC FINDINGS
• Histologic findings: disorganization of the proliferative zone, abnormalities within the hypertrophic zone, abnormal formation of the primary and secondary spongiosa

TREATMENT
• Achondrodysplasia—considered a normal abnormality in some (chondrodystrophic) breeds
• Surgery—usually of little benefit for nonselected chondrodysplasia
• Corrective osteotomy to realign limb(s) or joint(s)—may have limited benefit

MEDICATIONS

DRUGS
• Analgesics and anti-inflammatory agents—palliative use warranted; may try buffered or enteric-coated aspirin (10–25 mg/kg PO q8h or q12h), caroprofen (2.2 mg/kg PO q12h), etodolac (10–15 mg/kg PO once daily), phenylbutazone (3–7 mg/kg PO q8h, total dose < 800 mg/day), meclofenamic acid (0.5 mg/kg PO q12h), or piroxicam (0.3 mg/kg PO q24h for 3 days; then every other day)
• Chondroprotective agents—polysulfated glycosaminoglycans, glucosamine, and chondroitin sulfate; may have limited benefit in preventing articular cartilage changes

CONTRAINDICATIONS/POSSIBLE INTERACTIONS
N/A

FOLLOW-UP

PREVENTION/AVOIDANCE
• Do not repeat dam–sire breedings that resulted in affected offspring.
• Discourage breeding affected animals.

POSSIBLE COMPLICATIONS
Intra-articular and periarticular joint structures—degenerate owing to abnormal conformation of the appendicular skeleton; leads to altered biomechanics; results in poor quality of life

EXPECTED COURSE AND PROGNOSIS
• Depend on severity

MISCELLANEOUS

SYNONYMS
Dwarfism

Suggested Reading
Sande RD, Bingel SA. Animal models of dwarfism. Vet Clin North Am Small Anim Pract 1982;13:71.
Author Peter D. Schwarz
Consulting Editor Peter D. Schwarz

DISEASES

OSTEOCHONDROSIS

 BASICS

DEFINITION
A pathologic process in growing cartilage, primarily characterized by a disturbance of endochondral ossification that leads to excessive retention of cartilage

PATHOPHYSIOLOGY
• Cells of the immature articular joint cartilage and growth plates do not differentiate normally.
• The process of endochondral ossification is retarded, but the cartilage continues to grow, resulting in abnormally thick regions that are less resistant to mechanical stress.
• Bilateral disease common
• Most commonly affected joints—shoulder (caudocentral humeral head); elbow (medial aspect humeral condyle); stifle (femoral condyle: lateral more often than medial); hock (ridge of the talus: medial more common than lateral)
• Other reported locations—femoral head; dorsal rim of the acetabulum; glenoid cavity (scapula); patella; distal radius; medial malleolus; cranial end plate of the sacrum; vertebral articular facets; cervical vertebrae Immature Joint Cartilage
• Nutrition maintained by diffusion of nutrients from the synovial fluid
• Thickened cartilage results in impaired metabolism, leading to degeneration and necrosis of the poorly supplied cells
• Fissure within the thickened cartilage—may result from mechanical stress; eventually leads to the formation of a cartilage flap, or OCD; may cause lameness
• Lameness (pain)—becomes evident once synovial fluid establishes contact with subchondral bone; affected by cartilage breakdown products released into the synovial fluid; inflammation
Retention of Cartilage in Growth Plates
• Usually does not lead to necrosis, probably owing to nutrition provided by vessels within the cartilage
• May lead to slippage and asymmetric growth; most marked in the distal ulnar physis

SYSTEMS AFFECTED
Musculoskeletal

GENETICS
• Polygenetic transmission—expression determined by an interaction of genetic and environmental factors
• Heritability index—depends on breed; 0.25–0.45

INCIDENCE/PREVALENCE
Frequent and serious problem in many dog breeds

GEOGRAPHIC DISTRIBUTION
N/A

SIGNALMENT

Species
• Dogs
• Demonstrated clinically—horses; pigs; broiler chickens; turkeys; humans

Breed Predilections
Large and giant breeds—great Danes, Labrador retrievers, Newfoundlands, rottweilers, Bernese mountain dogs, English setters; Old English sheepdogs

MEAN AGE AND RANGE
• Onset of clinical signs—typically 4–8 months
• Diagnosis—generally 4–18 months
• Symptoms of secondary DJD—any age

PREDOMINANT SEX
• Shoulder—males (2:1)
• Elbow, stifle, and hock—none

SIGNS

General Comments
• Depend on the affected joint(s) and concurrent DJD

Historical Findings
Lameness—most common; sudden or insidious in onset; one or more limbs; becomes worse after exercise; duration of several weeks to months; slight, moderate, or severe; patient may support little weight on the affected limb.

Physical Examination Findings
• Pain—usually elicited on palpation by flexing, extending, or rotating the involved joint
• Generally a weight-bearing lameness
• Joint effusion with capsular distention—common with OCD of elbow, stifle, and hock
• Muscle atrophy—consistent finding with chronic lameness
• Hock OCD—hyperextension of the tarsocrural joint

CAUSES
• Developmental
• Nutritional

RISK FACTORS
• Diet containing three times the recommended calcium levels
• Rapid growth and weight gain

 DIAGNOSIS

DIFFERENTIAL DIAGNOSIS
• Intra-articular (osteochondral) fractures
• Elbow dysplasia
• Panosteitis

CBC/BIOCHEMISTRY/URINALYSIS
N/A

OTHER LABORATORY TESTS
N/A

IMAGING

Radiography
• Standard craniocaudal and mediolateral views—necessary for all involved joints
• Appears as flattening of the subchondral bone or as a subchondral lucency
• Cannot be differentiated from OCD
• Sclerosis of the underlying bone—common in chronic OCD lesions; may see flap if it is calcified
• Calcified bodies within the joint (joint mice)—indicate dislodged cartilage flap
• Contralateral joint—comparison; check for involvement
• Oblique views—may improve visualization, especially for hock, elbow, and shoulder lesions
• Skyline views of the talar ridges of the hock joint—help identify medial and lateral lesions

CT and MRI
• Useful for visualizing extent of subchondral lesions
• Not reliable for detecting a loose cartilage flap

Positive Contrast Arthrography
Useful for differentiating from OCD of the shoulder

DIAGNOSTIC PROCEDURES
• Joint tap and analysis of synovial fluid—confirms involvement; should note straw-colored fluid with normal to decreased viscosity; from cytology, should note

< 10,000 nucleated cells/μL (> 90% should be mononuclear cells)
• Arthroscopy—minimally invasive; excellent method for differentiating from OCD and for corrective treatment

PATHOLOGIC FINDINGS
• Articular cartilage—initially may appear yellowish
• Retention of articular cartilage extending into subchondral bone surrounded by increased amount of trabecular bone
• Clefts between the underlying trabecular bone and the degenerated and necrotic deep layer of the overlying thickened (retained) cartilage

TREATMENT

APPROPRIATE HEALTH CARE
Not treatable

NURSING CARE
• Cryotherapy (ice packing) of affected joint—immediately postsurgery; 15–20 min three times a day for 3–5 days
• Range-of-motion exercises—initiated as soon as patient can tolerate

ACTIVITY
• Restricted
• Avoid hard concussive activities (e.g., running on concrete).

DIET
• Weight control—important for decreasing load and, therefore, the stress on the affected joint(s)

CLIENT EDUCATION
• Discuss the heritability of the disease.
• Warn client that DJD may develop.
• Discuss the influence of excessive intake of nutrients that promote rapid growth.

SURGICAL CONSIDERATIONS
• Nonsurgical condition
• May progress to OCD as the patient grows
• Arthrotomy or arthroscopy—indicated for most OCD patients
• Shoulder—indicated for all OCD lesions; exploratory procedure indicated for pain and lameness with radiographic evidence of osteochondrosis
• Elbow—indicated for all OCD lesions; indicated to assess for other conditions (see Elbow Dysplasia)

• Stifle—controversial; patients develop DJD even with procedure; arthroscopy may improve the recovery rate and long-term function.
• Hock—remove osteochondral flap; controversial; all patients develop severe DJD even with procedure; attempt to reattach the flap to the underlying subchondral bone, if warranted.

MEDICATIONS

DRUGS OF CHOICE
Anti-inflammatory drugs (NSAIDs) and analgesics—may be used to symptomatically treat associated DJD; do not promote healing of the cartilage flap (thus surgery is still indicated)

CONTRAINDICATIONS
Avoid corticosteroids owing to potential side effects and articular cartilage damage associated with long-term use.

PRECAUTIONS
• NSAIDs—gastrointestinal irritation may preclude their use.

POSSIBLE INTERACTIONS
N/A

ALTERNATIVE DRUGS
Chondroprotective drugs (e.g., polysulfated glycosaminoglycans, glucosamine, and chondroitin sulfate)—may help limit cartilage damage and degeneration; may help alleviate pain and inflammation

FOLLOW-UP

PATIENT MONITORING
• Periodic monitoring until patient is skeletally mature—recommended to assess progression to an OCD lesion
• Postsurgery—limit activity for 4–6 weeks; encourage early, active movement of the affected joint(s).
• Yearly examinations—recommended to assess progression of DJD

PREVENTION/AVOIDANCE
• Discourage breeding of patients.
• Do not repeat dam–sire breedings that resulted in affected offspring.
• Restricted weight gain and growth in young dogs—may decrease incidence

POSSIBLE COMPLICATIONS
N/A

EXPECTED COURSE AND PROGNOSIS
• Shoulder—good to excellent prognosis for return to full function; minimal osteoarthritis development
• Elbow, stifle, and hock—fair to guarded prognosis; depends on size of lesion (most important), DJD, and age at diagnosis and treatment; progressive osteoarthritis development, even after surgery

MISCELLANEOUS

ASSOCIATED CONDITIONS
N/A

AGE-RELATED FACTORS
N/A

ZOONOTIC POTENTIAL
N/A

PREGNANCY
N/A

SEE ALSO
Elbow Dysplasia

ABBREVIATIONS
• DJD = degenerative joint disease
• OCD = osteochondritis dissecans

Suggested Reading
Fox SM, Walker AM. The etiopathogenesis of osteochondrosis. Vet Med 1993;88:116–122.
Olsson SE. Lameness in the dog: a review of lesion causing osteoarthrosis of the shoulder, elbow, hip, stifle and hock joints. Proceedings of the American Animal Hospital Association, 1975;42:363–370.
Olsson SE. Osteochondritis dissecans in dogs: a study of pathogenesis, clinical signs, pathologic changes, natural course and sequelae [Abstract]. J Am Vet Radiol Soc 1973;14:4.
Author Peter D. Schwarz
Consulting Editor Peter D. Schwarz

OSTEOMYELITIS

 BASICS

DEFINITION

An acute or chronic inflammation of bone and the associated soft tissue elements of marrow, endosteum, periosteum and vascular channels that is usually caused by bacteria and rarely by fungi and other microorganisms

PATHOPHYSIOLOGY

• Hematogenously disseminated micro-organisms—may localize in metaphyseal bone of young animals and vertebrae of adults; cause osteomyelitis when tissue defense mechanisms have been compromised • Direct inoculation of bone with pathogenic bacteria—may not initiate infection unless there is concurrent tissue injury, bone necrosis, sequestration, fracture instability, altered tissue defenses, foreign material, or surgical implants • Once bone infection is established, bacteria may persist by adhering to implants and sequestra. • Bio-film—made up of slime produced by staphylococci and other bacteria together with host-derived proteins, cellular debris, and carbohydrate; enshrouds bacterial colonies; provides protection from antimicrobial drugs and host defenses; induces some bacteria to transform to more virulent strains that are more resistant to antimicrobial drugs • Fracture instability exacerbates infection; resorption of bone owing to infection and instability causes widening of the fracture gap and implant loosening, contributing to persistence of infection.

SYSTEMS AFFECTED

Musculoskeletal

GENETICS

Autosomal recessive mode of inheritance—suspected in border collies with neutropenia and hematogenous disease

INCIDENCE/PREVALENCE

• Prevalence after open reduction and internal fixation of closed fractures—usually < 1% • Prevalence after trauma and open fracture—unknown; relatively common • Hematogenous disease in young dogs—uncommon • Diskospondylitis in adult dogs and cats and fungal disease—not uncommon

GEOGRAPHIC DISTRIBUTION

• *Actinomyces* infections—regions of sharp grass awns: California, Florida, UK, and Australia • Blastomycosis—central and eastern regions of the U.S: Great Lakes region and the Mississippi and Ohio River valleys • Coccidioidomycosis—southwestern U.S., Mexico, and Central and South America • Histoplasmosis—Ohio, Missouri, and Mississippi River valleys and tributaries

SIGNALMENT

Species

Dogs and cats

Breed Predilections

• German shepherds—*Aspergillus* infection, possibly owing to a breed-related immunodeficiency • Large-breed dogs—blastomycosis • Border collies with neutropenia and Irish setters with leukocyte adhesion protein deficiency—hematogenous disease

Mean Age and Range

Hematogenous metaphyseal infection—young dogs

Predominant Sex

Male dogs—for post-traumatic infection; blastomycosis

SIGNS

General Comments

• Acute postoperative wound infections after orthopedic surgery—may be indistinguishable from acute condition; may progress to chronic disease • Most patients have chronic disease at time of examination and diagnosis.

Historical Findings

• Episodes of lameness • Draining tracts • Persistent ulcers • Previous trauma • Fracture or surgery—post-traumatic disease • Affected vertebrae or intervertebral disks (dogs)—may note hind limb weakness and difficulty in rising • Travel to regions endemic for mycotic infections—fungal infection

Physical Examination Findings

• Acute hematogenous disease (dogs)—sudden onset of systemic illness; pyrexia; lethargy; limb pain; local signs of acute inflammation • Chronic condition—usually associated with chronic draining tracts, nonhealing ulcers, pain, secondary muscle atrophy, and joint stiffness • Unhealed fractures with concurrent infection—may note instability, crepitus, and limb deformity • Fungal infections—may see limb swelling, lameness, and intermittently draining tracts • Bone infections of the spine—may cause pain and neurologic deficits (e.g., paresis and paralysis)

CAUSES

• Open fracture • Traumatic injury • Open reduction and internal fixation of closed fracture • Elective orthopedic surgery • Prosthetic joint implant • Gunshot wound • Penetrating foreign body • Bite and claw wounds • Extension to bone of soft tissue infection—periodontitis; rhinitis; otitis media; paronychia • Hematogenous infection • Staphylococci—cause approximately 50% of bone infections; often monomicrobial infections • Polymicrobial infection—common; may contain mixtures of aerobic gram-negative bacteria;

• Anaerobic bacteria—difficult to isolate; involved in up to 60% of bone infections; include *Actinomyces, Clostridium, Peptostreptococcus, Bacteroides,* and *Fusobacterium* • Fungal infection—*Coccidioides immitis; Blastomyces dermatitidis; Histoplasma capsulatum; Cryptococcus neoformans; Aspergillus*

RISK FACTORS

• Open fracture and bone contamination • Soft tissue trauma • Bite and claw wounds • Migrating foreign body • Orthopedic surgery • Prosthetic orthopedic implant • Cortical bone allograft • Immunodeficiency

 DIAGNOSIS

DIFFERENTIAL DIAGNOSIS

• Neoplasia • Bone cysts • Delayed fracture union as a result of instability • Hypertrophic osteodystrophy • Secondary hypertrophic osteopathy • Medullary bone infarction

CBC/BIOCHEMISTRY/URINALYSIS

Hemogram—inflammatory left shift usually evident only with acute disease

OTHER LABORATORY TESTS

Serology—confirms some fungal infections

IMAGING

Radiology

• Acute disease—bone architecture normal; see only soft tissue swelling • Chronic disease—sequestra (dead piece of cortical bone); reactive periosteal new bone; involucrum formation (shell of new bone surrounding sequestrum); bone resorption • Bone resorption—widening of fracture gaps; cortical thinning; generalized osteopenia; implant loosening • Contrast films—may help delineate sinuses and radiolucent foreign bodies; inject water-soluble contrast media through a Foley catheter into the sinuses.

Other

• Ultrasonography—localize large accumulations of fluid; guide fluid sampling by needle aspiration • Scintigraphy—^{99m}Tc-labeled methylene diphosphonate; highly sensitive for detecting skeletal lesions; not specific for osteomyelitis

DIAGNOSTIC PROCEDURES

• Fluid aspirates or Jamshidi-needle tissue biopsies—collected from focus of infection by sterile techniques; cultured aerobically and anaerobically; identify microorganisms; determine in vitro antimicrobial drug susceptibility

• Open surgical biopsy—indicated when needle aspirates are negative or when débridement is necessary for treatment; culture samples of necrotic tissue, sequestra, implants, and foreign material; histopathologic examination for suspected fungal infection and to rule out neoplasia
• Fluid and tissue samples for anaerobic culture—immediately place into appropriate medium (e.g., reduced Cary-Blair anaerobic transport medium).
• Pus from draining tracts—culture is misleading; tracts are colonized by skin organisms and gram-negative bacteria.
• Blood cultures—may be positive with acute disease

PATHOLOGIC FINDINGS
• Bone sequestration—virtually diagnostic
• Inflammation and necrosis of bone and the adjacent tissues—pyogenic bacteria
• Cytologic or histopathologic examination of smears or sections—usually leads to diagnosis of fungal infection; special fungal stains (methenamine silver; PAS) for microorganism identification

TREATMENT

APPROPRIATE HEALTH CARE
• Inpatient—surgical débridement, drainage, culturing, irrigation, and wound management until infection begins to resolve; infected fractures (surgical stabilization)
• Outpatient—long-term oral antimicrobial drug therapy

NURSING CARE
• Depends on severity, location, and degree of associated soft tissue injury
• Take care to prevent contamination by the pathogen to other patients in the hospital.

ACTIVITY
Restricted—with any danger of a pathologic fracture developing; with a unhealed fracture

DIET
No restriction

CLIENT EDUCATION
• Warn the client about the expense of treatment, the likelihood of recurrence, the problems with sequestration, the need for repeated surgical intervention, and the long duration of therapy.
• Discuss the prognosis.

SURGICAL CONSIDERATIONS
• Chronic disease—surgical débridement; removal of sequestrum; establishment of drainage
• Infected stable fracture—leave pre-existing internal fixation implants in place during healing.

• Infected unstable fracture—remove implants; stabilize with an external skeletal fixator.
• Bone deficits—graft with autologous cancellous bone after infection has abated and granulation tissue has filled the wound.
• Large segmental deficits in long bones—bridge by Ilizarov technique of bone segment transport.
• Localized chronic infection—may be amenable to resolution by amputation (tail, digit, limb) or en bloc resection (sternum, thoracic wall, mandible, maxilla) and primary wound closure
• Remove all implants after the fracture has healed; bacteria harbored by implant-associated biofilm lead to recurrence.

MEDICATIONS

DRUGS OF CHOICE
• Antimicrobial drugs—depend on in vitro determination of susceptibility of microorganisms; also consider possible toxicity, frequency and route of administration, and expense; most penetrate normal and infected bone well; must be given for 4–8 weeks
• Staphylococci (dogs)—usually *S. intermedius*, which are resistant to penicillin because of β-lactamase production; highly susceptible to cloxacillin, amoxicillin-clavulanate, cefazolin, and clindamycin
• Anaerobes—more are sensitive to metronidazole and clindamycin.
• Aminoglycosides and quinolones (ciprofloxacin and enrofloxacin)—effective against gram-negative aerobic bacteria
• Quinolones—may give orally; not nephrotoxic; to protect against resistance, use only for infections caused by gram-negative organisms or *Pseudomonas* that are resistant to other oral antimicrobial drugs.
• Chronic disease—continuous local delivery of antimicrobial drugs by antibiotic-impregnated methylmethacrylate beads
• Itraconazole—5–10 mg/kg PO q24h; given continuously, may control disseminated aspergillosis for up to 2 years

CONTRAINDICATIONS
Quinolones—do not give to young patients; experimentally induce articular cartilage lesions in immature dogs

PRECAUTIONS
Aminoglycosides—may cause nephrotoxicity, especially in dehydrated patients and with electrolyte losses or pre-existing renal disease

POSSIBLE INTERACTIONS
N/A

ALTERNATIVE DRUGS
Identify other antimicrobial drugs by repeating cultures and susceptibility determination if the

infection becomes unresponsive to the initial agent.

FOLLOW-UP

PATIENT MONITORING
• Radiography—every 4–6 weeks; determine bone healing • Reculture bone—suspected persistent infection

PREVENTION/AVOIDANCE
N/A

POSSIBLE COMPLICATIONS
• Recurrence • Chronic disease—may result in limb deformity, impaired function, fracture disease, or neurologic deficits • Malignant neoplasia—rare sequela to chronic infection of fractures repaired by internal fixation

EXPECTED COURSE AND PROGNOSIS
• Acute infection and chronic bacterial diskospondylitis—may be cured by 4–8 weeks of antimicrobial drug therapy if there is limited bone necrosis and no fracture • Chronic disease—resolution with antimicrobial drug therapy alone unlikely; provide appropriate surgical treatment. • Recurrence of chronic infection—evident by return of lameness or draining tracts; may occur weeks, months, or years after the last treatment; may require repeated sequestrectomy, debridement, microbiologic culturing, drainage, fracture stabilization, bone grafting, or implant removal

MISCELLANEOUS

ASSOCIATED CONDITIONS
N/A

AGE-RELATED FACTORS
N/A

ZOONOTIC POTENTIAL
N/A

PREGNANCY
N/A

SYNONYMS
Bone infection

SEE ALSO
• Diskospondylitis • Fungal Infections

Suggested Reading

Johnson KA. Osteomyelitis. In: Birchard SJ, Sherding RG, eds. Saunders manual of small animal practice. Philadelphia: Saunders, 1994:1091–1095.

Johnson KA. Osteomyelitis in dogs and cats. J Am Vet Med Assoc 1994;205:1882–1887.

Author Kenneth A. Johnson

Consulting Editor Peter D. Schwarz

DISEASES

OSTEOSARCOMA

BASICS

DEFINITION
• Most common primary bone tumor in dogs
• Typically affects the appendicular skeleton of large- to giant-breed dogs
• Malignant, with microscopic lung metastases in > 90% of dogs at the time of diagnosis
• Cats—less common; less malignant than in dogs

Pathophysiology
Chronic low-grade bone trauma in large dogs—hypothesized as a cause

Systems Affected
• Musculoskeletal—appendicular skeleton (metaphyseal region of the distal radius, proximal humerus, distal femur, and proximal tibia) most commonly affected in dogs; may also occur in the axial skeleton
• Respiratory—most common metastatic site is the lungs

Genetics
• Does not appear to be heritable; although breed predilections do occur
• Breed size and rate of maturity may be more important than breed or family line.

Incidence/Prevalence
• Dogs—accounts for up to 85% of all primary bone tumors
• Cats—most common primary bone tumor; accounts for < 7% of all reported malignancies

Geographic Distribution
N/A

SIGNALMENT
Species
Dogs and cats

Breed Predilections
• Dogs—large to giant breeds
• Cats—domestic shorthair

Mean Age and Range
• Dogs—bimodal peak at 2 years and 7 years; reported as young as 6 months
• Cats—mean age, 8.5 years; range, 4–18 years

Predominant Sex
• Dogs—males predominate (1.2:1) in most reports
• Cats—both males and females

SIGNS
Historical Findings
• Vary
• Lesions may be subtle—key features: localized swelling, a palpable mass, or pain
• Swelling, lameness, and pain common
• Other complaints—inappetence and lethargy

Physical Examination Findings
• Depend on site
• A firm, painful swelling of the affected site common
• Degree of lameness—varies from mild to non–weight bearing
• Pathologic fracture rare

CAUSES
Unknown in both species

RISK FACTORS
• Dogs—large to giant breeds; metallic implants at fracture repair sites; history of exposure to ionizing radiation
• Cats—unknown

DIAGNOSIS

DIFFERENTIAL DIAGNOSIS
• Other primary or metastatic bone tumor
• Fungal or bacterial osteomyelitis

CBC/BIOCHEMISTRY/URINALYSIS
No consistent abnormalities identified

OTHER LABORATORY TESTS
N/A

IMAGING
Radiographs—Primary Site
• Take at least two views.
• Typical findings—bony lysis; proliferation in the metaphyseal region of long bones
• Marked soft tissue swelling common
• Does not usually involve both sides of a joint cavity

Radiographs—Thoracic
• Always take three views, although metastatic disease is seen in < 10% of patients at the time of examination.
• Metastatic lesions—typically discrete, round, soft-tissue density nodules

Nuclear Bone Scans
• May be useful for identifying bony or soft tissue metastatic disease earlier than via radiography
• Will not distinguish between sites of previous trauma or inflammation and metastatic neoplasia

DIAGNOSTIC PROCEDURES
• Cytologic examination of bone aspirate—may yield diagnosis
• Bone biopsy—gold standard for diagnosis

PATHOLOGIC FINDINGS
• Gross—mild to severe destruction of cortical bone with new bone proliferation
• Histologic—malignant population of mesenchymal cells that are plump and polygonal to spindyloid in shape; osteoid production is diagnostic.
• Parosteal (juxtacortical)—soft tissue variant; may be less aggressive than other forms

TREATMENT

APPROPRIATE HEALTH CARE
• Diagnostic evaluation—outpatient
• Surgery and the first chemotherapy treatment—inpatient
• Subsequent chemotherapy—outpatient

NURSING CARE
Manage pain as needed (see Alternative Drugs).

ACTIVITY
Restricted after surgery until adequate healing has occurred

DIET
N/A

CLIENT EDUCATION
• Warn client that the long-term prognosis is poor; achievable goals should be to relieve discomfort and prolong a good quality of life.
• Prepare clients for possible chemotherapy-induced side effects.

SURGICAL CONSIDERATIONS

Dogs
Appendicular Sites
• Amputation of affected limb—forequarter or hip disarticulation
• Limb-salvage therapy—available at a limited number of referral hospitals
• Adjuvant chemotherapy—recommended after either surgical procedure
Axial Sites
• Aggressive surgical excision
• Chemotherapy—after surgery recommended
Metastatectomy
• Pulmonary metastasectomy—has been described

Cats
Appendicular Sites
• Amputation of affected limb
• Adjuvant therapy may not be necessary.
Axial Sites
• Attempt aggressive surgical excision—depending on site of lesion
• Local recurrence—main reason for treatment failure

Both Species
Inoperable neoplasms—radiotherapy offers marked pain relief.

MEDICATIONS

DRUGS OF CHOICE
• Definitive treatment
• Postsurgical chemotherapy with a platinum-based drug—current standard of care
• Cisplatin—70 mg/m² IV every 3 weeks; must be given with saline-induced diuresis to prevent nephrotoxicity; begin diuresis (18.3 mL/kg/hr) for 4 hr; administer chemotherapy over 20 min; then continue diuresis for another 2 hr; will cause vomiting within 2 hr of administration (give butorphanol at 0.4 mg/kg IM 20 min before cisplatin administration to minimize)
• Carboplatin—300 mg/m² IV every 3 weeks; more expensive and less toxic than cisplatin; use in cats

CONTRAINDICATIONS
• Pre-existing renal dysfunction—do not treat with platinum-based drugs.
• Cisplatin—do not give to cats.

PRECAUTIONS
• Avoid aluminum or metal-containing catheters and needle hubs because aluminum interferes with the activity of platinum-containing drugs.
• Seek advice before initiating therapy if you are unfamiliar with cytotoxic drugs.

POSSIBLE INTERACTIONS
N/A

ALTERNATIVE DRUGS
• Doxorubicin—either alone or in combination with cisplatin; not very effective when used alone
• Palliative treatment—pain management must be addressed for patients whose owners decline definitive treatment; manage with aspirin (20 mg/kg PO q8h), piroxicam (0.3 mg/kg PO q24h with food), or butorphanol (0.5–1.0 mg/kg PO q6h); consider fentanyl patches.

FOLLOW-UP

PATIENT MONITORING
• Monitor for myelosuppression 7–10 days after chemotherapy.
• Take thoracic radiographs every 2–3 months after surgery.
• Take radiographs of graft site every 2–3 months after surgery because local recurrence is possible after limb salvage.

PREVENTION/AVOIDANCE
N/A

POSSIBLE COMPLICATIONS
• Metastasis
• Hypertrophic osteopathy

EXPECTED COURSE AND PROGNOSIS

Dogs
• Median survival without treatment, with amputation alone, or with palliative radiotherapy alone—approximately 4 months
• Median survival with surgery and chemotherapy—10 months
• Mandibular osteosarcoma—less aggressive than other sites; 1-year survival with surgery alone—71% reported

Cats
• Appendicular—median survival with surgery: > 2 years
• Axial—median survival with surgery: 5.5 months

MISCELLANEOUS

ASSOCIATED CONDITIONS
N/A

AGE-RELATED FACTORS
N/A

ZOONOTIC POTENTIAL
None

PREGNANCY
Do not breed animals undergoing chemotherapy.

SYNONYM
Osteogenic sarcoma

SEE ALSO
• Chondrosarcoma, Bone
• Fibrosarcoma, Bone
• Hemangiosarcoma, Bone

Suggested Reading
Botettp WV, Patnaik AK, Schrader SC, et al. Osteosarcoma in cats: 22 cases (1974–1984). J Am Vet Med Assoc 1987;190:91–93.
Morrison WB. Cancer drug pharmacology and clinical experience. In: Morrison WB, ed. Cancer in dogs and cats: medical and surgical management. Baltimore: Williams & Wilkins, 1998:359–385.
Waters DJ, Cooley DM. Skeletal neoplasms. In: Morrison WB, ed. Cancer in dogs and cats: medical and surgical management. Baltimore: Williams & Wilkins, 1998:639–654.
Author Ruthanne Chun
Consulting Editor Wallace B. Morrison

OTITIS EXTERNA AND MEDIA

BASICS

DEFINITION
• Otis externa—inflammation of the external ear canal
• Otitis media—inflammation of the middle ear
• The terms are not diagnoses but descriptions of clinical signs.

PATHOPHYSIOLOGY
• Otis externa—chronic inflammation results in alterations in the normal environment of the canal; the external ear canal is lined with epithelium containing modified apocrine (cerumen) glands; the glands enlarge and produce excessive wax; the epidermis and dermis thicken and become fibrotic; thickened canal folds effectively reduce canal width; calcification of auricular cartilage is the end-stage result.
• Otitis media—often an extension of otitis externa through a ruptured tympanum; may occur without a membrane being ruptured; can occur from polyps or neoplasia within the middle ear

SYSTEMS AFFECTED
• Skin/Exocrine
• Nervous—inflammation of the vestibulo-cochlear nerve

GENETICS
N/A

INCIDENCE/PREVALENCE
N/A

GEOGRAPHIC DISTRIBUTION
N/A

SIGNALMENT
Species
Dogs and cats

Breed Predilections
• Pendulous-eared dogs, especially spaniels and retrievers
• Dogs with hirsute external canals—terriers and poodles
• Stenosis of the external ear canal is common in shar peis.

Mean Age And Range
N/A

Predominant Sex
None

SIGNS
General Comments
• Otitis externa—often a secondary symptom of an underlying disease
• Infection—purulent and malodorous exudate
• Inflammation—exudation, pain, pruritus, and erythema

• Chronic otitis externa (dogs)—results in tympanic membrane rupture (71%) and otitis media (82%)

Historical Findings
• Pain
• Head shaking
• Scratching at the pinnae
• Malodorous ears

Physical Examination Findings
• Redness and swelling of the external canal, leading to stenosis
• Scaling and exudation—may result in malodor and canal obstruction
• Cats—hold the pinna down or tilt the head
• Vestibular signs (with head tilt, nystagmus, anorexia, ataxia, and infrequent vomiting) indicate development of otitis media/interna.

CAUSES
Primary Causes
• Parasites (otitis externa)—*Otodectes cynotis, Demodex* spp., *Sarcoptes* and *Notoedres,* and *Otobius megnini*
• Hypersensitivities—atopy, food allergy, contact allergy, and systemic or local drug reaction
• Foreign bodies—plant awns
• Obstructions—neoplasia, polyps, cerumen gland hyperplasia, and accumulation of hair; may also be a secondary event
• Keratinization disorders and increased cerumen production—functional obstruction of the ear canal
• Autoimmune diseases—frequently affect the pinnae; sometime affect the external ear canal

Perpetuating Factors
• Secondary bacterial infections—common; *Staphylococcus intermedius* most often cultured from the horizontal canal in otitis externa; *Pseudomonas* spp, *Proteus* spp., *Corynebacterium* spp., and *E. coli* frequently reported; *Pseudomonas* spp. most often cultured in otitis media
• Infections—often mixed with, or entirely the result of, *Malassezia pachydermatis;* other yeast (*Candida*) or fungal species rare
• Progressive changes—canal hypertrophy, cerumen gland hyperplasia and adenitis, fibrosis, and cartilage calcification; cause recalcitrant otitis externa; prevent return to a normal ear canal even with proper treatment
• Otitis media—can produce symptoms on its own; can act as a reservoir for organisms, causing recurrent condition

RISK FACTORS
• Abnormal or breed-related conformation of the external canal (e.g., stenosis, hirsutism, and pendulous pinnae) restricts proper air flow into the canal.

• Excessive moisture (e.g., from swimming or frequent cleanings with improper solutions) can lead to infection; overzealous client compliance with recommendations for ear cleanings common
• Topical drug reaction and irritation and trauma from abrasive cleaning techniques
• Underlying systemic diseases produce abnormalities in the environment and ear canal immune response.

DIAGNOSIS

DIFFERENTIAL DIAGNOSIS
N/A

CBC/BIOCHEMISTRY/URINALYSIS
May indicate a primary underlying disease

OTHER LABORATORY TESTS
N/A

IMAGING
Bullae radiographs—otitis media

DIAGNOSTIC PROCEDURES
• Skin scrapings from the pinna—parasites
• Skin biopsy—autoimmune disease, neoplasia, or cerumen gland hyperplasia
• Culture of exudate—rarely assists in devising a treatment plan; reserve for resistant infection
• Microscopic examination of aural exudate—single most important diagnostic tool after complete examination of the ear canal
• Appearance of the exudate—yeast infections commonly produce a yellow-tan thick exudate; bacterial infections commonly produce a brownish black thin exudate; however, appearance does not allow an accurate diagnosis of the type of infection; microscopic examination necessary
• Infections within the canal can change with prolonged or recurrent therapy; repeat examination of aural exudate is required in chronic cases.

Microscopic Examination
• Preparations—make from both canals (the contents of the canals may not be the same); spread samples thinly on a glass microscope slide; examine both unstained and modified Wright-stained samples.
• Mites—presumptive diagnosis
• Type(s) of bacteria or yeast—assist in the choice of therapy
• Findings (types of organisms; WBCs)—note in the record; rank the number of organisms and cell types on a scale of 0–4 to allow treatment monitoring
• WBCs within the exudate—active infection; systemic antibiotic therapy may be warranted.

PATHOLOGIC FINDINGS
N/A

OTITIS EXTERNA AND MEDIA

TREATMENT

APPROPRIATE HEALTH CARE
Outpatient, unless severe vestibular signs are noted

NURSING CARE
N/A

ACTIVITY
No restrictions

DIET
No restrictions unless a food allergy is suspected

CLIENT EDUCATION
Teach clients, by demonstration, the proper method for cleaning ears.

SURGICAL CONSIDERATIONS
• Indicated when the canal is severely stenotic or obstructed or when neoplasia or a polyp is diagnosed
• Severe, unresponsive otitis media may require a bullae osteotomy.

MEDICATIONS

DRUGS OF CHOICE

Systemic
• Antibiotics—useful in severe cases of bacterial otitis externa; mandatory when the tympanum has ruptured; trimethoprim-potentiated sulfonamides (dosage varies by preparation), cephalexin (25 mg/kg q8–12h), enrofloxacin (2.5 mg/kg q12h), or clindamycin (10 mg/kg q12h)
• Antifungals—use with overwhelming yeast or fungal infection; ketoconazole (5–10 mg/kg q12h)
• Corticosteroids—reduce swelling and pain; reduce wax production; anti-inflammatory dosages of prednisone (0.25–0.5 mg/kg q12h); use sparingly and for short durations only
• Ivermectin—various external ear parasites; 300 µg/kg SC weekly for 4 weeks eliminates *Otodectes* infestation.

Topical
• Topical therapy paramount for resolution and control of otitis externa.
• First, completely clean the external ear canal of debris; complete flushing under general anesthesia reserved for uncooperative patients or severe cases, including otitis media
• Second, thoroughly clean the ear daily during initial therapy; then every 3–7 days once signs resolve

• Finally, apply appropriate topical medications frequently and in sufficient quantity to completely treat the entire canal.
• Not recommended—combination ointments (e.g., Otomax, Panalog, Liquachlor), which often accumulate and perpetuate the condition
• Recommended—antibacterial (e.g., gentocin) or antiyeast drops (miconazole), with or without corticosteroid; commercial ear cleansers with cerumenolytics, antiseptics, and astringents; Alocetic for routine cleaning or when the competence of the tympanic membrane is in question; chlorhexidine-containing solutions (e.g., Chlorhexiderm Flush, Hexadene Flush) for more severe cases when the tympanic membrane is intact (controversial)
• Cerumenolytics—dioctyl sodium sulfosuccinate or carbamide peroxide; emulsify waxes facilitating removal
• Antiseptics—acetic acid or chlorhexidine gluconate; reduce or eliminate infectious organisms
• Astringents—isopropyl alcohol, boric acid, or salicylic acid; reduce moisture
• Antibiotics, antifungals, and/or parasiticides—use only when presence of organism(s) has been confirmed.
• Ivermectin—effective for ear mites in cats, but recurrence rates higher than with other parasiticides; use only for large numbers of animals (kennels) or when a persistent carrier state is suspected
• Resistance to medications—perform a culture and sensitivity of the aural exudate; recently, suspensions of silver sulfadiazine and of enrofloxacin have been shown to be effective
• Generally, ingredients should be limited to those needed to treat a specific infection (i.e., antibiotics only for a bacterial infection).

CONTRAINDICATIONS
• Ivermectin—not FDA approved for treating ear mites; client disclosure and consent are paramount before administration; herding breeds (dogs) have increased sensitivity and should not be treated with this drug.
• Ruptured tympanum—use caution with topical cleansers and medications other than sterile saline or dilute acetic acid; potential for ototoxicity is a concern; controversial

PRECAUTIONS
• Use extreme caution when cleaning the external ear canals of all animals with severe and chronic otitis externa, because the tympanum can easily be ruptured.
• Postflushing vestibular complications are common in cats, although usually temporary; warn clients of possible complications and residual effects.

POSSIBLE INTERACTIONS
Several topical medications infrequently induce contact irritation or allergic response; re-evaluate all worsening cases

ALTERNATIVE DRUGS
N/A

FOLLOW-UP

PATIENT MONITORING
Repeat exudate examinations can assist in monitoring infection.

PREVENTION/AVOIDANCE
• Routine ear cleaning by the client
• Control of underlying diseases

POSSIBLE COMPLICATIONS
Uncontrolled otitis externa can lead to otitis media, deafness, vestibular disease, cellulitis, facial nerve paralysis, progression to otitis interna, and rarely meningoencephalitis.

EXPECTED COURSE AND PROGNOSIS
• Otitis externa—with proper therapy, most cases resolve in 3–4 weeks; failure to correct underlying primary cause results in recurrence.
• Perpetuating factors (e.g., stenosis of the ear canal and calcification of the auricular cartilage) will not resolve and may result in recurrence.
• Otitis media—may take 6+ weeks of systemic antibiotics until all signs have resolved and the tympanic membrane has healed

MISCELLANEOUS

ASSOCIATED CONDITIONS
N/A

AGE-RELATED FACTORS
N/A

ZOONOTIC POTENTIAL
Potenially *Sarcoptes* or *Notoedres* mite infestation and fungal infection

PREGNANCY
Do not use systemic glucocorticoids during pregnancy, if possible.

SYNONYMS
N/A

SEE ALSO
Causes

Suggested Reading
Griffin CE. Otitis externa and otitis media. In: Griffin CE, Griffin CE, Kwochka KW, MacDonald JM, eds. Current veterinary dermatology: the science and art of therapy. St. Louis: 1993.

Author Alexander H. Werner
Consulting Editor Karen Helton Rhodes

DISEASES

OTITIS MEDIA AND INTERNA

BASICS

DEFINITION
Inflammation of the middle (otitis media) and inner (otitis interna) ears most commonly caused by bacterial infection

PATHOPHYSIOLOGY
• Most often arises from extension of infection of the external ear through the tympanic membrane; may extend from the oral and nasopharyngeal cavities via the eustachian tube • Interna—may also result from hematogenous spread of a systemic infection

SYSTEMS AFFECTED
• Nervous—vestibulocochlear receptors in the inner ear and the facial nerve and sympathetic chain in the middle ear (peripheral) with possible extension of infection intracranially (central) • Ophthalmic—cornea and conjunctiva; from exposure and/or lack of tear production after nerve damage • Gastrointestinal—taste; from damage to the parasympathetic branch of the facial nerve (chordae tympani) supplying the ipsilateral rostral two thirds of the tongue

GENETICS
N/A

INCIDENCE/PREVALENCE
N/A

GEOGRAPHIC DISTRIBUTION
N/A

SIGNALMENT

Species
Dogs and cats

Breed Predilections
• Cocker spaniels and other long-eared breeds
• Poodles with chronic otitis or pharyngitis from dental disease

Mean Age and Range
Any age

Predominant Sex
N/A

SIGNS

General Comments
Related to the severity and extent of the infection; may range from none to those related to bulla discomfort and nervous system involvement

Historical Findings
• Pain when opening the mouth; reluctance to chew; shaking the head; pawing at the affected ear • Head tilt • Patient may lean, veer, or roll toward the side affected with peripheral vestibulitis. • Vestibular deficits—may be transient and episodic • Bilateral involvement—may note wide head excursions, truncal ataxia, and deafness

• Vomiting and nausea—may occur during the acute phase • Facial nerve damage—saliva and food dropping from the corner of the mouth; an inability to blink; ocular discharge • Anisocoria and/or protrusion of the third eyelid (Horners syndrome)—may be noted

Physical Examination Findings
• Evidence of aural erythema, discharge, and thick and stenotic canals support otitis externa. • Gray, dull, opaque, and bulging tympanic membrane on otoscopic examination indicates a middle ear exudate. • Dental tartar, gingivitis, tonsillitis, or pharyngitis—may be associated • Ipsilateral mandibular lymphadenopathy—may occur with severe infections • Pain—upon opening the mouth or bulla palpation may be detected. • Corneal ulcer—may be caused by inability to blink or a dry eye

Neurologic Examination Findings
• Damage to the associated neurologic structures depends on the severity and location.
• Vestibular portion of cranial nerve VIII—when vestibular portion is affected, there is always an ipsilateral head tilt.
• Bilateral damage of cranial nerve VIII—rare; patient is reluctant to move and may stay in a crouched posture with wide head excursions; physiologic nystagmus poor to absent
• Nystagmus—resting or positional and rotatory or horizontal; may be seen
• Vestibular strabismus—ipsilateral ventral deviation of eyeball with neck extension; may be noted
• Ipsilateral leaning, veering, falling, or rolling—may occur
• Facial nerve damage—ipsilateral paresis/paralysis of the ear, eyelids, lips, and nares; may be reduced tear production (indicated by the Schirmer tear test); with chronic facial nerve paralysis, contracture of the affected side of the face caused by fibrosis of the denervated muscles; deficits can be bilateral.
• Affected sympathetic chain—Horners syndrome; always miosis of the affected pupil; may note protrusion of the third eyelid, ptosis, and enophthalmos

CAUSES
• Bacteria—primary agents
• Yeast (*Malassezia* spp., *Candida* spp.) and *Aspergillus*—agents to consider
• Mites—predispose patient to secondary bacterial infections
• Unilateral disease—foreign bodies, trauma, polyps, and tumors (e.g., fibromas, squamous cell carcinoma, ceruminous gland carcinoma, and primary bone tumors)

RISK FACTORS
• Nasopharyngeal polyps and inner, middle, or outer ear neoplasia—may predispose patient to bacterial infection.
• Vigorous ear flush

• Ear cleaning solutions (e.g., chlorhexidine)—may be irritating to the middle and inner ear; avoid if the tympanum is ruptured.
• Inhalant anesthesia and traveling by airplane—change middle ear pressures

DIAGNOSIS

DIFFERENTIAL DIAGNOSIS
• Signs associated with congenital vestibular anomalies are present from birth.
• Hypothyroidism—may cause a polyneuropathy with a predilection for cranial nerves VII and VIII; abnormal thyroid profile (T_4, free T_4, TSH level or response) supports the diagnosis.
• Central vestibular diseases—differentiated by occurrence of lethargy, somnolence, stupor, and other brainstem signs
• Neoplasia and nasopharyngeal polyps—common causes of refractory and relapsing otitis media and interna; diagnosed by imaging of the head
• Thiamine deficiency (cats)—bilateral central vestibular signs; history of an all-fish diet or persistent anorexia helps the diagnosis.
• Metronidazole toxicity—bilateral central vestibular signs after high dosage or prolonged use
• Trauma—history and physical evidence of injury
• Idiopathic vestibular disease (old dogs and young to middle-aged cats), idiopathic facial paralysis, and idiopathic Horners syndrome—diagnoses made by exclusion

CBC/BIOCHEMISTRY/URINALYSIS
• Leukocytosis with a left shift—may be noted
• Globulins—may be high if infection is chronic
• Urinalysis—usually normal; pyuria and bacteriuria may be seen if the bacterial infection is hematogenous.

OTHER LABORATORY TESTS
• Blood and/or urine cultures—may be positive with a hematogenous source of infection
• Low T_4, free T_4 with a high TSH level, or inadequate elevation of T_4 levels after a TSH response test—hypothyroidism

IMAGING
• Bullae radiographs—tympanic bullae may appear cloudy if exudate is present; may see thickening of the bullae and petrous temporal bone with chronic disease; may see lysis of the bone with severe cases of osteomyelitis; may be normal
• CT and MRI—detailed evidence of fluid and soft tissue density within the middle ear and the extent of involvement of the adjacent structures; CT better at revealing associated

bony changes

DIAGNOSTIC PROCEDURES
• Myringotomy—insert a spinal needle (20 gauge; 2.5–3.5 in.) through the otoscope and tympanic membrane to aspirate middle ear fluid for cytologic examination and culture and sensitivity.
• BAER—test the functional integrity of the peripheral and central auditory pathways; detect any associated hearing loss
• CSF analysis—if neutrophilic pleocytosis and increased protein with intracranial extension of the infection are noted, perform culture and sensitivity

PATHOLOGIC FINDINGS
Purulent exudate within the middle ear cavity surrounded by a thickened bullae and microscopic evidence of degenerative neutrophils with intracellular bacteria characteristic

 TREATMENT

APPROPRIATE HEALTH CARE
• Inpatient—severe debilitating infection; neurologic signs
• Discharge stable patients, pending further diagnostics and surgery, if indicated.

NURSING CARE
• Fluid therapy—if unable to eat or drink owing to vomiting and disorientation
• Concurrent otitis externa—culture and clean the ear; use warm normal saline if the tympanum is ruptured; if a cleaning solution is used, follow with a thorough flush with normal saline; dry the ear canal with a cotton swab and low vacuum suction; astringents (e.g., Otic Domeboro or boric acid) can be effective.

ACTIVITY
Restrict with substantial vestibular signs to avoid injury.

DIET
• Vomiting from vestibulitis—withhold food and water for 12–24 hr
• Severe disorientation—hand feed and water small amounts frequently; elevate head to avoid aspiration pneumonia.

CLIENT EDUCATION
• Inform client that most bacterial infections resolve with an early aggressive course of broad-spectrum antibiotics and do not recur.
• Warn client that relapsing signs may occur and may require surgical drainage if bony structure changes and/or middle ear effusion are evident on imaging studies.

SURGICAL CONSIDERATIONS
• Reserve surgery for relapsing or nonresponsive patients.

• Do not rely on severity of neurologic signs as an indication for surgical intervention; reserve surgery for patients with evidence of middle ear exudate, osteomyelitis refractory to medical management, and nasopharyngeal polyps or neoplasia.
• Bullae osteotomy—allows drainage of the middle ear cavity
• Ear ablation through the horizontal ear canal—indicated when otitis media is associated with recurrent otitis externa or neoplasia
• Cytologic examination and culture and sensitivity of middle ear effusion and histopathologic evaluation of samples of abnormal tissue—perform at the time of surgery

 MEDICATIONS

DRUGS OF CHOICE
• Topical water-based or ophthalmic antibiotic solutions—chloramphenicol or a triple antibiotic preparation; preferred
• Antibiotics—long-term (6–8 weeks); broad-spectrum systemic agents; select on basis of culture and sensitivity, if available
• Penicillinase-resistant penicillin and cephalosporins—good initial drugs

CONTRAINDICATIONS
• Ruptured tympanum or associated neurologic deficits—avoid oil-based or irritating external ear preparations (e.g., chlorhexidine) and aminoglycosides, which are toxic to inner ear structures
• Otitis media or interna—topical and systemic corticosteroids contraindicated; may exacerbate the signs associated with infection

PRECAUTIONS
Avoid rigorously flushing the external ear; may result in or exacerbate signs of otitis media or interna.

POSSIBLE INTERACTIONS
N/A

ALTERNATIVE DRUGS
N/A

 FOLLOW-UP

PATIENT MONITORING
Evaluate for resolution of signs after 10–14 days or sooner if the patient is deteriorating.

PREVENTION/AVOIDANCE
• Routine ear cleaning and dental prophylaxis—may reduce chances of infection

POSSIBLE COMPLICATIONS
• Signs associated with vestibular and facial nerve damage or Horners syndrome—may remain • Severe infections—may spread to the brainstem • Osteomyelitis of the petrous temporal bone and middle ear cavity effusion—common sequela to severe, chronic infections • Bulla osteotomy—postoperative complications include Horners syndrome, facial paralysis, and onset or exacerbation of vestibular dysfunction. • Cats—consider avoiding bilateral bullae osteotomies in patients with bilateral effusions; may be an increased incidence of death after surgery.

EXPECTED COURSE AND PROGNOSIS
• Otitis media and interna—usually responsive to medical management • When medical management is ineffective, a surgical evaluation for lateral ear resection should be explored. • Vestibular signs—improvement in 2–6 weeks; more rapid in small dogs and in cats

 MISCELLANEOUS

ASSOCIATED CONDITIONS
N/A

AGE-RELATED FACTORS
Ear mites more common in kittens and puppies

ZOONOTIC POTENTIAL
N/A

PREGNANCY
N/A

SYNONYMS
Middle and inner ear infections

SEE ALSO
• Facial Nerve Paresis/Paralysis • Head Tilt (Vestibular Disease) • Horners Syndrome • Otitis Externa and Media

ABBREVIATIONS
• BAER = brainstem auditory-evoked response • CSF = cerebrospinal fluid • TSH = thyroid-stimulating hormone

Suggested Reading
Bruyette DS, Lorenz MD. Otitis externa and media: diagnostic and medical aspects. Semin Vet Med Surg Small Anim 1993;8:3–9.
Schunk KL, Averill DR. Peripheral vestibular syndrome in the dog: a review of 83 cases. J Am Vet Med Assoc 1983;182:1354–1358.
Author Richard J. Joseph
Consulting Editor Joane M. Parent

OVARIAN TUMORS

BASICS

OVERVIEW
• Epithelial (carcinoma), germ cell (dysgerminoma and teratoma), and sex-cord stromal (granulosa cell tumor, Sertoli-Leydig cell tumor, thecoma, and luteoma) tumors
• Dogs—rare (0.5%–1.2% of tumors); 40% carcinomas, 10% germ cell, and 50% sex-cord
• Cats—extremely rare (0.7%–3.6% of tumors); 15% germ cell and 85% sex-cord
• Metastasis common
• Some tumors produce hormones.

SIGNALMENT
• Dogs and cats
• Middle-aged to old animals
• Teratoma develops in young patients.

SIGNS
• Tumors that produce steroid hormones—anestrus; persistent estrus; pyometra; gynecomastia; bilaterally symmetrical alopecia; pancytopenia; masculinization
• Ascites or pleural effusion—occasionally
• Other signs associated with mass effects of the tumor

CAUSES & RISK FACTORS
Intact sexual status

DIAGNOSIS

DIFFERENTIAL DIAGNOSIS
• Other causes of abdominal effusion
• Other midabdominal mass

CBC/BIOCHEMISTRY/URINALYSIS
No consistent abnormalities

OTHER LABORATORY TESTS
N/A

IMAGING
• Abdominal radiography—may reveal unilateral or bilateral midabdominal mass at the caudal pole of the kidney or effusion
• Abdominal ultrasound—confirm abdominal radiographic findings
• Thoracic radiography—may reveal metastasis

DIAGNOSTIC PROCEDURES
• Cytologic evaluation of pleural or abdominal fluid—may be diagnostic for malignant effusion
• Histopathologic examination—necessary for definitive diagnosis

TREATMENT
• Ovariohysterectomy—treatment of choice for a solitary mass
• Peritoneal transplantation during surgical removal is possible.

MEDICATIONS

DRUGS

• Chemotherapy—little information for dogs and cats
• Cyclophosphamide, chlorambucil, lomustine, and bleomycin—successful treatment in one patient (dog)
• Cisplatin—successful treatment in three dogs

CONTRAINDICATIONS/POSSIBLE INTERACTIONS

Cisplatin—do not use in cats; do not use in dogs with renal disease.

 FOLLOW-UP

• Abdominal and thoracic radiography—every 3 months; monitor for recurrence and metastasis
• Ovariohysterectomy—prevention
• Prognosis—guarded
• Chemotherapy—has potential to lengthen survival

 MISCELLANEOUS

ASSOCIATED CONDITIONS

• Pyometra
• Ovarian cysts
• Cystic endometrial hyperplasia

Suggested Reading

Morrison WB. Cancer of the reproductive tract. In: Morrison WB, ed., Cancer in dogs and cats: medical and surgical management. Baltimore: Williams & Wilkins, 1998:581–590.

Patnaik AK, Greenlee PG. Canine ovarian neoplasms: a clinicopathologic study of 71 cases including histology of 12 granulosa cell tumors. Vet Pathol 1987;24:509–514.

Author Terrance A. Hamilton
Consulting Editor Wallace B. Morrison

PANCREATITIS

BASICS

DEFINITION
• Inflammation of the pancreas • Acute pancreatitis—inflammation of the pancreas that occurs abruptly with little or no permanent pathologic change • Chronic pancreatitis—continuing inflammatory disease that is often accompanied by irreversible morphologic change

PATHOPHYSIOLOGY
• Most defense mechanisms prevent pancreatic autodigestion by the enzymes it secretes. • Under select circumstances, these natural defenses fail; autodigestion occurs when these digestive enzymes are activated within acinar cells. • Local and systemic tissue injury is due to the activity of released pancreatic enzymes and a variety of inflammatory mediators such as kinins, free radicals, and complement factors.

SYSTEMS AFFECTED
• Gastrointestinal—altered GI motility (ileus) due to regional chemical peritonitis; local or generalized peritonitis due to enhanced vascular permeability; concurrent inflammatory bowel disease may be seen in cats. • Hepatobiliary—lesions due to shock, pancreatic enzyme injury, inflammatory cellular infiltrates, and intra/extrahepatic cholestasis • Respiratory—pulmonary edema or pleural effusion; adult respiratory distress syndrome is an uncommon but potentially fatal sequel with systemic complications • Cardiovascular—cardiac arrhythmias may result from release of myocardial depressant factor. • Hematologic—activation of the coagulation cascade and systemic consumptive coagulopathy (DIC) occur

INCIDENCE/PREVALENCE
• Unknown • Up to 1% of normal dogs have histologic evidence of pancreatitis. • Necropsy surveys suggest an increased prevalence in cats with cholangiohepatitis, hepatic lipidosis and inflammatory bowel disease.

SIGNALMENT

Species
Dogs and cats

Breed Predilections
• Miniature schnauzer • Miniature poodle • Cocker spaniel • Siamese cats

Mean Age and Range
• Acute pancreatitis is most common in middle-aged and old (>7 years) dogs; mean age at presentation is 6.5 years. • Mean age for acute pancreatitis in cats is 7.3 years.

Predominant Sex
Female—dogs

SIGNS

General Comments
• Dogs—GI tract signs • Cats—vague, nonspecific, and nonlocalizing

Historical Findings
• Lethargy/depression/anorexia—common in dogs and cats • Vomiting—common in dogs, less common in cats • Weight loss—common in cats • Dogs may exhibit abdominal pain. • Diarrhea—more frequently seen in dogs than cats

Physical Examination Findings
• Severe lethargy—both species • Dehydration—common; due to GI loss • Abdominal pain • Mass lesions may be palpable in both dogs and cats. • Fever—common in dogs; both fever and hypothermia reported in cats • Icterus—more common in cats • Less common systemic abnormalities include respiratory distress, bleeding disorders, and cardiac arrhythmias.

CAUSES
Usually unknown; possibilities include:
• Nutritional factors (e.g., hyperlipoproteinemia) • Pancreatic trauma/ischemia • Duodenal reflux • Drugs/toxins (see Contraindications) • Pancreatic duct obstruction • Hypercalcemia • Infectious agents—toxoplasmosis, feline infectious peritonitis (FIP)

RISK FACTORS
• Breed • Obesity in dogs • Concurrent disease in dogs (e.g., diabetes mellitus, hyperadrenocorticism, chronic renal failure, and neoplasia) • Recent drug administration (see Contraindications) • Concurrent hepatic/gut inflammatory disease • See Causes

DIAGNOSIS

DIFFERENTIAL DIAGNOSIS
Other causes of acute abdomen:
• GI disease (obstruction, foreign body, perforation, gastroenteritis, ulcer disease)—exclude with CBC/biochemistry/urinalysis, imaging, paracentesis, and endoscopy with biopsy • Splenic torsion—exclude with imaging • Hypoadrenocorticism—exclude with CBC/biochemistry/urinalysis, ACTH stimulation test • Urogenital disease (pyelonephritis, prostatitis or abscessation, pyometra, urinary tract rupture or obstruction, acute renal failure)—exclude with CBC/biochemistry/urinalysis, urine culture/sensitivity and imaging • Hepatobiliary disease (cholangiohepatitis)—exclude with CBC/biochemistry /urinalysis, bile acids, imaging, and biopsy • Abdominal neoplasia—exclude with imaging and cytology or biopsy

CBC/BIOCHEMISTRY/URINALYSIS
• CBC—in dogs often reveals hemoconcentra-tion, leukocytosis with a left shift, and toxic neutrophils; cats are more variable and may show neutrophilia (30%) and nonregenerative anemia (26%) • Serum biochemistries—often show prerenal azotemia, liver enzyme activities (ALT, ALP) are often high because of hepatic ischemia or exposure to pancreatic toxins; hyperbilirubinemia is more common in cats and is due to hepatocellular damage and intra/extrahepatic biliary obstruction; hyperglycemia is seen in dogs and cats with necrotizing pancreatitis due to hyperglucagonemia; may see mild hypoglycemia in dogs; cats with suppurative pancreatitis may be hypoglycemic; hypercholesterolemia and hypertriglyceridemia are common • Urinalysis—unremarkable

OTHER LABORATORY TESTS
• Serum amylase and lipase activities—may be elevated in dogs but are nonspecific; also increase with hepatic, renal, or neoplastic disease in the absence of pancreatitis; dexamethasone may increase serum lipase concentrations in dogs; lipase may be normal or high in cats; lipase activity is a more reliable marker for the diagnosis of canine pancreatitis; normal plasma lipase activity does not rule out disease • TLI assay—TLI is pancreatic specific, and serum concentrations may be increased with acute pancreatitis in dogs and cats; serum TLI tends to peak before and decreases more rapidly than amylase and lipase in dogs; reduced glomerular filtration may also increase serum TLI; normal TLI assay results do not rule out pancreatitis. • ELISA for trypsinogen activation peptide (TAP)—acute pancreatitis stimulates intrapancreatic activation of trypsinogens, with the release of TAP into the serum; TAP is then eliminated from the body in the urine; a recent ELISA test detects TAP in urine and plasma but is not yet commercially available; this assay appears to be specific and rapid for the diagnosis of acute pancreatitis in the dog.

IMAGING
• Abdominal radiographs—may include increased soft tissue opacity in the right cranial abdominal compartment; loss of visceral detail ("ground glass appearance") due to abdominal effusion; static gas pattern in the proximal duodenum; widened angle between pyloric antrum and proximal duodenum • Thoracic radiographs—may be mild pleural effusion or more severe pulmonary complications • Abdominal ultrasound—nonhomogeneous solid or cystic mass lesions indicate pancreatic abscess; may be a pancreatic mass or altered echogenicity in the area of the pancreas; may see peritoneal effusion and extrahepatic biliary obstruction

DIAGNOSTIC PROCEDURES
Ultrasound-guided needle-aspiration biopsy may confirm a diagnosis.

PATHOLOGIC FINDINGS

• Gross findings (acute pancreatitis)—mild swelling with edematous pancreatitis; grayish yellow areas of pancreatic necrosis with varying amounts of hemorrhage with necrotizing pancreatitis • Gross findings (chronic pancreatitis)—pancreas is reduced in size, firm, gray, and irregular; may contain extensive adhesions to surrounding viscera • Microscopic changes (acute pancreatitis)— include edema, parenchymal necrosis, and neutrophilic cellular infiltrate with acute lesions • Microscopic changes (chronic pancreatitis)—pancreatic fibrosis around ducts, ductal epithelial hyperplasia, and mononuclear cellular infiltrate; inflammatory lesions may also be seen in the hepatic parenchyma and intestinal mucosa of cats

TREATMENT

APPROPRIATE HEALTH CARE

• Inpatient medical management • Aggressive IV fluid therapy • Fluid therapy goals—correct hypovolemia and maintain pancreatic microcirculation. • A balanced electrolyte solution such as lactated Ringer solution (LRS) is first-choice rehydration fluid • Correct initial dehydration (ml = % dehydration × weight in kg × 1000) and give over 4–6 hr. • May need colloids (oxyglobin, hetastarch) • Following replacement of deficits, give additional fluids to match maintenance requirements (2.5 × weight in kg) and on-going losses (estimated). • Potassium chloride (KCl) supplementation usually needed because of potassium loss in the vomitus; base potassium supplementation on measured serum levels (use 20 mEq of KCl/L of IV fluid if serum potassium levels are not known; do not administer faster than 0.5 mEq/kg/h)

ACTIVITY

Restrict

DIET

• NPO 3–5 days to reduce pancreatic secretions; failure to withhold oral intake for this minimum time may result in relapse; once no vomiting 24–48 hr, offer small volumes of water; if tolerated, begin small, frequent feedings of a carbohydrate (e.g., boiled rice); gradually introduce a protein source of high biologic value such as cottage cheese or lean meat. • Avoid high-protein and high-fat diets • Patients needing extended NPO may require jejun-ostomy enteral feeding or total parenteral nutrition.

CLIENT EDUCATION

• Discuss the need for extended hospitalization. • Discuss the expense of diagnosis and treatment. • Discuss possible short-term and long-term complications (see Associated Conditions).

SURGICAL CONSIDERATIONS

• May need surgery to remove pseudocysts, abscesses, or devitalized tissue seen with necrotizing pancreatitis. • May need laparotomy and pancreatic biopsy to confirm pancreatitis and/or rule out other, nonpancreatic diseases • Extrahepatic biliary obstruction from pancreatitis requires surgical correction.

MEDICATIONS

DRUGS OF CHOICE

• Corticosteroids only indicated in shock • Centrally acting antiemetics indicated with intractable vomiting—chlorpromazine (0.5 mg/kg IM or SC q8h) or prochlorperazine (0.1 mg/kg q8h) antibiotics if evidence of sepsis—penicillin G (20,000 U/kg q6h), ampicillin sodium (20 mg/kg q8h), and possibly aminoglycosides (gentamicin 3–4 mg/kg IV q12h) • Analgesics to relieve abdominal pain (butorphanol 0.4 mg/kg IV or SC q8h)

CONTRAINDICATIONS

• Anticholinergics (e.g., atropine) • Azathioprine• Chlorothiazide • Estrogens • Furosemide • Tetracycline

PRECAUTIONS

• Only use phenothiazine antiemetics in well-hydrated patients; these drugs have hypotensive properties.

FOLLOW-UP

PATIENT MONITORING

• Evaluate hydration status closely during first 24 h of therapy; twice daily check physical examination, body weight, hematocrit, total plasma protein, BUN, and urine output. • Evaluate the effectiveness of fluid therapy after 24 h and adjust flow rates and fluid composition accordingly; repeat biochemistries to assess electrolyte/acid–base status • Repeat plasma enzyme concentrations (lipase or TLI) after 48 h to evaluate the inflammatory process. • Watch closely for systemic complications involving a variety of organ systems; perform appropriate diagnostic tests as needed (see Associated Conditions). • Gradually taper fluids down to maintenance requirements if possible. • Gradually introduce oral alimentation as described above.

PREVENTION/AVOIDANCE

• Weight reduction if obese • Avoid high-fat diets. • Avoid drugs that may precipitate disease (see Contraindications).

POSSIBLE COMPLICATIONS

• Failed response to supportive therapy • Life-threatening associated conditions

EXPECTED COURSE AND PROGNOSIS

• Fair—most patients with edematous pancreatitis; these patients usually respond to appropriate symptomatic therapy; relapse or treatment failure is most common with premature oral alimentation. • More guarded to poor— patients with necrotizing pancreatitis and associated conditions

MISCELLANEOUS

ASSOCIATED CONDITIONS

Life-Threatening
• Pulmonary edema (e.g., adult respiratory distress syndrome) • Cardiac arrhythmias • Peritonitis • DIC • Feline hepatic lipidosis

Non–Life-Threatening
• Diabetes mellitus • EPI • Feline cholangiohepatitis • Feline inflammatory bowel disease

AGE-RELATED FACTORS

Most common in middle-aged animals.

SEE ALSO

• Amylase and Lipase • Acute Abdomen • Exocrine Pancreatic Insufficiency (EPI) • Trypsin-like Immunoreactivity (TLI)

ABBREVIATIONS

• ALT = alanine aminotransferase • ALP = alkaline phosphatase • DIC = disseminated intravascular coagulation • EPI = exocrine pancreatic insufficiency • FIP = feline infectious peritonitis • GI = gastrointestinal • NPO = nothing per os • TLI = trypsin-like immunoreactivity

Suggested Reading

Cook AK, Breitschwerdt EB, Levine JF, et al. Risk factors associated with acute pancreatitis in dogs: 101 cases (1985–1990). J Am Vet Med Assoc 1993;203:673–679.

Simpson KW. Current concepts of the pathogenesis and pathophysiology of acute pancreatitis in the dog and cat. Comp Contin Ed Pract Vet 1993;15:247–253.

Simpson KW. Acute pancreatitis. In: August JR, ed. Consultations in feline internal medicine. 3rd ed. Philadelphia: Saunders, 1997:91–98.

Author Albert E. Jergens
Consulting Editors Mitchell A. Crystal and Brett M. Feder

PANNICULITIS

BASICS

OVERVIEW
• An inflammation of the subcutaneous fat tissue
• Uncommon in dogs and cats
• Multiple causes
• Single or multiple subcutaneous nodules or draining tracts
• Usually involves the trunk
• The lipocyte (fat cell) is susceptible to trauma, ischemic disease, and inflammation from adjacent tissues.
• Histology—divided into lobular (involves the fat lobules), septal (involves the interlobular connective tissue septa), and diffuse (involves both lobular and interlobular septa) types
• Diffuse most common in dogs
• Septal most common in cats

SIGNALMENT
• No age, sex, or breed predilection
• Sterile nodular panniculitis—dachshunds are predisposed; collies and miniature poodles are at risk; can occur in any breed

SIGNS
• Lesions—usually occur over the trunk; most dogs have a single nodular lesion over the ventral or lateral trunk; may become cystic and develop draining tracts; may be painful before and just after rupturing; ulcerations often heal with crusting and scarring.
• Early cases of single or multifocal disease—nodules are freely movable underneath the skin; skin overlying the nodule is usually normal but may become erythematous or (less often) brown or yellow.
• Nodules—vary from a few millimeters to several centimeters in diameter; may be firm and well circumscribed or soft and poorly defined; as they enlarge and develop, may fix to the deep dermis (thus the overlying skin is not freely movable)
• Involved fat may necrose.
• Exudate—usually a small amount of oil discharge; yellow-brown to bloody
• Multiple lesions (dogs and cats)—systemic signs common (e.g., anorexia, pyrexia, lethargy, and depression)

CAUSES & RISK FACTORS
• Infectious—bacterial, fungal, atypical mycobacteria, infectious embolism
• Immune-mediated—lupus panniculitis, erythema nodosum
• Idiopathic—sterile nodular panniculitis
• Trauma
• Neoplastic—multicentric mast cell tumors, cutaneous lymphosarcoma
• Foreign bodies
• Postinjection—corticosteroids, vaccines, other subcutaneous injections

DIAGNOSIS

DIFFERENTIAL DIAGNOSIS

Deep Pyoderma
• More common than panniculitis
• More likely over pressure points
• May have associated lesions of superficial pyoderma (e.g., papules, pustules, and epidermal collarettes)
• Aspirates and impression smears—marked numbers of neutrophils with variable numbers of mononuclear cells and bacteria
• Culture/sensitivity and biopsies—confirm diagnosis

Cutaneous Cysts
• Usually nonpainful
• Well-demarcated
• Usually no inflammation
• Aspirates—amorphous debris; no inflammatory cells
• Biopsies—confirm diagnosis

Cutaneous Neoplasia
• Lipomas—soft; usually well demarcated
• No inflammation or draining tracts
• Aspirates—lipocytes; no inflammatory cells
• Biopsies—confirm diagnosis

Mast Cell Tumors/Cutaneous Lymphosarcoma
• Multifocal
• May affect the head, legs, and mucous membranes
• Often erythematous
• Variable presentations
• Aspirates—often suggestive
• Biopsies—confirm diagnosis

Sterile Nodular Panniculitis
- A diagnosis made by ruling out other causes of panniculitis
- Biopsies, cultures, and other diagnostic tests—as indicated by the clinical presentation

CBC/BIOCHEMISTRY/URINALYSIS
- Most cases have no abnormalities.
- Occasional regenerative left shift or eosinophilia
- Mild leukocytosis
- Mild normochromic, normocytic nonregenerative anemia

OTHER LABORATORY TESTS
- Antinuclear antibody
- Direct immunofluorescence testing
- Serum protein electrophoresis
- Serum lipase/amylase levels

IMAGING
Ultrasound—pancreatitis may be a contributing factor (rare)

DIAGNOSTIC PROCEDURES
- Bacterial culture and sensitivity testing—necessary for identifying primary or secondary bacteria
- Fungal and atypical mycobacteria culture
- Biopsies—negative cultures help diagnose sterile nodular panniculitis
- Special stains of histologic samples—help identify causative agent

PATHOLOGIC FINDINGS
- Surgical excisional biopsies—much more accurate than punch biopsy specimens in most cases; punch biopsies do not provide a deep enough sample to make the diagnosis.
- Histologic lesions—required to make a diagnosis of panniculitis; determine septal, lobular, or diffuse inflammatory infiltrate by neutrophils, histiocytes, plasma cells, lymphocytes, eosinophils, or multinucleated giant cells; identify necrosis, fibrosis, or vasculitis.

 TREATMENT
- Single lesions—cured with surgical excision
- Multiple lesions—require systemic medications

 MEDICATIONS
- Positive culture results require appropriate antifungal, antibacterial, or antimycobacterial treatment.
- Sterile nodular panniculitis—systemic treatment with steroids; prednisone (2.2 mg/kg daily) until lesions completely regress (36 weeks); after remission, gradually taper dosage over 2 weeks; occasionally may need slower taper to minimize chance of recurrence; many patients cured; some patients need low-dose alternate-day treatment to maintain remission.
- Oral vitamin E—may control mild cases
- Oral potassium iodide or azathioprine (1 mg/kg daily)—alternatives when steroids are contraindicated

 FOLLOW-UP
- Depends on type and duration of treatment
- Monitor CBC, platelet count, chemistry profile, and urinalysis if immune-suppressing agents or long-term glucocorticosteroids are used.

 MISCELLANEOUS

Suggested Reading
Scott DW, Miller WH, Griffin CE. Muller and Kirk's Small animal dermatology. 5th ed. Philadelphia: Saunders, 1995.
Author Kevin Shanley
Consulting Editor Karen Helton Rhodes

PANOSTEITIS

BASICS

DEFINITION
A self-limiting, painful condition affecting one or more of the long bones of young, medium- to large-breed dogs that is characterized clinically by lameness and radiographically by high density of the marrow cavity.

PATHOPHYSIOLOGY
• Cause unknown
• Attempts to isolate microorganisms have failed
• Metabolic, allergic, or endocrine aberrations—without support
• Pain—may be owing to disturbance of endosteal and periosteal elements, vascular congestion, or high intramedullary pressure

SYSTEMS AFFECTED
Musculoskeletal—lameness of variable intensity; may affect a single limb or become a shifting leg lameness

GENETICS
• No proven transmission
• Predominance of German shepherds in the affected population strongly suggests an inheritable basis.

INCIDENCE/PREVALENCE
No reliable estimates; common

GEOGRAPHIC DISTRIBUTION
N/A

SIGNALMENT

Species
Dogs

Breed Predilections
• German shepherds and German shepherd mixes—most commonly affected
• Medium to large breeds—most commonly affected

Mean Age and Range
• Usually 5–18 months of age
• As young as 2 months and as old as 5 years

Predominant Sex
Male

SIGNS

General Comments
Lameness—if no distinct abnormalities noted on physical examination or radiographs, repeat examinations 4-6 weeks later.

Historical Findings
• No associated trauma
• Lameness—varying intensity; usually involves the forelimbs initially; may affect the hind limbs; may see shifting leg lameness; may be non–weight bearing
• Severe disease—mild depression; inappetence; weight loss

Physical Examination Findings
• Pain—on deep palpation of the long bones (diaphysis) in an affected limb; distinguishing characteristic; palpate firmly along the entire shaft of each bone while carefully avoiding any pinching of nearby muscle.
• Bones—ulna most commonly affected; may affect radius, humerus, femur, and tibia (in decreasing order of frequency) either concurrently or subsequently
• May note low-grade fever
• May see muscle atrophy

CAUSES
Unknown

RISK FACTORS
Purebred German shepherd or German shepherd mix

DIAGNOSIS

DIFFERENTIAL DIAGNOSIS
• Always consider the diagnosis with lameness in a young German shepherd or German shepherd mix.
• May occur alone or with other juvenile orthopedic diseases
• Osteochondritis dissecans
• Fragmented medial coronoid process
• Un-united anconeal process
• Hip dysplasia
• Fractures and ligamentous injuries from unobserved trauma
• Shifting leg lameness—immune-mediated arthritides; Lyme disease; bacterial endocarditis

CBC/BIOCHEMISTRY/URINALYSIS
• Usually normal
• May note eosinophilia early in disease

OTHER LABORATORY TESTS
N/A

IMAGING
• Radiographic densities within the medulla of long bones—characteristic; confirm diagnosis
• Early, middle, and late radiographic lesions
• Early—trabecular pattern of the ends of the diaphysis becomes more prominent; may appear blurred; may see granular opacities
• Middle—patchy sclerotic opacities first around the nutrient foramen and later throughout the diaphysis; widened cortex; thickened periosteum with increased opacity
• Late—during resolution, diminished overall opacity of the medullary canal (toward normal); a coarse trabecular pattern and some granular opacity may remain; may be a period in which the medullary canal becomes more lucent than normal

DIAGNOSTIC PROCEDURES
Bone biopsy—occasionally indicated to rule out neoplasia and bacterial or fungal infections that have similar radiographic appearances

PATHOLOGIC FINDINGS
• Biopsy or necropsy—rarely performed because of excellent prognosis for recovery
• No gross pathologic lesions
• Degeneration of the marrow adipocytes

surrounding the nutrient foramen followed by proliferation of vascular stromal cells within the marrow sinusoids
• Osteoid formation and endosteal new bone formation—progress proximally and distally
• Vascular congestion—may accompany the proliferation of new bone, secondarily stimulating endosteal and periosteal reaction
• Remodeling of the endosteum—occurs during resolution; reestablishes normal endosteal and marrow architecture

 TREATMENT

APPROPRIATE HEALTH CARE
Outpatient

NURSING CARE
Maintenance and replacement fluid therapy—occasionally owing to prolonged periods of inappetence and pyrexia

ACTIVITY
• Limited—not shown to hasten recovery; lessens pain
• Moderate to severe disease—pain may cause self-limited movement leading to muscle atrophy.

DIET
N/A

CLIENT EDUCATION
• Warn client that patient may develop other juvenile orthopedic diseases.
• Inform client that signs of pain and lameness may last for several weeks.
• Warn client that recurrence of clinical signs is common up to 2 years of age.

SURGICAL CONSIDERATIONS
N/A

 MEDICATIONS

DRUGS OF CHOICE
NSAIDs

• Minimize pain; decrease inflammation
• Symptomatic therapy has no bearing on the duration of the disease.
• May try buffered or enteric-coated aspirin (10–25 mg/kg PO q8h or q12h), caroprofen (2.2 mg/kg PO q12h), etodolac (10–15 mg/kg PO q24h), phenylbutazone (3–7 mg/kg PO q8h, total dose < 800 mg/day), meclofenamic acid (0.5 mg/kg PO q12h), or piroxicam (0.3 mg/kg PO q24h for 3 days, then q48h)

Glucocorticoids
• May give antiinflammatory dosage—prednisone (0.1–0.5 mg/kg PO)
• Potential side affects well documented
• Goal for chronic use—low-dose and alternate-day therapy

CONTRAINDICATIONS
NSAIDs—gastrointestinal upset may preclude use.

PRECAUTIONS
• NSAIDs—most cause some degree of gastric ulceration.
• Acetaminophen—unsuitable; potential for toxicity

POSSIBLE INTERACTIONS
NSAIDs—do not use in conjunction with glucocorticoids; risk of gastrointestinal tract ulceration

ALTERNATIVE DRUGS
N/A

 FOLLOW-UP

PATIENT MONITORING
Recheck lameness every 2–4 weeks to detect more serious concurrent orthopedic problems.

PREVENTION/AVOIDANCE
N/A

POSSIBLE COMPLICATIONS
N/A

EXPECTED COURSE AND PROGNOSIS
• Self-limiting disease

• Treatment—symptomatic; appears to have no influence on duration of clinical signs.
• Multiple limb involvement—common
• Lameness—typically lasts from a few days to several weeks; may persist for months

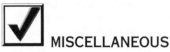 MISCELLANEOUS

ASSOCIATED CONDITIONS
N/A

AGE-RELATED FACTORS
Typically affects immature and young dogs

ZOONOTIC POTENTIAL
N/A

PREGNANCY
Females reported to be more susceptible to panosteitis during estrus; no proven relationship to reproductive hormones or pregnancy

SYNONYMS
• Enostosis
• Fibrous osteodystrophy
• Juvenile osteomyelitis
• Eosinophilic panosteitis

Suggested Reading
Brinker WO, Piermattei DL, Flo GL. Disease conditions in small animals. In: Brinker WO, Piermattei DL, Flo GL, eds. Handbook of small animal orthopedics and fracture treatment. 2nd ed. Philadelphia: Saunders 1990:547–550.

Halliwell WH. Tumorlike lesions of bone. In: Bojrab MJ, ed., Disease mechanisms in small animal surgery. 2nd ed. Philadelphia: Saunders 1993:932–933.

Manly PA, Romich JA. Miscellaneous orthopedic diseases. In: Slatter DH, ed., Textbook of small animal surgery. 2nd ed. Philadelphia: Saunders 1993:1984–1987.

Muir P, Dubielzig RR, Johnson KA. Panosteitis. Compend Contin Educ Pract Vet 1996;18:29–33.
Author Larry Carpenter
Consulting Editor Peter D. Schwarz

PAPILLEDEMA

BASICS

OVERVIEW
• Papilledema—swelling of optic disk secondary to increased intracranial pressure without discernable vision loss
• Optic disc EDEMA
• Swelling of the optic disk reflecting other pathologies—including optic neuritis
• Affects the ophthalmic and nervous systems

SIGNALMENT
Dogs and cats

SIGNS
Historical Findings
• Cerebral signs
• Disk edema per se produces no visual deficits.

Physical Examination Findings
• CNS signs
• Elevation and hyperemia of optic nerve head
• Blurring of optic disk margin
• Filling in of physiologic cup
• Pupillary light reflexes are normal.

CAUSES & RISK FACTORS
• Hydrocephalus
• Hepatic encephalopathy
• Neoplasm—primary or metastatic
• Distemper (dogs)
• FIP (cats)
• Systemic mycoses
• Toxoplasmosis
• Neosporum caninum
• Granulomatous meningoencephalomyelitis
• Trauma

DIAGNOSIS

DIFFERENTIAL DIAGNOSIS
Diseases causing optic disk swelling—optic neuritis; congential anomalies
• Optic neuritis–abnormal pupillary light reflexes

CBC/BIOCHEMISTRY/URINALYSIS
No specific abnormalities

OTHER LABORATORY TESTS
Specific viral, fungal or protozoal serologic testing

IMAGING
• Neuroimaging—CT or MRI
• Orbital ultrasound

DIAGNOSTIC PROCEDURES
CSF analysis—measure intracranial pressure

TREATMENT
• Resolve cause of increased intracranial pressure or orbital disease.
• Patients need critical monitoring.
• Hyperventilation—maintain $PaCO_2$ at 25–30 mm Hg

MEDICATIONS

DRUGS
• Mannitol—250 mg/kg IV over 20 min; repeated as necessary
• Furosemide (Lasix)—1 mg/kg IV q8h
• Corticosteroids—prednisone (0.5 mg/kg PO q12h) or dexamethasone SP *0.25 mg/kg IV q8–12h)

CONTRAINDICATIONS/POSSIBLE INTERACTIONS
• Mannitol—contraindicated with intracranial hemorrhage
• Beware of brain herniation.
• Systemic corticosteroids—do not use until infectious causes are ruled out.

FOLLOW-UP

Prognosis—depends on underlying disease

MISCELLANEOUS

ABBREVIATIONS
• CNS = central nervous system
• CSF = cerebrospinal fluid
• CT = computed tomography
• FIP = feline infectious peritonitis
• MRI = magnetic resonance imaging

Suggested Reading
Whiting AS, Johnson LN. Papilledema: clinical clues and differential diagnosis. Am Fam Physician 1994;5:1125–1134.
Author David Lipsitz
Consulting Editor Paul E. Miller

BASICS

OVERVIEW
• Papillomaviruses (PVs)—group of nonenveloped, double-stranded DNA viruses that induce proliferative cutaneous tumors in cats and dogs and mucosal tumors in dogs; each is host and fairly site-specific, with characteristic clinical and microscopic changes in infected tissues. • Tumors—papillomas, warts, or verrucae; generally benign; spontaneously regress; rarely may undergo conversion to SCC • Lesions—often multiple, well demarcated, and exophytic; sometimes hyperkeratotic plaques or with papules; may be deeply pigmented (black or brown), pink, tan, or white • Infection—inoculation through breaks in the epidermis or mucosal epithelium; iatrogenic transmission through use of contaminated instruments possible

SIGNALMENT
Dogs
• At least five types of PV may infect dogs. • Oral and ocular papillomas—generally seen in young animals (6 months to 4 years); however, any age may be affected • Cutaneous papillomas—any age • Miniature schnauzers and pugs—pigmented sessile papillomas generally manifest before 5 years of age

Cats
• Feline papillomatosis and Bowen's disease—old animals (7 years and up) • PV-induced lesions have been identified in kittens. • No breed predisposition

SIGNS
Historical Findings
• Dysphagia • Ptyalism • Reluctance to eat • Halitosis—dogs with oral papillomas

Physical Examination Findings
Dogs
• True cutaneous papillomas—rare; lesion is an exophytic, often pedunculated, papilliferous growth consisting of multiple fronds of epithelium; may be found anywhere on the body; rarely exceed 1 cm in diameter • Venereal warts—affect the lower genital tract; probably caused by a novel PV • Cutaneous inverted papillomas—rare; caused by a unique PV; lesions: generally found on the ventral trunk and abdomen, 1–2 cm in diameter, raised and firm, small pore opening to the skin surface • Familial form—rare; pugs and miniature schnauzers; up to 80 scaly, black plaques scattered on the ventral neck, trunk, and medial aspects of limbs (pigmented epidermal nevi and lentiginosis profusa)
Oral
• Multiple tumors (as many as 100) on the mucocutaneous junctions around the mouth, lips, tongue, palate, epiglottis, and upper esophagus and on the mucosa of the oro-

pharynx • Early papillomas—discrete, pale, smooth elevations of the mucosa; proceed to develop a filiform to cauliflower-like appearance • Lesions—may bleed and be ulcerated owing to trauma from teeth • Halitosis and discharge from the mouth—with secondary bacterial infection of traumatized lesions • Respiratory distress—rare; multiple tumors may obstruct the airway • The canine oral PV is believed to be the cause of some eyelid, corneal, and conjunctival papillomas.
Cats
• Exophytic papillomas—exceedingly rare • Cutaneous—multifocal to coalescing plaques of epidermal hyperplasia that may be pigmented or waxy and white • Lesions—persistent; may progress to SCC (Bowen's disease or multicentric SCC in situ) • SCC in situ lesions—well demarcated; deeply pigmented; erythematous; crusted; occasionally ulcerated; may progress to invasive SCC

CAUSES & RISK FACTORS
• Oral (dogs)—young and immunologically naive; recovered animals appear to be immune. • Cutaneous (dogs and cats)—immunosuppression (acquired, congenital, or iatrogenic from use of corticosteroids) facilitates all types of PV infection; defects in cell-mediated immunity thought to have a permissive effect on the persistence of PV-induced lesions

DIAGNOSIS

DIFFERENTIAL DIAGNOSIS
Dogs
• Oral cavity and oropharynx—fibromatous epulis; transmissible venereal tumor; if ulcerated, SCC • Cutaneous—sebaceous hyperplasias; cutaneous tags • Pigmented—melanomas • Inverted—intracutaneous cornifying epitheliomas

Cats
Multiple sessile, hyperkeratotic lesions—eosinophilic granulomas or plaques; actinic keratosis; cutaneous lesions of FeLV; multicentric SCC in situ; SCC

CBC/BIOCHEMISTRY/URINALYSIS N/A

OTHER LABORATORY TESTS N/A

IMAGING N/A

DIAGNOSTIC PROCEDURES
• Oral papillomatosis—gross appearance and physical examination findings generally provide the diagnosis; biopsy of one or two lesions may be used for confirmation. • Histopathology—generally required for cutaneous, venereal, and some ocular papillomas • Immunohistochemistry—avidin–biotin complex method to detect PV group–related antigens; dogs: helps make the diagnosis; cats: recommended for confirmation of diagnosis

TREATMENT
• Oral—self-limiting; lesions generally regress spontaneously. • Surgery to remove oral tumors (excision, cryosurgery, or electrosurgery)—airway is being occluded; patient is unable to eat comfortably; aesthetic reasons • Systemic corticosteroids—withdraw if severe or persistent oral or cutaneous disease reoccurs. • Persistent disease (dogs)—may treat with autovaccination; use heat-inactivated autogenous vaccine. • Cats—no efficacious therapy for chronic PV-induced skin lesions; SCC in situ lesions may respond to ^{90}Sr plesiotherapy.

MEDICATIONS N/A

FOLLOW-UP

PATIENT MONITORING
Monitor lesions carefully to detect signs (ulceration, purulent exudation, and rapid growth) of malignant transformation to SCC.

PREVENTION/AVOIDANCE
• Separate dogs with oral papillomatosis from susceptible animals. • Commercial kennels with outbreaks of oral papillomatosis—may use autogenous vaccines • Live canine oral PV vaccine—reported to induce hyperplastic epithelial tumors and SCC at vaccination sites; latency period 11–34 months

EXPECTED COURSE AND PROGNOSIS
• Dogs—prognosis usually good; incubation period 1–8 weeks; regression usually occurs at 1–5 months; lesions may persist for 24 months or more. • Cats—long-term prognosis for chronic papillomatosis and Bowen disease uncertain

MISCELLANEOUS

ZOONOTIC POTENTIAL
None

ABBREVIATIONS
• FeLV = feline leukemia virus • SCC = squamous cell carcinoma

Suggested Reading
Sundberg JP. Papillomaviruses. In: Castro AE, Heuscele WP, eds. Veterinary diagnostic virology. St. Louis: Mosby, 1992:148–150.
Authors Suzette M. LeClerc and Edward G. Clark
Consulting Editor Stephen C. Barr

PARAGONIMIASIS

BASICS

OVERVIEW
Paraonimus kellicotti—lung fluke; trematode that may inhabit the lungs of a variety of mammals; only species of importance to dogs and cats in the U.S.

Fluke Life Cycle
• Adults in the lung—release operculated eggs into the bronchial tree that are subsequently coughed up, swallowed, and shed in the feces
• Eggs in an aquatic environment—after 2–3 weeks of development, short-lived, ciliated miracidia emerge and must find a suitable snail intermediate within 24 hr or perish; amphibious snails (*Pomatiopsis* spp.) serve as the first intermediate host.
• Miracidia—initiate a complex asexual reproductive phase in snail tissue; produce large numbers of free-swimming cercariae
• Cercariae—penetrate through the exoskeleton of the crayfish (*Cambarus* spp.; the second intermediate host) and encyst as metacercaria
• Metacercariae—await ingestion by the final host; locate in the crayfish heart muscle; become infective to the final host in several weeks; an immature fluke exists within the cyst wall at this time; after ingestion, excyst in the small intestine
• Young flukes—penetrate the intestinal wall into the peritoneal cavity; migrate across the diaphragm to the pleural cavity; migrate in lung tissue for 3–4 weeks before pairing up; migration may be marked by small hemorrhages that progress to small scars; after pairing up, two adults are generally found within individual cysts; cysts are radiographically visible 4 weeks after infection.
• Mature flukes—found in fibrous pulmonary cysts 5–6 weeks after infection, at which time patency occurs; cysts are usually found close to the lung surface and appear as nodular, elevated masses 1–2 cm beneath the pleura; small thick flukes (1 × 0.5 cm); reddish brown when alive
• Hosts—like most flukes, adults not host specific; *P. kellicotti* found in a number of mammals; mink regarded as preferred; reservoirs include muskrat, opossum, raccoon, skunk, bobcat, and fox

SIGNALMENT
• Most common in cats, dogs, and other mammalian hosts 6 months of age and older
• No breed or gender predilection recognized

SIGNS
• Respiratory—typically mild; persistent cough
• Lung sounds—usually normal unless important pathologic changes develop; likely to be more severe during the migratory and growth phases as the flukes establish themselves
• With heavy infection—slightest exertion initiates a cough; hemoptysis sometimes seen at this stage
• Death—owing to pulmonary hemorrhage or secondary infection after simultaneous entry of a number of flukes into the lungs
• Pneumothorax—may result if subpleural cysts rupture

CAUSES & RISK FACTORS
• Ingestion of crayfish–infected with *P. kellicotti metacercariae*
• Geographic location
• Louisiana and Great Lakes region—high incidence of mammalian host infection; reported in most states in the eastern U.S.

DIAGNOSIS

DIFFRENTIAL DIAGNOSIS
For the circumscribed pulmonary soft tissue densities seen on radiographs—abscessation; primary or metastatic pulmonary neoplasia; congenital pulmonary anomaly

CBC/BIOCHEMISTRY/URINALYSIS
• May note eosinophilia
• Serum chemistry profile and urinalysis unremarkable

OTHER LABORATORY TESTS
N/A

IMAGING
Thoracic radiography—make diagnosis, particularly when eggs are not being passed; fluke-containing cysts seen as circumscribed pulmonary soft tissue densities; rarely, cysts are radiolucent (air bubble appearance); this "signet ring" is pathognomonic for *Paragonimus* infection.

DIAGNOSTIC PROCEDURES
• Routine fecal flotation or fecal sedimentation procedure—find characteristic operculated eggs; eggs of many fluke species sink in flotation solution
• Aspirated fluid obtained by transtracheal wash or tracheobronchial lavage via bronchoscopy—may identify eggs
• *Paragonimus* eggs—yellow-brown; have an operculum set into a characteristic collar-like thickening

TREATMENT
• Directed at killing the flukes contained within the pulmonary cysts
• Pulmonary lesions—resolve within 2 months after successful treatment; may persist if they are several years old

MEDICATIONS

DRUGS
• Fenbendazole and albendazole—effective; 25 mg/kg PO q12h for 14–21 days
• Praziquantel—effective; 25 mg/kg PO q8h for 3 days

CONTRAINDICATIONS/POSSIBLE INTERACTIONS
N/A

FOLLOW-UP
• Thoracic radiography and periodic fecal examination—monitor progress
• Clinical improvement and reversal of respiratory signs—most patients
• Nodular radiographic lesions—resolve within 2 months of successful treatment

MISCELLANEOUS

Suggested Reading
Bowman DD, Frongillo MK, Johnson RC, et al. Evaluation of praziquantel for treatment of experimentally induced paragonimiasis in dogs and cats. Am J Vet Res 1991;52:68–71.
Author Johnny D. Hoskins
Consulting Editor Eleanor C. Hawkins

BASICS

OVERVIEW
• Phimosis—inability to protrude the penis beyond the preputial orifice
• Paraphimosis—penis protrudes from the preputial orifice and cannot be returned to its normal position

SIGNALMENT
• Dogs and cats
• German shepherds and golden retrievers—observed congenital preputial stenosis, possibly hereditary

SIGNS
• Phimosis—may be undetected until patient is unsuccessful in attempts to copulate; severe defects in the neonate interfere with urination; may cause pooling of urine in preputial cavity, which may cause balanoposthitis, leading to septicemia; persistent and painful penile erection in the absence of sexual stimulation
• Paraphimosis—short duration: only sign may be licking of an exteriorized penis; after some hours of exposure: may see ischemic necrosis and urethral obstruction; edema and swelling may make differentiation from phimosis difficult.

CAUSES & RISK FACTORS
• Phimosis—caused by an abnormally small preputial orifice; may be congenital or acquired (e.g., caused by injury or disease); may be associated with a persistent penile or preputial frenulum, a thin band of connective tissue joining the penis and prepuce along the ventral glans
• Paraphimosis—usually associated with erection and/or copulation; hair surrounding the preputial orifice is trapped against the surface of the penis, especially the bulbus glandis, preventing retraction; moderately stenotic preputial orifice may contribute; injuries; os penis fractures; priapism
• Priapism—dogs and cats; cause often unknown; trauma common in the history; one report on cats noted 6 of 7 cases were Siamese.

DIAGNOSIS

DIFFERENTIAL DIAGNOSIS
Paraphimosis—exposure of the glans penis caused by abnormality of the retractor penis muscles or preputial muscles, large preputial opening, short prepuce, or priapism

CBC/BIOCEMISTRY/URINALYSIS
• Usually normal
• Phimosis in neonates—may note severe balanoposthitis and evidence of septicemia (e.g., leukocytosis, neutrophilia progressing to neutropenia, positive urine cultures)

OTHER LABORATORY TESTS
N/A

IMAGING
N/A

DIAGNOSTIC PROCEDURES
N/A

TREATMENT

Phimosis
• Surgical enlargement of the preputial orifice
• Persistent penile frenulum (dogs)—remove the band of tissue holding the glans penis to the parietal lamina of prepuce.

Paraphimosis
• Requires immediate treatment—after 24 hr, tissue damage and urethral obstruction may necessitate penile amputation; goal is to replace the penis in a normal position.
• Indwelling urinary catheter—if urethral patency is in question
• Remove foreign objects.
• Lubricate the penis.
• Apply compresses of hypertonic glucose solutions.
• Surgically enlarge the preputial orifice, if necessary.

• Penile amputation and perineal urethrostomy—indicated for cats with difficulty urinating
• Abdominal compression bandage and indwelling urinary catheter—maintain the penis within the prepuce; may also reduce localized edema

MEDICATIONS

DRUGS
Antibiotic ointments—maintain treatment; prevent adhesions between the penis and prepuce

CONTRAINDICATIONS/POSSIBLE INTERACTIONS
N/A

FOLLOW-UP
N/A

MISCELLANEOUS

Suggested Reading

Burke TJ. Small animal reproduction and infertility. Philadelphia: Lea & Febiger, 1986.
Feldman EC, Nelson RW. Canine and feline endocrinology and reproduction. Philadelphia: Saunders, 1987:692–693.
Gunn-Moore DA, Brown PJ, Holt PE, Gruffydd-Jones T. Priapism in seven cats. J Sm Anim Pract 1995;36:262–266.
Author Rolf E. Larsen
Consulting Editor Sara K. Lyle

PARVOVIRAL INFECTION—DOGS

BASICS

DEFINITION
• CPV-2 infection is an acute systemic illness characterized by hemorrhagic enteritis.
• Often fatal in pups, who may collapse in a "shock-like" state and die suddenly without enteric signs, after only a brief period of malaise. • The myocardial form, observed in pups during the early outbreaks when the dog population was fully susceptible, is now rare.
• Most pups are now protected against neonatal infection by maternal antibodies.
• Monoclonal antibodies have revealed antigenic changes in CPV-2 since its emergence in 1978. • The original virus is now virtually extinct in the domestic dog population. • The viruses currently circulating in dogs, designated CPV-2a and CPV-2b, have been genetically stable since 1984.
• These viruses are more virulent than the original isolates, and case mortality rates appear to be higher than in the earliest outbreaks. • Most of the clinical literature is based on the response of dogs to CPV-2 and should be reevaluated in light of the emergence and dominance of the newer types in dogs. • As with rabies variants, the antigenic changes in CPV-2 do not affect the ability of various vaccines to protect dogs.

PATHOPHYSIOLOGY
• CPV-2 is very closely related to feline panleukopenia virus (FPV) and several other parvoviruses that infect carnivores. • Parvoviruses, including CPV-2, require actively dividing cells for growth. • After ingestion of virus, there is a 2- to 4-day period of viremia, with concomitant growth in lymphatic tissues throughout the body. • Early lymphatic infection is accompanied by lymphopenia and precedes intestinal infection and clinical signs. • By the third postinfection (PI) day, the rapidly dividing crypt cells of the small intestine are infected. • Viral shedding in the feces starts ~3–4 days PI, and peaks about when clinical signs first appear.
• Virus ceases to be shed in detectible amounts by PI days 8–12. • Absorption of bacterial endotoxins from the damaged intestinal mucosa is believed to play a role in CPV-2 disease. • Intensity of illness appears to be related to the viral dose and the antigenic type (CPV-2 vs. CPV-2a, CPV-2b).

SYSTEMS AFFECTED
• Cardiovascular—myocarditis with sudden death (now rare) • Gastrointestinal—small intestinal crypt cells and adjacent mucosal epithelium; severe hemorrhagic diarrhea, vomiting, dehydration; hypovolemic and septic/endotoxic shock • Hemic/Lymphatic/Immune—thymus, lymph nodes, spleen, Peyer's patches.

GENETICS
• Unknown

INCIDENCE/PREVALENCE
• Most common in breeding kennels, animal shelters, pet stores, or wherever pups are reared. • Rates vary.

GEOGRAPHIC DISTRIBUTION
Worldwide

SIGNALMENT

Species
Dog

Breed Predilections
Rottweilers, Doberman pinschers, and English springer spaniels are reported to be at exceptional risk of severe disease.

Mean Age and Range
• Illness may occur at any age. • Most severe illness occurs in pups 6–16 weeks of age.

Predominant Sex
N/A

SIGNS

General Comments
Suspect CPV-2 infection whenever pups have an enteric illness, especially with sudden onset of lethargy, vomiting, and/or diarrhea.

Historical Findings
• Sudden onset of bloody diarrhea, anorexia, and repeated episodes of vomiting • Rapid weight loss • Some pups may collapse in a shock-like state and die without enteric signs. • In breeding kennels, several littermate pups may become ill simultaneously or within a short period of time. • Occasionally, one or two pups in a litter have minimal or no signs, followed by the death of littermates that presumably encounter greater amounts of virus.

Physical Examination Findings
• Dehydration, weight loss, and abdominal discomfort are consistent features. • Often there is severe hemorrhagic diarrhea. • Fluid-filled intestinal loops may be palpated. • Occasionally enlarged mesenteric lymph nodes are palpable. • May be fever or hypothermia

RISK FACTORS
• Dogs from kennels, animal shelters, pet shops, or elsewhere where dogs have congregated are at greatest risk. • Pups <4 months of age are at higher risk of severe infection.
• Copathogens such as parasites, viruses, and certain bacterial species (e.g., *Campylobacter* spp., *Clostridium* spp.) hypothesized to exacerbate illness • Severe, often fatal, parvoviral infections have been demonstrated in pups exposed simultaneously to CPV-2 and canine coronavirus. • Crowding and poor sanitation increases the risk of infection, especially in kennels or animal shelters. • Certain distemper vaccines (e.g., vaccine virus grown in canine cell cultures) reportedly have increased the risk of severe disease in pups exposed simultaneously to CPV-2 and distemper vaccines.

DIAGNOSIS

DIFFERENTIAL DIAGNOSIS
• Canine coronavirus infection • Salmonellosis; colibacillosis; other enteric bacterial infections • Gastrointestinal foreign bodies • Gastrointestinal parasites • Hemorrhagic gastroenteritis • Intussusception • Toxin ingestion

CBC/BIOCHEMISTRY/URINALYSIS
• Lymphopenia—characteristic of CPV-2 infection; commonly occurs between PI days 4 and 6 • Severely affected dogs often exhibit severe neutropenia concurrently with the onset of intestinal damage. • Hemograms are an important part of the diagnostic regimen.
• Leukocytosis is common during recovery.
• Serum chemistry profiles help assess electrolyte disturbances (especially hypokalemia), presence of azotemia associated with dehydration, panhypoproteinemia, and hypoglycemia.

OTHER LABORATORY TESTS
Serologic tests are not diagnostic because dogs often have high titers from vaccination and/or maternal antibodies.

IMAGING
• If done as part of the diagnostic workup, abdominal radiographs often reveal a generalized small intestinal ileus; exercise caution to prevent misdiagnosis of an intestinal obstruction. • Unfortunately, many parvoviral enteritis cases are diagnosed only after exploratory surgery. • To complicate matters, intussusceptions occur uncommonly in dogs with parvoviral enteritis.

DIAGNOSTIC PROCEDURES
• May detect virus in stool or intestinal contents at the onset of disease and for 2–4 days afterward by use of commercial solid-phase ELISA assays in which sensitivity and specificity appear high. • Electron microscopy is another method of detecting virus during the early stages of infection. • Virus may be identified in tissue samples by immunofluorescence or immunoperoxidase staining. • Samples for virus detection should be submitted during the acute phase of infection; ship specimens refrigerated, not frozen.

PARVOVIRAL INFECTION—DOGS

PATHOLOGIC FINDINGS
• Gross changes include subserosal congestion and hemorrhage or frank hemorrhage into the small intestinal lumen. • Some dogs exhibit intestines that are empty or contain yellow or blood-tinged fluid. • Mesenteric lymph nodes are often enlarged and edematous, with hemorrhages in the cortex.
• Thymic atrophy is common in young dogs.
• Pulmonary edema and hydropericardium may be the only gross change in pups with myocarditis and acute heart failure (now rarely seen).
• Histopathology reveals intestinal inflammation and necrosis, with severe villus atrophy.
• Pups that die with the cardiac form typically have focal areas of lymphocytic infiltration and necrosis in the myocardium.

TREATMENT

APPROPRIATE HEALTH CARE
• Symptomatic and supportive (refer to sections on treatment of acute vomiting, acute diarrhea, and hemorrhagic gastroenteritis).
• Intensity depends on the severity of signs on examination.
• Goals are to mollify the intestinal tract, restore and maintain fluid and electrolyte balance, and resolve shock, sepsis, and endotoxemia.
• Prompt, intensive inpatient care favors treatment success.
• Proper, strict isolation procedures are essential.
• Exercise care to prevent spread of CPV-2, a very stable virus.

NURSING CARE
• Hospitalize patients and monitor for dehydration and electrolyte imbalance.
• Hydration and electrolyte replacement are essential to treatment success in severely ill dogs.
• Fluids are usually supplemented with potassium chloride, 5% dextrose, and possibly sodium bicarbonate (if severe metabolic acidosis).

ACTIVITY
Restrict until symptoms abate.

DIET
• Withhold food and water until clinical signs (i.e. vomiting and diarrhea) are resolved.
• Give recovering pups highly digestible, low-fat nourishment.

CLIENT EDUCATION
• Inform about the need for thorough disinfection, especially if other dogs are on the premises.
• A 1:30 dilution of bleach (5% sodium hypochlorite) destroys CPV-2 in a few minutes.
• Strict sanitation is essential.
• If possible, isolate pups until they reach 3 months of age.
• Pups can be infected with virulent virus before any vaccine will engender immunity.
• CPV-2 is shed for less than 2 weeks after infection; no carrier state has been substantiated.

SURGICAL CONSIDERATIONS
• Exercise caution to prevent misdiagnosis of an intestinal obstruction.
• Although uncommon, intussusceptions can occur in dogs with parvoviral enteritis.

MEDICATIONS
Refer to sections on treatment and management of acute vomiting, acute diarrhea, and hemorrhagic gastroenteritis.

DRUGS OF CHOICE
Additional recommended drugs include parenteral antibiotics (ampicillin and gentamicin), short-acting soluble corticosteroids (dexamethasone sodium phosphate or prednisolone sodium succinate), and antiemetics (e.g., metoclopramide).

CONTRAINDICATIONS
N/A

PRECAUTIONS
N/A
Gentamicin can cause renal toxicity in dehydrated pups.

POSSIBLE INTERACTIONS
N/A

ALTERNATIVE DRUGS
N/A

FOLLOW-UP

PATIENT MONITORING
N/A

PREVENTION/AVOIDANCE
• Inactivated and live vaccines are available for prophylaxis. • Inactivated vaccines engender protection from disease but do not interrupt transmission. • Immunization is uncertain if pups have maternal antibodies. • About 75% of pups vaccinated with efficacious products will have developed immunity at 12 weeks of age. • Vaccination is not an effective control method in contaminated environments. • Vaccines have not been shown to cause clinical disease; if dogs develop signs of infection within 5 days of vaccination, they were exposed to virulent virus about the time they were vaccinated. • Vaccines differ in their capacity to immunize pups with maternal antibodies.
• Control of CPV-2 requires efficacious vaccines, pup isolation, and stringent hygiene.

POSSIBLE COMPLICATIONS
• Septicemia/endotoxemia • Secondary bacterial pneumonia • Intussusception

EXPECTED COURSE AND PROGNOSIS
• Prognosis is guarded in severely affected pups. • Prognosis is good for dogs that receive prompt initial treatment and survive the initial crisis of illness.

MISCELLANEOUS

ASSOCIATED CONDITIONS
N/A

AGE-RELATED FACTORS
Pups < 6 months of age suffer a higher rate of severe illness.

ZOONOTIC POTENTIAL
N/A

PREGNANCY
No in utero infections have been reported in field cases.

SYNONYMS
N/A

SEE ALSO
• Diarrhea, Acute • Vomiting, Acute • Gastroenteritis, Hemorrhagic

ABBREVIATIONS
• CPV-2 = canine parvovirus type 2 • FPV = feline panleukopenia virus

Suggested Reading
Pollock RHV, Carmichael LE. Canine viral enteritis. In: Greene CE, ed. Infectious diseases of the dog and cat. Philadelphia: WB Saunders, 1990:268–279.
Pollock RHV, Parrish CR. Canine parvovirus. In: Olsen RG, Krakowa S, Blakeslee JR, eds. Boca Raton, FL: CRC Press, 1985:145–177.
Zimmer JF. Clinical management of acute gastroenteritis including virus-induced enteritis. In: Kirk RW, ed. Current veterinary therapy—small animal practice, VIII. Philadelphia: Saunders, 1983:171–1177.
Author Leland Carmichael
Consulting Editors Brett M. Feder and Mitchell A. Crystal

DISEASES

PATELLAR LUXATION

BASICS

DEFINITION
Medial or lateral displacement of the patella from its normal anatomic position in the femoral trochlea

PATHOPHYSIOLOGY
• May be mild to severe; different degrees of clinical and pathologic changes; classified into grades I–IV
• Common musculoskeletal changes—tibial rotation on its long axis; bowing of the distal and proximal tibia; shallow to absent femoral trochlea; dysplasia of the femoral and tibial epiphysis; displacement of the quadriceps muscle group

SYSTEMS AFFECTED
Musculoskeletal

Genetics
• Recessive, polygenic, and multifocal inheritances proposed
• Hereditary factor in Devon rex cats

INCIDENCE/PREVALENCE
• One of the most common stifle joint abnormalities in dogs
• Medial—> 75% of cases
• Bilateral involvement—50% of cases
• Uncommon in cats, but may be more common than suspected because most affected cats are not lame

GEOGRAPHIC DISTRIBUTION
N/A

SIGNALMENT

Species
• Predominately dogs
• Rarely cats

BREED PREDILECTIONS
• Most common in toy and miniature dog breeds
• Dogs—miniature and toy poodles; Yorkshire terriers; Pomeranians; Pekingese; Chihuahuas; Boston terriers

Mean Age and Range
Clinical signs—may develop soon after birth; generally after 4 months of age

PREDOMINANT SEX
Risk for females 1.5 times that for males

SIGNS

General Comments
Depend on grade (severity), amount of degenerative arthritis, chronicity of disease, and occurrence of other stifle joint abnormalities (e.g., cruciate ligament rupture)

Historical Findings
• Persistent abnormal hindlimb carriage and function in neonates and puppies
• Occasional skipping or intermittent hindlimb lameness—worsens in young to mature dogs
• Sudden signs of lameness—owing to minor trauma or worsening DJD in mature animals

Physical Examination Findings
• Grade I—patella can be manually luxated; patella reduces when pressure is released.
• Grade II—patella can be manually luxated or can spontaneously luxate with flexion of the stifle joint; patella remains luxated until it is manually reduced or the patient extends the joint and derotates the tibia in the opposite direction of luxation.
• Grades I and II—patient intermittently carries the affected limb with the stifle joint flexed.
• Grade III—patella remains luxated most of the time but can be manually reduced with the stifle joint in extension; flexion and extension of the stifle joint results in reluxation of the patella.
• Grade IV—patella is permanently luxated and cannot be manually repositioned; may be up to 90° of rotation of the proximal tibial plateau; shallow or missing femoral trochlear; displacement of quadriceps muscle group in the direction of luxation
• Grades III and IV—crouching, bowlegged (genu varum) or knock-kneed (genu valgum) stance for medial or lateral luxations, respectively; most of the body weight is transferred to the front limbs.
• Pain—may be elicited with chondromalacia of the patella or femoral trochlea

CAUSES
• Congenital
• Traumatic

RISK FACTORS
• Coxa vara—decreased femoral neck–femoral shaft axis; associated with medial luxation
• Coxa valga—increased femoral neck–femoral shaft axis; associated with lateral luxation

• Excessive anteversion—forward inclination of the femoral head and neck

DIAGNOSIS

DIFFERENTIAL DIAGNOSIS
• Cranial cruciate ligament rupture—distinguished by palpation of cranial drawer motion; concurrent in 15%–20% of cases
• Avulsion fracture of the tibial tubercle—causes laxity of the quadriceps mechanism; results in patella instability
• Rupture of the patellar tendon—causes proximal displacement of the patella and instability
• Malunion and malalignment of fractures of the femur or tibia—may result in displacement of the quadriceps muscle group
• Craniodorsal hip luxation—often concurrent with grade I luxation owing to laxity of the quadriceps muscle group; laxity spontaneously resolves after reduction of the hip luxation.

CBC/BIOCHEMISTRY/URINALYSIS
N/A

OTHER LABORATORY TESTS
N/A

IMAGING
• Craniocaudal and mediolateral radiographs of the stifle joint—indicated for all grade III and IV luxations; include the joint above (hip) and below (hock) to detect bowing and/or torsion of the femur and tibia.
• Skyline radiographs of the femoral trochlea—help determine its shape (shallow, flattened, or convex)

DIAGNOSTIC PROCEDURES
Arthrocentesis and synovial fluid analysis—slightly increase in mononuclear cells (generally < 2000 cells/ml)

PATHOLOGIC FINDINGS
• Gross—cartilage wear lesions of the patella and femoral trochlea; osteophytes at the joint capsule–bone interface; joint capsule redundancy on the side opposite of luxation; fibrosis and contracture on the side of luxation
• Microscopic—cartilage fibrillation and loss of glycosaminoglycan content; synovitis

PATELLAR LUXATION

TREATMENT

APPROPRIATE HEALTH CARE
• Outpatient—all grade I and some grade II luxations
• Inpatient (surgery)—most grade II and all grade III and IV luxations

NURSING CARE
• Cryotherapy (ice packing)—initiated immediately after surgery; 15–20 min every 8 hr for 3–5 days
• Range-of-motion exercises of the stifle joint—as soon as tolerated

ACTIVITY
Normal to restricted, depending on severity

DIET
Weight control—important for decreasing the load and, therefore, stress on the stifle joint

CLIENT EDUCATION
• Discuss the heritability of the condition.
• Warn client of the possibility of DJD development.
• Inform client of the increased risk of cranial cruciate ligament disease.
• Warn client that the condition could worsen over time (e.g., from grade I to grade II).

SURGICAL CONSIDERATIONS
• Bone deformity (e.g., shallow trochlea or tibial tubercle deviation)—requires surgical bone reconstruction; assumed in all grade II or higher luxations
• Trochleoplasty—arthroplastic procedure; deepen trochlear sulcus
• Trochlear sulcoplasty—curettage technique; remove hyaline cartilage and cancellous bone to deepen the sulcus; fibrocartilage eventually resurfaces the trochlea.
• Recession sulcoplasty—taco shell technique; remove a V-shaped wedge; preserves the hyaline cartilage; after the trochlea is deepened, the osteochondral bone wedge is replaced; creates a new sulcus composed of hyaline cartilage; preferred technique for most patients
• Trochlear chondroplasty—cartilage flap technique; useful only in young patients (< 6 months); create a distally based cartilage flap; remove subchondral bone beneath it; replace flap to line the new sulcus; preserves hyaline cartilage to cover the bottom of the sulcus; fibrocartilage covers the sides.
• Transposition of the tibial tubercle—realign the longitudinal axis of the quadriceps mechanism so that it is centered over the femoral trochlea; osteotomize the tibia

tubercle, transpose it opposite the direction of luxation, and stabilize it with pins and a tension band wire.
• Imbrication of the joint capsule and supporting soft tissues on the side opposite the luxation—helps pull the patella over
• Desmotomy or releasing incision—made on the side toward which the patella is luxated
• Patellar and tibial antirotational suture ligaments—reinforce stretched supporting soft tissue structures
• Corrective osteotomy—realigns the longitudinal axis of the hindlimb; generally indicated in only grade III and IV luxations

MEDICATIONS

DRUGS OF CHOICE
NSAIDs—minimize pain; decrease inflammation; may try buffered or enteric-coated aspirin (10–25 mg/kg PO q8h or q12h), caroprofen (2.2 mg/kg PO q12h), etodolac (10–15 mg/kg PO once daily), phenylbutazone (3–7 mg/kg PO q8h, total dose < 800 mg/day), meclofenamic acid (0.5 mg/kg PO q12h), or piroxicam (0.3 mg/kg PO q24h for 3 days, then every other day)

CONTRAINDICATIONS
Avoid corticosteroids because of potential side effects and articular cartilage damage associated with long-term use.

PRECAUTIONS
NSAIDs—gastrointestinal irritation may preclude their use.

POSSIBLE INTERACTIONS
N/A

ALTERNATIVE DRUGS
Chondroprotective drugs (e.g., polysulfated glycosaminoglycans, glucosamine, and chondroitin sulfate)—may help limit cartilage damage and degeneration

FOLLOW-UP

PATIENT MONITORING
• Post-trochleoplasty—encourage early, active use of the limb.
• Limit exercise for 4 weeks; prevent jumping.
• Onset of an acute non-weight-bearing lameness—may indicate cranial cruciate ligament disease
• Yearly examinations—to assess progression

PREVENTION/AVOIDANCE
• Discourage breeding of affected animals.
• Do not repeat dam–sire breedings that result in affected offspring.

POSSIBLE COMPLICATIONS
Recurrence after surgical stabilization—reported to be as high as 48%; usually of a lower grade than the original luxation

EXPECTED COURSE AND PROGNOSIS
• With surgical treatment—> 90% of patients are free from lameness and clinical dysfunction.
• DJD—radiographic evidence in almost all affected stifle joints

MISCELLANEOUS

ASSOCIATED CONDITIONS
Cranial cruciate ligament disease

AGE-RELATED FACTORS
N/A

ZOONOTIC POTENTIAL
N/A

PREGNANCY
N/A

SEE ALSO
Arthritis (Osteoarthritis)

ABBREVIATION
DJD = degenerative joint disease

Suggested Reading
Arnoczky S, Tarvin G. Surgical repair of patella luxations and fractures. In: Bojrab MJ, ed. Current techniques in small animal surgery. 4th ed. Philadelphia: Lea & Febiger, 1998;1237–1244.
Brinker WO, Piermattei DL, Flo GL. Patellar luxations. In: Brinker WO, Piermattei DL, Flo GL, eds. Handbook of small animal orthopedics and fracture repair. 3rd ed. Philadelphia, Saunders, 1997;516–534.
Slocum B, Slocum TD. Patella luxation. In: Bojrab MJ, ed. Current techniques in small animal surgery. 4th ed. Philadelphia: Lea & Febiger, 1998;1222–1236.
Willauer C, Vasseur P. Clinical results of surgical correction of medial luxation of the patella in dogs. Vet Surg 1987;16:31–36.
Author Peter D. Schwarz
Consulting Editor Peter D. Schwarz

PATENT DUCTUS ARTERIOSUS

BASICS

DEFINITION
PDA represents a persistent patency of the fetal ductus arteriosus connecting the descending aorta to the pulmonary artery.

PATHOPHYSIOLOGY
Flow across a PDA is typically from the aorta to pulmonary artery (left to right). The hemodynamic consequences depend on the magnitude of the shunt, the pulmonary vascular resistance, and intercurrent heart defects. Small shunt volumes are well tolerated; moderate-to-large shunt volumes cause left-sided CHF from volume overload. Much less frequently, a large-diameter PDA causes pulmonary vascular injury, high pulmonary vascular resistance, pulmonary hypertension, and reversal of the shunt (Eisenmenger's physiology or "reversed" PDA), with bidirectional shunting across the PDA. Patients affected with right-to-left shunting suffer from arterial desaturation and hypoxia-triggered polycythemia.

SYSTEMS AFFECTED
• Cardiovascular—volume overload (left-to-right shunt) or pulmonary vascular disease and polycythemia (right-to-left shunt) • Respiratory—if pulmonary edema develops • Hemic/Lymph/Immune—if polycythemia develops

GENETICS
Genetically transmitted (polygenic model) defect in many canine breeds, including the miniature poodle, collie, Maltese, Shetland sheepdog, German shepherd, cocker spaniel, Pomeranian, and Labrador retriever.

INCIDENCE/PREVALENCE
Second most common congenital heart defect in dogs; prevalence estimated to be 6.5–8 cases per 1000 live births.

SIGNALMENT

Species
Dogs and cats

Breed Predilections
See genetics

Mean Age and Range
• Vast majority identified during the initial vaccination sequence • Onset of signs related to CHF—weeks to many years

Predominant Sex
Dogs—females predisposed

SIGNS

General Comments
• Onset of reversed PDA—quite sudden in dogs (usually before 4 months of age); can develop more gradually in cats • No significant documentation that shunt reversal begins after 6 months of age, but signs related to reversed shunting may be overlooked; onset of related

problems has been reported in dogs older than 5 years of age.

Historical Findings
• Respiratory distress, coughing, exercise intolerance • Stunted growth • Right-to-left shunting PDA—exertional rear limb weakness and complications of polycythemia and hyperviscosity (seizures or sudden death related to arrhythmias or right to left embolus) • Signs usually precipitated by exercise

Physical Examination Findings
• Typically, continuous, machinery-type murmur loudest over pulmonary artery at the left craniodorsal cardiac base; localized in some dogs; murmur may be loud over the manubrium sterni in small dogs; often a concurrent systolic murmur of mitral regurgitation at the left apex • Loud murmurs—associated with a palpable precordial thrill • Arterial pulses—hyperkinetic ("waterhammer") • Caudoventral displacement of the ventricular apex • Tachypnea, respiratory distress, and inspiratory crackle—may indicate left-sided CHF • Rapid, irregular cardiac rhythm with variable-intensity arterial pulses if atrial fibrillation develops • In right-to-left shunting ("reversed") PDA findings differ—no continuous murmur, normal arterial pulses, and a prominent right ventricular impulse; may be a systolic ejection murmur and a tympanic, or split, second heart sound; may be a prominent jugular pulse • Classic feature of right-to-left shunting PDA is differential cyanosis: pink cranial, but cyanotic caudal, mucous membranes; in severe secondary polycythemia, the cranial mucous membranes may also be cyanotic.

CAUSES
Congenital heart disease genetically predisposed in most cases

RISK FACTORS
Genetic predisposition in dogs; risk factors in cats are unknown.

DIAGNOSIS

DIFFERENTIAL DIAGNOSIS
• Principal auscultatory differentials are congenital aortic stenosis with aortic insufficiency (to-and-fro systolic/diastolic murmur) and ventricular septal defect with aortic valve prolapse into the defect (causing both systolic and diastolic murmurs). • Very rare causes of continuous murmurs—arteriovenous fistula of the lung or related to thyroid neoplasia, aorticopulmonary communication, rupture of the aorta into the right atrium or right ventricle, and coronary artery fistula • Simplified by completing a workup that includes Doppler echocardiography

CBC/BIOCHEMISTRY/URINALYSIS
Usually normal unless right-to-left shunting;

then may be variable degrees of polycythemia (PCV 58–80%)

OTHER BLOOD TESTS
Reversed PDA—low femoral arterial pO_2, comparable to a pO_2 obtained by careful puncture of the carotid or brachial artery using a 25-gauge needle

IMAGING

Thoracic Radiographic Findings
• Lateral projection—variable degrees of left heart enlargement; typically pulmonary over-circulation; frequently the lobar pulmonary veins are larger than the attendant arteries, related to high left atrial pressure or incipient heart failure • Dorsoventral view (preferable to accentuate the aorta) demonstrates cardiac elongation (left ventricular enlargement), left auricular enlargement (2 to 3 o'clock lateral bulge), and dilation of the descending aorta (called a "ductus bump"); the main pulmonary artery is dilated. • Left-sided CHF—evident as distended pulmonary veins, increased interstitial/alveolar densities • Reversed PDA—heart usually normal sized, but the contour of the right cardiac border is more prominent on the DV view, and the pulmonary circulation appears normal to reduced; the main pulmonary artery and proximal lobar branches are dilated; a ductus bump generally is seen on the DV view.

Echocardiographic Findings
• Left atrium, left ventricle, and main pulmonary artery are dilated; right ventricle is normal, except in cats in which it is more likely to be hypertrophied to varying degrees; the ductal ampulla and the distal ductus can generally be imaged from the left cranial hemithorax. • Left ventricular systolic function (shortening fraction) is normal to reduced; may be markedly decreased in larger dogs with long-standing PDA • Doppler studies demonstrate continuous flow into the main pulmonary artery (from the ductus); often concurrent pulmonary insufficiency, related to dilation of the pulmonary artery and mitral regurgitation caused by left-sided cardiac dilatation; transmitral flow velocity and transaortic flow velocity are high because of increased volume; aortic velocities can be augmented substantially (up to 2.8 m/sec), mimicking findings of mild subvalvular aortic stenosis • Right-to-left shunting PDA—small left heart chambers, right atrial dilation, right ventricular hypertrophy, and dilation of the main and branch pulmonary arteries; contrast echocardiography is useful to confirm the diagnosis.

Angiographic Findings
• Echocardiography has completely supplanted angiography for the diagnosis. • Angiographic demarcation is useful during interventional procedures such as coil occlusion of the ductus; injection of contrast material into the descend-

ing aorta demonstrates whether the ductus is tapered or short and wide, information crucial to catheter-occlusion techniques.

DIAGNOSTIC PROCEDURES

Electrocardiography
• ECG—rarely needed for diagnosis of PDA; used to diagnose auscultable arrhythmias
• Atrial fibrillation—observed infrequently, related to marked dilatation of the left atrium
• Typical abnormalities include widened P waves (atrial enlargement) and increased-amplitude QRS complexes in the left caudal leads (II, aVF, III) and left precordial leads.

PATHOLOGIC FINDINGS
• Necropsy findings in left-to-right shunting PDA include pulmonary edema, cardiomegaly (left sided), and dilation of the aorta and pulmonary artery. • Right-to-left shunting PDA—right ventricular hypertrophy, dilation of the pulmonary artery, and prominent bronchial arteries; ductal diameter is invariably very wide, generally approaching that of the descending aorta.

TREATMENT

APPROPRIATE HEALTH CARE
• Manage pulmonary edema with furosemide and, if necessary, oxygen and cage rest; following stabilization, occlude the PDA promptly.
• Can schedule stable animals for elective surgery; but do not delay procedure; asymptomatic dogs as young as 7–8 weeks of age show no higher operative mortality than older dogs.
• Dogs with polycythemia caused by right-to-left shunting PDA—periodic phlebotomy to maintain the PCV < 65% (typically 62–65%).

DIET
Normal diet unless CHF, then restricted sodium intake.

CLIENT EDUCATION
• Surgery—do not delay; mortality is higher and left ventricular function impaired if clinical signs develop. • Echocardiography with Doppler is the best approach to identify concurrent defects. • Following successful surgery and a 2-week convalescence, the dog can be treated normally.

SURGICAL CONSIDERATIONS
• Surgery can generally proceed within 24–48 h of medical stabilization. • Standard therapy involves ductal ligation via left thoracotomy; surgical and perioperative mortality should be < 8% for all cases. • Catheter-delivered occlusion devices, including thrombogenic Gianturco coils that can occlude the ductus in some animals. • Never correct right-to-left PDA surgically; the right ventricle will not be able to eject against the pulmonary vascular resistance without the "pop-off" of the PDA.

MEDICATIONS

DRUGS OF CHOICE
• Treat pulmonary edema with furosemide (2–4 mg/kg q6–12 h PO, SQ, IM, or IV as required); can be discontinued when the PDA is closed • When surgery is not an option—prescribe furosemide, enalapril (0.5 mg/kg q12–24h PO), and digoxin (0.005 mg/kg q12h PO) to control CHF. • To control severe, life-threatening CHF—can use direct vasodilators such as hydralazine (1–2 mg/kg q12h PO) or sodium nitroprusside (1–5 µg/kg/min)

CONTRAINDICATIONS
• In left-to-right PDA—drugs that increase systemic vascular resistance and arterial blood pressure, except as needed for anesthesia and surgery • In right-to-left PDA—drugs that lead to systemic arterial vasodilation and reduce systemic arterial blood pressure

PRECAUTIONS
• Measure digoxin levels to ensure therapeutic, nontoxic concentrations. • Monitor arterial blood pressure, renal function, and serum electrolytes to identify problems related to diuretic and vasodilator therapies.

ALTERNATIVE DRUGS
• Prostaglandin inhibitors (e.g. indomethacin) do *not* close PDAs effectively in dogs. • Consider hydroxyurea to treat severe polycythemia unresponsive to phlebotomy; consult a specialist regarding use.

FOLLOW-UP

PATIENT MONITORING
• Postoperative—vital signs and dyspnea related to pneumothorax indicated postoperatively; provide analgesics for 24–48 hr.
• Cardiac auscultation postoperatively and at suture removal; if sounds are normal, no further follow-up or diagnostic studies required. • Persistent, continuous murmur indicates either incomplete closure of the ductus, recannulization (rule out infection), or a concurrent cardiac defect. Systolic murmurs variably heard postoperatively should abate by time of suture removal. Reinvestigate unexpected murmurs by Doppler echocardiography. When only partial ligation at surgery, consider referral to a cardiologist for coil occlusion. • Sudden illness, fever, or acute respiratory signs postoperatively—consider bacterial infection of the ligation site and recannulization of the ductus with hematogenous pneumonia; aggressive antibiotic therapy needed; consult surgical specialist or cardiologist

PREVENTION/AVOIDANCE

Do not breed affected animals.

POSSIBLE COMPLICATIONS
• Left-sided CHF • Cardiac arrhythmias
• Recannulization of the ductus • Perioperative death (from torn ductus), bleeding, or infection • Pulmonary vascular disease with pulmonary hypertension, reversed shunting, exercise intolerance, and polycythemia

EXPECTED COURSE AND PROGNOSIS
• Infrequently dogs remain asymptomatic for life. Unless the defect is closed, approximately 50–60% of dogs die from CHF within 1 year of diagnosis. PDA in an dog > 3 years should be evaluated on a case-by-case basis with appropriate consultation as needed. • Surgery performed prior to onset of moderate-to-severe CHF—excellent; approximately 5–8% surgical/perioperative mortality • Moderate-to-severe CHF is related to either left ventricular myocardial failure or atrial fibrillation—guarded; referral to a specialist advised • Dogs with right-to-left shunting PDA can live for several years but often die suddenly; infrequently, dogs live beyond 5 years of age (especially cocker spaniels). • Cats—varies from rapidly progressive left-sided CHF to gradual development of pulmonary vascular disease; even right-sided CHF can develop in cats with PDA and pulmonary vascular disease.

MISCELLANEOUS

ASSOCIATED CONDITIONS
Typically an isolated defect, but may occur in conjunction with other congenital heart lesions that are more likely in larger breeds.

PREGNANCY
Carries greater risk for CHF in pregnant bitches (and affected dogs should not be bred); offspring carry greater risk for large PDA or reversed shunting due to pulmonary vascular disease.

SYNONYMS
Persistently patent ductus arteriosus

SEE ALSO
• Congestive Heart Failure, Left-sided
• Murmurs, heart

ABBREVIATIONS
• PDA = patent ductus arteriosus
• CHF = congestive heart failure

Suggested Reading
Bonagura JD, Lehmkuhl LB. Congenital heart disease. In: Fox PR, Sisson D, Moise NS. Textbook of canine and feline cardiology. Philadelphia: Saunders. 1999:471–535.
Author John D. Bonagura
Consulting Editor Larry P. Tilley and Francis W. K. Smith, Jr.

PECTUS EXCAVATUM

BASICS

OVERVIEW
- Deformity of the sternum and costal cartilages that results in a dorsal to ventral narrowing of the chest, primarily in the caudal aspect
- May note secondary abnormalities of respiratory and cardiovascular function from restriction of ventilation and cardiac compression
- Most cases are congenital.
- Concurrent cardiac defects common
- Speculated that upper respiratory obstruction at a young age may cause abnormal respiratory gradients and subsequent pectus excavatum
- Some patients demonstrate swimmer syndrome—neonatal dogs lack the ability to posture properly and remain in sternal recumbency, which may lead to invagination of the sternum

SIGNALMENT
- Dogs and cats
- Brachycephalic breeds predisposed
- Most common age—4 weeks to 3 months

SIGNS
- Dyspnea
- Exercise intolerance
- Weight loss
- Hyperpnea
- Recurrent pulmonary infections
- Cough
- Vomiting
- Cyanosis
- Poor appetite
- Episodes of mild upper respiratory disease
- Thoracic defect—easily palpated or seen
- Respiratory problems—common; increased inspiratory effort; inspiratory stridor; moist rales (with infection)
- Cardiac murmurs associated with concurrent cardiac defects or compression of the heart common.
- Heart sounds—often muffled, especially over the right hemithorax
- No correlation between severity signs and the severity of anatomic or physiologic abnormalities
- Swimmer syndrome—possible; limbs not adducted properly; ambulation impaired

CAUSES & RISK FACTORS
- Genetic predisposition—may exist
- Puppies raised on surfaces enabling poor footing—may be predisposed to swimmer syndrome
- Dogs predisposed to respiratory obstructive processes—higher risk than others

DIAGNOSIS

DIFFERENTIAL DIAGNOSIS
- Numerous causes of dyspnea, cyanosis, hyperpnea, and cough
- Physical examination and radiographic evaluation—rule out the most common differentials
- Tracheal malformations or collapse
- Cardiac disease
- Electric cord bite
- Hemothorax
- Pyothorax
- Pneumonia
- Allergic bronchitis
- Stenotic nares
- Elongated soft palate

CBC/BIOCHEMISTRY/URINALYSIS
N/A

OTHER LABORATORY TESTS
N/A

IMAGING
- Radiographs—confirm the diagnosis; readily reveal deformities that cause decreased thoracic volume; cardiac malposition common (heart shifted to the left of midline and sometimes cranially); may note cardiac enlargement (may be artifact of malpositioning); may note evidence of concurrent disease in the lung fields; heart shadow shift to the left may expose the right hilus and encourage a diagnosis of pulmonary disease.
- Echocardiography—fully evaluate cardiac status; eliminate primary cardiac disease; detect possible concurrent cardiac defects

DIAGNOSTIC PROCEDURES
N/A

TREATMENT
- Surgery—only available modality
- Decision to repair deformities—made on the basis of clinical signs
- Mild disease (only a flat chest)—patient may become normal without surgical intervention; try manual medial compression of the thorax by the owners or with a splint.
- Moderate or severe disease—surgical candidate; frontosagittal and vertebral indexes provide objective criteria for determining severity.
- Technique—may be dictated by the age; young patient with a compliant sternum and ribs may do well with external coaptation; old patient with a less compliant thorax may need partial sternotomy.
- Surgery benefits patients with concurrent respiratory distress; benefits unknown with no respiratory distress but with moderate or severe deformity unknown
- Asymptomatic patient may develop respiratory distress; patients with clinical signs of disease may show progression.
- Puppies with swimmer syndrome—place on surfaces with excellent footing; careful toggling of front and rear legs may improve adduction.
- Brachycephalic breeds with concurrent upper airway problems—may benefit from surgery directed at these problems

MEDICATIONS

DRUGS
Treat underlying or secondary medical conditions.

CONTRAINDICATIONS/POSSIBLE INTERACTIONS
Anesthesia—patients require constant monitoring; respiratory support should be available.

FOLLOW-UP
- Examinations—dictated by clinical signs or when surgical intervention has been precluded
- No specific actions for avoiding disease; genetic factors may sometimes be involved.
- Progression of respiratory signs—may develop in asymptomatic or mildly symptomatic patients
- Prognosis—for all patients guarded; depends on properly timed and expertly administered intervention

MISCELLANEOUS

ASSOCIATED CONDITIONS
- Cardiac defects
- Swimmer syndrome

Suggested Reading
Boudrieau RJ, Fossum TW, Hartsfield SM, et al. Pectus excavatum in dogs and cats. Compend Contin Educ Pract Vet 1990; 12:341–355.
Author Justin H. Straus
Consulting Editor Eleanor C. Hawkins

BASICS

OVERVIEW
• An inherited disorder characterized by leukocyte nuclear hyposegmentation in the presence of a mature coarse chromatin pattern
• Limited breeding studies suggest autosomal dominant transmission of the anomaly in dogs and cats; however, autosomal dominant transmission with incomplete penetrance occurs in Australian shepherds.
• Heterozygous anomaly—usual phenotype; neutrophils resemble bands and metamyelocytes; not associated with immunodeficiency, predisposition to infection, or abnormalities of leukocyte function
• Homozygous anomaly—usually lethal in utero; survivors may have leukocytes with round to oval nuclei on stained blood smear.
• Skeletal abnormalities—homozygous anomaly and chondrodysplasia reported in one stillborn kitten; heterozygous anomaly and skeletal anomalies (chondrodysplasia and brachygnathia) reported in Samoyeds; not linked conclusively to Pelger-Huët anomaly in either species.

SIGNALMENT
Several breeds of dogs (e.g., American foxhounds, Australian shepherds, basenjis) and domestic shorthair cats

SIGNS
Historical Findings
Parents or siblings may be affected.

Physical Examination Findings
No abnormalities

CAUSES & RISK FACTORS
Genetic defect with probable autosomal dominant transmission (or proven autosomal dominant trait with incomplete penetrance in Australian shepherd dogs)

DIAGNOSIS

DIFFERENTIAL DIAGNOSIS
• Severe inflammation or bacterial infection often associated with toxic change of neutrophils
• FeLV or FIV infection in cats with altered cellular maturation
• Drug-induced alterations in cellular morphology, especially encountered with use of sulfa drugs
• Preleukemic maturation disturbances

CBC/BIOCHEMISTRY/URINALYSIS
• Serendipitous finding during WBC differential count
• On stained blood smear, nuclear hyposegmentation of neutrophils (persistent left shift without toxic changes), eosinophils, basophils, and monocytes

OTHER LABORATORY TESTS
None

IMAGING
None

OTHER DIAGNOSTIC PROCEDURES
• Bone marrow biopsy—stained smear reveals nuclear hyposegmentation of leukocytes and nuclear hypolobulation of megakaryocytes; blast cell count within reference intervals
• Hereditary nature of disease revealed by examination of blood smears from parents and siblings; if relatives are unavailable for study, demonstrated by prospective test mating

TREATMENT
None needed, because no associated clinical disease

MEDICATIONS

DRUGS
None

CONTRAINDICATIONS/POSSIBLE INTERACTIONS
None

FOLLOW-UP

PATIENT MONITORING
None

PREVENTION/AVOIDANCE
• Inform owner to avoid unnecessary laboratory testing or inappropriate drug administration in future.
• Provide genetic counseling to eliminate trait from breeding animals.
• Breed affected heterozygotes and select normal offspring for future matings to preserve desirable genetic lines.

POSSIBLE COMPLICATIONS
• When heterozygotes are bred, litter size may be small because homozygous phenotype is usually a lethal trait.
• Association with chondrodysplasia or other skeletal abnormalities not yet confirmed

EXPECTED COURSE AND PROGNOSIS
• Heterozygous anomaly—normal life span
• Homozygous anomaly—usually lethal (fetal resorption)

MISCELLANEOUS

ASSOCIATED CONDITIONS
Fetal resorption (homozygous embryos)

PREGNANCY
Fetal resorption (homozygous embryos)

ABBREVIAIONS
• FeLV = feline leukemia virus
• FIV = feline immunodeficiency virus

Suggested Reading
Ettinger SJ, Feldman EC. Textbook of veterinary internal medicine. 4th ed. Philadelphia: Saunders, 1994.
Author Kenneth S. Latimer
Contributing Editor Susan M. Cotter

PELVIC BLADDER

BASICS

OVERVIEW
Describes a condition in which the neck of the bladder is located extremely caudally in the pelvic canal and the urethra is shortened or displaced; most often associated with incontinence in young intact female dogs, but some dogs with pelvic bladder do not exhibit urinary incontinence

SIGNALMENT
• Dogs and rarely cats; the difference in prevalence between species is presumably because the cat has a longer urethra than a dog of similar size.
• May occur in dogs of both sexes, either intact or neutered, but primarily affects young intact female dogs (< 1 year of age); usually detected in male dogs after neutering

SIGNS
• Incontinence is usually intermittent, and there are voluntary urinations.
• Involuntary urine dribbles from the vulva or prepuce
• Urinary "soiling" of the perineum, tail, or caudal thighs; urine spots or pools of urine where the dog has been lying down or sleeping
• May be asymptomatic

CAUSES & RISK FACTORS
Incontinence that accompanies a pelvic bladder is attributed to two components of the disorder: (1) the extreme caudal displacement of the bladder into the pelvic canal, limiting bladder distension, and (2) the abnormal position of the urethra in these animals. The urethra takes on a variety of appearances, from short and dilated to S-shaped.

DIAGNOSIS

DIFFERENTIAL DIAGNOSIS
• Causes of intermittent or continuous incontinence—ectopic ureter, urethral incompetence, hormonal incontinence, urge incontinence, urinary tract infection, neurologic conditions, detrusor instability
• The level of incontinence caused by a pelvic bladder often exceeds that seen with urethral incompetence or hormone-responsive incontinence.

CBC/BIOCHEMISTRY/URINALYSIS
• Hematologic and biochemical analysis may be indicated in patients with polyuric disorders.
• Urinalysis may reveal evidence of urinary tract infection (e.g. pyuria, hematuria, and bacteriuria) or polyuria (e.g. low urine specific gravity).

OTHER LABORATORY TESTS
N/A

IMAGING
• Abdominal radiographs may reveal caudally displaced bladder; interpret cautiously if the bladder is not distended.
• Use contrast radiography in juvenile animals exhibiting urinary incontinence.
• Excretory urography also may allow visualization of the kidneys, ureteral terminations, urinary bladder, and urethra.
• Retrograde vaginourethrography allows visualization of the vaginal vault, urethra, and urinary bladder.
• Double-contrast cystourethrography may be required for full visualization of urinary bladder and urethra.
• After maximum dilation with infusion of carbon dioxide or contrast medium, most of the bladder remains within the pelvic canal.
• May be a short, widened urethra or a urethra with a prominently convoluted appearance
• Ultrasonography of the kidneys and urinary bladder can be used to identify uroliths, masses, hydronephrosis or hydroureter, and evidence of pyelonephritis.

DIAGNOSTIC PROCEDURES
• Neurologic examination—a cursory assessment of caudal spinal and peripheral nerve function is provided by examination of anal tone, tail tone, perineal sensation, and bulbospongiosus reflexes; results are normal.
• Urodynamic procedures—consider cystometrography and urethral pressure profilometry to evaluate urinary bladder and urethral function more objectively. Detrusor function is usually normal; however, higher threshold pressures may be generated at lower volumes. The functional urethral length is shortened, and intraurethral pressure is frequently decreased.

TREATMENT

• Usually outpatient
• Identify urinary tract infection and treat appropriately.
• Surgical procedures such as seromuscular flap, colposuspension, cystourethropexy, and Teflon or collagen implants have been described for the treatment of patients refractory to medical management. Treat patients refractory to medical management with a combination of α-adrenergic agonists and diethylstilbestrol before attempting surgical correction.

MEDICATIONS

DRUGS
• α-Adrenergic agonists (e.g., phenylpropanolamine, phenylephrine, pseudoephedrine) and/or estrogen (diethylstilbestrol) therapy
• Imipramine—a tricyclic antidepressant with α-agonist actions; provides an alternative method of treatment, but often needs to be administered in combination with phenylpropanolamine.

CONTRAINDICATIONS/POSSIBLE INTERACTIONS
Adrenergic agonists are contraindicated in animals with cardiac disease, renal disease, and hypertensive disorders.

FOLLOW-UP

PATIENT MONITORING
• Periodically, for urinary tract infection
• Patients receiving α-adrenergic agonists—adverse effects of the drug, including tachycardia, anxiety, and hypertension
• After seeing a therapeutic effect, slowly reduce the dosage and frequency of administration of medications to the minimum required.

POSSIBLE COMPLICATIONS
• Recurrent and ascending urinary tract infection
• Urine scald and perineal and ventral dermatitis
• Refractory and unmanageable incontinence

MISCELLANEOUS

ASSOCIATED CONDITIONS
• Urethral incompetence/urethral dysplasia
• Urinary tract infection

Suggested Reading
Lane IF, Lappin MR. Urinary incontinence and congenital urogenital anomalies in small animals. In: Kirk RW, Bonagura JD, eds. Current veterinary therapy XII. Philadelphia: Saunders, 1995:1022–1026.
Mahaffey MB, Barsanti JA, et al. Pelvic bladder in dogs without urinary incontinence. J Am Vet Med Assoc 1984;184(12):1477.
Author Mary Anna Labato
Consulting Editors Larry G. Adams and Carl A. Osborne

BASICS

OVERVIEW
• Very rare, autoimmune vesiculobullous severe ulcerative dermatosis of the skin and/or oral mucosa in dogs
• Forms—bullous (commonly identified) and chronic (rare)

SIGNALMENT
• Dogs
• Breed predilection—collies, Shetland sheepdogs, and (possibly) Doberman pinschers
• No age or sex predisposition

SIGNS

Bullous
• Cutaneous lesions—transient blisters, crusts, epidermal collarettes, and ulcerations
• Widespread distribution—mucous membranes, head, neck, axillae, ventral abdomen, groin, and feet (nailbed involvement or footpad ulceration); oral cavity and skin of the axillae and groin most frequently involved
• Onset often acute with severe signs
• Severely affected dogs—anorexia, depression, and pyrexia
• Pain and pruritus variable
• Signs similar to pemphigus vulgaris

Chronic Pemphigoid
• Clinically benign
• Lesions—confined to the axillae, groin, or isolated mucocutaneous areas
• Slow and chronic course

CAUSES & RISK FACTORS
• Deposit of an autoantibody ("pemphigoid antibody") directed against the antigen at the basement membrane zone of skin and mucosa; results in blister formation below the epidermis
• Sunlight may exacerbate lesions.

DIAGNOSIS

DIFFERENTIAL DIAGNOSIS
• Pemphigus vulgaris
• Systemic lupus erythematosus
• Erythema multiforme
• Toxic epidermal necrolysis
• Drug eruption
• Mycosis fungoides
• Lymphoreticular neoplasia
• Hidradenitis suppurativa
• Ulcerative stomatitis

CBC/BIOCHEMISTRY/URINALYSIS
Leukocytosis, neutrophilia, mild nonregenerative anemia, hypoalbuminemia, and hyperglobulinemia may be seen.

OTHER LABORATORY TESTS
• Antinuclear antibody titer normal
• Lupus erythematosus test negative

IMAGING
N/A

DIAGNOSTIC PROCEDURES
• Biopsies of lesions—subepidermal vesicle formation with inflammatory infiltrates of granulocytes and mononuclear cells; no acantholysis
• Direct immunofluorescence usually negative if positive, dermoepidermal junction pattern
• Bacteriologic culture—identification and drug sensitivity of secondary bacteria

TREATMENT

• Supportive inpatient care if serious systemic signs or secondary infections occur
• Subsequent outpatient treatment; frequent hospital rechecks and monitoring every 1–4 weeks
• Low-fat diet—avoids pancreatitis secondary to corticosteroid and possible azathioprine therapy
• Avoid sunlight—UV light may exacerbate lesions.

Bullous
• Immunosuppressive agents
• Antibiotics for common secondary bacterial infections
• Gentle soaks/cleansing with antibacterial shampoos or povidone iodine and water

Chronic
• Immunosuppressive therapy
• Topical or intralesional corticosteroids

MEDICATIONS

DRUGS

Corticosteroids
• Prednisone or prednisolone—1.1–3.3 mg/kg PO q12h
• Higher doses are probably necessary, but side effects are likely and need to be monitored.

Cytotoxic Agents
• Required by many patients to achieve control, owing to intolerable side effects of high-dose corticosteroids or failure to achieve or maintain remission with corticosteroids alone
• Work synergistically with corticosteroids to reduce side effects
• Azathioprine—2.2 mg/kg PO q24h; then q48h
• Chlorambucil—0.1 mg/kg PO q24h; then q48h
• Cyclophosphamide—50 mg/m² BSA q48h
• 6-Mercaptopurine—2.2 mg/kg PO q24h; then q48h
• Dapsone—1 mg/kg PO q8h; then as needed; rarely used

Crysotherapy with Prednisone
• Aurothioglucose—administer a test dose of 1 mg IM (animals < 25 kg) or 5 mg IM (animals > 25 kg) 1st week; 2 mg IM (animals < 25 kg) or 10 mg IM (animals > 25 kg) 2nd week; then 1 mg/kg IM weekly until a clinical response is noted (usually a lag phase of 6–8 weeks); then 1 mg/kg IM every 2–4 weeks for maintenance
• Auranofin—0.1–0.2 mg/kg PO q12–24h

CONTRAINDICATIONS/POSSIBLE INTERACTIONS
• Corticosteroids—polyuria, polydipsia, polyphagia, temperament changes, hepatotoxicity
• Corticosteroid and azathioprine—pancreatitis
• Cytotoxic drugs—leukopenia, thrombocytopenia, nephrotoxicity, hepatotoxicity
• Chrysotherapy—nephrotoxicity, dermatitis, stomatitis, and allergic reactions
• Cyclophosphamide—hemorrhagic cystitis
• Immunosuppression—may predispose patient to Demodex, cutaneous and systemic fungal and bacterial infections

FOLLOW-UP

PATIENT MONITORING
Monitor often for signs of immunosuppression or progression of disease and medication side effects (reported, hematologic studies, and serum biochemistry).

EXPECTED COURSE AND PROGNOSIS

Bullous
• May be fatal if untreated
• Treatment must be aggressive; side effects may affect quality of life.
• Lifelong treatment and monitoring of side effects are usually necessary.
• Secondary infections cause morbidity and possible mortality.
• Some patients may not respond to therapy.

Chronic
• Fair prognosis
• Mild, chronic disease treated with relatively low doses of systemic glucocorticoids; some patients can be treated with topical glucocorticoids alone.

MISCELLANEOUS

Suggested Reading
Scott DW, Miller WH, Griffin CE. Bullous pemphigoid. In: Muller & Kirk's small animal dermatology. 5th ed. Philadelphia: Saunders, 1995:573–578.
Author Margaret S. Swartout
Consulting Editor Karen Helton Rhodes

DISEASES

BASICS

OVERVIEW
• A group of autoimmune dermatoses characterized by varying degrees of ulceration, crusting, and pustule and vesicle formation • Affects the skin and sometimes mucous membranes

PATHOPHYSIOLOGY
• Tissue-bound autoantibody directed at inter-epidermal cell antigen is deposited within the intercellular spaces, causing epidermal cell separation and cell rounding (acantholysis). • Severity of ulceration and disease—related to depth of autoantibody deposition within the skin • Types—foliaceus, vulgaris, erythematosus, and vegetans • Foliaceus—autoantibody deposition in the superficial layers of the epidermis • Vulgaris—lesions more severe; mediated by autoantibody deposition just above the basement membrane zone; results in deeper ulcer formation

SYSTEMS AFFECTED
Skin/Exocrine—autoantibody is tissue-bound

GENETICS
N/A

INCIDENCE/PREVALENCE
• Uncommon group of diseases • Foliaceus—most common type • Erythematosus—relatively common; may be a more benign variant of pemphigus foliaceus or may be a crossover syndrome of pemphigus and lupus erythematosus • Vulgaris—second most common type; the most severe form • Vegetans—rarest type; possibly a relatively benign variant of pemphigus vulgaris

GEOGRAPHIC DISTRIBUTION
N/A

SIGNALMENT
Species
• Foliaceus, erythematosus, and vulgaris—dogs and cats • Vegetans—dogs only

Breed Predilections
• Foliaceus—akitas, bearded collies, chow chows, dachshunds, Doberman pinschers, Finnish spitzes, Newfoundlands, and schipperkes. • Erythematosus—collies, German shepherds, and Shetland sheepdogs

Mean Age and Range
Usually middle-aged to old animals

Predominant Sex
None

SIGNS
Foliaceus
• Scales, crust, pustules, epidermal collarettes, erosions, erythema, alopecia, and footpad hyperkeratosis with fissuring • Occasional vesicles are transient. • Common involvement—head, ears and footpads; often becomes generalized • Mucosal and mucocutaneous lesions uncommon • Cats—nipple and nailbed involvement common • Sometimes lymphadenopathy, edema, depression, fever, and lameness (if footpads involved); however, patients are often in good health. • Variable pain and pruritus • Secondary bacterial infection possible

Erythematosus
• As for pemphigus foliaceus • Lesions usually confined to head, face, and footpads • mucocutaneous depigmentation more common than with other forms.

Vulgaris
• Ulcerative lesions, erosions, epidermal collarettes, blisters, and crusts • More severe than pemphigus foliaceus and erythematosus • Affects mucous membranes, mucocutaneous junctions, and skin; may become generalized • Oral ulceration frequent • Axillae and groin areas often involved • Positive Nikolsky sign (new or extended erosive lesion created when lateral pressure is applied to the skin near an existing lesion) • Variable pruritus and pain • Anorexia, depression, and fever • Secondary bacterial infections common

Vegetans
• Pustule groups become eruptive papillomatous lesions and vegetative masses that ooze. • Oral involvement has not been noted. • No systemic illness

CAUSES
Unknown

RISK FACTORS
Unknown

DIAGNOSIS

DIFFERENTIAL DIAGNOSIS
Foliaceus
• Bacterial folliculitis • Dermatophytosis • Demodicosis • Candidiasis • Keratinization disorders • Lupus erythematosus • Pemphigus erythematosus • Subcorneal pustular dermatosis • Drug eruption • Zinc-responsive dermatitis • Dermatomyositis • Tyrosinemia • Mycosis fungoides • Lymphoreticular malignancies • Metabolic epidermal necrosis • Sterile eosinophilic pustulosis • Linear IgA dermatosis

Erythematosus
• Pemphigus foliaceus • Systemic lupus erythematosus • Discoid lupus erythematosus • Nasal pyoderma • Demodicosis • Dermatophytosis • Epidermolysis bullosa simplex • Uveodermatologic syndrome

Vulgaris
• Bullous pemphigoid • Systemic lupus erythematosus • Toxic epidermal necrolysis • Drug eruption • Mycosis fungoides • Lymphoreticular neoplasia • Ulcerative stomatitis causes • Erythema multiforme

Vegetans
• Pemphigus vulgaris • Bacterial folliculitis • Pemphigus foliaceus • Lichenoid dermatoses • Cutaneous neoplasia

CBC/BIOCHEMISTRY/URINALYSIS
• Abnormalities uncommon • Leukocytosis and hyperglobulinemia sometimes noted

OTHER LABORATORY TESTS
• Antinuclear antibody—may be weakly positive in pemphigus erythematosus only

IMAGING
N/A

DIAGNOSTIC PROCEDURES
• Cytology of aspirates or impression smears of pustules or crusts—acantholytic cells and neutrophils • Bacteriologic culture—identify secondary bacterial infections

PATHOLOGIC FINDINGS
• Biopsies of lesional or perilesional skin—acantholysis and intraepidermal clefting; microabscess or pustule formation; surface acantholytic keratinocytes • Location of epidermal lesions—varies with disease; pemphigus foliaceous and erythematosus have subcorneal or intragranular clefting and acantholysis; pemphigus vulgaris and vegetans have suprabasilar clefting. • Immunopathology of biopsied skin via immunofluorescent antibody assays or immunohistochemical testing—may demonstrate positive staining in the intercellular spaces in 50%–90% of cases; results can be affected by concurrent or previous corticosteroid (or other immunosuppressive drug) administration; indirect immunofluorescence usually negative; pemphigus erythematosus may demonstrate staining of basement membranes and intercellular spaces.

TREATMENT

APPROPRIATE HEALTH CARE
• Initial inpatient supportive therapy for severely affected patients • Outpatient treatment with initial frequent hospital visits (every 1–3 weeks); taper to every 1–3 months remission is achieved and the patient is on maintenance medical regime.

NURSING CARE
Severely affected patients may need antibiotics and soaks.

ACTIVITY
N/A

DIET
Low-fat—to avoid pancreatitis predisposed by corticosteroids and (possibly) azathioprine therapy

CLIENT EDUCATION
Advise client that the patient should avoid the sun, because UV light may exacerbate lesions.

SURGICAL CONSIDERATIONS
N/A

MEDICATIONS

DRUGS
Pemphigus Vulgaris and Foliaceus
Corticosteroids
• Prednisone or prednisolone—1.1–2.2 mg/kg/day PO divided q12h to initiate control
• Minimum maintenance—0.5 mg/kg PO q48h
• Taper dosage at 2–4-week intervals by 5–10 mg per week.
Cytotoxic Agents
• More than half of patients require the addition of other immunomodulating drugs.
• Generally work synergistically with prednisone, allowing reduction in dose and side effects of the corticosteroid
• Azathioprine—2.2 mg/kg PO q24h, then q48h (dogs); infrequently used in cats, owing to potential for marked bone marrow suppression; feline dose 1 mg/kg q24–48h
• Chlorambucil—0.2 mg /kg daily; best choice for cats
• Cyclophosphamide—50 mg/m² PO BSA q48h (dogs)
• Cyclosporine—15–27 mg/kg daily PO; limited application
• Dapsone—1 mg/kg PO q8h; then as needed (dogs); limited application
Chrysotherapy
• Often used in conjunction with prednisone
• Aurothioglucose—administer a test dose of 1 mg IM (animals < 25 kg) or 5 mg IM (animals > 25 kg) 1st week; 2 mg IM (animals < 25 kg) or 10 mg IM (animals > 25 kg) 2nd week; then 1 mg/kg IM weekly until a clinical response is noted (generally a lag phase of 6–8 weeks); then 1 mg/kg IM every 2–4 weeks for maintenance
• Aranofin—0.1–0.2 mg/kg PO q12–24h

Pemphigus Erythematosus and Vegetans

• Oral prednisone or prednisolone—1.1 mg/kg PO q24h; then q48h; then to the lowest maintenance dose possible; may be stopped when in remission
• Topical steroids may be sufficient in mild cases.

CONTRAINDICATIONS
N/A

PRECAUTIONS
• Corticosteroids—polyuria, polydipsia, polyphagia, temperament changes, diabetes mellitus, pancreatitis, and hepatotoxicity
• Azathioprine—pancreatitis
• Cytotoxic drugs—leukopenia, thrombocytopenia, nephrotoxicity, and hepatotoxicity
• Chrysotherapy—leukopenia, thrombocytopenia, nephrotoxicity, dermatitis, stomatitis, and allergic reactions
• Cyclophosphamide—hemorrhagic cystitis
• Immunosuppression—can predispose animal to *Demodex*, cutaneous and systemic bacterial and fungal infection

POSSIBLE INTERACTIONS
N/A

ALTERNATIVE DRUGS
Alternative Corticosteroids
• Use instead of prednisone if undesirable side effects or poor response occur
• Methylprednisolone—0.8–1.5 mg/kg PO q12h; for patients that tolerate prednisone poorly
• Triamcinolone—0.2–0.3 mg/kg PO q12h; then 0.05–0.1 mg/kg q48–72h
• Glucocorticoid pulse therapy—11 mg/kg IV methylprednisolone sodium succinate for 3 consecutive days to induce remission; limited application

Topical Steroids
• Hydrocortisone cream
• More potent topical corticosteroids—0.1% betamethasone valerate, fluocinolone acetonide, or 0.1% triamcinonide; q12h; then q24–48h

Miscellaneous
Tetracycline and niacinamide—500 mg PO q8h (dogs > 10 kg); half doses for dogs < 10 kg; limited application

FOLLOW-UP

PATIENT MONITORING
• Monitor response to therapy • Monitor for medication side effects—routine hematology and serum biochemistry, especially patients on high doses of corticosteroids, cytotoxic drugs, or chrysotherapy; check every 1–3 weeks; then every 1–3 months when in remission.

PREVENTION/AVOIDANCE
N/A

POSSIBLE COMPLICATIONS
N/A

EXPECTED COURSE AND PROGNOSIS
Pemphigus Vulgaris and Foliaceus
• Therapy with corticosteroids and cytotoxic drugs needed • Patients may require medication for life. • Monitoring necessary • Side effects of medications may affect quality of life. • May be fatal if untreated (especially pemphigus vulgaris) • Secondary infections cause morbidity and possible mortality (especially pemphigus vulgaris).

Pemphigus Erythematosus and Vegetans
• Relatively benign and self-limiting.
• Oral corticosteroids may eventually be tapered to low maintenance doses; may be stopped in some patients
• Dermatosis develops if untreated; systemic symptoms rare
• Prognosis fair

MISCELLANEOUS

ASSOCIATED CONDITIONS
N/A

AGE-RELATED FACTORS
N/A

ZOONOTIC POTENTIAL
None

PREGNANCY
Avoid steroids and cytotoxic drugs during pregnancy.

SYNONYMS
None

Suggested Reading
Ackerman LJ. Immune-mediated skin diseases. In: Morgan RV, ed. Handbook of small animal practice. 3rd ed. Philadelphia: Saunders, 1997:941–943.
Angarano DW. Autoimmune dermatosis. In: Nesbitt GH, ed. Contemporary issues in small animal practice: dermatology. New York: Churchill Livingston, 1987:79–94.
Rosenkrantz WS. Pemphigus foliaceous. In: Griffin CE, Knochka KW, MacDonald JM, et al., eds., Current veterinary dermatology. St. Louis: Mosby, 1993:141–148.
Author Margaret S. Swartout
Consulting Editor Karen Helton Rhodes

DISEASES

PERIANAL FISTULA

 BASICS

OVERVIEW
• Characterized by multiple chronic fistulous tracts or ulcerating sinuses involving the perianal region
• Cause—Not known; apocrine gland inflammation (hidradenitis suppurativa), impaction and infection of the anal sinuses and crypts, infection of the circumanal glands and hair follicles, and anal sacculitis have all been implicated.
• An association with colitis in German shepherd dogs has been proposed.
• The gastrointestinal system becomes involved when excessive scar tissue formation around the anus results in tenesmus, dyschezia, or other problems associated with defecation.
• Self-mutilation can be a major problem.

SIGNALMENT
• Dogs
• German shepherd dog and Irish setter most commonly affected breeds
• Mean age, 7 years; range, 7 months to 12 years
• No gender predisposition reported; sexually intact dogs have a higher prevalence.
• A genetic basis has been proposed but not proven.

SIGNS
• Vary with the severity and extent of involvement
• Dyschezia
• Tenesmus
• Hematochezia
• Constipation
• Diarrhea
• Malodorous mucopurulent anal discharge
• Painful tail movements
• Licking and self-mutilation
• Reluctance to sit, posturing difficulties, and personality changes
• Fecal incontinence
• Anorexia
• Weight loss
• Perianal fistulous tracts

CAUSES & RISK FACTORS
• Low tail carriage and a broad tail base—proposed risk factors predisposing the dog to inflammation and infection because of poor ventilation, accumulation of feces, moisture, and secretions
• High density of apocrine sweat glands in the cutaneous zone of the anal canal of German shepherd dogs
• Hidradenitis suppurativa may be associated with immune or endocrine dysfunction, genetic factors, and poor hygiene.

 DIAGNOSIS

DIFFERENTIAL DIAGNOSIS
• Chronic anal sac abscess
• Perianal adenoma or adenocarcinoma with ulceration and drainage
• Rectal fistula

CBC/BIOCHEMISTRY/URINALYSIS
• Usually normal
• Patients with inflammation may have an inflammatory leukogram.

OTHER LABORATORY TESTS
N/A

IMAGING
N/A

DIAGNOSTIC PROCEDURES
• Presumptive diagnosis—based on clinical signs and results of physical examination
• Definitive diagnosis—made by biopsy of the affected area
• Colonoscopy with biopsy may reveal associated colitis

 TREATMENT

• Surgery is considered the most effective treatment if medical therapy is unsuccessful.
• Which surgical method to use is quite controversial; none of those currently used consistently resolves the problem.
• Surgical options include electrosurgery, cryo-surgery, surgical debridement with fulguration by chemical cautery, exteriorization and fulguration by electrocautery, surgical resection, radical excision of the rectal ring, tail setting, tail amputation, and laser surgery.
• Perform anal sacculectomy with the above-selected procedure.
• Each technique has advantages and disadvantages that must be weighed when making a choice.
• Primary objective of surgery is complete removal or destruction of diseased tissue while preserving normal tissue and function.
• Multiple procedures may be necessary for complete resolution.

NURSING CARE
- Clipping hair from the affected area
- Daily antiseptic lavage
- Systemic and topical antibiotics
- Hydrotherapy
- Elevation of the tail
- Analgesics
- Dietary modification—stool softeners if pain/tenesmus; fiber-enhanced or hypoallergenic diet if associated colitis/proctitis
- Postoperative nursing care may also include warm-packing the affected area.

MEDICATIONS

DRUGS
- Cyclosporine (2–3 mg/kg PO q24h × 12 weeks)—most dogs improve; up to 50% may clear completely; 50% still require surgery because of inadequate clearing of fistulas or anal stricture.
- Unsuccessful medical treatment can be detrimental by delaying surgery.
- Antibiotics and analgesics may be indicated in some cases.
- Corticosteroids (2 mg/kg PO q12h) and a hypoallergenic diet for 6 weeks may yield partial or complete resolution (about 33% of cases); most dogs do not improve; corticosteroid side effects are common.

CONTRAINDICATIONS/POSSIBLE INTERACTIONS
Corticosteroids are contraindicated when infection is probable.

FOLLOW-UP

PATIENT MONITORING
- Assess cyclosporine levels every 3 weeks; appropriate levels are 200–300 ng/mL.
- Reexamine after surgery to assess healing, signs of recurrence, and associated complications.

POSSIBLE COMPLICATIONS
- Recurrence
- Failure to heal
- Dehiscence of surgical site
- Tenesmus
- Fecal incontinence
- Anal stricture
- Flatulence
- The incidence of postoperative complications is directly related to severity of disease.

EXPECTED COURSE/PROGNOSIS
- Guarded for complete resolution except in mildly affected patients
- Clients often become frustrated with the difficulty of attaining definitive resolution.

MISCELLANEOUS

ASSOCIATED CONDITIONS
Constipation and/or obstipation can develop.

AGE-RELATED FACTORS
N/A

ZOONOTIC POTENTIAL
N/A

PREGNANCY
Caution with drug use (cyclosporine, corticosteroids) and surgery

SEE ALSO
- Colitis and Proctitis
- Constipation and Obstipation
- Dyschezia and Hematochezia

ABBREVIATIONS
N/A

Suggested Reading

Harkin KR, Walshaw R, Mullaney TP. Association of perianal fistula and colitis in the German shepherd dog: response to high-dose prednisone and dietary therapy. J Am Anim Hosp Assoc 1996;32:515–520.

Matthews KA, Sukhiani HR. OL27–400 (cyclosporin) treatment of canine perianal fistulas: a prospective, randomized, double-blind, controlled study. Proceedings, 6th Ann ACVS Symposium, San Francisco, CA, 1997:15–16.

Matthiesen DT, Marretta SM. Diseases of the anus and rectum. In: Slatter D, ed. Textbook of small animal surgery. 2nd ed. Philadelphia: Saunders, 1993;627–644.

van Ee RT. Perianal fistulas. In: Bojrab MJ, ed. Disease mechanisms in small animal surgery. 2nd ed. Philadelphia: Lea & Febiger, 1993;285–286.

Author James L. Cook

Consulting Editors Mitchell A. Crystal and Brett M. Feder

DISEASES

PERICARDIAL EFFUSION

BASICS

DEFINITION
Abnormally high volume of fluid within the pericardial sac; cardiac tamponade is clinical result of hemodynamic compromise.

PATHOPHYSIOLOGY
Accumulate of effusion exceeds elastic, or stretching, capabilities of the pericardial sac; further accumulation leads to high intrapericardial pressure. Cardiac tamponade occurs when intrapericardial pressure exceeds cardiac diastolic filling pressure. The right atrium and right ventricle normally have the lowest cardiac filling pressure and are predominantly affected. The resultant reduction in cardiac filling (pre-load reduction) diminishes forward blood flow (low cardiac output). In animals with chronic pericardial disease, low cardiac output activates compensatory mechanisms that lead to fluid accumulation. Congestive signs are typically manifested as right-sided CHF. Animals with acutely developing effusions typically exhibit signs of weakness or collapse.

SYSTEMS AFFECTED
• Cardiovascular—signs of low cardiac output and CHF • Hepatobiliary—chronic passive congestion with mildly to moderately high liver enzymes • Renal/Urologic—prerenal azotemia • Respiratory—tachypnea or pleural effusion

GENETICS
N/A

INCIDENCE/PREVALENCE
N/A

GEOGRAPHIC DISTRIBUTION
N/A

SIGNALMENT
Species
Dogs and cats

Breed Predispositions
Golden retrievers and German shepherd are predisposed to right atrial hemangiosarcoma and idiopathic effusion.

Mean Age and Range
Middle-aged to old dogs are predisposed.

Predominant Sex
Male dogs are predisposed to idiopathic effusion.

SIGNS
General Comments
Chronic pericardial effusion often causes ascites without a cardiac murmur.

Historical Findings
• Lethargy • Anorexia • Weakness • Exercise intolerance • Abdominal distension • Syncope or collapse

Physical Examination Findings
Acute pericardial effusion
• Pallor • Slow capillary refill time • Weak arterial pulses • Weakness, syncope, collapse • Tachypnea • Tachycardia
Chronic pericardial effusion
• Jugular vein distension • Ascites • Muffled heart sounds • Weak arterial pulses • Pulsus paradoxus • Pallor • Slow capillary refill time • Weakness • Tachypnea • Tachycardia

CAUSES
• Neoplasia—hemangiosarcoma, heart-base tumor (chemodectoma), thyroid carcinoma, mesothelioma, metastatic neoplasia and lymphoma (cats) • Idiopathic—benign or hemorrhagic • Coagulopathy—intoxication with vitamin K antagonist rodenticide, thrombocytopenia, other coagulopathies • Infection—feline infectious peritonitis, coccidioidomycosis, bacterial pericarditis • Congenital disorders—peritoneopericardial hernia • Left atrial tear or cardiac trauma • CHF • Foreign body

RISK FACTORS
N/A

DIAGNOSIS

DIFFERENTIAL DIAGNOSIS
• CHF secondary to other causes (e.g., chronic valvular disease and cardiomyopathy), hepatic failure, abdominal neoplasm with hemorrhage, protein-losing nephropathy or enteropathy
• Usually cardiac murmur or gallop in animals with heart failure caused by cardiomyopathy or valvular disease • Other causes of ascites (e.g., hepatic failure, hypoproteinemia, intra-abdominal neoplasia, and hemorrhage caused by coagulopathy)—characteristically cause remarkable abnormalities on CBC and biochemistry profile and typically lack jugular venous distension. Examination of the jugular vein can be extremely helpful in differentiating these conditions from heart failure.

CBC/BIOCHEMISTRY/URINALYSIS
• CBC—usually normal, but may be anemia in animals with hemangiosarcoma, lymphoma, or coagulopathy • Red cell morphology may be abnormal (e.g., nucleated red blood cells, schistocytes, and acanthocytes); may be thrombocytopenia in animals with hemangiosarcoma • Biochemistry profile—often normal; may be mild to moderately high liver enzymes (in animals with chronic passive hepatic congestion), mild azotemia (typically prerenal), and mild electrolyte abnormalities (e.g., hyponatremia, hypochloremia, and hyperkalemia) • Urinalysis—usually normal with normal renal concentrating ability unless a diuretic has been administered

OTHER LABORATORY TESTS
• Clotting times (e.g., activated partial thromboplastin time and one-stage prothrombin time)—prolonged in animals with vitamin K antagonist rodenticide intoxication
• Feline infectious peritonitis titers may be high in cats.
• Cats with lymphoma may be feline leukemia virus positive.

IMAGING
Thoracic Radiographic Findings
• Mild-to-severe cardiac enlargement; cardiac silhouette often globoid and often very sharp edges on the dorsoventral view because of lack of cardiac motion artifact
• Mild-to-moderate pleural effusion in some patients
• Ascites in many patients
• Large caudal vena cava in some patients

Echocardiography
• Superior diagnostic test to confirm diagnosis
• Echo-free space clearly identified between the pericardium and the epicardial surface of the heart
• Often demonstrates the cause of pericardial effusion in patients with neoplasia (e.g., right atrial hemangiosarcoma and heart base tumor around aorta) or peritoneopericardial hernia

Pneumopericardiography
• May identify mass lesions
• Inferior to echocardiography in diagnostic accuracy
• Images often difficult to interpret without extensive experience with this technique

DIAGNOSTIC PROCEDURES
Electrocardiographic Findings
• Sinus tachycardia in many patients; occasionally ventricular or supraventricular arrhythmias
• Low-voltage QRS complexes (< 1 mV in leads I, II, III, aVR, aVL, and aVF), ST segment elevation, and electrical alternans in some patients
• Electrical alternans, a regular (1 to 1 or 2 to 1) variation in QRS-T wave height or morphology, results from the heart swinging back and forth within the pericardial sac.

TREATMENT

APPROPRIATE HEALTH CARE
Cardiac tamponade indicates immediate pericardiocentesis; if uncomfortable with this technique of pericardiocentesis, referral to individuals with competence in this technique is strongly advised; repeated pericardiocentesis may be needed; surgery may be indicated in selected patients

PERICARDIOCENTESIS

• Place the patient in sternal recumbency. Clip hair coat on the right thorax between the 3rd and 8th intercostal space from above the costochondral junction ventrally to the sternum. Right side of the thorax is preferred over the left because less likelihood of coronary artery laceration. Simultaneous ECG monitoring is advised to detect arrhythmias due to contact between the needle or catheter and the myocardium. Echocardiography is useful to identify the best intercostal space; if no echocardiography, perform pericardiocentesis at the 5th intercostal space just below the costochondral junction. After aseptic skin preparation and local anesthetic block with lidocaine, advance a long (= 2 cm), large (=18 gauge) catheter into the pericardial sac; may obtain a small amount of clear pleural fluid before advancement of the catheter into the pericardial sac. In dogs, pericardial effusion is usually hemorrhagic, but some patients have a serous or serosanguineous effusion. Remove as much effusion as possible. If arrhythmias develop, reposition the needle or catheter.
• Unless patient has active hemorrhage into the pericardial sac, the effusion obtained by pericardiocentesis should not clot and should have a packed cell volume that differs from that of peripheral blood. The supernatant of the effusion is often xanthochromic.

NURSING CARE

Unless the patient has marked dehydration, fluids are generally not required or recommended for chronic pericardial effusion. Mild volume expansion may be useful in selected animals with acute pericardial effusion due to intrapericardial hemorrhage—0.45 NaCl with 2.5% dextrose is preferred by some; infusion volume is usually one half of calculated maintenance fluid requirement. Administer oxygen to dogs with tachypnea or signs of hemodynamic instability.

SURGICAL CONSIDERATIONS

• Pericardiectomy may be useful in the treatment of chemodectoma or heart-base tumor.
• If idiopathic—may respond to pericardiocentesis; pericardiectomy is indicated if it recurs.
• Surgery and chemotherapy are generally ineffective in the treatment of right atrial hemangiosarcoma.

MEDICATIONS

DRUGS OF CHOICE

• Should not be used in place of pericardiocentesis

• Diuretics—may help reduce ascites but can lead to progressive azotemia and renal dysfunction and worsen the patient's weakness; can use diuretics such as furosemide or spironolactone if client refuses pericardiocentesis, but in low dosage, with caution; generally not advised
• Vitamin K—indicated for patients with rodenticide anticoagulant intoxication
• Appropriate antibiotics—indicated for infection by susceptible organism causing infectious pericarditis
• Chemotherapy—may be useful to treat effusion caused by lymphosarcoma; usually ineffective in the treatment of atrial hemangiosarcoma and heart-base tumor

CONTRAINDICATIONS

Digitalis, vasodilators, and angiotensin converting enzyme inhibitors—reported to be relatively or absolutely contraindicated

PRECAUTIONS

Diuretic administration often leads to weakness and prerenal azotemia.

POSSIBLE INTERACTIONS

N/A

ALTERNATIVE DRUGS

• Systemic or intrapericardial chemotherapy may be attempted to treat right atrial hemangiosarcoma; generally ineffective
• Corticosteroids by systemic or intrapericardial administration—may be useful in selected patients with idiopathic pericardial effusion
• Azathioprine at a dosage of 1 mg/kg PO q24h for 3 months—can be considered for recurrent idiopathic pericardial effusion; not commonly used and, like steroids, has not been evaluated in prospective trials to confirm efficacy in idiopathic pericardial effusion

FOLLOW-UP

PATIENT MONITORING

• ECG—advised during first 24 h because pericardiocentesis often leads to ventricular arrhythmias • Pericardial effusion may recur at any stage; examination and echocardiography at 10–14 days and every 2–4 months recommended to detect idiopathic pericardial effusion

PREVENTION/AVOIDANCE

N/A

POSSIBLE COMPLICATIONS

• Hypotension or shock • Pneumothorax, arrhythmias, and myocardial injury secondary to pericardiocentesis

EXPECTED COURSE AND PROGNOSIS

• Right atrial hemangiosarcoma—poor; tumor is highly malignant, usually not resectable at

the time of diagnosis, minimally responsive to chemotherapy; pericardectomy may result in exsanguination. • Chemodectoma—fair; slow-growing tumors, late to metastasize; pericardectomy often resolves clinical signs; reported survival of up to 3 years has been reported following pericardectomy. • Prognosis is good with idiopathic pericardial effusion—good; approximately 50% of cases resolve after 1 or 2 pericardiocenteses; pericardectomy is generally curative in persistent cases.

MISCELLANEOUS

ASSOCIATED CONDITION

Hemangiosarcoma of the spleen

AGE-RELATED FACTORS

• Idiopathic pericardial effusion may be more common in middle-aged to elderly dogs.
• Hemangiosarcoma and heart-base tumors are more common in elderly dogs.

ZOONOTIC POTENTIAL

Coccidioidomycosis

PREGNANCY

N/A

SYNONYMS

• Cardiac tamponade
• Pericardial tamponade
• Pericarditis

SEE ALSO

• Anticoagulant Rodenticide Toxicity
• Atrial tear
• Chemodectoma
• Coccidioidomycosis
• Pericarditis
• Feline Infectious Peritonitis
• Hemangiosarcoma, Liver and Spleen
• Myocardial Tumors

ABBREVIATIONS

CHF = congestive heart failure

Suggested Reading

Miller MW, Sisson DD. Pericardial disorders. In: Ettinger SJ, Feldman EC, eds. Textbook of veterinary internal medicine. 4th ed. Philadelphia: Saunders, 1995:1032–1045.

Sisson D, Thomas WP. Pericardial disease and cardiac tumors. In: Fox PR, Sisson D, Moise NS, eds. Textbook of canine and feline cardiology. 2nd ed. Philadelphia: Saunders, 1999:679–702.

Smith FWK Jr, Rush JE. Diagnosis and treatment of pericardial effusion. In: Bonagura JD, ed. Kirk's current veterinary therapy XIII. Philadelphia: Saunders, 1999:772–777.

Author John E. Rush

Consulting Editors Larry P. Tilley and Francis W. K. Smith, Jr.

DISEASES

PERICARDITIS

BASICS

OVERVIEW
• Inflammatory condition of the parietal (pericardial sac) and/or visceral (epicardium) pericardium; clinical syndromes caused by pericardial effusion, constrictive pericarditis, inflammatory extension to surrounding tissues (pleural, myocardium), or the underlying cause of the pericarditis • In dogs—most commonly seen as idiopathic hemorrhagic pericarditis, is a mild inflammatory condition that can lead to life-threatening pericardial effusion and tamponade

SIGNALMENT
• Dogs and cats • Idiopathic hemorrhagic pericarditis more common in young to middle-aged, medium to large-breed dogs (e.g., great Pyrenees, Great Dane, Saint Bernard, golden retriever); males predisposed • Others depend on the underlying disease.

SIGNS
• Cats—rarely seen on examination. • Dogs—usually caused by low cardiac output and right heart failure secondary to cardiac tamponade (i.e., anorexia, weakness, collapse, ascites, dyspnea, diminished pulse strength, tachycardia, muffled heart sounds, jugular distension or pulsation); similar to those often seen in animals with constrictive pericarditis and pericardial effusion, which may coexist (constrictive-effusive pericarditis).

CAUSES & RISK FACTORS
• Idiopathic hemorrhagic pericarditis—unknown • Pericarditis in dogs—blunt or penetrating trauma and bacterial or fungal infection (e.g., tuberculosis, coccidioidomycosis, actinomycosis, nocardiosis, and infection with *Pasteurella* spp) • Cats—pericarditis unusual but occurs as a consequence of trauma or infection; associated infectious agents include FIP, *Staphylococcus aureus*, *Escherichia coli*, *Streptococcus*, *Actinomyces*, *Cryptococcus*, and possibly *Toxoplasma*.

DIAGNOSIS

DIFFERENTIAL DIAGNOSIS
• Other causes of pericardial effusion (e.g., neoplasia, left atrial rupture, right-sided CHF, peritoneal-pericardial diaphragmatic hernia, and pericardial cysts)
• Other causes of right-sided CHF (e.g., cardiomyopathy, myocarditis, tricuspid or pulmonary valve disease, congenital heart disease, and severe left-sided CHF) • Other causes of abdominal effusion (e.g., neoplastic effusion, hemorrhage, and hypoproteinemia)
• Other causes of weakened arterial pulses or collapse (e.g., cardiomyopathy, shock, hypoadrenocorticism, arrhythmias, saddle thrombus, and aortic stenosis) • May be concealed by multisystemic signs relating to the underlying disease

CBC/BIOCHEMISTRY/URINALYSIS
Leukocytosis in some animals with a systemic inflammatory condition, but not dogs with idiopathic hemorrhagic pericarditis

IMAGING
Thoracic Radiography
• May suggest pericardial effusion (rounded cardiac silhouette), particularly when chronic effusion allows slow but marked expansion of the pericardium; absence of this finding does not rule out pericardial effusion or pericarditis • May see radiodense foreign objects • Intrapericardial injection of gas after pericardiocentesis (pneumopericardiography) may reveal space-occupying lesions; neoplastic lesions may be difficult to distinguish from granulomas or cysts.

Echocardiography
Two-dimensional echocardiography is preferred for evaluation of effusion, cardiac tamponade, and neoplasia; diagnosis by direct visualization.

Cardiac Catheterization
Constrictive pericardial physiology is difficult to diagnose but recognized by simultaneous pressure measurements from the right and left ventricles showing pressure equalization of the two sides at an elevated end-diastolic pressure. Atrial tracings show a rapid drop in pressure in early diastole followed by an early rise to plateau at an elevated end-diastolic pressure.

DIAGNOSTIC PROCEDURES
Electrocardiographic Findings
May see small QRS complexes, electrical alternans, S-T segment elevation, and arrhythmias

Fluid Analysis
Cytologic examination of pericardial effusion—usually not helpful because it cannot differentiate the most common causes, neoplastic and idiopathic; can potentially reveal an etiologic agent and rule out a suppurative process; cytologic evaluation of effusion or pericardial biopsy provides the definitive diagnosis of pericarditis.

Other Procedures
• If an infectious agent is suspected, aerobic and anaerobic cultures of the effusion are indicated. • Histopathologic examination of the pericardium.

TREATMENT
• Pericardiocentesis and partial pericardectomy for severe effusion. Right heart failure (R-CHF) may cause or result from pericardial effusion; medical treatment of R-CHF is appropriate in the former. Effusion due to idiopathic pericarditis in dogs may subside after one or more pericardiocenteses. For pericardial effusion, thoracic exploration with partial pericardectomy prevents effusions from limiting cardiac function and allows surgical debridement, retrieval of specimens for histopathologic examination, removal of foreign objects, and evaluation for neoplastic or granulomatous disease. • Constrictive pericarditis with extensive involvement of the epicardium may require epicardial stripping to relieve the constriction and relieve adhesions between the epicardium and pericardium; this is a difficult procedure with high mortality.

MEDICATIONS

DRUGS
• Treat infectious disease with chemotherapeutic agents determined through culture and sensitivity testing. • Steroid administration in dogs with idiopathic hemorrhagic pericarditis has been recommended, but efficacy is unknown; this is also true of azathioprine recommended at 1.0 mg/kg q24h for 3 months.

CONTRAINDICATIONS/POSSIBLE INTERACTIONS
• Fluid therapy exacerbates R-CHF • Diuretics and preload reducers—relatively contraindicated in animals with cardiac tamponade • Steroids may exacerbate an infection.

FOLLOW-UP
Pericardial effusion may recur if the pericardium is intact. Occasionally, clinically important pleural effusion may occur after pericardectomy; echocardiography or thoracic radiography is recommended.

MISCELLANEOUS

ABBREVIATIONS
• R-CHF = right-sided congestive heart failure.
• FIP = feline infectious pericarditis.

Suggested Reading
Miller MW, Sisson DD. Pericardial disorders. In: Ettinger SJ, Feldman EC, eds. Textbook of veterinary internal medicine. 4th ed. Philadelphia: Saunders, 2000:923–936.
Author Donald J. Brown
Consulting Editors Larry P. Tilley and Francis W. K. Smith, Jr.

BASICS

OVERVIEW
• Results from a defect in the musculature of the pelvic diaphragm
• Allows herniation of retroperitoneal fat or pelvic viscera through the pelvic diaphragm
• Organ systems potentially involved—GI, musculoskeletal, urologic, reproductive

SIGNALMENT
• Much more common in dogs than cats
• Almost exclusively (95%) male dogs
• Usually older than 5 years of age
• Boston terriers, collies, boxers, Pekingese, and mongrels overrepresented

SIGNS

Historical Findings
• Tenesmus
• Stranguria/dysuria if prostate or bladder entrapment
• Painful defecation
• Flatulence
• Fecal or urinary incontinence (rare)

Physical Examination Findings
• Fluctuant perineal swelling—unilateral or bilateral
• Defect in pelvic diaphragm palpable per rectum

CAUSES & RISK FACTORS
• Unknown
• Suggested causes include congenital pelvic muscle weakness, gonadal hormone imbalance, prostatic disease, chronic constipation/tenesmus, concurrent rectal disease (diverticulum, sacculation, deviation)

DIAGNOSIS

DIFFERENTIAL DIAGNOSIS
• Perianal or perineal neoplasia is usually a firm irregular swelling.
• Anal sac disease (abscess, cellulitis) is usually painful and localized to the anal sacs.

CBC/BIOCHEMISTRY/URINALYSIS
• No consistent changes
• Complete laboratory analysis recommended to look for concurrent diseases in older patients.
• May be azotemic if urinary obstruction is due to bladder entrapment

OTHER LABORATORY TESTS
N/A

IMAGING
• Plain radiographs document extent of rectal/colonic dilatation.
• GI contrast radiography differentiates rectal deviation from rectal sacculation or diverticulum.
• Contrast cystography demonstrates bladder entrapment.
• Ultrasonography (abdominal, perineal) may demonstrate prostatic, bladder, and/or GI entrapment.

DIAGNOSTIC PROCEDURES
N/A

TREATMENT
• Inpatient surgical management; not an emergency unless bladder or GI entrapment with obstruction
• Surgery indicated to reduce hernia and repair muscular defect.
• Internal obturator flap herniorrhaphy technique has the lowest recurrence rate.
• May use semitendinosus muscle flap to repair large ventral hernias, especially when other surgeries have failed
• Can perform colopexy/cystopexy in conjunction with, or independent of, herniorrhaphy to prevent herniation of rectum and urinary bladder, respectively
• Concurrent castration is recommended.
• High-fiber diet may help obtain a soft, formed stool; if colonic fecal overdistension occurs with bulk-fiber diets, a low-residue diet is indicated.
• Warn owners that underlying cause may not be corrected by surgery.

MEDICATIONS

DRUGS
• Use stool softeners as needed to maintain a soft, formed stool, and thus reduce straining.
• Perioperative prophylactic antibiotics are justified; choose one with broad-spectrum activity against gram-negative organisms.

CONTRAINDICATIONS/POSSIBLE INTERACTIONS
N/A

FOLLOW-UP

PREVENTION/AVOIDANCE
Early neutering of male dogs reduces risk.

POSSIBLE COMPLICATIONS
Immediate postsurgical complications include infection, fecal incontinence, sciatic nerve entrapment, and rectal prolapse.

EXPECTED COURSE AND PROGNOSIS
Overall recurrence rate 10–50% following repair

MISCELLANEOUS

ASSOCIATED CONDITIONS
• Megacolon
• Prostatic disease
• Dyschezia
• Tenesmus

ABBREVIATION
GI = gastrointestinal

Suggested Reading
Anderson MA, Constantinescu GM, Mann FA. Perineal hernia repair in the dog. In: Bojrab MJ, ed., Current techniques in small animal surgery. 4th ed. Philadelphia: Williams & Wilkins, 1998:555–564.
Author Bradford C. Dixon
Consulting Editors Mitchell A. Crystal and Brett M. Feder

PERIPHERAL EDEMA

 BASICS

DEFINITION
Edema is focal or diffuse excessive accumulation of tissue fluid within the interstitium; often at gravitative surfaces, whether localized or generalized

PATHOPHYSIOLOGY
• High capillary hydrostatic pressure
• Increased capillary permeability
• Lymphatic drainage abnormality
• Low plasma colloid osmotic pressure

SYSTEMS AFFECTED
• Skin/Exocrine
• Musculoskeletal

SIGNALMENT
Dogs and cats of any breed, age, and sex

SIGNS

Historical Findings
• Allergic or other immune, cardiac, hepatic or other organic disease
• Trauma
• Exposure to toxic (venomous) or infectious agents such as ticks or other arachnids

Physical Examination Findings
• Unexplained weight gain may be noted initially, otherwise early detection is unlikely.
• Noninflammatory subcutaneous edema is often first recognized at the dependent thorax or abdomen or distal limbs.
• Inflammatory edema may be noted in nondependent foci of the interstitium

CAUSES

Localized or Single-Limb Edema
• High capillary hydrostatic pressure
• Venous or arterial obstruction, e.g., thrombosis or postcaval syndrome
• Arteriovenous fistula
• Increased capillary permeability
• Focal or multifocal immune, infectious, or toxic (chemical or biologic) insults (e.g., snake bite or bee sting)
• Trauma
• Burns
• Lymphatic obstruction
• Sterile (juvenile pyoderma) or infectious lymphangitis
• Primary or metastatic neoplastic invasion of lymphatic tissue
• Congenital aplasia or dysgenesis of the lymphatic system

Regional or Generalized Edema
• High capillary hydrostatic pressure
• Congestive heart failure (CHF)
• Cardiac tamponade
• Cranial or caudal vena caval thrombosis

• Renal failure and hypernatremia (salt retention)
• Paralysis or prolonged recumbency with subsequent failure of the venous pump
• Tourniquet effect of a bandage
• Increased capillary permeability
• Systemic immune, infectious, or toxic insults (e.g., sepsis or vasculitis)
• Lymphatic abnormalities
• Acquired regional traumatic, immune, infectious or neoplastic process
• Congenital aplasia or other lymphatic dysgenesis
• Low plasma colloid osmotic pressure
• Protein-losing disease (e.g., nephrotic syndrome or intestinal lymphangiectasia)
• Failure to produce protein (e.g., cirrhosis)
• Exudative protein loss (e.g., severe burn)

RISK FACTORS
Variable

 DIAGNOSIS

DIFFERENTIAL DIAGNOSIS
• Peripheral edema secondary to myxedema or inflammation is typically nonpitting.
• Bilateral forelimb edema with jugular venous distension implies cranial vena caval syndrome.
• Bilateral rear limb edema with or without ascites implies either hypoalbuminemia or caudal vena caval obstruction.
• Fore and/or rear limb edema with jugular venous distension—hydrothorax and/or ascites implies cardiac disease.
• Focal edema with bruit and fremitus implies an arteriovenous fistula.
• Focal edema with erythema may be secondary to an insect or other bite.
• Multifocal or diffuse edema with petechiation and/or ecchymosis may be associated with a coagulopathy or vasculitis.

CBC/BIOCHEMISTRY/URINALYSIS
• Leukocytosis suggests inflammatory or infectious disease.
• Thrombocytopenia may be secondary to vasculitis (e.g., Rocky Mountain spotted fever [RMSF]), systemic lupus erythematosus (SLE), or a coagulopathy (e.g., disseminated intravascular coagulation [DIC]).
• Panhypoproteinemia is consistent with gastrointestinal disease, but diarrhea is not an obligatory clinical sign.
• Panhypoproteinemia and hypocholesterolemia are seen with intestinal lymphangiectasia.
• Hypoalbuminemia may occur with hepatic failure.

• Hypoalbuminemia with proteinuria suggests glomerular disease.
• Hypoalbuminemia with proteinuria and hypercholesterolemia in an edematous patient defines nephrotic syndrome.

OTHER LABORATORY TESTS
• Antithrombin III assay indicated in conditions with albumin loss
• Further delineate thrombocytopenia with a bone marrow biopsy, antinuclear antibody (ANA), *Ehrlichia* and RMSF titers, and a coagulation profile.
• Panhypoproteinemia may dictate a need for intestinal biopsy.
• Hypoalbuminemia may warrant liver function testing, (e.g., bile acids test, hepatic or renal biopsy)
• Confirm proteinuria with a urine protein: creatinine ratio.
• Bacterial and fungal cultures of blind fistulae may prove useful.
• Fungal or other titers of infectious disease may be warranted.
• Pleural or peritoneal fluid analysis is suggested if effusion present.
• Low resting thyroid hormone (T_4) should be elaborated with a thyrotropin-releasing hormone (TRH) stimulation test, free T_4 by equilibrium dialysis, or thyroid-stimulating hormone (TSH) concentration.

IMAGING
• Suspected heart disease necessitates thoracic radiographs and echocardiogram.
• Angiography (e.g., venacavagram) may help define a vascular obstruction.
• Diagnostic ultrasound may help to delineate a vascular occlusion.
• Thermography and perfusion scans (e.g., scintigraphy) are esoteric but have been used to diagnose occlusive vascular disease.

DIAGNOSTIC PROCEDURES
• Fine-needle aspiration of an affected area for cytology and culture may be helpful.
• Biopsy and deep culture may help define an underlying cause for edema.

 TREATMENT

• Intervention—depends on the cause of the edema
• Diuretics—generally contraindicated in patients with noncardiogenic edema
• Pressure bandages (e.g., Robert Jones splint) used with variable success, especially for primary lymphedema
• Good nursing care required to prevent decubital ulceration in recumbent patients

• Maintain a patent airway and provide cardiovascular support in type I hypersensitivity reactions
• Surgery such as lymphangioplasty, thrombectomy, or lymphaticovenous shunt may be palliative.
• Amputation of the edematous limb is sometimes indicated.
• Arteriovenous fistulae may be treated by various surgical methods.

MEDICATIONS

DRUGS OF CHOICE
• Anaphylaxis—epinephrine (1 mg/mL) at 0.01 mL/kg IM or SC to a maximum of 0.02–0.05 mL; prednisone sodium succinate 10–30 mg/kg IV; antihistamines are of equivocal benefit once anaphylaxis ensues
• Lymphedema—benzopyrone use yields variable results in veterinary medicine; rutin, 50 mg/kg PO q8h, was mixed with food for cats with chylothorax.
• Cardiogenic edema—combinations of positive or negative inotropes, vasodilators, and diuretics common in patients with CHF
• Immune-mediated edema requires immunosuppressive therapy (e.g., prednisone and cyclophosphamide)
• Vasculitis and edema secondary to rickettsial disease typically respond to tetracycline (22 mg/kg PO q8h) or doxycycline (5 mg/kg PO q12h).
• Edema in association with other infectious agents requires antifungal therapy or antibiotic therapy (ideally dictated by culture and sensitivity)
• Myxedema secondary to hypothyroidism should respond gradually to T_4 supplementation.
• Edema associated with toxic insults may be slowed with antidotes (e.g., antivenom).
• Anticoagulant therapy (e.g., heparin and warfarin) may benefit patients with DIC or AT cIII depletion, respectively.
• Vascular volume expanders such as hydroxyethyl starch or plasma often benefit patients with low plasma oncotic pressure; very low dose furosemide in a constant-rate infusion of 0.1 mg/kg/h has been effective in conjunction with a volume expander

CONTRAINDICATIONS
• Diuretics generally aggravate edema of noncardiogenic origin.
• Steroids may worsen edema secondary to infectious disease.
• Epinephrine—generally contraindicated in shock except in anaphylaxis
• Propranolol (β-blocker)—contraindicated in patients predisposed to bronchospasm

PRECAUTIONS
• Avoid IM injections in patients with thrombocytopenia.
• Taper patients on long-term steroid therapy so that endogenous steroid production resumes.
• Use epinephrine cautiously in patients predisposed to ventricular fibrillation.
• Use enalapril cautiously in patients with renal disease.
• Long-term antibiotic therapy may facilitate a superinfection by a fungus (e.g., *Candida*) or resistant bacteria.
• Monitor anticoagulants closely to avoid fatal hemorrhage.

POSSIBLE INTERACTIONS
N/A

ALTERNATIVE DRUGS
N/A

FOLLOW-UP

PATIENT MONITORING
• Repeat complete blood counts, chemistries, and urine protein:creatinine ratios for blood dyscrasias and serum and urine protein concentrations, respectively
• Weekly assessment of prothrombin or partial thromboplastin time for patients on warfarin or heparin, respectively
• Serial biopsies of affected tissue such as kidney in glomerulonephritis may help to prognosticate.
• Repeat cultures or acute and convalescing titers for patients suffering from an infectious disease
• Periodic T_4 assay for patients receiving thyroid supplementation

POSSIBLE COMPLICATIONS
• Decubital ulceration
• Fatal hemorrhage
• Fatal thrombosis
• Refractory cardiac, gastrointestinal, hepatic, or renal failure
• Malnutrition
• Cerebral edema and herniation
• Resistant infection and sepsis

MISCELLANEOUS

ASSOCIATED CONDITIONS
Pericardial, pleural, or peritoneal effusion

AGE-RELATED FACTORS
Vascular anomalies or primary lymphedema are generally documented in juvenile patients (e.g., anasarca)

ZOONOTIC POTENTIAL
• Recent tick exposure is a common element in pets and their owners who may suffer simultaneously from rickettsial disease.
• Certain protozoal (*Leishmania*), fungal (*Sporothrix*), and bacterial (*Brucella*) organisms may transfer to people via direct contact.

PREGNANCY
Brucellosis has been associated with vulvar edema, necrotizing vasculitis, and embryonic death or fetal abortion.

SYNONYMS
N/A

SEE ALSO
• Albumin, Hypoalbuminemia
• Ascites
• Chylothorax
• Cirrhosis and Fibrosis of the liver
• Globulins
• Lipids, Hyperlipidemia
• Lymphedema
• Proteinuria
• Thrombocytopenia
• Vasculitis, Cutaneous
• Vasculitis, Systemic

ABBREVIATIONS
• AT III = antithrombin III
• RMSF = Rocky Mountain spotted fever
• T_4 = thyroid hormone
• TRH = thyrotropin-releasing hormone
• TSH = thyroid-stimulating hormone

Suggested Reading
Bright JM. Peripheral edema. In: Ettinger SJ, Feldman EC, eds. Textbook of veterinary internal medicine. 4th ed. Philadelphia: Saunders, 1995:100–103.
Fossum TW, King LA, Miller MW, et al. Lymphedema. Clinical signs, diagnosis and treatment. J Vet Int Med 1992;6:312–319.
Fossum TW, Miller MW. Lymphedema. Etiopathogenesis. J Vet Int Med 1992;6:283–293.
Guyton AC, Hall JE. The microcirculation and the lymphatic system: capillary fluid exchange, interstitial fluid, and lymph flow and the body fluid compartments: extracellular and intracellular fluids; interstitial fluid and edema. In: Textbook of medical physiology. 9th ed. Philadelphia: Saunders, 1996:308–311.
Suter FP, Fox PR. Peripheral vascular disease. In: Ettinger SJ, Feldman EC, eds. Textbook of veterinary internal medicine. 4th ed. Philadelphia: Saunders, 1995.

Author Marc Elie
Consulting Editors Larry P. Tilley and Francis W. K. Smith, Jr.

DISEASES

PERIPHERAL NEUROPATHIES (POLYNEUROPATHIES)

BASICS

DEFINITION
Diseases that affect many peripheral motor, sensory, autonomic, and/or cranial nerves, in any combination

PATHOPHYSIOLOGY
• Inherited or acquired • Primary pathological process—destruction or degeneration of the ventral horn cells (neuronopathy), primary demyelination, or axonal degeneration (with secondary demyelination)

SYSTEMS AFFECTED
• Nervous—primarily peripheral nervous system; possible involvement of the cranial nerves • Other organ systems—many may be involved in the primary disease process.

GENETICS
• Most inherited as autosomal recessive disorders. • Spinal muscular atrophy in Brittany spaniels—autosomal dominant disorder

INCIDENCE/PREVALENCE
• Inherited—rare • Peripheral nerve involvement in metabolic and neoplastic diseases—incidence unknown • Inflammatory—uncommon; coonhound paralysis most frequently encountered (somewhat seasonal prevalence: highest in fall and early winter)

GEOGRAPHIC DISTRIBUTION
• Coonhound paralysis—confined to North and Central America and parts of South America. • Distal denervating disease—most common in dogs in the UK; not reported elsewhere • Other polyneuropathies—no evidence of a geographical distribution

SIGNALMENT

Species
Dogs and cats

Breed Predilections
INHERITED
Spinal Muscular Atrophy
• Brittany spaniels, Swedish Lapland dogs, English pointers, German shepherds, rottweilers • Progressive neuronopathy—cairn terriers
Axonopathies
• Giant axonal neuropathy—German shepherds • Progressive axonopathy—boxers • Primary hyperoxaluria—domestic shorthair cats • Laryngeal paralysis—polyneuropathy complex—Dalmatians and rottweilers • Distal polyneuropathy—Birman cats • Distal sensorimotor polyneuropathy—rottweilers
Demyelination
Hypertrophic neuropathy—Tibetan mastiffs
Lysosomal Storage Diseases
• Globoid cell leukodystrophy—West Highland whites, cairn terriers, domestic shorthair kittens • G_{M1} gangliosidosis type II—Siamese and mixed-breed cats • Sphingomyelinosis—Siamese cats • Ceroid lipofuscinosis—English setters, Chihuahuas, Siamese

cats • Sensory neuropathy—long-haired dachshunds, English pointers, border collies
ACQUIRED
• Coonhound paralysis—because of their use, coonhounds have a higher incidence than other breeds. • Clinical diabetic polyneuropathy—more common in cats than dogs • Insulinomas—German shepherds, boxers, Irish setters, standard poodles, and collies

Mean Age and Range
INHERITED
• Usually begin at < 6 months of age • Feline hyperchylomicronemia—usually > 8 months • Feline hyperoxaluria—5–9 months • Rottweiler distal polyneuropathy—> 1 year • Giant axonal neuropathy in German shepherds—14–16 months • Intermediate and chronic forms of spinal muscular atrophy in heterozygote Brittany spaniels—6–12 months
ACQUIRED
• Secondary to neoplasia and insulinoma-associated hypoglycemia—tend to occur in middle-aged and old animals • Neospora polyradiculoneuritis—most commonly seen in dogs < 6 months of age; highest incidence 2–4 months

Predominant Sex
N/A

SIGNS

Historical Findings
INHERITED
• Most—slow, progressive; generalized weakness, muscle tremors, muscle atrophy, often with a plantigrade/palmigrade stance and gait • Sensory neuropathies—may see self-mutilation or ataxia • Lysosomal storage diseases—evidence of slowly progressive CNS involvement common; head tremors, ataxia, dysmetria, seizures, blindness, dementia, and depression • Giant axonal neuropathy of German shepherds—rapidly progressive generalized weakness (< 3 weeks)
ACQUIRED
• Rapid or slow progression • Rapidly progressive course—an initial stiff, stilted gait, leading to progressive generalized paresis or paralysis (coonhound paralysis, distal denervating disease) • Slowly progressive course—generalized weakness and muscle atrophy; in the distal polyneuropathies (diabetic cat), a plantigrade stance • Dysautonomia—primarily an acute onset (< 48 hr) of depression, anorexia, constipation, third eyelid protrusion, vomiting, and urinary incontinence • Metabolic—owner reports the non-neurologic clinical signs associated with the initiating defect. • Paraneoplastic—primary tumor may be clinically silent at the time of presentation.

Physical Examination Findings
• Motor and sensorimotor—tetraparesis to tetraplegia, hyporeflexia to areflexia, hypotonia to atonia, and muscle atrophy classic; muscle tremors common • Sensory—proprioceptive deficits; hyposthenia to anesthesia, without muscle atrophy or hyporeflexia (except in

boxers) • Hypothyroidism—associated with generalized polyneuropathy, laryngeal paralysis, megaesophagus, facial nerve paralysis, and peripheral vestibular disease • Lysosomal storage diseases—hepatosplenomegaly common • Paraneoplastic—may be evidence of neoplasia • Dysautonomia—dry rhinarium, xerostomia, low tear production, bradycardia, and anal areflexia • Primary feline hyperchylomicronemia—lipid granulomata, which can be palpated under the skin and in the abdomen, common • Primary hyperoxaluria (cats)—enlarged, painful kidneys on abdominal palpation • Cranial nerve abnormalities (including dysphonia and aphonia)—variable

CAUSES

Acquired
• Immune—primary or secondary; may be seen with SLE or other immune diseases (e.g., polymyositis, glomerulonephritis, polyarthritis, and pemphigus) • Metabolic—diabetes mellitus (cats), hypothyroidism, and insulinoma; may be associated with (adeno) carcinomas, malignant melanoma, mast cell tumor, osteosarcoma, multiple myeloma, or lymphosarcoma • Infectious—*Neospora caninum;* FeLV • Cancer drugs—vincristine; vinblastine; cisplatin; colchicine • Toxic—thallium; organophosphates; carbon tetrachloride; lindane • Idiopathic

RISK FACTORS
Development of associated specific diseases (metabolic, immune, neoplastic) or exposure to associated specific drugs/toxins or causal factors (raccoon saliva)

DIAGNOSIS

DIFFERENTIAL DIAGNOSIS
• Acute—botulism; tick paralysis; acute disseminated or multifocal myelopathies • Chronic—polymyopathy; chronic disseminated or multifocal myelopathies

CBC/BIOCHEMISTRY/URINALYSIS
• Standard laboratory tests—do not reflect occurrence of polyneuropathy; often indicate possible underlying metabolic or neoplastic disease • High serum creatine kinase—indicates an accompanying myopathy

OTHER LABORATORY TESTS
• None with respect to the actual polyneuropathy • ANA, lupus erythematosus preparation, and Coombs test—assist in the diagnosis of immune disease • Low TSH stimulation test, low T_4, low free T_4, and high endogenous TSH—hypothyroidism • Amended insulin:glucose ratio—> 30 supports the diagnosis of an insulinoma • Serology—assists in the diagnosis of *N. caninum* and FeLV infection • Low specific leukocyte lysosomal enzymes—indicate specific storage diseases • High plasma epinephrine and norepinephrine levels—dysautonomia • High serum cholesterol, triglycerides, and very low density

PERIPHERAL NEUROPATHIES (POLYNEUROPATHIES)

lipoprotein—hyperchylomicronemia • Hyperoxaluria and L-glyceric aciduria—seen in primary hyperoxaluria (cats) • Monoclonal gammopathy—multiple myeloma

IMAGING
• Thoracic and abdominal radiographs—important in the diagnosis of megaesophagus; demonstrate ileus, bladder atony, constipation, and delayed gastric emptying in dysautonomia • Radiography and ultrasound—help the search for a neoplastic cause

DIAGNOSTIC PROCEDURES
• Electrophysiology (EMG, motor and sensory nerve conduction and action potential amplitudes, and late wave studies)—cornerstone for diagnosis • Lumbar CSF analysis—valuable in diagnosing nerve root involvement • Muscle biopsy—confirms evidence of denervation (myofiber angular atrophy type I and II) • Peripheral nerve biopsy—further delineates disease process

PATHOLOGIC FINDINGS
• Degrees of axonal degeneration, demyelination, and/or neuronal cell body degeneration depends on the specific condition. • Anatomic distribution of the lesion along the peripheral nerves (proximal, distal or widespread) depends on the specific condition.

TREATMENT

APPROPRIATE HEALTH CARE
• Usually outpatient • Inpatient—observe acute polyradiculoneuropathies closely for respiratory failure in the early progressive phase of disease.

NURSING CARE
• Dysautonomia—may require intensive IV fluid therapy and/or parenteral feeding • Physiotherapy—an excellent ancillary treatment

ACTIVITY
No restrictions, if ambulatory

DIET
• Generally no special management, unless megaesophagus or dysphagia occurs • Hyperchylomicronemia—low-fat diet alone can resolve the polyneuropathy within 2–3 months. • Paralysis—make sure the patient can reach food and water. • Regurgitation and/or vomiting (e.g., in dysautonomia)—temporarily halt oral intake. • Diabetes mellitus—important to carefully monitor food intake

CLIENT EDUCATION
• Inform client that treatment of the primary cause may not lead to reversal of the peripheral nerve signs, and, in some cases, deterioration will continue. • Inform client that many polyneuropathies are idiopathic, despite extensive diagnostic workup.

SURGICAL CONSIDERATIONS
Paraneoplastic—treat the primary tumor via surgery, chemotherapy, or radiation.

MEDICATIONS

DRUGS OF CHOICE
• Inherited—most are untreatable. • Acquired—principal goal is usually to treat the primary cause, if identified, with the hope that the secondary polyneuropathy will improve or resolve after appropriate therapy; not always successful • Chronic progressive or relapsing—most likely of immune origin; may improve with long-term immunosuppressive corticosteroid therapy (prednisone at 1–2 mg/kg PO q12h), azathioprine (2.2 mg/kg PO q24h), or cyclophosphamide (50 mg/m² q48h); response of individual patient variable • SLE-related—treat as for chronic progressive or relapsing polyneuropathy. • Neoplasia—immunosuppressive corticosteroid therapy may improve the polyneuropathy without specific action against the primary tumor. • *Neospora*-associated polyradiculoneuritis—best treated with clindamycin (5.5 mg/kg PO q12h); efficacy is questionable. • Dysautonomia—treat symptomatically with IV fluid therapy, artificial tears, metoclopramide (0.2–0.4 mg/kg PO q8h), bethanechol (cats: 0.5–2.5 mg SC q12h or 2.5–10 mg PO q6–8h; dogs: 0.5–15 mg SC q12h or 2.5–30 mg PO q6–8h), and physostigmine eye drops.

CONTRAINDICATIONS
Corticosteroid therapy—contraindicated in *Neospora*-associated polyradiculoneuritis and coonhound paralysis

PRECAUTIONS
N/A

POSSIBLE INTERACTIONS
N/A

ALTERNATIVE DRUGS
N/A

FOLLOW-UP

PATIENT MONITORING
Repeat neurologic examinations.

PREVENTION/AVOIDANCE
• Avoid breeding patients with inherited or *Neospora*-associated (placental transfer of the organism from the bitch) diseases. • Avoid contact with raccoons for dogs with a previous history of coonhound paralysis.

POSSIBLE COMPLICATIONS
• Inherited—continued neurologic deterioration, eventually leading to inability to successfully ambulate • Acute or chronic progressive—severe muscle atrophy and resultant pressure sores; urinary tract

infection; muscle fibrosis and contracture; aspiration pneumonia

EXPECTED COURSE AND PROGNOSIS
• Purely demyelinating conditions have a more rapid course of improvement than those involving axonal degeneration (the majority), which can take months for partial or complete recovery, if at all. • Inherited—most have a poor to hopeless prognosis for any recovery of peripheral nerve function (except hyperchylomicronemia in cats). • Acute polyradiculoneuritis (coonhound paralysis)—good long-term prognosis; may take weeks to months to recover ambulation • Metabolic—fair to good prognosis with successful treatment of the primary metabolic abnormality; insulinomas have a high recurrence rate. • Other acquired—most show continued deterioration despite treatment; guarded to poor prognosis; sometimes progression is slow and insidious over many months or years.

MISCELLANEOUS

ASSOCIATED CONDITIONS
N/A

AGE-RELATED FACTORS
N/A

ZOONOTIC POTENTIAL
N/A

PREGNANCY
• Metabolic—some have a significant affect on pregnant patients • High-dose corticosteroids and other immunosuppressive agents—contraindicated during pregnancy

SYNONYMS
N/A

SEE ALSO
See Causes

ABBREVIATIONS
• ANA = antinuclear antibody • CSF = cerebrospinal fluid • EMG = electromyography • FeLV = feline leukemia virus • SLE = systemic lupus erythematosus • TSH = thyroid-stimulating hormone

Suggested Reading
Cuddon PA. Feline neuromuscular diseases. Feline Pract 1994;22:7–13.
Cummings JF. Canine inflammatory polyneuropathies. In: Kirk RW, Bonagura JD, eds. Current veterinary therapy XI. Small animal practice. Philadelphia: Saunders, 1992:1034–1037.
Duncan ID. Peripheral neuropathy in the dog and cat. Prog Vet Neurol 1991;2:111–128.
Towell TL, Shell LC. Endocrinopathies that affect peripheral nerves of cats and dogs. Compend Contin Educ Pract Vet 1994;16:157–161.
Author Paul A. Cuddon
Consulting Editor Joane M. Parent

PERIRENAL PSEUDOCYSTS

BASICS

OVERVIEW
Capsulogenic renal cyst, capsular cyst, pararenal pseudocyst, capsular hydronephrosis, perirenal cyst, and *perirenal pseudocyst* are terms used to describe renomegaly caused by accumulation of fluid between the kidney and its surrounding capsule. One or both kidneys are affected.

SIGNALMENT
- Primarily old male cats (>8 years)
- When detected in young cats, the disease is usually unilateral.
- Rare in dogs; the difference in prevalence between species may be related to the prominent network of subcapsular veins that characterize feline kidneys.

SIGNS
- Maybe none
- Nonpainful, large abdomen common
- Signs of concomitant renal failure in some animals

CAUSES & RISK FACTORS
- Cause of perirenal accumulation of fluid— not completely understood; a dynamic, not a static, process
- Evaluation of the pseudocyst fluid may aid understanding of the pathophysiologic mechanisms.
- Transudate-type fluid may accumulate because of high capillary hydrostatic pressure or lymphatic obstruction. Some cats have histopathologic evidence of renal fibrosis, but it is not known whether progressive renal parenchymal contraction occludes lymphatics and blood vessels, promoting transudation of fluid.
- Perirenal accumulation of transudate can also result from ruptured renal cysts.
- Accumulation of perirenal urine may indicate disruption of the renal pelvis or proximal ureter.
- Accumulation of blood in pseudocysts can result from external trauma, surgery, neoplastic erosion of blood vessels, rupture of aneurysms, coagulopathies, or paracentesis.

DIAGNOSIS

DIFFERENTIAL DIAGNOSIS
- Causes of renomegaly include renal neoplasia, hydronephrosis, polycystic kidney disease (common), feline infectious peritonitis, and mycotic or bacterial nephritis (less common).
- Ascites and enlargement of other abdominal organs can cause nonpainful distension.

CBC/BIOCHEMISTRY/URINALYSIS
- Results unremarkable unless animal has renal insufficiency
- Azotemia and inappropriately low urinary specific gravity (<1.035) indicate concomitant renal failure.

OTHER LABORATORY TESTS
N/A

IMAGING
- Renomegaly is commonly detected by survey radiography.
- Excretory urography and ultrasonography delineate normal or small kidneys beneath an abnormally wide intracapsular space.

DIAGNOSTIC PROCEDURES
Examination of aspirate of intracapsular material may reveal a modified transudate (acellular, low-protein fluid), hemorrhage, or urine (fluid creatinine concentration several times higher than serum creatinine concentration).

TREATMENT
- Perirenal pseudocysts are not immediately life-threatening.
- Some animals need no treatment, but monitor renal function so that treatment can be considered if it declines. Capsulectomy or peritoneal fenestration is generally associated with a short-term favorable outcome.
- Long-term response unknown
- Avoid nephrectomy to preserve maximal renal function
- Decompress by paracentesis with a needle and syringe for temporary relief.
- Pseudocysts usually refill in 1–2 weeks; paracentesis can then be repeated.
- Some patients require treatment for concomitant renal failure.

MEDICATIONS

DRUGS
Consider appropriate antimicrobic (i.e., lipid soluble antibiotic chosen on the basis of antimicrobial susceptibility) if the pseudocyst becomes infected.

CONTRAINDICATIONS/POSSIBLE INTERACTIONS
N/A

FOLLOW-UP
- Monitor patients periodically (every 2–6 months) for development of renal failure.
- Short-term prognosis—appears favorable after capsulectomy in patients with no evidence of renal dysfunction
- Long-term prognosis—not known because it is not known whether perirenal pseudocysts are associated with underlying lesions in the renal parenchyma that may be progressive.

MISCELLANEOUS

Suggested Reading

Lulich JP, Osborne CA, Polzin DJ. Cystic diseases of the kidney. In: Osborne CA, Finco DR, eds. Canine and feline nephrology and urology. Philadelphia: Williams & Wilkins, 1995:460–483.

Authors Jody P. Lulich and Carl A Osborne
Consulting Editors Larry G. Adams and Carl A. Osborne

PERITONEOPERICARDIAL DIAPHRAGMATIC HERNIA

 BASICS

OVERVIEW
- Embryologic malformation of the ventral midline allowing communication between the pericardial and peritoneal cavities
- May be associated with other congenital malformations including congenital malformations, sternal deformities (especially in cats), cranial abdominal hernia, and ventricular septal defects
- Signs may be due to large amounts of abdominal viscera compressing the heart or lungs and incarceration of abdominal organs (e.g., liver and small bowel).

SIGNALMENT
- Dogs and cats
- Age when clinical signs first occur varies; more than one-third of patients are 4 years of age or older.
- Weimaraners and Persians may be predisposed.
- No evidence that lesions are hereditary, but have been reported in littermates.

SIGNS
General Comments
Depend on the nature and amount of abdominal contents that herniate

Historical Findings
- Vomiting
- Diarrhea
- Weight loss
- Abdominal pain
- Coughing
- Dyspnea

Physical Examination Findings
- Muffled heart sounds
- Displaced or attenuated apical cardiac impulse
- Palpable sternal deformity or cranial abdominal hernia
- Cardiac tamponade and signs of right-sided congestive heart failure (rare)

CAUSES & RISK FACTORS
- Embryologic malformation
- Prenatal injury of the septum transversum and pleuroperitoneal folds

 DIAGNOSIS

DIFFERENTIAL DIAGNOSIS
- Never an acquired traumatic defect because no natural direct communication exists between the peritoneal and pericardial cavities after birth
- Pericardial effusion

CBC/BIOCHEMISTRY/URINALYSIS
No associated hematologic or biochemical alterations

OTHER LABORATORY TESTS
N/A

Imaging
- Radiographic findings depend on size of defect and amount of herniated abdominal contents; caudal heart border and diaphragm may overlap; thoracic radiographs may show an "empty" abdomen and possible multiple radiographic densities
- Barium series may demonstrate bowel loops crossing the diaphragm and within the pericardial sac.
- Nonselective angiography outlines the cardiac chambers within the large cardiac silhouette.
- Echocardiography gives a definitive diagnosis.

Diagnostic Procedures
ECG may show small complexes if abdominal contents have herniated or marked effusion is present.

 TREATMENT

Surgical closure of the hernia after returning viable organs to their normal location is usually curative.

 MEDICATIONS

DRUGS
- Myocardial contractility is unaffected in most patients; drugs for improving cardiac output are not indicated.
- Can give symptomatic treatment based on nature and amount of abdominal contents that are herniated

CONTRAINDICATIONS/POSSIBLE INTERACTIONS
Drugs that reduce ventricular afterload (e.g., arteriolar vasodilators) or preload (e.g., venous dilators and diuretics) are not useful and can cause reduction of ventricular filling, hypotension, and low cardiac output.

 FOLLOW-UP

Prognosis after surgery is excellent in animals with no other significant congenital anomalies or complicating factors.

 MISCELLANEOUS

Suggested Reading

Kienle RD. Pericardial disease and cardiac neoplasia. In: Kittleson MD. Kienle RD, eds. Small animal cardiovascular medicine. St. Louis: Mosby, 1999:413.

Neiger R. Peritoneopericardial diaphragmatic hernia in cats. Compend Contin Educ 1996:461–479.

Author Larry P. Tilley

Consulting Editors Larry P. Tilley and Francis W. K. Smith, Jr.

DISEASES

PERITONITIS

BASICS

DEFINITION
An inflammatory process involving the serous membrane of the abdominal cavity

PATHOPHYSIOLOGY
• Insult to the peritoneal cavity, whether localized or generalized, leads to an inflammatory process characterized by vasodilation, cellular infiltration, stimulation of pain fibers, and development of adhesions.
• Extent and severity depend on type of insult.

SYSTEMS AFFECTED
• Gastrointestinal
• Cardiovascular
• Renal/Urologic
• Hemic/Lymphatic/Immune

GENETICS
N/A

INCIDENCE/PREVALENCE
N/A

GEOGRAPHIC DISTRIBUTION
N/A

SIGNALMENT
Species
Dogs and cats

Breed Predilections
None

Mean Age and Range
None

Predominant Sex
None

SIGNS
• Abdominal pain—localized or generalized; patient usually resents palpation
• A "praying" position—for relief; similar to that sometimes seen with pancreatitis
• Vomiting common
• Hypotension and shock—may develop rapidly
• Tachycardia—often noted; a variety of arrhythmias may be detected.
• Fever—not consistent; when noted with other signs of peritonitis suggests bacterial contamination of the abdominal cavity

CAUSES
Primary Peritonitis
• Uncommon
• Results from direct infection through hematogenous spread of the causative agent (e.g., FIP)

Secondary Peritonitis
• Predominant form
• Results from disruption of the abdominal cavity or hollow viscus
• Septic or chemical contamination—from dehiscence of surgical sites, penetrating abdominal wounds, blunt abdominal trauma, severe pancreatitis, pyometra, liver, or prostatic abscesses; also rupture of the gallbladder, urinary bladder, or bile duct

RISK FACTORS
• Trauma
• Gastrointestinal surgery
• Undetected abscess of liver, pancreas, prostate, uterine stump

DIAGNOSIS

DIFFERENTIAL DIAGNOSIS
Other causes of abdominal pain or distention, sepsis, and shock

CBC/BIOCHEMISTRY/URINALYSIS
• Neutrophilic leukocytosis most common finding; may be a left shift; degenerative left shift or development of neutropenia may portend a worsening prognosis.
• Hemoconcentration common
• Hypoproteinemia—owing to exudation of albumin
• Hypokalemia
• Azotemia
• Metabolic acidosis
• Hypoglycemia—may indicate sepsis

OTHER LABORATORY TESTS
N/A

IMAGING
Ultrasound
May identify free fluid within the abdomen; abscesses of the pancreas, liver, or prostate; and rupture of the gallbladder

Radiography
• Findings inconsistent and depend on cause
• Loss of abdominal detail (ground-glass appearance—suggests fluid in the abdominal cavity; do not confuse with dehydration or lack of intra-abdominal fat
• Standing lateral view—may see free fluid line
• Left lateral recumbent view with a horizontal beam—may see free gas within the abdominal cavity
• Generalized ileus associated with free abdominal gas and a visible fluid line—may support the diagnosis; consider other causes of ileus

• Contrast procedures—usually not warranted; may complicate management if contrast material enters the abdominal cavity; avoid barium if gastrointestinal perforation is suspected.

DIAGNOSTIC PROCEDURES
• Abdominocentesis and DPL—safe and reliable
• Paracentesis—empty urinary bladder; aseptically prepare centesis site; use a 22-gauge needle or Teflon catheter to penetrate the abdominal cavity; sometimes a few drops of abdominal fluid may be recovered; if not successful, use a 3-mL syringe to apply gentle negative pressure; tap all four quadrants (i.e., four separate needle punctures).
• DPL—if abdominal fluid not recovered by paracentesis; empty urinary bladder; aseptically prepare site; gravity infuse 20 mL/kg warm sterile saline into the abdominal cavity; may gently roll patient from side to side to increase recovery of the lavage fluid; no need to recover entire amount of infused fluid
• Cytology—collect samples into EDTA tubes; note color and clarity of the fluid and clarity and presence of fibrin before submitting to the laboratory.
• Culture and sensitivity—collect samples into sterile clot tubes.
• Suspected chemical peritonitis—analyze abdominal fluid for BUN and creatinine (to detect urine leakage), amylase (for pancreatitis), alkaline phosphatase (for intestinal trauma), and bilirubin (for bile leakage).
• Suspected FIP—may submit abdominal fluid for protein electrophoresis and globulin determination.

PATHOLOGIC FINDINGS
N/A

TREATMENT

APPROPRIATE HEALTH CARE
Inpatient—intensive monitoring; supportive care

NURSING CARE
Intravenous Fluid Therapy
• Critical for restoration of hemodynamic disturbances and correction of electrolyte and acid–base abnormalities
• Balanced electrolyte solution—lactated Ringer's solution or Normosol-R usually acceptable

• Potassium and glucose—may need to supplement
• Replacement rate—may initially be as high as 45 mL/kg/hr (cats) and 90 mL/kg/hr (dogs); adjust rate frequently as patient status changes; if supplemented with potassium, the rate should not exceed 0.5 mEq/kg/hr of potassium.

ACTIVITY
Usually limited as a result of hospitalization and confinement

DIET
• Dictated by cause, when identified, and any concurrent conditions (e.g., heart disease)
• Feeding tube, if necessary, may be placed for nutritional support (e.g., esophagostomy, gastrostomy, enterostomy).
• Adequate nutrition—essential to optimize outcome

CLIENT EDUCATION
• Advise client of the high rate of morbidity and, in some cases, mortality.
• Inform client that extensive monitoring and intensive care may be costly.

SURGICAL CONSIDERATIONS
• Decision to treat medically or surgically—dictated by cause (if known), patient's response to initial treatment, and owner's financial constraints
• Mild cases that seem to respond to medical therapy—surgery may not be required.
• Known bacterial contamination or suspected chemical peritonitis—surgical intervention necessary
• Inform clients who decline surgery of the possible consequences; even with surgical attention, many animals will succumb.
• Exploratory laparotomy—prepare skin in anticipation of a large surgical field; if source of infection can be identified, remove or correct it; collect fluid sample for gram staining; use monofilament absorbable or nonabsorbable suture within the abdomen (avoid multifilament nonabsorbable suture and catgut); before closing, thoroughly lavage the abdomen with 200–300 ml/kg sterile saline solution, warmed to body temperature.
• Leaving the abdomen open or closed—determined by degree of contamination, ability to remove all debris, severity of the illness, and anticipation of septic complications; closed: use a routine closure; open: partially close and apply a sterile laparotomy pad and secure bandaging; consult a detailed surgical text for management of open peritoneal drainage.

MEDICATIONS

DRUGS OF CHOICE
• Antimicrobials—broad-spectrum (against gram-positive and gram-negative, aerobic, and anaerobic organisms); when possible, based on culture and sensitivity
• Results of culture and sensitivity pending—try a combination of an aminoglycoside (e.g., amikacin, gentamicin) and a cephalosporin (e.g., cefazolin) or a penicillin (e.g., ampicillin)
• Ampicillin sodium—22 mg/kg IV q8h
• Gentamicin—2–3 mg/kg IV q8h
• Pain control—consider if indicated.

CONTRAINDICATIONS
• Glucocorticoids and NSAIDs—use is controversial

PRECAUTIONS
• Aminoglycosides—use with caution if renal function is impaired.
• Adequate hydration—essential to enhance safety of these drugs

POSSIBLE INTERACTIONS
N/A

ALTERNATIVE DRUGS
Fluoroquinolone—enrofloxacin or orbifloxacin; substitute for an aminoglycoside, especially with impaired renal function

FOLLOW-UP

PATIENT MONITORING
• Fluid balance, electrolyte balance, acid–base status—monitor closely
• Frequency of monitoring—varies with patient's condition and response to treatment
• CBC, chemistry profile, urinalysis—every 1–2 days during periods of intensive monitoring, even in patients who are responding

PREVENTION/AVOIDANCE
Prevention—difficult except when specific risk factors are identified (e.g., pyometra)

POSSIBLE COMPLICATIONS
• If underlying cause is not identified and managed, patient is at risk for complications.
• Open peritoneal drainage—herniation of abdominal contents
• Adhesions

EXPECTED COURSE AND PROGNOSIS
• Prognosis—depends on rapid identification and successful management of the underlying cause and appropriate follow-up care
• Septic peritonitis—open peritoneal drainage may improve survival.

MISCELLANEOUS

ASSOCIATED CONDITIONS
N/A

AGE-RELATED FACTORS
N/A

ZOONOTIC POTENTIAL
N/A

PREGNANCY
N/A

SEE ALSO
Sepsis and Bacteremia

ABBREVIATIONS
• DPL = diagnostic peritoneal lavage
• FIP = feline infectious peritonitis

Suggested Reading
Greenfield CL, Walshaw R. Open peritoneal drainage for treatment of contaminated peritoneal cavity and septic peritonitis in dogs and cats: 24 cases (1980–1986). J Am Vet Med Assoc 1987;191:100–105.
Seim HB. Management of peritonitis. In: Bonagura JD, ed., Current veterinary therapy XII. Philadelphia: Saunders, 1995:764–770.
Author Sharon K. Fooshee
Consulting Editor Stephen C. Barr

DISEASES

PERSISTENT RIGHT AORTIC ARCH

BASICS

OVERVIEW
• Entrapment of the esophagus by a persistent right 4th aortic arch on the right, the base of the heart and pulmonary artery centrally, and ductus or ligamentum arteriosum on the left and dorsally
• Causes megaesophagus cranial to the obstruction at the base of the heart

SIGNALMENT
Seen most commonly in the German shepherd, Irish setter, and Boston terrier

SIGNS
• Regurgitation of undigested solid food in animals < 6 months old
• Malnourishment in many patients
• Time between eating and regurgitation varies
• Signs of aspiration pneumonia (e.g., cough and tachypnea or dyspnea) in some patients

CAUSES & RISK FACTORS
N/A

DIAGNOSIS

DIFFERENTIAL DIAGNOSIS
• Other vascular ring anomalies such as double aortic arch (rare)
• Congenital megaesophagus
• Stricture, diverticulum, or esophageal foreign body
• Esophageal motility disorder in shar-pei

CBC/BIOCHEMISTRY/URINALYSIS
• Results usually normal
• High WBC in some patients with aspiration pneumonia

OTHER LABORATORY TESTS
N/A

IMAGING
• Thoracic radiographs show food-filled cranial esophagus or signs of aspiration pneumonia in some patients.
• Contrast esophagram confirms megaesophagus extending to the heart base.
• Can use fluoroscopy to differentiate esophageal motility disorders
• May need angiography to differentiate between specific vascular ring anomalies

DIAGNOSTIC PROCEDURES

Endoscopy
Can use esophagoscopy to differentiate esophageal motility disorders

TREATMENT
• Surgical correction of the vascular entrapment; may need medical management of concurrent aspiration pneumonia
• May also need feeding procedures for megaesophagus

MEDICATIONS

DRUGS
• Patient with aspiration pneumonia may need supportive care with oxygen.
• Use broad-spectrum antibiotics such as enrofloxacin (2.5 mg/kg PO q12h) and amoxicillin (10–15 mg/kg PO q12h) in animals with aspiration pneumonia.

CONTRAINDICATIONS/POSSIBLE INTERACTIONS
N/A

FOLLOW-UP
• Prognosis for resolution of the problem, even after surgery, is guarded to poor.
• Complications of malnourishment and aspiration pneumonia are common and severe.
• Esophageal function is often permanently compromised.

MISCELLANEOUS

SEE ALSO
Double Aortic Arch

Suggested Reading
Bonagura JD, Lehmkuhl LB. Congenital heart disease. In: Fox PR, Sisson D, Moise NS, eds. Textbook of canine and feline cardiology. Philadelphia: Saunders, 1999: 471–535.

Author Carroll Loyer
Consulting Editors Larry P. Tilley and Francis W. K. Smith, Jr.

DISEASES

PHEOCHROMOCYTOMA

BASICS

DEFINITION
• Tumor of the adrenergic portion of the sympathetic nervous system • Tumors arise from chromaffin cells of the adrenal medulla and rarely from extraadrenal chromaffin cells (paragangliomas).

PATHOPHYSIOLOGY
• Most commonly involve the adrenal medulla; the vast majority are unilateral. • Can vary in size from small nodules 0.5 cm in diameter to large, space-occupying intraabdominal masses; the larger the tumor the more frequently there are related clinical signs. • Approximately 50% are classified as malignant because of either local tissue invasion or distant metastasis. • Distant metastasis is most commonly observed in the liver, lungs, spleen, kidney, brain, and bone; metastasis to regional lymph nodes is also frequent. • Pheochromocytomas produce clinical signs by direct invasion of adjacent structures (kidney, aorta, or caudal vena cava) and by production of epinephrine, norepinephrine, and less commonly dopamine. • The predominant clinical signs result from α_1-mediated vasoconstriction and β_1-mediated cardiac chronotropic and inotropic effects that cause systemic hypertension or tachyarrhythmias.

SYSTEMS AFFECTED
• Cardiovascular • Respiratory • Behavior • Neuromuscular • Renal/Urologic • Gastrointestinal • Ophthalmic

INCIDENCE/PREVALENCE
Uncommon disease in dogs; rare in cats

SIGNALMENT

Species
Dogs and cats

Breed Predilections
None

Mean Age and Range
• Median age is 11 years; range is 1–26 years of age • The great majority of affected dogs are ≥7 years old.

SIGNS

General Comments
Difficult to diagnose antemortem; 48–85% of reported pheochromocytomas have been identified unexpectedly during necropsy examination or exploratory surgery.

Historical Findings
• Clinical signs are often episodic or acute. • Common presenting signs are (in decreasing order of frequency) generalized weakness, collapse, anorexia, lethargy/depression, vomiting, tachypnea, and polyuria/polydipsia. • Less common presenting complaints are diarrhea, weight loss, rear limb edema, abdominal distension, epistaxis, acute blindness, pacing,
and seizures.

Physical Examination Findings
• Related to excessive catecholamine release or tumor invasion of adjacent structures; abnormalities not always present • Respiratory—tachypnea is one of the most common; dyspnea or abnormal lung sounds are less commonly observed. • Cardiovascular—tachycardia or cardiac arrhythmias are very common; epistaxis is occasionally noted; some patients present in cardiovascular shock. • Neuromuscular—weakness, loss of muscle mass, shaking, muscle tremors, and rarely seizures • Ocular—blindness, retinal detachment, retinal hemorrhage, and tortuous retinal vessels may occur in dogs with prolonged or severe hypertension.

CAUSES
Pheochromocytomas are chromaffin cell tumors.

DIAGNOSIS

DIFFERENTIAL DIAGNOSIS
• Primary differentials include causes of systemic hypertension such as renal disease, hyperadrenocorticism, hyperthyroidism, primary hyperaldosteronism, and essential hypertension. • Hyperadrenocorticism can closely mimic, and may occur simultaneously with, pheochromocytomas.

CBC/BIOCHEMISTRY/URINALYSIS
• Decreased plasma volume may result in an increased PCV; also some evidence indicates that catecholamines may cause increased kidney erythropoietin release. • Any anemia is usually mild and nonregenerative and is thought to be secondary to chronic disease or chronic low-grade hemorrhage. • A mature neutrophilic leukocytosis is the most common leukogram abnormality. • The most common serum biochemistry abnormality is elevated liver enzymes; no apparent correlation exists between elevated liver enzymes and hepatic metastasis. • Hypercholesterolemia is frequently noted. • Proteinuria, seen in up to 50% of patients, results from hypertensive glomerulonephropathy.

OTHER LABORATORY TESTS
• In humans, a diagnosis of pheochromocytoma is confirmed by demonstrating elevated levels of serum or urine catecholamines and their metabolites. • In veterinary medicine, these tests are rarely done because of their technical difficulty, expense, and unavailability and the lack of documented normal reference values. • Quantification of urinary catecholamines and their metabolites from a 24-h urine collection is the preferred method of confirming a diagnosis of pheochromocytoma in humans. • Test sensitivity is greatly enhanced by assays for urinary catecholamines (dopamine, epinephrine, and norepinephrine) and
their metabolites (metanephrine, normetanephrine and vanillylmandelic acid). • Urine must be acidified (pH < 3.0) and kept cold during collection and transport to the laboratory.

Phentolamine Suppression Test
• Phentolamine is an intravenous α-receptor antagonist that lowers blood pressure by inhibiting catecholamine-mediated vasoconstriction; test can only be performed if patient is hypertensive. • After obtaining a baseline blood pressure, administer 0.5–1.5 mg of phentolamine as an IV bolus; measure blood pressure every 30 sec for 3 min, then every minute for 7 min. • If the patients' blood pressure decreases by at least 35 mm Hg systolic or 25 mm Hg diastolic and the decrease lasts for a minimum of 5 min, the result is considered positive; in humans, the test has been associated with a large number of false positives.

Abdominal Radiography
• A cranial abdominal mass has been detected in up to 56% of patients; ~7% of pheochromocytomas have had radiographically detectable calcification. • Tumor extension into the adjacent kidney or liver lobule may cause abnormalities in their radiographic contours.

Thoracic Radiography
• Common thoracic abnormalities are generalized cardiomegaly, right or left ventricular enlargement, and pulmonary edema or congestion; thoracic radiographs are also indicated to evaluate for metastatic disease. • Pulmonary metastasis has been detected radiographically in approximately 11% of evaluated patients; in one study, 50% of pulmonary metastatic lesions were not detected on radiographs.

Abdominal Ultrasonography
• An abdominal mass was identified in 50–83% of patients evaluated with ultrasound; the origin of the mass frequently cannot be identified. • Pheochromocytomas are usually unilateral; the contralateral adrenal gland usually is normal in size, shape, and echo texture. • Ultrasonography is relatively sensitive for identifying tumor invasion of the caudal vena cava and other adjacent structures and for detecting intraabdominal metastasis; however, in one study, tumor invasion of adjacent tissues was missed in 75% of affected animals examined.

OTHER IMAGING MODALITIES
Computed tomography (CT scan) and magnetic resonance imaging (MRI) are very sensitive imaging methods for detection of adrenal masses and intraabdominal metastasis.

DIAGNOSTIC PROCEDURES

Arterial Blood Pressure
Identification of systemic hypertension (systolic blood pressure > 160 mm Hg, diastolic > 100 mm Hg) is highly variable in canine patients with pheochromocytoma; therefore, normal blood pressure does not rule out a diagnosis of pheochromocytoma.

Electrocardiography (ECG)
Sinus tachycardia is the most common ECG abnormality; ventricular premature contractions are less commonly observed.

Adrenal Testing
Hyperadrenocorticism is one of the primary differential diagnoses for patients with clinical signs consistent with a pheochromocytoma. In addition, hyperadrenocorticism reportedly occurs concurrently in up to 20% of canine patients with pheochromocytomas.

PATHOLOGIC FINDINGS
• Grossly, pheochromocytomas are dark-red to tan, and multinodular. • They arise from the adrenal medulla; the surrounding adrenal cortex is compressed into a thin surrounding shell of tissue. • Histologically, pheochromocytomas are composed of round to cuboidal cells with granular eosinophilic cytoplasm. • Immunohistochemical staining of tumor tissues with chromogranin A or synaptophysin will allow differentiation of pheochromocytomas.

TREATMENT

APPROPRIATE HEALTH CARE
• Surgical removal of the tumor is the only treatment modality that may be curative. • Surgical exploration and biopsy are usually required for a definitive diagnosis. • Medical therapy is most commonly used to stabilize patients prior to surgery or in patients with nonresectable or metastatic tumors; medical therapy is only palliative and can be conducted on an outpatient basis. • Patients that are presented in a hypertensive crisis represent a diagnostic and therapeutic challenge; these patients require intensive emergency and critical care.

CLIENT EDUCATION
Survival times of > 1–3 years are possible following successful surgical tumor removal, even in dogs with tumor invasion of adjacent tissues or blood vessels; however, perioperative mortality rates of close to 50% have been reported.

SURGICAL CONSIDERATIONS
Preoperative Care
• Severe hypertension and cardiac arrhythmias are life-threatening complications that commonly develop during anesthetic induction and tumor removal in patients with pheochromocytomas. • Marked hypotension commonly develops following tumor removal. • Phenoxybenzamine, a noncompetitive adrenergic α antagonist is given for 2–3 weeks prior to surgery; the initial dosage is 0.25 mg/kg BID; the dosage can be incrementally increased until the patient's clinical signs and blood pressure are controlled; the maximum dosage is 1.5 mg/kg BID in canines and 0.5 mg/kg BID in cats.

COMPLICATIONS AND PATIENT MONITORING
• Common complications—hypertension, severe tachycardia, other cardiac arrhythmias, and hypovolemia/hypotension • Closely monitor the ECG, central venous pressure (CVP) and blood pressure. Hypertension can be treated with phentolamine (0.02–0.1 mg/kg IV to effect) or sodium nitroprusside (0.5–15 mg/kg/min constant-rate IV infusion); sodium nitroprusside is a direct-acting vasodilator with an immediate onset and a short duration of activity. • Cardiac arrhythmias and severe tachycardia—common problems; usually respond to β-blocking agents such as propranolol (0.03–0.1 mg/kg IV to effect) or esmolol (0.5 mg/kg slow IV bolus followed by 0.05–0.2 mg/kg/min IV infusion) • Hypotension and hypovolemia may develop following tumor removal or secondary to uncontrolled hemorrhage; hypotension is best treated by volume expansion with IV fluid therapy; adequacy of fluid therapy is based on normalization of blood pressure and maintaining the patient's CVP between 5 and 10 mm H_2O.

Anesthesia
• The anesthetic protocol should include agents that do not directly or indirectly cause the release of catecholamines or sensitize tissues to their effects. • Appropriate drugs are diazepam, oxymorphone, midazolam, and acepromazine (low dosage) or combinations of the above. • Atropine or glycopyrrolate should not be a routine part of the preinduction protocol because they can predispose the patient to life-threatening tachycardia. • Anesthetic induction should be as stress-free as possible; emergency drugs (phentolamine, sodium nitroprusside, propranolol, esmolol, and lidocaine) should be readily available, and the appropriate dosages and/or infusion rates predetermined. • Anesthesia is induced with a narcotic agent or propofol; propofol should be used cautiously because it occasionally causes histamine release that can induce tumor catecholamine secretion. • Maintain anesthesia with isoflurane, since it causes less sensitization of the myocardium to catecholamines than does halothane.

Surgery
• The surgeon should be prepared to do an adrenalectomy, nephrectomy, and thrombectomy even if the preoperative evaluation showed no evidence of tumor invasion of adjacent organs or vessels. • Arterial blood pressure typically increases dramatically when the tumor is manipulated and falls acutely following tumor removal.

MEDICATIONS

CONTRAINDICATIONS
• Metoclopramide can cause tumor catecholamine secretion and thus initiate a hypertensive crisis. • Anesthetic agents—

morphine, morphine, meperidine, xylazine, and ketamine

PRECAUTIONS
See Anesthetic Considerations.

ALTERNATIVE DRUGS
• α-Methyltyrosine has been used to reduce catecholamine secretion and ameliorate clinical signs in humans with inoperable or metastatic disease; it inhibits tyrosine hydroxylase, the rate-limiting enzyme in catecholamine synthesis; this drug has not been used in dogs or cats

FOLLOW-UP

PATIENT MONITORING
• Blood pressure and CVP—closely in the immediate postoperative period (24–72 h) • Blood pressure and ECG—at least monthly in patients being treated long-term for ongoing hypertension and/or cardiac arrhythmias

POSSIBLE COMPLICATIONS
Postoperative—intraabdominal hemorrhage, hypotension, peritonitis, sepsis, or unresolved hypertension

EXPECTED COURSE AND PROGNOSIS
• Survival times > 3 years have been reported in dogs following tumor removal. • Prognosis in general is guarded and is commonly adversely affected by concurrent diseases.

MISCELLANEOUS

ASSOCIATED CONDITIONS
• Most dogs with pheochromocytomas have concurrent organ dysfunction, neoplasms, or other diseases. • Hyperadrenocorticism has been observed in up to 20% of dogs with pheochromocytomas.

SEE ALSO
• Systemic Hypertension
• Hyperadrenocorticism

Suggested Readings
Barthez PB, Marks SL, Woo J, et al. Pheochromocytoma in dogs: 61 cases (1984–1995). JVIM 1997;11:272–278.

Gilson SD, Withrow SJ, Orton EC. Surgical treatment of pheochromocytoma: technique, complications, and results in six dogs. Vet Surg 1994;23:195–200.

Gilson SD, Withrow SJ, Wheeler SL, Twedt DC. Pheochromocytoma in 50 dogs. JVIM 1994;8:228–232.

Maher ER, McNeil EA. Pheochromocytoma in dogs and cats. Vet Clin North Am Small Anim Pract 1997; 27:359–380.

Author John W. Tyler
Consulting Editor Deborah S. Greco

PHOSPHOFRUCTOKINASE DEFICIENCY

BASICS

OVERVIEW
- Phosphofructokinase is the most important rate-controlling enzyme in glycolysis and RBCs; intensely exercising skeletal muscles depend heavily on anaerobic glycolysis for energy.
- Affected dogs have compensated hemolytic anemia and mild myopathy caused by markedly reduced total phosphofructokinase activity in both tissues.
- Anemia develops because of insufficient generation of ATP to maintain normal RBC shape, ionic composition, and deformability and because RBCs from affected dogs are alkaline fragile and lyse when blood pH is slightly high.

SIGNALMENT
- English springer spaniels and American cocker spaniels
- Transmitted as an autosomal recessive trait
- Affected homozygous animals generally not recognized as abnormal before 1 year of age

SIGNS
- Some animals exhibit mild clinical signs that go unrecognized for years; others regularly exhibit episodes of severe illness.
- Depression or weakness concomitant with episodes of red to brown pigmenturia; hemoglobinuria less likely to be recognized in female dogs, because of the sex difference in urination pattern
- Mild lethargy with slight fever during mild hemolytic episodes
- Marked lethargy, weakness, pale or icteric mucous membranes, mild hepatosplenomegaly, muscle wasting, and fever as high as 41°C (106°F) possible during severe hemolytic crises
- Intravascular hemolysis can be caused by hyperventilation-induced alkalemia associated with exercise or excitement.
- Signs of muscle dysfunction—usually limited to exercise intolerance and slightly diminished muscle mass, but muscle cramping and severe progressive myopathy can occur
- Heterozygous carrier animals appear clinically normal.

CAUSES & RISK FACTORS
Deficiency of the muscle-type subunit of phosphofructokinase—markedly reduced total activity in RBCs and skeletal muscle

DIAGNOSIS

DIFFERENTIAL DIAGNOSIS
- Other causes of hemolytic anemia—immune-mediated hemolytic anemia, hemobartonellosis, babesiosis, Heinz body hemolytic anemia, microangiopathic hemolytic anemia, and pyruvate kinase deficiency.
- Affected dogs—negative Coombs test, no parasites or Heinz bodies in stained blood films, seronegative for *Babesia* spp., and no evidence of DIC or heartworm disease
- Differentiated from pyruvate kinase deficiency by specific enzyme assays or DNA test

CBC/BIOCHEMISTRY/URINALYSIS
- Persistent compensated hemolytic anemia
- MCV usually 80–90 fL
- Reticulocyte counts generally 10–30%
- PCV values generally 30–40%; during hemolytic crises may decrease to ≤ 15%
- Bilirubinuria—often markedly high in male dogs
- Hemoglobinuria in association with episodes of intravascular hemolysis
- Serum—slightly high potassium, magnesium, calcium, urea, AST, total protein, and globulin; slightly to moderately high pyruvate kinase, LDH, ALP, iron, and bilirubin; markedly high bilirubin in association with a hemolytic crisis; markedly high urea and creatinine if renal failure develops secondary to hemoglobin nephrosis or shock

OTHER LABORATORY TESTS
- Measure RBC phosphofructokinase activity—easily identify affected animals older than 3 months; heterozygous carrier dogs have approximately one-half normal activity.
- Perform DNA test by PCR technology—clearly differentiate normal and carrier animals of any age.

IMAGING
N/A

DIAGNOSTIC PROCEDURES
N/A

TREATMENT

• Bone marrow transplantation is the only cure.
• In patients with severe intravascular hemolysis, IV fluid therapy minimizes the chance of acute renal failure.
• Blood transfusions usually not needed, but should be given if anemia becomes life-threatening

MEDICATIONS

DRUGS

For fever that often accompanies intravascular hemolysis and potentiates hemolytic crisis—aspirin (10 mg/kg PO q12h) or dipyrone (0.055 mL of 50% solution/kg SC q8h).

CONTRAINDICATIONS/POSSIBLE INTERACTIONS

None

FOLLOW-UP

• Infrequently, affected dogs may die during a hemolytic crises because of anemia or renal failure.
• Affected animals can have a normal life span if properly managed.
• Owners should avoid placing affected dogs in stressful situations or subjecting them to strenuous exercise, excitement, or high environmental temperatures.

MISCELLANEOUS

ABBREVIATIONS

• ALP = alkaline phosphatase
• AST = aspartate aminotransferase
• DIC = disseminated intravascular coagulation
• LDH = lactate dehydrogenase
• MCV = mean cell volume
• PCR = polymerase chain reaction
• PCV = packed cell volume

Suggested Reading

Harvey JW. Congenital erythrocyte enzyme deficiencies. Vet Clin North Am Small Anim Pract 1996;26:1003–1011.

Author John W. Harvey
Consulting editor Susan M. Cotter

PHYCOMYCOSIS (PYTHIOSIS)

BASICS

DEFINITION
• Pythiosis is an infectious disease affecting primarily the GI system or skin of dogs, cats, horses, cattle, and man.
• Caused by the aquatic pathogen, *Pythium insidiosum,* a protistan organism classified in the class Oomycetes
• The horse and the dog are the most common species affected.

PATHOPHYSIOLOGY
• Exposure to *Pythium* by water containing infective zoospores that are released into warm, swampy aquatic environments (e.g., along the Gulf Coast in the summer); these motile spores can chemotactically orient themselves toward certain aquatic plants and animal hair; when animals enter such an environment zoospores rapidly orient toward their hair and may infect damaged skin or mucosa.
• *P. insidiosum* is considered pathogenic rather than opportunistic because immune suppression is apparently not required for infection.
• The organism causes chronic pyogranulomatous disease that manifests in the GI tract by segmental transmural thickening of the stomach, small intestine, colon, or rarely, the esophagus.
• *Pythium*-induced local thromboembolic events may lead to bowel wall ischemia and GI perforation.

SYSTEMS AFFECTED
• Usually affects only one system in a patient; GI and cutaneous forms are most common.
• GI—system most commonly affected in dogs; rare in other species; may affect the stomach and proximal small intestine, the distal small intestine and proximal colon, or rarely, the esophagus
• Skin—most commonly affected in cats, horses, and cattle; sporadically in dogs
• Ophthalmic (keratitis)—rare manifestation
• Ophthalmic (retrobulbar) and respiratory (nasopharyngeal) disease—reported in cats
• Multisystemic disseminated disease—rare

GENETICS
• Large-breed dogs are most often affected.
• May reflect an increased likelihood of environmental exposure rather than a genetic predisposition

INCIDENCE/PREVALENCE
• Depends on geographic distribution
• Dogs are usually exposed to infective zoospores in the summer and are presented for clinical disease in the fall or early winter months.

GEOGRAPHIC DISTRIBUTION
• Disease caused by *P. insidiosum* occurs primarily in tropical and subtropical areas of the world.
• Reported in Australia, Brazil, Burma, Colombia, Costa Rica, Indonesia, Japan, New Guinea, Thailand, and the United States
• In the United States pythiosis occurs most commonly in states bordering the Gulf of Mexico; most reported cases are from Louisiana, Texas, and Florida; it occurs sporadically throughout the warmer and temperate regions of the country.

SIGNALMENT

Species
Canine, equine, and feline (less common in cats)

Breed Predilections
• Large-breed dogs, especially dogs used in hunting or field trial work near water
• Labrador retrievers are overrepresented in many studies of GI pythiosis.
• German shepherds may be predisposed to cutaneous pythiosis.
• Cats—none

Mean Age and Range
Animals less than 3 years old are most likely to be infected.

Predominant Sex
Males are affected more often than females.

SIGNS

General Comments
Affected dogs are not usually systemically ill or anorectic until late in the disease course.

Historical Findings
• Chronic weight loss and intermittent vomiting—most common
• Diarrhea—may be evident if the colon or a large segment of the small intestine is affected
• Regurgitation—in rare esophageal disease
• Cutaneous disease—nodules that ulcerate and drain

Physical Examination Findings
GI Pythiosis
• Emaciation—common
• Palpable abdominal mass in the cranial abdomen—common
• Malaise—uncommon, despite severe weight loss
• Fever—occasionally noted
• Signs of systemic illness and/or abdominal pain—when intestinal obstruction, infarction, or perforation occurs
Cutaneous pythiosis
• Cutaneous lesions—may occur anywhere on the body; slightly pruritic, poorly defined nodules that soon become ulcerated
• Multiple tracts draining a serosanguinous or purulent exudate may be present.

• Rarely, cutaneous disease may be present in a dog with GI involvement.

CAUSES
Pythium insidiosum

RISK FACTORS
• Environmental exposure to swampy areas with warm water containing zoospores
• Outdoor activities (e.g., hunting or field trials)

DIAGNOSIS

DIFFERENTIAL DIAGNOSIS

GI Pythiosis
• Proximal small intestinal obstructive disease (e.g., foreign body)
• Histoplasmosis
• GI lymphosarcoma
• Other GI neoplasia
• Inflammatory bowel disease
• Zygomycosis—*Mucor, Absidia,* or *Rhizopus* infection
• *Basidiobolus* or *Conidiobolus* infections
• Prototheocosis
• Idiopathic pyogranulomatous disease
• Histiocytic or idiopathic colitis

Cutaneous Pythiosis
• Nodular bacterial skin diseases (e.g., actinomycosis, mycobacteriosis, botryomycosis, brucellosis, or *Rhodococcus equi* infection)
• Mycotic skin diseases (e.g., cryptococcosis, coccidioidomycosis, sporotrichosis, basidiobolomycosis, conidiobolomycosis, phaeohyphomycosis, hyalohyphomycosis, eumycotic mycetoma, and dermatophytic mycetoma)
• Prototheocosis or nodular leishmaniasis
• Noninfectious pyogranulomatous disease (e.g., foreign body reaction, idiopathic nodular panniculitis, sebaceous nodular adenitis, and canine cutaneous sterile pyogranuloma/granuloma syndrome)
• Cutaneous neoplasia
• Systemic vasculitis and cutaneous embolic disease

CBC/BIOCHEMISTRY/URINALYSIS
• Findings nonspecific
• Anemia of chronic disease and leukocytosis consistent with stress have been reported.
• May see hypoalbuminemia in chronically affected dogs or when GI ulceration is present; hypokalemia, hyponatremia, hypochloremia, and metabolic alkalosis in dogs with proximal duodenal obstruction
• Hypercalcemia reported in a single case

OTHER LABORATORY TESTS
Serologic testing—a sensitive, specific ELISA test was developed but is not yet commercially available.

IMAGING
• Abdominal radiography—may see an obstructive pattern or proximal small intestinal thickening
• Abdominal ultrasonography—may reveal segmental transmural thickening of the stomach, proximal small intestine, or ileocolic junction; may see granulomas or enlarged lymph nodes in the mesentery

DIAGNOSTIC PROCEDURES
• Biopsy of affected GI tissue or skin
• Must base definitive diagnosis on culture and/or histologic identification of the organism
• An immunoperoxidase stain can definitively identify *Pythium* in histologic sections
• Culture on Sabouraud's media or vegetable extract agar is not difficult from tissue; do not chill the tissue sample.

PATHOLOGIC FINDINGS
• Severe annular thickening of segmental portions of bowel with obstruction of the intestinal lumen
• Granulomatous thickening of the mesentery with mesenteric lymphadenopathy and multiple adhesions
• Histologically the canine GI form of the disease is characterized by mucosal ulceration, lymphoplasmacytic and eosinophilic inflammation in the lamina propria, and granulomatous inflammation within the submucosa and muscularis; irregularly branching, rarely septate hyphae with thick walls will stain positively with special fungal stains.

TREATMENT

APPROPRIATE HEALTH CARE
Treatment of choice is wide surgical excision; unfortunately, most dogs do not see a veterinarian until complete excision is not possible; these patients often require intensive and expensive inpatient medical and surgical treatment.

NURSING CARE
Supportive care should include fluid (with appropriate potassium supplementation) and antibiotics as indicated.

ACTIVITY
Limited

DIET
Highly digestible, caloric, dense

CLIENT EDUCATION
Treatment is expensive, and rate of response is not well established (guarded to poor prognosis).

SURGICAL CONSIDERATIONS
• Attempt wide surgical excision to obtain 5- to 6-cm margins even if medical therapy is contemplated.
• Dogs often improve after obstructive lesions are removed, even if significant disease is still grossly evident.

MEDICATIONS

DRUGS OF CHOICE
Itraconazole (10 mg/kg PO daily)—most extensively evaluated; must give with food

CONTRAINDICATIONS
Possibly corticosteroids

PRECAUTIONS
• Do not use azole drugs in patients with severe liver disease.
• Anorexia, increased liver enzymes, and cutaneous vasculitis are the most common adverse affects of itraconazole and the other azole drugs.

POSSIBLE INTERACTIONS
Antacids and anticonvulsants may decrease blood levels of itraconazole.

ALTERNATIVE DRUGS
• ABLC—(1–2 mg/kg, dog; 0.5–1 mg/kg , cat; IV 3×/week) for 12 treatments; total dose of 12–24 mg in dogs; not tested in cats; dilute in 5% dextrose to a concentration of 1 mg/mL and give IV over 30–60 min.
• Do not use ABLC in azotemic or hypokalemic patients.
• Side effects of ABLC (e.g., chills, trembling, fever, anorexia, and vomiting)—may see during infusion; if so, slow the infusion rate; nephrotoxicity is low, and diuresis is not required.
• Terbinafine has been used in humans.

FOLLOW-UP

PATIENT MONITORING
• Evaluate liver enzymes monthly while on itraconazole.
• Evaluate serum BUN, creatinine, and potassium before each dose of ABLC.
• Abdominal ultrasonography is useful in reevaluating intestinal lesions.
• Medical management may reduce nonresectable lesions to the point that they become resectable.

PREVENTION/AVOIDANCE
Monitor for signs of recurrence.

POSSIBLE COMPLICATIONS
Acute peritonitis and death from GI thrombosis and perforation

EXPECTED COURSE AND PROGNOSIS
• Without medical management—prognosis poor; <5% of dogs are alive 3 months after diagnosis.
• Itraconazole treatment—approximately 20% of dogs are cured.
• A minimum of 2 months of therapy is usually required before improvement becomes obvious.
• At least 6 months of therapy is usually required in dogs responding.
• Prognosis with ABLC treatment is being evaluated; preliminary results are promising.

MISCELLANEOUS

ASSOCIATED CONDITIONS
None

AGE-RELATED FACTORS
Young animals are predisposed.

ZOONOTIC POTENTIAL
• Infections in people are very rare and are from a common environmental source.
• No direct transmission from animal to man

PREGNANCY
Azole antifungals are teratogenic; do not use in pregnant animals.

SYNONYMS
Phycomycosis, swamp cancer

SEE ALSO
N/A

ABBREVIATIONS
• ABLC = Amphotericin B Lipid Complex
• GI = gastrointestinal

Suggested Reading
Bissonnette EW, Sharp NJH, Dykstra MH, et al. Nasal and retrobulbar mass in a cat caused by *Pythium* insidiosum. J Med Vet Mycol 1991;29:39–44.
Patton CS, Hake R, Newton J, Toal RL. Esophagitis due to Pythium insidiosum infection in two dogs. J Vet Intern Med 1996;10:139–142.
Taboada J, Merchant SR. Protozoal and miscellaneous infections. In: Ettinger SJ, Feldman EC, eds. Textbook of veterinary internal medicine. Philadelphia: Saunders, 1994: 384–397.
Taboada J. Systemic mycoses. In: Morgan RV, ed. Handbook of small animal practice. Philadelphia: Saunders, 1997:1113–1126.
Taboada J, Werner BE, Legendre AM. Successful management of gastrointestinal pythiosis with itraconazole in two dogs. J Vet Intern Med 1994;8:176 (Abstract).
Authors Joseph Taboada and Amy Grooters
Consulting Editors Brett M. Feder and Mitchell A.Crystal

PHYSALOPTERA

 BASICS

OVERVIEW
• Stomach worm, *Physaloptera* spp., of dogs, cats
• Gastritis caused by small number of parasites, even single-worm infections
• No extraintestinal involvement
• Infective larvae carried by coprophagous grubs, beetles, and other bugs.

SIGNALMENT
Dogs and cats; any age or sex

SIGNS
• Vomiting
• Small 2.5- to 5-cm worms with cuticular collars and spiral tails seen in vomitus

CAUSES & RISK FACTORS
Physaloptera, spirurid worms, transmitted as infective larvae in coprophagous beetles, bugs, or transport hosts such as birds, rodents, and frogs

 DIAGNOSIS

DIFFERENTIAL DIAGNOSIS
• Other spirurid infections (e.g., *Spirocerca,* the esophageal worm) produce similar eggs and may cause projectile vomiting.
• Viral, bacterial infections
• Foreign objects in the stomach
• Noxious substances accidentally ingested

CBC/BIOCHEMISTRY/URINALYSIS
Usually normal

OTHER LABORATORY TESTS
N/A

IMAGING
Abdominal radiography, including contrast studies, to eliminate other causes of vomiting

DIAGNOSTIC PROCEDURES
• Fecal examination for ovoid-to-ellipsoidal eggs 30–40 × 20 μm, thick-shelled, larvated
• Endoscopy—adult worms seen with gastroscopy; worm retrieval and identification

 TREATMENT

Outpatient treatment

 MEDICATIONS

With no migration beyond the stomach wall, use adulticide anthelmintics with release in stomach.

DRUGS
• Fenbendazole 50 mg/kg PO q24h for 5 days
• Dichlorvos packets/tabs as single dose or biweekly
• Medication to reduce gastritis—histamine H$_2$-antagonists (e.g., famotidine 0.5 mg/kg PO q24h); sucralfate 0.25–1 g PO q8–12h in the dog; 0.25 g PO q8–12h in the cat

CONTRAINDICATIONS/POSSIBLE INTERACTIONS
• Do not give organophosphates to heartworm-positive dogs or cats.
• Do not give dichlorvos concurrently with other organophosphates such as insecticides.

 FOLLOW-UP

Fecal examination after 2 weeks to determine drug effect.

 MISCELLANEOUS

Suggested Reading
Corwin RM, Green SE. Gastrointestinal parasitism in the dog and cat. In: Jones BD, ed. Canine and feline gastroenterology. Philadelphia: Saunders, 1986:487–509.
Author Robert M. Corwin
Consulting Editors Brett M. Feder and Mitchell A. Crystal

BASICS

DEFINITION
Ingestion of nonfood items

PATHOPHYSIOLOGY
• Most cases not caused by disease, but anemia and gastrointestinal (GI) or hepatic disease may lead to ingestion of nonfood items.
• Unknown

SYSTEMS AFFECTED
GI—obstruction from foreign objects, vomiting, and/or diarrhea can occur.

SIGNALMENT
Dogs and cats

SIGNS

Historical Findings
Ingestion of nonfood items (e.g., dogs: rocks and feces; cats: cat litter, fabrics, and plastics)

Physical Examination Findings
• Pallor and weakness if anemia
• Thin body condition if a maldigestive/malabsorptive process
• Neurologic signs if neurologic disease

CAUSES
• Behavioral—compulsive or stereotypic behavior
• Anemia—iron deficiency, other
• Maldigestion/malabsorption (e.g., EPI)
• Hunger
• Neurologic disease—primary CNS, portosystemic shunt

RISK FACTORS
• Underlying disease predisposing to anemia, maldigestion, or malabsorption
• Confinement of dogs in barren yards with no environmental stimulation or enrichment—especially predisposes to coprophagia
• Early weaned oriental-breed cats on low-roughage diets with no access to prey or grass are most at risk for wool eating.

DIAGNOSIS

DIFFERENTIAL DIAGNOSIS
Licking behaviors may indicate nausea; differentiate by observation.

CBC/BIOCHEMISTRY/URINALYSIS
May see anemia, hypoproteinemia (maldigestion/malabsorption), or changes representative of a portosystemic shunt (microcytosis, target cells, hypoalbuminemia, decreased BUN, ammonium biurate crystalluria)

OTHER LABORATORY TESTS

• Test any anemic cat for feline leukemia virus (FeLV) and feline immunodeficiency virus (FIV).
• Trypsin-like immunoreactivity testing should be performed if EPI is suspected.
• Test fasting and 2-h postprandial serum bile acids if a portosystemic shunt is suspected.

IMAGING
Survey abdominal radiography and abdominal ultrasonography—may help rule out some foreign bodies in the GI tract; may demonstrate microhepatica if a portosystemic shunt exists

DIAGNOSTIC PROCEDURES
Upper GI endoscopy if a foreign body is suspected in this location

TREATMENT

• Treat any underlying disease.
• When no pathologic cause exists—(1) limit access to nonfood items to prevent ingestion, (2) find a safe substitute that the animal can ingest with impunity, and (3) change the animal's motivation to ingest the nonfood item.
• Dogs—can keep indoors and walk on a leash to prevent rock chewing and coprophagia
• Can remove plastic from the cat's environment and store away woolen clothes
• Applying a pungent or bitter taste to objects may discourage consumption.
• May give cats a high-roughage diet, tough meat to chew, or a garden of grass or catnip to graze on

MEDICATIONS

The animal's motivation can be changed by administering psychoactive drugs or punishment.

DRUGS OF CHOICE
• Clomipramine (1–3 mg/kg PO q24h)—a tricyclic antidepressant, serotonin reuptake blocker
• Cyproheptadine (4 mg/cat PO q24h)—an appetite stimulant, serotonin antagonist

CONTRAINDICATIONS
N/A

PRECAUTIONS
N/A

POSSIBLE INTERACTIONS
N/A

ALTERNATIVE DRUGS
N/A

FOLLOW-UP

PATIENT MONITORING
• Contact the owner in 10–14 days to confirm compliance and determine if the pica has abated.
• If dietary and management changes did not markedly improve the problem, prescribe further diagnostic work and/or medication.

POSSIBLE COMPLICATIONS
GI complications—foreign bodies, diarrhea, vomiting

MISCELLANEOUS

ASSOCIATED CONDITIONS
N/A

AGE-RELATED FACTORS
Chewing and sometimes swallowing objects is normal puppy behavior; the mouth is the best instrument the dog can use to feel and taste its environment during its exploratory period.

ZOONOTIC POTENTIAL
N/A

PREGNANCY
N/A

SYNONYMS
• Depraved appetite
• Wool chewing
• Wool sucking
• Coprophagia

SEE ALSO
• Gastrointestinal Foreign Bodies
• Coprophagia

ABBREVIATIONS
• EPI = exocrine pancreatic insufficiency
• FeLV = feline leukemia virus
• FIV = feline immunodeficiency virus
• GI = gastrointestinal

Suggested Reading
Bradshaw JWS. The behaviour of the domestic cat. Oxon, UK: C.A.B. International, 1992:200–203.
Houpt KA. Domestic animal behavior for veterinarians and animal scientists. Ames: Iowa State University Press, 1991:310–312.
Author Katherine A. Houpt
Consulting Editors Mitchell A. Crystal and Brett M. Feder

DISEASES

PLAGUE (*YERSINIA PESTIS*)

BASICS

OVERVIEW
• *Yersinia pestis*—gram-negative, bipolar staining rod; an Enterobacteriaceae; reservoir includes wild rodents (sylvatic), ground squirrels, prairie dogs, rabbits, bobcats, coyotes
• Occurs worldwide
• U.S.—reported cases from New Mexico, Arizona, California, Colorado, Idaho, Nevada, Oregon, Texas, Utah, Washington, Wyoming, and Hawaii
• Common from May to October
• Infected vectors (fleas) transmit the bacterium in bite.
• Bacteria—rapidly migrate from skin lymphatics to regional lymph nodes; survive phagocytosis (because of capsule protection) and multiply in lymph nodes; phagocytic cells rupture and organism is resistant to further phagocytosis.
• Infection—fever and painful lymphadenopathy (bubo); intense local inflammation results in bubonic plague; intermittent bacteremia; lymph nodes may rupture; may become septicemic with or without lymph node involvement
• Cats—highly susceptible to infection; severe fatal disease
• Dogs—naturally resistant to infection

SIGNALMENT
Cats and rarely dogs

SIGNS
Dogs—may exhibit mild febrile signs and depression

Bubonic (Cats)
• Most common form
• Incubation period—2–7 days after flea bite or after eating infected rodent
• Duration of illness variable
• Buboes—head and neck; marked lymphadenopathy (hemorrhagic, necrotic, edematous); if patient survives long enough, lymph nodes abscess, rupture, and drain through fistula tracts to skin.
• Fever—39.5–40.5°C (103–105°F)
• Depression
• Vomiting/diarrhea
• Dehydration
• Enlarged tonsils
• Anorexia
• Ocular discharge
• Weight loss
• Ataxia
• Coma
• Oral ulcers

Septicemic (Cats)
• Rare
• Septicemia without lymphadenopathy or abscess formation

• Other signs same as for bubonic

CAUSES & RISK FACTORS
• Hunter (outdoor) cats—greater risk of contacting wild rodent populations and rodent fleas
• Travel to endemic areas—western United States and Hawaii
• Environment—homes or pet with heavy flea infestation; homes with large nearby rodent population (e.g., garbage food source or wood pile)

DIAGNOSIS

DIFFERENTIAL DIAGNOSIS
Fight wound abscess—*Pasteurella multocida; Staphylococcus aureus*

CBC/BIOCHEMISTRY/URINALYSIS
• Leukocytosis with left shift and marked toxic changes
• Thrombocytopenia—with DIC
• High liver enzyme activity and hyperbilirubinemia

OTHER LABORATORY TESTS
• Serology—Communicable Disease Center and/or state health department; cats and dogs develop high passive hemagglutinating titers to fraction 1A (capsule antigen) 8–12 days postinfection; may see fourfold rise in titer between acute and convalescent serum samples; high titers persist > 1 year in surviving animals.
• Prolonged clotting times—with DIC

IMAGING N/A

DIAGNOSTIC PROCEDURES
• Culture isolation—by reference laboratory; definitive (large numbers of gram-negative coccobacilli with bipolar staining); samples from antemortem clinical material (abscess, lymph node, peripheral blood) before treatment is given or from postmortem tissue (lymph node, abscess, liver, spleen)
• Florescent antibody test—quick presumptive method for identifying infected animals; samples same as for culture

PATHOLOGIC FINDINGS
• Acutely ill cats—few lesions; enlarged lymph nodes (buboes) on head and neck; enlarged liver and spleen
• Lymph nodes—destruction of normal architecture; hemorrhagic necrosis; extracellular bacteria

TREATMENT
• Inpatient
• High mortality if not treated early
• Treat aggressively with intravenous fluids to counteract septicemia.

• Treat DIC, if indicated.
• Treat patient for fleas.

MEDICATIONS

DRUGS
• Treat all suspect cases empirically until laboratory confirmation is obtained.
• Systemic antimicrobials—use in all patients except those with lung involvement (such patients should be euthanized because of high zoonotic potential).
• Tetracyclines—oxytetracyclines, tetracycline, chlortetracycline; 25 mg/kg PO q8h for 10 days; parenteral, 7.5 mg/kg q12h
• Doxycycline—effectiveness not established but probably effective
• Chloramphenicol—30–50 mg/kg PO q8h
• Gentamicin, trimethoprim-sulfamethoxazole, and kanamycin—use if the other listed drugs cannot be used.

CONTRAINDICATIONS/POSSIBLE INTERACTIONS N/A

FOLLOW-UP

PATIENT MONITORING
DIC—common later in infection, if disease not treated early

PREVENTION/AVOIDANCE
• Limit travel with pet to avoid endemic areas. • Endemic areas—keep pet on a leash to limit/control exposure to wild rodents and their fleas; periodically spray or dust pet and home for flea control. • Neuter cats—limit hunting behavior and wild rodent exposure. • Rodents—eliminate animals and their habitats near houses and outbuildings (e.g., wood piles, garbage piles); store food in rodent-proof containers.

EXPECTED COURSE AND PROGNOSIS
Prognosis—poor if not treated early

MISCELLANEOUS

ZOONOTIC POTENTIAL
High; do not mistake for bite abscesses or tularemia.

ABBREVIATION
DIC = disseminated intravascular coagulation

Suggested Reading
Rollag OJ, Skeels MR, Nims LJ, et al. Feline plague in New Mexico: report of five cases. J Am Vet Med Assoc 1981;179:1381–1383.

Author Patrick L. McDonough
Consulting Editor Stephen C. Barr

PLASMA CELL GINGIVITIS AND PHARYNGITIS

BASICS

OVERVIEW
An uninhibited, excessive immune inflammatory response affecting the oral cavity in cats

SIGNALMENT
• Cat
• Purebred breeds predisposed—Abyssinian, Persian, Himalayan, Burmese, Siamese, and Somali

SIGNS
• Ptyalism
• Halitosis
• Dysphagia
• Anorexia—prefers soft food
• Weight loss
• Scruffy haircoat
• Erythematous, ulcerative, proliferative lesions affecting the gingiva, glossopalatine arches, tongue, lips, buccal mucosa, and/or the hard palate
• Gingival inflammation completely surrounds the tooth, compared with gingivitis, which usually only occurs on the buccal and labial surfaces.
• May extend to the glossopharyngeal arches as well as the palate

CAUSES & RISK FACTORS
• Cause unknown; bacterial, viral, and immunologic etiologies suspected
• Significant findings of feline coronavirus in one study
• Immunosuppression from FeLV or FIV can also lead to nonresponsive infections; most affected cats are negative for FeLV and FIV.

DIAGNOSIS

DIFFERENTIAL DIAGNOSIS
• Periodontal disease
• Oral malignancy
• Eosinophilic granuloma complex

CBC/BIOCHEMISTRY/URINALYSIS
• Polyclonal gammopathy secondary to antibody production following bacterial invasion into periodontal tissues
• Leukocytosis and eosinophilia may be present.

OTHER LABORATORY TESTS
N/A

IMAGING
Intraoral radiographs to evaluate periodontal disease and feline oral odontoclastic resorptions

DIAGNOSTIC PROCEDURES
Biopsy (especially unilateral lesions) to rule out neoplasia—primarily squamous cell carcinoma

TREATMENT

• First-line therapy involves teeth cleaning above and below the gingiva as well as strict home care and treatment (extraction) for teeth affected with grades 3 and 4 periodontal disease and/or feline odontoclastic resorptive lesions.
• Currently, the only treatment that consistently delivers 60–80% (depending on the study) cure without the use of follow-up medications is extraction of all teeth distal to the canines.
• To aid the extractions; flap all quadrants and use a high-speed bur with water spray to remove a trough of bone where the roots were, thus removing most of the keratinized gingiva, periodontal ligament, and periradicular alveolar bone; before suturing, "smooth down" the alveolar socket to remove sharp edges.
• If patients do not respond to extraction of the teeth distal to the canines, remove all teeth; when extracting the teeth, pay meticulous attention to removing all tooth substance; take intraoral radiographs before and after surgery; postoperative application of fluocinonide 0.05% (Lidex Gel) to the gingival margin helps in the healing process.

MEDICATIONS

DRUGS
• Medication and other therapies have been used with limited long-term success; lack of permanent response to conventional oral hygiene, antibiotics, antiinflammatory drugs, and immunosuppressives is typical.

• Antibiotics—clindamycin (5 mg/kg q12h), metronidazole, amoxicillin, ampicillin, enrofloxacin, tetracycline
• Corticosteroids—prednisone (2 mg/kg initially daily, followed by every other day); methylprednisolone acetate 2 mg/kg q7–30 days) may also help control inflammation.
• Gold Salts Solganol (Shering)—1 mg/kg IM every week until improvement (up to 4 months), then every 14–35 days
• Chlorambucil—2 mg/m² orally every other day or 20 mg/m² every other week
• Bovine Lactoferrin (40 mg/kg) applied to the oral mucous membranes
• CO_2 laser to remove the inflamed tissue
• Megestrol acetate 1 mg/kg
• Levamisole
• Cyclophosphamide
• Cyclosporine

CONTRAINDICATIONS/POSSIBLE INTERACTIONS
N/A

FOLLOW-UP
N/A

MISCELLANEOUS

ABBREVIATIONS
FeLV = feline leukemia virus
FIV = feline immunodeficiency virus

Suggested Reading
Harvey CE, Emily PP. Small animal dentistry. St. Louis: CV Mosby, 1993.
Wiggs RB, Lobrise HB. Veterinary dentistry: principles and practice. Lippincott-Raven, 1997.

Author Jan Bellows
Consulting Editor Jan Bellows

DISEASES

PLASMACYTOMA, MUCOCUTANEOUS

 BASICS

OVERVIEW
• Tumor of plasma cell origin
• Rapid development
• May be a subtype of extramedullary plasmacytoma that is a primary tumor of soft tissue origin or may be metastasis of primary osseous multiple myeloma

SIGNALMENT
• Dogs and rarely cats
• Most common in mixed-breed dogs and cocker spaniels
• Age at diagnosis (dogs)—mean, 9.7 years; median, 10.5 years
• Both sexes affected equally

SIGNS
• Usually raised or ulcerated solid nodule, 0.25–6.0 cm in diameter
• Tumor of the lips—typically small
• Usually solitary
• Rarely polypoid
• Common locations—mouth, feet, trunk, and ears
• Occasionally occurs with multiple myeloma or lymphosarcoma, developing together or at different times
• Systemic signs rare

CAUSES & RISK FACTORS
Unknown

 DIAGNOSIS

DIFFERENTIAL DIAGNOSIS
• Other round cell tumors—lymphosarcoma; mast cell tumor; histiocytoma; transmissible venereal tumor
• Poorly differentiated carcinoma
• Amelanotic melanoma
• Biopsy—distinguishes from other tumors

CBC/BIOCHEMISTRY/URINALYSIS
Usually normal, unless patient has multiple myeloma or lymphosarcoma

OTHER LABORATORY TESTS
N/A

IMAGING
No evidence of metastasis or bony lysis will be seen.

DIAGNOSTIC PROCEDURES
• Cytologic examination of fine-needle aspirate—reveals moderate to marked cellularity; round to polyhedral individual tumor cells with discrete margins and prominent anisocytosis and anisokaryosis; round to oval nuclei with fine to coarse chromatin and no visible nucleoli; cytoplasm stains lightly basophilic.
• Histologic—usually well circumscribed and easily identifiable

 TREATMENT
• Occasionally invasive—aggressive surgical excision recommended
• Radiotherapy—successful in some patients

PLASMACYTOMA, MUCOCUTANEOUS

MEDICATIONS

DRUGS
Chemotherapy not recommended

CONTRAINDICATIONS/POSSIBLE INTERACTIONS
N/A

FOLLOW-UP

PATIENT MONITORING
Usually none, unless accompanied by multiple myeloma or lymphosarcoma

EXPECTED COURSE AND PROGNOSIS
Excellent in most patients

MISCELLANEOUS

ASSOCIATED CONDITIONS
• Multiple myeloma
• Lymphosarcoma (lymphoma)—dogs
• Cats—may note systemic amyloidosis

SEE ALSO
• Amyloidosis
• Lymphosarcoma—dogs
• Multiple Myeloma

Suggested Reading
Rakich PM, Latimer KS, Weiss R, Steffens WL. Mucocutaneous plasmacytomas in dogs. 75 cases (1980–1987). J Am Vet Med Assoc 1989;194:803–810.
Author Wallace B. Morrison
Consulting Editor Wallace B. Morrison

PLEURAL EFFUSION

 BASICS

DEFINITION
Abnormal accumulation of fluid within the pleural cavity

PATHOPHYSIOLOGY
• More than normal production or less than normal resorption of fluid • Alterations in hydrostatic and oncotic pressures or vascular permeability and lymphatic function may contribute to fluid accumulation.

SYSTEMS AFFECTED
• Respiratory • Cardiovascular

GENETICS
N/A

INCIDENCE/PREVALENCE
N/A

GEOGRAPHIC DISTRIBUTION
N/A

SIGNALMENT
Species
Dogs and cats

Breed Predilections
Varies with underlying cause

Mean Age and Range
Varies with underlying cause

Predominant Sex
Varies with underlying cause

SIGNS
General Comments
Depend on the fluid volume, rapidity of fluid accumulation, and the underlying cause

Historical Findings
• Dyspnea • Tachypnea • Orthopnea • Open-mouth breathing • Cyanosis • Exercise intolerance • Lethargy • Inappetence • Cough

Physical Examination Findings
• Dyspnea—respirations often shallow and rapid • Muffled or inaudible heart and lung sounds ventrally • Preservation of breath sounds dorsally • Dullness ventrally on thoracic percussion

CAUSES
High Hydrostatic Pressure
• CHF • Overhydration • Intrathoracic neoplasia

Low Oncotic Pressure
Hypoalbuminemia—protein-losing enteropathy, protein-losing nephropathy, and liver disease

Vascular or Lymphatic Abnormality
• Infectious—bacterial, viral, or fungal • Neoplasia (e.g., mediastinal lymphosarcoma, thymoma, mesothelioma, primary lung tumor, and metastatic disease) • Chylothorax (e.g., from lymphangiectasia, CHF, cranial vena

cava obstruction, neoplasia, fungal, heartworms, diaphragmatic hernia, lung lobe torsion, and trauma) • Diaphragmatic hernia • Hemothorax (e.g., from trauma, neoplasia, and coagulopathy) • Lung lobe torsion • Pulmonary thromboembolism • Pancreatitis

RISK FACTORS
N/A

 DIAGNOSIS

DIFFERENTIAL DIAGNOSIS
• Historical or physical evidence of external trauma—consider hemothorax or diaphragmatic hernia
• Fever suggests an inflammatory, infectious, or neoplastic cause.
• Murmurs, gallops, or arrhythmias combined with jugular venous distension or pulsation suggest an underlying cardiac cause.
• Concurrent ascites suggests FIP, CHF (mainly dogs), severe hypoalbuminemia, diaphragmatic hernia, disseminated neoplasia, or pancreatitis.
• In cats, decreased compressibility of the cranial thorax suggests a cranial mediastinal mass.
• Concurrent ocular changes (e.g., chorioretinitis and uveitis) suggest FIP or fungal disease.

CBC/BIOCHEMISTRY/URINALYSIS
• Hemogram results may be abnormal in patients with pyothorax, FIP, neoplasia, or lung lobe torsion.
• Severe hypoalbuminemia (generally < 1 g/dL to cause effusion) suggests protein-losing enteropathy, protein-losing nephropathy, or liver disease.
• Hyperglobulinemia (polyclonal) suggests FIP.

OTHER LABORATORY TESTS
• Fluid analysis should include physical characteristics (i.e., color, clarity, odor, clots), pH, glucose, total protein, total nucleated cell count, and cytologic examination; Table 1 provides characteristics of various pleural fluid types and their disease associations.
• Can also classify pleural effusions on the basis of LDH concentration in the fluid; in cats the LDH concentration in transudates is < 200 IU/L and in exudates > 200 IU/L.
• Pleural fluid pH < 6.9 suggests pyothorax in cats.
• Glucose concentration in pleural fluid usually parallels levels in serum. In cats, pyothorax and malignancy lower pleural fluid glucose concentration relative to serum glucose concentration; thus pleural fluid with a normal pH and low glucose concentration suggests malignancy in cats.
• Serologic tests for feline leukemia virus (if patient has mediastinal lymphosarcoma), feline immunodeficiency virus (if patient has

pyothorax), and coronavirus (if FIP is suspected) are available.
• Cardiac disease suspected—consider a heartworm test in dogs and cats and a thyroid and taurine evaluation in cats.
• Infection suspected—do a bacterial culture and sensitivity test and consider special stains. (e.g., gram and acid-fast stains) of the fluid
• FIP suspected—consider protein electrophoresis of the fluid; γ-globulin level > 32% of total protein strongly predicts a diagnosis of FIP.
• Chyle suspected—do an ether clearance test or Sudan stain of the pleural fluid, and triglyceride and cholesterol evaluations of the fluid and serum.

IMAGING
Radiographic Findings
• Used to confirm pleural effusion; should not be performed until after thoracocentesis in dyspneic patients with evidence of pleural effusion on physical examination
• Evidence of pleural effusion includes separation of lung borders away from the thoracic wall and sternum by fluid density in the pleural space, fluid-filled interlobar fissure lines, loss or blurring of the cardiac and diaphragmatic borders, blunting of the lung margins at the costophrenic angles (ventrodorsal view), and widening of the mediastinum (ventrodorsal view).
• Rounding of the caudal lung lobe borders (lateral view)—most common in patients with fibrosing pleuritis caused by chylothorax, pyothorax, or FIP
• Unilateral effusion—most common in patients with chylothorax and pyothorax; hemothorax, pulmonary neoplasia, diaphragmatic hernias, and lung lobe torsion
• Evaluate postthoracocentesis radiographs carefully for cardiomegaly, intrapulmonary lesions, mediastinal masses, diaphragmatic hernia, lung lobe torsion, and evidence of trauma (e.g., rib fractures).
• Can diagnose a diaphragmatic hernia with positive-contrast peritoneography
• Can evaluate the thoracic duct by positive contrast lymphangiography

Echocardiographic Findings
• Ultrasonographic evaluation of the thorax is recommended whenever cardiac disease, a diaphragmatic hernia, or cranial mediastinal mass is suspected.
• Echocardiography is easiest to perform before thoracocentesis, provided the patient is stable.

DIAGNOSTIC PROCEDURES
• Thoracocentesis—allows characterization of the fluid type and determination of potential underlying cause
• Exploratory thoracotomy—to obtain biopsy specimens of lung, lymph nodes, or pleura, if indicated

TREATMENT

• First, thoracocentesis to relieve respiratory distress; if the patient is stable after thoracocentesis, outpatient treatment may be possible for some diseases. Most patients are hospitalized because they require intensive management such as indwelling chest tubes (e.g., patients with pyothorax) or thoracic surgery.
• Preventing fluid reaccumulation requires treatment based on a definitive diagnosis.
• Surgery is indicated for management of some neoplasias, diaphragmatic hernia repair, lymphangiectasia (i.e., thoracic duct ligation), foreign body removal, and lung lobectomy for lung lobe torsion.

MEDICATIONS

DRUGS OF CHOICE

• Treatment varies with specific disease
• Diuretics generally reserved for patients with diseases causing fluid retention and volume overload (e.g., CHF)

CONTRAINDICATIONS

N/A

PRECAUTIONS

• Drugs that depress respirations or decrease blood pressure

• Inappropriate use of diuretics predisposes the patient to dehydration and electrolyte disturbances without eliminating the effusion.

POSSIBLE INTERACTIONS

N/A

ALTERNATIVE DRUGS

N/A

FOLLOW-UP

PATIENT MONITORING

Radiographic evaluation key to assessment of treatment in most patients

PREVENTION/AVOIDANCE

N/A

POSSIBLE COMPLICATIONS

Death due to respiratory compromise

EXPECTED COURSE AND PROGNOSIS

Varies with underlying cause, but usually guarded to poor

MISCELLANEOUS

ASSOCIATED CONDITIONS

N/A

AGE-RELATED FACTORS

N/A

ZOONOTIC POTENTIAL

N/A

PREGNANCY

N/A

SYNONYMS

• May use hydrothorax for transudates and modified transudates • Pyothorax = empyema = septic pleuritis

SEE ALSO

See Causes

ABBREVIATIONS

• CHF = congestive heart failure • FIP = feline infectious peritonitis • LDH = lactate dehydrogenase

Suggested Reading

Bauer T, Woodfield JA. Pleura and pleural space disorders. In: Ettinger SJ, Feldman EC, eds. Textbook of veterinary internal medicine, vol 1. 4th ed. Philadelphia: Saunders, 1995:817–829.

Fossum TW. Pleural effusion. In: Birchard SJ, Sherding RG, eds. Saunders manual of small animal practice. Philadelphia: Saunders, 1994:580–586.

Padrid P. Pulmonary diagnostics. In: August JR, ed. Consultations in feline internal medicine 3. Philadelphia: Saunders, 1997: 292–302.

Sherding RG. Disease of the pleural cavity. In: Sherding RG, ed. The cat: diseases and clinical management. 2nd ed. New York: Churchill Livingstone, 1994:1053–1083.

Authors Linda B. Lehmkuhl and Francis W. K. Smith, Jr.

Consulting Editors Larry P. Tilley and Francis W. K. Smith, Jr.

Table 1.

		Transudate	Modified Transudate	Nonseptic Exudate	Septic Exudate	Chyle	Hemorrhage
Color		Colorless to pale yellow	Yellow or pink	Yellow or pink	Yellow to red-brown	Milky white	Red
Turbidity		Clear	Clear to cloudy	Clear to cloudy; fibrin	Cloudy to opaque; fibrin	Opaque	Opaque
Protein (g/dl)		<1.5	2.5–5.0	3.0–8.0	3.0–7.0	2.5–6.0	>3.0
Nucleated cells/µl		<1,000	1,000–7,000 (LSA up to 100,000)	5,000–20,000 (LSA up to 100,000)	5,000–300,000	1,000–20,000	Similar to peripheral blood
Cytology		Mostly mesothelial cells	Mostly macrophages and mesothelial cells; few nondegenerate PMN; neoplastic cells in some cases	Mostly nondegenerate PMN and macrophages; neoplastic cells in some cases	Mostly degenerate PMN, also macrophages; bacteria	Small lymphocytes, PMN, and macrophages	Mostly RBC; macrophages with erythrophagocytosis
Disease associations		Hypoalbuminemia (protein-losing nephropathy, protein-losing enteropathy, or liver disease); early CHF	CHF; neoplasia; diaphragmatic hernia; pancreatitis	FIP; neoplasia; diaphragmatic hernia; lung lobe torsion	Pyothorax	Lymphangiectasia, CHF, cranial vena cava obstruction, neoplasia, fungal, dirofilariasis, diaphragmatic hernia, lung lobe torsion, trauma	Trauma, coagulopathy, neoplasia, lung lobe torsion

Characterization of Pleural Fluid

Modified from Sherding RG. Diseases of the pleural cavity, In: Sherding RG, ed. The cat: diseases and clinical management. 2nd ed. New York: Churchill Livingstone, 1994; 1061.

PNEUMOCYSTOSIS

BASICS

OVERVIEW
• *Pneumocystis carinii*—saprophyte of the mammalian respiratory tract is whose life cycle completed in the alveolar spaces; classified as an atypical fungal organism based on analysis of nucleic acids
• Infections—dogs, clinical; cats, subclinical; usually confined to the respiratory tract; a reported case of disseminated disease in a dog
• Transmission—infected to susceptible animal within a species; strain differences may account for the lack of interspecies transmission.

SIGNALMENT
• Dogs
• No clinical infections reported in cats
• Dachshunds < 6 months of age—majority of reported cases; suspected as having a congenital immunodeficiency
• Shetland sheepdogs and Cavalier King Charles spaniels—clinical disease also reported
• Animals with predilection for impaired immunity seem to carry an increased risk for overgrowth of the organism (e.g., the very young or very old).

SIGNS
• Gradual weight loss despite good appetite
• Respiratory difficulty progressing over 1–4 weeks
• Exercise intolerance—often a primary complaint
• Coughing
• Vomiting and diarrhea—occasionally noted
• Cachexia
• Slight fever
• Dyspnea
• Tachycardia
• Marked dry respiratory sounds on thoracic auscultation
• Cyanosis—with severe infection

CAUSES & RISK FACTORS
• *P. carinii*
• Humans—increased risk with immuno-deficiency (HIV); stress; immunosuppressive therapy; concurrent pulmonary infection
• Dogs—factors that affect human risk may play a role

DIAGNOSIS

DIFFERENTIAL DIAGNOSIS
• Infectious tracheobronchitis
• Bacterial and mycotic pneumonitis
• Congestive heart failure

CBC/BIOCHEMISTRY/URINALYSIS
• Changes usually nonspecific
• Leukocytosis with neutrophilia and a left shift
• Eosinophilia and monocytosis
• Erythrocytosis—secondary to chronic hypoxemia

OTHER LABORATORY TESTS
• Arterial blood gases—impaired gas exchange with hypoxemia, hypocapnia, and an increase in blood pH
• Antigens to *P. carinii*—may be detected in sputum by ELISA or fluorescent antibody tests
• Serologic tests—available for human serum; uncertain value for dogs

IMAGING

Thoracic Radiographs
• May show a mixed alveolar and interstitial pattern
• Cor pulmonale—may result in tracheal elevation, right-sided heart enlargement, and pulmonary arterial enlargement
• Solitary lesions, unilateral changes, cavitary lesions, pneumothorax, or lobar infiltrate may be seen.

DIAGNOSTIC PROCEDURES
• Pulse oximetry—low arterial oxygen saturation
• Transtracheal aspiration, gastric contents, bronchoalveolar lavage, and oropharyngeal secretions—identify organism
• Lung aspirate or lung biopsy—most reliable diagnostic procedures; carry the greatest risk for complications
• Impression smears may be made before tissue fixation.

PATHOLOGIC FINDINGS
• Lungs—firm, consolidated, and pale brown or gray; fluid not expressed from cut surfaces; do not collapse when the chest cavity is opened; small amounts of pleural fluid may be noted.
• Right heart—may find some degree of enlargement
• Alveolar spaces—may be filled with amorphous, foamy, eosinophilic material with a honeycombed appearance; macrophages; few neutrophils; septa may be thickened and fibrosed; trophozoites and cyst stages may be identified.

TREATMENT
• Inpatient—oxygen administration for hypoxemic patients; decrease exposure of immunocompromised patients to other pathogens
• Nebulization with chemotherapeutic drugs may provide some benefits.
• Cage rest or restricted exercise
• Intravenous fluids as deemed necessary

MEDICATIONS

DRUGS
• Trimethoprim-sulfonamide—15mg/kg PO q6h for 2 weeks
• Pentamidine isethionate—4mg/kg IM q24h for 2 weeks
• Carbutamide—50mg/kg IM q12h for 3 weeks
• Drug combinations—dapsone and pyrimethamine; trimethoprim and atovaquone

CONTRAINDICATIONS/POSSIBLE INTERACTIONS
Pentamidine isethionate—impaired renal function, hepatic dysfunction, hypoglycemia, hypotension, hypocalcemia, urticaria, and hematologic disorders; localized pain at the injection site

FOLLOW-UP

PATIENT MONITORING
• Serial blood gases and thoracic radiographs—provide valuable prognostic information; monitor response to therapy.
• Pentamidine isethionate—check BUN and glucose daily; discontinue or decrease dosage if azotemia or other complications are noted.
• Monitor for resolution of cough and dyspnea.
• Clinical course variable

MISCELLANEOUS

ZOONOTIC POTENTIAL
Little to none

ABBREVIATION
ELISA = enzyme-linked immunoabsorbent assay

Suggested Reading
Lobetti RG, Leisewitz AL, Spencer JA. *Pneumocystis carinii* in the miniature dachshund: case report and literature review. J Small Anim Pract 1996;37:280–285.
Author Tania N. Davey
Consulting Editor Stephen C. Barr

DISEASES

PNEUMONIA, ALLERGIC—DOGS

 BASICS

DEFINITION
The fully developed inflammatory response to antigens in lung parenchyma characterized by exudation of cells and fluid into lung interstitium, conducting airways, and alveolar spaces

PATHOPHYSIOLOGY
• Immunologic basis—supporting evidence generally accepted; mechanisms involved not yet clarified
• Evolution of disease—likely determined by characteristics of antigens, the host response, and the regulation of that response
• Three disease patterns—eosinophilic pneumonitis, allergic bronchitis, and pulmonary eosinophilic granulomatosis
• Antigens enter the lower respiratory tract primarily by the inhalation route and less commonly by the hematogenous route.
• Chronic exposure to antigens—elicits a humoral and cellular immune response
• Allergic or hypersensitivity pulmonary disorders—associated with an abnormal humoral antibody response and a cell-mediated immunoregulatory defect
• Immunoglobulin classes involved—IgE, IgG, and others
• High numbers of activated macrophages and T-lymphocytes and depressed suppressor T-cell activity—alter cell-mediated immunity
• Inflammatory infiltration—of lung interstitium and alveolar spaces
• Severely affected patients develop marked granulomatous disease.
• Occult heartworm disease with pneumonitis—microfilaria become entrapped in the pulmonary circulation.
• Allergic bronchial disease—response to infection or colonization of the airways with a fungal organism, usually *Aspergillus* spp.
• Mortality—associated with severe hypoxemia (e.g., low arterial oxygen concentration) and (rarely) severe hemoptysis

SYSTEMS AFFECTED
• Respiratory
• Cardiovascular—may see cor pulmonale

GENETICS
N/A

INCIDENCE/PREVALENCE
N/A

GEOGRAPHIC DISTRIBUTION
Widespread

SIGNALMENT
Species
Dogs
Breed Predilection
None
Mean Age and Range
All ages
Predominant Sex
None

SIGNS
General Comments
• Extremely variable, depending on the severity
Historical Findings
• Cough—unresponsive to antibacterial therapy
• Fever
• Labored breathing
• Exercise intolerance
• Anorexia
• Lethargy
• Weight loss
Physical Examination Findings
• Cough
• Fever
• Dyspnea
• Abnormal breath sounds on auscultation—increased intensity of bronchial breath sounds; crackles; wheezes
• Weight loss
• Peripheral lymphadenopathy—rare

CAUSES
• Aeroallergens—spores or hyphae from fungi and actinomycetes; pollen; insect antigens
• Parasitic antigens—heartworm microfilaria

RISK FACTORS
• Living in a heartworm endemic area without receiving preventive medication
• Dusty or moldy environment

 DIAGNOSIS

DIFFERENTIAL DIAGNOSIS
• Parasitic pneumonia—capillariasis; paragonimiasis; dirofilariasis
• Fungal pneumonia—histoplasmosis; blastomycosis; coccidioidomycosis cryptococcosis
• For eosinophilic pneumonitis—bacterial pneumonia; viral pneumonia (e.g., canine distemper virus and canine adenovirus); rickettsial pneumonia (e.g., ehrlichiosis and Rocky Mountain spotted fever); protozoal pneumonia (e.g., toxoplasmosis); congestive heart failure
• For allergic bronchitis—infectious tracheobronchitis; chronic bronchitis
• For pulmonary eosinophilic granulomatosis—neoplasia (including lymphomatoid granulomatosis); pulmonary abscess; bronchial foreign body

CBC/BIOCHEMISTRY/URINALYSIS
• Inflammatory leukogram—neutrophilic leukocytosis with or without a left shift, eosinophilia, basophilia, or monocytosis
• Hyperglobulinemia—suggests occult dirofilariasis

OTHER LABORATORY TESTS
Arterial Blood Gas Analysis
• Values correlate well with the degree of physiologic disruption; sensitive monitor of patient's progress during treatment
• Hypoxemia—mild or moderate, $PaO_2 < 80$ torr on room air; severe $PaO_2 < 60$ torr on room air

Other
• Heartworm microfilaria and antigen tests—positive results suggest pulmonary hypertension associated with dirofilariasis or eosinophilic pneumonitis associated with microfilaria trapped in the lung.
• Protein electrophoresis—β-globulin spike (hyperbetaglobulinemia) often found with occult dirofilariasis

IMAGING
• Radiographic findings depend on extent and severity of disease.
• Thoracic radiographs—help document the severity of pulmonary artery disease; reveal interstitial pneumonitis in dogs with dirofilariasis
• Eosinophilic pneumonitis—linear or miliary interstitial pattern that resemble changes seen with early pulmonary edema or fungal pneumonia; alveolar pattern characterized by increased pulmonary densities with indistinct margins in severely affected patients; tortuous, large pulmonary arteries and right-sided cardiomegaly in patients with dirofilariasis
• Allergic or eosinophilic bronchitis—bronchial pattern with bronchi extending into the periphery of the lung (tram/railroad track and donut signs)
• Eosinophilic granuloma—multiple nodular lesions of variable sizes in different lung lobes; patchy, focal alveolar densities; tracheobronchial lymphadenopathy

DIAGNOSTIC PROCEDURES
• Cytologic examination of aspirates, washings, or brushings—definitive diagnosis; eosinophilic inflammation predominates; may note other types of inflammatory cells; carefully examine specimens for antigenic sources (e.g., parasites, fungi, or neoplasia).

- Transtracheal washing
- Bronchoscopy
- Bronchoalveolar lavage—with or without bronchoscope
- Fine-needle lung aspiration and examination
- Intradermal skin testing—may identify allergens
- Fecal examinations—routine flotation, direct smear, sediment examination, and Baermann technique; when negative, respiratory parasitic infection less likely

PATHOLOGIC FINDINGS
- Gross—diffuse, patchy, or nodular firm lesions; usually pale or mottled
- Histopathologic—eosinophilic, lymphocytic, and macrophagic infiltration of alveolar walls and alveolar spaces; as the disease progresses, interstitial infiltrative process becomes fibrotic with obliteration of alveolar spaces and granulomas may be dispersed within the interstitial fibrosis.

 TREATMENT

APPROPRIATE HEALTH CARE
Inpatient—recommended with multisystemic signs (e.g., anorexia, weight loss, or lethargy)

NURSING CARE
- Dehydration—hinders mucociliary clearance and secretion mobilization; maintain normal systemic hydration with a balanced multielectrolyte solution.
- Supplemental oxygen—for respiratory distress

ACTIVITY
Restricted during treatment (inpatient or outpatient)

DIET
Ensure normal intake.

CLIENT EDUCATION
Warn client that morbidity and mortality are associated with severe hypoxemia.

SURGICAL CONSIDERATIONS
May remove lung lobes with large granulomas

 MEDICATIONS

DRUGS OF CHOICE
- Corticosteroids—prednisolone or prednisone at 2–4 mg/kg/day until clinical signs begin to resolve; then taper

- Heartworm adulticidal therapy—for heartworm-positive patient; initiate after the patient has been stabilized with corticosteroids and rest.
- Itraconazole or ketoconazole—may be used with confirmed allergic bronchopulmonary fungal infection, which is a rare condition; use antifungal drugs only if the fungal infection is confirmed by cytologic examination or culture.

CONTRAINDICATIONS
N/A

PRECAUTIONS
N/A

POSSIBLE INTERACTIONS
N/A

ALTERNATIVE DRUGS
- Other immunosuppressive drugs (e.g., cyclophosphamide, azathioprine, and mercaptopurine)—may use when corticosteroids are contraindicated or have been ineffective
- Bronchodilators—may be helpful, particularly if wheezes are ausculted or labored respiratory effort is observed; see Asthma, Bronchitis—Cats and/or Bronchitis, Chronic (COPD)

 FOLLOW-UP

PATIENT MONITORING
- Arterial blood gases—most sensitive monitor of progress
- Auscult patient thoroughly several times daily.
- Thoracic radiographs—improve more slowly than the clinical appearance

PREVENTION/AVOIDANCE
- Routine heartworm-prevention medication
- Change patient's environment if an aeroallergen is suspected.

POSSIBLE COMPLICATIONS
Pulmonary thromboembolism—patients treated with adulticide for dirofilariasis

EXPECTED COURSE AND PROGNOSIS
- If primary allergen is identified and eliminated—prognosis good
- If allergen is not identified—prognosis for control good; many patients require long-term treatment with steroids.
- Heartworm infection—prognosis depends on severity of pulmonary hypertension, cor pulmonale, and thromboembolism
- Eosinophilic granulomatosis—prognosis guarded; often progressive

 MISCELLANEOUS

ASSOCIATED CONDITIONS
- Dirofilariasis
- Bronchopulmonary fungal infection

AGE-RELATED FACTORS
N/A

ZOONOTIC POTENTIAL
N/A

PREGNANCY
Corticosteroids and other immunosuppressive drugs are contraindicated in pregnant animals.

SYNONYMS
- Allergic bronchitis
- Chronic eosinophilic bronchitis
- Bronchitic pulmonary eosinophilia
- Allergic bronchopulmonary aspergillosis
- Allergic alveolitis
- Eosinophilic pneumonitis
- Eosinophilic pneumonia
- Hypersensitivity pneumonitis
- Eosinophilic pulmonary granulomatosis
- Extrinsic allergic alveolitis
- Occult heartworm pneumonia
- Parasitic pulmonary eosinophilia
- Pulmonary infiltrates with eosinophilia (PIE)

SEE ALSO
- Cough
- Dyspnea, Tachypnea, and Panting
- Heartworm Disease
- Lymphomatoid Granulomatosis
- Respiratory Parasites

Suggested Reading

Bauer T. Pulmonary hypersensitivity disorders. In: Kirk RW, ed. Current veterinary therapy X. Philadelphia: Saunders, 1989:369–376.

Calvert CA, Rawlings CA. Pulmonary manifestations of heartworm disease. Vet Clin North Am Small Anim Pract 1985;15:991–1009.

Clavert CA. Eosinophilic pulmonary granulomatosis. In: Kirk RW, Bonagura JD, eds. Current veterinary therapy XI. Philadelphia: Saunders, 1992:813–816.

Hawkins EC. Tracheal wash and bronchoalveolar lavage in the management of respiratory disease. In: Kirk RW, Bonagura JD, eds. Current veterinary therapy XI. Philadelphia: Saunders, 1992:795–800.

Kuehn NF, Roudebush P. Allergic lung disease. In: Allen DG, ed. Small animal medicine. Philadelphia: Lippincott, 1991: 423–432.

Author Philip Roudebush
Consulting Editor Eleanor C. Hawkins

PNEUMONIA, ASPIRATION

 BASICS

OVERVIEW
• Inflammation of the lungs caused by inhaled material (e.g., oral ingesta, regurgitated material, and vomitus) and subsequent pulmonary dysfunction; develops when laryngeal reflexes function improperly or are overwhelmed; thus a consequence of an underlying problem
• Pulmonary dysfunction—caused by a combination of factors; (1) obstruction–large particles obstruct large airways, causing acute respiratory distress (extremely rare); particulates cause direct obstruction of small airways and indirect obstruction from bronchospasm and the production of mucus and exudate; (2) Aspiration of gastric acid—results in marked damage to the respiratory epithelium; may cause bronchospasm and occasionally ARDS; (3) Bacterial pneumonia—common component in regurgitated material, food, or pharyngeal flora; may initiate an immediate infection or a secondary infection occurring later in the course of disease

SIGNALMENT
Dogs more commonly affected than cats

SIGNS
• May be peracute, acute, or chronic
• Cough
• Respiratory distress
• Tachypnea
• Fever
• Cyanosis
• Exercise intolerance
• Nasal discharge
• Depend on underlying cause
• Regurgitation
• Vomiting
• Dysphagia
• Altered consciousness—depression, post-ictus, dementia, sedation, and anesthesia
• Stertor

CAUSES & RISK FACTORS
• Pharyngeal abnormalities—local paralysis (e.g., idiopathic, focal myasthenia gravis, and traumatic nerve damage); generalized neuromuscular disease; cricopharyngeal motor dysfunction; anatomic malformations; post operative laryngoplasty
• Esophageal abnormalities
• Megaesophagus*
• Reflux esophagitis
• Esophageal obstruction—mass, foreign body, stricture
• Bronchoesophageal fistula
• Altered consciousness
• Sedation
• Anesthesia—during or recovery from
• Postictus
• Forebrain disease
• Severe metabolic disturbance
• Iatrogenic cause
• Force feeding
• Tube feeding—improper technique; misplacement of tube
• Mineral oil administration

 DIAGNOSIS

DIFFERENTIAL DIAGNOSIS
• Bacterial pneumonia—component of cases; may develop for reasons other than the overt aspiration of foreign material
• Lung lobe abscess—consolidated appearance radiographically; may be a sequela to aspiration pneumonia, bacterial pneumonia, or foreign body

CBC/BIOCHEMISTRY/URINALYSIS
• Neutrophilic leukocytosis with a left shift
• WBC count—may be normal
• Nonregenerative anemia associated with inflammatory disease

OTHER LABORATORY TESTS
• Arterial blood gas analysis—hypoxemia expected; $PaCO_2$ generally low but may be high with large airway obstruction or systemic neuromuscular disease
• Other tests—pursue underlying cause; antiacetylcholine antibodies for suspected myasthenia gravis; ANA, thyroid function, or adrenal function for suspected polyneuropathy

IMAGING
• Thoracic radiography—bronchoalveolar pattern most severe in the gravity-dependent lung lobes (e.g., right middle and cranial and left middle); may take up to 24 hr for pattern to develop after acute aspiration; scrutinize for evidence of esophageal or mediastinal disease.
• Contrast swallowing study—ideally with fluoroscopy; provides evidence of swallowing or esophageal dysfunction that may predispose the patient to aspiration

DIAGNOSTIC PROCEDURES
• Tracheal wash—collect material for bacterial culture and sensitivity testing; collect before administering antibiotics; infection often caused by multiple organisms with unpredictable susceptibility
• Bronchoscopy—suspected large airway obstruction based on breathing pattern, auscultation, or radiographic findings
• Appropriate tests to investigate underlying causes

PNEUMONIA, ASPIRATION

TREATMENT

- Oxygen—respiratory distress; if distress persists, provide ventilatory support.
- Intravenous fluids—indicated for shock or dehydration or if oral intake is withheld
- Oral intake—withhold until primary problem identified and managed, particularly in acutely affected, unstable patients
- Cage rest—for respiratory distress
- Do not allow patient to remain laterally recumbent on one side for more than 2 hr.
- Once stable, mild exercise may assist in productive cough and airway clearance.
- Nebulization and coupage—recommended for consolidation or if resolution is proceeding slowly
- Airway suction—indicated only if aspiration is observed (e.g., during recovery from anesthesia)
- Lavage—contraindicated; forces material deeper into lungs; any gastric acid neutralized in seconds

MEDICATIONS

DRUGS

- Antibiotic therapy—as for bacterial pneumonia; ideally, withhold until an airway specimen is collected; continue for 10 days after resolution of clinical and radiographic signs
- Bronchodilators (e.g., theophylline and terbutaline)—may improve breathing with acute aspiration, with ausculted wheezing, and in cats; continue if beneficial
- Short-acting corticosteroids—may be administered once to combat inflammation with peracute life-threatening aspiration

CONTRAINDICATIONS/POSSIBLE INTERACTIONS

- Diuretics—contraindicated
- Corticosteroids—generally contraindicated; predispose patient to infection
- Fluoroquinolone antibiotics and chloramphenicol—may prolong clearance of theophylline-derivative bronchodilators, resulting in signs of toxicity

FOLLOW-UP

PATIENT MONITORING

- Radiographs, blood gas analysis, and clinical signs—monitor response to treatment.
- Radiographs—evaluate every 3–7 days initially to determine appropriateness of treatment; then every 1–2 weeks
- Signs do not resolve or suddenly worsen—possible recurrence of aspiration or a secondary infection; repeat diagnostic evaluation, including examination of tracheal wash.

PREVENTION/AVOIDANCE

The underlying cause must be identified and managed.

POSSIBLE COMPLICATIONS

- Secondary infection common
- ARDS—may develop, particularly after aspiration of gastric acid
- Abscessation or foreign body granuloma rare

EXPECTED COURSE AND PROGNOSIS

- Prognosis—depends on severity of signs when patient is examined and the ability to correct the underlying problem
- Acute, severe aspiration—can be fatal
- Recurrence—likely if underlying cause is not or cannot be addressed

MISCELLANEOUS

SEE ALSO

- Acute Respiratory Distress Syndrome (ARDS)
- Megaesophagus
- Pneumonia, Bacterial

ABBREVIATIONS

- ANA = antinuclear antibody
- ARDS = acute respiratory distress syndrome

Suggested Reading

Hawkins EC. Aspiration pneumonia. In: Bonagura JD, Kirk RW, eds. Current veterinary therapy XII. Philadelphia: Saunders, 1995:915–919.

Author Eleanor C. Hawkins
Consulting Editor Eleanor C. Hawkins

DISEASES

PNEUMONIA, BACTERIAL

 BASICS

DEFINITION
The fully developed inflammatory response to virulent bacteria in lung parenchyma characterized by exudation of cells and fluid into conduction airways and alveolar spaces

PATHOPHYSIOLOGY
• Bacteria—enter the lower respiratory tract primarily by the inhalation or aspiration routes; enter less commonly by the hematogenous route; infections incite an overt inflammatory reaction. • Tracheobronchial tree and lungs—normally not continuously sterile • Oropharyngeal bacteria—frequently aspirated; may be present for an unknown interval in the normal tracheobronchial tree and lung; have the potential to cause or complicate respiratory infection; cloud interpretation of airway and lung cultures • Respiratory infection—development depends on the complex interplay of many factors: size, inoculation site, number of organisms and their virulence, and resistance of the host • Viral infections—alter bacterial colonization patterns; increase bacterial adherence to respiratory epithelium; reduce mucociliary clearance and phagocytosis; thus may allow resident bacteria to invade the lower respiratory tract • Exudative phase—inflammatory hyperemia; serous exudation of high protein fluid into interstitial and alveolar spaces • Leukocytic emigration phase—leukocytes infiltrate the airways and alveoli; consolidation, ischemia, tissue necrosis, and atelectasis owing to bronchial occlusion, obstructive bronchiolitis, and impaired collateral ventilation • Mortality—associated with severe hypoxemia (low arterial oxygen concentration) and sepsis

SYSTEMS AFFECTED
Respiratory—primary or secondary infection

GENETICS N/A

INCIDENCE/PREVALENCE N/A

GEOGRAPHIC DISTRIBUTION
Widespread

SIGNALMENT
Species
More common in dogs than cats
Breed Predilection
Dogs—sporting breeds, hounds, working breeds, and mixed breeds > 12 kg
Mean Age and Range
Dogs—range 1 month to 15 years; many < 1 year old
Predominant Sex
Dogs—60% males

SIGNS
Historical Findings
• Cough • Fever • Labored breathing • Exercise intolerance • Anorexia and weight loss • Lethargy • Nasal discharge
Physical Examination Findings
• Cough • Fever • Dyspnea • Abnormal breath sounds on auscultation—increased intensity or bronchial breath sounds, crackles, and wheezes • Weight loss • Serous or mucopurulent nasal discharge • Lethargy • Dehydration

CAUSES
Dogs
• *Bordetella bronchiseptica* and *Streptococcus zooepidemicus*—primary bacterial pathogens • Isolates—most thought to be opportunistic invaders; usually one or two bacterial pathogens; but may see three or more; gram-negative species and *Mycoplasma* spp. predominate in single and mixed infections. • *B. bronchiseptica, Escherichia coli, Klebsiella pneumoniae, Pasteurella multocida, Staphylococcus* spp., *Streptococcus* spp., *Mycoplasma* spp., and *Pseudomonas aeruginosa*—most common isolates • Anaerobic bacteria—found in pulmonary abscesses and aspiration pneumonia
Cats
• Bacterial pathogens—poorly documented; *B. bronchiseptica* and *Pasteurella* spp. most frequently reported • Carrier state—may exist; periods of shedding *B. bronchiseptica* after stress; infected queens may not shed organism prepartum but begin shedding postpartum, serving as a source of infection for kittens.

RISK FACTORS
• Pre-existing viral, mycoplasmal, parasitic, or fungal respiratory infection • Regurgitation, dysphagia, or vomiting • Reduced level of consciousness—stupor, coma, and anesthesia • Thoracic trauma or surgery • Bronchial foreign body • Bronchiectasis • Administration of certain drugs—aspirin and digoxin • Immunosuppressive therapy—chemotherapy and glucocorticoids • Severe metabolic disorders—uremia, diabetes mellitus, hyperadrenocorticism, and hypoadrenocorticism • Functional or anatomic defects—tracheal hypoplasia, cleft palate, primary ciliary dyskinesia, megaesophagus, laryngeal paralysis, and collapsed trachea • Urinary tract infection • Intravenous catheter placement • Protein–calorie malnutrition • Immunodeficiency • Phagocyte dysfunction—FeLV and diabetes mellitus • Complement deficiency—rare • Selective IgA deficiency • Combined T cell and B cell dysfunction—rare

 DIAGNOSIS

DIFFERENTIAL DIAGNOSIS
• Viral pneumonia—canine distemper virus and canine adenovirus • Rickettsial pneumonia—ehrlichiosis and Rocky Mountain spotted fever • Protozoal pneumonia—toxoplasmosis • Parasitic pneumonia—capillariasis, paragonimiasis, and dirofilariasis • Fungal pneumonia—histoplasmosis, blastomycosis, coccidioidomycosis, and cryptococcosis • Bacterial or fungal rhinitis • Chronic sinusitis • Pharyngitis • Tonsillitis • Infectious tracheobronchitis • Pulmonary abscess • Pleural infection—pyothorax • Bronchial foreign body

CBC/BIOCHEMISTRY/URINALYSIS
Inflammatory leukogram—neutrophilic leukocytosis with or without a left shift; absence does not rule out the diagnosis.

OTHER LABORATORY TESTS
• Arterial blood gas analysis—values correlate well with the degree of physiologic disruption; sensitive monitor of progress during treatment; PaO_2 < 80 torr on room air, mild or moderate hypoxemia; PaO_2 < 60 torr on room air, severe hypoxemia • Blood culture—may help identify causal agent

IMAGING
Thoracic radiography
Alveolar pattern characterized by increased pulmonary densities (margins indistinct; air bronchograms or lobar consolidation); patchy or lobar alveolar pattern with a cranial ventral lung lobe distribution

DIAGNOSTIC PROCEDURES
• Microbiologic and cytologic examinations—aspirates, washings, or brushings; definitive diagnosis • Samples—transtracheal washing, bronchoscopy, bronchoalveolar lavage (with or without bronchoscope), or fine-needle lung aspiration • Septic inflammation with degenerate neutrophils predominates • Recent antibiotic administration—nonseptic inflammation likely • Bacteria—visible microscopically in < 50% of affected dogs; always culture specimens, even if no bacteria are seen on cytologic examination.

PATHOLOGIC FINDINGS
Gross
• Irregular consolidation in cranioventral regions • Consolidated lung—varies from dark red to gray-pink to more gray, depending on age of patient and nature of the process

• Palpable firmness of the tissue—single most important gross criterion

Histopathologic
• Nidus of inflammation—bronchiolar–alveolar junction
• Early—bronchioles and adjacent alveoli filled with neutrophils and an admixture of cell debris, fibrin, and macrophages; necrotic to hyperplastic epithelium
• Later—neutrophilic, fibrinous, hemorrhagic, or necrotizing inflammation, depending on virulence of bacteria and host response

TREATMENT

APPROPRIATE HEALTH CARE
Inpatient—recommended with multisystemic signs (e.g., anorexia, high fever, weight loss, and lethargy)

NURSING CARE
• Maintain normal systemic hydration—important to aid mucociliary clearance and secretion mobilization; use a balanced multielectrolyte solution.
• Nebulization with bland aerosols—results in more rapid resolution if used in conjunction with physiotherapy and antibacterials
• Physiotherapy—mild forced exercise, chest wall coupage, tracheal manipulation to stimulate mild cough, and postural drainage; may enhance clearance of secretions; always do immediately after nebulization; avoid allowing the patient to lie in one position for a prolonged time.
• Oxygen therapy—for respiratory distress

ACTIVITY
Restrict during treatment (inpatient or outpatient), except as part of physiotherapy after aerosolization.

DIET
• Ensure normal intake with food high in protein and energy density
• Enteral or parenteral nutritional support—indicated in severely ill patients

CLIENT EDUCATION
Warn client that morbidity and mortality are associated with severe hypoxemia and sepsis.

SURGICAL CONSIDERATIONS
Surgery (lung lobectomy)—may be indicated with pulmonary abscessation or bronchopulmonary foreign body with secondary pneumonia; may be indicated if unresponsive to conventional treatment and disease is limited to one or two lobes

MEDICATIONS

DRUGS OF CHOICE

Antimicrobials
• Gram-positive cocci—ampicillin;, ampicillin-sulbactam; amoxicillin; amoxicillin-clavulanic acid; chloramphenicol; erythromycin; gentamicin; trimethoprim-sulfonamide; first-generation cephalosporins
• Gram-negative rods—amikacin; chloramphenicol; gentamicin; trimethoprim-sulfonamide; fluoroquinolones; carboxypenicillins
• Bordetella—tetracyclines; amikacin; chloramphenicol; gentamicin; enrofloxacin; kanamycin
• Anaerobes—amoxicillin-clavulanic acid; chloramphenicol; metronidazole; clindamycin
• Continue treatment for at least 10 days beyond clinical resolution; usually a total of 3 weeks or longer

CONTRAINDICATIONS
Anticholinergics and antihistamines—may thicken secretions and inhibit mucokinesis and exudate removal from airways

PRECAUTIONS
Antitussives—use with caution and only for short intervals to control intractable cough; potent, centrally acting agents may inhibit mucokinesis and exudate removal from airways.

POSSIBLE INTERACTIONS N/A

ALTERNATIVE DRUGS
Expectorants—recommended by some clinicians; no objective evidence that they increase mucokinesis or mobilization of secretions

FOLLOW-UP

PATIENT MONITORING
• Arterial blood gases—most sensitive monitor of progress • Auscultate patient thoroughly several times daily. • Thoracic radiographs—improve more slowly than the clinical appearance

PREVENTION/AVOIDANCE
• Vaccination—against upper respiratory viruses; against B. bronchiseptica if a dog is boarded or exposed to large numbers of other animals • Catteries—environmental strategies to lower population density and improve hygiene help control outbreaks of bordetellosis.

POSSIBLE COMPLICATIONS
Young dogs infected with B. bronchiseptica may develop chronic bronchitis.

EXPECTED COURSE AND PROGNOSIS

• Prognosis—good with aggressive anti-bacterial and supportive therapy; more guarded in young animals, patients with immunodeficiency, and patients that are debilitated or have severe underlying disease
• Prolonged infection—potential for chronic bronchitis or bronchiectasis in any patient

MISCELLANEOUS

ASSOCIATED CONDITIONS
• Frequently develops secondary to underlying metabolic diseases—hyperadrenocorticism; diabetes mellitus; uremia • Frequently develops secondary to underlying functional or anatomic abnormalities—cleft palate; tracheal hypoplasia; primary ciliary dyskinesia; collapsed trachea; laryngeal paralysis; megaesophagus • Bronchiectasis—both predisposing factor and potential complication

AGE-RELATED FACTORS
• Young puppies and kittens—may have a poorer prognosis; puppies often develop long-term complications (e.g., chronic bronchitis).
• Underlying functional and anatomic problems and immunodeficiencies—suspect in young patients

ZOONOTIC POTENTIAL N/A

PREGNANCY
Bitches or queens infected with B. bronchiseptica—may transmit infection to neonates

SEE ALSO
• Pneumonia, Aspiration • Bordetellosis—Cats • Tracheobronchitis, Infectious—Dogs

ABBREVIATION
FeLV = feline leukemia virus

Suggested Reading
Hawkins EC. Tracheal wash and bronchoalveolar lavage in the management of respiratory disease. In: Kirk RW, Bonagura JD, eds. Current veterinary therapy XI. Philadelphia: Saunders, 1992:795–800.
Jameson PH, King LA, Lappin MR, et al. Comparison of clinical signs, diagnostic findings, organisms isolated, and clinical outcome in dogs with bacterial pneumonia: 93 cases (1986–1991). J Am Vet Med Assoc 1995;206:206–209.
Roudebush P. Infectious pneumonia. In: Kirk RW, Bonagura JD, eds. Current veterinary therapy XI. Philadelphia: Saunders, 1992:228–236.
Author Philip Roudebush
Consulting Editor Eleanor C. Hawkins

DISEASES

PNEUMONIA, FUNGAL

 BASICS

DEFINITION
Inflammation of the pulmonary interstitial, lymphatic, and peribronchial tissues caused by deep mycotic infection

PATHOPHYSIOLOGY
• Mycelial fungal elements—inhaled from contaminated soil; organisms then colonize the lungs • Dimorphic fungi—grow in the yeast phase at body temperature • Systemic dissemination of yeast common in dogs and cats • Clinical signs determined by organ systems affected • Pulmonary interstitial involvement—may cause hypoxia • Airway involvement—may cause cough • Cell-mediated immunity—important response to fungal infection; leads to pyogranulomatous inflammation

SYSTEMS AFFECTED
• Depend on the specific fungal disease (see also chapters dealing with specific fungi) • Blastomycosis—about 85% of dogs and cats have respiratory involvement; diffuse interstitial or bronchial pneumonia most common; solitary mass lesions seen; tracheobronchial lymphadenopathy may contribute to cough; nasal infection occasionally detected • Histoplasmosis—diffuse interstitial pneumonia common, especially in cats; tachypnea or dyspnea seen in only 50% of cats and < 50% of dogs; perihilar or mediastinal lymphadenopathy often contributes to cough. • Coccidioidomycosis—diffuse interstitial or bronchial pneumonia common in dogs but less common in cats; perihilar or mediastinal lymphadenopathy common • Cryptococcosis—nasal involvement most common in cats; lungs usually subclinically affected by small multifocal granulomas in dogs • Systemic aspergillosis—pneumonia noted only in systemically affected patients and usually involves *Aspergilli terreus; A. fumigatus* more common with rhinitis

GENETICS
Breed susceptibilities may be related to defects in cell-mediated immunity.

INCIDENCE/PREVALENCE
Depends on geographic distribution

GEOGRAPHIC DISTRIBUTION
• Blastomycosis—endemic in U.S. Southeast and Midwest along the Mississippi, Ohio, Missouri, and Tennessee rivers and southern Great Lakes; also in southern Midatlantic states • Histoplasmosis—similar to but more widely distributed than *Blastomycosis;* pockets of disease in Texas, Oklahoma, and California

• Coccidioidomycosis—U.S. Southwest from Texas to California • Cryptococcosis and aspergillosis—sporadically throughout the U.S.

SIGNALMENT

Species
Dogs and less commonly in cats

Breed Predilection
• Systemic mycosis—large-breed dogs kept outdoors or used for hunting or field trials; Doberman pinschers and rottweilers may be predisposed to more severe disseminated disease. • Cryptococcosis—cocker spaniels may be overrepresented. • Systemic aspergillosis—German shepherds may be overrepresented.

Mean Age And Range
• Young animals (< 4 years) predisposed • Any age may be affected.

Predominant Sex
Males affected 2–4 times more often than females

SIGNS

General Comments
• Depend primarily on the organ systems involved • Multisystemic illness apparent

Historical Findings
• Chronic weight loss and inappetence • Fever • Oculonasal discharge • Coughing—may be prominent; seen inconsistently even with marked pulmonary disease • Dyspnea or exercise intolerance common • Labored breathing—more common in cats; sign of severe disease in both dogs and cats • Acute blindness or blepharospasm—if eyes are affected • Cutaneous nodules—uncommon until draining tracts appear • Lameness—common if the feet are affected or if osteomyelitis develops

Physical Examination Findings
• Depression and emaciation—may note in chronically affected patients • Fever—about 50% of patients • Harsh, loud breath sound—common on auscultation • Crackles—may be prominent, especially in cats • Cough—may be induced on tracheal palpation • Dyspnea—at rest with severe disease • Blastomycosis—multiple cutaneous and subcutaneous nodules with draining tracts; uveitis; granulomatous retinal detachment common • Coccidioidomycosis (dogs)—severe pain caused by osteomyelitis common • Histoplasmosis (dogs)—emaciation and diarrhea (often bloody) prominent

CAUSES
• *Blastomyces dermatitidis*—lungs primary route of infection
• *Histoplasma capsulatum*—lungs and possibly gastrointestinal tract primary routes of infection

• *Coccidioides immitis*—lungs primary route of infection
• *Cryptococcus neoformans*—nasal cavity primary route of infection with direct extension into the eyes or CNS
• *Aspergillus* spp.—nasal cavity and lungs primary routes of infection

RISK FACTORS
• Blastomycosis, histoplasmosis, and cryptococcosis—environmental exposure to soils rich in organic matter; exposure to bird droppings or other fecal matter may predispose patient to blastomycosis and cryptococcosis
• Coccidioidomycosis—environmental exposure to sandy, alkaline soil after periods of rainfall; outdoor activities (hunting and field trials); immunosuppression (especially poor cell-mediated immunity) may contribute to systemic spread of fungal infection; test cats for FeLV and FIV.
• Prednisone—may markedly worsen the disease
• Antineoplastic chemotherapy
• Lymphoreticular neoplasia

 DIAGNOSIS

DIFFERENTIAL DIAGNOSIS
• Parasitic pneumonia
• Bacterial pneumonia
• Chronic bronchial disease
• Metastatic neoplasia
• Lymphoreticular and histiocytic neoplasia
• Eosinophilic lung disease
• Lymphomatoid granulomatosis
• Idiopathic pyogranulomatous disease
• FIP or other vasculitic disease
• Pulmonary edema

CBC/BIOCHEMISTRY/URINALYSIS
• Depend on the systems affected
• Moderate leukocytosis with or without a left shift
• Lymphopenia common
• Leukopenia—may note with histoplasmosis
• Thrombocytopenia and nonregenerative anemia common
• Hyperglobulinemia and hypoalbuminemia common
• Hypercalcemia—occasionally
• Liver enzymes—more likely to be high with histoplasmosis
• Urinalysis usually normal
• Proteinuria—may detect
• Organisms—may see in urine (rarely) if the kidneys or lower urinary tract is affected

OTHER LABORATORY TESTS
• Serologic testing—yields both false-positive and false-negative results; high incidence of seropositivity may represent previous or subclinical infection in endemic areas.

• Latex agglutination test—for capsular antigen; highly reliable for cryptococcosis
• Cytologic or histologic identification of the organism—definitive diagnosis
• Culture—not usually necessary; may be difficult

IMAGING
• Thoracic radiography—diffuse nodular interstitial and peribronchial infiltrates; nodular densities may coalesce to granulomatous masses with indistinct edges; tracheobronchial lymphadenopathy common; large focal granulomas more likely in cats than in dogs
• Appendicular or axial skeleton radiography—osteolysis with periosteal proliferation; soft tissue swelling
• Abdominal ultrasonography—may reveal granulomas or large lymph nodes
• Ocular ultrasonography—may reveal a retrobulbar mass

DIAGNOSTIC PROCEDURES
• Impression smear or aspirate of a skin nodule—most likely to yield organisms
• Fine-needle aspirate of the lung—more likely to be diagnostic than transtracheal aspirate or bronchoalveolar lavage specimen
• Lymph node aspirate or biopsy
• CSF tap—with cryptococcosis
• Examination of bone marrow or splenic aspirate—with histoplasmosis
• Biopsy—may be needed

PATHOLOGIC FINDINGS
• Pyogranulomatous inflammation
• Organisms—usually seen with blastomycosis, histoplasmosis, and cryptococcosis; sometimes difficult to find coccidioidomycosis

TREATMENT

APPROPRIATE HEALTH CARE
• Outpatient—if patient is still eating
• Inpatient evaluation and treatment—dehydration, anorexia, and severe hypoxia

NURSING CARE
Administration of fluids, potassium, oxygen, and antibiotics as needed

ACTIVITY
Restricted

DIET
• Feed high-protein, calorically dense food.
• Histoplasmosis accompanied by marked gastrointestinal involvement—highly digestible food

CLIENT EDUCATION
• Inform client that < 70% of dogs and a smaller percentage of cats are likely to respond to treatment.
• Warn client that treatment is expensive and

will probably be necessary for at least 2 months
• Advise client to clean areas in the environment with high organic matter or feces

SURGICAL CONSIDERATIONS
None

MEDICATIONS

DRUGS OF CHOICE
• Itraconazole—5–10 mg/kg PO daily; most often used first; must be given with food
• Amphotericin B—0.5 mg/kg (dogs) or 0.25 mg/kg (cats) IV 3 times a week to a total dose of 8 mg/kg if used alone or 4 mg/kg if used with an azole drug (e.g., itraconazole); administer in 200–500 mL of D_5W; best used with itraconazole or ketoconazole for severely affected patients
• Amphotericin B—alternative; 0.5–0.8 mg/kg 2–3 times per week; to reduce nephrotoxicity, may give subcutaneously diluted in 0.45% saline/2.5% dextrose solution (400 mL for cats, 500 mL for dogs < 20 kg, 1000 mL for dogs > 20 kg)
• Fluconazole—10 mg/kg PO q12h; drug of choice for cryptococcosis and patients with CNS or urinary tract involvement

CONTRAINDICATIONS
Corticosteroids

PRECAUTIONS
• Azole drugs—do not use with severe liver disease.
• Amphotericin B—do not use in azotemic or dehydrated patients; stop use if BUN > 50 mg/dL or creatinine > 3.0 mg/dL.
• Itraconazole and the other azole drugs—anorexia; increase in liver enzymes; cutaneous vasculitis

POSSIBLE INTERACTIONS
• Antacids and anticonvulsants—may lower the blood concentration of itraconazole

ALTERNATIVE DRUGS
• Ketoconazole—10–30 mg/kg; may be effective; longer treatment is necessary; relapse common
• Lipid-complexed amphotericin B—1–2 mg/kg IV q48h for 12 treatments; nephrotoxicity low; diuresis not required

FOLLOW-UP

PATIENT MONITORING
• Liver enzymes—evaluated monthly while patient is on itraconazole, fluconazole, or ketoconazole. • BUN and creatinine—measure before each dose of amphotericin B. • Thoracic radiographs—re-evaluate before discontinuing treatment.

PREVENTION/AVOIDANCE
Monitor for signs of recurrence

POSSIBLE COMPLICATIONS
• Blindness is usually permanent. • Renal failure from amphotericin B

EXPECTED COURSE AND PROGNOSIS
• Blastomycosis—requires a minimum of 2 months of treatment; 60%–70% of dogs are cured by itraconazole; those not cured usually relapse. • Others—continued until 1 month past remission • Systemic aspergillosis—prognosis not as good as for other causes • Relapse—may occur up to 1 year after treatment

MISCELLANEOUS

ASSOCIATED CONDITIONS
None

AGE-RELATED FACTORS
Young animals predisposed

ZOONOTIC POTENTIAL
• Infections in people—primarily from a common environmental source; no direct transmission from animals to humans, except by penetrating wounds contaminated by the organism

PREGNANCY
• Fungal abortion possible • Azole antifungals—teratogenic; do not use in pregnant animals.

SEE ALSO
• Aspergillosis • Blastomycosis • Coccidioidomycosis • Cryptococcosis • Histoplasmosis

ABBREVIATIONS
• CSF = cerebrospinal fluid • FeLV = feline leukemia virus • FIP = feline infectious peritonitis • FIV = feline immunodeficiency virus

Suggested Reading

Greene CE, ed. Infectious diseases of the dog and cat. 2nd ed. Philadelphia: Saunders, 1998.

Taboada J. Systemic mycoses. In: Morgan RV, ed. Handbook of small animal practice. 3rd ed. Philadelphia: Saunders, 1997: 1113–1126.

Wolf AM. Antifungal agents. In: August JR, ed. Consultations in feline internal medicine 2. Philadelphia: Saunders, 1994.

Wolf AM, Troy GC. Deep mycotic diseases. In: Ettinger SJ, Feldman EC, eds. Textbook of veterinary internal medicine. 4th ed. Philadelphia: Saunders, 1995:439–463.

Author Joseph Taboada
Consulting Editor Eleanor C. Hawkins

DISEASES

PNEUMOTHORAX

BASICS

DEFINITION
• Accumulation of air or gas within the pleural space that can be classified as spontaneous (nontraumatic) or traumatic • Spontaneous—further subdivided into primary (idiopathic) and secondary (resulting from underlying pulmonary disease) • Tension—may have spontaneous or traumatic cause; results in a life-threatening increase in intrathoracic pressure

PATHOPHYSIOLOGY
• Normally, the intrapleural space is a potential space, and intrapleural pressure is subatmospheric; a small amount of fluid within the normal pleural space forms a cohesive bond between the lungs and the thoracic wall.
• Intrapleural space filled with air—cohesive bond lost; the normal elastic recoil of the lungs causes collapse from the thoracic wall as the thorax expands. • Respiratory compromise—secondary to decreased tidal volume and hypoxia; diffusion impairment; ventilation–perfusion mismatch; intrapulmonary shunting of blood • Initial physiologic responses—tachypnea followed by hyperventilation decreases the arterial CO_2 and increases the arterial pH; as alveoli collapse, PAO_2 decreases, causing vasoconstriction, which reduces perfusion to poorly ventilated areas.
• Generalized pulmonary hypoxic vasoconstriction and mechanical collapse of pulmonary vessels—increases pulmonary arterial pressure and right heart work; as intrapleural pressure increases, compensatory mechanisms fail, arterial oxygen decreases, arterial CO_2 increases, the patient becomes severely acidotic, and death may ensue. • Tension—a flap of pulmonary parenchymal tissue acts as a one-way valve, allowing entry of air into the pleural space during inspiration but preventing its escape during expiration; the thorax becomes fixed in maximal expansion, and patient loses the ability to compensate. • Cardiovascular effects—compression and collapse of the venae cava secondary to loss of negative intrapleural pressure; decrease in venous return

SYSTEMS AFFECTED
• Respiratory
• Cardiovascular

GENETICS
N/A

INCIDENCE/PREVALENCE
• Traumatic—most common type in dogs; occurs in 11%–18% of dogs and cats examined for vehicular trauma

GEOGRAPHIC DISTRIBUTION
N/A

SIGNALMENT
Species
Dogs and cats

Breed Predilections
Spontaneous—rottweilers may be over-represented; most affected dogs have a deep-chested conformation.

Mean Age and Range
Spontaneous—most common in middle-aged and old animals

Predominant Sex
None

SIGNS
Historical Findings
• Traumatic—recent history of trauma; often acute dyspnea • Spontaneous—insidious or acute onset; may note dyspnea and tachypnea developing over days to months; low exercise tolerance; may note history of previous lung or thoracic disease (secondary spontaneous)

Physical Examination Findings
• Dyspnea—degree depends on severity of lung collapse and the rate of progression
• Tachypnea and anxiety—most common findings • Frothy blood—may exude from nose and mouth • Cyanosis, pale mucous membranes, and open-mouth breathing—severely affected patients • Tension—may note barrel-shaped thoracic cavity, minimal respiratory excursions, and tachycardia
• Abdominal breathing—apparent
• Auscultation—decreased vesicular lung sounds dorsally; may note muffled heart sounds • Percussion—hyperresonant chest wall; tympanic with tension pneumothorax
• Open pneumothorax—may note external wounds of the thorax • Closed pneumothorax—may note evidence of blunt trauma
• Cervical subcutaneous emphysema—may occur with laceration of the trachea or esophagus

CAUSES
Traumatic
• External forces—gun shot; vehicular accidents; bite or stab wounds
• Iatrogenic—chest tube removal; thoracocentesis; thoracotomy complications; excessive PPV
• Pneumomediastinum—rupture of mediastinal pleura owing to esophageal perforation or tracheal laceration or avulsion

Spontaneous
• Primary—unknown; has not been well-documented in dogs or cats
• Secondary—destruction of pulmonary parenchyma leading to pulmonary cavitation and necrosis of visceral pleura; caused by bullous emphysema, bacterial pneumonia, parasitic or mycotic granuloma, dirofilariasis, invasive thymoma, bronchogenic carcinoma, pulmonary abscess, foreign body, or congenital pulmonary cysts

RISK FACTORS
• Traumatic—free-roaming dogs and cats more likely to sustain trauma
• Spontaneous—previous pulmonary disease or pneumothorax

DIAGNOSIS

DIFFERENTIAL DIAGNOSIS
• Restrictive pulmonary diseases
• Diaphragmatic hernia
• Pleural effusion
• Hemothorax, chylothorax, pyothorax, and hydrothorax

CBC/BIOCHEMISTRY/URINALYSIS
• Stress leukogram and leukocytosis—with bacterial infection
• High liver enzymes—secondary to trauma or hypoxia
• Urinalysis—usually normal

OTHER LABORATORY TESTS
Arterial blood gas analysis—may reveal hypoxemia, hypocapnia or hypercapnia, respiratory alkalosis, or respiratory or metabolic acidosis; depends on magnitude of disorder and ability of patient to compensate

IMAGING
Radiography
• Perform only after patient is stabilized.
• Lateral and dorsoventral positioning—may be less stressful
• Retraction of lung margins from thoracic wall and partial pulmonary collapse
• Lateral view—heart appears elevated off the sternum
• Unilateral tension pneumothorax—mediastinal shift away from the side of high intrapleural pressure
• Evaluate pulmonary parenchyma only after expansion of the lungs after thoracocentesis.
• Traumatic—traumatic bullae or areas of consolidation (contusion); radiopaque, penetrating foreign objects (e.g., pellets and bullets); signs of trauma (e.g., pleural effusion and rib fractures)
• Spontaneous—primary: infrequently, cavitary lesions, bullae, or subpleural blebs; secondary: pulmonary parenchymal disease (e.g., pneumonia, neoplasia, and dirofilariasis)

DIAGNOSTIC PROCEDURES
• Thoracocentesis—diagnostic test of choice; perform as a therapeutic measure before all other diagnostic tests in dyspneic patients
• Thoracoscopy—evaluate pleural space and pulmonary surface
• Bronchoscopy—locate lacerations of the trachea or main bronchi

PATHOLOGIC FINDINGS
• Depend on underlying cause
• Histopathologic examination of the lungs with bullous emphysema—may reveal

subpleural alveolar emphysema, pleural fibrosis, multifocal pulmonary atelectasis, smooth muscle hypertrophy of bronchioles, and bronchiolitis
• Gross inspection of lungs—may reveal pulmonary blebs

TREATMENT

APPROPRIATE HEALTH CARE
• Inpatient—for treatment and observation until stable
• Traumatic—temporarily close pleurocutaneous fistulae with sterile antibiotic ointment and gauze; close surgically after stabilization
• No dyspnea and stable—evacuation of air unnecessary (air will eventually be resorbed)
• With dyspnea—evacuate pleural air immediately; needle thoracocentesis using butterfly or intravenous catheter, three-way stop cock, and extension set; tube thoracostomy with severe and active pneumothorax; perform at an aseptically prepared site on the dorsal two thirds of the thorax between the seventh and ninth rib spaces; lateral recumbency position often makes evacuation of air more efficient; tube thoracostomy recommended if more than two thoracocenteses are necessary within 24 hr
• Continuous negative-pressure pleural drainage by thoracostomy tubes is recommended if pleural air rapidly reaccumulates.
• Heimlich valves—limited because the flutter device often becomes occluded; small patients may not generate enough intrathoracic pressure to evacuate the chest.
• Exploratory thoracotomy—consider if disorder and clinical signs persist > 2–5 days, if more than two episodes recur after proper treatment, or with radiographic evidence that the source of the leakage can be surgically resected (e.g., pulmonary blebs and bullae)
• Treatment may require the use of a trocar into the pleural space to relieve high intrapleural pressure before the thoracostomy tube is placed.

NURSING CARE
• Intravenous fluid therapy—trauma patients in cardiovascular shock
• Supportive care of primary causes (e.g., trauma)—wound cleaning, ongoing fluid therapy, turning the patient to prevent decubital ulcers, enteral nutritional support
• Oxygen administration—for dyspnea and hypoxemia; will not alone take the place of adequate air evacuation from the pleural space
• Other supportive care depends on the primary cause

ACTIVITY
Cage rest—recommended to enhance healing of pulmonary tissue

DIET
Trauma patients benefit from early enteral feeding (within 12 hr) to enhance tissue repair.

CLIENT EDUCATION
Discuss clinical signs of recurrence and advise immediate return if pneumothorax recurs.

SURGICAL CONSIDERATIONS
• Identify site of air leakage—flood the pleural cavity with saline solution; confirm by bubbles rising from the site of the fistula
• Median sternotomy—often necessary because source of the bronchopleural fistula is often unknown and multiple lesions are common
• Large lacerations—may require sutures
• Neoplastic lesions—usually require lobectomy
• Pulmonary blebs—resect
• Abrasion of the visceral pleura with a dry sponge (mechanical pleurodesis) and resection of apical blebs may prevent recurrence of spontaneous pneumothorax secondary to bullous emphysema.

MEDICATIONS

DRUGS OF CHOICE
• Spontaneous—antibiotics for pneumonia; chemotherapy for neoplasia; adulticide for dirofilariasis
• Anesthetic agents—if required, use drugs that allow rapid control of the airway by endotracheal intubation (e.g., ketamine and diazepam, thiobarbiturates).

CONTRAINDICATIONS
Avoid heavy sedation in critical patients.

PRECAUTIONS
• Drugs that suppress respiration (e.g., narcotics)—use with caution; watch for signs of hypoventilation (high $PaCO_2$, low PaO_2); may need PPV

POSSIBLE INTERACTIONS
N/A

ALTERNATIVE DRUGS
N/A

FOLLOW-UP

PATIENT MONITORING
• Respiratory rate and character, mucous membrane color, and heart rate—monitor hourly for the first 24–48 hr; pulse oximetry aids in the continuous monitoring of hemoglobin oxygen saturation. • ECG—detect

arrhythmia; recommended for trauma • Serial radiographic evaluation and blood gas analyses—reveal effectiveness of pleural air evacuation and re-expansion of lungs; may find pulmonary bullae • Thoracostomy tubes—may be removed if ≤ 10 mL of air is removed in 12 hr

PREVENTION/AVOIDANCE
• Do not allow dogs to roam free. • Avoid excessively high airway pressures (> 25–30 cm H_2O) during PPV to prevent barotrauma.

POSSIBLE COMPLICATIONS
Re-expansion (noncardiogenic) pulmonary edema may occur; the incidence unknown, reported in cats after surgery to repair diaphragmatic hernia

EXPECTED COURSE AND PROGNOSIS
• Traumatic—full recovery expected with conservative management (e.g., thoracocentesis or thoracostomy tubes) in most patients; prognosis good if injury is not massive and recognition and treatment are prompt • Spontaneous—recurrence rates high (up to 100% of patients treated by thoracocentesis alone, up to 81% of patients treated by thoracostomy tubes); surgical treatment with pleurodesis recommended to reduce the recurrence rate (25% of patients treated by surgical resection of lesion) if disorder does not resolve within 48 hr of conservative management

MISCELLANEOUS

ASSOCIATED CONDITIONS
N/A

AGE-RELATED FACTORS
N/A

ZOONOTIC POTENTIAL
N/A

PREGNANCY
N/A

ABBREVIATION
PPV = positive pressure ventilation

Suggested Reading
Dramek BA, Caywood DD. Pneumothorax. Vet Clin North Am Sm Anim Pract 1987;17:285–300.
Holstinger RH, Ellison GW. Spontaneous pneumothorax. Compend Contin Educ Pract Vet 1995;17:197–210.
Valentine A, Smeak D, Allen D, et al. Spontaneous pnuemothorax in dogs. Compend Contin Educ Pract Vet 1996;18:53–62.
Author Cynthia C. Ramsey
Consulting Editor Eleanor C. Hawkins

POLIOENCEPHALOMYELITIS—CATS

 BASICS

DEFINITION
• Nonsuppurative meningoencephalomyelitis of unknown cause
• Neurons in the thoracic spinal cord appear preferentially affected.
• Lesions are also seen in the cervical and lumbar spinal cord, brainstem, and cerebrum.
• Axonal degeneration and demyelination in ventral and lateral funiculi of spinal cord occurs secondary to neuronal necrosis.

SIGNALMENT
• Domestic shorthair cats and a few purebreds
• Age range—2 months to 6.5 years
• Females more commonly affected than males

SIGNS
• Vary with location of CNS lesion
• Chronic, progressive incoordination of hind or all four limbs
• Seizures in a few patients

CAUSES & RISK FACTORS
Viral cause suspected but not proven

 DIAGNOSIS

DIFFERENTIAL DIAGNOSIS
• FIP
• Toxoplasmosis
• Fungal infection
• Bacterial infection

CBC/BIOCHEMISTRY/URINALYSIS
• Laboratory changes not well characterized
• Nonspecific changes (e.g., leukopenia and nonregenerative anemia) rare

OTHER LABORATORY TESTS
N/A

IMAGING
N/A

DIAGNOSTIC PROCEDURES
• Mononuclear pleocytosis with mild to moderately high CSF protein (few data)
• Serum or CSF antibody titers—not thoroughly evaluated

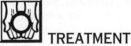 TREATMENT

Not attempted in any of the reported cases

MEDICATIONS

DRUGS
• No drug therapy used in reported cases.
• Because lesions are nonsuppurative, steroid therapy may palliate clinical signs, at least temporarily.

CONTRAINDICATIONS/POSSIBLE INTERACTIONS
N/A

 FOLLOW-UP
N/A

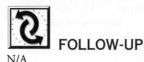 **MISCELLANEOUS**

ABBREVIATIONS
• CSF = cerebrospinal fluid
• FIP = feline infectious peritonitis

Suggested Reading
Hoff EJ, Vandevelde M. Nonsuppurative encephalomyelitis in cats suggestive of a viral origin. Vet Pathol 1981;18:170–180.
Vandevelde M, Braund KG. Polioencephalitis in cats. Vet Pathol 1979;16:420–427.
Author Karen Dyer Inzana
Consulting Editor Joane M. Parent

POLYARTHRITIS, EROSIVE, IMMUNE-MEDIATED

 BASICS

DEFINITION
An immune-mediated inflammatory disease of joints that results in erosion of articular cartilage

PATHOPHYSIOLOGY
• Pathogenesis—involves a type III hypersensitivity reaction; immune complexes are deposited within the synovial membrane; leads to an inflammatory response and complement activation
• Destructive enzymes—released from inflammatory cells, synoviocytes, and chondrocytes; damage the articular cartilage, leading to erosive changes
• RA—associated with an abnormal antigenic response to host immunoglobulin
• EPG and FCPP—offending antigens unknown

SYSTEMS AFFECTED
Musculoskeletal—diarthrodial joints

GENETICS
• Not known to be hereditary

INCIDENCE/PREVALENCE
Rare

GEOGRAPHIC DISTRIBUTION
N/A

SIGNALMENT
Species
• Dogs—RA; EPG
• Cats—FCPP

Breed Predilections
• Small or toy breeds (dogs)—more susceptible to RA
• Greyhounds—only breed known to be susceptible to EPG

Mean Age and Range
• RA (dogs)—young to middle-aged (8 months to 8 years)
• EPG—young greyhounds more susceptible (3–30 months)
• FCPP (cats)—onset at 1.5–4.5 years of age

Predominant Sex
FCPP—reported to affect only male cats

SIGNS
General Comments
• Nonerosive and erosive forms of immune mediated inflammatory disease initially appears similar

Historical Findings
• Dogs and cats—typically, acute onset of a single- or multiple-limb lameness
• Cats—may note a more insidious onset; may note shifting leg lameness
• Joint swelling—may be evident, especially in the carpi and tarsi
• Usually no history of trauma
• May also note vomiting, diarrhea, anorexia, and pyrexia
• Often cyclic—may appear to respond to antibiotic therapy, but may be undergoing spontaneous remission

Physical Examination Findings
• Stiffness of gait, lameness, decreased range of motion, crepitus, and joint swelling and pain in one or more joints
• Joint instability and subluxation—depend on duration of disease
• Lameness—mild weight-bearing to more severe non–weight-bearing
• Diarthrodial joints—all may be affected; RA and FCPP usually affect the carpi, tarsi, and phalangeal joints; EPG usually affects the carpi, tarsi, elbow, stifle, and hip.

CAUSES
• Unknown
• Immunologic mechanism likely
• *Mycoplasma spumans* (EPG)—cultured from one affected greyhound; not isolated in other patients
• FeLV and FeSFV—linked to cats with FCPP

RISK FACTORS
N/A

 DIAGNOSIS

DIFFERENTIAL DIAGNOSIS
• Idiopathic polyarthritis
• Infectious arthritis
• Systemic lupus erythematosus
• Reactive polyarthritis
• Neoplasia
• Osteoarthritis—primary or secondary

CBC/BIOCHEMISTRY/URINALYSIS
• Usually normal
• Hemogram—may note leukocytosis, neutrophilia, and hyperfibrinogenemia

OTHER LABORATORY TESTS
• Rheumatoid factor—positive in only about 25% of RA patients
• Coombs test and antinuclear antibody titer—normal
• Serum titers for *Borrelia, Ehrlichia,* and *Rickettsia*—should be normal
• Serologic evidence of FeSFV—found in all FCPP patients
• Serologic evidence of FeLV exposure—found in 50% or fewer FCPP patients

IMAGING
Radiography
• Severe disease—joint capsular distension; osteophytosis; soft tissue thickening; narrowed joint spaces; subchondral sclerosis
• Cyst-like lucencies—occasionally seen in subchondral bone
• Chronic disease—subluxation, luxation, and obvious joint deformity

DIAGNOSTIC PROCEDURES
• Arthrocentesis and synovial fluid analysis—essential for diagnosis
• Synovial fluid—typically cloudy with normal viscosity; large number of nondegenerate neutrophils (20,000–200,000 cells/ mL); submit for bacterial culture and sensitivity.
• Biopsy of synovial tissue—helps make the diagnosis; rules out other arthritides and neoplasia

PATHOLOGIC FINDINGS
• Erosion of articular cartilage—particularly near the periphery at synovial attachments
• Eburnation and sclerosis of subchondral bone with full-thickness cartilage loss—chronic disease
• Synovial membrane—grossly thickened; may see villous projections
• Granulation tissue (pannus)—may invade the margins of articular cartilage
• Enthesiophytes—at joint capsular attachments and adjacent to the joint
• Histopathology of the synovial membrane—typically reveals villous synovial hyperplasia, hypertrophy, and a lymphoplasmacytic inflammatory infiltrate
• Synovial fluid—cloudy; increased volume

 TREATMENT

APPROPRIATE HEALTH CARE
Usually outpatient

NURSING CARE
• Physical therapy—range-of-motion exercises, massage, and swimming; may be indicated for severe disease
• Bandages and/or splints—to prevent further breakdown of the joint; may be indicated for severe disease with greatly compromised ambulation

POLYARTHRITIS, EROSIVE, IMMUNE-MEDIATED

ACTIVITY
Limited to minimize aggravation of clinical signs

DIET
Weight reduction—decrease stress placed on affected joints

CLIENT EDUCATION
Warn client of the poor prognosis for cure and complete resolution.

SURGICAL CONSIDERATIONS
• Healing rates—may be long and protracted; range of recovery levels
• Surgery—generally not recommended as a good treatment option
• Arthroplasty—total hip replacement, femoral head ostectomy; may consider
• Arthrodesis—in selective cases of joint pain and joint instability; carpus: generally yields the best results; shoulder, elbow, stifle, or hock: less predictable results

MEDICATIONS

DRUGS OF CHOICE

RA
• NSAIDs (dogs)—unrewarding
• Prednisone—1.5–2.0 mg/kg PO q12h for 10–14 days as initial therapy; slowly taper over several weeks to 1.0 mg/kg PO q48h if synovial fluid cell counts return to < 4000 cells/mL and mononuclear cells predominate; add cytotoxic drugs if clinical signs persist or synovial fluid analysis is abnormal.
• Combination of glucocorticoids and cytotoxic drugs—recommended for synergistic effect; may try cyclophosphamide, azathioprine, 6-mercaptopurine, or methotrexate
• Cyclophosphamide—patient < 10 kg: 2.5 mg/kg; patient 10–50 kg: 2.0 mg/kg; patient > 50 kg 1.75 mg/kg; agent given orally every 24 hr for 4 consecutive days of each week; can give concurrently with prednisone
• Azathioprine or 6- mercaptopurine—2.0 mg/kg PO for 14–21 days; then q48h; give prednisone as for cyclophosphamide, but on alternating days
• Remission—usually induced by combination chemotherapy within 2–16 weeks; determined by resolution of clinical signs and confirmation of a normal synovial fluid analysis
• Discontinue cytotoxic drugs 1–3 months after remission is achieved.
• Maintaining remission—alternate-day glucocorticoid therapy (prednisone, 1.0 mg/kg

PO) is generally successful; clinical signs or synovial effusion recurs: may require long-term cytotoxic drug therapy; clinical signs do not recur after 2–3 months: may stop the glucocorticoid; clinical signs recur after glucocorticoid is stopped: continue treatment.
• Aurothiomalate (chrysotherapy)—1 mg/kg IM weekly; successfully alleviates symptoms

EPG
• Treatment is unrewarding.
• Antibiotics, NSAIDs, glucocorticoids, cytotoxic drugs, and polysulfated glycosaminoglycan (Adequan)—fail to induce remission

FCPP
• Treatment may help slow progression.
• Prednisone (2 mg/kg q12h) and cyclophosphamide (2.5 mg/kg q24h)—typically used as described for RA

CONTRAINDICATIONS
• Cytotoxic drugs—do not use with chronic infections or bone marrow suppression (cats with FCPP).
• Chrysotherapy—do not use with renal disease owing to nephrotoxicity.

PRECAUTIONS
• Glucocorticoids—long-term use may lead to Cushing disease.
• Cytotoxic drugs—frequently induce bone marrow suppression; monitor CBC; if leukocyte count < 6000 cells/mL and platelet count < 125,000 cells/mL: reduce dose by one-quarter; if leukocyte < 4000 cells/mL and platelet < 100,000 cells/mL: discontinue for 1 week, then reinstitute at three-quarters dose when counts return to normal.
• Thiopurines generally cause bone marrow suppression at 2–6 weeks; cyclophosphamide, at several months.
• Cyclophosphamide—limit to < 4 months; sterile hemorrhagic cystitis may develop; immediately discontinue if symptoms occur.

POSSIBLE INTERACTIONS
None known

ALTERNATIVE DRUGS
See Drugs of Choice

FOLLOW-UP

PATIENT MONITORING
• Treatment is often frustrating and requires frequent re-evaluation.
• Clinical deterioration—requires a change in drug selection or dosage or surgical intervention

PREVENTION/AVOIDANCE
N/A

POSSIBLE COMPLICATIONS
N/A

EXPECTED COURSE AND PROGNOSIS
• Progression likely
• Long-term prognosis poor
• Cure is not expected; remission is the goal.

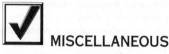

MISCELLANEOUS

ASSOCIATED CONDITIONS
N/A

AGE-RELATED FACTORS
N/A

ZOONOTIC POTENTIAL
N/A

PREGNANCY
N/A

SEE ALSO
Polyarthritis, Nonerosive Immune-Mediated

ABBREVIATIONS
• EPG = erosive polyarthritis of greyhounds
• FCPP = feline chronic progressive polyarthritis
• FeLV = feline leukemia virus
• FeSFV = feline syncytium-forming virus
• RA = rheumatoid arthritis

Suggested Reading
Beale BS. Arthropathies. In: Bloomberg MS, Taylor RT, Dee J, eds. Canine sports medicine and surgery. Philadelphia: Saunders, 1998:517–532.

Goring RL, Beale BS. Immune mediated arthritides. In: Bojrab MJ, ed. Disease mechanisms in small animal surgery. Philadelphia: Lea & Febiger, 1993:742–750.

Pedersen NC. Joint diseases of dogs and cats. In: Ettinger SJ, ed. Textbook of veterinary internal medicine. 3rd ed. Philadelphia: Saunders, 1989:2329–2377.

Author Brian S. Beale
Consulting Editor Peter D. Schwarz

DISEASES

POLYARTHRITIS, NONEROSIVE, IMMUNE-MEDIATED

BASICS

DEFINITION
An immune-mediated inflammatory disease of joints that does not cause erosive change; includes idiopathic polyarthritis, SLE, polyarthritis associated with chronic disease (chronic infectious, neoplastic, or enteropathic disease), polyarthritis–polymyositis syndrome, polyarthritis–meningitis syndrome, polyarteritis nodosa, familial renal amyloidosis in Chinese shar pei dogs, lymphocytic–plasmacytic synovitis, villonodular synovitis, juvenile-onset polyarthritis of akitas, and the proliferative form of FCPP

PATHOPHYSIOLOGY
• Pathogenesis—involves a type III hypersensitivity reaction; immune complexes deposited within the synovial membrane; inflammatory response and complement activation ensue, leading to clinical signs of arthritis
• SLE—nuclear material from various cells becomes antigenic, leading to formation of autoantibodies (antinuclear antibody).

SYSTEMS AFFECTED
Musculoskeletal—diarthrodial joints

GENETICS
Not known to be hereditary

INCIDENCE/PREVALENCE
• Idiopathic—most common form in dogs
• Other forms uncommon

GEOGRAPHIC DISTRIBUTION
N/A

SIGNALMENT

Species
Dogs and cats

BREED PREDILECTIONS
• Idiopathic—large- (more common) and small-breed dogs; uncommon in cats; German shepherds, Doberman pinschers, retrievers, spaniels, pointers, toy poodles, lhaso apsos, Yorkshire terriers, and Chihuahuas over-represented
• SLE—tendency to affect large-breed dogs; collies, German shepherds, poodles, beagles, and Shetland sheepdogs
• Secondary to administration of sulfa drugs—increased sensitivity in Doberman pinschers
• Polyarthritis–meningitis syndrome—reported in weimaraners, German shorthaired pointers, boxers, Bernese mountain dogs, and Japanese akitas
• Amyloidosis and synovitis—prominent features of a syndrome affecting young shar pei dogs
• Juvenile onset—polyarthritis reported in akitas

MEAN AGE AND RANGE
Dogs—young to middle-aged

PREDOMINANT SEX
FCPP—male cats only

SIGNS

General Comments
• Nonerosive and erosive forms of immune mediated inflammatory disease initally appears similar

Historical Findings
• Dogs and cats—acute onset; single- or multiple-limb lameness
• Lameness—may shift from leg to leg
• Usually no history of trauma
• May also note vomiting, diarrhea, anorexia, pyrexia, polyuria, or polydipsia
• May note signs associated with systemic disease (pyometra, prostatitis, or diskospodylitis) or neoplastic disease
• Often cyclic—may appear to respond to antibiotic therapy, but may be undergoing spontaneous remission
• Disease may develop when patient is being treated with (sulfur-containing) antibiotics.

Physical Examination Findings
• Stiffness of gait, lameness, decreased range of motion, crepitus, and joint swelling and pain in one or more joints
• Lameness—mild weight-bearing to more severe non–weight-bearing
• Diarthrodial joints—all may be affected; usually stifle, elbow, carpus, and tarsus

CAUSES
• Unknown for most
• Immunologic mechanism likely
• Chronic—associated with antigenic stimulation along with concurrent gastrointestinal disease, neoplasia, urinary tract infection, periodontitis, bacterial endocarditis, heartworm disease, pyometra, chronic otitis media or externa, fungal infections, and chronic *Actinomyces* infections
• May occur secondary to a hypersensitivity reaction involving the deposition of drug–antibody complexes in blood vessels of the synovium; suspected antibiotics include sulfas, cephalosporins, lincomycin, erythromycin, and penicillins.
• FeLV and FeSFV—linked to FCPP

RISK FACTORS
N/A

DIAGNOSIS

DIFFERENTIAL DIAGNOSIS
• Early erosive polyarthritides
• Infectious arthritis
• Joint trauma
• Polymyositis

CBC/BIOCHEMISTRY/URINALYSIS
• Usually normal
• Hemogram—may show leukocytosis, neutrophilia, and hyperfibrinogenemia
• Hematologic abnormalities (e.g., thrombocytopenia and hemolytic anemia)—seen in only 10%–20% of patients with SLE

OTHER LABORATORY TESTS
• Positive lupus erythematous preparation or positive antinuclear antibody test—dogs with SLE
• Serum titers (*Borrelia, Ehrlichia,* and *Rickettsia*)—should be normal
• Serological evidence of FeSFV—found in all FCPP patients
• Serologic evidence of FeLV exposure—found in 50% or fewer FCPP patients

IMAGING
• Primary radiographic change—joint capsular distension
• May see enthesiophytosis in prolonged or recurrent disease

DIAGNOSTIC PROCEDURES
• Arthrocentesis and synovial fluid analysis—essential for diagnosis
• Synovial fluid—typically appears cloudy with normal viscosity; large increase in nondegenerate neutrophils (20,000–200,000 cells/mL); submit for bacterial culture and sensitivity
• Synovial biopsy—may help diagnosis

POLYARTHRITIS, NONEROSIVE, IMMUNE-MEDIATED

PATHOLOGIC FINDINGS
• The joint capsule—may by thickened; synovial effusion
• Synovial hypertrophy and hyperplasia—associated with a mononuclear cell infiltrate
• Neutrophils—seen in the synovial tissues owing to chemotaxis

TREATMENT

APPROPRIATE HEALTH CARE
Usually outpatient

NURSING CARE
• Physical therapy—range-of-motion exercises, massage, and swimming; may be indicated for severe disease
• Bandages and/or splints—to prevent further breakdown of the joint; may be indicated for severe disease with compromised ambulation

ACTIVITY
Limited to minimize aggravation of clinical signs

DIET
Weight reduction—decrease stress placed on affected joints

CLIENT EDUCATION
Warn client of the poor prognosis for cure and complete resolution.

SURGICAL CONSIDERATIONS
N/A

MEDICATIONS

DRUGS OF CHOICE
• Typical therapy—initial trial of glucocorticoids; if poor response, then combination chemotherapy (glucocorticoids and cytotoxic drugs)
• Eliminate underlying causes if possible—chronic disease; offending antibiotic
• Complete remission—usually achieved in 2–16 weeks; determined by resolution of clinical signs and confirmation of normal synovial fluid analysis
• Recurrence rate—30%–50% once therapy is discontinued
• Prednisone—1.5–2.0 mg/kg PO q12h for 10–14 days as initial treatment; synovial fluid cell counts < 4000 cells/mL and mononuclear cells predominate: slowly taper over several weeks to 1.0 mg/kg PO q48h; clinical signs persist or abnormal synovial fluid analysis: add cytotoxic agents; no clinical signs after 2–3 months of alternate-day therapy: discontinue
• Combination of glucocorticoids and cytotoxic—recommended for synergistic effect; may try cyclophosphamide and the thiopurines (azathioprine and 6-mercaptopurine)
• Cyclophosphamide—patient < 10 kg: 2.5 mg/kg; patient 10–50 kg: 2.0 mg/kg; patient > 50 kg: 1.75 mg/kg; agent given orally every 24 hr for 4 consecutive days of each week; given concurrently with prednisone (as described above; some clinicians reduce the total daily dose by half)
• Azathioprine or 6-mercaptopurine—2.0 mg/kg PO q24h for 14–21 days, then q48h; given concurrently with prednisone as for cyclophosphamide, but on alternating days
• Discontinue cytotoxic drugs 1–3 months after remission is achieved.
• Maintaining remission—alternate-day glucocorticoid therapy (prednisone, 1.0 mg/kg PO) is generally successful; clinical signs or synovial neutrophilia recur: long-term cytotoxic drug therapy may be necessary; clinical signs do not recur after 2–3 months: may stop the glucocorticoid; clinical signs recur after glucocorticoid is stopped: continue treatment.

FCPP
• Treatment may help slow progression.
• Prednisone (2 mg/kg q12h) and cyclophosphamide (2.5 mg/kg)—typically used as described above

CONTRAINDICATIONS
Do not use cytotoxic drugs with chronic infections or bone marrow suppression (cats with FCPP).

PRECAUTIONS
• Glucocorticoids—long-term use may lead to iatrogenic Cushing disease.
• Cytotoxic drugs—frequently induce bone marrow suppression; monitor CBC weekly (see Polyarthritis, Erosive Immune-mediated).

POSSIBLE INTERACTIONS
None known

ALTERNATIVE DRUGS
See Drugs of Choice

FOLLOW-UP

PATIENT MONITORING
Clinical deterioration—indicates a change in drug selection or dosage

PREVENTION/AVOIDANCE
N/A

POSSIBLE COMPLICATIONS
N/A

EXPECTED COURSE AND PROGNOSIS
• Recurrence—seen intermittently
• SLE and FCPP—progression common; guarded prognosis
• Other forms—good prognosis

MISCELLANEOUS

ASSOCIATED CONDITIONS
N/A

AGE-RELATED FACTORS
N/A

ZOONOTIC POTENTIAL
N/A

PREGNANCY
N/A

ABBREVIATIONS
• FCPP = feline chronic progressive polyarthritis
• FeLV = feline leukemia virus
• FeSFV = feline syncytium-forming virus
• SLE = systemic lupus erythematous

Suggested Reading
Beale BS. Arthropathies. In: Bloomberg MS, Taylor RT, Dee J, eds. Canine sports medicine and surgery. Philadelphia: Saunders, 1998:517–532.
Goring RL, Beale BS. Immune mediated arthritides. In: Bojrab, MJ, ed. Disease mechanisms in small animal surgery. Philadelphia: Lea & Febiger, 1993:742–750.
Pedersen NC. Joint diseases of dogs and cats. In: Ettinger SJ, ed. Textbook of veterinary internal medicine. 3rd ed. Philadelphia: Saunders, 1989:2329–2377.
Author Brian S. Beale
Consulting Editor Peter D. Schwarz

DISEASES

POLYCYSTIC KIDNEY DISEASE

BASICS

OVERVIEW
A disorder in which large portions of normally differentiated renal parenchyma are displaced by multiple cysts; renal cysts develop in pre-existing nephrons and collecting ducts; both kidneys are invariably involved, probably because the disease is inherited.

SIGNALMENT
• Persian and other long-haired cats are affected more commonly than other breeds.
• Dog breeds affected include cairn terriers and beagles.

SIGNS
• Cysts often remain undetected until they become large and numerous enough to contribute to renal failure or abdominal enlargement; thus patients typically are clinically normal during initial stages of cyst formation and growth.
• May detect bosselated (lumpy) kidneys by abdominal palpation
• Most renal cysts are not painful when palpated, but acute secondary infection of cysts may be associated with rapid distension of the renal capsule and pain.

CAUSES & RISK FACTORS
• Believed to be inherited; however, lack of genealogic information often precludes a precise diagnosis of inherited disease in most adult dogs and cats with multiple renal cysts.
• The stimuli for renal cyst formation remains obscure; genetic, endogenous, and environmental factors appear to influence the process.
• Endogenous compounds hypothesized to stimulate cellular hyperplasia and contribute to cyst development include parathyroid hormone, vasopressin, cAMP, and endotoxins of enteric microbes.
• Cystogenic chemicals include diphenylthiazole, nordihydroguaiarectic acid, diphenylamine, trichlorophenoxyacetic acid, and long-acting corticosteroids.

DIAGNOSIS

DIFFERENTIAL DIAGNOSIS
• Other multicystic diseases of the kidneys
• Glomerulocystic disease of collie
• Renal cystadenocarcinoma associated with nodular fibrosis in German shepherd dogs
• Renal cysts associated with chronic renal failure or renal dysplasia
• Noncystic causes of renomegaly
• Renal neoplasia
• Hydronephrosis

• Perirenal pseudocysts
• Feline infectious peritonitis
• Mycotic or bacterial nephritis

CBC/BIOCHEMISTRY/URINALYSIS
• Results usually unremarkable unless patient has renal insufficiency
• Hematuria is rare.

OTHER LABORATORY TESTS
• Cyst fluid can be clear, cloudy, or hemorrhagic, and the fluid from different cysts in the same kidney can differ.
• Bacterial culture of cyst fluid helps in diagnosing concomitant infection.

IMAGING

Radiography
Survey radiography and intravenous urography are insensitive methods of confirming cystic disease.

Ultrasonography
• Reveals anechoic cavitating lesions characterized by sharply marginated smooth walls and distal enhancement, which are diagnostic
• Reveals hypoechoic cystic cavities in some patients with cysts that are infected with bacteria
• Used to detect cysts in other organs (e.g., liver), which helps to differentiate polycystic kidney disease from acquired multicystic disorders of the kidneys

DIAGNOSTIC PROCEDURES
Evaluation of fine-needle aspirates of the kidney may allow differentiation of cystic disease from other diseases that cause renomegaly.

TREATMENT

• Usually not immediately life-threatening, but bacterial nephritis and cyst involvement warrants immediate measures to prevent sepsis and mortality
• Spontaneous resolution of cysts is not documented in dogs or cats; with time, most cysts increase in size and number, often compressing adjacent normally functioning renal parenchyma.
• Elimination of renal cysts and associated renal parenchymal lesions is not yet feasible; treatment is often limited to minimizing the pathophysiologic consequences of renal cyst formation (i.e., renal failure, renal infection, hematuria, and pain).
• Can use percutaneous aspiration of fluid from large renal cysts to minimize pain and compression of adjacent normal renal parenchyma. This procedure is impractical for kidneys with hundreds of cysts. Periodic aspiration of fluid (weekly to biweekly) is needed to maintain reduced cyst volume.

• Some patients may require treatment for concomitant renal failure.
• Avoid nephrectomy but may consider if infected cysts are associated with sepsis

MEDICATIONS

DRUGS
• Bacterial infection of cysts has been observed in cats. Unless infection is accompanied by pyelonephritis, bacteria may not be observed in urine. Consider parenchymal infection when renal cysts are associated with renal pain and fever, even in absence of bacteriuria.
• Treatment of infected cysts requires special consideration. The acidic nature of cyst fluid and its containment by an epithelial barrier might inhibit establishment of bactericidal concentrations of commonly used acidic antibiotics (e.g., cephalosporins and penicillins) within cystic lumens. Alkaline, lipid-soluble antibiotics (e.g., trimethoprim-sulfonamide combinations, enrofloxacin, chloramphenicol, tetracycline, and clindamycin), which penetrate epithelial barriers and become ionized and trapped in cyst lumens, have been recommended for humans with infected cysts and should be considered for veterinary patients.

CONTRAINDICATIONS AND POSSIBLE INTERACTIONS
N/A

FOLLOW-UP

• Monitor patients every 2–6 months for associated disease (e.g., renal failure, renal infection, and pain).
• In the absence of sepsis, the short-term prognosis appears to be favorable without treatment.
• The long-term prognosis for patients with polycystic kidney disease often depends on the severity and progression of renal failure.

MISCELLANEOUS

Suggested Reading
Lulich JP, Osborne CA, Polzin DJ. Cystic diseases of the kidney. In: Osborne CA, Finco DR, eds. Canine and feline nephrology and urology. Baltimore: Williams & Wilkins, 1995:460–470.
Authors Jody P. Lulich and Carl A. Osborne
Consulting Editors Larry G. Adams and Carl A. Osborne

BASICS

OVERVIEW
Myeloproliferative disorder that results in high blood viscosity secondary to an increased RBC mass

SIGNALMENT
• Dogs and cats
• Primarily old animals

SIGNS
• Gradual in onset; runs a chronic course
• Depression
• Anorexia
• Weakness
• Polydipsia and polyuria
• Erythema of skin and mucous membranes
• Dilated and tortuous retinal blood vessels
• Splenomegaly and hepatomegaly uncommon

CAUSES & RISK FACTORS
Unknown

DIAGNOSIS

DIFFERENTIAL DIAGNOSIS
• Severe dehydration
• Renal neoplasia
• Chronic pyelonephritis
• Hyperadrenocorticism
• Androgen stimulation
• Pulmonary disease
• Cardiac disease with right-to-left shunts

CBC/BIOCHEMISTRY/URINALYSIS
• High PCV
• Absolute increase in RBC mass
• Prerenal azotemia possible
• Leukocytosis in 50% of dogs

OTHER LABORATORY TESTS
• PaO$_2$—normal
• Serum erythropoietin concentration—low to zero
• Cytologic examination of bone marrow and core biopsy

IMAGING
• Radiography—assess kidneys and cardiopulmonary system
• Abdominal ultrasonography—assess kidneys and adrenal glands
• Echocardiography—evaluate for right-to-left cardiac shunts
• Intravenous pyelogram—assess kidneys
• Imaging studies—normal in affected animals

DIAGNOSTIC PROCEDURES
• Bone marrow biopsy
• Electrocardiography—assess heart disease

TREATMENT

• Phlebotomy and concurrent replacement with intravenous isotonic fluids—quick relief of signs during clinical crisis
• Hydroxyurea—inhibit intracellular DNA synthesis and retard bone marrow proliferation

MEDICATIONS

DRUGS
Hydroxyurea—40–50 mg/kg divided twice daily; titrate to response and toxicity (dogs and cats)

CONTRAINDICATIONS/POSSIBLE INTERACTIONS
Hydroxyurea—potentially myelosuppressive; frequent blood monitoring advised

FOLLOW-UP

Periodic re-examinations—CBC and platelet count to monitor toxic effects of hydroxyurea on bone marrow

MISCELLANEOUS

SEE ALSO
Polycythemia

ABBREVIATION
PCV = packed cell volume

Suggested Reading
Hamilton TA. The leukemias. In: Morrison WB, ed. Cancer in dogs and cats: medical and surgical management. Baltimore: Williams & Wilkins, 1998:721–729.

Morrison WB. Polycythemia. In: Ettinger SJ, Feldman EC, eds., Textbook of veterinary internal medicine. 4th ed. Philadelphia: Saunders, 1995;197–199.

Author Wallace B. Morrison
Consulting Editor Wallace B. Morrison

POLYPHAGIA

BASICS

DEFINITION
Increased food intake

PATHOPHYSIOLOGY
- Failure to assimilate or loss of nutrients (e.g., maldigestion/malabsorption syndromes such as EPI)
- Inability to use nutrients (e.g., diabetes mellitus, poor quality diets, GI parasites)
- Hypoglycemia (e.g., insulinoma, insulin overdose)
- Increased metabolic rate or demand (e.g., hyperthyroidism, cold environments, pregnancy, lactation)
- Psychologic or learned behaviors (e.g., palatable diets, competition, drugs such as anticonvulsants or glucocorticoids)

SYSTEMS AFFECTED
- Musculoskeletal—overweight patients are susceptible to arthritis and other orthopedic problems.
- Integument—obese animals, especially cats, are susceptible to dermatitis.
- Respiratory—obesity exacerbates dyspnea in patients with respiratory disease.
- Cardiovascular—obesity can worsen clinical cardiac disease.

SIGNALMENT
Dogs and cats

SIGNS

Historical Findings
- Eating more frequently and/or a greater quantity than normal
- Weight loss may occur with certain disease states (e.g., EPI, diabetes mellitus, hyperthyroidism).
- PU/PD occurs in some patients (diabetes mellitus, hyperthyroidism, hyperadrenocorticism).

Physical Examination Findings
Patients may have excessive body fat, but those with an underlying medical problem (e.g., EPI, diabetes mellitus, hyperthyroidism) may be thin.

CAUSES

Physiologic
- Pregnancy
- Lactation
- Growth
- Response to a cold environment
- Increased exercise

Pathologic
- Diabetes mellitus
- Hyperthyroidism—cats
- Hyperadrenocorticism—dogs
- EPI
- GI parasites
- Insulinoma
- Insulin overdose
- Lymphangiectasia
- Growth hormone–secreting pituitary tumor
- Megaesophagus
- Lymphocytic plasmacytic enteritis—cats; uncommon
- Neoplasms of the brain—rare
- GI neoplasms—rare

Iatrogenic
- Corticosteroids
- Progestins
- Benzodiazepines
- Anticonvulsants
- Palatable food/overfeeding
- Poor diets
- Competition for food

RISK FACTORS
See Causes.

DIAGNOSIS

DIFFERENTIAL DIAGNOSIS
PU/PD (excessive trips to food/water area)—differentiate by observation.

CBC/BIOCHEMISTRY/URINALYSIS
- Neutrophilia, monocytosis, lymphopenia, and eosinopenia with hyperadrenocorticism, and in patients receiving corticosteroids
- Hyperglycemia with diabetes mellitus, growth hormone–secreting pituitary tumors (cats, insulin-resistant diabetes mellitus) and hyperadrenocorticism (mild)
- Hypercholesterolemia with recent food intake, hyperadrenocorticism, and diabetes mellitus, and in patients receiving corticosteroids
- High ALP and ALT activity with hyperadrenocorticism (dogs), hyperthyroidism (cats), and diabetes mellitus, and in patients receiving corticosteroids
- Hypoproteinemia with protein-losing enteropathies (e.g., lymphangiectasia, IBD)
- Hypoglycemia in patients with insulinoma or insulin overdose
- Low urine specific gravity with diabetes mellitus, hyperthyroidism, and hyperadrenocorticism, and in patients receiving corticosteroids
- Glucosuria $\pm$ ketonuria with diabetes mellitus

OTHER LABORATORY TESTS
- Fecal examination to rule out GI parasites
- Serum TLI to rule in or out EPI
- Total serum T_4 to rule out hyperthyroidism (cats); T_3 suppression testing if hyperthyroidism is suspected but serum total T_4 is normal
- Low-dose dexamethasone suppression and/or ACTH stimulation to rule out hyperadrenocorticism; plasma ACTH level or high-dose dexamethasone suppression testing to differentiate pituitary-dependent hyperadrenocorticism from adrenal tumor if hyperadrenocorticism is confirmed with the low-dose dexamethasone suppression test or ACTH stimulation test
- Serum insulin levels in hypoglycemic patients to rule out insulinoma

IMAGING
- Abdominal radiology may demonstrate

hepatomegaly associated with hyperadreno-corticism, diabetes mellitus, and corticosteroid administration.

• Thoracic radiology may demonstrate mega-esophagus.

• Abdominal ultrasonography may demonstrate an adrenal mass or bilateral adrenomegaly (hyperadrenocorticism), hepatomegaly (hyperadrenocorticism, diabetes mellitus, and corticosteroid administration), bowel wall thickening or bowel wall layering disruption (IBD, lymphoma, lymphangiectasia), and pancreatic masses (insulinoma).

DIAGNOSTIC PROCEDURES
Endoscopy with biopsy of the upper GI tract to rule GI diseases

TREATMENT
• Usually outpatient medical management
• Polyphagia without weight gain or with weight loss is more likely due to a medical problem; evaluate the animal prior to food restriction/manipulation.
• Once pathologic causes of polyphagia have been excluded, limit the amount of food available, feed a reduced-calorie diet, or increase exercise if obesity or weight gain is present.
• The average animal's daily caloric need can be estimated by the formula 30 × weight (kg) + 70.
• Chew toys can be used as a substitute for food.

MEDICATIONS

DRUGS OF CHOICE
(See specific disease chapters for detailed therapy)
• Diabetes mellitus—insulin, complex carbohydrate diet
• Hyperthyroidism—radioactive ^{131}I therapy, thyroidectomy or methimazole (Tapazole)
• Hyperadrenocorticism—options include

$o'p'$DDD (Mitotane, Lysodren), selegiline (Deprenyl, Anipryl), and ketoconazole (Nizoral)
• EPI—pancreatic enzyme replacement
• GI parasitism—anthelminthics
• Insulinoma—frequent feeding of small meals, surgery, corticosteroids, diazoxide, somatostatin
• Megaesophagus—upright feedings, cisapride
• GI disease—varies with disease process
• Drug-induced—attempt to taper or discontinue drug.
• If a compulsive eating disorder is suspected, can use drugs such as clomipramine or amitriptyline (1–3 mg/kg PO q12h)

CONTRAINDICATIONS
N/A

PRECAUTIONS
N/A

POSSIBLE INTERACTIONS
N/A

ALTERNATIVE DRUGS
N/A

FOLLOW-UP

PATIENT MONITORING
In patients with nonpathologic causes of polyphagia—body weight; make appropriate adjustments in the number of calories fed.

POSSIBLE COMPLICATIONS
• Obesity in nonpathologic polyphagia
• Weight loss/emaciation in pathologic causes of polyphagia
• Worsening of respiratory or cardiovascular disease processes in obese patient

MISCELLANEOUS

ASSOCIATED CONDITIONS
Obesity

AGE-RELATED FACTORS

N/A

ZOONOTIC POTENTIAL
N/A

PREGNANCY
A normal physiologic response to pregnancy

SYNONYMS
• Hyperphagia
• Eating disorder

SEE ALSO
• Specific causes
• Obesity

ABBREVIATIONS
• ACTH = adrenocorticotropic hormone
• ALP = alkaline phosphatase
• ALT = alanine aminotransferase
• EPI = exocrine pancreatic insufficiency
• GI = gastrointestinal
• IBD = inflammatory bowel disease
• PU/PD = polyuria/polydipsia
• TLI = trypsin-like immunoreactivity

Suggested Reading

Bradshaw JWS. The behaviour of the domestic cat. Oxon, U.K.: C.A.B. International, 1992:219.

Crystal MA. Polyphagic weight loss. In: The feline patient. Essentials of diagnosis and treatment. Philadelphia: Williams & Wilkins, 1998:81–83.

Houpt KA. Domestic animal behavior for veterinarians and animal scientists. Ames: Iowa State University Press, 1991:408.

Monroe WE. Anorexia and polyphagia. In: Ettinger SJ, Feldman EC, eds. Textbook of veterinary internal medicine. Philadelphia: Saunders, 1995:18–21.

Scarlett JM, Donoghue S, Saidla J, Wills J. Overweight cats: prevalence and risk factors. J Obes 1994;18:S22-S28.

Author Katherine A. Houpt
Consulting Editors Mitchell A. Crystal and Brett M. Feder

PORTOSYSTEMIC SHUNT

BASICS

DEFINITION
• Congenital PSVA—venous malformations bridging the portal and systemic circulations that permit portal blood to circumvent the liver (hepatofugal circulation); may be intra-hepatic or extrahepatic; most are single vessels; patients may also have portal venous hypo-plasia external to or within the liver. • APSS—develops subsequent to portal hypertension; typically multiple; represents normally present but unused vascular channels bridging the splanchnic and systemic circulations; lack of valves in the portal vein permits circulatory accommodation through the shunt. • Portal hypertension—usually associated with hepatic fibrosis or cirrhosis, portal venous thrombo-embolism, stricture, or hypoplasia, and (rarely) congenital or acquired hepatic arteriovenous fistula (which arterializes the portal circulation)

PATHOPHYSIOLOGY
• Hepatofugal circulation—eliminates hep-atocellular cleansing of portal blood that contains toxins derived from the gut • May lead to episodic development of hepatic encephalopathy associated with ingestion of high-protein food, gastrointestinal bleeding, azotemia, electrolyte disturbances, blood transfusion, infections, and administration of certain drugs • Compromised hepatic per-fusion and lack of hepatatrophic factors—result in microhepatia • Hyperammonemia and impaired transformation of uric acid to water-soluble allantoin—result in ammonium urate crystalluria or calculi

SYSTEMS AFFECTED
• Nervous—episodic hepatic encephalopathy • Gastrointestinal—intermittent inappetence; vomiting; diarrhea; pica; ptyalism (cats) • Uro-genital—ammonium urate urolithiasis; PSVA: large kidneys, ammonium urate crystalluria, calculi, 50% of affected male dogs are cryptor-chid. • Hemic/Lymph/Immune—poikilo-cytosis; target cells; erythrocytic microcytosis • Ocular (PSVA)—golden iris color in non-blue-eyed, non-Persian cats • Musculoskeletal (PSVA)—failure to grow; unthrifty appearance

GENETICS
• Basis unknown • Kindreds affected (PSVA)—miniature schnauzers; Irish wolfhounds; Old English sheepdogs; cairn terriers; Yorkshire terriers

INCIDENCE/PREVALENCE
• Incidence (PSVA)—greatest in purebred dogs and mixed-breed cats • Prevalence—unknown

GEOGRAPHIC DISTRIBUTION
PSVA—reported in North America, Japan, England, and Australia

SIGNALMENT

Species
Dogs and cats

Breed Predilection
APSS—depends on underlying cause
PSVA
• Higher risk in purebred dogs and mixed breed cats • Especially common in Yorkshire terriers • Small-breed dogs and cats—extrahepatic shunt common • Large-breed dogs—intrahepatic shunt common

Mean Age and Range
PSVA—usually noted in young animals; range 4 weeks to 12 years

Predominant Sex
N/A

SIGNS

General Comments
• Represent sequela of impaired hepatic function • Episodic hepatic encephalop-athy—predominates; episodes transiently improve after rehydration and treatment with broad-spectrum antibiotics and lactulose • Affected cats—initially thought to have an upper respiratory infection based on the display of ptyalism • PSVA—usually noted at initial feeding of puppy or kitten food; stunted growth common

Historical Findings
CNS Signs
• Anorexia • Lethargy • Episodic weakness • Pacing • Ataxia • Disorientation • Head pressing • Blindness • Behavioral changes—aggression (cats); vocalization; hallucinations • Seizures • Coma
Gastrointestinal Signs
• Inappetence • Vomiting • Diarrhea • Pica
Urinary Signs
• Polyuria or polydipsia • Ammonium urate crystalluria—pollakiuria dysuria; hematuria; urethral; (rare) ureteral obstruction

Physical Examination Findings
• PSVA—normal appearance; stunted stature; microhepatia; hepatic encephalopathy; golden or copper irises in non-blue-eyed and non-Persian cats; ascites and edema rare • APSS—depend on chronicity of underlying disorder causing portal hypertension; ascites and edema common (often wax and wane in severity)

CAUSES
• PSVA—congenital malformations • APSS—portal hypertension owing to hepatic fibrosis or cirrhosis, impaired portal perfusion of splanch-nic segment of portal vein (thromboembolism, stricture, strangulation), hepatic arteriovenous fistula causing arterialization of the portal venous system (see Hypertension, Portal)

RISK FACTORS
• PSVA—purebred dogs, especially terrier type breeds; particular kindreds may be affected. • APSS—chronic liver diseases; portal thrombi; other prehepatic causes of portal hypertension

DIAGNOSIS

DIFFERENTIAL DIAGNOSIS
• CNS signs—infectious disorders (e.g., FIP, canine distemper, toxoplasmosis, FeLV-related infections); toxicities (e.g., lead, mushrooms, recreational drugs); hydrocephalus; idiopathic epilepsy; metabolic disorders (e.g., severe hypo-glycemia, hypokalemia or hyperkalemia, hypo-calcemia) • Gastrointestinal signs—bowel obstruction; dietary indiscretion; foreign body ingestion; inflammatory bowel disease • Uri-nary tract signs—bacterial urinary tract infection; urolithiasis • Polyuria or poly-dipsia—disorders of urine concentration (e.g., diabetes insipidus, abnormal adrenal function, hypercalcemia, primary polydipsia) • Primary liver disease—distinguished via diagnostic imaging and liver biopsy • Abnormal liver function that suggests PSVA but with no demonstrable macroscopic shunt—hepatoportal microvascular dysplasia

CBC/BIOCHEMISTRY/URINALYSIS
• CBC—microcytosis; mild nonregenerative anemia; poikilocytosis (cats); target cells (dogs) • Biochemistry—low BUN, creatinine, glu-cose, and cholesterol common; liver enzyme activity variable (ALP usually high in young patients owing to bone isoenzyme); bilirubin normal with PSVA but may be high with APSS; hypoalbuminemia common with APSS but inconsistent and mild with PSVA • Uri-nalysis—hyposthenuria or isosthenuria, ammonium urate crystalluria, hematuria, pyuria, and proteinuria owing to mechanical inflammation and infection secondary to metabolic stones

OTHER LABORATORY TESTS
• Total serum bile acids—sensitive indicators; random fasting values may be within normal reference range; 2-hr postprandial values mark-edly high (usually > 100 μmol/L) • Blood ammonia values—sensitive indicators; less reliable than total serum bile acids because of analytic problems • Ammonia tolerance testing—more reliable than random ammonia values; samples cannot be stored, frozen, or mailed for analysis. • Cytologic and physico-chemical analysis—abdominal effusion; pure transudate or modified transudate with chronic liver disease

IMAGING

Abdominal Radiography
• Microhepatia—PSVA: common in dogs, less consistent in cats; APSS: common in most dogs, variable in cats • Renomegaly (PSVA) • Abdominal effusion (APSS) • Ammonium urate calculi—radiolucent unless surrounded by other minerals

Radiographic Portovenography
• Contrast injection into a mesenteric or splenic vein, splenic pulp, or venous phase of cranial mesenteric angiogram • Gold standard

for confirming diagnosis • May reveal portal thrombi causing APSS

Abdominal Ultrasonography

PSVA
• Subjective estimation of microhepatia, hypervascularity, and observation of the shunting vessel • Color-flow Doppler—assists in shunt localization • Intrahepatic shunts—most easily imaged • Renomegaly • Renal and cystic calculi (ammonium biurate urolithiasis) common

APSS
• Liver size depends on underlying cause. • Altered parenchymal and biliary tract echogenicity • Portosystemic collaterals adjacent to kidneys or spleen • Abdominal effusion—easily detected. • Ammonium urate calculi in renal pelvis or bladder • Intrahepatic arteriovenous fistula—pulsating vascular structure within an enlarged liver lobe, along with abdominal effusion, and APSS • Color-flow Doppler—portal thrombi

Colorectal Scintigraphy
• Sensitive noninvasive • Confirms diagnosis; cannot differentiate between PSVA and APSS • Administer technetium 99m pertechnetate rectally; image with gamma camera to determine rate of isotope appearance in liver versus heart; calculate shunt fraction (< 15% is normal).

DIAGNOSTIC PROCEDURES
Liver biopsy

PATHOLOGIC FINDINGS

PSVA
• Gross—small, smooth-surfaced liver; shunting vessel may be difficult to verify at autopsy. • Microscopic—small nonperfused portal venules; increased portal lymphatics; multiple cross-sections of portal arterioles; scattered lipogranulomas; hepatocellular atrophy

APSS
• Gross—small, irregularly contoured liver; regenerative nodules with associated chronic hepatopathy • Microscopic—depends on underlying disease

 TREATMENT

APPROPRIATE HEALTH CARE
Inpatient—severe signs of hepatic encephalopathy; for supportive care

NURSING CARE

Hepatic Encephalopathy
• Eliminate causal factors—dehydration; azotemia; gastrointestinal bleeding; high-protein foods; infection (urinary tract, other); treatment with certain drugs • Protein-restricted diet—dogs: dairy and soy protein may perform better than meat and fish proteins; cats: require balanced, meat-based protein • Increase dietary protein tolerance by concurrent treatment with lactulose (0.5–1 mL/ kg PO q8–12h; dose based on production of two to three soft stools daily), metro-

nidazole (7.5 mg/kg PO q8–12h), and/or neomycin (22 mg/kg PO q12h).

Hepatic Coma
• Discontinue oral medications. • Parenteral fluids—with APSS use sodium-restricted agents; avoid alkalinization (augments ammonia toxicity). • Dextrose—supplementation commonly needed; 2.5%–5.0% • Potassium chloride—supplement at 20 mEq/L fluids (not to exceed 0.5 mEq/kg/hr) • Cleansing enemas with warmed isotonic fluids—until free of feces • Retention enemas—15 mL/kg; with lactulose (1:2 dilution with water) and neomycin (10–15 mg/kg)

SURGICAL CONSIDERATIONS
• Surgical ligation—PSVA • Goal—total ligation of anomalous vessel; often only partial ligation can be safely done (judged by effects on splanchnic circulation and portal venous pressure during the procedure); surgical assessment of extent of ligation may be inaccurate. • Alternative ligation with amaroid constrictor band—removes immediate surgical concern of overligation • Hepatic encephalopathy signs—resolve before surgery • Intrahepatic PSVA—most difficult to ligate; without portogram, ligation of the wrong vessel is possible. • Postoperative complications—portal venous thrombi; severe portal hypertension; mesenteric ischemia; seizures; sepsis; acute pancreatitis; hemorrhage • Intraoperative hypothermia—especially problematic in very small patients • Emergency surgery to remove ligature may be necessary. • Abdominal effusion—common after shunt ligation; alone does not indicate pathologic portal hypertension • Postoperative monitoring essential—96 hr

 MEDICATIONS

DRUG(S) OF CHOICE
See Nursing Care

CONTRAINDICATIONS
Avoid medications that rely on hepatic biotransformation or excretion and that react with the GABA–benzodiazepine receptor.

PRECAUTIONS
Certain sedatives may promote hepatic encephalopathy—benzodiazepine; tranquilizers

POSSIBLE INTERACTIONS
N/A

ALTERNATIVE DRUGS
N/A

 FOLLOW-UP

PATIENT MONITORING

PSVA
• Postsurgery—continue management of hepatic encephalopathy for 2–4 weeks or

indefinitely, depending on extent of ligation and individual response. • Evaluate completeness of ligation noninvasively by colorectal scintigraphy. • Partial ligation may eventually completely occlude • Amaroid constrictor bands may provide full ligation within just a few days.

PREVENTION/AVOIDANCE
APSS—treat underlying disease.

POSSIBLE COMPLICATIONS
• Dogs (PSVA)—may note only transient improvement after surgical ligation; most patients do well with only partial ligation; increased risk for small white dogs (especially Maltese) • Ligation of PSVA—may lead to APSS if portal hypertension is created

EXPECTED COURSE AND PROGNOSIS
• Partial or complete shunt ligation (PSVA)—usually good clinical outcome • Total serum bile acids—often do not normalize even with complete ligation, owing to associated hepatoportal microvascular dysplasia • Cats (PSVA)—prognosis after surgery not as good as for dog; clinical signs may recur with APSS formation. • No presurgical method to predict postoperative prognosis

 MISCELLANEOUS

ASSOCIATED CONDITIONS
• Cryptorchidism (dogs) • Copper-colored iris (cats) • Ammonium urate urolithiasis • Hepatic encephalopathy

AGE-RELATED FACTORS
PSVA—surgical outcome may be good in young and old patients.

ZOONOTIC POTENTIAL
N/A

PREGNANCY
PSVA—affected dogs can carry litters to term.

SYNONYMS
• Portocaval shunt • Portovascular anastomosis

SEE ALSO
• Hepatic Encephalopathy • Hypertension, Portal

ABBREVIATIONS
• ALP = alkaline phosphatase • APSS = acquired portosystemic shunt • FeLV = feline leukemia virus • FIP = feline infectious peritonitis • GABA = γ-aminobutyric acid • PSVA = portosystemic vascular anomaly

Suggested Reading
Center SA. Hepatic vascular diseases. In: Guilford WG, Center SA, Strombeck DR, et al., eds. Strombeck's small animal gastroenterology. 3rd ed. Philadelphia: Saunders, 1996:802–846.
Author Susan E. Johnson
Consulting Editor Sharon A. Center

POXVIRUS INFECTION—CATS

BASICS

OVERVIEW
• Member of the genus *Orthopoxvirus,* family Poxviridae
• Enveloped DNA virus, resistant to drying (viable for years) but readily inactivated by most disinfectants
• Geographically limited to Eurasia
• Relatively common

SIGNALMENT
• Cats—domestic and exotic
• No age, sex, or breed predisposition

SIGNS
• Skin lesions—multiple, circular; dominant feature; usually develop on head, neck, or forelimbs
• Primary lesions—crusted papules, plaques, nodules, crateriform ulcers, or areas of cellulitis or abscesses
• Secondary lesions—erythematous nodules that ulcerate and crust; often widespread; develop after 1–3 weeks
• Pruritus variable
• Systemic—20% of cases; anorexia; lethargy; pyrexia; vomiting; diarrhea; oculonasal discharge; conjunctivitis; pneumonia

CAUSES & RISK FACTORS
• Reservoir host—wild rodents
• Infection thought to be acquired during hunting; most common in young adults and active hunters, often from rural environment
• Lesions—often develop at the site of a bite wound (presumably inflicted by the prey animal carrying the virus)
• Most cases occur in autumn, when small wild mammals are at maximum population and most active.
• Severe cutaneous and systemic signs with poor prognosis are frequently associated with immunosuppression (iatrogenic or co-infection with FeLV or FIV).
• Cat-to-cat transmission—rare; causes only subclinical infection

DIAGNOSIS

DIFFERENTIAL DIAGNOSIS
• Bacterial and fungal infections
• Eosinophilic granuloma complex
• Neoplasia—particularly mast cell tumor; lymphosarcoma
• Miliary dermatitis

CBC/BIOCHEMISTRY/URINALYSIS
Noncontributory

OTHER LABORATORY TESTS
Serologic testing—demonstrate rising titers; hemagglutination inhibition, virus neutralizing, complement fixation, or ELISA; titers may remain high for months or years.

IMAGING
N/A

DIAGNOSTIC PROCEDURES
• Virus isolation from scab material—definitive diagnosis; 90% positive
• Electron microscopy of extracts of scab, biopsy, or exudate—rapid presumptive diagnosis; 70% positive
• Skin biopsy—characteristic histologic changes of epidermal hyperplasia and hypertrophy; multilocular vesicle and ulceration; large eosinophilic intracytoplasmic inclusion bodies

TREATMENT
• No specific treatment
• Supportive (antibiotics, fluids) when necessary
• Elizabethan collar—to prevent self-induced damage

MEDICATIONS

DRUGS
Antibiotics—prevent secondary infections

CONTRAINDICATIONS/POSSIBLE INTERACTIONS
Immunosuppressive agents (e.g., glucocorticoids and megestrol acetate)—absolutely contraindicated because they can induce fatal systemic disease

FOLLOW-UP

PREVENTION/AVOIDANCE
• Natural reservoir host is possibly small rodents; cats infected incidentally
• Vaccines—none available; vaccinia virus may be considered for valuable zoo collections, but its effects in nondomestic cats have not been investigated

EXPECTED COURSE AND PROGNOSIS
• Most cats recover spontaneously in 1–2 months.
• Healing may be delayed by secondary bacterial skin infection.
• Prognosis is poor with severe respiratory or pulmonary involvement.

MISCELLANEOUS

ZOONOTIC POTENTIAL
• Rare human pox virus infections have been linked to contact with infected cats with skin lesions; use basic hygiene precautions (disposable gloves) when handling infected cats.
• May cause painful skin lesion and severe systemic illness, particularly in the very young or elderly, people with a pre-existing skin condition, and the immunodeficient.

ABBREVIATIONS
• ELISA = enzyme-linked immunoadsorbent assay
• FeLV = feline leukemia virus
• FIV = feline immunodeficiency virus

Suggested Reading
Gaskell RM, Bennett M. Feline poxvirus infection. In: Chandler EA, Gaskell CJ, Gaskell RM, eds. Feline medicine and therapeutics. Oxford, UK: Blackwell Scientific, 1994:515–520.

Author J. Paul Woods
Consulting Editor Stephen C. Barr

PROLAPSED GLAND OF THE THIRD EYELID (CHERRY EYE)

BASICS

OVERVIEW
• Gland of the third eyelid—normally anchored by a fibrous attachment to the periorbita beneath the third eyelid
• Weak attachment—several breeds of dogs and cats; predisposes animals to unilateral or bilateral prolapse

SIGNALMENT
• Dogs and cats
• Dogs—usually in young dogs (aged 6 months to 2 years); common breeds: cocker spaniels, bulldogs, beagles, bloodhounds, lhasa apsos, shih tzus, other brachycephalic breeds
• Cats—rare; occurs in Burmese and Persians

SIGNS
• Oval, hyperemic mass protruding from behind the leading edge of the third eyelid
• May be unilateral or bilateral
• May see accompanying epiphora, hyperemic conjunctiva, or blepharospasm
• Additional swelling and hyperemia caused by environmental irritation and desiccation of the exposed gland

CAUSES & RISK FACTORS
• Congenital weakness of the attachment of the gland of the third eyelid
• Inheritance unknown.

DIAGNOSIS

DIFFERENTIAL DIAGNOSIS
• Scrolled or everted cartilage of the third eyelid—seen in Wiemaraners, Great Danes, German short-haired pointers, and other breeds in which the T-shaped cartilage of the third eyelid is rolled away from the surface of the eye instead of conforming to the surface of the cornea
• Neoplasia of the third eyelid—usually seen in old animals; may see squamous cell carcinoma, lymphosarcoma, or fibrosarcoma; may be origin of adenoma or adenocarcinoma; small incisional biopsy is indicated in old patients (> 7–9 years) to differentiate.
• Orbital fat prolapse—may dissect anteriorly between the conjunctiva and globe; occasionally occurs in the medial canthus and simulates a prolapsed gland of the third eyelid

CBC/BIOCHEMISTRY/URINALYSIS
N/A

OTHER LABORATORY TESTS
N/A

IMAGING
N/A

DIAGNOSTIC PROCEDURES
N/A

TREATMENT
• Surgical replacement of the gland—see Suggested Reading
• Excision of the gland—avoid; gland produces up to 50% of the aqueous tear film; puts patient at substantial risk for developing KCS at it ages
• Elizabethan collar—recommended to prevent self-trauma

MEDICATIONS

DRUGS
Topical anti-inflammatory medications—may be used before and after surgery to lessen swelling

CONTRAINDICATIONS/POSSIBLE INTERACTIONS
N/A

FOLLOW-UP
• Recurrence—5%–20%, depending on the surgical procedure; re-replacement of the gland is encouraged.
• If unilateral, warn client that the other gland may develop a prolapse and that no preventive procedure or medication exists.

MISCELLANEOUS

SYNONYM
Cherry Eye

ABBREVIATION
KCS = keratoconjunctivitis sicca

Suggested Reading
Stanley RG, Kaswan RL. Modification of the orbital rim anchorage method for surgical replacement of the gland of the third eyelid in dogs. J Am Vet Med Assoc 1994;205:1412–1414.

Author Brian C. Gilger
Consulting Editor Paul E. Miller

PROPTOSIS

BASICS

OVERVIEW
• Forward displacement of the globe, with the eyelids situated caudal to the eyeball
• Frequently associated with trauma to the head and usually occurs peracutely
• Potentially vision threatening
• May cause bradycardia secondary to traction on the retrobulbar muscles and the associated oculocardiac reflex (regulated through the trigeminal and vagus nerves)

SIGNALMENT
• More common in the brachycephalic breeds due to the prominence of the eyes, relatively shallow orbits, and large palpebral fissures
• May occur in any species or breed if the traumatic force is severe enough

SIGNS
General Comments
Globe situated anterior to the eyelids so that the eyelids are entrapped posterior to the eyeball

Possible Accompanying Signs
• Abnormalities in pupil size—dilated or constricted
• Corneal ulceration and/or desiccation
• Intraocular inflammation
• Fractures of the bony orbit or other parts of the skull
• Subconjunctival or intraocular hemorrhage
• Rupture of the globe
• Brain trauma
• Trauma to the contralateral eye
• Shock
• Other signs associated with trauma

Associated Signs After Repositioning
• Dorsolateral strabismus—due to rupture of the inferior oblique and medial rectus muscles
• Blindness
• Dilated pupil
• Decreased tear production
• Corneal desiccation

CAUSES & RISK FACTORS
• Trauma—primary cause; relatively minor force in brachiocephalic breeds; usually severe force in dolichocephalic and mesocephalic breeds
• Retrobulbar tumor or severe cellulitis or other infection—rare

DIAGNOSIS

DIFFERENTIAL DIAGNOSIS
• Buphthalmia—enlargement of the globe; rarely acute; eyelids still positioned correctly, but may not be able to close completely over the globe
• Exophthalmia—may be defined as forward displacement of the globe; eyelids positioned correctly; may be acute; rarely peracute; eye cannot be retropulsed due to a mass effect (e.g., neoplasia, retrobulbar polymyositis, infection, or cellulitis) in the retrobulbar tissues.

CBC/BIOCHEMISTRY/URINALYSIS
Normal, unless secondary to trauma

OTHER LABORATORY TESTS
N/A

IMAGING
Skull radiographs—may show fractures owing to trauma

DIAGNOSTIC PROCEDURES
N/A

TREATMENT

• Keep the cornea lubricated.
• Assess the patient systemically before performing surgery on the globe.
• Treat primary condition, as necessary.
• Treat shock and head trauma, if necessary.

Repositioning the Globe
• Perform as soon as possible or once the patient is stable after obvious infection, rupture, or desiccation of the globe or severed optic nerve.
• Performed under sedation and local anesthesia or, if the patient is stable, under general anesthesia
• Preplace two or three temporary tarsorrhaphy mattress sutures through the eyelids, exiting at the lid margins, crossing across to the other lid, entering at the lid margin, and reversing the procedure.
• Lateral canthotomy—may ease tension on the eyelids and allow easier suture placement
• While protecting the globe (a lubricated scalpel blade handle can serve this function), tie the preplaced sutures and reposition the globe; suture the lateral canthotomy closed.

MEDICATIONS

DRUGS
• Systemic and topical broad-spectrum antibiotics—until sutures are removed
• Systemic corticosteroids—usually used at least initially; may be continued on a chronic basis with marked periorbital and retrobulbar swelling
• Topical corticosteroids—may be used with associated intraocular inflammation (uveitis) or hyphema, as long as no corneal or conjunctival ulcers exist
• Topical atropine—for intraocular inflam-

mation or hyphema; relieve ciliary spasm and lower the risk of synechiae

CONTRAINDICATIONS/POSSIBLE INTERACTIONS
• Topical corticosteroids—do not use with ulcerations.
• Systemic corticosteroids—do not use with retrobulbar infection.

FOLLOW-UP

PATIENT MONITORING
• Suture removal—usually done sequentially, rather than all at once, starting 10–14 days after repositioning. Integrity of the globe, vision, and cornea—reassessed 10–14 days after surgery

POSSIBLE COMPLICATIONS
• Most patients retain a dorsolateral strabismus, which may improve with time. • Schirmer tear tests—perform after suture removal; may note decreased tear production • Neurotrophic keratitis with chronic ulceration secondary to corneal denervation

EXPECTED COURSE AND PROGNOSIS
• Most affected eyes can be salvaged; majority caused by trauma will be blind (more common in the dolichocephalic than in the brachycephalic breeds). • Normal retinal vessels and optic nerve, normal IOP, and a short time from occurrence to repair—relatively favorable prognosis for maintaining vision • Positive menace response or direct or consensual pupillary light reflex originating from the injured eye—good prognosis for maintaining vision • Pupil size at the time of the injury—not necessarily an accurate prognostic indicator; mydriasis may be the result of trauma to the optic nerve (if permanent, results in blindness) or damage to the oculomotor nerve (does not affect vision) • Miosis—does not necessarily indicate a good prognosis for vision; most likely cause is uveitis (if severe enough, pupillary constriction occurs even with retinal or optic nerve damage)

MISCELLANEOUS

SEE ALSO
Orbital Diseases (Exophthalmus, Enophthalmus, Strabismus)

ABBREVIATION
IOP = intraocular pressure

Suggested Reading
Slatter D. Fundamentals of veterinary ophthalmology. 2nd ed. Philadelphia: Saunders, 1990.
Author Stephanie L. Smedes
Consulting Editor Paul E. Miller

BASICS

OVERVIEW
Prostatic and periprostatic cysts are single or multiple, epithelial-lined, serosanguineous fluid-filled structures. The cysts are usually large and are attached to, or in the region of, the prostate gland. Although the cause is rarely known, obstruction of prostatic ducts ("retention cyst"), expansion of microscopic cysts of benign prostatic hyperplasia, and, rarely, resolution of a hematoma, have been considered.

SIGNALMENT
Adult male intact dogs; age range 2–12 years, mean age 7.5 years

SIGNS
• Dysuria
• Tenesmus
• Urethral discharge
• Abdominal distension

CAUSES AND RISK FACTORS
Androgenic hormones

DIAGNOSIS

DIFFERENTIAL DIAGNOSIS
• Prostatic abscess
• Distended urinary bladder
• Prostatic neoplasia
• Results of cytologic examination of fluid and ultrasonographic examination usually rule out these diseases. Prostatic neoplasia is occasionally associated with cystic areas

within the prostate. The cysts can become secondarily infected, so detection of bacteria should not be overinterpreted.

CBC/BIOCHEMISTRY/URINALYSIS
No abnormalities expected

OTHER LABORATORY TESTS
• Cytologic examination of cyst fluid (often collected by ultrasound-guided, fine-needle aspiration) usually reveals serosanguineous fluid.
• Culture the fluid for bacteria, since it can become infected secondarily.

IMAGING
• Contrast urocystography and ultrasonography will differentiate intraprostatic from extraprostatic locations.
• Detection of calcified cysts by survey radiography (rare) is diagnostic for osteocollagenous prostatic retention cyst.

OTHER DIAGNOSTIC PROCEDURES
N/A

TREATMENT
• If cysts are large, infected, or causing clinical signs, complete surgical excision (if possible) is the treatment of choice. If surgical excision is not feasible, biopsy and marsupialize the cyst wall. Concomitant castration is recommended to reduce the development of nonneoplastic prostatic disease.
• If the cysts are small, castration is the treatment of choice. Reevaluate after castration to confirm resolution of the cyst(s).

MEDICATIONS

DRUGS
N/A

CONTRAINDICATIONS/POSSIBLE INTERACTIONS
N/A

FOLLOW-UP
• Ultrasonographic examination at 2- to 4-week intervals after castration to follow resolution of small cysts
• Evaluation 2 weeks after surgery may be adequate if no complications arise. If a drainage procedure is used, periodic evaluations (biweekly after discharge from the hospital) are recommended.
• Postoperative urinary incontinence and ascending infection are common potential sequelae of marsupialization; a guarded prognosis is warranted if complete cyst resection is not possible.

MISCELLANEOUS

Suggested Reading

Weaver AD. Discrete prostatic (paraprostatic) cysts in the dog. Vet Rec 1978;102:435–440.
Author Laine A. Cowan
Consulting Editors Larry G. Adams and Carl A. Osborne

PROSTATITIS AND PROSTATIC ABSCESS

BASICS

DEFINITION
Subdivided into acute bacterial prostatitis, chronic bacterial prostatitis, and prostatic abscess; fungal and granulomatous prostatitis are extremely rare. Acute and chronic prostatitis refer to the inflammatory process and are differentiated by clinical signs. Prostatic abscess is intraprostatic parenchymal accumulation of purulent inflammatory reactants.

PATHOPHYSIOLOGY
• Bacteria usually gain access to the prostate gland by ascending the urethra and overcoming the lower urinary tract host defense mechanisms. Most intact male dogs with bacterial urinary tract infection have the same bacteria present in the prostate gland. However, dogs with prostatic inflammation may have a prostatic infection without evidence of bacteria or inflammation in their urine. • Incomplete resolution of acute bacterial prostatitis can lead to chronic bacterial prostatitis or abscess formation; however, most dogs with chronic bacterial prostatitis do not have a history of urinary tract or prostatic infection. • Intraprostatic accumulation of prostatic secretions (e.g., in animals with cystic benign prostatic hyperplasia or squamous metaplasia) can become secondarily infected, resulting in chronic bacterial prostatitis or prostatic abscess.

SYSTEMS AFFECTED
• Renal/Urologic—the remainder of the urinary tract can be infected by extension of the urinary tract infection. • Reproductive—alterations in prostatic fluid in dogs with bacterial prostatitis can cause infertility. • Gastrointestinal—dogs with acute bacterial prostatitis or abscess often have tenesmus when the prostate gland is large or tender. • Hepatobiliary—some dogs with prostatic abscess have hyperbilirubinemia and high alkaline phosphatase (ALP). Liver alterations probably result from sepsis and the resulting cholestasis. • Peritoneum—focal or generalized peritonitis can develop in animals with prostatic abscessation.

GENETICS
No known genetic basis

INCIDENCE/PREVALENCE
Since many dogs with chronic bacterial prostatitis are asymptomatic, the prevalence is difficult to determine. Among surveys of dogs with prostatic disease, infection was present in 40%.

GEOGRAPHIC DISTRIBUTION
N/A

SIGNALMENT

Species
Dogs

Breed Predilections
Any breed can be affected; higher prevalence in doberman pinschers than in other breeds

Mean Age and Range
• Dogs with bacterial prostatitis usually are middle-aged • Mean age, 7–11 years; range, 1–16 years

Predominant Sex
Intact male dogs

SIGNS

Common Signs
• Lethargy • Blood or pus dripping from the urethra independent of urination • Tenesmus • Pyrexia • Pain

Less Common Signs
• Shock • Stiff hind limb gait • Preputial or hind limb edema
Clinical signs are useful in differentiating chronic bacterial prostatitis from acute bacterial prostatitis and prostatic abscess.
• Dogs with chronic bacterial prostatitis are often asymptomatic. • Dogs with acute bacterial prostatitis are systemically ill, usually depressed, and febrile, and the prostate gland is tender on palpation. • Dogs with prostatic abscess usually have signs similar to those with acute bacterial prostatitis and prostatomegaly. Occasionally, these dogs may have extremes of signs—they can be asymptomatic or be in septic shock; occasionally, prostatic abscess impinges on the urethra and causes stranguria.

CAUSES
• Bacterial urinary tract infection in an intact dog usually results in concomitant prostatic infection. • Gonadal infection (e.g., *Brucella canis*) is less common than urinary tract infection. • Systemic mycotic pathogens are rare.

RISK FACTORS
• Impaired host immunity—e.g., corticosteroid administration, diabetes mellitus, urinary retention, urolithiasis, and lower urinary tract anatomic abnormality • High urinary/urethral bacterial numbers—e.g., caused by catheterization • Intraprostatic accumulation of prostatic secretions, such as cystic benign prostatic hypertrophy or squamous metaplasia, may become infected secondarily.

DIAGNOSIS

DIFFERENTIAL DIAGNOSIS
• Noninfectious prostatic disease—e.g., benign prostatic hypertrophy, neoplasia, prostatic cysts, and periprostatic or perirectal masses or cysts • Disease that causes tenesmus—e.g., large intestinal disease • Rectal and abdominal palpation helps localize the problem to the prostate gland. Can rule out benign prostatic hypertrophy, cysts, and neoplasia on the basis of results of ultrasonography and cytologic examination or histopathologic evaluation of the prostate gland.

CBC/BIOCHEMISTRY/URINALYSIS
• Chronic bacterial prostatitis—hematuria, pyuria, and bacteriuria in some patients • Acute bacterial prostatitis—pyuria and bacteriuria ± hematuria in most animals; neutrophilic leukocytosis ± left shift and neutrophil toxicity • Abscess—pyuria and bacteriuria, ± hematuria in most animals; neutrophilic leukocytosis with a regenerative left shift, high ALP and bilirubin, and hypoglycemia

OTHER LABORATORY TESTS
Prostatic fluid evaluation by cytologic examination and bacterial culture confirms the diagnosis of bacterial prostatitis.

IMAGING
Ultrasonographic evaluation of the prostate gland helps differentiate cavitary (i.e., abscess) from noncavitary (i.e., acute bacterial prostatitis and chronic bacterial prostatitis) bacterial prostatic diseases noninvasively.

DIAGNOSTIC PROCEDURES
• Use prostatic wash techniques cautiously in patients with acute bacterial prostatitis or prostatic abscess; sepsis or abscess rupture can result. • Examination of an ultrasound-guided, fine-needle aspiration of a cystic region in the prostate may be used to confirm an abscess if no ejaculate can be obtained, but fine-needle aspiration can also rupture an abscess. If a prostatic abscess is suspected, avoid percutaneous needle biopsy. • In dogs with prostatic abscess that are not systemically ill—a preoperative cystometrogram and urethral pressure profile may yield baseline measurements for use if the dog develops urinary incontinence after surgery.

PATHOLOGIC FINDINGS
• Biopsies are rarely indicated in animals with acute bacterial prostatitis or chronic bacterial prostatitis. • Acute bacterial prostatitis—purulent inflammation may be multifocal or centered on the acini or it may invade the stroma; if the prostatic ducts are occluded during resolution of the acute inflammation, multifocal, walled-off, chronic bacterial prostatitis may result; alternatively, the acute inflammation may cause scarring. • Chronic bacterial prostatitis—the disease process is usually focal or multifocal; the diagnostic histologic lesion may be missed if a small sample is obtained. The typical eosinophilic staining of the columnar epithelium is lost. The acinar lumina and periacinar tissue contain debris and are infiltrated with various numbers of neutrophils and macrophages. • Prostatic abscess—multifocal accumulations of purulent exudate in the prostatic parenchyma

PROSTATITIS AND PROSTATIC ABSCESS

TREATMENT

APPROPRIATE HEALTH CARE
Treat dogs with chronic bacterial prostatitis as outpatients. Hospitalization is required because dogs with acute bacterial prostatitis are systemically ill, and dogs with abscesses require surgery.

NURSING CARE
Patients with acute bacterial prostatitis or prostatic abscess usually require parenteral fluid support. If in shock, administer a shock dose (90 mL/kg for 1 h) of isotonic fluids (0.9% NaCl or lactated Ringer solution). If the patient is hypoglycemic, add glucose to the fluids. Treatment for septic shock (including flunixine and dexamethasone) may be necessary.

ACTIVITY
• No restrictions necessary • Dogs may be infertile; do not breed until infection resolves.

DIET
N/A

CLIENT EDUCATION
• Acute and chronic prostatitis can become recurrent problems—manifested as chronic bacterial prostatitis or abscess • Prostatic abscessation can be life-threatening—e.g., sepsis and shock • Postoperative urinary incontinence and recurrent infection are common; repeat surgery may be necessary in dogs with prostatic abscess.

SURGICAL CONSIDERATIONS
• Penrose tube drainage, marsupialization, and partial or complete prostatectomy procedures have been recommended; the latter two require special surgical expertise. Preliminary reports on the use of an ultrasonic surgical aspirator (for subtotal prostatectomy in dogs with prostatic abscesses) are promising. Although surgical drainage is essential for treatment of prostatic abscess, problems are associated with each surgical option. • Many of these dogs are poor anesthetic candidates because of sepsis. • To lessen the likelihood of recurrence, castrate dogs with prostatic infection—after infection resolves in patients with acute bacterial prostatitis or chronic bacterial prostatitis

MEDICATIONS

DRUGS OF CHOICE
• Patients with chronic bacterial prostatitis—chosen antibiotic must be able to enter the prostatic lumen and be chosen on the basis of in vitro susceptibility testing; usually, trimethoprim/sulfonamides or fluoroquinolones are the drugs of choice (since *Escherichia coli* is the most common organism); a minimum of 4 weeks of antimicrobial administration is necessary. • Patients with acute bacterial prostatitis—a similar antimicrobial choice is appropriate while awaiting the results of the bacterial susceptibility; penetration into the prostate gland is not as great a concern; usually, a 3-week regimen suffices. • Patients with acute bacterial prostatitis and prostatic abscess—dogs are usually systemically ill and may be septic; parenteral antibiotics are indicated until the dog is stable; a minimum of 8 weeks of antimicrobial administration is indicated for dogs with prostatic abscess • Patients with tenesmus—a stool softener such as psyllium can be used

CONTRAINDICATIONS
Estrogens and androgens may cause prostatic squamous metaplasia or enlargement, respectively.

PRECAUTIONS
• In sensitive dogs, long-term sulfonamide administration may lead to keratoconjunctivitis sicca. • An adverse reaction to sulfonamide drugs, characterized by a cutaneous or lupus-like syndrome, has occurred in a small number of doberman pinschers.

POSSIBLE INTERACTIONS
None

ALTERNATIVE DRUGS
• If the bacteria are not sensitive to the drugs listed, other antimicrobials that enter the prostate gland include chloramphenicol, erythromycin, and clindamycin. • Colloids ± hypertonic saline may be used to treat septic shock.

FOLLOW-UP

PATIENT MONITORING
• Because of the problem of recurrent infection, repeat prostatic fluid culture is indicated 1, 4, and 8 weeks after completion of the antimicrobial regimen. • Reevaluate dogs treated for prostatic abscess should be reevaluated every 2 weeks until the problem resolves: ultrasound imaging, urine analysis, prostatic fluid analysis, and a CBC are usually indicated at each reevaluation.

PREVENTION/AVOIDANCE
Castration, by causing prostatic involution, is the best method of preventing recurrence.

POSSIBLE COMPLICATIONS
• Recurrent urinary tract infections • Urinary incontinence—primarily associated with prostatic abscess • Infected stoma or edema—associated with some prostatic drainage procedures

EXPECTED COURSE AND PROGNOSIS
• Aside from the potential for recurrent prostatic infection, acute and chronic bacterial prostatitis usually respond well to treatment. • Dogs with prostatic abscesses often need prolonged follow-up and reassessment. • Some dogs that are incontinent immediately after surgery may regain partial or complete urinary control with drug therapy.

MISCELLANEOUS

ASSOCIATED CONDITIONS
Urinary tract infection, urocystolithiasis, and chronic glucocorticoid exposure (iatrogenic or hyperadrenocorticism) may be associated with chronic bacterial prostatitis.

AGE-RELATED FACTORS
Sexually mature dogs

ZOONOTIC POTENTIAL
Brucella canis has been isolated from dogs with prostatic infection (rare).

PREGNANCY
N/A

SYNONYMS
None

SEE ALSO
• Benign Prostatic Hyperplasia • Dysuria and Pollakiuria • Hematuria • Incontinence, Urinary • Lower Urinary Tract Infection • Prostatic Cysts • Prostatomegaly • Pyelonephritis • Pyuria• Urine Retention, Functional • Urinary Tract Obstruction

ABBREVIATIONS
ALP = alkaline phosphatase

Suggested Reading

Feeney DA, Johnston GR, Klausner JS, et al. Canine prostatic disease—comparison of ultrasonographic appearance with morphologic and microbiologic findings: 30 cases (1981–1985). J Am Vet Med Assoc 1987;190:1027–1034.

Krawiec DR, Heflin D. Study of prostatic disease in dogs: 177 cases (1981–1986) J Am Vet Med Assoc 1992;200:1119–1122.

Mullen HS, Matthiesen DT, Scavelli TD. Results of surgery and postoperative complications in 92 dogs treated for prostatic abscessation by a multiple penrose drain technique. J Am Anim Hosp Assoc 1990;26:369–379.

Rawlings CA, Crowell WA, Barsanti JA, et al. Intracapsular subtotal prostatectomy in normal dogs: use of an ultrasonic surgical aspirator. Vet Surg 1994;23:182–189.

Author Laine A. Cowan
Consulting Editors Larry G. Adams and Carl A. Osborne

PROTEIN-LOSING ENTEROPATHY

 BASICS

DEFINITION
• A group of diseases characterized by excessive loss of serum proteins into the intestinal tract
• The diseases associated with PLE include primary gastrointestinal diseases and generalized disorders such as congestive heart failure, nephrotic syndrome, and metastatic neoplasia.

PATHOPHYSIOLOGY
• The intestines serve as a route for catabolism of serum proteins.
• The capillaries in the intestinal mucosa have large fenestrations that allow macromolecules to enter the interstitial space.
• Once they leak into the gastrointestinal tract through these fenestrations, serum proteins are rapidly digested into constituent amino acids that can be reabsorbed and used for synthesis of new proteins.
• In the dog, two-thirds of normal protein loss occurs through the small intestine.
• If this normal protein loss is accelerated by mucosal disease processes or by obstruction of lymphatic outflow from the intestines, protein (both albumin and globulin) is lost.
• In response to increased protein loss through the intestines, the liver increases production of albumin, but the liver cannot increase albumin synthesis to more than twice normal production.
• When protein loss exceeds protein synthesis, hypoproteinemia results. • Hypoproteinemia causes decreased plasma oncotic pressure, which alters body fluid hemodynamics and leads to peripheral edema or body cavity effusions.

SYSTEMS AFFECTED
• Gastrointestinal—diarrhea, vomiting, ascites
• Respiratory—pleural effusion, dyspnea
• Skin/exocrine—subcutaneous edema

GENETICS
Breeds of dogs with a familial predisposition for intestinal lymphangiectasia include soft-coated wheaten terrier, basenji, and lundehund.

INCIDENCE/PREVALENCE
True incidence unknown

GEOGRAPHIC DISTRIBUTION
N/A

SIGNALMENT

Species
Dogs and cats

Breed Predilection
See Genetics

• Increased prevalence for intestinal lymphangiectasia has been reported in Yorkshire terriers.

Mean Age and Range
Any age

Predominant Sex
None

SIGNS

General comments
Clinical signs are variable.

Historical findings
• Diarrhea (chronic, intermittent, watery to semisolid), weight loss, and lethargy—most frequently reported
• Vomiting—uncommon

Physical Examination Findings
• Ascites, dependent edema, and dyspnea from pleural effusion are detected with marked hypoproteinemia.
• Abdominal palpation may reveal thickened bowel loops.

CAUSES

Disorders of Lymphatics
• Intestinal lymphangiectasia
• Neoplasia (lymphosarcoma)
• Granuloma of the small bowel or mesentery
• Congestive heart failure—constrictive pericarditis, Budd-Chiari syndrome

Diseases Associated with Increased Mucosal Permeability or Mucosal Ulceration
• Lymphoplasmacytic enteritis
• Intestinal neoplasia—lymphosarcoma, carcinoma
• Acute or chronic enteritis
• Intussusception—especially chronic
• Chronic foreign body
• Ulcerative gastritis/enteritis
• Histoplasmosis
• Granulomatous enteritis
• Intestinal parasitism—hookworms, whipworms, coccidia
• Hemorrhagic gastroenteritis
• Immune-mediated diseases—food allergies, eosinophilic gastroenteritis, gluten-induced enteropathies

RISK FACTORS
• Disorders of lymphatics
• Heart disease
• Gastrointestinal disease

 DIAGNOSIS

DIFFERENTIAL DIAGNOSIS
• Must differentiate from other causes of hypoproteinemia

• Severe hepatic disease causes reduced hepatic synthesis of albumin; globulin level is often normal or high.
• Glomerulonephritis or renal amyloidosis causes excessive loss of albumin.
• Should detect proteinuria by urinalysis; globulin level usually normal
• Acute or chronic blood loss
• Inadequate protein intake (i.e., starvation) is a rare cause of hypoproteinemia.

CBC/BIOCHEMISTRY/URINALYSIS
• May be anemia
• Lymphopenia is seen with lymphangiectasia.
• Hypoalbuminemia and hypoglobulinemia (panhypoproteinemia)
• Hypocalcemia—secondary to hypoalbuminemia
• May be hypocholesterolemia
• Urinalysis should be normal.

OTHER LABORATORY TESTS
• Perform three to five fecal examinations to rule out parasitism; they should be negative.
• Serum protein electrophoresis can quantitate and identify protein loss; gastrointestinal protein loss is characterized by loss of albumin and globulins; liver disease is characterized by low levels of albumin with normal or high globulins, and renal disease characteristically causes hypoalbuminemia with normal serum globulins.
• Can determine urinary protein:creatinine ratio to rule out proteinuria.
• Serum bile acids (pre- and postprandial) to assess hepatic function
• Specific gastrointestinal function tests—Sudan stains to detect steatorrhea, oral D-xylose test to detect poor absorption of carbohydrates, and plasma turbidity test to detect abnormal fat absorption
• Cytologic examination of feces and rectal mucosal smears may reveal histoplasmosis.
• Can measure fecal α_1-antiprotease, a plasma protein that resists proteolytic degradation in the gastrointestinal tract; concentration should be high with PLE.

IMAGING
• Take survey thoracic and abdominal radiographs to rule out causes of PLE such as cardiac disease, fungal disease, and intestinal obstruction.
• Perform cardiac ultrasound to rule out cardiac disease.
• Perform upper gastrointestinal contrast study to look for infiltrative bowel diseases or masses.
• Can use radioactive labels to document protein loss through the gastrointestinal tract; the gold standard has been ^{51}Cr-labeled albumin; other radioactive labels used successfully include ^{51}Cr-labeled EDTA and ^{111}In-labeled transferrin.

PROTEIN-LOSING ENTEROPATHY

DIAGNOSTIC PROCEDURES
• Endoscopy allows mucosal visualization and biopsy.
• Laparotomy allows visualization of dilated intestinal lymphatics and biopsy of intestines (full-thickness) and lymph nodes.

PATHOLOGIC FINDINGS

Intestinal Lymphangiectasia
• Gross—visualization of dilated lymphatics in the mesentery and on the serosal surface of intestines; may see yellow-white nodules and foamy granular deposits adjacent to lymphatics
• Histopathologic—a ballooning distortion of villi caused by markedly dilated lacteals; the villi can be edematous, and some have a blunted appearance; mucosal edema is usually present, and diffuse or multifocal accumulations of lymphocytes and plasma cells can be identified in the lamina propria.

Lymphoplasmacytic Enteritis
Histopathologic—infiltration of the lamina propria with lymphocytes and plasma cells; villous atrophy may be present; inflammation should be characterized as mild, moderate, or severe.

Intestinal Lymphosarcoma
• Gross—diffuse or segmental thickening of loops of intestine; mesenteric lymphadenopathy is often observed.
• Histopathologic—diffuse infiltration of the lamina propria and submucosa with neoplastic lymphocytes

Histoplasmosis
• Gross—may include thickened loops of intestine, mesenteric lymphadenopathy, hepatomegaly, and splenomegaly
• Histopathologic—*Histoplasma capsulatum* organisms within macrophages in the lamina propria and submucosa

TREATMENT

APPROPRIATE HEALTH CARE
Most can be treated as outpatients.

NURSING CARE
• Can give plasma transfusions, hetastarch, or dextran to increase plasma oncotic pressure when clinical signs from edema or effusion are severe
• Administer these agents at a dose of 6–20 mL/kg IV; the infusion rate should not exceed 2.5–5 mL/kg/h.

ACTIVITY
Normal

DIET
Usually modified, depending on the underlying cause of PLE

CLIENT EDUCATION
Prepare clients for long-term therapy; spontaneous cures are rare.

SURGICAL CONSIDERATIONS
• Hypoalbuminemia increases postoperative morbidity because of slow wound healing.
• Some causes of PLE (e.g., intestinal neoplasia, intussusception, chronic foreign body) require surgical intervention.

MEDICATIONS

DRUGS OF CHOICE
• Can use diuretics such as furosemide to control edema and pleural effusion, although they do not work well because of decreased plasma oncotic pressure
• Treat intestinal lymphangiectasia, the most common lesion in PLE, by feeding a low-fat diet.
• Can use corticosteroids if dietary therapy is unsuccessful or if no underlying cause for intestinal lymphangiectasia can be found
• Intestinal lymphosarcoma treatment includes the use of chemotherapeutic agents.
• Lymphoplasmacytic enteritis treatment includes dietary modification and immunosuppressive agents.
• Antibiotics such as metronidazole, sulfasalazine, or tylosin may be effective.
• Treat eosinophilic gastroenteritis by feeding a hypoallergenic diet and administering corticosteroids.
• Treat gluten-induced enteropathy by feeding a high-protein diet with exclusion of glutens that are contained in wheat, rye, barley, oats, and buckwheat; alternatively, corticosteroids or other immunosuppressive agents can be used.

CONTRAINDICATIONS
N/A

PRECAUTIONS
N/A

POSSIBLE INTERACTIONS
N/A

ALTERNATIVE DRUGS
N/A

FOLLOW-UP

PATIENT MONITORING
Check body weight, serum protein concentration, and evidence of recurrent clinical signs (pleural effusion, ascites, and/or edema) every 7–14 days.

PREVENTION/AVOIDANCE
N/A

POSSIBLE COMPLICATIONS
• Respiratory difficulty from pleural effusion
• Severe protein-calorie malnutrition
• Intractable diarrhea
• Prognosis is guarded; primary disease often cannot be cured.

EXPECTED COURSE AND PROGNOSIS
Varies considerably with underlying cause

MISCELLANEOUS

ASSOCIATED CONDITIONS
Soft-coated wheaten terriers may have protein-losing nephropathy in conjunction with PLE.

AGE-RELATED FACTORS
N/A

ZOONOTIC POTENTIAL
Histoplasmosis, hookworms, and coccidia are potentially zoonotic to humans.

PREGNANCY
N/A

SYNONYMS
N/A

ABBREVIATION
PLE = protein-losing enteropathy

Suggested Reading
Berry CR, Guilford WG, Koblik PD, et al. Scintigraphic evaluation of four dogs with protein-losing enteropathy using [111]Indium-labeled transferrin. Vet Radiol Ultrasound 1997;38:221–225.
Fossum TW. Protein-losing enteropathy. Semin Vet Med Surg (Small Anim) 1989;4:219–225.
Fossum TW, Sherding RG, Zack PM, et al. Intestinal lymphangiectasia associated with chylothorax in two dogs. J Am Vet Med Assoc 1987;190:61–64.
Hall EJ, Batt RM. Enhanced intestinal permeability to ^{51}Cr-labeled EDTA in dogs with small intestinal disease. J Am Vet Med Assoc 1990;196:91–95.
Tams TR, Twedt DC. Canine protein-losing gastroenteropathy syndrome. Compend Contin Educ Pract Vet 1981;3:105–114.
Author Mollyann Holland
Consulting Editors Brett M. Feder and Mitchell A. Crystal

PROTOTHECOSIS

BASICS

OVERVIEW
• *Prototheca wickerhamii* and *P. zopfii*—single-celled achlorophyllous blue-green algae (Chlorophyta) that can cause disease in warm-blooded animals
• Humans and cats—usually localized infection of the skin or gastrointestinal tract
• Dogs—usually widely disseminated disease

SIGNALMENT
• Dogs and cats—uncommon
• Dogs—medium-large, middle-aged females most frequently affected

SIGNS

Historical Findings
Dogs
• Intermittent and chronic bloody diarrhea
• Chronic weight loss
• Blindness
• Neurologic disease
• Cutaneous lesions
Cats
Chronic cutaneous or mucous membrane ulceration with few systemic signs

Physical Examination Findings
Dogs
• Depend on organ system involvement
• Most often disseminated
• Hemorrhagic colitis
• Severe weight loss
• Debilitation
• Blindness with posterior segment disease and/or retinal granulomas and/or detached retinas not infrequent
• CNS—depression, ataxia, vestibular signs, and paresis may be seen.
• Ragged ulcers and crusts found on the extremities and mucosal surfaces—a few cases with cutaneous infection
Cats
Large cutaneous nodules on the limbs or face

CAUSES & RISK FACTORS
• Dogs—usually *P. zopfii*; one reported case of *P. wickerhamii* infection
• Cats—usually *P. wickerhamii*
• Basis for the pathogenicity of Prototheca unknown
• Organism—ecological niche is raw and treated sewage; survive as contaminants of water, soil, and food; occasionally isolated from fresh fecal samples from healthy individuals
• Dogs and humans—depressed cell-mediated immunity may predispose to gastrointestinal and disseminated infections with *P. zopfii.*
• Cats—no known predisposing factors

DIAGNOSIS

DIFFERENTIAL DIAGNOSIS
• Systemic—systemic mycoses
• Cutaneous—systemic and subcutaneous mycoses; mycobacterioses

CBC/BIOCHEMISTRY/URINALYSIS
• Dogs—often normal; depends on organ system affected; organism occasionally seen in urine sediment
• Cats—almost always normal

OTHER LABORATORY TESTS
CSF tap—may find pleocytosis with mononuclear cells; increased protein; organisms

IMAGING
N/A

DIAGNOSITIC PROCEDURES

Cytology
• Most common definitively diagnostic test; use Wright-Giemsa stain
• Rectal or colonic mucosa, anterior chamber aspirations, CSF taps, cutaneous aspirations
• Organisms—unicellular, nonpigmented, oval; 1.5–16 μm in diameter; cell walls often appear folded; diagnostic characteristic is endospore formation with internal septation in two planes.

Histopathology
Biopsy specimens—identification of organisms may be diagnostic; special stains (GMS or PAS) or IFA stains used at the CDC

Culture
• Grow on Sabouraud dextrose agar at 25–37°C (77–97°F) in 2 to 7 days; or on blood agar.
• Specific identification accomplished by IFA at the CDC.

PATHOLOGIC FINDINGS

Dogs
• Small granulomatous foci—may be found in many organs, especially kidneys
• Colonic muscularis and myocardium
• Nodular thickening of the gastrointestinal mucosa with ulceration
• Granulomas—poorly organized; mixed with other inflammatory cells
• Organisms—contained within macrophages and multinucleate giant cells; may be masses in the colon and kidney with minimal inflammatory response; may be masses in all layers and subjacent fascia and muscle of cutaneous lesions (ulceration frequent)

Cats
Cutaneous masses—localized; extend deep into subcutaneous tissues; consist of granulomatous inflammation and mixed cell inflammation; made up primarily by organisms

TREATMENT
• Dogs—depends on organ system(s) involved
• Cats—excision of localized cutaneous masses is primary therapeutic modality.

MEDICATIONS

DRUGS
• Amphotericin B—use for localized disease after surgical excision; 0.25–0.5 mg/kg IV 3 times weekly or until a total dose of 8 mg/kg; or lipid formulation; concurrent administration of tetracyclines may provide synergistic effect; lipid formulations may be more efficacious and less toxic for cutaneous disease; reported effective for ocular disease
• Ketoconazole, fluconazole, and itraconazole—may use in conjunction with amphotericin B, as consolidation treatment, or as sole agents for less life-threatening disease
• Alternative treatments—clotrimazole (locally for *P. wickerhamii*); potassium iodide

CONTRAINDICATIONS/POSSIBLE INTERACTIONS
N/A

FOLLOW-UP

EXPECTED COURSE AND PROGNOSIS
• Difficult to eradicate with drug therapy
• No well-defined therapeutic protocol
• Dogs—prognosis guarded to grave
• Cats—prognosis fair to good for cutaneous disease if lesions can be completely excised

MISCELLANEOUS

ZOONOTIC POTENTIAL
None recorded

ABBREVIATIONS
• CSF = cerebrospinal fluid
• GMS = Gomori methenamine silver
• IFA = immunofluorescent antibody test
• PAS = periodic acid–Schiff

Suggested Reading
Greene CE. Protothecosis. In. Greene CE, ed. Infectious diseases of the dog and cat. Philadelphia: Saunders, 1998:430–435.
Author Carol S. Foil
Consulting Editor Stephen C. Barr

PSEUDORABIES VIRUS INFECTION

BASICS

OVERVIEW
• Uncommon but highly fatal disease of dogs and cats, usually occurring in animals that have contact with swine
• Characterized by sudden death, often without characteristic signs or with signs that include hypersalivation, intense pruritus, and neurologic changes

SIGNALMENT
• Domestic and exotic dogs and cats
• Other domestic animals—swine, cattle, sheep, and goats
• Primarily farm dogs and cats, with no breed or age predilection

SIGNS
• Sudden death
• Hypersalivation
• Rapid and labored breathing
• Fever
• Vomiting
• Neurologic—depression and lethargy, ataxia, convulsions, reluctance to move, recumbency, intense pruritus and self-mutilation, coma, and death

CAUSES & RISK FACTORS
• Pseudorabies virus (herpesvirus suid)—an α-herpesvirus
• Contact with swine
• Eating contaminated, uncooked meat or offal from swine
• Ingestion of infected rats

DIAGNOSIS

DIFFERENTIAL DIAGNOSIS
• Rabies—in the furious form, affected dog or cat will attack anything that moves; no pruritus or sudden death; immunofluorescent antibody test of brain positive
• Canine distemper—no hypersalivation, sudden death, or personality change; respiratory and gastrointestinal signs common
• Poisoning (organophosphate, lead, strychnine, inorganic arsenic)—no pruritus or personality change; history of exposure to toxin; signs consistent with toxicity

CBC/BIOCHEMISTRY/URINALYSIS
No characteristic changes

OTHER LABORATORY TESTS
Serologic assays—reveal pseudorabies virus antibodies if an animal recovers

IMAGING
N/A

DIAGNOSTIC PROCEDURES
• Immunofluorescent antibody test—brain tissue
• Viral isolation—affected tissues
• Animal (rabbit) inoculation

PATHOLOGIC FINDINGS
• Severe skin lesions—caused by self-mutilation from intense pruritus
• Histopathologic examination—glial and ganglion cells of neurologic tissues reveal Cowdry type A intranuclear inclusion bodies
• Nonsupporative meningoencephalitis in the medulla oblongata

TREATMENT

• Dogs and cats—no known effective treatment
• General supportive therapy and prevention of self-injury indicated

MEDICATIONS

DRUG(S)
• None specific
• Antiherpetic antivirals—not evaluated for dogs and cats
• Rapid course makes successful use of antiviral drugs unlikely.

CONTRAINDICATIONS/POSSIBLE INTERACTIONS
None

FOLLOW-UP

PREVENTION/AVOIDANCE
• Avoid contact with infected swine, the reservoir host.
• Avoid ingestion of contaminated pork.
• Avoid ingestion of infected rats.
• Cat-to-cat and dog-to-dog transmission usually does not occur.

EXPECTED COURSE AND PROGNOSIS
• Classic (cats)—60% of cases; lasts 24–36 hr; almost invariably fatal
• Atypical (cats)—40% of cases; lasts > 36 hr; almost invariably fatal

MISCELLANEOUS

ZOONOTIC POTENTIAL
Mild potential for human infection; take precautions when treating infected animals and handling infected tissues and fluids.

Suggested Reading
Gustafson DP. Pseudorabies (Aujeszky's disease, mad itch, infectious bulbar paralysis). In: Holzworth J, ed. Diseases of the cat. Philadelphia: Saunders, 1987:242–246.
Author Fred W. Scott
Consulting Editor Stephen C. Barr

PUG ENCEPHALITIS (MENINGOENCEPHALITIS)

BASICS

OVERVIEW
• One of the breed-restricted encephalitis defined by highly characteristic morphologic features
• Similar to the described necrotizing encephalitis of Maltese dogs
• Differs from necrotizing encephalitis of Yorkshire terriers by clinical and pathologic features
• Sporadic disease; known for many years; occurs worldwide
• A genetic basis is probable.
• Affects the CNS

SIGNALMENT
• Pug dogs
• Age range—6 months to 7 years

SIGNS
• Generalized seizures—most common; may be the only sign at the beginning of the disease
• Typical for cortical involvement—circling, blindness
• Cervical rigidity sometimes seen

CAUSES & RISK FACTORS
• Unknown
• An infectious agent might be suspected.

DIAGNOSIS

DIFFERENTIAL DIAGNOSIS
Neoplasia and other inflammatory or infectious diseases

CBC/BIOCHEMISTRY/URINALYSIS
Usually normal

OTHER LABORATORY TESTS
N/A

IMAGING
CT and MRI (brain)—nonspecific changes; may help support the clinical diagnosis considering breed and age

DIAGNOSTIC PROCEDURES
• CSF analysis—pleocytosis (200–550 leukocytes/mm³) with mononuclear cells; lymphocytes predominating cell population; mild protein elevation
• Brain biopsy—should help confirm or support the diagnosis in vivo

PATHOLOGIC FINDINGS
• Extensive necrosis and nonsuppurative inflammation of the cerebral gray and white matter
• Inflammatory changes are severe.

TREATMENT
• Inpatient or outpatient
• No specific treatment known
• Supportive only—prevent seizures

MEDICATIONS

DRUGS
• None specific
• Seizures—phenobarbital (2–8 mg/kg PO q12h); monitor serum concentrations.
• Inflammatory response—corticosteroids; prednisolone or prednisone (1–2 mg/kg PO q24h for the first 1–2 weeks; then taper dosage slowly)

CONTRAINDICATIONS/POSSIBLE INTERACTIONS
N/A

FOLLOW-UP

PATIENT MONITORING
• Monitor serum concentration of phenobarbital.
• Perform regular clinical and neurologic examinations.

PREVENTION/AVOIDANCE
N/A

POSSIBLE COMPLICATIONS
N/A

EXPECTED COURSE AND PROGNOSIS
• May be acute
• Status epilepticus may develop.
• Often chronic for months or even years, but neurologic signs are progressive.
• Prognosis—guarded

MISCELLANEOUS

ASSOCIATED CONDITIONS
In one patient, myocardial necrosis was seen in addition to the encephalitic lesions.

PREGNANCY
• Report of three patients in Japan with a history of pregnancy before onset of clinical signs
• Other more extended studies report patients of both sexes.

SEE ALSO
• Necrotizing Encephalitis of Yorkshire Terriers
• Necrotizing Meningoencephalitis of Maltese Dogs
• Seizures (Convulsions, Status Epilepticus)—Dogs

ABBREVIATION
CSF = cerebrospinal fluid

Suggested Reading
Cordy DR, Holliday TA. A necrotizing meningoencephalitis of pug dogs. Vet Pathol 1989;26:191–194.
Author Andrea Tipold
Consulting Editor Joane M. Parent

PULMONARY CONTUSIONS

BASICS

OVERVIEW
• Hemorrhage in the lung parenchyma caused by tearing and crushing during direct trauma to the thorax • Relatively small volumes of blood in the lungs may markedly compromise lung function by causing ventilation–perfusion mismatch. • In patients in shock with capillary damage, the hemorrhage may later be accompanied by pulmonary edema after fluid resuscitation.

SIGNALMENT
• Dogs and cats • No specific breed, age, or sex predilection

SIGNS
• Historical findings consistent with blunt trauma • Tachypnea • Abnormal respiratory effort • Postural adaptations to respiratory distress • Cyanotic or pale mucous membranes • Auscultation of harsh bronchovesicular sounds or crackles • Expectoration of blood or blood-tinged fluid

CAUSES & RISK FACTORS
• Blunt trauma • Motor vehicle accidents • Falls from a height • Abuse—beating • Coagulopathy • von Willebrand factor deficiency

DIAGNOSIS

DIFFERENTIAL DIAGNOSIS
• Hemothorax—may cause dull lung sounds; may see pleural effusion on thoracic radiographs
• Pneumothorax—may cause dull lung sounds; may see pleural air on thoracic radiographs
• Diaphragmatic hernia—distinguished radiographically
• Coagulopathy—may cause pulmonary hemorrhage; distinguished by coagulation testing and platelet count
• Acute onset of pulmonary hemorrhage—may be a feature of some neoplasms (e.g., hemangiosarcoma); occasionally accompanies pulmonary infarction associated with bacterial endocarditis and heartworm disease

CBC/BIOCHEMISTRY/URINALYSIS
• CBC—may reveal anemia or mature neutrophilia
• Serum biochemistry profile—may demonstrate hypoproteinemia, indicating blood loss; may reveal damage to other organ systems
• Urinalysis—usually normal

OTHER LABORATORY TESTS
N/A

IMAGING
Thoracic radiographs—usually reveals patchy areas of alveolar pattern, focal or asymmetrical; always perform in trauma patients to rule out hemothorax, pneumothorax, and diaphragmatic hernia.

DIAGNOSTIC PROCEDURES
• Examination of transtracheal wash—may demonstrate excessive numbers of erythrocytes and macrophages; culture to monitor for development of a superimposed bacterial infection.
• Pulse oximetry or arterial blood gas analysis—may confirm hypoxemia

TREATMENT
• Usually inpatient for stabilization
• Support respiratory function, stabilize cardiovascular function, and resuscitate if necessary.
• Assess and treat injuries to other organ systems.
• Restrict activity, minimize stress, and observe carefully for deterioration of respiratory function during the first 24 hr after trauma.
• Respiratory support—oxygen supplementation for hypoxemia; intubation and PPV in severely affected patients; nebulization of saline to facilitate clearance of respiratory secretions; coupage and physical therapy to facilitate clearance of respiratory secretions
• Shock—fluids may be required to support cardiovascular function; if possible, be conservative with fluid administration because it may lead to deterioration of pulmonary function by creating and exacerbating pulmonary edema; to minimize edema development, consider synthetic colloids with hypoproteinemia.
• Blood or plasma transfusion—consider if hemorrhage has caused anemia or with a coagulopathy
• Nutritional support—if needed to maintain body condition and immune status

MEDICATIONS

DRUGS
Low-dose diuretics—furosemide (0.5–2 mg/kg IV, IM); when hemorrhage is accompanied by edema and respiratory distress is severe

CONTRAINDICATIONS/POSSIBLE INTERACTIONS
Diuretics—no value in the early stages and may, in fact, be harmful; cause diuresis and decrease intravascular volume, which is contraindicated for shock; after fluid resuscitation, some pulmonary edema may accompany hemorrhage, and the edema and respiratory distress may be responsive.

FOLLOW-UP

PATIENT MONITORING
• Monitor respiratory rate and effort, mucous membrane color, heart rate and pulse quality, and lung sounds • Measure PCV and total solids and perform pulse oximetry and arterial blood gas analysis for 24 hr. • Monitor ECG frequently to detect ventricular arrhythmias.
• Radiographs—repeated in 48 hr to ensure that the contusions are resolving.

PREVENTION AND AVOIDANCE
Rely on appropriate restriction of the animal to prevent exposure to trauma

POSSIBLE COMPLICATIONS
• Bacterial pneumonia—owing to systemic immunosuppression, reduced pulmonary defenses, and aspiration of gastrointestinal tract contents • Development of a moist productive cough and failure improve within 48 hr—suspect pneumonia • Patients with severe shock may develop ARDS (less common)

EXPECTED COURSE AND PROGNOSIS
• Usually deterioration of respiratory function occurs during the initial 12–24 hr after trauma, and then gradually improves • Marked clinical improvement in respiratory status generally occurs within 48 hr, with a more gradual resolution of radiographic lesions. • If patients fails to improve after 48 hr, evaluate for complications or concurrent disease.

MISCELLANEOUS

ASSOCIATED CONDITIONS
• Fractured ribs • Flail chest • Ruptured trachea, bronchi, or esophagus • Cardiac arrhythmias—ventricular • Other possible complications of trauma

ABBREVIATIONS
• ARDS = acute respiratory distress syndrome
• PCV = packed cell volume
• PPV = positive pressure ventilation

Suggested Reading
Hackner SG. The emergency management of traumatic pulmonary contusions. Compend Contin Educ Pract Vet 1995;17:677–686.

Author Lesley G. King
Consulting Editor Eleanor C. Hawkins

PULMONARY EDEMA

BASICS

DEFINITION
An accumulation of extravascular fluid in the pulmonary interstitial and alveolar spaces

PATHOPHYSIOLOGY
In normal lungs, fluid exudes from the pulmonary capillaries into the interstitial space and returns to the circulation via the pulmonary lymphatic vessels, a dynamic process that depends upon capillary and interstitial hydrostatic and oncotic pressures and capillary and alveolar epithelial permeability. When fluid formation exceeds fluid removal by the lymphatic vessels, pulmonary edema results. When edema becomes clinically important, pulmonary gas exchange is impaired, and clinical signs develop.

SYSTEMS AFFECTED
• Respiratory
• Cardiovascular

GENETICS
N/A

INCIDENCE/PREVALENCE
N/A

GEOGRAPHIC DISTRIBUTION
N/A

SIGNALMENT
Species
Dogs and cats

Breed Predispositions
None

Mean Age and Range
• Immature and mature animals with cardiac disease
• Animals of any age affected by noncardiac causes

Predominant Sex
N/A

SIGNS
General Comments
Clinical signs depend upon the cause and severity of edema and the rapidity of onset.

Historical Findings
• Tachypnea
• Dyspnea
• Dry cough (uncommon in cats)
• Open-mouth breathing (common in cats)

Physical Examination Findings
• May be no auscultable abnormalities

• Crackles at end inspiration
• Crackles and wheezes during inspiration and expiration
• Pink-tinged, frothy secretions from nares and mouth (end stage)
• Cardiac murmurs, gallops, and arrhythmias (patients with cardiogenic pulmonary edema)

CAUSES
High Capillary Hydrostatic Pressure
• Cardiogenic—cardiomyopathy (i.e., dilated, hypertrophic, intermediate, and restrictive), mitral valvular endocardiosis, ruptured chordae tendineae, thyrotoxicosis, endocarditis, aortic valve disease, patent ductus arteriosus, ventricular septal defect, and arrhythmias
• Noncardiogenic—overzealous intravenous fluid administration

Low Capillary Oncotic Pressure
• Hypoproteinemia
• Overzealous IV fluid administration

High Capillary or Alveolar Epithelial Permeability
• Pneumonia
• Toxins (e.g., smoke, gastric contents, and snake venom)
• Heatstroke, disseminated intravascular coagulation
• Near-drowning
• Circulating endotoxins

High Negative Intrathoracic or Interstitial Pressure
• Upper airway obstruction
• Reexpansion of atelectatic lung

Unknown Mechanisms
Neurogenic (e.g., seizures, head trauma, and electrocution)

RISK FACTORS
Heart disease

DIAGNOSIS

DIFFERENTIAL DIAGNOSIS
• Must differentiate from other causes of coughing or dyspnea such as upper airway obstruction, tracheitis, bronchitis, pneumonia, heartworm disease, collapsing trachea, respiratory foreign body, and neoplasia; thoracic radiographs and hematologic testing help exclude these.
• Many patients with cardiogenic pulmonary edema have other signs of heart disease (e.g., murmur, arrhythmias, and tachycardia).

• The character of the cough (i.e., dry versus moist) and dyspnea (i.e., expiratory versus inspiratory) may better define the cause of the clinical signs.

CBC/BIOCHEMISTRY/URINALYSIS
• Help evaluate noncardiogenic causes of pulmonary edema
• Generally normal in patients with cardiogenic edema; may see stress leukogram, prerenal azotemia, and high liver enzymes because of passive congestion or poor forward cardiac output

OTHER LABORATORY TESTS
Arterial blood gas analysis documents hypoxemia, but does not correlate well with the severity of pulmonary edema.

IMAGING
Thoracic Radiographic Findings
• Signs of pulmonary edema vary with the severity and cause of the edema.
• An interstitial or alveolar lung pattern is characteristic of pulmonary edema.
• Cardiogenic pulmonary edema—often associated with cardiomegaly (most often left atrium or auricular appendage) and pulmonary venous enlargement; early edema in dogs is often situated in the hilar region; becomes diffuse in patients with advanced heart failure; usually symmetrical, but may start out in the right caudal lung lobe; usually patchy and diffuse in cats
• Neurogenic pulmonary edema—often situated in the caudal lung field

Echocardiography
May confirm cardiac disease but cannot identify pulmonary edema

DIAGNOSTIC PROCEDURES
• Pulmonary capillary wedge pressure, an indicator of left atrial pressure, can be measured with a Swan-Ganz catheter temporarily "wedged" in the pulmonary artery; usually high pressure (> 20–25 mm Hg) in patients with cardiogenic pulmonary edema
• Central venous pressure not always high in animals with left heart failure

PATHOLOGIC FINDINGS
• Fluid accumulates in the pulmonary interstitium and alveoli; lungs usually normal color but often heavy and "wet"
• Lungs may not collapse completely when the thorax is opened.
• May see white or pink-tinged froth in the trachea and small airways

PULMONARY EDEMA

TREATMENT

APPROPRIATE HEALTH CARE
• Whether to treat the patient as an inpatient or outpatient depends on the degree of respiratory compromise and the underlying cause of the edema.
• If respiratory distress—minimal handling and supplemental oxygen (< 50%) are indicated; postpone diagnostic tests until the patient's condition is more stable; intubate and ventilate if necessary.

NURSING CARE
• Oxygen therapy as needed
• Fluid therapy in animals with pulmonary edema is challenging. Hypovolemic patients in heart failure are hard to manage with parenteral fluid therapy. Small volumes of isotonic saline solutions may be most appropriate for volume replacement if plasma cannot be used. Once circulating volumes are restored, low sodium (0.45% NaCl in 2.5% dextrose) or sodium-free (D5W) fluids can maintain hydration without further increasing total body sodium. Monitor patients closely for worsening edema by auscultation and thoracic radiography. Central venous or pulmonary capillary wedge pressures—may use to assist with fluid management; neither should be relied upon exclusively

ACTIVITY
Cage rest or exercise restriction is recommended until the edema resolves.

DIET
Restrict sodium (< 13 mg/kg/day; < 90 mg/100 g of dry food) in patients with cardiogenic edema.

CLIENT EDUCATION
Cardiogenic pulmonary edema signals advanced heart disease; long-term prognosis is guarded to poor. Many patients respond well to initial medical management, but the owner must monitor closely for the earliest signs of dyspnea, tachypnea, or coughing (dogs) that might signal recurrence.

SURGICAL CONSIDERATIONS
Pulmonary edema treated and resolved prior to anesthesia

MEDICATIONS

DRUGS OF CHOICE

To Reduce Edema
• Diuretics (e.g., furosemide, hydrochlorothiazide, and spironolactone)
• Vasodilators (e.g., nitroglycerin, nitroprusside, and enalapril)

To Improve Oxygen Delivery to Alveoli (May Be Useful)
Bronchodilators (e.g., aminophylline, theophylline, terbutaline)

To Reduce Anxiety (Use Only If Necessary)
• Morphine (dogs only)
• Acepromazine
• Diazepam

To Increase Capillary Oncotic Pressure (Noncardiogenic Pulmonary Edema)
• Plasma
• Intravenous colloids (e.g., dextran and hetastarch)

To Treat Increased Capillary Permeability (Noncardiogenic Pulmonary Edema)
• Treat the underlying cause.
• Consider corticosteroids.

CONTRAINDICATIONS
• Unless specifically indicated, drugs with negative inotropic actions in animals with cardiogenic pulmonary edema
• Morphine in patients with neurogenic pulmonary edema

PRECAUTIONS
Reduced cardiac output, hypotension, and prerenal azotemia may occur with overzealous use of a diuretic or vasodilator.

POSSIBLE INTERACTIONS
N/A

ALTERNATIVE DRUGS
Addition of a thiazide diuretic or spironolactone to furosemide may benefit patients with refractory cardiogenic pulmonary edema.

FOLLOW-UP

PATIENT MONITORING
Thoracic radiographs to assess treatment

PREVENTION/AVOIDANCE
N/A

POSSIBLE COMPLICATIONS

Cardiogenic Pulmonary Edema
• Often recurs since the inciting cause is rarely eliminated.
• Response to treatment is a good indicator of short-term prognosis.

EXPECTED COURSE AND PROGNOSIS
• Long-term—guarded with cardiogenic edema because underlying disease generally cannot be cured; exception: some forms of congenital heart disease
• Noncardiogenic edema—quite variable; depends on the underlying cause; often good, if underlying cause can be corrected

MISCELLANEOUS

ASSOCIATED CONDITIONS
N/A

AGE-RELATED FACTORS
N/A

ZOONOTIC POTENTIAL
N/A

PREGNANCY
N/A

SYNONYMS
Pulmonary congestion

SEE ALSO
• Congestive Heart Failure, Left-Sided
• Cough
• Dyspnea
• Pulmonary Edema, Noncardiogenic

ABBREVIATION
D5W = 5% dextrose in water

Suggested reading

Cooke K, Snyder P. Fluid therapy in the cardiac patient. Vet Clin North Am 1998;28(3)663–676.
Harpster N. Pulmonary edema. In: Kirk RW, ed. Current veterinary therapy X. Philadelphia: Saunders, 1989:385–392.
Ware W, Bonagura JB. Pulmonary edema. In: Fox PR, Sisson D, Moise NS. eds. Textbook of canine and feline cardiology. Philadelphia: Saunders, 1999:251–264.
Author Patti S. Snyder
Consulting Editors Larry P. Tilley and Francis W. K. Smith, Jr.

DISEASES

PULMONARY EDEMA, NONCARDIOGENIC

 BASICS

DEFINITION
The accumulation of edema fluid in the pulmonary interstitium and alveoli, in the absence of heart disease

PATHOPHYSIOLOGY
• Common cause of all forms—increased pulmonary vascular permeability, which is associated with leakage of fluid into the interstitium and alveoli; if severe, may be followed by an inflammatory response and accumulation of neutrophils and macrophages in the interstitium and alveoli
• Several mechanisms may contribute to changes in pulmonary vascular permeability.
• Profound but transient increases in pulmonary arterial pressure caused by massive sympathetic discharge
• Systemic release of catecholamines—may lead to systemic vasoconstriction, temporarily shunting blood into the pulmonary circulation and leading to transient pulmonary circulatory overload and endothelial damage; probably occurs in patients with neurogenic edema, electric cord bites, and upper airway obstruction
• Increased intrathoracic negative pressure induced by inspiratory attempts against an airway obstruction
• Pulmonary manifestation of a generalized inflammatory response—systemic inflammatory response syndrome; develops in patients with sepsis or pancreatitis
• For all forms, the inciting insult may trigger a cascade inflammatory response that often worsens over 24-hr after the initial episode.
• Severity of clinical manifestation—varies, ranging from mild to severe; the most seriously affected patients may progress from normal to death in as little as a couple of hours after the incident.

SYSTEMS AFFECTED
• Respiratory
• Hemic/Lymphatic/Immune—if severe and causing respiratory failure, may be associated with DIC
• Cardiovascular—hypotension, tachycardia, and shock
• Renal/Urologic—acute renal failure

GENETICS
Unknown

INCIDENCE/PREVALENCE
Uncommon

GEOGRAPHIC DISTRIBUTION
N/A

SIGNALMENT
Species
Mainly dogs, occasionally cats

Breed Predilection
None specific; brachycephalic dogs are more prone to airway obstruction.

Mean Age and Range
• Higher incidence in puppies < 1 year old
• Young—associated with strangulation, head trauma, and electric cord bites
• Old—associated with laryngeal obstruction and neoplasia

Predominant Sex
None

SIGNS
General Comments
Vary, depending on underlying cause and severity

Historical Findings
• Predisposing cause—airway obstruction; electric cord bite
• Acute onset of dyspnea

Physical Examination Findings
• Mild to severe dyspnea
• Increased respiratory rate and effort; open-mouthed breathing
• Postural adaptations to respiratory distress (severe)
• Unwillingness to lie down
• Pale or cyanotic mucous membranes (severe)
• Harsh sounds (early, mild) or generalized crackles (late, severe) on auscultation
• Expectoration of pink froth or bubbles; in severely affected, intubated patient, may note large volumes of bloody fluid flowing out through the endotracheal tube
• Normal cardiac auscultation; may note arrhythmias; tachycardia common

CAUSES
• Upper airway obstruction—laryngeal paralysis; choke-chain injury; mass; abscess
• Electric cord bite
• Acute neurologic disease—head trauma; prolonged seizures
• Smoke inhalation
• Systemic inflammatory response syndrome—sepsis; endotoxemia; pancreatitis
• Anaphylaxis (cats)

RISK FACTORS
• Hypoproteinemia
• Crystalloid fluid resuscitation

 DIAGNOSIS

DIFFERENTIAL DIAGNOSIS
• Cardiogenic pulmonary edema
• Pulmonary infection—bacterial, viral, or fungal pneumonia
• Pulmonary neoplasia
• Pulmonary hemorrhage
• Pulmonary thromboembolism

CBC/BIOCHEMISTRY/URINALYSIS
• Leukocytosis but possibly leukopenia and thrombocytopenia—owing to neutrophil sequestration in the lung and platelet consumption
• Biochemistries—usually normal; may note hypoalbuminemia owing to pulmonary protein loss; mild hyperglycemia reported
• Urinalysis—usually normal

OTHER LABORATORY TESTS
• Arterial blood gas analysis—usually demonstrates mild to severe hypoxemia and hypocapnia; results are not specific but indicate the severity of pulmonary dysfunction.
• Coagulation testing (severely affected patients)—may reveal mild to moderate prolongation of PT and PTT because of consumption and DIC

IMAGING
• Thoracic radiographs—vital; may simply reveal prominent interstitial pattern with mild or early disease; may note alveolar infiltrates with moderate or severe disease; alveolar infiltrates in the dorsocaudal lung fields common; alveolar infiltrates may be seen in other lung fields, are often asymmetrical, and demonstrate predominant right-sided involvement.
• Echocardiography—rule out cardiogenic pulmonary edema

DIAGNOSTIC PROCEDURES
• Pulse oximetry—noninvasive, continuous monitoring of arterial hemoglobin saturation; provides information about the severity and progression of pulmonary dysfunction
• Pulmonary artery wedge pressure—confirms noncardiogenic origin

PATHOLOGIC FINDINGS
• Lungs—may be heavy, red, or congested; may fail to collapse; may exhibit a wet cut surface; may note foam in the major airways
• Histopathologic—depend on severity of the insult; early, mild: may note eosinophilic amorphous material filling the alveoli or may be near normal because fluid removed in processing; severe: alveolar hyaline membranes, alveolitis, and interstitial inflamma-

tory infiltrates with neutrophils and macrophages evident and accompanied by atelectasis, vascular congestion, and hemorrhage; may be found in only hours after a severe insult

TREATMENT

APPROPRIATE HEALTH CARE
• Inpatient vs. outpatient—depends on the severity of clinical manifestation of respiratory dysfunction; depends on the underlying cause of disease (e.g., dogs with upper airway obstruction or severe seizures may require hospitalization)
• Make every effort to resolve and treat the underlying cause (e.g., relieve airway obstruction or treat seizures).
• Mild to moderate—patients generally improve on their own within 24–48 hr with complete resolution; offer support of pulmonary and cardiovascular function while the lung repairs.
• Severe—difficult to treat; may require PPV because of respiratory failure; many die despite extensive supportive care.

NURSING CARE
• Minimize stress in dyspneic animals.
• Oxygen therapy—vital in moderate to severe disease; administer via a mask or hood, nasal catheter, or oxygen cage; inspired oxygen concentration depends on the severity of disease; most patients do well on 40%–50% oxygen, but severe disease may require 80%–100% to sustain life
• Severe—may require PPV and PEEP
• Fluid therapy with a balanced electrolyte—give as replacement solution with dehydration or shock
• Plasma or synthetic colloids—consider with hypoproteinemia; improve oncotic pressure, minimizing movement of fluid into the lungs

ACTIVITY
Dog with moderate to severe hypoxia and respiratory distress—rest and minimal stress vital for minimizing oxygen requirements

DIET
N/A

CLIENT EDUCATION
• Warn client that the condition may worsen before improving.
• Inform client that severe disease which progresses rapidly to fulminant pulmonary edema and respiratory failure, is associated with a very poor prognosis.

SURGICAL CONSIDERATIONS
Relevant only for treating the underlying cause

MEDICATIONS

DRUGS OF CHOICE
• Damaged endothelium in the pulmonary vasculature—no specific treatment available
• Inflammatory response—generated by a variety of mediators and cascades; cannot be blocked by one specific anti-inflammatory drug that leads to resolution of the edema
• Diuretics—often ineffective; edema caused by changes in permeability not high hydrostatic pressure; may use furosemide cautiously in boluses of 0.5–2 mg/kg IV, IM or at 0.1–1 mg/kg/hr IV in a continuous infusion.
• Corticosteroids—minimize swellings with upper airway obstruction; generally ineffective for pulmonary inflammatory response; may predispose patients to infectious complications (e.g., bacterial pneumonia); if used, recommend an anti-inflammatory dosage (dexamethasone sodium phosphate at 0.1–0.2 mg/kg IV)

CONTRAINDICATIONS
N/A

PRECAUTIONS
Diuretics (e.g., furosemide)—excessive use may cause dehydration and a marked decrease in intravascular volume with minimal resolution of edema; low intravascular volume may exacerbate cardiovascular collapse or shock.

POSSIBLE INTERACTIONS
N/A

ALTERNATIVE DRUGS
N/A

FOLLOW-UP

PATIENT MONITORING
• Observe respiratory rate and pattern and auscultate frequently (every 2–4 hr) for the first 24–48 hr, depending on severity of disease.
• Assess pulmonary function by pulse oximetry or arterial blood gas analysis (initially every 2–4 hr) with dyspnea.
• Perform PCV and total solids and evaluate mucous membranes, pulse quality, heart rate, and urine output every 2–4 hr to assess cardiovascular status and progression to shock.

PREVENTION/AVOIDANCE
• Avoid contact with electric wire.
• Correct airway obstruction.
• Treat seizures or high intracranial pressure.

POSSIBLE COMPLICATIONS
Usually none if patient recovers from the acute crisis

EXPECTED COURSE AND PROGNOSIS
• mild to moderate—uneventful resolution of signs in 24–72 hr; no specific treatment required except for oxygen and careful fluid supplementation
• Overall survival rates—80%–100%
• Long-term prognosis—excellent for recovered patients

MISCELLANEOUS

ASSOCIATED CONDITIONS
Acute respiratory distress syndrome

AGE-RELATED FACTORS
N/A

ZOONOTIC POTENTIAL
N/A

PREGNANCY
N/A

SYNONYMS
• Shock lung
• Traumatic wet lung
• Acute alveolar failure
• Capillary leak syndrome
• Progressive respiratory distress
• Congestive atelectasis
• Hemorrhagic lung syndrome

SEE ALSO
Acute respiratory distress syndrome (ARDS)

ABBREVIATIONS
• DIC = disseminated intravascular coagulation
• PCV = packed cell volume
• PEEP = positive end-expiratory pressure
• PPV = positive pressure ventilation
• PT = prothrombin time
• PTT = partial thromboplastin time

Suggested Reading
Drobatz KJ, Concannon K. Noncardiogenic pulmonary edema. Compend Contin Educ Pract Vet 1994;16:333–346.
Drobatz KJ, Saunders HM, Pugh C, Hendricks JC. Noncardiogenic pulmonary edema 26 cases (1987–1993). J Am Vet Med Assoc 1995;206:1732–1736.
Kerr LY. Pulmonary edema secondary to upper airway obstruction in the dog: a review of nine cases. J Am Anim Hosp Assoc 1989;25:207–212.
Kolata RJ, Burrows CF. The clinical features of injury by chewing electrical cords in dogs and cats. J Am Anim Hosp Assoc 1981;17:219–222.
Author Lesley G. King
Consulting Editor Eleanor C. Hawkins

PULMONARY FIBROSIS

 BASICS

OVERVIEW
• Fibrosis of the lung interstitium
• Affects pulmonary mechanics, alters ventilation–perfusion ratios, and leads to chronic tachypnea
• End result of previous lung injury; may be preceded by multifocal alveolitis
• The initiating causes—unknown; in humans > 100 known agents can incite alveolar inflammation

SIGNALMENT
• Dogs and cats
• West Highland white terriers and other terriers predisposed
• Affected animals usually old

SIGNS

Historical Findings
• Open-mouth breathing
• Exercise intolerance
• Cough

Physical Examination Findings
• Dyspnea
• Increased respiratory rate and effort
• Cyanosis
• Auscultation—reveals bilateral end-inspiratory and early expiratory crackles

CAUSES & RISK FACTORS
• Usually idiopathic
• Viral infections—canine distemper; adenovirus; parainfluenza
• Toxins or drugs—paraquat; kerosene; nitrofurantoin
• Oxygen toxicosis
• Acute pancreatitis

 DIAGNOSIS

DIFFERENTIAL DIAGNOSIS
• Generalized cardiogenic pulmonary edema—accompanied by left-sided heart enlargement and pulmonary venous distention; response to diuretic expected
• Fungal pneumonia and metastatic neoplasia—associated with an interstitial pattern; usually diagnosed by results of cytologic examination and culture of transtracheal wash or bronchoalveolar lavage

specimen and by identification of organisms or neoplastic cells from other affected organs
• Obesity, end expiration, and poor film quality—cause increase in lung density

CBC/BIOCHEMISTRY/URINALYSIS
Polycythemia caused by chronic hypoxemia

OTHER LABORATORY TESTS
N/A

IMAGING
• Radiography—bilateral, diffuse increase in interstitial pattern; right-sided cardiomegaly may be caused by chronic lung disease.
• Echocardiography—may document right heart enlargement
• Doppler echocardiography—may demonstrate pulmonary hypertension

DIAGNOSTIC PROCEDURES
• Arterial blood gas measurements—hypoxemia and high alveolar–arterial oxygen difference
• Cytologic examination of bronchoalveolar lavage specimen—nontoxic neutrophil count exceeding 20% of cells in dogs with alveolitis or fibrosis
• Bacterial, *Mycoplasma,* and fungal cultures—no growth
• Open lung biopsy—proliferative interstitial pneumonia

PATHOLOGIC FINDINGS
• Proliferation of atypical and multinucleated alveolar epithelial cells
• Thickening of interalveolar septa
• Intra-alveolar hemorrhage and edema
• Intracapillary and intra-alveolar fibrin deposits
• Macrophages and alveolar epithelial cells in alveolar lumina
• Masson trichrome staining—reveals increase in interalveolar septal collagen

 TREATMENT

• Inpatient if oxygen is needed
• Goals—control signs and enhance quality of life; manifestations of disorder do not occur until pulmonary gas exchange is severely compromised.
• Obesity—may impair diaphragmatic function; may cause early, small airway closure; may impede ventilation; weight loss lessens signs of respiratory impairment.
• Eliminate exposure to dusts or fumes.

 MEDICATIONS

DRUGS
• Immunosuppressive dosage of prednisone—1 mg/kg PO q12h for 2 weeks; then taper over the next month; recommended if no underlying infection; most beneficial early in the course of disease
• Concurrent use of azathioprine—may offer additional benefit
• Bronchodilators—may diminish signs
• Administer oxygen during acute exacerbation.

CONTRAINDICATIONS/POSSIBLE INTERACTIONS
• Steroids—may predispose patient to overt infection; not advised unless bacterial and fungal cultures are negative.
• Nonselective β blockers—may cause bronchoconstriction
• Diuretics—decrease pulmonary clearance mechanisms owing to airway dehydration; may predispose patient to infection

 FOLLOW-UP

• Monitor with serial arterial blood gas measurements and cytologic examination of bronchoalveolar lavage specimens.
• Progressive condition with a guarded prognosis
• Pulmonary hypertension and right heart failure—may develop with any severe, chronic lung disease
• Bullous emphysema and spontaneous pneumothorax—may develop as a result of severe alveolar damage

 MISCELLANEOUS

Suggested Reading
Bonagura JD, Hamlin RL, Gaber CE. Chronic respiratory disease in the dog. In: Kirk RW, ed. Current veterinary therapy X. Philadelphia: Saunders, 1989:361–368.
Author Rosemary A. Henik
Consulting Editor Eleanor C. Hawkins

PULMONARY MINERALIZATIONS

BASICS

OVERVIEW
- Both calcification and ossification and may be generalized or localized
- Discrete—if individual mineral deposits can be identified
- Diffuse—preclude identification of individual deposits
- Calcification—dystrophic or metastatic; dystrophic: occurs secondary to tissue degeneration or inflammation; metastatic: occurs secondary to metabolic disease; may be normal (e.g., the pleura in old dogs or premature calcification of the tracheal and bronchial cartilages in chondrodystrophic breeds); often a sign of inactivity of a lesion, thus most focal calcifications are functionally unimportant
- Ossification—also called heterotopic bone formation; calcification of a bony matrix; pulmonary ossification in the form of small, multiple nodules (osteomas) common in normal dogs
- Generalized pulmonary mineralizations of unknown cause—reported in dogs and cats under descriptive terms: pulmonary alveolar microlithiasis or pumice stone lung, bronchiolar microlithiasis, idiopathic pulmonary calcification or ossification

SIGNALMENT
Older dogs and cats

SIGNS

Historical Findings
- None if focal pulmonary mineralization is incidental finding
- Exercise intolerance
- Cough

Physical Examination Findings
- Dyspnea
- High respiratory rate and abnormal effort
- Cyanosis
- Abnormal breath sounds
- Pleural effusion

CAUSES & RISK FACTORS
- Often idiopathic

- Metastatic calcification—secondary to metabolic disease that induces high serum calcium concentration and/or bone resorption (e.g., hyperadrenocorticism, primary or secondary hyperparathyroidism, hypervitaminosis D, and renal failure)
- Hyperadrenocorticism—may cause dystrophic mineralization owing to the gluconeogenic and catabolic effects of high cortisol on proteins; calcium binds to the organic matrix of the abnormal proteins.
- Alveolar and bronchial microlith—may be secondary to exudative or granulomatous lung disease

DIAGNOSIS

DIFFERENTIAL DIAGNOSIS
- Dystrophic calcification secondary to chronic pulmonary inflammatory disease
- Atypical pulmonary neoplasia
- Histoplasmosis or tuberculosis granuloma—usually with hilar lymph node calcification
- Alveolar microlithiasis
- Barium sulfate aspiration
- Interstitial pulmonary edema—will respond to diuretic; differentiated by bone scintigraphy

CBC/BIOCHEMISTRY/URINALYSIS
- Hypercalcemia—with hyperparathyroidism, neoplasia, or hypervitaminosis D
- Polycythemia—with chronic hypoxemia
- Stress leukogram, low urine specific gravity, and high ALP—may see in dogs with hyperadrenocorticism

OTHER LABORATORY TESTS
Arterial blood gas measurements—may note hypoxemia

IMAGING
Thoracic radiographs—generalized or localized, discrete or diffuse abnormalities, ranging from an unstructured interstitial pattern to mineralized nodules within the pulmonary parenchyma

DIAGNOSTIC PROCEDURES
- Cytologic examination of transtracheal wash or bronchoalveolar lavage specimen—reveals inflammatory cells with underlying inflammation or infection; microliths appear as nonstaining crystalline concretions.

- Bacterial and fungal cultures—results depend on underlying cause
- Delayed bone phase scintigraphy (^{99m}Tc-methylene diphosphonate)—generalized pulmonary uptake if sufficient osteoid is being produced
- Lung biopsy—firm, noncompressible, and variably resistant to blunt dissection because of mineralizations

TREATMENT
None indicated if localized form found in asymptomatic patient

MEDICATIONS

DRUGS
- Bronchodilators—relief of dyspnea and respiratory muscle fatigue
- Antimicrobial or antifungal—with positive bacterial or fungal culture
- Treat underlying metabolic disease—mitotane for hyperadrenocorticism; chemotherapy for neoplasia

CONTRAINDICATIONS/POSSIBLE INTERACTIONS
Fluid loading—may exacerbate dyspnea and right heart failure

FOLLOW-UP
Pleural effusion, chronic obstructive bronchitis, or emphysematous bullae—may develop owing to severe, chronic pulmonary disease

MISCELLANEOUS

ABBREVIATION
ALP = alkaline phosphatase

Suggested Reading
Suter PF, Lord PF. Thoracic radiography: a text atlas of thoracic diseases of the dog and cat. Wettswil, Switzerland: Author, 1984.

Author Rosemary A. Henik
Consulting Editor Eleanor C. Hawkins

PULMONARY THROMBOEMBOLISM

 BASICS

DEFINITION
Develops when a thrombus lodges in the pulmonary arterial tree and occludes blood flow to the lung served by that artery

PATHOPHYSIOLOGY
• Pulmonary thromboemboli associated with heartworm disease occur in situ in the pulmonary vessels; in most other instances, the origin of the thrombus is unclear.
• Potential sites of origin include the right atrium, vena cava, jugular veins, and femoral or mesenteric veins; these venous thrombi are carried in the bloodstream to the lungs where they lodge in the pulmonary circulation.
• Abnormal blood flow (stasis), vascular endothelial damage, and altered coagulability (hypercoagulable state) are believed to predispose to thrombus formation.
• In most patients, pulmonary thromboembolism is a complicating feature of another primary disease process.

SYSTEMS AFFECTED
• Respiratory—diminished pulmonary blood flow leads to arterial hypoxemia and dyspnea
• Cardiovascular—pulmonary hypertension may result, leading to right ventricular enlargement and right ventricular failure

GENETICS
N/A

INCIDENCE/PREVALENCE
• Not known—likelihood of pulmonary thromboembolism increases in animals with abnormal coagulation or severe systemic disease
• Uncommon diagnosis in dogs; rare diagnosis in cats

GEOGRAPHIC DISTRIBUTION
N/A

SIGNALMENT

Species
Dogs and cats

Breed Predilections
No predisposition; disease may be more common in medium- and large-breed dogs

Mean Age and Range
More frequently seen in mature and old dogs

Predominant Sex
N/A

SIGNS

Historical Findings
• Often reflect the primary disease
• Occasionally the reason for initial examination; in such a patient, peracute dyspnea, collapse, cough or hemoptysis, weakness, and inability to sleep or get comfortable may be historical complaints.

Physical Examination Findings
• Tachypnea and dyspnea in most animals
• Tachycardia, weak arterial pulses, jugular vein distension, pale or cyanotic mucous membranes, delayed capillary refill time, and split second heart sound in some animals

CAUSES
• Heartworm disease
• Neoplasia
• Hyperadrenocorticism (Cushing's disease)
• Protein-losing nephropathy (renal loss of antithrombin III)
• Cardiac disease
• Immune-mediated hemolytic anemia
• Pancreatitis
• Orthopedic trauma or surgery
• Sepsis
• Disseminated intravascular coagulopathy
• Liver disease

RISK FACTORS
• Coagulopathy, especially any hypercoagulable state
• Diseases listed under "Causes" are associated
• Estrogen administration and airplane travel may be causative.

 DIAGNOSIS

DIFFERENTIAL DIAGNOSIS
• Other diseases that cause clinically important dyspnea and hypoxemia without profound radiographic findings include upper airway obstruction, laryngeal paralysis, and diffuse airway disease processes (e.g., toxin inhalation and interstitial pneumonia).
• Upper airway obstruction often manifests as inspiratory dyspnea; lung sounds often loudest over the trachea or larynx
• Should be a leading diagnostic consideration in a patient with acute onset of dyspnea and a disease known to be associated with pulmonary thromboembolism

CBC/BIOCHEMISTRY/URINALYSIS
• Results often reflect the underlying disease.
• Leukocytosis may develop.

OTHER LABORATORY TESTS
• Arterial blood gases often show arterial hypoxemia ($PaO_2 < 65$ mm Hg) and low $PaCO_2$ with respiratory alkalosis.
• Metabolic and respiratory acidosis may develop in severely affected patients.
• Coagulation profile may show high fibrin degradation products, high fibrinogen, or alterations in one-stage PT and activated PTT.

IMAGING

Thoracic Radiographic Findings
Normal or pulmonary artery enlargement or pruning, cardiomegaly, interstitial and alveolar lung patterns, small-volume pleural effusion, or areas of regional hyperlucency

Echocardiographic Findings
Right ventricular enlargement, an enlarged pulmonary artery segment, or diminished size of the left ventricular cavity in some patients; infrequently a thrombus is imaged in the right heart or the pulmonary artery

Angiographic Findings and Radionuclide Studies
• Usually required for definitive diagnosis
• Right-sided cardiac catheterization with pulmonary angiography may permit identification of an intravascular thrombus or regions of reduced pulmonary blood flow; nonselective angiography has a low level of diagnostic success, especially in medium- and large-breed dogs
• Combined ventilation and perfusion scans with radioisotopes permit identification of well-ventilated lung regions that do not receive blood flow; when thoracic radiographs are nearly normal, a perfusion scan alone may suffice.

DIAGNOSTIC PROCEDURES

Electrocardiography
• Acute cor pulmonale—right axis deviation, P pulmonale, ST segment deviation, large T waves
• Arrhythmias

PATHOLOGIC FINDINGS
• Thrombi in the major branches of the pulmonary arteries in most patients

• Some patients exhibit multiple smaller thrombi in small vessels of the pulmonary arteries, eventually leading to marked respiratory dysfunction and death.

TREATMENT

APPROPRIATE HEALTH CARE
Always treat patients suspected of having pulmonary thromboembolism as inpatients until hypoxemia is resolved.

NURSING CARE
• Administer IV fluids cautiously unless preexisting volume depletion exists; they may contribute to the development of right-sided congestive heart failure.
• Administer oxygen if dyspnea exists and/or $PaO_2 < 65$ mm Hg.

ACTIVITY
Restrict to prevent worsening hypoxemia or syncope.

DIET
N/A

CLIENT EDUCATION
• Alert client that disease is often fatal; further episodes are likely unless an underlying cause is identified and corrected; sudden death is not unusual.
• Treatment with anticoagulant medications can lead to bleeding; frequent reevaluation of clotting times (e.g., PT and PTT) is needed for successful management; anticoagulant administration may be required for several months even after resolution of the causative disease.

SURGICAL CONSIDERATIONS
Requires cardiopulmonary bypass and is not available at most institutions; even if available, extrapolation from human literature suggests probable high surgical mortality

MEDICATIONS

DRUGS OF CHOICE
• Always identify and treat the underlying disease; if this is unlikely to be successful, aggressive efforts to treat pulmonary thromboembolism will probably be in vain.

• Heparin may help prevent further thrombi from developing; low dosages are probably inadequate for management; a dosage of 200–300 units/kg SC q8h is indicated.
• Thrombolytic drug administration (e.g., streptokinase and tissue plasminogen activator) may also be useful; these drugs are expensive and carry a higher risk of bleeding complications.
• Warfarin—usually indicated for long-term treatment (0.1 mg/kg q24h), with dosage adjustments to maintain a PT 1.5–2 times the baseline value

CONTRAINDICATIONS
N/A

PRECAUTIONS
Warfarin—interacts with many other drugs; degree of anticoagulation may change after giving these drugs; dose titration may be difficult in patients with diseases that result in coagulopathy. Review the mechanism of action and pharmacology of the antithrombotic drugs before use.

POSSIBLE INTERACTIONS
N/A

ALTERNATIVE DRUGS
N/A

FOLLOW-UP

PATIENT MONITORING
• Serial arterial blood gases—may help determine improvement in respiratory function
• PT every 3 days initially for adjusting warfarin dosage to achieve a PT 1.5–2 times the baseline value. International normalization ratios are recommended to minimize the effects of test kit variability on PT results. Check weekly after an effective dosage is achieved (typically no sooner than 2 weeks).

PREVENTION/AVOIDANCE
• Activity may improve venous blood flow and prevent development of venous thrombi in immobile patients with severe systemic disease.
• Aspirin may have some preventive role but is inadequate as treatment.
• Heparin may be administered to animals predisposed to the development of pulmonary thromboembolism (200 units/kg IV initially and 75 units/kg SC q4–8h).

POSSIBLE COMPLICATIONS
Clinically important bleeding complications may arise in patients treated with anticoagulant drugs. Bleeding may occur from any organ system. Anticipate active bleeding or anemia necessitating blood or plasma transfusion and have blood products readily available.

EXPECTED COURSE AND PROGNOSIS
Generally guarded to poor; depends on resolution of the precipitating cause. For irreversible diseases (e.g., some neoplasias and advanced protein-losing nephropathy), it is poor long-term; somewhat better for patients with trauma or sepsis

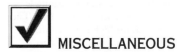

MISCELLANEOUS

ASSOCIATED CONDITIONS
See Causes and Risk Factors

AGE-RELATED FACTORS
N/A

ZOONOTIC POTENTIAL
N/A

PREGNANCY
N/A

SYNONYMS
Pulmonary embolism, PTE

SEE ALSO
• Immune-mediated Hemolytic Anemia
• Hyperadrenocorticism (Cushing's Disease)
• Nephrotic Syndrome
• Heartworm Disease
• Sepsis and Bacteremia
• Disseminated Intravascular Coagulation

ABBREVIATIONS
• PT = prothrombin time
• PTT = partial thromboplastin time

Suggested Reading

Hawkins EC. Diseases of the lower respiratory system. In: Ettinger SJ, Feldman EC, eds. Textbook of veterinary internal medicine. 4th ed. Philadelphia: Saunders, 1995: 767–811.

LaRue MJ, Murtaugh RJ. Pulmonary thromboembolism in dogs: 47 cases (1986–1987). J Am Vet Med Assoc 1990;197:1368–1372.

Author John E. Rush

Consulting Editors Larry P. Tilley and Francis W. K. Smith, Jr.

DISEASES

PULMONIC STENOSIS

BASICS

DEFINITION
Congenital narrowing of the right ventricular outflow tract, obstructing the passage of flow from the right ventricle to the pulmonary artery; usually valvular, but may be subvalvular or supravalvular

PATHOPHYSIOLOGY
The stenosis causes a pressure overload of the right ventricle, resulting in hypertrophy. The right ventricle develops high systolic pressures to overcome the stenosis, whose magnitude correlates with the severity of the stenosis. The difference between the high right ventricular pressure and the normal pulmonary artery pressure (i.e., the pressure gradient) is often used to describe the severity of the stenosis. Hypertrophy of the right ventricle increases the risk of ischemia and arrhythmias, and the geometric changes in right ventricular shape may result in secondary tricuspid insufficiency. With exercise, the right ventricle may be unable to increase stroke volume adequately. Tricuspid insufficiency with or without myocardial failure of the right ventricle may lead to high right atrial pressures, and R-CHF. A concurrent atrial septal defect or patent foramen ovale may cause right-to-left shunting, especially with exercise, which may result in cyanosis on exertion. Mild pulmonic stenosis usually produces no significant hemodynamic effects apart from an ejection murmur.

SYSTEMS AFFECTED
• Cardiovascular—R-CHF, arrhythmias
• Hepatobiliary—hepatomegaly with R-CHF
• Nervous—cerebral hypoperfusion during exercise

GENETICS
Inherited defect in beagles; polygenic mode of transmission suggested

INCIDENCE/PREVALENCE
• Most surveys show PS to be the third most common congenital cardiac defect in dogs, comprised 21% of congenital heart defects in one study
• Uncommon in cats, especially as an isolated defect; comprised 3% of congenital heart defects in one study

GEOGRAPHIC DISTRIBUTION
N/A

SIGNALMENT
Species
Dogs and cats

Breed Predilections
English bulldog, Scottish terrier, wirehaired fox terrier, miniature schnauzer, West Highland white terrier, Chihuahua, Samoyed, mastiff, cocker spaniel, beagle, boxer

Mean Age and Range
Present from birth and may be detected as a murmur in puppies; if murmur is not detected, affected animals may not be identified until clinical signs develop later in life.

Predominant Sex
Noted only in English bulldogs—a predilection for males

SIGNS
General Comments
• Mild stenosis—usually no clinical signs
• Severely affected patients—may develop CHF, exertional syncope, or sudden death

Historical Findings
• Abdominal distension
• Dyspnea
• Exertional syncope, exercise intolerance or sudden death
• Asymptomatic

Physical Examination Findings
• Systolic murmur loudest over the left heart base; may radiate widely
• Murmur—midsystolic or holosystolic, and crescendo–decrescendo
• Louder murmurs with a precordial thrill—generally associated with more severe stenosis
• Arrhythmias may occur; the heart rate may be high in CHF.
• Other signs of CHF include ascites, jugular venous distension, and tachypnea.

CAUSES
Congenital

RISK FACTORS
N/A

DIAGNOSIS

DIFFERENTIAL DIAGNOSIS
Similar Murmurs May Be Found with
• Aortic stenosis
• Ventricular or atrial septal defects with marked left-to-right shunting
• Tetralogy of Fallot

R-CHF Associated with a Murmur May Be Seen With
• Acquired valvular disease (endocardiosis)
• Dilated cardiomyopathy

CBC/BIOCHEMISTRY/URINALYSIS
Generally unremarkable

OTHER LABORATORY TESTS
N/A

IMAGING
Radiographic findings
• Thoracic radiographs usually show right-sided cardiac enlargement, with a poststenotic pulmonary artery bulge visible on the dorso-ventral view at 1–2 o'clock.
• The caudal vena cava may be wide, and ascites may be present with or without pleural effusion in congestive failure.

Echocardiographic Findings
• Right ventricular hypertrophy, with flattening of the interventricular septum and a "figure-of-eight" appearance on short axis views in severe cases
• Can usually image the site of the stenosis, but may be more difficult when the valve is hypoplastic. Dysplastic pulmonic valves appear as thickened echodense leaflets; fused leaflets have abnormal motion with systolic doming; discrete subvalvular or supravalvular stenoses may appear as a localized hyperechoic narrowing.
• Localized hypertrophy may be seen in the right ventricular infundibular region.
• May see poststenotic dilation of the pulmonary artery

Doppler Echocardiography
• Can use spectral Doppler to measure the elevated pulmonary artery flow velocity to calculate the pressure gradient across the stenosis. Pressure gradients under 50 mm Hg generally represent mild stenosis; those over 100 mm Hg, severe stenosis.
• Color-flow Doppler may reveal tricuspid regurgitation.

Angiography
• Selective cardiac angiography can help identify the precise morphologic abnormalities prior to surgery; may image dysplastic valves and hypertrophy of the infundibulum and supravalvular crest more clearly
• Useful in identifying pulmonic stenosis caused by an anomalous coronary artery encircling the right ventricular outflow tract, which may affect the choice of therapy; recommended for English bulldogs because this anomaly is reported frequently

DIAGNOSTIC PROCEDURES
Electrocardiography
• QRS complex waveform changes include deep S waves in leads I, II, III, and aVF and right axis deviation.

• Atrial fibrillation may occur with severe right atrial enlargement.

Cardiac Catheterization
Pressure measurement by this technique is rarely necessary for diagnosis; pressure gradients can be assessed noninvasively with Doppler echocardiography.

PATHOLOGIC FINDINGS
• Various forms exist; most result in right ventricular hypertrophy and poststenotic dilation of the pulmonary artery; infundibular hypertrophy may occur proximal to the obstruction.
• Hypoplastic pulmonic valve, with thickened leaflets ("dysplastic pulmonic valve")
• Normal pulmonic valve annulus with fused commissures
• Anomalous coronary arteries
• Discrete supravalvular or subvalvular stenosis, with possible concurrent tricuspid dysplasia
• Fibromuscular bands dividing the right ventricular inflow and outflow tracts ("double-chambered right ventricle")

 TREATMENT

APPROPRIATE HEALTH CARE
Most managed as outpatients; initial hospitalization of those with severe CHF may be better.

Nursing Care
Rarely, pleural effusions may need draining; ascites is usually treated medically.

Activity
Exercise should be restricted in cases with syncope or congestive failure, and severe exertion should be avoided in asymptomatic cases with severe stenosis.

Diet
Low-salt diets may benefit those with refractory ascites.

Client Education
• Mildly affected animals may lead normal lives.
• Severely affected patients may benefit from interventions such as balloon catheter dilation or surgery; prognosis is guarded once congestive signs develop.
• Do not breed affected animals.

Surgical Considerations
• Balloon catheter dilation—relatively safe procedure that involves passing a catheter across the stenosis and inflating a balloon to dilate the obstruction; in many cases, the pressure gradient is significantly reduced, especially when the lesion is caused by fused commissures; less successful with dysplastic or hypoplastic valves and contraindicated with anomalous coronary arteries
• Alternative surgical techniques include valvulotomy or patch-graft procedures; mortality rates tend to be higher than with balloon valvuloplasty.

 MEDICATIONS

DRUGS OF CHOICE
If signs of CHF, treat ascites with furosemide (2–4 mg/kg PO q8–12h); in refractory failure, it may be worth adding spironolactone (1–2 mg/kg PO q12h); treat atrial fibrillation with digoxin (0.22 mg/m$_2$ PO q12h).

CONTRAINDICATIONS
Vasodilators (e.g. hydralazine, enalapril) may cause hypotension without relieving the stenosis and are best avoided.

PRECAUTIONS
Take care to avoid overuse of diuretics; administer intravenous fluids (when required) cautiously to avoid exacerbating congestive signs.

POSSIBLE INTERACTIONS
N/A

ALTERNATIVE DRUGS
N/A

 FOLLOW-UP

PATIENT MONITORING
Use serial echocardiograms to follow the pressure gradient and cardiac chamber size.

PREVENTION/AVOIDANCE
Do not breed affected animals.

POSSIBLE COMPLICATIONS
• R-CHF
• Arrhythmias
• Exercise intolerance
• Exertional syncope
• Sudden death

EXPECTED COURSE AND PROGNOSIS
• Mildly affected animals may remain asymptomatic with a normal life span.
• Severely affected animals have a guarded prognosis because they may develop CHF or sudden death; clinical signs are generally more common in animals over 1 year of age.

 MISCELLANEOUS

ASSOCIATED CONDITIONS
• Ventricular septal defects, atrial septal defects, and patent foramen ovale
• English bulldogs described with a single right coronary artery from which an anomalous left main coronary artery arises and then encircles and constricts the base of the pulmonic valve

AGE-RELATED FACTORS
Defect and murmur are present from birth.

ZOONOTIC POTENTIAL
N/A

PREGNANCY
Do not breed affected animals.

SYNONYMS
Pulmonary stenosis

SEE ALSO
• R-CHF
• Murmurs, Heart

ABBREVIATIONS
• PS = pulmonic stenosis
• R-CHF = right-sided congestive heart failure

Suggested Reading
Bonagura JD, Darke PGG. Congenital heart disease. In: Ettinger SJ, ed. Textbook of veterinary internal medicine. 4th ed. Philadelphia: Saunders, 1995:892–943.
Buchanan JW. Pulmonic stenosis caused by single coronary artery in dogs: four cases (1965–1984). J Am Vet Med Assoc 1990;196:115–120.
Fingland RB, Bonagura JD, Myer CW. Pulmonic stenosis in the dog: 29 cases (1975–1984). J Am Vet Med Assoc 1986;189:218–226.
Martin MWS, Godman M, Luis Fuentes V, et al. Assessment of balloon pulmonary valvuloplasty in six dogs. J Small Anim Pract 1992;33:443–449.
Orton EC, Bruecker KA, McCracken TO. An open patch-graft technique for correction of pulmonic stenosis in the dog. Vet Surg 1990;19:148–154.

Author Virginia Luis Fuentes
Consulting Editors Larry P. Tilley and Francis W. K. Smith, Jr.

PUPPY STRANGLES (JUVENILE CELLULITIS)

BASICS

OVERVIEW
• An uncommon granulomatous and pustular disorder of puppies
• Rarely seen in adult dogs
• The face, pinnae, and submandibular lymph nodes are the most common sites.
• Immunopathogenesis unknown

SIGNALMENT
• Dogs
• Age range—usually between 3 weeks and 4 months
• Predisposed breeds—golden retrievers, dachshunds, and Gordon setters

SIGNS
• Acutely swollen face (eyelids, lips, and muzzle)
• Submandibular lymphadenopathy
• A marked pustular and exudative dermatitis, which frequently fistulates, develops within 24–48 hr.
• Purulent otitis externa
• Lesions often become crusted.
• Affected skin is usually painful.
• Lethargy—50% of cases
• Anorexia, pyrexia, and a sterile suppurative arthritis—25% of cases
• A sterile pyogranulomatous panniculitis (rare) over the trunk, preputial, or perianal area; lesions may appear as fluctuant subcutaneous nodules that fistulate.

CAUSES & RISK FACTORS
• Cause and pathogenesis unknown
• An immune dysfunction with a heritable cause is suspected.

DIAGNOSIS

DIFFERENTIAL DIAGNOSIS
• Staphylococcal dermatitis
• Demodicosis
• Drug eruption
• Deep fungal infection

CBC/BIOCHEMISTRY/URINALYSIS
No specific changes noted

OTHER LABORATORY TESTS
• Cytology—pyogranulomatous inflammation with no microorganisms; nondegenerate neutrophils
• Culture—sterile

IMAGING
N/A

DIAGNOSTIC PROCEDURES
• Skin biopsy
• Multiple discrete or confluent granulomas and pyogranulomas—clusters of large epithelioid macrophages and neutrophils
• Sebaceous glands and apocrine glands may be obliterated.
• Suppurative changes in the dermis—predominate in later stages
• Panniculitis

TREATMENT
• Early and aggressive therapy, because scarring may be severe
• Topical therapy—may be soothing and palliative; adjunct to corticosteroids

Puppy Strangles (Juvenile Cellulitis)

 MEDICATIONS

DRUGS
• Corticosteroids—high doses required; prednisone (2.2 mg/kg divided twice daily for at least 2 weeks)
• Do not taper too rapidly.
• Chemotherapeutics—rare resistant cases
• Adult dogs with panniculitis may require longer therapy.
• Antibiotics—if there is evidence of secondary bacterial infection; as an adjunct therapy with immunosuppressive doses of steroids

CONTRAINDICATIONS/POSSIBLE INTERACTIONS
None

 FOLLOW-UP
• Most cases do not recur.
• Scarring may be a problem, especially around the eyes.

 MISCELLANEOUS

Suggested Reading
Scott DW, Miller WH, Griffin CE. eds. Muller & Kirk's small animal dermatology. Philadelphia: Saunders, 1995:938–941.
Author Karen Helton Rhodes
Consulting Editor Karen Helton Rhodes

PYELONEPHRITIS

BASICS

DEFINITION
A microbial colonization of the upper urinary tract including the renal pelvis, collecting diverticula, renal parenchyma, and ureters; because it is not usually limited to the renal pelvis and parenchyma, a more descriptive term is *upper urinary tract infection;* this chapter is limited to bacterial pyelonephritis.

PATHOPHYSIOLOGY
• Infection of any portion of the urinary tract usually requires some impairment of normal host defenses against urinary tract infection (see chapter on lower urinary tract infection); normal defenses against ascending urinary tract infection include mucosal defense barriers, ureteral peristalsis, ureterovesical flap valves, and an extensive renal blood supply. Pyelonephritis usually occurs by ascension of microbes causing lower urinary tract infection. In dogs and cats, hematogenous seeding of the kidneys does not usually cause pyelonephritis. Regardless of the route of infection, an upper urinary tract infection is frequently accompanied by lower urinary tract infection.
• Can develop secondarily to infection of metabolic nephroliths; upper urinary tract infection with urease-producing bacteria can predispose to formation of struvite nephroliths.
• Obstruction of an infected kidney or ureter can cause septicemia (so-called urosepsis).

SYSTEMS AFFECTED
• Renal/Urologic
• Can cause urosepsis, thus affecting any body system

GENETICS
N/A

INCIDENCE/PREVALENCE
• Unknown
• Probably occurs much more commonly than is recognized clinically, because many animals with pyelonephritis are asymptomatic or have signs limited to lower urinary tract infection.

GEOGRAPHIC DISTRIBUTION
N/A

SIGNALMENT

Species
Dogs affected more commonly than cats

Breed Predilections
N/A

Mean Age and Range
Mean age of affected dogs and cats unknown; dogs of any age can be affected.

Predominant Sex
Unknown; dogs—urinary tract infection affects more females than males; cats—urinary tract infection is uncommon and occurs with similar frequency in males and females

SIGNS

General Comments
Many patients are asymptomatic or have signs of lower urinary tract infection only

Historical Findings
• None
• Polyuria/polydipsia (PU/PD)
• Abdominal or lumbar pain
• Signs associated with lower urinary tract infection—e.g., dysuria, pollakiuria, stranguria, hematuria, and malodorous or discolored urine

Physical Examination Findings
• None
• Pain upon palpation of kidneys
• Fever

CAUSES
Usually, ascending urinary tract infection caused by aerobic bacteria; most common isolates are *Escherichia coli* and *Staphylococcus* spp.; other bacteria, including *Proteus, Streptococcus, Klebsiella, Enterobacter,* and *Pseudomonas* spp., which frequently infect the lower urinary tract, may ascend into the upper urinary tract. Anaerobic bacteria, ureaplasma, and fungi rarely infect the upper urinary tract.

RISK FACTORS
• Ectopic ureters, vesicoureteral reflux, congenital renal dysplasia, and lower urinary tract infection; conditions that predispose to urinary tract infection—e.g., diabetes mellitus, hyperadrenocorticism, exogenous steroid administration, renal failure, urethral catheterization, urine retention, uroliths, urinary tract neoplasia, perineal urethrostomy
• In cats with experimentally induced lower urinary tract disease, indwelling urinary catheters combined with administration of exogenous steroids frequently resulted in pyelonephritis.

DIAGNOSIS

DIFFERENTIAL DIAGNOSIS
• Clinical diagnosis of pyelonephritis is usually presumptive, based on results from CBC, biochemical analysis, urinalysis, urine culture, and diagnostic imaging; definitive diagnosis is not usually required for planning treatment.
• Since many dogs and cats lack specific symptoms attributable to pyelonephritis, any patient with urinary tract infection could potentially have pyelonephritis; the best methods for differentiating between upper and lower urinary tract infection are ultrasonography or excretory urography.
• Consider the possibility of pyelonephritis since patients are frequently asymptomatic; consider as a differential diagnosis for dogs or cats with fever of unknown origin, PU/PD, chronic renal failure, or lumbar/abdominal pain.

CBC/BIOCHEMISTRY/URINALYSIS
• CBC—results often normal with chronic pyelonephritis; leukocytosis and neutrophilia with a left shift detected in some patients
• Biochemistry—usually normal unless chronic pyelonephritis leads to chronic renal failure (azotemia with an inappropriate urinary specific gravity)
• Urinalysis reveals hematuria, pyuria, proteinuria, bacteriuria, and leukocyte casts in some animals. Leukocyte casts are diagnostic for renal inflammation and usually result from pyelonephritis. Observe dilute urine specific gravity in patients with nephrogenic diabetes insipidus, which may occur secondary to pyelonephritis. Absence of abnormalities does not rule out pyelonephritis.

OTHER LABORATORY TESTS
• Quantitative urine culture to confirm urinary tract infection; see chapter on lower urinary tract infection for interpretation.
• Dogs with chronic pyelonephritis may have a negative urine culture and require multiple urine cultures to confirm urinary tract infection.

IMAGING
• Ultrasonography or excretory urography are the best methods for presumptively differentiating between upper and lower urinary tract infection. Experimentally, ultrasonography is more useful than excretory urography for identification of mild-to-moderate acute pyelonephritis.
• Ultrasonographic findings supporting pyelonephritis include dilation of the renal pelvis and proximal ureter and a hyperechoic mucosal margin line within the renal pelvis and/or proximal ureter.
• Excretory urography may reveal dilation and blunting of the renal pelvis with lack of filling of the collecting diverticula, dilation of the proximal ureter, decreased opacity of the nephrogram phase and of the contrast media in the collecting system.
• In patients with acute pyelonephritis, the kidneys may be large; in patients with chronic pyelonephritis, the kidneys may be small with an irregular surface contour.
• Concomitant nephroliths detected in some patients by survey radiography, ultrasonography, or excretory urography

DIAGNOSTIC PROCEDURES
• Definitive diagnosis requires urine cultures obtained from the renal pelvis or parenchyma or histopathology from a renal biopsy. Pyelocentesis can be performed percutaneously using ultrasound guidance or during exploratory surgery; can obtain specimen for culture from the renal pelvis (or from nephroliths) during nephrotomy

• To confirm the diagnosis the biopsy specimen must include the renal cortex and medulla; thus renal biopsy should be performed by open surgery and only if necessary.

• May have a patchy distribution and can be missed by needle biopsy.

PATHOLOGIC FINDINGS

• Kidneys affected by chronic pyelonephritis have areas of infarction and scarring on the capsular surface in some animals. The renal pelvis and collecting diverticula may be dilated and distorted from chronic infection and inflammation. Purulent exudate is occasionally noted in the renal pelvis.

• Histologic findings include papillitis, pyelitis, interstitial nephritis, and leukocyte casts in tubular lumens.

TREATMENT

APPROPRIATE HEALTH CARE

Outpatient unless animal has septicemia or renal failure

NURSING CARE

N/A

ACTIVITY

Unlimited

DIET

Modification recommended in animals with concomitant chronic renal failure or nephrolithiasis

CLIENT EDUCATION

• Recurrent pyelonephritis may be asymptomatic. Unresolved chronic pyelonephritis may lead to chronic renal failure; diagnostic follow-up is important to document resolution of pyelonephritis.

• In patients with nephroliths, resolution is unlikely unless the nephroliths are removed.

SURGICAL CONSIDERATIONS

• Complete obstruction of the upper urinary tract of a patient with pyelonephritis may result in urosepsis and should be corrected by surgery (or lithotripsy for nephroliths).

• Infected nephroliths—surgically remove, medically dissolve (struvite), or fragment by extracorporeal shock wave lithotripsy; use periprocedural antibiotics to reduce the risk of urosepsis when manipulating infected nephroliths

• Unilateral nephrectomy is not effective for elimination of suspected unilateral pyelonephritis.

MEDICATIONS

DRUGS OF CHOICE

• Base antibiotic selection on urine culture and sensitivity testing.

• Antibiotics should be bactericidal, achieve good serum and urine concentrations, and not be nephrotoxic.

• High serum and urinary antibiotic concentrations do not necessarily ensure high tissue concentrations in the renal medulla; thus chronic pyelonephritis may be difficult to eradicate.

• Give orally administered antibiotics at full therapeutic dosages for 4–6 weeks.

• Do not use drugs that achieve good concentrations in urine but poor concentrations in serum (e.g., nitrofurantoin).

CONTRAINDICATIONS

Do not use aminoglycosides unless no other alternatives exist on the basis of urine culture and sensitivity testing.

PRECAUTIONS

Trimethoprim/sulfa combinations can cause side effects (keratoconjunctivitis sicca, blood dyscrasias, polyarthritis) when administered for more than 4 weeks.

POSSIBLE INTERACTIONS

N/A

ALTERNATIVE DRUGS

N/A

FOLLOW-UP

PATIENT MONITORING

Do urine cultures and urinalysis during antibiotic administration (~ 5–7 days into treatment) and 1 and 4 weeks after antibiotics are finished.

PREVENTION/AVOIDANCE

Eliminate factors predisposing to urinary tract infection; correct ectopic ureters.

POSSIBLE COMPLICATIONS

Renal failure, recurrent pyelonephritis, struvite nephrolithiasis, septicemia, septic shock, metastatic infection (e.g., endocarditis, polyarthritis)

EXPECTED COURSE AND PROGNOSIS

• Patients with pyelonephritis—fair to good, with a return to normal health unless the patient also has nephrolithiasis, chronic renal failure, or some other underlying cause for urinary tract infection (e.g., obstruction or neoplasia)

• Established infection of the renal medulla may be difficult to resolve because of poor tissue penetration of antibiotics.

• Patients with chronic renal failure caused by pyelonephritis—determined by the severity and rate of progression of the chronic renal failure

• Recurrent pyelonephritis is likely if infected nephroliths are not removed.

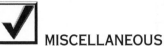

MISCELLANEOUS

ASSOCIATED CONDITIONS

Hyperadrenocorticism, exogenous glucocorticoid administration, and diabetes mellitus are associated with lower urinary tract infection, which can ascend into the ureters and kidneys.

AGE-RELATED FACTORS

N/A

ZOONOTIC POTENTIAL

N/A

PREGNANCY

Use antibiotics that are safe for the pregnant bitch or queen.

SYNONYMS

Upper urinary tract infection, pyelitis

SEE ALSO

• Lower Urinary Tract Infection
• Nephrolithiasis
• Renal Failure, Chronic
• Urinary Tract Obstruction
• Urolithiasis, Struvite—Canine
• Urolithiasis, Struvite—Feline

ABBREVIATIONS

PU/PD = polyuria and polydipsia

Suggested Reading

Allen TA, Jaenke RS. Pyelonephritis in the dog. Compend Contin Educ Pract Vet 1985;7:421–428.

Lees GE, Forrester SD. Update: bacterial urinary tract infections. In: Kirk RW, Bonagura JD, eds. Current Veterinary Therapy. XI Philadelphia: WB Saunders, 1992:909–914.

Lulich JP, Osborne CA. Fungal urinary tract infections. In: Kirk RW, Bonagura JD, eds. Current veterinary therapy. XI Philadelphia: WB Saunders, 1992:914–919.

Lulich JP, Osborne CA. Bacterial infections of the urinary tract. In: Ettinger SJ, Feldman EC, eds. Textbook of veterinary internal medicine. 4th ed. Philadelphia: WB Saunders, 1995:1775–1788.

Neuwirth L, Mahaffey M, Crowell W, et al. Comparison of excretory urography and ultrasonography for detection of experimentally induced pyelonephritis in dogs. Am J Vet Res 1993;54:660–669.

Author Larry G. Adams
Consulting Editors Larry G. Adams and Carl A. Osborne

DISEASES

PYODERMA

 BASICS

DEFINITION
Bacterial infection of the skin

PATHOPHYSIOLOGY
Skin infections occur when the surface integrity of the skin has been broken, the skin has become macerated by chronic exposure to moisture, normal bacterial flora have been altered, circulation has been impaired, or immunocompetency has been compromised.

SYSTEMS AFFECTED
Skin/Exocrine

GENETICS
N/A

INCIDENCE/PREVALENCE
• Dogs—very common
• Cats—uncommon

GEOGRAPHIC DISTRIBUTION
N/A

SIGNALMENT
Species
Dogs and cats
Breed Predilections
• Breeds with short coats, skin folds, or pressure calluses
• German shepherds develop a severe, deep pyoderma that may only partially respond to antibiotics and frequently relapses.
Mean Age and Range
Age of onset usually related to underlying cause
Predominant Sex
N/A

SIGNS
General Comments
• Superficial—usually involves the trunk; extent of lesions may be obscured by the hair coat.
• Deep—often affects the chin, bridge of the nose, pressure points, and feet; may be generalized

Historical Findings
• Acute or gradual onset
• Variable pruritus—underlying cause may be pruritic or the staphylococcal infection itself may be pruritic

Physical Examination Findings
• Papules
• Pustules
• Hemorrhagic bullae
• Crusts
• Epidermal collarettes
• Circular erythematous or hyperpigmented spots
• Target lesions
• Alopecia, moth-eaten hair coat
• Scaling
• Lichenification
• Abscess
• Furunculosis, cellulitis

CAUSES
• *Staphylococcus intermedius*—most frequent
• *Pasteurella multocida*—an important pathogen in cats
• Deep—may be complicated by gram-negative organisms (e.g., *E. coli, Proteus* spp., *Pseudomonas* spp.)
• Rarely caused by higher bacteria (e.g., *Actinomyces, Nocardia, Mycobacteria, Actinobacillus*)

RISK FACTORS
• Allergy—flea; atopy; food; contact
• Parasites—especially *Demodex*
• Fungal infection—dermatophyte
• Endocrine disease—hypothyroidism; hyperadrenocorticism; sex hormone imbalance
• Immune incompetency—glucocorticoids; young animals
• Seborrhea—acne; schnauzer comedo syndrome
• Conformation—short coat; skin folds
• Trauma—pressure points; grooming; scratching; rooting behavior; irritants
• Foreign body—foxtail; grass awn

 DIAGNOSIS

DIFFERENTIAL DIAGNOSIS
• Allergy—pruritus usually precedes the rash; pruritus will not resolve with resolution of the pyoderma.

• Endocrine problem causing a relapsing pyoderma—consider if pruritus resolves with resolution of the pyoderma; reports of polydipsia, polyuria, pendulous abdomen, lethargy, weight gain, and/or signs of feminization
• Flea allergy or atopy—may be seasonal
• Pustular disease—superficial staphylococcal pyoderma; dermatophytosis; demodicosis; pemphigus foliaceus; and subcorneal pustular dermatosis
• Furunculosis—deep staphylococcal pyoderma; higher bacterial infection; demodicosis; dermatophytosis; opportunistic fungal infections; deep fungal infections; panniculitis; and zinc-responsive dermatosis
• Superficial pyoderma in short-coated breeds is often misdiagnosed as urticaria, because of the acute onset of pruritic papules misdiagnosed as hives.

CBC/BIOCHEMISTRY/URINALYSIS
• Superficial—normal or may reflect the underlying cause (e.g., anemia owing to hypothyroidism; stress leukogram and high serum alkaline phosphatase owing to Cushing disease; eosinophilia owing to parasitism)
• Generalized, deep—may show leukocytosis with a left shift and hyperglobulinemia; also changes related to the underlying cause

OTHER LABORATORY TESTS
N/A

IMAGING
N/A

DIAGNOSTIC PROCEDURES
• Skin scrapings, dermatophyte culture, intradermal allergy testing, hypoallergenic food trial, endocrine tests—identify the underlying cause
• Skin biopsy
• Direct smear from intact pustule—neutrophils engulfing bacteria
• Cytology—differentiate pemphigus foliaceus (acantholytic keratinocytes) and deep fungal infections (blastomycosis, cryptococcosis) from pyodermas; of tissue grains may identify filamentous organisms characteristic of higher bacteria

Culture
• Usually positive for *S. intermedius*
• Other gram-negative organisms besides staphylococci and higher bacteria may be cultured from deep pyodermas.
• Contents of an intact pustule—most reliable results
• Punch biopsy obtained by sterile technique—if no pustules are noted; more likely to get false-negative results
• Freshly expressed exudate from a draining tract or beneath a crust—may yield the pathogen or a contaminant; least reliable method

PATHOLOGIC FINDINGS
• Subcorneal pustules
• Intraepidermal neutrophilic microabscesses
• Perifolliculitis
• Folliculitis
• Furunculosis
• Nodular to diffuse dermatitis
• Panniculitis
• Inflammatory reaction—suppurative or pyogranulomatous
• Tissue grains within pyogranulomas—observed most often with *Staphylococcus, Actinomyces, Actinobacillus,* and *Nocardia*
• Special stains—identify gram-negative bacteria or acid-fast organisms

TREATMENT

APPROPRIATE HEALTH CARE
Usually outpatient, except for severe, generalized deep pyodermas

NURSING CARE
• Severe, generalized, deep—may require IV fluids, parenteral antibiotics, or daily whirlpool baths
• Benzoyl peroxide or chlorhexidine shampoos—remove surface debris
• Whirlpool baths—deep pyodermas; remove crusted exudate; encourage drainage

ACTIVITY
No restriction

DIET
• Hypoallergenic if secondary to food allergy; otherwise a high-quality, well-balanced dog food
• Avoid high-protein, poor-quality "bargain" diets and excessive supplementation.

CLIENT EDUCATION
N/A

SURGICAL CONSIDERATIONS
Fold pyodermas require surgical correction to prevent recurrence.

MEDICATIONS

DRUGS OF CHOICE
• *S. intermedius* isolates—usually susceptible to cephalosporins, cloxacillin, oxacillin, methicillin, amoxicillin-clavulanate, erythromycin, and chloramphenicol; somewhat less responsive to lincomycin and trimethoprim-sulfonamide; frequently resistant to amoxicillin, ampicillin, penicillin, tetracycline, and sulfonamides
• Amoxicillin-clavulanate—most isolates of *Staphylococcus* and *P. multocida* susceptible; generally effective for skin infections in cats
• Superficial—initially may be treated empirically with one of the antibiotics listed above
• Recurrent, resistant, or deep—base antibiotic therapy on culture and sensitivity testing
• Multiple organisms with different antibiotic sensitivities—choose antibiotic on basis of staphylococcal susceptibility

CONTRAINDICATIONS
Steroids—will encourage resistance and recurrence even when used concurrently with antibiotics

PRECAUTIONS
• Erythromycin, lincomycin, and oxacillin—vomiting; administer with small amount of food
• Gentamicin and kanamycin—renal toxicity usually precludes their prolonged systemic use.
• Trimethoprim-sulfa—associated with keratoconjunctivitis sicca, fever, hepatotoxicity, polyarthritis, and hematologic abnormalities
• Chloramphenicol—use with caution in cats; may cause mild, reversible anemia in dogs

POSSIBLE INTERACTIONS
Trimethoprim-sulfa—may lead to low thyroid test results

ALTERNATIVE DRUGS
Staphage lysate, staphoid AB, or autogenous bacterins—may improve antibiotic efficacy and decrease recurrence in a small percentage of cases

FOLLOW-UP

PATIENT MONITORING
Administer antibiotics for a minimum of 2 weeks beyond clinical cure; this is usually about 1 month for superficial pyodermas, and 2–3+ months for deep pyodermas.

PREVENTION/AVOIDANCE
• Routine bathing with benzoyl peroxide or chlorhexidine shampoos—may help prevent recurrences
• Some cases that continue to relapse may be managed with subliminal inhibitory concentrations of antibiotics (long-term/low-dose).
• Padded bedding—may ease pressure point pyodermas
• Topical benzoyl peroxide gel or mupirocin ointment may be helpful adjunct therapies

POSSIBLE COMPLICATIONS
Bacteremia and septicemia

EXPECTED COURSE AND PROGNOSIS
Likely to be recurrent or nonresponsive if underlying cause is not identified and effectively managed

MISCELLANEOUS

ASSOCIATED CONDITIONS
N/A

AGE-RELATED FACTORS
• Impetigo—affects young dogs before puberty; associated with poor husbandry; often requires only topical therapy
• Superficial pustular dermatitis—occurs in kittens; associated with overzealous "mouthing" by the queen
• Pyoderma secondary to atopy—usually begins at 1–3 years of age
• Pyoderma secondary to endocrine disorders—usually begins in middle adulthood

ZOONOTIC POTENTIAL
• Cutaneus tuberculosis—rare
• Feline leprosy—unknown

PREGNANCY
N/A

SEE ALSO
• Acne—Cats
• Acne—Dogs
• Interdigital Dermatitis
• Perianal Fistula
• Pododermatitis

Suggested Reading
Muller GH, Kirk RW, Scott DW. Small animal dermatology. 4th ed. Philadelphia: Saunders, 1989.

Authors Ellen C. Codner and Karen Helton Rhodes

Consulting Editor Karen Helton Rhodes

PYOMETRA AND CYSTIC ENDOMETRIAL HYPERPLASIA

BASICS

DEFINITION
• Cystic endometrial hyperplasia—hormonally mediated, progressive pathologic change in the uterine lining
• Pyometra—secondary to cystic endometrial hyperplasia; develops when bacterial invasion of the abnormal endometrium leads to intraluminal accumulation of purulent exudate

PATHOPHYSIOLOGY
• Normal cycling bitches—2-month diestrus, with ovarian secretion of progesterone after every estrus
• Repeated exposure of the endometrium to high concentrations of estrogen followed by high concentrations of progesterone without pregnancy—leads to cystic endometrial hyperplasia
• Bacteria—secretions provide excellent media for growth; ascend from the vagina through the partially open cervix during proestrus and estrus; normal vaginal flora; *Escherichia coli* most common isolate

SYSTEMS AFFECTED
• Reproductive
• Renal/Urologic
• Hemic/Lymphatic/Immune
• Hepatobiliary

GENETICS
No predisposition known

INCIDENCE/PREVALENCE
Incidence—accurate assessment cannot be made because most dogs and cats in the U.S. undergo elective ovariohysterectomy.

GEOGRAPHIC DISTRIBUTION
N/A

SIGNALMENT
Species
Dogs and cats

Breed Predilections
N/A

Mean Age and Range
• Usually > 6 years old
• Young animals—especially if treated with exogenous estrogen or progestogen
• Dogs—usually diagnosed 1–12 weeks after estrus
• Cats—onset relative to estrus more variable
• Pyometra of the uterine stump in spayed animals—may develop any time after ovariohysterectomy

Breed Predilections
• None known

Predominant Sex
N/A

SIGNS

Historical Findings
Closed cervix—signs systemic illness, progressing to signs of septicemia and shock

Physical Examination Findings
• Uterus—palpably large; careful palpation may allow determination of size; overly aggressive palpation may induce rupture; with open cervix, may not be palpably large
• Vaginal discharge—depends on cervical patency; sanguinous to mucopurulent
• Depression and lethargy
• Anorexia
• Polyuria and polydipsia
• Vomiting
• Abdominal distension

CAUSES
• Dogs—the unique, repeated exposure of the endometrium to estrogen followed by exposure to progesterone
• Cats—may be the result of estrogen at estrus followed by a progestational phase, caused by induction of ovulation by coitus or other (as yet undefined) stimuli

RISK FACTORS
• Old, nulliparous females may be predisposed.
• Pharmacologic use of estrogen (mismate) shots during midstrus to early diestrus
• No correlation with pseudopregnancy in dogs

DIAGNOSIS

DIFFERENTIAL DIAGNOSIS
• Pregnancy
• Other causes of polyuria and polydipsia—diabetes mellitus; hyperadrenocorticism; primary renal disease
• Severe vaginal disease

CBC/BIOCHEMISTRY/URINALYSIS
• Neutrophilia—immature; more severe with closed cervix
• Mild, normocytic, normochromic anemia
• Hyperglobulinemia and hyperproteinemia
• Azotemia
• ALT and ALP—high with septicemia or severe dehydration
• Electrolyte disturbances—depend on clinical course
• Urinalysis—sample collected by catheterization of the urinary bladder (least traumatic and most diagnostically accurate)

OTHER LABORATORY TESTS
• Cytologic examination of vaginal discharge—regenerative polymorphonuclear cells and bacteria; may be indistinguishable from the purulent discharge associated with vaginal disease (e.g., vaginitis, vaginal mass, foreign object, and vaginal anatomic anomaly)
• Bacterial culture and sensitivity test of vaginal discharge—not helpful in confirming diagnosis (bacteria cultured are usually normal vaginal flora); is useful in determining appropriate antibiotic use
• Serologic testing for *Brucella canis*—rapid slide agglutination test used as a screen; sensitive but not specific; if positive, recheck by an agar gel immunodiffusion test (Cornell University Diagnostic Laboratory, 607-253-3900) or bacterial culture of whole blood, lymph node aspirate, or vaginal discharge.

IMAGING

Radiography
• Detect a large uterus
• Rule out pregnancy—45 days after ovulation; 43–54 days after breeding
• Pyometra—uterus may appear as a distended, tubular structure in the caudal ventral abdomen.

Ultrasonography
• Assess size of uterus and extent of cystic endometrial hyperplasia; nature of uterine contents
• Rule out pregnancy—20–24 days ovulation
• Normal uterine wall—not visible as a distinct entity
• Pyometra or cystic endometrial hyperplasia—associated with a thickened uterine wall and intraluminal fluid
• Pyometra—may occur with pregnancy in dogs (rare)

DIAGNOSTIC PROCEDURES
Vaginoscopy—indicated only in dogs with purulent vulvar discharge and no apparent uterine enlargement; allows determination of site of origin of the vaginal discharge; not possible in cats

PATHOLOGIC FINDINGS
• Endometrium (dogs and cats)—described as cobblestone (either condition)
• Cystic endometrial surface—covered by malodorous, mucopurulent exudate; thickened because of increased endometrial gland size and cystic gland distension

TREATMENT

APPROPRIATE HEALTH CARE
• Inpatient
• Pyometra—life-threatening condition if the cervix is closed

PYOMETRA AND CYSTIC ENDOMETRIAL HYPERPLASIA

NURSING CARE
Supportive care—immediate intravenous fluid administration and antibiotics

ACTIVITY
N/A

DIET
N/A

CLIENT EDUCATION
• Inform client that ovariohysterectomy is the preferred treatment.
• Recommend medical treatment only for valuable breeding animals; warn client that nonprogestational, estrus-suppressing drugs must be given for life.
• Warn client that medical treatment of closed-cervix pyometra can be associated with uterine rupture and peritonitis (see Precautions).
• Inform client that medical treatment probably does not cure underlying cystic endometrial hyperplasia in patients with either open- or closed-cervix pyometra but may enable some affected bitches to reproduce.

SURGICAL CONSIDERATIONS
• Pyometra (open and closed cervix)—ovariohysterectomy preferred treatment; chronic progressive disease
• Closed-cervix pyometra—use caution during ovariohysterectomy; enlarged uterus may be friable.
• Uterine rupture or leakage of purulent material from the uterine stump—repeated lavage of the peritoneal cavity with sterile saline

MEDICATIONS

DRUGS OF CHOICE

Antibiotics
• Empirical, pending results of bacterial culture and sensitivity test
• All patients with pyometra
• Common choices—ampicillin (20 mg/kg PO q8h); enrofloxacin (Baytril; 2.5 mg/kg PO q12h)

PGF$_{2\alpha}$
• Recommended dosages for only the native compound; dosages for analogues not well defined
• Cats—0.1–0.5 mg/kg SC q24h for 2–5 days until the size of the uterus nears normal
Dogs
• Administered at 0.05–0.25 mg/kg SC q24h for 2–7 days until the uterus nears normal size as determined by palpation, radiography, or ultrasound
• In luteal phase (serum progesterone > 2 ng/mL)—may use 0.05–0.25 mg/kg SC q12h for 4 days
• Once-daily dosing—causes smooth muscle contractions and subsequent uterine evacuation

• Twice-daily dosing—causes luteolysis and a subsequent decrease in serum progesterone concentration
• Re-evaluate patient 2–4 weeks after discontinuation; if the uterus has increased in size or the patient still has marked vaginal discharge, the protocol can be repeated.
• Ovariohysterectomy—performed in patients refractory to prostaglandin

CONTRAINDICATIONS
• PGF$_{2\alpha}$ with closed-cervix pyometra—strong myometrial contractions may cause uterine rupture or force purulent exudate through the uterine tubes, causing secondary peritonitis.
• PGF$_{2\alpha}$ in a valuable breeding animal—always rule out pregnancy before administering.

PRECAUTIONS
• PGF$_{2\alpha}$—not approved for use in dogs and cats
• Side effects of PGF$_{2\alpha}$—referable to contraction of smooth muscle; hypersalivation emesis; defecation; intense grooming of the flanks and vulva (cats); appear within minutes of injection; subside within 30–60 min; severity diminishes throughout the treatment regimen; may be diminished by diluting the drug with an equal volume of sterile saline before subcutaneous injection and by walking dogs for 20–30 min after injection

POSSIBLE INTERACTIONS
N/A

ALTERNATIVE DRUGS
• Drugs that enhance the immune response (e.g., estrogens) or induce myometrial contractility (e.g., oxytocin and ergot alkaloids)—unreliable
• Antibiotics—not efficacious as sole treatment unless the uterus is of normal size and the serum progesterone is < 2 ng/mL

FOLLOW-UP

PATIENT MONITORING
• Discharge from the hospital—when the uterus is of near normal size and clinical signs have lessened in severity or disappeared; re-evaluation in 2–4 weeks
• Antibiotics—administration continued for 3–4 weeks
• Vaginal discharge—may persist for up to 4 weeks
• Serial CBC—WBC count rises precipitously after ovariohysterectomy, because bone marrow continues to release polymorphonuclear neutrophils into the bloodstream, from which they can no longer enter the uterus (the sink of inflammation for these conditions).

PREVENTION/AVOIDANCE
• Next proestrus—obtain a specimen of the anterior vagina for bacterial culture using a guarded culture swab.
• Treat bitch with an appropriate antibiotic for 3 weeks.
• Breed in that season—the gravid uterus may be less susceptible to re-infection; bitch with underlying cystic endometrial hyperplasia has limited breeding life (best to get the desired number of pups as soon as possible); bitch not more likely to clear the disease spontaneously if allowed to cycle without being bred

POSSIBLE COMPLICATIONS
Bitch may enter estrus sooner after treatment than anticipated—medical treatment induced premature luteolysis.

EXPECTED COURSE AND PROGNOSIS
Dogs—underlying cystic endometrial hyperplasia still exists; predisposed to recurrence; breed patient to desired stud dogs in a timely manner; recommend ovariohysterectomy as soon as breeding life is over; use of subfertile stud dogs not recommended

MISCELLANEOUS

ASSOCIATED CONDITIONS
Pyometra of the uterine stump in spayed animals—may develop any time after ovariohysterectomy; may be associated with an ovarian remnant

AGE-RELATED FACTORS
N/A

ZOONOTIC POTENTIAL
N/A

PREGNANCY
PGF$_{2\alpha}$—always rule out pregnancy before administration to valuable breeding animals; effective pregnancy-terminating agent

ABBREVIATIONS
• ALP = alkaline phosphatase
• ALT = alanine transferase
• PGF$_{2\alpha}$ = prostaglondin F$_{2\alpha}$

Suggested Reading
Hardy RM, Osborne CA. Canine pyometra: pathophysiology, diagnosis and treatment of uterine and extrauterine lesions. J Am Anim Hosp Assoc 1974;10:245–268.
Author Margaret V. Root
Consulting Editor Sara K. Lyle

PYOTHORAX

 BASICS

DEFINITION
Accumulation of pus within the pleural cavity, usually associated with infection

PATHOPHYSIOLOGY
• Infectious—generally arises from transpulmonary, transesophageal, or transthoracic inoculation of bacteria into the pleural space, with subsequent suppurative pleuritis
• Dogs—commonly associated causes: inhaled grass awn or other foreign object and penetrating wound to the thorax
• Cats—most common cause: penetrating bite wound
• Secondary to systemic infection or pneumonia—uncommon

SYSTEMS AFFECTED
• Respiratory
• Hemic/Lymphatic/Immune
• Renal/Urologic—protein-losing glomerulopathy

GENETICS
N/A

INCIDENCE/PREVALENCE
N/A

GEOGRAPHIC DISTRIBUTION
N/A

SIGNALMENT
Species
Dogs and cats

Breed Predilections
• Dogs—hunting and sporting breeds
• Cats—domestic shorthair

Mean Age And Range
N/A

Predominant Sex
• Dogs—none
• Cats—males, because of tendency to fight

SIGNS
General Comments
• Often insidious in nature, with few clinical signs until late in the course of disease
• Respiratory compromise—often not severe until the disease is advanced

Historical Findings
• Diminished activity
• Collapse after exercising and slow recovery
• Weight loss and partial anorexia.
• Temporary improvement with antibiotic therapy
• Confirm history of fights or puncture wounds

Physical Examination Findings
• Tachypnea—usually apparent; may be mild and not associated with dyspnea

• Cachexia—often observed
• Cough—may be observed
• Pyrexia—usually low-grade, may be observed
• Thoracic auscultation—may reveal muffled heart sounds, diminished lung sounds ventrally, and amplified lung sounds dorsally
• Cats—may show few clinical signs before onset of apparently acute respiratory distress, collapse, and septic shock
• Injury to the thoracic wall—may not be apparent or may be healed at the time of examination
• Perform thorough palpation and inspection of the thorax for evidence of scarring or fibrosis.

CAUSES
• Infectious—dogs: *Actinomyces* spp., *Nocardia* spp., *Bacteroides* spp., *Corynebacterium, Escherichia coli,* fungal agents, and *Streptococcus* spp.; cats: oral commensals (e.g., *Pasteurella multocida* and *Bacteroides* spp.) most common; frequency of isolation of these organisms may vary geographically
• Neoplastic—rarely intrathoracic tumors secondary to tumor necrosis

RISK FACTORS
• Dogs—hunting, field trials, and other strenuous outdoor sporting activities
• Cats—outdoor lifestyle and fighting

 DIAGNOSIS

DIFFERENTIAL DIAGNOSIS
Other pleural effusions—chylothorax and hemothorax; nonseptic exudates (FIP or neoplasia); transudative effusions; differentiated via cytologic examination

CBC/BIOCHEMISTRY/URINALYSIS
• Marked neutrophilic leukocytosis with a (usually regenerative) left shift, monocytosis, and anemia of chronic disease
• Regenerative anemia—may be seen with substantial hemorrhage into the pleural cavity
• Biochemistry—often normal
• Possible hyperglobulinemia—owing to inflammation
• Hypoalbuminemia—from renal loss
• Mildly high ALP
• Prerenal azotemia—may note if the patient is dehydrated
• Organ-specific changes—if other organs are secondarily infected (e.g., pyelonephritis and hepatitis)
• Proteinuria—possible with glomerulopathy

OTHER LABORATORY TESTS
• Serologic test for fungus may be positive.
• Cats—may be FeLV or FIV positive; test

IMAGING
• Radiography—unilateral or bilateral pleural

effusion with pleural fissure lines; abscesses within the pulmonary parenchyma possible
• Ultrasonography—pleural effusion; may show marked amount of fibrinous deposition in the pleural space

DIAGNOSTIC PROCEDURES
Thoracocentesis
• Cytologic evaluation—often necessary to confirm the diagnosis, because many effusions appear grossly hemorrhagic
• Gram stains—may facilitate early identification of pathogenic organisms
• Sulfa granules (small accumulations of purulent debris) in the exudate—characteristic of infection by filamentous organisms (e.g., *Actinomyces* and *Nocardia*)
• Organisms may be seen in the fluid samples, often within neutrophils.
• Degenerative neutrophils abundant
• The effusion is often malodorous/putrid, especially in cats.

Microbiology
• Culture all fluid samples aerobically and anaerobically.
• Many of the filamentous, microaerophilic, and anaerobic organisms are slow-growing, so cultures should be maintained for 2–4 weeks
• Sulfa granules—maceration may enhance culturing; contain higher concentrations of bacteria
• Fungal organisms—culture depends on history and geographic location.
• Urine samples—culture with suspected pyelonephritis.

PATHOLOGIC FINDINGS
• Fibrinous and suppurative pleuritis, with or without pulmonary abscessation
• Glomerulonephritis

 TREATMENT

APPROPRIATE HEALTH CARE
• Inpatient—often for several weeks
• Treat like any abscess; drainage is critical, without which resolution is highly unlikely.

NURSING CARE
• Continuous evacuation via tube thoracostomy with low-pressure suction through a perforated tube; use a large-bore tube to minimize occlusion; continue until net drainage is < 2–3 mL/kg/day and intracellular bacteria are no longer visible on gram stain; drainage may be slightly higher with red rubber tubes, because they are more irritating.
• Cats—usually require general anesthesia for tube placement
• Dogs with severe respiratory compromise—may substitute local anesthesia and regional analgesia for general anesthesia
• Periodic thoracic radiography—ensure

bilateral tube placement is not necessary, tube placement is adequate, and there is no pocketing or loculation of exudate; determine any primary pulmonary pathologic change that may not have been apparent on initial examination.
• Thoracic lavage—every 6–8 hr with warm, sterile saline; may help break down consolidated debris
• Coupage (rapid thoracic percussion)—may help remove consolidated debris
• Repeat bacterial culture if the patient fails to improve.

ACTIVITY
• Inpatient—encourage the patient to exercise lightly (10 min every 6–8 hr); promote ventilatory efforts; help break down pleural adhesions
• After discharge—gradually increase exercise over 2–4 months

DIET
• High-calorie food
• Protein replacement is usually unnecessary.

CLIENT EDUCATION
Warn client that the duration of treatment (inpatient and outpatient) is long and expensive.

SURGICAL CONSIDERATIONS
• Surgery—associated with higher mortality; contraindicated unless the patient has pulmonary abscessation, pleural fibrosis, lung-lobe torsion, or extensive loculation of the pus that limits effective thoracic drainage
• Identified foreign body via thoracic imaging (radiography, ultrasound, CT, or MRI)—thoracotomy and retrieval indicated; grass awns are rarely found even during surgery; attempted surgical retrieval is not recommended unless foreign body visualized via imaging.
• Surgery may be indicated if pus is restricted to mediastinum.

MEDICATIONS

DRUGS OF CHOICE
Antimicrobials
• Ultimately, choice determined by in vitro results of sensitivity testing
• Suspected specific pathogen—may initiate treatment before culture results are available; choose on the basis of common antibiotic sensitivities of particular organisms; *Actinomyces* spp. and *Bacteroides* (non-*fragilis*) spp. often susceptible to amoxicillin; *Nocardia* spp. often susceptible to potentiated sulfonamides; obligate anaerobic bacteria (including *B. fragilis*) susceptible to amoxicillin-clavulanic acid, chloramphenicol, and usually metronidazole; *Pasteurella* spp. often susceptible to potentiated penicillins

• Ampicillin or amoxicillin with a β-lactamase inhibitor—good initial choice for most patients; ampicillin and sulbactam (20 mg/kg IV q8h) followed by amoxicillin-clavulanic acid (25 mg/kg PO q8h) when medications can be given orally
• Trimethoprim-sulfa, aminoglycosides, and quinolones—generally ineffective
• Multiple antibiotics occasionally necessary
• Dosages are generally high (e.g., amoxicillin 40 mg/kg PO q8h) to allow adequate distribution into the pleural cavity; may need to continue drug for several months and occasionally indefinitely

Analgesics
• Generally not required
• With severe discomfort—may use intrapleural anesthesia (e.g., bupivacaine mixed with the lavage fluid)

CONTRAINDICATIONS
Glucocorticoids and immunosuppressive agents—avoid with infectious pyothorax

PRECAUTIONS
Potentiated sulfas—may be associated with keratoconjunctivitis sicca, polyarthropathy, hypothyroidism, thrombocytopenia, and anemia, especially with prolonged use

POSSIBLE INTERACTIONS
N/A

ALTERNATIVE DRUGS
No specific suspected organism and culture and sensitivity results pending—use amoxicillin owing to its high efficacy against anaerobic bacteria and low probability of complications or toxicity; may consider clindamycin

FOLLOW-UP

PATIENT MONITORING
• Measure net thoracic fluid production—determine when thoracic drains may be removed
• Evaluate thoracic radiographs—ensure adequate evacuation of fluid
• Antibiotics—continue for 1 month after the patient is clinically normal, the hemogram is normal, and there is no radiographic evidence of fluid reaccumulation; average duration of therapy is 3–4 months but may continue for 6–12 months or longer
• Assess CBC and radiographs monthly—residual radiographic changes may be permanent, but fluid should be absent.

PREVENTION AND AVOIDANCE
Avoid activity that predisposes the animal to the disease (often not practical).

POSSIBLE COMPLICATIONS
• Incorrect insertion of the drainage tube—may prevent adequate drainage or produce

pneumothorax; too proximal a placement may put pressure on the brachial arteries and veins, resulting in unilateral limb edema or lameness; lung laceration during placement
• Persistent, recurrent pyothorax—compartmentalization of pus; premature discontinuation of treatment
• Chronic fibrosing pleuritis and poor performance upon apparent recovery—may be treated surgically on occasion
• Persistent mediastinitis

EXPECTED COURSE AND PROGNOSIS
• With aggressive management—prognosis fair to excellent
• With repeated intermittent antibiotic therapy only or with inadequate drainage—prognosis poor
• Return to performance—depends on chronicity of disease and level of management

MISCELLANEOUS

ASSOCIATED CONDITIONS
• Retroperitoneal abscessation and diskospondylitis caused by migration of a foreign body through the diaphragm into the retroperitoneal space—occasionally seen • Glomerulonephropathy

AGE-RELATED FACTORS
N/A

ZOONOTIC POTENTIAL
Fungal infection during in vitro isolation

PREGNANCY
N/A

SYNONYMS
• Empyema • Suppurative pleuritis • Pleurisy

SEE ALSO
• Chylothorax • Dyspnea, Tachypnea, and Panting • Pleural Effusion

ABBREVIATIONS
• ALP = alkaline phosphatase • FeLV = feline leukemia virus • FIP = feline infectious peritonitis • FIV = feline immunodeficiency virus

Suggested Reading
Bauer TG, Woodfield JA. Mediastinal, pleural, and extrapleural diseases. In: Ettinger SJ, Feldman EC, eds. Textbook of small animal internal medicine. 4th ed. Philadelphia: Saunders, 1995:812–842.
Edwards DF. Actinomycosis and nocardiosis. In: Greene CE, ed. Infectious diseases of the dog and cat. 2nd ed. Philadelphia: Saunders, 1998:303–313.
Greene CE. Pleural infections. In: Greene CE, ed. Infectious diseases of the dog and cat. 2nd ed. Philadelphia: Saunders, 1998:592–594.
Author Mark Rishniw
Consulting Editor Eleanor C. Hawkins

DISEASES

PYRETHRIN AND PYRETHROID TOXICOSIS

BASICS

OVERVIEW
• Insecticides • Pyrethrins—natural; derived from *Chrysanthemum cinerariaefolium* and related plant species • Pyrethroids—synthetic; include allethrin, cypermethrin, deltamethrin, fenvalerate, fluvalinate, permethrin, phenothrin, and tetramethrin • Affect the nervous system—reversibly prolong sodium conductance in nerve axons, resulting in repetitive nerve discharges; enhanced effect in hypothermic mammals and cold-blooded animals

SIGNALMENT
Adverse reactions occur more frequently in cats; small dogs; and young, old, sick, or debilitated animals.

SIGNS
• Result from immune-mediated allergic hypersensitivity and anaphylactic reactions, genetic-based idiosyncratic reactions, and neurotoxic reactions; may be challenging to differentiate among these • Mild—hypersalivation; paw flicking; ear twitching; mild depression; vomiting; diarrhea • Moderate to serious—protracted vomiting and diarrhea; marked depression; ataxia; muscle tremors (must be differentiated from paw flicking and ear twitching) • Extreme dermal or oral overdose—may produce seizures or death • Cats—especially sensitive to concentrated permethrin-containing products labeled for use on dogs; may develop muscle tremors, ataxia, seizures, and death within hours • Allergic reactions—urticaria; hyperemia; pruritus; anaphylaxis; shock; respiratory distress; (rarely) death • Idiosyncratic reactions—not allergic; resemble toxic reactions at much lower doses • Death—thoroughly investigate to rule out predisposing underlying conditions

CAUSES & RISK FACTORS
• Cats—more sensitive; less-efficient metabolic pathways, extensive grooming habits, and long haircoats that can retain large quantities of topically applied product
• Patients with subnormal body temperatures after anesthesia or sedation—predisposed to clinical signs

DIAGNOSIS

DIFFERENTIAL DIAGNOSIS
• Exposure history (amount and frequency of product usage), type and severity of clinical signs, and onset and duration of clinical signs—must be consistent before a tentative diagnosis can be made
• Organophosphorous compounds, carbamate, or D-limonene toxicosis

• With sudden death—flea bite anemia, cardiomyopathy, or hyperthyroidism
• Anaphylactic and idiosyncratic reactions

CBC/BIOCHEMISTRY/URINALYSIS
N/A

OTHER LABORATORY TESTS
• Pyrethrins—analytical tests for detection in tissues or fluids not generally available
• Pyrethroids—some types can be detected in tissues to confirm exposure.
• Cholinesterase activity—not reduced; may rule out exposure to organophosphate or carbamate insecticides

IMAGING
N/A

DIAGNOSTIC PROCEDURES
N/A

PATHOLOGIC FINDINGS
N/A

TREATMENT
• Adverse reactions (salivation, paw flicking, and ear twitching)—often mild and self-limiting
• Patient saturated with spray products—dry with a warmed towel; brush.
• Continued mild signs—bathe at home with a mild hand dishwashing detergent.
• Progression to tremors and ataxia—hospitalize
• Seriously affected patient—fluid support with balanced electrolyte solution recommended
• Symptomatic patient within 1–2 hr of ingestion—gastric lavage with patient under sedation and an endotracheal tube in place; use a large-bore stomach tube; repeat flushing until clear water is seen draining from the stomach tube.
• Maintenance of a normal body temperature—critical

MEDICATIONS

DRUGS
• Minor tremors—diazepam (0.05–1.0 mg/kg IV) or phenobarbital (3.0–30 mg/kg IV to effect, low dosage in cats)
• Severe, uncontrollable tremors or seizures—especially for cats exposed to permethrin; methocarbamol (Robaxin-V injectable at 55–220 mg/kg IV not to exceed 330 mg/kg/day; administer one-half dose rapidly IV, wait until the patient begins to relax, continue administration to effect)
• Large ingestion or dermal overdose of a pyrethroid (e.g., permethrin on cats)—

activated charcoal (2.0 g/kg PO or by stomach tube) containing sorbitol as a cathartic
• Emetics—rarely warranted; most formulations are rapidly absorbed liquids containing water, various alcohols, or hydrocarbon solvents; do not use with hydrocarbon solvent exposure (potential for aspiration); if indicated, if the patient is asymptomatic, and if it is within 1–2 hr of ingestion: induced with 3% hydrogen peroxide (2.2 mL/kg, maximum 45 mL) after feeding

CONTRAINDICATIONS/POSSIBLE INTERACTIONS
• Atropine sulfate—not antidotal; avoid; may can cause tachycardia, CNS stimulation, disorientation, drowsiness, respiratory depression, and even seizures
• Judiciously avoid hypothermia.

FOLLOW-UP

PREVENTION/AVOIDANCE
• Proper application of flea-control products—greatly reduces incidence of adverse reactions; correct dose of most sprays: 1–2 pumps of a typical trigger sprayer per pound body weight
• Reduction of salivation by sensitive cats (sprays)—spray onto a grooming brush; evenly brush through haircoat. • Liquids—term *dip* common; never submerge animal; pour on body; sponge to cover dry areas.
• Premise products—do not apply topically unless labeled for such use; after treating house or yard, do not allow animal in the area until product has dried and environment has been ventilated. • Do not apply dog-only products on cats.

EXPECTED COURSE AND PROGNOSIS
• Hypersalivation—may recur for several days after use of flea-control product when patient (especially cat) grooms itself
• Most clinical signs (mild to severe) resolve within 24–72 hr.

MISCELLANEOUS

SEE ALSO
• Organophosphate and Carbamate Toxicity
• Poisoning (Intoxication)

Suggested Reading
Hansen SR, Villar D, Buck WB, et. al. Pyrethrins and pyrethroids in dogs and cats. Compend Contin Educ Pract Vet 1994;16:707–713.

Authors Steven R. Hansen and Elizabeth A. Curry-Galvin

Consulting Editor Gary D. Osweiler

PYRUVATE KINASE DEFICIENCY

BASICS

OVERVIEW
• RBCs require energy in the form of ATP for maintenance of shape, deformability, active membrane transport, and limited synthetic activities; mature RBCs lack mitochondria and depend on anaerobic glycolysis for ATP generation.
• PK catalyzes an important rate-controlling, ATP-generating step in glycolysis; consequently, energy metabolism is markedly impaired in PK-deficient RBCs, resulting in shortened RBC life-span and anemia; bone marrow attempts to compensate by erythroid hyperplasia, with marked reticulocytosis in peripheral blood.

SIGNALMENT
• Autosomal recessive trait recognized in basenjis, beagles, West Highland white terriers, Cairn terriers, American Eskimo dogs, and Abyssinian cats
• Affected homozygous animals generally not recognized as abnormal until several months of age or until adulthood

SIGNS
• Exercise intolerance
• Pale mucous membranes
• Tachycardia
• Systolic heart murmurs
• Often splenomegaly or hepatomegaly
• Icterus rarely seen
• Affected dogs may be slightly smaller than normal for their breed and age and may exhibit weakness and muscle wasting.
• Heterozygous carriers asymptomatic

CAUSES & RISK FACTORS
• RBCs from normal adult dogs exhibit only one PK isozyme (the R-type).
• Basenji dogs—a single base deletion of the PK-L allele, which encodes for the L-type isozyme in hepatocytes and the R-type isozyme in RBCs
• Specific molecular defects in other breeds of dogs and in cats have not been reported.

DIAGNOSIS

DIFFERENTIAL DIAGNOSIS
• Other causes of hemolytic anemia—immune-mediated hemolytic anemia, hemobartonellosis, babesiosis, Heinz body hemolytic anemia, microangiopathic hemolytic anemia, and phosphofructokinase deficiency.
• Affected dogs—negative Coombs test, no parasites or Heinz bodies in stained blood films, seronegative for *Babesia* spp., and no evidence of DIC or heartworm disease
• In contrast to phosphofructokinase, affected dogs do not exhibit episodes of intravascular hemolysis and hemoglobinuria; these deficiencies are differentiated by specific enzyme assays or DNA tests.

CBC/BIOCHEMISTRY/URINALYSIS
• Macrocytic hypochromic anemia, with PCV values of 16%–28% and uncorrected reticulocyte counts of 15%–50%
• Normal or slightly high leukocyte counts with mature neutrophilia
• Normal to slightly high platelet count
• Moderate to marked polychromasia, anisocytosis, and numerous nucleated RBCs on stained blood films
• Poikilocytosis in some animals, especially in splenectomized dogs
• Possible abnormal clinical chemistry findings, such as hyperferremia, mild hyperbilirubinemia, and slightly high ALT and ALP activities; dogs with liver failure may have hypoalbuminemia
• Normal urinalysis, except for bilirubinuria in dogs

OTHER LABORATORY TESTS
• Total RBC PK activity—low value diagnostic in cats and some dogs; many affected dogs have normal or high activities because of the expression of a M_2 isozyme that does not normally occur in mature RBCs; approximately 50% of normal in heterozygous animals
• Additional assays (e.g., enzyme heat stability test, measurement of RBC glycolytic intermediates, electrophoresis of isozymes, and enzyme immunoprecipitation)—to reach a diagnosis in dogs whose total enzyme activity is not low
• DNA diagnostic test—for screening basenji dogs and in other breeds with an identical defect

IMAGING
N/A

DIAGNOSTIC PROCEDURES
N/A

TREATMENT
Affected animals can only be cured by bone marrow transplantation.

MEDICATIONS

DRUGS OF CHOICE
Although not adequately evaluated, long-term treatment with iron-chelating drugs, such as deferoxamine mesylate, might prolong the life expectancy of affected animals.

CONTRAINDICATIONS/POSSIBLE INTERACTIONS
None

FOLLOW-UP
• Hepatic iron overload—develops in affected dogs; can result in cirrhosis
• Myelofibrosis and osteosclerosis—develop in affected dogs with age; thus most die by 4 years of age as a result of bone marrow or liver failure.
• Severe anemia with minimal reticulocytosis or abnormal liver function tests and ascites secondary to hypoalbuminemia indicate the terminal stage of the disease in dogs.
• The long-term consequences of this deficiency in cats have not been reported.

MISCELLANEOUS

ABBREVIATIONS
• ALP = alkaline phosphatase
• ALT = alanine aminotransferase
• DIC = disseminated intravascular coagulation
• PCV = packed cell volume
• PK = pyruvate kinase

Suggested Reading
Harvey JW. Congenital erythrocyte enzyme deficiencies. Vet Clin North Am Small Anim Pract 1996;26:1003–1011.
Author John W. Harvey
Consulting Editor Susan M. Cotter

DISEASES

Q FEVER

BASICS

OVERVIEW
• Caused by the zoonotic rickettsia *Coxiella burnetii*
• Infection—most commonly by inhalation or ingestion of organisms while feeding on infected body fluids (urine, feces, milk, or parturient discharges), tissues (especially placenta), or carcasses of infected animal reservoir hosts (cattle, sheep, goats); can occur after tick exposure (many species of ticks implicated)
• Lungs—thought to be main portal of entry to systemic circulation
• Organism replicates in vascular endothelium; causes widespread vasculitis; severity depends on the pathogenicity of the strain of organism; vasculitis results in necrosis and hemorrhage in lungs, liver, and CNS
• An extended latent period exists after recovery until chronic immune-complex phenomena develop; organism reactivated out of the latent state during parturition, resulting in large numbers entering the placenta, parturient fluids, urine, feces, and milk
• Endemic worldwide

SIGNALMENT
Cats and dogs

SIGNS

Historical Findings
• Fever
• Lethargy
• Depression
• Anorexia
• Abortion—especially cats
• Ataxia and seizures—especially dogs

Physical Examination Findings
• Usually asymptomatic
• Multifocal neurologic signs—dogs

CAUSES & RISK FACTORS
• *C. burnetii*
• Exposure to infected animals (especially following parturition) and ticks

DIAGNOSIS

DIFFERENTIAL DIAGNOSIS
• Cats—other causes of abortion: infections (viral rhinotracheitis, panleukopenia, FeLV, toxoplasmosis, bacteria including coliforms, *Streptococci, Staphylococci, Salmonellae*); fetal defects; maternal problems (nutrition, genital tract abnormalities); environmental stress; endocrine disorders (hypoluteidism)
• Dogs—other causes of encephalitis

CBC/BIOCHEMISTRY/URINALYSIS
Nonspecific

OTHER LABORATORY TESTS

Serology
• Collect 2–3 mL of serum and refrigerate, for organism identification.
• Collect tissue sample (e.g., placenta) and refrigerate, for animal inoculation.
• Tests available from the New Mexico Department of Agriculture, Veterinary Diagnostic Services, 700 Camino de Salud NE, Albuquerque, NM 87106

IMAGING
N/A

DIAGNOSTIC PROCEDURES
N/A

TREATMENT
• Alert client of possible zoonotic risk.
• Inpatient—avoids zoonotic risk to client
• Wear gloves and masks when treating an infected animal or when attending an aborting cat.

MEDICATIONS

DRUGS

• Tetracycline—22 mg/kg PO q8h for 2 weeks
• Doxycycline—20 mg/kg PO q12h for 1 week
• Enrofloxacin—10 mg/kg PO q12h for 1 week; should be effective but no clinical reports; effective in vitro

CONTRAINDICATIONS/POSSIBLE INTERACTIONS

N/A

FOLLOW-UP

• Difficult to determine success of therapy because many animals spontaneously improve
• Even asymptomatic cases should be aggressively treated because of the zoonotic potential.
• Utility of predicting success of therapy based on serologic improvement unknown

MISCELLANEOUS

ZOONOTIC POTENTIAL

• Major zoonotic potential
• By the time a diagnosis is made in a cat or dog, human exposure and infection has occurred
• Instruct owners and people in contact with the pet to seek medical advice immediately.
• Humans contract the disease by inhalation of infected aerosols (e.g., after parturition); children commonly infected from ingestion of raw milk but are usually asymptomatic
• Previous urban outbreaks have been related to exposure to infected cats.
• Incubation period from time of contact until the first signs of illness—5–32 days.
• Person-to-person transmission possible

Suggested Reading

Greene CE, Breitschwerdt EB. Rocky mountain spotted fever, Q fever, and typhus. In: Greene CE, ed. Infectious diseases of the dog and cat. 2nd ed. Philadelphia: Saunders, 1998:155–165.

Author Stephen C. Barr
Consulting Editor Stephen C. Barr

DISEASES

RABIES

BASICS

DEFINITION
A severe, invariably fatal, viral polioencephalitis of warm-blooded animals, including humans

PATHOPHYSIOLOGY
Virus—enters body through a wound (usually from a bite of rabid animal) or via mucous membranes; replicates in myocytes; spreads to the neuromuscular junction and neurotendinal spindles; travels to the CNS via intra-axonal fluid within peripheral nerves; spreads throughout the CNS; finally spreads centrifugally within peripheral, sensory, and motor neurons

SYSTEMS AFFECTED
• Nervous—clinical encephalitis, either paralytic or furious
• Salivary glands—contain large quantities of infectious virus particles that are shed in saliva

GENETICS
None

INCIDENCE/PREVALENCE
• Incidence of disease within infected animals, high (approaches 100%)
• Prevalence—overall low; can be significant in enzootic areas; especially high in underdeveloped countries where vaccination of dogs and cats is not routinely carried out

GEOGRAPHIC DISTRIBUTION
• Worldwide
• Exceptions—British Isles, Australia, New Zealand, Hawaii, Japan, and parts of Scandinavia
• Species adapted strains—specific geographic distributions within endemic countries

SIGNALMENT

Species
• All warm-blooded animals, including dogs, cats, and humans
• U.S.—four strains endemic within fox, raccoon, skunk, and bat populations, all four strains can be transmitted to dogs and cats.

Breed Predilections
None

Mean Age and Range
None, but adult animals that come in contact with wildlife at most risk

Predominant Sex
None

SIGNS

General Comments
• Quite variable; atypical presentation is the rule rather than the exception.
• Three progressive stages of disease—prodromal; furious; and paralytic

Historical Findings
• Change in attitude—solitude; apprehension, nervousness, anxiety; unusual shyness or aggressiveness
• Erratic behavior—biting or snapping; licking or chewing at sight of wound; biting at cage; wandering and roaming; excitability; irritability; viciousness
• Disorientation
• Muscular—incoordination; seizures; paralysis
• Change in tone of bark
• Excess salivation or frothing

Physical Examination Findings
• All or some of the historical findings
• Mandibular and laryngeal paralysis, with dropped jaw
• Inability to swallow
• Hypersalivation
• Fever

CAUSES
Rabies virus—a single-stranded RNA virus; genus *Lyssavirus;* family Rhabdoviridae

RISK FACTORS
• Exposure to wildlife, especially skunks, raccoons, bats, and foxes
• Lack of adequate vaccination against rabies
• Bite or scratch wounds from unvaccinated dogs, cats, or wildlife
• Exposure to aerosols in bat caves
• Immunocompromised animal—use of modified live virus rabies vaccine

DIAGNOSIS

DIFFERENTIAL DIAGNOSIS
• Must seriously consider rabies for any dog or cat showing unusual mood or behavior changes or exhibiting any unaccountable neurologic signs; **CAUTION:** handle with considerable care to prevent possible transmission of the virus to individuals caring for or treating the animal.
• Any neurologic disease—brain tumor; viral encephalitis

• Head wound—identify lesions from wound
• Laryngeal paralysis
• Choking
• Pseudorabies virus infection

CBC/BIOCHEMISTRY/URINALYSIS
No characteristic hematologic or biochemical changes

OTHER LABORATORY TESTS
N/A

IMAGING
N/A

DIAGNOSTIC PROCEDURES
• CSF—minimal increased protein and leukocyte counts may be seen.
• DFA test of nervous tissue—rapid and sensitive test; collect brain, head, or entire body of a small animal that has died or has been euthanatized; chill sample immediately; submit to a state-approved laboratory for rabies diagnosis; **CAUTION:** use extreme care when collecting, handling, and shipping these specimens.
• DFA test of dermal tissue—skin biopsy of the sensory vibrissae of the maxillary area, including deeper subcutaneous hair follicles

PATHOLOGIC FINDINGS
• Gross changes—generally absent, despite dramatic neurologic disease
• Histopathologic changes—acute to chronic polioencephalitis; gradual increase in the severity of the nonsuppurative inflammatory process in the CNS as disease progresses; large neurons within the brain may contain the classic intracytoplasmic inclusions (Negri bodies).

TREATMENT

APPROPRIATE HEALTH CARE
Strictly inpatient

NURSING CARE
Administer with extreme caution.

ACTIVITY
• Confine to secured quarantine area with clearly posted signs indicating suspected rabies.
• Runs or cages should be locked; only designated people should have access.
• Feed and water without opening the cage or run door.

DIET
Soft, moist food; most patients will not eat.

CLIENT EDUCATION
• Thoroughly inform client of the seriousness of rabies to the animal and the zoonotic potential.
• Ask client about any human exposure (e.g., contact, bite) and strongly urge client to see a physician immediately.
• Local public health official must be notified.

SURGICAL CONSIDERATIONS
• Generally none
• Skin biopsy—may help establish ante-mortem diagnosis; must be confirmed by identification from CNS tissue

MEDICATIONS

DRUGS OF CHOICE
• No treatment
• Once the diagnosis is certain, euthanasia is indicated.

CONTRAINDICATIONS
None

PRECAUTIONS
N/A

POSSIBLE INTERACTIONS
N/A

ALTERNATIVE DRUGS
N/A

FOLLOW-UP

PATIENT MONITORING
• All suspected rabies patients should be securely isolated and monitored for any development of mood change, attitude change, or clinical signs that might suggest the diagnosis.
• An apparently healthy dog or cat that bites or scratches a person should be monitored for a period of 10 days; if no signs of illness occur in the animal within 10 days, the person has had no exposure to the virus; dogs and cats do not shed the virus for more than 3 days before development of clinical disease.
• An unvaccinated dog or cat that is bitten or exposed to a known rabid animal must be quarantined for up to 6 months or according to local or state regulations.

PREVENTION/AVOIDANCE
• Vaccines (dogs and cats)—vaccinate according to standard recommendations and state and local requirements; all dogs and cats with any potential exposure to wildlife or other dogs; vaccinate after 12 weeks of age; then 12 months later; then every 3 years using a vaccine approved for 3 years; use only inactivated vaccines for cats.
• Rabies-free countries—entering dogs and cats are quarantined for long periods, usually 6 months.
• Disinfection—any contaminated area, cage, food dish, or instrument must be thoroughly disinfected; use a 1:32 dilution (4 ounces per gallon) of household bleach to quickly inactivate the virus.

POSSIBLE COMPLICATIONS
From paralysis or attitude changes

EXPECTED COURSE AND PROGNOSIS
• Prognosis—grave; almost invariably fatal
• All dogs and cats with clinical infection will succumb within 7–10 days of onset of clinical signs.

MISCELLANEOUS

ASSOCIATED CONDITIONS
None

AGE-RELATED FACTORS
None

ZOONOTIC POTENTIAL
• Extreme
• Humans must avoid being bitten by a rabid animal or an asymptomatic animal that is incubating the disease.
• Rabies cases must be strictly quarantined and confined to prevent exposure to humans and other animals.
• Local and state regulations must be adhered to carefully and completely.

PREGNANCY
Infection during pregnancy will be fatal to dam.

SYNONYMS
Rage

ABBREVIATIONS
• CSF = cerebrospinal fluid
• DFA = direct immunofluorescent antibody

Suggested Reading

Barr MC, Olsen CW, Scott FW. Feline viral diseases. In: Ettinger SJ, Feldman EC, eds. Veterinary internal medicine. Philadelphia: Saunders; 1995:409–439.

Eng TR, Fishbein DB. National Study Group on rabies. Epidemiologic factors, clinical findings, and vaccination status of rabies in cats and dogs in the United States in 1988. J Am Vet Med Assoc 1990;197:201–209.

Greene CE, Dreesen DW. Rabies. In: Greene CE, ed. Infectious diseases of the dog and cat. 2nd ed. Philadelphia: Saunders, 1998:114–126.

Jenkins SR, Auslander M, Johnson RH, et al. Compendium of animal rabies control, 1998. J Am Vet Med Assoc 1998;212:213–217.

Krebs JW, Strine TW, Smith JS, et al. Rabies surveillance in the United States during 1993. J Am Vet Med Assoc 1994;205: 1695–1709.

Author Fred W. Scott
Consulting Editor Stephen C. Barr

RECTAL AND ANAL PROLAPSE

 BASICS

OVERVIEW
• An anal prolapse (partial prolapse) is a protrusion of rectal mucosa through the external anal orifice.
• A double layer of the rectum that protrudes through the anal canal is a rectal prolapse (complete prolapse).

SIGNALMENT
• Dogs and cats
• Any age, sex, or breed
• High prevalence for young, parasitized dogs or cats with diarrhea

SIGNS
• Persistent tenesmus
• Tubular hyperemic mass protruding from the anus

CAUSES & RISK FACTORS
• Gastrointestinal parasitism
• Cystitis
• Prostatitis
• Dystocia
• Perineal hernia
• Prostatic hypertrophy
• Colitis
• Constipation/obstipation
• Rectal foreign body
• Proctitis
• Rectal or anal tumors
• Urolithiasis
• Tenesmus following perineal or urogenital surgery

 DIAGNOSIS

DIFFERENTIAL DIAGNOSIS
• Intussusception—rule out by passing a blunt probe between the mass and the anus (the probe should not penetrate more than 1–2 cm before contacting the fornix; if the probe easily passes 5–6 cm, then suspect prolapsed intussusception) or by abdominal ultrasound (look for increased intestinal layering)
• Neoplasia—rule out by palpation, fine-needle aspiration and cytology, and/or biopsy and histopathology

CBC/BIOCHEMISTRY/URINALYSIS
• *Usually* normal
• Inflammatory or stress leukogram may be present.

OTHER LABORATORY TESTS
Fecal examination may confirm parasitism.

IMAGING
• Abdominal radiography and ultrasonography—usually normal
• Abdominal radiography—may demonstrate foreign body, prostatomegaly, cystic calculi, or colonic fecal distention
• Abdominal ultrasonography—may demonstrate prostatomegaly, cystic calculi, bladder wall-thickening, or intussusception

DIAGNOSTIC PROCEDURES
• Rectal examination to palpate for perineal hernias
• Colonoscopy may help evaluate recurrent prolapse for an underlying cause.

PATHOLOGIC FINDINGS
Assess viability of the prolapsed tissue by surface appearance and tissue temperature—vital tissue appears swollen and hyperemic, and red blood exudes from the cut surface; devitalized tissue appears dark purple or black, and dark cyanotic blood exudes from the cut surface; ulcerations may be present.

 TREATMENT

APPROPRIATE HEALTH CARE
• Must identify and treat underlying cause
• Conservative medical management—gently replace prolapsed tissue through the anus with the use of lubricants; osmotic agents may help if severe swelling exists.
• Use of an epidural may facilitate treatment and relieve discomfort.
• Adjunctive use of a purse string suture may aid in retention and prevent postreduction recurrence; place the suture to allow room for defecation.
• Decrease straining with stool softeners.
• Loperamide recommended to increase sphincter tone and decrease tenesmus
• Colopexy recommended for recurrent viable prolapses
• When prolapse is devitalized, amputation and rectal anastomosis are recommended.

 MEDICATIONS

DRUGS OF CHOICE
• Appropriate anesthetic/analgesics as needed
• Topical agents to aid in reduction—50% dextrose solution and KY Jelly
• Stool softeners—docusate sodium (dogs, 50–200 mg PO q8–12h; cats, 50 mg PO q12–24h) or lactulose (10 g/15 mL of solution, 1 mL/4.5 kg q8–12h to effect)
• Agents to increase sphincter tone and decrease tenesmus—loperamide (dogs 0.1–0.2 mg/kg PO q8–12h; cats 0.08–0.16 mg/kg PO q12h)

CONTRAINDICATIONS/POSSIBLE INTERACTIONS
N/A

 FOLLOW-UP

PATIENT MONITORING
Purse string removal in 5–7 days

POSSLBLE COMPLICATIONS
• Recurrence—especially if uncontrolled underlying problem exists
• Postoperative—may include anastomosis dehiscence within 5–7 days postoperatively or rectal stricture

 MISCELLANEOUS

ASSOCIATED CONDITIONS
Intestinal parasitism

SEE ALSO
• Dyschezia and Hematochezia
• Colitis and Proctitis
• Intussusception

Suggested Reading
Burrows CF, Ellison GE. Recto anal disease. In: Ettinger SJ, Feldman EC, eds. Textbook of veterinary internal medicine. 3rd ed. Philadelphia: Saunders, 1989:1559–1568.
Matthiesen DT, Manfra-Marretta S. Diseases of the anus. In Slatter DH, ed. Textbook of small animal surgery. 2nd ed. Philadelphia: Saunders, 1993:627–645.
Author Michelle J. Waschak
Consulting Editors Mitchell A. Crystal and Brett M. Feder

BASICS

OVERVIEW
• Pathologic, fibrotic narrowing or constriction of the rectal canal • Excessive fibrous connective tissue formation results from wound healing, chronic inflammation, or neoplastic invasion. • Maturation of this scar tissue causes narrowing of the rectal luminal diameter. • Gastrointestinal function is compromised because of outflow obstruction.

SIGNALMENT
• Dogs and cats • No age, breed, or gender predilection reported • No genetic basis reported

SIGNS
• Vary with severity of the lesion • Dyschezia • Tenesmus • Constipation • Large bowel diarrhea • Secondary megacolon can develop.

CAUSES & RISK FACTORS
• Inflammatory—rectoanal abscess, anal sacculitis, perianal fistulas, proctitis, foreign body, fungal infection (histoplasmosis, pythiosis) • Traumatic—lacerations • Neoplastic—rectal adenocarcinoma, leiomyoma, rectal polyps • Iatrogenic—rectal anastomosis, rectal mass excision, rectal biopsy • Congenital—atresia ani

DIAGNOSIS

DIFFERENTIAL DIAGNOSIS
• Space-occupying processes that lead to diminished rectal capacity (extraluminal rectal compression [e.g., prostatic disease, pelvic fractures], intraluminal rectal obstruction [e.g., pseudocoprostasis, foreign body]) and functional constriction (rectal muscle spasms) • Differentiate by rectal palpation and imaging.

CBC/BIOCHEMISTRY/URINALYSIS
• Usually normal
• Patients with inflammation or infection may have an inflammatory leukogram.

OTHER LABORATORY TESTS
N/A

IMAGING
• Survey abdominal radiography and contrast studies (e.g., barium, air, or double-contrast enema and barium gastrointestinal series) may reveal consistent narrowing of the rectal luminal diameter.
• Contrast radiography requires adequate patient preparation (warm water enemas ± polyethylene glycol [GoLytely] 30–50 mL/kg PO 12 and 6 h prior to procedure) followed by instillation of 10 mL of barium/kg through a balloon catheter.

• A combination of air and barium allows the best visualization of the colonic mucosa; lesions in close proximity to the rectum may be difficult to delineate.
• Abdominal ultrasonography may reveal thickening and altered architecture if infiltrative rectocolonic disease is present (e.g., pythiosis, neoplasia).

DIAGNOSTIC PROCEDURES
• Digital rectal palpation to characterize and determine the extent and location of the stricture
• Proctoscopy/colonoscopy may be useful to visualize a stricture, determine the extent of the lesion, and procure a biopsy specimen.
• Colonic scrapings may aid in cytological diagnosis of fungal (histoplasmosis) and neoplastic diseases.
• Biopsy and evaluate the lesion histopathologically to classify the disease process and prognosis.

TREATMENT
• Resolve the underlying cause before specifically treating the stricture when possible.
• Direct medical treatment at either palliation by use of stool softeners and enemas or the elimination of infective agents or inflammatory conditions.
• Give fluid therapy to attain/maximize hydration prior to administering an enema to constipated or obstipated patients.
• Anesthesia may be necessary for enema administration.
• Surgical treatment ranges from balloon dilation or bougienage for benign superficial strictures to partial or complete resection for more extensive lesions (see references for greater detail).
• Radiotherapy and/or chemotherapy may benefit the treatment of some neoplasms.

MEDICATIONS

DRUGS OF CHOICE
• Stool softeners—docusate sodium (dogs, 50–200 mg PO q8–12h; cats, 50 mg PO q12–24h), lactulose (10 g/15 mL of solution, 1 mL/4.5 kg q8–12h to effect)
• Corticosteroids—can use prednisone to treat noninfectious inflammatory conditions (dosage, 0.5–1 mg/kg PO q24h or divided q12h) and after balloon dilation or bougienage to prevent restricture.
• Antineoplastic chemotherapeutic agents may be indicated for various neoplasms.
• Give antifungal therapy if fungal infection present.

• Appropriate perioperative antimicrobial therapy has been advocated in conjunction with medical or surgical therapy; chose one with a Gram-negative spectrum (e.g., cefoxitin sodium [Mefoxin] 30 mg/kg IV).

CONTRAINDICATIONS/POSSIBLE INTERACTIONS
• Corticosteroids when infection is possible
• Corticosteroids may adversely affect healing after surgical correction of the stricture.

FOLLOW-UP

PATIENT MONITORING
• Resolution or recurrence of clinical signs
• Patients with neoplastic lesions—recurrence and metastatic disease

POSSIBLE COMPLICATIONS
• Medical treatment—can include inefficacy, diarrhea, and adverse effects of medications
• Surgical treatment—fecal incontinence, secondary stricture formation, and wound dehiscence

EXPECTED COURSE AND PROGNOSIS
• Varies with the severity of the stricture • Patients with benign strictures that are readily managed medically or with balloon dilation, bougienage, or resection may have a good long-term outcome. • Most patients with recognizable clinical signs have a guarded to poor prognosis for complete resolution.

MISCELLANEOUS

AGE-RELATED FACTORS
Atresia ani is seen within weeks of birth.

SEE ALSO
• Colitis and Proctitis • Constipation and Obstipation • Dyschezia and Hematochezia • Histoplasmosis • Perianal Fistula • Pythiosis • Rectoanal Polyps

Suggested Reading
Biery DN. The large bowel. In: Thrall DE, ed. Textbook of veterinary diagnostic radiology. Philadelphia: Saunders, 1986:513–514.
Matthiesen DT, Marretta SM. Diseases of the rectum and anus. In: Slatter D, ed. Textbook of small animal surgery. 2nd ed. Philadelphia: Saunders, 1993:627–644.
Niebauer GW. Rectoanal disease. In: Bojrab MJ, ed. Disease mechanisms in small animal surgery. 2nd ed. Philadelphia: Lea & Febiger, 1993:271–284.
Authors James L. Cook and Michelle J. Waschak
Consulting Editors Mitchell A. Crystal and Brett M. Feder

DISEASES

RECTOANAL POLYPS

 BASICS

OVERVIEW
• Benign growths of the rectoanal mucosa that typically occur within 3 cm of the anus
• Histopathologic evaluation typically reveals adenomas (common) or papillomas (uncommon).

SIGNALMENT
• Dogs and cats
• Middle-aged to old
• No sex predilection

SIGNS
• Blood-tinged or mucous-covered feces
• Feces usually formed; rarely, large bowel diarrhea
• Tenesmus
• Soft, pedunculated, and possibly friable mass may be seen or palpated rectally; single polyps are typical, but multiple polyps can occur.
• Rectal or polyp prolapse

CAUSES & RISK FACTORS
Unknown

 DIAGNOSIS

DIFFERENTIAL DIAGNOSIS
• Adenocarcinoma
• Leiomyoma
• Lymphoma
• Rectal or anal prolapse

CBC/BIOCHEMISTRY/URINALYSIS
• Usually normal
• One report of paraneoplastic leukocytosis

OTHER LABORATORY TESTS
N/A

IMAGING
N/A

DIAGNOSTIC PROCEDURES
• Colonoscopy—recommended to evaluate the entire rectum and colon for additional polyps
• Typical polyp appearance—a raised, sessile mass with a smooth surface; can be stalked or have a granular surface
• Histopathologic examination of excised tissue is required for definitive diagnosis.
• Cytological examination of polyp aspirate or scrapping may help the initial diagnosis.

PATHOLOGIC FINDINGS
• Adenomatous polyp
• Adenomatous hyperplasia
• Uncommonly papilloma

 TREATMENT

• Surgical excision is the treatment of choice.
• Mass may be exteriorized directly through the anus and removed with submucosal resection.
• A dorsal rectal or ventral abdominal approach is rarely required.
• Since rectal polyps rarely invade the muscularis mucosa, can remove small or pedunculated tumors by local excision

MEDICATIONS

DRUGS
• Appropriate perioperative antibiotics are recommended (e.g., cefoxitin sodium [Mefoxin] 30 mg/kg IV).
• Stool softeners may help decrease tenesmus—docusate sodium (dogs, 50–200 mg PO q8–12h; cats, 50 mg PO q12–24h) or docusate calcium (dogs, 50–100 mg PO q12–24h; cats, 50 mg PO q12–24h)

ALTERNATIVE DRUGS
Alternative stool softeners—lactulose (1 mL/4.5 kg PO q8h to effect)

CONTRAINDICATIONS/POSSIBLE INTERACTIONS
N/A

 FOLLOW-UP

PATIENT MONITORING
Reexamination of excision site 14 days after surgery and again at 3 and 6 months to ensure absence of recurrence or stricture

POSSIBLE COMPLICATIONS
• Recurrence
• Rectal stricture (rare)

EXPECTED COURSE AND PROGNOSIS
• Excellent prognosis for cure
• Recurrence occasionally seen

 MISCELLANEOUS

SEE ALSO
• Adenocarcinoma, Anal Sac/Perianal/Rectal
• Dyschezia and Hematochezia
• Rectal Prolapse

Suggested Reading

Leib MS, Matz ME. Diseases of the large intestine. In: Ettinger SJ, Feldman EC, eds. Textbook of veterinary internal medicine. Philadelphia: Saunders, 1995:1232–1260.

Matthiesen DT, Manafra-Marretta S. Diseases of the anus. In: Slatter DH, ed. Textbook of small animal surgery. 2nd ed. Philadelphia: Saunders, 1993:627–645.

Author Michelle Joy Waschak
Consulting Editors Mitchell A. Crystal and Brett M. Feder

RENAL DISEASE, CONGENITAL AND DEVELOPMENTAL

BASICS

DEFINITIONS
• Functional or morphologic abnormalities resulting from heritable (genetic) or acquired disease processes affecting differentiation and growth of the developing kidney before or shortly after birth • Renal agenesis—complete absence of one or both kidneys • Renal dysplasia—disorganized renal parenchymal development • Renal ectopia—congenital malposition of one or both kidneys; ectopic kidneys may be fused. • Glomerulopathy—glomerular disease of any type • Tubulointerstitial nephropathy—a noninflammatory disorder of renal tubules and interstitium • Polycystic renal disease—characterized by formation of multiple, variable-sized cysts throughout the renal medulla and cortex • Renal telangiectasia—characterized by multifocal vascular malformations involving the kidneys and other organs • Renal amyloidosis—the extracellular deposition of amyloid in glomerular capillaries, glomeruli, and interstitium • Nephroblastoma—a congenital renal neoplasm arising from the pluripotent metanephric blastema • Multifocal renal cystadenocarcinoma—a hereditary renal neoplasm in dogs • Fanconi's syndrome—a generalized renal tubular functional anomaly characterized by impaired reabsorption of glucose, phosphate, electrolytes, amino acids, and uric acid • Primary renal glucosuria—an isolated functional defect in renal tubular reabsorption of glucose. • Cystinuria—excessive urinary excretion of cystine because of an isolated functional defect in renal tubular reabsorption of cystine and other dibasic amino acids • Hyperuricuria—excessive urinary excretion of uric acid, sodium urate, or ammonium urate caused by impaired hepatic conversion of uric acid to allantoin and enhanced renal tubular secretion of uric acid • Primary hyperoxaluria—a disorder characterized by intermittent hyperoxaluria, L-glyceric aciduria, oxalate nephropathy, and acute renal failure • Congenital nephrogenic diabetes insipidus—a disorder of renal concentrating ability, caused by diminished renal responsiveness to antidiuretic hormone

PATHOPHYSIOLOGY
• Many congenital and developmental renal disorders are caused by genetic abnormalities that disrupt the normal sequential and coordinated development and interaction of multiple embryonic tissues involved in formation of the mature kidney. • Congenital and developmental renal disorders may also be caused by nongenetic factors affecting the developing kidney before or shortly after birth.

SYSTEMS AFFECTED
Renal/Urologic

GENETICS
Familial renal disorders have been reported in the following breeds of dogs and cats:
• Renal agenesis in beagle and Doberman pinscher dogs • Renal dysplasia in chow chow, keeshond, Lhasa apso, miniature schnauzer, shih tzu, soft-coated wheaten terrier, and standard poodle dogs • Glomerulopathy in Bernese mountain dog, samoyed, Doberman pinscher, cocker spaniel, greyhound, rottweiler, and soft-coated wheaten terrier dogs • Tubulointerstitial nephropathy in Norwegian elkhound dogs • Polycystic renal disease in beagle and Cairn terrier dogs and Persian and domestic longhaired cats • Renal telangiectasia in Welsh corgi dogs • Renal amyloidosis in Abyssinian, oriental shorthaired, and Siamese cats and in shar-pei dogs • Renal cystadenocarcinoma in German shepherd dogs • Fanconi's syndrome in basenji dogs • Primary renal glucosuria in Norwegian elkhound dogs • Cystinuria in basset hound, bulldog, dachshund, Irish terrier, and Newfoundland dogs and in domestic cats • Hyperuricuria in dalmation and English bulldog dogs • Primary hyperoxaluria in domestic shorthaired cats and in Tibetan spaniel dogs

INCIDENCE/PREVALENCE
Uncommon, but disorders caused by genetic factors occur more frequently in related animals from more than one generation than in the general population.

GEOGRAPHIC DISTRIBUTION
N/A

SIGNALMENT

Species
Dogs and cats

Breed Predilections
Sporadic cases of congenital/developmental renal disease can occur without a familial predisposition in any breed of dog or cat.

Mean Age and Range
Most patients are < 5 years old at time of diagnosis

Predominant Sex
• Familial cystinuria primarily in male dogs • Samoyed hereditary glomerulopathy more common in males than females; Newfoundlands have both genders affected. • Familial glomerulonephropathy of Bernese mountain dogs more in females than males

SIGNS

General Comments
Most congenital and developmental disorders cannot be distinguished from noncongenital/developmental renal diseases on the basis of history or physical examination.

Historical Findings
• Indicate chronic renal failure • Some glomerulopathies associated with abdominal distension, edema, or other signs of the nephrotic syndrome • Abdominal distension in some patients with polycystic kidneys or renal neoplasms • Hematuria in some patients with renal telangiectasia or renal neoplasms • Apparent abdominal pain in some patients with renal telangiectasia • Patients with unilateral renal agenesis, ectopic kidneys, and isolated renal tubular transport defects are frequently asymptomatic.

Physical Examination Findings
• Those associated with chronic renal failure • Ascites or pitting edema in some patients with protein-losing glomerulopathies or amyloidosis • Renomegaly or abdominal mass lesions in some patients with polycystic kidneys, renal neoplasms, or fused ectopic kidneys • Renal pain in some patients with renal telangiectasia

CAUSES

Nonhereditary
• Infectious agents—feline panleukopenia virus and canine herpesvirus infection associated with renal dysplasia • Drugs—corticosteroids, diphenylamine, and biphenyls associated with polycystic kidneys; chlorambucil and sodium arsenate associated with renal agenesis • Dietary factors—hypo- or hypervitaminosis A associated with renal ectopia

RISK FACTORS
See factors listed under Causes.

DIAGNOSIS

DIFFERENTIAL DIAGNOSIS
• Rule out noncongenital and nondevelopmental causes of primary renal disease. • Rule out nonrenal causes of hematuria, proteinuria, glucosuria, abdominal distention, or ascites.

CBC/BIOCHEMISTRY/URINALYSIS
• Nonregenerative anemia in patients with chronic renal failure • Azotemia and urine specific gravity < 1.030 in dogs and < 1.035 in cats if renal failure develops • Proteinuria, hypoalbuminemia, and hypercholesterolemia in patients with the nephrotic syndrome • Normoglycemic glucosuria in animals with Fanconi's syndrome or primary renal glucosuria • Hematuria in patients with congenital renal neoplasia or renal telangiectasia • Cystine crystalluria in patients with cystinuria • Urate crystalluria in patients with hyperuricuria

OTHER LABORATORY TESTS
See chapters describing specific renal diseases, clinical syndromes, clinical problems, or laboratory test abnormalities

IMAGING
Survey abdominal radiography, renal ultrasonography, and excretory urography are important means of identifying and

RENAL DISEASE, CONGENITAL AND DEVELOPMENTAL

characterizing congenital and developmental renal disorders.

DIAGNOSTIC PROCEDURES

Consider light microscopic evaluation of kidney biopsy specimens from patients with morphologic or functional abnormalities of the kidney for which a definitive diagnosis has not been established by other, less invasive means.

PATHOLOGIC FINDINGS

• Congenital and developmental renal disorders may be associated with various combinations of primary, compensatory, and degenerative lesions. Conversely, some functional disorders may not be associated with alterations in renal morphology. • Renal dysplasia—end-stage kidneys; primary lesions include immature ("fetal") glomeruli, persistent mesenchyme, persistent metanephric ducts, atypical tubular epithelium, and dysontogenic metaplasia; primary lesions usually associated with, and may be obscured by, secondary degenerative, inflammatory, and compensatory lesions • Glomerulopathies—usually normal-to-small kidneys; most hereditary glomerulopathies are characterized by a primary membranoproliferative glomerulonephritis with variable degrees of tubulointerstitial disease, but cystic atrophic membranous glomerulopathy is the characteristic lesion in affected rottweilers. • Tubulointerstitial nephropathy—end-stage kidneys; renal lesions include periglomerular fibrosis, parietal epithelial cell hyperplasia and hypertrophy, interstitial fibrosis, and interstitial mononuclear cell infiltrate. • Polycystic renal disease—see specific chapter • Renal amyloidosis—see specific chapter • Renal telangiectasia—lesions include multiple, variable-sized, red-black, blood-filled nodules in the renal cortex and medulla, interstitial fibrosis, interstitial mononuclear cell infiltrate, and hydronephrosis. • Nephroblastoma—unilateral renal mass; microscopically characterized by both embryonic mesenchymal and epithelial tissue components • Multifocal renal cystadenocarcinoma—bilaterally large kidneys with irregular protruding cystic structures or multifocal neoplastic renal tubular epithelial cell proliferations; often associated with cutaneous nodular dermatofibrosis and multiple uterine leiomyomas • Renal ectopia—kidneys may be located in the retroperitoneal space of the pelvic canal, iliac fossa, or abdomen; fused kidneys assume a variety of shapes; horseshoe kidneys are symmetrically fused along the medial border of either pole. • Fanconi's syndrome—inconsistent microscopic findings of tubular atrophy, interstitial fibrosis, tubular cell karyomegaly, and acute papillary necrosis • Primary hyperoxaluria—large, irregularly-shaped kidneys; microscopic lesions include renal tubular deposition of calcium oxalate crystals and variable interstitial and periglomerular fibrosis.

TREATMENT

• The nature of congenital and developmental renal disorders often precludes specific treatment.
• Supportive or symptomatic treatment may improve quality of life and minimize progression in patients with renal dysfunction.
• Base treatment options on clinical signs and appropriate laboratory evaluations.
• Refer to chapters describing specific renal diseases, clinical syndromes, clinical problems, or laboratory test abnormalities.

MEDICATIONS

DRUGS OF CHOICE

Refer to chapters describing specific renal diseases, clinical syndromes, clinical problems, or laboratory abnormalities.

CONTRAINDICATIONS

Avoid potentially nephrotoxic drugs (e.g., gentamicin) or anesthetic agents that decrease renal function (e.g., methoxyflurane) when possible.

PRECAUTIONS

Avoid drugs requiring renal excretion in patients with renal failure; if necessary, modify dosage regimens to compensate for decreased renal clearance of drugs and other metabolites.

POSSIBLE INTERACTIONS
N/A

ALTERNATIVE DRUGS
N/A

FOLLOW-UP

PATIENT MONITORING

Refer to chapters describing specific renal diseases, clinical syndromes, clinical problems, or laboratory test abnormality.

PREVENTION/AVOIDANCE

Congenital and developmental renal disorders are irreversible, so control lies in their prevention. Always consider early identification and correction of predisposing factors (genetic and nongenetic) that may affect future offspring.

POSSIBLE COMPLICATIONS

• Acute or chronic renal failure • Nephrotic syndrome • Urolithiasis • Hydronephrosis • Urinary tract infection

EXPECTED COURSE AND PROGNOSIS

• Highly variable; depends on the specific disorder, the extent of primary lesions, and the severity of renal dysfunction • Most congenital and developmental disorders are irreversible and may result in advanced chronic renal failure, but some patients with mild-to-moderate renal dysfunction may remain stable for long periods. • Patients with some disorders (e.g., unilateral renal agenesis, renal ectopia, cystinuria, hyperuricuria, primary renal glucosuria) may remain asymptomatic unless disorder is complicated by urolithiasis, urinary tract infection, or other disease processes that promote progressive renal dysfunction.

MISCELLANEOUS

ASSOCIATED CONDITIONS

• Polycystic renal disease associated with hepatic biliary cysts • Cystinuria and hyperuricuria associated with formation of uroliths • Amyloidosis in Chinese shar peis associated with intermittent pyrexia or swelling of the hocks • Renal neoplasms associated with hypertrophic osteoarthropathy, polycythemia, or other paraneoplastic syndromes

AGE-RELATED FACTORS
N/A

ZOONOTIC POTENTIAL
N/A

PREGNANCY
N/A

SYNONYMS
Familial renal disease, juvenile renal disease

SEE ALSO
• Amyloidosis • Anemia of Chronic Renal Disease • Fanconi's Syndrome • Hematuria • Hyperparathyroidism, renal secondary • Nephrotic syndrome • Oliguria/anuria • Polycystic kidneys • Polydipsia/polyuria • Renal failure, acute • Renal failure, chronic • Renal tubular acidosis • Renomegaly • Urolithiasis, cystine

ABBREVIATIONS
N/A

Suggested Reading

Finco DR. Inherited and congenital renal disorders. In: Osborne CA, Finco DR, eds. Canine and feline nephrology and urology. 2nd ed. Baltimore: Williams & Wilkins, 1995: 471–483.

Kruger JM, Osborne CA, Lulich JP, et al. The urinary system. In: Hoskins JD, ed. Veterinary pediatrics. 2nd ed. Philadelphia: WB Saunders, 1996:399–426.

Authors John M. Kruger, Carl A. Osborne, and Scott D. Fitzgerald

Consulting Editors Larry G. Adams and Carl A. Osborne

RENAL FAILURE, ACUTE

BASICS

DEFINITION

Acute renal failure (ARF) is a syndrome characterized by sudden onset of filtration failure by the kidneys, accumulation of uremic toxins, and dysregulation of fluid, electrolyte, and acid–base balance. It is potentially reversible if diagnosed quickly and treated aggressively. Although postrenal azotemia fulfills these criteria, the following discussion refers to intrinsic acute renal failure.

PATHOPHYSIOLOGY

Initiated by ischemia, nephrotoxins, or intrinsic renal disease; renal excretory failure is perpetuated by multiple factors including (1) reduced glomerular surface area and permeability, (2) low renal blood flow, (3) intratubular obstruction by tubular debris, (4) cellular and interstitial edema, and (5) "backleak" of filtrate across damaged tubular epithelia; resolution occurs by renal regeneration and repair

SYSTEMS AFFECTED

• Renal • Gastrointestinal • Nervous • Respiratory • Musculoskeletal • Hemic/Lymph/ Immune

INCIDENCE/PREVALENCE

• Prevalence is substantially lower than that of chronic renal failure (CRF). • Prevalence may increase in the fall and winter with greater exposure of animals to antifreeze containing ethylene glycol.

SIGNALMENT

Species
Dogs and cats

Breed Predilections
None

Mean Age and Range
Older animals at greater risk

SIGNS

Historical Findings
Sudden onset of anorexia, listlessness, vomiting (± blood), diarrhea (± blood), halitosis, ataxia, seizures, known toxin exposure, recent medical or surgical conditions, and oliguria/ anuria or polyuria

Physical Examination Findings
Normal body condition and haircoat (no evidence of chronicity), depression, dehydration (sometimes overhydration), variable scleral injection, oral ulceration, glossitis, necrosis of the tongue, uremic breath, hypothermia, fever, tachypnea, bradycardia, nonpalpable urinary bladder, and large, painful, firm, kidneys

CAUSES

Hemodynamic/Hypoperfusion
Shock, malignant hypertension, heart failure, thromboembolism (e.g., disseminated intravas-

cular coagulation [DIC], vasculitis, and transfusion reaction), heatstroke, excessive vasoconstriction (e.g., administration of nonsteroidal antiinflammatory drug [NSAID]), excessive vasodilation (e.g., administration of angiotensin-converting enzyme [ACE] inhibitor or antihypertensive drug), and prolonged anesthesia

Nephrotoxic
Administration of antimicrobials (e.g., aminoglycoside, sulfonamide, and cephalosporin), amphotericin B, chemotherapeutic agent (e.g., cisplatin and doxorubicin), thiacetarsamide, NSAIDs, radiographic contrast agents, ethylene glycol, heavy metals (e.g., lead, mercury, arsenic, and thallium), insect or snake venom, heme pigment, or calcium

Intrinsic and Systemic Disease
Leptospirosis, immune-mediated glomerulonephritis and arteritis, septicemia, DIC, hepatic failure, heat stroke, transfusion reaction, bacterial endocarditis, pyelonephritis, cortical necrosis, and lymphosarcoma

RISK FACTORS

• Endogenous—preexisting renal disease, dehydration, hypovolemia, hypotension, advanced age, concurrent disease, hyponatremia, hypokalemia, hypocalcemia, and acidosis • Exogenous—drugs (e.g., furosemide, NSAIDs, prolonged anesthesia, and aminoglycoside), diet (e.g., low sodium, high or low protein), prolonged surgery, trauma, multiple organ disease, and high environmental temperature

DIAGNOSIS

DIFFERENTIAL DIAGNOSIS

• Prerenal azotemia—oliguria, concentrated urine specific gravity (dogs, ≥1.030; cats, ≥1.035), correctable with fluid repletion • Postrenal azotemia—anuria, dysuria, stranguria, large bladder, urethral obstruction, and uroperitoneum • CRF—polyuria, polydipsia, chronic history of illness, loss of body condition, and anemia • Prerenal on CRF—clinical and laboratory features of CRF but partially correctable with fluid repletion • Prerenal on ARF—acute-onset uremia, partially correctable with fluid repletion • Hypoadrenocorticism— hyponatremia, hyperkalemia, and "flat" ACTH stimulation test • Pancreatitis—markedly high serum lipase, cranial abdominal pain, large nonhomogeneous pancreas (ultrasound), high trypsinlike immunoreactivity, hyperbilirubinemia, and high liver enzyme activity • Hepatorenal syndrome—clinical and laboratory evidence of hepatic failure

CBC/BIOCHEMISTRY/URINALYSIS

• Normal or high PCV, variable leukocytosis, and lymphopenia • Progressive (moderate to severe) increases in BUN, creatinine, and phosphate; variably high potassium and glucose;

and variably low bicarbonate and calcium • Inability to concentrate urine (≥1.020), mild-to-moderate proteinuria, glucosuria; variably high number of casts, WBCs, RBCs, and tubular epithelial cells; variable bacteriuria and crystalluria (calcium oxalate)

OTHER LABORATORY TESTS

• Enzymuria—high urinary a-glutamyl transpeptidase, N-acetyl-β-D-glucosaminidase predicts early nephrotoxic tubular damage in some patients • Metabolic acidosis common; mixed disorders may occur • Leptospirosis titer—≥1:3200 or rising if patient infected • Ethylene glycol concentration— positive if patient poisoned

IMAGING

• Routine and contrast radiography—kidneys are normal to large, with smooth contours.
• Ultrasonography—hyperechoic kidneys suggest ethylene glycol toxicity.

DIAGNOSTIC PROCEDURES

• Catheterize to monitor urine output—helps establish the diagnosis and formulates treatment and prognosis: anuria, ≤ 0.1 mL/kg/h; oliguria, ≤ 0.25 mL/kg/h; nonoliguria, ≥ 2 mL/kg/h • Percutaneous renal biopsy—helps establish the cause, severity, and potential reversibility of injury; later in the course of disease (4-6 weeks) it may help predict ongoing renal repair and permanence of renal damage.

PATHOLOGIC FINDINGS

Nephrosis or nephritis, interstitial edema, and lack of interstitial fibrosis; the subacute stage is characterized by attenuated epithelium, interstitial fibrosis and mineralization, cellular infiltration, and variable tubular regeneration

TREATMENT

APPROPRIATE HEALTH CARE

Inpatient management; eliminate inciting insults; discontinue nephrotoxic drugs; establish and maintain hemodynamic stability; ameliorate life-threatening fluid imbalances, biochemical abnormalities, and uremic toxicities; induce emesis; institute gastric lavage and administer activated charcoal, cathartics, and specific antidotes to patients with acute poisoning; early hemodialysis can eliminate dialyzable toxins.

NURSING CARE

• Hypovolemia—correct estimated fluid deficits with normal (0.9%) saline or balanced polyionic solution within 4–6 h; replace blood losses by whole blood transfusion; once the patient is hydrated, ongoing fluid requirements are provided by 5% dextrose for insensible requirements (approximately 20–25 mL/kg/ day) and balanced electrolyte solution equal to urinary and other losses (i.e., vomiting and diarrhea). • Hypervolemia—stop fluid administration and eliminate excess fluid by diuretic administration or dialysis

DIET

• Restrict oral intake until vomiting subsides. For most patients, endogenous fat stores supply requisite calories during early phases of dietary restriction; thereafter moderately protein-restricted diets or enteral feeding solutions are used to control azotemia and supply caloric requirements. • Parenteral nutrition (vomiting animals)—provide caloric requirements by 30–50% dextrose and 20% emulsified lipid solution; protein requirements (dogs, 3–4 g/100 kcal; cats, 5–6 g/100 kcal) provided by 8.5% amino acid mixture via central venous catheter • Enteral feeding (anorectic, nonvomiting animals)—caloric and protein requirements supplied by blended commercial prescription renal diet or commercial formulated liquid diet (e.g., Renal Care); enteral feedings can be force-fed or given by nasoesophageal, pharyngostomy, gastrostomy, or enterostomy tube.

CLIENT EDUCATION

Inform of the poor prognosis for complete recovery, potential for morbid complications of treatment (e.g., fluid overload, sepsis, and multiple organ failure), expense of prolonged hospitalization, alternatives to conventional medical management (i.e., peritoneal dialysis, hemodialysis, and renal transplantation), and zoonotic potential of leptospirosis

SURGICAL CONSIDERATIONS

Renal transplantation may provide long-term survival for patients (particularly cats) with fulminating ARF.

MEDICATIONS

DRUGS OF CHOICE

Inadequate Urine Production

• Ensure patient is fluid-volume-replete; provide additional isonatric fluid to achieve mild (3–5%) volume expansion; failure to induce diuresis by fluid replacement indicates severe parenchymal damage or underestimation of fluid deficit; if fluid-replete, administer diuretics and/or dopamine. • Hypertonic mannitol (10–20%)—0.5–1.0 g/kg IV over 15–30 min; if effective, continue as intermittent IV bolus q4–6h or 1.0–2.0 mg/kg/min IV continuous-rate infusion (CRI); if ineffective, discontinue • Furosemide (alternative or subsequent to mannitol)—2–6 mg/kg IV; if effective, continue q8h; if ineffective, discontinue or combine with dopamine • Dopamine—1–5 μg/kg/min IV in 5% dextrose as CRI; synergistic with furosemide; if effective, continue as CRI; if ineffective, combine with furosemide or discontinue • If these treatments fail to induce diuresis within 4–6 h, consider dialysis.

Acid–Base Disorders

Administer bicarbonate if serum bicarbonate ≤ 15 mEq/L; bicarbonate replacement: mEq = bicarbonate deficit × body weight (kg) × 0.3; give half IV over 30 min and the remainder over 4–6 h; then reassess

Hyperkalemia

See Potassium, Hyperkalemia

Vomiting

• NPO until vomiting subsides • Reduce gastric acid production—cimetidine (2.5–5.0 mg/kg IV q8–12h) or ranitidine (2 mg/kg IV q8–12h) or omeprazole (0.7–2.0 mg/kg PO q24h [dogs]) • Mucosal protectant—sucralfate (0.5–1.0 g PO q6–8h) • Antiemetics—metoclopramide (0.2–0.5 mg/kg IV or IM q6–8h)

CONTRAINDICATIONS

Avoid nephrotoxic agents

PRECAUTIONS

Modify dosages of all drugs that require renal metabolism or elimination.

POSSIBLE INTERACTIONS

Metoclopramide may impair the effects of dopamine.

ALTERNATIVE DRUGS

Control of vomiting—chlorpromazine (0.5 mg/kg IM q6–12h), prochlorperazine (0.1–0.2 mg/kg IM q6–8h), or trimethobenzamide (3.0 mg/kg IM q6–8h) can be used to treat vomiting but is associated with CNS depression, vasodilatation, and hypotension.

Peritoneal or Hemodialysis

• Dialysis can stabilize the patient until renal function is restored; without dialysis, most oliguric patients die before renal repair can occur. • Specific indications include severe oliguria or anuria, life-threatening fluid overload, life-threatening electrolyte or acid–base disturbance, BUN ≥ 100 mg/dL, serum creatinine ≥ 10 mg/dL, clinical course refractory to conservative treatment for more than 24 h, and poisoning with a dialyzable toxin.

FOLLOW-UP

PATIENT MONITORING

Fluid, electrolyte, and acid–base balances; body weight; urine output; and clinical status; daily

PREVENTION/AVOIDANCE

Anticipate the potential for ARF in patients that are hemodynamically unstable, receiving nephrotoxic drugs, have multiple organ failure, or are undergoing prolonged anesthesia and surgery; maintenance of hydration, mild saline volume expansion, and administration of mannitol may be preventive.

POSSIBLE COMPLICATIONS

Seizures, coma, cardiac arrhythmias, congestive heart failure, pulmonary edema, uremic pneumonitis, gastrointestinal bleeding, hypovolemic shock, sepsis, cardiopulmonary arrest, and death

EXPECTED COURSE AND PROGNOSIS

• Nonoliguric ARF—milder than oliguric; recovery may occur over 3–6 weeks, but the prognosis remains guarded to unfavorable. • Oliguric ARF—predicts extensive renal injury, is difficult to manage, and has a poor prognosis for recovery; recovery signaled by a sudden (and often excessive) increase in urine production and a sluggish and incomplete return of renal function over 4–12 weeks; dialysis extends the potential for renal regeneration and repair. • Anuric ARF—generally fatal; dialysis required for renal repair; recovery of renal function is usually incomplete • Oligoanuric ARF with multiple organ failure—uniformly fatal

MISCELLANEOUS

ZOONOTIC POTENTIAL

Leptospirosis has infectious and zoonotic potential; avoid contact with infective urine.

PREGNANCY

A rare complication of pregnancy in animals; promoted by acute metritis, pyometra, and postpartum sepsis or hemorrhage

SYNONYMS

Acute tubular necrosis, acute uremia, lower nephron nephrosis, and vasomotor nephropathy

SEE ALSO

• Oliguria and Anuria
• Creatinine and BUN—Azotemia and Uremia
• Renal Failure, Chronic

ABBREVIATIONS

• ACE = angiotensin-converting enzyme
• ARF = acute renal failure
• CRF = chronic renal failure
• CRI = continuous-rate infusion
• DIC = disseminated intravascular coagulation

Suggested Reading

Grauer GF, Lane IF. Acute renal failure. In: Ettinger SJ, Feldman EC, eds. Textbook of veterinary internal medicine. 4th ed. Philadelphia: Saunders 1995:1720–1733.
Author Larry D. Cowgill
Consulting Editors Larry G. Adams and Carl A. Osborne

DISEASES

RENAL FAILURE, CHRONIC

 BASICS

DEFINITION
Azotemia and urine specific gravity < 1.030 in dogs and < 1.035 in cats; results from primary renal disease that has persisted for months to years; characterized by irreversible renal dysfunction that tends to deteriorate progressively over months to years.

PATHOPHYSIOLOGY
More than approximately 75% reduction in functional renal mass results in impaired urine-concentrating ability (leading to polyuria and polydipsia [PU/PD]) and retention of nitrogenous waste products of protein catabolism (leading to azotemia). Severe chronic renal failure (CRF) results in uremia. Decreased erythropoietin and calcitriol production by the kidneys results in hypoproliferative anemia and renal secondary hyperparathyroidism, respectively.

SYSTEMS AFFECTED
• Renal/Urologic—impaired renal function leading to PU/PD and signs of uremia • Nervous, Gastrointestinal, Musculoskeletal, and other body systems—secondarily affected by uremia • Hemic/Lymph/Immune—anemia

GENETICS
Inherited in the following breeds (mode of inheritance, known or suspected, indicated in parentheses):
• Abyssinian cats (autosomal dominant with incomplete penetrance) • Persian cats (autosomal dominant) • Bull terrier (autosomal dominant) • Cairn terrier (autosomal recessive) • German shepherd (autosomal dominant) • Samoyed (X-linked dominant) • English cocker spaniel (autosomal recessive)

INCIDENCE /PREVALENCE
• Reportedly 9 cases per 1000 dogs examined and 16 cases per 1000 cats examined • Prevalence increases with age—in animals >15 years of age, reportedly 57 per 1000 dogs examined and 153 per 1000 cats examined

GEOGRAPHIC DISTRIBUTION
N/A

SIGNALMENT

Species
Dogs and cats

Breed Predilections
All breeds of dogs and cats are affected. Familial renal disease resulting in CRF has been reported in basenji, beagle, bull terrier, Cairn terrier, chow chow, Doberman pincher, English cocker spaniel, German shepherd, golden retriever, Lhasa apso, miniature schnauzer, Norwegian elkhound, rottweiler, samoyed, Chinese shar pei, shih tzu, soft-coated wheaten terrier, standard poodle, and Abyssinian cats.

Mean Age and Range
Mean age at diagnosis is approximately 7 years in dogs and 9 years in cats. Animals of any age can be affected, but prevalence increases with increasing age.

Predominant Sex
None

SIGNS

General Comments
Clinical signs are related to the severity of renal dysfunction and presence or absence of complications such as hypertension. Cats with mild CRF may be asymptomatic. An animal with stable CRF may decompensate, resulting in a uremic crisis.

Historical Findings
• PU/PD (less frequent in cats than dogs) • Anorexia • Lethargy • Vomiting • Weight loss • Nocturia • Constipation • Diarrhea • Acute blindness—because of hypertension • Seizures or coma—late • Cats may also have ptyalism and muscle weakness with cervical ventroflexion—because of hypokalemic myopathy

Physical Examination Findings
• Small, irregular kidneys (or enlarged kidneys secondary to polycystic kidney disease or lymphoma) • Dehydration • Cachexia • Mucous membrane pallor • Oral ulceration • Uremic breath odor • Constipation • Hypertensive retinopathy • Renal osteodystrophy

CAUSES
• Most are idiopathic, and the disease is termed *chronic generalized nephropathy.* • Include familial and congenital renal disease, nephrotoxins, hypercalcemia, hypokalemic nephropathy, glomerulonephritis, amyloidosis, pyelonephritis, polycystic kidney disease, nephroliths, chronic urinary obstruction, drugs, lymphoma, leptospirosis (following acute renal failure), FIP (cats), and, possibly, diabetes mellitus.

RISK FACTORS
Aging, hypercalcemia, hypokalemia (cats), hypertension, urinary tract infection, diabetes mellitus

 DIAGNOSIS

DIFFERENTIAL DIAGNOSIS
• See chapter on polyuria/polydipsia for differential diagnosis.
• Azotemia—includes causes of prerenal and postrenal azotemia, acute renal failure, and hypoadrenocorticism
• Prerenal azotemia—characterized by azotemia with urine specific gravity > 1.030 in dogs and > 1.035 in cats
• Postrenal azotemia—characterized by azotemia with obstruction or rupture of the excretory system

• Acute renal failure—differentiated by normal renal size, cylindruria, lack of indications of chronicity (e.g., nonregenerative anemia and renal secondary hyperparathyroidism), and recent nephrotoxin exposure or hypotensive episode
• Hypoadrenocorticism—characterized by hyponatremia, hyperkalemia with decreased cortisol response to ACTH stimulation

CBC/BIOCHEMISTRY/URINALYSIS
• Nonregenerative anemia
• Azotemia (high BUN and creatinine), hyperphosphatemia, acidosis (low total CO_2), hyperamylasemia, hyperlipasemia, hypokalemia or hyperkalemia, and hypercalcemia or hypocalcemia
• Urine specific gravity < 1.030 in dogs and < 1.035 in cats; mild proteinuria

OTHER LABORATORY TESTS
Urinary protein:creatinine ratio to determine magnitude of proteinuria

IMAGING
• Abdominal radiographs may demonstrate small kidneys (or large kidneys secondary to polycystic kidney disease or lymphoma).
• Ultrasound demonstrates small kidneys and hyperechoic renal parenchyma with less apparent distinction between the cortex and medulla in some animals. Animals with lymphoma often have renomegaly with hypoechoic renal parenchyma. See also Congenital/Developmental Renal Disorders, Pyelonephritis, Nephrolithiasis, Hydronephrosis, and Polycystic Kidneys.

DIAGNOSTIC PROCEDURES
• Direct or indirect blood pressure determinations indicated to detect hypertension
• Renal biopsy helpful in selected patients to document underlying cause; especially in patients with glomerular disease, familial renal disease, lymphoma, and FIP, but renal biopsy not indicated in most dogs and cats

PATHOLOGIC FINDINGS
• Gross findings—small kidneys with a lumpy or granular surface; renal capsule frequently adheres to the renal parenchyma.
• Histopathologic findings—frequently nonspecific; chronic generalized nephropathy or end-stage kidneys; findings are specific for diseases causing CRF in some patients.

 TREATMENT

APPROPRIATE HEALTH CARE
Patients with compensated CRF may be managed as outpatients; patients in uremic crisis should be managed as inpatients.

NURSING CARE
• Patients in uremic crisis—correct fluid and electrolyte deficits with intravenous fluid

therapy (e.g. lactated Ringer solution); correct dehydration over 2–6 h to prevent additional renal injury from ischemia
• Subcutaneous fluid therapy (daily or every other day) may benefit patients with moderate-to-severe CRF.

ACTIVITY
Unrestricted

DIET
• Reduced dietary protein, phosphorus, and sodium with adequate buffering capacity (alkalinizing diet); supplemental n-3 fatty acids may be beneficial.
• Recommendations for animals with mild-to-moderate renal failure are controversial; some authors suggest protein restriction not required until the patient has moderate-to-severe renal failure
• Free access to fresh water at all times

CLIENT EDUCATION
• Tends to progress to terminal CRF over months to years
• Heritability of familial renal diseases

SURGICAL CONSIDERATIONS
• Avoid hypotension during anesthesia to prevent additional renal injury.
• Renal transplantation has been successfully performed in dogs and cats with advanced disease.

MEDICATIONS

DRUGS OF CHOICE

Uremic Crisis
• Cimetidine (dogs, 10 mg/kg IV initial dose followed by 5 mg/kg IV q8–12 h; cats, 2.5–5 mg/kg IV q8–12 h) to minimize nausea and vomiting
• Potassium chloride in IV fluids or potassium gluconate PO (2–6 mEq/cat/day) as needed to correct hypokalemia

Compensated CRF
• Famotidine (dogs, 0.5–1 mg/kg PO q24h; cats, 5 mg/cat PO q48 h) to minimize nausea
• Potassium gluconate (2–6 mEq/cat/day PO) as needed for hypokalemia
• Intestinal phosphate binders (e.g., aluminum carbonate, 30–100 mg/kg/day PO with meals) as needed to correct hyperphosphatemia (see Renal Secondary Hyperparathyroidism)
• Calcitriol (see Renal Secondary Hyperparathyroidism)
• Erythropoietin (see Anemia of Chronic Renal Disease)
• Angiotensin-converting enzyme (ACE) inhibitors (e.g., enalapril 0.5 mg/kg PO q24 h) or amlodipine (dogs, 0.1 mg/kg PO q24h; cats 0.18 mg/kg or 0.625–1.25 mg/cat PO q24 h) as needed for hypertension
• Oxazepam (2.5 mg/cat PO) as needed to increase appetite

CONTRAINDICATIONS
Avoid nephrotoxic drugs (aminoglycosides, cisplatin, amphotericin B) and corticosteroids

PRECAUTIONS
• Reduce dosage or prolong dosing interval of drugs eliminated by the kidneys, including cimetidine, enalapril, ranitidine, and metoclopramide.
• Use ACE inhibitors with caution; monitor patient for worsening of azotemia or proteinuria
• Use caution with NSAIDs

POSSIBLE INTERACTIONS
Cimetidine or trimethoprim may cause artifactual increases in the serum creatinine concentration by reducing tubular secretion in dogs with CRF.

ALTERNATIVE DRUGS
• Metoclopramide (0.2–0.4 mg PO or SC q6–8h) can be used in addition to H_2-receptor antagonists to treat uremic vomiting.
• Ranitidine (0.5–2 mg/kg PO or IV q12h) or cimetidine (5 mg/kg q8–12h for dogs; 2.5–5 mg/kg q8–12h for cats) may be used instead of famotidine for uremic gastritis.
• Hemodialysis and renal transplantation are available at selected referral hospitals.

FOLLOW-UP

PATIENT MONITORING
Dogs and cats with CRF should be monitored at regular intervals, depending on therapy and severity of disease; initially weekly for patients receiving calcitriol or erythropoietin; reevaluate patients with mild-to-moderate CRF every 1–3 months.

PREVENTION/AVOIDANCE
Do not breed animals with familial renal disease.

POSSIBLE COMPLICATIONS
Systemic hypertension, uremic stomatitis, gastroenteritis, anemia, secondary urinary tract infection

EXPECTED COURSE AND PROGNOSIS
• Short-term—depends on severity • Long-term—guarded to poor because CRF tends to be progressive over months to years

MISCELLANEOUS

ASSOCIATED CONDITIONS
• Hyperthyroidism in cats • Urinary tract infection • Systemic hypertension

AGE-RELATED FACTORS
Increased incidence in older animals; normal renal function decreases with aging.

ZOONOTIC POTENTIAL
None

PREGNANCY
Patients with mild CRF may maintain pregnancy; those with moderate-to-severe disease may be infertile or have spontaneous abortions; breeding of female patients not recommended

SYNONYMS
• Kidney failure • Chronic renal disease

SEE ALSO
• Anemia of Chronic Renal Disease
• Congenital/Developmental Renal Disorders
• Creatinine and Blood Urea Nitrogen (BUN)—Azotemia and Uremia
• Hydronephrosis • Hyperparathyroidism, Renal Secondary • Hypertension, Systemic
• Nephrolithiasis • Polycystic Kidneys
• Polyuria/Polydipsia • Pyelonephritis • Renal Failure—Acute • Urinary Tract Obstruction

ABBREVIATIONS
• ACE = angiotensin-converting enzyme
• CRF = chronic renal failure • FIP = feline infectious peritonitis • NSAID = nonsteroidal antiinflammatory drug • PU/PD = polyuria/polydipsia

Suggested Reading

Brown SA, Barsanti JA, Finco DR. Medical management of canine chronic renal failure. In: Kirk RW, Bonagura JD, eds. Current veterinary therapy. XI Philadelphia: WB Saunders, 1992:842–847.

DiBartola SP. Familial renal disease in dogs and cats. In: Ettinger SJ, Feldman EC, eds. Textbook of veterinary internal medicine. 4th ed. Philadelphia: WB Saunders, 1995:1796–1801.

Gregory CR. Renal transplantation in cats. Compend Contin Educ Pract Vet 1993;15:1325–1339.

Polzin DJ, Osborne CA, Adams LG, Lulich JP. Medical management of feline chronic renal failure. In: Kirk RW, Bonagura JD, eds. Current veterinary therapy. XI Philadelphia: WB Saunders, 1992:848–853.

Polzin DJ, Osborne CA, Bartges JW, et al. Chronic renal failure. In: Ettinger SJ, Feldman EC, eds. Textbook of veterinary internal medicine. 4th ed. Philadelphia: WB Saunders, 1995:1734–1760.

Author Larry G. Adams
Consulting Editors Larry G. Adams and Carl A. Osborne

DISEASES

RENAL TUBULAR ACIDOSIS

BASICS

OVERVIEW
A rare syndrome that refers to the development of metabolic acidosis because of either reduced bicarbonate reabsorption from the proximal renal tubule (proximal or type 2 renal tubular acidosis) or reduced hydrogen ion secretion in the distal tubule (distal or type 1 renal tubular acidosis); proximal renal tubular acidosis has not been documented as an isolated entity in dogs but has been observed as part of Fanconi's syndrome; the following discussion is limited to distal renal tubular acidosis.

SIGNALMENT
• Reported in 5 dogs and 3 cats
• No apparent breed or sex predilection
• Age range at time of diagnosis, 1–8 years

SIGNS
• Anorexia and lethargy—most common
• Others depend on the presence or absence of associated diseases (e.g., pyelonephritis).
• Panting
• Weakness—related to hypokalemia
• Polyuria
• Polydipsia
• Vomiting
• Weight loss
• Hematuria
• Dysuria—related to urolithiasis
• Fever

CAUSES & RISK FACTORS
• Associated with distal renal tubular acidosis in human beings: primary (i.e., inherited), secondary to other inherited diseases (e.g., Ehlers-Danlos syndrome), toxins and drugs (e.g., amphotericin B), altered calcium metabolism causing nephrocalcinosis (e.g., hypervitaminosis D), autoimmune and hypergammaglobulinemic disorders (e.g., multiple myeloma, systemic lupus erythematosus) and tubulointerstitial nephropathies
• In cats, distal renal tubular acidosis has been associated with pyelonephritis (two cases) and hepatic lipidosis (one case).
• In dogs, all clinical reports of distal renal tubular acidosis appeared to be idiopathic; struvite urolithiasis (one case) occurred secondary to distal renal tubular acidosis; distal renal tubular acidosis has also been caused by experimentally induced renal ischemia.

DIAGNOSIS

DIFFERENTIAL DIAGNOSIS
Consider other diseases that may cause a normal anion gap metabolic acidosis (e.g. diarrhea).

CBC/BIOCHEMISTRY/URINALYSIS
• Vary depending on associated diseases
• Hypokalemia (because of increased renal excretion) in some animals; may be severe enough to cause muscle weakness
• Alkaline urine—pH > 6.0, assuming urinary tract infection is absent

OTHER LABORATORY TESTS
Blood gas analysis and evaluation of serum electrolytes reveals normal anion gap metabolic acidosis.

IMAGING
May detect uroliths radiographically

DIAGNOSTIC PROCEDURES
The key diagnostic feature is normal anion gap metabolic acidosis accompanied by an inappropriately alkaline urine pH (> 6.0). In some patients in which no nonrenal cause for a normal anion gap metabolic acidosis can be found and the urine pH is 6.0 (or very close to it), an acid load may be required to demonstrate distal renal tubular acidosis—administer ammonium chloride (200 mg/kg PO, dogs); drain the bladder hourly; urinary pH (measured by a pH meter) should decrease to < 6.0 (often < 5.5) within 3–6 h; avoid this test if severe acidosis

TREATMENT

• Individualize depending on the nature and severity of associated conditions.
• Typically, less bicarbonate is needed to resolve metabolic acidosis associated with distal renal tubular acidosis than is needed to resolve acidosis associated with proximal renal tubular acidosis.
• Hypokalemia may resolve with bicarbonate administration alone, or potassium supplementation may be required.

MEDICATIONS

DRUGS
• Sodium bicarbonate—10–50 mg/kg q8–12h PO
• Potassium supplementation—potassium gluconate 2–8 mEq/day divided q12h PO (cats); 2–44 mEq/day divided q12h PO (dogs, depending on body size), if required

CONTRAINDICATIONS/POSSIBLE INTERACTIONS
N/A

FOLLOW-UP

• Serial blood gas analyses every 3–5 days until acid–base status has normalized
• Monitor serum electrolytes, particularly potassium, as needed
• Long-term prognosis depends on the nature and severity of associated conditions; may be reasonably good in patients without other diseases and that respond well to bicarbonate therapy, but little information exists on the long-term course of this disease

MISCELLANEOUS

SEE ALSO
• Acidosis, Metabolic
• Potassium, Hypokalemia

Suggested Reading
Mueller DL, Jergens AE. Renal tubular acidosis. Compend Contin Educ 1991;13:435–444.
Author Darcy H. Shaw
Contributing Editors Larry G. Adams and Carl A. Osborne

REOVIRUS INFECTIONS

BASICS

OVERVIEW
• Respiratory enteric orphan virus (reovirus)—genus in the family Reovirus; nonenveloped, double-stranded RNA virus; isolated from respiratory and enteric tracts; not associated with any known disease (hence *orphan*)
• Ubiquitous in geographic distribution and host range, virtually every species of mammal, including humans
• Virus—infects mature epithelial cells on luminal tips of the intestinal villi; causes cellular destruction, resulting in villous atrophy (similar to rotavirus and coronavirus)
• Loss of absorptive capability and loss of brush border enzymes (e.g., disaccharidases) leads to osmotic diarrhea.

SIGNALMENT
Dogs and cats

SIGNS

Dogs
• Conjunctivitis
• Rhinitis
• Tracheobronchitis—minor role
• Pneumonia
• Diarrhea
• Encephalitis—rare

Cats
• Generally mild disease
• Respiratory illness
• Conjunctivitis
• Gingivitis
• Ataxia
• Diarrhea

CAUSES & RISK FACTORS
• Predominantly excreted from respiratory and digestive tract; acquired by inhalation and oral ingestion

• Infection common; specific disease has not been reproduced.
• Other viral pathogens—infections observed repeatedly; speculated that reovirus may have an immunosuppressive effect that aggravates such infections

DIAGNOSIS

DIFFERENTIAL DIAGNOSIS
• Canine viral enteritis—canine parvovirus; canine coronavirus; canine astrovirus; canine calicivirus; canine herpesvirus; canine distemper virus; canine rotavirus
• Canine infectious tracheobronchitis—canine parainfluenza; *Bordetella bronchiseptica;* mycoplasmas canine adenovirus types 1 and 2; canine herpesvirus; canine distemper virus
• Feline upper respiratory disease—feline rhinotracheitis virus; feline calicivirus; *Chlamydia;* mycoplasma; bacterial infection

CBC/BIOCHEMISTRY/URINALYSIS
Noncontributory

OTHER LABORATORY TESTS
• Virus isolation—cytopathic effect slow to develop
• Histopathology—large intracytoplasmic inclusion bodies

IMAGING
N/A

DIAGNOSTIC PROCEDURES
N/A

TREATMENT
• Doubtful that reovirus is an important pathogen

• No vaccines developed
• Other control measures ignored

MEDICATIONS

DRUGS
N/A

CONTRAINDICATIONS/POSSIBLE INTERACTIONS
N/A

FOLLOW-UP
N/A

MISCELLANEOUS

ZOONOTIC POTENTIAL
• Infection can spread among individuals of the same or different species.
• The role (if any) that animals serve as a reservoir for virus or as a possible source of human infection unknown
• Humans—by early childhood, the vast majority demonstrate serologic evidence of past reovirus infection; difficult to link to disease; majority of infections must be asymptomatic or blend imperceptibly with minor respiratory and gastrointestinal illness of infancy and early childhood

Suggested Reading
Thein P, Scheid R. Mammalian reoviral infections. In: Steele JH, ed. CRC handbook series in zoonoses. Vol. 2: Viral zoonoses. Boca Raton, FL: CRC, 1981:191–216.
Author J. Paul Woods
Consulting Editor Stephen C. Barr

DISEASES

RESPIRATORY PARASITES

 BASICS

DEFINITION
Helminths and arthropods that reside in the respiratory tract or pulmonary vessels of dogs and cats

PATHOPHYSIOLOGY
Infestation with parasites causes irritant allergic rhinitis, bronchitis, pneumonitis, or arteritis, depending on the location of the organism within the respiratory system.

SYSTEMS AFFECTED
• Respiratory
• Cardiovascular
• Hepatic—with hepatopulmonary migration of some parasites

GENETICS
N/A

INCIDENCE/PREVALENCE
Depends on parasite

GEOGRAPHIC DISTRIBUTION
• *Pneumonyssoides caninum*—worldwide
• *Oslerus (Filaroides) osleri*—worldwide
• *Filaroides hirthi*—North America
• *Filaroides milksi*—North America; Europe
• *Aelurostrongylus abstrusus*—worldwide
• *Capillaria aerophila*—North America
• *Crenosoma vulpis*—worldwide
• *Angiostrongylus vasorum*—Europe; Africa; Asia
• *Dirofilaria immitis*—worldwide
• *Paragonimus kellicotti*—North America
• *Eucoleus boehmi*—North America

SIGNALMENT

Species
Dogs and Cats

Breed Predilections
None

Mean Age and Range
N/A

Predominant Sex
N/A

SIGNS

General Comments
• Three basic categories—upper respiratory, lower respiratory, and vascular; based on location and lifestyle of parasite
• Often insidious and chronic, with few clinical signs
• Respiratory compromise often not severe

Historical Findings
• Upper respiratory—sneezing; nasal discharge (serous, sanguinous); reverse sneezing; nasal irritation or rubbing
• Lower respiratory—chronic coughing nonresponsive to empirical treatment
• Vascular—chronic coughing; fatigue; weight-loss; tachypnea; living in or traveling through an endemic heartworm area

Physical Examination Findings
• Upper respiratory—similar to historical findings; variable
• Lower respiratory—elicitable cough; occasionally harsh lung sounds; often cause coughing in cats
• Vascular—elicitable cough; possibly heart murmur; occasional split second heart sound (with pulmonary hypertension)

CAUSES
• Upper respiratory—*Pneumonyssus caninum* (nasal mites); *Eucoleus boehmi; Crenosoma vulpis*
• Lower respiratory—dogs and cats: *Capillaria aerophila* (rare in cats), *Paragonimus kellicotti* (lung fluke); dogs: *Filaroides osleri (Oslerus osleri), Filaroides hirthi, Filaroides milksi, Crenosoma vulpis;* cats: *Aelurostrongylus abstrusus*
• Vascular—dogs and cats: *Dirofilaria immitis* (heartworm); dogs: *Angiostrongylus vasorum*

RISK FACTORS
• Depends on the specific parasite—some have intermediate or paratenic hosts that must be ingested by the definitive host, putting scavenging animals at higher risk
• *Crenosoma vulpis*—snails
• *Paragonimus kellicotti*—snails; crabs; shellfish
• *Aelurostrongylus abstrusus*—snails and slugs; transport hosts: rodents, frogs, lizards, birds
• *Dirofilaria immitis*—mosquitoes
• Multianimal households with unhygienic living conditions—allows fecal–oral or direct-contact transmission

 DIAGNOSIS

DIFFERENTIAL DIAGNOSIS
• Upper respiratory—other causes of epistaxis, rhinitis, or sinusitis (see specific topics)
• Lower respiratory—allergic bronchitis (nonparasitic); chronic bronchitis; infectious tracheobronchitis; allergic pneumonitis; bronchopneumonia; granulomatous pneumonia; pulmonary granulomatosis; hepatopulmonary migration of enteric helminths
• Vascular—pneumonitis; pulmonary arterial hypertension; pneumonia; severe left heart failure; right heart failure

CBC/BIOCHEMISTRY/URINALYSIS
• CBC—variable; may note eosinophilia, basophilia (especially with heartworm disease), neutrophilia, and monocytosis
• Biochemistry—often normal; high liver enzyme activity with some parasites during early stages as a result of hepatic migration if burden is substantial.
• Urinalysis—normal; may see proteinuria with heartworm disease

OTHER LABORATORY TESTS
• Hematologic examination for microfilaria—Difil Test and Knott test
• Serologic testing—antigen detection via ELISA for *Dirofilaria* (e.g., CITE test, Dirocheck, ad VetRed); antibody testing for feline dirofilariasis

IMAGING
• Thoracic radiography—often unrewarding; generalized interstitial pattern; tortuous pulmonary arteries with vascular parasites; granulomatous masses (especially right caudal lobe) with *Paragonimus*
• Echocardiography—may be helpful with vascular parasites; may see worms within main pulmonary artery and right ventricle

DIAGNOSTIC PROCEDURES
Sputum examination—may reveal eggs or larvae (L-1)

Fecal Examination
• Lung flukes, *Capillaria,* and *Eucoleus*—may shed eggs into the feces
• Other lungworm eggs—usually hatch within the respiratory system; necessary to extract larva from feces via the Baermann method
• *Angiostrongylus* eggs and larvae—may be found in feces
• Multiple examinations often necessary; negative results do not rule out infection.

Rhinoscopy/Bronchoscopy
• Upper respiratory—examination via retrograde pharyngoscopy or rhinoscopy with antegrade flushing of anesthetic gas; often allows visualization of nasal mites; retrograde nasal lavage and cytological examination of fluid may be helpful.
• Lower respiratory—may see tracheal and bronchial parasites and parasitic nodules; occasionally may be removed for definitive identification; bronchoalveolar lavage may allow extraction of larvae or worms from alveoli.
• May attempt anthelmintic response therapeutic trial

PATHOLOGIC FINDINGS
• Upper respiratory—may find nasal mites or worms in sinuses and nasal cavity
• Lower respiratory—may see pulmonary nodules throughout the parenchyma or within bronchi
• Vascular—may see heartworms within pulmonary vessels and cardiac chambers; may see arteritis of end arteries; may see arterioles with myointimal proliferation; may note thromboemboli

TREATMENT

APPROPRIATE HEALTH CARE
• Outpatient—upper and lower respiratory parasites; may need repeated examinations to monitor response
• Inpatient—usually necessary for heartworm adulticide treatment

ACTIVITY
• No restrictions unless severe pulmonary dysfunction occurs with upper or lower respiratory parasites
• Restricted after treatment for heartworm

DIET
No special restrictions

CLIENT EDUCATION
• Explain that treatment response and duration depends on the type of parasite.
• Warn client of the risk of recurrence in dogs that maintain lifestyles conducive to transmission of the parasites (e.g., hunting, sporting dogs, and multidog households).

SURGICAL CONSIDERATIONS
N/A

MEDICATIONS

DRUGS OF CHOICE
• Anthelminthics—few studies confirm efficacy; most data anecdotal
• *Pneumonyssoides caninum*—ivermectin at 200–400 μg/kg SC, PO for 2 treatments 2 weeks apart; **NOTE:** not registered for use in dogs at this dosage; dosage contraindicated in collies, collie breeds, and Australian shepherds because of high incidence of toxicity; try pyrethrin/pyrethroid inhalation (e.g., Shelltox Ministrips) instead
• *Aelurostrongylus abstrusus*—fenbendazole at 50 mg/kg PO q24h for 4 days, repeat after 10 days; ivermectin at 200 μg/kg SC q24h for 3 days or PO for 5 days; **NOTE:** ivermectin not registered for use in cats at this dosage
• Other upper and lower respiratory—fenbendazole at 50–100 mg/kg PO q24h for 7–14 days or longer with evidence of persistent infestation; variable success with ivermectin at 200 μg/kg every week for 2–4 treatments
• *Crenosoma vulpis*—reported to be susceptible to diethylcarbamazine (dosage unknown), fendendazole at 50 mg/kg PO q24h for 7 days
• *Paragonimus kellicotti*—praziquantel at 25 mg/kg PO, SC for 3 days; fenbendazole at 50–100 mg/kg PO q24h for 10–14 days
• *Angiostrongylus vasorum*—mebendazole for 5 days (dosage unknown)
• *Dirofilaria immitus*—see Heartworm

Disease–dogs and heartworm disease–cats
• Anti-inflammatory agents—generally not required; may reduce efficacy of anthelminthic

CONTRAINDICATIONS
Ivermectin—not registered for use in dogs or cats other than for heartworm prophylaxis; contraindicated at dosages > 50 μg/kg in breeds with known increased sensitivity (collies, collie breeds, and Australian shepherds)

PRECAUTIONS
Ivermectin—use caution when considering treatment with ivermectin; after administration at 200 μg/kg, observe for adverse side effects for 4–6 hr.

POSSIBLE INTERACTIONS
N/A

ALTERNATIVE DRUGS
N/A

FOLLOW-UP

PATIENT MONITORING
• Serial fecal Baermann larval extractions or examination for eggs—some anthelminthics may suppress egg or larval production in some species.
• Repeating bronchoscopic examination—may help assess efficacy of treatment for lower respiratory parasites
• Resolution of clinical signs—suggests response to treatment; does not indicate complete clearance of parasites
• Peripheral eosinophilia, if noted initially, may subside with treatment.
• See Heartworm Disease–dogs and heartworm disease–cats recommendations concerning dirofilariasis.

PREVENTION AND AVOIDANCE
• Avoid activity that predisposes to infestations (often not practical).
• Avoid contact with wildlife reservoirs (especially wild canides).
• Consider prophylactic treatment for heartworm.

POSSIBLE COMPLICATIONS
• Chronic pulmonary damage—possible with persistent and heavy lower respiratory parasite burdens
• Infestations rarely fatal
• Pulmonary hypertension and right-heart failure—may occur with heartworm disease
• Angiostrongylus infestations—may cause coagulopathies

EXPECTED COURSE AND PROGNOSIS
• With aggressive management—prognosis usually fair to excellent; variable
• Return to performance—depends on chronicity of disease and level of chronic pulmonary damage by lower respiratory parasites
• Recurrence possible

MISCELLANEOUS

ASSOCIATED CONDITIONS
N/A

AGE-RELATED FACTORS
N/A

ZOONOTIC POTENTIAL
N/A

PREGNANCY
N/A

SYNONYMS
• Lungworm infestation—*Aelurostrongylus, Angiostrongylus, Capillaria, Crenosoma, Filaroides, Paragonimus*
• Nasal mite infestation—*Pneumonyssus caninum*
• Heartworm disease, dirofilariasis—*Dirofilaria immitus*

SEE ALSO
• Heartworm Disease—Cats
• Heartworm Disease—Dogs
• Paragonimiasis • Pneumonia, Allergic

ABBREVIATION
ELISA = enzyme-linked immunoadsorbent assay

Suggested Reading
American Heartworm Society. Recommendations for the diagnosis and management of heartworm (*Dirofilaria immitus*) infection. American heartworm society bulletin 1993;19:1–8.
Foreyt WJ. Veterinary parasitology reference manual. Pulman: Washington State University, Board of Regents, 1989.
Marks SL, Moore MP, Rishniw M. Pneumonyssus caninum: the canine nasal mite. Compend Contin Educ Pract Vet 1994;16:577–582.
Shaw DH, Conboy GA, Hogan PM, et. al. Eosionophilic bronchitis caused by crenosoma vulpis infection in dogs. Can Vet J 1996;37:361–363.
Soulsby EJL. Helminths, arthropods and protozoa of domesticated animals. 7th ed. Philadelphia: Lea & Febiger, 1982.
Urquhart GM, Armour J, Duncan JL, et al. Veterinary parasitology. UK: Longman Scientific, 1987.
Author Mark Rishniw
Consulting Editor Eleanor C. Hawkins

DISEASES

RETAINED PLACENTA

BASICS

OVERVIEW
• Dogs—placenta retained beyond the immediate postpartum period; placentae usually passed within 15 min of birth of a puppy; may develop acute metritis secondary to retained placenta
• Cats—may retain placentae for days without signs of illness
• Extremely uncommon

SIGNALMENT
• Dogs—most common in toy dog breeds
• Cats—rare

SIGNS

Historical Findings
• Recent parturition
• Continued vulvar discharge of lochia
• Owner may note number of placentae passed; not always reliable

Physical Examination Findings
• Green lochia vulvar discharge
• Palpation of firm mass in uterus—not always possible

CAUSES & RISK FACTORS
• Toy breed
• Large litter size
• Dystocia

DIAGNOSIS

DIFFERENTIAL DIAGNOSIS
• Postpartum metritis—physical examination and vaginal cytologic examination show no signs of infection with uncomplicated condition; may develop concurrently
• Retained fetus—differentiated by radiography or ultrasonography

CBC/BIOCHEMISTRY/URINALYSIS
• Usually normal when uncomplicated

OTHER LABORATORY TESTS
Vaginal cytologic examination—parabasal epithelial cells; may note erythrocytes; biliverdin clumps

IMAGING
Ultrasonography—echogenic but nonfetal mass within the uterus

DIAGNOSTIC PROCEDURES
Celiotomy or hysterotomy—may be required for diagnosis

TREATMENT
• Outpatient for healthy bitch or queen
• Instruct owner to monitor temperature and observe for signs of systemic illness.
• Ovariohysterectomy—curative; recommend if future breeding is not a consideration
• Surgical removal—indicated if medical treatment is unsuccessful and the bitch develops metritis

MEDICATIONS

• Oxytocin—known or suspected condition in otherwise healthy cats and dogs; dogs, 0.5 U/kg IM up to 20 U; cats, 0.5–3.0 U IM)
• Metritis—treat accordingly (see Metritis)

CONTRAINDICATIONS/POSSIBLE INTERACTIONS

Do not give progestational drugs.

 FOLLOW-UP

• Monitor temperature and physical condition.
• Acute metritis (dogs)—may develop if the placenta is not passed; fair to good prognosis for recovery with treatment
• Prognosis for future reproduction—good without metritis; fair to poor with metritis

 MISCELLANEOUS

Suggested Reading

Feldman EC, Nelson RW. Canine and feline endocrinology and reproduction, 2nd ed. Philadelphia: Saunders, 1996:586–675.

Author Joni L. Freshman
Consulting Editor Sara K. Lyle

RETINAL DETACHMENT

 BASICS

DEFINITION
Any separation of the neural retina from the RPE at the outer segment–neuroepithelium interface

PATHOPHYSIOLOGY
• Subretinal space—potential space between the RPE and neural retina in which fluid or exudates accumulate • Characterized by its etiopathogenesis—one or a combination of rhegmatogenous (retinal tear), subretinal exudation, or traction
Rhegmatogenous
• A tear that may be related to age, cataracts, or retinal degeneration • Allows vitreous to move into the subretinal space and results in detachment • Probably the predominant type that occurs in association with cataracts and after cataract surgery • Usually requires some vitreous abnormality (e.g., liquefaction)
Exudative
• Fluid accumulates in the subretinal space because of breakdown of the blood–retinal barrier. • Fluid—may be serous, hemorrhagic, or exudative (e.g., granulomatous in patients with blastomycosis chorioretinitis) • Hematogenous pathogenetic factors—common • Vasculitis, hypertension, and hyperviscosity—may cause serous detachment with or without hemorrhage

Traction
• Traction on the retina—usually by fibrous or fibrovascular tissue; raises the retina from the underlying RPE • Occurs after trauma or inflammation

SYSTEMS AFFECTED
• Ophthalmic—retina • Nervous—vision may be severely compromised or permanently lost.

GENETICS
• Depends on cause—dogs with hereditary cataracts or lens luxations may develop rhegmatogenous detachment.

INCIDENCE/PREVALENCE
• Exudative—most common in dogs and cats • Rhegmatogenous—more common in dogs than in cats because of the greater prevalence of cataracts and cataract surgery

GEOGRAPHIC DISTRIBUTION
N/A

SIGNALMENT
Species
Dogs and cats

Breed Predilections
• Depends on cause • Terrier breeds—predisposed to primary lens luxation, which may contribute to retinal tear and detachment with or without surgery • Breeds that develop cataracts • Shih tzus—appear to be predisposed to spontaneous rhegmatogenous detachments owing to abnormal vitreous (significant vitreous liquefaction)

Mean Age and Range
• Depends on cause • More common in old patients—cataracts and systemic diseases (e.g., hypertension, neoplasia, and immune-mediated disease) are often age-related.

Predominant Sex
N/A

SIGNS
• Blindness or reduced vision • Dilated pupil with slow or no pupillary light reflex • Blood vessels or a membrane is usually observed easily through the pupil just behind the lens. • Vitreous abnormalities—liquefaction, hemorrhage, or syneresis (liquefaction); common • Interruption or alteration of the course of blood vessels owing to retinal elevation • With clear subretinal fluid—vessels may cast shadows on the tapetum or RPE. • Depend on any underlying systemic diseases • See Chorioretinitis for signs of inflammation.

CAUSES
• Bilateral—suggests a systemic problem • Toxic—idiosyncratic reactions to drugs (e.g., trimethoprim-sulfa in dogs, griseofulvin in cats)
Degenerative
• End-stage progressive retinal atrophy (degeneration)—may lead to retinal hole formation and detachment • Chronic glaucoma with globe stretching and retinal thinning
Anomalous
• Optic nerve colobomas—Collie eye anomaly • Multiple ocular anomalies—akitas or any breed • Severe retinal dysplasia—oculoskeletal dysplasia in Labrador retrievers, English springer spaniels, and Bedlington terriers • RPE dysplasia—Australian shepherds • Congenital ocular defect—any young animal; congenital or juvenile retinal detachment
Metabolic
• Systemic hypertension • Hypothyroidism • Hyperviscosity • Polycythemia • Hypoxia with hemorrhagic complications • Dogs—renal failure or pheochromocytoma with systemic hypertension, hypothyroidism, hypercholesterolemia, and hyperproteinemia (e.g., with multiple myeloma) • Bilateral (cats)—probably most often caused by systemic hypertension either as a primary condition or secondary to renal failure or hyperthyroidism
Neoplastic
• Any primary or metastatic neoplasm • Commonly associated with multiple myeloma, lymphosarcoma, granulomatous meningoencephalitis, and intraocular masses—ciliary body adenocarcinoma or melanoma
Infectious
• Infectious retinitis or chorioretinitis—may cause focal or diffuse detachment

• Infection may extend from or to the CNS—see Chorioretinitis.
Immune–mediated/Inflammatory
• Immune complex disease—may cause vasculitis or inflammation that may result in exudative detachment
• Dogs—SLE; uveodermatologic syndrome
• Cats—periarteritis nodosa; SLE
Idiopathic
• If all other causes are ruled out, including retinal tears
• Idiopathic steroid-responsive detachment—reported in giant-breed dogs
Trauma
• Bilateral—probably never occurs
• Penetrating injury or foreign body that causes retinal tears or intraocular hemorrhage—may cause partial or complete detachment
• Severe blunt trauma with inflammation or hemorrhage
• Surgical trauma—may contribute to retinal tearing

RISK FACTORS
• Systemic hypertension
• Old age
• Hypermature cataracts
• Luxated lenses
• Extracapsular or intracapsular lens extraction

 DIAGNOSIS

DIFFERENTIAL DIAGNOSIS
• Ophthalmic examination—usually sufficient for diagnosis
• Blindness or impaired vision—optic neuritis; glaucoma; cataracts; progressive retinal atrophy; SARDS; CNS disease
• Dilated pupil with slow or absent pupillary light reflexes—glaucoma; oculomotor nerve lesion; optic neuritis; progressive retinal atrophy; SARDS
• Membrane or vessels associated with or behind lens—persistent tunica vasculosa lentis; persistent pupillary membranes; fibrovascular membrane secondary to intraocular neoplasia or inflammation

CBC/BIOCHEMISTRY/URINALYSIS
• Typically normal if the problem is confined to the eye
• Abnormalities consistent with an associated systemic disease process

OTHER LABORATORY TESTS
• Depend on suspected systemic problem
• Protein electrophoresis
• Documentation of Bence-Jones protein in urine
• Coagulation profile
• Bacterial culture of ocular or body fluids
• Thyroid hormone measurement (cats)

RETINAL DETACHMENT

• Serologic testing for infectious diseases—see Chorioretinitis.

IMAGING
• Thoracic radiograph—search for lymphadenopathy, metastatic disease, or infiltrates consistent with infectious agents.
• Radiographs of the spine—may reveal bony changes consistent with multiple myeloma
• Ocular ultrasound—identify retinal detachments, intraocular masses, and sometimes lens luxations; especially helpful if the ocular media is not clear
• Cardiac ultrasound (cats)—may be indicated with hypertensive retinopathy

DIAGNOSTIC PROCEDURES
• Single or repeated blood pressure measurement—may reveal hypertension; mean arterial pressure in dogs and cats usually < 160 mm Hg
• CSF tap—indicated with signs of CNS disease or optic neuritis
• Vitreocentesis or subretinal fluid aspirate—may be performed if other diagnostic tests failed to yield a cause and an infectious agent or neoplasia is suspected; may aggravate the inflammation or induce hemorrhage, which may lessen the chance of the retina reattaching and restoring vision

PATHOLOGIC FINDINGS
• Retina separated from the RPE and underlying choroid
• May note masses or subretinal exudate
• Chronic—results in retinal atrophy and a tombstone appearance to the RPE

TREATMENT

APPROPRIATE HEALTH CARE
• Depends on the physical condition of the patient
• Usually outpatient
• Acute blindness—vision may be restored if the underlying cause is rapidly identified and treated; make every attempt to determine the cause.
• Degeneration occurs rapidly—provide therapy, whether surgical or medical, as soon as possible after diagnosis.
• Rhegmatogenous—an ophthalmologist may be able to provide surgical treatment.

NURSING CARE
As appropriate for any associated systemic disease; see Retinal Degeneration.

ACTIVITY
• Restrict until reattachment has occurred.
• Supervise irreversibly blind patients.

DIET
N/A

CLIENT EDUCATION
• Explain that retinal detachment (especially if bilateral) may be a sign of systemic disease, so diagnostic testing is important.
• Inform client that retinal detachment associated with lens luxation or cataract surgery has a bilateral potential, so both eyes should be observed closely.
• Inform client that retinal detachments may be reversible with return of vision if the underlying cause is treated and the detachment is caught early.
• Advise client that blind pets, especially cats, can adapt remarkably well and live a good quality life (see Retinal Degeneration).

SURGICAL CONSIDERATIONS
• Rhegmatogenous—may be surgically repaired; refer patient to an ophthalmologist.
• Laser retinopexy—may reverse detachments associated with optic disk colobomas with Collie eye anomaly

MEDICATIONS

DRUGS OF CHOICE
• Depend on underlying systemic causes, which should be identified and treated appropriately
• Systemic prednisone—2 mg/kg divided q12h for 3–10 days, then taper; if systemic mycosis is ruled out and the detachment is believed to be immune-mediated; may facilitate retinal reattachment; for immune-mediated disease, taper medications very slowly over months.
• Antiinflammatory doses of prednisone—0.5 mg/kg, then taper; may be useful for exudative detachments of an infectious nature as long as the underlying disease is being definitively treated

CONTRAINDICATIONS
Systemic corticosteroids—do not use unless systemic mycosis is ruled out or is being definitively treated.

PRECAUTIONS
N/A

POSSIBLE INTERACTIONS
N/A

ALTERNATIVE DRUGS
• Chemotherapeutic agents—suggested for treatment of neoplastic conditions (e.g., lymphosarcoma or multiple myeloma)
• Azathioprine (dogs)—2 mg/kg preoperatively q24h initially, then 0.5–1 mg/kg q48h; to control inflammation; may be required in addition to steroids for uveodermatologic syndrome or idiopathic immune-mediated detachment; avoid in cats.

FOLLOW-UP

PATIENT MONITORING
• Depends on underlying cause and type of medical treatment • Azathioprine—obtain an initial CBC, then every 1–2 weeks for the first 1–3 months; monitor every 1–2 months for bone marrow suppression (if noted, reduce the dose or discontinue).

PREVENTION/AVOIDANCE
N/A

POSSIBLE COMPLICATIONS
• Permanent blindness • Cataracts • Glaucoma
• Chronic ocular pain • Death if secondary to a systemic disease process

EXPECTED COURSE AND PROGNOSIS
• Prognosis for vision in with complete detachment—guarded • Blindness—may develop in days to weeks even if reattachment occurs (earlier with exudative than with serous detachments). • Vision may return if the underlying cause is removed and reattachment occurs. • Focal or multifocal chorioretinitis—does not markedly impair vision; will leave scars • Systemic disease or neoplasia with ocular manifestations—may influence the prognosis for life

MISCELLANEOUS

ASSOCIATED CONDITIONS
• Exudative—systemic disease • Cataracts
• Trauma • Traction and/or rhegmatogenous—vitreal hemorrhage or inflammation

AGE-RELATED FACTORS
N/A

ZOONOTIC POTENTIAL
N/A

PREGNANCY
N/A

SEE ALSO
• Blind Quiet Eye • Chorioretinitis • Retinal Degeneration

ABBREVIATIONS
• CSF = cerebrospinal fluid • RPE = retinal pigment epithelium • SARDS = sudden acquired retinal degeneration syndrome
• SLE = systemic lupus erythematosus

Suggested Reading
Gelatt KN ed. Veterinary ophthalmology. 2nd ed. Philadelphia: Lea & Febiger, 1991.
Millichamp NJ, Dziezyc J. Small animal ophthalmology. Vet Clin North Am Small Anim Pract 1990;20:564–877.
Author Patricia J. Smith
Consulting Editor Paul E. Miller

RHABDOMYOMA

 ## BASICS

OVERVIEW
• An extremely rare, benign, striated muscle tumor that occurs only half as frequently as its malignant counterpart
• Cardiac—usual site; probably congenital; exhibits no potential for malignant transformation
• Extracardiac—very rare; reported in the tongue and larynx in dogs and pinna in cats

SIGNALMENT
• Dogs and cats
• Extracardiac—affects mostly middle-aged animals
• No sex or breed predilections identified

SIGNS
• Cardiac—none
• Extracardiac—localized swelling

CAUSES & RISK FACTORS
Unknown

 ## DIAGNOSIS

DIFFERENTIAL DIAGNOSIS

Cardiac
• Rhabdomyosarcoma
• Lymphosarcoma
• Hemangioma or hemangiosarcoma
• Fibroma or fibrosarcoma
• Chondroma
• Myxoma
• Myxofibroma
• Mesothelioma
• Neurofibroma
• Teratoma
• Lipofibroma
• Lymphangioendothelioma
• Mixed spindle cell sarcoma

Extracardiac
• Rhabdomyosarcoma
• Lipoma or liposarcoma
• Mast cell tumor
• Fibrosarcoma
• Nonneoplastic, inflammatory disease

CBC/BIOCHEMISTRY/URINALYSIS
Normal

OTHER LABORATORY TESTS
N/A

IMAGING
• Radiography—generally reveals soft tissue density; not helpful with extracardiac form
• Echocardiography (cardiac)—may reveal a pedunculated mass or an infiltrative mass, most often affecting the cardiac ventricles; the interventricular septum appears to be the most common site.

DIAGNOSTIC PROCEDURES
• ECG—arrhythmias may be noted
• Biopsy

PATHOLOGIC FINDINGS
• Cytologic examination of an aspirate—occasionally suggests a mesenchymal neoplasm; usually does not afford a definitive diagnosis
• Useful immunohistochemical markers—actin, desmin, and myoglobin; differentiate striated muscle neoplasms from other spindle cell neoplasms.
• Embryonic disease—actin is considered the most reliable marker because embryonic rhabdomyoblasts stain positive for actin before staining positive for desmin.
• May be difficult to differentiate from other eosinophilic granular cell neoplasms

 ## TREATMENT
• Cardiac—none
• Extracardiac—surgical excision

 ## MEDICATIONS

DRUG(S)
N/A

CONTRAINDICATIONS/ POSSIBLE INTERACTIONS
N/A

 ## FOLLOW-UP
• Evaluate monthly for the first 3 months; then at 3–6-month intervals for another year.
• Cardiac—cardiac decompensation progressing to congestive heart failure may develop.

 ## MISCELLANEOUS

Suggested Reading
Moulton JE. Tumors in domestic animals. 3rd ed. Berkeley: University of California Press, 1990.
Reams Rivera RY, Carlton WW. Lingual rhabdomyoma in a dog. J Compend Pathol 1992;106:83–87.
Author James P. Thompson
Consulting Editor Wallace B. Morrison

BASICS

OVERVIEW
• A malignant tumor derived from striated muscle (adult variety) or embryonic, pluripotent mesenchymal cells (juvenile variety)
• Most common striated muscle tumor in animals, but represents < 1% of spontaneous neoplasms
• Typically shows diffuse and infiltrative growth characteristics
• Aggressive and widespread metastasis

SIGNALMENT
• Dogs and cats
• Adult variety—middle-age to old animals
• Juvenile variety—young dogs
• No sex or breed predilection

SIGNS
• Large, diffuse, soft tissue mass generally of skeletal muscle
• Reported in laryngeal and cardiac locations
• May metastasize within the primary muscle (multiple nodules)

CAUSES & RISK FACTORS
Unknown

DIAGNOSIS

DIFFERENTIAL DIAGNOSIS

Skeletal Muscle Location
• Fibrosarcoma
• Mast cell neoplasia
• Rhabdomyoma
• Lipoma, infiltrative lipoma, or liposarcoma

Laryngeal Location
• Squamous cell carcinoma
• Adenocarcinoma
• Undifferentiated carcinoma
• Osteosarcoma
• Chondrosarcoma
• Fibrosarcoma
• Myxochondroma
• Leiomyoma
• Oncocytoma
• Melanoma

Cardiac Location
• Hemangiosarcoma
• Chemodectoma
• Rhabdomyoma
• Ectopic thyroid tumor
• Ectopic parathyroid tumor
• Lymphoma
• Metastatic neoplasia

CBC/BIOCHEMISTRY/URINALYSIS
• Usually normal
• May cause hypoglycemia

OTHER LABORATORY TESTS
N/A

IMAGING
Dense, soft tissue mass

DIAGNOSTIC PROCEDURES
Cytologic examination—reveals a malignant mesenchymal neoplasm; usually does not provide a definitive diagnosis (requires histopathologic examination)

PATHOLOGIC FINDINGS
• Two varieties based on histomorphologic features
• Adult—large, pleomorphic, elongated tumor cells that may have cross-striation and eosinophilic cytoplasm
• Juvenile—embryonal and alveolar features
• Transmission electron microscopy—may be required for definitive diagnosis
• Immunohistologic examination—may be required for definitive diagnosis; useful markers: actin, desmin, and myoglobin

TREATMENT
• Surgical excision—difficult because of invasiveness
• Amputation of an affected limb—consider
• Radiotherapy—may be helpful

MEDICATIONS

DRUGS
• Chemotherapy—may provide palliation; no specific regimens evaluated
• A 21-day protocol—may be useful; doxorubicin (cats, 20 mg/m² IV; dogs, 30 mg/m² IV on day 0); cyclophosphamide (50 mg/m² PO on days 3, 4, 5, and 6); vincristine (0.5 mg/m² IV on days 7 and 14)

CONTRAINDICATIONS/POSSIBLE INTERACTIONS
Chemotherapy—may be myelosuppressive and cause gastrointestinal toxicity; very important to monitor carefully; do not use without prior experience.

FOLLOW-UP
Physical examination, thoracic radiography, and abdominal ultrasound—monthly for 3 months; then every 3–6 months

MISCELLANEOUS

Suggested Readings
Kim DY, Hodgin EC, Cho DY, et al. Juvenile rhabdomyosarcomas in two dogs. Vet Pathol 1996;33:447–450.
Author James P. Thompson
Consulting Editor Wallace B. Morrison

DISEASES

RHABDOMYOSARCOMA, URINARY BLADDER

BASICS

OVERVIEW
• A malignant tumor derived from pluripotent or striated myoblastic cells of mesenchymal origin that surround the developing Müllerian or Wolffian ducts
• Metastasis—extension to visceral organs and lymph nodes occurs; prevalence not clearly defined
• Constitutes < 1% of all bladder tumors

SIGNALMENT
• Most occur in female, large-breed dogs < 18 months of age
• St. Bernard—may be overrepresented
• Cats—very rare

SIGNS
• Predominantly consistent with lower urinary tract disease
• Hematuria
• Stranguria
• Pollakiuria
• Urine retention possible

CAUSES & RISK FACTORS
Unknown

DIAGNOSIS

DIFFERENTIAL DIAGNOSIS
• Bacterial cystitis
• Urocystolithiasis
• Transitional cell carcinoma
• Squamous cell carcinoma
• Fibroma or fibrosarcoma
• Bladder polyps
• Granulomatous urethritis

CBC/BIOCHEMISTRY/URINALYSIS
• Usually normal
• Urinalysis—usually reveals hematuria
• Cytologic examination of urine sediment—may find cellular pleomorphism and cross-striations consistent with rhabdomyosarcoma

OTHER LABORATORY TESTS
N/A

IMAGING
• Bladder ultrasonography or double-contrast cystourethrography
• Intravenous pyelography—evaluate any trigonal mass; assess the ureters and renal pelves

DIAGNOSTIC PROCEDURES
N/A

TREATMENT
• Surgical excision—difficult because of invasiveness
• Surgical resection—may be enhanced by bladder submucosal saline injection to aid in establishing a dissection plane

RHABDOMYOSARCOMA, URINARY BLADDER

MEDICATIONS

DRUGS
• Adjuvant chemotherapy—recommended; assist in control or elimination of residual neoplastic disease after surgical resection
• A 21-day cycle—used successfully; doxorubicin (30 mg/m^2 IV on day 0) and cyclophosphamide (75 mg/m^2 PO on days 3, 4, 5, and 6); administer a total of four cycles; tumor cell growth indicates clear evidence of chemotherapy resistance.

CONTRAINDICATIONS/POSSIBLE INTERACTIONS
Chemotherapy may be toxic; seek advice before initiating treatment if you are unfamiliar with cytotoxic drugs.

FOLLOW-UP
• Evaluate every 21 days during chemotherapy and every 3–6 months thereafter; include a physical examination, CBC, serum biochemistry profile, and urinalysis.
• Thoracic radiography and abdominal ultrasonography—every 3–6 months during the first year after surgery

MISCELLANEOUS

ASSOCIATED CONDITIONS
• Hypertrophic osteopathy—occasionally
• Concurrent bacterial cystitis common; choose antibiotics on the basis of bacterial culture and sensitivity testing.

SYNONYMS
• Botryoid rhabdomyosarcoma (i.e., grapelike appearance)
• Embryonal rhabdomyosarcoma

Suggested Reading
Morrison WB. Cancers of the urinary tract. In: Morrison WB, ed. Cancer in dogs and cats: medical and surgical management. Baltimore: Williams & Wilkins, 1998: 569–579.
Senior DF, Lawrence DT, Gunson C, et al. Successful treatment of botryoid rhabdomyosarcoma in the bladder of a dog. J Am Anim Hosp Assoc 1993;29:386–390.
Author James P. Thompson
Consulting Editor Wallace B. Morrison

DISEASES

RHINITIS AND SINUSITIS

BASICS

DEFINITION
• Rhinitis—inflammation of the mucous membrane of the nose • Sinusitis—inflammation of the associated paranasal sinuses • Rhinosinusitis—coined term, because one rarely occurs without the other

PATHOPHYSIOLOGY
• May be acute or chronic, noninfectious or infectious • Patients seen in clinics usually have chronic disease. • All causes are often complicated by opportunistic secondary microbial invasion. • Associated mucosal vascular congestion and friability, excessive mucus gland secretion, neutrophil chemotaxis, and nasolacrimal duct obstruction—lead to congestion, obstructed airflow, sneezing, epistaxis, nasal discharge (mucopurulent), and epiphora • Turbinate and facial bone destruction—may develop with neoplastic or fungal disease

SYSTEMS AFFECTED
• Respiratory—nasolacrimal drainage • Nervous—CNS involvement via ethmoidal invasion

GENETICS
Unknown

INCIDENCE/PREVALENCE
• Viral upper respiratory infection—common in cats • Nasal tumors and foreign bodies—seen occasionally • Primary bacterial rhinosinusitis—extremely rare

GEOGRAPHIC DISTRIBUTION
N/A

SIGNALMENT

Species
Dogs and cats

Breed Predilections
Brachycephalic cats—more prone to chronic viral rhinitis than other cats

Mean Age and Range
• Infectious, foreign body, and congenital disease—young dogs and cats • Allergic rhinitis—middle-aged animals • Tumor and dental disease—old animals

Predominant Sex
None

SIGNS

Historical Findings
• Sneezing • Nasal discharge • Epistaxis • Pawing at the nose • Anosmia and inappetence—common in cats with sinusitis

Physical Examination Findings
• Nasal discharge—unilateral suggests foreign body, tooth root abscess, or neoplasm • Epistaxis—suggests fungal or neoplastic disease; tooth root abscesses and foreign body erosion

may bleed; violent sneezing may cause traumatic epistaxis. • Diminished nasal airflow—unilateral or bilateral • Ocular discharge—serous with nasolacrimal obstruction; mucoid with viral or chlamydial rhinitis • Mandibular lymphadenopathy • Frontal and facial bone deformity—fungal or neoplastic disease

CAUSES

Infectious
• Viral—cats: herpes (type 1) and calicivirus; dogs: herpes, adenovirus (types I and II), and parainfluenza viruses • *Chlamydia psittaci*—cats • Fungal—*Cryptococcus neoformans* most common in cats; *Aspergillus fumigatus* most common in dogs; *Blastomycosis*, rhinosporidiosis, and penicilliosis rarely seen • Bacterial—primary bacterial rare, often secondary to a breach of the mucosal barrier from trauma, foreign body, or viral infection; *Pasteurella multocida* common; *Bordetella bronchiseptica, Staphylococcus, Pseudomonas,* and *E. coli* have been cultured. • Parasitic—*Cuterebriasis* in cats; *Pneumonyssoides caninum* in dogs (often reverse sneezing)

Noninfectious
• Less common than infectious • Facial trauma • Foreign body—mostly inhaled vegetable matter (e.g., grass and seeds); penetrating objects (e.g., bullets and teeth from fights); objects refluxed from the nasopharynx (e.g., sticks) • Allergic or irritant—inhaled pollen, mold, dusty litter, or cigarette smoke • Dental disease—periapical abscess of the canine incisors; carnassial abscess generally fistulates laterally through the cheek. • Oronasal fistula—congenital palatal defect; fistula caused by extraction of canine incisors • Nasal and nasopharyngeal polyps—most common in young cats • Neoplasia—nasal lymphoma most common nasal tumor in cats, with or without FIV; adenocarcinoma most common nasal tumor in dogs; squamous cell carcinoma, osteosarcoma, chondrosarcoma, and fibrosarcoma also seen

RISK FACTORS
• Dolichocephalic dogs—prone to fungal and neoplastic disease • Brachycephalic cats—prone to chronic viral rhinosinusitis • Toy breed dogs—prone to severe periodontal disease

DIAGNOSIS

DIFFERENTIAL DIAGNOSIS
Epistaxis—coagulopathy or hypertension

CBC/BIOCHEMISTRY/URINALYSIS
• Hemogram—may reflect chronic inflammation and blood loss anemia • Serum chemistry panel and urinalysis—usually normal

OTHER LABORATORY TESTS
• FeLV and FIV serologic testing—determine causes of immunosuppression • Serum *Aspergillus* titer • Cryptococcal antigen titer

IMAGING
• Skull series radiology—must be taken under general anesthesia • Intraoral dental films—excellent for cats and toy breed dogs; use nonscreen film for tabletop technique. • All patients with nasal discharge (e.g., hemorrhagic, mucous, or serous) have fluid density that obscures nasal detail. • Bony lysis or proliferation of the turbinate and facial bones—most important radiographic finding, consistent with fungal and neoplastic invasion • Assess the apical roots of the canine incisors. • Soft tissue masses—rarely seen on standard radiographs as distinct from surrounding secretions

DIAGNOSTIC PROCEDURES
• Coagulation studies—include activated clotting and mucosal bleeding time; perform before tissue sampling • Blind biopsy—core biopsy harvested by a modified urinary catheter as described below (see Cytology) or with a Tru-Cut biopsy needle passed nasally; may use small alligator or endoscopic clamshell biopsy forceps to grasp tissue • With blind techniques, never pass instruments near the cribiform plate

Cytology
• Nasal swab or flush—rarely yields diagnostic sample • Diagnostic sample—generally requires a traumatic flush technique, such as passing a bevel-pointed, stiff, polypropylene urinary catheter nasally, rapidly inserting the point into the area of interest, and flushing out the debris • New methylene blue—identify the capsule of *C. neoformans*

Endoscopy
• Rostral rhinoscopy with an otoscope speculum only—provides a view of the most rostral rhinarium, rarely a site of lesions • Small-bore, rigid fiberoptic arthroscope or cystoscope, especially under continuous saline flushing through the sheath—provides excellent visualization to the level of the ethmoid turbinates; allows visual guidance of biopsy or foreign body retrieval instruments • Destructive rhinitis—characterized by the loss of the scroll-like turbinate structure; typically found with chronic infection secondary to foreign body or tooth root abscess and with aspergillosis; may see fungal plaques; friable mucosa bleeds easily; hence, continuous saline lavage through the endoscope sheath is required for visualization. • Caudal rhinoscopy—involves using a dental mirror and rostral retraction of the soft palate with a spay hook; retroflexed bronchoscope may provide visual inspection of the nasopharynx to the level of the caudal choanae, allowing for directed biopsy of any lesions; neoplasms generally seen as masses protruding from between the turbinals or occupying the caudal choanal lumina

Exploratory Rhinotomy
• Most invasive, but also most informative, diagnostic procedure • Ventral rhinotomy—provides excellent exposure and cosmesis in dogs • Dorsal rhinotomy and frontal sinusotomy—cats and brachycephalic dogs • Culture and biopsy samples may be harvested.
• Complete turbinectomy—often required; reserved for progressive disease that cannot be otherwise diagnosed or controlled

TREATMENT

APPROPRIATE HEALTH CARE
Depends on underlying cause

NURSING CARE
Humidification of environment—often helps mobilize nasal discharge; enhances patient comfort

ACTIVITY
No change

DIET
No change

CLIENT EDUCATION
• Warn client that a cure is unlikely with chronic viral sinusitis, that the goal of treatment is to control the more severe clinical signs with medication, or possibly surgery, and that treatment is probably life-long. • Discuss the contagious potential of some of the infectious causes (e.g., calicivirus in a cattery).

SURGICAL CONSIDERATIONS
• Rhinotomy and turbinectomy—refractory patients; remove infected tissue or foreign body • Nasopharyngeal polyp removal in cats • Surgical excision—alone not considered effective treatment for nasal tumors in dogs; indicated only when combined with radiotherapy; orthovoltage radiotherapy must be preceded by surgical debulking; megavoltage and cobalt radiotherapy are effective without surgery. • Mesenchymal neoplasms (e.g., osteosarcoma) carry a poor prognosis, with or without surgical excision.

MEDICATIONS

DRUGS OF CHOICE

Antibiotics
• Improvement noted in most patients, irrespective of the underlying cause • Secondary bacterial infection—may cause many clinical signs • Relapse inevitable with cessation of treatment • Systemic therapy—4–6 weeks may be indicated to help prevent deep colonization by the resident flora • Low-dose, once-daily treatment—may be continued indefinitely to maintain remission in some patients; never a substitute for a thorough diagnostic evaluation • Selection based on results of nasal culture or empirically
• Cefadroxil—dogs: 22 mg/kg q12h; cats: 22 mg/kg q24h • Trimethoprim sulfadoxine—dogs and cats: 15 mg/kg q12h • Chloramphenicol—dogs: 50 mg/kg q12h; cats: 12.5–20 mg/kg q12h • Suspected *Chlamydia*—tetracycline (dogs and cats) at 15–20 mg/kg q8h or doxycycline (dogs and cats) at 3–5 mg/kg q12h

Other
• Allergic rhinitis—corticosteroids: prednisone (dogs and cats) at 0.5–1.0 mg/kg q12–24 h; and antihistamines: hydroxyzine (dogs) 1-mg/kg q6–8h • Nasal lymphoma—chemotherapeutically as any multicentric lymphoma • Cryptosporidiosis in cats and aspergillosis in dogs—itraconazole: dogs, 2.5 mg/kg q12h; cats 5 mg/kg q12h administered systemically • *Aspergillus* and *Penicillium* infections in dogs—local flushing of enilconazole or clotrimazole via surgically placed tubing in the frontal sinus • *Aspergillus* infection in dogs—nonsurgical intranasal infusion of clotrimazole for 1 hr of contact throughout the nasal cavity and frontal sinuses

CONTRAINDICATIONS
Do not use topical clotrimazole in dogs with disruption of the cribriform plate.

PRECAUTIONS
• Systemic antifungals—may cause hepatopathy • Tetracyclines—may damage the tooth buds in young animals

POSSIBLE INTERACTIONS
N/A

ALTERNATIVE DRUGS
Anectdotal reports of response to low-dose human α-interferon (30 IU PO q24h) in cats with viral rhinosinusitis

FOLLOW-UP

PATIENT MONITORING
Clinical assessment and monitoring for relapse of clinical signs

PREVENTION/AVOIDANCE
• Remove chronically infected cats from the cattery. • Prevent exposure to bird feces (risk factor for aspergillosis).

POSSIBLE COMPLICATIONS
• Extension of infection into the brain

EXPECTED COURSE AND PROGNOSIS
• Prognosis—depends on cause and chronicity • Trauma and foreign body—prognosis good to excellent • Viral infection—prognosis fair to good; many cats become chronically infected. • Fungal infection—prognosis guarded to fair, depending on invasiveness (e.g., grave with CNS signs) • Neoplasms—prognosis grave to poor; cats with lymphoma may survive 8–10 months with chemotherapy; cats tend to have a better prognosis with surgery and orthovoltage irradiation than do dogs.

MISCELLANEOUS

ASSOCIATED CONDITIONS
N/A

AGE-RELATED FACTORS
• Most of the infectious causes are found in young animals. • Neoplasms—more common in old animals

ZOONOTIC POTENTIAL
None documented for any of the fungal rhinitides

PREGNANCY
Antifungal drugs are teratogenic.

SEE ALSO
• Adenocarcinoma, nasal • Aspergillosis • Cryptococcosis • Epistaxis • Nasal and Nasopharyngeal Polyps • Nasal Discharge (Sneezing, Reverse Sneezing, Gagging) • Nasopharyngeal Stenosis • Respiratory Parasites • Tracheobronchitis, Infectious—Dogs

ABBREVIATIONS
• FeLV = feline leukemia virus • FIV = feline immunodeficiency virus

Suggested Reading
August JR. Chronic sneezing. In: August JR, ed., Consultations in feline medicine (2). Philadelphia: Saunders, 1994:273–277.
Greene CE. Upper respiratory tract infections. In: Greene CE, ed. Infectious diseases of the dog and cat. 2nd ed. Philadelphia: Saunders, 1998:583–585.
Kuehn NF, Roudebush P. Nasal discharge. In: Allen DG, ed. Small animal medicine. Philadelphia: Lippincott, 1991:383–395.
Mathews KG, Koblik PD, Richardson EF, et al. Computed tomographic assessment of noninvasive intranasal infusions in dogs with fungal rhinitis. Vet Surg 1996;25:309–319.
Ogilvie GK, Moore AS. Managing the veterinary cancer patient. Trenton, NJ: Veterinary Learning Systems, 1996.
Author Robert A. Mason
Consulting Editor Eleanor C. Hawkins

DISEASES

RHINOSPORIDIOSIS

 BASICS

OVERVIEW
- A rare chronic fungal infection of the mucous membranes of dogs; generally forms a cauliflower-like mass that often protrudes from the nostril
- Respiratory system affected
- Worldwide distribution
- Endemic areas—Argentina, Sri Lanka, and India
- U.S.—most infections have been reported in the southern states.

SIGNALMENT
- Reported in 13 dogs, 7 of which were males
- No apparent breed predilection
- Not reported in cats

SIGNS
- Anterior nasal cavity—most common site
- Sneezing, epistaxis, and stertorous breathing—most prominent
- Mass—often seen protruding from the nostril; usually single and polypoid; may be lobulated or sessile; surface may have white or yellowish superficial flecks, which are fungal sporangia.
- Humans—reported sites: vagina, penis, conjunctival sac, and ears

CAUSES & RISK FACTORS
- *Rhinosporidium seeberi*
- Suspected that stagnant fresh water and arid environment increase likelihood of occurrence

 DIAGNOSIS

DIFFERENTIAL DIAGNOSIS
- Nasal neoplasia
- Nasal inflammatory polyp

CBC/BIOCHEMISTRY/URINALYSIS
Usually normal

OTHER LABORATORY TESTS
None

IMAGING
Radiographs of nasal cavity—generally normal; mass located in the anterior nasal cavity and does not invade turbinates

DIAGNOSTIC PROCEDURES
Impression smears—reveal organisms from nasal mass; use new methylene blue stain.

PATHOLOGIC FINDINGS

Histopathology
- Examination of mass—papillomatous hyperplasia; ulceration of the epithelium; fibrovascular stroma
- Identification of the organism is diagnostic.
- An intense inflammatory reaction will be seen if organisms are released into the surrounding tissues.

 TREATMENT

- Good nursing care important; anorexia and dehydration not typically reported
- Cage confinement or other means of exercise restriction—helpful if epistaxis occurs
- Surgical excision of the mass—treatment of choice; approach through the external nares or rhinotomy; failure to remove the entire mass will likely result in regrowth.

MEDICATIONS

DRUG

Dapsone—used to treat humans; report of use in one dog (1.1 mg/kg PO q8–12h) with favorable response but no cure

CONTRAINDICATIONS/POSSIBLE INTERACTIONS

Dapsone (dogs)—hepatotoxicity; anemia; neutropenia; thrombocytopenia; gastrointestinal signs; skin reactions

 FOLLOW-UP

If surgical approach was through the external nasal orifice, monitor patient closely for regrowth; difficult to remove the entire mass

 MISCELLANEOUS

ZOONOTIC POTENTIAL

• No known risk of direct transmission to humans by handling of infected dogs
• Organism is infectious to humans.

Suggested Reading

Breitschwerdt EB, Castellano MC. Rhinosporidiosis. In: Greene CE, ed. Infectious diseases of the dog and cat. Philadelphia: Saunders, 1998:402–404.

Author Gary D. Norsworthy
Consulting Editor Stephen C. Barr

ROCKY MOUNTAIN SPOTTED FEVER

 BASICS

DEFINITION
• A tick-borne rickettsial disease, caused by *Rickettsia rickettsii,* that affects dogs and is considered the most important rickettsial disease in humans
• Other as yet undefined rickettsial organisms may also cause clinical signs in dogs.

PATHOPHYSIOLOGY
• Vector—American dog tick (*Dermacentor variabilis*), found east of the Great Plains; wood tick (*D. andersoni*), found from the Cascades to the Rocky Mountains
• Transmission—via the saliva of the vector or blood transfusion; tick must be attached for 5–20 hr to infect host (humans, dogs, and cats) or reservoir host (rodents and dogs).
• Incubation period—2 days to 2 weeks
• Infection—organism invades and multiplies in vascular endothelium; causes microvascular hemorrhage, platelet aggregation (thrombocytopenia), vasoconstriction, increased vascular permeability, increased plasma loss into the interstitial space (organ swelling), hypotension, and eventually DIC and shock; leads to widespread vasculitis in organs with endarterial circulation (cause of clinical signs)

SYSTEMS AFFECTED
• Multisystemic involvement
• Hemic/Lymphatic/Immune—bleeding tendency from thrombocytopenia, vasculitis, lymphadenopathy, splenomegaly
• Musculoskeletal—joint pain
• Ophthalmic—conjunctivitis, scleral injection
• Nervous—stupor, seizures, vestibular deficits, coma, cervical pain
• Respiratory—dyspnea, cough
• Skin/Exocrine—edema of extremities, face
• Cardiovascular—vasculitis, hypotension, shock

GENETICS
N/A

INCIDENCE/PREVALENCE
• Tick season—late March to the end of September
• Prevalence—overall infections in ticks < 2%; varies by geographic locality

GEOGRAPHIC DISTRIBUTION
• North and South America
• U.S.—no accurate data for dogs; similar distribution as for humans: eastern seaboard states (especially the Carolinas), Mississippi River valley, and south-central states (Texas, Oklahoma, Kansas)

SIGNALMENT
Species
Dogs

Breed Predilections
• Purebred dogs seem more prone to developing clinical illness than do mixed-breed dogs.
• German shepherds—more common

Mean Age and Range
Any age

Predominant Sex
None

SIGNS
Historical Findings
• Fever—within 2–3 days of tick attachment
• Lethargy
• Depression
• Anorexia
• Swelling (edema)—lips, scrotum, prepuce, ears, extremities
• Stiff gait—especially with scrotal or prepucial swelling
• Spontaneous bleeding—sneezing, epistaxis
• Respiratory distress
• Neurologic—ataxia, head tilt
• Ocular pain

Physical Examination Findings
• Both clinical and subclinical illness occur.
• Clinical—variable in severity; lasts 2–4 weeks untreated
• Ticks may still be present in acute cases.
• Pyrexia
• Cutaneous lesions—edema of face, limbs, prepuce, scrotum
• Conjunctivitis
• Scleral injection
• Respiratory—dyspnea, exercise intolerance resulting from pneumonitis, increased bronchovesicular sounds
• Generalized lymphadenopathy
• Neurologic—vestibular dysfunction, altered mental status, seizures
• Myalgia/ arthralgia
• Petechia
• Ecchymoses—ocular, oral, genital regions; 20% of patients
• Hemorrhagic diathesis—epistaxis, melena, hematuria; in severe cases
• Cardiac arrhythmias—sudden death
• DIC and death from shock—in severe acute cases

CAUSES
R. rickettsii

RISK FACTORS
Exposure to ticks

 DIAGNOSIS

DIFFERENTIAL DIAGNOSIS
• Canine ehrlichiosis—*Ehrlichia canis;* not seasonal; can be clinically indistinguishable from Rocky Mountain spotted fever (especially acute cases); differentiate with

serologic testing; both respond to same treatment.
• Immune-mediated thrombocytopenia—not usually associated with fever or lymphadenopathy; differentiate with serologic testing; may treat for both until results are known
• Systemic lupus erythematosus—antinuclear antibody titer usually negative with Rocky Mountain spotted fever; serologic testing diagnostic
• Brucellosis—scrotal edema; serologic testing diagnostic

CBC/BIOCHEMISTRY/URINALYSIS
CBC
• Thrombocytopenia
• Megathrombocytosis mild anemia (normochromic, normocytic), mild leukopenia (early in infection), leukocytosis (and monocytosis)—as disease becomes more chronic

Biochemistry
• Usually nonspecific
• Mild increases in ALT, ALP, BUN, creatinine, and total bilirubin (rare)
• Hypercholesterolemia—consistently found; cause unknown
• Hypoalbuminemia—from vascular endothelial damage
• Azotemia
• Hyponatremia
• Hypochloremia
• Metabolic acidosis

Urinalysis
• Proteinuria—with or without azotemia; from glomerular/tubular damage
• Hematuria—coagulation defects

OTHER LABORATORY TESTS
• Serum titers—take 2–3 weeks to rise; may be negative in very acute cases
• Paired titers—perform 3 weeks apart; four-fold increase between acute and convalescent titers; avoid misdiagnosis because of considerable cross-reactivity with other rickettsial organisms
• High titers can be detected for up to 1 year after treatment.

IMAGING
N/A

DIAGNOSTIC PROCEDURES
• Direct immunofluorescence—skin biopsies obtained by local anesthesia and punch biopsies from affected lesions; detect rickettsial antigens as early as 3–4 days postinfection
• CSF—often normal; may show an increase in protein and nucleated cells

PATHOLOGIC FINDINGS
• Widespread petechia, splenomegaly, and generalized hemorrhagic lymphadenopathy
• Necrotizing vasculitis with perivascular cell infiltration (mononuclear and neutrophilic)
• Vascular lesions—most prominent in the skin, kidneys, myocardium, meninges, retina,

pancreas, gastrointestinal tract, and urinary bladder
• Hepatic and focal myocardial necrosis, nodular gliosis in the brain, and interstitial pneumonia common
• Special stains—to identify organisms

TREATMENT

APPROPRIATE HEALTH CARE
Inpatient until stable and showing response to treatment

NURSING CARE
• Dehydration—balanced electrolyte solution; use cautiously because of increased vascular permeability and expanded extracellular fluid volume (exacerbating cerebral and pulmonary edema)
• Anemia—blood transfusion
• Hemorrhage from thrombocytopenia—platelet-rich plasma or a blood transfusion

ACTIVITY
Restricted

DIET N/A

CLIENT EDUCATION
• Prognosis—good in acute cases with appropriate and prompt therapy • Response occurs within hours of treatment. • If treatment is not instituted until CNS signs occur or later in the disease process, mortality is high; patient with CNS signs may die within hours.

SURGICAL CONSIDERATIONS
• If surgery is required for other reasons, blood transfusion may be needed to correct anemia and/or thrombocytopenia.

MEDICATIONS

DRUGS OF CHOICE
• Doxycycline—synthetic derivative of tetracycline, 10 mg/kg PO q12h for 10 days; or IV for 5 days if patient is vomiting
• Prednisone—concurrent use; anti-inflammatory or immunosuppressive dose; given early in course of disease does not seem to be detrimental to the clinical recovery

CONTRAINDICATIONS
• Tetracyclines (or derivatives)—do not use in patients < 6 months because of permanent yellowing of the teeth.
• Renal insufficiency—do not use tetracycline; doxycycline may be given (also excreted via the gastrointestinal tract).
• Enrofloxacin—avoid in young dogs because articular cartilage damage can occur (preceded by lameness); gastrointestinal upset (vomiting, anorexia)

PRECAUTIONS
Chloramphenicol
• Avoid if serologic confirmation will be conducted after treatment has started; reduces titers to a greater extent than will tetracyclines
• Warn client of public health risks; directly interferes with heme and bone marrow synthesis
• Avoid use in dogs with thrombocytopenia, pancytopenia, or anemia.

POSSIBLE INTERACTIONS
None

ALTERNATIVE DRUGS
• Tetracyclines, chloramphenicol, and enrofloxacin—equally efficacious if used early
• Oxytetracycline and tetracycline—22 mg/kg PO q8h for 14 days; effective and less expensive
• Chloramphenicol—puppies < 6 months of age; 20 mg/kg PO q8h for 14 days; recommended to avoid yellow discoloration of erupting teeth
• Enrofloxacin—3 mg/kg PO q8h for 7 days

FOLLOW-UP

PATIENT MONITORING
Monitor platelet count every 3 days until normal.

PREVENTION/AVOIDANCE
• Control tick infestation on dogs—use dips or sprays containing dichlorvos, chlorfenvinphos, dioxathion, propoxur, or carbaryl
• Flea and tick collars—may reduce reinfestation; reliability is unproven.
• Avoid tick-infested areas.
• Environment—tick eradication impossible; organism maintained in rodents and other reservoir hosts
• Removing ticks by hand—use gloves (see Zoonotic Potential); ensure mouth parts are removed, because a foreign body reaction is likely to result if they are left in place.

COMPLICATIONS N/A

EXPECTED COURSE AND PROGNOSIS
• Early antibiotic treatment—reduces fever and albumin extravasation and improves patient's attitude within 24–48 hr
• Platelet counts—repeat every 3 days after initiating treatment until within normal range; should return to normal within 2–4 days after initiating treatment
• Serologic titers—lower in treated than in untreated dogs; titers remain positive during convalescence.
• Naturally infected dogs never seem to become reinfected.
• Acute cases—excellent prognosis with appropriate treatment
• With CNS disease—poor prognosis

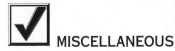

MISCELLANEOUS

ASSOCIATED CONDITIONS
None

AGE-RELATED FACTORS
None

ZOONOTIC POTENTIAL
• Incidence (humans)—dropping in the U.S.; mid-1992–mid-1993: 300 cases; earlier incidence: up to 1000 cases/year
• Mainly young adults and children infected
• Source of infection (humans)—from ticks that are transferred from dogs; not from dogs directly; when removing infected ticks from dogs
• Major clinical signs (humans)—mimic those in dogs; mainly fever and headache; neurologic signs occur later; skin rash appreciated in only 50% of patients
• Treatment with tetracyclines results in a rapid recovery.

PREGNANCY N/A

ABBREVIATIONS
• ALP = alkaline phosphatase
• ALT = alanine aminotransferase
• CSF = cerebrospinal fluid
• DIC = disseminated intravascular coagulation

Suggested Reading
Breitschwerdt EB, Davidson MG, Aucoin DP, et al. Efficacy of chloramphenicol, enrofloxacin, and tetracycline for treatment of experimental Rocky Mountain spotted fever in dogs. Antimicrob Agents Chemother 1991;35:2375–2381.
Breitschwerdt EB, Davidson MG, Hegarty BC, et al. Prednisolone at anti-inflammatory or immunosuppressive dosages in conjunction with doxycycline does not potentiate the severity of *Rickettsia rickettsii* infection in dogs. Antimicrob Agents Chemother 1997;41:141–147.
Greene CE, Breitschwerdt EB. Rocky Mountain spotted fever, Q fever, and typhus. In: Greene CE, ed. Infectious diseases of the dog and cat. 2nd ed. Philadelphia: Saunders, 1998;155–165.
Greene CE, Burgdorfer W, Cavagnolo R, et al. Rocky Mountain spotted fever in dogs and its differentiation from canine ehrlichiosis. J Am Vet Med Assoc 1985;186:465–472.
Hibler SC, Hoskins JD, Greene CE. Rickettsial infections in dogs. Part I: Rocky Mountain spotted fever and *Coxiella* infections. Compend Contin Educ Pract Vet 1985;7:856–865.

Author Stephen C. Barr
Consulting Editor Stephen C. Barr

DISEASES

RODENTICIDE ANTICOAGULANT POISONING

BASICS

DEFINITION
Coagulopathy caused by reduced vitamin K_1–dependent clotting factors in the circulation after exposure to anticoagulant rodenticides

PATHOPHYSIOLOGY
• Inhibits vitamin K_1 epoxide reductase, due to diaphorase, and possibly other enzymes involved in the reduction of vitamin K_1 epoxide to vitamin K_1
• Vitamin K_1—required for carboxylation of clotting factors II, VI, IX, and X; uncarboxylated clotting factors cannot bind calcium and thus are unable to participate in clot formation.

SYSTEMS AFFECTED
Hemic/Lymphatic/Immune—depletion of activated clotting factors, causing hemorrhage

GENETICS
N/A

INCIDENCE/PREVALENCE
Common—many baits are sold over the counter and widely used in homes.

GEOGRAPHIC DISTRIBUTION
None

SIGNALMENT
• Dogs and cats
• No breed, age, or sex predilections

SIGNS

General Comments
• May be slightly more prevalent in the spring and fall when rodenticide products are used

Historical Findings
• Use of anticoagulant rodenticides
• Dyspnea
• Bleeding

Physical Examination Findings
• Hematomas—often ventral and at venipuncture sites
• Muffled heart or lung sounds
• Pale mucous membranes
• Lethargy
• Depression

CAUSES
• Exposure to anticoagulant rodenticide products
• First-generation coumarin anticoagulants (e.g., warfarin, pindone)—largely replaced by more potent second-generation anticoagulants
• Second-generation anticoagulants (e.g., brodifacoum, bromadiolone, diphacinone, and chlorphacinone)—generally more toxic and persist much longer before excretion than are first-generation agents
• Difenthialone (D-Cease)—highly toxic to rats and mice (0.52 mg/kg and 0.47 mg/kg, respectively); less toxic to dogs (LD_{50} 4 mg/kg) than are brodifacoum (LD_{50} 0.25–2.5 mg/kg), bromadiolone (LD_{50} 11–20 mg/kg), chlorophacinone (LD_{50} 50–100 mg/kg), and warfarin (LD_{50} 20–50 mg/kg); similar to diphacinone (LD_{50} 3–7.5 mg/kg); cats, LD_{50} > 16 mg/kg; concentration in baits lower (0.0025%; 25 ppm) than that of other second-generation rodenticide baits (0.005%; 50 ppm), so dogs and cats may tolerate higher intakes.

RISK FACTORS
• Small doses over several days more dangerous than a single large dose; either type of exposure may cause toxicosis.
• Secondary toxicosis by consumption of poisoned rodents—unlikely

DIAGNOSIS

DIFFERENTIAL DIAGNOSES
• DIC
• Congenital clotting factor deficiencies

CBC/BIOCHEMISTRY/URINALYSIS
Anemia—with marked hemorrhage

OTHER LABORATORY TESTS
• ACT > 150 sec—supports coagulopathy
• Prolonged PT and PTT—support exposure to rodenticide; PT affected earlier than is PTT.
• Analysis of blood or liver—confirm exposure to a specific product

IMAGING
Thoracic radiography—may detect hemothorax or hemopericardium

DIAGNOSTIC PROCEDURES
Thoracentesis—dyspneic patients; may confirm hemothorax

PATHOLOGIC FINDINGS
• Free blood in the thoracic cavity, lungs, and abdominal cavity—common
• Hemorrhage into the cranial vault, gastrointestinal tract, and urinary tract—less common; may occur both subcutaneously and intramuscularly

RODENTICIDE ANTICOAGULANT POISONING

TREATMENT

APPROPRIATE HEALTH CARE
• Inpatient—acute crisis
• Outpatient—consider once the coagulopathy is stabilized

NURSING CARE
Fresh whole blood or plasma transfusion—may be required with hemorrhaging; provides immediate access to vitamin K–dependent clotting factors; whole blood may be preferred with severe anemia from acute or chronic blood loss.

ACTIVITY
Confine patient during the early stages; activity enhances blood loss.

DIET
No recognized effect

CLIENT EDUCATION
Warn client that re-exposure could be a serious problem.

SURGICAL CONSIDERATIONS
• Thoracentesis—may be important for removing free thoracic blood, which causes dyspnea and respiratory failure
• Must correct coagulopathy before surgery

MEDICATIONS

DRUGS OF CHOICE
Vitamin K_1—2.5–5.0 mg/kg PO q24h 5 days to 6 weeks (depending on the specific product); bioavailability enhanced by the concurrent feeding of a small amount of fat, such as canned dog food
• Vitamin K_1 administration—continued for 3–4 weeks with suspected second-generation anticoagulant toxicosis

CONTRAINDICATIONS
• Vitamin K_3—not efficacious in the treatment of anticoagulant rodenticide toxicosis; contraindicated
• Intravenous vitamin K_1—reported anaphylactic reactions; avoid this route of administration.

PRECAUTIONS
• Avoid unnecessary surgical procedures and parenteral injections.
• Use the smallest possible needle when giving an injections or collecting samples.

POSSIBLE INTERACTIONS
Sulfonamides and phenylbutazone—may displace anticoagulant rodenticides from plasma binding sites, leading to more free toxicant and toxicosis

ALTERNATIVE DRUGS
None

FOLLOW-UP

PATIENT MONITORING
ACT and PT—assess efficacy of therapy; monitoring continued 3–5 days after discontinuation of treatment

PREVENTION/AVOIDANCE
Do not allow animals access to anticoagulant rodenticides.

POSSIBLE COMPLICATIONS
May note secondary bacterial pneumonia after intrapulmonary hemorrhage

EXPECTED COURSE AND PROGNOSIS
• Patient survives the first 48 hr of acute coagulopathy—prognosis improves

MISCELLANEOUS

ASSOCIATED CONDITIONS
N/A

AGE-RELATED FACTORS
N/A

ZOONOTIC POTENTIAL
N/A

PREGNANCY
Chlorophacinone—may pass into amniotic fluid and on to the fetuses of an exposed pregnant bitch; similar concerns for feeding affected milk to pups

SEE ALSO
Poisoning (Intoxication)

ABBREVIATIONS
• ACT = activated clotting time
• DIC = disseminated intravascular coagulation
• PPT = partial thromboplastin time
• PT = prothrombin time

Suggested Reading
Murphy M, Gerken D. The anticoagulant rodenticides. In: Kirk RW, Bonagura J., eds. Current veterinary therapy X. Philadelphia: Saunders, 1989:143–146.
Author Michael J. Murphy
Consulting Editor Gary D. Osweiler

ROTAVIRUS INFECTIONS

BASICS

OVERVIEW
• Nonenveloped, double-stranded RNA virus; *rota* (Latin; "wheel") for shape of the capsid; genus within the family Reoviridae; relatively resistant to environmental destruction (acid and lipid solvents); unique double-capsid protects virus from inactivation in the upper gastrointestinal tract.
• Wide host range, identified in almost every species investigated
• Most significant cause of severe gastroenteritis in young children (< 2 years) and animals throughout the world
• Transmission—fecal–oral contamination
• Infection—affects mature epithelial cells on luminal tips of the intestinal villi; causes swelling, degeneration, and desquamation; denuded villi contract; results in villous atrophy with loss of absorptive capability and loss of brush border enzymes (e.g., disaccharidases); leads to osmotic diarrhea

SIGNALMENT
• Dogs and cats
• Pups < 12 weeks old and more often < 2 weeks old—diarrhea
• Kittens and young cats (<6 months of age)—more susceptible to infection

SIGNS
• Dogs—most infections subclinical or limited to relatively mild, nonspecific watery to mucoid diarrhea, anorexia, and lethargy; rare fatalities reported
• Cats—primarily subclinical or mild diarrhea; with co-infections or in stressed conditions, more severe clinical disease may occur.

CAUSES & RISK FACTORS
• Rotavirus
• Young animals with immature immune systems at increased risk

DIAGNOSIS

DIFFERENTIAL DIAGNOSIS
• Canine viral enteritis—canine parvovirus; canine coronavirus; canine astrovirus; canine calicivirus; canine herpesvirus; canine distemper virus; canine reovirus
• Feline viral enteritis—feline parvovirus (feline panleukopenia virus); FeLV; feline coronavirus; feline astrovirus; feline calicivirus
• Other causes of enteritis—bacteria (e.g., *Salmonella, Campylobacter, Clostridium*); fungi; protozoa; parasites; foreign bodies; intussusception; allergies; toxicants

CBC/BIOCHEMISTRY/URINALYSIS
Noncontributory

OTHER LABORATORY TESTS
• Serology—not recommended; most animals (e.g., 85% of dogs) carry antibodies owing to previous exposure or from passive antibody immunization transfer from the bitch or queen; must demonstrate fourfold difference in acute and convalescent serum samples
• Direct electron microscopy—detects virus in feces; rapid; lack of sensitivity
• Immunoelectron microscopy—more sensitive and specific than direct electron microscopy; not commonly available
• ELISA—detect common group rotavirus antigen in feces; Rotazyme (Abbott Laboratories, North Chicago, IL)
• Virus isolation
• Polymerase chain reaction—being developed

IMAGING
N/A

DIAGNOSTIC PROCEDURES
Histology—swollen small intestinal villi; mild infiltration by macrophages and neutrophils; virus detected by fluorescent antibody test

TREATMENT
• Symptomatic for diarrhea—fluids, electrolytes, and dietary restriction
• Antibiotic therapy not indicated
• Principal protection—probably antibodies in milk of immune bitch or queen

MEDICATIONS

DRUGS
N/A

CONTRAINDICATIONS/POSSIBLE INTERACTIONS
N/A

FOLLOW-UP
N/A

MISCELLANEOUS

ZOONOTIC POTENTIAL
• Rotaviruses not host-specific; thus affected puppy or kitten may pose a potential human health hazard, particularly for infants.
• Exercise care when handling fecal material from pets with diarrhea.
• Humans—diarrhea; infants in developed countries: high morbidity and low mortality (attributed to fluid therapy); infants and young children in developing countries: leading cause of life-threatening diarrhea

ABBREVIATIONS
• ELISA = enzyme-linked immunoabsorbent assay
• FeLV = feline leukemia virus

Suggested Reading
Hoskins JD. Canine viral enteritis. In: Greene CE, ed. Infectious diseases of the dog and cat. 2nd ed. Philadelphia: Saunders, 1998:40–49.
Pedersen NC. Feline rotavirus. In: Appel M, ed. Virus infections of carnivores. New York: Elsevier Science, 1987:259–260.
Author J. Paul Woods
Consulting Editor Stephen C. Barr

BASICS

OVERVIEW
• Ascariasis of dogs, especially pups, is caused by *Toxocara canis*, and, of cats, by *Toxocara cati*; both host species are infected by *Toxascaris leonina*.
• These are relatively large, robust worms up to 10–12 cm long, so distension of the small intestine often leads to colic, interference with gut motility, and inability to use food.
• Because of transplacental transmission to fetuses, pups may be born with a developing worm burden.
• Over first month of life, infected neonatal pups may rapidly debilitate with abdominal pain, prior to appearance of eggs in stools.
• Kittens may be similarly affected by trans-colostral transmission.
• Older pups and kittens may become infected by ingesting infective eggs disseminated on premises by dams with postgestational infections.
• *Toxascaris* may be transmitted by eggs or by predation of transport hosts (rodents) infected with dormant infective larvae.

SIGNALMENT
Dogs and cats; clinically especially important in pups and kittens

SIGNS

Historical Findings
• Abdominal distension
• Colic
• Cachexia
• Poor nursing or appetite
• Scant feces
• Coughing—due to larval migration
• Whole litter may be affected

Physical Examination Findings
• Weakness, loss of condition, cachexia
• Abdominal distension—often with distended intestines palpable

CAUSES & RISK FACTORS
• *Toxocara* infection
• Infected bitch or queen
• Food or environment contaminated with feces
• Concurrent enteric infections

DIAGNOSIS

DIFFERENTIAL DIAGNOSIS
• Hookworm infection
• *Strongyloides* infection

CBC/BIOCHEMISTRY/URINALYSIS
Usually normal

OTHER LABORATORY TESTS
N/A

IMAGING
N/A

DIAGNOSTIC PROCEDURES
• Fecal egg examination of pups, kittens >3 weeks of age
• *Toxocara* egg—spherical, with pitted outer shell membrane, single dark cell (zygote filling interior), 80–85 μm *(T. canis)*, ~ 75 μm *(T. cati)*
• *Toxascaris* egg—ovoid, with smooth exterior shell membrane, 1- or 2-cell, not filling interior, light cytoplasm, 80 × 70 μm
• Necropsy findings of siblings that have died of similar signs

TREATMENT
• Acute severe cases—inpatients; supplement with intravenous fluids
• Educate client to possibility of sudden death or chronic debilitation.
• Treat bitch or queen with adulticide/larvicide anthelmintic (fenbendazole) to decrease likelihood of subsequent litter and mature maternal infections.

MEDICATIONS

DRUGS

Adulticide/Larvicide Anthelmintics
• Fenbendazole 50 mg/kg PO q24h for 5 days
• Milbemycin oxime tabs monthly

Adulticide Anthelmintics
• Dichlorvos twice monthly
• Febantel + praziquantel tablets for cats; febantel + praziquantel + pyrantel pamoate tablets for dogs
• Ivermectin + pyrantel pamoate monthly
• Pyrantel pamoate twice monthly

CONTRAINDICATIONS/POSSIBLE INTERACTIONS
• Organophosphates in heartworm-positive patients
• Do not give dichlorvos concurrently with other organophosphates such as insecticides.

FOLLOW-UP
Monitor fecal egg counts posttreatment.

MISCELLANEOUS

AGE-RELATED FACTORS
Greater clinical concern in neonates

ZOONOTIC POTENTIAL
Visceral larva migrans may follow ingestion of infective eggs.

SYNONYMS
Ascariasis

Suggested Reading
Bowman DD, ed. Georgi's parasitology for veterinarians. 6th ed. Philadelphia: Saunders, 1994:203–206.
Author Robert M. Corwin
Consulting Editors Brett M. Feder and Mitchell A. Crystal

SALMON POISONING DISEASE

 BASICS

OVERVIEW
• Infection with the rickettsial organism *Neorickettsia helminthoeca*
• Organism—invades small intestinal epithelium and associated lymphoid tissue; systemic infection eventually develops.
• Occurs in the northern Pacific rim of the U.S.

SIGNALMENT
• Dogs of all ages
• No sex or breed predisposition

SIGNS
• Diarrhea
• Vomiting
• Lymphadenopathy
• Nasal and ocular discharge
• Fever

CAUSES & RISK FACTORS
• Ingestion of raw fish containing the trematode vector or *Neorickettsia helminthoeca* organisms
• Eating raw fish in an endemic area is a risk factor.

 DIAGNOSIS

DIFFERENTIAL DIAGNOSIS
• Poisoning
• Canine parvovirus type 2
• Ehrlichiosis
• Canine distemper

CBC/BIOCHEMISTRY/URINALYSIS
No specific findings

OTHER LABORATORY TESTS
N/A

IMAGING
N/A

DIAGNOSTIC PROCEDURES
• Giemsa-stain—aspirate of enlarged lymph node; reveals intracytoplasmic rickettsial bodies
• Fecal examination—reveal operculated eggs of the trematode *Nanophyetus salmincola*

PATHOLOGIC FINDINGS
• Changes in lymphoid tissue—enlarged, yellowish, prominent white foci
• Intestinal contents—frequently contain free blood

 TREATMENT

• Inpatient—acutely ill patients
• Treat as for canine ehrlichiosis.
• Supportive therapy—fluids with electrolytes; basic measures to control diarrhea

SALMON POISONING DISEASE

MEDICATIONS

DRUGS
• Oxytetracycline—7.5–10 mg/kg IV q12h for 14 days; 20 mg/kg PO q12h
• Tetracycline—15–20 mg/kg PO q8h for 14 days
• Chloramphenicol—40–50 mg/kg PO q8h for 14 days
• Praziquantel—20–30 mg/kg SC or PO q24h for 3 days to kill flukes

FOLLOW-UP

PATIENT MONITORING
Monitor hydration, electrolytes, acid–base balance, and body temperature.

PREVENTION /AVOIDANCE
• Prevent animals from eating raw fish.
• Inform client of necessity to act quickly and consider other dogs that may have eaten the same raw fish.

EXPECTED COURSE AND PROGNOSIS
• Animals likely to succumb within 5–10 days of infection unless treated.
• With early diagnosis and treatment—prognosis good
• Untreated—often fatal

MISCELLANEOUS

ASSOCIATED CONDITIONS
• Elokomin fluke fever agent—similar rickettsia; causes a more mild form of the disease
• Infection with *Nanophyetus salmincola* does not itself cause severe clinical disease.

ZOONOTIC POTENTIAL
No reported risk to humans

Suggested Reading
Gorham JR, Foreyt WJ. Salmon poisoning disease. In: Greene CE, ed. Infectious diseases of the dog and cat. 2nd ed. Philadelphia: Saunders, 1998:135–139.
Author Johnny D. Hoskins
Consulting Editor Stephen C. Barr

SALMONELLOSIS

BASICS

DEFINITION
A bacterial disease that causes enteritis, septicemia, and abortions and is caused by many different serotypes of *Salmonella*

PATHOPHYSIOLOGY
• *Salmonella*—a gram-negative bacterium; colonizes the small intestine (ileum); adheres to and invades the enterocytes; eventually enters and multiplies in the lamina propria and local mesenteric lymph nodes; cytotoxin (cell death) and enterotoxin (increases cAMP) are produced; inflammation occurs; and prostaglandin synthesis ensues; results in secretory diarrhea and mucosal sloughing • Uncomplicated gastroenteritis—organisms are stopped at the mesenteric lymph node stage; patient has only diarrhea, vomiting, and dehydration • Bacteremia and septicemia following gastroenteritis—more serious disease; focal extraintestinal infections (abortion, joint disease) or endotoxemia may result; may lead to organ infarction, generalized thrombosis, DIC, and death • Some patients recover from the septicemic form but suffer prolonged recovery as a result of their debilitated state.

SYSTEMS AFFECTED
• Gastrointestinal—enterocolitis; inflammation, mucosal sloughing, secretory diarrhea • Systemic disease (e.g., bacteremia, focal infections, septicemia)—multiorgan infarction, thrombosis, abscesses, meningitis, osteomyelitis, abortion

GENETICS
Genetic susceptibility not well known

INCIDENCE/PREVALENCE
• True incidence unknown • Most infections subclinical • Dogs—clinical disease most often seen in the young and pregnant; fecal/rectal swab survey of clinically normal domestic pets, boarding kennels, and veterinary hospitals shows incidences of 30%, 16.7%, and 21.5%, respectively. • Cats—have a high natural resistance; stressed hospitalized animals at high risk; fecal survey of normal cats and cats from a research colony shows incidences of 18% and 10.6%, respectively; pandemics of salmonellosis in migrating songbirds (usually *typhimurium*) in spring create epidemics in bird-hunting cats.

GEOGRAPHIC DISTRIBUTION
Worldwide

SIGNALMENT

Species
Dogs and cats

Breed Predilections
None

Mean Age and Range
• Dogs—clinical disease manifests in neonatal/immature puppies and in pregnant bitches; most adult carrier dogs clinically normal • Cats—adults highly resistant

Predominant Sex
N/A

SIGNS

General Comments
Disease severity—subclinical (carrier state: *Salmonella* shed in stool) to mild, moderate, and severe clinical cases in neonatal and stressed adult dogs and cats; subclinical infection more common than clinical disease (rare)

Historical Findings
• Diarrhea • Vomiting • Fever • Malaise • Anorexia • Vaginal discharge/abortion—dogs • Chronic febrile illness—persistent fever, anorexia, malaise without diarrhea

Physical Examination Findings
• Asymptomatic carrier states—no clinical signs • Gastroenteritis—anorexia; malaise/lethargy; depression fever (39–40°C; 102–104°F); diarrhea with mucus and/or blood; progressive dehydration; abdominal pain; tenesmus; pale mucous membranes; mesenteric lymphadenopathy; weight loss • Gastroenteritis with bacteremia and septicemia, septic shock, or endotoxemia—pale mucous membranes; weakness; cardiovascular collapse; tachycardia; tachypnea • Focal extraintestinal infections—conjunctivitis; uterus/abortion; cellulitis; pyothorax • Cats—may exhibit syndrome of a chronic febrile illness (without gastrointestinal signs); persistent fever; prolonged illness with vague, nonspecific clinical signs; and left shift on leukogram • Recovering patients—may exhibit chronic intermittent diarrhea for 3–4 weeks; may shed *Salmonella* in stool for 6 weeks or longer

CAUSES
• Any one of more than 2000 serotypes of salmonellae • Two or more simultaneous serotypes in a host animal not uncommon

RISK FACTORS

Disease Agent
Salmonella serotype—virulence factors, infectious dose, and route of exposure • Host factors that increase susceptibility • Age—neonatal/young dogs and cats; immature immune system • Overall health status—debilitated young animals or adults: other concurrent disease, parasitism; young animals: immature gastrointestinal tract, poorly developed normal microbial flora • Disrupted gastrointestinal bacteria flora (adult cats)—antimicrobial treatment; subsequent exposure to salmonellae during hospitalization

Environmental Factors
• Coprophagia spreads infection. • Dehydrated (dry) pet food—known to harbor salmonellae; semimoist foods (e.g., kibble and dog biscuits) usually not as risky • Grooming habits—may result in *Salmonella*-contaminated hair coat, which contaminates cage or run environment, feed and water dishes • Dense population—research colony, boarded animals, shelter/pound animals; overcrowded housing; unsanitary conditions; exposure to other infected (or carrier) animals—buildup of *Salmonella* in the environment; more efficient fecal–oral cycling; high opportunity for fecal exposure; stress factors

Hunting/Stray Animals
• Scavenging for food—exposure to garbage, contaminated food/water, dead animals • Exposure to other infected (or carrier) animals

Hospitalized Animals
Nosocomial exposure (plus stress) or activation (by stress) of pre-existing asymptomatic (carrier) *Salmonella* infection, especially in animals treated with antimicrobial drugs

DIAGNOSIS

DIFFERENTIAL DIAGNOSIS
• Acute gastroenteritis—vomiting, diarrhea, infectious enteritis; differentiate by serology and/or culture • Viral gastroenteritis—feline panleukopenia, FeLV, FIV, feline enteric coronavirus, canine enteric coronavirus, canine parvovirus, rotavirus, canine distemper • Bacterial gastroenteritis—*E. coli, Campylobacter jejuni, Yersinia enterocolitica* • Bacterial overgrowth syndrome—*Clostridium difficile, Clostridium perfringens* • Parasites—helminths (hookworms, ascarids, whipworms, strongyloides); protozoa (*Giardia, Coccidia, Cryptosporidia*); Rickettsiae; salmon poisoning • Acute gastritis—erosions or ulcers • Dietary-induced distress—overeating, abrupt changes, starvation, thirst, allergy or food intolerance, indiscretions (foreign material, garbage) • Drug or toxin-induced distress • Extraintestinal disorders/metabolic disease

CBC/BIOCHEMISTRY/URINALYSIS
• CBC—variable; depends on stage of illness • Neutropenia initially • Left shift with toxic neutrophils • Nonregenerative anemia • Lymphopenia • Thrombocytopenia • Hypoalbuminemia • Electrolyte imbalances

OTHER LABORATORY TESTS N/A

IMAGING N/A

DIAGNOSTIC PROCEDURES
• Fecal/rectal culture—positive; special media needed
• Fecal leukocytes—positive
• Blood cultures—positive in patients with bacteremia
• Joint fluid—may be culture-positive

• Subclinical carrier states—chronic; intermittent fecal culture positive (> 6 weeks)
• **NOTE:** use of antimicrobials in a patient before sampling may produce false-negative cultures.

PATHOLOGIC FINDINGS
• Gross lesions—only in severely affected patients
• Cultures of ileum, mesenteric lymph node, liver/spleen, and bone marrow—positive

TREATMENT

APPROPRIATE HEALTH CARE
• Outpatient—uncomplicated gastroenteritis (without bacteremia) and carrier states
• Inpatient—with bacteremia/septicemia and for gastroenteritis in neonatal/immature animals that are rapidly debilitated by diarrhea

NURSING CARE
• Varies according to severity of illness—assess percentages of dehydration, body weight, ongoing fluid loss, shock, PCV/total protein, electrolytes, acid–base status

Uncomplicated Gastroenteritis
• Supportive care—fluid and electrolyte replacement
• Parenteral, balanced, polyionic isotonic solution (lactated Ringer's)
• Oral fluids—hypertonic glucose solutions; for secretory diarrhea
• Plasma transfusions—if serum albumin < 2 g/dL

Neonates, Aged, and Debilitated Animals
• Plasma transfusions
• Supportive care—as outlined above

ACTIVITY
• Isolate inpatients—all patients in acute stages may shed large numbers of salmonellae in the stool.
• Restrict activity with cage rest, monitor, and provide warmth—acutely ill, bacteremic/septicemic, and chronically ill animals.

DIET
Restrict food 24–48 hr; gradually introduce a highly digestible, low-fat diet.

CLIENT EDUCATION
Instruct client to wash hands frequently and to restrict access to patient in acute stages of the disease; large numbers of salmonellae may be shed in the stool.

SURGICAL CONSIDERATIONS N/A

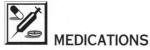

MEDICATIONS

DRUGS OF CHOICE

Asymptomatic Carrier State
• Antimicrobials—contraindicated
• Quinolone drugs—demonstrated clearing of carrier states in humans; more controlled trials in animals needed

Uncomplicated Gastroenteritis
• Antimicrobials not indicated
• Locally acting intestinal adsorbents and protectants

Neonates, Aged, and Debilitated Animals
• Glucocorticoids—shown to reduce mortality in endotoxic shock
• Antimicrobial therapy—indicated; culture and susceptibility testing/MIC necessary to assess drug-resistance problems
• Trimethoprim-sulfa—15 mg/kg PO or SC q12h
• Enrofloxacin—5 mg/kg PO or IM q12h
• Norfloxacin—22 mg/kg PO q12h
• Chloramphenicol—dogs: 50 mg/kg PO, IV, IM, or SC q8h; cats: 50 mg/kg total PO, IV, IM, or SC q12h

CONTRAINDICATIONS
None

PRECAUTIONS
• Chloramphenicol and trimethoprim-sulfa—use cautiously in neonatal and pregnant patients.
• Fluoroquinolones—avoid use in pregnant, neonatal, or growing animals (medium-sized dogs < 8 months of age; large or giant breeds < 12–18 months of age) because of cartilage lesions.

POSSIBLE INTERACTIONS N/A

ALTERNATIVE DRUGS N/A

FOLLOW-UP

PATIENT MONITORING
• Fecal culture—repeat monthly for few months to assess development of carrier state
• Other animals—monitor for secondary spread of infection • Advise client to contact veterinarian if patient shows signs of recurring disease.

PREVENTION/AVOIDANCE
• Keep animals healthy—proper nutrition; no raw meat; vaccinate for other infectious diseases; clean and disinfect cages, runs, and food and water dishes frequently; store food and feeding utensils properly • Reduce over-crowding—pounds, shelters, kennels, catteries, and research colonies • New arrivals—isolate and screen; monitor for sickness before mixing

with other animals. • Important to protect animals being treated with antimicrobial drugs from exposure to a salmonella-contaminated environment (e.g., an animal hospital)

POSSIBLE COMPLICATIONS
• Spread of infection not uncommon within household to other animals or humans • Development of chronic infection with diarrhea
• Recurrence of disease with stress

EXPECTED COURSE AND PROGNOSIS
• Uncomplicated gastroenteritis—prognosis excellent; frequently self-limited; patients recover with good nursing care. • Recovered animals may shed *Salmonella* intermittently for months or longer as a recovered carrier. • Neonatal, aged, stressed animals—can develop septicemia and systemic disease; can be severe and debilitating; may lead to death if untreated

MISCELLANEOUS

ASSOCIATED CONDITIONS N/A

AGE-RELATED FACTORS
Clinical disease is frequently seen in neonatal and aged animals.

ZOONOTIC POTENTIAL
• High potential, especially in children, elderly, immunosuppressed, and antimicrobial drug users • Acutely ill animals shed large numbers of salmonellae in stool. • Grooming habits allow rapid contamination of animal's fur and environment. • Isolation is needed.

PREGNANCY
• May complicate disease • Abortion—may be a sequela to infection • Antimicrobial therapy—take into account the effect on the fetus.

SYNONYMS
Songbird fever

ABBREVIATIONS
• DIC = disseminated intravascular coagulation • FeLV = feline leukemia virus • FIV = feline immunodeficiency virus • MIC = minimal inhibitory concentration • PCV = packed cell volume

Suggested Reading
Dow SW, Jones RL, Henik RA, Husted PW. Clinical features of salmonellosis in cats: six cases (1981–1986). J Am Vet Med Assoc 1989;194:1464–1466.
Greene CE. Salmonellosis. In: Greene CE, ed. Infectious diseases of the dog and cat. Philadelphia: Saunders, 1998:235–240
Morse EV, Duncan MA. Canine salmonellosis: prevalence, epizootiology, signs, and public health significance. J Am Vet Med Assoc 1975;167:817–820.
Author Patrick L. McDonough
Consulting Editor Stephen C. Barr

BASICS

OVERVIEW
• A nonseasonal, intensely pruritic, highly contagious parasitic skin disease of dogs caused by infestation with the mite *Sarcoptes scabiei* var. *canis*
• Mites burrow through the stratum corneum and cause intense pruritus by mechanical irritation, production of irritating byproducts, and secretion of allergenic substances that produce a hypersensitivity reaction in sensitized dogs.

SIGNALMENT
Dogs of all ages and breeds

SIGNS
• Nonseasonal, extremely intense pruritus
• Alopecia and erythematous rash—elbows, hocks, ventral abdomen, and chest
• Lesions on ear margins—vary from barely perceptible scaling to alopecia or crusts; ear canals not affected
• Chronic—periocular and truncal alopecia; secondary crusts, excoriations, and pyoderma
• Possible peripheral lymphadenopathy
• Frequently bathed dogs—chronic pruritus but no skin lesions
• Dogs—often minimal or no response to anti-inflammatory doses of steroids
• Multiple dog households—more than one dog usually shows signs.

CAUSES & RISK FACTORS
• Exposure to a carrier dog 2–6 weeks before development of symptoms
• Living outside (roaming dogs)
• Boarded at kennel
• Visits to veterinarian's office
• Visits to groomer
• Residence at animal shelter

DIAGNOSIS

DIFFERENTIAL DIAGNOSIS
• Food allergy
• Atopy
• *Malassezia* dermatitis
• Flea-allergic dermatitis
• *Cheyletiella*
• Pyoderma
• Demodicosis
• Contact allergy
• *Pelodera* dermatitis
• Pruritic impetigo

CBC/BIOCHEMISTRY/URINALYSIS
N/A

OTHER LABORATORY TESTS
• ELISA technique—identify *Sarcoptes*-infested dogs; early studies show good results
• Commercial tests not available

IMAGING
N/A

DIAGNOSTIC PROCEDURES
• Positive pinnal-pedal reflex—rubbing the ear margin between the thumb and forefinger should induce the dog to scratch with the ipsilateral hind leg; occurs in 75%–90% of cases
• Superficial skin scrapings—positive in only 20% of cases
• Fecal flotation—occasionally reveals mites or ova
• Favorable response to scabicidal treatment—most common method for tentative diagnosis
• Any dog with nonseasonal pruritus that responds poorly to steroids should be treated with a scabicide (even if skin scrape results are negative) to definitively rule out sarcoptic mange.

TREATMENT
• Scabicidal dips—the entire dog must be treated; treatment failures often linked to owner's reluctance to apply dip to the patient's face and ears; do not let the patient get wet between treatments.
• All in-contact dogs—should be treated, even those with no clinical signs; may be asymptomatic carriers
• Thoroughly clean and treat environment; *Sarcoptes* mites can survive for up to 3 weeks.

MEDICATIONS

DRUGS
• Ivermectin—highly effective; 0.2–0.4 mg/kg SC or PO every 1–2 weeks for 2–4 treatments; do not use in herding breeds.
• Milbemycin (Interceptor)—effective when used at 0.75 mg/kg PO q24h; may be effective at 2 mg/kg PO every week for 3 weeks
• Amitraz (Mitaban) dip—250 ppm; may be effective at every 1–2 weeks for 3 treatments; make sure entire body is covered, including the face and ears.
• Whole-body rinse solution—2%–3% solution of lime sulfur (LymDip) or organophosphate (Paramite) dip; apply for 5–6 weeks; make sure entire body is covered, including the face and ears.
• Topical antiseborrheic therapy in conjunction with scabicidal therapy helps speed clinical resolution of the lesions.
• Systemic antibiotics—may be needed for 21 days or longer to resolve any secondary pyoderma
• Antihistamines or low-dose glucocorticoids (0.5 mg/kg q12h for 1st week of treatment), if mites were identified; may pruritus

diminish more quickly.

CONTRAINDICATIONS/POSSIBLE INTERACTIONS
Ivermectin—use with extreme caution in collies, Shetland sheepdogs, old English sheepdogs, Australian shepherds, and their crossbreeds; toxicity is more likely to occur in herding-type breeds.

FOLLOW-UP
• It can take as long as 4–6 weeks for the intense pruritus and clinical signs to resolve, owing to the hypersensitivity reaction.
• Topical treatments are prone to failure, owing to incomplete application of the treatment solution.
• Reinfection can occur if the contact with infected animals continues.

MISCELLANEOUS

ASSOCIATED CONDITIONS
• Always consider sarcoptic mange as a possible cause of pruritus in allergic dogs that cease to responsive to steroid therapy.
• Approximately 30% of dogs with *Sarcoptes* infections will also react to house dust mite antigens.

ZOONOTIC POTENTIAL
People who come in close contact with an affected dog may develop a pruritic, papular rash on their arms, chest, or abdomen; human lesions are usually transient and should resolve spontaneously after the affected animal has been treated; if the lesions persist, clients should seek advice from their dermatologist.

ABBREVIATION
ELISA = enzyme-linked immunoadsorbent assay

Suggested Reading
De Jaham C, Henry CJ. Treatment of canine sarcoptic mange using milbemycin oxime. Can Vet J 1995;36;42–43.
Griffin CE. Scabies. In: Griffin CE, Kwochka KW, MacDonald JM, eds. Current veterinary dermatology: the science and art of therapy. St. Louis: Mosby, 1993:85–89.
Authors Linda Medleau and Keith A. Hnilica
Consulting Editor Karen Helton Rhodes

SCHIFF-SHERRINGTON PHENOMENON

BASICS

OVERVIEW
• Thoracic limb extension associated with hind limb paralysis after acute and usually severe spinal cord lesion cranial to L2 and caudal to the cervical intumescence
• Posture—caused by the release of the border cells, interneurons located in the lumbar spinal cord (mainly L2–4) and normally inhibiting the extensor motor neurons of the cervical intumescence

SIGNALMENT
• Any dog suffering from a severe thoracolumbar spinal cord injury

SIGNS
• Forelimbs—rigidly extended; normal gait and postural reactions (because the lesion is caudal to the cervical intumescence)
• Hindlimbs—depend on the severity and location of the lesion; usually upper motor neuron in type, but may be lower motor neuron

CAUSES & RISK FACTORS
Road accident and intervertebral disk disease—most common

DIAGNOSIS

DIFFERENTIAL DIAGNOSIS
• Decerebrate rigidity—observed with brain disease in which all four limbs are rigid and upper motor neuron dysfunction occurs in all limbs; patient is unconscious.
• Decerebellate rigidity—observed with cerebellar disease in which the forelimbs are rigid but the hind limbs are flexed; consciousness may be normal but is usually altered.
• Cervical spinal cord injury—may have extensor hypertonia in the forelimbs; upper motor neuron and proprioceptive deficits of limbs are also seen.

CBC/BIOCHEMISTRY/URINALYSIS
N/A

OTHER LABORATORY TESTS
N/A

IMAGING
Radiology (myelography, CT, MRI)—demonstrate the thoracolumbar spinal lesion

DIAGNOSTIC PROCEDURES
N/A

TREATMENT
• Directed toward the underlying thoracolumbar lesion
• No specific treatment available
• Condition resolves if adequate spinal cord function is restored.

MEDICATIONS

DRUGS
As indicated for underlying spinal cord disease

CONTRAINDICATIONS/POSSIBLE INTERACTIONS
N/A

FOLLOW-UP
• Posture may persist for days to weeks; not an indication of a hopeless prognosis
• With rapid and aggressive treatment, the patient may recover, especially if there is pain perception caudal to the lesion.

✓ MISCELLANEOUS

Suggested Reading
de Lahunta A. Veterinary neuroanatomy and clinical neurology. 2nd ed. Philadelphia: Saunders, 1983.
Author Mary O. Smith
Consulting Editor Joane M. Parent

SCHWANNOMA

 BASICS

OVERVIEW
• Tumors of nerve sheath origin, arising from Schwann cells
• Peripheral nerve sheath tumor—proposed term to include schwannomas, neurofibromas, and neurofibrosarcomas, because all arise from the same cell

SIGNALMENT
• Dogs and rarely cats
• Dogs—mean age, 8.7 years
• No breed predilection
• Slight male predisposition (1.4:1)

SIGNS
• Chronic, progressive forelimb lameness and muscle atrophy—most common
• Hind limbs—may be primarily affected; less common
• Peripheral neuropathy (self-mutilation)—occasionally
• Palpable mass—> 50% of patients
• Horner's syndrome—with cervical involvement

CAUSES & RISK FACTORS
None identified

 DIAGNOSIS

DIFFERENTIAL DIAGNOSIS
• Orthopedic disease
• Other neurologic disease—intervertebral disk disease
• Other neoplasia—lymphoma

CBC/BIOCHEMISTRY/URINALYSIS
Usually normal

OTHER LABORATORY TESTS
CSF analysis—usually unrewarding

IMAGING
• Plain radiography—rarely helpful
• Myelography—may be helpful with dorsal or ventral nerve root involvement
• CT or MRI—provides the most information regarding extent and location of disease

DIAGNOSTIC PROCEDURES
Electromyography—consistently reveals abnormal, spontaneous electrical activity in muscles of the affected limb

 TREATMENT

• Surgical excision—treatment of choice
• Distal mass—limb may still be functional after excision.
• Amputation—usually required
• Laminectomy—necessary with nerve root involvement
• Local recurrence after surgery common
• Radiotherapy—deserves further evaluation

 MEDICATIONS

DRUGS
• Chemotherapy—no successful management described
• Corticosteroids—may help reduce peritumoral edema; may temporarily relieve clinical signs

CONTRAINDICATIONS/POSSIBLE INTERACTIONS
N/A

 FOLLOW-UP

EXPECTED COURSE AND PROGNOSIS
• Recurrence after surgical excision—common; up to 72% of cases
• The more distal the tumor, the better the possibility of a surgical cure.
• Median disease-free interval with brachial or lumbosacral plexus involvement—7.5 months
• Median disease-free interval with dorsal or ventral nerve root involvement—1 month
• Metastasize—(rarely) to regional lymph nodes or lungs

 MISCELLANEOUS

ABBREVIATION
CSF = cerebrospinal fluid

Suggested Reading

Brehm DM, Vite CH, Steinberg HS, et al. A retrospective evaluation of 51 cases of peripheral nerve sheath tumors in the dog. J Am Anim Hosp Assoc 1995;31:349–359.
Morrison WB. Cancer affecting the nervous system. In: Morrison WB, ed. Cancer in dogs and cats: medical and surgical management. Baltimore: Williams & Wilkins, 1998:655–665.
Author Ruthanne Chun
Consulting Editor Wallace B. Morrison

BASICS

OVERVIEW
• An inflammatory disease process directed against the cutaneous adnexal structures (sebaceous glands)
• May be genetically inherited, immune-mediated, or metabolic
• Initial defect—a keratinization disorder or an abnormality in lipid metabolism (accumulation of toxic intermediate metabolites)

SIGNALMENT
• Young adult to middle-aged dogs
• Two forms—one in long-coated and one in short-coated breeds
• Predisposed—standard poodles, akitas, Samoyeds, and vizslas

SIGNS

Long-Coated Breeds
• Symmetrical, partial alopecia
• Dull brittle hair
• Tightly adherent silver-white scale
• Follicular casts around hair shaft
• Small tufts of matted hair
• Lesions—often first observed along dorsal midline and dorsum of the head
• Severe—secondary bacterial folliculitis, pruritus, and malodor
• Akitas—often relatively severely affected

Short-Coated Breeds
• Alopecia—moth-eaten, circular, or diffuse
• Mild scaling
• Affects the trunk, head, and ears
• Secondary bacterial folliculitis rare

CAUSES & RISK FACTORS
Mode of inheritance is being studied.

 DIAGNOSIS

DIFFERENTIAL DIAGNOSIS
• Primary seborrhea—keratinization disorder
• Bacterial folliculitis
• Demodicosis
• Dermatophytosis
• Endocrine skin disease

CBC/BIOCHEMISTRY/URINALYSIS
N/A

OTHER LABORATORY TESTS
N/A

IMAGING
N/A

DIAGNOSTIC PROCEDURES
• Skin scrapings—normal
• Dermatophyte culture—negative
• Endocrine function tests—normal
• Skin biopsies

PATHOLOGIC FINDINGS
• Nodular granulomatous to pyogranulomatous inflammatory reaction at the level of the sebaceous glands
• Orthokeratotic hyperkeratosis and follicular cast formation; more prominent in long-coated breeds
• Advanced—complete loss of sebaceous glands; periadnexal fibrosis
• Destruction of entire hair follicle and adnexal unit rare

 TREATMENT

• Clinical signs may wax and wane irrespective of treatment.
• Controlled studies have not been done to document efficacy of any therapy.
• Results extremely variable; response may depend on severity of disease at the time of diagnosis.
• Akita—breed most refractory to treatment

 MEDICATIONS

DRUGS
• Propylene glycol and water—50–75% mixture; spray every 24 hr to affected areas
• Baby oil—soak affected areas for 1 hr; follow with multiple shampoos to remove oil and scales
• Derm Cap (1 extra-strength) and evening primrose oil (500 mg)—q12h PO; possible side effects include vomiting, diarrhea, and flatulence.
• Isotretinoin (Accutane)—1 mg/kg q12h PO; reduce to 1 mg/kg q24h after 1 month and to 1 mg/kg q48h after 2 months; continue as needed for maintenance.
• Cyclosporine (Sandimmune)—5 mg/kg q12h PO; side effects include vomiting, diarrhea, gingival hyperplasia, hirsutism, papillomatous skin lesions, increased incidence of infections, nephrotoxicity, and hepatotoxicity.
• Bactericidal antibiotics and Sulf-Oxydex shampoo—for secondary bacterial folliculitis

CONTRAINDICATIONS/POSSIBLE INTERACTIONS
N/A

 FOLLOW-UP

Urge owners to register affected dogs so that mode of inheritance can be determined.

✓ MISCELLANEOUS

Suggested Reading
Rosser EJ. Sebaceous adenitis. In: Griffin CE, Kwochka KW, MacDonald JM, eds. Current veterinary dermatology. St. Louis: Mosby, 1993:211–214.
Authors Ellen C. Codner and Karen Helton Rhodes
Consulting Editor Karen Helton Rhodes

DISEASES

SEMINOMA

BASICS

OVERVIEW
- Benign, unilateral, solitary tumor of the testis
- Usually < 2 cm in diameter; often difficult to palpate
- Exists in 1 in 9 dogs > 4 years; 71% not detected by physical examination
- One-third found in a cryptorchid testis; extrascrotal tumors more common in the right testis

SIGNALMENT
- Usually old male dogs
- Mean age, 10 years
- No breed predisposition
- Cats—extremely rare; one reported case of malignant tumor with metastasis

SIGNS
- Usually none
- Palpable testicular mass in 29% of cases
- Rarely associated with feminization from estrogen excess (see Sertoli Cell Tumor)

CAUSES & RISK FACTORS
Cryptorchidism

DIAGNOSIS

DIFFERENTIAL DIAGNOSIS
- Sertoli cell tumor
- Interstitial cell tumor

CBC/BIOCHEMISTRY/URINALYSIS
Usually normal unless evidence of male feminization syndrome

OTHER LABORATORY TESTS
N/A

IMAGING
Ultrasound—tumors < 3 cm in diameter usually hypoechoic; > 5 cm in diameter usually mixed echo pattern

DIAGNOSTIC PROCEDURES
- Castration
- Histopathologic examination

TREATMENT
- Castration
- Radiotherapy—reported effective in patients with regional metastasis

MEDICATIONS

DRUGS
N/A

CONTRAINDICATIONS/POSSIBLE INTERACTIONS
N/A

FOLLOW-UP

PREVENTION/AVOIDANCE
N/A

POSSIBLE COMPLICATIONS
None likely

EXPECTED COURSE AND PROGNOSIS
- After castration—recovery usually complete; prognosis excellent
- Usually benign; occasional metastasis to regional lymph nodes, visceral organs, lungs, and other sites

MISCELLANEOUS

ASSOCIATED CONDITIONS
- Prostate disease
- Perianal adenoma
- Perineal hernia

Suggested Reading

McDonald RK, Walker M, Legendre AM, et al. Radiotherapy of metastatic seminoma in the dog. J Vet Intern Med 1988;2:103–107.

Morrison WB. Cancers of the reproductive tract. In: Morrison WB, ed. Cancer in dogs and cats: medical and surgical management. Baltimore: Williams & Wilkins, 1998: 581–590.

Author Wallace B. Morrison
Consulting Editor Wallace B. Morrison

SERTOLI CELL TUMOR

 BASICS

OVERVIEW
• Common testicular tumor in dogs
• Between 10% and 14% are malignant and metastasize to regional lymph nodes and other abdominal and thoracic organs.

SIGNALMENT
• Old male dogs
• Cats—extremely rare; two reported cases of malignant tumor with metastasis

SIGNS
• Unilaterally large testicle with atrophy of the unaffected testicle
• Feminization syndrome—gynecomastia; galactorrhea; atrophy of penis; pendulous prepuce; attraction to other male dogs; standing in the female position to urinate
• Squamous metaplasia of the prostate and prostatomegaly—occasionally
• Dermatologic changes—nonpruritic alopecia; thinning of the haircoat; hyperpigmentation
• Abdominal mass—if patient is cryptorchid
• Inguinal location possible

CAUSES & RISK FACTORS
Cryptorchid testicles are 13–13.6 times more likely to develop neoplasia than are scrotally located testicles.

 DIAGNOSIS

DIFFERENTIAL DIAGNOSIS
• Interstitial cell tumor
• Seminoma
• Hyperadrenocorticism
• Hypothyroidism
• More likely to have an abdominal location than other testicular tumors; high testicular temperature in the abdominal location may destroy spermatogenic cells and leave Sertoli cells unregulated.

CBC/BIOCHEMISTRY/URINALYSIS
Nonregenerative anemia, leukopenia, and thrombocytopenia associated with hyperestrogenism

OTHER LABORATORY TESTS
• Serum estradiol concentration high in most patients
• Serum progesterone concentration high in most patients

IMAGING
Variable echotexture on ultrasound

DIAGNOSTIC PROCEDURES
Castration and histopathologic examination of appropriate tissue

 TREATMENT

• Castration

 MEDICATIONS

DRUGS
N/A

CONTRAINDICATIONS/POSSIBLE INTERACTIONS
N/A

 FOLLOW-UP

PATIENT MONITORING
N/A

PREVENTION/AVOIDANCE
N/A

POSSIBLE COMPLICATIONS
None unless associated with surgery or estrogen excess

EXPECTED COURSE AND PROGNOSIS
• Good in most patients
• Guarded if severe cytopenias develop because of hyperestrogenism

 MISCELLANEOUS

ASSOCIATED CONDITIONS
• 25–29% of dogs with Sertoli cell tumor develop male feminization syndrome.
• About 70% of intra-abdominal testicular tumors in dogs are associated with male feminization syndrome.
• Hyperestrogenism can cause hematopoietic failure.

Suggested Reading
Metzger FL, Hattel AL, White DG. Hematuria, hyperestrogenemia, and hyperprogesteronemia due to a sertoli-cell tumor in a bilaterally cryptorchid dog. Canine Pract 1993;18:32–35.
Morrison WB. Cancers of the reproductive tract. In: Morrison WB, ed. Cancer in dogs and cats: medical and surgical management. Baltimore: Williams & Wilkins 1998: 581–590.

Author Wallace B. Morrison
Consulting Editor Wallace B. Morrison

DISEASES

SEX HORMONE–RESPONSIVE DERMATOSES

BASICS

DEFINITION
Uncommon alopecias and dermatoses suspected to result from an imbalance of sex hormones; often defined on the basis of stimulatory response to sex hormone therapy

SIGNALMENT
See Causes

SIGNS
• Alopecia—localized alopecia more common than generalized; initially involves the perineum, ventrum, thighs, and cervical areas; later involves the caudodorsal back and flank; flank alopecia may be the first or only sign in some patients with hyperestrogenism and may be seasonal in some spayed females.
• Fur—may be soft or dry and brittle.
• Nipples, mammary glands, vulva, prepuce, testicles, ovaries, and prostate—often abnormal
• Secondary seborrhea, pruritus, pyoderma, comedones, ceruminous otitis externa, and hyperpigmentation—variable
• Tail gland hyperplasia and perianal gland hyperplasia with macular melanosis—dogs with testicular tumors
• Urinary incontinence—estrogen- and testosterone-responsive conditions

CAUSES & RISK FACTORS

Estrogen-Responsive—Females (Ovarian Imbalance II)
• Possible deficiency or imbalance of estrogen; serum estradiol concentrations may be normal
• Inadequate production of adrenal sex hormones
• Cutaneous defect in the sex hormone receptor/metabolism system
• Rare in dogs
• Extremely rare in cats
• Predisposed breeds—dachshunds and boxers
• Primarily seen in young adults
• May occur after ovariohysterectomy in noncycling, intact females
• Occasionally seen during pseudopregnancy
• Variant—cyclical flank alopecia and hyperpigmentation; noted in Airedales, boxers, and English bulldogs; may worsen in winter

Hyperestrogenism—Females (Ovarian Imbalance I)
• Estrogen excess or imbalance owing to cystic ovaries, ovarian tumors (rare), or exogenous estrogen overdose
• Abnormal peripheral conversion of sex hormones
• Ectopic production of sex hormones
• Animals with normal serum estrogen concentrations may have increased numbers of estrogen receptors in the skin.
• Rare in dogs
• Extremely rare in cats

• English bulldogs may be predisposed to cystic ovaries.
• Generally, middle-aged and old intact female dogs

Hyperestrogenism—Male Dogs with Testicular Tumors
• Estrogen excess (or rarely hyperprogesteronism) owing to Sertoli cell tumor (most common), seminoma, or interstitial cell tumor (rarely)
• Cryptorchidism predisposes animals to the formation of testicular tumors.
• Intact males; usually middle-aged or older
• Predisposed breeds—boxers, Shetland sheepdogs, Weimaraners, German shepherds, Cairn terriers, Pekingese, and collies
• Associated with male pseudohermaphrodism in miniature schnauzers

Hyperandrogenism Associated with Testicular Tumors
Androgen-producing testicular tumors (especially interstitial cell tumors) in intact male dogs

Idiopathic Male Feminizing Syndrome
• Undetermined
• Serum sex hormone concentrations normal
• Blockage of androgen receptors in the skin may prevent attachment of testosterone.
• Intact, middle-aged male dogs.

Testosterone-Responsive—Males
• Rare
• Old castrated male dogs
• Afghan hounds over-represented;
• Extremely rare in cats
• Suspected hypoandrogenism or a possible defect in the skin sex hormone–receptor system

Castration Responsive
• Intact males with normal testicles
• Estradiol, testosterone, and progesterone—variably high, low, or normal
• Onset 1–4 years or older
• Predisposed breeds—chow chows, Samoyeds, keeshonds, Pomeranians, huskies, malamutes, and miniature poodles

Adrenal Sex Hormone Imbalance (Adrenal Hyperplasia-like Syndrome)
• Adrenal enzyme (21-hydroxylase) deficiency resulting in excessive adrenal androgen or progesterone secretion
• Males and females, intact or neutered.
• Onset 1–5 years of age
• Pomeranians predisposed

DIAGNOSIS

DIFFERENTIAL DIAGNOSIS
• Hypothyroidism and hyperadrenocorticism—critical to rule out first; these diseases generally cause truncal alopecia first; **REMEMBER:** sex hormones can change the affinity of binding proteins, so that the

baseline total T_4 can be normal or above normal in dogs with hyperandrogenemia or hypoestrogenemia.
• Growth hormone–responsive/adrenal hyperplasia dermatosis
• Follicular dysplasia
• Dachshunds—pattern baldness
• Keratinization disorders
• Allergic skin disease

CBC/BIOCHEMISTRY/URINALYSIS
• Usually unremarkable
• Bone marrow hypoplasia or aplasia are noted occasionally in states of estrogen excess, owing to testicular tumors in male and hyperestrogenism in female dogs

OTHER LABORATORY TESTS
• Serum estrogen/estradiol concentrations—sometimes high (30%–40% of patients) with hyperestrogenism of female dogs, hyperestrogenism in male dogs with testicular tumors, and castration-responsive dermatosis; rarely helpful in estrogen-responsive dermatosis, because serum estradiol 17β concentrations in spayed females are similar to intact females
• Serum testosterone and progesterone—sometimes elevated in animals with castration-responsive dermatosis; occasionally elevated with hyperestrogenism (ovarian imbalance) in female dogs
• Serum sex hormone concentrations—often normal, treat according to the suspected diagnosis based on clinical signs; by ruling out other disorders, and by noting the response to therapy.

Combined ACTH Stimulation and Adrenal Reproductive Hormone Test
• Obtain plasma and serum before injection; administer ACTH (cosyntropin 0.5 IU/kg IV or ACTH gel 0.22 USP U/kg IM); obtain plasma and serum 1 hr later (and a 2-hr sample if ACTH gel is used)
• Partial deficiency of 21-hydroxylase enzyme results in accumulation of steroid precursors (e.g., progesterone, 17-hydroxyprogesterone, androstenedione, and DHEAS), resulting in dermatosis of Pomeranians and other breeds; clinically similar to growth hormone–responsive dermatosis

GnRH (Cystorelin) Response Test
• Demonstrates response of gonads to stimulation
• Especially useful when basal hormones are normal
• Determine baseline serum estradiol, testosterone, and progesterone before injection; administer GnRH (0.22 mg/kg IV); obtain serum samples 1–2 hr later; determine levels of the three sex hormones; values vary with lab.

SEX HORMONE–RESPONSIVE DERMATOSES

IMAGING
Radiography, ultrasonography, and laparoscopy—detect cystic ovaries, ovarian tumors, testicular tumors (scrotal and abdominal), sublumbar lymphadenopathy, and possible thoracic metastases of malignant tumors

DIAGNOSTIC PROCEDURES
• Preputial cytology—may demonstrate cornification of cells (similar to bitch in estrus) in advanced patients with testicular feminizing tumors
• Skin biopsy

PATHOLOGIC FINDINGS
• General endocrinopathy findings (see above)—all syndromes, except hyperandrogenism owing to testicular tumors
• Perivascular dermatitis—may be seen in pruritic animals (male feminizing syndrome, hyperestrogenism of female dogs)
• Sebaceous glands—relatively spared in estrogen-responsive dermatosis of female dogs and in testosterone-responsive dermatosis of male dogs
• Hair follicles—hypereosinophilic tricholemmal keratinization ("flame follicles") may be seen with castration-responsive dermatosis

TREATMENT
• Cryptorchid animals—do not breed (prevention and avoidance of problems); neuter when young
• Exploratory laparotomy—diagnosis and treatment (e.g., ovariohysterectomy and castration) for ovarian cysts and tumors and abdominal testicular tumors
• Castration—castration-responsive dermatosis and scrotal testicular tumors
• Discontinue excessive exogenous estrogen administration

MEDICATIONS

DRUGS OF CHOICE

Estrogen-Responsive Dermatosis
• Spayed females—DES at 0.02 mg/kg (maximum, 1 mg) PO q24h for 14–21 days; stop for 1 week; repeat cycle until hair regrowth; then give 2–3 times weekly to maintain hair coat; discontinue during estrus and resume maintenance when estrus subsides; if no response, try methyltestosterone (see below) or milbolerone (at 30 μg [dogs < 11 kg] or 50 μg [dogs 11–23 kg]) until hair regrowth and then taper to maintenance
• Intact females—DES (5 mg PO q24h) until bloody discharge; if no response after 7 days, double the dose; give until proestrus day 2 (maximum, 14 days total) until sanguineous

vaginal discharge and vulvar edema are noted; then for 2 days more; then LH (5 mg IM) on day 5 of proestrus; then FSH on days 9 and 11 of proestrus
• Alternative treatment—FSH (0.75 mg/kg IM daily) until signs of estrus appear

Testosterone Responsive (Males)/Some Estrogen Responsive (Female Dogs)
• Methyltestosterone—0.5–1.0 mg/kg (maximum, 30 mg) PO q48h until response; may take 1–3 months; after hair regrowth is complete, 2–3 times/week for maintenance;
• Respositol testosterone (2 mg/kg [maximum, 30 mg[IM every 1–4 months) as needed to maintain normal hair coat

Hyperestrogenism—Female Dogs
• Consider o,p'-DDD (Lysodren) or L-deprenyl.
• Alternative treatments—GnRH or hCG
• Tamoxifen—may be useful

Other Conditions
• Castration-responsive alopecia—may respond to hCG (50 IU/kg IM twice weekly for 6 weeks) or testosterone (see above) if castration is not possible
• Adrenal 21-hydroxylase enzyme deficiency—o,p'-DDD (Lysodren) if adrenal sex hormones are high; beginning dose 15–25 mg/kg PO q24h for 7 days; maintenance doses (15–25 mg/kg PO every 5–14 days) titrated to maintain post-ACTH-stimulation cortisol within the baseline range

General Treatment
• Topical antiseborrheic therapy—conditions with associated keratinization defects and comedones
• Antibiotics—associated pyodermas
• Prednisone—for pruritus if infections and bone marrow suppression have been ruled out; 0.5 mg/kg PO q12h for 5–7 days; then 0.5 mg q24h for 5–7 days; then 0.5 mg/kg q48h for 7 days

CONTRAINDICATIONS
N/A

POSSIBLE INTERACTIONS
N/A

FOLLOW-UP

PATIENT MONITORING
• DES supplementation—CBC for bone marrow hypoplasia or aplasia every 2 weeks for the first month; then every 3–6 months
• Testosterone supplementation—serum biochemistry with an emphasis on liver enzymes every 3–4 weeks for the first 3 months; every 4–6 months
• o,p'-DDD—electrolytes with ACTH-stimulation testing every 3 months

POSSIBLE COMPLICATIONS
• Estrogen—bone marrow hypoplasia (uncommon); aplasia (uncommon); signs of estrus (rare)
• methyltestosterone—cholangiohepatitis (rare); behavior changes (uncommon); seborrhea oleosa
• o,p'-DDD—potential toxicities (e.g., vomiting, diarrhea, collapse, and iatrogenic hypoadrenocorticism)
• Tamoxifen—vulva swelling; discontinue until signs of estrus are gone.

EXPECTED COURSE AND PROGNOSIS
• Estrogen responsive—regrowth of hair may take about 3 months and may be transient
• Female hyperestrogenism—improvement should occur within 3–6 months after ovariohysterectomy
• Estrogen- and androgen-secreting tumors—resolution of signs noted within 3–6 months of castration; bone marrow aplasia associated with hyperestrogenism usually does not respond to castration, and the prognosis for recovery is grave; relapse after a positive response to castration may indicate metastasis, and if confirmed, the prognosis is poor
• Castration responsive—response noted 2–4 months after castration
• Testosterone therapy—may result in hair regrowth in 4–12 weeks
• Adrenal sex hormone imbalance—response seen 4–12 weeks after adrenal hyperplasia therapy with o,p'-DDD

MISCELLANEOUS

ABBREVIATIONS
• DES = diethylstilbestrol
• DHEAS = dehydroepiandrosterone sulfate
• FSH = follicle-stimulating hormone
• GnRH = gonadotropin-releasing hormone
• hCG = human chorionic gonadotropin
• LH = luteinizing hormone
• o,p'-DDD = 1,1-(o,p'-dichlorodiphenyl)-2,2-dichloroethane

Suggested Reading
Schmeitzel LP. Sex hormone-related and growth hormone-related alopecias. Vet Clin North Am Small Anim Pract 1990;20:1579–1601.
Author Margaret S. Swartout
Consulting Editor Karen Helton Rhodes

DISEASES

SEXUAL DEVELOPMENT DISORDERS

BASICS

DEFINITION
• Errors in the establishment of chromosomal, gonadal, or phenotypic sex that cause abnormal sexual differentiation
• Variety of patterns from ambiguous genitalia to apparently normal genitalia with sterility

PATHOPHYSIOLOGY
Normal sexual differentiation—establishment of chromosomal sex at fertilization (either XX or XY), development of gonadal sex, and development of phenotypic sex

Chromosomal
• XXY (Klinefelter's) syndrome—79, XXY; hypoplastic testes; phenotypic male (normal to hypoplastic genitalia); dogs and cats (some tortoiseshell males)
• XO (Turner's) syndrome—77, XO; dysgenetic ovaries; phenotypic female; infantile genitalia; dogs and cats
• XXX syndrome—79, XXX; ovaries without follicles; female phenotype; high FSH and LH; dogs
• True hermaphrodite chimera—XX/XY or XX/XXY; ovarian and testicular tissue; phenotypic sex depends on amount of testicular tissue; dogs and cats
• XX/XY chimera with testes and XY/XY chimera—vary from phenotypic female with abnormal genitalia to male with possible fertility; dogs and cats (some tortoiseshell males)
• Gonadal differentiation—determined by the sex chromosome constitution; *Sry* (located on the Y chromosome) encodes a protein that initiates testis differentiation; without *Sry*, ovarian differentiation occurs.

Disagreement Between Chromosomal and Gonadal
• XX sex reversal, XX true hermaphrodite—ovaries and testes; phenotypic female or partially masculinized female phenotype; varies from normal to abnormal vulva and normal-sized to large clitoris, uterus, oviducts, epididymis, and vas deferens; rarely fertile
• XX males—testes, usually cryptorchid; epididymis, vas deferens, prostate, and uterus; hypoplastic penis and prepuce; dogs only
• Phenotypic sex differentiation (tubular reproductive tract and external genitalia)—depends on gonadal sex; basic embryonic plan is female; male phenotype only with testes that are capable of secreting müllerian-inhibiting substance and testosterone

Phenotypic
• Chromosomal and gonadal sex agree; internal or external genitalia ambiguous
• Female pseudohermaphrodite—XX; ovaries; masculinized genitalia (mild clitoral enlargement to nearly normal male genitalia); caused by sex steroid administration during pregnancy; dogs only
• Male pseudohermaphrodite—XY; testes; some degree of internal or external genitalia female
• PMDS—all wolffian and müllerian duct derivatives present; usually normal penis, prepuce, and scrotum; dogs and cats
• Hypospadias—abnormal location of urinary orifice (from glans penis to perineum); external genitalia unambiguous; dogs
• Testicular feminization—XY; testes (often abdominal); no wolffian or müllerian duct derivatives; vulva externally; cats

SYSTEMS AFFECTED
• Reproductive—anomalies of the gonads, tubular tract, and external genitalia
• Renal/Urologic—occasionally affected (e.g., incontinence, hematuria, and cystitis)
• Skin/Exocrine—perivulvar dermatitis (hypoplastic vulva); perineal or peripreputial dermatitis (hypospadias); hyperpigmentation (testicular neoplasia)

GENETICS
• Chromosomal—usually caused by random events during gamete formation or early embryonic development
• Gonadal—XX sex-reversal in American cocker spaniels inherited as an autosomal recessive trait; similar familial disorders in German shorthaired pointers, English cocker spaniels, beagles, Chinese pugs, Kerry blue terriers, Weimaraners (breeding trials needed to confirm mode of inheritance)
• Phenotypic—PMDS in miniature schnauzers inherited as an autosomal recessive trait with expression limited to XY individuals; hypospadias considered inherited in Boston terriers; testicular feminization (cats only) probably X-linked

INCIDENCE/PREVALENCE
• Generally rare
• In affected breeds—may be common within families or even within the breed as a whole

GEOGRAPHIC DISTRIBUTION
N/A

SIGNALMENT

Species
Dogs and cats

Breed Predilections
Dogs—American cocker spaniels; English cocker spaniels; beagles; German shorthaired pointers; Weimaraners; Chinese pugs; Kerry blue terriers; basset hounds; miniature schnauzers; Boston terriers

Mean Age and Range
• Disorders congenital; defects present at birth
• Individuals with normal external genitalia may not be identified until breeding age or at routine gonadectomy.

Predominant Sex
Found in both phenotypic females and phenotypic males

SIGNS

General Comments
• Depend on the type of disorder
• Listed here are the possible findings for any of the conditions; not all occur with each specific disorder

Historical Findings
• Failure to cycle
• Infertility and sterility (male or female)
• Vulva or prepuce and penis—abnormal size, shape, or location
• Urine stream—abnormal location
• Male attracted to other males
• Urinary incontinence
• Vulvar discharge

Physical Examination Findings
• Vulva normal or hypoplastic
• Clitoris large; os clitoris
• Perivulvar dermatitis and vulvar discharge
• Testes scrotal, unilateral, or bilateral cryptorchid
• Penis and prepuce normal or hypoplastic
• Urethral meatus normal or abnormal location
• Dermatologic signs of hyperestrogenism in males
• Abdominal mass

CAUSES
• Congenital—heritable or nonheritable
• Exogenous steroid hormone administration during gestation

RISK FACTORS
Androgen or progestogen administration during pregnancy (female pseudohermaphrodite)

DIAGNOSIS

DIFFERENTIAL DIAGNOSIS

Unambiguous Genitalia
• Infertility (female)—male infertility; mistimed breeding; subclinical cystic endometrial hyperplasia; hypothyroidism

SEXUAL DEVELOPMENT DISORDERS

• Failure to cycle (female)—silent heat; hypothyroidism; hypercortisolism; previous gonadectomy
• Infertility (male)—female infertility; mistimed breeding; exogenous drug use affecting fertility; orchitis or epididymitis; testicular degeneration or hypoplasia; prostatitis

CBC/BIOCHEMISTRY/URINALYSIS
• Usually normal
• Urinalysis—may reveal evidence of cystitis with anatomic abnormalities that affect the location of the urethral meatus

OTHER LABORATORY TESTS
• Sex steroid hormones (progesterone, testosterone, and estradiol)—generally below the normal range; may be normal with some mild disorders (patient not sterile)
• Karyotyping—required to define chromosomal sex

IMAGING
• Routine radiography and ultrasonography—may be of diagnostic value for suspected abdominal mass (e.g., testicular neoplasia) in phenotypic females or males or with signs referable to pyometra (uterus present with female pseudohermaphrodite or PMDS)
• Contrast studies of the lower urogenital tract—may be useful in diagnosing female pseudohermaphrodites

DIAGNOSTIC PROCEDURES
N/A

PATHOLOGIC FINDINGS
Gross
• All patients—a precise description of the external genitalia, with particular attention given to the size and location of the vulva or prepuce, existence of the clitoris or penis, and position of the urinary orifice
• Most patients with no identified chromosomal abnormalities—exploratory laparotomy to determine the location and morphology of the gonads and internal genitalia

Histopathologic
• Examination of all tissues removed—paramount for defining the type of disorder
• Gonads—vary from nearly normal architecture to dysgenetic or a combination of ovotestis
• Essential to describe the components of the müllerian and/or wolffian duct system, if found

 TREATMENT

APPROPRIATE HEALTH CARE
• Usually outpatient
• Inpatient—exploratory laparotomy

NURSING CARE
Phenotypic females with perivulvar dermatitis secondary to a hypoplastic vulva and phenotypic males with hypospadias—local therapy for improvement of dermatologic sequelae, as necessary (see Dermatoses, Erosive or Ulcerative)

ACTIVITY
N/A

DIET
N/A

CLIENT EDUCATION
• Advise client to allow sterilization of affected individuals.
• Advise client to remove carriers of heritable disorders from the breeding program.

SURGICAL CONSIDERATIONS
• Gonadectomy and hysterectomy (if a uterus is found)—recommended
• Amputation of an enlarged clitoris—recommended when the mucosal surface is repeatedly traumatized
• Reconstructive surgery of the prepuce and malformed penis—dogs; may be necessary with XX male syndrome or hypospadias

 MEDICATIONS

DRUG(S) OF CHOICE
N/A

CONTRAINDICATIONS
Avoid androgen or progestogen use during pregnancy.

PRECAUTIONS
N/A

POSSIBLE INTERACTIONS
N/A

ALTERNATIVE DRUGS
N/A

 FOLLOW-UP

PATIENT MONITORING
N/A

PREVENTION/AVOIDANCE
• Sterilize individuals with heritable disorders.
• Remove carriers of heritable disorders from the breeding program.

POSSIBLE COMPLICATIONS
• Infertility
• Sterility
• Urinary tract problems—incontinence; cystitis
• Testicular neoplasia
• Pyometra

EXPECTED COURSE AND PROGNOSIS
N/A

 MISCELLANEOUS

ASSOCIATED CONDITIONS
N/A

AGE-RELATED FACTORS
Patients not diagnosed at an early age—pyometra (e.g., PMDS; female pseudohermaphrodite); testicular neoplasia (e.g., PMDS; testicular feminization; XX sex reversal)

ZOONOTIC POTENTIAL
N/A

PREGNANCY
N/A

SYNONYMS
• Hermaphrodites
• Pseudohermaphrodites
• Intersexes
• Klinefelter syndrome
• Turner syndrome

SEE ALSO
Cryptorchidism

ABBREVIATIONS
• FSH = follicle-stimulating hormone
• LH = luteinizing hormone
• PMDS = persistent müllerian duct syndrome

Suggested Reading
Meyers-Wallen VN. Genetics of sexual differentiation and anomalies in dogs and cats. J Reprod Fert Suppl 1993;47:441–452.
Meyers-Wallen VN, Patterson DF. Disorders of sexual development in dogs and cats. In: Current veterinary therapy X. Philadelphia: Saunders, 1989:1261–1269.
Meyers-Wallen VN, Patterson DF. Disorders of sexual development in the dog. In: Current therapy in theriogenology. 2nd ed. Philadelphia: Saunders, 1986:567–574.
Authors Sara K. Lyle and Vickie N. Meyers-Wallen
Consulting Editor Sara K. Lyle

SHAKER SYNDROME (GENERALIZED TREMOR SYNDROME)

 BASICS

OVERVIEW
Whole body tremor

SIGNALMENT
• Dogs
• Most often in young to middle-aged dogs
• Dogs with white hair coats (e.g., Maltese and West Highland white terriers)—historically have been overrepresented; but disease found in dogs with other coat colors
• Both sexes affected

SIGNS
• Diffuse body tremoring
• Initially, can be confused with signs of apprehension or hypothermia

CAUSES & RISK FACTORS
Most often associated with mild inflammatory CNS disease

 DIAGNOSIS

DIFFERENTIAL DIAGNOSIS
Other causes of weakness, apprehension, hypothermia, and seizure

CBC/BIOCHEMISTRY/URINALYSIS
Usually normal

OTHER LABORATORY TESTS
N/A

IMAGING
N/A

OTHER DIAGNOSTIC PROCEDURES
CSF analysis—mild (< 20 WBC $\times$ 10/L) monocytic or lymphocytic pleocytosis with normal protein content in most patients; can be normal

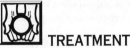 TREATMENT

Inpatient or outpatient

SHAKER SYNDROME (GENERALIZED TREMOR SYNDROME)

 MEDICATIONS

DRUGS
• Corticosteroids—reduce the inflammatory response; prednisolone or prednisone (1–2 mg/kg divided q12h) for the first 1–2 weeks
• Depending on clinical response, taper dosage slowly (usually over 4–6 months); assess periodically for clinical deterioration; if dosage is reduced too rapidly, clinical signs may recur, necessitating reinduction of initial dosage
• Many patients do not require further treatment.

CONTRAINDICATIONS/POSSIBLE INTERACTIONS
Corticosteroids—may be contraindicated with infectious encephalitis

 FOLLOW-UP

PATIENT MONITORING
Weekly evaluations for approximately 1 month; then monthly until corticosteroids are discontinued

PREVENTION/AVOIDANCE
N/A

POSSIBLE COMPLICATIONS
N/A

EXPECTED COURSE AND PROGNOSIS
• Clinical signs usually subside in 3–7 days from onset of steroid treatment.
• In some patients, recurrence necessitates reinstitution of corticosteroids.
• A small percentage of patients require every-other-day, low-dose corticosteroids, indefinitely, to maintain remission.

 MISCELLANEOUS

SYNONYMS
• Idiopathic Cerebellitis
• Shaker Syndrome

SEE ALSO
Tremors

ABBREVIATION
CSF = cerebrospinal fluid

Suggested Reading
Bagley RS, Kornegay JN, Wheeler SJ, et al. Generalized tremors in Maltese: clinical findings in seven cases. J Am Anim Hosp Assoc 1993;29:141–145.
Wagner SO, Podell M, Fenner WR. Generalized tremors in dogs: 24 cases (1984–1995). J Vet Med Assoc 1997;211:731–735
Author Rodney S. Bagley
Consulting Editor Joane M. Parent

DISEASES

SHOULDER, LIGAMENT, AND TENDON CONDITIONS

 BASICS

DEFINITION
• Make up the majority of causes for lameness in the canine shoulder joint, excluding osteochondritis dissecans lesions

PATHOPHYSIOLOGY
Bicipital Tenosynovitis
• Strain injury to the tendon of the biceps brachii • Mechanism of injury—direct trauma; indirect trauma (more common) • Pathological changes—from partial disruption of the tendon to chronic inflammatory changes, including dystrophic calcification • Proliferation of the fibrous connective tissue and adhesions between the tendon and the sheath—limit motion; cause pain
Fibrotic Contracture of the Infraspinatus Muscle
• Primary muscle–tendon disorder—not a neuropathy • Fibrous tissue—replaces normal muscle–tendon unit architecture • Loss of elasticity • Functional shortening of the muscle and tendon • Degeneration and atrophy of affected muscle • Partial muscle disruption—likely caused by direct or indirect trauma
Other
• Rupture of the biceps brachii tendon of origin—strain injury or disruption of the tendinous fibers at or near the junction with the supraglenoid tubercle of the scapula • Mineralization of the supraspinatus tendon—degenerative condition; granular grayish white calcium deposited between the fibers of the tendon; unknown cause; probably the result of overuse and indirect trauma • Avulsion or fracture of the supraspinatus tendon—overuse injury; variable amount of bone is avulsed from the greater tubercle of the proximal humerus

SYSTEMS AFFECTED
Musculoskeletal

INCIDENCE/PREVALENCE
Common cause of forelimb lameness

SIGNALMENT
Species
Dogs

Breed Predilections
Medium- to large-breed dogs

Mean Age and Range
• Skeletally mature dogs ≥ 1 year of age • Usually 3–7 years of age

SIGNS
General Comments
• Depend on the severity and chronicity of the disease • Atrophy of the spinati muscles—consistent finding for all conditions
Historical Findings
• Bicipital tenosynovitis—onset usually insidious; often of several months' duration; may be a traumatic incident as the inciting cause; subtle, intermittent lameness that worsens with exercise • Rupture of the biceps brachii tendon of origin—similar to bicipital tenosynovitis; may have acute onset owing to a known traumatic event; usually subtle, chronic lameness that worsens with exercise • Mineralization of the supraspinatus tendon—onset usually insidious; chronic lameness that worsens with activity • Avulsion/fracture of the supraspinatus tendon—similar to mineralization of supraspinatus tendon • Fibrotic contracture of the infraspinatus muscle—usually sudden onset during a period of outdoor exercise (e.g., hunting); shoulder lameness and tenderness gradually disappears within 2 weeks; condition results in chronic, persistent lameness 3–4 weeks later, which is not particularly painful

Physical Examination Findings
• Bicipital tenosynovitis—short and limited swing phase of gait owing to pain on extension and flexion of the shoulder; pain inconsistently demonstrated on manipulation of shoulder; pain most evident by applying deep digital pressure over the tendon in the intertubercular groove region while simultaneously flexing the shoulder and extending the elbow • Rupture of the biceps brachii tendon—similar • Mineralization of the supraspinatus tendon—similar; manipulations often do not produce pain; may palpate firm swelling over the greater tubercle • Avulsion or fracture of the supraspinatus tendon—similar to mineralization of the supraspinatus tendon
Fibrotic Contracture of the Infraspinatus Muscle—Usually not painful on manipulation • Internal rotation (pronation) of the shoulder joint—patient incapable; when forced, caudal aspect of the scapula elevates off the trunk and becomes more prominent. • When patient is standing—elbow adducted; paw abducted and outwardly rotated • When patient is walking—lower limb swings in a lateral arc (circumduction) as the paw is advanced during the stride. • Marked atrophy of the infraspinatus muscle on palpation

CAUSES
• Indirect or direct trauma—likely • Strain injury (indirect trauma)—most common

RISK FACTORS
• Overexertion • Poor conditioning before performing athletic activities • Obesity

 DIAGNOSIS

DIFFERENTIAL DIAGNOSIS
• Luxation or subluxation of the shoulder joint—often a history of trauma with an acute onset of lameness; often severe lameness with marked pain on manipulation of the shoulder joint • Osteosarcoma of the proximal humerus—progressive lameness with varying degrees of pain on manipulation of the shoulder; may note swelling and tenderness of the proximal humerus • Brachial plexus nerve sheath tumor—slow, insidious, progressive lameness over a period of months; marked atrophy of the spinati muscles with chronic disease; may feel a firm mass deep in the axillary region that is painful to digital pressure

IMAGING
Radiology
• Required for differentiation • Craniocaudal and mediolateral views necessary for all patients
Bicipital Tenosynovitis
• Generally normal
• Mediolateral view (chronic disease)—reveals bony reaction on the supraglenoid tubercle, dystrophic calcification of the bicipital tendon, sclerosis of the floor of the intertubercular groove, and osteophytes in the intertubercular groove • Hyperflexed CP-CD or CD-CP view (tangential) of the intertubercular groove—important for identifying the location of calcification; CP-CD view taken with patient in sternal recumbency (radiographic cassette placed on top of the forearm) with the elbow hyperflexed; CD-CP view taken with patient in dorsal recumbency with the shoulder joint hyperflexed and the limb rotated externally approximately 30°; position the radiographic tube directly over the scapulohumeral joint.
Rupture of the Biceps Brachii Tendon of Origin—to externally rotate shoulder joint
• Normal • Chronic disease—may see bony, irregular reaction on the supraglenoid tubercle
Mineralization of the Supraspinatus Tendon
• Mediolateral view—generally reveals calcification • Occurs cranial and immediately medial to the greater tubercle of the proximal humerus • Superimposition on the greater tubercle of the humerus—requires high-quality images • Tangential or skyline view of the intertubercular region of the proximal humerus—as for bicipital tenosynovitis; eliminates superimposition; allows distinction from calcification of the biceps brachii tendon • Density(ies)—smooth or irregular; multiple lesions common. • Often bilateral radiographically but rarely produces bilateral lameness
Avulsion or Fracture of the Supraspinatus Tendon
• Similar to mineralization of the supraspinatus tendon • Bone fragment—origin may be seen as a defect in the greater tubercle of the humerus; generally not as radiographically dense as that identified with mineralization of the supraspinatus tendon
Fibrotic Contracture of the Infraspinatus Muscle
Radiographically normal
Ultrasonography
• May help identify bicipital tenosynovitis and rupture of the biceps brachii tendon of origin
Contrast Arthrography
• Helps identify bicipital tenosynovitis • Useful for determining the location of calcific densities near the intertubercular groove • Incomplete filling of the tendon sheath—may indi-

cate proliferative inflammatory synovitis and adhesions between the tendon sheath and intertubercular groove

DIAGNOSTIC PROCEDURES
• Joint tap and analysis of synovial fluid—identify intra-articular disease; fluid should be straw colored with normal to decreased viscosity; cytologic evaluation: $< 10,000$ nucleated cells/μl ($> 90\%$ are mononuclear cells)
• Arthroscopic exploration of the shoulder joint—diagnose bicipital tenosynovitis and rupture of the biceps brachii tendon of origin; confirm lack of intra-articular disease

PATHOLOGIC FINDINGS
• Bicipital tenosynovitis—grossly, mineralization of the biceps tendon; osteophytosis of the intertubercular groove; proliferative synovitis; and fibrous adhesions between the biceps tendon and its synovial sheath; histologically, synovial proliferation, edema, fibrosis, dystrophic mineralization, and lymphocytic-plasmocytic infiltration of the tendon and synovium • Rupture of the biceps brachii tendon of origin—grossly, partial to complete rupture of the biceps tendon at its insertion on the supraglenoid tubercle, proliferative synovitis, and fibrous adhesions between the biceps tendon and its synovial sheath; histologically, synovial proliferation, edema, fibrosis, and occasional dystrophic mineralization • Mineralization of the supraspinatus tendon—grossly, tendon often looks normal, but longitudinal incision reveals numerous pockets of mineralized debris within the fibers; histologically, chondromucinous stromal degeneration of the tendon with multiple foci of dystrophic mineralization • Avulsion or fracture of the supraspinatus tendon—grossly, tendon often looks normal, but longitudinal incision reveals bone fragment(s) surrounded by a fibrous tissue capsule; usually see a corresponding bony defect in the greater tubercle • Fibrotic contracture of the infraspinatus muscle—grossly, atrophied, fibrotic, and contracted muscle, normal tendon, and (commonly) adhesions to the underlying joint capsule; histologically, degeneration, atrophy, and fibroplasia within the damaged muscle

TREATMENT

APPROPRIATE HEALTH CARE
• Outpatient—early diagnosis • Inpatient—chronic, severe disease requires surgical intervention. • Bicipital tenosynovitis—50%–75% success with medical treatment; requires surgery with evidence of chronic changes and failure of medical management • Rupture of the biceps brachii tendon of origin generally requires surgery • Mineralization of the supraspinatus tendon—may be an incidental finding; requires surgery after excluding other causes of lameness and medical treatment • Avulsion or fracture of the supraspinatus tendon—often requires surgery because of persistent bone fragment irritation of the tendon • Fibrotic contracture of the

infraspinatus muscle—requires surgery

NURSING CARE
• Cryotherapy (ice packing)—immediately postsurgery; helps reduce inflammation and swelling at the surgery site; performed 15–20 min every 8 hr for 3–5 days • Regional massage and range-of-motion exercises—improve flexibility; decrease muscle atrophy

ACTIVITY
• Medical treatment—requires strict confinement for 4–6 weeks; activity; premature return to normal likely exacerbates signs and induces a chronic state. • Postsurgery—depends on procedure performed

DIET
Weight control—decrease the load applied to the painful joint

SURGICAL CONSIDERATIONS
• Bicipital tenosynovitis—recommended with poor response to medical treatment and chronic disease; goal: eliminate movement of the biceps tendon within the inflamed synovial sheath by performing a tenodesis of the bicipital tendon; remove the tendon from its origin on the scapular supraglenoid tubercle and reattach it to the proximal lateral aspect of the humerus. • Rupture of the biceps brachii tendon of origin—tenodesis is the treatment of choice; reattach tendon to the proximal lateral aspect of the humerus using either a screw and spiked washer or passing the tendon through a bone tunnel and suturing it to the supraspinatus tendon. • Mineralization of the supraspinatus tendon—longitudinally incise the tendon; remove the calcium deposits; • Avulsion or fracture of the supraspinatus tendon—remove the bone fragment(s) • Fibrotic contracture of the infraspinatus muscle—tenotomy and excision of part of the tendon of insertion often feel a distinct pop after excision of the last adhesio, which allows complete range of motion of the shoulder joint

MEDICATIONS

DRUGS OF CHOICE

Biciptial Tenosynovitis
• Intra-articular injection of a corticosteroid—initial treatment of choice • Systemic treatment (NSAIDs or steroids)—not as effective • Do not inject into a septic joint; perform complete synovial fluid analysis if any doubt. • Prednisolone acetate—20–40 mg, depending on size • Lameness markedly improved but not eliminated—give a second injection in 3–6 weeks. • Incomplete resolution—recommend surgery

NSAIDs and Analgesics
• May be used for symptomatic treatment • May try buffered or enteric-coated aspirin (10–25 mg/kg PO q8h or q12h), caroprofen (2.2 mg/kg PO q12h), etodolac (10–15 mg/kg PO q24h), phenylbutazone (3–7 mg/kg PO q8h, total dose < 800 mg/day), meclofenamic acid (0.5 mg/kg PO q12h), or piroxicam (0.3

mg/kg PO q24h for 3 days, then every other day)

CONTRAINDICATIONS
• Avoid corticosteroids because of the potential side effects and articular cartilage damage associated with long-term use. • Direct injection of a corticosteroid into the biceps tendon—may promote further tendon disruption and eventual rupture

PRECAUTIONS
NSAIDs—gastrointestinal irritation may preclude use.

ALTERNATIVE DRUGS
Chondroprotective drugs (e.g., polysulfated glycosaminoglycans, glucosamine, and chondroitin sulfate)—may help limit associated cartilage damage and degeneration

FOLLOW-UP

PATIENT MONITORING
• Most patients require a minimum of 1–2 months of rehabilitation after treatment.

EXPECTED COURSE AND PROGNOSIS
• Medically managed bicipital tenosynovitis—often successful after one or two treatments (50%–75% of cases) with no chronic changes • Surgically treated bicipital tenosynovitis—good to excellent results (90% of cases); recovery to full function may take 2–8 months • Surgically treated tenodesis of the bicipital brachii tendon—good to excellent prognosis; $> 85\%$ of patients show improved return to function. • Surgically treated mineralization of the supraspinatus tendon—good to excellent prognosis; recurrence possible but uncommon • Surgically treated avulsion or fracture of the supraspinatus tendon—good to excellent prognosis; recurrence possible but uncommon • Surgically treated fibrotic contracture of the infraspinatus muscle—good to excellent prognosis; patients uniformly return to normal limb function.

MISCELLANEOUS

Suggested Reading

Flo GL, Middleton D. Mineralization of the supraspinatus tendons in dogs. J Am Vet Med Assoc 1990;197:95–97.

Rivers B, Wallace L, Johnston GR. Biceps tenosynovitis in the dog: radiographic and sonographic findings. Vet Comp Orthop Trauma 1992;5:51–57.

Stobie D, Wallace LJ, Lipowitz AJ, et al. Chronic bicipital tenosynovitis in dogs: 29 cases (1985–1992). J Am Vet Med Assoc 1995;207:201–207.

Author Peter D. Schwarz
Consulting Editor Peter D. Schwarz

DISEASES

SJÖGREN SYNDROME

 BASICS

OVERVIEW
• A systemic autoimmune disease characterized by keratoconjunctivitis sicca, xerostomia, and lymphoplasmacytic adenitis
• Underlying mechanism unknown; however, autoantibodies directed against glandular tissues have been identified.
• Associated with other autoimmune or immune-mediated diseases, such as rheumatoid arthritis and pemphigus

SIGNALMENT
• Higher incidence in several canine breeds—English bulldogs, West Highland white terriers, and miniature schnauzers
• Chronic disease of adult dogs
• Cats unaffected

SIGNS
Historical Findings
• Adult onset
• Conjunctivitis and keratitis
• Keratitis sicca most prominent clinical feature

Physical Examination Findings
• Blepharospasm
• Conjunctival hyperemia
• Corneal lesions (opacity to ulceration)
• Gingivitis
• Stomatitis

CAUSES & RISK FACTORS
• Possible genetic predisposition in breeds with high incidence
• Develops concurrently with other immune-mediated and autoimmune diseases

 DIAGNOSIS

DIFFERENTIAL DIAGNOSIS
• Other causes of keratoconjunctivitis sicca—canine distemper, trauma, and drug toxicities
• Keratoconjunctivitis sicca associated with other immune-mediated diseases—atopy, lymphocytic thyroiditis, polymyositis, systemic lupus erythematosus, rheumatoid arthritis, and pemphigoid diseases

CBC/BIOCHEMISTRY/URINALYSIS
Normal

OTHER LABORATORY TESTS
• Hypergammaglobulinemia revealed by serum protein electrophoresis
• Positive antinuclear antibody test
• Positive lupus erythematosus cell test
• Positive rheumatoid factor test
• Positive indirect fluorescent antibody test for autoantibodies

IMAGING
N/A

DIAGNOSTIC PROCEDURES
Schirmer tear test (0–5 mm/min)

PATHOLOGIC FINDINGS
• Histopathologic changes in salivary glands—lymphoplasmacytic adenitis
• Conjunctival biopsy—reveals conjunctivitis

 TREATMENT

• Directed at controlling keratoconjunctivitis sicca
• Any concurrent disease must be medically managed
• May include administration of anti-inflammatory or immunosuppressive drugs
• Surgical management of keratoconjunctivitis sicca indicated in animals that fail to respond to medical treatment

MEDICATIONS

DRUGS
• Topical tear preparations
• Appropriate topical antibiotics for secondary bacterial infection
• Immunosuppressive or anti-inflammatory drugs
• For more aggressive medical treatment and surgical intervention, see Keratoconjunctivitis Sicca.

CONTRAINDICATIONS/POSSIBLE INTERACTIONS
Use of topical steroids in patients with acute keratoconjunctivitis sicca may cause corneal ulceration and is, therefore, not recommended.

 FOLLOW-UP

• Re-examine patients weekly until kerato-conjunctivitis sicca controlled
• Additional monitoring may be indicated to manage underlying or concurrent disease.
• Immunosuppressive drugs—monitor patients every other week for possible side effects.
• Prognosis variable and depends on existence of concurrent disease

 MISCELLANEOUS

SEE ALSO
Keratoconjunctivitis Sicca (KCS)

Suggested Reading
Quimby FW, Schwartz RS, Poskitt T, et al. A disorder of dogs resembling Sjögren's syndrome. Clin Immunol Immunopathol 1979;12:471–476.
Author Paul W. Snyder
Consulting Editor Susan M. Cotter

SMALL INTESTINAL BACTERIA OVERGROWTH (SIBO)

BASICS

DEFINITION
• A syndrome in which an increased number of bacteria in the small intestine causes small intestinal dysfunction
• Almost any bacteria may be responsible, and usually multiple species are present; the species may change with time.
• SIBO has been defined as $>10^4$ anaerobic and/or $>10^5$ total bacterial colony-forming units (CFUs)/mL of fasting intestinal fluid; these criteria are now controversial in dogs.
• Simply having more bacteria than expected may differ from SIBO (having too many bacteria plus signs of small intestinal dysfunction); SIBO differs from colonization of the alimentary tract by known pathogenic bacteria with virulence factors (i.e., *Salmonella* spp., *Campylobacter jejuni*, etc.) or overgrowth of toxigenic *Clostridium perfringens* in the colon.

PATHOPHYSIOLOGY
• Bacteria are constantly ingested with food and/or saliva.
• Most are destroyed by gastric acid or antibacterial factors in the small intestine (e.g., pancreatic enzymes).
• Bacteria that survive are eliminated from the small intestine by normal intestinal motility.
• When these natural defenses fail and excessive bacteria persist in the upper small intestine, they may cause pathology even though they are not obligate pathogens.
• Because the species and numbers of bacteria in the small intestine may vary between and even within patients, pathophysiology is not consistent.
• Purported mechanisms include deconjugation of bile acids, dehydroxylation of fatty acids, formation of alcohols, and destruction of brush border enzymes.
• Anaerobic bacteria (e.g., *Bacteroides* spp. and *Clostridium* spp.) have been considered more likely to cause pathology than many aerobic bacteria; SIBO can cause protein-losing enteropathy.

SYSTEMS AFFECTED
• Gastrointestinal—normal absorptive function is disrupted, resulting in weight loss with or without diarrhea or vomiting.
• Hepatobiliary—the portal vein carries bacterial toxins and other substances from the small intestines into the liver.

GENETICS
• No genetic basis has been established.
• Some breeds (German shepherds, shar peis) appear to be at increased risk.
• Decreased serum IgA concentrations have purportedly been associated with SIBO.

INCIDENCE/PREVALENCE
Unknown

GEOGRAPHIC DISTRIBUTION
N/A

SIGNALMENT

Species
• Dogs
• Cats—unknown; clinically normal cats can have $>10^5$ bacteria/mL in fasted small intestines.

Breed Predilections
Subjectively, German shepherds and shar peis have an increased incidence.

Mean Age And Range
• Unknown
• Identified in dogs <1 year of age and >8 years of age

Predominant Sex
N/A

SIGNS AND SYMPTOMS

General Comments
Can cause signs of small intestinal dysfunction

Historical Findings
• Weight loss may occur despite a reasonable appetite—principal sign
• Small bowel diarrhea (e.g., no mucus or blood in the feces, no tenesmus)—common
• Vomiting and borborygmus—occasional/variable
• May wax and wane or be consistent

Physical Examination Findings
• Weight loss and poor condition
• May be evidence of diarrhea
• Intestinal thickening is unexpected unless other infiltrative intestinal disease is also present.
• Signs typical of infection (i.e., fever, depression) are unexpected.

CAUSES
• Idiopathic
• Altered small intestinal anatomy—blind or stagnant loops, partial obstruction
• Exocrine pancreatic insufficiency (EPI)—approximately 70% of dogs with EPI have concurrent SIBO.
• Hypochlorhydria or achlorhydria—spontaneous or iatrogenic
• Immunodeficiency and preexisting intestinal disease—suggested, but unproven

RISK FACTORS
Not clearly identified; the following are suspected:
• Serum IgA deficiency
• Intestinal disease (e.g., inflammatory bowel disease [IBD], dietary intolerance, parasites) that affects local defense mechanisms

DIAGNOSIS

DIFFERENTIAL DIAGNOSIS
• Maldigestion—EPI
• Malabsorption due to any cause—IBD, alimentary lymphoma, lymphangiectasia, dietary intolerance/allergy, giardiasis, whether protein losing or not; IBD may mimic and/or be associated with SIBO.
• Intestinal parasites (especially *Giardia*)

CBC/BIOCHEMISTRY/URINALYSIS
• Usually normal
• Hypoalbuminemia—rare; when present, it suggests particularly severe intestinal disease and warrants an aggressive diagnostic and therapeutic approach.

OTHER LABORATORY TESTS

Serum Cobalamin and Folate
• Serum folate may be increased and cobalamin concentrations decreased.
• High specificity, low sensitivity—some dogs with symptomatic SIBO have normal serum folate and cobalamin concentrations.

Breath Hydrogen Analysis
• Typically performed in institutions
• Some false-negative and false-positive results occur.

Unconjugated Serum Bile Acids
Under investigation; seems to hold promise

IMAGING
N/A—may reveal an underlying cause, such as intestinal mass or partial obstruction

DIAGNOSTIC PROCEDURES

Quantitated Culture
• Aerobic and anaerobic bacteria from fasted, upper intestinal fluid—the "gold standard"
• Difficult to perform
• Recent work suggests the criterion of $>10^4$ anaerobic or $>10^5$ total bacteria/mL of intestinal fluid may be too low, leading to false-positive results.
• False negatives also believed to occur

Therapeutic Trials
• Treat for SIBO and observe the results.
• Simple and inexpensive
• Main difficulty—interpreting the results; more than one disease (e.g., IBD plus SIBO, dietary intolerance plus SIBO) may be present, and lack of clinical response to antibiotics might lead to incorrect conclusion that SIBO is absent; incorrect antibiotic selection might also cause failure of clinical response.

PATHOLOGIC FINDINGS
• No evidence seen at surgery or endoscopy
• Histopathology and cytology of small intestinal mucosa—typically unremarkable

SMALL INTESTINAL BACTERIA OVERGROWTH (SIBO)

TREATMENT

APPROPRIATE HEALTH CARE
• Outpatient medical management
• Results/improvement may take days to weeks.

NURSING CARE
• Usually none
• Supportive care for emaciated or hypoalbuminemic patients is rarely needed.

ACTIVITY
Unrestricted

DIET
• Highly digestible, restricted in fat
• Antigen-restricted diets recommended if concurrent dietary intolerance/allergy is suspected.

CLIENT EDUCATION
• Some patients show clinical improvement in days—the diarrhea stops.
• Some patients require weeks of therapy before demonstrating improvement—treat for at least 3–4 weeks before concluding therapy is ineffective.
• Any concurrent or predisposing diseases (e.g., IBD, EPI, dietary intolerance/allergy, alimentary tract neoplasia, partial obstruction, etc) must also be treated.
• Continual or repeated treatment is often required; rarely permanent resolution with one course of therapy

SURGICAL CONSIDERATIONS
Indicated for a partial obstruction, diverticulum, or intestinal mass

MEDICATIONS

DRUGS OF CHOICE
• Broad-spectrum, orally administered antibiotics effective against both aerobic and anaerobic bacteria are preferred.
• Since the species of bacteria in the affected intestine can apparently change over time, culture and sensitivity are not necessarily useful unless the patient failed to respond to previous appropriate therapy.
• Tetracycline (20 mg/kg PO q12h)—good initial choice; do not administer with food (calcium in the diet chelates the tetracycline and renders it ineffective).
• Tylosin (40–80 mg/kg/day PO divided q12h)—often useful; usually a powder (designed to be used in poultry) administered in the food; can be used long-term; very safe; may approximate the dose by giving 1/4th tsp BID to dogs >15 kg, 1/8th tsp to dogs 7–15 kg, and 1/16th tsp to dogs <7 kg

• Drugs that do not kill anaerobic bacteria (e.g., neomycin) may be less effective.

CONTRAINDICATIONS
N/A

PRECAUTIONS
• Must use tetracycline carefully in patients with significant hepatic disease
• Avoid tetracyclines in very young patients.
• Renal disease can occur with high doses of tetracyclines.
• Tetracyclines may cause fever, abdominal pain, hair loss, and depression in cats.

POSSIBLE INTERACTIONS
N/A

ALTERNATIVE DRUGS
• Amoxicillin (20 mg/kg PO q12h) or clavamox (22 mg/kg PO q12h)—often acceptable
• Metronidazole (10–15 mg/kg PO q12h)—used to treat SIBO because of its activity against anaerobic bacteria; may also have immunomodulatory effects, possibly helpful in treating IBD; has not seemed as effective as tetracycline in some cases
• Dogs with EPI plus SIBO—appropriate supplementation of pancreatic enzymes with a low-fat diet is usually efficacious; concurrent therapy for SIBO is indicated if enzyme replacement plus a low-fat diet does not resolve diarrhea and/or weight loss.

FOLLOW-UP

PATIENT MONITORING
• Body weight and (in hypoproteinemic patients) serum albumin concentration—most important parameters; improvement suggests effective therapy
• Diarrhea should also resolve.
• If diarrhea persists despite improved body weight and/or increased serum albumin concentration, investigation for concurrent intestinal disease is indicated.
• Weight ± serum albumin every 7–14 days, until patients is clearly improving

PREVENTION/AVOIDANCE
N/A

POSSIBLE COMPLICATIONS
Although unproven, SIBO may predispose or cause IBD in some dogs.

EXPECTED COURSE AND PROGNOSIS
• SIBO without complicating diseases (e.g., IBD, lymphoma)—prognosis with therapy usually good
• Best results expected if treated before severe secondary intestinal disease (see below) occurs

MISCELLANEOUS

ASSOCIATED CONDITIONS
• SIBO might cause IBD in some patients (unproven).
• Consider the possibility of concurrent EPI.

AGE-RELATED FACTORS
N/A

ZOONOTIC POTENTIAL
N/A

PREGNANCY
Avoid tetracyclines and metronidazole, especially during early pregnancy.

SYNONYMS
N/A

SEE ALSO
• Inflammatory Bowel Disease
• Exocrine Pancreatic Insufficiency
• Cobalamin and Folate
• Trypsin-like Immunoreactivity
• Diarrhea, Chronic
• Lymphoma
• *Giardia*

ABBREVIATIONS
• EPI = exocrine pancreatic insufficiency
• IBD = inflammatory bowel disease
• SIBO = intestinal (small) bacterial overgrowth

Suggested Reading
Batt RM, Barnes A, Rutgers HC, Carter SD. Relative IgA deficiency and small intestinal bacterial overgrowth in German shepherd dogs. Res Vet Sci 1991;50:106–111.
Davenport DJ. Small intestinal bacterial overgrowth—need for a new definition? Proc 14th ACVIM Forum 1996;16:346–347.
Rutgers HC, Batt RM, Elwood CM, Lamport A. Small intestinal bacterial overgrowth in dogs with chronic intestinal disease. J Am Vet Med Assoc 1995;206(2):187–193.
Simpson KW. Small intestinal bacterial overgrowth. Letter to the editor. J Am Vet Med Assoc 1994;205(3):405–407.
Willard MD, Simpson RB, Fossum TW, et al. Characterization of naturally developing small intestinal bacterial overgrowth in 16 German shepherd dogs. J Am Vet Med Assoc 1994;204(8):1201–1206.

Author Michael D. Willard
Consulting Editors Mitchell A. Crystal and Brett M. Feder

SMOKE INHALATION

BASICS

OVERVIEW
• Injury occurs as a result of direct heat damage to the upper airway and nasal mucosa; inhalation of carbon monoxide, which decreases tissue oxygen delivery by preferentially binding to hemoglobin; inhalation of other toxins (e.g., oxidants and aldehydes) that directly irritate the airway, and inhalation of particulate matter that adheres to the airways and alveoli.
• Extent of damage—depends the degree and duration of exposure and the material that was burning
• Dogs and cats may have serious lung injury with little cutaneous or oral evidence of burning.
• Lung reaction—initially bronchoconstriction, airway edema, and mucus production; then an inflammatory response, necrotizing tracheobronchitis, and pulmonary fluid accumulation owing to increased capillary permeability
• Superimposed bacterial infections—common cause of morbidity late in the disease; most patients show progression of lung dysfunction in the initial 2–3 days after exposure

SIGNALMENT
Dogs and cats

SIGNS
• Historical findings consistent with exposure
• Patient may have a smoky odor.
• Tachypnea and increased depth of respiration
• Inspiratory effort that suggests upper airway obstruction by edema
• Postural adaptations to respiratory distress
• Mucous membranes—may be cherry red owing to carbon monoxyhemoglobin, pale, or cyanotic
• Auscultation of wheezes, harsh bronchovesicular sounds, or crackles
• Cough

CAUSES & RISK FACTORS
Exposure to smoke, usually because of being trapped in a burning building

DIAGNOSIS

DIFFERENTIAL DIAGNOSIS
N/A

CBC/BIOCHEMISTRY/URINALYSIS
• Neutropenia—poor prognostic sign; indicates neutrophil sequestration in the lungs
• Thrombocytopenia—may suggest platelet sequestration or consumption
• Serum chemistry profile—may reveal hypoxic damage to other organ systems (e.g., kidneys or liver)
• Urinalysis—usually normal

OTHER LABORATORY TESTS
N/A

IMAGING
Thoracic radiographs—always take to establish a baseline; findings vary from normal to a bronchointerstitial or alveolar pattern; cranioventral alveolar infiltrates suggest aspiration pneumonia.

DIAGNOSTIC PROCEDURES
• Cytologic examination and culture of a transtracheal wash specimen—perform for suspected superimposed bacterial tracheobronchitis or pneumonia; results usually reveal an acute suppurative reaction with excessive mucus, neutrophils, and alveolar macrophages; bacteria may be seen, but the absence of obvious bacteria does not rule out a bacterial infection.
• Pulse oximetry or arterial blood gas analysis—may confirm hypoxemia; of less value for determining tissue oxygen delivery when carbon monoxyhemoglobin occurs
• Bronchoscopy—may demonstrate the severity of airway damage; bronchoalveolar lavage allows collection of appropriate samples for cytologic examination or culture.

TREATMENT
• Initial management—stabilization of respiratory function; establishment of a patent airway; severe upper airway edema or obstruction may require intubation or tracheostomy.
• Oxygen—administer immediately after rescue from the fire to displace carbon monoxide from hemoglobin; use the highest available concentration for at least 1 hr; deliver by mask, hood, cage, or nasal line; after elimination of carbon monoxy-hemoglobin, continue supplementation at 40%–60% as needed.
• Fluid administration—may be required with shock to support cardiovascular function but should be conservative, if possible, to minimize pulmonary edema; use synthetic colloids (e.g., hetastarch) with hypoproteinemia; high requirements with extensive dermal burns (usually considerable loss of fluid and protein from the skin surface)
• Blood or plasma transfusions—may be necessary
• Nebulization of saline—facilitate clearance of respiratory secretions
• Coupage and physical therapy—facilitate clearance of respiratory secretions
• Nutritional support—if needed to maintain body condition and immune status

MEDICATIONS

DRUGS
• Suspected bacterial infection—consider broad-spectrum antibiotics after appropriate specimens for bacterial culture have been obtained.
• Severe edema—may try diuretics (e.g., furosemide at 0.5–2 mg/kg IV, IM), but usually of little benefit; single early dose of corticosteroids may decrease airway edema

CONTRAINDICATIONS/POSSIBLE INTERACTIONS
• Diuretics—may decrease the intravascular volume without a major beneficial effect on airway function or pulmonary edema
• Corticosteroids—use only if absolutely necessary; may predispose the patient to bacterial infection

FOLLOW-UP

PATIENT MONITORING
• Carefully monitor respiratory rate and effort, mucous membrane color, heart rate and pulse quality, auscultation of the lungs, and PCV and total solids for 24–72 hr.
• Repeat radiographs in 48 hr—ensure condition is resolving; monitor for bacterial pneumonia
• Pulse oximetry and arterial blood gas analysis—as needed to monitor the degree of hypoxemia and response to treatment

POSSIBLE COMPLICATIONS
• Bacterial tracheobronchitis or pneumonia—owing to systemic immunosuppression and reduced pulmonary defenses, including poor mucociliary clearance
• Moist productive cough, fever, and failure to improve within 48 hr—provokes suspicion of pneumonia
• Profound, generalized pulmonary inflammatory response or severe systemic inflammatory response syndrome—may develop ARDS

EXPECTED COURSE AND PROGNOSIS
• Most patients deteriorate during the initial 24–48 hr after trauma and then gradually improve, unless they develop bacterial pneumonia or ARDS.
• Severe burns or organ injury—associated with a poor prognosis

MISCELLANEOUS

ABBREVIATIONS
• ARDS = acute respiratory response syndrome
• PCV = packed cell volume

Suggested Reading
Saxon WD, Kirby R. Treatment of acute burn injury and smoke inhalation. In: Kirk RW, Bonagura JD, eds. Kirk's current veterinary therapy XI. Philadelphia: Saunders, 1992:146–154.
Author Lesley G. King
Consulting Editor Eleanor C. Hawkins.

SNAKE VENOM TOXICITY—CORAL SNAKES

 BASICS

OVERVIEW

Coral Snakes

• Two clinically important subspecies in North America—*Micrurus fulvius fulvius*, eastern coral snake (North Carolina to the north; southern Florida to the south; West of the Mississippi River) and *M. fulvius tenere*, Texas coral snake (west of Mississippi; in Arkansas, Louisiana, and Texas)
• Family Elapidae—fixed front fangs
• Color pattern—bands fully encircling the body; red, yellow, and black; distinguished from the harmless tricolored king snake by the arrangement of the bands: if yellow (caution) and red (danger) color bands touch, then stay clear; relatively small head; black snout; round pupils

Bites

• Relatively uncommon—snake's reclusive behavior and nocturnal habits
• Often occur on the lip
• Onset of clinical signs may be delayed several hours (up to 18 hr) after envenomation.
• Victims develop bulbar paralysis
• Primary cause of death—respiratory collapse

SIGNALMENT
Dogs and cats

SIGNS
• Bulbar paralysis—affecting cranial motor nerves, respiratory tract, and skeletal muscles; acute flaccid quadriplegia
• Salivation—caused by dysphagia
• Dyspnea
• Dysphonia
• Hyporeflexive spinal reflexes

CAUSES & RISK FACTORS
Size of the snake

 DIAGNOSIS

DIFFERENTIAL DIAGNOSIS
• Myasthenia gravis
• Botulism
• Polyradiculoneuritis
• Tick bite paralysis

CBC/BIOCHEMISTRY/URINALYSIS
• Hemolysis
• RBC burring
• May note high creatine kinase
• Hemoglobinuria

OTHER LABORATORY TESTS
N/A

IMAGING
N/A

DIAGNOSTIC PROCEDURES
N/A

 TREATMENT

• Inpatient—hospitalized for a minimum of 48 hr
• Specific antivenin available (*M. fulvius*)—equine origin (Wyeth); cross-reactivity for both subspecies
• First aid—generally avoid; most effective measure is rapid transport to a veterinary facility for antivenin administration; **CAUTION:** do not wait for onset of clinical signs.
• Antivenin unavailable—provide ventilatory support for several days in a critical care facility.

 MEDICATIONS

DRUGS
• *M. fulvius* antivenin (Wyeth)—indicated if the history includes recent coral snake interaction; evidence of puncture wounds; clinical signs consistent with coral snake envenomation; administer 1–2 vials; additional vials may be necessary (technique same as for pit viper antivenin).
• Broad-spectrum antibiotic for 7–10 days

CONTRAINDICATIONS/POSSIBLE INTERACTIONS
• Corticosteroids—not indicated
• Observe the same precautions outlined for pit viper antivenin administration (see Snake Venom Toxicity—Pit Vipers)

 FOLLOW-UP
Clinical signs may last 1–1.5 weeks.

✔ MISCELLANEOUS

Suggested Reading
Peterson M, Meerdink G. Venomous bites and stings. In: Kirk RW, ed., Current veterinary therapy X. Philadelphia: Saunders, 1989:177–186.
Author Michael E. Peterson
Consulting Editor Gary D. Osweiler

SNAKE VENOM TOXICITY—PIT VIPERS

BASICS

OVERVIEW
• Pit vipers—*Crotalus* spp. (rattlesnakes), *Sistrurus* spp. (pigmy rattlesnakes and massassauga), and *Agkistrodon* spp. (copper-heads and cottonmouth water moccasins); retractable fangs; heat-seeking pit between the nostril and eye; triangular-shaped head
• Range—throughout the continental U.S.
• Toxicity—considered hematoxic; several species have subpopulations with lethal neurotoxic components (e.g., Mojave rattlesnake); general ranking of severity: (1) rattlesnakes, (2) moccasins, (3) copperheads
• Venom—enzymes: hyaluronidase and phospholipase A (cause local tissue injury) and others that interfere with the coagulation cascade (cause major coagulation defects); nonenzymatic polypeptides: affect the cardiovascular and respiratory systems
• Bite—85% of victims have altered laboratory values and clinically important swelling; severe hypotension from pooling of blood within the splanchnic (dogs) or pulmonary (cats) vessels; fluid loss from the vascular compartment secondary to severe peripheral edema

SIGNALMENT
Dogs and cats

SIGNS
General Comments
May be delayed for 8 hr after envenomation
Historical Findings
• Outdoors, rural setting
• Owner saw bite or heard snake.
Physical Examination Findings
• Puncture wounds on head and forelimbs in most animals
• Local tissue swelling and pain surrounding bite site
• Bruising, with possible necrosis and sloughing of bite site tissue
• Ecchymosis and petechiation of tissues and mucous membranes
• Hypotension and shock
• Tachycardia
• Shallow respiration
• Depression and lethargy
• Nausea and excessive salivation

CAUSES & RISK FACTORS
Snake-associated
• Toxic peptide fraction:enzyme fraction ratio—higher in spring; lower in fall; high in very young snakes
• Amount of venom production since last bite
• Aggressiveness and motivation of snake
Victim-associated
• Bite site—bites to tongue and torso are of major concern.
• Size of victim
• Elapsed time between bite and initiation of treatment
• Activity level of victim after the bite—activity increases absorption of venom.

DIAGNOSIS

DIFFERENTIAL DIAGNOSIS
• Angioedema secondary to insect envenomation
• Blunt trauma
• Penetrating wound
• Animal bite
• Penetration of foreign body
• Draining abscess

CBC/BIOCHEMISTRY/URINALYSIS
• Hemoconcentration
• Burring of RBCs within first 24 hr
• Thrombocytopenia
• Hypokalemia
• High creatine kinase
• Hematuria or myoglobinuria

OTHER LABORATORY TESTS
Clotting tests—may note prolonged ACT, PT, and PTT; may note high FDP

IMAGING
N/A

DIAGNOSTIC PROCEDURES
ECG—may detect ventricular arrhythmia, especially in severely depressed patients

TREATMENT
• Tissue reaction around the bite site—not a reliable indicator of systemic toxicity
• Bite location—may affect uptake of venom; bites to tongue and torso are of major concern.
• First aid measures—calming patient; transporting quickly to a veterinary facility
• Intravenous fluids—correct hypotension

MEDICATIONS

DRUGS
• Antivenin (Crotalidae polyvalent, equine origin)—1 vial mixed with 200 mL crystalloid fluids administered slowly IV with careful monitoring of the inner pinna for onset of hyperemia (indicator of possible allergic reaction)
• Allergic reaction—stop antivenin; give diphenhydramine; after 5 min, restart antivenin infusion at a slower rate

CONTRAINDICATIONS/POSSIBLE INTERACTIONS
• Corticosteroids—of no value
• DMSO—enhances uptake and spread of venom
• Heparin—do not use.

FOLLOW-UP
• Repeated laboratory analysis—6 hr after admission to hospital
• Clinical signs—may last 1–1.5 weeks

MISCELLANEOUS

ABBREVIATIONS
• ACT = activated clotting time
• DMSO = dimethyl sulfoxide
• FDP = fibrin degradation products
• PT = prothrombin time
• PTT = partial thromboplastin time

Suggested Reading
Peterson M, Meerdink G. Venomous bites and stings. In: Kirk RW, Bonagura D, eds. Current veterinary therapy X. Philadelphia: Saunders, 1989:177–186.
Author Michael E. Peterson
Consulting Editor Gary D. Osweiler

BASICS

OVERVIEW
• Spermatocele—a cystic distension of the efferent ductules or epididymis containing spermatozoa, usually associated with loss of patency of the duct
• Sperm granuloma—the granulomatous inflammatory reaction that develops when spermatozoa escape from the efferent ductules or epididymal duct into the surrounding tissue; clinically important when bilateral obstruction of the duct system leads to azoospermia

SIGNALMENT
N/A

SIGNS
• Suspected in azoospermic dog with normal-sized testicles
• Rarely associated with pain or visible or palpable lesions

CAUSES & RISK FACTORS
• Trauma causing a break in the epididymal duct—releases sperm antigens into the surrounding tissue
• Adenomyosis—invasion of the epithelial lining cells of the epididymis into the muscular layers; may be a factor; associated with excess estrogenic stimulation
• Epithelial hyperplasia of the epididymis—may be a precursor of adenomyosis; not often seen in dogs < 2.5 years old; noted to some degree in 75% of dogs > 7.75 years old; risk increases with age.
• Complication of vasectomy—especially when surgical technique was not meticulous
• Congenital anomaly

DIAGNOSIS

DIFFERENTIAL DIAGNOSIS
• Azoospermia (dogs)—testicular degeneration; hypoplasia; retrograde ejaculation
• Scrotal signs (e.g., pain and palpable lesions; dogs)—epididymitis; orchitis; scrotal dermatitis

CBC/BIOCHEMISTRY/URINALYSIS
• Urinalysis (cystocentesis) after ejaculation—rule out retrograde ejaculation
• CBC and biochemistry profile–usually normal

OTHER LABORATORY TESTS
• Assay for canine FSH—high concentration associated with degeneration and hypoplasia; normal concentration in azoospermic dogs with normal-sized testicles associated with bilateral blockage of the epididymis or retrograde ejaculation

IMAGING
N/A

DIAGNOSTIC PROCEDURES
Surgical testicular biopsy—reveals epididymis; spermatoceles appear as yellow cysts within the epididymis.

PATHOLOGIC FINDINGS
Histologic examination of testicular specimen—complete spermatogenesis in an azoospermic dog indicates blockage.

TREATMENT
• Azoospermic dogs—rarely spontaneously recover
• Bilateral blockage of the epididymis—probably not treatable except by micro-surgical anastomosis of the ductus deferens to the cystic structure or patent segment of the epididymis; few attempts have been made to perform this procedure in dogs.

MEDICATIONS
None recognized as effective in unblocking the duct system.

DRUGS
N/A

FOLLOW-UP
N/A

MISCELLANEOUS

ABBREVIATION
FSH = follicle-stimulating hormone

Suggested Reading
Althouse GC, Evans LE, Hopkins SM. Episodic scrotal mutilation with concurrent bilateral sperm granuloma in a dog. J Am Vet Med Assoc 1993;202:776–778.
Mayenco Aguirre AM, Garcia Fernandez P, Sanchez Muela M. Sperm granuloma in the dog: complication of vasectomy. J Sm Anim Pract 1996;37:392–393.
McEntee K. Reproductive pathology of do-mestic animals. New York: Academic Press, 1990;309–332.
Author Rolf E. Larsen
Consulting Editor Sara K. Lyle

BASICS

OVERVIEW
• Black widow spider—*Latrodectus* spp.; females toxic; 2–2.5 cm in length; shiny black; red or orange hourglass mark on the ventral abdomen; immature females brown with red to orange stripes that change into the hourglass shape as she darkens to black and ages
• Bites—may be dry (no venom injected)
• Range—genus found in every state except Alaska; often found around buildings and human habitation
• Venom—contains α-latrotoxin, a potent neurotoxin; opens cation-selective channels at the presynaptic nerve terminal; causes massive release of acetylcholine and norepinephrine, which causes sustained muscular spasms

SIGNALMENT
Dogs and cats

SIGNS

Historical Findings
• Usually sudden onset
• May be delayed several days with mild envenomation

Physical Examination Findings
Dogs
• Progressive muscle fasciculations
• Severe pain
• Cramping of large muscle masses
• Abdominal rigidity without tenderness
• Marked restlessness, writhing, and contorted spasms
• Hypertension and tachycardia anticipated
• May note bronchorrhea, hypersalivation, hyperesthesia, lymph node tenderness, regional numbness, facial swelling (*Latrodectus* facies)
• Rhabdomyolysis possible
Cats
• Early, marked paralysis
• Severe pain—manifested by howling and loud vocalizations

• Excessive salivation and restlessness
• Vomiting—not unusual to vomit up the spider
• Diarrhea
• Muscle tremors and cramping
• Ataxia and inability to stand—becomes adynamic and atonic
• Respiratory collapse
• Death without antivenin

CAUSES & RISK FACTORS
• Very young or old age—increased risk
• Systemic hypertension—increased risk

DIAGNOSIS

DIFFERENTIAL DIAGNOSIS
• Back pain from disk disease
• Acute abdomen

CBC/BIOCHEMISTRY/URINALYSIS
• Leukocytosis
• High creatine kinase—with severe muscle spasms
• Albuminuria

OTHER LABORATORY TESTS
Normal stool hemoccult test

IMAGING
Normal abdominal radiographs

DIAGNOSTIC PROCEDURES
N/A

TREATMENT
• Inpatient—supportive care
• Monitor respiratory status.

MEDICATIONS

DRUGS
• Antivenin (Lyovac (latrodectus), equine origin)—1 vial mixed with 100 mL crystalloid solution IV given slowly with monitoring of

the inner ear pinna for evidence of hyperemia (indicator of allergic response); dose usually sufficient for response within 30 min; with proper use, reactions are rare.
• Allergic reaction—stop antivenin; diphenhydramine; after 5–10 min, restart antivenin at a slower rate
• Muscle spasms and severe pain—controlled by careful intravenous administration of narcotics or benzodiazepines at lowest effective dosage to avoid respiratory depression; methocarbamol (Robaxin) relieves muscle spasms but has no effect on hypertension or respiratory depression.
• Intractable hypertension—sodium nitroprusside

CONTRAINDICATIONS/POSSIBLE INTERACTIONS
Intravenous fluids with hypertension

FOLLOW-UP
• Weekly monitoring of the wound site until healed
• Prognosis—uncertain for days; cats, usually fatal without antivenin
• Weakness, fatigue, and insomnia—may persist for months

MISCELLANEOUS

Suggested Reading
Peterson ME, Meerdink G. Venomous bites and stings. In: Kirk RW, Bonagura D, eds. Current veterinary therapy X. Philadelphia: Saunders, 1989:177–186.
Author Michael E. Peterson
Consulting Editor Gary D. Osweiler

SPIDER VENOM TOXICOSIS—BROWN RECLUSE FAMILY

 ## BASICS

OVERVIEW
• Brown recluse family—*Loxosceles* spp.; 8–15 mm in body size; legs 2–3 cm long; violin-shaped pattern on cephalothorax with the neck of the fiddle extending caudally; active at night
• Distribution—found throughout the southern U.S. and up the Mississippi River valley to southern Wisconsin
• Bites—usually occur when spider becomes trapped in bedding; induce necrotic arachnidism, an indolent dermatonecrotic lesion mediated by the venom enzyme sphingo-myelinase D, direct hemolysis of erythrocytes, platelet aggregation, renal failure, coagulopathy, and death

SIGNALMENT
Dogs and cats

SIGNS
• Local pain and stinging (may last 6–8 hr); followed by pruritus and soreness
• Classic target lesion—ischemic area with a dark central eschar on an uneven erythematous background; after 2–5 weeks, central eschar may slough, leaving a deep, nonhealing ulcer that usually spares muscle tissue.
• Less common—hemolytic anemia with hemoglobinuria in the first 24 hr
• Other possible systemic manifestations within the first 2–3 days after envenomation—fever; chills; rash; weakness; leukocytosis; nausea; arthralgia

CAUSES & RISK FACTORS
N/A

 ## DIAGNOSIS

DIFFERENTIAL DIAGNOSIS
• Bacterial or mycobacterial infection
• Decubitus ulcer
• Third-degree burn
• Hemolytic anemia
• Jaundice
• Thrombocytopenia
• Ehrlichiosis
• RBC parasitism

CBC/BIOCHEMISTRY/URINALYSIS
• Anemia
• Leukocytosis
• Thrombocytopenia
• Hemoglobinuria

OTHER LABORATORY TESTS
Coagulation profile—may reveal prolonged clotting times

IMAGING
N/A

DIAGNOSTIC PROCEDURES
N/A

 ## TREATMENT
• Supportive care—fluid therapy; presumptive treatment of bacterial superinfection; (rarely) blood transfusion
• Mild, local envenomation—usually responds to cool compresses
• Necrotic lesions—may need débridement after erythema has subsided
• Severe envenomation—may require skin grafting after the lesion reaches full maturity

 ## MEDICATIONS

DRUGS
• Dapsone (dogs)—1 mg/kg q8h for 10 days; for dermatonecrotic lesions; a leukocyte inhibitor; minimizes inflammatory component of the envenomation; repeat, if needed.
• Cats—author has no experience using dapsone in cats.
• Antibiotics—patients not treated with dapsone

CONTRAINDICATIONS/ POSSIBLE INTERACTIONS
• Dapsone—may cause hypersensitivity and methemoglobinemia in patients with G6PD deficiency
• Do not use heat—exacerbates condition

 ## FOLLOW-UP
Monitor wound site weekly until healed.

 ## MISCELLANEOUS

ABBREVIATION
G6PD = glucose-6-phosphate dehydrogenase

Suggested Reading
Peterson ME, Meerdink G. Bites and stings of venomous animals. In: Kirk RW, ed. Current veterinary therapy X. Philadelphia: Saunders, 1989:177–186.
Author Michael E. Peterson
Consulting Editor Gary D. Osweiler

SPLENIC TORSION

BASICS

OVERVIEW
• May occur as a separate entity in association with gastric dilatation-volvulus syndrome
• Acute or chronic
• Pathophysiology—unknown
• Systems affected—Hemic/Lymphatic/Immune and Cardiovascular
• Isolated splenic torsion uncommon

SIGNALMENT
• More common in large-breed, deep-chested dogs, such as German shepherds and Great Danes
• No sex predilection

SIGNS

Historical Findings
• Acute—cardiovascular collapse and abdominal pain
• Chronic—intermittent anorexia, vomiting, weight loss, and possibly hemoglobinuria

Physical Examination Findings
• Pale mucous membranes, tachycardia, and other signs of hypoperfusion
• Palpable abdominal mass

CAUSES & RISK FACTORS
• Large breed and deep chest (dogs)
• Prior stretching of gastrosplenic, phrenicosplenic, and splenocolic ligaments
• Historical gastric dilatation
• Excessive exercise, rolling, and retching may contribute

DIAGNOSIS

DIFFERENTIAL DIAGNOSIS
• Other splenic disease (e.g., neoplasia and immune-mediated disease)
• Acute gastrointestinal disease with abdominal pain
• Other causes of intravascular hemolysis

CBC/BIOCHEMISTRY/URINALYSIS
• Anemia
• Thrombocytopenia
• Leukocytosis
• High liver enzyme values
• Hemoglobulinuria

OTHER LABORATORY TESTS
Coagulation test—DIC (prolonged prothrombin time, partial thromboplastin time, and fibrin split products) because of accelerated consumption

IMAGING

Abdominal Radiography
• Cranial or midabdominal mass may be seen.
• Spleen may be abnormally located.

Abdominal Ultrasound
• Splenic congestion
• Dilated splenic veins
• Splenic infarction

DIAGNOSTIC PROCEDURES
ECG—may show ventricular arrhythmias

PATHOLOGIC FINDINGS
Splenic congestion and infarction

TREATMENT
• Surgical emergency
• After adequate cardiovascular stabilization, a splenectomy should be performed without untwisting the splenic pedicle.
• A permanent gastropexy should also be performed because of the association with gastric dilatation volvulus syndrome.
• A splenic specimen should be submitted for histopathologic examination.
• Fluid support and cardiovascular monitoring indicated after splenectomy

MEDICATIONS

DRUGS
• No specific drugs required
• Postoperative pain relief advised
• Heparin (75 IU/kg SC q8h) or plasma transfusion may be considered if DIC documented

CONTRAINDICATIONS/POSSIBLE INTERACTIONS
None

FOLLOW-UP
Surgical correction considered curative

MISCELLANEOUS

ABBREVIATION
DIC = disseminated intravascular coagulation

Suggested Reading
Hurley RE, Stone MS. Isolated torsion of the splenic pedicle in a dog. J Am Anim Hosp Assoc 1994;30:119–122.
Author Elizabeth Rozanski
Consulting Editor Susan M. Cotter

BASICS

OVERVIEW
• Degenerative, noninflammatory condition of the vertebral column characterized by the production of osteophytes along the ventral, lateral, and dorsolateral aspects of the vertebral endplates
• Most common location—dogs: thoracolumbar spine in the area of the anticlinal vertebra and the upper lumbar vertebrae; cats: thoracic vertebrae reported in 68% of asymptomatic domestic cats

SIGNALMENT
• Dogs and cats
• Dogs—commonly seen in large breeds, especially German shepherds; also boxers, Airedale terriers, and cocker spaniels
• Occurrence increases with age; 50% of dogs by 6 years and 75% by 9 years; may be evident in young dogs with an inherited predisposition
• Females affected more than males.

SIGNS
General Comments
• Patients are typically asymptomatic; lesions of minor clinical importance
• Pain may follow fracture of bony spurs or bridges.

Historical Findings
• Stiffness
• Restricted motion
• Pain

Physical Examination Findings
Neurologic deficits referable to the spinal cord or nerve root compression unusual

CAUSES & RISK FACTORS
• Repeated microtrauma
• Major trauma
• Inherited predisposition

DIAGNOSIS

DIFFERENTIAL DIAGNOSIS
• Diskospondylitis—differentiated by radiographic evidence of end-plate lysis
• Spinal osteoarthritis—degeneration of the articular facet joints

CBC/BIOCHEMISTRY/URINALYSIS
Normal

OTHER LABORATORY TESTS
N/A

IMAGING
Spinal radiography—initially shows osteophytes as triangular projections several millimeters from the edge of the vertebral body; with progression, they appear to bridge the intervertebral space; true ankylosis rare

DIAGNOSTIC PROCEDURES
Myelography and CT or MRI—for unusual cases; demonstrate an atypical dorsal osteophyte compressing the spinal cord or nerve roots or encroaching on critical soft tissue structures

TREATMENT

• Inform owner that the condition is usually an asymptomatic, incidental finding and is probably not responsible for the clinical signs.
• Back pain or neurologic deficits—perform a neurodiagnostic evaluation of the spine in consideration of surgical intervention.
• Spondylosis—treat as outpatient with strict rest and analgesic administration or possibly acupuncture.
• Obesity—recommend a weight-reduction program.

MEDICATIONS

DRUGS
Use only when the patient is exhibiting signs.

NSAIDs
• Preferred to steroids in dogs unless the patient has neurologic deficits, because of fewer side effects
• Administer after feeding and in combination with an antacid (cimetidine at 6–10 mg/kg PO q8h or ranitidine at 1–2 mg/kg PO q12h) or a gastrointestinal protector (misoprostol at 3–5 μg/kg PO q6–8h) to reduce the possibility of gastrointestinal ulceration
• Carprofen (Rimadyl)—2.2mg/kg PO q12h in dogs

• Phenylbutazone—11–22 mg/kg PO for maximum daily dose of 80 mg in dogs
• Naproxen—2 mg/kg PO q48h for maximum daily dose of 75 mg in dogs
• Aspirin—dogs: buffered, enteric-coated aspirin (e.g., Ascriptin or Ecotrin) at 10–20 mg/kg q8–12h); adult cats: a baby aspirin or one-quarter of a 325-mg aspirin tablet every 3 days
• Other NSAIDs should be used cautiously, because they are more likely to cause gastrointestinal ulceration.
• Acetaminophen (Tylenol)—5 mg/kg PO q12h PO in dogs only; non-NSAID analgesic

Corticosteroids
• Prednisone—0.5–1.0 mg/kg divided q12h; taper to alternate days or less, if possible
• Use only in patients with neurologic deficits.

CONTRAINDICATIONS/POSSIBLE INTERACTIONS
• Acetaminophen (Tylenol)—do not use in cats.
• Avoid prolonged administration of NSAIDs or combinations of NSAIDs and steroids because of risk of gastrointestinal ulceration.

FOLLOW-UP

• Gradually return the animal to normal activity after signs have subsided for several weeks.
• Relapse can occur with strenuous activity.

MISCELLANEOUS

Suggested Reading
Romatowski J. Spondylosis deformans in the dog. Compend Contin Educ Pract Vet 1986;8:531–536.
Author Richard J. Joseph
Consulting Editor Joane M. Parent

SPOROTRICHOSIS

BASICS

OVERVIEW
- A zoonotic fungal disease that may affect the integument or lymphatics or be generalized
- Caused by the virtually ubiquitous dimorphic fungus *Sporothrix schenckii,* which typically infects via direct inoculation; direct inoculation not a requirement

SIGNALMENT
- Cats, dogs, and humans
- Dogs—more commonly seen in hunting dogs because of the increased likelihood of puncture wounds associated with thorns or splinters
- Cats—intact male cats that roam outdoors and fight because of the increased likelihood of puncture wounds and acquiring the disease from their opponents

SIGNS

Historical Findings
- Previous trauma or puncture wound in the affected area—variable finding
- Poor response to previous antibacterial therapy

Physical Examination Findings
- Cutaneous form—dog: associated with numerous nodules, which may drain or crust, typically affecting the head or trunk; cat: lesions often initially appear as wounds or abscesses, mimicking wounds associated with fighting, found on the head, lumbar region, or distal limbs
- Cutaneolymphatic form—usually an extension of the cutaneous form; spreads via the lymphatics, resulting in new nodules and draining tracts or crusts; lymphadenopathy common
- Disseminated form—associated with the systemic signs of malaise and fever; consider the potential of an underlying immunosuppressive disease as a contributing factor

CAUSES & RISK FACTORS
- Animals exposed to soil rich in decaying organic debris appear to be predisposed.
- Puncture wounds associated with foreign bodies provide an increased opportunity for infection in dogs; cat scratches provide a similar opportunity in roaming cats.
- Immunosuppressive disease—risk factor for the disseminated form

DIAGNOSIS

DIFFERENTIAL DIAGNOSIS
- Various bacterial and fungal diseases— consider when symptoms include a nodular granulomatous disease and draining tracts
- Neoplastic conditions
- Parasitic infections (*Demodex* or *Pelodera*)

CBC/BIOCHEMISTRY/URINALYSIS
N/A

OTHER LABORATORY TESTS
N/A

IMAGING
N/A

DIAGNOSTIC PROCEDURES
- **REMEMBER:** this is a zoonotic disease and proper precautions should be taken to prevent infection; absence of a break in the skin does not protect against the disease.
- Cytology of the exudate and staining—cats: often the only test necessary to confirm infection; cigar- to round-shaped yeast may be found intracellularly or free in the exudate; dogs: special fungal stains (PAS or GMS) may aid in the diagnosis; a negative finding does not rule out the disease
- Cultures of the deeply affected tissue— often require surgery to obtain an adequate sample; alert the laboratory that sporotrichosis is a differential diagnosis; secondary bacterial infections common

TREATMENT
- Remember the zoonotic potential when treating patients.
- Sometimes outpatient treatment may be considered.

MEDICATIONS

DRUGS
SSKI
- Treatment of choice—dogs: 40 mg/kg PO q8h with food; cats: 20 mg/kg PO q12h with food
- Continue for 30 days after resolution of the clinical lesions.
- Dogs—if signs of iodism are noted (dry hair coat, excessive scales, nasal or ocular discharge, vomiting, depression, or collapse), discontinue for 1 week; mild symptoms, reinitiate at the same dose; severe or recurrent symptoms, consider other drugs

- Cats—signs of iodism (depression, vomiting, anorexia, twitching, hypothermia, and cardiovascular collapse) are more common; if noted, discontinue; use other drugs

Ketoconazole and Itraconazole
- Shown encouraging results for fungal diseases in cats and dogs
- Dogs—ketoconazole: 15mg/kg PO q12h, preferably with an acidic meal (e.g., tomato juice), until 1 month after clinical resolution; resolution should occur within approximately 3 months; side effects relatively mild, anorexia most common; acute hepatopathy, pruritus, alopecia, and lightening of the hair color reported
- Cats—ketoconazole: 5–10 mg/kg PO q12–24h, or itraconazole 10mg/kg/day preferably with an acidic meal until 1 month after clinical resolution; side effects include gastrointestinal disturbances, depression, fever, jaundice, and neurologic signs; may be necessary to alternate drugs

CONTRAINDICATIONS/POSSIBLE INTERACTIONS
N/A

FOLLOW-UP

PATIENT MONITORING
Re-evaluate every 2 to 4 weeks for clinical signs and side effects associated with treatment.

PREVENTION/AVOIDANCE
Although difficult, try to determine the source of the original infection to prevent repeat infections.

EXPECTED COURSE AND PROGNOSIS
Unresponsive to therapy—not unexpected; consider alternative treatment or combined treatment regimens (SSKI and ketoconazole); itraconazole relatively untested but promising

MISCELLANEOUS

ZOONOTIC POTENTIAL
Zoonotic; proper precautions and client education are of paramount importance.

ABBREVIATION
SSKI = supersaturated potassium iodide

Suggested Reading
Scott DW, Miller WH, Griffin CE. Muller and Kirk's small animal dermatology. 5th ed. Philadelphia: Saunders, 1995.
Author Dunbar Gram
Consulting Editor Karen Helton Rhodes

SQUAMOUS CELL CARCINOMA, DIGIT

 BASICS

OVERVIEW
• Malignant tumor arising from the subungual epithelium
• Cats—metastasis to one or multiple digits from other cutaneous sites reported
• Dogs—most common digital tumor

SIGNALMENT
• Dogs and rarely cats
• Large breeds and black dogs—predisposed; particularly standard poodles and Labrador retrievers
• Median age, 10 years; may occur in dogs as young as 4 years old

SIGNS
• Swelling of digit—reason for examination
• May note ulceration
• Multiple digits—rarely in dogs; may be seen in cats as part of a metastatic process
• Lymph node and lung metastasis—reported; uncommon at the time of examination

CAUSES & RISK FACTORS
• Cause—unknown
• Risk factors—hereditary; black skin pigmentation

 DIAGNOSIS

DIFFERENTIAL DIAGNOSIS
• Nail bed infection
• Other tumors—melanoma; soft tissue sarcomas; mast cell tumor

CBC/BIOCHEMISTRY/URINALYSIS
N/A

OTHER LABORATORY TESTS
N/A

IMAGING
• Thoracic radiographs—important to rule out metastatic disease; results typically normal at the time of diagnosis
• Radiographs of the affected foot—reveal lysis of the third phalanx of the affected digit in 75% of patients

DIAGNOSTIC PROCEDURES
• Wedge biopsy of abnormal tissue—required to confirm diagnosis
• Lymph node biopsy—may be indicated

 TREATMENT

• Amputation of the affected digit at the level of the metacarpal (or metatarsal) phalangeal joint—treatment of choice
• Complete surgical excision of the primary lesion and no evidence of metastasis—no additional treatment required

 MEDICATIONS

DRUGS
• Multiple affected digits owing to metastasis (cats)—surgery not an option because digits from multiple limbs are generally affected; pain control with piroxicam (0.3 mg/kg q24–28h) may offer temporary relief; benefit of chemotherapy unknown

CONTRAINDICATIONS/POSSIBLE INTERACTIONS
None

 FOLLOW-UP

• Survival with complete surgical excision and no evidence of metastatic disease—1 year, 76%; 2 years, 43%
• Recurrence not anticipated
• Metastasis uncommon

 MISCELLANEOUS

Suggested Reading

O'Brien MG, Berg J, Engler SJ. Treatment by digital amputation of subungual squamous cell carcinoma in dogs: 21 cases (1987–1988). J Am Vet Med Assoc 1992;201:759–761.
Thomas RC, Fox LE. Tumors of the skin and subcutis. In: Morrison WB, ed. Cancer in dogs and cats: medical and surgical management. Baltimore: Williams & Wilkins, 1998:489–510.
Author Robyn E. Elmslie
Consulting Editor Wallace B. Morrison

SQUAMOUS CELL CARCINOMA, EAR

BASICS

OVERVIEW
- Malignant tumor arising from the squamous epithelium of the skin of the pinnae
- Occasionally involves the ear canal
- Most are very invasive but very slow to metastasize.
- Most common in animals that have had high exposure to sunlight

SIGNALMENT
- Cats and rarely dogs
- Common in cats with white or light-colored fur and skin
- Mean age at time of diagnosis—12 years (range, 7–24 years)

SIGNS
- Lesions develop slowly over months to years.
- Precancerous stage—characterized by crusty eczematous lesions of the edge of the pinnae that flare up and regress repeatedly
- Proliferation and ulceration of the ear—signal the true cancerous phase; ear becomes extensively disfigured if left untreated.
- Metastatic disease uncommon

CAUSES & RISK FACTORS
- Prolonged sunlight exposure—important cause
- White fur and light skin pigmentation—risk factors

DIAGNOSIS

DIFFERENTIAL DIAGNOSIS
- Classic clinical findings—help differentiate from other neoplastic conditions
- Lesions on the pinnae caused by vasculitis or cryoglobulinemia—may resemble squamous cell carcinoma

CBC/BIOCHEMISTRY/URINALYSIS
N/A

OTHER LABORATORY TESTS
N/A

IMAGING
Thoracic radiographs—may help definitely rule out the rare pulmonary metastasis

DIAGNOSTIC PROCEDURES
- Biopsy of pinna—confirm diagnosis
- Cytologic—evaluate lymph nodes; may help definitively rule out metastasis

PATHOLOGIC FINDINGS
Distinguished microscopically by characteristic groups of epithelial cells and keratinizing cells forming keratin pearls

TREATMENT

- Aggressive surgical excision—required; must amputate the pinnae below the demarcation of unhealthy tissue
- Histologic evaluation of the surgical margins—essential to assess completeness of surgical excision
- Photodynamic therapy—alternative to amputation; results less predictable; more than one treatment often required
- Cryosurgery—successful for small lesions
- Hyperthermia—reported to be beneficial

MEDICATIONS

DRUGS
- Etretinate—0.75–1 mg/kg q24h; used successfully to prevent progression of precancerous lesions
- Vitamin E—400–600 IU PO q12h; may be beneficial to prevent or delay progression of precancerous lesions
- Bleomycin—10–20 IU/m² SC once per week; has been used systemically to treat advanced disease
- Chemotherapy—benefit not yet established

CONTRAINDICATIONS/POSSIBLE INTERACTIONS
None

FOLLOW-UP

- Limit sun exposure—may prevent development of new lesions
- Sunscreen and tattooing—useful for preventing development of new lesions
- Early treatment of crusting lesions on the ears by cryosurgery or surgical excision is recommended.
- Prognosis—good if complete surgical excision is achieved

✓ MISCELLANEOUS

Suggested Reading

Dorn CR, Taylor D. Sunlight exposure and the risk of developing cutaneous and oral squamous cell carcinoma in white cats. J Natl Cancer Inst 1971;46:1073–1078.

Thomas RC, Fox LE. Tumors of the skin and subcutis. In: Morrison WB, ed. Cancer in dogs and cats: medical and surgical management. Baltimore: Williams & Wilkins, 1998:589–610.

Author Robyn E. Elmslie
Consulting Editor Wallace B. Morrison

SQUAMOUS CELL CARCINOMA, GINGIVA

BASICS

OVERVIEW
• Progressive, rapid (weeks), local invasion of neoplastic epithelial cells within the oral cavity in dogs and cats
• The most common oral malignancy in cats and second most common in dogs
• Highly invasive to the bone with a nonencapsulated, raised, irregular, ulcerated, or necrotic surface
• Metastasis—rare; spread to lymph nodes more common than to the lungs
• Cause of death—secondary to local recurrence, dysphagia, and subsequent cachexia

SIGNALMENT
• Dogs and cats
• Mean age (dogs and cats)—10.5 years (range, 3–15 years)
• More common in medium- and large-breed dogs

SIGNS

Historical Findings
• Excessive salivation
• Dysphagia
• Halitosis
• Bloody oral discharge
• Weight loss

Physical Examination Findings
• Loose teeth
• Facial deformity
• Cervical lymphadenmegaly—occasionally
• Rostral mandible—most common site

CAUSES & RISK FACTORS
None identified

DIAGNOSIS

DIFFERENTIAL DIAGNOSIS
• Other oral malignancy
• Epulis
• Abscess
• Benign polyp

CBC/BIOCHEMISTRY/URINALYSIS
Usually normal

OTHER LABORATORY TESTS
Cytologic evaluation—obtain impression smear from an incisional biopsy specimen (wedge); may yield diagnosis

IMAGING
• Skull radiography—evaluate bone involvement deep to the mass.
• Thoracic radiography—detect pulmonary metastasis (uncommon).

DIAGNOSTIC PROCEDURES
Large, deep tissue biopsy (down to bone)—required to sufficiently differentiate from other oral malignancies

TREATMENT
• Radical surgical excision—required (e.g., hemimandibulectomy); usually well-tolerated by patient; survival improves when excisional margins are free of neoplastic cells; margins of at least 2 cm necessary
• Cryosurgery—indicated for small lesions minimally adherent to the bone
• Inpatient radiotherapy—considerable long-term control if inoperable; most plans attempt 40–60 Gy over 3–6 weeks; combined with low-dose cisplatin chemotherapy improves overall survival; combined with hyperthermia does not improve overall survival; complications common in cats (mucositis, anorexia, and dehydration requiring aggressive supportive care)
• Soft foods—may be recommended to prevent tumor ulceration or after radical oral excision

MEDICATIONS

DRUGS
• Cisplatin (dogs)—60–70 mg/m^2 IV once every 3–4 weeks for four treatments; provides marked palliation of clinical signs; response depends on severity of the localized or metastatic lesion; nephrotoxic must use with saline diuresis (18.3 mL/kg/hr IV over 6 hr; give cisplatin after 4 hr)
• Butorphanol—0.4 mg/kg IM; before and after cisplatin; reduces emesis
• Local control (palliation) by intralesionally administered cisplatin has been reported.

CONTRAINDICATIONS/POSSIBLE INTERACTIONS
• Cisplatin—never use in cats.
• Chemotherapy may be toxic; seek advice if unfamiliar with cytotoxic drugs.

FOLLOW-UP
• Survival after excision (dogs)—1 year, 25%–45%; 2-year, 20%–35%
• Median survival after excision (dogs)—7–11 months; survival improves when excisional margins are free of neoplastic cells.
• Survivals after excision and radiotherapy (dogs)—mean, 7 months; median 8 months; range, 0–27 months
• Survival after excision (cats)—mean, 2.5 months; median, 14 months; range, 0–36 months
• Median survival after excision and radiotherapy (cats)—14 months; range, 1–36 months
• Cause of death—related to local recurrence and secondary anorexia and cachexia
• Overall prognosis—poor in cats because most tumors are locally invasive and diagnosed late in the course of disease

MISCELLANEOUS

Suggested Reading
Hutson CA, Willauer CC, Walder EJ, et al. Treatment of mandibular squamous cell carcinoma in cats by use of mandibulectomy and radiotherapy: seven cases (1987–1989). J Am Vet Med Assoc 1992;201:777–781.
Oakes MG, Lewis DD, Hedlund CS, et al. Canine oral neoplasia. Compend Contin Educ Pract Vet 1993;15:15–31.
Author Kevin A. Hahn
Consulting Editor Wallace B. Morrison

SQUAMOUS CELL CARCINOMA, LUNG

BASICS

OVERVIEW
• Rare primary tumor of bronchial epithelial origin with squamous metaplasia (epidermoid carcinoma)
• Commonly develops in the right caudal lung lobe in dogs and the left caudal lung lobe in cats
• High metastatic potential, especially if regional lymph nodes are positive

SIGNALMENT
• Dogs and cats
• Mean age—dogs, 11 years; cats, 12 years
• No breed predilection

SIGNS

Historical Findings
• Sometimes none
• Harsh, nonproductive cough
• Dyspnea
• Lethargy or exercise intolerance
• Cachexia and weight loss
• Lameness—resulting from bone metastasis

Physical Examination Findings
• Tachypnea
• Wheeze
• Hemoptysis
• Hypertrophic osteopathy
• Neuromyopathy and paraplegia
• Digital lesions (metastasis) in cats

CAUSES & RISK FACTORS
Approximately 74% of patients come from an urban environment.

DIAGNOSIS

DIFFERENTIAL DIAGNOSIS
• Bronchogenic cysts
• Bullae and blebs
• Abscesses
• Paragonimus
• Eosinophilic lung disease
• Other primary lung neoplasm
• Metastatic pulmonary neoplasm
• Aspiration pneumonia

CBC/BIOCHEMISTRY/URINALYSIS
• Neutrophilic leukocytosis
• Hypercalcemia rare

OTHER LABORATORY TESTS
Cytology—examination of tissue obtained by endoscopic bronchial brushing or fine-needle aspiration; may provide tentative diagnosis

IMAGING
• Survey thoracic radiographs—solitary mass arising from a single focus most common appearance
• Right caudal lung lobes in dogs and the left caudal lung lobe in cats common
• Margins—well circumscribed; sharp demarcation from other surrounding normal parenchyma
• Arises from larger bronchi
• Trachea or mainstem bronchi—displaced or compressed
• Partial or complete airway obstruction and peripheral atelectasis

DIAGNOSTIC PROCEDURES
Tissue biopsy—definitive diagnosis

TREATMENT
• Surgery—wide and complete resection of affected lung lobe; best opportunity for long-term control; examine tracheobronchial lymph nodes; manually palpate all remaining lung lobes; biopsy of lymph nodes advised, even if they appear normal; removal is best, but frequently difficult and thus not often done
• Chemotherapy—best to start when there is residual disease that can be measured on radiographs or ultrasound; may administer before or after surgery; best to have some tumor present so it is possible to evaluate response

MEDICATIONS

DRUGS
• Cisplatin—60 mg/m² IV every 3 or 4 weeks for four treatments; nephrotoxic, so must use with saline diuresis (18.3 mL/kg/hr IV over 6 hr; give cisplatin after 4 hr
• Butorphanol—0.4 mg/kg IM before and after cisplatin; reduces emesis
• Doxorubicin—dogs > 10 kg: 30 mg/m² IV once every 2 weeks for five treatments; dogs < 10 kg and cats: 1 mg/kg; has provided marked palliation

CONTRAINDICATIONS/POSSIBLE INTERACTIONS
• Cisplatin—never use in cats.
• Chemotherapy may be toxic; seek advice before treatment if you are unfamiliar with cytotoxic drugs.

FOLLOW-UP
• Survival if left untreated or with evidence of metastatic disease—usually < 3 months
• Median survival with complete excision of primary tumor and tracheobronchial lymph nodes negative for neoplastic cells (dogs and cats)—> 300 days
• Median survival with incomplete surgical excision of primary tumor or tracheobronchial lymph nodes positive for neoplastic cells (dogs and cats)—< 75 days
• Pleural effusion—poor prognosis

MISCELLANEOUS

Suggested Reading
Frazier DL, Hahn KA. Cancer chemotherapeutics. In: Hahn KA, Richardson RC, eds., Cancer chemotherapy, a veterinary handbook. Baltimore: Williams & Wilkins, 1995:77–150.
Hahn KA, Anderson TA. Tumors of the respiratory tract. In: Bonagura JD, ed. Kirk's current veterinary therapy XIII. Philadelphia: Saunders, 1998:500–505.
Author Kevin A. Hahn
Consulting Editor Wallace B. Morrison

SQUAMOUS CELL CARCINOMA, NASAL PLANUM

BASICS

OVERVIEW
• Malignant tumor of squamous epithelial cells of the nasal planum
• Locally invasive and rarely metastasizes

SIGNALMENT
• Common in cats; rare in dogs
• Mean age—cats, 8.5–12.1 years; dogs, 9–10 years
• No reported sex or breed predilection
• More likely to develop in animals with a lightly pigmented nose

SIGNS
• Slow progression
• May begin as superficial crusting and scabbing, progress to carcinoma in situ, and develop into superficial and then invasive erosive carcinoma
• Dogs—sneezing; epistaxis; swelling of planum

CAUSES & RISK FACTORS
• Exposure to ultraviolet light
• Absence of protective pigment

DIAGNOSIS

DIFFERENTIAL DIAGNOSIS
Biopsy—differentiate from immune-mediated disease, eosinophilic granuloma complex, and other neoplasms

CBC/BIOCHEMISTRY/URINALYSIS
Usually normal

OTHER LABORATORY TESTS
N/A

IMAGING
Thoracic radiographs—evaluate for metastasis (rare)

DIAGNOSTIC PROCEDURES
• Fluorescent nuclear antibody test—detect metastasis
• Cytologic—fine-needle aspirate of large lymph nodes; detect metastasis

PATHOLOGIC FINDINGS
• Lesions—may vary in appearance depending on stage of disease; typically ulcerative not proliferative
• Histopathologic—characterized by irregular masses or cords of epidermal cells that proliferate downward into the dermis
• Keratin formation, horn pearls, desmosomes, mitotic figures, and cellular atypia—frequent

TREATMENT
• Superficial—surgery, cryosurgery, irradiation, or photodynamic therapy
• Etretinate—synthetic retinoid; may be useful for early precancerous lesions
• Invasive—requires radical surgical excision and adjunctive radiotherapy
• Immediate postoperative nutritional support may be required, especially for cats.

MEDICATIONS

DRUGS
Chemotherapy—not yet evaluated

CONTRAINDICATIONS/POSSIBLE INTERACTIONS
N/A

FOLLOW-UP

PATIENT MONITORING
• Physical examination and thoracic radiography—1, 3, 6, 9, 12, 18, and 24 months after treatment
• Biopsy—any suspicious lesion

PREVENTION/AVOIDANCE
• Limit sun exposure, especially between 10:00 A.M. and 2:00 P.M.
• Yearly tattoos on nonpigmented areas may be helpful.
• Sunscreens ineffective

POSSIBLE COMPLICATIONS
N/A

EXPECTED COURSE AND PROGNOSIS
• Survival with radiotherapy alone (cats)—mean, 17.7 months; 1 year, 61.5% with 81.8% recurrence
• Mean survival with surgery alone (cats)—18 months with 37.5%–50% recurrence
• Recurrence with radiotherapy alone (8 dogs)—100%; mean time to recurrence, 2.9 months
• Dogs—surgery alone may be curative if the lesions are superficial.
• Prognosis—good for small, noninvasive tumors; guarded for invasive tumors

MISCELLANEOUS

ASSOCIATED CONDITION
Secondary bacterial infection

Suggested Reading
Thomas RC, Fox LE. Tumors of the skin and subcutis. In: Morrison WB, ed. Cancer in dogs and cats: medical and surgical management. Philadelphia: Williams & Wilkins, 1998:489–510.
Author Joanne C. Graham
Consulting Editor Wallace B. Morrison

SQUAMOUS CELL CARCINOMA, NASAL AND PARANASAL SINUSES

BASICS

OVERVIEW
• Progressive local invasion of neoplastic keratinizing and nonkeratinizing squamous epithelium arising from within the nasal and paranasal sinuses
• Keratinizing—tend to arise from the nasal area
• Nonkeratinizing—tend to arise from the frontal sinus region
• Transitional (intermediate) in a nonkeratinizing form—classified as undifferentiated
• Slowly progressive (months)
• Commonly bilateral
• Approximately 35% of patients have extension to the brain and seizures; usually nonkeratinizing tumors
• Prevalence (nasal neoplasia)—0.3%–8% of all tumors in dogs and cats
• Keratinizing and nonkeratinizing—28.5% of all nasal neoplasia in dogs
• Only adenocarcinomas occur more frequently.

SIGNALMENT
• More common in dogs than in cats
• Dogs—median age, 9.5 years (range, 3–16 years); male predilection for keratinizing form (3.4:1)

SIGNS

Historical Findings
• Intermittent and progressive unilateral to bilateral epistaxis—median duration, 3 months
• Epiphora
• Sneezing
• Halitosis
• Anorexia
• Seizures secondary to cranial invasion

Physical Examination Findings
• Noninfectious nasal discharge
• Facial deformity or exophthalmia
• Pain on nasal or paranasal sinus examination

CAUSES & RISK FACTORS
Unknown

DIAGNOSIS

DIFFERENTIAL DIAGNOSIS
• Bacterial sinusitis—uncommon
• Viral infection—cats
• Cryptococcosis—cats
• Aspergillosis
• Foreign body
• Trauma
• Tooth root abscess
• Oronasal fistula
• Coagulopathy

CBC/BIOCHEMISTRY/URINALYSIS
Usually normal

OTHER LABORATORY TESTS
Cytologic and bacterial examination—rarely helpful

IMAGING
• Skull radiographs—reveal typical pattern of asymmetrical destruction of caudal turbinates; superimposition of a soft tissue mass; may see fluid density in the frontal sinuses secondary to outflow obstruction
• Thoracic radiographs—detect pulmonary metastasis (uncommon)
• CT or MRI—best method for observing integrity of cribriform plate or orbital invasion

DIAGNOSTIC PROCEDURES
• Deep tissue biopsy—necessary for definitive diagnosis
• Bacterial culture—often positive
• Rhinoscopy—reveals soft, friable, fleshy mass; tumor often obscured by exudate; avoid progressing caudally into the cribriform plate.

TREATMENT
• Surgery alone—not curative
• Turbinectomy—may be performed before external (teletherapy) or internal (brachytherapy) irradiation
• Inpatient radiotherapy—60–80 Gy; with or without surgery; best clinical control in dogs

SQUAMOUS CELL CARCINOMA, NASAL AND PARANASAL SINUSES

 MEDICATIONS

DRUGS
• Cisplatin—60–70 mg/m², IV once every 3 weeks for four treatments; may be a good option; nephrotoxic, so must use with saline diuresis (18.3 mL/kg/hr IV over 6 hr; give cisplatin after 4 hr)
• Butorphanol—0.4 mg/kg IM; before and after cisplatin will reduce emesis

CONTRAINDICATIONS/POSSIBLE INTERACTIONS
• Cisplatin—never use in cats
• Chemotherapy may be toxic; seek advice before initiating treatment if you are unfamiliar with cytotoxic drugs.

 FOLLOW-UP

PATIENT MONITORING
Skull radiography, CT, and MRI—when signs recur

POSSIBLE COMPLICATIONS
• Rhinitis—after turbinectomy and radiotherapy; usually subsides in 1–2 months
• Secondary fungal rhinitis—occasionally after turbinectomy

EXPECTED COURSE AND PROGNOSIS
• Median survival if left untreated—3–5 months
• Survival with radiotherapy—1 year, 38%–57% (dogs and cats); 2 years, 30%–48% (dogs); median 8–25 months (dogs); median, 1–36 months (cats)
• Median survival after cisplatin (dogs)—22 weeks; may provide marked palliation of clinical signs
• Local recurrence with extension to the brain—common; brain involvement is a poor prognostic sign.

 MISCELLANEOUS

Suggested Reading
Adams WM, Withrow SJ, Walshaw R, et al. Radiotherapy of malignant nasal tumors in 67 dogs. J Am Vet Med Assoc 1987;191:311–315.
Patnaik AK. Canine sinonasal neoplasms: clinicopathological study of 285 cases. J Am Anim Hosp Assoc 1989;25:103–114.
Theon AP, Peaston AE, Madewell BR, et al. Irradiation of nonlymphoproliferative neoplasms of the nasal cavity and paranasal sinuses in 16 cats. J Am Vet Med Assoc 1994;204:78–83.
Author Kevin A. Hahn
Consulting Editor Wallace B. Morrison

DISEASES

SQUAMOUS CELL CARCINOMA, SKIN

 BASICS

DEFINITION
• Malignant tumor of squamous epithelium
• Bowen disease (cats)—multicentric squamous cell carcinoma in situ

Pathophysiology
Metastasis—to any site; more commonly to regional lymph nodes and lungs

Systems Affected
Skin/Exocrine—skin and metastatic sites

Genetics
Unknown

Incidence/Prevalence
Represents 9%–25% of all skin tumors in cats and 4%–18% in dogs

Geographic Distribution
More prevalent in sunny climates and high altitudes (high ultraviolet light exposure)

SIGNALMENT

Species
Dogs and cats

Breed Predilection
• Cats—none reported; patients often have light or unpigmented skin.
• Dogs—Scottish terriers, Pekingese, boxers, poodles, Norwegian elkhounds, Dalmatians, beagles, whippets, and white English bull terriers may be predisposed; large breeds with black skin and haircoats may be predisposed to multiple squamous cell carcinoma involving the digits.

Mean Age and Range
• Dogs—9 years
• Cats—9–12.4 years

Predominant Sex
None

SIGNS

Historical Findings
• Crusts, ulcer, or mass that may have been present for months and unresponsive to conservative treatment
• Bowen disease (cats)—skin becomes pigmented; ulcer forms in the center; followed by a painful scabby lesion that may expand peripherally

• Lips, nose, and pinna involvement—may start out as a shallow crusting lesion that progresses to a deep ulcer
• Facial skin involvement (cats)
• Nail bed involvement (dogs)

Physical Examination Findings
• Proliferative or erosive skin lesions
• Most common sites—cats: nasal planum, eyelids, lips, and pinna; dogs: toes, scrotum, nose, legs, and anus
• Flank and abdomen involvement
• Bowen disease (cats)—may note 2 to > 30 lesions on the head, digits, neck, thorax, shoulders, and ventral abdomen; hair in the lesion epilates easily; crusts cling to the epilated hair shaft.

CAUSES
• Unknown
• Exposure to ultraviolet irradiation

RISK FACTORS
• Prolonged exposure to ultraviolet light
• Light or nonpigmented skin
• Previous thermal injury—burn scar

 DIAGNOSIS

DIFFERENTIAL DIAGNOSIS
• Often misdiagnosed as draining abscesses or infected wounds on the basis of gross appearance
• Digit involvement—sometimes confused with nail bed infection and osteomyelitis
• Biopsy and histopathology—distinguish from eosinophilic granuloma complex, immune-mediated disease, mast cell tumor, and cutaneous lymphosarcoma

CBC/BIOCHEMISTRY/URINALYSIS
Usually normal

OTHER LABORATORY TESTS
None

IMAGING
• Thoracic radiography—detects lung metastasis
• Abdominal radiography—evaluates and monitors sublumbar lymph nodes, if clinically relevant
• Radiography of extremities—with digital tumor; determines extent of underlying bone involvement

DIAGNOSTIC PROCEDURES
• Cytologic examination—fine-needle aspirate; evaluate large lymph nodes for metastasis
• Biopsy—needed to confirm diagnosis

PATHOLOGIC FINDINGS

Gross
• Ulcerative tumors—most common; may appear shallow and crusted and progress to deep craters
• Proliferative tumors—may have a cauliflower-like appearance; may ulcerate and bleed easily
• Bowen disease—painful ulcers that scab over and expand peripherally to reach more than 4 cm in diameter

Histopathologic
• Cords or irregular masses of epidermal cells infiltrating into the dermis and subcutis
• Large numbers of horn (keratin) pearls in well-differentiated tumors
• Desmosomes and mitotic figures common
• Bowen disease—dysplastic, highly ordered keratinocytes proliferate, replacing normal epidermis, but do not penetrate the basement membrane into the surrounding dermis.

Squamous Cell Carcinoma, Skin

TREATMENT

APPROPRIATE HEALTH CARE
• Invasive tumors—inpatient; require aggressive surgical excision or radiotherapy
• Superficial tumors—surgery, cryosurgery, photodynamic therapy, or irradiation
• Topical synthetic retinoids—may be useful for early superficial lesions

NURSING CARE
Interventional parenteral nutrition (feeding tube)—with nasal planum resection

ACTIVITY
• Dictated by the location of the tumor and the type of treatment
• Generally limit until sutures are removed, if surgery has been done

DIET
Normal

CLIENT EDUCATION
• Inform client about the benefit of early diagnosis and treatment.
• Discuss risk factors associated with the development of the tumor (ultraviolet light exposure).

SURGICAL CONSIDERATIONS
• Wide surgical excision—treatment of choice; skin flaps and body wall reconstruction sometimes required
• Digit involvement—amputation
• Pinna involvement—may require partial or total resection
• Invasive tumors of the nares—removal of the nasal planum recommended
• Radiotherapy—recommended for inoperable tumors or as adjunct to surgery

MEDICATIONS

DRUGS OF CHOICE
• Adjunctive chemotherapy—recommended with incomplete surgical excision, non-resectable mass, and metastasis
• Cisplatin (dogs), carboplatin, and mitoxantrone—reported to induce partial and complete remission; generally of short duration; small number of patients
• Intralesional sustained-release chemotherapeutic gel implants (dogs)—contain either 5-fluorouracil or cisplatin; effective

CONTRAINDICATIONS
• Cisplatin—do not use in cats, causes severe hydrothorax, pulmonary edema, and death; do not use in dogs with concurrent renal disease, potentially nephrotoxic
• 5-Fluorouracil—contraindicated in cats

PRECAUTIONS
Chemotherapeutics—follow published guidelines and protocols for safe use; be familiar with potential side effects.

POSSIBLE INTERACTIONS
None

ALTERNATIVE DRUGS
Topical synthetic retinoids—may be useful for early superficial lesions

FOLLOW-UP

PATIENT MONITORING
• Physical examination and radiography—1, 3, 6, 9, 12, 18, and 24 months after treatment or if the owner thinks the tumor is recurring
• Thoracic and abdominal radiography—at each recheck examination, if the lesion is on the caudal portion of the patient

PREVENTION/AVOIDANCE
• Limit sun exposure, especially between the hours of 10:00 A.M. and 2:00 P.M.
• Yearly tattoos on nonpigmented areas may be helpful.
• Sunscreens—usually licked off by the patient; may help in some areas (e.g., pinna)

POSSIBLE COMPLICATIONS
N/A

EXPECTED COURSE AND PROGNOSIS
Prognosis—good with superficial lesions that receive appropriate treatment; guarded with invasive lesions and those involving the nail bed or digit

MISCELLANEOUS

ASSOCIATED CONDITIONS
N/A

AGE RELATED FACTORS
N/A

ZOONOTIC POTENTIAL
N/A

PREGNANCY
N/A

SEE ALSO
Squamous Cell Carcinoma, Nasal Planum

ABBREVIATIONS
N/A

Suggested reading

Himsel CA, Richardson RC, Craig JA. Cisplatin chemotherapy for metastatic squamous cell carcinoma in two dogs. J Am Vet Med Assoc 1986;189:1575–1578.

Marks S. Clinical evaluation of etretinate (Tegison) for the treatment of preneoplastic and early neoplastic cutaneous squamous cell carcinoma in dogs. Vet Can Soc Newslett 1990;14:4–5.

O'Brien MG, Berg J, Engler SJ. Treatment by digital amputation of subungual squamous cell carcinoma in dogs: 21 cases (1987–1988). J Am Vet Med Assoc 1992;201:759–761.

Peaston AE, Leach MW, Higgins RJ. Photodynamic therapy for nasal and aural squamous cell carcinoma in cats. J Am Vet Med Assoc 1993;202:1261–1265.

Thomas RC, Fox LE. Tumors of the skin and subcutis. In: Morrison WB, ed. Cancer in dogs and cats: medical and surgical management. Baltimore: Williams & Wilkins, 1998:489–510.

Author Joanne C. Graham
Consulting Editor Wallace B. Morrison

DISEASES

SQUAMOUS CELL CARCINOMA, TONGUE

BASICS

OVERVIEW
• Rare tumor that occurs more commonly in cats than in dogs
• Cats—most commonly located on the ventrolateral surface of the body of the tongue at the level of the reflection of the frenulum
• Dogs—most commonly located on the dorsum of the tongue
• Usually grows rapidly
• Highly metastatic by way of lymphatic vessels to regional lymph nodes and lungs (37%–43% at examination)

SIGNALMENT
• Most dogs and cats middle-aged or old (> 7 years)
• No breed predilection in dogs

SIGNS

Historical Findings
• Excessive salivation
• Halitosis
• Dysphagia
• Bloody oral discharge
• Weight loss

Physical Examination Findings
• Tongue mass—may be small, white, cauliflower-like, nodular lesions with a broad base on examination
• Loose teeth
• Facial deformity
• Cervical lymphadenomegaly—occasionally

CAUSES & RISK FACTORS
None identified

DIAGNOSIS

DIFFERENTIAL DIAGNOSIS
• Other lingual malignancy
• Epulis
• Abscess
• Benign polyp

CBC/BIOCHEMISTRY/URINALYSIS
Usually normal

OTHER LABORATORY TESTS
Cytologic—impression smear obtained from an incisional biopsy specimen (wedge); may yield diagnosis

IMAGING
• Skull radiography—rarely demonstrates bone involvement deep to the mass
• Thoracic radiographs—required to evaluate lungs for metastasis

DIAGNOSTIC PROCEDURES
• Extensive physical examination of the cervical region—detect lymphadenomegaly (mandibular and retropharyngeal nodes)
• Deep tissue biopsy—necessary for definitive diagnosis

TREATMENT

• Surgical—most are inoperable; aggressive excision may be warranted; function of the tongue after recuperation is usually acceptable
• Postsurgical care (e.g., gastrotomy tube) by owner often required
• Partial glossectomy—may be performed on the rostral half (mobile tongue) or longitudinal half of the tongue (40%–60% removed); more than 50% of patients have incomplete surgical margins.
• Other surgical methods (e.g., electrocautery and cryosurgery)—do not offer any additional advantage to conventional excision.
• Cervical lymphadenectomy—rarely curative; perform only for diagnosis or before adjuvant therapy.
• Response to radiotherapy—poor (< 7 weeks)

MEDICATIONS

DRUGS
• Chemotherapy—no effective agents available for local or systemic control

CONTRAINDICATIONS/POSSIBLE INTERACTIONS
Chemotherapy may be toxic; seek advice before initiating treatment if you are unfamiliar with cytotoxic drugs.

FOLLOW-UP

• Prognosis—grave, owing to extensive local disease and high rate of metastasis
• Few patients survive > 6 months after diagnosis
• Survival after surgical excision—1 year, < 25%
• Survival with incomplete resection and mitoxantrone chemotherapy (1 dog)—27 months
• Survival with incomplete resection and localized radiotherapy combined with cisplatin chemotherapy (1 dog)—6 weeks
• Cause of death—secondary to local recurrence, dysphagia, and subsequent cachexia

✓ MISCELLANEOUS

Suggested Reading
Carpenter LG, Withrow SJ, Powers BE, et al. Squamous cell carcinoma of the tongue in 10 dogs. J Am Anim Hosp Assoc 1993;29:17–24.
Evans SM, Shofer F. Canine oral nontonsillar squamous cell carcinoma: prognostic factors for recurrence and survival following orthovoltage radiation therapy. Vet Radiol 1988;29:133–137.
Author Kevin A. Hahn
Consulting Editor Wallace B. Morrison

SQUAMOUS CELL CARCINOMA, TONSIL

 BASICS

OVERVIEW
• Rapid and progressive local invasion by cords of neoplastic squamous epithelium arising from the tonsillar fossa into tonsillar lymphoid tissue
• Local extension common
• Quick to metastasize to lymph nodes (> 98%), lungs (> 63%), and other distant organs (>20)
• Composes 20%–25% of all oral tumors and 50% of all intraoral tumors in dogs and cats
• Commonly unilateral, affecting the right more than the left tonsil

SIGNALMENT
• Middle-aged or old (range, 2.5–17 years) dogs and cats
• No known breed or sex predilection

SIGNS
Historical Findings
• Excessive salivation
• Halitosis
• Dysphagia
• Bloody oral discharge
• Weight loss

Physical Examination Findings
• Abnormally large tonsil (oral mass)
• Cervical lymphadenomegaly possible

CAUSES & RISK FACTORS
• Exact cause unknown
• Ten times more common in animals living in an urban environment than in those living in a rural environment

 DIAGNOSIS

DIFFERENTIAL DIAGNOSIS
• Lymphoma
• Abscess
• Salivary gland tumor
• Metastatic neoplasm
• Mast cell tumor
• Tonsillitis

CBC/BIOCHEMISTRY/URINALYSIS
Usually normal

OTHER LABORATORY TESTS
Cytologic—impression smear obtained from an incisional biopsy specimen (wedge); may yield diagnosis

IMAGING
• Skull radiography—rarely demonstrates bone involvement deep to the mass
• Thoracic radiography—detect lung metastasis
• Cervical radiography—evaluate retropharyngeal lymph nodes

DIAGNOSTIC PROCEDURES
• Thorough physical examination of the cervical region—detect abnormally large, regional lymph nodes (e.g., mandibular and retropharyngeal)
• Large, deep tissue biopsy—required to sufficiently differentiate from other oral malignancies

 TREATMENT

• Surgery—most are inoperable; aggressive excision may be warranted in patients with airway obstruction; tonsillectomy, when done, should be bilateral.
• Postoperative care (e.g., gastrotomy tube) by owner is often required.
• Other surgical methods (e.g., electrocautery and cryosurgery)—no advantage over conventional excision
• Cervical lymphadenectomy—rarely curative; perform only for diagnosis or before adjuvant therapy.
• Regional radiotherapy—response poor (< 7 weeks)

 MEDICATIONS

DRUGS
Chemotherapy—no effective agents available for local or systemic control; no anecdotal reports of cisplatin or bleomycin having been used with limited success

CONTRAINDICATIONS/POSSIBLE INTERACTIONS
Chemotherapy may be toxic; seek advice before initiating treatment if you are unfamiliar with cytotoxic drugs.

 FOLLOW-UP

• Prognosis—grave owing to extensive local disease and high rate of metastasis; few patients survive > 6 months after diagnosis
• Local recurrence common with regional extension to tongue, pharynx, and lymph nodes
• Median survival after localized radiotherapy (dogs)—110 days
• Median survival after systemic chemotherapy (dogs)—60–130 days
• Median survival after localized radiotherapy combined with systemic chemotherapy (e.g., doxorubicin and cisplatin; dogs)—270 days
• Survival after surgical excision (dogs)—1 year, < 10%
• Metastasis—common on examination; leading cause of death regardless of treatment

 MISCELLANEOUS

Suggested Reading
Brooks MB, Matus RE, Leifer CE, et al. Chemotherapy versus chemotherapy plus radiotherapy in the treatment of tonsillar squamous cell carcinoma in the dog. J Vet Intern Med 1988;2:206–211.
Postorino-Reeves NC, Turrel JM, Withrow SJ. Oral squamous cell carcinoma in the cat. J Am Anim Hosp Assoc 1993;29:438–441.
Author Kevin A. Hahn
Consulting Editor Wallace B. Morrison

DISEASES

STAPHYLOCOCCAL INFECTIONS

BASICS

OVERVIEW
• *Staphylococcus*—gram-positive, facultatively anaerobic, spherical bacteria; *staphyle* (Greek; "bunch of grapes") from characteristic microscopic arrangement in clusters; produces a variety of infections characterized by pus formation involving all tissues of the body; can produce toxins (superantigens) that exert profound systemic signs (fever, hypotension, shock, multiorgan failure, death)
• Ubiquitous; live free in environment and as commensal parasites of skin and upper respiratory tract
• Pathogenic and nonpathogenic strains; wide spectrum of virulence, host range, and site specificities; not strictly host or site specific
• Pathogenic strains—possess extracellular toxins and enzymes (e.g., coagulase, staphylokinase, hemolysin, epidermolysins); staphylocoagulase in more pathogenic strains (e.g., *S. Aureus, S. intermedius*)

SIGNALMENT
• Dogs and cats
• Very young—susceptible because of incomplete, developing immunity
• Old, debilitated—susceptible because of impaired host defenses
• Immunocompromised—more susceptible

SIGNS
• Fever
• Anorexia
• Pain
• Can affect every organ system
• Abscesses and infections of the skin, eyes, ears, respiratory system, genitourinary tract, skeleton, and joints—common
• Dogs—pyoderma; otitis externa; cystitis; prostatitis; pneumonia; abscesses; osteomyelitis; discospondylitis; arthritis; mastitis; bacteremia; endocarditis; wound infections; toxic shock syndrome
• Cats—abscesses; oral infections; otitis externa; conjunctivitis; metritis; cholangiohepatitis; cystitis; bacteremia

CAUSES & RISK FACTORS
• Opportunistic pathogens
• Disease—from disturbance of the natural host–parasite equilibrium when local and general defense mechanisms are significantly lowered (e.g., chronic debilitating diseases)
• Secondary infection—allergies (atopy, food, fleas); endocrinopathies (hypothyroidism, hyperadrenocorticism); parasites (demodicosis); seborrhea
• Burns or wounds—complications
• Transmission—airborne organisms; carriers; and direct contact (droplet nuclei)

DIAGNOSIS

DIFFERENTIAL DIAGNOSIS
• Dermatitis—allergies, seborrhea, immune-mediated
• Other infectious causes—viruses, bacteria, fungi, *Rickettsia*, protozoa
• Neoplasia
• Immune-mediated diseases

CBC/BIOCHEMISTRY/URINALYSIS
• Normal or high WBCs
• Biochemistry—may suggest underlying cause (e.g., hypothyroidism, hyperadrenocorticism)
• Urinalysis—pyuria (with or without bacteruria) with cystitis

OTHER LABORATORY TESTS
• Direct microscopy
• Gram stain
• Cytology—neutrophils and cocci singly or in pairs, short chains, or irregular clusters
• Culture—avoid superficial contamination; collect samples by aspiration, wash, or biopsy; do not overinterpret a positive isolation; organisms can be isolated from normal animals.
• Organisms survive up to 48 hr in clinical specimens when kept cool (4°C; 40°F), particularly on swabs containing a holding medium
• Antibiotic susceptibility testing

STAPHYLOCOCCAL INFECTIONS

IMAGING
Radiology—osteolytic and osteoproliferative lesions with osteomyelitis; interstitial or alveolar pulmonary pattern with pneumonia; radiodense uroliths (struvite)

DIAGNOSTIC PROCEDURES
CSF—if meningitis or discospondylitis suspected

PATHOLOGIC FINDINGS
Characteristic abscess lesion—necrotic tissue, fibrin, and a large number of neutrophils

TREATMENT

• Properly handle and dispose of contaminated objects.
• Organism resistant to many environmental insults and common disinfectants
• Topical antibacterial cleaning of wounds and pyoderma—may be beneficial

MEDICATIONS

DRUGS
• Antibiotic resistance—great propensity owing to production of β-lactamase, which inactivates penicillins; may carry plasmids (segments of genetic material that may carry genes for antimicrobial resistance) that can be transferred to other strains of staphylococci or species of bacteria
• History of previous antimicrobial therapy for staphylococcal infection—culture and antibiotic susceptibility testing indicated
• Nonpenicillinase-producing strains—penicillin G at 10,000–20,000 U/kg IM, SC q12–24h or penicillin V at 8–30 mg/kg PO q8h
• Penicillinase-producing strains—use penicillinase-resistant drugs
• First-generation cephalosporins—rarely resistant; cephalexin at 22 mg/kg PO q8h; cefadroxil at 22 mg/kg PO q8–12h
• β-lactamase-resistant synthetic penicillins—rarely resistant; oxacillin at 22–40 mg/kg PO q8h; dicloxacillin, and clavulanic acid-potentiated amoxicillin at 12.5–25 mg/kg PO q8–12h
• Gentamicin—rarely resistant; 2–4 mg/kg IV, IM, SC q8h
• Enrofloxacin—rarely resistant; 2.5–5 mg/kg PO, IM q12h
• Trimethoprim-potentiated sulfonamides—infrequently resistant; 30 mg/kg IV, PO q12h
• Chloramphenicol—infrequently resistant; 40–50 mg/kg IV, IM, SC, PO q8–12h
• Penicillin allergy—try cephalosporin, clindamycin, or vancomycin

CONTRAINDICATIONS/POSSIBLE INTERACTIONS
Avoid immunosuppressive drugs.

FOLLOW-UP
N/A

MISCELLANEOUS

ZOONOTIC POTENTIAL
• Possibile
• Most people and pets carry their own pathogenic staphylococcal flora; disease not caused by mere exposure

ABBREVIATION
CSF = cerebrospinal fluid

Suggested Reading
Cox HU. Staphylococcal infections. In: Greene CE, ed. Infectious diseases of the dog and cat. Philadelphia: Saunders, 1998:214–217.
Author J. Paul Woods
Consulting Editor Stephen C. Barr

STEROID HEPATOPATHY

BASICS

DEFINITION
Reversible vacuolar change in hepatocytes in dogs, associated with glucocorticoid treatment, hyperadrenocorticism (iatrogenic or spontaneous), or chronic illnesses in other organ systems; typified by high ALP activity without signs of hepatic insufficiency

PATHOPHYSIOLOGY
• Glucocorticoids—cause reversible glycogen accumulation in hepatocytes within 2–3 days after administration; injectable and reposital forms usually induce more severe changes than do oral forms; topical, ocular, cutaneous, and aural administration may also produce an effect • Cell swelling—leads to parenchymal enlargement and hepatomegaly • Response (dogs)—marked individual variation related to the type, route, dosage, duration of treatment, and individual sensitivity; may develop even with low-dose, short-term oral medication • May develop with systemic diseases not related to glucocorticoid exposure or hyperadrenocorticism • Association with significant nonhepatobiliary health problems that involve inflammation—suggests a relationship with stress (endogenous glucocorticoid release) or acute phase reactants

SYSTEMS AFFECTED
• Hepatobiliary—variable impairment of hepatic function • Systemic effects of glucocorticoids

GENETICS
N/A

INCIDENCE/PREVALENCE
• Dogs—common; occurs in up to 33% of patients undergoing liver biopsy; many patients identified through laboratory and imaging studies. Cats—extremely rare; usually hepatic lipidosis

GEOGRAPHIC DISTRIBUTION
N/A

SIGNALMENT

Species
Dogs and rarely cats

Breed Predilections
Breeds predisposed to hyperadrenocorticism (dachshunds, poodles, beagles, boxers, Boston terriers) and hyperlipidemia

Mean Age and Range
• Middle-age to old dogs—when caused by spontaneous hyperadrenocorticism (> 75% older than 9 years); when caused by chronic inflammation or neoplasia • Dogs of any age—iatrogenic disease subsequent to glucocorticoid administration • Young dogs—idiopathic hyperlipidemia

Predominant Sex
N/A

SIGNS

General Comments
• Often related to multisystemic effects of glucocorticoids or another systemic illness causing stress • Rarely note signs of hepatic disease or failure

Historical Findings
• Glucocorticoid excess—polydipsia and polyuria; polyphagia; endocrine alopecia; abdominal distention; muscle weakness; panting; lethargy • Other causes—depend on the affected system

Physical Examination Findings
• Hepatomegaly • Relate to glucocorticoid excess or the underlying disease; depend on severity and duration • Adrenal overproduction of sex hormones—endocrine alopecia with hyperpigmentation

CAUSES
• Glucocorticoid administration • Hyperadrenocorticism • Other adrenal gland hyperfunction—overproduction of sex hormones • Systemic diseases associated with an acute-phase response or stress—severe dental disease; inflammatory bowel disease; chronic pancreatitis; systemic neoplasia (especially lymphoma); chronic infections (urinary tract, skin); hypothyroidism; inborn errors of lipid metabolism (lipid and glycogen accumulate in hepatocytes)

RISK FACTORS
• Pharmacologic doses of glucocorticoids • Breeds at risk for hyperadrenocorticism • Spontaneous hyperadrenocorticism—pituitary-dependent or functional adrenal mass • Other systemic conditions—see Causes • Breeds at risk for hyperlipidemia—schnauzers, shelties, beagles

DIAGNOSIS

DIFFERENTIAL DIAGNOSIS
• Most other diffuse hepatopathies (especially those causing hepatomegaly and high serum hepatic enzyme activities)—passive congestion; neoplasia (primary or metastatic to the liver); inflammatory disease; anticonvulsant hepatopathy; hepatocellular swelling associated with diabetes mellitus (lipid vacuolation) • Distinguishing features—normal serum total bilirubin concentration; normal to mild abnormalities in hepatic function tests (total serum bile acids concentrations); homogenous hyperechoic liver on ultrasonography; characteristic morphologic findings on hepatic fine-needle aspiration and biopsy • If laboratory and clinical signs are compatible with the disorder and another underlying cause is not evident or the patient is symptomatic for hyperadrenocorticism, assess the pituitary–adrenal axis. • Thorough physical assessment—essential; strong association with chronic illness

CBC/BIOCHEMISTRY/URINALYSIS

CBC
• Depends on underlying disease • Nonregenerative anemia—chronic inflammatory disease or hypothyroidism • Relative polycythemia—hyperadrenocorticism • Stress leukogram—hyperadrenocorticism; treatment with glucocorticoids; stress of other illness • Thrombocytosis—hyperadrenocorticism

Biochemistry
• ALP and GGT—markedly high serum activities; GGT activity usually parallels that of ALP and cannot differentiate from other disorders • ALT and AST—moderate increase • Serum albumin and total bilirubin—usually normal; high bilirubin is unusual and indicates another hepatobiliary or hemolytic disease process. • Hypercholesterolemia—hyperadrenocorticism; some in-born errors of lipid metabolism; hypothyroidism; pancreatitis

OTHER LABORATORY TESTS
• Total serum bile acids—may be normal or slightly to moderately high (up to ~ 75 μmol/L) • Ammonia tolerance test—usually normal • ALP glucocorticoid isoenzyme—always high in dogs with hyperadrenocorticism; also high in affected dogs without associated hyperadrenocorticism; sensitive for ruling out hyperadrenocorticism but cannot differentiate causes • Pituitary–adrenal axis—evaluated with ACTH-response test or dexamethasone-suppression tests; document and differentiate types of hyperadrenocorticism • High urine cortisol:creatinine ratio—suggests hyperadrenocorticism; less reliable than ACTH-response test or LDDST (spurious increases may occur in stressed patients) • ACTH-stimulation test—blunted in patients receiving glucocorticoids • Thyroid testing—rule out hypothyroidism

IMAGING
• Abdominal radiography—reveals hepatomegaly and other underlying conditions • Thoracic radiography—evaluated for lymphadenopathy or metastatic disease when hyperadrenocorticism is not noted; provides evidence of other primary disease process • Abdominal ultrasonography—reveals hepatomegaly and diffuse or multifocal hyperechoic hepatic parenchyma; with multifocal disease, may observe a nodular-like pattern; may disclose evidence of underlying primary visceral disease, mesenteric lymphadenopathy, and adrenal size (often enlarged in stressed dogs)

DIAGNOSTIC PROCEDURES

• Hepatic aspiration cytology—23- or 25-gauge, 2.5–3.75-cm (1–1.5-in) needle; may aspirate diffusely enlarged liver without ultrasonography; aspirate representative regions with multifocal echogenic pattern, sampling tissue with different echogenicity. • Hepatic biopsy—verify vacuolar change; exclude primary hepatic disease if other systemic diagnoses have not been made; method: ultrasound-guided needle, laparoscopy, or laparotomy • Cytologic evaluation—may note inflammatory infiltrates, neoplasia, and obvious vacuolar or rarefied appearance of hepatocellular cytosol; expect bile in hepatocytes and canalicular casts between hepatocytes with severe disease • Tissue evaluation—with suspected suppuration, initiate microbial culture (aerobic and anaerobic bacterial; fungal, if appropriate); special stains: PAS with and without amylase to discern glycogen • Coagulation assessment—PT, APTT, ACT, fibrinogen, PIVKA, and mucosal bleeding time; indicated before liver biopsy

PATHOLOGIC FINDINGS

• Gross—variable; normal liver; mild to moderate hepatomegaly; mild surface irregularity; loss of normal lobular pattern • Microscopic—abnormalities usually pathognomonic; marked vacuolization and ballooning of hepatocytes in a centrilobular or diffuse distribution; mild hepatic necrosis; extramedullary hematopoiesis ; small focal aggregates of neutrophils

 TREATMENT

APPROPRIATE HEALTH CARE

Outpatient—common; for underlying disease

ACTIVITY

Normal

DIET

Hyperlipidemia and pancreatitis—fat restriction

CLIENT EDUCATION

• Inform clients that the clinical signs are related to multisystemic effects of glucocorticoids or associated disease. • Inform client that liver failure is not expected. • Instruct client to stop glucocorticoid administration in any form.

SURGICAL CONSIDERATIONS

• Depend on underlying conditions
• Adrenocortical masses may be resected

 MEDICATIONS

DRUGS OF CHOICE

• Pituitary-dependent hyperadrenocorticism—usually treated medically once diagnosis is confirmed; o,p'-DDD (mitotane, Lysodren), ketoconazole, or L-deprenyl • Depend on underlying disease • Management of causal inflammatory conditions that may require immunosuppressive or anti-inflammatory medications—use very low dosages of glucocorticoids combined with other medications (see Alternative Drugs). • Neoplasia—tumor resection and/or chemotherapy • Dental disease—antibiotic therapy; appropriate dental procedures • Pyelonephritis, chronic *Staphylococcus intermedius* dermatitis, or other infectious disorder—long-term antimicrobial treatment based on results of microbial culture and sensitivity tests • Hypothyroidism—supplemental thyroxin

CONTRAINDICATIONS

Avoid hepatotoxic drugs.

PRECAUTIONS

Glucocorticoids—use caution when administering glucocorticoids to all patients; use an alternate-day protocol to reduce the severity of the disorder and the influence on the pituitary–adrenal axis; use caution when administering to dogs with inborn errors of lipid metabolism (schnauzers are at greatest risk of developing severe disease)

POSSIBLE INTERACTIONS N/A

ALTERNATIVE DRUGS

• Metronidazole, azathioprine, chlorambucil, and cyclophosphamide—may be considered for patients with immune-mediated disorders managed with glucocorticoids

 FOLLOW-UP

PATIENT MONITORING

• Hepatomegaly—abdominal palpation and radiography • Normalizing enzymes—biochemistry • Hyperadrenocorticism—ACTH-stimulation test to assess treatment efficacy • Neoplasia—repeat physical examinations and imaging studies • Control of infection—repeating cultures (e.g., urine) • Hyperlipidemia—plasma lipemia, triglycerides, and cholesterol

PREVENTION/AVOIDANCE

• Limit administration of glucocorticoids to confirmed conditions requiring antiinflammatory or immunosuppressive therapy. • Use alternate-day therapy and titrate to the lowest effective dose to minimize risk.

POSSIBLE COMPLICATIONS

Numerous—related to multisystemic effects of glucocorticoids and associated conditions

EXPECTED COURSE AND PROGNOSIS

• Some patients do not develop disorder even with chronic glucocorticoid therapy. • Some patients develop very high serum enzymes and disorder persisting for weeks even after short-term glucocorticoid therapy. • The laboratory and hepatic morphologic abnormalities are completely reversible.

 MISCELLANEOUS

ASSOCIATED CONDITIONS

• Spontaneous hyperadrenocorticism—pituitary- or adrenal-dependent • Diabetes mellitus • Pulmonary thromboembolism • Urinary tract infections • Myopathy • Neuropathy • Hyperlipidemia • Inflammatory bowel disease • Dental disease • Hypothyroidism • Neoplasia • Chronic pancreatitis

AGE-RELATED FACTORS

• Associated spontaneous hyperadrenocorticism (dogs)—usually middle-aged to old • Depend on underlying disease

ZOONOTIC POTENTIAL N/A

PREGNANCY

Reproductive failure with glucocorticoid excess—testicular atrophy; abnormal estrus

SYNONYMS

• Glucocorticoid hepatopathy • Corticosteroid hepatopathy • Vacuolar change • Vacuolar hepatopathy

SEE ALSO

• Hyperadrenocorticism (Cushing Disease)
• Lipids, Hyperlipidemia • Storage Diseases, Glycogen

ABBREVIATIONS

• ACT = activated clotting time • ALP = alkaline phosphatase • ALT = alanine amino transferase • APTT = activated partial thromboplastin time • AST = aspartate aminotransferase • GGT = gamma-glutamyltransferase • LDDST = low-dose dexamethasone-suppression test • PIVKA = proteins invoked by vitamin K absence or antagonism • PT = prothrombin time

Suggested Reading

Center SA. Hepatic Lipidosis, Glucocortizoid Hepathopathy, Vacuolar Hepatopathy, Storage Disorders, Amyloidosis, and Iron Toxicity in Guilford GW, Center, SA, Strombeck DR, et al., eds., Small animal gastroenterology. Philadelphia:Sanders, 1996:766–801.

Author Keith P. Richter
Consulting Editor Sharon A. Center

STEROID-RESPONSIVE MENINGITIS-ARTERITIS (SRMA)—DOGS

BASICS

OVERVIEW
• May be acute or protracted
• Lesions—most impressive in CNS, affecting the meninges and the meningeal arteries; also see vascular changes in the heart, liver, kidney, and gastrointestinal system
• Genetic factors—may play a role; suspected in beagle colonies
• Worldwide occurrence

SIGNALMENT
• Dogs
• Beagles, Bernese mountain dogs, toller retrievers, and boxers predisposed; every breed can be affected.
• Affects mostly young adult dogs of both sexes; age range 5–18 months

SIGNS
• Classical (acute)—hyperesthesia; cervical rigidity; stiff gait; fever of up to 42°C (107.6°F)
• Protracted—further neurologic deficits, usually reflecting a spinal cord or multifocal lesion

CAUSES & RISK FACTORS
• Cause unknown
• Pathologic and laboratory data and marked response to steroids—suggest an immune-mediated disease related to a dysregulation of IgA production
• Epidemiologic observations—altered immune response may be triggered by an environmental factor, possibly of infectious nature

DIAGNOSIS

DIFFERENTIAL DIAGNOSIS
• Acute—bacterial meningitis; tumors of the meninges (histiocytosis, meningioma, lymphosarcoma)
• Protracted—bacterial meningitis; tumors of the meninges (histiocytosis, meningioma, lymphosarcoma); viral encephalitides; granulomatous meningoencephalitis; protozoal infections

CBC/BIOCHEMISTRY/URINALYSIS
• Acute—leukocytosis with neutrophilia and left shift; high erythrocyte sedimentation rate
• Protracted—CBC noncontributory

OTHER LABORATORY TESTS
• IgA levels (serum and CSF)—usually high; strongly supports the diagnosis, especially with protracted disease

IMAGING
Myelography or CT—exclude tumors

DIAGNOSTIC PROCEDURES

CSF Analysis
• Acute—mild to clear elevation of protein; pleocytosis with several hundreds to thousands of leukocytes, predominantly polymorphonuclear cells
• Protracted—normal or slightly high protein; mild to moderate pleocytosis with mixed cell population or with a predominance of mononuclear cells

PATHOLOGIC FINDINGS

Acute
• Marked meningitis with invasion of macrophages, plasma cells, lymphocytes, and varying numbers of polymorphonuclear cells, mostly in the meninges of the cervical region
• Lesions of the meningeal arteries—more degenerative with perivascular inflammation

Protracted
• Marked fibrous thickening and focal mineralization of the leptomeninges
• Arterial walls—many are thickened with considerable stenosis owing to cellular proliferation of the intima and fibrosis.

TREATMENT
• Inpatient—at onset, fluid therapy and ice packs useful for high body temperature
• Outpatient—after initial treatment; owners may dispense medication.
• Regular controls—must be initiated; inform owner about side effects of long-term steroid treatment.
• Activity—do not alter (prevention of muscle atrophy).

MEDICATIONS

DRUGS
• Initial signs and pleocytosis of the CSF mild—NSAIDs; carefully monitor the patient.
• First relapse or symptoms become worse with massive pleocytosis in the CSF—start long-term treatment (6 months) with prednisolone (4 mg/kg PO q24h for 1–2 days; then taper slowly); re-examine patient (including a CSF tap and blood profile) every 4–6 weeks after the initiation of therapy
• Neurologic examination and CSF become normal—reduce steroid dose
• Persistent pleocytosis—continue same steroid dosage
• Treatment may be stopped after about 6 months.
• Immunosuppressive drugs (purine analogs)—azathioprine (1.5 mg/kg PO q48h) if patient does not respond well to prednisolone alone; used in combination

• Consider protecting patient against ulceration in the gastrointestinal tract.

CONTRAINDICATIONS/POSSIBLE INTERACTIONS
• Corticosteroids—high-dose treatment can lead to serious complications; nonlife threatening side effects (polyuria, polydipsia, polyphagia and weight gain); not tolerated in about 5% of dogs

FOLLOW-UP

PATIENT MONITORING
Clinical control examinations—every 4–6 weeks; include blood examination and CSF collection; until steroids discontinued

PREVENTION/AVOIDANCE
Strictly control treatment schedule to prevent frequent relapses.

POSSIBLE COMPLICATIONS
• Hypoxic lesions of the spinal cord or the brain—protracted disease; may result in gait abnormalities and seizures
• Side effects of immunosuppressive treatment—bacterial infections; bleeding in the gastrointestinal tract; pancreatitis

EXPECTED COURSE AND PROGNOSIS
• Acute—prognosis relatively good in young dogs and with early aggressive therapy
• Protracted cases with frequent relapses—prognosis guarded; controlled studies note about 60% of dogs are cured after immunosuppressive treatment

MISCELLANEOUS

ASSOCIATED CONDITIONS
In rare cases, arthritis

AGE-RELATED FACTORS
Old animals do not tolerate long-term steroid treatment well; but condition is rare in dogs > 5 years of age.

PREGNANCY
Avoid pregnancy during treatment.

SYNONYMS
• Beagle pain syndrome
• Corticosteroid-responsive meningomyelitis
• Canine juvenile polyarteritis syndrome
• Aseptic meningitis

ABBREVIATION
CSF = cerebrospinal fluid

Suggested Reading
Tipold A, Jaggy A. Steroid-responsive meningitis-arteritis in dogs—long-term study of 32 cases. J Small Anim Pract 1994;35:311–316.

Author Andrea Tipold
Consulting Editor Joane M. Parent

BASICS

OVERVIEW
• Also known as glycogenoses; rare inherited disorders characterized by abnormal glycogen metabolism owing to defective or deficient enzyme activity controlling glycogen metabolism
• Tissue glycogen accumulation—leads to organ enlargement and dysfunction; primarily affects liver, heart, skeletal muscle, kidney, and CNS
• Impaired hepatic glycogen mobilization—produces symptomatic hypoglycemia
• Classification—according to type of enzymatic defect and primary organ(s) involved; > 12 in humans; 4 in dogs (types Ia, II, III, and VII); 1 in cats (type IV)

SIGNALMENT
• Clinical signs manifest in juveniles, days to several months after birth
• Type Ia (von Gierke disease)—litter mate Maltese puppies
• Type II (Pompe disease)—Laplands; onset beginning at 6 months of age
• Type III (Cori disease)—young female German shepherds
• Type IV—Norwegian Forest cats; may be stillborn; may fade shortly after birth; may manifest signs at 5–7 months of age
• Type VII—English springer spaniels 2–9 years of age
• No known sex predilection
• Autosomal recessive inheritance—Norwegian forest cats, English springer spaniels, and Laplands; suspected for Maltese and German shepherds

SIGNS
• Depend on enzymatic defect
• Type Ia (Maltese puppies)—failure to thrive; mental depression; hypoglycemia; abdominal distension; hepatomegaly; die or euthanized by 47 days of age
• Type II (Laplands)—vomiting and regurgitation related to megaesophagus; progressive muscle weakness; cardiac changes; die < 2 years of age
• Type III (German shepherds)—depression; weakness; failure to grow; abdominal distension from hepatomegaly; mild hypoglycemia
• Type IV (Norwegian forest cats)—often dies in the perinatal period; intermittent fevers generalized muscle tremors muscle atrophy weakness progressing to tetraplegia; sudden death from myocardial degeneration and terminal dysrhythmia

• Type VII (English springer spaniels)—compensated hemolytic anemia; episodic intravascular hemolysis; hemoglobinuria; one patient developed a progressive myopathy at 11 years of age.

CAUSES & RISK FACTORS
• Type Ia—glucose-6-phosphatase deficiency
• Type II—acid-α-glucosidase-deficient activity
• Type III—amylo-1,6-glucosidase deficiency
• Type IV—glycogen branching enzyme (α-1,4-D-glucan) deficiency
• Type VII—phosphofructokinase deficiency

DIAGNOSIS

DIFFERENTIAL DIAGNOSIS
• High index of suspicion required for diagnosis
• Breed affiliation
• Other causes of juvenile hypoglycemia—malnutrition; endoparasitism; transient fasting hypoglycemia; portosystemic vascular anomaly
• Other causes of muscular weakness—infectious; endocrinopathy; immune-mediated; hypokalemia

CBC/BIOCHEMISTRY/URINALYSIS
• Types I and III—hypoglycemia
• Type VII—anemia; reticulocytosis; pigmenturia

OTHER LABORATORY TESTS
• Type IV—PCR carrier test (developed for Norwegian forest cats); available at Michigan State University (517-432-4071)
• Type VII—in vitro erythrocyte testing

IMAGING
• Type II—thoracic radiography; may show cardiomegaly and megaesophagus
• Types Ia and III—abdominal radiography; may reveal hepatomegaly
• Abdominal ultrasonography—may reveal hepatomegaly and echogenic changes suggesting hepatic glycogen deposition
• Types II and IV—echocardiography; may reveal cardiac changes

DIAGNOSTIC PROCEDURES
• Tissue enzyme analysis and glycogen determination—definitive diagnosis
• Electromyography
• Electrocardiography

PATHOLOGIC FINDINGS
• Type Ia—emaciation; massive hepatomegaly; glycogen accumulation in liver and kidney

• Type II—glycogen accumulation in skeletal, smooth, and cardiac muscle
• Type III—hepatomegaly owing to glycogen; also in skeletal muscle
• Type IV—generalized muscle atrophy; glycogen accumulation in skeletal muscle, CNS and peripheral nervous system
• Type VII—polysaccharide deposits in skeletal muscle

TREATMENT
• Supportive care
• Types I and III—may require intravenous dextrose for resolution of hypoglycemic crisis; high-carbohydrate diet to control hypoglycemia

MEDICATIONS

DRUG(S)
N/A

CONTRAINDICATIONS/POSSIBLE INTERACTIONS
N/A

FOLLOW-UP
• Monitor for hypoglycemia.
• Cull parents from breeding programs.
• Prognosis—poor; most patients die or are euthanized owing to progressive deterioration.

MISCELLANEOUS

SEE ALSO
• Mucopolysaccharidosis (MPS)
• Storage Diseases, Lysosomal

ABBREVIATION
PCR = polymerase chain reaction

Suggested Reading
Brix AE, Howerth EW, et al. Glycogen storage disease type Ia in two littermate Maltese puppies. Vet Pathol 1995;32:460–465.
Harvey JW, Calderwood MB. Polysaccharide storage myopathy in canine phosphofructokinase deficiency (type VII glycogen storage disease) Vet Pathol 1990;27:1–8.
Walvoort HC. Glycogen storage disease type II in the Lapland dog. Vet Q 1985; 7:187–190.
Author Angelyn M. Cornetta
Consulting Editor Sharon A. Center

DISEASES

STORAGE DISEASES, LYSOSOMAL

  BASICS

OVERVIEW
• Rare inherited disorders caused by partial or complete deficiency of a lysosomal enzyme or an enzyme-activator protein, which leads to intracytoplasmic accumulation (storage) of the substrate of that enzyme
• Storage products—proteins, carbohydrates, lipids, or a combination
• Many different types are reported in both dogs and cats.
• Inheritance is usually autosomal recessive or X-linked.

SIGNALMENT
• Dogs—German short-haired pointers, English setters, beagle, cairn terriers, bluetick hounds, West Highland terriers, and Sidney silky terriers
• Cats—Siamese, Korats, and domestic shorthair cats
• Most affected animals are < 1 year old.

SIGNS

General Comments
• Vary with the severity of the enzyme deficiency
• Carrier animals can be affected with a milder form of the disease.
• Many organ systems are affected, but neurologic signs tend to predominate.

Historical Findings
• Affected animals usually normal at birth
• Fail to thrive
• Manifest a variety of neurologic signs within the first few months of life that suggest multifocal neurologic disease

Physical Examination Findings
• Cerebellar dysfunction common
• Other neurologic—ataxia; exercise intolerance; seizures; behavioral changes; visual deficits
• Non-neurologic—may see organomegaly or skeletal malformations

CAUSES & RISK FACTORS
• Genetic—deletion or mutation involving a single gene that causes an absolute or partial deficiency of a lysosomal enzyme or activator protein; deficient production of enzymes that do not have normal biological activity
• Susceptible breed

 DIAGNOSIS

DIFFERENTIAL DIAGNOSIS
• Metabolic encephalopathy—usually episodic clinical signs; results of hemogram, biochemistry analysis, and urinalysis are often diagnostic.
• Toxicities—acute onset of clinical signs; history of exposure
• Cerebellar hypoplasia—onset at 3–6 weeks of age; nonprogressive
• Cerebellar abiotrophy—deficits limited to the cerebellum; may be difficult to differentiate in the early stages without specific tests
• Prenatal or neonatal infections (especially viral) resulting in meningoencephalomyelitis—differentiated by CSF analysis; may be other signs, such as chorioretinitis
• Metabolic diseases—especially organic and amino acidurias

CBC/BIOCHEMISTRY/URINALYSIS
• Regular blood smears—cytoplasmic vacuolation of leukocytes caused by the accumulation of storage products
• Urine—may find abnormal accumulation of substances (e.g., oligosaccharide in α-mannosidosis)

OTHER LABORATORY TESTS
N/A

IMAGING
N/A

DIAGNOSTIC PROCEDURES
Specific diagnosis is made by demonstrating low enzyme activity in preparations of serum, brain, viscera, leukocytes, or skin fibroblasts.

 TREATMENT

• Outpatient—unless severe deficits preclude nursing care at home
• Activity—restrict to safe areas; avoid stairs.
• Diet and fluids—ensure proper intake (patients are often debilitated); parenteral fluid therapy and enteral or parenteral nutritional support may be needed with severe disease
• Bone marrow transplantation—used experimentally with some success
• Gene therapy—may offer hope for specific treatment
• Primary treatment—preventative; control of breeding; genetic counseling
• Patients may be at high risk of developing secondary infection; monitor closely; initiate appropriate treatment if infection develops.

 MEDICATIONS

DRUGS
N/A

CONTRAINDICATIONS/POSSIBLE INTERACTIONS
N/A

 FOLLOW-UP

• Progressive and ultimately fatal
• Pedigree analysis—may be useful in diagnosis; important for identification of potential carrier animals

 MISCELLANEOUS

ABBREVIATION
CSF = cerebrospinal fluid

Suggested Reading
Evans RJ. Lysosomal storage diseases in dogs and cats. J Small Anim Pract 1989;30:144–150.
Wood PA. Lysosomal storage diseases. In: August JR, ed. Consultations in feline internal medicine. Philadelphia: WB Saunders, 1991:497–501.
Author Mary O. Smith
Consulting Editor Joane M. Parent

BASICS

OVERVIEW
• *Streptococcus*—gram-positive, nonmotile, spherical bacteria; grow in pairs or chains; commensal organisms; normal flora of the upper respiratory tract, oropharynx, lower genital tract, and skin; under appropriate conditions, capable of infecting all areas of body; primary infections involve respiratory, circulatory, integumentary, urogenital, or central nervous systems; frequent secondary invader of body tissues
• Classified by ability to hemolyze RBCs and produce zone on blood agar plates around bacterial colony—α-hemolytic (green zone of partial hemolysis); β-hemolytic (clear zone of hemolysis); γ-hemolytic (no change; non-hemolytic); β-hemolytic usually more pathogenic than α-hemolytic, which is more pathogenic than nonhemolytic strains
• Hemolytic strains further subdivided by antigenic differences in cell wall carbohydrates—Lancefield serogroups A–H and K–T (e.g., group G *S. canis*); some groups more likely to be associated with disease, depending on species (e.g., group G associated with cats and dogs; group A associated with humans)
• Produce exotoxins—streptolysins (hemolysins), streptokinases, deoxyribonucleases, and hyaluronidases

SIGNALMENT
• Dogs and cats
• Very young—more prone to infection because of incomplete, developing immunity; particularly kittens born to primiparous queen

SIGNS
• Vary with site of infection and host immunocompetence
• Weakness
• Coughing
• Dyspnea
• Fever
• Hematemesis
• Hematuria
• Lymphadenopathy
• Dogs—septicemia; endometritis; vaginitis; mastitis; fading puppies; abortion; urinary tract infection; pyelonephritis; pneumonia; necrotizing fasciitis; streptococcal shock syndrome
• Cats—septicemia; peritonitis; cervical lymphadenitis; pharyngitis; tonsillitis; fading kitten

CAUSES & RISK FACTORS
• Age, exposure, and immune response—important for determining disease
• Virulence—depends on cellular products, surface components, and related substances
• Opportunistic—wounds, trauma, surgical procedures, viral infections, or immuno-suppressive conditions
• FeLV, FIP, immunodeficiency, respiratory viral infections, feline lower urinary tract disease—predisposing conditions
• Maternal antibodies generally protect puppies and kittens against clinical disease.
• Carrier state occurs

DIAGNOSIS

DIFFERENTIAL DIAGNOSIS
Other infectious causes—viruses, bacteria, fungi, *Rickettsia,* protozoa

CBC/BIOCHEMISTRY/URINALYSIS
• Normal or high WBCs with neutrophilic inflammatory response with a left shift or degenerative left shift
• Cocci—may be found in circulating neutrophils in overwhelming sepsis
• Biochemistry—may suggest predisposing conditions
• Urinalysis—pyuria (with or without bacteriuria) with cystitis

OTHER LABORATORY TESTS
• Direct microscopy
• Gram stain—of exudates; reveals chains of and single gram-positive cocci
• Culture—affected tissues; exudate or needle aspirates; confirms diagnosis
• Antibiotic susceptibility testing

IMAGING
Radiographs—interstitial or alveolar pulmonary pattern with pneumonia; radiodense uroliths (struvite)

DIAGNOSTIC PROCEDURES
N/A

PATHOLOGIC FINDINGS
• Acute inflammation—gross or microscopic abscesses
• Septicemia—postmortem reveals omphalophlebitis, peritonitis, hepatitis, pneumonia, and myocarditis.

TREATMENT
• Good nursing care
• Rehydrate.
• Drain and flush abscess.
• Debride necrotic tissue.

MEDICATIONS

DRUGS
• Penicillin—first choice; penicillin G at 10,000–20,000 U/kg IM, SC q12–24h or penicillin V at 8–30 mg/kg PO q8h
• Ampicillin—20–30 mg/kg IV, IM, SC, PO q8h; alone or in combination with gentamicin at 2–4 mg/kg IV, IM, SC q8h; for group B
• Prophylactic treatment—all kittens born to primiparous queens indicated for neonatal infections

CONTRAINDICATIONS/POSSIBLE INTERACTIONS
Avoid immunosuppressive drugs

FOLLOW-UP

PREVENTION/AVOIDANCE
• Avoid overcrowding and poor environmental sanitation
• Prevention in newborns—dipping navel and umbilical cord in 2% tincture of iodine.
• Prevention in colonies—avoid overcrowding; maintain clean feeders; segregate infected animals.

MISCELLANEOUS

ZOONOTIC POTENTIAL
• Dogs and cats may show no clinical signs with group A streptococci but may serve as a reservoir for human infection.
• Streptococci isolated from people are usually of human not animal origin.

ABBREVIATIONS
• FeLV = feline leukemia virus
• FIP = feline infectious peritonitis

Suggested Reading
Greene CE, Prescott JF. Streptococcal and other gram-positive bacterial infections. In: Greene CE, ed. Infectious diseases of the dog and cat. Philadelphia: Saunders, 1998:205–214.
Author J. Paul Woods
Consulting Editor Stephen C. Barr

BASICS

OVERVIEW
• Neonatal infection of paramucosa of small intestine by *Strongyloides canis and S. felis (stercoralis)* associated with acute and chronic diarrhea
• Transcolostral transmission to neonates, skin penetration by infective larvae, or ingestion of infective larvae; may persist by autoinfection
• Relatively host-specific; possibly transmission to humans
• *Strongyloides tumefaciens* in cats causes adenomatous mass in colon

SIGNALMENT
• Dogs and cats
• Neonatal diarrhea of pups and kittens with transcolostral transmission

SIGNS

Historical Findings
• Neonatal diarrhea or constipation
• Dermatitis

Physical Examination Findings
• Debilitated pups or kittens
• Dermatitis

CAUSES & RISK FACTORS
• Transcolostral transmission
• Possibility of autoinfection
• Skin penetration by infective larvae

 DIAGNOSIS

DIFFERENTIAL DIAGNOSIS
• *Toxocara* infections
• Viral infections

CBC/BIOCHEMISTRY/URINALYSIS
Usually normal

OTHER LABORATORY TESTS
N/A

IMAGING
N/A

DIAGNOSTIC PROCEDURES
Fecal examination for small (∼ 50 μm long), larvated eggs

 TREATMENT

Usually outpatient unless intravenous fluid supplementation needed for dehydration

 MEDICATIONS

DRUGS
Adulticide/larvicide recommended for neonatal infection of small intestine with possible respiratory migration by infective larvae

• Fenbendazole 50 mg/kg PO q24h PO for 5 days
• Ivermectin 50 μg/kg PO as single dose (extralabel use)

CONTRAINDICATIONS/POSSIBLE INTERACTIONS
Difficulty with administration of efficacious anthelmintic

 FOLLOW-UP

Fecal examination for *Strongyloides* larvae or eggs posttreatment

 MISCELLANEOUS

ZOONOTIC POTENTIAL
Humans may experience dermatitis and severe abdominal discomfort

Suggested Reading
Bowman DD, ed. Georgi's parasitology for veterinarians. 6th ed. Philadelphia: Saunders. 1994;154–158.
Author Robert M. Corwin
Consulting Editors Brett M. Feder and Mitchell A. Crystal

BASICS

OVERVIEW
• Strychnine—potent convulsant; alkaloid toxin; derived from the seeds of *Strychnos nux-vomica* and *S. ignatii;* used to kill rats, moles, gophers, and predators
• Rapid absorption
• Onset of clinical signs—10 min to 2 hr
• Effects—reversibly blocks the binding of the inhibitory neurotransmitter glycine; results in an unchecked reflex stimulation; eliminated as hepatic metabolites and as the parent compound in the urine
• Cause of death—apnea and hypoxia owing to rigidity of the respiration muscles
• Baits—containing > 0.5% strychnine limited to use by certified applicators; containing < 0.5% strychnine available to the general public

SIGNALMENT
Dogs and cats

SIGNS
• Violent tetanic seizures—may be initiated by physical, visible, or auditory stimuli
• Extensor rigidity
• Muscle stiffness
• Opisthotonus
• Tachycardia
• Hyperthermia
• Apnea
• Vomiting—rare

CAUSES & RISK FACTORS
• Malicious poisoning—fairly common
• Direct exposure to baits—more common in dogs than other species
• Relay toxicoses by the ingestion of poisoned rodents and birds has occurred.
• LD_{50}—dogs, > 0.2 mg/kg; cats, 0.5 mg/kg

DIAGNOSIS

DIFFERENTIAL DIAGNOSES
• Other toxicants—lead; nicotine; amphetamines; metaldehyde; chocolate; zinc phosphide; tremorogenic mycotoxins; antidepressants; 4-aminopyridine; cocaine; pyrethrins or pyrethroids; 1080 (fluoroacetate); caffeine; LSD; organochlorine insecticides

• Systemic diseases—uremia; hepatic failure; neoplasia; hypoglycemia; encephalitides; heat stroke; trauma; ischemia; tetanus

CBC/BIOCHEMISTRY/URINALYSIS
• High creatine kinase and lactate dehydrogenase
• Myoglobinuria

OTHER LABORATORY TESTS
• Analysis of stomach content, liver, kidney, or urine—reveal strychnine; if death is too rapid, kidney and urine are negative
• Blood gases—reveal acidosis

IMAGING
N/A

DIAGNOSTIC PROCEDURES
• **CAUTION:** do not induce a seizure with a stimulus; it is *not* diagnostic and may be lethal.
• Blood pressure—may reveal systemic hypertension

PATHOLOGIC FINDINGS
• Associated with trauma from the seizure activity
• Baits—often found in the stomach contents; may be color-coded red or green

TREATMENT

GENERAL LIFE SUPPORT
• Inpatient—may require treatment for as long as 48 hr
• Primary goals—prevent asphyxia; control seizures; may require complete anesthesia and artificial respiration
• Keep patient in a quiet, dimly lit room.
• Cool water baths—with hyperthermia

DECONTAMINATION
• Lessens duration and severity of signs
• Gastric or enterogastric lavage—lessens absorption
• Fluid diuresis—enhances elimination; normal saline with 5% mannitol (7 mg/kg/hr)
• Emesis—do not induce unless it is within minutes of the ingestion and the patient is asymptomatic

MEDICATIONS

DRUGS
• Decontamination—activated charcoal (2 g/kg); cathartic (sorbitol at 2.1 g/kg or magnesium sulfate at 0.5 g/kg)
• Seizure control—diazepam (may not be effective); pentobarbital (to effect); glycerol guaiacolate (110 mg/kg IV, repeated as needed); methocarbamol (150 mg/kg IV, repeated at 90 mg/kg as needed); inhalation anesthesia
• Urinary acidification—ammonium chloride (150 mg/kg); enhances elimination

CONTRAINDICATIONS/POSSIBLE INTERACTIONS
• Do not acidify with ammonium chloride if the patient is acidotic.
• Do not use ketamine.
• Do not use morphine.

FOLLOW-UP
• Monitor for secondary renal damage from myoglobinuria and possible tubular cast development.
• Prognosis—guarded until seizures are controlled; good after seizures are controlled

MISCELLANEOUS

SEE ALSO
Poisoning (Intoxication)

Suggested Reading
Osweiler GD. Strychnine poisoning. In: Kirk RW, ed., Current veterinary therapy VIII. Philadelphia: Saunders, 1983:98–100.
Author Jeffery O. Hall
Consulting Editor Gary D. Osweiler

SUBINVOLUTION OF PLACENTAL SITES

BASICS

OVERVIEW
- Failure or delay of normal postpartum uterine involution
- Failure of eosinophilic masses of collagen at placental sites to slough at 3–4 weeks postpartum
- Failure of fetal trophoblastic cells to regress normally; instead, they invade the maternal myometrium.
- Cause—unknown; hormonal or uterine basis not suspected

SIGNALMENT
- Dogs only
- Bitches < 3 years
- Seen with first litter
- No breed predilections

SIGNS

Historical Findings
- Patient presented 6–12 weeks postpartum
- Serosanguineous vulvar discharge beyond 6 weeks postpartum
- No systemic signs

Physical Examination Findings
- Serosanguineous vulvar discharge
- Firm, spherical structure within uterus on abdominal palpation

CAUSES & RISK FACTORS
- Unknown
- Hormonal—unlikely, because only some of the placental sites may be involved
- Uterine disease—unlikely, because of high first litter prevalence

DIAGNOSIS

DIFFERENTIAL DIAGNOSIS
- Metritis—differentiated by vaginal cytology and physical examination
- Vaginitis—differentiated by vaginal cytology
- Vaginal neoplasia—differentiated by vaginal cytology and vaginal endoscopy
- Uterine neoplasia—differentiated by ultrasonography or exploratory laparotomy

- Cystitis—differentiated by vaginal cytology and urinalysis
- Coagulopathy—differentiated by clotting times
- Trauma
- Endogenous estrogen stimulation—bitch with an extremely shortened interestrous interval
- Exogenous estrogen stimulation

CBC/BIOCHEMISTRY/URINALYSIS
- Usually normal

OTHER LABORATORY TESTS
- Serology for *Brucella canis* negative

IMAGING
Uterine ultrasonography—focal uterine wall thickening; echogenic fluid in the lumen

DIAGNOSTIC PROCEDURES
- Vaginal cytologic examination—key for diagnosis; reveals erythrocytes and parabasal epithelial cells; may note pathognomonic trophoblastic cells
- Guarded anterior vaginal culture—if vaginal cytologic examination or hemogram supports a diagnosis of secondary metritis

PATHOLOGIC FINDINGS
- Gross—sites characterized by a thickened, hemorrhagic area that may be nodular
- Histopathologic—definitive diagnosis; eosinophilic collagen masses with trophoblasts extending into the myometrium

TREATMENT
- Usually outpatient
- Spontaneous remission—occurs before or at next cycle
- Medical—for rare development of anemia, metritis, or peritonitis
- Severely affected patients—may require blood transfusion (rare)
- Warn owner of the rare possibility of excessive hemorrhage; instruct owner to monitor mucous membrane color.
- Ovariohysterectomy—curative; treatment of choice if future breeding not desired
- Surgical curettage of subinvoluted sites— may also be performed

MEDICATIONS

DRUGS
Generally not successful

CONTRAINDICATIONS/POSSIBLE INTERACTIONS
- Ecbolics—may cause uterine rupture
- Progestational drugs—increase the risk of metritis, which may mimic pyometra

FOLLOW-UP

PATIENT MONITORING
- Mucous membrane color and amount of discharge
- Packed cell volume—if anemia is a concern
- Changes in discharge color or odor ands vaginal cytologic examination and culture— diagnose secondary infection

POSSIBLE COMPLICATIONS
Infection, blood-loss anemia, or uterine rupture—rare

EXPECTED COURSE AND PROGNOSIS
- Spontaneous resolution—the norm
- Recurrence—not expected
- Prognosis for future reproduction— excellent with spontaneous resolution

MISCELLANEOUS

Suggested Reading
Johnston SD. Subinvolution of placental sites. In: Kirk RW, ed. Current veterinary therapy IX. Philadelphia: Saunders, 1986;1231–1233.
Wheeler SL. Subinvolution of placental sites in the bitch. In: Morrow DA, ed. Current therapy in theriogenology 2. Philadelphia: Saunders, 1986;513–515.
Author Joni L. Freshman
Consulting Editor Sara K. Lyle

BASICS

OVERVIEW
- A rare canine disorder
- Usually a cutaneous marker for advanced hepatic disease or concurrent hepatic disease and diabetes mellitus
- Rarely associated with a glucagon-secreting pancreatic tumor
- Lesions—pathogenesis unclear; result of keratinocyte degeneration and necrosis; hyperglucagonemia, hypoaminoacidemia, zinc and essential fatty acid deficiencies believed to play a direct or indirect role

SYSTEMS AFFECTED
- Skin/Exocrine—eroded, erythematous, and crusting lesions around the mouth and eyes and on the legs, feet, and genitalia
- Hepatobiliary—hepatic cirrhosis or vacuolar hepatopathy with parenchymal collapse and nodular hyperplasia
- Endocrine/Metabolic—glucagon-secreting pancreatic tumor

SIGNALMENT
- Dogs
- No breed predilection
- Often old dogs
- Males more likely affected

SIGNS
- Skin lesions—usually precede clinical evidence of internal disease by weeks or months; usually the presenting complaint; consist of erythema, crusts, and erosions or ulcerations affecting the muzzle, mucocutaneous areas of the face, distal limbs, feet, and external genitalia
- Footpads—usually hyperkeratotic and affected with fissures and ulcerations; pain associated with walking
- Secondary bacterial and/or fungal infections—often associated with footpad lesions

CAUSES & RISK FACTORS
- Specific cause unknown
- Keratinocyte degeneration and necrosis—probably result from cellular starvation or other nutritional imbalance
- Nutritional imbalance—probably hypoaminoacidemia or deficiencies in essential fatty acids and zinc; owing to metabolic abnormalities caused by high serum glucagon levels, liver dysfunction, or a combination
- No risk factors have been identified.

DIAGNOSIS

DIFFERENTIAL DIAGNOSIS
- Pemphigus foliaceus
- Systemic lupus erythematosus
- Zinc-responsive dermatosis
- Toxic epidermal necrolysis
- Drug eruption
- Distal extremity erythema and footpad hyperkeratosis—unique; strongly suggest the diagnosis

CBC/BIOCHEMISTRY/URINALYS
- Anemia—may be noted; usually normocytic, normochromic, and nonregenerative
- RBC abnormalities—polychromasia; anisocytosis; poikilocytosis; and target cells
- ALP, ALT, and AST—high activity
- Total bilirubin and bile acid levels—high
- BSP retention
- Biochemistry abnormalities are not seen in dogs with glucagon-secreting tumors.
- Most patients develop borderline or frank hyperglycemia.

OTHER LABORATORY TESTS
- Elevated plasma glucagon levels—consistently present with glucagon-secreting tumors; variably observed with chronic hepatic disorders
- Hypoaminoacidemia common
- High insulin levels may be noted.

IMAGING
Abdominal radiography and ultrasonography—usually unremarkable with glucagon-secreting pancreatic tumors; abnormalities compatible with hepatic cirrhosis or vacuolar hepatopathy and nodular hyperplasia seen with advanced liver disease

DIAGNOSTIC PROCEDURES
Skin biopsies—important diagnostic tool; sample early lesions because chronic lesions rarely show the unique epidermal edema

PATHOLOGIC FINDINGS
- Skin biopsies—diffuse parakeratotic hyperkeratosis with high-level intracellular and intercellular epidermal edema are unique; irregular epidermal hyperplasia and mild superficial perivascular dermatitis
- Chronic lesions—marked parakeratotic hyperkeratosis and epidermal hyperplasia; also noted with zinc deficiency

TREATMENT
- Usually as outpatients
- Patients with signs of liver failure may need to be hospitalized for supportive care.
- Surgical excision of glucagon-secreting tumors—can be curative if diagnosis is made before metastasis; unfortunately, this is rarely the case.
- Most cases are associated with chronic irreversible liver disease.
- Inform clients that this disorder indicates concurrent severe internal disease with a poor prognosis.
- Hydrotherapy and shampoos—help remove crusts; lessen pruritus and pain

MEDICATIONS

DRUGS
- Specific treatment—attempt to correct the underlying disease; not usually accomplished
- Nonspecific symptomatic therapy—antibiotics and antifungal drugs for secondary skin infections
- Glucocorticoids—improve skin lesions; may induce a diabetic crisis because patients are either prediabetic or overtly diabetic at diagnosis; may induce ascites if patient has chronic severe liver disease; prednisone or prednisolone: usual initial dosage of 0.5–1.0 mg/kg daily; maintain at lowest possible alternate-day dosage
- Zinc sulfate or gluconate—10 mg/kg daily; results unrewarding
- Essential fatty acids—not beneficial

CONTRAINDICATIONS/POSSIBLE INTERACTIONS
N/A

FOLLOW-UP

PATIENT MONITORING N/A

PREVENTION/AVOIDANCE N/A

POSSIBLE COMPLICATIONS
- Liver failure
- Secondary bacterial and/or fungal skin infections

EXPECTED COURSE AND PROGNOSIS
Prognosis poor; survival time reported as 5 months after development of skin lesions

MISCELLANEOUS

ASSOCIATED CONDITIONS
Diabetes mellitus—usually nonketoacidotic

SYNONYMS
- Hepatiocutaneous syndrome
- Necrolytic migratory erythema
- Metabolic epidermal necrosis
- Canine diabetic dermatosis

ABBREVIATIONS
- ALP = alkaline phosphatase
- ALT = alanine aminotransferase
- AST = aspartate aminotransferase
- BSP = sulfobromophthalein

Suggested Reading
Scott DW, Miller WH, Griffin GE. Endocrine and metabolic diseases. In: Muller & Kirk's small animal dermatology. 5th ed. Philadelphia: Saunders, 1995:706–710.
Author Sheila M. F. Torres
Consulting Editor Karen Helton Rhodes

DISEASES

SYNOVIAL CELL SARCOMA

 BASICS

OVERVIEW
• Malignant neoplasm believed to arise from primitive mesenchymal precursor cells outside the synovial membrane of joints and bursa; precursor cells have the ability to differentiate into epithelial or fibroblastic cells; thus tumor may have components of both epithelial and mesenchymal neoplasia.
• Highly locally invasive; potential to metastasize in > 40% of cases
• Most common sites—appendicular skeleton, specifically elbow, stifle, and scapulohumeral regions

SIGNALMENT
• Dogs—large-breed dogs of either sex; median age, 9 years
• Cats—rarely reported

SIGNS
• Slowly progressive lameness
• Palpable mass
• Weight loss
• Anorexia

CAUSES & RISK FACTORS
Unknown

 DIAGNOSIS

DIFFERENTIAL DIAGNOSIS
• Other primary neoplasia—chondrosarcoma; fibrosarcoma; osteosarcoma
• Metastatic neoplasia—prostatic carcinoma
• Other primary bone diseases—osteoarthritis; osteomyelitis

CBC/BIOCHEMISTRY/URINALYSIS
No consistent abnormalities

OTHER LABORATORY TESTS
N/A

IMAGING
• Radiographs of the primary lesion—show both bone and joint involvement; increased soft tissue opacity in and around the involved joints common; may note periosteal reaction
• Thoracic radiographs—screen for metastatic disease

DIAGNOSTIC PROCEDURES
• Biopsy—definitive diagnosis; ideally, obtain both soft tissue and bony components for histologic evaluation.
• Regional lymph nodes—palpate; obtain fine-needle aspirates, if possible.

 TREATMENT

Radical surgical excision (amputation)—treatment of choice

 MEDICATIONS

DRUGS
• Chemotherapy—definitive regimen not described; isolated case reports of response to doxorubicin and cyclophosphamide; no evidence that treatment adjuvant to surgery is indicated.
• Pain management—NSAIDs, as necessary

CONTRAINDICATIONS/POSSIBLE INTERACTIONS
N/A

 FOLLOW-UP

PATIENT MONITORING
Monitor for local recurrence and pulmonary metastatic disease—every 2–3 months for the first year; every 6 months thereafter

EXPECTED COURSE AND PROGNOSIS
• Clinical course—may be protracted over months to years
• Localized disease—prognosis excellent; median survival > 48 months
• Median survival with amputation alone—17 months
• Metastatic disease, specific histologic criteria (e.g., high mitotic rate, high percent tumor necrosis, and high nuclear pleomorphism), and positive immunocytochemical staining for cytokeratin—prognosis poor; median survival, < 4 months

 MISCELLANEOUS

PREGNANCY
Do not breed animals who are undergoing chemotherapy.

Suggested Reading
Vail DM, Powers BE, Getzy DM, et al. Evaluation of prognostic factors for dogs with synovial sarcoma: 36 cases (1986–1991). J Am Vet Med Assoc 1994;205:1300–1307.

Author Ruthanne Chun
Consulting Editor Wallace B. Morrison

TAPEWORMS (CESTODIASIS)

BASICS

OVERVIEW
• Tapeworm infections of small intestine with *Taenia* spp., esp. *T. pisiformis* of dogs and *T. taeniaeformis* of cats, and *Dipylidium caninum* of dogs and cats
• Taeniids are transmitted by predation of rabbits or rodents; *Dipylidium* is flea-vectored, with flea maggots picking up tapeworm eggs in dog or cat feces, and transmitted by adult fleas ingested by dogs or cats.
• No apparent harm done to host, but may result in mild perianal pruritus

SIGNALMENT
Dogs and cats

SIGNS
• Chains of segments or single segments in feces
• Dragging or rubbing anus on ground because of perianal pruritus with *Dipylidium*
• Segments pasted to perianal skin

CAUSES & RISK FACTORS
• Taeniid infections—eating viscera of rabbits, rodents
• *Dipylidium* infections—fleas in environment

DIAGNOSIS

DIFFERENTIAL DIAGNOSIS
Anal sac impaction

CBC/BIOCHEMISTRY/URINALYSIS
Normal

OTHER LABORATORY TESTS
N/A

IMAGING
N/A

DIAGNOSTIC PROCEDURES
• *Dipylidium*—Scotch tape pressed to perianal skin for egg packets; single egg ~50 μm diameter; pale yellow, hexacanth embryo
• *Taenia*—eggs spherical, brown, ~30–35 μm; hexacanth embryo (six apparent hooks on embryo)

TREATMENT
• Outpatient
• Discuss need for flea control to prevent recurrence of *Dipylidium*.

MEDICATIONS

DRUGS
• Fenbendazole effective at 50 mg/kg PO q24h for 5 days for taeniid infections
• Praziquantel 5 mg/kg PO once for *Taenia, Dipylidium;* praziquantel/pyrantel pamoate for cats; praziquantel/pyrantel pamoate/febantel for dogs
• Epsiprantel 5.5 mg/kg PO for dogs, 2.8 mg/kg PO cats, for *Taenia, Dipylidium*
• Flea control necessary for control of *Dipylidium*

CONTRAINDICATIONS/POSSIBLE INTERACTIONS
Do not use praziquantel or epsiprantel for puppies or kittens < 4 weeks old.

FOLLOW-UP
Fecal examination for tapeworm segments

MISCELLANEOUS

ZOONOTIC POTENTIAL
Children may be at risk for *Dipylidium* infections.

SYNONYMS
Cestodiasis

Suggested Reading
Bowman DD, ed. Georgi's parasitology for veterinarians. 6th ed. Philadelphia: Saunders, 1994:137–150.
Author Robert M. Corwin
Consulting Editors Brett M. Feder and Mitchell A. Crystal

TAURINE DEFICIENCY

 ## BASICS

OVERVIEW
• Taurine is an essential amino acid in the diet of cats; they must conjugate bile acids with taurine and cannot synthesize enough to cope with this obligatory loss, so diets deficient in taurine cause taurine deficiency in cats. All cat food manufacturers add taurine to their feline diets. Taurine is not an essential amino acid in dogs and so most canine diets do not contain added taurine.
• Taurine is found throughout the body, with highest concentrations in excitable tissues (e.g., myocardium, CNS, and retina), where its exact function remains a mystery. It probably helps maintain osmolar gradients and may help regulate calcium movement. Taurine is actively concentrated in myocardial cells by a membrane pump that is under the influence of catecholamines.
• Taurine deficiency results in retinal degeneration and myocardial failure (i.e., decreased myocardial contractility), a condition commonly termed dilated cardiomyopathy (DCM), which has been identified in domestic cats, foxes, and some dogs. In each, the myocardial failure was fully or partially reversible with dietary taurine supplementation.

SIGNALMENT
• Cats—DCM due to taurine deficiency is rare because taurine is added to most cat foods.
• Dogs—American cocker spaniels with DCM are almost uniformly taurine-deficient; most golden retrievers with DCM are probably taurine-deficient. Many dogs with DCM that are members of breeds that do not commonly get DCM or mixed breed dogs with DCM have a low plasma taurine concentration.

SIGNS
See Cardiomyopathy, Dilated (Cats and Dogs)

CAUSES & RISK FACTORS
• Cats fed home-cooked diets (e.g., vegetarian or boiled-meat diets) are at risk; occasionally a cat with DCM that is on a commercial diet will have a low plasma taurine concentration.
• Only risk factor known for dogs is breed.

 ## DIAGNOSIS

DIFFERENTIAL DIAGNOSIS
Idiopathic dilated cardiomyopathy or myocardial failure due to another cause; see Cardiomyopathy, Dilated (Cats and Dogs)

CBC/BIOCHEMISTRY/URINALYSIS
No characteristic abnormalities

OTHER LABORATORY TESTS
• Obtain a heparinized blood sample, place it on ice, and centrifuge within 30 min. Do not allow clotting because platelets are rich in taurine. Avoid hemolysis. A plasma taurine concentration below 50–60 nmoles/mL is too low in dogs and cats. Heparinized whole-blood can also be analyzed; a whole blood concentration below 300 nmoles/mL is too low.
• Prolonged fasting in cats can produce a low plasma taurine concentration; the whole-blood concentration stays within the normal range longer.

IMAGING
Myocardial failure is diagnosed by identifying an increase in end-systolic diameter, usually with a compensatory smaller increase in end-diastolic diameter and a reduced shortening fraction on an echocardiogram.

DIAGNOSTIC PROCEDURES
Examine any taurine-deficient patient for central retinal degeneration.

 ## TREATMENT

• Use conventional heart failure therapy until taurine supplementation has caused significant echocardiographic and clinical improvement; drug therapy can usually be discontinued after 3–6 months of taurine supplementation in both dogs and cats.
• Most cats in heart failure do better if they are sent home, as long as the owner can provide good nursing care.

 ## MEDICATIONS

DRUGS OF CHOICE
• Supplement taurine (250 mg PO q12h, cats; 250–1000 mg PO q12h, dogs), usually for life
• Taurine supplements—can obtain from health food stores without a prescription; they are relatively inexpensive.
• Carnitine supplementation (1 g PO q12h)—also recommended for American cocker spaniels.

CONTRAINDICATIONS/POSSIBLE INTERACTIONS
No known adverse effects of taurine supplementation; excess taurine is eliminated in the urine

 ## FOLLOW-UP

Routine examinations for a patient with heart failure; repeat echocardiogram in 3–6 months to document improvement. If no improvement, can discontinue taurine supplementation

 ## MISCELLANEOUS

ABBREVIATIONS
DCM = dilated cardiomyopathy

Suggested Reading
Kittleson MD, Keene B, Pion PD, Loyer CG, and the MUST Study Investigators. Results of the Multicenter Spaniel Trial (MUST): taurine- and carnitine-responsive dilated cardiomyopathy in American cocker spaniels with decreased plasma taurine concentration. J Vet Int Med 1997;11(4):204–211.
Kramer GA, Kittleson MD, Fox PR, et al. Plasma taurine concentrations in normal dogs and in dogs with heart disease. J Vet Int Med 1995;9:253–258.
Pion PD, Kittleson MD, Rogers QR, Morris JG. Myocardial failure in cats associated with low plasma taurine: a reversible cardiomyopathy. Science 1987;237:764–768.
Author Mark D. Kittleson
Consulting Editors Larry P. Tilley and Francis W. K. Smith, Jr.

TESTICULAR DEGENERATION AND HYPOPLASIA

 BASICS

OVERVIEW
• Degeneration—histologic changes in the testes after puberty; may be differentiated from hypoplasia by the increased thickness of the basement membrane in the degenerated testis
• Hypoplasia—a variety of histologic lesions thought to be congenital (although often not obvious until after puberty) or heritable

SIGNALMENT
• Dogs and cats
• Dogs—any age or breed; hypoplasia, generally young; degeneration, generally old
• Tortoiseshell cats—may be fertile; usually linked with sex chromosome abnormalities (see Sexual Development Disorders)

SIGNS
• Infertility
• Reduced spermatozoa (or no spermatozoa) in the ejaculate
• Hypoplasia (dogs)—rarely any physical signs other than small testes
• Degeneration (dogs)—any previous serotal or testicular lesion can be related.

CAUSES & RISK FACTORS
Degeneration
• Heat
• Irradiation
• Metals—lead salts; cadmium; organic mercurial compounds
• Nitrogen-containing and halogenated compounds
• Other toxins
• Orchitis
• Steroid hormones—estrogen secreted by a Sertoli cell tumor
• Other hormonal abnormalities—hypothyroidism; hypocortisolism; hyperadrenocorticism
• Increasing age—6.3% of beagles maintained to 7.75 years had incomplete spermatogenesis
• Arterial sclerosis
• Some chemotherapeutic agents—cimetidine; ketoconazole; nitrofurans).
• Any previous scrotal or testicular lesion may be related.

Hypoplasia
• Klinefelter (XXY) syndrome
• Hypogonadotropic hypogonadism—may be acquired from traumatic or neoplastic lesion of the pituitary

 DIAGNOSIS

DIFFERENTIAL DIAGNOSIS
• Degeneration—old, azoospermic or severely oligospermic previously fertile dogs with small testes
• Hypoplasia—young, azoospermic, never-fertile dogs with small testes
• Spermatocele
• Sperm granuloma
• Orchitis
• Neoplasia
• Ejaculatory failure—retrograde ejaculation

CBC/BIOCHEMISTRY/URINALYSIS
N/A

OTHER LABORATORY TESTS
Canine FSH assay—differentiate from blockage (spermatocele); high concentration indicates incomplete spermatogenesis associated with hypoplasia or degeneration.

IMAGING
Ultrasonography—testicular size; homogeneity of the parenchyma

DIAGNOSTIC PROCEDURES
• Semen evaluation—primary diagnostic procedure; dog: always obtained by use of an artificial vagina or collection cone; cat: obtained by electroejaculation, when available; collect two ejaculates on separate days; establish azoospermia or oligospermia
• Testicular biopsy (for azoospermia)—fine-needle: identify long spermatids and spermatozoa; Tru-Cut (tissue plug) or open incision: most complete histopathologic diagnosis; fix tissue for sectioning in Bouin or Zenker fixative.
• Karyotype—identify extra X chromosome or other numerical or structural chromosome anomaly

PATHOLOGIC FINDINGS
• Normal spermatogenesis—indicates blockage in azoospermic dogs
• Basement membrane thickness—differentiates hypoplasia from degeneration

 TREATMENT
• Degeneration linked to pituitary, adrenal gland, thyroid gland, or other metabolic disruption—goal is to correct the underlying cause.
• No specific diagnosis—may try gonadotropic hormones; rare anecdotal success

 MEDICATIONS

DRUGS
• hCG—500 IU SC 2 times a week
• eCG—20 IU/kg SC 3 times a week

CONTRAINDICATIONS/POSSIBLE INTERACTIONS
N/A

 FOLLOW-UP

PATIENT MONITORING
Suspected testicular degeneration (dogs)—a repeat semen analysis performed at least 60 days after correcting any identified underlying cause is needed before reversibility can be assessed.

EXPECTED COURSE AND PROGNOSIS
• Hypoplasia (dogs)—prognosis for fertility poor
• Degeneration (dogs)—prognosis for fertility depends on the cause, site, and extent of injury; usually guarded to poor

 MISCELLANEOUS

SEE ALSO
• Infertility, Male—Dogs
• Sexual Development Disorders
• Spermatocele/Sperm Granuloma

ABBREVIATIONS
• eCG = equine chorionic gonadotropin
• FSH = follicle-stimulating hormone
• hCG = human chorionic gonadotropin

Suggested Reading
Axner E, Strom B, Linde-Forsberg C, et al., Reproductive disorders in 10 domestic male cats. J Sm Anim Pract 1996;37:394–401.
McEntee K. Reproductive pathology of domestic animals. San Diego: Academic Press, 1990:262–263.
Author Rolf E. Larsen
Consulting Editor Sara K. Lyle

DISEASES

TETANUS

BASICS

OVERVIEW
• *Clostridium tetani*—an obligate, anaerobic, spore-forming, gram-positive rod found in soil and as part of the normal bacterial flora of the intestinal tract of mammals with a predilection for contaminated, necrotic, anaerobic wounds (puncture, surgery, lacerations, burns, frostbite, open fractures, abrasions)
• Germi-nating spores—in wounds produce potent exotoxin tetanospasmin (tetanus toxin); resistant to disinfectants and to the effects of environmental exposure
• Found worldwide, especially in the tropics.

SIGNALMENT
• Dogs—occasionally
• Cats—rarely

SIGNS

Historical Findings
• Appear a few days to few months after spores enter wound (fracture, surgery, and puncture)
• Wound—often necrotic; but may have healed over

Physical Examination Findings
Localized
• Mild rigidity of muscles or leg nearest the site of spore inoculation (wound)
• Stiffness of (hind) limbs; stilted gait; mild weakness and incoordination
• Can resolve spontaneously—reflects partial immunity to tetanospasmin
• Can be prodromal to generalized disease—when enough toxin gains access to CNS

Progressive/Generalized
• Tail—stretches out; progressive tetany of muscles to point of sawhorse appearance
• Convulsions (clonic)—limbs; whole body (opisthotonus); pain during contractions
• Difficulty breathing—dyspnea
• Difficulty opening jaws—lockjaw, trismus
• Difficulty eating—dysphagia
• Eyes—lids retract (visus sardonicus); third eyelid prolapses when head is touched; eyeballs recede into orbit (enophthalmos)
• Wrinkled forehead
• Erect ears
• Grinning appearance—commissure of lips retracted
• Salivation
• Fever, painful urination (dysuria) and constipation—may be seen
• Tetanic muscle spasms—from stimulation (sudden movement, sound, touch)
• Death—during spasm of laryngeal and respiratory muscles (fatal acute asphyxia); when respiratory muscles are sufficiently paralyzed

CAUSES & RISK FACTORS
• Unattended wounds (e.g., punctures, surgical, compound bone fractures)—portal of entry for spores
• Outdoor pets—greater opportunity for acquiring wounds

DIAGNOSIS

DIFFERENTIAL DIAGNOSIS
Intoxications mimicking tetanus—lead and strychnine poisoning

CBC/BIOCHEMISTRY/URINALYSIS
• Initial leukopenia; switch to moderate leukocytosis; then gradual return to normal range
• AST and CPK—some increase; result of muscle damage during later stages of disease
• Urinalysis—essentially normal; high myoglobin from muscles damaged by constant excitation

OTHER LABORATORY TESTS
• Serology—antitetanus antibody often undetectable in serum
• Culture—wounds and serum; usually unrewarding to culture for *C. tetani* or to detect toxin (by mouse neutralization); CSF and blood cultures for bacterial pathogens of meningitis

IMAGING N/A

DIAGNOSTIC PROCEDURES N/A

PATHOLOGIC FINDINGS
None of significance; may find a healed-over wound, sometimes containing a foreign body

TREATMENT

• Inpatient—good supportive and constant nursing care important; prolonged period (3–4 weeks)
• Feeding—patients often have difficulty in prehending food unless helped; pay particular attention to what consistency of food the patient easily ingests; placement of a gastrotomy tube may be necessary; force feeding or feeding with a stomach tube may exacerbate tetanic state, so not advised
• Hydration—maintain with oral water; if inadequate, give a balanced intravenous fluid
• Keep patient in darkened, quiet area; do not disturb.
• Keep patient on soft bedding; prevent decubital ulcers.
• Airway and ventilation—assess; may be necessary to perform endotracheal intubation; tracheostomy may be necessary later.
• Urinary and fecal retention—may occur as a result of hypertonic anal and urethral sphincters; urinary catheterization and enemas (to relieve constipation) may be necessary.

MEDICATIONS

DRUGS

Sedation

• To control reflex spasms and convulsions
• Phenothiazines—drugs of choice; chlorpromazine; with or without barbiturates (e.g., phenobarbital)
• Heart rate—may drop when phenothiazines are used in combination; if < 60 beats/min, reverse the bradycardia with glycopyrrolate.

• Diazepam—alternative to phenobarbital Tetanus
• First test for hypersensitivity reaction.
• Human tetanus immunoglobulin—administer 500–3000 U IM at multiple sites, especially proximal to wound; or use or equine tetanus antitoxin (10,000 U IV).
• Administer adsorbed tetanus toxoid intramuscularly.

Antibiotics

• Have no effect against toxin already bound to nerves
• Penicillin—administer systemically and locally into the wound; 20,000 IU/kg q12h for 5 days; use crystalline penicillin on the first day and procaine penicillin thereafter.

CONTRAINDICATIONS/POSSIBLE INTERACTIONS

• Avoid glucocorticoids and atropine.
• Avoid narcotics—depress respiratory center

FOLLOW-UP

PATIENT MONITORING

• Prevent decubital ulcers and peripheral nerve palsies—cautiously move stabilized patient.
• Monitor blood pressure and ECG.

PREVENTION/AVOIDANCE

• Vaccinate—tetanus toxoid
• Prevent skin wound trauma—clear runs and yards of wire, glass, etc.
• Wound management—early and thorough irrigation with hydrogen peroxide; debridement, draining, especially in known tetanus-prone wounds
• Penicillin—administer for minimum of 3 days for all deep contaminated wounds

EXPECTED COURSE AND PROGNOSIS

• Prognosis—depends on number of factors; the more toxin bound to nerves, the poorer the prognosis; improve by removing source of additional toxin (debriding and cleaning wound).
• Course of recovery—slow; requires rehabilitation to regain full use of limbs; most recover in 1 week; some have a course of 3–4 weeks; unattended disease usually fatal

MISCELLANEOUS

ZOONOTIC POTENTIAL

None, but tetanus spores ubiquitous in environment

ABBREVIATIONS

• AST = aspartate aminotransferase
• CPK = creatine phosphokinase
• CSF = cerebrospinal fluid

Suggested Reading
Greene CE. Tetanus. In: Greene CE, ed. Infectious diseases of the dog and cat. Philadelphia: Saunders, 1998:267–273.
Author Patrick L. McDonough
Consulting Editor Stephen C. Barr

TETRALOGY OF FALLOT

BASICS

OVERVIEW
• A congenital cardiac malformation that consists of a VSD, pulmonic stenosis, an overriding aorta, and right ventricular hypertrophy. The aorta straddles the malalignment VSD (Figure 1). The VSD is usually large, with an area that equals or exceeds that of the open aortic valve. The essential developmental abnormality is probably a cranial deviation of a component of the infundibular septum; the other defects are secondary. Some reserve the term for malformations that strictly fulfill the above criteria; others apply it more liberally to include patients that have a VSD and right ventricular outflow tract obstruction.
• Hemodynamics are determined primarily by the size of the VSD and the severity of right ventricular outflow tract obstruction. A large VSD allows equilibration of left and right ventricular pressures, with shunt direction determined by the relationship between peripheral vascular resistance and the resistance to right ventricular ejection. Severe right ventricular outflow tract obstruction results in a right-to-left shunt with cyanosis and compensatory erythrocytosis as prominent clinical features.

• An uncommon congenital defect, but the most common congenital cardiac malformation that causes cyanosis in dogs and cats

SIGNALMENT
• Dogs and cats—uncommon in both
• English bulldogs and keeshonds predisposed

SIGNS

Historical Findings
• Weakness
• Syncope
• Shortness of breath

Physical Examination Findings
• A systolic ejection murmur at the left heart base, caused by right ventricular outflow tract obstruction in most patients; some with hyperviscosity and severe pulmonary stenosis do not have murmurs.
• Cyanosis—in most patients; degree of cyanosis depends on the direction and volume of shunt. If right ventricular outflow tract obstruction is mild, the direction of the shunt may be left to right; in this case, cyanosis is absent and the pathophysiology is that of an isolated VSD.
• Arterial pulses usually normal
• Congestive heart failure occurs rarely, possibly because the right ventricle can unload into the left.

CAUSES & RISK FACTORS
Congenital; polygenic inheritance of a continuum of conotruncal defects that includes tetralogy of Fallot has been shown in keeshonds. Genetic and environmental factors probably contribute to development of naturally occurring disorder.

DIAGNOSIS

DIFFERENTIAL DIAGNOSIS
• Pulmonic stenosis, aortic stenosis, ventricular septal defect, and atrial septal defect can all cause left basilar ejection murmurs.
• Patients with severe pulmonic stenosis and a right-to-left atrial level shunt may have similar findings on physical examination.
• Other anatomic right-to-left shunts (PDA or VSD with pulmonary hypertension) do not typically cause murmurs; differential cyanosis (mucous membranes in head are pink and those in caudal portions of body are cyanotic) are observed if a PDA shunts right to left.

CBC/BIOCHEMISTRY/URINALYSIS
• Compensatory erythrocytosis if the shunt is right to left.
• Other clinicopathologic findings usually normal

OTHER LABORATORY TESTS
N/A

IMAGING

Thoracic Radiographic Findings
• Variable degree of right ventricular enlargement
• Ascending aorta may be prominent.
• Pulmonary vessels are small.

Echocardiographic Findings
• Right ventricular hypertrophy
• Large VSD visualized directly
• Straddling of the VSD by the aorta
• Narrow infundibulum and/or abnormal pulmonic valve
• Doppler evidence of pulmonic stenosis
• Contrast echocardiography delineates a right-to-left shunt.

Angiocardiography
• Reveals malalignment VSD, right ventricular hypertrophy, pulmonic stenosis, and direction of shunt
• Nonselective angiography may confirm the diagnosis in small animals.

DIAGNOSTIC PROCEDURES

Electrocardiographic Findings
• Right ventricular hypertrophy pattern in most dogs and cats
• Various intraventricular conduction disturbances observed in cats

Oximetry
Used to confirm peripheral desaturation of hemoglobin

TREATMENT
• Most can be treated as outpatients.
• Exercise restriction recommended
• Definitive surgical correction requires cardiopulmonary bypass.
• Palliative surgical procedures that enhance pulmonary blood flow have been attempted.
• Treat erythrocytosis by periodic phlebotomy to maintain a PCV of 62–68%.

MEDICATIONS

DRUGS
Nonselective β-adrenergic antagonists such as propranolol may be palliative; they act as negative inotropes and prevent the physiologic drop in peripheral vascular resistance that occurs during exercise. These hemodynamic effects serve to limit right-to-left shunting. Propranolol may also favorably affect the oxyhemoglobin dissociation curve.

CONTRAINDICATIONS/POSSIBLE INTERACTIONS
Vasodilators contraindicated

FOLLOW-UP
• Monitor PCV every 1–3 months.
• Breeding affected animals not advised
• Bacterial endocarditis, neurologic complications associated with erythrocytosis, arrhythmias, and sudden death are potential sequelae.
• Prognosis is poor; most patients with clinical signs live less than 1 year, although survivals > 3 years have been documented.

MISCELLANEOUS

ABBREVIATIONS
• PDA = patent ductus arteriosus
• VSD = ventricular septal defect

Suggested Reading
Kittleson MD. Tetralogy of Fallot. In Kittleson MD, Kienle RD, eds. Small animal cardiovascular medicine. St. Louis: Mosby, 1998:240–247.
Author Jonathan A. Abbott
Consulting Editors Larry P. Tilley, Francis W. K. Smith, Jr.

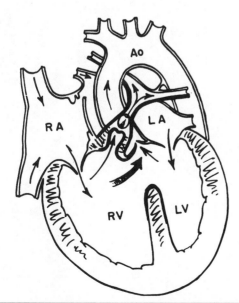

Figure 1.

Classic tetralogy of Fallot. RA = right atrium, LA = left atrium, RV = right ventricle, LV = left ventricle, AO = aorta. (From Roberts W. Adult congential heart disease. Philadelphia: F.A. Davis Co., 1987, with permission.)

THROMBOCYTOPATHIES

 BASICS

OVERVIEW
• Acquired or hereditary defects that can affect any of the main functions of the platelets, including activation, adhesion, and aggregation
• Affected animals typically have normal platelet counts but have spontaneous bleeding; mucosal bleeding is the most common sign.

SIGNALMENT
• Hereditary platelet function defects diagnosed at all ages, but may first appear in young animals when excessive bleeding occurs with loss of deciduous teeth
• Acquired defects—any breed of dog or cat
• Von Willebrand disease—many breeds of dogs and rarely cats (see von Willebrand Disease)
• Thromboasthenic thrombopathia—otter hounds
• Basset hound hereditary thrombopathia—widespread in this breed
• Spitz thrombopathia—Spitz
• Type I Glanzmann thromboasthenia—Great Pyrenees
• Platelet function defect—gray collies with cyclic hematopoiesis
• Chediak-Higashi syndrome—cats

SIGNS
• Spontaneous bleeding in some animals, often associated with mucosal surfaces
• Frequent epistaxis
• Auricular hematomas in basset hounds with hereditary thrombopathia
• Prolonged bleeding in some animals during diagnostic or surgical procedures

CAUSES & RISK FACTORS

Acquired
• Drugs—anesthetics, antibiotics, antihistamines, anti-inflammatories, and heparin; NSAIDs (e.g., aspirin) inhibit platelet function by preventing the formation of thromboxane A_2, a potent platelet agonist.
• Secondary to systemic disease—renal azotemia, pancreatitis, liver disease, immune-mediated thrombocytopenia, and neoplastic disorders (both hematopoietic and nonhematopoietic neoplasms)

Hereditary
• Von Willebrand disease—a deficiency of von Willebrand's factor, which is critical for platelet adhesion
• Canine thromboasthenic thrombopathia in otter hounds—a deficiency of the platelet glycoproteins necessary for fibrinogen-induced aggregation
• Basset hound hereditary thrombopathia and Spitz thrombopathy—platelet aggregation defects
• Aggregation defect caused by lack of the fibrinogen receptor—great Pyrenees with type I Glanzmann thrombasthenia
• Aggregation defect caused by lack of normal constituents in the platelet dense granules—gray collies with cyclic hematopoiesis and Chediak-Higashi syndrome.

 DIAGNOSIS

DIFFERENTIAL DIAGNOSIS
Other acquired or hereditary bleeding disorders characterized by bleeding that is more severe than the bleeding seen in most animals with acquired or hereditary platelet function defects

CBC/BIOCHEMISTRY/URINALYSIS
• Anemia, if bleeding is severe; regenerative or nonregenerative
• Platelet counts typically normal in dogs with thrombocytopathies, but low counts seen in some otter hounds with thrombo-asthenic thrombopathy
• Giant platelets in some dogs with thrombo-asthenic thrombopathy
• Large pink cytoplasmic granules in granulocytes with or without granules in monocytes in cats with Chediak-Higashi syndrome
• Biochemical profile—no specific changes

OTHER LABORATORY TESTS
• Von Willebrand disease assay—in animals suspected of having this disease
• Thyroid function evaluation—in dogs suspected of having von Willebrand disease; concurrent hypothyroidism in some animals

• Platelet function testing—in select laboratories to characterize hereditary platelet function defects
• Coagulation tests (PT and APTT)—to eliminate DIC or a vitamin K antagonist from the differential diagnosis; APTT may be prolonged in some animals with von Willebrand disease.

IMAGING
N/A

DIAGNOSTIC PROCEDURES
Mucosal bleeding time—platelet function defects; normal buccal mucosal bleeding time measured by a two-blade, spring-loaded device (Simplate II Organon Teknika Corp., Durham, NC) in normal dogs is 1.7–4.2 min

 TREATMENT

• Many affected animals have spontaneous bleeding that is not life-threatening.
• If a factor such as von Willebrand factor is low, give whole blood or plasma (cryoprecipitate of fresh frozen plasma is preferred) to replace the deficient factor.
• Restrict activity during a bleeding episode.
• Before surgery, identify animals with platelet function defects by mucosal bleeding time or cuticle bleeding to allow preparation to prevent excessive bleeding during the procedure.
• In animals with acquired platelet function disorders, treat the underlying disease process or remove the offending agent

 MEDICATIONS

DRUGS
• Give desmopressin acetate (1 μg/kg [0.01 mL/kg] SC or IV diluted in 20 mL saline administered over 10 min) to dogs with von Willebrand disease during a bleeding episode; administration of this drug to normal dogs increases von Willebrand factor.
• Give DDAVP to normal dogs 30 min before collection of blood for transfusion to dogs with von Willebrand disease.
• Provide thyroid supplementation for dogs with hypothyroidism and concurrent von Willebrand disease (efficacy of this treatment has recently been questioned)

CONTRAINDICATIONS/POSSIBLE INTERACTIONS
Do not use NSAIDs because they inhibit platelet function.

 FOLLOW-UP

• Take special precautions when performing surgical procedures on these animals.
• Make owner aware that animals with hereditary platelet function defects may have recurring bleeding episodes, but fatal bleeds are uncommon.
• If a hereditary defect is identified, do not use the animal for breeding.

 MISCELLANEOUS

SEE ALSO
Von Willebrand Disease

ABBREVIATIONS
• DDAVP = 1 deamino-8-D-arginine vasopressin
• DIC = disseminated intravascular coagulation
• PT = prothrombin time
• APTT = activated partial thromboplastin time

Suggested Reading
Reagan WJ. Rebar AH. Platelet disorders. In: Ettinger SL, Feldman EC, eds. Textbook of veterinary internal medicine. 4th ed. Philadelphia: Saunders, 1995:1964–1976.
Author William J. Reagan
Consulting Editor Susan M. Cotter

THROMBOCYTOPENIA, PRIMARY IMMUNE-MEDIATED (IMT)

 BASICS

DEFINITION
Immune-mediated destruction of platelets with no identifiable cause

PATHOPHYSIOLOGY
Autoantibodies (primarily IgG) bound to the platelet surface result in premature platelet destruction by macrophages.

SYSTEMS AFFECTED
• Skin/Exocrine • Gastrointestinal • Respiratory • Ophthalmic • Renal/Urologic

GENETICS
• Predisposition is suggested by high disease prevalence in several breeds. • Mode of inheritance is complex and poorly understood.

INCIDENCE/PREVALENCE
• Common in dogs: 5% of hospital admissions in one study; reported incidence is 3 to 18%. • Rare in cats

GEOGRAPHIC DISTRIBUTION
• No regional differences • Regional variations in the prevalence of infectious causes of thrombocytopenia, especially rickettsial and heartworm diseases, influence the likelihood that a patient with thrombocytopenia has primary IMT.

SIGNALMENT

Species
• Common in dogs • Rare in cats

Breed Predilection
• Cocker spaniels, poodles, and Old English sheepdogs • Any breed, including crossbreeds, can be affected.

Mean Age and Range
• Most common in middle-aged dogs • Reported age range is 8 months to 15 years.

Predominant Sex
Females, spayed or intact, are affected twice as frequently as males.

SIGNS

Historical Findings
• Anorexia, lethargy, weakness • Epistaxis, hematochezia, mucosal hemorrhages

Physical Examination Findings
• Lethargy and weakness • Mucosal and cutaneous petechia and ecchymoses • Hyphema • Retinal hemorrhages • Melena • Hematemesis • Epistaxis • Mucous membrane pallor • Central nervous system or intraocular hemorrhage can lead to neurologic signs or blindness, respectively. • Fever, hepatosplenomegaly, and lymphadenomegaly are unusual in dogs with primary IMT.

CAUSES
• Unknown • In dogs, may occur with SLE and secondary to drug administration (potentially any drug, but especially potentiated sulfonamide antibiotics), neoplasia (especially lymphoma), dirofilariasis, and ehrlichiosis • In cats, may occur secondary to FeLV or FIV infection

RISK FACTORS
May be preceded by vaccination or a stressful event

 DIAGNOSIS

DIFFERENTIAL DIAGNOSIS
• Diagnosis is made by excluding other causes of thrombocytopenia; the extent to which other causes of thrombocytopenia can or need to be definitively excluded varies; in many cases, history, physical examination, and results of screening blood tests (see CBC/Biochemistry/Urinalysis) are sufficient to establish a working diagnosis. • Response to treatment can be used for diagnostic confirmation. • DIC—to rule out, perform a coagulation profile • Hemorrhage (especially owing to anticoagulant rodenticide toxicity) may cause mild to moderate thrombocytopenia but will not cause petechial hemorrhages; coagulation testing can investigate anticoagulant rodenticide toxicity. • Secondary IMT—investigate history of drug exposure, heartworm status, *Ehrlichia* titers, and evidence of lymphadenopathy or hepatosplenomegaly; response to doxycycline treatment can be used to investigate ehrlichiosis. • Other signs of SLE (e.g., mucocutaneous ulceration, polyarthritis, polymyositis, protein-losing nephropathy) should prompt ANA and LE tests. • Vasculitis (ehrlichiosis, Rocky Mountain spotted fever, leptospirosis, sepsis, systemic mycoses)—fever and evidence of renal and/or liver disease on chemistry profile are more consistent with ehrlichiosis, Rocky Mountain spotted fever, leptospirosis, sepsis, or systemic mycosis; titers and response to doxycycline can be used to investigate rickettsial disease; titers and response to ampicillin can be used to investigate leptospirosis; clinical signs, blood and urine cultures, and response to broad-spectrum antibiotics can be used to investigate bacterial sepsis; thoracic radiographs, serology, and cytology can be used to investigate systemic mycoses. • Hemangiosarcoma—abdominal palpation (splenomegaly), ultrasonography, coagulation profile • Snake envenomation—history • Splenomegaly causes only mild thrombocytopenia (not < 100,000/μL); diagnose by abdominal palpation, radiographs, and ultrasonography. • Bone marrow disease can cause thrombocytopenia of variable severity; neutropenia or nonregenerative anemia in a patient with thrombocytopenia should prompt consideration of bone marrow aspiration or core biopsy. • Estrogen toxicity—history, palpate testes, bone marrow aspirates • Greyhounds have lower platelet counts than other breeds. • Pseudothrombocytopenia can be caused by platelet clumping, presence of many large platelets (especially in Cavalier King Charles spaniels), or inappropriate automated hematology analyzer settings; thrombocytopenia should always be verified by blood smear evaluation. • The most common causes of thrombocytopenia in cats are infectious diseases (FeLV, FIV, toxoplasmosis, hemobartonellosis), neoplasia (especially lymphoproliferative and myeloproliferative disease), and thromboembolism secondary to underlying cardiac disease; test for FeLV, FIV, and *Haemobartonella*; *Ehrlichia risticii* titers, because infection in cats may lead to thrombocytopenia; doxycycline treatment trial for *Haemobartonellosis* and ehrlichiosis; bone marrow aspiration or core biopsy if bone marrow disease is suspected from the CBC

CBC/BIOCHEMISTRY/URINALYSIS
• Peripheral blood smear evaluation enables rapid in-house assessment of platelet numbers, although a CBC is necessary to quantify its severity. • Dogs with primary IMT usually have marked thrombocytopenia (platelets < 50,000/μL). • High mean platelet volume or presence of large platelets on blood smear evaluation indicates that bone marrow production of platelets is increased. • Low mean platelet volume (microthrombocytosis) suggests IMT. • Some patients will have neutrophilia. • Neutropenia suggests bone marrow disease or sepsis. • Anemia may occur from hemorrhage or concurrent immune-mediated hemolytic anemia and will be regenerative if there has been sufficient time (5–7 days) for the bone marrow to respond. • Many fragmented red blood cells (schistocytes or schizocytes) support DIC, hemangiosarcoma, or heartworm disease as the cause. • Autoagglutination or numerous spherocytes support a diagnosis of immune-mediated hemolytic anemia; thrombocytopenia in these patients is likely to be owing to either IMT or DIC • Biochemical profile is usually normal, although liver enzymes are often mildly to moderately high in dogs with concurrent AIHA. • Hematuria may be present.

OTHER LABORATORY TESTS
• The utility of tests for antiplatelet autoantibodies in dogs with thrombocytopenia is uncertain. • The platelet factor 3 test is not specific for IMT. • Megakaryocyte immunofluorescence is not highly sensitive, and its specificity is uncertain. • Increased platelet-bound IgG is a highly sensitive but nonspecific test. • Coagulation profiles can be done to investigate DIC and anticoagulant rodenticide toxicity. • Antinuclear antibody and lupus erythematosus tests are indicated in patients with clinical signs and laboratory abnormalities that support SLE. • Serology for ehrlichiosis, Rocky Mountain spotted fever, dirofilariasis, and leptospirosis may be indicated.

IMAGING
Radiographs and ultrasound can be obtained to investigate other causes of thrombocytopenia, such as hemangiosarcoma, lymphoma, hemorrhage, and systemic mycosis.

DIAGNOSTIC PROCEDURES
• Bone marrow evaluation is not routinely necessary. • Indications for bone marrow aspiration or core biopsy include neutropenia, presence of blast cells on blood smear evaluation, nonregenerative anemia, history of exposure to exogenous estrogens, or thrombo-

THROMBOCYTOPENIA, PRIMARY IMMUNE-MEDIATED (IMT)

cytopenia that is refractory to immunosuppressive therapy. • Response to immunosuppressive treatment can be used for diagnostic confirmation of primary IMT. • A doxycycline treatment trial can be used in patients suspected of having rickettsial infections. • Doxycyclines and corticosteroids can be administered concurrently to treat both IMT and rickettsial infections

PATHOLOGIC FINDINGS
• Petechial and ecchymotic hemorrhages on the skin and mucosal and serosal surfaces
• Hemorrhage into the eyes and respiratory, gastrointestinal, urogenital, or central nervous system • Megakaryocytic and erythroid hyperplasia evident from bone marrow histology • Lymphoid hyperplasia, platelet phagocytosis, and extramedullary hematopoiesis seen on splenic histology

TREATMENT

APPROPRIATE HEALTH CARE
Treat outpatient unless hemorrhaging is severe or other diagnostic procedures are required.

NURSING CARE
• Hypovolemia or anemia can be managed by administration of crystalloid or colloid solutions, packed red blood cells, or whole blood.
• Platelet transfusions are rarely necessary, and multiple units of platelets must be administered to have any appreciable effect on platelet numbers.

DIET
N/A

CLIENT EDUCATION
• Strict rest is important to minimize hemorrhage. • Animals with severe hemorrhage, seizures, or changes in mental status should be brought to the hospital for monitoring.
• Unnecessary medications and NSAIDs should be avoided.

SURGICAL CONSIDERATIONS
• Splenectomy is an option for dogs refractory to other treatments. • Increased risk of bleeding in dogs with < 30,000 platelets/μL.

MEDICATIONS

DRUGS OF CHOICE
• Corticosteroids—prednisone or prednisolone at an induction dose of 1–3 mg/kg q12h or dexamethasone at an induction dose of 0.1–0.6 mg/kg q24h • Other immunosuppressive medications are often combined with corticosteroids for initial treatment of primary IMT in dogs; whether this improves treatment success is uncertain. • The majority of dogs with IMT will attain a platelet count > 50,000–100,000/μL within 7 days of commencing corticosteroid treatment or other immunosuppressive

medications. • Failure of patients to respond to initial treatment should prompt reconsideration of the diagnosis. • Treatment options for dogs refractory to initial treatment include increasing the dose of corticosteroid or using an alternate corticosteroid: vincristine (0.02 mg/kg slow IV push or diluted in normal saline and administered over 4–6 hr), cyclophosphamide (200 mg/kg PO or IV weekly), azathioprine (2 mg/kg PO q24h induction dose), danazol (5 mg/kg PO q12h), cyclosporine (10 mg/kg PO q24h, drug monitoring advised), human immunoglobulin concentrate (0.5–1.5 g/kg IV over 2–4 hr), or splenectomy. • Once the platelet count normalizes, taper immunosuppressive medications to cessation over 4–6 months
• Sucralfate and antacids can be administered if gastric ulceration is suspected. • Cats usually respond well to immunosuppressive doses of prednisone or prednisolone (1–3 mg/kg PO q12h).

CONTRAINDICATIONS
NSAIDs

PRECAUTIONS
• Any unnecessary medications should be discontinued, because they may induce secondary IMT. • High-dose corticosteroids may cause gastrointestinal ulceration; dexamethasone may be more ulcerogenic than is prednisone. • Long-term treatment with corticosteroids can result in iatrogenic hyperadrenocorticism. • Excessive immunosuppression can predispose to infections by opportunistic pathogens. • Cytotoxic medications can cause bone marrow suppression. • Dose tapering too rapidly after remission may predispose to recurrence.

POSSIBLE INTERACTIONS
Combination therapy causes increasing immunosuppression, which can predispose to opportunistic infections.

ALTERNATIVE DRUGS
See Drugs of Choice.

FOLLOW-UP

PATIENT MONITORING
• Platelet count daily to every few days until platelet numbers exceed 50,000/μL, then weekly until platelet numbers normalize (in some patients the platelet count may never return to normal range) • Platelet counts should be performed weekly or every 2 weeks during the period of drug dose tapering.
• Animals with severe hemorrhage, seizures, or changes in mental status should be brought to the hospital for monitoring.

PREVENTION/AVOIDANCE
• Whether MLV vaccination will induce recurrence is uncertain; unnecessary vaccinations should be avoided. • Minimize stress that may initiate recurrence. • If medications are suspected to have caused secon-

dary IMT, they should never again be administered to the patient.

POSSIBLE COMPLICATIONS
• Death from hemorrhagic shock or central nervous system hemorrhage • Gastrointestinal ulceration

EXPECTED COURSE AND PROGNOSIS
• Most dogs with primary IMT will have platelet count increases to < 50,000–100,000/μL within 7–10 days of starting corticosteroid treatment, either alone or in conjunction with other immunosuppressive medications. • Approximately 50% of dogs with primary IMT will experience only one episode of disease. • Approximately 50% of dogs will experience recurrence. • The mortality rate for dogs is ~ 30%

MISCELLANEOUS

ASSOCIATED CONDITIONS
Approximately 20% of dogs with primary IMT also have AIHA.

AGE-RELATED FACTORS
None

ZOONOTIC POTENTIAL
None

PREGNANCY
Use of immunosuppressive drugs may cause fetal damage or abortion.

SYNONYMS
• Idiopathic thrombocytopenic purpura (ITP)
• Autoimmune thrombocytopenia • Autoimmune thrombocytopenic purpura (ATP)

SEE ALSO
• Anemia, Immune-mediated • Disseminated Intravascular Coagulation (DIC) • Ehrlichiosis
• Thrombocytopenia

ABBREVIATIONS
• AIHA = autoimmune hemolytic anemia
• ANA = antinuclear antibody • DIC = disseminated intravascular coagulation • FeLV = feline leukemia virus • FIV = feline immunodeficiency virus • LE = lupus erythematosus • MLV = modified live virus
• SLE = systemic lupus erythematosus

Suggested Reading

Breitschwerdt EB. Infectious thrombocytopenia in dogs. Compend Contin Educ Pract Vet 1988;10:1177–1190.
Jordan HL, Grindem CB, Breitschwerdt EB. Thrombocytopenia in cats: a retrospective study of 41 cases. J Vet Intern Med 1993;7:261–265.
Lewis DC. Management of refractory immune thrombocytopenia. ACVIM Proc 1997;15:94–96.
Lewis DC, Meyers KM. Canine idiopathic thrombocytopenic purpura. J Vet Intern Med 1996;10:207–218.
Author David C. Lewis
Consulting Editor Susan M. Cotter

DISEASES

THYMOMA

BASICS

OVERVIEW
• Originates from thymic epithelium
• Infiltrated with mature lymphocytes

SIGNALMENT
• Rare in dogs and cats
• Most common in medium- and large-breed dogs
• Dogs—mean age, 9 years
• Cats—mean age, 10 years

SIGNS
• Coughing
• Tachypnea
• Dyspnea
• Swelling of the head, neck, or forelimbs—cranial caval syndrome
• Muscle weakness and megaesophagus—caused by myasthenia gravis

CAUSE & RISK AFACTORS
N/A

DIAGNOSIS

DIFFERENTIAL DIAGNOSIS
• Lymphoma
• Branchial cyst
• Ectopic thyroid carcinoma
• Chemodectoma
• Mesothelioma

CBC/BIOCHEMISTRY/URINALYSIS
Lymphocytosis—occasionally

OTHER LABORATORY TESTS
N/A

IMAGING
Thoracic radiographs—may reveal a cranial mediastinal mass, pleural effusion, and megaesophagus

DIAGNOSTIC PROCEDURES
• Cytologic—shows mature lymphocytes and epithelial cells
• Evaluate for myasthenia gravis—patients with signs of muscle weakness, dysphagia, or regurgitation

TREATMENT

• Inpatient
• Surgical excision—treatment of choice; tends to be highly invasive and difficult to resect in dogs and less invasive and easier to remove in cats; use an intercostal approach for small masses and a sternotomy for large masses.
• Radiotherapy—potentially beneficial by reducing the lymphoid component of the mass

MEDICATIONS

DRUGS
• Chemotherapy—little information available
• Prednisone (20 mg/m² q48h) and cyclo-phosphamide (50–100 mg/m² q48h)—used in a very limited number of patients, two of which had a partial remission
• Myasthenia gravis—treat with prednisone and anticholinesterase drugs until the tumor can be removed.

CONTRAINDICATIONS/POSSIBLE INTERACTIONS
Immunosuppressive drugs—do not use to treat myasthenia gravis with aspiration pneumonia.

 FOLLOW-UP

• Thoracic radiography—every 3 months; monitor for recurrence
• Cure—possible if tumor is surgically resectable
• Prognosis—poor with nonresectable tumor

 MISCELLANEOUS

ASSOCIATED CONDITIONS
Concurrent nonthymic tumors, polymyositis, and other autoimmune diseases—20%–40% of patients

SEE ALSO
Myasthenia Gravis

Suggested Reading
Atwater SW, Powers BE, Park RD, et al. Thymoma in dogs: 23 cases (1980–1991). J Am Vet Med Assoc 1994;205:1007–1013.

Morrison WB. Nonpulmonary intrathoracic cancer. In: Morrison WB, ed. Cancer in dogs and cats: medical and surgical management. Baltimore: Williams & Wilkins, 1998:537–550.

Author Terrance A. Hamilton
Consulting Editor Wallace B. Morrison

DISEASES

TICK BITE PARALYSIS

BASICS

DEFINITION
Flaccid, lower motor neuron paralysis caused by salivary neurotoxins from certain species of female ticks

PATHOPHYSIOLOGY
• Tick—injects salivary neurotoxins that probably interfere with the depolarization/acetylcholine release mechanism in the presynaptic nerve terminal, leading to reduction in the release of acetylcholine
• *Ixodes holocyclus* tick infestation—neurotoxin depends strongly on temperature; one adult tick is sufficient to cause neurologic signs, but a large larval or nymphal *Ixodes* tick infestation can also induce signs.
• Signs—occur 6–9 days after initial tick attachment
• Not all infested animals develop tick paralysis; not all adult female ticks produce the toxin.

SYSTEMS AFFECTED
• Nervous—peripheral nervous system and the neuromuscular junction most affected by the neurotoxin; cranial nerves can become involved, including the vagal, facial, and trigeminal nerves; sympathetic system also affected
• Respiratory—may see paralysis of the intercostal muscles and diaphragm; caudal brainstem respiratory center may be affected

GENETICS
No genetic basis

INCIDENCE/PREVALENCE
• North America and Australia—somewhat seasonal (more prevalent in the summer months); in the warmer areas (southern U.S.; northern Australia) may become a year-round problem
• Overall incidence—low in the U.S.; higher in Australia

GEOGRAPHIC DISTRIBUTION
• U.S.—*Dermacentor variabilis:* wide distribution over the eastern two-thirds of the country and in California and Oregon; *D. andersoni:* from the Cascades to the Rocky Mountains; *Amblyomma americanum:* from Texas and Missouri to the Atlantic Coast; *A. maculatum:* high temperature and humidity of the Atlantic and Gulf of Mexico seaboards
• Australia—limited to the coastal areas of the east; especially associated with areas of bush and scrub

SIGNALMENT

Species
• Australia—dogs and cats
• U.S.—dogs; cats appear to be resistant

Breed Predilections
None

Mean Age and Range
Any age

Predominant Sex
N/A

SIGNS

Historical Findings
• Patient walked in a wooded area approximately 1 week before onset of signs.
• Onset—gradual; starts with unsteadiness and weakness in the pelvic limbs

Physical Examination Findings
Non-Ixodes Tick
• Once neurologic signs appear, there is rapid ascending lower motor neuron paresis to paralysis.
• Patient becomes recumbent in 1–3 days, with hyporeflexia to areflexia and hypotonia to atonia.
• Pain sensation preserved
• Cranial nerve dysfunction—not a prominent feature; may note facial weakness and reduced jaw tone; sometimes dysphonia and dysphagia early in the course
• Respiratory paralysis—uncommon in the U.S.; may occur in severely affected patients
• Urination and defecation usually normal
Ixodes Tick
• Neurologic signs—much more severe and rapidly progressive; ascending motor weakness can progress to paralysis within a few hours.
• Sialosis, megaesophagus, and vomiting or regurgitation characteristic
• Sympathetic nervous system—mydriatic and poorly responsive pupils; hypertension; tachyarrhythmias; high pulmonary capillary hydrostatic pressure; pulmonary edema.
• Caudal medullary respiratory center—additive to the peripheral pulmonary changes, causing progressive fall in respiratory rate without a change in tidal volume, resulting in hypoxia, hypercapnia, and respiratory acidosis
• Respiratory muscle paralysis—much more prevalent; dogs and cats progress to dyspnea, cyanosis, and respiratory paralysis within 1–2 days if not treated.

CAUSES

United States
• *D. variabilis*—common wood tick
• *D. andersoni*—Rocky Mountain wood tick
• *A. americanum*—lone star tick
• *A. maculatum*—Gulf Coast tick

Australia
I. holocyclus—secretes a far more potent neurotoxin than that of the North American species

RISK FACTORS
• Environments that harbor ticks

DIAGNOSIS

DIFFERENTIAL DIAGNOSIS
• Botulism
• Acute polyneuropathy
• Coonhound paralysis
• Acute polyradiculoneuritis
• Distal denervating disease
• Generalized (diffuse) or multifocal myelopathy

CBC/BIOCHEMISTRY/URINALYSIS
Normal

OTHER LABORATORY TESTS
Arterial blood gases—severely affected patients; low PaO_2, high $PaCO_2$, and low pH

IMAGING
Thoracic radiography (*Ixodes* tick)—megaesophagus

DIAGNOSTIC PROCEDURES
• Thoroughly search for a tick—head, neck, body and limbs, ear canals, mouth, rectum, vagina, prepuce, and in between the digits and foot pads; immediately remove tick.
• Electrodiagnostics (electromyogram)—normal insertion activity and an absence of spontaneous myofiber activity (no fibrillations and positive sharp waves); lack of motor unit

action potentials; motor nerve stimulation is followed by either a dramatic decrease in amplitude or a complete absence of compound muscle action potentials.

PATHOLOGIC FINDINGS
N/A

TREATMENT

APPROPRIATE HEALTH CARE
Inpatient—any neurologic dysfunction suggesting tick paralysis; hospitalize until either a tick is found and removed or appropriate treatment to kill a hidden tick is performed.

NURSING CARE
• Inpatient supportive care—essential until patient begins to show signs of recovery
• Oxygen cage—hypoventilation and hypoxia
• Artificial ventilation—respiratory failure
• Intravenous fluid therapy—generally not required unless recovery is prolonged

ACTIVITY
• Keep patient in a quiet environment.
• *Ixodes* tick paralysis—keep patient in a cool, air-conditioned area; toxin is temperature-sensitive; avoid activity to prevent increase in body temperature.

DIET
• Withhold food and water if patient has dysphagia or vomiting/regurgitation.

CLIENT EDUCATION
• Non-*Ixodes* tick—inform client that good nursing care is essential, although the patient's recovery is rapid after removal of ticks.
• *Ixodes* tick—warn client that signs often continue to worsen despite tick removal; thus more aggressive treatment to neutralize the toxin must be undertaken.

SURGICAL CONSIDERATIONS
N/A

MEDICATIONS

DRUGS OF CHOICE
• U.S.—if the tick cannot be found, dip the patient in an insecticidal bath; often the only treatment needed

• Australia—must neutralize circulating toxin via hyperimmune serum (0.5–1 mg/kg IV), depending on severity of clinical signs; if severe, phenoxybenzamine, an α-adrenergic antagonist (1 mg/kg IV diluted in saline and given slowly over 20 min) appears to be beneficial in relieving the sympathetic effects; acepromazine (0.5–1 mg/kg IV) can be used as an alternative (it has α-adrenergic blocking effects).

CONTRAINDICATIONS
• Drugs that interfere with neuromuscular transmission are contraindicated (e.g., tetracyclines, aminoglycosides, and procaine penicillin).
• *Ixodes* tick—atropine contraindicated in the advanced stages of disease or with marked bradycardia

PRECAUTIONS
Ixodes tick—administer intravenous fluids at a very slow rate to avoid further complications of pulmonary congestion

POSSIBLE INTERACTIONS
N/A

ALTERNATIVE DRUGS
N/A

FOLLOW-UP

PATIENT MONITORING
• Non-*Ixodes* tick—reassess neurologic status after tick removal at least daily—should see rapid improvement in muscle strength in animals
• *Ixodes* tick—monitor neurologic status and respiratory and cardiovascular functions continuously and intensively even after tick removal, because of the residual effect of neurotoxin.

PREVENTION/AVOIDANCE
• Vigilantly check for ticks after exposure (at least every 2–3 days); signs do not occur for 4–6 days after tick attachment.
• Weekly insecticidal baths or the use of insecticide-impregnated collars helps.
• Short-term acquired immunity develops after exposure to *Ixodes* neurotoxin.

POSSIBLE COMPLICATIONS
No long-term complications if the patient survives the acute effects of the toxin

EXPECTED COURSE AND PROGNOSIS
• Non-*Ixodes* tick—prognosis good to excellent if ticks are removed; recovery occurs in 1–3 days.
• *Ixodes* tick—prognosis often guarded; recovery prolonged; death in 1–2 days without treatment

MISCELLANEOUS

ASSOCIATED CONDITIONS
N/A

AGE-RELATED FACTORS
N/A

ZOONOTIC POTENTIAL
Although humans can acquire the disease by being bitten by the same ticks (especially in Australia), tick paralysis is not transmitted to humans from affected pets.

PREGNANCY
Unknown

SEE ALSO
• Coonhound Paralysis (Idiopathic Polyradiculoneuritis)
• Peripheral Neuropathies (Polyneuropathies)

Suggested Reading
Braund KG. Clinical syndromes in veterinary neurology. 2nd ed. St. Louis: Mosby, 1994.
Ilkiw JE. Tick paralysis in Australia. In: Kirk RW, ed. Current veterinary therapy VIII. Small animal practice. Philadelphia: Saunders, 1983:691–693.
Malik R., Farrow BRH. Tick paralysis in North America and Australia. Vet Clin North Am 1991;21:157–171.
Author Paul A. Cuddon
Consulting Editor Joane M. Parent

DISEASES

TICKS AND TICK CONTROL

BASICS

DEFINITION
• Dogs and cats may be parasitized by hard ticks of the family Ixodidae.
• Ectoparasites that feed only on the blood of their hosts; arthropods; closely related to scorpions, spiders, and mites
• Transmitted microbial pathogens—protozoa, helminths, fungi, bacteria, rickettsiae, and viruses
• May cause toxicosis, hypersensitivity, paralysis, and blood-loss anemia

PATHOPHYSIOLOGY
• Hard ticks—four life stages: egg, larva, nymph, and adult; larvae and nymphs must feed to repletion before detaching and molting; as adult female ixodid ticks engorge, they may increase their weight by more than 100-fold; after detachment females may lay thousands of eggs.
• Blood-loss anemia—from heavy infestations
• Damage to the integument—tick mouth parts cut through the host's skin; bites are generally painless; local irritation and infection may occur.
• Salivary secretion of neurotoxins—may lead to systemic signs (tick paralysis); local action may cause impaired hemostasis and immune suppression.
• Pathogens—acquired when ticks feed on infected reservoir hosts (often rodents and small feral mammals); sometimes transovarial transmission occurs and infected eggs hatch and produce infected larvae; greatest potential for systemic disease occurs when infections acquired in early life stages are transmitted to new hosts when the next stage feeds; may affect virtually any organ system
• Transmission of pathogens and toxins—often requires periods of attachment from hours to days; the essentially painless bite allows adequate feeding times.

SYSTEMS AFFECTED
• Skin/Exocrine—irritation secondary to bite
• Hemic/Lymphatic/Immune—blood-loss anemia
• Nervous—neurotoxin-induced paralysis

Genetics
N/A

INCIDENCE/PREVALENCE
N/A

GEOGRAPHIC DISTRIBUTION
• Strong geographic specificities exist for some tick species; thus geographic prevalence of associated diseases
• *Ixodes scapularis*—Lyme disease; midwest, northeast, and parts of the southeast
• *Ixodes pacificus*—western coastal states
• *Rhipicephalus sanguineus*—found throughout the continental U.S.; but canine ehrlichiosis and babesiosis most common in the southeast

SIGNALMENT

Species
• Dogs and cats
• Cats are thought to be quite efficient at removing ticks, but tick attachment and subsequent tick-vectored diseases are routinely diagnosed.

Breed Predilections
None

Mean Age and Range
None

Predominant Sex
None

SIGNS
• Attached ticks or tick feeding cavities from which ticks have detached may be seen on the skin.
• Associated tick-borne diseases (borreliosis, ehrlichiosis, babesiosis, Rocky Mountain spotted fever, and others)—vary with the organ system(s) affected
• Irritation caused by ticks and subsequent self-trauma—may lead to pyotraumatic dermatitis ("hot spots") in dogs

CAUSES
• Direct contact with questing ticks
• Ticks—attracted to hosts by motion, variation in light patterns, warmth, presence of carbon dioxide, and host-associated odors

RISK FACTORS
• Large hunting breeds (dogs)—considered to be at high risk, because they are likely to come in contact with environments harboring questing ticks
• Domestic animals—can be in close contact with ticks owing to encroachment of ticks into suburban environments and expansion of suburban environment into surrounding forests, prairies, and coast line areas

DIAGNOSIS

• Ticks—examine the skin for attached ticks or tick feeding cavities
• Tick-borne diseases—evaluate epidemiologic considerations for each disease, history of tick parasitism, and complete clinical examination

DIFFERENTIAL DIAGNOSIS
N/A

CBC/BIOCHEMISTRY/URINALYSIS
N/A

OTHER LABORATORY TESTS
N/A

IMAGING
N/A

DIAGNOSTIC PROCEDURES
N/A

PATHOLOGIC FINDINGS
N/A

TREATMENT

APPROPRIATE HEALTH CARE
• Outpatient after removal of ticks
• Removal—do as soon as possible to limit time available for neurotoxin or pathogen transmission; grasp ticks close to the skin with fine-pointed tweezers and gently pull free; species with short, strong mouth parts (e.g., *Dermacentor*) usually pull free with host skin attached; species with long, fragile mouth parts (e.g., *Ixodes*) often leave fragments of mouth parts embedded in the feeding cavity.

NURSING CARE
Wash feeding cavity with soap and water; generally sufficient to prevent local inflammation or secondary infection

ACTIVITY
N/A

DIET
N/A

CLIENT EDUCATION
Inform client that application of hot matches, Vaseline, or other materials not only fails to cause tick detachment but allows for longer periods of attachment and feeding.

SURGICAL CONSIDERATIONS
N/A

MEDICATIONS

DRUGS OF CHOICE
See Prevention/Avoidance

CONTRAINDICATIONS
N/A

PRECAUTIONS
N/A

POSSIBLE INTERACTIONS
N/A

ALTERNATIVE DRUGS
N/A

FOLLOW-UP

PATIENT MONITORING
N/A

PREVENTION/AVOIDANCE
• Avoid environments that harbor ticks; may be difficult except for pets kept strictly indoors
• Tick control—essential to realize that this does not always equal control of tick-borne diseases; often the goal is the perceived absence of ticks on the host animal.
• Pets—owners report complete tick control even though there may be some period of attachment and tick feeding or live ticks may spend some time crawling on the animal after they have been exposed to lethal levels of an acaricide; immature ticks of some species (*R. sanguineous* and *I. scapularis*) may be undetected because of their minute size.
• Tick-borne pathogens—may be transmitted very rapidly (viruses) or may require several hours (*Rickettsia rickettsii*) or days (*Borrelia burgdorferi*)

Insecticides and Acaricides
• In the U.S., the EPA licenses agents as effective against various species of pests.
• Control—inferred as providing control of diseases carried by that species; although this may be correct in some or all cases, veterinarians should be sophisticated enough to require demonstration of efficacy in prevention of disease transmission before accepting a disease-control claim at face value; challenging because ticks are widely dispersed in the environment, spend a relatively short time on their hosts, posses great reproductive capacities, and have long lifetimes
• Acaricidal collars (Preventic) and spot treatment (Frontline)—have gained wide use; ease of application is as important as efficacy; direct marketing to pet owners of veterinarian-dispensed products has been a major factor in shifting tick control away from OTC formulations

• Bathing, spraying, or powdering with appropriate organophosphate- or pyrethrin-containing products has become far less common with the advent of new convenient and effective products.

POSSIBLE COMPLICATIONS
Tick-borne diseases or tick paralysis

EXPECTED COURSE AND PROGNOSIS
N/A

MISCELLANEOUS

ASSOCIATED CONDITIONS
• Canine babesiosis—vectored by *R. sanguineous;* caused by protozoan parasite *Babesia canis;* infects canine RBCs, leading to sludging in capillaries and destruction in the spleen
• Rocky Mountain spotted fever—vectored by *Dermacentor variabilis;* caused by *R. rickettsii;* invades vascular endothelial tissues, leading to necrotizing vasculitis
• Canine ehrlichiosis—vectored by *R. sanguineous;* caused by *Ehrlichia canis;* infects mononuclear cells and platelets
• Granulocytic ehrlichiosis—emerging disease; caused by *E. equi* (also called *E. phagocytophila*); infects granulocytes, leading to nonspecific signs and fever
• Lyme disease—vectored by *I. scapularis* and *I. pacificus;* caused by *Borrelia burgdorferi;* dogs may develop fevers associated with arthritis or syndromes leading to complete heart block, protein-loosing nephropathy, and neurologic abnormalities.
• Canine hepatozoonosis—caused by protozoal organism *Hepatozoon canis* after the dog ingests an infected *R. sanguineous;* cysts and pyogranulomas in the muscles and other tissues associated with myositis and renal failure, often leading to death in chronic cases
• Tick paralysis—caused by a neurotoxin; affects acetylcholine synthesis and/or liberation at the neuromuscular junction of the host animal; signs (typified by ascending flaccid paralysis often initially affecting the pelvic limbs) develop 5–9 days after tick attachment.

Vaccines
• Currently for "prevention" of only Lyme disease; two types for dogs: whole-cell, killed bacterin (since 1990) and Osp A (since 1996)
• Safety and efficacy—peer-reviewed published data for dogs naturally exposed to *B. burgdorferi* available only for bacterin; 1969 dogs received a total of 4033 doses of bacterin during a 20-month period; 4498 control dogs were not vaccinated; immunization was found

to be safe regardless of previous history of Lyme disease or exposure to *B. burgdorferi;* 38 (1.9%) of vaccinated dogs had minor reactions that resolved without complications immediately or within 72 hr after vaccination; cumulative incidence of Lyme disease was 1.0% in vaccinated dogs and 4.7% in control dogs; 40% of vaccinated dogs had serologic evidence of infection with *B. burgdorferi* before vaccination but the incidence of Lyme disease was only 2%; incidence of Lyme disease in infected control dogs was 4.8%; thus vaccination of infected dogs was associated with about a 50% decrease in the incidence of Lyme disease; some clinical experiences have not shown this high degree of efficacy and have reported potentially harmful side affects (e.g., immune-mediated phenomena).

AGE-RELATED FACTORS
N/A

ZOONOTIC POTENTIAL
• Ticks may parasitize many different species of mammals, birds, and reptiles at different stages in their developmental cycles; infections acquired in early life stages may be transmitted when ticks feed again in the next stage.
• Humans, if parasitized, may be exposed to babesiosis, Rocky Mountain spotted fever, ehrlichiosis, borreliosis, or tick paralysis.

PREGNANCY
N/A

SYNONYMS
Acariasis

SEE ALSO
• Babesiosis
• Ehrlichiosis
• Hepatozoonosis
• Lyme Disease (Borreliosis)
• Rocky Mountain Spotted Fever
• Tick Bite Paralysis

Suggested reading
Hoskins JD, ed. Tick-transmitted disease, Vet Clin North Am 1991:21.
Levy SA, Barthold SW, Dombach DM, et al. Canine borreliosis. Compend Continuing Education 1993;15:833–848.
Levy SA, Lissman BA, Ficke CM. Performance of a *Borrelia burgdorferi* bacterin in borreliosis endemic areas. J Am Vet Med Assoc 1993;202:1834–1838.
Sonenshine DE. Biology of ticks. Vol. 2. New York: Oxford University Press, 1993.
Author Steven A. Levy
Consulting Editor Karen Helton Rhodes

DISEASES

TOAD VENOM TOXICOSIS

BASICS

OVERVIEW
- Two species of primary concern—Colorado River toad (*Bufo alvarius*) and marine toad (*B. marinus*); marine toad more toxic; both can be fatal.
- Toads—most active during periods of high humidity (the monsoon season of late summer in the desert Southwest for Colorado River toads); most encounters occur during the evening, night, or early morning.
- Toxin—produced from the parotid glands; defensive; rapidly absorbed across the victim's mucous membranes; contains several major components: indole alkyl amines (similar to the street drug LSD), cardiac glycosides, and noncardiac sterols

SIGNALMENT
Primarily dogs; rarely, ferrets and cats

SIGNS
General Comments
Rapid onset
Historical Findings
- Crying and pawing at the mouth
- Ataxia or stiff gaited
- Seizures
Physical Examination Findings
- Profuse hypersalivation
- Hyperexcitability with vocalization
- Brick red buccal mucous membranes
- Hyperthermia
- Collapse
- Marked cardiac ventricular arrhythmia—less common with Colorado River toad intoxication
- Cyanosis
- Dyspnea

CAUSES & RISK FACTORS
- Living in proximity to toads
- Moist, warm, outside environment
- Outdoor animal

DIAGNOSIS

DIFFERENTIAL DIAGNOSIS
Caustics or other oral irritants

CBC/BIOCHEMISTRY/URINALYSIS
May note hyperkalemia

OTHER LABORATORY TESTS
N/A

IMAGING
N/A

DIAGNOSTIC PROCEDURES
Electrocardiogram—may reveal ventricular arrhythmias

TREATMENT
- Marine toad intoxication—medical emergency; death common
- Decontamination—flush mouth with copious quantities of water for 5–10 min.
- Hyperthermia (> 40.6°C; 105°F)—provide a cool bath; remove patient from bath once temperature reaches 39.4°C (103°F).
- Rapid evaluation of cardiac activity necessary

MEDICATIONS

DRUGS

• Atropine—0.04 mg/kg IM, SC; reduces the amount of salivation; helps prevent aspiration; use with bradycardia, heart block, or other sinoatrial node alterations as a result of the digitalis-like effect of the toxin
• Propranolol (Inderal)—2 mg/kg IV (see Contraindications); rapid administration may be required to combat tachyarrhythmias; may be repeated in 20 min; may need continuous intravenous infusion (0.02–0.2 mg/kg) for persistent arrhythmias
• Anesthesia with pentobarbital (dogs)—increases tolerance to intoxication

CONTRAINDICATIONS/POSSIBLE INTERACTIONS

• Cardiac disease or bronchial asthma—patient may not tolerate the generally recommended high dose of propranolol; try propranolol at 0.5 mg/kg as a slow IV bolus; monitor cardiac rhythm and stop injection when it normalizes.
• Anesthetics (e.g., pentobarbital)—may depress function of an already compromised myocardium; use with caution.

FOLLOW-UP

• Continuous electrocardiographic monitoring—recommended until the patient is fully recovered
• Colorado River toad intoxication—patients usually normal within 30 min of onset of treatment; death relatively uncommon if treated; do not underestimate the risk of secondary heatstroke.
• Marine toad intoxication—medical emergency; death common

MISCELLANEOUS

Suggested Reading

Palumbo NE, Perri SF. Toad poisoning. In: Kirk RW, ed. Current veterinary therapy VIII. Philadelphia: Saunders, 1983:160–162.
Author Michael E. Peterson
Consulting Editor Gary D. Osweiler

TOOTH FRACTURE

 BASICS

DEFINITION
• Traumatic tooth injuries may involve fracture of enamel, dentine, and cement or damage to the periodontium.
• May involve the crown and root of the affected tooth
• Classified as uncomplicated if they do not involve pulpal exposure and complicated if the pulp is exposed by the fracture line

PATHOPHYSIOLOGY
• Untreated pulpal exposure invariably leads to pulpitis and eventually pulpal necrosis and periapical pathology.
• Pulpitis and pulpal necrosis may also occur with uncomplicated fractures, particularly if the fracture line is close to the pulp chamber, which exposes a large number of wide-diameter dentinal tubules and allows communication between the pulp and the external environment.

SYSTEMS AFFECTED
Oral cavity initially, but may lead to lesions of multiple internal organs

GENETICS
N/A

INCIDENCE/PREVALENCE
N/A

GEOGRAPHIC DISTRIBUTION
N/A

SIGNALMENT
Species
Dogs and cats

Breed Predilections
None

Mean Age and Range
Any age

Predominant Sex
None

SIGNS
Crown Fractures
• Clinical loss of tooth crown substance; may affect enamel only, or enamel and dentin; fracture line may be transverse or oblique.

• Uncomplicated fractures with the fracture line close to the pulp chamber—pale pink pulp is visible through the dentin; gentle exploring will not allow the explorer into the pulp cavity.
• In complicated crown fractures, the pulp chamber is open and readily accessed with an explorer.
• The fresh complicated fracture is associated with hemorrhage from the pulp.
• Older fractures may exhibit a necrotic pulp; clinically the pulp chamber is filled with dark necrotic material, and the tooth is often discolored.

Root Fractures
• May occur at any point along the root surface; often in combination with fracture of the crown, but may occur in isolation
• Fracture line may be transverse or oblique; segments may remain aligned or be displaced.
• Clinical signs indicating a possible root fracture include pain on closure of the mouth or during open mouth breathing.
• Abnormal horizontal or vertical mobility of a periodontally sound tooth may raise suspicion of a root fracture.

CAUSES & RISK FACTORS
Generally the result of a traumatic incident (e.g., road traffic accident, blunt blow to the face, chewing on hard objects)

 DIAGNOSIS

DIFFERENTIAL DIAGNOSIS
• Crown fracture—none
• Root fracture—luxation; definitive diagnosis of root fractures is by radiography.

CBC/BIOCHEMISTRY/URINALYSIS
N/A

OTHER LABORATORY TESTS
N/A

IMAGING
• Radiographs are mandatory.
• Intraoral radiographic technique and dental intraoral film are recommended.
• Radiographs reveal the full extent of the lesion and allow treatment planning.

• Radiographs are required for adequate performance of endodontic procedures and monitoring treatment outcome.

DIAGNOSTIC PROCEDURES
N/A

PATHOLOGIC FINDINGS
Untreated pulpal exposure invariably leads to pulpitis and eventual pulpal necrosis and periapical pathology.

 TREATMENT

Uncomplicated Crown Fractures
Remove sharp edges with a bur and seal the exposed dentin tubules with a suitable liner or restorative material.

Complicated Crown Fractures
All require endodontic therapy if the tooth is to be maintained; extraction is preferable to no treatment at all.

Mature Tooth
• Recent fracture in the mature tooth with the pulp still vital—two options exist, partial pulpectomy and direct pulp capping (vital pulpotomy) followed by restoration or conventional root canal therapy and restoration.
• For partial pulpectomy and direct pulp capping to succeed, ideally the procedure should be carried out within hours of the injury.
• Tell the client at the beginning that the procedure may not be the final treatment—the tooth may require conventional root canal treatment later if the pulp becomes necrotic.
• When the pulp is already chronically inflamed or necrotic, conventional root canal therapy and restoration are the treatment of choice if the tooth is periodontally sound.

Immature Tooth
• A vital pulp is required for continued root development; so long as the pulp is vital the treatment of choice is partial pulpectomy and direct pulp capping, followed by restoration.
• If the pulp is necrotic, no further root development will occur; necrotic immature teeth need endodontic treatment to be maintained; remove the necrotic tissue and pack the root

canal with calcium hydroxide paste; some apexogenesis (physiologic event, continued root development) and apexification (closure of the apex, induced by treatment) can be stimulated if this procedure is performed; change the calcium hydroxide every 6 months until the apex is closed when a conventional root canal is performed.
• Immature teeth may be present in the mature animal if trauma to the developing teeth caused pulp necrosis; treat such teeth as you would any immature teeth.

Root Fractures

• Treatment of crown and root fractures depends on how far below the gum margin the fracture line extends.
• If the fracture line does not involve the pulp and does not extend more than 4–5 mm below the gum, restorative dentistry can be performed; if the fracture extends more than 5 mm below the gum margin and involves the pulp, the tooth should usually be extracted.
• The fracture level determines the choice of treatment for horizontal root fractures; a fracture in the apical region carries a better prognosis than one close to the gingival margin.
• A horizontal fracture of the coronal part of the root usually mandates tooth extraction; the main exception is the lower canine, since jaw stability and strength depend on the canine roots.
• If the root is periodontally sound it must receive endodontic treatment after removal of the coronal portion; horizontal midroot and apical fractures will heal if the tooth is immobilized; horizontal root fractures can heal by means of a dentinocemental callus, a fibrous union, or an osteofibrous union.
• If the pulp of the coronal fragment becomes necrotic the fracture will not heal; endodontic treatment of the coronal segment is indicated; the apical segment may be left in situ if there is no radiographic evidence of periapical pathology; if radiographic evidence of periapical pathology exists, remove the apical segment.

MEDICATIONS

DRUGS OF CHOICE
A broad-spectrum bacteriocidal antibiotic drug is recommended; a 5- to 7-day course is sufficient.

CONTRAINDICATIONS/POSSIBLE INTERACTIONS
None

PRECAUTIONS
None

POSSIBLE INTERACTIONS
None

ALTERNATIVE DRUGS
None

FOLLOW-UP

PATIENT MONITORING
• Check a partial pulpectomy and direct pulp-capping procedure with postoperative radiographs after 6 and 12 months, or at intervals determined by clinical signs, to detect pulp death and consequent periapical changes indicating the need for root canal treatment.
• Check the outcome of conventional root canal therapy radiographically 6–12 months postoperatively; evidence of periapical pathology at this time indicates the need for further endodontic therapy or extraction of the tooth; further endodontic therapy consists of redoing the root canal therapy, often in conjunction with surgical endodontics.
• Check root fractures radiographically 6–12 months postoperatively.
• Check uncomplicated fractures postoperatively with radiographs at 4–6 months to assess periapical status.

PREVENTION/AVOIDANCE
• Avoid situations in which teeth are likely to be damaged; keep animal from chewing on hard objects such as rocks.
• To avoid complications, institute treatment within hours of injury.

POSSIBLE COMPLICATIONS
• Untreated pulpal exposure invariably leads to pulpitis and eventual pulpal necrosis and periapical pathology.
• Arrested development of immature teeth

EXPECTED COURSE AND PROGNOSIS
Vary with vitality of the pulp, location of the fracture, and whether the tooth is mature or immature; see Treatment section for detailed discussion.

MISCELLANEOUS

ASSOCIATED CONDITIONS
None

AGE-RELATED FACTORS
Treatment of mature and immature teeth differs; see Treatment section.

ZOONOTIC POTENTIAL
None

PREGNANCY
N/A

SYNONYMS
None

SEE ALSO
N/A

ABBREVIATIONS
None

Suggested Reading
Gorrel C, Penman S, Emily P. Handbook of small animal oral emergencies. New York: Pergamon Press, 1993.
Gorrel C, Robinson J. Endodontic therapy. In: Crossley, Penman, eds. Manual of small animal dentistry. Gloucester, UK: British Veterinary Dental Association, 1995
Author Cecilia Gorrel
Consulting Editor Jan Bellows

DISEASES

TOOTH LUXATION/AVULSION

 BASICS

OVERVIEW
• Luxation of a tooth can be either vertical (i.e., an intrusion or extrusion) or lateral.
• An intrusion occurs when the tooth is pushed apically into the alveolar bone.
• An extrusion occurs when the tooth is dislocated vertically partially out of the alveolus.
• Lateral luxation—the affected tooth is tipped in either a labial or a palatal/lingual direction; can occur when trauma pushes the crown in one direction and the root in the opposite direction; always associated with a fracture of the lingual or labial alveolar bone plate that allows the tooth to luxate rather than fracture
• An avulsed tooth has been totally luxated from its alveolus.

SIGNALMENT
Dog and cats

SIGNS
• Intrusion—tooth appears shorter than normal; no tooth mobility detected
• Extrusion—tooth appears longer than normal and is mobile both vertically and horizontally
• Lateral luxation—tooth crown is displaced in either a labial or palatal/lingual direction
• Avulsion—intact tooth is totally displaced from its alveolus

CAUSES & RISK FACTORS
• Luxation/avulsion—usually results from a traumatic incident (e.g., road traffic accident or dog fight)
• The trauma causes injury to the periodontium, thus allowing abnormal tooth mobility and malpositioning.
• The upper canine tooth is the most commonly luxated/avulsed tooth.
• Advanced periodontitis will predispose

 DIAGNOSIS

DIFFERENTIAL DIAGNOSIS
• Luxation—root fracture where the coronal segment is displaced
• Avulsion—tooth lost due to severe periodontitis

CBC/BIOCHEMISTRY/URINALYSIS
Noncontributory

OTHER LABORATORY TESTS
N/A

IMAGING
General
• Radiographs are mandatory.
• Intraoral radiographic technique and dental X-ray film are required.

Radiographic Findings
• Intrusion—narrowing of the periodontal ligament space in the apical region
• Extrusion—widening of the periodontal ligament, especially in the apical section
• Lateral luxation—widening and narrowing of the periodontal ligament space and fracture of the alveolar bone plate
• Avulsion—empty but intact alveolus

 TREATMENT

• Replace and fix the tooth in its normal position; bond with acrylic splints and fine ligature wire—an effective method of achieving stabilization and occlusal alignment.
• Handle the avulsed tooth only by its crown and rinse gently with sterile saline solution; if severely contaminated, the tooth root can be gently cleaned with sterile gauze swabs moistened with saline.
• Be gentle; tooth handling should be kept to a minimum; it is essential not to remove the periodontal ligament from the root; a viable periodontal ligament is necessary for healing
• Replace the tooth in its bony socket; there is usually no need to remove the blood clot from the alveolus; the tooth is just firmly placed in its bony socket and fixed in that position.
• Contraindications for repositioning a luxated or avulsed tooth are deciduous teeth, severe periodontitis caries or resorptive lesion.
• The two most important factors determining the result of treatment are the length of time the avulsed tooth has been out of its bony socket and the medium in which the tooth has been stored during this period.
• The sooner an avulsed tooth is reimplanted the better the prognosis; optimal results are achieved if the tooth is reimplanted within 30 min of avulsion; do not let the avulsed tooth dry prior to reimplantation; the best medium for storing an avulsed tooth is saline; if not available, use milk.
• Advise clients to place the tooth in either saline or milk and bring the affected animal in for treatment as quickly as possible.
• The appliance for fixation is usually left in place for 4–6 weeks; maintain oral hygiene during this period; a water pick or curved-tip syringe is used to flush debris from between the splint, teeth, and soft tissue; rinsing the oral cavity with chlorhexidine solution is also useful.
• The appliances are removed with pliers or high-speed drill; at this stage the tooth should be stable or very slightly mobile; take radiographs; if the tooth is still loose, reimplantation has failed and it should be extracted.

MEDICATIONS

DRUGS
• Use of a broad-spectrum bacteriocidal antibiotic is recommended; if oral hygiene is maintained, only a short course is necessary.
• If no oral hygiene measures are possible, antibiotics may be indicated throughout the period of fixation.
• Daily rinsing with 0.12% chlorhexidine gluconate solution will diminish the need for prolonged administration of antibiotics.

CONTRAINDICATIONS/POSSIBLE INTERACTIONS
N/A

FOLLOW-UP
• An avulsed tooth invariably develops pulpal necrosis; the tooth must receive endodontic therapy to prevent development of periapical pathology.
• Best to perform endodontic therapy when the appliance is removed
• External root resorption and ankylosis commonly follow reimplantation.
• Luxated teeth often suffer pulp necrosis; check at regular intervals.
• Signs of pulp pathology (e.g., tooth discoloration or radiographic evidence of periapical pathology) are indications for endodontic treatment.

MISCELLANEOUS

Suggested Reading

Gorrel C, Penman S, Emily P. Handbook of small animal oral emergencies. New York: Pergamon Press, 1993.
Gorrel C, Robinson J. Endodontic therapy. In: Crossley, Penman, eds. Manual of small animal dentistry. Br Vet Dent Assoc 1995: 168–181.

Author Cecilia Gorrel
Consulting Editor Jan Bellows

TOOTH ROOT ABSCESS (APICAL ABSCESS)

BASICS

OVERVIEW
- An abscess is a localized collection of pus in a cavity formed by the disintegration of tissues.
- Can divide into "acute" and chronic phases on the basis of severity of pain and presence or absence of systemic signs and symptoms
- Accumulation of inflammatory cells at the apex of a nonvital tooth—periapical abscess
- Acute exacerbation of a chronic periapical abscess is called a *phoenix abscess*.
- An abscess spreads along the pathway of least resistance from the tooth apex, resulting in osteomyelitis and, if perforated through the cortex, a cellulitis that can burst through the skin to create a cutaneous sinus.
- Systemic spread of bacteria (bacteremia and pyemia) can affect other organ systems.

SIGNALMENT
Species
- Dogs and cats
- Can occur in deciduous and permanent dentition
- Usually occurs in active animals that bite or chew a lot
- Can involve any teeth; canines and carnassial teeth are most commonly affected.

SIGNS
- Tooth is visibly broken—90% of cases
- Tooth may appear discolored.
- Tooth is not sensitive to cold or hot liquids or foods—**Note:** acute tooth fracture with pulp exposure would be sensitive.

- Facial swelling
- Cutaneous sinus exuding pus
- Facial sensitivity may be slight.
- Increased accumulation of plaque and calculus on the affected side of the mouth
- Animal does not want to chew, especially on the affected side.
- Tooth may be asymptomatic for a long time but will be affected sooner or later.
- Tooth may be sensitive to percussion.
- A deep "vertical" periodontal pocket may extend to the apex of the affected tooth.
- Putrid smell
- Tooth may be loose and painful on palpation.
- May have facial lymphadenitis
- Sinusitis—maxillary sinus is most commonly affected.

CAUSES & RISK FACTORS
- Any pulpal trauma
- Direct blow causing fracture of the crown of severe pulpitis and pulpal necrosis
- Defense (fighting)—the canines are most commonly affected.
- Chewing hard objects (e.g., bones, hooves, rocks, wood, especially with knots)—carnassials are most commonly affected)
- Malocclusive trauma
- "Tugging" rags with puppies
- Previous surgical repair to an area around the dentition—bone plating for fracture repair
- Bacteria—the pulp can be affected by bacteria from dental caries, exposed dentinal tubules
- Septicemia—documented in humans but not yet proven in animals

- Thermal heat resulting in pulpal necrosis—electrical cord burns
- Immature patients (<18 months)
- Small animals on long-term corticosteroids
- Diabetes or Cushing's disease

DIAGNOSIS

DIFFERENTIAL DIAGNOSIS
- Feline odontoclastic resorptive lesions—radiographs show no apical lucency or abscessation.
- Squamous cell carcinoma and fibrosarcoma—rapidly growing and invasive; displace and increase mobility of the teeth.
- Cementomas—radiographically show enlarged apical roots with a thin radiolucent zone continuous with the periodontal ligament
- Ameloblastoma—displaces and increases mobility to the teeth; slowly enlarges
- Cysts—radiographs usually show a very large lytic area; can mimic apical abscesses and apical abscesses can become cystic (radicular cysts, apical periodontal granulomas); conventional endodontic treatment is unsuccessful; primordial cyst occurs at the site of a congenitally missing tooth and radiographically has a round oval radiolucency with a thin radiopaque border.
- Dentigerous cyst—occurs from the follicular cyst of an impacted or embedded tooth (usually the first premolars in dogs); radiographs show a tooth within the cyst.

TOOTH ROOT ABSCESS (APICAL ABSCESS)

CBC/BIOCHEMISTRY/URINALYSIS
CBC may show a leucocytosis and/or a mild regenerative anemia.

OTHER LABORATORY TESTS
N/A

IMAGING
• Key diagnostic aid—demonstrates thickening of the apical periodontal ligament; ill-defined radiolucency; shows bone loss at the apex as the lesion becomes chronic
• As the lesion progresses, radiographic lesions consistent with osteomyelitis and cellulitis occur.
• If fistulation has occurred, can place a gutta percha cone into the sinus and take a radiograph to identify the affected tooth

DIAGNOSTIC PROCEDURES
• Surgical removal of the abscess site (surgical endodontics) or extraction
• Endodontic treatment evaluation in 6 months to a year

PATHOLOGIC FINDINGS
• Apical area has a central area of liquefaction necrosis containing disintegrating neutrophils and cellular debris, surrounded by macrophages, lymphocytes, and plasma cells; can see bacteria
• Chronic changes as above, but tracts lead away from the central lesion and can be lined with epithelium; may be osteomyelitis and cellulitis lesions or the outer portion of granulation tissue becomes fibrotic and a capsule develops (radicular cyst and or a periapical periodontal granuloma)

TREATMENT
• Drainage and elimination of the focus of infection
• Extraction of the tooth involved, with curettage of the apical infected area
• Endodontic treatment of the involved tooth
• Surgical endodontic treatment of the involved tooth if the apical lesion is large
• Chronic conditions require surgical removal of the granulation tissue and curettage of the tract.
• After treatment, cold packs on the area will help reduce inflammation.
• Complete rest for a few days
• Give nothing hard to chew for a few days.

MEDICATIONS

DRUGS
• Antibiotics preoperatively to prevent systemic spread of infection
• Broad-spectrum antibiotic postoperatively for 7–10 days
• Analgesics preoperatively, intraoperatively, and postoperatively for 3–4 days
• If a surgical endodontic treatment or an extraction was performed; a protective collar may be required.

CONTRAINDICATIONS/POSSIBLE INTERACTIONS
N/A

FOLLOW-UP
• Recheck 10 days postoperatively.
• General examination of the area; percussion to test for sensitivity, healing of the extraction or surgical endodontic site, and integrity of the endodontic access fillings
• Recheck in 6 months to a year; repeat radiographs to see if the lesion has resolved (in endodontic treatment).
• Avoid traumatic injuries (e.g., letting the dog chase cars).
• Eliminate bones, hooves, and other chewable hard objects.
• Stop throwing rocks or wood for the dog to retrieve.
• Decrease fighting.
• Curtail bite work—avoid handler sleeves that have tears or hole in them
• Check the mouth regularly for broken or discolored teeth.

MISCELLANEOUS

Suggested Reading
Ingle JI, Tainto JF. Endodontics. Philadelphia: Lea & Febiger, 1985:419–445.
Neville BW, Damm DD, Allen CM, Bouguot JE. Oral & maxillofacial pathology. Philadelphia: Saunders, 1995:96–121.
Author James M. G. Anthony
Consulting Editor Jan Bellows

DISEASES

TOXOPLASMOSIS

BASICS

DEFINITION
Toxoplasma gondii—an obligate intracellular coccidian protozoan parasite that infects nearly all mammals; Felidae the definitive hosts; all other warm-blooded animals are intermediate hosts.

PATHOPHYSIOLOGY
• Severity and manifestation—depend on location and degree of tissue injury caused by tissue cysts • Infection—acquired by ingestion of tissue cysts or oocysts; organisms spread to extraintestinal organs via blood or lymph; results in focal necrosis to many organs (heart, eye, CNS) • Acute disseminated infection rarely fatal • Chronic disease—tissue cysts form; low-grade disease; usually not clinically apparent unless immunosuppression or concomitant illness allows organism to proliferate, causing an acute inflammatory response • Clinical disease—often associated with other infections that cause severe immunosuppression (e.g., canine distemper, FIP, and FeLV).

SYSTEMS AFFECTED
• Multisystemic—usually the same in cats and dogs • Ophthalmic—approximately 80% of affected cats have evidence of intraocular inflammation, most commonly uveitis.

GENETICS N/A

INCIDENCE/PREVALENCE
• Approximately 30% of cats and up to 50% of people serologically positive for *T. gondii* • Most animals asymptomatic

GEOGRAPHIC DISTRIBUTION
Worldwide

SIGNALMENT
Species
Cats more commonly symptomatic than dogs
Breed Predilections
None
Mean Age and Range
In one study, mean age 4 years; range 2 weeks to 16 years
Predominant Sex
Male cats—more common

SIGNS
General Comments
• Determined mainly by site and extent of organ damage • Acute—at the time of initial infection • Chronic—reactivation of encysted infection; caused by immunosuppression

Historical Findings
• Nonspecific signs of lethargy, depression, and anorexia
• Weight loss
• Fever

• Ocular discharge, photophobia, miotic pupils (cats)
• Respiratory distress
• Neurologic—ataxia; seizures; tremors; paresis/paralysis; cranial nerve deficits
• Digestive tract—vomiting; diarrhea; abdominal pain; jaundice
• Stillborn kittens

Physical Examination Findings
Cats
• Most severe in transplacentally infected kittens, which may be stillborn or die before weaning
• Surviving kittens—anorexia; lethargy; high fever unresponsive to antibiotics; reflect necrosis/inflammation of lungs (dyspnea, increased respiratory noises), liver (icterus, abdominal enlargement from ascites), and CNS (encephalopathic)
• Respiratory and gastrointestinal (postnatal)—most common; anorexia; lethargy; high fever unresponsive to antibiotics; dyspnea; weight loss; icterus; vomiting; diarrhea; abdominal effusion
• Neurologic (postnatal)—seen in < 10% of patients; blindness; stupor; incoordination; circling; torticollis; anisocoria; seizures
• Ocular signs (postnatal)—common; uveitis (aqueous flare, hyphema, mydriasis); iritis; detached retina; iridocyclitis; keratic precipitates
• Rapid course—acutely affected patient with CNS and/or respiratory involvement
• Slow course—patients with reactivation of chronic infection
Dogs
• Young—usually generalized infection; fever; weight loss; anorexia; tonsillitis; dyspnea; diarrhea; vomiting
• Old—tend to localized infections; mainly associated with neural and muscular systems
• Neurologic—quite variable; usually reflect diffuse neurologic inflammation; seizures; tremors; ataxia; paresis; paralysis; muscle weakness; and tetraparesis
• Ocular—rare; similar to those found in cats
• Cardiac involvement—occurs; usually not clinically apparent

CAUSES
T. gondii

RISK FACTORS
Immunosuppression—may predispose to infection or reactivation: FeLV, FIV, FIP, hemobartonellosis, canine distemper, and glucocorticoid or antitumor chemotherapy

DIAGNOSIS

DIFFERENTIAL DIAGNOSIS
Cats
• Intraocular disease (anterior uveitis)—FIP;

FeLV; FIV; immune-mediated; trauma; lens-induced; corneal ulceration with reflex uveitis
• Dyspnea (respiratory signs)—asthma; cardiogenic; pneumonia (bacterial, fungal, parasitic); neoplasia; heartworm disease; pleural disease (effusions); diaphragmatic hernia; chest wall injury
• Neurologic (causes of meningoencephalitis)—viral (FIP, rabies, pseudorabies); fungal (cryptococcosis, blastomycosis, histoplasmosis); parasitic (cuterebriasis, coenurosis, aberrant heartworm migration); bacterial; idiopathic disease (feline polioencephalomyelitis)
Dogs
• Often associated with other immunosuppressive diseases—e.g., signs of distemper may be seen.
• Neurologic—usually in very young dogs; differentiate from *Neospora caninum* (both produce CNS and neuromuscular disease)
• Consider other conditions causing multifocal signs—infectious or inflammatory toxicity; metabolic disease

CBC/BIOCHEMISTRY/URINALYSIS
CBC (Cats)
• Most show mild normocytic normochromic anemia.
• Leukopenia—approximately 50% of patients with severe disease; mainly owing to lymphopenia
• Neutropenia—alone or in addition to lymphopenia and a degenerative left shift
• Leukocytosis—may occur during recovery

Biochemistry
• ALT and AST—marked increase in most patients
• Hypoalbuminemia
• Cats—icterus seen in approximately 25% of patients; mildly low serum calcium concentrations often seen with pancreatitis; amylase levels unreliable

Urinalysis (Cats)
• Mild proteinuria—small proportion of patients
• Bilirubinuria—especially with icterus

OTHER LABORATORY TESTS
Serology
• IgM, IgG, and antigen serum titers—most definitive information from one sample; determine type of infection (active, recent, chronic) with a follow-up sample taken 3 weeks later; titers available from Veterinary Diagnostic Laboratory, College of Veterinary Medicine, Colorado State University, Fort Collins, CO 80523
• IgM—single serologic titer of choice for diagnosis of active infection; elevated 2 weeks postinfection (usually coincides with onset of clinical signs); persists for a maximum of 3 months; then falls; prolonged titer: reactivation or delay in antibody class shift to

IgG (result of immunosuppression from FeLV or FIV infection or steroid therapy)
• IgG—titers rise 2–4 weeks postinfection; persist > 1 year; single high titer not diagnostic for active infection; fourfold increase over a 3-week period suggests active infection
• Antigen—positive 1–4 weeks postinfection; because it remains positive during active or chronically persistent infections, does not add much to antibody titer results

IMAGING
Radiographs—may see mixed pattern of patchy alveolar and interstitial pulmonary infiltrates, pleural and abdominal effusions, and hepatomegaly

DIAGNOSTIC PROCEDURES
• CSF—high leukocyte count (both mononuclear cells and neutrophils) and protein in encephalopathic patients
• Cytology—organism rarely detected in body fluids during acute infection (CSF, pleural or peritoneal effusions); broncho-alveolar lavage effective in identifying organisms in affected cats with signs of pulmonary involvement
• Fecal—evaluation with Sheather sugar solution may be diagnostic; fecal oocyst shedding rarely occurs during clinical disease; oocysts may be detected on routine examination in asymptomatic cats but are morphologically indistinguishable from *Hammondia* spp. and *Besnoitia;* distinguish organisms via mouse inoculation

PATHOLOGIC FINDINGS
• Necrotic foci—up to 1 cm; most often in liver, pancreas, mesenteric lymph nodes, and lungs; necrosis of brain (1-cm areas of discoloration)
• Ulcers and granulomas—may be seen in stomach and small intestine

TREATMENT

APPROPRIATE HEALTH CARE
• Usually outpatient
• Inpatient—severe disease; patient cannot maintain adequate nutrition or hydration.
• Confine—patients with neurologic signs

NURSING CARE
Dehydration—intravenous fluids

ACTIVITY N/A

DIET N/A

CLIENT EDUCATION
• Cats—prognosis guarded in patients needing therapy; response to therapy inconsistent
• Neonates and severely immunocompromised animals—prognosis worse

SURGICAL CONSIDERATIONS N/A

MEDICATIONS

DRUGS OF CHOICE
• Clindamycin—25–50 mg/kg PO or IM daily, divided into two doses, for at least 2 weeks after clinical signs clear
• 1% prednisone drops—every 8 hours for 2 weeks for uveitis; use concurrently

CONTRAINDICATIONS N/A

PRECAUTIONS
Clindamycin—anorexia, vomiting, and diarrhea (dose dependent)

POSSIBLE INTERACTIONS
None

ALTERNATIVE DRUGS
• Sulfadiazine (30 mg/kg PO q12h) in combination with pyrimethamine (0.5 mg/kg PO q12h) for 2 weeks; can cause depression, anemia, leukopenia, and thrombocytopenia, especially in cats.
• Folinic acid (5 mg/day) or brewer's yeast (100 mg/kg/day)—correct bone marrow suppression caused by sulfadiazine/pyrimethamine therapy

FOLLOW-UP

PATIENT MONITORING
Clindamycin
• Examine 2 days after initiation treatment—clinical signs (fever, hyperesthesia, anorexia, uveitis) should begin to resolve; uveitis should resolve completely within 1 week. • Examine 2 weeks after initiation of treatment—assess neuromuscular deficits; should partially resolve (some deficits permanent owing to CNS or peripheral neuromuscular damage) • Examine 2 weeks after owner-reported resolution of signs—assess discontinuing treatment; some neuromuscular deficits permanent;

PREVENTION/AVOIDANCE
Cats
• Diet—prevent ingestion of raw meat, bones, viscera, or unpasteurized milk (especially goat's milk); or mechanical vectors (flies, cockroaches); feed only well-cooked meat. • Behavior—prevent free roaming to hunt prey (birds, rodents) or to enter buildings where food-producing animals are housed.

POSSIBLE COMPLICATIONS N/A

EXPECTED COURSE AND PROGNOSIS
• Prognosis—guarded; varied response to drug treatment • Acute—prompt and aggressive therapy often successful • Residual deficits (especially neurologic) cannot be predicted until after a course of therapy.

• Ocular disease—usually responds to appropriate therapy • Severe muscular or neurologic disease—usually chronic debility

MISCELLANEOUS

ASSOCIATED CONDITIONS
• Young dogs—distemper • Cats—FeLV, FIP, and FIV; FIV infection does not affect clinical outcome or the ability of the animal to mount a protective immune response to subsequent reinfection.

AGE-RELATED FACTORS
Disease worse in neonates

ZOONOTIC POTENTIAL
• Considerable • Cats—healthy animal with a positive antibody titer poses little danger to humans; animal with no antibody titer at more risk of becoming infected, shedding oocysts in the feces, and constituting a risk to humans • Avoid contact with oocysts or tissue cysts—do not feed raw meat; wash hands and surfaces (cutting boards) after preparing raw meat; boil drinking water if source is unreliable; keep sandboxes covered to prevent cats from defecating in them; wear gloves when gardening; wash hands and vegetables before eating to avoid contact with oocyst soil contamination; empty cat litter boxes daily (oocysts need at least 24 hr to become infective); disinfect litter boxes with boiling water; control stray cat population to avoid oocyst contamination of environment.
• Pregnant women—avoid all contact with a cat that is excreting oocysts in feces; avoid contact with soil and cat litter; do not handle or eat raw meat (to kill organism, cook to 66°C; 150°F).

PREGNANCY
• Parasitemia during pregnancy—spread of organism to fetus; probably does not happen unless first-time infection of dam occurs during pregnancy (as with humans)
• Placental transmission rare

ABBREVIATIONS
• ALT = alanine aminotransferase
• AST = aspartate aminotransferase
• FeLV = feline leukemia virus
• FIP = feline infectious peritonitis
• FIV = feline immunodeficiency virus

Suggested Reading
Dubey JP. Toxoplasmosis. J Am Vet Med Assoc 1994;205:1593–1598.
Dubey JP, Lappin MR. Toxoplasmosis and neosporosis. In: Greene CE, ed. Infectious diseases of the dog and cat. Philadelphia: Saunders, 1998:493–509.
Author Stephen C. Barr
Consulting Editor Stephen C. Barr

DISEASES

TRACHEAL COLLAPSE

BASICS

DEFINITION
• Dynamic reduction in the luminal diameter of the large conducting airway with respiration • May involve the cervical trachea, the intrathoracic trachea, or both segments • Compression of the trachea or bronchi as a result of hilar lymphadenopathy or external mass lesions—not considered part of this condition

PATHOPHYSIOLOGY
• Hypocellular tracheal cartilage—identified in some patients • Lack of chondroitin sulfate and/or decreased glycoproteins within the cartilage matrix—results in a reduction in bound water and loss of turgidity in the cartilage • Abnormalities in the cartilage structure—may represent defects in chondrogenesis associated with primary genetic influences, nutritional deficiencies, or possibly degenerative changes caused by longstanding airway disease • Collapse—weak cartilage allows flattening of the tracheal ring structure; trachea collapses in a dorsoventral direction when pressures change within the airway lumen. • Increased tension on the trachealis dorsalis muscle or neurogenic atrophy of the muscle—causes stretching of the dorsal tracheal membrane with protrusion into the airway lumen • Coughing—mechanical trauma to the tracheal mucosa from collapse of the dorsal tracheal membrane exacerbates airway edema and inflammation and may lead to pseudomembrane formation. • Abnormal pressure gradients develop along the trachea during inspiration, which lead to increased inspiratory effort and dynamic collapse of the airway. • Chronic increase in respiratory effort—may lead to secondary abnormalities in laryngeal structure and function • Upper airway obstruction—worsens clinical signs • High intrapleural pressure during expiration—leads to collapse of the intrathoracic trachea • Small airway disease—increases pressure gradient and potentiates collapse; may be perpetuated by chronic cough and airway inflammation, leading to more widespread pulmonary dysfunction

SYSTEMS AFFECTED
• Respiratory—lower respiratory tract infection or inflammation owing to poor clearance of secretions and bacteria • Cardiovascular—pulmonary hypertension • Nervous—may be involved when syncope develops from hypoxia or a vasovagal reflex associated with cough

GENETICS
Unknown

INCIDENCE/PREVALENCE
Common clinical entity

GEOGRAPHIC DISTRIBUTION
Worldwide

SIGNALMENT
Species
Primarily dogs, rarely cats

Breed Predilections
• Miniature poodles, Yorkshire terriers, Chihuahuas, Pomeranians, and other small and toy breeds • Occasionally seen in young, large-breed dogs

Mean Age and Range
• Middle-aged to elderly—onset of signs at 4–14 years of age
• Severely affected animals < 1 year of age

Predominant Sex
None

SIGNS
Historical Findings
• Usually worsened by excitement, heat, humidity, exercise, or obesity
• Dry honking cough
• May have chronic history of intermittent coughing or difficulty breathing
• Retching—often observed; from an attempt to clear respiratory secretions from the larynx
• Tachypnea, exercise intolerance, and/or respiratory distress—common
• Cyanosis or syncope—may see in severely affected individuals

Physical Examination Findings
• Increased tracheal sensitivity—virtually always seen
• Dyspnea—inspiratory dyspnea with cervical collapse; expiratory with intrathoracic collapse
• Wheezing or musical tracheal sounds when ausculting over a region of narrowed trachea
• An end-expiratory snap—may be heard when large segments of the intrathoracic airway collapse during forceful expiration
• Wheezes or crackles—indicate concurrent small airway disease
• Mitral insufficiency murmurs—often found concurrently in small-breed dogs
• Congestive heart failure (dogs)—typically exhibit a rapid heart rate
• Normal to low heart rate and/or marked sinus arrhythmia—more common in dogs with tracheal collapse, unless marked respiratory distress occurs
• Loud second heart sound—suggests pulmonary hypertension
• Hepatomegaly—common; cause unknown

CAUSES
• Congenital, nutritional, or familial defects of chondrogenesis
• Chronic small airway disease

RISK FACTORS
• Obesity
• Pulmonary infection
• Upper airway obstruction

DIAGNOSIS

DIFFERENTIAL DIAGNOSIS
• Infectious tracheobronchitis
• Tracheal or laryngeal obstruction
• Chronic bronchitis
• Pneumonia—viral, bacterial, fungal, parasitic, eosinophilic
• Congestive heart failure
• Bronchiectasis

CBC/BIOCHEMISTRY/URINALYSIS
• CBC—may show an inflammatory leukogram secondary to chronic stress or pneumonia

OTHER LABORATORY TESTS
N/A

IMAGING
Thoracic Radiography
• Collapse identified in 60% of affected patients
• Inspiratory radiographs—show cervical collapse
• Expiratory radiographs—show tracheal collapse; may also note collapse of the mainstem bronchus and ballooning of the cervical trachea
• Bronchitis, pneumonia, or bronchiectasis—may be identified
• Right-sided heart enlargement—may be seen secondary to chronic pulmonary disease and cor pulmonale

Fluoroscopy
Dynamic collapse of the cervical or intrathoracic trachea and/or dorsal tracheal membrane—may be more easily identified after induction of cough

DIAGNOSTIC PROCEDURES
Tracheal Wash
Use oral intubation (rather than the transtracheal approach) and a sterile catheter when obtaining samples for cytologic examination and bacterial culture and sensitivity.

Bronchoscopy
• Grade severity of collapse; identify small airway disease.
• Grade I—slight protrusion of the dorsal tracheal membrane into the airway lumen; diameter reduced by < 25%
• Grade II—reduction of the tracheal lumen by 50%
• Grade III—reduction of the tracheal lumen by 75%; trachealis muscle brushing the tracheal mucosa
• Grade IV—tracheal rings flattened; < 10% of the tracheal lumen can be seen; may note a double lumen trachea when the trachealis muscle contacts the ventral surface of the trachea and the rings have bowed dorsally

• Submit airway samples for cytologic examination and bacterial culture and sensitivity testing; specific cultures for *Mycoplasma* are recommended.

Cytology
• Sepsis and suppuration along with marked bacterial growth of a pathogen—suggests pulmonary infection
• Neutrophils without intracellular bacteria or marked bacterial growth—indicates airway inflammation

PATHOLOGIC FINDINGS
• Trachealis muscle—greatly elongated
• Cartilage rings—flattened
• May note tracheal inflammation or pseudomembrane formation
• Hypocellularity of the cartilage with low glycoproteins and chondroitin sulfate—may be noted via histopathologic examination or electron microscopy
• May see changes associated with chronic obstructive pulmonary disease

TREATMENT

APPROPRIATE HEALTH CARE
• Outpatient—stable patients
• Inpatient—oxygen therapy and heavy sedation for severe dyspnea

NURSING CARE
Oxygen therapy and heavy sedation—severely dyspneic patients

ACTIVITY
• Severely limited until patient is stable
• During management of disease—gentle exercise recommended to encourage weight loss

DIET
• Most affected dogs improve after losing weight.
• Institute weight-loss program with a high-fiber reducing diet.
• Feed 60% of total daily requirement of calories; use a slow weight-loss program designed to achieve 1%–2% weight loss per week.

CLIENT EDUCATION
• Warn client that obesity, overexcitement, and humid conditions may precipitate a crisis.
• Advise client to use a harness instead of a collar.

SURGICAL CONSIDERATIONS
• Upper airway obstructive disorder (e.g., laryngeal paralysis, everted laryngeal saccule)—may improve after corrective surgery
• Placement of C-shaped stents in selected patients (primarily with cervical collapse) by a skilled surgeon—shown to improve quality of life and reduce clinical signs when adequate stabilization of the airway can be achieved and when chronic pulmonary changes do not limit resolution of disease
• Consider likelihood of complications after surgery (e.g., persistent cough, dyspnea, or laryngeal paralysis); some patients may require a permanent tracheostomy.

MEDICATIONS

DRUGS OF CHOICE
• Sedation and cough suppression—butorphanol (0.05 mg/kg SC); addition of acepromazine (0.025 mg/kg SC) may enhance sedative effects and further reduce the cough reflex; narcotic cough suppressants (butorphanol at 0.5–1.0 mg/kg PO q4–8h or hydrocodone at 0.22 mg/kg PO q4–8h) effective for chronic treatment
• Dilation of small airways and lowering pressure gradients with lower airway disease—sustained-release Theo-Dur tablets (10–20 mg/kg q12h), Slo-bid Gyro-Caps (25 mg/kg q12h), or terbutaline (1.25–5.0 mg/dog q8–12h); bronchodilators have no effect on tracheal diameter.
• Reduction of bronchial inflammation—prednisone (0.5–1.0 mg/kg PO q12h; taper to q48h) may help.

CONTRAINDICATIONS
None

PRECAUTIONS
• Theo-Dur—use tablets and not sprinkles; sprinkles have poor bioavailability.
• Do not initially use generic sustained-release theophylline products because of unknown pharmacokinetic properties.
• Avoid long-term steroid use because of the propensity for weight gain and diseases associated with immunosuppression.

POSSIBLE INTERACTIONS
• Theophylline metabolism—increased by concurrent treatment with ketoconazole or phenobarbital, which results in inadequate plasma concentration; decreased by fluoroquinolones (e.g., enrofloxacin), erythromycin, cimetidine, steroids, β-blockers, mexiletine, and thiabendazole, which results in toxic plasma concentration and gastrointestinal upset, nervousness, or tachycardia; adjust dosages when concurrent use is necessary.
• Theophylline bioavailability and pharmacokinetics—affected by congestive heart failure, cor pulmonale, and liver disease; affected by use of a high-fiber diet; pay careful attention to dosage to avoid undesirable side effects.

ALTERNATIVE DRUGS
Robitussin DM—may provide palliation

FOLLOW-UP

PATIENT MONITORING
• Body weight • Exercise tolerance • Pattern of respiration • Incidence of cough

PREVENTION/AVOIDANCE
• Avoid obesity in breeds commonly afflicted.
• Avoid heat and humidity. • Use harnesses.

POSSIBLE COMPLICATIONS
Intractable dyspnea leading to respiratory failure or euthanasia

EXPECTED COURSE AND PROGNOSIS
• Combinations of medications along with weight control may reduce clinical signs. • Surgery—may benefit some patients, primarily those with cervical collapse • Patient will cough throughout life. • Prognosis—based on bronchoscopic evidence of airway obstruction

MISCELLANEOUS

ASSOCIATED CONDITIONS
• Chronic bronchitis • Laryngeal paralysis
• Everted laryngeal saccules • Pulmonary hypertension • Breeds of dogs that develop tracheal collapse also commonly have mitral insufficiency.

AGE-RELATED FACTORS
N/A

ZOONOTIC
N/A

PREGNANCY
N/A

SYNONYMS
N/A

SEE ALSO
Bronchitis, Chronic (COPD)

Suggested Reading
Buback JL, Boothe HW, Hobson HP. Surgical treatment of tracheal collapse in dogs: 90 cases (1983–1993). J Am Vet Med Assoc 1996;308:380–384.
Hedlund CS. Tracheal collapse. Probl Vet Med 1991;3:229–238.
McKiernan BC. Current uses and hazards of bronchodilator therapy. In Kirk RW, Bonagura JD, eds. Current veterinary therapy XI. Philadelphia: Saunders, 1992:660–668.
White RAS, Williams JM. Tracheal collapse. Is there really a role for surgery? A survey of 100 cases. J Small Anim Pract 1994;35:191–196.
Author Lynelle Johnson
Consulting Editor Eleanor C. Hawkins

DISEASES

TRACHEOBRONCHITIS, INFECTIOUS—DOGS

BASICS

DEFINITION
Any contagious respiratory disease of dogs that is manifested by coughing and seemingly not caused by canine distemper virus

PATHOPHYSIOLOGY
Pathogenesis usually involves an injury to the respiratory epithelium, viral infection, or both followed by invasion of the damaged tissue by bacterial, fungal, mycoplasmal, parasitic, or other virulent organisms, resulting in further damage and clinical signs.

SYSTEMS AFFECTED
Respiratory—primarily affected unless associated with sepsis or congenital anomaly

GENETICS
N/A

INCIDENCE/PREVALENCE
Occurs most commonly in places where dogs of varying ages and susceptibility congregate, often under less than ideal hygienic conditions

GEOGRAPHIC DISTRIBUTION
Worldwide

SIGNALMENT

Species
Dogs

Breed Predilections
None

Mean Age and Range
• Most severe in puppies 6 weeks to 6 months old
• May develop in dogs of all ages and often with pre-existing subclinical airway disease (e.g., congenital anomaly, chronic bronchitis, and bronchiectasis)

Predominant Sex
None

SIGNS

General Comments
• Related to the degree of respiratory tract damage and age of the affected dog
• May be nonexistent, mild, or severe with pneumonia
• Most viral, bacterial, and mycoplasmal agents spread rapidly from seemingly healthy dogs to others in the same environment; signs usually begin about 4 days after exposure to the infecting agent(s).

Historical Findings
• Uncomplicated—cough in an otherwise healthy animal is characteristic; may be dry and hacking, soft and dry, moist and hacking, or paroxysmal, followed by gagging or expectoration of mucus; excitement, exercise, changes in temperature or humidity of the inspired air, and gentle pressure (eg. from collar) on the trachea induce a paroxysm of coughing.
• Severe—affect on appetite severe; cough (when noted) is moist and productive; may see lethargy, anorexia, dyspnea, and exercise intolerance

Physical Examination Findings
• Uncomplicated—cough readily induced with tracheal pressure; lung sounds often normal; otherwise healthy
• Severe—may detect constant, low-grade, or fluctuating fever (39.4–40.0°C; 103–104°F); may detect increased intensity of normal lung sounds, crackles, or (less frequently) wheezes

CAUSES
• Viral—canine distemper virus; CAV-2; CPI; CAV-1; canine reovirus type 1, 2, or 3; canine herpesvirus
• CAV-2 and CPI—may damage respiratory epithelium to such an extent that invasion by various bacteria and mycoplasmas causes severe airway disease
• Bacterial—*Bordetella bronchiseptica,** with no other respiratory pathogens, produces clinical signs indistinguishable from other bacterial causes; *Pseudomonas, Escherichia coli, Klebsiella, Pasteurella, Streptococcus, Mycoplasma,* and other species equally likely

RISK FACTORS
• Less than ideal hygienic conditions—seen in some pet shops, humane society shelters, research facilities, and boarding and training kennels
• Coexisting subclinical airway disease—congenital anomalies; chronic bronchitis; bronchiectasis

DIAGNOSIS

DIFFERENTIAL DIAGNOSIS
• The diagnosis is usually provisionally established by eliminating noninfectious causes of coughing.
• Numerous organisms that infect the lungs
• History that reveals a source of exposure
• Patient's vaccination status
• See Cough.

CBC/BIOCHEMISTRY/URINALYSIS
• Early mild leukopenia (5000–6000 cells/dL)—may be detected; suggests viral cause
• Neutrophilic leukocytosis with a left shift—frequently found with severe pneumonia
• Serum chemistry profile and urinalysis—usually normal

OTHER LABORATORY TESTS
Arterial blood gas analysis—may be useful with pneumonia

IMAGING
• Radiographs—unremarkable with uncomplicated disease; of value primarily to rule out noninfectious causes of a cough
• Thoracic radiographs—severe: may demonstrate an interstitial and alveolar lung pattern with a cranioventral distribution typical of bacterial pneumonia; may see a diffuse interstitial lung pattern typical of viral pneumonia; may note a mixed lung pattern (e.g., combination of alveolar, interstitial, and peribronchial lung patterns)

DIAGNOSTIC PROCEDURES
• With suspected severe disease—perform transtracheal washing or tracheobronchial lavage via bronchoscopy.
• Antimicrobial sensitivity pattern of cultured bacteria—identification aids markedly in providing an effective treatment plan

PATHOLOGIC FINDINGS
• CPI—causes few to no clinical signs; lungs of infected dogs 6–10 days after exposure may contain petechia hemorrhages that are evenly distributed over the surfaces; detected by immunofluorescence in columnar epithelial cells of the bronchi and bronchioles 6–10 days after aerosol exposure
• CAV-2—lesions confined to the respiratory system; large intranuclear inclusion bodies found in bronchial epithelial cells and alveolar septal cells; clinical signs tend to be mild and short-lasting; lesions persist for at least a month after infection.
• Bordetellosis and severe bacterial infection—evidence of purulent bronchitis, tracheitis, and rhinitis with hyperemia and enlargement of the bronchial, mediastinal, and retropharyngeal lymph nodes; may see large numbers of gram-positive or -negative organisms in the mucus of the tracheal and bronchial epithelium

TREATMENT

APPROPRIATE HEALTH CARE
• Outpatient—strongly recommended for uncomplicated disease
• Inpatient—strongly recommended for complicated disease and/or pneumonia

NURSING CARE
Fluid administration—indicated for complicated disease and/or pneumonia

ACTIVITY
Enforce rest—for at least 14–21 days with uncomplicated disease; for at least the duration of radiographic evidence of pneumonia

DIET
Good-quality canned or dry commercial food

CLIENT EDUCATION
• Encourage client to isolate patient from other animals; infected dogs can transmit the agent(s) before onset of clinical signs and afterward until immunity develops.
• Inform client that patients with uncomplicated disease should respond to treatment in 10–14 days.
• Inform client that once infection spreads in a kennel, it can be controlled by evacuation for 1–2 weeks and disinfecting with commonly used chemicals, such as sodium hypochlorite (1:30 dilution), chlorhexidine, and benzalkonium.

SURGICAL CONSIDERATIONS
N/A

MEDICATIONS

DRUGS OF CHOICE
• Amoxicillin/clavulanic acid (12.5–25 mg/kg PO q12h) or doxycycline (5 mg/kg PO q12h)—initial treatment of uncomplicated disease
• Gentamicin (2–4 mg/kg IV, IM, SC q6–8h) or amikacin (6.5 mg/kg IV, IM, SC q8h) and a first-generation cephalosporin (cefazolin, 20–35 mg/kg IV, IM q8h) or enrofloxacin (2.5–5 mg/kg PO, IM, IV ql2h)—usually effective for severe disease
• Antimicrobial therapy—continue for at least 10 days beyond radiographic resolution.
• *B. bronchiseptica* and other resistant species—some antimicrobials may not reach adequate therapeutic concentrations in the lumen of the lower respiratory tract, so oral or parenteral administration may have limited effectiveness; nebulization with kanamycin (250 mg), gentamicin (50 mg), or polymyxin B (333,000 IU) may eliminate species when administered daily for 3–5 days.
• Butorphanol (0.55 mg/kg PO q8–12h) or hydrocodone bitartrate (0.22 mg/kg PO q6–8h)—effective suppression of dry, nonproductive cough
• Bronchodilators (e.g., Theo-Dur, 10–25 mg/kg PO q12h)—may use to control bronchospasm; made clinically apparent by wheezing

CONTRAINDICATIONS
Do not use cough suppressants with pneumonia.

PRECAUTIONS
None

POSSIBLE INTERACTIONS
N/A

ALTERNATIVE DRUGS
None

FOLLOW-UP

PATIENT MONITORING
• Uncomplicated disease—should respond to treatment in 10–14 days; if patient continues to cough 14 days or more after establishment of an adequate treatment plan, question the diagnosis of uncomplicated disease.
• Severe disease—repeat thoracic radiography until at least 14 days beyond resolution of all clinical signs

PREVENTION/AVOIDANCE
Shedding of the causative agent(s) of infectious tracheobronchitis in respiratory secretions of dogs undoubtedly accounts for the persistence of this problem in kennels, animal shelters, boarding facilities, and veterinary hospitals.

Viral and Bacterial Vaccines
• Available to control the principal agents involved
• *B. bronchiseptica* and CPI vaccine—may vaccinate puppies intranasally with as early as 2–4 weeks of age without interference from maternal antibody and follow with annual revaccination; may vaccinate mature dogs with a one-dose intranasal vaccination (at the same time as their puppies or when they receive their annual vaccinations)
• Inactivated *B. bronchiseptica* parenteral vaccine—administered as two doses, 2–4 weeks apart; initial vaccination of puppies is recommended at or about 6–8 weeks of age; revaccinate at 4 months of age.

POSSIBLE COMPLICATIONS
N/A

EXPECTED COURSE AND PROGNOSIS
• Natural course of uncomplicated disease, if untreated—10–14 days; simple restriction of exercise and prevention of excitement shortens the course.
• Typical course of severe disease—2–6 weeks; patients that die often developed severe pneumonia that affected multiple lung lobes.

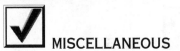

MISCELLANEOUS

ASSOCIATED CONDITIONS
May accompany other respiratory tract anomalies

AGE-RELATED FACTORS
Most severe in puppies 6 weeks to 6 months old and in puppies from commercial pet shops and humane society shelters

ZOONOTIC POTENTIAL
None

PREGNANCY
High risk in dogs on extensive medical treatment; especially risky for the developing puppies

SYNONYMS
Kennel cough—uncomplicated disease

ABBREVIATIONS
• CAV = canine adenovirus
• CPI = canine parainfluenza

Suggested Reading
Bemis DA. Bordetella and mycoplasma respiratory infection in dogs. Vet Clin North Am Small Anim Pract 1992;22:1173–1186.
Ford RB, Vaden SL. Canine infectious tracheobronchitis. In: Greene CE, ed. Infectious diseases of the dog and cat. Philadelphia: Saunders, 1990:259–265.
Hoskins JD, Taboada J. Specific treatment of infectious causes of respiratory disease in dogs and cats. Vet Med 1994;89:443–452.
Padrid P. Chronic lower airway disease in the dog and cat. Probl Vet Med 1992;4:320–344.
Author Johnny D. Hoskins
Consulting Editor Eleanor Hawkins

TRANSITIONAL CELL CARCINOMA, RENAL, BLADDER, URETHRA

BASICS

DEFINITION
Malignancy arising from the transitional epithelium of the kidney, ureters, urinary bladder, urethra, prostate, or vagina

PATHOPHYSIOLOGY
Flea-control products and cyclophosphamide—possible causal agents

SYSTEMS AFFECTED
Renal/Urologic
• Kidneys—less commonly affected than other renal sites; may be primary site
• Urinary bladder (may include ureters)—trigone most commonly affected site in dogs; local invasion of the distal ureter also common; may lead to postrenal azotemia; apex more often affected than is the trigone in cats
• Urethra—second most common site in dogs; may find urethral obstruction and postrenal azotemia
Other
• Reproductive—vagina less commonly affected but may be primary site; prostate may be involved by local invasion or may be primary site.
• Metastatic sites—regional lymph nodes and lungs most common
• Paraneoplastic organ involvement—hypertrophic osteopathy has been reported secondary to transitional cell carcinoma of the urinary bladder.

GENETICS
N/A

INCIDENCE/PREVALENCE
• Dogs—< 1% of all reported malignancies
• Rare in cats

GEOGRAPHIC DISTRIBUTION
N/A

SIGNALMENT
Middle-aged to old, spayed, female small-breed dogs most commonly reported

Species
Dogs and cats

Breed Predilections
• Dogs—Scottish terriers, west Highland white terriers, Shetland sheepdogs, American Eskimo dogs, and dachshunds; may occur in any breed
• Cats—none

Mean Age and Range
• Dogs—8 years; range, 1–15+ years
• Cats—7 years; range, 3–16 years

Predominant Sex
Female

SIGNS

General Comments
Similar to those of bacterial urinary tract infection; for patients showing temporary or no response to appropriate antibiotics, consider transitional cell carcinoma; may temporarily respond to antibiotic therapy

Historical Findings
• Recurrent stranguria, pollakiuria, hematuria, dysuria, urinary incontinence, or any combination

Physical Examination Findings
• Often normal
• Mass—occasionally palpable in the caudal abdomen and urinary bladder region
• Urethral or vaginal—may be palpable on rectal examination
• Enlarged intrapelvic or sublumbar lymph nodes—rarely palpable

CAUSES
• Dogs—see Risk Factors
• Cats—unknown

RISK FACTORS
Dogs—obesity, environmental carcinogens; chronic exposure to flea-control products, and long-term or a large bolus dose of cyclophosphamide

DIAGNOSIS

DIFFERENTIAL DIAGNOSIS
• Urinary tract infection
• Urolithiasis
• Vaginitis
• Prostatitis
• Other primary neoplasia or metastatic neoplasia

CBC/BIOCHEMISTRY/URINALYSIS
• Usually normal
• Biochemistry—may show signs of renal and/or postrenal azotemia with ureteral or urethral obstruction
• Urinalysis—often reveals epithelial cells with multiple criteria of malignancy; interpret cytologic examination with caution if the sample is inflammatory, because epithelial cells may exhibit criteria of malignancy in the presence of inflammation.
• Avoid cystocentesis because seeding of tumor cells along needle tract is probable.

OTHER LABORATORY TESTS
Urine culture and sensitivity testing—indicated because concurrent urinary tract infection is common

IMAGING
• Thoracic radiography—metastatic patterns: multiple well-defined interstitial nodules, interstitial pattern more pronounced than normal, and alveolar infiltrates; up to 37% of dogs have metastatic disease at the time of examination.
• Abdominal radiography—probably will not reveal specific urinary bladder disease unless the mass is mineralized (rare); may reveal sublumbar lymphadenomegaly
• Double-contrast cystography—dogs: lesion(s) usually at trigone of the urinary bladder; cats lesion(s) usually at the apex of the urinary bladder
• Intravenous pyelography, voiding urethrogram, or vaginogram—sometimes indicated
• Ultrasonography—helps identify location and extent of disease; excellent for monitoring response to treatment

TRANSITIONAL CELL CARCINOMA, RENAL, BLADDER, URETHRA

DIAGNOSTIC PROCEDURES
- Biopsy—gold standard for definitive diagnosis
- Exploratory laparotomy—reasonable method for obtaining specimens of the primary tumor and regional lymph nodes
- Cystoscopy—less invasive way to view lesions and retrieve specimens
- Ultrasound-guided biopsy—not recommended, because seeding of the biopsy tract with viable tumor cells is likely

PATHOLOGIC FINDINGS
- Irregular to diffuse thickening of the urinary bladder mucosa
- Metastasis possible

TREATMENT

APPROPRIATE HEALTH CARE
- Outpatient—stable patients
- Radiotherapy (intraoperative and fractionated)—reported to result in longer survival times and better local control than chemotherapy; potential side effects: urinary bladder stricture and fibrosis with urinary incontinence

NURSING CARE
N/A

ACTIVITY
Normal

DIET
Normal, unless concurrent renal failure

CLIENT EDUCATION
- Warn client that the long-term prognosis is poor but palliation is often attainable.
- Inform client that the tumor is not usually surgically resectable in dogs.

SURGICAL CONSIDERATIONS
- Highly exfoliative and highly transplantable tumor; multiple reports of surgically induced seeding; replace all surgical instruments and gloves after contact with the tumor.
- Surgery may result in a cure if the mass is surgically resectable.
- Wide surgical margins necessary; up to 50% of the urinary bladder may be resected with minimal loss of function.
- Tube cystostomy placement—may greatly prolong survival times by bypassing urethral obstruction

MEDICATIONS

DRUGS OF CHOICE
- Piroxicam (Feldene)—0.3 mg/kg PO q24h with food; reported to have activity in up to 20% of cases
- Cisplatin—50–70 mg/m^2 IV every 3 weeks; conventional agent; reported activity not > 20%
- Other agents (doxorubicin, mitoxantrone, and doxorubicin/cyclophosphamide combination) may have activity.

CONTRAINDICATIONS
- Piroxicam—do not use with known gastrointestinal erosions or ulcers; do not use with renal insufficiency; not evaluated in cats
- Cisplatin—do not use in cats; do not use with renal insufficiency.

PRECAUTIONS
- Cisplatin or piroxicam (dogs)—monitor for renal insufficiency; patients may have renal damage caused by hydroureter, hydronephrosis, or pyelonephritis.
- Seek advice before initiating treatment if you are unfamiliar with cytotoxic drugs.

POSSIBLE INTERACTIONS
- Cisplatin and piroxicam—do not use concurrently because of the risk of cumulative nephrotoxicity.
- Cisplatin—do not use concurrently with other nephrotoxic drugs.

ALTERNATIVE DRUGS
Antibiotics—administered as necessary

FOLLOW-UP

PATIENT MONITORING
- Contrast cystography or ultrasonography—every 6–8 weeks; assess response to treatment.
- Thoracic radiography—every 2–3 months; detect metastatic disease

PREVENTION/AVOIDANCE
N/A

POSSIBLE COMPLICATIONS
- Urethral or ureteral obstruction and renal failure
- Metastatic disease to regional lymph nodes, lungs, or bone
- Recurrent urinary tract infection
- Urinary incontinence
- Myelosuppression or gastrointestinal toxicity secondary to chemotherapy
- Gastrointestinal ulceration secondary to piroxicam therapy

EXPECTED COURSE AND PROGNOSIS
- Long-term prognosis grave
- Progressive disease probable
- Median survival—no treatment, 4–6 months; with treatment, 6–12 months

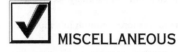

MISCELLANEOUS

ASSOCIATED CONDITIONS
- Recurrent urinary tract infection
- Paraneoplastic hypertrophic osteopathy

AGE-RELATED FACTORS
N/A

ZOONOTIC POTENTIAL
N/A

PREGNANCY
N/A

SEE ALSO
N/A

ABBREVIATIONS
N/A

Suggested Reading
Chun R, Knapp DW, Widmer WR, et al. Cisplatin treatment of transitional cell carcinoma of the urinary bladder in dogs: 18 cases (1983–1993). J Am Vet Med Assoc 1996;209:1588–1591.

Morrison WB. Cancers of the urinary tract. In: Morrison WB, ed. Cancer in dogs and cats: medical and surgical management. Baltimore: Williams & Wilkins, 1998:569–579.

Author Ruthanne Chun
Consulting Editor Wallace B. Morrison

TRANSMISSIBLE VENEREAL TUMOR

BASICS

OVERVIEW
• Sexually transmitted, naturally occurring tumor
• Appears to be more common in temperate areas and large cities

SIGNALMENT
Young, intact dogs of either sex

SIGNS
• Red, friable, lobulated mass on the mucosa of the vagina or penis
• Oral mucosa may also be affected.
• Blood dripping from the prepuce or vagina
• Excessive licking of the genital area
• Tumor protrusion

CAUSES & RISK FACTORS
• Direct transplantation of tumor cells onto abraded mucosa, either by coitus or oral transmission
• Intact, free-roaming dogs—at greater than average risk

DIAGNOSIS

DIFFERENTIAL DIAGNOSIS
• Other neoplasms—squamous cell carcinoma; cutaneous lymphoma
• Vaginal hyperplasia

CBC/BIOCHEMISTRY/URINALYSIS
• Usually normal
• Free-catch urine—hematuria and abnormal cells may be noted.

OTHER LABORATORY TESTS
N/A

IMAGING
• Thoracic radiographs—part of a thorough staging procedure; although rarely metastatic
• Abdominal radiography or ultrasonography—may be useful in staging

DIAGNOSTIC PROCEDURES
• Careful palpation of regional lymph nodes
• Examination of impression smears or aspirate of the tumor—reveals homogenous sheets of round to oval cells with prominent nucleoli, scant cytoplasm, and multiple clear cytoplasmic vacuoles
• Biopsy—provides definitive diagnosis

TREATMENT
• May spontaneously regress; treatment recommended because spontaneous remission is not reliable.
• Surgical excision of small tumors—often followed by recurrence
• Radiotherapy alone—may be curative
• Medical treatment with vincristine—usually curative

MEDICATIONS

DRUGS
• Vincristine sulfate—0.5–0.7 mg/m² IV once weekly for 2 weeks beyond complete resolution of gross disease
• Partial or no remission—try doxorubicin (30 mg/m² IV every 3 weeks)

CONTRAINDICATIONS/POSSIBLE INTERACTIONS
• Myelosuppression secondary to vincristine or doxorubicin administration
• Doxorubicin—may be cardiotoxic; use with caution once a cumulative dose of 150 mg/m² is reached.
• Vincristine and doxorubicin—tissue sloughing if administered perivascularly; always administer through a patent IV catheter.
• Seek advice before initiating treatment if you are unfamiliar with cytotoxic drugs.

FOLLOW-UP

PATIENT MONITORING
CBC and platelet count—before each chemotherapy treatment

PREVENTION/AVOIDANCE
• Spay or neuter
• Prevent animals from roaming free.

POSSIBLE COMPLICATIONS
• Tumor recurrence after incomplete surgical excision or reexposure
• Metastatic disease uncommon

EXPECTED COURSE AND PROGNOSIS
Usually an excellent response to treatment (primarily chemotherapy or radiotherapy) and an excellent prognosis

MISCELLANEOUS

PREGNANCY
• Do not treat pregnant animals with chemotherapy.
• Animals may be infected with transmissible veneral tumor during coitus.

Suggested Reading
Brown NO, Calvert C, MacEwen EG. Chemotherapeutic management of transmissible venereal tumors in 30 dogs. J Am Vet Med Assoc 1980;176:983–986.
Morrison WB. Cancers of the reproductive tract. In: Morrison WB, ed. Cancer in dogs and cats: medical and surgical management. Baltimore: Williams & Wilkins, 1998:581–590.
Author Ruthanne Chun
Consulting Editor Wallace B. Morrison

BASICS

OVERVIEW
• Traumatic myocarditis is the term applied to the syndrome of arrhythmias that sometimes complicates blunt trauma; it is a misnomer, because myocardial lesions (if present) are more likely to take the form of necrosis than inflammation.
• Direct cardiac injury is not required for development of posttraumatic arrhythmia; extracardiac conditions are likely to have equal or greater etiologic importance.
• Ventricular tachyarrhythmias occur in most affected patients; supraventricular arrhythmias and bradyarrhythmias are uncommon. Ventricular rhythms that complicate blunt trauma are often relatively slow and detected only during pauses in the sinus rhythm; they are most appropriately referred to as AIVRs. The QRS complexes are wide and bizarre; the rate is > 100 bpm but generally < 160 bpm. Usually, these rhythms are electrically and hemodynamically benign.
• Dangerous ventricular tachycardias can also complicate blunt trauma and can also evolve from seemingly benign AIVRs, compromising perfusion and placing the patient at risk for sudden death.

SIGNALMENT
Dogs, rarely cats

SIGNS

Historical Findings
• Trauma, most often from road accidents
• Arrhythmias often noticed 24–48 h after trauma

Physical Examination Findings
• Arrhythmias may be inapparent if the rate of an AIVR closely matches the sinus rate.
• Rapid, irregular rhythms in some patients
• Signs of poor peripheral perfusion (e.g., weakness, pale mucous membranes, and weak femoral pulses) in patients with rapid, poorly tolerated ventricular rhythms

CAUSES & RISK FACTORS
• Blunt trauma
• Hypoxia
• Autonomic imbalance
• Electrolyte derangements
• Acid–base disturbances

DIAGNOSIS

DIFFERENTIAL DIAGNOSIS
AIVRs should be differentiated from ventricular tachycardia.
• AIVRs—usually initiated by late diastolic ventricular (escape) complexes or fusion complexes; heart rate is generally 100–160 bpm.
• Ventricular tachycardia—usually initiated by a ventricular premature complex; heart rates exceed 160 bpm.

CBC/BIOCHEMISTRY/URINALYSIS
• Creatine kinase, liver enzymes, and lactic dehydrogenase often high because of organ trauma
• Electrolyte derangements (particularly hypokalemia and hypomagnesemia) predispose to ventricular arrhythmia

OTHER LABORATORY TESTS
N/A

IMAGING

Thoracic Radiographic Findings
Evidence of trauma, including pneumothorax, rib fractures, and pulmonary contusion in some patients

DIAGNOSTIC PROCEDURES

Electrocardiographic Findings
• Ventricular arrhythmias, as previously discussed

TREATMENT
• Treat extracardiac conditions including pain, electrolyte derangements, and hypoxia, which can predispose to ventricular arrhythmia, if possible.
• Thoracic radiographs for all patients with blunt trauma; identify and remedy disorders such as pneumothorax.
• The need for antiarrhythmic therapy is predicated on clinical signs and the electrocardiographic character of the arrhythmia; pharmacologic suppression of AIVR is usually unnecessary.
• Fluid therapy for shock

MEDICATIONS

DRUGS
• First treat rapid ventricular rhythms or those associated with hemodynamic compromise with lidocaine (2 mg/kg boluses IV); a total of 8 mg/kg can be administered over 10–12 min. Start a lidocaine infusion (25–75 (μg/kg/min) once the rhythm is stabilized with lidocaine boluses.
• If lidocaine administration fails to convert to sinus rhythm, try procainamide, β-blockers such as esmolol or propranolol, or even class III agents such as bretylium.
• Consider DC conversion while animal is under anesthesia or heavy sedation, to treat rapid, hemodynamically unstable, ventricular rhythms that do not respond to drug therapy.
• Antiarrhythmic agents are not necessarily benign; they can worsen existing arrhythmias and provide a substrate for development of new arrhythmias (proarrhythmia); weigh the relative risk or benefit carefully at every step.

CONTRAINDICATIONS/POSSIBLE INTERACTIONS
N/A

FOLLOW-UP
• ECG monitoring of animals with arrhythmias is recommended; generally, the arrhythmias that complicate blunt trauma are self-limiting and resolve within 48–72 h.
• If antiarrhythmic therapy deemed necessary, it can often be discontinued after 2–5 days.
• Although dangerous arrhythmias occasionally complicate blunt trauma, the prognosis usually depends on the severity of extracardiac injury.

MISCELLANEOUS

SEE ALSO
• Shock, Cardiogenic
• Idioventricular Rhythm
• Ventricular Tachycardia

ABBREVIATIONS
• AIVR = accelerated idioventricular rhythm
• DC = direct current

Suggested Reading
Abbott JA. Traumatic myocarditis. In: Bonagura JD, ed. Current veterinary therapy XII. Philadelphia: Saunders, 1995: 846–830.

Author Jonathan A. Abbott
Consulting Editors Larry P. Tilley and Francis W. K. Smith, Jr.

DISEASES

TRIGEMINAL NEURITIS

BASICS

OVERVIEW
• Acute onset of inability to close the jaw owing to bilateral dysfunction of the mandibular branch of the trigeminal nerves
• Nerve injury—from bilateral nonsuppurative neuritis, demyelination, and (occasionally) fiber degeneration of all branches of trigeminal nerve and ganglion

SIGNALMENT
• Primarily adult dogs
• Rare in cats

SIGNS
• Acute onset of a dropped jaw
• Inability to close the mouth
• Drooling
• Difficulty in prehending food
• Messy eating
• No apparent deficits in sensory perception
• Swallowing intact

CAUSES & RISK FACTORS
• Unknown
• Possibly immune-mediated

DIAGNOSIS

DIFFERENTIAL DIAGNOSIS
• Musculoskeletal disorders of the temporomandibular joints and jaw—differentiated by history of trauma and pain and physical examination findings
• Rabies—always initially consider until there is sufficient evidence to rule it out.
• Neoplasia—both mandibular nerves secondary to myelomonocytic leukemia, lymphosarcoma, and neurofibrosarcoma reported; usually does not have an acute onset
• Masticatory muscle myositis—trismus; jaw is difficult to open.

CBC/BIOCHEMISTRY/URINALYSIS
Usually normal

OTHER LABORATORY TESTS
N/A

IMAGING
N/A

DIAGNOSTIC PROCEDURES
• No specific test
• Skull radiography, examination of bone marrow aspirate, and muscle biopsy—rule out the differentials

TREATMENT
• Outpatient if owner is able to help the patient eat and drink
• Patient cannot prehend and move food and water to the throat; requires help when eating and drinking
• Patient is able to lap and swallow food offered by a large syringe placed in the corner of mouth with the head slightly elevated.
• Fluids—administer subcutaneously; may be necessary to maintain hydration
• Pharyngostomy or gastrostomy tubes—rarely necessary to maintain adequate food intake

MEDICATIONS

DRUGS OF CHOICE
Corticosteroids—anti-inflammatory dosage may speed recovery

CONTRAINDICATIONS/POSSIBLE INTERACTIONS
Steroids—use with caution; dehydration may develop from steroid-induced polyuria and polydipsia in a patient that relies on its owner for water intake.

FOLLOW-UP
• Self-limiting disorder
• Full recovery in 2–4 weeks
• Occasional masticatory muscle atrophy but without trismus

MISCELLANEOUS

Suggested Reading
de Lahunta A. Veterinary neuroanatomy and clinical neurology. 2nd ed. Philadelphia: Saunders, 1983.
Author T. Mark Neer
Consulting Editor Joane M. Parent

BASICS

OVERVIEW
• *Francisella tularensis*—small gram-negative coccobacillus; type A, more virulent, found in rabbits and ticks; type B, waterborne, found in rodents and ticks; in North America principally found in wild lagomorphs (cottontail, jack, snowshoe) and rodents (moles, squirrels, muskrats, beavers); facultative intracellular parasite; survives and grows in liver-producing granulomas and/or abscesses • Peak occurrence—late spring; June–August; December • Northern Hemisphere—absent from United Kingdom, Africa, South America, Australia; in U.S. most cases found in Missouri, Alaska, Oklahoma, South Dakota, Tennessee, Kansas, Colorado, Illinois, Utah, and Maine. • Infection—ingestion of tissue or body fluids of an infected mammal or contaminated water; bitten by blood-sucking arthropod (tick), flies, mites, midges, fleas, or mosquitos; few bacteria needed to infect cats through skin, airways, or conjunctiva; larger number required to infect through the gastrointestinal tract • Skin contact—organism multiplies locally (papule) 3–5 days after contact; ulcerates 2–4 days later; spreads via lymphatics to regional LN and bloodstream; results in septicemia (lung, liver, spleen, LN, bone marrow) • Ingestion—may involve lymphadenopathy of cervical and mesenteric LN followed by septicemic spread; distribution of lesions to face, oral cavity, tonsils, intestines, and LN • Acute disease—2–7 days after contact with organism

SIGNALMENT
• Cats—occasionally • Dogs—rarely

SIGNS
• Sudden onset of anorexia, lethargy, fever (40–41°C; 104–106°F) • Enlarged palpable submandibular and cervical LN • Tender abdomen, palpable mesenteric LN, hepatomegaly—depending on stage of disease • Multifocal white patches or ulcers along glossopalatine arches and tongue • Icterus

CAUSES & RISK FACTORS
• Organism—all *Francisella* biogroups may infect cats but may differ in virulence; some cats may have mild infection
• Hunter or outdoor cats in endemic areas
• Infected wildlife in the area of hunting activity
• Exposure to infected blood-sucking parasites

DIAGNOSIS

DIFFERENTIAL DIAGNOSIS
• Any acute disease state manifested by acute lymphadenopathy, malaise, oral ulceration, and fatal outcome—consider tularemia
• Bubonic plague (*Yersinia pestis*)—western U.S.
• Pseudotuberculosis (*Yersinia pseudotuberculosis*)—usually vomiting and diarrhea

CBC/BIOCHEMISTRY/URINALYSIS
• Initially severe panleukopenia; then leukocytosis with left shift, toxic neutrophils, thrombocytopenia
• Hyperbilirubinemia
• Hyponatremia
• Hypoglycemia
• Alanine aminotransferase—elevated
• Bilirubinuria
• Hematuria

OTHER LABORATORY TESTS
Serology with tube agglutination or ELISA—possible; difficult to perform, except in reference laboratory

IMAGING N/A

DIAGNOSTIC PROCEDURES
• Direct smear—lesion or biopsy; difficult to see organism on Gram staining
• Cultural isolation—by reference laboratory; blood, pleural fluid, LN aspirate onto cysteine- or cystine-containing media; not recoverable on routine laboratory media; CAUTION: use extreme care when working with infected specimens or isolates
• Direct fluorescent antibody testing—clinical materials or tissues; rapid assay of infection status

PATHOLOGIC FINDINGS
• Multifocal white patches or ulcers along glossopalatine arches and tongue
• Oral, tonsillar ulceration
• Lymphadenopathy of cervical, retropharyngeal, or submandibular LN with abscessation
• Diffuse intestinal lesions
• Mesenteric lymphadenopathy, hepatosplenomegaly and icterus

TREATMENT
• Inpatient with good nursing care
• Early treatment important to prevent high mortality
• Treat for ectoparasites.

MEDICATIONS

DRUGS
• Treat all cases empirically until laboratory confirmation obtained

Cats
• Little information available on the efficacy of antimicrobials because of high mortality if patient not treated early
• Early treatment with amoxicillin (20 mg/kg PO q8h for 5–7 days or 20 mg/kg IM or SC q12h for 5 days) in combination with gentamicin (4.4 mg/kg IM or SC q12h once and then q24h thereafter until a clinical response or until 7 days) has been successful.

CONTRAINDICATIONS/POSSIBLE INTERACTIONS N/A

FOLLOW-UP

PATIENT MONITORING
Monitor for DIC—may occur late in the infection

PREVENTION/AVOIDANCE
• Travel with pet—avoid endemic areas
• Endemic areas—confine animals to control exposure to and ingestion of wildlife and their ectoparasites (ticks); ecoparasite control by periodic spraying or dusting of animal and pastures • Neuter cats—limit hunting behavior and wildlife exposure • Take precautions to limit contamination of food and water with carcasses of infected wildlife.

EXPECTED COURSE AND PROGNOSIS
Prognosis poor if not treated early; prognosis poor if mesenteric LN palpable

MISCELLANEOUS

ZOONOTIC POTENTIAL
• High • All personnel in contact with patient or body fluids must use face mask, gloves, and gowns to avoid infection. • Isolate patients
• Do not mistake for bite abscess in cats or plague

SYNONYMS
• Rabbit fever • Deerfly fever • Market men's disease

ABBREVIATIONS
• DIC = disseminated intravascular coagulation • ELISA = enzyme-linked immunosorbent assay • LN = lymph node(s)

Suggested Reading
Rohrbach BW. Tularemia. J Am Vet Med Assoc 1988;193:428–432.
Author Patrick L. McDonough
Consulting Editor Stephen C. Barr

DISEASES

TUMORAL CALCINOSIS

BASICS

OVERVIEW
Ectopic deposition of calcium salts in soft tissue and in periarticular areas

SIGNALMENT
• Usually young, large-breed dogs
• German shepherds < 2 years old—more than half of reported patients

SIGNS
• One or more hard, well-circumscribed, nonpainful swellings in the cervical region, foot pads, or mouth
• None, unless location interferes with function

CAUSES & RISK FACTORS
Cause and pathogenesis obscure; several theories advanced but none satisfactorily explains development in all anatomic areas

DIAGNOSIS

DIFFERENTIAL DIAGNOSIS
• Mineralized neoplasm
• Mineralized abscess

CBC/BIOCHEMISTRY/URINALYSIS
Not affected

OTHER LABORATORY TESTS
N/A

IMAGING
Radiography—reveals calcified mass

DIAGNOSTIC PROCEDURES
N/A

TREATMENT
Surgical excision recommended

MEDICATIONS

DRUGS
N/A

CONTRAINDICATIONS/POSSIBLE INTERACTIONS
N/A

FOLLOW-UP

PATIENT MONITORING
Usually not required

PREVENTION/AVOIDANCE
N/A

POSSIBLE COMPLICATIONS
Usually none

EXPECTED COURSE AND PROGNOSIS
Usually good after surgical excision

MISCELLANEOUS

ASSOCIATED CONDITIONS
Identical lesions are seen with chronic renal failure, uremia, and primary hyperparathyroidism.

SYNONYMS
• Lipocalcinosis
• Calcinosis circumscripta
• Apocrine cystic calcinosis
• Tumoral lipocalcinosis
• Hip stone

Suggested Reading
Marks SL, Bellah JR, Wells M. Resolution of quadriparesis caused by cervical tumoral calcinosis in a dog. J Am Anim Hosp Assoc 1992;27:72–76.

Author Wallace B. Morrison
Consulting Editor Wallace B. Morrison

TYZZER DISEASE

BASICS

OVERVIEW
• *Clostridium piliformis* (formally *Bacillus piliformis*)—gram-negative bacterium; 0.5 × 10–40 μm in size; an obligate intracellular pathogen
• Infection—organism thought to initially proliferate in intestinal epithelial cells; spreads to the liver via the hepatic portal vein; hepatic colonization associated with multifocal periportal hepatic necrosis

SIGNALMENT
• Dogs and cats
• Any age; young at higher risk
• Rodents—clinically affected

SIGNS
• Rapid onset of lethargy, depression, anorexia, abdominal discomfort, hepatomegaly, and abdominal distention; followed by hypothermia
• Death—within 24–48 hr
• Fecal matter—diarrhea infrequent; small amounts of pasty feces more common

CAUSES & RISK FACTORS
• *C. piliformis*
• Contact with rodents—may be a risk factor
• Neonates and immunocompromised animals (e.g., distemper, FeLV, feline panleukopenia, familial hyperlipo-proteinemia)—seem to be at greatest risk

DIAGNOSIS

DIFFERENTIAL DIAGNOSIS
• Diagnosis usually made at necropsy—rapid and highly fatal disease diagnosis
• Distinguished from other causes of sudden death and acute hepatitis

CBC/BIOCHEMISTRY/URINAYSIS
• ALT—marked elevations in blood samples taken shortly before death

OTHER LABORATORY TESTS
• Serology—identify latent infections in rodent colonies; could be used to investigate illness in dogs and cats
• Isolation of organism—requires inoculation of mice, embryonating eggs, or cell culture

IMAGING
N/A

DIAGNOSTIC PROCEDURES
N/A

PATHOLOGIC FINDINGS
Gross
• Multifocal whitish gray to hemorrhagic foci throughout the liver; may also occur in other viscera
• Focal myocarditis, thickening and congestion of the intestine, mesenteric lymphadenopathy—reported
Histologic
• Multifocal hepatic necrosis
• Necrotic ileitis or colitis
• Intracellular filamentous organisms—usually numerous; difficult to visualize with H&E; require silver stains (e.g., modified-Steiner or Warthin-Starry)

TREATMENT
• None effective

MEDICATIONS

DRUGS
None

CONTRAINDICATIONS/POSSIBLE INTERACTIONS
None

FOLLOW UP

PREVENTION/AVOIDANCE
• Avoid predisposing factors—may limit disease

MISCELLANEOUS

ABBREVIATIONS
• ALT = alanine aminotransferase
• FeLV = feline leukemia virus
• H&E = hematoxylin and eosin

Suggested Reading
Jones BR, Green CE. Tyzzer's disease. In: Greene CE, ed. Infectious diseases of the dog and cat. Philadelphia: Saunders, 1998:242–243.
Author Kenneth W. Simpson
Consulting Editor Stephen C. Barr

DISEASES

URETEROLITHIASIS

BASICS

OVERVIEW
Occurrence of a urolith (calculus) within a ureter; most ureteroliths originate in the renal pelves and so commonly occur in association with nephroliths. Most uroliths that enter the ureter continue to the bladder without impedance, but uroliths may cause partial or complete obstruction of the ureter, resulting in dilation of the proximal ureter and renal pelves and subsequent destruction of renal parenchyma.

SIGNALMENT
• Dogs and cats
• Breed, age, and sex predispositions vary with type of nephrolith.
• See Nephrolithiasis

SIGNS
• May be initially asymptomatic
• Pain (ureteral colic) during passage of ureteroliths or following acute ureteral obstruction
• Renomegaly if ureteral obstruction leads to hydronephrosis
• Unilateral ureteral obstruction results in azotemia and uremic clinical signs only when the function of the contralateral kidney is compromised.
• Signs referable to a lower urinary tract infection and septicemia may be present concurrently.
• Ureteral rupture may occur, resulting in urine accumulation in the retroperitoneal space.

CAUSES & RISK FACTORS
• For a list of causes, see chapters on each urolith type.
• Prior treatment of nephroliths by extra-corporeal shock wave lithotripsy (ESWL), medical dissolution, or surgery to remove nephroliths may be additional risk factors.

DIAGNOSIS

DIFFERENTIAL DIAGNOSIS
• Consider in all cases of renal failure, unilateral or bilateral renomegaly, abdominal pain, or fluid accumulation in the retroperitoneal space
• Radiopacities on abdominal radiographs that may be confused with ureteroliths include particulate fecal material in the colon, mammary gland nipples, peritoneoliths, calcified lymph nodes, and mineralization of the renal pelvis.
• Radiolucent ureteroliths may be difficult to differentiate from ureteral blood clots. Other causes of ureteral obstruction include intraluminal tumors, ureteroceles, ureteral strictures (following surgery or trauma), and extraluminal compression. Hydroureter and hydronephrosis may occur because of ureteral ectopia, pyelonephritis, and obstruction of the ureteral opening at the trigone, most commonly due to transitional cell carcinoma of the bladder.

CBC/BIOCHEMISTRY/URINALYSIS
These tests evaluate renal function and screen for concurrent disease before the treatment of ureterolithiasis. They do not directly contribute to the diagnosis of ureterolithiasis. Urinalysis, serum calcium concentration, and fractional excretion of electrolytes may permit estimation of urolith composition pending results of definitive analysis.

OTHER LABORATORY TESTS
• Submit all retrieved ureteroliths for quantitative analysis to determine appropriate preventive strategies.
• Patients (other than dalmatians and bull-dogs) with urate stones should be evaluated for portosystemic shunts.

IMAGING
• Radiopaque ureteroliths may be visualized with survey radiographs. If obstruction and hydronephrosis have occurred, renomegaly may be apparent. If ureteral rupture occurs, contrast in the retroperitoneal space may be lost.
• Small uroliths may not be visualized on radiographs even if they are radiopaque.
• When ureteroliths are suspected, but cannot be documented, an intravenous urogram may help to identify the obstruction and will also distinguish ureteral rupture from retroperitoneal hemorrhage. In many instances the damaged tubules do not concentrate dye adequately, resulting in poor delineation of the ureter; in these cases contrast injection by nephropyelocentesis may be useful.
• Ultrasound is valuable for detecting hydronephrosis or hydroureter.
• Changes suggesting pyelonephritis may also be observed by ultrasound. The dilated proximal ureter may be traced to the ureterolith and thus allow direct observation of it.
• Ureteroliths in the middle or distal ureter are less frequently observed sonographically.

DIAGNOSTIC PROCEDURES
• Nuclear scintigraphy has been advocated to determine each kidney's contribution to the total GFR, but since GFR measurements cannot be used to predict the functional recovery possible following the relief of obstruction, nuclear scintigraphy alone should not determine whether or not to preserve or surgically remove a kidney.
• Voiding urohydropropulsion may be performed to retrieve ureteroliths that have spontaneously passed into the bladder or to collect ureterolith fragments following ESWL.

PATHOLOGIC FINDINGS
• Gross changes in the kidney—progressive dilation of the pelves and calyces; in advanced cases, the kidney may be transformed into a thin-walled sac with only a thin shell of atrophic cortical parenchyma; ureteral dilation proximal to the site of obstruction is typical

• Microscopic changes—begin with dilation of the tubules, which then atrophy, separate, and are replaced by diffuse cortical fibrosis; the glomeruli are relatively well preserved in the residual cortical tissue.

 TREATMENT

• Remove ureteroliths that are causing obstruction (i.e., causing hydronephrosis or hydroureter) or which have not moved on sequential radiographs.
• Ureteroliths in dogs have been successfully treated with ESWL.
• Surgical techniques recommended for removal of ureteroliths vary, depending on the site of obstruction, the presence or absence of infection, and the degree of function of the associated kidney. Ureteroneocystotomy may be performed for ureteroliths in the middle and distal ureter: the ureter proximal to the obstruction is excised and reimplanted into the bladder. Ureteroliths in the proximal ureter are removed by ureterotomy. Concurrent placement of a nephrostomy catheter is recommended. Performance of a ureterotomy or ureteroneocystotomy requires experience in microsurgical techniques, particularly in cats. When the contralateral kidney functions normally or when severe hydronephrosis or pyelonephritis is present in the affected kidney, ureteronephrectomy may be appropriate.

 MEDICATIONS

DRUGS OF CHOICE
• Medical dissolution is largely ineffective.
• Therapy aimed at prevention of recurrent disease is imperative following relief of obstruction.

CONTRAINDICATIONS/POSSIBLE INTERACTIONS
• Medical therapy designed to promote the dissolution or prevent the recurrence of uroliths is not totally benign. Some patients will not tolerate the high salt concentration, protein restriction, acidification, or related management procedures that may be required. Take particular care in patients with high metabolic demands, such as growth or lactation, and in animals with congestive heart failure or renal failure.
• Attempts to prevent one type of urolith may promote formation of a second type.

 FOLLOW-UP

PATIENT MONITORING
Following successful removal of ureteroliths, recheck every 3–6 months for recurrence of uroliths and to ensure owner compliance with preventive measures; urinalysis, radiographs (or ultrasound) and a urine culture are usually appropriate.

PREVENTION/AVOIDANCE
• Elimination of factors predisposing to the development of urolithiasis
• Specific therapy depends on the mineral composition of the urolith. Refer to chapters on individual urolith types for appropriate preventive measures.

POSSIBLE COMPLICATIONS
Hydronephrosis, renal failure, recurrent urinary tract infection, pyelonephritis, sepsis, ureteral rupture

EXPECTED COURSE AND PROGNOSIS
Highly variable; if unilateral disease is present and recurrence is prevented, the prognosis is good.

 MISCELLANEOUS

ASSOCIATED CONDITIONS
Commonly associated with uroliths elsewhere in the urinary tract, especially nephroliths

AGE-RELATED FACTORS
Geriatric dogs that are poor surgical candidates may be treated with ESWL.

PREGNANCY
A contraindication to ESWL

SEE ALSO
• Nephrolithiasis
• Renal Failure, Chronic
• Hydronephrosis
• Pyelonephritis
• Urinary Tract Obstruction
• Urolithiasis, Calcium Oxalate
• Urolithiasis, Calcium Phosphate
• Urolithiasis, Cystine
• Urolithiasis, Struvite—Cats
• Urolithiasis, Struvite—Dogs
• Urolithiasis, Urate
• Urolithiasis, Xanthine

ABBREVIATIONS
• ESWL = extracorporeal shock wave lithotripsy
• GFR = glomerular filtration rate

Suggested Reading

Stone EA. Surgical management of urinary tract disease: ureteral calculi in cats and urinary bladder neoplasia in dogs Compend Contin Educ Pract Vet 1997;19(Suppl 3):62–68.

Authors Harriet M. Syme and Larry G. Adams

Consulting Editors Larry G. Adams and Carl A. Osborne

URETHRAL PROLAPSE

 ## BASICS

OVERVIEW
- Occurs when the mucosal lining of the distal portion of the urethra prolapses through the external urethral orifice
- Exact pathophysiology unknown; see Causes and Risk Factors
- Systems affected include urinary, reproductive (bleeding may sometimes only occur during penile erection), and hemic/lymph/immune (blood loss can be severe enough to cause anemia, especially in smaller breeds of dogs).

SIGNALMENT
- Dogs
- Most common in English bulldogs and Boston terriers
- Mean age, 18 months; range, 4 months to 5 years
- Male dogs only

SIGNS

Historical Findings
- Intermittent or persistent bleeding from the urethra independent of urination
- Intermittent or persistent licking of the penis
- Depending on the underlying cause, dysuria and pollakiuria caused by concomitant disorders may also be present.

Physical Examination Findings
- Red to purple, pea-sized, doughnut-shaped mass protruding from the distal end of the penis
- Pale mucous membranes if bleeding is severe
- Uroliths may be palpable in the urinary bladder or urethra.

CAUSES & RISK FACTORS
- May result from sexual excitement and/or unrelated disorders (e.g., infections, uroliths) of the lower urinary tract
- Increased intraabdominal pressure secondary to dysuria associated with urocystoliths may be a predisposing factor.
- Other proposed causes include abnormal development of the urethra with superimposed increased intraabdominal pressure as a consequence of brachycephalic airway syndrome, dysuria, or sexual activity. This increased intraabdominal pressure could impair venous return of blood through the pudendal veins, predisposing susceptible dogs to engorgement of the corpus spongiosum surrounding the distal urethra

 ## DIAGNOSIS

DIFFERENTIAL DIAGNOSIS
- Prostatic disease
- Persistent penile frenulum
- Fractures of the os penis
- Testicular disease
- Urethritis
- Urethroliths
- Coagulopathy

CBC/BIOCHEMISTRY/URINALYSIS
- CBC—may reveal regenerative anemia
- Serum biochemistries—usually normal
- May not detect significant hematuria in urine collected by cystocentesis, but a voided urine sample may reveal hematuria.

OTHER LABORATORY TESTS
Coagulation profile may rule out coagulopathy.

IMAGING
- Survey abdominal radiographs—useful to rule out radiodense uroliths and to evaluate the prostate gland
- Double-contrast cystography and positive-contrast urethrography—useful to rule out radiolucent uroliths, other urethral disorders, and prostatic disease
- Abdominal ultrasonography—useful to evaluate the prostate and urinary bladder further

DIAGNOSTIC PROCEDURES
- Ejaculation—useful to evaluate urethra during penile erection; some urethral prolapses are present only during penile erection.
- Evaluation of ejaculates may also facilitate evaluation of prostatic fluid for evidence of prostatic disease.

 ## TREATMENT

- May not be required if prolapsed urethra is asymptomatic or only associated with episodic bleeding
- If prolapsed urethra is present only during penile erection, consider castration prior to attempting surgical removal of prolapsed tissue; diethylstilbestrol given for 3–6 weeks after surgery may reduce frequency of erections.
- Consider surgery for patients with excessive bleeding, pain, or extensive ulceration and/or necrosis of the prolapsed tissue.
- If surgery is necessary, Elizabethan collars or similar restraint devices may be needed to prevent licking-induced trauma to the surgical site.
- Regardless of treatment chosen, advise the owner that recurrence is possible.
- Because brachycephalic breeds are at risk for this problem, use caution in choosing an anesthetic regimen; monitor brachycephalic breeds carefully during anesthesia to ensure maintenance of adequate oxygenation.

MEDICATIONS

DRUGS
• Bacterial urethritis warrants use of appropriate antibiotics.
• May need to consider using diethylstilbestrol for 3–6 weeks after surgery to reduce frequency of erections

CONTRAINDICATIONS/POSSIBLE INTERACTIONS
Because of the possibility of bone marrow suppression, consider risk:benefit ratios before giving estrogens, especially if patients are already anemic.

 FOLLOW-UP

PATIENT MONITORING
At least 7–10 days following surgery, for evidence of severe hemorrhage or recurrence of urethral prolapse

PREVENTION/AVOIDANCE
If urethral prolapse is associated with penile erection, advise owners to prevent contact with female dogs or other situations likely to cause penile erection.

POSSIBLE COMPLICATIONS
Advise owners that postsurgical recurrence of prolapse may occur, especially if no underlying cause has been detected and eliminated or controlled.

EXPECTED COURSE AND PROGNOSIS
• Some dogs may not require therapy; urethral prolapse is not associated with significant abnormalities.
• Other dogs may not have any further problems after castration and/or surgical correction of a prolapsed urethra.
• If the underlying cause(s) persists, postsurgical recurrence is common.

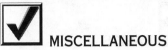 MISCELLANEOUS

ASSOCIATED CONDITIONS
• Concurrent urethritis is common.
• Concurrent urolithiasis may be a predisposing cause.
• May be present during, or worsened by, penile erection

Suggested Reading
Osborne CA, Sanderson SL. Medical management of urethral prolapse in male dogs. In: Bonagura JD, Kirk RW, eds. Current veterinary therapy XII. Philadelphia: Saunders, 1995:1027–1029.
Sinibaldi KR, Green RW. Surgical correction of prolapse of the male urethra in three English Bulldogs. J Am Anim Hosp Assoc 1973;9:450–453.
Authors Sherry L. Sanderson and Carl A. Osborne
Consulting Editors Larry G. Adams and Carl A. Osborne

DISEASES

UROLITHIASIS, CALCIUM OXALATE

BASICS

DEFINITION
Formation of calcium oxalate uroliths within the urinary tract and associated clinical conditions

PATHOPHYSIOLOGY
Presence of hypercalciuria, hyperoxaluria, hypocitraturia, and defective crystal growth inhibitors

Hypercalciuria
In dogs, normocalcemic hypercalciuria is thought to result from either intestinal hyper-absorption of calcium (so-called absorptive hypercalciuria) or reduced renal tubular reabsorption of calcium (so-called renal-leak hypercalciuria). Hypercalcemic hypercalciuria results from excessive glomerular filtration of mobilized calcium, which overwhelms normal renal tubular reabsorptive mechanisms (called resorptive hypercalciuria, since excessive bone resorption is associated with high serum calcium concentrations).

Hyperoxaluria
In humans, hyperoxaluria is associated with inherited abnormalities of excessive oxalate synthesis (i.e., primary hyperoxaluria), excess consumption of foods containing high quantities of oxalate or oxalate precursors, pyridoxine deficiency, and disorders associated with fat malabsorption.

Hypocitraturia
Urine citrate inhibits calcium oxalate urolith formation. By complexing with calcium ions to form the relatively soluble salt calcium citrate, citrate reduces the quantity of calcium available to bind with oxalate. In normal dogs, acidosis is associated with low urinary citrate excretion, whereas alkalosis promotes urinary citrate excretion.

Defective Crystal Growth Inhibitors
In addition to urinary concentration of calculogenic minerals, large-molecular-weight proteins in urine, such as nephrocalcin. have a profound ability to enhance solubility of calcium oxalate. Preliminary studies of urine obtained from dogs with calcium oxalate uroliths revealed that nephrocalcin had fewer carboxyglutamic acid residues than nephrocalcin isolated from normal dog urine.

SYSTEMS AFFECTED
Renal/urologic

GENETICS
N/A

INCIDENCE/PREVALENCE
In dogs, calcium oxalate accounts for approximately 30–35% of the uroliths removed from the lower urinary tract and 40% of those removed from the upper urinary tract. In cats, calcium oxalate accounts for approximately 45–55% of the uroliths removed from the lower urinary tract and 50% of those retrieved from the upper urinary tract.

GEOGRAPHIC DISTRIBUTION
Ubiquitous

SIGNALMENT

Species
Dogs and cats

Breed Predilections
• Dogs—in a large study, 44% of calcium oxalate uroliths came from three breeds: miniature schnauzer, Lhasa apso, and Yorkshire terrier.
• Cats—the two pure breeds of cat with the greatest number were Himalayan (9%) and Persian (9%).

Mean Age and Range
• All ages of dogs and cats are affected.
• Dogs—55%, 5–12 years
• Cats—53%, 4–9 years

Predominant Sex
Mostly male dogs (73%) and male cats (55%)

SIGNS

General Comments
• None in some animals
• Depend on location, size, and number of uroliths
• Animals with nephroliths are typically asymptomatic but may have persistent hematuria, ureteral obstruction, and subsequent hydronephrosis.

Historical Findings
Typical signs of urocystoliths or urethroliths include pollakiuria, dysuria, and hematuria.

Physical Examination Findings
• Detection of urocystoliths by abdominal or rectal palpation; failure to palpate uroliths does not exclude them from consideration.
• A thickened and contracted bladder wall palpable in some patients, especially in cats
• Large urinary bladder if patient has complete urethral obstruction

CAUSES
See Pathophysiology

RISK FACTORS
• Calcium supplements independent of meals
• Excessive dietary protein, sodium, and vitamin D promote hypercalciuria.
• Additional dietary oxalate (e.g., chocolate and peanuts) and ascorbic acid promote oxalate excretion.

• Exogenous or endogenous exposure to a high concentration of glucocorticoids, diets that promote formation of acidic urine, and furosemide promote hypercalciuria.
• Pyridoxine (vitamin B$_6$)-deficient diets promote hyperoxaluria.
• Consumption of dry diets is associated with a higher risk for calcium oxalate urolith formation than consumption of canned diets.

DIAGNOSIS

DIFFERENTIAL DIAGNOSIS
• Other common causes of hematuria, dysuria, and pollakiuria, with or without urethral obstruction, include urinary tract infection and lower urinary tract neoplasia.
• Other common radiodense uroliths including those composed of magnesium ammonium phosphate, calcium phosphate, and silica (dogs)

CBC/BIOCHEMISTRY/URINALYSIS
• Results usually unremarkable
• Urinary sediment evaluation may reveal calcium oxalate crystals, but absence of crystalluria does not exclude uroliths as a possibility.
• Hypercalcemia or azotemia (rare)

OTHER LABORATORY TESTS
Quantitative mineral analysis of uroliths retrieved during voiding, by voiding urohydropropulsion, by aspiration into a urinary catheter, or by cystoscopy or cystotomy

IMAGING
Calcium oxalate uroliths are radiodense and may be detected by survey radiography; intravenous urography or ultrasonography may be required to verify ureteral obstruction.

DIAGNOSTIC PROCEDURES
N/A

PATHOLOGIC FINDINGS
N/A

TREATMENT

APPROPRIATE HEALTH CARE
• Retrograde urohydropropulsion to flush urethral stones back into the urinary bladder or voiding urohydropropulsion to eliminate bladder and urethral stones can be performed on an outpatient basis. Voiding urohydropropulsion is contraindicated in patients with urethral obstruction.
• Shock wave lithotripsy and surgery require short periods of hospitalization.

UROLITHIASIS, CALCIUM OXALATE

NURSING CARE
N/A

ACTIVITY
Reduce during the period of tissue repair after surgery

DIET
• No reports of dissolution of calcium oxalate uroliths with special diets
• Hypercalcemia in cats without evidence of hyperparathyroidism or malignancy is sometimes minimized by use of Prescription Diet Feline w/d (Hill's).

CLIENT EDUCATION
• Urolith removal does not alter the factors responsible for their formation; eliminating risk factors is necessary to minimize recurrence.
• Approximately 60% of dogs with a normal serum calcium concentration reform uroliths within 3 years.
• Patients with hypercalcemia typically reform uroliths at a faster rate.

SURGICAL CONSIDERATIONS
• Medical dissolution of calcium oxalate uroliths remains a goal for the future.
• Consider surgical removal of uroliths from patients with obstruction or dysuria if they cannot be removed by nonsurgical methods (e.g., voiding urohydropropulsion, catheter retrieval) or if clinical signs cannot be alleviated by flushing uroliths back into the urinary bladder.
• In dogs (not cats), shock wave lithotripsy is an alternative to surgery for removal of nephroliths and ureteroliths.
• Consider parathyroidectomy for patients with primary hyperparathyroidism and hypercalcemia.

MEDICATIONS

DRUGS OF CHOICE
No available drugs effectively dissolve calcium oxalate uroliths.

CONTRAINDICATIONS
None

PRECAUTIONS
Steroids and furosemide promote calciuria.

POSSIBLE INTERACTIONS
N/A

ALTERNATIVE DRUGS
N/A

FOLLOW-UP

PATIENT MONITORING
• Postsurgical radiographs are essential to verify complete urolith removal.
• To prevent repeat surgery, do abdominal radiography every 3–5 months to detect urolith recurrence early. Small uroliths are easily removed by voiding urohydropropulsion or catheter retrieval.

PREVENTION/AVOIDANCE
• If patient is hypercalcemic, correct underlying cause.
• If patient is normocalcemic, consider diet with reduced oxalate, sodium, and protein that does not promote formation of acidic urine (Prescription Diet Canine u/d, Prescription Diet Feline c/d-oxl, Prescription Diet Feline k/d, or Prescription Diet Feline w/d, Hills Pet Products). Ideally, the diet should contain additional water (canned diets) and citrate, and have adequate phosphorus and magnesium. Avoid supplementation with vitamins C and D.
• Reevaluate patient 2–4 weeks after initiation of diet therapy to verify appropriate urine dilution (specific gravity < 1.020 for dogs and < 1.035 for cats), appropriate urine pH ($\geq$6.5), and amelioration of crystalluria. Do not use inappropriately collected or stored urine samples (e.g., urine collected by owners, refrigerated, or contaminated with debris) to monitor therapeutic efficacy. To promote less-concentrated urine consider canned formulations of food or add water to all types of food. If urine is acidic, consider additional potassium citrate (75 mg/kg PO q12h); adjust dosage to achieve a pH between 6.5 and 7.5. Vitamin B$_6$ (2–4 mg/kg PO q24–48h) may help minimize oxalate excretion, especially for animals fed homemade or pyridoxine-deficient diets.

POSSIBLE COMPLICATIONS
• Urocystoliths can pass into and obstruct the urethra in male dogs and cats, especially if the patient is dysuric; managed by retrograde urohydropropulsion
• Dogs that do not consume their daily requirement of the urolith prevention diet can develop various degrees of protein calorie malnutrition.
• Diet-associated hyperlipidemia develops in some patients. Miniature schnauzers with hereditary hyperlipidemia and predisposition to pancreatitis can develop pancreatitis when consuming the prevention diet, in which case Prescription Diet Canine w/d (Hills) can be

used as an alternative. This diet should be supplemented with potassium citrate as needed to maintain a urine pH between 6.5 and 7.5.

EXPECTED COURSE AND PROGNOSIS
• Approximately 60% of dogs with normal serum calcium concentration reform uroliths in 3 years. Treatment to minimize recurrence is helpful. Patients with hypercalcemia typically reform uroliths at a faster rate.
• Comparable data are not available for cats.

MISCELLANEOUS

ASSOCIATED CONDITIONS
Any condition predisposing to hypercalciuria (e.g., hyperadrenocorticism, acidemia, hypervitaminosis D, and hyperparathyroidism) or hyperoxaluria (e.g., vitamin B$_6$ deficiency, hereditary hyperoxaluria, and ingestion of chocolate and peanuts)

AGE-RELATED FACTORS
Rare in young animals

ZOONOTIC POTENTIAL
None

PREGNANCY
Diets used to prevent calcium oxalate uroliths are not appropriate.

SYNONYMS
Oxalate urolithiasis

SEE ALSO
Crystalluria

ABBREVIATIONS
N/A

Suggested Reading
Lulich JP, Osborne CA. Voiding urohydropropulsion: a nonsurgical technique for removal of urocystoliths. In: Bonagura JD, Kirk RW, eds. Current veterinary therapy XII. Philadelphia: Saunders, 1995; 1003–1006.
Lulich JP. Osborne CA, Felice L. Calcium oxalate urolithiasis: cause, detection and control. In: August JR, ed. Consultations in feline internal medicine. Philadelphia: Saunders, 1994;343–349.
Lulich JP, Osborne C, Thumchai R, et al. Management of canine calcium oxalate urolith recurrence. Compend Contin Educ Pract Vet. 1998;20:178–189.
Authors Jody P. Lulich and Carl A. Osborne
Consulting Editors Larry G. Adams and Carl A. Osborne

UROLITHIASIS, CALCIUM PHOSPHATE

BASICS

OVERVIEW
• Formation of calcium phosphate uroliths within the urinary tract and the associated clinical condition
• Calcium phosphate uroliths represent 1–2 % of uroliths from dogs and cats submitted to laboratories for analysis
• Calcium phosphate uroliths—commonly called apatite uroliths
• Hydroxyapatite and carbonate apatite are the most common forms; brushite and whitiockite are less common.
• A greater percentage of calcium phosphate uroliths are found in the kidneys than in the urinary bladder.

SIGNALMENT
• Dogs and cats
• Rarely detected in animals less than 1 year old
• No other distinguishing trends for breed, age, and gender in dogs or cats

SIGNS
• Depend on location, size, and number of uroliths
• None in some patients
• Typically, pollakiuria, dysuria, hematuria, and urethral obstruction
• Animals with nephroliths—typically asymptomatic but may have persistent hematuria

CAUSES & RISK FACTORS
• Calcium phosphate—commonly a minor component of struvite and calcium oxalate uroliths
• Pure calcium phosphate uroliths—usually associated with metabolic disorders such as primary hyperparathyroidism, renal tubular acidosis, and excessive dietary calcium and phosphorus
• Nephroliths, urocystoliths, and urethroliths composed of blood clots mineralized with calcium phosphate suggest dystrophic mineralization of tissue, in contrast to metastatic mineralization reflecting abnormal calcium and phosphorus metabolism.
• Other risk factors include concentrated urine, vitamin D supplements, and mineral supplements

DIAGNOSIS

DIFFERENTIAL DIAGNOSIS
• Other common causes of hematuria, dysuria, and pollakiuria, with or without urethral obstruction, include urinary tract infection and lower urinary tract neoplasia.
• Magnesium ammonium phosphate, calcium oxalate, cystine, and silica are other common radiodense uroliths.
• Metastatic or dystrophic mineralization of urinary tract parenchyma may resemble uroliths.

CBC/BIOCHEMISTRY/URINALYSIS
• Usually unremarkable
• Hypercalcemia or azotemia rarely detected; postrenal azotemia in some animals with complete obstruction
• Urinary sediment analysis reveals amorphous crystals in some patients; brushite (calcium hydrogen phosphate dihydrate) forms are elongated, lath-shaped crystals.

OTHER LABORATORY TESTS
• Quantitative analysis of retrieved uroliths necessary to confirm their mineral composition
• Serum concentrations of parathyroid hormone, parathyroid hormone–related peptide, and hydroxycholecalciferol may help establish underlying causes.

IMAGING
• Radiodense uroliths often detected by survey radiography
• Calcium phosphate uroliths may be detected by ultrasonography.

OTHER DIAGNOSTIC PROCEDURES
Calcium phosphate uroliths in the urethra and bladder may be detected by cystoscopy.

TREATMENT
• Medical dissolution of calcium phosphate uroliths remains a goal for the future.
• Can consider surgery for removal of clinically active uroliths
• Nonsurgical methods of removing uroliths from the lower urinary tract include voiding urohydropropulsion, aspiration into a urinary catheter, and lithotripsy.
• Correction of hyperparathyroidism or other causes of hypercalcemia should minimize further urolith formation.

MEDICATIONS

DRUGS
No effective medications available for dissolving calcium phosphate uroliths

CONTRAINDICATIONS/POSSIBLE INTERACTIONS
N/A

FOLLOW-UP

PATIENT MONITORING
• Radiography after surgery to verify complete urolith removal—essential
• Abdominal radiography or ultrasonography every 3–4 months to enhance early detection of urolith recurrence and prevent the need for repeat surgery
• Small uroliths are easily removed by voiding urohydropropulsion or catheter retrieval.

PREVENTION/AVOIDANCE
• A diet formulated to prevent formation of calcium oxalate uroliths may help prevent recurrence.
• Prescription Diet Canine U/D (Hill's Pet Nutrition) is formulated to reduce calcium excretion, is phosphorus-restricted, and reduces formation of concentrated urine.
• Because of the high moisture content of canned foods and their tendency to promote dilute urine, canned diets may be more effective than dry diets in preventing recurrence.

MISCELLANEOUS

SYNONYMS
Apatite uroliths

Suggested Reading
Kruger JM, Osborne CA, Lulich JP. Canine calcium oxalate uroliths: etiopathogenesis, diagnosis, management. Vet Clin North Am: Small Anim Pract 1999;29:141–159.
Lulich JP, Osborne CA, Bartges JW, et al. Canine lower urinary tract disorders. In: Ettinger S, Feldman EC, eds. Textbook of veterinary internal medicine. Philadelphia: Saunders, 1995:1833–1861.

Authors Jody P. Lulich and Carl A. Osborne
Consulting Editors Larry G. Adams and Carl A. Osborne

BASICS

OVERVIEW
• Formation of polycrystalline concretions (i.e., uroliths, calculi, or stones) composed of organic cystine in the urinary tract • Occurs in dogs and cats with cystinuria, an inborn error of metabolism characterized by abnormal transport of cystine and other amino acids by the renal tubules • Cystine—normally present in low concentrations in plasma; is freely filtered at the glomerulus, and most is actively reabsorbed in the proximal tubules; much less is reabsorbed from the glomerular filtrate by cystinuric dogs than by normal dogs, and some may even have net cystine secretion. • Cystine—relatively insoluble in acid urine; becomes more soluble in alkaline urine • Unless protein intake is severely restricted, cystinuric dogs have no detectable abnormalities associated with amino acid loss, with the exception of formation of cystine uroliths. The exact mechanism of cystine urolith formation is unknown. Because not all cystinuric dogs form uroliths, cystinuria is a predisposing, rather than a primary, cause of cystine urolith formation. • The precise mode of inheritance of canine cystinuria is unknown. In past years, this genetic disorder considered gender-linked in all affected breeds. However, cystinuria in Newfoundlands was recently reported to have a simple autosomal recessive pattern of transmission. In Newfoundlands, parents of cystinuric dogs are either cystinuric or carriers, although littermates may be cystinuric, cystinuric carriers, or normal.

SIGNALMENT
• Dogs and cats • Canine cystinuria primarily affects adult (mean age at diagnosis, 5 years; range, 3 months to 14 years) males but may also affect females. It occurs in many breeds, especially dachshund, English bulldog, Newfoundland, Staffordshire bull terrier, and Welsh corgi dogs. Cystine uroliths may be detected in Newfoundlands less than 1 year old. • Feline cystinuria primarily affects adult (mean age at diagnosis, 3.5 years; range, 4 months to 12 years) males and females; most commonly recognized in the domestic shorthair and Siamese breeds

SIGNS
• Depend on location, size, and number of uroliths; affected animals may be asymptomatic • Typical signs of urocystoliths include pollakiuria, dysuria, and hematuria. • Typical signs of urethroliths include pollakiuria, dysuria, and sometimes voiding of small smooth uroliths. Complete outflow obstruction may result in postrenal uremia. • Nephroliths are typically asymptomatic but may be associated with manifestations of hydronephrosis and renal insufficiency.

CAUSES & RISK FACTORS
Cystinuria is a risk factor.

Breed Predisposition
• In young and middle-age dogs with previous history of cystine urolithiasis—recurrence within 6–12 months following surgery unless prophylactic therapy is given • Urolith formation—enhanced by acidic urine, highly concentrated urine, incomplete and infrequent micturition

DIAGNOSIS

DIFFERENTIAL DIAGNOSIS
• Uroliths mimic other causes of pollakiuria, dysuria, hematuria, and/or outflow obstruction. • Differentiate from other types of uroliths, especially ammonium urate in English bulldogs, by urinalysis, radiography, and quantitative analysis of voided or retrieved uroliths.

CBC/BIOCHEMISTRY/URINALYSIS
• Cystine crystals are six-sided and are insoluble in acetic acid. • Positive urine cyanidenitroprusside test

OTHER LABORATORY TESTS
• Urinary amino acid profiles—reveal abnormal quantities of cystine and, in some dogs and cats, lysine, arginine, and ornithine • Quantitative mineral analysis of uroliths retrieved during voiding, by voiding urohydropropulsion, or by aspiration into a urinary catheter

IMAGING
• Radiography—the radiodensity of cystine uroliths compared with soft tissue is similar to that of struvite and silica, less than that of calcium oxalate and calcium phosphate, and greater than that of ammonium urate; when large enough, cystine uroliths can be detected by survey radiography. • Ultrasonography—can detect cystine uroliths, but does not provide information about the radiodensity or their shape

DIAGNOSTIC PROCEDURES
Urethrocystoscopy may detect cystine urethroliths and urocystoliths.

TREATMENT
• Medical dissolution of uroliths by a combination of N-(2-mercaptopropionyl)-glycine (2-MPG) and dietary therapy; prescription Diet Canine u/d (Hills) reduces urinary excretion of cystine, promotes formation of alkaline urine, and reduces urine concentration; it is used in conjunction with 2-MPG for urolith dissolution and is often effective alone in preventing recurrence of cystine uroliths. • Remove small urocystoliths by voiding urohydropropulsion or surgery.

MEDICATIONS

DRUGS

Urine Alkalinizers
• Consider for patients that have acidic urine despite dietary therapy and control of urease-positive urinary tract infections. • Data derived from studies in cystinuric humans suggest that dietary sodium may enhance cystinuria; thus potassium citrate may be preferable to sodium bicarbonate as a urine alkalinizer. Give enough potassium citrate (40–75 mg/kg q12h) to maintain a urine pH of 7.5.

Thiol-containing Drugs
• 2-MPG decreases the urine concentration of cystine by combining with cysteine to form cysteine-2-MPG, which is more soluble than cystine. • 2-MPG (Thiola-Mission Pharmacal) may be given at a dosage of 15–20 mg/kg q12h to dissolve canine cystine uroliths in conjunction with dietary therapy. In our hospital, mean dissolution time was 78 days (range, 11–211 days). • 2-MPG may be given at a lower dosage (5–10 mg/kg PO q12h) to prevent recurrent canine cystine uroliths, if dietary therapy is not optimal. • Drug-induced adverse events associated with 2-MGP are uncommon in dogs; they include reversible Coombs-positive spherocytic anemia, thrombocytopenia, and increased hepatic enzyme activity. • The efficacy and safety of 2-MPG has not been evaluated in cystinuric cats.

CONTRAINDICATIONS/POSSIBLE INTERACTIONS
N/A

FOLLOW-UP
• Prevention of recurrence with dietary management or 2-MPG • Monitor urolith dissolution at 30-day intervals by urinalysis and survey or contrast radiography or ultrasonography. • Although cystine uroliths tend to recur, recurrence does not happen in all cystinuric dogs and cats. • In some older dogs, the rate of recurrence declines as a consequence of a reduction in the magnitude of cystinuria.

MISCELLANEOUS

ABBREVIATION
2-MPG = N-(2-mercaptopropionyl)-glycine

Suggested Reading
Osborne CA, Sanderson SL, Lulich JP, et al. Canine cystine urolithiasis. Vet Clin North Am 1999;29:193–211.

Authors Carl A. Osborne, Jody P. Lulich, and Lisa Ulrich

Consulting Editors Larry G. Adams and Carl A. Osborne

UROLITHIASIS, STRUVITE—CATS

BASICS

DEFINITION
Struvite uroliths and struvite urethral plugs have physical and etiopathogenic differences; thus, these terms should not be used as synonyms. Struvite uroliths are polycrystalline concretions composed primarily of magnesium ammonium phosphate and small quantities of matrix. Struvite feline urethral plugs commonly are composed of large quantities of matrix mixed with magnesium ammonium phosphate. Some urethral plugs are composed primarily of organic matrix, sloughed tissue, blood, and/or inflammatory reactants.

PATHOPHYSIOLOGY
• See Urolithiasis, Struvite—Dogs
• The most commonly encountered form of naturally occurring feline urethral plugs contains relatively large quantities of matrix in addition to minerals, especially struvite. Risk factors associated with formation of MAP crystals contained in urethral plugs are similar to those associated with formation of struvite uroliths. Prevention or control of these risk factors should minimize the recurrence of the struvite component of urethral plugs. Specific causes and composition of urethral plug matrix have not yet been classified. One hypothesis is that plug matrix follows urinary tract infections, especially by viruses.

SYSTEMS AFFECTED
Renal/Urologic—upper and lower urinary tract

GENETICS
N/A

INCIDENCE/PREVALENCE
• The prevalence of feline struvite uroliths has been declining during the past decade in association with special diets designed to dissolve and prevent this type of stone.
• Currently, struvite makes up less than 40% of uroliths in the feline lower urinary tract. Of these, 95% are sterile.
• Struvite has been detected in less than 5% of feline nephroliths.
• Struvite remains the most common (80%) mineral in matrix-crystalline urethral plugs.

GEOGRAPHIC DISTRIBUTION
N/A

SIGNALMENT

Species
Cats (see Urolithiasis, Struvite—Dogs)

Breed Predilections
None

Mean Age and Range
• Mean age at time of diagnosis is 7 years (range, < 1 to 22 years).

• Sterile struvite uroliths do not affect immature cats; infection-induced struvite may occur in immature cats.

Predominant Sex
• Struvite uroliths are more common in females (55%) than males (45%).
• Struvite urethral plugs primarily affect males.

SIGNS

General Comments
• Affected cats may be asymptomatic.
• Depend on location, size, and number of uroliths.

Historical Findings
• Typical signs of urocystoliths include pollakiuria, dysuria, and hematuria.
• Typical signs of urethroliths include pollakiuria, dysuria, and sometimes voiding of small, smooth uroliths; signs of postrenal uremia (e.g., anorexia and vomiting) are found in some cats with outflow obstruction.
• Manifestations of renal insufficiency (polyuria and polydipsia) are found in some cats with nephroliths.
• Signs typical of outflow obstruction (e.g., dysuria, large painful urinary bladder, and signs of postrenal uremia) are found in cats with struvite urethral plugs.

Physical Examination Findings
• A thickened, firm, contracted bladder wall is found in some cats with urocystoliths.
• Detection of urocystoliths by palpation is unreliable.
• Urethral plugs or uroliths may be detected by examination of the distal penis and penile urethra.
• Outflow obstruction results in an enlarged urinary bladder and signs of postrenal uremia.

CAUSES
See Pathophysiology

RISK FACTORS
• For formation of sterile struvite uroliths—include mineral composition, energy content, and moisture content of diets; urine-alkalinizing metabolites in diets; quantity of diet consumed; ad libitum versus meal-feeding schedules; formation of concentrated urine; and retention of urine
• Elimination or control may result in dissolution of sterile struvite uroliths and prevention of their recurrence.
• Probable for infection-induced struvite urolithiasis—include urinary tract infection with urease-producing microbial pathogens, abnormalities in local host defenses that allow bacterial urinary tract infections (including perineal urethrostomies), and the quantity of urea (the substrate of urease) excreted in urine
• The normal small diameter of the distal urethra of male cats predisposes them to obstruction with plugs and uroliths.

DIAGNOSIS

DIFFERENTIAL DIAGNOSIS
• Uroliths mimic other causes of pollakiuria, dysuria, hematuria, and/or outflow obstruction.
• Differentiate struvite uroliths and urethral plugs from other types of uroliths by signalment, urinalysis, urine culture, radiography, ultrasonography, cystoscopy, and quantitative analysis of voided or retrieved uroliths or plugs.

CBC/BIOCHEMISTRY/URINALYSIS
• Complete outflow obstruction may cause postrenal azotemia (e.g., high BUN, creatinine, and phosphorus).
• Magnesium ammonium phosphate crystals typically appear as colorless, orthorhombic (having three unequal axes intersecting at right angles), coffinlike prisms. They often have three to eight sides.

OTHER LABORATORY TESTS
• Pretreatment quantitative bacterial urine cultures (preferably with specimen obtained by cystocentesis) yield bacterial urinary tract infections in only 1–3% of affected patients.
• Quantitative mineral analysis is the accepted standard of practice for uroliths and urethral plugs retrieved during voiding, by voiding urohydropropulsion, by aspiration into a urinary catheter, or by cystoscopy.
• Bacterial culture of inner portions of infection-induced struvite uroliths may be of value.

IMAGING

Radiography
• Struvite uroliths—radiodense; may be detected by survey radiography; some struvite urethral plugs may be detected by survey radiography.
• The size and number of uroliths are not a reliable index of probable efficacy of dissolution therapy.
• Contrast urethrocystography helps identify the site(s) of urethral obstruction and urethral strictures.

Ultrasonography
• Detects location, size, and number of uroliths, but does not indicate degree of radiodensity or shape of uroliths
• Determines precise location, size, and number of uroliths

DIAGNOSTIC PROCEDURES
Cystoscopy reveals location, number, size, and shape of urethroliths and urocystoliths.

PATHOLOGIC FINDINGS
Urethral plugs may contain red blood cells, white cells, transitional epithelial cells, bacteria, and/or viruses in addition to matrix and minerals.

TREATMENT

APPROPRIATE HEALTH CARE
• Retrograde urohydropropulsion to eliminate urethral stones, lavage to remove urethral plugs, voiding urohydropropulsion to eliminate bladder and urethral stones, and/or surgery require short periods of hospitalization.
• Medical dissolution of struvite uroliths is an outpatient strategy.

NURSING CARE
N/A

ACTIVITY
If dietary management is used, monitor outdoor activity.

DIET
• Sterile and infection-induced struvite urocystoliths and nephroliths may be dissolved by feeding a calculolytic diet (Prescription Diet Feline s/d; Hills Pet Nutrition).
• Continue diet therapy for 1 month after survey radiographic evidence of urolith dissolution.
• Struvite crystalluria may be minimized by feeding magnesium-restricted urine-acidifying diets.
• Canned (moist) foods help to reduce urine concentration of calculogenic metabolites and promote increased frequency of normal voiding.

CLIENT EDUCATION
• If dietary management is used, limit access to other foods and treats.
• Short-term (weeks to months) treatment with a calculolytic diet (Feline s/d) ± antibiotics as needed is effective in dissolving struvite uroliths. Avoid feeding calculolytic diets to immature cats.
• Owners of cats with infection-induced struvite urocystoliths must comply with dosage schedule for antibiotic therapy.

SURGICAL CONSIDERATIONS
• Ureteroliths cannot be dissolved. Consider surgery for persistent ureteroliths associated with morbidity.
• Urethroliths cannot be medically dissolved. Consider voiding urohydropropulsion to remove urethroliths or urethral plugs. Alternatively, move urethroliths into the bladder by retrograde urohydropropulsion.
• Immovable urethroliths, recurrent urethral plugs, or strictures of the distal urethra may require perineal urethrostomy.
• Nephroliths causing outflow obstruction, or associated with nonfunctioning kidneys cannot be dissolved medically.
• Consider surgical correction if uroliths are obstructing urine outflow, and/or if correctable abnormalities predisposing to recurrent

urinary tract infection are identified by radiography or other means.
• Uroliths and urethral plugs should be localized before considering surgical correction.

MEDICATIONS

DRUGS OF CHOICE
Dietary dissolution of infection-induced urocystoliths or nephroliths requires oral administration of appropriate antibiotics, chosen on the basis of bacterial culture and antimicrobial susceptibility tests. Give antibiotics at therapeutic dosages until the urinary tract infection is eradicated and no radiographic evidence of uroliths exists.

CONTRAINDICATIONS
Do not give urine acidifiers to azotemic patients or immature cats.

PRECAUTIONS
Azotemic patients are at increased risk for adverse drug events.

POSSIBLE INTERACTIONS
None

ALTERNATIVE DRUGS
None

FOLLOW-UP

PATIENT MONITORING
Check rate of urolith dissolution at monthly intervals by urinalysis, urine culture, survey or contrast radiography, or ultrasonography.

PREVENTION/AVOIDANCE
• Recurrent sterile struvite uroliths may be prevented by using acidifying, magnesium-restricted diets or urine acidifiers. Do not administer urine acidifiers with acidifying diets.
• Monitor patients whose urine has been acidified for calcium oxalate crystalluria. Change management protocol if persistent calcium oxalate crystalluria develops.
• In patients at risk for both struvite and calcium oxalate crystalluria, focus on preventing calcium oxalate uroliths. Struvite uroliths can be medically dissolved; recurrent calcium oxalate uroliths cannot be dissolved.
• Infection-induced struvite urolithiasis can be prevented by eradicating and controlling urinary tract infections. Use of magnesium-restricted, acidifying diets is an ancillary method of prevention.

POSSIBLE COMPLICATIONS
• Urocystoliths may pass into and obstruct the urethra of male cats, especially if the patient is persistently dysuric. Urethral obstruction may be managed by retrograde urohydropropulsion.
• Dysuria may be minimized by treatment of

bacterial urinary tract infection, and by administration of an anticholinergic drug (e.g., propantheline bromide 7.5 mg PO q3days).
• An indwelling transurethral catheter increases the risk for iatrogenic bacterial urinary tract infection and/or urethral stricture.

EXPECTED COURSE AND PROGNOSIS
In our hospital, the mean time for dissolution of feline sterile urocystoliths was 1 month (range, 2 weeks to 5 months). The mean time for dissolution of infection-induced struvite urocystoliths was 10 weeks (range, 9–12 weeks).

MISCELLANEOUS

ASSOCIATED CONDITIONS
Any disease that predisposes to bacterial urinary tract infection

AGE-RELATED FACTORS
Infection-induced struvite is the most common urolith in immature cats. Sterile struvite is rare in immature cats.

ZOONOTIC POTENTIAL
None

PREGNANCY
N/A

SYNONYMS
FUS, feline urological disease, feline lower urinary tract disease.

SEE ALSO
• Urolithiasis, Struvite—Dogs
• Lower Urinary Tract Infection
• Nephrolithiasis

ABBREVIATION
MAP = magnesium ammonium phosphate

Suggested Reading

Osborne CA, Lulich JP, Kruger JM, et al. Feline urethral plugs: etiology and pathophysiology. Vet Clin North Am 1996; 26:233–254

Osborne CA, Lulich JP, Thumchai R, et al. Feline urolithiasis: etiology and pathophysiology. Vet Clin North Am 1996; 26:217–232.

Osborne CA, Lulich JP, Thumchai R, et al. Diagnosis, medical treatment, and prognosis of feline urolithiasis. Vet Clin North Am 1996;26:589–628.

Osborne CA, Kruger JM, Lulich JP, et al. Feline lower urinary tract diseases. In: Ettinger SJ, Feldman EC, eds. Textbook of veterinary internal medicine. 5th ed, Philadelphia: Saunders, 1999.

Authors Carl A. Osborne, John M. Kruger, and Jody P. Lulich
Consulting Editors Larry G. Adams and Carl A. Osborne

DISEASES

UROLITHIASIS, STRUVITE—DOGS

BASICS

DEFINITION
Formation of polycrystalline concretions (i.e., uroliths, calculi, or stones) composed of MAP, or struvite, in the urinary tract.

PATHOPHYSIOLOGY

Infection-induced Struvite
• Urine must be supersaturated with MAP for struvite uroliths to form. MAP supersaturation of urine may be associated with several factors, including urinary tract infections with urease-producing microbes, alkaline urine, genetic predisposition, and diet. • If animals are affected by urinary tract infections caused by urease-producing microbes (especially species of *Staphylococcus, Proteus,* and *Ureaplasma*) and their urine contains sufficient urea, the result is a unique combination of concomitant elevations in the concentrations of ammonium and carbonate (CO_3^{2-}) in an alkaline environment. These conditions favor formation of uroliths containing struvite ($MgNH_4PO_4 \cdot 6H_2O$), calcium apatite [$Ca_{10}(PO_4)6(OH_2)_2$], and carbonate apatite [$Ca_{10}(PO_4)6CO_3$]. • Consumption of dietary protein in excess of the daily requirement for anabolism results in formation of urea from catabolism of amino acids. Hyperammonuria, hypercarbonaturia, and alkaluria mediated by microbial urease depend on the quantity of urea (the substrate of urease) in urine. • Abnormal urinary excretion of minerals as a result of enhanced glomerular filtration rate, reduced tubular reabsorption, or enhanced tubular secretion is not required for initiation and growth of infection-induced struvite uroliths; however, metabolic and anatomic abnormalities may indirectly induce struvite uroliths by predisposing to urinary tract infections.

Sterile Struvite
• Dietary or metabolic factors may be involved in the genesis of sterile struvite uroliths in these species. • Microbial urease is not involved in formation of sterile struvite uroliths.

SYSTEMS AFFECTED
Renal/Urologic

GENETICS
• The high incidence of struvite uroliths in some breeds of dogs such as miniature schnauzers suggests a familial tendency. We hypothesize that susceptible miniature schnauzers inherit some abnormality of local host defenses of the urinary tract that increases their susceptibility to urinary tract infection. • Sterile struvite uroliths were found in a family of English cocker spaniels.

INCIDENCE/PREVALENCE
Struvite uroliths account for approximately 50% of stones affecting the canine lower urinary tract and 33% of stones affecting the upper urinary tract.

GEOGRAPHIC DISTRIBUTION
Ubiquitous

SIGNALMENT

Species
Dogs (see Urolithiasis, Struvite—Cats)

Breed Predilections
• Miniature schnauzer, shih tzu, bichon frise, miniature poodle, cocker spaniel, and Lhasa apso • Any breed may be affected.

Mean Age and Range
• Mean age, 6 years (range, <1 to >19 years) • Most uroliths in immature dogs are infection-induced struvite.

Predominant Sex
More common in females (85%) than males (15%)

SIGNS

General Comments
• None in some dogs • Signs depend on location, size, and number of uroliths

Historical Findings
• Typical signs of urocystoliths include pollakiuria, dysuria, and hematuria; sometimes small, smooth uroliths are voided. • Typical signs of urethroliths include pollakiuria and dysuria; sometimes small, smooth uroliths are voided. • Nephroliths may be associated with manifestations of renal insufficiency. Obstruction to urine outflow with bacterial urinary tract infection may result in generalized pyelonephritis and septicemia.

Physical Examination Findings
• Uroliths may be palpated in the urinary bladder and urethra. • Obstruction of the urethra may cause enlargement of the urinary bladder. • Obstruction of a ureter may cause enlargement of the associated kidney. • Complete urine outflow obstruction combined with bacterial infection may cause ascending urinary tract infection, signs of renal failure, and signs of septicemia.

CAUSES
• Urinary tract disorders that predispose to infections with urease-producing bacteria, fungal pathogens, or ureaplasma in patients whose urine contains a large quantity of urea • Specific causes of sterile struvite uroliths are unknown.

RISK FACTORS
• Exogenous or endogenous exposure to high concentrations of glucocorticoids predispose to bacterial urinary tract infection. • Abnormal retention of urine • Alkaline urine decreases the solubility of struvite.

DIAGNOSIS

DIFFERENTIAL DIAGNOSIS
• Uroliths mimic other causes of pollakiuria, dysuria, hematuria, and/or outflow obstruction. • Differentiate from other types of uroliths by signalment, urinalysis, urine culture, radiography, and quantitative analysis of voided or retrieved uroliths.

CBC/BIOCHEMISTRY/URINALYSIS
• Complete outflow obstruction can cause postrenal azotemia (e.g., high BUN, creatinine, and phosphorus). • Magnesium ammonium phosphate crystals typically appear as colorless, orthorhombic (having three unequal axes intersecting at right angles), coffinlike prisms. They may have three to six or more sides and often have oblique ends.

OTHER LABORATORY TESTS
• Quantitative bacterial culture of urine, preferably collected by cystocentesis • Bacterial culture of inner portions of infection-induced struvite uroliths • Quantitative mineral analysis of uroliths retrieved during voiding, by voiding urohydropropulsion, by aspiration into a urinary catheter, or by cystoscopy

IMAGING
• Struvite uroliths are radiodense and may be detected by survey radiography. • Ultrasonography—can detect uroliths, but provides no information about their density or shape • Determine precise location, size, and number of uroliths; the size and number are not a reliable index of probable efficacy of dissolution therapy

DIAGNOSTIC PROCEDURES
N/A

PATHOLOGIC FINDINGS
N/A

TREATMENT

APPROPRIATE HEALTH CARE
• Retrograde urohydropropulsion to eliminate urethral stones, voiding urohydropropulsion to eliminate bladder and urethral stones, shock-wave lithotripsy, and/or surgery require short periods of hospitalization. • Medical dissolution of struvite uroliths is an outpatient strategy.

NURSING CARE
N/A

ACTIVITY
If dietary management is used, monitor outdoor activity.

DIET
• Infection-induced and sterile struvite

urocystoliths and nephroliths may be dissolved by feeding a calculolytic diet (Prescription Diet Canine s/d; Hills Pet Nutrition). • Continue calculolytic diet therapy for 1 month beyond survey radiographic evidence of urolith dissolution. • Avoid use of the protein-restricted diet in patients with protein-calorie malnutrition. The calculolytic diet is designed for short-term (weeks to months) dissolution therapy, rather than long-term (months to years) prophylactic therapy. If used, monitor the patient for evidence of protein malnutrition. Avoid prolonged feeding of the calculolytic diet to immature dogs.

CLIENT EDUCATION
• If dietary management is used, limit access to other foods and treats. • Short-term treatment with a calculolytic diet and administration of antibiotics has been effective in dissolving struvite uroliths. • Comply with dosage schedule for antibiotic therapy

SURGICAL CONSIDERATIONS
• Ureteroliths cannot be dissolved; consider surgery or shock-wave lithotripsy for persistent ureteroliths associated with morbidity. • Urethroliths cannot be medically dissolved; consider voiding urohydropropulsion if the urethroliths are likely to pass through the entire length of the urethra. Alternatively, move urethroliths into the bladder by retrograde urohydropropulsion. • Immovable urethroliths may require urethrotomy or urethrostomy. • Nephroliths causing outflow obstruction or associated with nonfunctioning kidneys cannot be dissolved medically. • Consider surgical correction if uroliths are obstructing urine outflow and/or if correctable abnormalities predisposing to recurrent urinary tract infection are identified by radiography or other means.

MEDICATIONS

DRUGS OF CHOICE
• Dietary dissolution of infection-induced urocystoliths or nephroliths requires oral administration of appropriate antibiotics, chosen on the basis of bacterial culture and antimicrobial susceptibility tests. Give antibiotics at therapeutic dosages until there is no radiographic evidence of uroliths and there is laboratory confirmation of eradication of urinary tract infection. • Patients with infection-induced struvite urocystoliths associated with persistent bacterial infection with urease-producing bacteria and refractory to dietary and antibiotic dissolution may be given AHA (Lithostat, Mission Pharmacal, 12.5 mg/kg PO q12 h). AHA is a urease inhibitor that blocks hydrolysis of urea to ammonia.

CONTRAINDICATIONS
AHA is teratogenic and should not be given to pregnant dogs.

PRECAUTIONS
• Diet-induced polyuria will reduce the concentration of antimicrobial drugs in urine; consider this fact when calculating antimicrobic dosages. • Prolonged administration of AHA at higher doses induces abnormalities in bilirubin metabolism in some dogs. • Higher doses of AHA may induce a reversible hemolytic anemia.

ALTERNATIVE DRUGS
N/A

FOLLOW-UP

PATIENT MONITORING
Rate of urolith dissolution at monthly intervals by urinalysis, urine culture, ultrasonography, and/or survey or contrast radiography

PREVENTION/AVOIDANCE
• Infection-induced struvite urolithiasis may be prevented by eradicating and controlling infections by urease-producing bacteria. • Recurrent sterile struvite uroliths may be prevented by use of acidifying, magnesium-restricted diets (Prescription Diet Canine c/d, Hills) or urine acidifiers. • Monitor patients whose urine has been acidified for calcium oxalate crystalluria. Change management protocol if persistent calcium oxalate crystalluria develops. • In patients at risk for both struvite and calcium oxalate crystalluria, focus on prevention of calcium oxalate uroliths—struvite uroliths can be medically dissolved if they recur; recurrent calcium oxalate uroliths cannot be dissolved.

POSSIBLE COMPLICATIONS
• Benefits and risks are associated with feeding struvitolytic diets. Not all patients qualify for dietary medical management, including those with (1) abnormal fluid accumulation, (2) azotemic primary renal failure, and (3) predispositions to pancreatitis. • Urocystoliths may pass into and obstruct the urethra of male dogs, especially if the patient is persistently dysuric. Urethral obstruction may be managed by retrograde urohydropropulsion. •Dysuria may be minimized by antimicrobic treatment of bacterial urinary tract infections and oral administration of anticholinergic drugs (e.g., propantheline). • Dogs that do not consume their daily requirement of the calculolytic diet may develop varying degrees of protein calorie malnutrition. This can be prevented by proper calculation of the daily dietary requirement and adjustment in the quantity of diet fed on the basis of serial physical examination. • Diet-associated polyuria will result in voiding increased urine volume. This may be associated with varying degrees of urinary incontinence in neutered female dogs with a predisposition to estrogen-responsive incontinence.

EXPECTED COURSE AND PROGNOSIS
• In our hospital, the mean time for dissolution of infection-induced urocystoliths was approx-

imately 3 months (range, 2 weeks to 7 months). The mean time for dissolution of infection-induced struvite nephroliths was 6 months (range, 2–10 months). The mean time for dissolution of sterile struvite urocystoliths was 6 weeks (range, 4–12 weeks). • Compliance with dietary recommendations is suggested by a reduced concentration of urea in serum (10 mg/dL), and a low urine specific gravity (1.004–1.014). • If uroliths increase in size during dietary management or do not begin to decrease in size after approximately 4–8 weeks of appropriate medical management, alternative methods should be considered. Difficulty in inducing complete dissolution of uroliths by creating urine undersaturated with struvite should prompt consideration that (1) the wrong mineral component was identified, (2) the nucleus of the uroliths has a different mineral composition than other portions of the urolith, and (3) the owner is not complying with medical recommendations.

MISCELLANEOUS

ASSOCIATED CONDITIONS
Any disease that predisposes to bacterial urinary tract infection

AGE-RELATED FACTORS
Infection-induced struvite is the most common form of urolith in immature dogs

ZOONOTIC POTENTIAL
None

PREGNANCY
• AHA is teratogenic • The calculolytic diet is not designed to sustain pregnancy.

SYNONYMS
Phosphate calculi, infections stones, urease stones, triple-phosphate stones

SEE ALSO
N/A

ABBREVIATIONS
• AHA = acetohydroxamic acid
• MAP = magnesium ammonium phosphate

Suggested Reading
Osborne CA, Lulich JP, Bartges JW, et al. Canine and feline urolithiasis: relationship of etiopathogenesis to treatment and prevention. In: Osborne CA, Finco DR, eds. Canine and feline nephrology and urology. Baltimore: Williams & Wilkins, 1995:798–888.

Osborne CA, Lulich JP, Polzin DJ, et al. Medical dissolution and prevention of canine struvite urolithiasis: twenty years of experience. Vet Clin North Am 1999;29:73–111.

Authors Carl A. Osborne, Jody P. Lulich, and David J. Polzin
Consulting Editors Larry G. Adams and Carl A. Osborne

UROLITHIASIS, URATE

 BASICS

DEFINITION
Uroliths composed of uric acid, sodium urate, or ammonium urate.

PATHOPHYSIOLOGY
• Impaired conversion of uric acid to allantoin causes high concentration of uric acid in serum and urine.

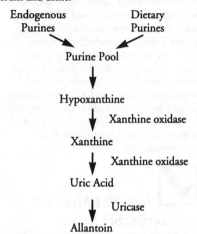

• Patients with portosystemic shunt may develop ammonium urate uroliths because of impaired metabolism of uric acid and ammonia.

SYSTEMS AFFECTED
Renal/urologic

GENETICS
Dalmatians have a breed predisposition to forming urate urolithiasis; The genetics of this condition are unknown.

INCIDENCE/PREVALENCE
Approximately 5–8% of uroliths retrieved from dogs and cats

GEOGRAPHIC DISTRIBUTION
N/A

SIGNALMENT
Species
Dogs and cats

Breed Predilections
Dalmatian, English bulldog, and breeds at risk for portosystemic shunt (e.g., Yorkshire terrier)

Mean Age and Range
• Mean age in patients without portosystemic shunt is 3.5 years (range, 0.5 to >10 years)
• Mean age in patients with portosystemic shunt is <1 year (range, 0.1 to >10 years).

Predominant Sex
• More common in male dogs without portosystemic shunt • No sex predilection in dogs with portosystemic shunt or cats

SIGNS
Historical Findings
• Hematuria • Dysuria • Possible hepatic encephalopathy in patients with portosystemic shunt

Physical Examination Findings
• Urethral obstruction • No signs in some patients

CAUSES
Rule out portosystemic shunt

RISK FACTORS
• High purine intake (glandular meat)
• Persistent aciduria in a predisposed animal.

 DIAGNOSIS

DIFFERENTIAL DIAGNOSIS
Other causes of lower or upper urinary tract disease

CBC/BIOCHEMISTRY/URINALYSIS
• Aciduria • Urate crystalluria • Azotemia in patients with urinary outflow obstruction
• Low BUN in patients with portosystemic shunt.

OTHER LABORATORY TESTS
Liver function tests such as bile acids have abnormal results in patients with portosystemic shunt.

IMAGING
• Urate uroliths may be radiolucent; may need intravenous pyelogram (IVP) to detect nephroliths or double contrast cystography to detect urocystoliths • Microhepatica in patients with portosystemic shunt • Ultrasonography may reveal small uroliths and portosystemic shunts.

DIAGNOSTIC PROCEDURES
Liver biopsy

PATHOLOGIC FINDINGS
In patients with portosystemic shunt, liver biopsy may reveal hepatic atrophy and/or dysplasia.

 TREATMENT

APPROPRIATE HEALTH CARE
Urethral or ureteral obstruction may require inpatient treatment. Urate uroliths can be dissolved on outpatient basis.

NURSING CARE
Fluid therapy to correct dehydration

ACTIVITY
Usually not restricted, except after surgery

DIET
For dissolution and prevention, a low-purine, urine-alkalinizing diet

CLIENT EDUCATION
Recurrence of uroliths is possible.

SURGICAL CONSIDERATIONS
• Cystotomy, urethrotomy, or nephrotomy to remove uroliths • Portosystemic shunt ligation

 MEDICATIONS

DRUGS OF CHOICE
Allopurinol (15 mg/kg PO q12h), a xanthine oxidase inhibitor, for dissolution (see algorithm 1)

CONTRAINDICATIONS
Glucocorticoids and other immunosuppressive drugs may promote hyperuricosuria.

PRECAUTIONS
Allopurinol is contraindicated in animals with renal failure.

POSSIBLE INTERACTIONS
Skin eruption with use of allopurinol and ampicillin

ALTERNATIVE DRUGS
N/A

 FOLLOW-UP

PATIENT MONITORING
See algorithm 2

PREVENTION/AVOIDANCE
Low-purine, urine-alkalinizing diet

POSSIBLE COMPLICATIONS
• Urethral obstruction • Uroliths likely to recur if no preventive measures

EXPECTED COURSE AND PROGNOSIS
• Medical dissolution takes an average of 4 weeks. • Medical dissolution usually not successful with portosystemic shunt

 MISCELLANEOUS

ASSOCIATED CONDITIONS
Portosystemic shunt

AGE-RELATED FACTORS
N/A

ZOONOTIC POTENTIAL
N/A

PREGNANCY
Low-protein diet is not recommended for pregnant or lactating animal.

SYNONYMS
N/A

SEE ALSO
• Urolithiasis, Xanthine • Portosystemic Shunt

ABBREVIATION
IVP = intravenous pyelogram

Suggested Reading

Bartges JW, Osborne CA, Felice LJ. Canine xanthine uroliths: risk factor management.

In: Kirk RW, Bonagura JD, eds. Current veterinary therapy XI. Philadelphia: WB Saunders, 1992:900–905.
Osborne CA, Lulich JP, Bartges JW, Polzin DJ. Metabolic uroliths in cats. In: Kirk RW, Bonagura JD, eds. Current veterinary ther-

apy XI. Philadelphia: WB Saunders, 1992:906–910.
Author Joseph W. Bartges
Consulting Editors Larry G. Adams and Carl A. Osborne

Figure 1.

Algorithm for Treatment of Urate Urocystolithiasis

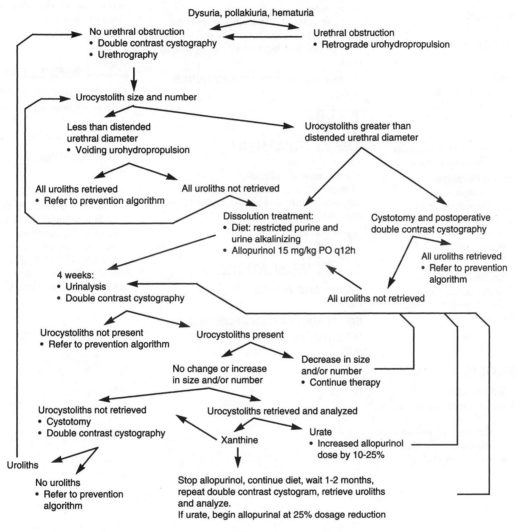

Figure 2.

Algorithm for Prevention of Urate Urocystolithiasis

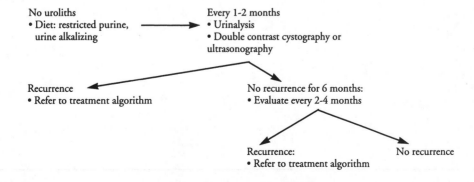

UROLITHIASIS, XANTHINE

BASICS

OVERVIEW
Xanthine is converted to uric acid by xanthine oxidase. Impaired conversion by allopurinol may cause hyperxanthinemia, xanthinuria, and xanthine uroliths.

SIGNALMENT
• Dogs and cats receiving allopurinol.
• Naturally occurring xanthine uroliths have been observed in young cats.

SIGNS

General Comments
Signs are related to anatomic location(s) of urolith(s). Affected animals may be asymptomatic.

Historical Findings
Typical signs of urocystoliths or urethroliths include pollakiuria, dysuria, and hematuria.

Physical Examination Findings
• Urocystoliths or urethroliths may be detected on abdominal or rectal palpation; failure to palpate uroliths does not exclude them from consideration.
• Large bladder if urethral obstruction is complete.

CAUSES AND RISK FACTORS
• Allopurinol administration, especially accompanied by high purine diet
• Hereditary xanthinuria

DIAGNOSIS

DIFFERENTIAL DIAGNOSIS
• Other cause of lower or upper urinary tract disease
• Differentiate from other types of uroliths—xanthine uroliths are radiolucent; xanthine crystals are yellow-brown, spherical

CBC/BIOCHEMISTRY/URINALYSIS
Results normal

OTHER LABORATORY TESTS
Quantitatively analyze urine sediment or uroliths. Xanthine crystals are yellow-brown, spherical.

IMAGING
• Xanthine uroliths are radiolucent and therefore are not detected on survey radiographs.
• Double contrast cystography, intravenous pyelography, or ultrasonography will identify uroliths and their location within the urinary tract.

OTHER DIAGNOSTIC PROCEDURES
N/A

TREATMENT
• Surgical removal
• Discontinue allopurinol.
• Low purine diet reduces amount of xanthine in urine and plasma. See urate urolithiasis.

MEDICATIONS

DRUGS AND FLUIDS
N/A

CONTRAINDICATIONS/POSSIBLE INTERACTIONS
N/A

FOLLOW-UP

• Monitor serial urinalyses and results of double contrast cystography or intravenous pyelography.
• If attempting to dissolve urate uroliths, discontinue allopurinol for 1–2 months and decrease dosage by 25% when reinstituted. Feed low-purine diet when using allopurinol
• Uroliths may recur.

MISCELLANEOUS

ASSOCIATED CONDITIONS
Urate urolithiasis, nephrolithiasis

SEE ALSO
Urolithiasis, Urate

ABBREVIATIONS
None

References
Bartges JW, Osborne CA, Felice LJ. Canine xanthine uroliths: risk factor management. In: Kirk RW, Bonagura JD, eds. Current veterinary therapy XI. Philadelphia: WB Saunders, 1992:900–905.
Author Joseph W. Bartges
Consulting Editors Larry G. Adams and Carl A. Osborne

BASICS

OVERVIEW
Failure of the uterine muscles to expel fetuses

Primary
• Uterine muscles do not contract normally at parturition
• Large-breed dog with an abnormally small litter—uterine contractions may not be induced

Secondary
• Pup not delivered within 2 hr
• May develop during a prolonged parturition or after dystocia with subsequent uterine muscle failure (see Dystocia)

SIGNALMENT
• Noted in some small breeds
• Seen in nervous, obese, older, and under-exercised females
• Possibly with small litters in all breeds

SIGNS
• Primary—lack of onset of parturition at the end of gestation; patient is bright and alert; may detect cervical dilation on vaginoscopy; may see small green-tinged vaginal discharge
• Secondary—patient usually has prolonged dystocia; may note one or two normal deliveries, after which labor ceases, even though there are more fetuses in the uterus

CAUSES & RISK FACTORS
• Primary—result of muscles that do not respond to hormonal stimuli; receptors that failed to develop; or hormones that are lacking, not released, or imbalanced; obesity and lack of exercise main causal factors
• Secondary—obstruction in the reproductive tract; absolute or relative fetal oversize; fetal deficiency of adrenocorticoid hormone; faulty fetal presentation, position, and posture
• Progesterone administration—mimics condition

DIAGNOSIS

DIFFERENTIAL DIAGNOSIS
• Primary—pseudopregnancy
• Secondary—obstructive dystocia

CBC/BIOCHEMISTRY/URINALYSIS
• Primary—normal; may be useful if cesarean section is indicated

• Secondary—may note low serum calcium and blood glucose

OTHER LABORATORY TESTS
Presumptive diagnosis—labor has not started after > 24 hr since the prepartum drop in rectal temperature or serum progesterone < 2 ng/mL for 36 hr.

IMAGING
• Radiography—number and disposition of the fetus(es)
• Ultrasonography—fetal stress and viability

DIAGNOSTIC PROCEDURES
N/A

TREATMENT

• True primary inertia—may not respond to medical treatment; immediate cesarean section indicated of ultrasonography documents fetal stress (HR < or 150 > 250 bpm)
• Medical treatment—contraindicated with obstructive dystocia and (rare) uterine rupture

MEDICATIONS

DRUGS

Oxytocin
• Small doses induce effective uterine contractions.
• Total dose—small breeds, 1–2 IU SC, IM; medium breeds, 3–4 IU SC, IM; large breeds, 5–6 IU SC, IM; may be repeated in 45 min
• No progress after two to three injections—surgery indicated
• May try adding 5–10 IU to 1 L 5% dextrose; administer intravenously at a maintenance dosage rate; if no effective contractions within 10–15 min, surgery indicated; if contractions are induced, wait 1–1.5 hr before performing surgery.

Other
• Calcium—2–10 mL slow IV bolus of 10% calcium gluconate; stop immediately if cardiac arrhythmias are detected.
• Glucose—10–20% dextrose in a slow intravenous infusion

CONTRAINDICATIONS/POSSIBLE INTERACTIONS
• Obstructive dystocia or uterine rupture (rare)
• Overtreatment with oxytocin—induces

nonproductive tetanic contractions
• Prostaglandins—may induce contractions; have not worked in author's experience

FOLLOW-UP

PATIENT MONITORING
• Successful medical treatment—make sure all placentae have passed.
• Evaluate dam for endocrine and reproductive tract disease, which may have been a predisposing factor.

PREVENTION/AVOIDANCE
Proper feeding and adequate exercise—prevent obesity during pregnancy.

POSSIBLE COMPLICATIONS
Death of pups—too much time elapses from time that labor should have started until treatment is initiated.

EXPECTED COURSE AND PROGNOSIS
• Primary—may recur at subsequent parturition dates
• Puppy survival—prognosis good if treatment is instituted on the date of expected parturition

MISCELLANEOUS

AGE-RELATED FACTORS
Relatively old bitches more prone

SEE ALSO
Dystocia

Suggested Reading
Davidson A. Periparturient problems in the bitch. Paper presented at the annual meetings of the Society of Theriogenology, 1997.
Johnston SD. Parturition and dystocia in the bitch. In: Morrow DA, ed., Current therapy in theriogenology 2. Philadelphia: Saunders, 1986:500–501.
Feldman EC, Nelson RW. Canine female reproduction. Canine and feline endocrinology and reproduction. Philadelphia: Saunders, 1987:399–480.
Author Klaas Post
Consulting Editor Sara K. Lyle

UTERINE TUMORS

BASICS

OVERVIEW
• Rare tumors, arising from the uterine smooth muscle and epithelial tissues
• Compose 0.3%–0.4% of tumors in dogs and 0.2%–1.5% in cats
• Dogs—usually benign; leiomyomas, 85%–90%; leiomyosarcoma, 10%; other types (e.g., carcinoma, fibroma, fibrosarcoma, lipoma) rare
• Cats—usually malignant (adenocarcinoma); include leiomyoma, leiomyosarcoma, fibrosarcoma, fibroma, and lipoma
• Metastasis—may occur with malignant forms

SIGNALMENT
• Dogs and cats
• No breed predilection reported
• Middle-aged to old animals usually affected

SIGNS
• Dogs—often clinically silent and discovered incidentally; vaginal discharge; pyometra; abdominal organ compression or secondary metastatic signs
• Cats—vaginal discharge; abnormal estrous cycles; polyuria; polydipsia; vomiting; abdominal distention; signs related to metastatic disease

CAUSES & RISK FACTORS
Intact sexual status

DIAGNOSIS

DIFFERENTIAL DIAGNOSIS
• Pyometra
• Other midcaudal abdominal masses

CBC/BIOCHEMISTRY/URINALYSIS
No specific abnormalities

OTHER LABORATORY TESTS
N/A

IMAGING
• Abdominal radiographs—may detect a midcaudal abdominal mass
• Thoracic radiographs—recommended; assess for metastasis
• Ultrasonography—may reveal uterine mass

DIAGNOSTIC PROCEDURES
• Cytologic evaluation—with abdominal effusion
• Histopathologic examination—necessary for definitive diagnosis

TREATMENT
Ovariohysterectomy—treatment of choice

MEDICATIONS

DRUGS
Doxorubicin, cisplatin, and carboplatin—rational choices for palliation of malignant or metastatic disease

CONTRAINDICATIONS/POSSIBLE INTERACTIONS
• Doxorubicin—carefully monitor patients with underlying cardiac disease; consider pretreatment and serial echocardiograms and ECG
• Cisplatin—do not use in dogs with pre-existing renal disease; do not use without appropriate and concurrent diuresis; do not use in cats (fatal).
• Chemotherapy may be toxic; seek advice if unfamiliar with these agents.

FOLLOW-UP

PATIENT MONITORING
• Malignant—consider thoracic and abdominal radiographs every 3 months.
• CBC, biochemical profile, and urinalysis (if using cisplatin)—perform before each chemotherapy treatment.

EXPECTED COURSE AND PROGNOSIS
Prognosis—excellent (cure) if benign; guarded if malignant; after chemotherapy, unknown

MISCELLANEOUS

ASSOCIATED CONDITIONS
Renal cystadenocarcinoma and nodular dermatofibrosis—reported in German shepherds with uterine leiomyoma

Suggested Reading
Klein MK. Tumors of the female reproductive system. In: Withrow SJ, MacEwen EG, eds. Small animal clinical oncology. 2nd ed. Philadelphia: Saunders, 1996:347–355.
Morrison WB. Cancers of the reproductive tract. In: Morrison WB, ed. Cancer in dogs and cats: medical and surgical management. Baltimore: Williams & Wilkins, 1998: 581–590.

Author Renee Al-Sarraf
Consulting Editor Wallace B. Morrison

BASICS

OVERVIEW
• The most common intraocular tumors in cats
• Usually arise from the anterior iridal surface with extension to the ciliary body and choroid
• Tend to be flat and diffuse, not nodular (unlike intraocular melanomas in dogs)
• Initially has a benign clinical and histologic appearance
• Unique feature—may develop metastatic disease up to several years later
• Metastasize to regional lymph nodes, numerous visceral organs (especially those in the abdominal cavity), lungs, and less commonly, the skeleton

SIGNALMENT
• No sex or breed predisposition
• May affect any age adult cat

SIGNS
Historical Findings
• Iris color change
• Secondary glaucoma leading to mydriasis or buphthalmia

Physical Examination Findings
• Iris surface—hyperpigmented
• Lesions—focal to diffuse; usually flat; slowly progressive; may involve one or both eyes
• Advanced disease—often see pigmented tumor cells in the aqueous; homogenously thickened iris
• May note drainage angle infiltration, which may result in secondary glaucoma

CAUSES & RISK FACTORS
N/A

DIAGNOSIS

DIFFERENTIAL DIAGNOSIS
• Most closely resembles iridal color change that results from chronic anterior uveitis
• Limbal melanomas—benign behavior; tend to be focal, superiorly located, flat to slightly raised limbal masses that do not invade the uveal tract unless they are very large

• Freckles on the surface of the iris that do not appear to change over time—may be benign pigmented lesions; more likely variants of iris melanoma
• Heterochromia irides—congenital, nonprogressive alteration in iridal pigmentation

CBC/BIOCHEMISTRY/URINALYSIS
Normal

OTHER LABORATORY TESTS
N/A

IMAGING
• Thoracic radiographs and abdominal ultrasonography—help determine extent of metastatic disease
• Recommended presurgically and every 6 months after the diagnosis

DIAGNOSTIC PROCEDURES
• Complete ophthalmic examination, including tonometry and gonioscopy
• Fine-needle aspiration of the iridal surface ("vacuuming")—advocated for cytologic confirmation; not beneficial for staging
• Iridal biopsy—may be performed, not beneficial for staging the disease
• Melanoma cells in the iridocorneal angle and ciliary venous plexus (even when small, superficial, freckle-like masses are identified and the eye is enucleated early) suggest that metastasis may occur before the development of invasive melanoma and secondary glaucoma.

TREATMENT
• Enucleation—recommended to lessen the likelihood of metastasis; controversial; often difficult for the owner to accept because the eye is visual and asymptomatic; use a gentle enucleation technique because enucleation has been associated with metastasis in human studies.
• Laser (diode) photoablation—has been used to treat freckle-like lesions with apparent success; no controlled or long-term follow-up studies

MEDICATIONS

DRUGS
N/A

CONTRAINDICATIONS/POSSIBLE INTERACTIONS
N/A

FOLLOW-UP

PATIENT MONITORING
• IOP—quarterly monitoring if surgical options are declined; mild elevation may be treated with carbonic anhydrase inhibitors (e.g., methazolamide at approximately 6 mg PO q12–24h); secondary glaucoma is best controlled by enucleation.
• Common metastasis sites—regional lymph nodes, lungs, and abdominal viscera; monitor periodically.

EXPECTED COURSE AND PROGNOSIS
• One long-term study shows that patients with early iris melanoma have no increased risk of life-threatening metastasis compared to controls, but patients with advanced lesions had dramatically shortened survival times.
• Prognosis—guarded, even with enucleation; metastasis may not become apparent for several years.

MISCELLANEOUS

SYNONYMS
• Iris melanoma
• Diffuse iris melanoma

ABBREVIATION
IOP = intraocular pressure

Sugested Reading
Dubielzig RR. Ocular neoplasia in small animals. Vet Clin North Am Small Anim Pract 1990;20:837–848.
Kalishman JB, Chappell RJ, Flood LA, Dubielzig RR, et al. A matche observational study of survival in cats with enucleation due to diffuse iris melanoma. Vet Ophthalmol. 1998;1:25–29.
Author Denise M. Lindley
Consulting Editor Paul E. Miller

UVEAL MELANOMAS—DOGS

BASICS

OVERVIEW
• Melanomas of the anterior uvea (e.g., iris and ciliary body) and posterior uvea (choroid)
• Most common primary intraocular neoplasm in dogs
• Usually benign and unilateral; often destructive to the eye
• Most often affect the anterior uvea
• Anterior uveal—4% rate of vascular metastasis to lungs and viscera
• Choroidal—do not metastasize

SIGNALMENT
• No breed or sex predilection
• Anterior uveal—average age 8–10 years
• Choroidal melanoma—average age 6.5 years
• Range—2 months to 17 years

SIGNS
Anterior Uveal
• Pigmented scleral or corneal mass
• Pigmented mass visible in the anterior chamber or posterior to the pupillary margin
• Irregular pupil
• Uveitis
• Glaucoma
• Hyphema
• No vision loss—unless mass obstructs the pupil or glaucoma has developed

Choroidal
• Often missed because of tumor location
• Posterior segment mass on funduscopy

CAUSES & RISK FACTORS
• Idiopathic
• Potential transformation of flat, pigmented iris freckles into melanomas

DIAGNOSIS

DIFFERENTIAL DIAGNOSIS
• Nonneoplastic uveal proliferations—iris freckles not raised
• Diffuse iris hyperpigmentation secondary to chronic uveitis
• Uveal cysts—transilluminate and may move freely within the eye, unlike melanomas
• Granulomatous masses
• Ocular perforation with uveal prolapse
• Other ocular neoplastic conditions
• Outward scrolling of pupillary margin owing to uveitis (ectropion uvea)

CBC/BIOCHEMISTRY/URINALYSIS
Usually normal

OTHER LABORATORY TESTS
N/A

IMAGING
Ultrasonography—may help determine the extent of the mass

DIAGNOSTIC PROCEDURES
• Slit-lamp biomicroscopy—determine size and location of mass
• Transillumination of mass
• Tonometry
• Indirect ophthalmoscopy—with or without concomitant scleral indentation
• Gonioscopy—evaluate drainage angle for tumor extension.
• Examination of fine-needle aspirate (infrequent)

PATHOLOGIC FINDINGS
• Usually restricted to the enucleated globe; biopsy not practical
• Two cell types usually seen—plump cells filled with melanin; spindle cells
• Benign appearance and low mitotic index (< 2 mitotic figures per high power field) common
• Mitotic index—most reliable criterion for malignancy; ≥ 4 for clinically malignant tumors
• When submitting eyes for histologic evaluation, request bleached tissue sections and mitotic index.

TREATMENT
• Usually benign, may opt to monitor every 3–6 months
• Counsel the client about enucleation; the procedure often causes the client emotional distress.
• Emphasize that the condition is unilateral, sparing the fellow eye, and that one-eyed animals function very well.
• Indications for enucleation—size of the mass increases rapidly; eye cannot be salvaged; mass spreads diffusely within the eye; visual function significantly impaired; extraocular invasion; secondary complications (e.g., glaucoma, signs of pain, and hemorrhage)
• Enucleation technique—use gentle surgical technique to prevent showering of tumor cells into the vascular circulation; exenterate the entire orbital contents, if extrascleral extension is noted.
• Other surgical treatments—infrequently used; sector iridectomy and iridocyclectomy of discrete small masses
• Laser treatment of small iris tumors—promising, recently developed procedure

MEDICATIONS

DRUGS
N/A

CONTRAINDICATIONS/POSSIBLE INTERACTIONS
N/A

FOLLOW-UP
• Postoperative thoracic and abdominal radiography or ultrasonography—at 6 and 12 months if the mitotic index is high or the patient has extrascleral, vascular, or optic nerve extension
• Evaluate the enucleation site for tumor recurrence.

MISCELLANEOUS

Suggested Reading
Wilcock BP, Peiffer RL. Morphology and behavior of primary ocular melanomas in 91 dogs. Vet Pathol 1986;23:418–424.
Author Terri L. McCalla
Consulting Editor Paul E. Miller

UVEODERMATOLOGIC SYNDROME (VKH)

BASICS

OVERVIEW
• Rare syndrome similar to Vogt-Koyanagi-Harada syndrome in humans
• Considered to be an autoimmune disorder resulting in concurrent granulomatous uveitis and depigmenting dermatitis and rare meningoencephalitis

SIGNALMENT
• Reported in dogs, especially akitas, Samoyeds, and Siberian huskies
• No apparent age or sex predilections

SIGNS
• Sudden-onset uveitis—may be painful and progress to blindness; concurrent or subsequent leukoderma of the nose, lips, and eyelids
• Footpads, scrotum, anus, and the hard palate may also become depigmented.
• Ulcerations may develop.
• Meningoencephalitis—reported (rare)

CAUSES & RISK FACTORS
• Thought to be an autoimmune disease; antiretinal antibodies have been found in affected dogs.
• Exposure to sunlight—exacerbates symptoms

DIAGNOSIS

DIFFERENTIAL DIAGNOSIS
• Immune-mediated skin diseases—pemphigus complex, systemic lupus erythematosus, and discoid lupus erythematosus, pemphigoid
• Neoplasia and numerous other inflammatory and infectious skin diseases that can cause depigmentation
• Skin biopsies, negative ANA titers, and a normal retinal examination—help differentiate these diseases

CBC/BIOCHEMISTRY/URINALYSIS
Usually normal

OTHER LABORATORY TESTS
N/A

IMAGING
N/A

DIAGNOSTIC PROCEDURES
• Biopsy and dermatopathology—best interpreted by a veterinarian experienced in detecting the sometimes subtle differences in pathologic patterns; early lesions have a lichenoid interface pattern with large histiocytes and pronounced pigmentary incontinence; hydropic degeneration of the epidermal basal cell rare
• Evaluate the retina.

TREATMENT
• Aggressive and rapid initiation of immunosuppressive therapy is recommended to prevent formation of posterior synechiae and secondary glaucoma, cataracts, or blindness.
• Retinal examinations—most important means of monitoring progress; improvement in dermatologic lesions may not reflect the retinal pathology.
• Enucleation—sometimes recommended because of pain

MEDICATIONS

DRUGS
• Corticosteroids—initial high doses of prednisone (1.1–2.2mg/kg PO q12–24h) and azathioprine (1.5–2.5 mg/kg PO q24h) recommended; taper dosages and frequencies to every other day for chronic use; some patients may improve with the initial use of prednisone alone, but the potential sequelae of delayed aggressive therapy warrants the additional use of azathioprine.
• Topical or subconjunctival steroids and cycloplegics—may be indicated with anterior uveitis

CONTRAINDICATIONS/POSSIBLE INTERACTIONS
Prednisone and azathioprine—anemia, leukopenia, thrombocytopenia, high serum alkaline phosphatase levels, vomiting, and pancreatitis; conduct biweekly serum chemistries and CBCs, including platelet counts, initially; decrease after the condition has stabilized and the dose and frequency have been tapered.

FOLLOW-UP
• Weekly or biweekly examinations including retinal evaluations—recommended initially for monitoring side effects associated with therapeutics; retinal examinations are important because improvement in dermatologic lesions may not indicate improvement in the retinal lesions.
• Azathioprine may be discontinued after a few months of therapy; prednisone may be necessary indefinitely.
• Iatrogenic hyperadrenocorticism—often a result of the steroid therapy

MISCELLANEOUS

ABBREVIATION
ANA = antinuclear antibody

Suggested Reading
Scott DW, Miller WH, Griffen CE. Small animal dermatology. 5th ed. Philadelphia: Saunders, 1995.
Author Dunbar Gram
Consulting Editor Karen Helton Rhodes

VACCINE-ASSOCIATED SARCOMA

BASICS

OVERVIEW
• Cats—vaccination may induce development of sarcoma (primarily fibrosarcoma) at the injection site, primarily in the muscle, skin, and subcutaneous tissues; malignant fibrous histiocytoma, osteosarcoma, rhabdomyosarcoma, and chondrosarcoma also associated
• FeLV and rabies vaccines—most common
• Interval from vaccination to tumor development—may be as short as several months
• Metastasis common
• Fibrosarcoma—prevalence in cats unknown; estimated at 20/100,000 cats

SIGNALMENT
Recognized only in cats

SIGNS
Firm, painless, subcutaneous swelling located at a previous vaccination site

CAUSES & RISK FACTORS
• Unknown; aluminum hydroxide, an adjuvant in many vaccines, suggested as a possibility
• Pathogenesis may be related to the degree of vaccine-induced inflammation.
• Exogenous retroviruses, FeLV, and feline sarcoma virus—not been isolated from tumors
• Vaccination for FeLV or rabies
• Risk from a single FeLV or rabies vaccination in the cervical or interscapular region—about 1.5 times higher than not receiving a vaccine at that site
• Risk from two vaccinations—approximately 2.3 times higher than not receiving a vaccine at that site
• Risk from three to four vaccinations—approximately 2.8 times higher
• Risk—higher with multidose vials
• No compelling evidence of difference in risk

between univalent and polyvalent vaccines; however, it appears prudent to vaccinate cats at different sites.
• No difference in risk among manufacturers has been observed.

DIAGNOSIS

DIFFERENTIAL DIAGNOSIS
• Vaccine-associated Arthus reaction
• Subcutaneous abscess
• Other benign or malignant tumors

CBC/BIOCHEMISTRY/URINALYSIS
Normal

OTHER LABORATORY TESTS
N/A

IMAGING
Regional and thoracic radiography—determine extent of disease and lung metastasis

OTHER DIAGNOSTIC PROCEDURES
• Cytologic examination of aspirate—suggests mesenchymal neoplasia
• Biopsy—necessary for definitive diagnosis

TREATMENT
• Wide surgical resection—necessary
• Amputation of affected limb—may be necessary
• Skip metastasis (tumor nodules separate from the primary tumor located in the same tissue compartment but outside the reactive/inflammatory zone surrounding the primary tumor)—may occur
• Radiotherapy—indicated with incomplete surgical removal
• Chemotherapy—may provide palliation for nonresectable tumors
• Inform owners of the benefits and risks of vaccinations.

MEDICATIONS

DRUGS
• No specific regimens evaluated
• A 21-day protocol—may be useful: doxorubicin (20 mg/m² IV) on day 0 and cyclophosphamide (50 mg/m² PO) on days 3, 4, 5, and 6; repeat every 21 days for five cycles; if no response after two cycles, tumor considered chemotherapy resistant

CONTRAINDICATIONS/POSSIBLE INTERACTIONS
N/A

FOLLOW-UP
• Evaluate monthly for the first 3 months after surgical resection; then every 3 months.
• CBC and platelet count—before each chemotherapy treatment

MISCELLANEOUS
Administer different vaccines at different sites; administer at sites amenable to surgical resection (e.g., hind limb) in case neoplasm develops.

ABBREVIATION
FeLV = feline leukemia virus

Suggested Reading
Kass PH, Barnes WG, Spangler WL, et al. Epidemiologic evidence for a causal relation between vaccination and fibrosarcoma tumorigenesis in cats. J Am Vet Med Assoc 1993;203:396–405.
Kass PH. Epidemiologic issues in the study of vaccine-associated sarcomas in cats. Feline Pract 1996;24:33.
Author James P. Thompson
Consulting Editor Wallace B. Morrison

Table 1

Abbreviated Vaccine-associated Sarcoma Task Force Recommendations

• Proceed with vaccine administration only after considering medical significance and zoonotic potential of the infectious agent, the patient's exposure risk, and germane legal requirements.
• Use of vaccines packaged in single-dose vials is encouraged.
• Report the occurrence of sarcoma or other adverse reaction to the vaccine manufacturer and to the *United States Pharmacopeia* (USP); information about the USP and a sample submission form can be found in J Am Vet Med Assoc 1996;208:361–363 (for additional reporting forms, call 800-487-7776).
• Standardize intrapractice vaccination protocols and document injection location, vaccine type, serial number, and manufacturer in the patient's medical record.
• Panleukopenia, feline herpesvirus type 1, and feline calicivirus (± *Chlamydia*) vaccines should be administered on the right shoulder and according to manufacturer's recommendations.
• Vaccines containing rabies antigen (plus any other antigen) should be administered on the right hind limb as distally as possible and according to manufacturer's recommendations.
• Vaccines containing FeLV antigen (plus any other antigen except rabies) should be administered on the left hind limb as distally as possible and according to manufacturer's recommendations.
• Record injection sites of other medications.

VAGINAL HYPERPLASIA AND PROLAPSE

BASICS

OVERVIEW
• Protrusion of spherical or donut-shaped mass from vulva during proestrus or estrus
• Type I—slight eversion of the vaginal floor but no protrusion through the vulva
• Type II—vaginal tissue prolapses through the vulvar opening
• Type III—donut-shaped eversion of the entire vaginal wall, including the urethral orifice, which can be seen ventrally on the prolapsed tissue
• Exaggerated response of vaginal mucosa to estrogen
• Despite the name, the change seen histopathologically is consistent with edema rather than hyperplasia or hypertrophy.
• Severe prolapse—may affect the urethra and prevent normal urination

SIGNALMENT
• Young (< 3 years of age), large-breed bitches
• Predisposed breeds—Labrador and Chesapeake Bay retrievers; boxers; bulldogs; mastiffs; German shepherds; St. Bernards; Airedale terriers; Weimeraners; springer spaniels; Walker hound
• Hereditary component probable

SIGNS

Historical Findings
• Onset of proestrus or estrus—rarely seen at parturition
• Licking of vulvar area
• Failure to allow copulation
• Dysuria
• Previous occurrence

Physical Examination Findings
• Protrusion of round, tongue-shaped, or donut-shaped tissue mass from the vulva
• Vaginal examination—locate lumen and urethral orifice; types I and II: lumen is dorsal to the prolapse; type III: lumen is central to the prolapse; urethral orifice is ventral to the prolapse with all three types.
• Tissue may be dry or necrotic

CAUSES & RISK FACTORS
• Estrogen stimulation
• Genetic predisposition

DIAGNOSIS

DIFFERENTIAL DIAGNOSIS
• Vaginal polyp—differentiated by vaginal examination
• Vaginal neoplasia—transmissible venerel tumor and leiomyoma; differentiated by signalment, stage of cycle, and vaginal examination

CBC/BIOCHEMISTRY/URINALYSIS
N/A

OTHER LABORATORY TESTS
N/A

IMAGING
N/A

DIAGNOSTIC PROCEDURES
Biospsy (old bitch)—differentiate from neoplasia

TREATMENT
• Outpatient; unless urethral obstruction
• Breeding—possible by artificial insemination
• Prolapsed tissue—keep clean and lubricated with sterile water-soluble lubricant.
• Elizabethan collar and clean indoor environment—minimize tissue trauma.
• Instruct client to monitor patient's ability to urinate.
• Regression—usually begins in late estrus; should be resolved during early diestrus
• Recurrence rate—66% at next cycle
• Ovariohysterectomy—prevents recurrence; may hasten resolution
• Severe condition—requires surgical reduction or resection; if possible, perform when the mass is beginning to regress; 25% recurrence at next cycle after surgery

MEDICATIONS

DRUGS
GnRH (2.2 µg/kg IM) or hCG (1000 IU IM)—if breeding not planned that cycle; may hasten ovulation and resolution; not effective if given after ovulation

CONTRAINDICATIONS/POSSIBLE INTERACTIONS
Avoid progestational drugs, because they can induce pyometra.

FOLLOW-UP

Patient Monitoring
Monitor health of prolapsed tissue and the ability to urinate

PREVENTION/AVOIDANCE
Ovariohysterectomy—recommended owing to genetic component and likelihood of recurrence

POSSIBLE COMPLICATIONS
Type III—may affect urethra and prevent normal urination

EXPECTED COURSE AND PROGNOSIS
• Medical treatment—prognosis for recovery good, except with urethra involvement
• Surgical intervention for type III—prognosis good

MISCELLANEOUS

ABBREVIATIONS
• GnRH = gonadotropin-releasing hormone
• hCG = human chorionic gonadotropin

Suggested Reading
Johnston SD. Vaginal prolapse. In: Kirk RW, ed. Current veterinary therapy X. Philadelphia: Saunders, 1989:1302–1305.
Wykes PM. Disease of the vagina and vulva in the bitch. In: Morrow DA, ed. Current therapy in theriogenology 2. Philadelphia: Saunders, 1986:476–481.
Author Joni L. Freshman
Consulting Editor Sara K. Lyle

VAGINAL MALFORMATIONS AND ACQUIRED LESIONS

BASICS

DEFINITION
• Altered anatomic architecture owing to congenital anomalies (imperforate hymen, dorsoventral septum, hymenal constriction, and cysts) and acquired conditions (vaginal hyperplasia, foreign bodies, strictures, adhesions, and neoplasia)

PATHOPHYSIOLOGY
Congenital
• Normal embryological development—the paired paramesonephric (müllerian) ducts fuse to form the uterine body, cervix, and vagina; urogenital sinus forms the vestibule, urethra, and urinary bladder; hymen (composed of the epithelial linings of the paramesonephric ducts and urogenital sinus and an interposed layer of mesoderm) normally disappears by birth
• Errors during embryonic development—imperforate hymens; dorsoventral septae, hymenal constrictions (including vestibulo-vaginal stenoses); cysts
Acquired
• Vaginal scarring—response to trauma or inflammation; with mature scarring, may note adhesions or strictures, which narrow the diameter of the vagina
• Vaginal hyperplasia—result of an exaggerated response of the vaginal mucosa to estrogen; effect produced is edema rather than hyperplasia or hypertrophy.
• Neoplastic processes—most common: extraluminal leiomyoma; usually old patients; no effect of ovarian status on occurrence

SYSTEMS AFFECTED
• Reproductive—principal effect: interference with natural mating and whelping; frequent concurrent problem: vaginitis
• Renal/Urologic—ascending urinary tract infections not uncommon; may note urinary incontinence in conjunction with congenital malformations of the hymenal area (inter-relationship not understood)
• Skin/Exocrine—usually see perivulvar dermatitis with secondary vaginitis or urinary incontinence

GENETICS
Congenital—heritable component may be suspected; no direct evidence

INCIDENCE/PREVALENCE
• Incidence (congenital)—unknown; conditions may be asymptomatic, especially if the female is never used for breeding.
• Prevalence (vaginal septa)—in one study, reported as 0.03% of all cases seen

SIGNALMENT
Breed Predilections
• Congenital—none identified

• Vaginal hyperplasia—large breeds more prone

Mean Age and Range
• Congenital lesion (e.g., imperforate hymen, stenosis, septa)—young (< 2 years of age) intact or spayed females
• Vaginal hyperplasia—young (< 2 years of age) intact females
• Acquired lesion (adhesions and strictures)—postpubertal females of any age
• Neoplasia—mean age, 10 years; ovarian status has no effect.

SIGNS
Historical Findings
• Vaginal discharge
• Excessive licking of vulva
• Frequent or inappropriate urination
• Stranguria or dyschezia
• Urinary incontinence
• Attractive to males
• Refuses mating
• Mass at vulvar labia

Physical Examination Findings
• Usually normal
• Evidence of vaginal discharge or perivulvar dermatitis common
• Hypoplastic vulva occasionally seen

CAUSES
• Congenital
• Inflammatory
• Hormonal
• Traumatic
• Neoplastic

RISK FACTORS
N/A

DIAGNOSIS

DIFFERENTIAL DIAGNOSIS
• Vaginitis—concurrent with many malformations; differentiated by vaginoscopy and positive contrast vaginography
• Urinary tract infection—differentiated by vaginal cytology and concurrent urinalysis on a sample collected by cystocentesis
• Pyometra—differentiated by CBC, biochemistry profiles, and abdominal ultrasonography

CBC/BIOCHEMISTRY/URINALYSIS
• CBC and biochemistry—usually normal
• Urinalysis—may show evidence of a secondary ascending urinary tract infection

OTHER LABORATORY TESTS
N/A

IMAGING
Positive-contrast Vaginography
• Defines vaginal vault to the cervix, urethra, cranial vestibule, and urinary bladder

• Defines the cervical canal and uterine lumen in intact patient in estrus
• Identifies strictures, septa, persistent hymens, masses, rectovaginal fistulas, urethrovaginal fistulas, vaginal rupture, and diverticular
• Patients should fast for 24 hr; give enema 2 hr before the procedure.
• Place patient under sedation or general anesthesia.
• Pass a balloon-tipped Foley catheter in the vestibule; inflate balloon; infuse aqueous iodinated contrast media (1 mL/kg); avoid overdistention and underdistention.
• Urinary incontinence—may require excretory urography to rule out ectopic ureters or an intrapelvically positioned bladder neck

Abdominal Ultrasonography
• Much of the vagina is not accessible owing to the bony pelvis
• Cranial vaginal masses—may occasionally be imaged
• Aid visualization by infusing saline into the vagina before examination.

DIAGNOSTIC PROCEDURES
• Order in which procedures are performed is important; they are listed here in the recommended order.
• Vaginal culture—identify secondary infections; guarded Culturette (Acculushure, Accu-Med) recommended to avoid contamination from the vestibule and caudal vagina (see Vaginal Discharge; Vaginitis)
• Vaginal cytology—identify stage of the estrous cycle; reveal inflammatory or neoplastic cells (see Breeding, Timing)
• Digital examination of the vestibule and caudal vagina—measure the diameter; identify caudal strictures or masses; occasionally requires sedation; note the size and conformation of the vulva; patient standing with abdomen supported; sedation or anesthesia may be required.
• Vaginoscopy—identify strictures, adhesions, septa, diverticula, masses, and foreign bodies; may use a variety of specula; a long (16–20 cm), hollow, rigid type (e.g., infant proctoscope) with either a fiberoptic or halogen light source recommended; match the speculum's diameter to size of the patient; postcervical fold normal (obscures visualization of the external os of the cervix)
• Imaging—when results of previous procedures suggest an anatomic abnormality; vaginography and/or ultrasonography

PATHOLOGIC FINDINGS
Congenital
• Imperforate hymen—thin fenestrated membrane, dorsoventral band(s), or a thick membrane at the vestibulovaginal junction;

simplest, most common defect; remainder of the genital tract normal
• Dorsoventral septum—oriented dorsoventrally in the vagina, cranial to the vestibulovaginal junction; may note a double cervix (most common variant), double vagina, or divided uterine fundus (rare)
• Hymenal constriction, vaginal hypoplasia, or vaginal aplasia—moderate to severe constriction at the vestibulovaginal junction (also called vestibulovaginal stenosis); vagina, cervix, uterus, vulva may be absent or hypoplastoc

Acquired
• Strictures and adhesions—may be identified anywhere in the vagina or vestibule; result of prior trauma and/or inflammation; persistent vaginitis, refusal to mate, dystocia, or problems with micturition common
• Vaginal hyperplasia and prolapse
• Vaginal neoplasia—usually leiomyoma; usually extraluminal in the wall of the vestibule; leiomyosarcomas, transmissible venereal tumors, lipomas, mast cell tumors, epidermoid carcinomas, squamous cell carcinomas, fibromas, fibrosarcomas, and invasive urinary tract carcinomas reported
• Foreign bodies—plant material, sticks, and swabs; occasionally found

TREATMENT

APPROPRIATE HEALTH CARE
• Usually outpatient, until nature of the defect is ascertained
• Inpatient—for positive contrast vaginography

NURSING CARE
Manual dilation—digitally or with a smooth rigid object; may attempt in patients that have an imperforate hymen or mild vestibulovaginal stenosis; may be performed in a sedated patient gradually over a course of several treatments; may be performed in an anesthetized patient at one time to maximal dilation; variable success; typically leads to reduction, but not complete resolution, of clinical signs

ACTIVITY
N/A

DIET
N/A

CLIENT EDUCATION
N/A

SURGICAL CONSIDERATIONS
• Resection, transection, excision—many minor congenital (e.g., imperforate hymen, small dorsoventral septa) and acquired lesions (small strictures or adhesions in the caudal portion of the vagina or masses)
• Episiotomy—usually required for adequate surgical access

• T-shaped vaginoplasty—described for vestibulovaginal stenoses; resection appears to provide superior results.
• Transendoscopic laser ablation—one report for correcting a dorsoventral septum in an English bulldog that subsequently bred and delivered four pups vaginally
• Ovariohysterectomy—patient has no breeding value; exhibits signs only during estrus
• Vaginal ablation (vaginectomy cranial to the external urethral orifice) and ovariohysterectomy—patient has no breeding value; concurrent severe, refractory vaginitis at all stages of the estrous cycle

MEDICATIONS

DRUGS OF CHOICE
• Concurrent vaginitis—common; usually resolves with correction of the anatomic defect; for severe condition, hasten resolution with appropriate local and antibiotic therapy (see Vaginitis).
• Stenotic lesions—corticosteroids (prednisone: 1 mg/kg PO q24h) used in conjunction with manual dilation in an attempt to prevent recurrence; high recurrence rates with or without steroids

CONTRAINDICATIONS
N/A

PRECAUTIONS
N/A

POSSIBLE INTERACTIONS
N/A

ALTERNATIVE DRUGS
N/A

FOLLOW-UP

PATIENT MONITORING
N/A

PREVENTION/AVOIDANCE
Congenital lesions—possibly inherited, but not confirmed; for a familial line with a high number of affected individuals, recommend sterilization of affected individuals and their parents.

POSSIBLE COMPLICATIONS
• Dystocia, urinary tract infections, incontinence, and vaginitis—with vaginal malformations; with patients that fail to respond to treatment
• Strictures and adhesions—may be postoperative complications of surgical procedures aimed at correcting abnormalities

EXPECTED COURSE AND PROGNOSIS
• Depend on the severity of the lesion and the

degree of inflammation after treatment
• Prognosis after treatment for imperforate hymens, short dorsoventral bands, or caudal strictures or adhesions—fair to good for improvement of clinical signs; fair to guarded for complete resolution of signs and normal fertility
• Prognosis for hymenal constrictions, vaginal hypoplasia or severe cranial strictures or adhesions—guarded to poor for complete resolution of signs and normal fertility; with concurrent severe vaginitis, the best recommendation is vaginal ablation.

MISCELLANEOUS

ASSOCIATED CONDITIONS
• Urinary tract infections
• Vaginitis
• Urinary incontinence

AGE-RELATED FACTORS
• Congenital—more likely in young bitches of any ovarian status
• Vaginal hyperplasia—more likely in young intact bitches
• Neoplasia of the vagina or vestibule—more likely in old bitches of any ovarian status

ZOONOTIC POTENTIAL
N/A

PREGNANCY
• Some patients may be bred by artificial insemination; the possibility for a vaginal delivery is unlikely.
• Warn owner that an elective cesarean section would probably be required.

SEE ALSO
• Transmissible Venereal Tumor
• Vaginal Discharge
• Vaginal Hyperplasia and Prolapse
• Vaginitis

Suggested Reading
Holt PE, Sayle B. Congenital vestibulo-vaginal stenosis in the bitch. J Small Anim Pract 1981;22:67–75.
Kyles AE, Vaden S, Hardie EM, Stone EA. Vestibulovaginal stenosis in dogs: 18 cases (1987–1995). J Am Vet Med Assoc 1996;209:1889–1893.
Root MV, Johnston SD, Johnston GR. Vaginal septa in dogs: 15 cases (1983–1992) J Am Vet Med Assoc 1995;206:56–58.
Wykes PM, Soderberg SF. Disorders of the canine vagina. In: Morgan RV, ed., Handbook of small animal practice. 2nd ed. New York: Churchill Livingstone, 1992:661–666.

Authors Bruce E. Eilts and Margaret V. Root Kustritz
Consulting Editor Sara K. Lyle

VAGINAL TUMORS

BASICS

OVERVIEW
• Second most common reproductive tumor, composing 2.4%–3.0% of all tumors in dogs
• Dogs—86% benign smooth muscle tumors (e.g., leiomyoma, fibroleiomyoma, and fibroma); lipoma, transmissible venereal tumor, mast cell tumor, squamous cell carcinoma, leiomyosarcoma, hemangiosarcoma, osteosarcoma, or extension of primary urinary tract carcinomas also reported
• Cats—extremely rare; usually of smooth muscle origin
• Hormonal influence—speculated to be involved in the etiopathogenesis

SIGNALMENT
• Dogs—mean age, 10.2–11.2 years
• Cats—no data available

SIGNS

Dogs
• Extraluminal—slow-growing perineal mass; vulvar discharge; dysuria; pollakiuria; vulvar licking; dystocia
• Intraluminal—mass protruding from the vulva (often at estrus); vulvar discharge; stranguria; dysuria; tenesmus

Cats
• Firm mass
• Constipation

CAUSES & RISK FACTORS
• Intact sexual status
• Nulliparous bitches more commonly affected

DIAGNOSIS

DIFFERENTIAL DIAGNOSIS
• Vaginal prolapse
• Urethral neoplasia
• Uterine prolapse
• Clitoral hypertrophy
• Vaginal polyp
• Vaginal abscess
• Vaginal hematoma

CBC/BIOCHEMISTRY/URINALYSIS
No consistent abnormalities

OTHER LABORATORY TESTS
N/A

IMAGING
• Abdominal radiography—may detect cranial extension of a mass
• Ultrasonography, vaginography, and urethrocystography—may help delineate mass

DIAGNOSTIC PROCEDURES
• Vaginoscopy with cytologic examination of an aspirate—may help determine cell type
• Histopathologic examination—often necessary for definitive diagnosis

PATHOLOGIC FINDINGS
• Intraluminal—vestibular wall; protruding into the vulva; may occur singularly or as multiple masses
• Extraluminal—vestibular roof; causing a bulging of the perineum

TREATMENT
• Surgical excision and concurrent ovariohysterectomy—treatment of choice
• Postoperative radiotherapy—may be of benefit for sarcoma
• Laser surgery with radiotherapy—reported anecdotally

MEDICATIONS

DRUGS
• Postoperative therapy—no standard established
• Doxorubicin, cisplatin, or carboplatin—rational choice to palliate malignant or metastatic disease

CONTRAINDICATIONS/POSSIBLE INTERACTIONS
• Doxorubicin—carefully monitor with underlying cardiac disease; consider pretreatment and serial echocardiograms and ECG
• Cisplatin—do not use in cats (fatal); do not use in dogs with renal disease; always use appropriate and concurrent diuresis.
• Chemotherapy may be toxic; seek advice if you are unfamiliar with chemotherapeutic drugs.

FOLLOW-UP

PATIENT MONITORING
• Thoracic and abdominal radiographs—consider every 3 months if tumor is malignant.
• CBC (doxorubicin, cisplatin, carboplatin), biochemical profile (cisplatin), urinalysis (cisplatin)—perform before each chemotherapy treatment

EXPECTED OUTCOME AND PROGNOSIS
• Prognosis—good with complete excision; guarded if incomplete excision; poor with metastatic disease; poor with carcinoma or squamous cell tumor
• Recurrence—15% (leiomyoma) without concurrent ovariohysterectomy

MISCELLANEOUS
• Dogs—may be an incidental finding at necropsy
• Cats—reported concurrent cystic ovaries and mammary gland adenocarcinoma

Suggested Reading
Manithaiudom K, Johnston SD. Clinical approach to vaginal/vestibular masses in the bitch. Vet Clin North Am Small Anim Pract 1991;21:509–521.
Morrison WB. Cancers of the reproductive tract. In: Morrison WB, ed. Cancer in dogs and cats: medical and surgical management. Baltimore, Williams & Wilkins, 1998: 581–590.
Author Renee Al-Sarraf
Consulting Editor Wallace B. Morrison

VAGINITIS

BASICS

DEFINITION
Inflammation of the vagina or vestibule

PATHOPHYSIOLOGY
• Primary bacterial or viral—not common
• Generally involves a predisposing factor—anomaly; chemical irritation; neoplasia; vaginal trauma; foreign body
• Other sources of discharge—uterus; clitoris; perivulvar skin; urinary tract

SYSTEMS AFFECTED
Reproductive

GENETICS
N/A

INCIDENCE/PREVALENCE
• Not common
• Reported as 7 in 1000 cases in a 5-year period

GEOGRAPHIC DISTRIBUTION
N/A

SIGNALMENT
Species
Primarily dogs

Breed Predilections
None

Mean Age and Range
• Anomalies and prepubertal vaginitis—suspect in prepubertal bitches
• May occur at any age, in any breed, or with any ovarian status

Predominant Sex
N/A

SIGNS
Historical Findings
• Discharge from the vulva
• Pollakiuria
• Vaginal licking
• Spotting
• Scooting
• Attracting males

Physical Examination Findings
• Discharge from the vagina
• Possibly, inflamed vulva and vagina

CAUSES
• Prepubertal vagina*
• Foreign bodies*
• Urinary tract infections
• Vaginal trauma

• Urine or feces contamination in patients with congenital anomaly
• May be incited by acquired problems
• Urine contamination in patients with ectopic ureters
• Incontinence owing to hypoestrogenism
• Vaginal neoplasia—transmissible venereal tumor; leiomyoma
• Bacterial—*Pasteurella; Streptococcus; E. coli; Pseudomonas; Mycoplasma; Chlamydia; Brucella canis*
• Viral—herpes
• Vaginal hematoma
• Vaginal abscess
• Exogenous androgens
• Vestibulovaginal stricture
• Zinc toxicity reported

RISK FACTORS
• Clitoral hypertrophy caused by exogenous androgens
• Alteration of normal vaginal bacterial flora owing to administration of prophylactic antibiotics that allow overgrowth of pathogenic species
• Anomalies in prepubertal bitches

DIAGNOSIS

DIFFERENTIAL DIAGNOSES
• History and signalment—establish risk of anomaly; possibility of prepubertal vaginitis
• Normal serosanguinous discharge—during proestrus; sometimes continues into estrus
• Slight purulent exudate—may be normal in early diestrus; usually see neutrophils on cytologic examination
• Normal postpartum discharge—for up to 6–8 weeks; odorless, dark brown or bloody discharge; substantial amounts are normal for up to 4 weeks.
• Subinvolution of the placental sites—when discharge lasts longer than 6–8 weeks postpartum
• Urinary tract infection
• Foreign body
• Pyometra
• Metritis
• Retained placentas
• Clitoral hypertrophy
• Embryonic or fetal death
• Urine or feces contamination owing to congenital anomaly or acquired condition
• Perivulvar dermatitis—may appear as vaginal discharge
• Urine contamination with ectopic ureter

• Incontinence owing to hypoestrogenism
• Normal mucus discharge during pregnancy
• Vaginal neoplasia—transmissible venereal tumor; leiomyoma
• Vaginal trauma
• Vaginal hematoma
• Vaginal abscess
• Ovarian neoplasia
• Zinc toxicity

CBC/BIOCHEMISTRY/URINALYSIS
• Routine laboratory tests usually within normal limits
• Voided urine samples—may note inflammatory cells

OTHER LABORATORY TESTS
• Serum progesterone concentration—determines if patient is in diestrus; slight diestrual discharge may be normal; high concentration increases possibility of pyometra or pregnancy.
• Rapid slide agglutination test—help rule out *Brucella canis*

IMAGING
• Contrast radiography of the vagina—rule out vaginal neoplasia; foreign body; vestibulovaginal, urethrovaginal, and rectovaginal stricture
• Ultrasonography—aid in identifying some intraluminal vaginal masses; distend the vagina with saline to greatly enhance visualization.

DIAGNOSTIC PROCEDURES
Vaginal Culture
• Guarded Culturette
• Perform before any other vaginal procedure.
• Only 5% of normal bitches that were cultured repeatedly had negative cultures.
• Most common vaginal isolates from normal and infertile bitches—*Pasteurella; Streptococcus*
• Less common isolates—*E. coli; Staphylococcus*
• Most common mixed culture—*Pasteurella, Streptococcus,* and *E. coli*
• Most common pure culture—*Pasteurella*
• More organisms usually grow during estrus than at other stages of the estrous cycle, but the types do not change.

Vaginal Cytologic Examination
• Determine if the discharge is pus, blood, or feces
• Septic inflammation—seen in older patients
• Extent of cornification—determines the estrogen influence; helps establish if the patient is in proestrus or estrus and if the discharge is normal

Vaginoscopy
• Detect an anomaly, band, mass, foreign body, hematoma, abscess, or inflamed vagina or vestibule
• Endoscope—may be needed to see anterior vagina
• Cannot normally see cervix by endoscopy, except possibly in large dogs
• Determine the most cranial origin of the discharge—differentiate uterus from vaginal and vestibular sources

Other
• Digital examination of the vagina—identify vaginal anomalies such as bands, strictures, or persistent hymen; palpate tumors
• Biopsy of vaginal masses—rule out neoplasia.

PATHOLOGIC FINDINGS
N/A

 TREATMENT

APPROPRIATE HEALTH CARE
• Usually outpatients
• Inpatient—surgical management of anatomic anomalies, foreign bodies, or neoplasia

NURSING CARE
N/A

ACTIVITY
Not altered

DIET
Not altered

CLIENT EDUCATION
• Inform client that prepubertal vaginitis normally resolves after the first estrus and that antibiotic therapy is not needed.
• Inform client that vaginitis in adults is often associated with a correctable predisposing factor.
• Discuss ovariohysterectomy and isolation of patients infected with *B. canis.*
• Inform client that exogenous androgens and estrogens must be removed.

SURGICAL CONSIDERATIONS
• Remove or treat any inciting causes—foreign body; neoplasia; anomaly
• Vaginectomy—has been used in refractory patients

 MEDICATIONS

DRUGS OF CHOICE
Primary
• Appropriate systemic antibiotics—normally eradicates susceptible bacteria within 24 hr
• Vaginal douches—0.05% chlorhexidine, 0.5% povidone-iodine, or 0.2% nitrofurazone; twice daily until the discharge resolves; reported to be beneficial
Prepubertal
• Estrus induction—may be helpful; long-term effects not documented
• DES—5 mg PO q24h for up to 7 days; count day 1 of bleeding as day 1 of induced cycle; continue treatment for an additional 2 days; may help persistent condition in patients that were spayed before puberty

CONTRAINDICATIONS
Many antibiotics are contraindicated during pregnancy.

PRECAUTIONS
Estrogens given during diestrus increase the chance of pyometra.

POSSIBLE INTERACTIONS
• Exogenous estrogen administered during diestrus
• Exogenous androgen

ALTERNATIVE DRUGS
Prepubertal—estrus induction with DES may help refractory cases; long-term effects not documented

 FOLLOW-UP

PATIENT MONITORING
• Prepubertal patients—re-examine after the first estrus or physical maturity.
• Mature patients with no predisposing factors—re-examine after a 14-day course of antibiotics.
• If condition persists—re-evaluate for an underlying or another cause; perform another vaginal bacterial culture and sensitivity test

PREVENTION/AVOIDANCE
Because some cases become refractory after the patient is spayed, there may be some rationale for delaying ovariohysterectomy until after the first estrus in prepubertal patients with a chronic condition

POSSIBLE COMPLICATIONS
N/A

EXPECTED COURSE AND PROGNOSIS
• Prepubertal—normally resolves after the first estrus
• Adults—usually resolves if the causative factor is removed; antibiotic therapy and vaginal douches may hasten recovery of uncomplicated chronic cases to within 2 weeks.

 MISCELLANEOUS

ASSOCIATED CONDITIONS
N/A

AGE-RELATED FACTORS
Puppies—prepubertal vaginitis, anomalies, and ectopic ureters

ZOONOTIC POTENTIAL
B. canis—rare in patients with vaginitis, but should be considered

PREGNANCY
Many antibiotics are contraindicated during pregnancy.

SEE ALSO
See Causes

ABBREVIATION
DES = diethylstilbestrol

Suggested Reading
Bjurström L, Linde-Forsberg C. Long-term study of aerobic bacteria of the genital tract in breeding bitches. Am J Vet Res 1992;53:665–669.
Holt PE, Sayle, B. Congenital vestibulovaginal stenosis in the bitch. J Small Anim Prac 1988;22:67–75.
Johnson CA. Diagnosis and treatment of chronic vaginitis in the bitch. Vet Clin North Am Small Anim Prac 1991;21:523–531.
Strom B, Linde-Forsberg C. Effects of ampicillin and trimethoprim-sulfamethoxazole on the vaginal bacterial-flora of bitches. Am J Vet Res 1993;54:891–896.
van Duijkeren E. Significance of the vaginal bacterial flora in the bitch: a review. Vet Rec 1992;131:367–369.
Wykes PM, Soderberg SF. Disorders of the canine vagina. In: Morgan RV, ed. Handbook of small animal practice. 2nd ed. New York: Churchill Livingstone, 1992:661–666.
Author Bruce E. Eilts
Consulting Editor Sara K. Lyle

DISEASES

VASCULITIS, CUTANEOUS

 BASICS

OVERVIEW
• An inflammation of blood vessels with a neutrophilic (leukocytoclastic/nonleukocyto-clastic), lymphocytic, rarely eosinophilic, granulomatous, or mixed cell types
• Pathomechanisms—type III (immune complex) and type I (immediate) reactions

SIGNALMENT
• Any age, breed, or sex may be affected.
• Dachshunds and rottweilers may be predisposed.
• Varies depending on cause

SIGNS
• Palpable purpura
• Hemorrhagic bullae
• Necrosis and "punched-out" ulcers
• Affects the extremities (paws, pinnae, lips, tail and oral mucosa) and may be painful
• Anorexia, depression, pyrexia, pitting edema of the extremities, polyarthropathy, and myopathy—depend on the underlying cause

CAUSES & RISK FACTORS
• Systemic lupus erythematosus
• Cold agglutinin disease
• Frostbite
• Disseminated intravascular coagulopathy
• Lymphoreticular neoplasia
• Drug reactions
• Postvaccine reaction
• Spider bites
• Immune-mediated disease
• Erythema nodosum–like panniculitis
• Rheumatoid arthritis
• Rocky Mountain spotted fever
• Staphylococcal hypersensitivity

 DIAGNOSIS

DIFFERENTIAL DIAGNOSIS
• See Causes & Risk Factors
• Ear margin seborrhea, chemical and thermal burns, toxic epidermal necrolysis, erythema multiforme, and sepsis—biopsy representative lesions for histopathologic examination

CBC/BIOCHEMISTRY/URINALYSIS
Usually normal

OTHER LABORATORY TESTS
• Sepsis, disseminated intravascular coagulation, systemic lupus erythematosus, Rocky Mountain spotted fever, and rheumatoid arthritis—abnormalities may be noted
• Consider serologic testing for parasitic and infectious disease in high-risk areas.
• Consider immunodiagnostics—ANA titer, Coombs test and cold agglutinin tests

IMAGING
N/A

DIAGNOSTIC PROCEDURES
• Skin scrapings—possible demodicosis (with secondary sepsis)
• Biopsy of early lesion—submit to a dermatopathologist; findings depend on the underlying cause, but usually include neutrophilic (leukocytoclastic/nonleukocyto-clastic), lymphocytic, eosinophilic, or granulomatous, mixed cells in and around the vessels; vascular necrosis and fibrin thrombi may be prominent; perivascular hemorrhage and edema may occur.
• Vasculitis—preform representative cultures (blood, urine, skin, etc.) if CBC, chemistry screen, or urinalysis reveal systemic disease

 TREATMENT

• Underlying disease—first priority in clinical management
• No systemic abnormalities—treat as out-patient with no alterations in food or water intake
• Systemic disease—inpatient care must be recommended
• Inform owner that the prognosis is guarded until a cause is found; prognosis is based on the cause.

 MEDICATIONS

DRUGS
• First line of therapy while awaiting histo-pathology results, if no drug reaction is suspected—antibiotics
• Immune-mediated disease with concurrent vasculitis—prednisone (2–4 mg/kg q24h)
• No known underlying cause or prednisolone alone does not work—try dapsone (1 mg/kg q8h) or sulfasalazine (20–40 mg/kg q8h)
• Vasculitis—pentoxifylline; published doses vary; 400 mg q24–48h has been recommended
• Alkylating agents including chlorambucil and azathioprine have been added to regimens to decease the need for corticosteroids.

CONTRAINDICATIONS/POSSIBLE INTERACTIONS
• Dapsone and sulfasalazine—not recommended with pre-existing renal disease, hepatic disease, or blood dyscrasias
• Sulfasalazine—not recommended with pre-existing or borderline keratoconjunctivitis sicca; use with caution in cats; may displace highly protein-bound drugs (e.g., methotrexate, warfarin, phenylbutazone, thiazide diuretics, salicylates, probenecid, and phenytoin); bioavailability decreased by antacids; may decrease bioavailability of folic acid or digoxin; blood levels may be decreased if concurrently administering ferrous sulfate or other iron salts
• Pentoxifylline—may increase prothrombin times; may decrease blood pressure

 FOLLOW-UP

• Patients receiving prednisolone or dapsone—initially monitor every 2 weeks with a CBC, chemistry screen, and urinalysis; if a specific underlying disease is found, then monitor appropriately.
• If no underlying disease is found, vasculitis may be difficult to treat and the prognosis is guarded.
• Immunosuppressive therapies should always be reduced to the lowest possible therapeutic dose.

 MISCELLANEOUS

PREGNANCY
• Corticosteroids and dapsone—do not use in pregnant animals.
• Sulfasalazine—use during pregnancy only when absolutely necessary.

ABBREVIATION
ANA = antinuclear antibody

Suggested Reading
Greek JS. New therapeutics in dermatology. Vet Med 1996.
Mueller GH, Kirk RW, Scott DW, eds. Small animal dermatology. 4th ed. Philadelphia: Saunders, 1989.
Authors Karen A. Kuhl and Jean S. Greek
Consulting Editor Karen Helton Rhodes

BASICS

OVERVIEW

• Blood vessel inflammation caused by endothelial injury or extension of adjacent inflammation or infection • Endothelial damage by infectious agent, parasite infestation, endotoxin, or immune complex deposition initiates local inflammation, neutrophil accumulation, and complement activation. Neutrophils release lysosomal enzymes leading to necrosis of vessel wall, thrombosis, and hemorrhage. In humans and dogs with polyarteritis nodosa, intimal proliferation and vessel wall degeneration and necrosis predominate and lead to hemorrhage, thrombosis, and necrosis of involved vessels and adjacent tissues in most patients. • Nondermal vasculitis (e.g., renal, hepatic, and serosal surfaces of body cavities) may be the mechanism leading to development of clinically apparent signs of systemic disease (e.g., polyarthritis and proteinuria) without causing obvious external lesions.

SIGNALMENT

Dogs and cats

SIGNS

Historical Findings

• Provocative drug (e.g., penicillin, sulfonamides, streptomycin, and hydralazine) given to sensitized animal • Exposure to ticks • Poor dirofilariasis prophylaxis in endemic area

Physical Examination Findings

• Swelling • Ulceration • Necrosis of affected skin, especially mucous membranes, mucocutaneous junctions, pinnae edges, and footpads • Systemic signs reflecting organ involvement (e.g., hepatic, renal, and CNS) • Systemic signs of illness (e.g., lethargy, lymphadenopathy, pyrexia, vague signs of pain, and weight loss) • Cutaneous lesions of polyarteritis nodosa (subcutaneous nodules—less common in dogs than in people) • Signs associated with underlying infectious or immune-related disease (e.g., thrombocytopenia and polyarthropathy)

CAUSES & RISK FACTORS

Infectious

• Parasitic (i.e., heart and pulmonary arteries)—*Dirofilaria immitis, Angiostrongylus vasorum* • Viral—e.g., feline infectious peritonitis and canine corona virus infection • Rickettsial—e.g., Rocky Mountain spotted fever and ehrlichiosis • Bacterial—sepsis

Immune-Related

• Systemic lupus erythematosus • Rheumatoid arthritis–like arthropathy • Lupus-like drug reaction • Type III hypersensitivities (e.g., to food, sulfonamides, and penicillin) • Polyarteritis nodosa • Neoplasia • Uremia

DIAGNOSIS

DIFFERENTIAL DIAGNOSIS

• Cutaneous signs developing after administration of medication implicate drug reaction (usually not immediate, may develop after days or weeks). • Vasculitis associated with polyarthropathy and pyrexia implicates immune or infectious cause. • Cold hemagglutinin disease suggested by distribution of cyanotic or necrotic lesions (nose, ears, toes, tail tip, prepuce) and history of exposure to cold.

CBC/BIOCHEMISTRY/URINALYSIS

Results depend on underlying disease

OTHER LABORATORY TESTS

• Serologic tests may aid diagnosis of tick-related (i.e., rickettsial) disease • ANA titer positive in patient with SLE, may also be positive in patients with other systemic illnesses • Occult heartworm test positive in patient with dirofilariasis • *Angiostrongylus* infestation diagnosed by fecal examination and cytologic examination of tracheal wash

IMAGING

Radiographs help diagnose dirofilariasis and *Angiostrongylus* infection.

DIAGNOSTIC PROCEDURES

• Skin biopsy specimen from edge of developing lesion may be diagnostic for vasculitis but may not reveal cause. • Immunofluorescence test of skin biopsy specimen may rule out pemphigus and pemphigoid diseases. • If allergic response is suspected, resolution of signs upon discontinuation of suspect medication or food supports diagnosis.

TREATMENT

• Usually resolution of underlying condition and supportive care • If untreatable or unknown underlying condition—glucocorticoid, immunosuppressive (e.g., cyclophosphamide, azathioprine), and other drugs (e.g., dapsone and sulfasalazine) are occasionally effective, but clinical trials of efficacy have not been reported in animals.

MEDICATIONS

DRUGS

• Infectious or immune-related—treat underlying disease (see specific condition); supportive care

• Lupus-like drug reactions—discontinue drug; supportive care • Type III hypersensitivity—discontinue drug; supportive care • Polyarteritis nodosa—glucocorticoids and cyclophosphamide (unknown value) • "Idiopathic" vasculitis—if other causes have been ruled out, administer dapsone (1 mg/kg PO q8h for 14 days, then 1 mg/kg PO q12h for 14 days, then 1 mg/kg PO q24 h; may eventually be decreased to q48h to maintain remission); alternative—sulfasalazine (45 mg/kg PO q8h). Neither drug's effectiveness is well documented. Pentoxifylline has been used in limited numbers of cases at doses of 400 mg q 24 to 48 hours. Immunosuppressive doses of corticosteroids may be helpful in idiopathic cases.

CONTRAINDICATIONS/POSSIBLE INTERACTIONS

• Do not administer sulfasalazine to patients sensitive to sulfonamides. • Pentoxifylline is a methylxanthine derivative and may reduce blood pressure.

FOLLOW-UP

• Patients undergoing treatment with dapsone—monitor CBC and liver enzymes for side effects (e.g., hemolytic anemia, methemoglobinemia, and hepatopathy) • Patients undergoing treatment with sulfasalazine—monitor for keratoconjunctivitis sicca, blood dyscrasias, and hepatopathy

✓ MISCELLANEOUS

SEE ALSO

• Leukocytoclastic vasculitis • Lupus erythematosus, systemic • Pemphigus • Vasculitis, cutaneous

ABBREVIATIONS

• ANA = antinuclear antibody • SLE = systemic lupus erythematosus

Suggested Reading

Greek, JS. New therapeutics in dermatology. Vet Med Nov 1996;90.

Suter PF, Fox PR. Peripheral vascular disease. In: Ettinger SJ, Feldman EC, eds. Textbook of veterinary internal medicine. 4th ed. Philadelphia: Saunders, 1995:1068–1083.

Author Jean S. Greek

Consulting Editors Larry P. Tilley and Francis W. K. Smith, Jr.

VENTRICULAR SEPTAL DEFECT

BASICS

DEFINITION
An anomalous communication between the two ventricles (Figure 1). The defect may be in the inlet, outlet, muscular, or membranous septum. Most VSDs in small animals are perimembranous and subcristal.

PATHOPHYSIOLOGY
• A VSD results in a pulmonary systemic shunt—direction and volume of the shunt are determined by the size of the defect, the relationship of the pulmonary and systemic vascular resistances, and the presence of other anomalies
• Most VSDs in dogs and cats are small and therefore restrictive (i.e., the difference between left and right ventricular pressures is maintained). Moderate-sized VSDs have an area > 40% of the area of the open aortic valve; they are only partially restrictive and result in various degrees of right ventricular hypertension. Large VSDs—area as large or larger than the open aortic valve; they are nonrestrictive, and right ventricular pressure is necessarily systemic. Only moderate and large defects impose a pressure load upon the right ventricle.
• In a patient with normal resistance to right ventricular ejection, the direction of the shunt is left to right, which increases pulmonary venous return and imposes a volume load on the left atrium and ventricle. With large shunts, left ventricular congestive failure can develop.
• Generally, the left ventricle unloads into the pulmonary arterial system during systole; unless the defect is of moderate size or large, the right ventricle is spared.

SYSTEMS AFFECTED
• Respiratory—if pulmonary edema develops
• Cardiovascular—theoretically, a large shunt could result in pulmonary vascular disease, pulmonary hypertension, and shunt reversal (i.e., Eisenmenger's syndrome). This is uncommon in small animals; if shunt reversal, usually early in life

GENETICS
Breed predispositions recognized; no genetic transmission established.

INCIDENCE/PREVALENCE
One of the most common congenital cardiac malformations in cats, comprising 15% of cases with congenital cardiac defects in one study. Less common in dogs, occurring in 10% of cases with congenital cardiac defects in one study

GEOGRAPHIC DISTRIBUTION
N/A

SIGNALMENT

Species
Dogs and cats

Breed Predilections
English bulldog; possibly, English springer spaniel, Brittany spaniel, chow chow, Newfoundland, and samoyed

Mean Age and Range
Most defects detected during routine examination of puppies and kittens.

Predominant Sex
N/A

SIGNS

Historical Findings
• Usually asymptomatic
• Clinical signs of left ventricular failure include dyspnea, exercise intolerance, syncope, and cough.

Physical Examination Findings
• Systolic murmur with a restrictive VSD. Murmur—typically loud, band-shaped, and heard best over the right hemithorax; may be a softer, midsystolic murmur of functional pulmonic stenosis heard over the left heart base; a diastolic decrescendo murmur results if the VSD undermines anatomic support of the aortic valve, causing aortic regurgitation. Patients with right-to-left shunts generally have no murmurs.
• Split second heart sound in some patients
• Femoral pulses usually normal
• Mucous membranes—pink, unless pulmonary hypertension causes a right-to-left shunt and arterial hypoxemia
• Tachycardia, dyspnea, and crackles may be evident if left ventricular failure occurs.

CAUSES
Congenital; may have a genetic basis

RISK FACTORS
N/A

DIAGNOSIS

DIFFERENTIAL DIAGNOSIS
• Other congenital cardiac malformations that cause systolic murmurs include atrioventricular valve dysplasia, aortic or pulmonary stenosis, and complex malformations such as tetralogy of Fallot.
• The "to-and-fro" murmur that results when aortic valve regurgitation complicates a VSD must be distinguished from the continuous murmur of patent ductus arteriosus.
• Generally, diagnosis of congenital cardiac malformations requires echocardiographic evaluation including Doppler studies.

CBC/BIOCHEMISTRY/URINALYSIS
• Results usually normal
• Uncommon right-to-left shunting results in compensatory erythrocytosis.

• Patients with severe CHF may have prerenal azotemia.

OTHER LABORATORY TESTS
N/A

IMAGING

Thoracic Radiography
• Radiographic appearance is determined by the size and direction of the shunt. Thoracic radiographs may be normal if the VSD is small. Larger defects cause various degrees of left or even generalized cardiac enlargement. Pulmonary hyperperfusion with prominence of the main pulmonary artery segment may be apparent. CHF is manifest as pulmonary edema.
• Patients with right-to-left shunts have right-sided cardiomegaly; the pulmonary arteries are large proximally but distally attenuated, and the pulmonary veins are small because of reduced pulmonary perfusion.

Echocardiography
• Two-dimensional echocardiographic study may demonstrate left atrial enlargement with left ventricular dilation and hypertrophy. Systolic myocardial function is usually preserved. Right ventricular hypertrophy is apparent only if the defect is moderate-sized or large or the VSD is one aspect of a complex malformation. The defect can sometimes be seen directly. Evaluate echocardiographic images critically; the artifact of "septal drop-out" is very common.
• Generally, the diagnosis is confirmed by Doppler interrogation of the interventricular septum. If the defect is restrictive, spectral Doppler reveals a discrete, high-velocity systolic jet. The shunt may be seen directly by color-flow Doppler.
• Contrast echocardiography may help in the diagnosis of a right-to-left VSD.

Cardiac Catheterization
Selective cardiac catheterization allows visualization of the defect by contrast angiocardiography and calculation of the shunt fraction (QP/QS) and pulmonary vascular resistance.

OTHER DIAGNOSTIC PROCEDURES

Electrocardiographic Findings
• Evidence of left atrial enlargement, left ventricular hypertrophy, or even right ventricular hypertrophy in some animals
• Right ventricular enlargement pattern in most animals if the shunt is right-to-left because of pulmonary hypertension or pulmonic stenosis.

PATHOLOGIC FINDINGS
Size of the defect determines the degree of chamber enlargement and hypertrophy; pulmonary edema and possibly ascites are seen in patients with CHF.

VENTRICULAR SEPTAL DEFECT

TREATMENT

APPROPRIATE HEALTH CARE
Clinical signs are related to CHF; most patients can be treated as outpatients.

NURSING CARE
N/A

ACTIVITY
Restrict if animal has CHF; need not restrict asymptomatic patients with small defects

DIET
Moderate sodium restriction recommended for patients with CHF

CLIENT EDUCATION
Definitive surgical correction is not widely available; if CHF develops, it is terminal, even with palliative care.

SURGICAL CONSIDERATIONS
Consider definitive surgical repair of the defect during cardiopulmonary bypass for moderate and large defects in which the QP/QS exceeds 2.5. Cardiopulmonary bypass is presently performed at a small number of veterinary centers. Consider pulmonary artery banding as a palliative procedure for patients with moderate or large shunts and CHF.

MEDICATIONS

DRUGS OF CHOICE
• Furosemide, enalapril, and digoxin—recommended for animals with CHF (see Congestive Heart Failure, Left-Sided)
• Consider using angiotensin-converting enzyme (ACE) inhibitors for patients with echocardiographic evidence of left atrial and ventricular volume overload, even in the absence of clinical signs.

CONTRAINDICATIONS
Vasodilators—contraindicated or used only with great caution in patients with complex malformations that include stenotic lesions.

PRECAUTIONS
ACE inhibitors and digoxin must be used cautiously if patient has renal dysfunction.

POSSIBLE INTERACTIONS
N/A

ALTERNATIVE DRUGS
N/A

FOLLOW-UP

PATIENT MONITORING
Periodic echocardiographic or radiographic evaluation suggested for patients without clinical signs

PREVENTION/AVOIDANCE
Breeding affected animals is not recommended.

POSSIBLE COMPLICATIONS
• Left ventricular congestive failure
• Bacterial endocarditis
• Pulmonary hypertension
• Arrhythmias

EXPECTED COURSE AND PROGNOSIS
• Patients with small shunts may have a normal life span; isolated, restrictive VSDs usually do not cause clinical signs.
• Concurrent anomalies such as pulmonic stenosis or aortic insufficiency worsen the prognosis.
• Patients with overt CHF may live 6–18 months with medical treatment.
• The development of pulmonary hypertension and shunt reversal is uncommon.

MISCELLANEOUS

ASSOCIATED CONDITIONS
• VSD may be one component of complex malformations such as tetralogy of Fallot.
• Aortic valve insufficiency resulting from a poorly supported aortic valve complicates the condition in some patients.
• Inlet VSD in cats may be associated with an atrial septal defect and tricuspid valve dysplasia as part of an endocardial cushion defect.

AGE-RELATED FACTORS
The murmur of VSD becomes apparent shortly after birth, when pulmonary vascular resistance drops.

ZOONOTIC POTENTIAL
N/A

PREGNANCY
High risk in patients with large defects; breeding affected animals is not recommended.

SYNONYMS
Interventricular septal defect

SEE ALSO
• CHF, Left-Sided
• Tetralogy of Fallot

ABBREVIATIONS
• ACE = angiotensin-converting enzyme
• CHF = congestive heart failure
• VSD = ventricular septal defect

Suggested Reading

Bonagura JD, Darke PG. Congenital heart disease. In: Ettinger SJ, Feldman EC, eds., Textbook of veterinary internal medicine—diseases of the dog and cat. 4th ed. Philadelphia: Saunders, 1995:892–943.
Bonagura JD, Lehmkuhl LB. Congenital heart disease. In: Fox PR, Sisson D, Moise NS, eds., Textbook of canine and feline cardiology. Philadelphia: Saunders, 1999: 471–535.

Author Jonathan A. Abbott

Consulting Editors Larry P. Tilley and Francis W. K. Smith, Jr.

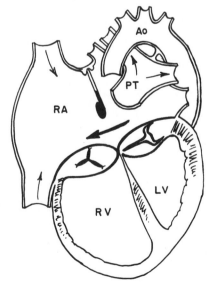

Figure 1.

Ventricular Septal Defect. The defect is an unobstructed communication. Right ventricular hypertrophy and pulmonary hypertension are associated. Left-to-right shunting is shown. RA = right atrium, LA = left atrium, RV = right ventricle, LV = left ventricle, AO = aorta, PT = pulmonary trunk. (From Roberts W. Adult Congenital Heart Disease. Philadelphia: FA Davis, 1987, with permission.)

DISEASES

VESICOURACHAL DIVERTICULA

BASICS

OVERVIEW
• A common congenital anomaly of the urinary bladder that occurs when the portion of the urachus (i.e., a fetal conduit that allows passage of urine from the bladder to the placenta) located at the bladder vertex fails to close; the result is a blind diverticulum of variable size that protrudes from the bladder vertex.
• Other characteristics include congenital microscopic diverticula (microscopic lumens that may persist at the bladder vertex).
• Acquired macroscopic diverticula develop after the onset of concurrent but unrelated acquired lower urinary tract diseases; presumably, urethral obstruction or detrusor hyperactivity induced by inflammation causes high intraluminal pressure and subsequent enlargement of microscopic diverticula.
• Congenital macroscopic diverticula, most likely caused by impaired urine outflow, develop before or soon after birth and persist indefinitely.

SIGNALMENT
• Dogs and cats
• Frequently encountered in cats with acquired lower urinary tract diseases; twice as common in male cats as in female cats
• No breed or age predisposition

SIGNS
• Depend on concomitant disorders predisposing to formation of macroscopic vesicourachal diverticula
• Hematuria, dysuria, pollakiuria, or signs of urethral obstruction in some patients with concurrent acquired lower urinary tract diseases

CAUSES & RISK FACTORS
• Of persistent congenital microscopic diverticula—unknown
• Congenital microscopic diverticula—risk factors for acquired macroscopic diverticula
• Diseases associated with increased bladder intraluminal pressure (e.g., bacterial urinary tract infection, uroliths, urethral plugs, and idiopathic disease) —risk factors for acquired macroscopic diverticula

DIAGNOSIS

DIFFERENTIAL DIAGNOSIS
• Persistent (or patent) urachus—characterized by inappropriate loss of urine through the umbilicus
• Persistent urachal ligaments are nonpatent fibrous remnants of the urachus, connecting the bladder vertex to the umbilicus.
• Urachal cysts are focal accumulations of fluid in isolated segments of a persistent urachus. They may be aseptic or septic.

CBC/BIOCHEMISTRY/URINALYSIS
• Abnormal findings related to the underlying disorder that causes vesicourachal diverticula, unless complicated by concurrent acquired lower urinary tract diseases.
• Abnormal findings related to secondary urinary tract infection.

OTHER LABORATORY TESTS
N/A

IMAGING
• Congenital and acquired macroscopic diverticula—best identified by positive-contrast urethrocystography
• Radiographs obtained with the bladder completely, then partially distended with contrast medium, may facilitate detection of small diverticula.

DIAGNOSTIC PROCEDURES
N/A

PATHOLOGIC FINDINGS
• Extramural macroscopic diverticula appear as convex or conical luminal projections from the bladder vertex.
• Intramural microscopic diverticula appear as transitional epithelium-lined lumens persisting at the bladder vertex from the level of the submucosa to subserosa.

TREATMENT
• Many macroscopic diverticula in cats (and probably dogs) are acquired and self-limiting if the underlying disease is eliminated.
• Direct treatment efforts toward eliminating underlying cause(s) of lower urinary tract disease.
• Consider diverticulectomy if a macroscopic diverticulum persists in a patient with persistent or recurrent bacterial urinary tract infection despite appropriate antimicrobial therapy.

VESICOURACHAL DIVERTICULA

 MEDICATIONS

DRUGS
N/A

CONTRAINDICATIONS/POSSIBLE INTERACTIONS
N/A

 FOLLOW-UP

PATIENT MONITORING
If bacterial urinary tract infection persists or recurs despite proper antimicrobial therapy, the status of the diverticulum should be reevaluated by contrast radiography.

PREVENTION/AVOIDANCE
Avoid diagnostic procedures or treatments that alter normal host urinary tract defenses and predispose to urinary tract infection.

POSSIBLE COMPLICATIONS
Persistent congenital macroscopic diverticula are risk factors for recurrent bacterial urinary tract infection.

EXPECTED COURSE AND PROGNOSIS
• Congenital microscopic diverticula are usually clinically silent unless complicated by concurrent lower urinary tract disease.
• Acquired macroscopic diverticula typically heal in 2–3 weeks after amelioration of clinical signs of lower urinary tract disease.
• Diverticulectomy and appropriate antimicrobial therapy usually resolve recurrent urinary tract infection in patients with persistent congenital macroscopic diverticula.

 MISCELLANEOUS

ASSOCIATED CONDITIONS
• Persistent congenital macroscopic diverticula are potential risk factors for recurrent bacterial urinary tract infection.
• Acquired macroscopic diverticula are typically encountered in patients with concurrent lower urinary tract diseases.

SEE ALSO
• Feline Lower Urinary Tract Disease
• Lower Urinary Tract Infection

Suggested Reading
Osborne CA, Johnston GR, Kruger JM, et al. Etiopathogenesis and biological behavior of feline vesicourachal diverticula. Vet Clin North Am 1987;17:697.
Authors John M. Kruger and Carl A. Osborne
Consulting Editors Larry G. Adams and Carl A. Osborne

DISEASES

VESTIBULAR DISEASE, GERIATRIC—DOGS

 BASICS

DEFINITION
Acute nonprogressive disturbance of the peripheral vestibular system in old dogs

PATHOPHYSIOLOGY
• Unknown
• Suspected abnormal flow of the endolymphatic fluid in the semicircular canals of the inner ear secondary to disturbance in production, circulation, or absorption of the fluid
• Possible intoxication of the vestibular receptors or inflammation of the vestibular portion of the vestibulocochlear nerve (cranial nerve VIII)
• Often incorrectly referred to as a stroke (disease is neither central in location nor suspected to be vascular or ischemic in origin)

SYSTEMS AFFECTED
Nervous—peripheral vestibular system

GENETICS
N/A

INCIDENCE/PREVALENCE
• Common, sporadic, acquired disease of old dogs

GEOGRAPHIC DISTRIBUTION
N/A

SIGNALMENT

Species
Dogs

Breed Predilections
• None reported
• Seems to occur more frequently in medium-to-large breeds

Mean Age and Range
Geriatric; patients usually > 8 years old

Predominant Sex
N/A

SIGNS

General Comments
• Strictly of peripheral vestibular dysfunction
• Severe disease—do not incorrectly attribute the signs (especially the gait) to a CNS location.

Historical Findings
• Sudden onset of imbalance, disorientation, reluctance to stand, and (usually) head tilt and irregular eye movements
• May be preceded or accompanied by nausea and vomiting

Physical Examination Findings
• Head tilt—mild to marked; directed toward the side of the lesion; occasionally bilateral disease with erratic side-to-side movements with or without mild tilt in the direction of the more severely affected side
• Abnormal nystagmus (resting or positional)—in early stages common; either horizontal or rotatory with the fast phase always in a direction opposite to the head tilt; with bilateral disease, may be mild with depressed or absent physiologic eye movements (e.g., normal vestibular nystagmus or conjugate eye movements)
• Mild to marked disorientation and vestibular ataxia with a tendency to lean or fall in the direction of the head tilt
• Strength and proprioception normal; with severe disease, patient may be reluctant to stand, making assessment of gait difficult; with bilateral disease, noticeable base-wide stance.

CAUSES
Unknown

RISK FACTORS
N/A

 DIAGNOSIS

DIFFERENTIAL DIAGNOSIS
• Primarily distinguished by the acute onset and rapid improvement without specific treatment
• Otitis media and interna—most challenging differentials; distinguished by concurrent ipsilateral facial (cranial nerve VII) paresis or paralysis, deafness, or Horner syndrome; otitis externa with ruptured tympanic membrane supports otitis media and interna.
• Ototoxic drugs—eliminated by history
• Trauma—may cause similar acute changes; differentiated by history, results of physical examination, and other neurologic deficits
• Hypothyroid neuropathy—not as acute in onset; associated with clinical signs of hypothyroidism and possible cranial nerve VII deficit

CBC/BIOCHEMISTRY/URINALYSIS
• Generally normal
• Hemoconcentration secondary to dehydration
• Unrelated concurrent disorders (e.g., renal and hepatic disease) associated with old age may cause other laboratory abnormalities.

OTHER LABORATORY TESTS
N/A

IMAGING
• Usually none
• Radiographs of bullae—may be required to rule out otitis media and interna

DIAGNOSTIC PROCEDURES
BAER—may help to rule out otitis media and interna; only the vestibular portion of cranial nerve VIII should be affected

PATHOLOGIC FINDINGS
None reported

VESTIBULAR DISEASE, GERIATRIC—DOGS

TREATMENT

APPROPRIATE HEALTH CARE
• Usually outpatient
• Severe disease—patients that cannot ambulate or require intravenous fluid support should be hospitalized during the initial stages.

NURSING CARE
• Treatment supportive, including rehydration and maintenance intravenous fluids if required.
• Keep recumbent patients warm and dry using soft, absorbent bedding.
• Severe disease—physical therapy, including passive manipulation of limbs and moving body to alternate sides, may be required initially.

ACTIVITY
Restrict activity as required by the degree of disorientation and vestibular ataxia.

DIET
• No modification usually required
• Nausea, vomiting, and severe disorientation—initially withhold oral intake.

CLIENT EDUCATION
Reassure client that although the initial signs can be alarming and incapacitating, the prognosis for rapid improvement and recovery is excellent.

SURGICAL CONSIDERATIONS
N/A

MEDICATIONS

DRUGS OF CHOICE
• Sedatives—for severe disorientation and ataxia; diazepam (2–10 mg/dog PO q8h)
• Antiemetic drugs or drugs against motion sickness—may be beneficial; dimenhydrinate (4–8 mg/kg PO, IM, IV q8h)

• Glucocorticoids—do not alter the course of the disease; not recommended, especially in old patients whose fluid intake may be low
• Antibiotics—advised when otitis media and interna cannot be ruled out; trimethoprim-sulfa (15 mg/kg PO q12h or 30 mg/kg PO q12–24h); first-generation cephalosporin (e.g., cephalexin 10–30 mg/kg PO q6–12h); amoxicillin/clavulanic acid (12.5–25 mg/kg PO q12h)

CONTRAINDICATIONS
N/A

PRECAUTIONS
N/A

POSSIBLE INTERACTIONS
N/A

ALTERNATIVE DRUGS
N/A

FOLLOW-UP

PATIENT MONITORING
• Neurologic examination of outpatient—repeat 2–3 days later to confirm stabilization and initial improvement.
• Discharge inpatient when it is able to ambulate and resume eating and drinking.

PREVENTION/AVOIDANCE
N/A

POSSIBLE COMPLICATIONS
Fluid and electrolyte imbalances and decompensation of renal insufficiency (if exists)—may follow vomiting and/or insufficient fluid and food intake

EXPECTED COURSE AND PROGNOSIS
• Improvement of clinical signs within approximately 72 hr with resolution of vomiting and improvement of nystagmus and vestibular ataxia

• Head tilt and ataxia—significant improvement usually occurs over 7–10 days; if not noted, evaluate patient for other causes of peripheral vestibular disease; mild head tilt may persist.
• Most patients return to normal within 2–3 weeks.
• Recurrence—rarely mild, brief return of signs with stress (e.g., anesthesia); repeat episodes on the same or opposite side uncommon

MISCELLANEOUS

ASSOCIATED CONDITIONS
N/A

AGE-RELATED FACTORS
Only geriatric dogs affected

ZOONOTIC POTENTIAL
N/A

PREGNANCY
N/A

SYNONYMS
• Canine idiopathic vestibular disease
• Old dog vestibular syndrome

SEE ALSO
• Head Tilt (Vestibular Disease)
• Otitis Media and Interna

ABBREVIATION
BAER = brainstem auditory-evoked response

Suggested Reading
de Lahunta A. Veterinary neuroanatomy and clinical neurology. 2nd ed. Philadelphia: Saunders, 1983.
Oliver JE, Lorenz MD, Kornegay JN. Handbook of veterinary neurology, 3rd ed. Philadelphia: WB Saunders, 1997:222–223.
Parent JM, Cochrane SM. Head tilt. In: Allen DG, ed., Small animal medicine. Philadelphia: Lippincott, 1991:753–759.
Author Susan M. Cochrane
Consulting Editor Joane M. Parent

VESTIBULAR DISEASE, IDIOPATHIC—CATS

BASICS

DEFINITION
Acute nonprogressive disturbance of the peripheral vestibular system of cats

PATHOPHYSIOLOGY
• Unknown
• Suspected abnormal flow of the endolymphatic fluid in the semicircular canals of the inner ear, secondary to a disturbance in the production, circulation, or absorption of the fluid
• Possible intoxication of the vestibular receptors or inflammation of the vestibular portion of the vestibulocochlear nerve (cranial nerve VIII)

SYSTEMS AFFECTED
Nervous—peripheral vestibular system

Genetics
N/A

Incidence/Prevalence
• Common, sporadic acquired disease
• None reported

Geographic Distribution
N/A

SIGNALMENT

Species
Cats

Breed Predilections
N/A

Mean Age and Range
Any age; rarely observed in cats < 1 year old

Predominant Sex
N/A

SIGNS

General Comments
Limited to signs associated with peripheral vestibular disturbance

Historical Findings
Sudden onset of severe disorientation, falling and rolling, leaning, vocalizing, and crouched posture with tendency to panic when picked up

Physical Examination Findings
• Head tilt—always toward the side of the lesion; occasionally bilateral disease with wide, side-to-side excursion of the head, with or without a mild tilt toward the most severely affected side
• Resting nystagmus—usually horizontal; may be rotatory with the fast phase always in direction opposite to the head tilt; with bilateral disease, the abnormal nystagmus mild or absent and diminished to absent physiologic nystagmus or conjugate eye movements
• Vestibular ataxia with tendency to roll and fall toward the side of the head tilt
• Preservation of strength and normal proprioception; with bilateral disease, patient may be reluctant to ambulate, preferring to stay in a crouched posture or having wide abduction of the limbs

CAUSES
• Unknown
• Previous upper respiratory tract infection—suspected in some patients; relationship not confirmed; limited necropsy data show no evidence of inflammation.

RISK FACTORS
• Reports of an increase in cases in the summer and early fall, possibly after outbreaks of upper respiratory disease; not been proven; disease occurs throughout the year.

DIAGNOSIS

DIFFERENTIAL DIAGNOSIS
• Diagnosis made on the basis of peripheral vestibular signs that improve rapidly without specific treatment
• Otitis media and interna (bacterial and parasitic)—most challenging differentials; distinguished by concurrent ipsilateral facial nerve (cranial nerve VII) paresis or paralysis, Horner syndrome, deafness, ruptured tympanic membrane, otitis externa, and radiographic changes in tympanic bulla; signs usually not as acute or severe at onset and not self-limiting
• Nasopharyngeal polyp(s)—may cause unilateral and bilateral peripheral vestibular signs; concurrent tympanic bulla involvement characteristic; signs usually not as acute and severe at onset and not self-limiting
• Blue-tailed lizard ingestion—southeastern U.S.; thought to produce a similar acute, unilateral, peripheral vestibular syndrome; vomiting, salivation, irritability, and trembling also noted; most patients recover without specific treatment.
• Aminoglycoside toxicity, especially streptomycin—may cause acute unilateral or bilateral peripheral vestibular syndrome or hearing loss; differentiated by history of drug use

CBC/BIOCHEMISTRY/URINALYSIS
Normal

OTHER LABORATORY TESTS
None required

VESTIBULAR DISEASE, IDIOPATHIC—CATS

IMAGING
• None usually necessary
• Radiographs of tympanic bullae—occasionally required to rule out otitis media and interna

DIAGNOSTIC PROCEDURES
• BAER—may help rule out other causes (e.g., otitis media and interna; nasopharyngeal polyps)
• Hearing test—should be intact; disease limited to the vestibular apparatus

PATHOLOGIC FINDINGS
None reported

TREATMENT

APPROPRIATE HEALTH CARE
• Usually outpatient
• Inpatient—severely affected patient may require a short period of hospitalization for supportive care.

NURSING CARE
• Treatment supportive only
• Severe disease—may require initial intravenous or subcutaneous fluids; maintain patient in quiet, well-padded cage initially.

ACTIVITY
Restricted according to the degree of disorientation and ataxia

DIET
• No specific changes or restrictions required
• Patient may be initially reluctant to eat and drink, possibly because of the disorientation or nausea.

CLIENT EDUCATION
Reassure client that, despite initial alarming and incapacitating signs, the prognosis for rapid and complete recovery is excellent.

SURGICAL CONSIDERATIONS
N/A

MEDICATIONS

DRUGS OF CHOICE
• Sedatives—for severe disorientation and rolling; diazepam (1–5 mg/cat PO q8–12h) and acepromazine (0.05–0.10 mg/kg IM, SC, IV; to a maximum of 1 mg)
• Antiemetic drugs and drugs against motion sickness—usually ineffective
• Glucocorticoids—do not alter the course of the disease; not recommended
• Antibiotics—have been recommended in the acute phase if otitis media and interna cannot be ruled out; trimethoprim-sulfa (30 mg/kg PO q12–24h); a first-generation cephalosporin (e.g., cephalexin (10–30 mg/kg PO q6–12h); amoxicillin/clavulanic acid (62.5 mg/cat PO q12h)

CONTRAINDICATIONS
N/A

PRECAUTIONS
N/A

POSSIBLE INTERACTIONS
N/A

ALTERNATIVE DRUGS
N/A

FOLLOW-UP

PATIENT MONITORING
• Neurologic examination of outpatient—repeat in approximately 72 hr to confirm stabilization and initial improvement.
• Discharge inpatient when it is able to ambulate and resume eating and drinking.

PREVENTION/AVOIDANCE
N/A

POSSIBLE COMPLICATIONS
• Uncommon
• Dehydration and electrolyte imbalance (rare)

EXPECTED COURSE AND PROGNOSIS
• Marked improvement especially in the resting nystagmus within 72 hr, with progressive improvement of the gait and head tilt
• Patients usually normal within 2–3 weeks
• Head tilt—final sign to resolve; mild residual tilt may remain.
• If signs do not improve rapidly, other causes of vestibular disease should be pursued.
• Rarely recurs; mild head tilt and ataxia may temporarily return with stress (e.g., general anesthesia).

MISCELLANEOUS

ASSOCIATED CONDITIONS
N/A

AGE-RELATED FACTORS
N/A

ZOONOTIC POTENTIAL
N/A

PREGNANCY
N/A

SYNONYMS
• Feline vestibular syndrome
• Idiopathic vestibular neuropathy

SEE ALSO
• Head Tilt (Vestibular Disease)
• Otitis Media and Interna

ABBREVIATION
BAER = brainstem auditory-evoked response

Suggested Reading
de Lahunta A. Veterinary neuroanatomy and clinical neurology. Philadelphia: Saunders, 1983.
Oliver JE, Lorenz MD. Handbook of veterinary neurologic diagnosis. Philadelphia: WB Saunders, 1993.
Parent JM, Cochrane SM. Head tilt. In: Allen DG, ed. Small animal medicine. Philadelphia: Lippincott, 1991:753–759.
Author Susan M. Cochrane
Consulting Editor Joane M. Parent

VITAMIN A TOXICITY

 BASICS

OVERVIEW
• Skeletal disease that occurs after excessive intake of vitamin A
• High concentrations of vitamin A—inhibits intramembranous and endochondral ossification, resulting in dystrophic calcification of the skeleton

SIGNALMENT
• Cats aged 2–9 years
• No breed or sex predilections recognized

SIGNS
Historical Findings
• Daily diet high in liver or vitamin A supplementation (e.g., liver or cod liver oil) for > 14 weeks
• Lethargy
• Anorexia
• Weight loss

Physical Examination Findings
• Resentment of handling
• Marsupial-like sitting position with the forelimbs raised
• Weight-bearing lameness—most notable in the forelimbs, as osseous proliferation impinges on spinal nerves
• Cutaneous hypersensitivity or hyposensitivity over the cervical and forelimb regions
• Cervical, joint, and/or spinal stiffness
• Unkempt hair coat from inability to groom
• Constipation

CAUSES & RISK FACTORS
• Diet that includes large amounts of raw liver (usually beef or sheep)
• Excessive intake of vitamin A supplement—cod liver oil can contain > 1000 IU/mL of vitamin A.

 DIAGNOSIS

DIFFERENTIAL DIAGNOSIS
• Osteomyelitis
• Multiple cartilaginous exostoses
• Neoplasia

CBC/BIOCHEMISTRY/URINALYSIS
• Neutrophilic leukocytosis with stress leukogram
• Stress-induced hyperglycemia

OTHER LABORATORY TESTS
N/A

IMAGING
Radiography—new bone formation involving the cervical vertebrae (often extending from C1 to T2), the sternum, and the costal cartilages; new periosteal bone formation on metaphyses or surrounding joints; bony arthrodesis of joints

DIAGNOSTIC PROCEDURES
N/A

 TREATMENT

• Stop feeding patient raw liver or supplementing with vitamin A.
• Use a balanced commercial cat food.

VITAMIN A TOXICITY

 MEDICATIONS

DRUGS

Analgesics intended for cats—as required

CONTRAINDICATIONS/POSSIBLE INTERACTIONS

Avoid NSAIDs, except for aspirin (cats)

 FOLLOW-UP

• Mature cats—reversal of most signs, except those related to bony arthrodesis
• Young cats—permanent retardation of long-bone growth; appositional bone formation returns to normal.
• Skeletal improvement—detected by radiographic and clinical changes
• Plasma concentrations of vitamin A—decrease to normal within a few weeks after dietary change; may note high vitamin A content of the liver for years

 MISCELLANEOUS

SEE ALSO

Poisoning (Intoxication)

Suggested Reading

Fry PD. Hypervitaminosis A in the cat. Vet Int 1989;1:16–31.
Goldman AL. Hypervitaminosis A in a cat. J Am Vet Med Assoc 1992;200:1970–1972.
Seawright AA, English PB. Hypervitaminosis A and deforming cervical spondylosis of the cat. J Compend Pathol 1967;77:29–39.
Author Johnny D. Hoskins
Consulting Editor Gary D. Osweiler

DISEASES

VITAMIN D TOXICITY

BASICS

DEFINITION
Abnormal accumulation of vitamin D in the body, most commonly from ingesting vitamin D–containing rodenticides or other preparation or oversupplementation

PATHOPHYSIOLOGY
• Cholecalciferol—fat-soluble vitamin; absorbed through chylomicrons and transported to the liver, where it is metabolized to 25-hydroxycholecalciferol, the major circulating metabolite during vitamin D excess; further metabolism occurs in the kidney, where calcitriol is produced.
• Cholecalciferol and 25-hydroxycholecalciferol—limited biological activity
• Calcitriol—most potent cholecalciferol metabolite in terms of enhancing calcium resorption from bone and intestinal calcium uptake
• Excessive ingestion—increased intestinal absorption of calcium; stimulated bone resorption; increased renal tubular reabsorption of calcium; results in hypercalcemia (serum calcium > 12 mg/dL) and associated dystrophic calcification

SYSTEMS AFFECTED
• Renal/Urologic—renal failure; dystrophic calcification
• Gastrointestinal—vomiting; dystrophic calcification
• Cardiovascular—arrhythmias; dystrophic calcification
• Nervous—seizures; other neurobehavioral effects resulting from hypercalcemia

GENETICS
N/A

INCIDENCE/PREVALENCE
• Cholecalciferol-based rodenticide toxicosis—common cause of poisoning in dogs and cats
• Incidence unknown

GEOGRAPHIC DISTRIBUTION
N/A

SIGNALMENT

Species
• Dogs and cats
• Other species

Breed Predilections
• Cholecalciferol-based rodenticide toxicosis—none reported; small dogs (adults < 12 kg) make up majority of reported canine cases.
• Chronic vitamin oversupplementation by owners—giant-breed dogs and cats

Mean Age and Range
All ages

Predominant Sex
N/A

SIGNS

General Comments
• Generally develop within 12–36 hr postingestion

Historical Findings
• Vomiting
• CNS depression
• Anorexia
• Polydipsia
• Polyuria
• Diarrhea

Physical Examination Findings
• Gastrointestinal and pulmonary hemorrhage—apparently because of dystrophic calcification
• Renal pain on palpation
• Bradycardia or other cardiac arrhythmias

CAUSES
• Excessive ingestion—most frequently in the form of cholecalciferol-based rodenticides or vitamin supplements
• National Research Council recommended daily requirement of vitamin D for growing dogs—22 IU/kg
• Dogs—daily vitamin D administration at 2,000–4,000 IU/kg for 1–2 weeks may cause toxicosis.
• Cats—prolonged ingestion of markedly high dietary vitamin D levels (60,000 IU/kg diet) reported to induce toxicity.
• Cholecalciferol-containing rodenticides (0.075%)—brand names Quintox, Rampage, Ortho Rat-B-Gone, and Ortho Mouse-B-Gone; reported toxicosis in dogs after ingestion of 2–3 mg cholecalciferol/kg body weight

RISK FACTORS
Pre-existing renal disease may predispose animal.

DIAGNOSIS

DIFFERENTIAL DIAGNOSIS
• Diagnosis—depends on history of exposure, development of consistent clinical signs, and a high vitamin D blood concentration and/or hypercalcemia
• Hypercalcemia—cholecalciferol-based rodenticide poisoning; hypercalcemia; cancer (paraneoplastic); hypoadrenocorticism; primary renal failure; primary hyperparathyroidism; hemoconcentration (hyperproteinemia); disuse osteoporosis; may be normal in juveniles
• Gastrointestinal and pulmonary hemorrhage—may be an apparent result of dystrophic calcification; should not lead to a misdiagnosis of anticoagulant rodenticide toxicosis when the identity of the ingested rodenticide is in question; vitamin D toxicity results in hypercalcemia, whereas anticoag-

ulant rodenticide toxicity induces altered clotting profiles.

CBC/BIOCHEMISTRY/URINALYSIS
• Calcium—hypercalcemia (serum calcium > 12 mg/dL) within 12 hr postingestion of a cholecalciferol-based rodenticide; determine baseline serum calcium for all cases of potentially toxic ingestion; levels likely to be within normal limits for up to several hours postingestion, even when potentially lethal doses are consumed
• Hyperphosphatemia—within 24 hr postingestion of a cholecalciferol-based rodenticide
• Hyperproteinemia
• Azotemia
• Urinalyses—may note hyposthenuria, proteinuria, and glucosuria
• Urine sediment examination—occasionally reveals leukocytes, erythrocytes, and casts in variable numbers
• Increased urinary excretion of NAG—sensitive marker of renal proximal tubular damage; occurs after toxicity
• May note metabolic acidosis

OTHER LABORATORY TESTS
• Total kidney calcium concentrations—may be higher than normal
• High serum concentrations of cholecalciferol and its primary metabolites (25-hydroxycholecalciferol, 24,25-dihydroxycholecalciferol, and/or 1,25-dihydroxycholecalciferol)—support the diagnosis

IMAGING
Radiology—may note mineralization of the kidneys, gastrointestinal tract, lungs, and other organs

DIAGNOSTIC PROCEDURES
May note electrocardiographic abnormalities (e.g., bradycardia)

PATHOLOGIC FINDINGS
• May note diffuse hemorrhage in the gastric mucosa, duodenum, and jejunum
• Necrosis and mineralization of the myocardium and arterial intima
• Mineralization of glomerular capillary walls, renal cortical tubular basement membranes, Bowman capsules, and stomach mucosa reported

TREATMENT

APPROPRIATE HEALTH CARE
• Acute accidental ingestion of vitamin D supplement (< 25,000 IU/kg)—none required
• Asymptomatic patients—clinical examination, baseline serum chemistries, initiation of gastrointestinal tract decontamination initiated

VITAMIN D TOXICITY

• Symptomatic patients—inpatient until serum calcium has normalized

Emetics

• Minimal exposure or substantial delay in transporting patient to hospital
• Initially, owner-administered
• Syrup of ipecac (dogs, 1–2 mL/kg; cats, 3.3 mL/kg) and 3% hydrogen peroxide (5–25 mL/5 kg)
• Usually initiate vomiting within 5–15 min; if patient has not vomited by 15 min, a single repeat dose recommended
• Warn client that prolonged vomiting and depression may occur.

NURSING CARE

• Fluid and electrolyte imbalances—correct
• Calciuresis—may enhance by intravenous 0.9 % sodium chloride
• Early diuresis—strongly recommended for immature patients, patients with pre-existing renal disease, and all patients that have ingested doses likely to cause renal damage
• Severe uremia or hypercalcemia—may use a peritoneal dialysis with a calcium-free dialysate to lower serum calcium concentrations, even if other methods have failed

ACTIVITY
N/A

DIET
Significant exposure—low calcium; milk, other dairy products, and calcium supplements contraindicated

CLIENT EDUCATION

• Encourage client to prevent any additional exposure to animals or children within the home.
• Discuss the need for aggressive therapy directed toward gastrointestinal tract decontamination and control of hypercalcemia

SURGICAL CONSIDERATIONS
N/A

MEDICATIONS

DRUGS OF CHOICE
Rarely required—seizure control, treatment of arrhythmias, and other symptomatic therapies

Decontaminate Gastrointestinal Tract
• Emetic and activated charcoal along with a saline or osmotic cathartic
• Apomorphine—generally limited to dogs; 0.03 mg/kg IV or 0.04 mg/kg IM
• Xylazine—1.1 mg/kg IM, SC; somewhat effective as an emetic in cats
• Activated charcoal powder (1–4 g/kg) combined with a saline (magnesium or sodium sulfate at 250 mg/kg) cathartic as a

suspension in water (10 times volume)—administered orally or by gastric tube

Reduce Hypercalcemia
• Furosemide—2–5 mg/kg PO q8–12h
• Prednisone—2 mg/kg PO q12h
• Salmon calcitonin—4–6 IU/kg SC q2–3h; until serum calcium levels normalize; may need increasing doses (up to 10–20 IU/kg) for refractory patients
• Furosemide (2–4.5 mg/kg PO q8–12h) and prednisone (2 mg/kg PO q12h)—for maintenance after serum calcium has stabilized

CONTRAINDICATIONS

• Calcium-containing fluids
• Emetics—with convulsing patients

PRECAUTIONS

• Xylazine—may aggravate respiratory depression and result in vagal-mediated slowing of the heart rate; yohimbine (0.1 mg/kg IV) effectively reverses xylazine-induced depression, bradycardia, and hypotension.
• Constipation—occasionally associated with activated charcoals; warn client that dark black stools and diarrhea are common.
• Prolonged calcitonin therapy (humans)—usually of value in cholecalciferol toxicosis; occasionally results in tachyphylaxis or anaphylactic reactions
• Prednisone and adrenocortical suppression—not expected; to lessen the likelihood, gradually taper doses toward the end of the 2–4-week treatment period.

POSSIBLE INTERACTIONS
N/A

ALTERNATIVE DRUGS
N/A

FOLLOW-UP

PATIENT MONITORING

• Serum calcium and BUN—measured 1, 2, and 3 days after clinically important exposure; if hypercalcemia is noted or the patient is still symptomatic, further diuresis and additional therapies may be indicated.
• Vitamin D-induced hypercalcemia—often persists for several weeks, necessitating long-term management

PREVENTION/AVOIDANCE

• Restricted access to cholecalciferol-based rodenticides
• Avoid diets that are unusually high in vitamin D.

POSSIBLE COMPLICATIONS

• Chronic renal failure
• Subclinical renal, cardiovascular, and gastrointestinal damage—owing to dystrophic calcification

EXPECTED COURSE AND PROGNOSIS

• Depend on severity and duration of the hypercalcemia
• Without hypercalcemia—excellent prognosis
• Unresponsive hypercalcemia after aggressive treatment—poor prognosis

MISCELLANEOUS

ASSOCIATED CONDITIONS
N/A

AGE-RELATED FACTORS
Distinguish from normal juvenile hypercalcemia.

ZOONOTIC POTENTIAL
None, but human poisoning is also possible.

PREGNANCY
Teratogenic effects (e.g., aortic and cardiac lesions)—reported in humans and rodents

SYNONYMS
Cholecalciferol toxicosis

SEE ALSO
• Poisoning (Intoxication)

ABBREVIATION
NAG = N-acetyl-β-D-glucosaminidase

Suggested Reading
Dorman DC. Anticoagulant, cholecalciferol and bromethalin-based rodenticides. Vet Clin North Am Sm Anim Pract 1990;20:339–352.

Gunther R, Felice LJ, Nelson RK, Franson AM. Toxicity of a vitamin D_3 rodenticide to dogs. J Am Vet Med Assoc 1988;193:211–214.

Livezey KL, Dorman DC, Hooser SB, Buck WB. Hypercalcemia induced by vitamin D_3 toxicosis in two dogs. Compend Anim Pract 1991;16:26–32.

Moore FM, Kudisch M, Richter K, Faggella A. Hypercalcemia associated with rodenticide poisoning in three cats. J Am Vet Med Assoc 1988;193:1099–1100.

Morita T, Awakura T, Shimada A, et al. Vitamin D toxicosis in cats: natural outbreak and experimental study. J Vet Med Sci 1995;57:831–837.

Author David C. Dorman
Consulting Editor Gary D. Osweiler

VON WILLEBRAND DISEASE

BASICS

DEFINITION
• A complex inherited defect of hemostasis related to defects in synthesis or function of vWF
• The most common inherited bleeding disorder in dogs

PATHOPHYSIOLOGY
• vWF—a large, multimeric glycoprotein consisting of identical subunits that are synthesized mostly by endothelial cells; circulates in the plasma as a macromolecular complex with factor VIII and is required for platelet adhesion to subendothelium and for stabilizing and preventing rapid clearance of factor VIII from the circulation
• Various defects in the vWF gene may cause deficient synthesis of vWF or production of dysfunctional or unstable forms of vWF; these defects may cause platelet function defects and delayed coagulation of blood.

SYSTEMS AFFECTED
Hemic/Lymph/Immune—bleeding diathesis with hemorrhages seen in a variety of organs but especially at surgical sites and mucosal surfaces

GENETICS
• An autosomal trait with a pattern of incomplete dominance in most dogs
• Described as autosomal recessive disease in Scottish terriers and Chesapeake Bay retrievers

INCIDENCE/PREVALENCE
Prevalence of a low concentration of vWF—extremely variable in different breeds; reported estimates of 68%–73% in Doberman pinschers, 18%–28% in Shetland sheepdogs, and 16%–30% in Scottish terriers

GEOGRAPHIC DISTRIBUTION
None

SIGNALMENT

Species
• Dogs
• Rare in cats

Breed Predilections
• Described in at least 60 breeds of dogs
• Breeds with a known high prevalence—Airedale terriers, Bassett hounds, dachshunds, Doberman pinschers, German shepherds, golden retrievers, keeshonds, Manchester terriers, miniature schnauzers, Pembroke Welsh corgis, rottweilers, Shetland sheepdogs, Scottish terriers, and standard poodles

Mean Age and Range
Present from birth

Predominant Sex
Males and females affected

SIGNS

General Comments
Can be subclinical or manifested as a bleeding diathesis, most commonly as a consequence of surgery, toenail clipping, or some form of injury.

Historical Findings
• Previous abnormal bleeding associated with teething or disproportionate hemorrhage associated with minor injury
• Many dogs survive ear cropping or tail docking without serious bleeding.

Physical Examination Findings
• Gastrointestinal bleeding
• Hematuria
• Bleeding around gums at teething
• Epistaxis
• Vaginal or penile bleeding
• Petechiae are uncommon, despite the platelet function defect.

CAUSES
• Divided into three classifications
• Type I—low vWF concentration but all sizes of multimers detected; most common pattern; clinical severity varies; typical of Doberman pinschers, Airedales, and the one-third of shelties with detectable vWF
• Type II—selective depletion of high molecular weight multimers; uncommon form described in a family of German shorthaired pointers
• Type III—severe deficiency of vWF with virtually undetectable multimers of vWF; typical of the defect in Scottish terriers, Chesapeake Bay retrievers, and about two-thirds of affected Shetland sheepdogs

RISK FACTORS
Hypothyroidism may exacerbate the bleeding tendency in affected animals.

DIAGNOSIS

DIFFERENTIAL DIAGNOSIS
• Classic hemophilia—defective synthesis of factor VIII is usually associated with much lower factor VIII activity and with a more severe bleeding tendency, including spontaneous hemorrhages in body cavities, deep muscle masses, and joints.
• Other inherited or acquired hemostatic defects

CBC/BIOCHEMISTRY/URINALYSIS
• Anemia proportional to the degree of blood loss
• Neutrophilia and mild left shift secondary to hemorrhage
• Mild reticulocytosis
• Normal platelet count

OTHER LABORATORY TESTS
• PT—normal
• APTT—normal in most dogs, even those with severe deficiency of vWF
• vWF assay—the test of choice for diagnosis; normal range reported as 60%–72% of normal reference pools of dogs; reference method is the Laurell rocket electroimmunoassay, but a reliable ELISA method is available (Zymtec, Iatric Corp., Tempe, AZ): < 7% indicates either a homozygous defect or severe (penetrant) heterozygous animal, 7%–50% usually indicates heterozygous animal (either asymptomatic carrier or bleeder), < 30% indicates animal is more likely to have a hemorrhagic tendency

IMAGING
N/A

DIAGNOSTIC PROCEDURES
Buccal mucosal bleeding time—useful in predicting bleeding problems in dogs suspected of being affected; use of a gauze strip tied around the maxilla to cause venous engorgement in the folded-back upper lip increases the sensitivity of the test; normal bleeding time for this method is 1.7–4.2 min (mean, 2.6 min); bleeding time does not identify all animals at risk for abnormal bleeding after surgery.

PATHOLOGIC FINDINGS
Hemorrhage is the only associated abnormality, which can occur at any site but most commonly occurs at sites of injury and mucosal surfaces.

WHIPWORMS (TRICURIASIS)

MEDICATIONS

DRUGS
• Fenbendazole 50 mg/kg PO q24h for 3–5 days; second course of treatment in 3 months
• Febantel/praziquantel/pyrantel pamoate
• Dichlorvos given twice, 3–4 weeks apart
• Milbemycin oxime monthly

CONTRAINDICATIONS/POSSIBLE INTERACTIONS
• Organophosphates in heartworm-positive dogs
• Do not give dichlorvos concurrently with other organophosphates such as insecticides.

FOLLOW-UP
Fecal examination for trichurid eggs 3–4 weeks following treatment

MISCELLANEOUS

SYNONYMS
Trichuriasis

Suggested Reading
Bowman DD, ed. Georgi's parasitology for veterinarians. 6th ed. Philadelphia: Saunders, 1994:226–229.
Author Robert M. Corwin
Consulting Editors Brett M. Feder and Mitchell A. Crystal

DISEASES

WOBBLER SYNDROME (CERVICAL VERTEBRAL INSTABILITY)

BASICS

DEFINITION
• Encompasses compressive spinal cord lesions affecting the cervical spine (primarily caudal) in large- and giant-breed dogs; may be disk related or vertebral related
• Disk related—mature dogs; arising from type II disk herniation with accompanying vertebral ligamentous hypertrophy, presumably caused by joint instability; C5–6 and C6–7 primarily involved; C3–4 and C4–5 may be involved.
• Vertebral-related—young dogs; arising from developmental abnormalities causing malformation and malarticulation of the vertebral column; all cervical joints may be affected.

PATHOPHYSIOLOGY
Compression of the cervical spinal cord

SYSTEMS AFFECTED
Nervous

GENETICS
No inheritance specifically identified, but many factors may be under genetic control

INCIDENCE/PREVALENCE
Reported in numerous breeds of large dogs

GEOGRAPHIC DISTRIBUTION
N/A

SIGNALMENT

Species
Dogs

Breed Predilections
• Disk related—Doberman pinschers
• Vertebral related—Great Danes

Mean Age and Range
• Disk related—mature, > 2 years old; most patients > 5 years
• Vertebral related—young, generally < 2 years old

Predominant Sex
N/A

SIGNS

General Comments
Highly variable, depending on the degree of compression and duration of lesion

Historical Findings
• Acute or chronic onset
• Progressive or nonprogressive nature

Physical Examination Findings
• Variable neck pain
• Difficulty rising to a standing posture
• Variable muscle atrophy, especially in forelimbs
• Worn toenails
• Ataxia—involves all four limbs but to a lesser degree in the forelimbs; normal, decreased, or absent postural reactions in all four limbs; lower or upper motor neuron signs in forelimbs and upper motor neuron signs in hind limbs
• Pain perception usually intact

CAUSES
• Disk-related—disk degeneration or vertebral instability
• Vertebral-related—nutritionally related malformation or malarticulation

RISK FACTORS
• Disk-related—none specifically identified
• Vertebral related—large, rapidly growing dogs

DIAGNOSIS

DIFFERENTIAL DIAGNOSIS
• Disk-related—trauma, diskospondylitis, primary disk disease, neoplasia, and inflammatory spinal cord diseases; differentiated by breed incidence, results of CSF analysis, and radiographic studies
• Vertebral-related—same as for disk related; juvenile orthopedic diseases

CBC/BIOCHEMISTRY/URINALYSIS
Usually normal

OTHER LABORATORY TESTS
N/A

IMAGING

Survey Cervical Radiography
• Disk-related—may be normal or show narrowing of the disk space suggesting disk herniation
Vertebral-related—may show abnormal articular facet shape or density, subluxation, malformed vertebral bodies, stenosis of the vertebral canal, and misshapen dorsal spinal processes

Myelography
• Disk-related—soft tissue compression of the spinal cord by the dorsal annulus of the disk, dorsal longitudinal ligament, and dorsal ligamentum flavum
• Vertebral-related—compression of the spinal cord owing to proliferation of the articular facets, remodeling of vertebral bodies, and other bony causes of stenosis of the spinal canal

DIAGNOSTIC PROCEDURES
CSF analysis—may be normal or show high protein owing to compressive degeneration of the spinal cord

PATHOLOGIC FINDINGS
• White and gray matter necrosis at the level of compression
• Wallerian-type degeneration of white matter above and below area of compression

WOBBLER SYNDROME (CERVICAL VERTEBRAL INSTABILITY)

TREATMENT

APPROPRIATE HEALTH CARE
Inpatient—requires surgery

NURSING CARE
• Nonambulatory—keep patient on soft bedding (synthetic fleece) to avoid bed sores.
• Bladder catheterization—avoids manual expression and urine scalding
• Passive and active manipulation of the limbs to avoid ankylosis

ACTIVITY
Limit to avoid exacerbation of the condition

DIET
Vertebral related disease—discontinue excessive use of dietary supplements; control food intake

CLIENT EDUCATION
• Depending on the chronicity of the disease, inform client that neurologic deficits may remain.
• Inform client that the goal of treatment is to stop the progression.
• Advise client that physiotherapy is usually required to maximize return of function.

SURGICAL CONSIDERATIONS

Decompression
• Ventral spondylectomy—best suited for solitary lesions compressing from the floor of the spinal canal; disk-related disease
• Dorsal laminectomy—best for multiple sites of involvement or when compression is mainly from the roof of the spinal canal; disk-related and developmental diseases

Other
• Fenestration—prevents additional sites of involvement; disk-related disease
• Stabilization/fusion—controversial for disk-related caudal cervical compression; advocates: primary lesion is unstable, which should be stabilized; opponents: stabilization without decompression does nothing for the compressive lesion and may actually precipitate additional damage at the disk spaces on either side of the fused space

MEDICATIONS

DRUG OF CHOICE
Glucocorticosteroids—in combination with surgery, the most advantageous therapeutic approach; without surgery, useful only in mildly affected patients

CONTRAINDICATIONS
N/A

PRECAUTIONS
Observe for signs of gastroenteritis and cystitis.

POSSIBLE INTERACTIONS
N/A

ALTERNATIVE DRUGS
N/A

FOLLOW-UP

PATIENT MONITORING
• Repeat neurologic examinations—as necessary to evaluate response to treatment

PREVENTION/AVOIDANCE
• Limit running and jumping
• Avoid collar; use body harness instead

POSSIBLE COMPLICATIONS
Disk related—adjacent sites may become involved.

EXPECTED COURSE AND PROGNOSIS
• Acute—immediate aggressive treatment necessary for best outcome
• Chronic progressive—the earlier surgery is performed, the better the outcome; paralyzed patients often cannot be helped.

MISCELLANEOUS

ASSOCIATED CONDITIONS
N/A

AGE-RELATED FACTORS
• Disk-related—old dogs
• Developmental related—young dogs

ZOONOTIC POTENTIAL
N/A

PREGNANCY
N/A

SYNONYMS
• Disk related—spondylolisthesis; vertebral subluxation; caudal cervical spondylopathy; cervical spondylopathy
• Vertebral related—vertebral stenosis; cervical vertebral stenotic myelopathy; cervical spondylopathy

SEE ALSO
• Intervertebral Disk Disease, Cervical
• Osteochondrosis

ABBREVIATION
BAER = brainstem auditory-evoked response

Suggested Reading
Braund KG. Degenerative and developmental diseases. In: Oliver JE, Hoerlein BF, Mayhew IG, eds. Veterinary neurology. Philadelphia: Saunders, 1987:185–215.
de Lahunta A. Veterinary neuroanatomy and clinical neurology. 2nd ed. Philadelphia: Saunders, 1983.
Oliver JE, Lorenz MD, Kornegay JN. Handbook of veterinary neurology. 3rd ed. Philadelphia: Saunders, 1997.
Summers BA, Cummings JF, de Lahunta. Veterinary neuropathology. St. Louis: Mosby. 1995.
Author Patricia J. Luttgen
Consulting Editor Joane M. Parent

DISEASES

ZINC TOXICITY

BASICS

OVERVIEW
• Toxicity from the ingestion of zinc ointment or zinc-containing objects
• Causes severe intravascular hemolysis and gastrointestinal irritation; may cause multiple organ failure (e.g., renal, hepatic, and cardiac), DIC, and cardiopulmonary arrest

SIGNALMENT
Most frequently reported in dogs

SIGNS
• Pale mucous membranes
• Hemoglobinuria
• Hematuria
• Anorexia
• Vomiting
• Diarrhea
• Icterus

CAUSES & RISK FACTORS
Ingestion of zinc-containing objects—nuts from transport cages and plumbing parts; zinc oxide ointment; game pieces from board games; pennies minted after 1982

DIAGNOSIS

DIFFERENTIAL DIAGNOSIS
• Autoimmune hemolytic anemia
• Babesia
• Onion toxicity
• Caval syndrome
• A radiographically apparent metallic object in the gastrointestinal tract—strongly supports diagnosis; may help differentiate from other diseases

CBC/BIOCHEMISTRY/URINALYSIS
• Severe intravascular hemolytic anemia
• High nucleated RBC counts
• Basophilic stippling
• Target cells
• Polychromasia
• High BUN, creatinine, ALP, and ALT—may indicate multiple organ failure

OTHER LABORATORY TESTS
• High serum zinc concentration—normal in dogs, 0.7–2.0 μg/mL
• Coagulation panel—may indicate DIC (prolonged PT and PTT, hypofibrinogenemia, thrombocytopenia, and high FDP)

IMAGING
Abdominal radiography—may reveal metallic object in the gastrointestinal tract

DIAGNOSTIC PROCEDURES
ECG—may reveal arrhythmias and ST-segment abnormalities

TREATMENT

• Rapid removal of the zinc object by endoscopy or laparotomy—imperative
• Maintain hydration—acute renal failure is a serious sequelae
• Severe intravascular hemolysis—may require blood transfusion
• Inform client about the hazards of ingesting zinc-containing objects (especially pennies minted after 1982).
• Advise client to avoid using zinc oxide ointments.

MEDICATIONS

DRUGS
• Heparin—150 U/kg SC q6h; for DIC
• H_2-receptor blockers—cimetidine, ranitidine; may help reduce stomach acidity and the rate of release of zinc
• CaEDTA—100 mg/kg diluted in 5% dextrose SC, divided into four doses per day; may be given for zinc chelation

CONTRAINDICATIONS/POSSIBLE INTERACTIONS
Avoid aminoglycoside antibiotics and other potential nephrotoxins—risk of acute renal failure

FOLLOW-UP

PATIENT MONITORING
• ECG—monitor for evidence of arrhythmias and ST-segment alterations.
• Coagulation profile, BUN, creatinine, ALP, and ALT–monitor for the first 72 hr after zinc removal

EXPECTED COURSE AND PROGNOSIS
• Multiple organ failure and cardiopulmonary arrest—potential outcomes
• Rapid removal of the source of zinc—may provide progressive improvement over 48–72 hr; complete recovery possible

MISCELLANEOUS

SEE ALSO
Poisoning (Intoxication)

ABBREVIATIONS
• ALP = alkaline phosphatase
• ALT = alanine aminotransferase
• DIC = disseminated intravascular coagulation
• FDP = fibrin degradation products
• PT = prothrombin time
• PTT = partial thromboplastin time

Suggested Reading
Ogden L. Zinc toxicosis. In: Kirk RW, Bonagura JD, eds. Current veterinary therapy XI. Philadelphia: Saunders, 1992:197–200.
Author Kathryn M. Meurs
Consulting Editor Gary D. Osweiler

APPENDICES

APPENDIX I

NORMAL REFERENCE RANGES FOR LABORATORY TESTS

Table I-A.

Normal Hematologic Values			
Test	Units	Dogs	Cats
WBC	$10 \times 3/mm^3$	6.0–17.0	5.5–19.5
RBC	$10 \times 6/mm^3$	5.5–8.5	6.0–10
Hemoglobin	g/dl	12.0–18.0	9.5–15
Hematocrit	%	37.0–55.0	29–45
MCV	fl	60.0–77.0	41.0–54
MCH	pg	19.5–26	13.3–17.5
MCHC	%	32.0–36.0	31–36
Platelet count (automated)	$10 \times 3/mm^3$	200–500	150–600
Platelet count (manual)	$10 \times 3/mm^3$	164–510	230–680
Neutrophils	%	60–77	35–75
	Absolute	3000–11,500	2500–12,500
Bands	%	0–3	0–3
	Absolute	0–510	0–585
Lymphocytes	%	12–30	20–55
	Absolute	1000–4800	1500–7000
Monocytes	%	3–10	1–4
	Absolute	180–1350	0–850
Eosinophils	%	2–10	2–12
	Absolute	1000–1250	0–1500
Basophils	%	0–1	0–1
	Absolute	0–100	0–100
Reticulocyte count	%	0.5–1.5	0.0–1.0
Corrected	%	0.0–1.0	0.0–1.0
Absolute	$/mm^3$	0–80000	0–50000

From Abbott Cell Dyne 3500; IDEXX Veterinary Services.
It is important to realize that normal values vary among individual laboratories.

Table I-B.

Normal Biochemical Values			
Test	*Units*	*Dogs*	*Cats*
Urea nitrogen (BUN)	mg/dl	7–27	15–34
Creatinine	mg/dl	0.4–1.8	0.8–2.3
Cholesterol	mg/dl	112–328	82–218
Glucose	mg/dl	60–125	70–150
Alkaline phosphatase (ALP)	IU/L	10–150	0–62
Alanine aminotransferase (ALT)	IU/L	5–60	28–76
Aspartate aminotransferase (AST)	IU/L	5–55	5–55
Total protein	g/dl	5.1–7.8	5.9–8.5
Albumin	g/dl	2.6–4.3	2.4–4.1
Globulin	g/dl	2.3–4.5	3.4–5.2
A-G ratio		0.75–1.9	0.6–1.5
Sodium	mEq/L	141–156	147–156
Potassium	mEq/L	4.0–5.6	3.9–5.3
Sodium-potassium ratio		27–40	> 27.0
Chloride	mEq/L	105–115	111–125
Total CO_2	mEq/L	17–24	13–25
Anion gap	mEq/L	12–24	13–27
Calcium	mg/dl	7.5–11.3	7.5–10.8
Phosphorus	mg/dl	2.1–6.3	3.0–7.0
Total bilirubin	mg/dl	0–0.4	0.0–0.4
Direct bilirubin	mg/dl	0.0–0.1	0.0–0.1
Indirect bilirubin	mg/dl	0–0.3	0.0–0.3
Lactate dehydrogenase (LDH)	IU/L	50–380	46–350
Creatine kinase (CK or CPK)	IU/L	10–200	64–440
Gamma glutamyl transferase (GGT)	IU/L	0–10	1–7
Uric acid	mg/dl	0–2	0–1
Amylase	IU/L	500–1500	500–1500
Lipase	U/L	100–500	10–195
Magnesium	mEq/L	1.8–2.4	1.8–2.4
Trigiycendes	mg/dl	20–150	20–90
Bile acids:			
Fasting	μmol/L	0.0–5.0	0.0–5.0
Postprandial	μmol/L	< 25	< 15
Random	μmol/L	< 25	< 15
Total iron	μg/dl	33–147	33–134
Unsaturated iron binding capacity	μg/dl	127–340	105–205
Total iron binding capacity	μg/dl	282–386	169–325

From Hitachi Chemistry Analyzer model 747 IDEXX Veterinary Services.
It is important to realize that normal values vary among individual laboratories.

Table I-C.

Conversion Table for Hematologic Units				
	Example values		Conversion factors	
Analyte	Traditional	SI*	Traditional to SI	SI to Traditional
Hemoglobin	15.0 g/dl	150 g/L	10	0.1
HCT or PCV	45%	0.45 L/L	0.01	100
Erythrocytes	$6.0 \times 10^6/mm^3$	$6.0 \times 10^{12}/L$	10^6	10^{-6}
MCV	$75 \mu^3$	75 fl	No change	No change
MCH	$25 \mu\mu g$	25 pg	No change	No change
MCHC	33 g/dl	330 g/L	10	0.1
WBC	$15.0 \times 10^3/mm^3$	$15.0 \times 10^9/L$	10^6	10^{-6}
Platelets	$250 \times 10^3/mm^3$	$250 \times 10^9/L$	10^6	10^{-6}

Système International d'Unités
Modified from Appendices. In: Bonagura JD, ed. Current veterinary therapy XIII Philadelphia: WB Saunders, 2000: 1209 (with permission).

Table I-D.

Conversion Table for Clinical Biochemical Units		
Analyte	Traditional unit (with examples)	Conversion factor	SI unit (with examples)
Alanine aminotransferase	0–40 U/L	1.00	0–40 U/L
Albumin	2.8–4.0 g/dl	10.0	28–40 g/L
Alkaline phosphatase	30–150 U/L	1.00	30–150 U/L
Ammonia	10–80 μg/dl	0.5871	5.9–47.0 μmol/L
Amylase	200–800 U/L	1.00	200–800 U/L
Aspartate aminotransferase	0–40 U/L	1.00	0–40 U/L
Bile acids (total)	0.3–2.3 μg/ml	2.45	0.74–5.64 μmol/L
Bilirubin	0.1–0.2 mg/dl	17.10	2–4 μmol/L
Calcium	8.8–10.3 mg/dl	0.2495	2.20–2.58 mmol/L
Carbon dioxide	22–28 mEq/L	1.00	22–28 mmol/L
Chloride	95–100 mEq/L	1.00	95–100 mmol/L
Cholesterol	100–265 mg/dl	0.0258	2.58–5.85 mmol/L
Copper	70–140 μg/dl	0.1574	11.0–22.0 μmol/L
Cortisol	2–10 μg/dl	27.59	55–280 nmol/L
Creatine kinase	0–130 U/L	1.00	0–130 U/L
Creatinine	0.6–1.2 mg/dl	88.40	50–110 μmol/L
Fibrinogen	200–400 mg/dl	0.01	2.0–4.0 g/L
Folic acid	3.5–11.0 μg/L	2.265	7.93–24.92 nmol/L
Glucose	70–110 mg/dl	0.05551	3.9–6.1 mmol/L
Iron	80–180 μg/dl	0.1791	14–32 μmol/L
Lactate	5–20 mg/dl	0.1110	0.5–2.0 mmol/L
Lead	150 μg/dl	0.04826	7.2 μmol/L
Lipase Sigma Tietz (37° C)	≤ 1 ST U/dl	280	≤ 280 U/L
Lipase Cherry Crandall (30° C)	0–160 U/L	1.00	0–160 U/L
Lipids (total)	400–850 mg/dl	0.01	4.0–8.5 g/L
Magnesium	1.8–3.0 mg/dl	0.4114	0.80–1.20 mmol/L
Mercury	≤ 1.0 μg/dl	49.85	≤ 50 nmol/L
Osmolality	280–300 mOsm/kg	1.00	280–300 mmol/kg
Phosphorus	2.5–5.0 mg/dl	0.3229	0.80–1.6 mmol/L
Potassium	3.5–5.0 mEq/L	1.0	3.5–5.0 mmol/L
Protein (total)	5–8 g/dl	10.0	50–80 g/L
Sodium	135–147 mEq/L	1.00	135–147 mmol/L
Testosterone	4.0–8.0 mg/ml	3.467	14.0–28.0 nmol/L
Thyroxine	1–4 μg/dl	12.87	13–51 nmol/L
Triglyceride	10–500 mg/dl	0.0113	0.11–5.65 mmol/L
Urea nitrogen	10–20 mg/dl	0.3570	3.6–7.1 nmol/L
Uric acid	3.6–7.7 mg/dl	59.44	214–458 μmol/L
Urobilinogen	0–4.0 mg/dl	16.9	0.0–6.8 μmol/L
Vitamin A	90 μg/dl	0.03491	3.1 μmol/L
Vitamin B_{12}	300–700 ng/L	0.738	221–516 pmol/L
Vitamin E	5.0–20.0 mg/L	2.32	11.6–46.4 μmol/L
D-xylose	30–40 mg/dl	0.06666	2.0–2.71 mmol/L
Zinc	75–120 μg/dl	0.1530	11.5–18.5 μmol/L

From Appendices. In: Bonagura JD, ed. Current veterinary therapy XIII. Philadelphia: WB Saunders, 2000: 1214 (with permission).

APPENDIX II

ENDOCRINE TESTING

Table II-A.

Endocrine Function Testing Protocols

ADRENAL GLAND DISORDERS

ACTH STIMULATION TEST

Dogs

Administer 20 IU ACTH gel IM or 0.25 mg synthetic ACTH IV or IM (Cortrosyn, Organon Pharmaceuticals, West Orange, NJ).
ACTH Gel
Serum samples should be obtained before and 2 hours after injection of ACTH for cortisol assay.
Synthetic ACTH
Serum samples should be obtained before and 1 hour after injection of ACTH for cortisol assay.

Cats

Administer 0.125 mg synthetic ACTH IV. Serum samples should be obtained before and 1 hour after injection of ACTH for cortisol assay.

Interpretation

Screening for Cushing's Disease
An exaggerated response to ACTH is consistent with Cushing's disease. High normal cut-off values differ slightly between laboratories.
Screening for Hypoadrenocorticism
Pre- and post-cortisol determinations < 1 μg/dl (30 nmol/L) is consistent with hypoadrenocorticism.
Monitoring Mitotane or Ketoconazole Therapy for Cushing's Disease
Pre- and post-cortisol determinations should be within the normal basal cortisol range.

LOW-DOSE DEXAMETHASONE SUPPRESSION TEST (LDDST)

Dogs

Administer 0.015 mg/kg dexamethasone (Azium) IV or IM. Obtain serum samples before and 4 and 8 hours after injection of dexamethasone for cortisol assay.

Cats

Administer 0.1 mg/kg dexamethasone (Azium) IV or IM. Obtain serum sample before and 4 and 8 hours after injection of dexamethasone for cortisol assay.

Interpretation

Three Basic Patterns
Lack of Suppression
All cortisol values remain above 1 μg/dl (30 nmol/L). This pattern is consistent with Cushing's disease.
Suppression
Cortisol values fall below 1 μg/dl (30 nmol/L) at 4 and 8 hours. This pattern suggests that the animal does not have Cushing's disease.
Escape from Suppression
Cortisol value falls below 1 μg/dl (30 nmol/L) at 4 hours and rises above 1 μg/dl at 8 hours. This pattern is consistent with pituitary-dependent Cushing's disease.

HIGH-DOSE DEXAMETHASONE SUPPRESSION TEST (HDDST)

Administer 1 mg/kg dexamethasone (Azium) IV or IM. Obtain serum samples before and 4 and 8 hours after injection of dexamethasone for cortisol assay.

Interpretation

Any cortisol determination that falls below 1.5 μg/dl (45 nmol/L) at any point during the 8-hour testing period is considered suppression. Suppression after a high dose of dexamethasone is consistent with pituitary-dependent Cushing's disease. Lack of suppression (all cortisol values remain above 1.5 μg/dl) is diagnostic of a pituitary or adrenal tumor.

THYROID GLAND DISORDERS

TSH STIMULATION TEST

Administer 0.5 U/kg TSH (maximum dose 5 U) IV. Obtain serum samples before and 6 hours after injection of TSH for T_4 determination.

Interpretation

Post-TSH T_4 levels < 3 μg/dl (35 nmol/L) is consistent with hypothyroidism.

TRH STIMULATION TEST

Administer 0.1 mg/kg TRH IV. Obtain serum samples before and 4 hours after TRH injection for T_4 determination.

Interpretation

An increase in T_4 concentration $< 50\%$ after TRH administration is consistent with hypothyroidism.

T3 SUPPRESSION TEST

Obtain a blood sample for determination of T_4 and T_3. The serum is removed and kept refrigerated or frozen. Administer T_3 (Cytomel, Smith, Kline, and French Laboratories) PO at a dosage of 25 μg/cat q8h for 2 days. On the morning of the third day, administer 25 μg of T_3, and 2–4 hours later obtain a second blood sample for T_3 and T_4 determinations. The basal (day 1) and postoral T_3 serum samples should be submitted to the laboratory together to avoid interassay variation.

Interpretation

Serum T_4 concentration after administration of T_3 $>$ than 1.5 μg/dl (20 nmol/L) is consistent with hyperthyroidism.

GASTRINOMA

SECRETIN STIMULATION TEST

Administer 2 units of secretin/kg IV. Take blood samples before administration of secretin and then 2, 5, 10, 15, and 30 minutes later. Assay the samples for gastrin.

Interpretation

Dogs with gastrinomas have a rise in gastrin levels after the injection of secretin. In three reported cases, two dogs had a rise in gastrin levels 2 times baseline 5 minutes after secretin injection, and one dog had a rise in gastrin levels 1.4 times baseline 5 minutes after secretin injection. Normal dogs have a decline in gastrin levels after administration of secretin.

CALCIUM CHALLENGE TEST

Administer 2 mg/kg of calcium gluconate IV over a 1-minute period or administer 5 mg/kg of calcium gluconate as an IV infusion over several hours.

Obtain a blood sample before calcium administration and then 15, 30, 60, 90, and 120 minutes after the calcium administration. Assay the samples for gastrin.

Interpretation

Two reported patients with gastrinoma had a doubling of the gastrin level 60 minutes after the calcium infusion.

SEX HORMONE DISORDERS

GN-RH STIMULATION TEST

Administer 0.5–1.0 μg of Gn-RH/kg IM. Obtain blood samples before Gn-RH administration and 1 hour later. Assay blood samples for testosterone.

Interpretation

Normal dogs have baseline testosterone levels between 0.5–5 ng/ml, and after administration of Gn-RH the testosterone levels rise above 5 ng/ml. Animals with hypoandrogenism have lower values.

HCG STIMULATION TEST

Administer 44 IU of hCG/kg IM. Obtain blood samples before hCG administration and 4 hours later. Assay blood samples for testosterone.

Interpretation

Normal dogs have baseline testosterone levels between 0.5–5 ng/ml, and after administration of hCG, the testosterone levels rise above 5 ng/ml. Animals with hypoandrogenism have lower values.

DIABETES INSIPIDUS

MODIFIED WATER DEPRIVATION TEST

Rule out other causes of polyuria and polydipsia (especially *byperadrenocorticism*). Begin water restriction 3 days before abrupt water deprivation.

Day 1   130–165 ml/kg/day
Day 2   100–125 ml/kg/day
Day 3   65–70 ml/kg/day (normal maintenance requirement)

The morning of the fourth day, discontinue food and water. Start the test. Weigh the patient and empty the bladder. Weigh at 1–2 hour intervals. Monitor carefully for dehydration and depression. When 5% of body weight is lost or azotemia develops, empty the bladder and check urine specific gravity. Consider plasma vasopressin determination at this point.

Interpretation

If the urine specific gravity is > 1.025 (dogs) or > 1.030 (cats), stop the test. The patient does not have diabetes insipidus. If the urine specific gravity is not > 1.025 (dogs) or > 1.030 (cats), administer 0.55 U/kg aqueous vasopressin IM (maximum dose 5 U). Empty the bladder and check urine specific gravity at 30, 60, and 120 minutes postadministration. If urine specific gravity increases $< 10\%$, nephrogenic diabetes insipidus is indicated; if it increases 10–50%, partial central diabetes insipidus is indicated; if it increases 50–800%, complete central diabetes insipidus is indicated.

Table II-B.

Tests of the Endocrine System*

Hormone	Unit	Dogs	Cats
Adrenocorticotrophic hormone, basal (ACTH, plasma)	pmol/L	2–15	1–20
Aldosterone[†] (plasma)			
Basal	pmol/L	14–957	194–388
Post-ACTH	pmol/L	197–2103	277–721
Cortisol (serum or plasma, urine)			
Basal	nmol/L	25–125	15–150
Post-ACTH	nmol/L	200–550	130–450
Post–low-close dexamethasone (0.01 or 0.015 mg/kg)	nmol/L	≤ 40	≤ 40
Post–high-dose dexamethasone (0.1 or 1.0 mg/kg)[‡]	nmol/L	≤ 40	≤ 40
Urinary cortisol-creatinine ratio	$\times 10^{-6}$	8–24[†], 10[§]	—
Insulin, basal (serum)	pmol/L	35–200	35–200
Intact parathormone[†] (serum)	pmol/L	2–13	0–4
Progesterone (serum or plasma, female)	mmol/L	≤ 3.0 in anestrus, proestrus	≤ 3.0 in anestrus, proestrus
		50–220 in diestrus, pregnancy	50–220 in diestrus, pregnancy
Testosterone (serum or plasma, male)	nmol/L	1–20	1–20
Thyroxine (T_4, serum)			
Basal	nmol/L	12–50	10–50
Post–thyroxine-stimulating hormone (TSH)	nmol/L	> 45	> 45
Triiodothyronine (T_3) suppression[‖]	nmol/L	—	≤ 20
Triiodothyronine, basal (T_3, serum)	nmol/L	0.7–2.3	0.5–2.0

*Prepared with the assistance of ME Peterson, The Animal Medical Center, New York, NY. Unless indicated otherwise, values in this table are adapted from Kemppainen RJ, Zerbe CA. Common endocrine diagnostic tests: normal values and interpretations. In: Kirk RW, ed. Current veterinary therapy X. Philadelphia: WB Saunders, 1989:961–968. Hormone determinations are variable between laboratories. The laboratory performing the analysis should provide reference values. Before submitting samples for hormone determinations, consult the laboratory for sample specifications, use of anticoagulants, and sample preservation. General sampling conditions are discussed in Reimers TJ. Guidelines for collection, storage, and transport of samples for hormone assay. In: Kirk RW, ed. Current veterinary therapy X. Philadelphia: WB Saunders, 1989:968–973. Factors that affect serum thyroid and adrenocortical hormone concentrations in dogs are discussed in Reimers TJ, Lawler DF, Sutaria PM, Correa MT, Erb HN. Effects of age, sex, and body size on serum concentrations of thyroid and adrenocortical hormones in dogs. Am J Vet Res 1990;51:454.
[†]Provided by RF Nachreiner, Animal Health Diagnostic Laboratory, Endocrine Diagnostic Section, Michigan State University.
[‡]This test is used after adrenocortical hyperfunction has been confirmed. It is used to differentiate adrenal tumor (where no suppression is seen) from pituitary-dependent cases (where suppression occurs but is variable).
[§]From Stolp R, Rijnberk A, Meiher JC, Croughs RJM. Urinary corticoids in the diagnosis of canine hyperadrenocorticism. Res Vet Sci 1983;34:141. Rijnberk A, van Wees A, Mol JA. Assessment of two tests for the diagnosis of canine hyperadrenocorticism. Vet Rec 1988;122:178–180.
[‖]From Peterson ME, Ferguson DC. Thyroid diseases. In: Ettinger SJ, ed. Textbook of veterinary internal medicine. Diseases of the dog and cat. 3rd ed. Philadelphia: WB Saunders, 1989:1632–1675.
From appendices In Bonagura J, ed. Kirk's current veterinary therapy XIII Philadelphia: WB Saunders, 2000; 1223 (with permission).

Table II-C.

| | Unit | | Conversion factors | |
Hormone	Traditional	SI	Traditional to SI	SI to Traditional
Aldosterone	ng/dl	pmol/L	27.7	0.036
Corticotrophin (ACTH)	pg/ml	pmol/L	0.22	4.51
Cortisol	μg/dl	mmol/L	27.59	0.36
β-endorphin	pg/ml	pmol/L	0.289	3.43
Epinephrine	pg/ml	pmol/L	5.46	0.183
Estrogen (estradiol)	pg/ml	pmol/L	3.67	0.273
Gastrin	pg/ml	ng/L	1.00	1.00
Glucagon	pg/ml	ng/L	1.00	1.00
Growth hormone (GH)	ng/ml	μg/L	1.00	1.00
Insulin	μU/ml	pmol/L	7.18	0.139
α-melanocyte–stimulating hormone (α-MSH)	pg/ml	pmol/L	0.601	1.66
Norepinephrine	pg/ml	nmol/L	0.006	169
Pancreatic polypeptide (PP)	mg/dl	mmol/L	0.239	4.18
Progesterone	ng/ml	mmol/L	3.18	0.315
Prolactin	ng/ml	μg/L	1.00	1.00
Renin	ng/ml//hr	ng/L/s	0.278	3.60
Somatostatin	pg/ml	pmol/L	0.611	1.64
Testosterone	ng/ml	nmol/L	3.47	0.288
Thyroxine (T_4)	μg/dl	nmol/L	12.87	0.078
Triiodothyronine (T_3)	ng/dl	nmol/L	0.0154	64.9
Vasoactive intestinal polypeptide (VIP)	pg/ml	pmol/L	0.301	3.33

Conversion Table for Hormone Assay Units

Contributed by ME Peterson, The Animal Medical Center, New York, NY.
From Appendices. In: Bonagura JD, ed. Current veterinary therapy XIII. Philadelphia: WB Saunders, 2000: 1223 (with permission).

APPENDIX III

APPROXIMATE NORMAL RANGES FOR COMMON MEASUREMENTS IN DOGS AND CATS

	Dog	Cat
Heart rate (bpm)	60–180	140–220
Capillary refill time	< 2 sec	< 2 sec
Body temperature	99.5–102.5° F	100.5–102.5° F
	37.5–39.2° C	38.1–39.2° C
Mean arterial pressure (mm Hg)	90–120	100–150
Blood volume (ml/kg)	75–90	47–66
Cardiac output		
(ml/kg/min)	100–200	167 ± 39
(L/M²/min)	4.72 ± 1.09	
Systemic resistance		
(mm Hg/ml/kg/min)	0.64 ± 0.16	
(dynes/sec/cm)	2162 ± 458	
Mean pulmonary arterial pressure (mm Hg)	14 ± 3	
Central venous pressure (cm H_2O)	3 ± 4	
Pulmonary artery occlusion pressure (mm Hg)	5 ± 2	
Urine output	1–2 ml/kg/hr	1–2 ml/kg/hr
Breathing rate (breaths/min)	10–30	24–42
Minute ventilation (ml/kg/min)	170–350	200–350
Oxygen delivery		
(ml/kg/min)	29 ± 8	
(ml/M²/min)	815 ± 234	
Oxygen consumption		
(ml/kg/min)	4–11	3–8
(ml/M²/min)	198 ± 53	
Arterial P_{O_2} (mm Hg)	85–105	100–115
Arterial S_{O_2}	> 95	> 95
Arterial P_{CO_2} (mm Hg)	30–44	28–35
Arterial pH	7.36–7.46	7.34–7.43
Bicarbonate (mEq/L)	20–25	17–21
Base deficit (mEq/L)	0 to −4	−1 to −8
Total plasma proteins (g/dl)	6.0–8.0	6.8–8.3
Albumin (g/dl)	2.5–3.5	1.9–3.9
Packed cell volume (%)	37–55	29–48
Hemoglobin (g/dl)	12–18	9–15.1
Sodium (mEq/L)	145–154	151–158
Potassium (mEq/L)	4.1–5.3	3.6–4.9
Chloride (mEq/L)	105–116	113–121
Total CO_2 (mEq/L)	16–26	15–21

Modified from Aldrich J, Haskins SC. Monitoring the critically ill patient. In: Current veterinary therapy XII. Philadelphia: WB Saunders, 1995;98–105 (with permission).

APPENDIX IV

NORMAL VALUES FOR THE CANINE AND FELINE ELECTROCARDIOGRAM

RATE

Dog	60 to 140 beats/min for giant breeds	
	70 to 160 beats/min for adult dogs	
	Up to 180 beats/min for toy breeds	
	Up to 220 beats/min for puppies	
Cat	Range: 120 to 240 beats/min	
	Mean: 197 beats/min	

RHYTHM

Dog   Normal sinus rhythm
Sinus arrhythmia
Wandering SA pacemaker
Cat   Normal sinus rhythm
Sinus tachycardia (physiologic reaction to excitement)

MEASUREMENTS (lead II, 50 mm/second, 1 cm = 1 mv)

Dog
- P wave-   Width: maximum, 0.04 second; 0.05 second in giant breeds
         Height: maximum, 0.4 mv
- P-R interval-   Width: 0.06 to 0. 13 second
- QRS complex- Width: maximum, 0.05 second in small breeds
               maximum, 0.06 second in large breeds
         Height of R wave[a]: maximum, 3.0 mv in large breeds
                          maximum, 2.5 mv in small breeds
- S-T segment- No depression: not more than 0.2 mv
         No elevation: not more than 0.15 mv
- T wave-   Can be positive, negative, or biphasic
         Not greater than one-fourth amplitude of R wave
         Amplitude range ± 0.05–1.0 mv in any lead
- Q-T interval- Width: 0.15 to 0.25 second at normal heart rate; varies with heart rate (faster rates have shorter Q-T intervals and vice versa)

Cat
- P wave-   Width: maximum, 0.04 second
         Height: maximum, 0.2 mv
- P-R interval-   Width: 0.05 to 0.09 second
- QRS complex- Width: maximum, 0.04 second
         Height of R wave: maximum, 0.9 mv
- S-T segment- No depression or elevation
- T wave-   Can be positive, negative, or biphasic—most often positive
         Maximum amplitude: 0.3 mv
- Q-T interval- Width: 0.12 to 0.18 second at normal heart rate (range 0.07 to 0.20 second); varies with heart rate (faster rates have shorter Q-T intervals and vice versa)

MEAN ELECTRICAL AXIS (frontal plane)

Dog   +40 to +100 degrees
Cat   0 to +160 degrees (not valid in many cats)

PRECORDIAL CHEST LEADS (values of special importance)

Dog CV_5RL (rV_2): T wave positive, R wave not greater than 3.0 mv
CV_6LL (V_2): S wave not greater than 0.8 mv, R wave not greater than 3.0 mv[a]
CV_6LU (V_4): S wave not greater than 0.7 mv, R wave not greater than 3.0 mv[a]
V_{10}: negative QRS complex, T wave negative except in Chihuahua
Cat CV_6LL (V_2): R wave not greater than 1.0 mv
CV_6LU (V_4): R wave not greater than 1.0 mv
V_{10}: T wave negative, R/Q not greater than 1.0 mv

[a]Not valid for thin, deep-chested dogs under 2 years of age.
Source: Tilley, L.P.: *Essentials of Canine and Feline Electrocardiography, Interpretation and Treatment*. 3rd edition. Baltimore: Williams and Wilkins, 1992, with permission.

CLINICAL TOXICOSIS—SYSTEMS AFFECTED AND CLINICAL EFFECTS

Neurological Toxicants

Excitation or simulation of nervous system
  Amphetamine
  Aminopyridine
  Caffeine
  Cyanide
  Ergot (Claviceps spp.)
  Fluoroacetate
  Lead
  Metaldehyde
  Moonseed (Menispermum canadense)
  Mycotoxins
  Nicotine
  Organochlorine insecticides
  Organophosphate insecticides
  Phenols and chlorophenols
  Strychnine
  Theobromine
  Theophylline
  Water hemlock (Cicuta spp.)
Depression, coma
  Alcohols
  Antihistamines
  Barbiturates
  Carbon monoxide
  Hydrocarbons, aliphatic
  Hydrocarbons, aromatic
  Hydrocarbons, halogenated
  Lead
  Mercury
  Morphine derivatives
  Salicylates
  Snake venoms
Loss of motor control
  Botulinum
  Buckeye (Aesculus spp.)
  Carbon disulfide
  Curare
  Ergot
  Ethylene glycol
  Hexachlorophene
  Lead
  Nicotine
  Organophosphates
  Triaryl phosphates
Autonomic stimulation
  Atropine
  Carbarnate insecticides
  Fly mushroom (Amanita muscaria)
  Organophosphate insecticides
Behavioral changes
  Belladonna alkaloids
  Ergot
  Lead
  Lysergic acid diethylamide (LSD)
  Marijuana
  Morning glory
  Nutmeg
  Opium derivatives
  Organochlorine insecticides
  Periwinkle
  Peyote

Gastrointestinal Toxicants

Stomatitis, pharyngitis
  Acids and alkalies
  Aldehydes
  Chromium salts
  Fertilizer
  Mercuric salts
  Detergents
  Petroleum distillates
  Phenol
Salivation
  Amanita muscaria
  Ammonia
  Cresol
  Metaldehyde
  Nicotine
  Organophosphates
  Thallium
Dry mouth
  Amphetamine
  Antihistamine
  Atropine
  Belladonna
  Opiates
Gastroenteritis
  Amanita spp.
  Antimony
  Arsenic
  Barium
  Bismuth
  Cantharidin
  Copper salts
  Croton oil
  Detergents, soaps, sanitizers
  Digitalis toxins
  Iron
  Lead
  Mercury
  Mushrooms
  Phenoxy herbicides
  Phosphorus
  Plants (see Appendix VII)
  Staphylococcus toxin
  Thallium
  Zinc phosphide

Hepatotoxins

Acetaminophen
Aflatoxin
Amanita phalloides
Blue-green algae
Coal tar derivatives
Copper
Halogenated hydrocarbons
Iron
Petroleum distillates
Phosphorus

Nephrotoxins

Inadvertent nephrotoxins
  Aldehydes
  Amanita mushrooms
  Arsenic
  Bismuth
  Cadmium
  Cresols
  Dichromate
  Ethylene glycol
  Halogenated hydrocarbons
  Mercury
  Ochratoxin
  Oxalates
  Petroleum distillates
  Phenols
  Thallium
  Turpentine
  Volatile oils (e.g., penny-royal oil or oil of juniper)
Nephrotoxic drugs
  Acetaminophen
  Amphotericin B
  Bacitracin
  Gentamicin
  Kanamycin
  Neomycin
  Polymyxin B
  Sulfonamides
  Vancomycin

Blood Toxicants

Methemoglobin
  Acetaminophen
  Aniline derivatives
  Chlorate
  Copper
  Methylene blue
  Nitrite
  Nitrobenzene
Hemolysis
  Acetaminophen*
  Aniline
  Arsine
  Chlorates
  Copper
  Methylene blue*
  Nitrobenzene
  Onions
  Snake venoms
  Turpentine
  Red maple leaves
Aplastic anemia, leukopenia, thrombo-cytopenia
  Arsenicals
  Aspirin
  Benzene
  Chloramphenicol
  Cytostatic agents
  Estrogens
  Phenylbutazone
  Toluene
  Trichlorethylene
Coagulopathy
  Aflatoxin
  Aspirin
  Coumarin rodenticides

*Especially in cats

Phosphorus
Sulfonamides

Cardiovascular Toxicants

Tachycardia and arrhythmias
  Adrenalin
  Aminophylline
  Amphetamine
  Aminoglycoside antibiotics
  Atropine
  Caffeine
  Cyanide
  Dinitrophenol
  Fluorocarbons
  Nicotine
  Thallium
Bradycardia
  Barium
  Cardiac glycosides
  Digitalis
  Morphine
  Opiates
  Oleander
  Red squill
Myocardial damage
  Amanita phalloides
  Barium
  Carbon monoxide
  Oleander
  Phosphorus
  Thallium
Vascular necrosis

Ergot
Lead
Mercury
Selenium

Respiratory Toxicants

Air pollutants (nitrogen dioxide, sulfur dioxide)
Allergens
Ammonia
ANTU rodenticide
Chlorine
Gasoline, kerosene
Organophosphate insecticides
Ozone
Paraquat herbicide
Thallium

Ocular Toxicants

Mydriasis
  Amanita mushrooms
  Atropine
  Belladonna
  Methanol
Miosis
  Heroin
  Morphine
  Nicotine
  Organophosphates
Optic neuropathy
  Arsenicals
  Lead

Mercury
Methanol
Thallium
Vitamin A

General Signs

Fever
  Atropine
  Carbon monoxide
  Dinitrophenol
  Lead
  Metaldehyde
  Organochlorine insecticides
Hypothermia
  Alcohol
  Arsenic
  Barbiturates
  Heroin
  Morphine
  Oxalates
  Phenols
Cyanosis
  Carbon dioxide
  Hydrogen sulfide
  Nitrite
  Paraquat
Pink skin color
  Arsenic
  Carbon monoxide
  Cyanide
  Mercury
  Thallium

From Osweiler G. A brief guide to clinical toxicosis in small animals. In: Kirk RW, ed. Current veterinary therapy IX. Philadelphia: WB Saunders, 1986:132–135 (with permission).

APPENDIX VI

TOXIC AGENTS AND THEIR SYSTEMIC ANTIDOTES—DOSAGE AND METHOD OF TREATMENT

Toxic agent	Systemic antidote	Dosage and method of treatment
Acetaminophen	N-acetylcysteine (Mucomyst, Mead Johnson)	150 mg/kg loading dose PO or IV, then 50 mg/kg q4h for 17–20 additional doses
Amphetamines	Chlorpromazine	1 mg/kg IM or IV; administer only half dosage if barbiturates have been given; blocks excitation
Arsenic, mercury, and other heavy metals except cadmium, lead, silver, selenium, and thallium	Dimercaprol (BAL, Hynson, Wescott & Dunning)	10% solution in oil; give small animals 2.5–5.0 mg/kg IM q6h for 2 days then q12h for the next 10 days or until recovery. (Note: With severe acute poisoning, 5 mg/kg should be given only on the first day.)
	D-penicillamine (Cuprimine, Merck)	Developed for chronic mercury poisoning, now seems most promising drug; no reports on dosage in animals; give 3–4 mg/kg q6h
Atropine, belladonna alkaloids	Physostigmine salicylate	0.1–0.6 mg/kg (do not use neostigmine)
Barbiturates	Doxapram	2% solution; give small animals 3–5 mg/kg IV only (0.14–0.25 ml/kg); repeat as necessary. (Note: The above is reliable only when depression is mild; in animals with deeper levels of depression, ventilatory support [and oxygen] is preferable.)
Bromides	Chlorides (sodium or ammonium salts)	0.5–1.0 g PO daily for several days; hasten excretion
Carbon monoxide	Oxygen	Pure oxygen at normal or high pressure; artificial respiration; blood transfusion
Cholecalciferol	Calcitonin (Calcimar, Rorer Pharm)	4 IU/kg SC or IM q8h–q12h
Cholinergic agents	Atropine sulfate	0.02–0.04 mg/kg, as needed
Cholinesterase inhibitors	Atropine sulfate	0.2 mg/kg, repeated as needed for atropinization; treat cyanosis (if present) first; blocks only muscarinic effects: atropine in oil may be injected for prolonged effect. Avoid atropine intoxication!
Cholinergic agents and cholinesterase inhibitors (organophosphates, some carbarnates; but not carbaryl, morphine, succinylcholine, or carbam piloxime)	Pralidoxime chloride (2-PAM)	5% solution; 20–50 mg/kg IM or by slow IV (0.2–1.0 mg/kg) injection (maximum dose is 500 mg per minute), repeat as needed; 2-PAM alleviates nicotinic effect and regenerates cholinesterase; and phenothiazine tranquilizers are contraindicated
Copper	D-penicillamine (Cuprimine)	See arsenic
Coumarin-derivative anticoagulants	Vitamin K_1 (AquaMEPHYTON, 5-mg capsules or 1% emulsion, Merck; Vita K1, 25-mg capsules, Eschar)	Give 3–5 mg/kg SC or PO per day with canned food; treat 7 days for warfarin-type, treat 21–30 days for second-generation anticoagulant rodenticides; oral therapy more effacious than parenteral
	Fresh whole blood, fresh plasma, or fresh frozen plasma	Blood transfusion, 10–25 ml/kg, as required
Curare	Neostigmine methylsulfate	Solution: 1:5000 or 1:2000 (1 ml = 0.2 or 0.5 mg/ml): dosage is 0.005 mg/5 kg SC; follow with IV injection of atropine (0.04 mg/kg)
	Edrophonium chloride (Tensilon, Roche)	1% solution: give 0.05–1.0 mg/kg IV
	Ventilatory support	
Cyanide	Methemoglobin (sodium nitrite is used to form methemoglobin)	1% solution of sodium nitrite; dosage is 16 mg/kg IV (1.6 ml/kg)
	Sodium thiosulfate	Follow with 20% solution of sodium thiosulfate at dosage of 30–40 mg/kg (0.15–0.2 ml/kg) IV; if treatment is repeated, use only sodium thiosulfate. (Note: both of the above may be given simultaneously as follows: 0.5 ml/kg of combination consisting of 10 g sodium nitrite, 15 g sodium thiosulfate distilled water q.s. to 250 ml; dosage may be repeated once; if further treatment is required, give only 20% solution thiosulfate at 0.2 ml/kg.)
Digitalis glycosides, oleander, and Bufo toads	Potassium chloride	Dogs: 0.5–2.0 g PO in divided doses or, in serious cases, aa diluted solution given IV by slow drip (ECG monitoring is essential)
	Diphenylhydantoin	25 mg per minute IV, until ventricular arrhythmias are controlled
	Propranolol (β-blocker)	0.5–1.0 mg/kg IV or IM as needed to control cardiac arrhythmias (ECG monitoring is essential)
	Atropine sulfate	0.02–0.04 mg/kg as needed for cholinergic and arrhythmia control
Fluoride	Calcium borogluconate	3–10 ml of 5–10% solution
Fluoroacetate (Compound 1080)	Glyceryl monoacetin (Sigma)	0.1–0.5 mg/kg IM hourly for several hours (total 2–4 mg/kg), or diluted (0.5–1.0% solution IV; danger of hemolysis); monoacetin is available only from chemical supply houses
	Acetamide	Animal may be protected if acetamide is given before or simultaneously with Compound 1080 (experimental)
	Pentobarbital	May protect against lethal dose (experimental). (Note: all treatments are generally unrewarding.)
Hallucinogens (LSD, phencyclidine hydrochloride [PCP])	Diazepam (Valium, Roche)	As needed—avoid respiratory depression (2–5 mg/kg)
Heparin	Protamine sulfate	1% solution; give 1.0–1.5 mg by slow IV injection to antagonize each 1 mg of heparin; reduce dose as time increases between heparin injection and start of treatment (after 30 minutes give only 0.5 mg)

TOXIC AGENTS AND THEIR SYSTEMIC ANTIDOTES—DOSAGE AND METHOD OF TREATMENT (CONT'D)

Iron salts	Deferoxamine mesylate (Desferal, Ciba)	Dosage for animals not yet established; dosage for humans is 5 g of 5% solution PO, then 20 mg/kg IM q4h–q6h; in case of shock, dosage is 40 mg/kg by IV drip over 4-hour period; may be repeated in 6 hours, then 15 mg/kg by drip q8h
Lead	Calcium disodium edetate (CaEDTA)	Maximum safe dosage is 75 mg/kg per 24 hours (only for severe case); EDTA is available in 20% solution; for IV drip, dilute in 5% glucose to 0.5%; for IM, add procaine to 20% solution to give 0.5% concentration of procaine
	EDTA and BAL	BAL is given as 10% solution in oil (a) In severe cases (CNS involvement with > 100 μg lead per 100 g whole blood), give 4 mg/kg BAL only as initial dose; follow after 4 hours, and q4h for 3–4 days, with BAL and EDTA (12.5 mg/kg) at separate IM sites; skip 2 or 3 days and then treat again for 3–4 days; (b) In subacute cases with < 100 μg lead per 100 g whole blood, give only 50 mg EDTA/kg per 24 hours for 3–5 days;
	Penicillamine (Cuprimine, Merck)	(c) May use after either treatment (a) or (b) with 100 mg/kg per day PO for 1–4 weeks
	Thiamine hydrochloride	Experimental to treat CNS signs; 5 mg/kg IV q12h for 1–2 weeks; give slowly and watch for untoward reactions
Metaldehyde	Diazepam (Valium, Roche)	2–5 mg/kg IV to control tremors
	Triflupromaize	0.2–2.0 mg/kg IV
	Pentobarbital	To effect
Methanol	Ethanol	Give 1.1 g/kg (4.4 ml/kg) of 25% solution IV; then give 0.5 g/kg (2.0 ml/kg) q4h for 4 days; to prevent or correct acidosis, use sodium bicarbonate 0.4 g/kg IV; activated charcoal, 5 g/kg PO if within 4 hours of ingestion
Methemoglobinemia-producing agents (nitrites, chlorates)	Methylene blue (not recommended for cats)	1% solution (maximum concentration); give by slow IV injection, 8.8 mg/kg (0.9 ml/kg), and repeat if necessary; to prevent fall in blood pressure in cases of nitrite poisoning, use a sympath omimetic drug (ephedrine or epinephrine)
Morphine and related drugs	Naloxone hydrochloride (Narcan, Endo)	0.1 mg/kg IV; do not repeat if respiration is not satisfactory
	Levallorphan tartrate (Lorfan, Roche)	Give IV 0.1–0.5 ml of solution containing 1 mg/ml. (Note: use either of the antidotes only in acute poisoning. Ventilatory support may be indicated. Activated charcoal is also indicated.)
Oxalates	Calcium	10% solution of calcium gluconate IV; give 3–20 ml (to control hypocalcemia)
Phenothiazine	Methamphetamine hydrochloride (Desoxyn, Abbot)	0.1–0.2 mg/kg; treatment for hypovolemic shock may be required.
	Diphenhydramine hydrochloride	For CNS depression, 2–5 mg/kg IV to treat extrapyramidal signs
Phytotoxins and botulin	Antitoxins not available commercially (attempt to obtain through Centers for Disease Control)	As indicated for specific antitoxins; examples of phytotoxins: ricin, abrin, robin, crotin
Plants		Treat signs as necessary (see appendix VII)
Red squill	Atropine sulfate, propranolol, potassium chloride	As for digitalis and oleander
Snake bite		
Rattlesnake	Antivenin (Wyeth),	Caution: equine origin; administer 1–2 vials IV, slowly, diluted in 250–500 ml of saline or lactated Ringer's solution; also adminis-
Copperhead	Trivalent Crotalidae	ter antihistamines; corticosteroids are contraindicated
Water moccasin	(Fort Dodge)	
Coral snake	(Wyeth)	Caution: equine origin; may be used as with pit viper antivenin
Spider bite		
Black widow	Antivenin (Merck)	Caution: equine origin; administer IV undiluted
	Dantrolene sodium (Dantrium, Norwich-Eaton)	For neurologic signs, 1 mg/kg IV, followed by 1 mg/kg PO q4h
Brown recluse	Dapsone	1 mg/kg q12h for 10 days
Strontium	Calcium salts	Usual dose of calcium borogluconate
	Ammonium chloride	0.2–0.5 g PO 3–4 times daily
Strychnine and brucine	Pentobarbital	Give IV, to effect; higher dose is usually required than that required for anesthesia; place animal in warm, quiet room
	Amobarbital	Give slowly IV, to effect; duration of sedation is usually 4–6 hours
	Methocarbamol (Robaxin, Robins)	10% solution; average first dosage is 149 mg/kg IV (range, 40–300 mg); repeat half dosage as needed
	Glyceryl guaiacolate (Geocolate, Summit Hill Labs)	110 mg/kg IV, 5% solution; repeat as necessary
	Diazepam (Valium, Roche)	2–5 mg/kg; controls convulsions
Thallium	Diphenylthiocarbazone	Dogs: 70 mg/kg PO q8h for 6 days; hastens elimination but is partially toxic
	Prussian blue	0.2 mg/kg PO in 3 divided doses daily
	Potassium chloride	Give simultaneously with thiocarbazone or Prussian blue, 2–6 g PO daily in divided doses

IM = intramuscularly; IV = intravenously; PO = orally; SC = subcutaneously; q = every; h = hour; q.s. = sufficient quantity; ECG = electrocardiogram; CNS = central nervous system.

From Bailey EM Jr, Garland T. Toxicologic emergencies. In: Murtaugh RJ, Kaplan PM, eds. Veterinary emergency and critical care medicine. St. Louis: Mosby, 1992:443–446.

APPENDIX VII

TOXIC PLANTS AND THEIR CLINICAL SIGNS—ANTIDOTES AND TREATMENTS

Plant and characteristics	Clinical signs	Antidotes and treatment
Angel's trumpet (Datura spp.) Garden annual with white trumpet-shaped flowers Whole plant toxic; highest in seeds	Thirst, GI atony, disturbed vision, delirium, hallucinations	Parasympatomimetic drugs
Autumn crocus (Colchicum autumnale) Houseplant Whole plant toxic; highest in bulbs	Burning sensation in throat and mouth, thirst, nausea, diarrhea	Fluids; analgesics and atropine to alleviate colic and diarrhea
Azalea (Rhododendron spp.) Garden, landscape plant Leaves and flowers are toxic Honey made from flower nectar is toxic	Burning sensation in mouth, salivation, emesis, diarrhea, muscular weakness, dimness of vision, bradycardia, arrhythmia, hypotension EMERGENCY CONDITION	Do not use emetics. Use activated charcoal. Fluid replacement and respiratory support are required. Treat heart block with isoproterenol.
Belladonna lily (Amaryllis spp.) Garden, potted plant Bulbs are most toxic	Nausea, diarrhea, hypotension, depression, liver damage	Gastric lavage, charcoal, fluids, and supportive treatment
Bittersweet (Celastrus spp.) Weed, vine with red berries Immature fruits are toxic	Gastric irritation, fever, diarrhea	Fluids
Bleeding heart (Dicentra spp.) Garden, woods, potted plant Toxicity of roots > leaves	Vomiting, diarrhea, convulsions or paralysis	Fluids and seizure control
Castor bean (Ricinus communis) Garden annual, grows to 2 m Seeds are 1 cm, dark and light mottled, and highly toxic	Latent period; colic, emesis, diarrhea, thirst	Emesis, charcoal, fluids, and electrolytes
Chinaberry tree (Melia azedarach) Ornamental tree in temperate to subtropical areas Fruit and bark are most toxic	Faintness, ataxia, mental confusion, intense gastritis, emesis, diarrhea	Fluid and electrolyte replacement
Christmas rose (Helleborus niger) Houseplant Entire plant is toxic	Pain in mouth and abdomen, nausea, emesis, colic, diarrhea, arrhythmia, hypotension	Gastric lavage or emesis; activated charcoal or saline cathartics to decontaminate the GI tract
Daphne (Daphne mezereum) Landscape shrub Entire plant is toxic	Vesication and edema of the lips and oral cavity, salivation, thirst, abdominal pain, emesis, hemorrhagic diarrhea	Fluid and electrolyte replacement
Delphinium or larkspur (Delphinium spp.) Outdoor garden, mountains; tall with blue flowers Toxicity of seeds > leaves	Trembling, ataxia, weakness, salivation	GI detoxication; physostigmine to treat muscarinic signs
English holly (Ilex spp.) Landscape plant Fruit is toxic	Nausea, vomiting, diarrhea	Fluid and electrolyte replacement
English ivy (Hedera helix) Houseplant Fruit and leaves	Salivation, thirst, emesis, gastroenteritis, diarrhea, dermatitis	Corticosteroids to treat dermal response; treat other signs symptomatically.
Foxglove (Digitalis purpurea) Outdoor gardens Entire plant (especially leaves)	Nausea, emesis, abdominal pain, diarrhea, bradycardia, arrhythmia with prolonged P-R interval and hyporkalemia	GI decontamination with activated charcoal or saline cathartics. Treat hyperkalemia and give lidocaine for ventricular arrhythmia.
Golden chain (Laburnum anagyroides) Landscape tree with long chains of yellow flowers Entire plant is toxic	Emesis, depression, weakness, incoordination, mydriasis, tachycardia	GI decontamination with lavage or emesis followed by activated charcoal
Horse chestnut or buckeye (Aesculus spp.) Landscape or forest tree; palmate leaves Nuts and twigs most toxic	Gastroententis, diarrhea, dehydration, electrolyte imbalance	Fluid and electrolyte replacement, demulcents, and therapy for gastroenteritis
Iris or flag (Iris spp.) Perennial garden flower Rootstock most toxic	Colic, nausea, vomiting, diarrhea	Fluid and electrolyte replacement

Plant and characteristics	Clinical signs	Antidotes and treatment
Irish potato (Solanum tuberosum) Vegetable garden Vines, green skin, and sprouts are toxic	Colic, diarrhea, salivation, ataxia, weakness, bradycardia, hypotension. Signs may vary from atropine-like to cholinsterase inhibition. Use antidotes accordingly and with caution.	GI decontamination. If atropine-like signs predominate, use physostigmine. If salivation and diarrhea are present, use atropine cautiously.
Jack-in-the-pulpit (Arisaema triphyllum) Woods and gardens of temperate zones Entire plant is toxic	Glossitis, pharyngitis, oral inflammation, edema, salivation	Irrigate mouth with water. Cool liquids or demulcents held in mouth may relieve signs.
Lantana (Lantana camara) Garden and wild in mild temperate to tropical areas; bright orange and yellow flowers Foliage and immature berries are toxic	Weakness, lethargy, vomiting, diarrhea, mydriasis, bradypnea. Advanced signs are cholestasis, bilirubinemia, and photosensitization.	GI decontamination, fluids, and respiratory support. Protect from sunlight and treat for hepatic insufficiency.
Lily, including Easter lily, tiger lily (Lilium spp.); daylily (Hemerocallis spp.)	Depression, oliguria, renal failure in cats as a result of toxic tubular necrosis	Prompt GI decontamination and supportive therapy for renal failure. Toxin presently is unknown.
Lily of the valley (Convallaria majalis) Garden ornamental Toxicity of seeds and flowers> leaves	Colic, vomiting, diarrhea, bradycardia, arrhythmia	Decontaminate GI tract with lavage and charcoal. Avoid emetics. Lidocaine to treat ventricular arrhythmias; treat as for other digitalis glycoside overdose, including correction of hyperkalemia.
Lupine (Lupinus spp.) Garden ornamental Toxicity of seeds > leaves	Salivation, ataxia, seizures, dyspnea	GI decontamination, control seizures
Mistletoe (Phoradendron spp.) Parasitic shrub on other trees Access to pets in homes at holiday time Leaves, stems, and berries are moderately toxic	Emesis, colic, diarrhea, mydriasis, hypovolemia	Fluid and electrolyte replacement; demulcents for gastroenteritis
Monkshood (Aconitum spp.) Perennial garden ornamental Entire plant is toxic	Glossitis, pharyngitis, salivation, nausea, emesis, impaired vision, bradycardia	GI decontamination, fluid and electrolyte replacement. Manage similar to digitalis glycoside overdose, with caution about potassium administration.
Moonseed (Menispermum canadense) Woody vine of forests Fruit is most toxic	Convulsions	Maintain airway and support respiration as needed. Control seizures with least medication possible (e.g., diazepam).
Morning glory (Ipomoea purpurea and I. tricolor) Garden annual, potted plant Seeds most toxic Occasionally used as hallucinogen	Nausea, mydriasis, hallucinations, decreased reflexes, diarrhea, hypotension	Activated charcoal, dark quiet surroundings, tranquilize with diazepam
Mountain laurel (Kalmia spp.) Native of eastern and southeastern woods, mountains Leaves and flowers are toxic Honey from nectar also toxic	Oral irritation, salivation, emesis, diarrhea, weakness, impaired vision, bradycardia, hypotension, AV block	Emetics are contraindicated. Use activated charcoal, fluid replacement, and respiratory support as needed. Isoproterenol to treat AV block as needed.
Narcissus, daffodil, jonquil (Narcissus spp.) Garden ornamental bulb Bulb is most toxic	Nausea, emesis, hypotension, diarrhea	Gastric lavage, charcoal, fluid replacement, supportive treatment for gastroenteritis
Nettle (Urtica diocia) Garden weed Hairs on leaves contain toxin that enters skin on contact	Oral irritation and pain, salivation, swelling and edema of nose and periocular areas or other areas of skin contact	Antihistamines and atropine may control appropriate signs. Local or systemic antiinflammatory supportive therapy to treat affected contact areas.
Oleander (Nerium oleander) Landscape shrub 1–3 m tall Whole plant is extremely toxic	Nausea, early signs of vomiting, colic, diarrhea; bradycardia and arrythmia with hyperkalemia develop soon after EMERGENCY CONDITION	Gastric lavage or induced emesis; activated charcoal or saline cathartics. Treat as for digitalis glycoside overdose, including correction of hyperkalemia. Lidocaine or other appropriate drugs for arrhythmia.
Philodendron (Monstera and Philodendron spp.) Houseplant Leaves are slightly to moderately toxic	Painful irritation, edema of lips, mouth, tongue, and throat; reported nephrotoxic to cats	Cool liquids or demulcents held in mouth may aid relief

TOXIC PLANTS AND THEIR CLINICAL SIGNS—ANTIDOTES AND TREATMENTS (CONTINUED)

Plant and Characteristics	Clinical signs	Antidotes and treatment
Poinsettia (Euphorbia pulcherrima) Garden or potted plant especially at Christmas holidays Sap of stem and leaves is mildly to moderately irritant or toxic	Irritation of mouth; may cause vomiting, diarrhea, and dermatitis	Demulcents and fluids to prevent dehydration
Rhubarb (Rheum rhaponicum) Garden plant Raw or canned Leaves are high in oxalates	Vomiting, diarrhea, and, occasionally, icterus. Renal failure develops from oxalate nephrosis.	Early GI decontamination is important. Demulcents and fluid replacement. Treat possible oxalate nephrosis.
Rosary pea or precatory bean (Abrus precatorius) Native of Caribbean islands Seeds (when broken or chewed) are highly toxic Illegal to import into United States	Nausea, vomiting, diarrhea, weakness, tachycardia, possible renal failure, coma, death	Emesis or lavage followed with charcoal, demulcents, fluids, and electrolytes. Vitamin C may improve survival.
Thorn apple or jimsonweed (Datura stramonium) Annual weed, some species are ornamental (D. metel) Entire plant is toxic, but seeds are most toxic and available Relatively common drug abuse plant used as hallucinogen	Thirst, disturbances of vision, delirium, mydriasis, gastrointestinal atony. Signs similar to atropine overdose.	Parasympathomimetic drug (e.g., physotigmine)
Tobacco (Nicotiana tabacum) Garden plant, weed, cigarettes Whole plant is toxic	Rapid onset of salivation, nausea, emesis, tremors, incoordination, and ataxia, followed by collapse and respiratory failure EMERGENCY CONDITION	Assist ventilation and vascular support first to save the animal. After respiration support, decontaminate the GI tract with lavage and activated charcoal.
Wisteria (Wisteria spp.) Woody vine or shrub with blue to white legume flowers Entire plant is toxic	Nausea, abdominal pain, prolonged vomiting	Antiemetics and fluid replacement therapy
Yellow jessamine (Gelsemium sempervirens) Mild temperate to subtropical climates Yellow trumpet-shaped flowers grow on evergreen vines	Abdominal pain, bradypnea, paresis, seizures, hypothermia	Symptomatic and supportive therapy of respiration and cardiovascular function. GI decontamination and fluid replacement therapy.
Yew (Taxus cuspidata and T. baccata) Evergreen landscape shrub with two-ranked flat needle Whole plant (except ripe fruit) is toxic	Acute onset or sudden death. Affected animals show trembling, muscle weakness, dyspnea, collapse, arrhythmia, and heart block.	Symptomatic and supportive therapy of respiration and cardiovascular function. GI decontamination and fluid replacement therapy.

Contributed by Gary Osweiler, College of Veterinary Medicine, Iowa State University, Ames, IA.

5-Minute Consult Drug Formulary

Drug Name (Trade or Other Names)	Pharmacology and Indications	Adverse Effects and Precautions	Dosing Information and Comments	Formulations	Dosage
Acepromazine (PromAce and many generic brands)	Phenothiazine tranquilizer. Inhibits action of dopamine as neurotransmitter. Used for sedation and preanesthetic purposes.	Phenothiazines can cause sedation as a common side effect. May lower seizure threshold and causes α-adrenergic blockade. Produces extrapyramidal side effects in some individuals.	Usually used as pre-anesthetic in combination with other drugs. When used as preanesthetic dose is ordinarily 0.02–0.2 mg/kg, IM, SC, IV.	5, 10, 25 mg tablet and 10 mg/mL injection.	Dog: 0.56–1.13 mg/kg PO q6–8h, or 0.02–0.1 mg/kg IV, IM, SC. Cat: 1.13–2.25 mg/kg PO q6–8h, or 0.02–0.1 mg/kg IM, SC, IV.
Acemannan (Acemannan immuno-stimulant)	Immunostimulant. A polysaccharide acetylated mannan extract from aloe. Proposed to stimulate T-cell activity in animals. It has been used to treat tumors in dogs and cats. It may stimulate TNF and other cytokine release.	No reported side effects.	After reconstitution, shake well to dissolve. Use within 4 hours after preparation. Beneficial effect is controversial. There has been a lack of demonstrated effect on lymphocyte blasto-genic response in cats.	10 mg vials reconstituted to 1 mg/mL.	Intraperitoneal (1 mg/kg) and intralesional injection (2 mg) every week for 6 treatments.
Acetaminophen (Tylenol, and many generic brands)	Analgesic agent. Exact mechanism of action is not known. *Not* a prostaglandin synthesis inhibitor.	Well-tolerated in dogs at doses listed. High doses have caused liver toxicity. Do *not* administer to cats.	Many OTC formulations available. Acetaminophen with codeine may have greater analgesic efficacy in some animals.	120, 160, 325, 500 mg tablets.	Dogs: 15 mg/kg, q8h, PO. Cats: not recommended.
Acetaminophen with codeine (Tylenol with codeine and many generic brands)	Same as above, except the opiate codeine is added to enhance analgesia.	See Codeine and Acetaminophen.	See Codeine and Acetaminophen.	Oral solution and tablets. Many forms, for example 300 mg acetaminophen plus either 15, 30, or 60 mg codeine.	Follow dosing recommendations for codeine.
Acetazolamide (Diamox)	Carbonic anhydrase inhibitor and diuretic; used primarily to lower intraocular pressure. (See also Dichlorphena-mide.)	Use cautiously in any animal sensitive to sulfonamides. Can produce hypokalemia in some patients. Do not use in patients with acidemia.	Usually used to treat glaucoma in combination with other agents.	125, 250 mg tablets.	5–10 mg/kg q8–12h PO. Glaucoma: 4–8 mg/kg q8–12h PO.
Acetylcysteine (Mucomyst)	Decreases viscosity of secretions. Used as mucolytic agent in eyes and in bronchial nebulizing solutions. However, as a donator of sulfhy-dral group, used as antidote for intoxications (for example, acetamino-phen toxicosis in cats).	May cause sensitization with prolonged topical administration. May react with certain materials in nebulizing equipment.	Available as agent for decreasing viscosity of respiratory secretions, but most common use is as a treatment for intoxications.	20% solution.	Antidote: 140 mg/kg (loading dose) then 70 mg/kg q4h IV or PO for 5 doses. Eye: 2% solution topically q2h.
Acetylsalicylic acid	See Aspirin.				
ACTH	See Corticotropin.				
Actinomycin D	See Dactinomycin.				
Activated charcoal	See Charcoal, Activated.				
Adequan	See Polysulfated glyco-saminoglycan (PSGAG).				
Albendazole (Valbazen)	Benzimidazole antiparasitic drug. Inhibits glucose uptake in parasites.	At approved doses there is a wide margin of safety. Adverse effects can include anorexia, lethargy, and bone marrow toxicity. At high doses has been associated with bone marrow toxicity (JAVMA 213: 44–46, 1998). Adverse effects are possible when administered for longer than 5 days.	Used primarily as anti-helmintic, but also has demonstrated efficacy for giardiasis.	113.6 mg/mL suspension and 300 mg/mL paste.	25–50 mg/kg q12h PO × 3 days. For giardia, use 25 mg/kg, q12h, × 2 days.

Drug Name (Trade or Other Names)	Pharmacology and Indications	Adverse Effects and Precautions	Dosing Information and Comments	Formulations	Dosage
Albuterol (Proventil, Ventolin)	β_2-adrenergic agonist. Bronchodilator. Stimulate β-2 receptors to relax bronchial smooth muscle. May also inhibit release of inflammatory mediators, especially from mast cells.	Causes excessive β-adrenergic stimulation at high doses (tachycardia, tremors). Arrhythmias occur at toxic doses. Avoid use in pregnant animals.	Doses are primarily derived from extrapolation of human dose. Well-controlled efficacy studies in veterinary medicine are not available. Onset of action is 15–30 min; duration of action may be as long as 8 hr.	2, 4, 5 mg tablets; 2 mg/5 mL syrup.	20–50 mcg/kg 4 times/day; or up to maximum of 100 mcg/kg 4 times daily.
Allopurinol (Lopurin, Zyloprim)	Decreases production of uric acid by inhibiting enzymes responsible for uric acid.	May cause skin reactions (hypersensitivity).	Used in people primarily for treating gout. In animals used to decrease formation of uric acid uroliths.	100, 300 mg tablets.	10 mg/kg q8h, then reduce to 10 mg/kg q24h.
Alumunium carbonate gel (Basalgel)	Antacid (neutralizes stomach acid), and phosphate binder in intestine.	Generally safe. May interact with other drugs administered orally.	Antacid doses are designed to neutralize stomach acid, but duration of acid suppression is short.	Capsules (equivalent to 500 mg aluminum hydroxide.)	10–30 mg/kg PO q8h (with meals).
Aluminium hydroxide gel (Amphogel)	Antacid (neutralizes stomach acid), and phosphate binder in intestine.	Generally safe. May interact with other drugs administered orally.	Antacid doses are designed to neutralize stomach acid, but duration of acid suppression is short.	64 mg/mL oral suspension; 600 mg tablet.	10–30 mg/kg PO q8h (with meals).
Amikacin (Amiglyde-V [veterinary] and Amikin [human])	Aminoglycoside antibacterial drug (inhibits protein synthesis). Mechanism is similar to other aminoglycosides (see Gentamicin), but may be more active than gentamicin.	May cause nephrotoxicosis with high doses or prolonged therapy. May also cause ototoxicity and vestibulotoxicity. (See Gentamicin.)	Once-daily doses are designed to maximize peak:MIC ratio. Consider therapeutic drug monitoring for chronic therapy. (See also Gentamicin.)	50, 250 mg/mL injection.	Dog, cat: 6.5 mg/kg, q8h, IV, IM, SC, or 20 mg/kg q24h, IV, IM, SC.
Aminopentamide (Centrine)	Antidiarrheal drug. Anticholinergic (blocks acetylcholine at parasympathetic synapse).	Use cautiously in animals with GI stasis or when anticholinergic drugs are contraindicated (e.g., glaucoma).	Dosing guidelines based on manufacturer's recommendation.	0.2 mg tablets; 0.5 mg/mL injection.	Dog: 0.01–0.03 mg/kg q8–12h IM SC PO. Cat: 0.1 mg/cat q8–12h IM SC PO.
Aminophylline (many [generic])	Bronchodilator. Aminophylline is a salt of theophylline, formulated to enhance oral absorption without gastric side effects. It is converted to theophylline after ingestion.	Causes excitement and possible cardiac effect with high concentrations. (See Theophylline.)	See also Theophylline. Therapeutic drug monitoring is recommended for chronic therapy.	100, 200 mg tablet; 25 mg/mL injection.	Dog: 10 mg/kg q8h PO, IM, IV. Cat: 6.6 mg/kg q12h PO.
6-Aminosalicylic acid	See Mesalamine, Olsalazine.				
Amitraz (Mitaban)	Antiparasite drug for ectoparasites. Used for treatment of mites, including Demodex. Inhibits monoamine oxidase in mites.	Causes sedation in dogs (α_2-agonist) which may be reversed by yohimbine or atipamezole. When high doses are used, other side effects reported include pruritus, PU/PD, bradycardia, hypothermia, hyperglycemia, and (rarely) seizures.	Manufacturer's dose should be used initially. But, for refractory cases, this dose has been exceeded to produce increased efficacy. Doses that have been used include: 0.025, 0.05, and 0.1% concentration applied 2× week and 0.125% solution applied to 1/2 body every day for 4 weeks to 5 months.	10.6 mL concentrated dip (19.9%).	10.6 mL per 7.5 L water (0.025% solution). Apply 3–6 topical treatments q14d. For refractory cases, this dose has been exceeded to produce increased efficacy. Doses that have been used include: 0.025, 0.05, and 0.1% concentration applied 2× week and 0.125% solution applied to 1/2 body every day for 4 weeks to 5 months.
Amitriptyline (Elavil)	Tricyclic antidepressant drug. Action is via inhibition of uptake of serotonin and other transmitters at presynaptic nerve terminals. Used in animals to treat variety of behavioral disorders, such as anxiety.	Multiple side effects are associated with tricyclic antidepressants such as antimuscarinic effects (dry mouth, rapid heart rate), and antihistamine effects (sedation).	Doses are primarily based on empiricism. There are no controlled efficacy trials available for animals. There is evidence for success treating idiopathic cystitis in cats	10, 25, 50, 75, 100, 150 mg tablets; 10 mg/mL injection.	Dog: 1–2 mg/kg, PO, q12–24h. cat: 5–10 mg per cat/day, PO; (cystitis): 2 mg/kg/day (2.5–7.5 mg/cat/day).

Drug Name (Trade or Other Names)	Pharmacology and Indications	Adverse Effects and Precautions	Dosing Information and Comments	Formulations	Dosage
	Used in cats for chronic idiopathic cystitis.	High doses can produce life-threatening cardio-toxicity. In cats, re-duced grooming, weight gain, and sedation are possible.	(JAVMA 213:1282–1286, 1998).		
Amlodipine besylate (Norvasc)	Calcium-channel blocking drug of the dihydropyridine class. Decreases calcium influx in cardiac and vascular smooth muscle. Its greatest effect is as a vasodila-tor. In cats and dogs it is used to treat hyper-tension.	Can cause hypotension and bradycardia. Use cautiously with other vasodilators.	In cats, efficacy has been established at 0.625 mg/cat once daily. If cats are large size (> 4.5 kg), or refractory, increase to higher dose (J Vet Int Med 12: 157–162, 1998).	2.5, 5, and 10 mg tablets.	Dogs: 2.5 mg/dog, or 0.1 mg/kg, once daily, PO. Cats: 0.625 mg/cat initially, PO once daily, and increase if needed to 1.25 mg/cat (average is 0.18 mg/kg).
Ammonium chloride (generic)	Urine acidifier	Do not use in patients with systemic acidemia. May be unpalatable when added to some animals food.	Doses are designed to maximize urine acidify-ing effect.	Available as crystals.	Dog: 100 mg/kg q12h PO. Cat: 800 mg/cat (approxi-mately 1/3 to 1/4 tsp) mixed with food daily.
Amoxicillin (Amoxi Tabs, Biomox, and other brands. [Omnipen, Principen, Totacillin are human forms])	β-lactam antibiotic. Inhibits bacterial cell wall synthesis. Gener-ally broad spectrum activity. Used for a variety of infections in all species.	Usually well-tolerated. Allergic reactions are possible. Diarrhea is common with oral doses.	Dose recommendations vary depending on the susceptibility of bacteria and location of infection. Generally, more frequent or higher doses needed for Gram-negative infections.	50, 100, 150, 200, 400 mg tablets. 250 and 500 mg capsules (human forms).	6.6–20 mg/kg q8–12h, PO.
Amoxicillin trihydrate (Amoxi-Tabs, Amoxi-drops, Amoxil, and others)	β-lactam antibiotic. Inhibits bacterial cell wall synthesis. Gener-ally broad spectrum activity, but resistance is common.	Use cautiously in animals allergic to penicillin-like drugs.	Dose requirements vary depending on susceptibility of bacteria.	50, 100, 200, 400 mg tablets. 50 mg/mL oral suspension.	6–20 mg/kg q8–12h PO.
Amoxicillin/Clavulanic acid (Clavamox)	β-lactam antibiotic + β-lactamase inhibitor (clavulanate/ clavulanic acid)	Same as amoxicillin.	Same as amoxicillin.	62.5, 125, 250, 375 mg tablet and 62.5 mg/mL suspension.	Dog: 12.5–25 mg/kg q12h PO. Cat: 62.5 mg/cat q12h PO. Consider administering these doses every 8 hr for Gram-negative infections.
Amphotericin B (Fungi-zone)	Antifungal drug. Fungi-cidal for systemic fungi, by damaging fungal membranes.	Produces a dose-related nephrotoxicosis. Also produces fever, phlebitis, and tremors.	Administer IV via slow infusion diluted in fluids, and monitor renal function closely. When preparing IV solution, do not mix with electro-lyte solutions (use D_5W, for example); administer NaCl fluid loading before therapy. (One study adminis-tered this drug sub-cutaneously: Aust Vet J 73:124, 1996)	50-mg injectable vial.	0.5 mg/kg IV (slow in fusion) q48h, to a cumulative dose of 4–8 mg/kg.
Amphotericin B (other formulations)	New formulations include amphotericin B lipid complex, Ampho-tericin B cholesteryl sulfate complex (Amphotec), and lipo-somal formulation of amphotericin B (AmBisome). These formulations have not been used regularly in veterinary medicine.				

Drug Name (Trade or Other Names)	Pharmacology and Indications	Adverse Effects and Precautions	Dosing Information and Comments	Formulations	Dosage
Ampicillin (Omnipen, Principen, others [human forms])	β-lactam antibiotic. Inhibits bacterial cell wall synthesis.	Use cautiously in animals allergic to penicillin-like drugs.	Dose requirements vary depending on susceptibility of bacteria. Absorbed approximately 50% less, compared to amoxicillin, when administered orally. Generally, more frequent or higher doses needed for Gram-negative infections.	250, 500 mg capsules; 125-, 250-, 500-mg vials of ampicillin sodium.	10–20 mg/kg q6–8h IV, IM, SC (ampicillin sodium); 20–40 mg/kg q8h PO.
Ampicillin + Sulbactam (Unasyn)	Ampicillin plus a β-lactamase inhibitor (sulbactam). Sulbactam has similar activity as clavulanate.	Same as ampicillin.	Same as amoxicillin + clavulanate.	2:1 combination for injection. 1.5- and 3-gram vials.	10–20 mg/kg IV, IM q8h.
Ampicillin trihydrate (Polyflex)	β-lactam antibiotic. Inhibits bacterial cell wall synthesis.	Use cautiously in animals allergic to penicillin-like drugs.	Absorption is slow and may not be sufficient for acute serious infection.	10, 25 mg vials for injection.	Dogs: 10–50 mg/kg q12–24h IM, SC. Cats: 10–20 mg/kg q12–24h IM, SC.
Amprolium (Amprol, Corid)	Antiprotozoal drug. Antagonizes thiamine in parasites. Used for treatment of coccidiosis, especially in puppies.	Toxicity observed only at high doses (CNS signs due to thiamine deficiency).	Usually administered as feed-additive to livestock. For dogs, 30 mL of 9.6% amprolium has been added to 3.8 Liters of drinking water for control of coccidiosis.	9.6% (9.6 grams/100 mL) oral solution. Soluble powder.	1.25 gm of 20% amprolium powder to daily feed, or 30 mL of 9.6% amprolium solution to 3.8 L of drinking water for 7 days.
Antacid drugs	(See Aluminum Hydroxide, Magnesium Hydroxide, Calcium Carbonate.)				
Apomorphine hydrochloride (generic)	Emetic drug. Causes emesis via dopamine release or direct effects on CRTZ.	Produces emesis before serious adverse effects occur. Use cautiously in cats that may be sensitive to opiates.	Consult local poison center or pharmacist for availability.	6 mg tablets.	0.02–0.04 mg/kg IV IM, 0.1 mg/kg SC, or instill 0.25 mg in conjunctiva of eye (dissolve 6 mg tablet in 1–2 mL of saline).
Ascorbic acid (Vitamin C)	Vitamin. Used as acidifier.	Toxicity only at very high doses.	Primarily used as nutritional supplement, but high doses have been used for treatment of certain diseases.	Various forms.	100–500 mg/animal/day (diet supplement), or 100 mg/animal q8h (urine acidification).
L-Asparaginase (Elspar)	Anticancer agent. Purified enzyme from *E. coli*. Used in lymphoma protocols. Depletes cancer cells of asparagine and interferes with protein synthesis.	Hypersensitivity, allergic reactions.	Usually used in combination with other drugs in cancer chemotherapy protocols.	10,000 U per vial for injection.	400 U/kg IM weekly or 10,000 U/m² weekly × 3 weeks.
Aspirin (many generic and brand names [Bufferin, Ascriptin])	Nonsteroidal anti-inflammatory drug. Anti-inflammatory action is generally considered to be caused by inhibition of prostaglandins. Used as analgesic, anti-inflammatory, and anti-platelet drug.	Narrow therapeutic index. High doses frequently cause vomiting. Other gastrointestinal effects can include ulceration and bleeding. Cats susceptible to salicylate intoxication because of slow clearance. Use cautiously in patients with coagulopathies because of platelet inhibition.	Analgesic and anti-inflammatory doses have primarily been derived from empiricism. Antiplatelet doses are lower because of prolonged effect of aspirin on platelets. When administering aspirin, buffered forms, or administration with food may decrease stomach irritation. Enteric-coated formulations are not recommended for dogs and cats.	81, 325 mg tablets.	Mild analgesia: (dog) 10 mg/kg, q12h. Anti-inflammatory: dog: 20–25 mg/kg q12h; cat: 10–20 mg/kg q48h. Antiplatelet: dog: 5–10 mg/kg q24–48h; cat: 80 mg q48h.

Drug Name (Trade or Other Names)	Pharmacology and Indications	Adverse Effects and Precautions	Dosing Information and Comments	Formulations	Dosage
Astemizole (Hismanal)	Antihistamine (H-1 blocking) drug. Primarily used for allergic disease; in people used as adjunct for asthma. This is one of the 2nd-generation antihistamines, which usually do not have the side effect of sedation as compared to other antihistamines.	Adverse effects have not been reported in small animals, but cardiotoxicity is a potential problem with high doses.	Available as tablets and oral suspension. Doses are primarily derived from extrapolation from human dose. Efficacy trials and dose titration have not been performed, but initial studies failed to demonstrate efficacy for pruritus in dogs.	10 mg tablets.	Dog: 0.2 mg/kg q24h, up to 1.0 mg/kg q12h PO.
Atenolol (Tenormin)	β-adrenergic blocker. Relatively selective for β$_1$-receptor. Used primarily as an antiarrhythmic, or other cardiovascular conditions to slow sinus rate.	Bradycardia and heart block are possible. May produce bronchospasm in sensitive patients.	Dosing precautions are similar to other β-blocking drugs. Atenolol is reported to be less affected by changes in hepatic metabolism than other β-blockers. Dose in animals based on AJVR 57: 1050–1053, 1996.	25, 50, 100 mg tablets; 25 mg/mL oral suspension; and 0.5 mg/mL ampules for injection.	Dog: 6.25–12.5 mg/dog q12h (or 0.25–1.0 mg/kg q12–24h). Cat: 6.25–12.5 mg/cat q12h (approx. 3 mg/kg).
Atipamezole (Antisedan)	α$_2$-antagonist. Used to reverse α$_2$-agonists such as medetomidine and xylazine.	Safe. Can cause some initial excitement in some animals shortly after reversal.	When used to reverse medetomidine, inject same volume as used for medetomidine.	5 mg/mL injection.	Inject same volume as used for medetomidine.
Atracurium (Tracurium)	Neuromuscular blocking agent (nondepolarizing). Competes with acetylcholine at neuromuscular end plate. Used primarily during anesthesia or other conditons in which it is necessary to inhibit muscle contractions.	Produces respiratory depression and paralysis. Neuromuscular blocking drugs have no effect on analgesia.	Administer only in situations in which careful control of respiration is possible. Doses may need to be individualized for optimum effect. Do not mix with alkalinizing solutions or lactated Ringer's solution.	10 mg/mL injection.	0.2 mg/kg IV initally, then 0.15 mg/kg q30min (or IV infusion at 3–8 mcg/kg/min).
Atropine (Many generic brands)	Anticholinergic agent (blocks acetylcholine effect at muscarinic receptor), parasympatholytic. Used primarily as adjunct to anesthesia or other procedures to increase heart rate, and decrease respiratory and gastrointestinal secretion. Also used as antidote for organophosphate intoxication.	Potent anticholinergic agent. Do not use in patients with glaucoma, intestinal ileus, gastroparesis, or tachycardia. Side effects of therapy include xerostomia, ileus, constipation, tachycardia, urine retention.	Used ordinarily as adjunct with anesthesia or other procedures. Do not mix with alkaline solutions.	400, 500, 540 mcg/mL injection; 15 mg/mL injection.	0.02–0.04 mg/kg q6–8h IV, IM, SC; 0.2–0.5 mg/kg (as needed) for organophosphate and carbamate toxicosis.
Auranofin (triethylphosphine gold) (Ridaura)	Used for gold therapy (crysotherapy). Mechanism of action is unknown, but may relate to immunosuppressive effect on lymphocytes. Used primarily for immune-mediated diseases.	Adverse effects include dermatitis, nephrotoxicity, and blood dyscrasias.	Use of this drug has not been evaluated in veterinary medicine. No controlled clinical trials are available to determine efficacy in animals. It has been suggested that this product (oral) is not as effective as injectable products such as aurothioglucose.	3 mg capsules.	0.1–0.2 mg/kg q12h PO.
Aurothioglucose (Solganol)	Used for gold therapy (crysotherapy). Mechanism of action is unknown, but may relate to immunosuppressive effect on lymphocytes. Used primarily for immune-mediated diseases (such as dermatologic disease).	Adverse effects include dermatitis, nephrotoxicity, and blood dyscrasias.	Use of this drug has not been evaluated in veterinary medicine. No controlled clinical trials are available to determine efficacy in animals. This drug is often used in combination with other immunosuppressive drugs such as corticosteroids.	50 mg/mL injection.	Dogs <10 kg: 1 mg IM first week, 2 mg IM second week, 1 mg/kg/week maintenance. Dogs >10 kg: 5 mg IM first week, 10 mg IM second week, 1 mg/kg/week maintenance. Cats 0.5–1 mg/cat q7d IM.

Drug Name (Trade or Other Names)	Pharmacology and Indications	Adverse Effects and Precautions	Dosing Information and Comments	Formulations	Dosage
Azathioprine (Imuran)	Thiopurine immunosuppressive drug. Acts to inhibit T-cell lymphocyte function. This drug is metabolized to 6-mercaptopurine, which may account for immunosuppressive effects. Used to treat various immune-mediated disease.	Bone marrow suppression is most serious concern. Cats particularly are susceptible. There has been some associaton with development of pancreatitis when administered with corticosteroids.	Usually used in combination with other immunosuppressive drugs (such as corticosteroids) to treat immune-mediated disease. Some evidence suggests that it is contraindicated in cats because of bone-marrow effects. Doses of 2.2 mg/kg to cats have produced toxicity.	50 mg tablets; 10 mg/mL for injection.	Dogs: 2 mg/kg q24h PO initially then 0.5–1 mg/kg q48h. Cats (use cautiously): 1 mg/kg, q48h, PO.
Azithromycin (Zithromax)	Azalide antibiotic. Similar mechanism of action as macrolides (erythromycin), which is to inhibit bacteria protein synthesis via inhibition of ribosome. Spectrum is primarily Gram-positive.	Has not been in common use in veterinary medicine to establish adverse effects. Vomiting is likely with high doses. Diarrhea may occur in some patients.	Azithromycin may be better tolerated than erythromycin. Primary difference from other antibiotics is the high intracellular concentrations achieved.	250 mg capsules, 250 and 600 mg tablets, 100 or 200 mg/5 mL oral suspension, and 500 mg vials for injection.	Dogs: 10 mg/kg, PO, once every 5 days, or 3.3 mg/kg, once daily for three days. Cats: 5 mg/kg, PO every other day.
AZT (Azothiouridine) See Zidovurdine.					
Bactrim (sulfamethoxazole + trimethoprim) See Trimethoprima-sulfonamide combinations.					
BAL	See Dimercaprol.				
Benazepril (Lotensin)	ACE-inhibitor. See Captopril and Enalapril for details. Used for hypertension and heart failure.	Similar to captopril and enalapril.	Dose is based on approved use in dogs in Europe and Canada. Monitor renal function and electrolytes 3–7 days after initiating therapy and periodically thereafter.	5,10, 20, 40 mg tablets.	Dog: 0.25 to 0.5 mg/kg q24h, PO. Cat: same.
Betamethasone (Celestone)	Potent, long-acting corticosteroid. Anti-inflammatory and immunosuppressive effects are approximately 30× more than cortisol. Anti-inflammatory effects are complex, but primarily via inhibition of inflammatory cells and suppression of expression of inflammatory mediators. Use is for treatment of inflammatory and immune-mediated disease.	Side effects from corticosteroids are many, and include polyphagia, polydipsia/polyuria, and HPA-axis suppression. Adverse effects include gastrointestinal ulceration, hepatopathy, diabetes, hyperlipidemia, decreased thyroid hormone, decreased protein synthesis and wound healing, and immunosuppression.	Dosing schedules are based on desired effect. Anti-inflammatory effects are seen at doses of 0.1–0.2 mg/kg, immunosuppressive effects at 0.2–0.5 mg/kg.	600 mcg (0.6 mg) tablets; 3 mg/mL sodium phosphate injection.	0.1–0.2 mg/kg q12–24h PO.
Bethanechol (Urecholine)	Muscarinic, cholinergic agonist. Parasympathomimetic. Stimulates gastric and intestinal motility, but primarily used to increase contraction of urinary bladder.	High doses of cholinergic agonists will increase motility of gastrointestinal tract and cause abdominal discomfort and diarrhea. Can cause circulatory depression in sensitive animals.	Administer injection SC only, not IV. Doses are derived from extrapolation of human doses or via empiricism. There are no well-controlled efficacy studies available for veterinary species.	5, 10, 25, 50 mg tablets; 5 mg/mL injection.	Dogs: 5–15 mg/dog q8h PO. Cats: 1.25–5 mg/cat q8h PO.
Bisacodyl (Dulcolax)	Laxative/cathartic. Acts via local stimulation of gastrointestinal motility, most likely by irritation of bowel. Used primarily as laxative or for procedures in which bowel evacuation is necessary.	Avoid use in patients with renal disease. Avoid overuse.	Available as OTC tablet. Doses are derived from extrapolation of human doses or via empiricism. There are no well-controlled efficacy studies available for veterinary species. Onset of action is approx. 1 hr.	5 mg tablets.	5 mg/animal q8–24h PO.

Drug Name (Trade or Other Names)	Pharmacology and Indications	Adverse Effects and Precautions	Dosing Information and Comments	Formulations	Dosage
Bismuth subsalicylate (Pepto Bismol)	Antidiarrhea agent and gastrointestinal protectant. Precise mechanism of action is unknown but antiprostaglandin action of salicylate component may be beneficial for enteritis. Bismuth component is efficacious for treating infections caused by spirochaete bacteria (*Helicobacter* gastritis).	Adverse effects are uncommon; however, salicylate component is absorbed systemically and overuse should be avoided in animals that cannot tolerate salicylates (such as cats and animals allergic to aspirin). Owners should be warned that bismuth will discolor stools.	Available as OTC product. Doses are derived from extrapolation of human doses or via empiricism. There are no well-controlled efficacy studies available for veterinary species.	Oral suspension. 262 mg/15 mL, or 525 mg/mL in extra strength formulation; 262 mg tablets.	1–3 ml/kg/day (in divided doses) PO.
Bismuth subcarbonate	Same as for bismuth subsalicylate.				0.3–3.0 gm q4h PO.
Bleomycin (Blenoxane)	Anticancer antibiotic agent. Used for treatment of various sarcomas and carcinomas. Exact mechanism of action is unknown, but may bind to DNA and prevent synthesis.	Causes local reaction at site of injection. Causes pulmonary toxicity in people as well as fever and chills, but side effects are not well documented in veterinary species.	Injectable solution usually used in combination with other anticancer agents. Consult anticancer protocols for details regarding use.	15 U vials for injection.	Dogs: 10 U/m² IV or SC for 3 days, then 10 units/m² weekly (maximum cumulative dose 200 U/m²).
Bromide	See Potassium bromide.				
BSP (Bromsulphalein)	See Sulfobromophthalein (BSP).				
Bunamidine hydrochloride (Scolaban)	Used as anticestodal agent. Primarily to treat tapeworm infections in dogs and cats. Mechanism of action is to damage integrity of protective integument on parasite.	Vomiting and diarrhea have occurred after use. Avoid use in young animals.	Do not break tablets. Administer tablets on empty stomach. Do not feed for 3 hr after administration.	400 mg tablet.	20–50 mg/kg PO.
Bupivacaine (Marcaine, and generic)	Local anesthetic. Inhibits nerve conduction via sodium channel blockade. Longer-acting and more potent than lidocaine or other local anesthetics.	Adverse effects rare with local infiltration. High doses absorbed systemically can cause nervous system signs (tremors and convulsions). After epidural administration respiratory paralysis is possible with high doses.	Used for local infiltration or infusion into epidural space. One may admix 0.1 mEq sodium bicarbonate per 10 mL solution to increase pH, decrease pain from injection, and increase onset. Use immediately after mixing with bicarbonate.	2.5 and 5 mg/mL solution injection.	1 mL of 0.5% solution per 10 cm for an epidural.
Buprenorphine (Buprenex [[Vetergesic in the UK])	Opioid analgesic. Partial μ-receptor agonist, κ-receptor antagonist. 25–50 × more potent than morphine. Buprenorphine may cause less respiratory depression than other opiates.	Adverse effects are similar to other opiate agonists, except there may be less respiratory depression. Dependency from chronic use may be less than with pure agonists.	Used for analgesia, often in combination with other analgesics or in conjunction with general anesthesia. Longer acting than morphine. Only partially reversed by naloxone.	0.3 mg/mL solution.	Dogs: 0.006–0.02 mg/kg IV, IM, SC, q4–8h. Cats: 0.005–0.01 mg/kg, IV, IM, q4–8h.
Buspirone (BuSpar)	Antianxiety agent. Acts to block release of serotonin by binding to presynaptic receptors. In veterinary medicine has been primarily used for treatment of urine spraying in cats.	Some cats show increased aggression; some cats show increased affection to owners.	Some efficacy trials suggest effectiveness for treating urine spraying in cats. There may be a lower relapse rate compared to other drugs.	5, 10 mg tablet.	2.5–5 mg/cat q24h, PO (may be increased to 5–7.5 mg per cat twice daily for some cats).
Busulfan (Myleran)	Anticancer agent. Bifunctional alkylating agent and acts to disrupt DNA of tumor cells. Used primarily for lymphoreticular neoplasia.	Leukopenia is most severe side effect.	Usually used in combination with other anticancer agents. Consult specific protocol for details.	2 mg tablets.	3–4 mg/m² q24h PO.

Drug Name (Trade or Other Names)	Pharmacology and Indications	Adverse Effects and Precautions	Dosing Information and Comments	Formulations	Dosage
Butorphanol (Torbutrol Torbugesic)	Opioid analgesic. κ-receptor agonist and weak μ-receptor antagonist. Butorphanol is used for perioperative analgesia, chronic pain, and as an antitussive agent.	Adverse effects are similar to other opioid analgesic drugs. Sedation is common at analgesic doses. Respiratory depression can occur with high doses. Dysphoric effects have been observed with these agonist/antagonist drugs.	Often used in combination with anesthetic agents or in conjunction with other analgesic drugs.	1, 5, 10 mg tablets. 0.5 or 10 mg/mL injection.	Dog: (antitussive): 0.055 mg/kg q6–12h SC or 0.55 mg/kg PO; (preanesthetic): 0.2–0.4 mg/kg IV, IM, SC (with acepromazine); (analgesic) 0.2–0.4 mg/kg q2–4h. Cats (analgesic): 0.2–0.8 mg/kg q2–6h, IV, SC or 1.5 mg/kg PO q4–8h.
Calcitriol (Rocaltrol, Calcijex)	Used to treat calcium deficiency and diseases such as hypocalcemia associated with hypoparathyroidism. Not indicated as Vitamin D supplement. Action is to increase calcium absorption in intestine.	Overdose can result in hypercalcemia.	Doses should be adjusted in each patient according to response and monitoring calcium plasma concentration.	Available as injection (Calcijex) and capsules (Rocaltrol). 0.25, 0.5 mcg capsules, 1 or 2 mcg/mL injection.	2.5–3 ng/kg (0.0025–0.003 mcg/kg) q24h PO.
Calcium carbonate (Many brands available: Titralac, Tums, generic)	Used as oral calcium supplement for hypocalcemia. Used as antacid to treat gastric hyperacidity and gastrointestinal ulcers. Neutralizes stomach acid. Also used as intestinal phosphate binder for hyperphosphatemia.	Few side effects. Increased calcium concentrations are possible. Drug interactions: Avoid use with oral fluoroquinolones (e.g., ciprofloxacin, enrofloxacin) as it may decrease their absorption.	Doses are primarily derived from extrapolation of human doses. When used as calcium supplement, doses should be adjusted according to serum calcium concentrations.	Many tablets or oral suspension, e.g., 650 mg tablets (contains 260 mg calcium ion).	5–10 mL of oral solution, q4–6h PO; for phosphate binder: 60–100 mg/kg/day in divided doses, PO.
Calcium chloride (generic)	Calcium supplement. Used in acute situations to supplement as electrolyte replacement or as a cardiotonic.	Overdose with calcium is possible. Do not administer IV solution SC, IM, because it may cause tissue necrosis.	Injection is (27.2 mg of calcium ion [1.36 mEq]) per ml. Usually used in emergency situations. Intracardiac administration has been performed, but avoid injections into the myocardium.	10% (100 mg/mL) solution.	0.1–0.3 mL/kg IV (slowly).
Calcium citrate (Citracal [OTC])	Calcium supplement. Used in treatment of hypocalcemia, such as with hypoparathyroidism.	Hypercalcemia possible with oversupplementation.	Doses should be adjusted according to serum calcium concentration.	950 mg tablets (contains 200 mg calcium ion).	Cats: 10–30 mg/kg q8h PO, (with meals).
Calcium disodium EDTA	See Edetate calcium disodium				
Calcium gluconate (Kalcinate, and generic)	Calcium supplement. Used in treatment of hypocalcemia, such as with hypoparathyroidism. Used in electrolyte deficiency.	Hypercalcemia possible with oversupplementation.	Injection is 97 mg (9.5 mg of calcium ion [0.47 mEq]) per mL. 500 mg tablets contain 45 mg of calcium ion. Avoid administration of IV solution IM or SC because it will cause tissue necrosis.	10% (100 mg/mL) injection.	0.5–1.5 mL/kg IV (slowly).
Calcium lactate (generic)	Generally same comments as for other calcium supplements.		Calcium lactate contains 130 mg of calcium ion per gram.	OTC tablets.	Dogs: 0.5–2.0 gm/dog/day PO (in divided doses). Cats: 0.2–0.5 gm/cat/day PO (in divided doses).
Captopril (Capoten)	Angiotensin-converting enzyme (ACE) inhibitor. Inhibits conversion of angiotensin I to angiotensin II. May have other vasodilating properties. Generally used to treat hypertension and congestive heart failure.	Hypotension possible with excessive doses. May cause azotemia in some patients, especially when administered with potent diuretics (furosemide). Drug interactions: Use cautiously with diuretics, potassium supplements. NSAIDs may diminish antihypertensive effect.	Monitor patients carefully to avoid hypotension. With all ACE-inhibitors, monitor electrolytes and renal function 3–7 days after initiating therapy and periodically thereafter. Use of captopril has been replaced by enalapril in many patients.	25 mg tablet.	Dogs: 0.5–2 mg/kg q8–12h PO. Cats: 3.12 to 6.25 mg/cat q8h PO.

Drug Name (Trade or Other Names)	Pharmacology and Indications	Adverse Effects and Precautions	Dosing Information and Comments	Formulations	Dosage
Carbenicillin (Geopen, Pyopen)	β-lactam antibiotic. Inhibits bacterial cell wall synthesis. Active against *Pseudomonas* and other Gram-negative bacteria.	Use cautiously in patients sensitive to penicillins (e.g., allergy).	Carbenicillin injection often is administered with an aminoglycoside. Do not mix with amino-glycosides prior to administration or inacti-vation will result.	1, 2, 5, 10, and 30 gram vials for injection.	40–50 mg/kg, and up to 100 mg/kg q6–8h, IV, IM, SC.
Carbenicillin indanyl sodium (Geocillin)	Same as for carbenicil-lin. Primary use is for treating infections of lower urinary tract.	Same as carbenicillin.	Oral formulation of carbenicillin, but attains concentrations that are only sufficient for treat-ing urinary tract infec-tions. Do not use for systemic infections.	500 mg tablets.	10 mg/kg q8h PO.
Carbimazole (Neomercazole)	Antithyroid drug similar to methimazole, but with perhaps fewer side effects.	See Methimazole.	Used in Europe. Clinical experience in U.S. is limited.	Available in Europe.	Cat: 5 mg/cat q8h PO; (induction), followed by 5 mg/cat q12h PO.
Carboplatin (Paraplatin)	Anticancer agent. Used for treating various carcinomas. Interrupts replication of DNA in tumor cells by cross-linking. Used for squamous cell carci-noma, and other carci-nomas, melanoma, osteosarcomas, and other sarcomas. Action is similar to cisplatin (see Cisplatin for further details).	Dose-limiting toxicosis is myelosuppression. May cause anemia, leukopenia, or throm-bocytopenia. Carbo-platin may induce renal toxicity. Compared to cisplatin, carboplatin is less emetogenic and less nephrotoxic. In cats, causes a dose-limiting neutropenia and thrombocytopenia (nadir at day 17).	Available for reconsti-tution for injection. Do not use with adminis-tration sets containing aluminum, because of incompatibility. Usually administered in specific anticancer protocols.	50 and 150 mg vial for injection.	Dogs: 300 mg/m² q3–4wks IV. Cats: 200–250 mg/m² every 4 weeks, IV.
Carprofen (Rimadyl [Zinecarp in the UK])	Analgesic agent. Used primarily for treatment of musculoskeletal pain. Although considered an NSAID, mechanism of action may involve mechanisms other than inhibition of prostaglan-din synthesis.	Appears to cause less incidence of gastro-intestinal ulceration and vomiting than other NSAIDs. In rare cases in dogs, carprofen has caused idiosyncratic acute hepatic toxicity. Highest incidence was in Labradors. Signs of toxicity appear 2–3 weeks after exposure. Do not use in cats.	Doses are based on clinical investigations in dogs with arthritis. Some dogs have been managed with once-daily dosing. Until safety studies are available, use is not recommended in cats. Injectable formulation available in the UK.	25, 75, and 100 mg tablets.	Dog: 2.2 mg/kg, q12h, PO. Cat: doses not available.
Cascara sagrada (many brands [e.g., Nature's Remedy])	Stimulant cathartic. Action is believed to be by local stimulation of bowel motility. Used as laxative to treat consti-pation or evacuate bowel for procedures.	Overuse can cause electrolyte losses.	Available in various OTC products.	100 and 325 mg tablets.	Dog: 1–5 mg/kg/day PO. Cat: 1–2 mg/cat/day.
Castor oil (generic)	Stimulant cathartic. Action is believed to be by local stimulation of bowel motility. Used as laxative to treat consti-pation or evacuate bowel for procedures.	Overuse can cause electrolyte losses. Castor oil has been known to stimulate premature labor in pregnancy.	Available as OTC product.	Oral liquid (100%).	Dog: 8–30 mL/day PO. Cat: 4–10 mL/day PO.

Drug Name (Trade or Other Names)	Pharmacology and Indications	Adverse Effects and Precautions	Dosing Information and Comments	Formulations	Dosage
Cefaclor (Ceclor)	Cephalosporin antibiotic. Action is similar to other β-lactam antibiotics, which is to inhibit synthesis of bacterial cell wall leading to cell death. Cephalosporins are divided into 1st, 2nd, or 3rd generation, depending on spectrum of activity. Consult package insert or specific reference for spectrum of activity of individual cephalosporin. Cefaclor is a 2nd-generation cephalosporin.	All cephalosporins are generally safe; however, sensitivity can occur in individuals (allergy). Rare bleeding disorders have been known to occur with some cephalosporins.	Used primarily when resistance has been demonstrated to 1st-generation cephalosporins.	250, 500 capsule and 25 mg/mL oral suspension.	4–20 mg/kg, q8h, PO.
Cefadroxil (Cefa-Tabs, Cefa-Drops)	See Cefaclor. Cefadroxil is a 1st-generation cephalosporin.	See Cefaclor. Cefadroxil has been known to cause vomiting after oral administration in dogs.	Spectrum of cefadroxil is similar to other 1st-generation cephalosporins. For susceptibility test, use cephalothin as test drug.	50 mg/mL oral suspension; 50, 100, 200, 1000 mg tablet.	Dog: 22 mg/kg q12h, up to 30 mg/kg q12h PO. Cat: 22 mg/kg q24h PO.
Cefazolin sodium (Ancef, Kefzol, and generic)	See Cefadroxil. Cefazolin is a 1st-generation cephalosporin.	See Cefaclor. For cefazolin, use cephalothin to test susceptibility.	Commonly used 1st-generation cephalosporin as injectable drug for prophylaxis for surgery as well as acute therapy for serious infections.	50 and 100 mg/50 mL for injection.	20–35 mg/kg q8h IV, IM. For perisurgical use: 22 mg/kg every 2 hr during surgery.
Cefdinir (Omnicef)	Oral 3rd-generation cephalosporin. Activity includes staphylococci, and many Gram-negative bacilli. Other characteristics are similar to other drugs in this class.	Similar to other oral cephalosporins.	Use in veterinary medicine has not been reported. Use and doses are extrapolated from human medicine.	300 mg capsules, 25 mg/mL oral suspension.	Dose not established. Human dose is 7 mg/kg q12h PO.
Cefixime (Suprax)	See Cefaclor. Cefixime is a 3rd-generation cephalosporin.	See Cefaclor.	Although not approved for veterinary use, pharmacokinetic studies in dogs have provided recommended doses.	20 mg/mL oral suspension and 200 and 400 mg tablets.	10 mg/kg q12h PO; for cystitis: 5 mg/kg q12–24h PO.
Cefotaxime (Claforan)	See Cefaclor. Cefotaxime is a 3rd-generation cephalosporin. Cefotaxime is used when resistance is encountered to other antibiotics, or when infection is in central nervous system.	See Cefaclor.	3rd-generation cephalosporin used when resistance encountered to 1st- and 2nd-generation cephalosporins.	500 mg; 1-, 2-, and 10-gm vials for injection.	Dog: 50 mg/kg, IV, IM, SC, q12h. Cat: 20–80 mg/kg q6h IV, IM.
Cefotetan (Cefotan)	See Cefaclor. Cefotetan is 2nd-generation cephalosporin.	See Cefaclor.	2nd-generation cephalosporin similar to cefoxitin, but may have longer half-life in dogs.	1-, 2-, and 10-gm vials for injection.	30 mg/kg, q8h, IV, SC.
Cefoxitin sodium (Mefoxin)	See Cefaclor. Cefoxitin is a 2nd-generation cephalosporin. May have increased activity against anaerobic bacteria.	See Cefaclor.	2nd-generation cephalosporin, which is often used when activity against anaerobic bacteria is desired.	1-, 2-, and 10-gm vials for injection.	30 mg/kg q6–8h IV.
Ceftazidime (Fortaz, Ceptaz, Tazicef)	3rd-generation cephalosporin. Ceftazidime has more activity than other cephalosporins against *Pseudomonas aeruginosa*.	See Cefaclor.	3rd-generation cephalosporin. May be reconstituted with 1% lidocaine for IM injection.	Vials (0.5, 1, 2, 6 gm) reconstituted to 280 mg/mL.	30 mg/kg q6h IV, IM.

Drug Name (Trade or Other Names)	Pharmacology and Indications	Adverse Effects and Precautions	Dosing Information and Comments	Formulations	Dosage
Ceftiofur (Naxcel [ceftiofur sodium]; Excenel [ceftiofur HCL]).	See Cefaclor. Ceftiofur is a unique cephalosporin that does not fit into a distinct class; however, its spectrum resembles many of the 3rd-generation cephalosporins.	See Cefaclor. Ceftiofur is primarily used only for urinary tract infections.	Available as powder for reconstitution prior to injection. After reconstitution stable for 7 days when refrigerated or 12 hrs at room temperature, or frozen for 8 weeks. Excenel is not approved for use in dogs.	50 mg/mL injection.	2.2–4.4 mg/kg, SC, q24h (for urinary tract infections).
Cephalexin (Keflex and generic forms)	See Cefaclor. Cephalexin is a 1st-generation cephalosporin.	See Cefaclor. For cephalexin, use cephalothin to test susceptibility.	Although not approved for veterinary use, trials in dogs with pyoderma show similar efficacy.	250, 500 mg capsules; 250, 500 mg tablets; 100 mg/mL or 125, 250 mg/5 mL oral suspension.	10–30 mg/kg q6–12h PO; for pyoderma, 22–35 mg/kg, q12h, PO.
Cephalothin sodium (Keflin)	See Cefaclor.	See Cefaclor.	1st-generation cephalosporin. Used as test drug for susceptibility tests of other 1st-generation cephalosporins.	1 and 2 gm vials for injection.	10–30 mg/kg q4–8h IV, IM.
Cephapirin (Cefadyl)	See Cefaclor. Cephapirin is a 1st-generation cephalosporin.	See Cefaclor.		500 mg, 1-, 2-, 4-gm vials for injection.	10–30 mg/kg q4–8h IV, IM.
Cephradine (Velosef)	See Cefaclor. Cephapirin is a 1st-generation cephalosporin.	See Cefaclor.		250, 500 mg capsules, and 250, 500 mg, 1 and 2 gm vials for injection.	10–25 mg/kg q6–8h PO.
Charcoal, activated (Acta Char, Charcodote, Toxiban, generic)	Adsorbent. Used primarily to adsorb drugs and toxins in intestine to prevent their absorption.	Not absorbed systemically. Safe for administration.	Available in variety of forms; usually used as treatment of poisoning. Many commercial preparations contain sorbitol, which acts as flavoring agent, and promotes intestinal catharsis.	Oral suspension.	1–4 gm/kg PO (granules); 6–12 mL/kg (suspension).
Chlorambucil (Leukeran)	Cytotoxic agent. Acts in similar manner as cyclophosphamide as alkylating agent. Used for treatment of various tumors and immunosuppressive therapy.	Myelosuppression is possible. Cystitis does not occur with chlorambucil as with cyclophosphamide.	Consult anticancer drug protocol for specific regimens.	2 mg tablet.	2–6 mg/m^2, or 0.1–0.2 mg/kg q24h initially, then q48h PO.
Chloramphenicol and Chloramphenicol palmitate (Chloromycetin, generic forms)	Antibacterial drug. Mechanism of action is via inhibition of protein synthesis via binding to ribosome. Broad spectrum of activity. Florfenicol acts via similar mechanism and has been substituted in some animals. (See Florfenicol section.)	Bone marrow suppression is possible with high doses, or prolonged treatment (especially in cats). Avoid use in pregnant or neonatal animals. Drug interactions with other drugs (e.g., barbiturates) possible because chloramphenicol will inhibit hepatic microsomal enzymes.	Chloramphenicol use based on susceptibility data. Chloramphenicol palmitate requires active enzymes and should not be administered to fasted (or anorectic) animal. *Note:* Some forms of chloramphenicol are no longer available in the U.S.	30 mg/mL oral suspension (palmitate), 250 mg capsules, and 100, 250, and 500 mg tablet.	Dog: 40–50 mg/kg q8h PO. Cat: 12.5–20 mg/kg q12h PO.
Chloramphenicol sodium succinate (Chloromycetin, generic)	Injection form of choramphenicol. Converted by liver to parent drug.	Same as chloramphenicol.	Injectable solution converted to chloramphenicol by hepatic metabolism.	100 mg/mL injection.	Dog: 40–50 mg/kg q6–8h IV, IM. Cat: 12.5–20 mg/cat q12h IV, IM.
Chlorothiazide (Diuril)	Thiazide diuretic. Inhibits sodium reabsorption in distal renal tubules. Used as diuretic and antihypertensive. Since it decreases renal excretion of calcium, it also has been used to treat calcium-containing uroliths.	Do not use in patient with elevated calcium. May cause electrolyte imbalance such as hypokalemia.	Not as effective as high-ceiling diuretics (such as furosemide).	250 and 500 mg tablets, 50 mg/mL oral suspension, and injection.	20–40 mg/kg q12h PO.

Drug Name (Trade or Other Names)	Pharmacology and Indications	Adverse Effects and Precautions	Dosing Information and Comments	Formulations	Dosage
Chlorpheniramine maleate (Chlortrimeton, Phenetron, and others)	Antihistamine (H-1 blocker). Blocks action of histamine on receptors. Also may have direct anti-inflammatory action. Used most often to prevent allergic reactions. Used for pruritus therapy in dogs and cats.	Sedation is most common side effect. Antimuscarinic effects (atropine-like effects) also are common.	Chlorpheniramine is included as ingredient in many OTC cough/cold and allergy medications.	4, 8 mg tablets.	Dog: 4–8 mg/dog q12h PO (up to a maximum of 0.5 mg/kg q12h). Cat: 2 mg/cat q12h PO.
Chlorpromazine (Thorazine)	Phenothiazine tranquilizer/antiemetic. Inhibits action of dopamine as neurotransmitter. Most often used as central antiemetic. Also used for sedation and preanesthetic purposes.	Causes sedation. May lower seizure threshold and causes α-adrenergic blockade. Produces extra-pyramidal side effects in some individuals.	Used for vomiting caused by toxins, drugs, or gastrointestinal disease. Higher doses than listed in dose section have been used with cancer chemotherapy (2 mg/kg q3h SC).	25 mg/mL injection solution.	0.5 mg/kg q6–8h IM, SC.
Chlortetracycline (generic)	Tetracycline antibacterial drug. Inhibits bacterial protein synthesis by interferring with peptide elongation by ribosome. Bacteriostatic agent with broad spectrum of activity.	Avoid use in young animals; may bind to bone and developing teeth. High doses have caused renal injury.	Broad-spectrum antibiotic. Used for routine infections and intracellular pathogens.	Powdered feed additive.	25 mg/kg q6–8h PO.
Chorionic gonadotropin	See Gonadotropin.				
Cimetidine (Tagamet [OTC and prescription])	Histamine-2 antagonist (H-2 blocker). Blocks histamine stimulation of gastric parietal cell to decrease gastric acid secretion. Used to treat ulcers and gastritis.	Adverse effects usually seen only with decreased renal clearance. In people, CNS signs may occur with high doses. *Drug interactions:* May increase concentrations of other drugs used concurrently (e.g., theophylline), because of inhibition of hepatic enzymes.	Precise doses needed to treat ulcers have not been established. Doses are derived from gastric secretory studies.	100, 150, 200, 300 mg tablets and 60 mg/mL injection.	10 mg/kg q6–8h IV, IM, PO (in renal failure, administer 2.5–5 mg/kg q12h IV, PO).
Ciprofloxacin (Cipro)	Fluoroquinolone antibacterial. Acts to inhibit DNA gyrase and inhibit cell DNA and RNA synthesis. Bactericidal. Broad antimicrobial activity.	Avoid use in dogs 4 weeks to 7 months of age. High concentrations may cause CNS toxicity, especially in animals with renal failure. Use cautiously in epileptic patients. Causes occasional vomiting. IV solution should be given slowly (over 30 min).	Doses are based on plasma concentrations needed to achieve sufficient plasma concentration above MIC. Efficacy studies have not been performed in dogs or cats. Ciprofloxacin is not absorbed orally as well as enrofloxacin.	250, 500, 750 mg tablet; 2 mg/mL injection.	10–20 mg/kg q24h PO, IV.
Cisapride (Propulsid [Prepulsid in Canada])	Prokinetic agent. Stimulates gastric and intestinal motility by either acetylcholine-action, activity on serotonin receptors, or direct effect on smooth muscle. Used for gastric reflux, gastroparesis, ileus, constipation.	Contraindicated in patients with gastrointestinal obstruction.	Doses are based on extrapolation from human doses, experimental studies and anecdotal evidence. Efficacy studies have have not been performed in dogs or cats.	10 mg tablet.	Dog: 0.1–0.5 mg/kg q8–12h, PO (as high as 0.5–1.0 mg/kg). Cat: 2.5–5 mg/cat q8–12h, PO (as high as 1 mg/kg q8h).

Drug Name (Trade or Other Names)	Pharmacology and Indications	Adverse Effects and Precautions	Dosing Information and Comments	Formulations	Dosage
Cisplatin (Platinol)	Anticancer agent. Used for treating various solid tumors, including osteosarcoma. Action is believed to be similar to bifunctional alkylating agents and interrupts replication of DNA in tumor cells.	Nephrotoxicity is the most limiting factor to cisplatin therapy. In cats, causes a dose-related, species-specific, primary pulmonary toxicosis. Vomiting may occur in dogs with administration. Transient thrombocytopenia may occur in dogs.	To avoid toxicity, fluid loading before administration using sodium chloride should be performed. Anti-emetic agents are often administered before therapy to decrease vomiting.	1 mg/mL injection.	Dogs only: 60–70 mg/m² q3–4wks IV (administer fluid for diuresis with therapy).
Clavamox	See Amoxicillin/ Clavulanic acid.				
Clavulanic acid	See Amoxicillin/ Clavulanic acid.				
Clemastine (Tavist, Contac 12 hr allergy, and generic)	Antihistamine (H-1 blocker). Blocks action of histamine on tissues. Used primarily for treatment of allergy. Some evidence suggests that clemastine is more effective than other antihistamines for pruritus in dogs.	Sedation is most common side effect.	Used for short-term treatment of pruritus in dogs. May be more efficacious when combined with other anti-inflammatory drugs. Tavist syrup contains 5.5% alcohol.	1.34 mg tablets (OTC), 2.64 mg tablets (Rx), and 0.134 mg/mL syrup.	Dog: 0.05–0.1 mg/kg q12h PO.
Clindamycin (Antirobe [veterinary], Cleocin [human])	Antibacterial drug of the lincosamide class (similar in action to macrolides). Inhibits bacterial protein synthesis via inhibition of bacterial ribosome. Primarily bacteriostatic, with spectrum of activity primarily against Gram-positive bacteria and anaerobes.	Generally well-tolerated in dogs and cats. Oral liquid product may be unpalatable to cats. Lincomycin and clindamycin may alter bacterial population in intestine and cause diarrhea; for this reason, do not administer to rodents or rabbits.	Most doses are based on manufacturer's drug approval data and efficacy trials. See dosing column for specific guidelines for different infections.	Oral liquid 25 mg/mL; 25, 75, and 150 mg capsule, and 150 mg/mL injection (Cleocin).	Dog: 11 mg/kg q12h PO, or 22 mg/kg q24h PO. Cat: 5.5 mg/kgq12h, or 11 mg/kg q24h (staphylococcal infections); 11 mg/kg q12h, or 22 mg/kg q24h, (anaerobic infections) PO. Toxoplasmosis: 12.5 mg/kg PO, q12h for 4 weeks.
Clofazimine (Lamprene)	Antimicrobial agent used to treat feline leprosy. Slow bactericidal effect on Mycybacterium leprae	Adverse effects have not been reported in cats. In people, the most serious adverse effects are gastrointestinal.	Doses based on empiricism or extrapolation of human studies.	50 and 100 mg capsule.	Cat: 1 mg/kg up to a maximum of 4 mg/kg/day PO.
Clomipramine (Clomicalm [veterinary]; Anafranil [human])	Tricyclic antidepressant drug (TCA). Used in people to treat anxiety and depression. Used in animals to treat variety of behavioral disorders, including obsessive-compulsive disorders and separation anxiety. Action is via inhibition of uptake of serotonin at presynaptic nerve terminals.	Reported adverse effects include: sedation, reduced appetite. Other side effects associated with TCAs are: antimuscarinic effects (dry mouth, rapid heart rate), and antihistamine effects (sedation). Overdoses can produce life-threatening cardiotoxicity.	When adjusting doses, one may initiate therapy with low dose and increase gradually. There may be a 2–4 week delay after initiation of therapy before beneficial effects are seen. (JAVMA 213: 1760–1766, 1998).	5, 20, 80 mg tablets (veterinary); 10, 25, 50 mg tablets (human).	Dog: 1–3 mg/kg/day, q12h PO. Cat: 1–5 mg per cat q12–24 hr PO.
Clonazepam (Klonopin)	Benzodiazepine. Action is to enhance inhibitory effects of GABA in CNS. Used for antiseizure action, sedation, and treatment of some behavioral disorders.	Side effects include sedation and polyphagia. Some animals may experience paradoxical excitement.	Doses are based primarily on reports from human medicine, empiricism, or experimental studies. No clinical efficacy studies have been performed in dogs or cats.	0.5, 1, and 2 mg tablet.	0.5 mg/kg q8–12h PO.

Drug Name (Trade or Other Names)	Pharmacology and Indications	Adverse Effects and Precautions	Dosing Information and Comments	Formulations	Dosage
Clorazepate (Tranxene)	Benzodiazepine. Action is to enhance inhibitory effects of GABA in CNS. Used for antiseizure action, sedation, and treatment of some behavioral disorders.	Side effects include sedation and poly-phagia. Some animals may experience para-doxical excitement.	Doses are based pri-marily on reports from human medicine, empiricism, or experi-mental studies. No clinical efficacy studies have been performed in dogs or cats. Clorazepate tablets degrade quickly in presence of light, heat, or moisture. Keep in original packaging or in tightly-sealed container.	3.75, 7.5, 11.25, 15, and 22.5 mg tablet.	2 mg/kg q12h PO.
Cloxacillin (Cloxapen, Orbenin, Tegopen)	β-lactam antibiotic. Inhibits bacterial cell wall synthesis. Spec-trum is limited to Gram-positive bacteria, espe-cially staphylococci.	Use cautiously in animals allergic to penicillin-like drugs.	Doses based on empir-icism or extrapolation from human studies. No clinical efficacy studies available for dogs or cats. Oral absorption is poor; administer if possible on empty stomach.	250, 500 mg capsules, 25 mg/mL oral solution.	20–40 mg/kg q8h PO.
Codeine (generic)	Opiate agonist. Mecha-nism is similar to mor-phine, except with approximately 1/10 potency of morphine. (see Morphine for other details.)	See Morphine.	Available as codeine phosphate and codeine sulfate oral tablets. Doses listed for anal-gesia are considered initial doses; individual patients may need higher doses, depend-ing on degree of toler-ance or pain threshold.	15, 30, 60 mg tablet, 5 mg/mL syrup, 3 mg/mL oral solution.	Analgesia: 0.5–1 mg/kg q4–6h PO. Antitussive: 0.1–0.3 mg/kg q4–6h PO.
Colchicine (generic)	Anti-inflammatory agent. Used primarily to treat gout. In animals, used to decrease fibro-sis and development of hepatic failure (possibly by inhibiting formation of collagen).	Do not administer to pregnant animals. Adverse effects are not well-documented in animals. Colchicine may cause dermititis in people.	Doses based on empir-icism. There are no well-controlled efficacy studies in veterinary species.	500, 600 mcg tablets and 500 mcg/mL ampule injection.	0.01–0.03 mg/kg q24h PO.
Colony-stimulating factor (Amgen)	Stimulates granulocyte development in bone marrow. Used primarily to regenerate blood cells to recover from cancer chemotherapy or other therapy.		Doses based on limited experimental informa-tion performed in dogs. (JAVMA 200: 1957, 1992)		2.5 mcg/kg q12h SC.
Corticotropin (ACTH) (Acthar)	Used for diagnostic purposes to evaluate adrenal gland function. Stimulates normal synthesis of cortisol from adrenal gland.	Adverse effects unlikely when used as single injection for diagnostic purposes.	Doses established by measuring normal adre-nal response in animals. See also Cosyntropin.	Gel 80 U/mL.	Response test: Collect pre-ACTH sample and inject 2.2 IU/kg IM. Collect post-ACTH sample at 2 hr in dogs and at 1 and 2 hr in cats.
Cosequin (glucosamine + chondroitin sulfate) (Cosequin)	Cosequin is brand name for combination of glucosamine HCl and chondroitin sulfate. According to manufac-turer, these compounds stimulate synthesis of synovial fluid and inhibit degradation and improve healing of articular cartilage. Used primarily for degenerative joint disease.	Adverse effects have not been reported, although hypersensi-tivity is possible.	Doses are based primarily on empiricism and manufacturer's recommendations. No published trials of efficacy are available.	Regular (RS) and double strength (DS) capsules.	Dogs: 1–2 RS capsules per day (2–4 capsules of DS for large dogs). Cat: 1 RS capsule daily.

Drug Name (Trade or Other Names)	Pharmacology and Indications	Adverse Effects and Precautions	Dosing Information and Comments	Formulations	Dosage
Cosyntropin (Cortrosyn)	Cosyntropin is a synthetic form of corticotropin (ACTH) used for diagnostic purposes only. In humans, it is preferred over corticotropin because it is less allergenic.	Same as for corticotropin.	Same as for corticotropin. Use for diagnostic purposes only; not intended for treatment of hypoadrenocorticism.	250 mcg per vial.	Response test: collect pre-ACTH sample and inject 5 mcg/kg IV (dog) or 0.125 mg IV (cat), and collect post sample at 30, 60 min.
Cyanocobalamin (Vitamin B$_{12}$) (many)	Vitamin B analogue.	Adverse effects rare except in high overdoses.	Same as for other Vitamin B preparations.	100 mcg/mL injection.	Dog: 100–200 mcg/day PO. Cat: 50–100 mcg/day PO.
Cyclophosphamide (Cytoxan, Neosar)	Cytotoxic agent. Bifunctional alkylating agent. Disrupts base-pairing and inhibits DNA and RNA synthesis. Cytotoxic for tumor cells and other rapidly dividing cells. Used primarily as adjunct for cancer chemotherapy and as immunosuppressive therapy.	Bone marrow suppression is most common adverse effect. Can produce severe neutropenia (that usually is reversible). Vomiting and diarrhea may occur in some patients. Dogs are susceptible to bladder toxicity (sterile hemorrhagic cystitis). May cause hair loss when used in some chemotherapeutic protocols.	Cyclophosphamide is usually administered with other drugs (other cancer drugs in cancer protocols or corticosteroids) when used for immunosuppressive therapy. Consult specific anticancer protocols for specific regimens.	25 mg/mL injection; 25, 50 mg tablet.	Anticancer: 50 mg/m^2 once daily 4 days/week PO, or 150–300 mg/m^2 IV, and repeat in 21 days. Immunosuppressive therapy: 50 mg/m^2 (approx. 2.2 mg/kg) q48h PO, or 2.2 mg/kg once daily for 4days/week. Cat: 6.25–12.5mg/cat once daily 4 days/week.
Cyclosporine (Cyclosporin-A) (Neoral; Sandimmune, Optimmune [ophthalmic]. Other name for cyclosporine is cyclosporin A)	Immunosuppressive drug. Suppresses induction of T-cell lymphocytes.	Can cause vomiting, diarrhea, anorexia. Nephrotoxicity may occur. In comparison to other immunosuppressive drugs, does not cause myelosuppression. Drug Interactions: Cimetidine, erythromycin, or ketoconazole may increase cyclosporine concentrations when used concurrently.	Adjust dose via monitoring if possible. Suggested trough blood concentration range (whole blood assay) is 300–400 ng/mL. Neoral oral products are absorbed more predictably than Sandimmune. Neoral may produce 50% higher blood concentrations in some patients. Oral solution can be diluted to make it more palatable. Topical cyclosporine has been used successfully as treatment for keratoconjunctivitis sicca.	Neoral: 25 and 100 microemulsion capsules; 100 mg/mL oral solution (for microemulsion). Sandimmune: 100 mg/mL oral solution; 25, 100 mg capsules. Optimune: 0.2% ointment.	Dog: 3–7 mg/kg q12h, PO. Cat: 3–5 mg/kg PO q12h.
Cyproheptadine (Periactin)	Phenothiazine with antihistamine and antiserotonin properties. Used as appetite stimulant (probably by altering serotonin activity in appetite center).	May cause increased appetite and weight gain.	Clinical studies have not been performed in veterinary medicine. Use is based primarily on empiricism and extrapolation from human results. Syrup contains 5% alcohol.	4 mg tablet; 2 mg/5 mL syrup.	Antihistamine: 1.1 mg/kg q8–12h PO. Appetite stimulant: 2 mg/cat PO.
Cytarabine (cytosine arabinoside) (Cytosar)	Anticancer agent. Exact mechanism is not known. Probably inhibits DNA synthesis. Used for lymphoma and leukemia protocols.	Bone marrow suppression. Causes vomiting and nausea.	Consult anticancer protocols for precise dosing regimens.	100 mg vial.	Dog (lymphoma): 100 mg/m^2 once daily, or 50 mg/m^2 twice daily for 4 days IV, SC. Cat: 100 mg/m^2 once daily for 2 days
Dacarbazine (DTIC)	Anticancer agent. Monofunctional alkylating agent. Used for melanoma.	Leukopenia, nausea, vomiting, diarrhea. Do not use in cats.	Consult anticancer protocol for specific regimens.	200 mg vial for injection.	200 mg/m^2 for 5 days q3wks IV; or 800–1000 mg/m^2, q3wks IV.
Danazol (Danocrine)	Gonadotropin inhibitor. Suppresses LH and FSH and estrogen synthesis. In people, used for endometriosis. May reduce destruction of platelets or RBC in immune-mediated disease.	May cause signs similar to other adrogenic drugs. Adverse effects have not been reported in animals. Gonadotropin inhibitor.	When used to treat autoimmune disease, usually used in conjunction with other drugs (e.g., corticosteroids).	50, 100, 200 mg capsules.	5–10 mg/kg q12h PO.

Drug Name (Trade or Other Names)	Pharmacology and Indications	Adverse Effects and Precautions	Dosing Information and Comments	Formulations	Dosage
Dantrolene (Dantrium)	Muscle relaxant. Inhibits calcium leakage from sarcoplasmic reticulum. In addition to muscle relaxation, it has been used for malignant hyperthermia. Also has been used to relax urethral muscle in cats.	Muscle relaxants can cause weakness in some animals.	Doses have been primarily extrapolated from experimental studies or extrapolation of human studies. No clinical trials available in veterinary medicine. Studies in which dantrolene relaxed urethra in cats used 1 mg/kg IV.	100 mg capsule, and 0.33 mg/mL injection.	For prevention of malignant hyperthermia: 2–3 mg/kg IV. Dog: 1–5 mg/kg q8h PO. Cat: 0.5–2 mg/kg q12h PO.
Dapsone (generic)	Antimicrobial drug used primarily for treatment of mycobacterium. May have some immuno-suppressive properties or inhibit function of inflammatory cells. Used primarily for dermatologic diseases in dogs and cats.	Hepatitis and blood dyscrasias may occur. Toxic dermatological reactions have been seen in people. *Drug interactions:* Do not administer with trimethoprim (may increase blood concentrations).	Doses are derived from extrapolation of human doses or empiricism. No well-controlled clinical studies have been performed in veterinary medicine.	25 and 100 mg tablets.	1.1 mg/kg q8–12h PO.
Darbazine (prochlorperazine + isopropamide) (Darbazine)	Combination product. Chlorpromazine is a central-acting dopamine antagonist (antiemetic); isopropamide is an anticholinergic drug (atropine-like effects). Used primarily to control vomiting in animals.	Side effects are attributed to each component. Prochlorperazine produces phenothiazine-like effects (see Acepromazine). Isopropamide produces anti-muscarinic effects (see Atropine). Use of anti-muscarinic drugs is contraindicated in animals with gastro-paresis and should be used cautiously in animals with diarrhea.	Doses are based on manufacturer's recommendations.	No. 1, 2, and 3 capsules.	Dog and cats: 0.14–0.2 mL/kg q12h SC. Dog 2–7 kg: 1–#1 capsule q12h PO. Dog 7–14 kg: 1–#2 capsule q12h PO. Dog > 14 kg: 1–#3 capsule q12h PO.
Deferoxamine (Desferal)	Chelating agent with strong affinity for tri-valent cations. Used to treat acute iron toxicosis. Indicated in cases of severe poisoning. Deferoxamine also has been used to chelate aluminum and facilitate removal.	Adverse effects have not been reported in animals. Allergic reactions and hearing problems have occurred in people.	100 mg of deferoxamine binds 8.5 mg of ferric iron. Monitor serum iron concentrations to determine severity of intoxication and success of therapy. Contact local poison control center for guidance. Successful therapy is indicated by monitoring urine color (orange-rose color change to urine indicates chelated iron is being eliminated).	500 mg vial for injection.	10 mg/kg IV, IM q2h for two doses, then 10 mg/kg q8h for 24 hr.
Deprenyl (L-deprenyl)	See Selegiline.				
DES	See Diethylistilbestrol.				
Desmopressin acetate (DDAVP) (DDAVP)	Synthetic peptide similar to antidiuretic hormone (ADH). Used as replacement therapy for patients with diabetes insipidus. Desmopressin also has been used for treatment of patients with mild to moderate von Willebrand's disease prior to surgery or other procedure that may cause bleeding.	No side effects reported. In people, it rarely has caused thrombotic events.	Desmopressin is used only for central diabetes insipidus. Duration of effect is variable (8–20 hours). It is ineffective for treatment of nephrogenic diabetes insipidus or polyuria from other causes. Intranasal product has been administered as eye drops in dogs. Onset of effect is within one hour. (JAVMA 205: 170, 1994; JAVMA 209: 1884, 1996). Oral tablets are available for humans.	4 and 15 mcg/mL injection and desmopressin acetate nasal solution 100 mcg/mL (0.01%) metered spray. Tablets 0.1 and 0.2 mg.	Diabetes insipidus: 2–4 drops (2 mcg) q12–24h intranasally or in eye. 0.05–0.1 mg q12h PO as needed. von Willebrand's disease treatment: 1 mcg/kg (0.01 mL/kg) SC, IV, diluted in 20 mL of saline administered over 10 min.

Drug Name (Trade or Other Names)	Pharmacology and Indications	Adverse Effects and Precautions	Dosing Information and Comments	Formulations	Dosage
Desoxycorticosterone pivalate (Percorte n-V, DOCP, or DOCA pivalate)	Mineralocorticoid. Used for adrenocortico-insufficiency (hypo-adrenocorticism). No glucocorticoid activity.	Excessive mineralo-corticoid effects with high doses.	Initial dose based on studies performed in clinical patients. Individual doses may be based on monitoring electrolytes in patients. Actual interval between doses may range from 14–35 days. (J Vet Intern Med 11: 43–49, 1997).	Injection.	1.5–2.2 mg/kg q25 days IM.
Detomidine (Dormosedan)	α_2-adrenergic agonist. More potent and more specific than xylazine. Used primarily for anesthesia and analgesia.	Potent α_2-agonist. Produces sedation and ataxia. Cardiac depression, heart block, and hypotension possible with high doses.	Doses not established for small animals; used primarily for horses.	10 mg/mL injection.	Doses not established for small animals.
Dexamethasone (Dexamethasone solution and dexa-methasone sodium phosphate) (Azium solution in polyethylene glycol. Sodium phosphate forms include: Dexaject SP, Dexavet, and Dexasone. Tablets include Decadron and generic)	Corticosteroid. Dexa-methasone has approx-imately 30× potency of cortisol. Multiple anti-inflammatory effects (see Betamethasone).	Multiple side effects. (See Betamethasone.)	Doses based on sever-ity of underlying disease (see Betamethasone). Dexamethasone is used for testing hyper-adrenocorticism. Low-dose-dexamethasone suppression test: dogs 0.01 mg/kg IV, cats 0.1 mg/kg IV, and collect sample at 0, 4 and 8 hours. For high-dose-dexamethasone suppression test: dogs 0.1 mg/kg, cats 1.0 mg/kg.	Azium solution, 2 mg/mL. Sodium phosphate forms are 3.33 mg/mL. 0.25, 0.5, 0.75, 1, 1.5, 2, 4, 6 mg tablets.	Anti-inflammatory: 0.07–0.15 mg/kg q 12–24h IV, IM, PO. For shock, spinal injury: 2.2–4.4 mg/kg IV (of sodium phosphate form). Dexamethasone suppression test: dogs 0.01 mg/kg IV, cats 0.1 mg/kg IV, and collect sample at 0, 4 and 8 hours.
Dextran (Dextran 70, Gentran 70)	Synthetic colloid used for volume expansion. High-molecular-weight fluid replacement. Primarily used for acute hypovolemia and shock.	Only limited use in veterinary medicine and adverse effects have not been reported. In people, coagulop-athies are possible because of decreased platelet function. Ana-phylactic shock also has occurred.	Used primarily in critical care situations. Delivered via constant rate infusion slowly. Monitor patient's cardiopulmonary status carefully during administration.	Injectable solution. 250, 500, 1000 mL.	10–20 mL/kg IV to effect.
Dextromethorphan (Benylin and others)	Centrally acting anti-tussive drug. Shares similar chemical struc-ture as opiates, but does not affect opiate receptors. Appears to directly affect cough receptor.	Adverse effects not reported in veterinary medicine. High over-dose may cause sedation.	Many OTC preparations that may contain other ingredients (e.g., anti-histamines, decongest-ants, and acetamino-phen).	Availabe in syrup, capsule, and tablet. Many OTC products.	0.5–2 mg/kg q6–8h PO.
Dextrose solution 5% (D₅W)	Sugar added to fluid solutions. Isotonic.	High doses produce pulmonary edema.	Commonly used fluid solution administered via constant rate infusion. *Not* a main-tenance solution.	Fluid solution for IV administration.	40–50 mL/kg q24h IV.
Diazepam (Valium and generic)	Benzodiazepine. Central-acting CNS depressant. Mecha-nism of action appears to be via potentiation of GABA-receptor medi-ated effects in CNS. Used for sedation, an-esthetic adjunct, anti-convulsant, and behav-ioral disorders. Diaze-pam metabolized to desmethyldiazepam (nordiazepam) and oxazepam.	Sedation is most com-mon side effect. May cause paradoxical excitement in dogs. Causes polyphagia. In cats, idiopathic fatal hepatic necrosis has been reported.	Clearance in dogs is many times faster than people (half-life in dogs less than 1 hr) requires frequent administration. For treatment of status epilepticus, may be administered IV or rectally. Avoid admin-istration IM.	2, 5 mg tablet. 5 mg/mL solution for injection.	Preanesthetic: 0.5 mg/kg IV. Status epilepticus: 0.5 mg/kg IV, 1 mg/kg rectal; repeat if necessary. Appetite stimulant (cat): 0.2 mg/kg IV. For behavior treatment in cats: 1–4 mg per cat q12–24 hr PO.
Dichlorophene	Vermiplex (see Toluene)				

Drug Name (Trade or Other Names)	Pharmacology and Indications	Adverse Effects and Precautions	Dosing Information and Comments	Formulations	Dosage
Dichlorphenamide (Daranide)	Carbonic anhydrase inhibitor. Diuretic. Acts to inhibit enzyme that forms hydrogen and bicarbonate ions. Reduces plasma bicarbonate concentration, producing systemic metabolic acidosis and alkaline diuresis. Primarily used to treat glaucoma.	Sulfonamide derivative. Use cautiously in animals sensitive to sulfonamides. Hypokalemia may occur in some patients. Severe metabolic acidosis is rare.	Dichlorphenamide is not used as diuretic, but is most commonly employed to treat glaucoma. May be combined with other antiglaucoma agents.	50 mg tablet.	3–5 mg/kg q8–12h PO.
Dichlorvos (Task)	Antiparasitic drug, used primarily to treat hookworms, roundworms, whipworms. Kills parasites by anticholinesterase action.	Do not use in heartworm-positive patients. Overdoses can cause organophosphate intoxication. (Treat with 2-PAM, atropine).	Doses based on manufacturer's recommendations.	10, 25 mg tablet.	Dog: 26.4–33 mg/kg PO. Cat: 11 mg/kg PO.
Dicloxacillin (Dynapen)	β-lactam, antibiotic. Inhibits bacterial cell wall synthesis. Spectrum is limited to Gram-positive bacteria, especially staphylococci.	Use cautiously in animals allergic to penicillin-like drugs.	No clinical efficacy studies available for dogs or cats. In dogs, oral absorption is very low and may not be suitable for therapy (JVPT 21: 414–417, 1998). Administer, if possible, on empty stomach.	125, 250, 500 mg capsules, 12.5 mg/mL oral suspension.	11–55 mg/kg q8h PO.
Diethylcarbarnazine (DEC) (Caricide, Filaribits)	Heartworm preventative. For action, see Piperazine.	Safe in all species. Reactions can occur in animals with positive microfilaria.	Doses based on manufacturer's recommendations. Specific protocols for heartworm administration may be based on region of country.	Chewable tablets. 50, 50, 60, 180, 200, 400 mg tablet.	Heartworm prophylaxis: 6.6 mg/kg q24h PO.
Diethylstilbestrol (DES) (DES, generic [no longer manufactured in US, but available from compounding pharmacist])	Synthetic estrogen compound. Used for estrogen replacement in animals. DES is most commonly used to treat estrogen-responsive incontinence in dogs. Also has been used to induce abortion in dogs.	Side effects may occur that are caused by excess estrogen. Estrogen therapy may increase risk of pyometra and estrogen-sensitive tumors.	Doses listed are for treating urinary incontinence, and vary depending on response. Titrate dose to individual patients. Although used to induce abortion, it was *not* efficacious in one study that administered 75 mcg/kg.	1, 5 mg tablet; 50 mg/mL injection.	Dog: 0. 1–1.0 mg/dog q24h PO. Cat: 0.05–0.1 mg/cat q24h PO.
Difloxacin hydrochloride (Dicural)	Fluoroquinolone antibacterial drug. Acts via inhibition of DNA gyrase in bacteria to inhibit DNA and RNA synthesis. Bactericidal with broad spectrum of activity. Used for variety of infections, including skin infections, wound infections, and pneumonia.	Adverse effects include: seizures in epileptic animals, arthropathy in young animals, vomiting at high doses. *Drug interactions:* May increase concentrations of theophylline if used concurrently. Coadministration with di- and trivalent cations (e.g., sucralfate) may decrease absorption.	Dose range can be used to adjust dose, depending on severity of infection and susceptibility of bacteria. Bacteria with low MIC can be treated with low dose; susceptible bacteria with higher MIC should be treated with higher dose. Difloxacin is primarily eliminated in feces rather than urine (urine is < 5% of clearance). Sarafloxacin is an active desmethyl metabolite.	11.4, 45.4, and 136 mg tablet.	5–10 mg/kg q24h, PO (see dosing information guidelines).

Drug Name (Trade or Other Names)	Pharmacology and Indications	Adverse Effects and Precautions	Dosing Information and Comments	Formulations	Dosage
Digitoxin (Crystodigin [no longer available from some distributors])	Cardiac ionotropic agent. Increases cardiac contractility and decreases heart rate. Mechanism is via inactivation of cardiac muscle sodium-potassium ATPase. Beneficial effects for heart failure may occur via neuroendocrine effects (alters sensitivity of baroreceptors).	Digitalis glycosides have narrow therapeutic index. May cause variety of arrhythmias in patients (e.g., heart block, ventricular tachycardia). Causes vomiting, anorexia, diarrhea. Adverse effects potentiated by hypokalemia, reduced by hyperkalemia.	Used in heart failure for ionotropic effect and decrease heart rate. Used in supraventricular arrhythmias to decrease ventricular response to atrial stimulation. May be used with other cardiac drugs. Monitor concentrations in patients to determine optimum therapy.	0.05, 0.1 mg tablet.	0.02–0.03 mg/kg q8h PO.
Digoxin (Lanoxin, Cardoxin)	Cardiac ionotropic agent. Increases cardiac contractility and decreases heart rate. Mechanism is via inactivation of cardiac muscle sodium-potassium ATPase. Beneficial effects for heart failure may occur via neuroendocrine effects (alters sensitivity of baroreceptors). Used in heart failure for ionotropic effect and to decrease heart rate. Used in supraventricular arrhythmias to decrease ventricular response to atrial stimulation.	Digitalis glycosides have narrow therapeutic index. May cause variety of arrhythmias in patients (e.g., heart block, ventricular tachycardia). Causes vomiting, anorexia, diarrhea. Adverse effects potentiated by hypokalemia, reduced by hyperkalemia. Some breeds of dogs (Dobermans) and cats more sensitive to adverse effects.	Monitor patients carefully. Optimum plasma concentration is 1–2 ng/mL. Adverse effects common at concentration above 3.5 ng/mL. When dosing, calculate dose on lean body weight. Doses should be 10% less for elixir, because of increased absorption.	0.0625, 0.125, 0.25 mg tablet; 0.05, 0.15 mg/mL elixir.	Dog: < 20 kg body weight: 0.01 mg/kg q12h; > 20 kg use 0.22 mg/m^2 q12h PO (subtract 10% for elixir). Dog (rapid digitalization): 0.0055–0.011 mg/kg q1h IV to effect. Cat: 0.08–0.01 mg/kg q48h PO (approximately 1/4 of a 0.125 mg tablet/cat).
Dihydrotachysterol (Vitamin D) (Hytakerol, DHT)	Vitamin D analogue. Used as treatment of hypocalcemia, especially hypoparathyroidism associated with thyroidectomy. Vitamin D promotes absorption and utilization of calcium.	Overdose may cause hypercalcemia. Avoid use in pregnant animals because it may cause fetal abnormalities. Use cautiously with high doses of calcium-containing preparations.	Available as oral solution, tablets, and capsules. Doses for individual patients should be adjusted by monitoring serum calcium concentrations.	0. 125 mg tablet; 0.5 mg/ml oral liquid.	0.01 mg/kg/day PO; for acute treatment, administer 0.02 mg/kg initially, then 0.01–0.02 mg/kg q24–48h PO, thereafter.
Diltiazem (Cardizem, Dilacor)	Calcium-channel blocking drug. Blocks calcium entry into cells via blockade of slow channel. Produces vasodilation, negative chronotropic effects. Used for supraventricular arrhythmias in dogs; hypertrophic cardiomyopathy in cats.	Hypotension, cardiac depression, bradycardia, AV block. May cause anorexia in some patients.	Diltiazem preferred over verapamil in patients with heart failure, because of less cardiac suppression. Note that "XR , SR, or CD" refers to slow-release formulations. Usually, for slow-release form, doses are higher, but administered less often, such as once daily.	30, 60, 90, 120 mg tablets. 5 mg/mL injection. Extended release capsules are 60, 90, 120, 180, 240, 300 mg.	Dog: 0.5–1.5 mg/kg q8h PO, 0.25 mg/kg over 2 min IV (repeat if necessary). Cat: 1.75–2.4 mg/kg q8h PO. For Dilacor XR or Cardizem, CD dose is 10 mg/kg, once daily, PO. Dilacor capsules contain 60-mg tablets for dosing cats.
Dimenhydrinate (Dramamine, [Gravol in Canada])	Antihistamine drug. Converted to active diphenhydramine. (See Chlorpheniramine.)	See Chlorpheniramine.	See Chlorpheniramine. There have been no clinical studies on the use of dimenhydrinate. It is primarily used empirically for treatment of vomiting.	50 mg tablets; and 50 mg/mL injection.	Dog: 4–8 mg/kg q8h PO, IM, IV. Cat: 12.5 mg/cat q8h IV IM PO.
Dimercaprol (BAL) (BAL in oil)	Chelating agent. Used to treat lead, gold, arsenic toxicity.	Adverse effects not reported in veterinary medicine. In people, sterile absesses occur at injection site. High doses have caused seizures, drowsiness, and vomiting.	Use as soon as possible after intoxicant exposure. Alkalinization of urine will increase toxin removal. For lead intoxication, may be used with edetate calcium.	Injection.	4 mg/kg q4h IM.
Dinoprost tromethamine	See Prostaglandin F$_{2\alpha}$ 5 mg/mL injection				

Drug Name (Trade or Other Names)	Pharmacology and Indications	Adverse Effects and Precautions	Dosing Information and Comments	Formulations	Dosage
Dioctyl calcium sulfosuccinate	See Docusate calcium.				
Dioctyl sodium sulfosuccinate	See Docusate sodium.				
Diphenhydramine (Benadryl)	Antihistamine (see Chlorpheniramine)	See Chlorpheniramine.	Antihistamine used primarily for allergic disease in animals.	Available OTC. 2.5 mg/ml elixir, 25, 50 mg capsule and tablets. 50 mg/mL injection.	2–4 mg/kg mg/kg q6–8h, PO, or 1 mg/kg IM, IV. (For dogs administer 25–50 mg/dog q8h IV IM PO.)
Diphenoxylate (Lomotil)	Opiate agonist. Stimulates smooth muscle segmentation in intestine, as well as electrolyte absorption. Used for acute treatment of nonspecific diarrhea.	Adverse effects have not been reported in veterinary medicine. Diphenoxylate is poorly absorbed systemically and produces few systemic side effects. Excessive use can cause constipation.	Doses are based primarily on empiricism or extrapolation of human dose. Clinical studies have not been performed in animals. Contains atropine, but dose is not high enough for significant systemic effects.	2.5 mg.	Dog: 0.1–0.2 mg/kg q8–12h PO. Cat: 0.05–0.1 mg/kg q12h PO.
Diphenylhydantoin	See Phenytoin.				
Diphosphonate disodium edidronate	See Etidronate disodium.				
Dipyridamole (Persantine)	Platelet inhibitor. Mechanism of action is attributed to increased levels of cAMP in platelet, which decreases platelet activation. Indicated primarily to prevent thromboembolism.	Adverse effects have not been reported in animals.	Used primarily in people to prevent thromboembolism. Use in animals has not been reported. When used in people, it is combined with other antithrombotic agents (e.g., warfarin).	25, 50, 75 mg tablets; 5 mg/mL injection.	4–10 mg/kg q24h PO.
Dipyrone	No longer available commercially. (Previous use in animals was at: 28 mg/kg q8h IV, IM, SC.)				
Disopyramide (Norpace [Rhythmodan in Canada])	Antiarrhythmic agent of Class I. Depresses myocardial electrophysiologic conduction rate.	Adverse effects have not been reported in animals. High doses may cause cardiac arrhythmias.	Not commonly used in veterinary medicine. Other antiarrhythmic drugs are preferred.	100, 150 mg capsules (10 mg/mL injection in Canada only).	6–15 mg/kg q8h PO.
Disophenol (DNP)	Injectable antihookworm compound. Withdrawn from market by manufacturer.	Adverse effects are rare at recommended doses. Signs of toxicosis are tachycardia, polypnea, and hyperthermia.	Doses based on clinical studies in dogs and cats.	No longer available.	10 mg/kg (0.22 mL/kg) SC, once.
Dithiazine iodide (Dizan)	Microfilaricidal drug for dogs. Also effective for hookworms, roundworms, and whipworms.	Adverse effects are rare. Causes vomiting in some dogs. Causes discoloration of feces.	Before ivermectin and similar drugs, this was the only microfilaricidal agent for dogs. Not commonly used.	10, 50, 100, 200 mg tablets.	Heartworm: 6.6–11 mg/kg q24h PO for 7–10 days. For other parasites: 22 mg/kg PO.
Divalproex sodium	Depakote, Epival. Equivalent to Valproic acid (see Valproic acid).				
Dobutamine (Dobutrex)	Adrenergic agonist. Action is primarily to stimulate myocardium via action on cardiac β_1-receptors. Increases heart contraction, without increase in heart rate. Some action may occur via α-receptors. Primarily used for acute treatment of heart failure.	May cause tachycardia and ventricular arrhythmias at high doses, or in sensitive individuals.	Dobutamine has a very rapid elimination half-life (minutes) and therefore must be administered via carefully monitored constant rate infusion. When mixing, avoid alkalinizing solutions. Usually dilute in 5% dextrose solution (e.g., 250 mg in 1 L 5% dextrose).	250 mg/20 mL vial for injection. (12.5 mg/mL)	Dog: 5–20 mcg/kg/min IV infusion. Cat: 0.5–2 mcg/kg/min IV infusion.

Drug Name (Trade or Other Names)	Pharmacology and Indications	Adverse Effects and Precautions	Dosing Information and Comments	Formulations	Dosage
Docusate calcium (Surfak, Doxidan)	Stool softener (surfactant). Acts to decrease surface tension to allow more water to accumulate in the stool.	No adverse effects reported in animals. In people high doses have caused abdominal discomfort.	Doses are based on extrapolations from humans, or empiricism. No clinical studies reported for animals. Docusate calcium products may contain stimulant cathartic phenolphthalein, which should be used cautiously in cats.	60 mg tablets (and many others).	Dog: 50–100 mg per dog q12–24h PO. Cat: 50 mg per cat q12–24h PO.
Docusate sodium (Colace, Doxan, Doss; many OTC brands)	See Docusate calcium.	See Docusate calcium.	See Docusate calcium.	50, 100 mg capsule, 10 mg/mL liquid.	Dog: 50–200 mg per dog q8–12h PO. Cat: 50 mg per cat q12–24h PO.
Domperidone (Motilium)	Motility modifier (similar to metoclopramide)	See metoclopramide.	Not available in U.S., only in Canada.	Not available in US.	2–5 mg/animal PO.
Dopamine (Intropin)	Adrenergic agonist. Action is primarily to stimulate myocardium via action on cardiac β_1-receptors. There is some suggestion that dopamine increases renal perfusion via action on renal dopaminergic receptors, however, clinical evidence for beneficial effect is lacking.	May cause tachycardia and ventricular arrhythmias at high doses, or in sensitive individuals.	Dopamine has a very rapid elimination half-life (minutes), and therefore must be administered via carefully monitored constant-rate infusion. When mixing, avoid alkalinizing solutions. Administer in 5% dextrose solution, or LRS. Mix 200–400 mg in 250 to 500 mL of fluid.	40, 80, or 160 mg/mL.	Dog, cat: 2–10 mcg/kg/min IV infusion.
Doxapram (Dopram)	Respiratory stimulant via action on carotid chemoreceptors and subsequent stimulation of respiratory center. Used to treat respiratory depression, or to stimulate respiration post-anesthesia. May also increase cardiac output.	Adverse effects not reported in animals. Cardiovascular effects and convulsions have occurred with high doses in people. Contraindicated in newborn infants, because it contains benzyl alcohol as vehicle.	Used for short-term treatment only. No longer available from manufacturer.	20 mg/mL injection.	5–10 mg/kg IV neonate: 1–5 mg SC, sublingual, or via umbilical vein.
Doxorubicin (Adriamycin)	Anticancer agent. Acts to intercalate between bases on DNA, disrupting DNA and RNA synthesis in tumor cell. Doxorubicin also may affect tumor cell membranes. Used for treatment of various neoplasia, including lymphoma.	Most common acute effect is anorexia, vomiting, and diarrhea. Dose-related toxicity also includes bone marrow suppression, hair loss (in certain breeds), and cardiotoxicity. Cardiotoxicity limits the total dose administered (usually do not exceed 200 mg/m²).	Regimen listed may differ for various tumors. Consult specific anticancer protocol for guidelines. Dose must be infused IV (over 20–30 min). Animals may require antiemetic and antihistamine (diphenhydramine) prior to therapy. Monitor ECG during therapy. Dose according to body weight may be more effective for small dogs.	2 mg/mL injection.	30 mg/m², IV q21 days, or: > 20 kg use 30 mg/m² and < 20 kg use 1 mg/kg. Cats: 1 mg/kg IV, q3weeks.
Doxycycline (Vibramycin, and generic forms)	Tetracycline antibiotic. Mechanism of action of tetracyclines is to bind to 30S ribosomal subunit and inhibit protein synthesis. Usually bacteriostatic. Broad spectrum of activity including bacteria, some protozoa, Rickettsia, Ehrlichia.	Severe adverse reactions not reported with doxycycline. Tetracyclines in general may cause renal tubular necrosis at high doses. Tetracyclines can affect bone and teeth formation in young animals. *Drug interactions:* Tetracyclines bind to calcium-containing compounds, which decreases oral absorption.	Many pharmacokinetic and experimental studies have been conducted in small animals, but no clinical studies. Ordinarily considered the drug of choice for Rickettsia and Ehrlichia infections in dogs. Doxycycline IV infusion is stable for only 12 hr at room temperature and 72 hr if refrigerated.	10 mg/mL oral suspension, 100 mg tablet, 100 mg injection vial.	3–5 mg/kg q12h PO IV, or 10 mg/kg q24h PO. For Rickettsia in dogs: 5 mg/kg q12h.

Drug Name (Trade or Other Names)	Pharmacology and Indications	Adverse Effects and Precautions	Dosing Information and Comments	Formulations	Dosage
Edetate calcium disodium (CaNa₂EDTA) (Calcium disodium versenate)	Chelating agent. Indicated for treatment of acute and chronic lead poisoning. Sometimes used in combination with dimercaprol.	No adverse effects reported in animals. In people, allergic reactions (release of histamine) occurs after IV administration.	May be used with dimercaprol. Equally effective when administered IV or IM, but IM injection may be painful. Ensure adequate urine flow before the first dose.	20 mg/mL injection.	25 mg/kg q6h SC, IM, IV for 2–5 days.
Edrophonium (Tensilon, and others)	Cholinesterase inhibitor. Causes cholinergic effects by inhibiting metabolism of acetylcholine. Very short-acting and ordinarily is only used for diagnostic purposes (e.g., for myasthenia gravis. Also has been used to reverse neuromuscular blockade of nondepolarizing agents (pancuronium).	Short-acting and side effects are minimal. Excessive muscarinic/cholinergic effects may occur with high doses (counteract with atropine).	Usually used only for determination of diagnosis of myasthenia gravis in patients. Too short-acting to be used for therapy.	10 mg/mL injection.	Dog: 0.11–0.22 mg/kg IV. Cat: 2.5 mg/cat IV.
Enalapril (Enacard, Vasotec)	ACE-inhibitor (see Captopril for details). Used for vasodilation and treatment of heart failure. Primarily used in dogs, but may benefit some cats in heart failure.	(See Captopril.) May cause azotemia in some patients; carefully monitor patients receiving high doses of diuretics. Drug interactions: Use cautiously with other hypotensive drugs and diuretics. NSAIDs may decrease vasodilating effects. Do not use in cats with uncomplicated hypertrophic cardiomyopathy.	Doses are based on clinical trials conducted in dogs by manufacturer. For dogs, start with once/daily administration and increase to q12h if needed. Other drugs used for treatment of heart failure may be used concurrently. With all ACE-inhibitors, monitor electrolytes and renal function 3–7 days after initiating therapy and periodically thereafter.	2.5, 5, 10, 20 mg tablet.	Dog: 0.5 mg/kg q12–24h PO. Cat: 0.25–0.5 mg/kg q12–24h PO.
Enflurane (Ethrane)	Inhalent anesthetic.	Adverse effects (not related to anesthesia) not reported in animals.	Titrate dose for each individual with anesthetic monitoring.	Available as solution for inhalation.	Induction: 2–3% maintenance: 1.5–3%.
Enilconazole (Imaverol, Clina-Farm-EC)	Azole antifungal agent, for topical use only. Like other azoles, inhibit membrane synthesis (ergosterol) in fungus. Highly effective for dermatophytes.	Administered topically. Adverse effects have not been reported.	Imaverol® is available only in Canada as 10% emulsion. In the U.S. Clinafarm EC® is available for use in poultry units as 13.8% solution. Dilute solution to at least 50:1 and apply topically every 3–4 days for 2–3 weeks. Enilconazole also has been instilled as 1:1 dilution into nasal sinus for nasal aspergillosis.	10% or 13.8% emulsion.	Nasal aspergillosis: 10 mg/kg q12h instilled into nasal sinus for 14 days (10% solution diluted 50/50 with water). Dermatophytes: dilute 10% solution to 0.2% and wash lesion with solution 4 times at 3–4 day intervals
Enrofloxacin (Baytril)	Fluoroquinolone antibacterial drug. Acts via inhibition of DNA gyrase in bacteria to inhibit DNA and RNA synthesis. Bactericidal. Broad spectrum of activity.	Adverse effects include: seizures in epileptic animals, arthropathy in dogs 4–28 weeks of age, vomiting in dogs and cats at high doses. Drug interactions: May increase concentrations of theophylline if used concurrently. Coadministration with di- and trivalent cations (e.g., sucralfate) may decrease absorption.	Low dose of 5 mg/kg/day is used for sensitive organisms with MIC of 0.12 mcg/mL or less, or urinary tract infection; dose of 5–10 mg/kg/day is used for organisms with MIC of 0.12–0.5 mcg/mL; dose of 10–20 mg/kg/day is used for organisms with MIC of 0.5–1.0 mcg/mL. Solution is not approved for IV use, but has been administered via this route safely if given slowly.	68, 22.7 mg, and 5.7 mg tablet. Taste Tabs are 22.7 and 68 mg. 22.7 mg/mL injection.	5–20 mg/kg/day (see dosing information guidelines).

Drug Name (Trade or Other Names)	Pharmacology and Indications	Adverse Effects and Precautions	Dosing Information and Comments	Formulations	Dosage
Ephedrine (many, generic)	Adrenergic agonist. Agonist on α- and β$_1$-adrenergic receptors, but not β$_2$-receptors. Used as vasopressor, e.g., administered during anesthesia. CNS stimulant. Also has been used to treat urinary incontinence because of action on bladder sphincter muscle.	Adverse effects related to excessive adrenergic activity (e.g., peripheral vasoconstriction, and tachycardia).	Used primarily in acute situations to increase blood pressure and urinary incontinence in dogs.	25, 50 mg/mL injection.	Urinary incontinence: 4 mg/kg, or 12.5–50 mg/dog q8–12h PO (2–4 mg/kg for cats). Vasopressor: 0.75 mg/kg, IM, SC, repeat as needed.
Epinephrine (Adrenaline and generic forms)	Adrenergic agonist. Nonselectively stimulates α- and β$_2$-adrenergic receptors. Used primarily for emergency situations to treat cardiopulmonary arrest and anaphylactic shock.	Overdose will cause excessive vasoconstriction and hypertensions. High doses can cause ventricular arrhythmias. When high doses are used for cardiopulmonary arrest, an electrical defibrillator should be available.	Doses are based on experimental studies, primarily in dogs. Clinical studies are not available. IV doses are ordinarily used, but endotracheal administration is acceptable when intravenous access is not available. Intraosseous route also has been used and doses are equivalent to IV. When endotracheal route is used, the dose is higher and duration of effect may be longer than IV administration. There appears to be no advantage to intracardiac injection compared to IV administration.	1 mg/mL (1:1,000) injection solution.	Cardiac arrest: 10–20 mcg/kg, IV; or 200 mcg/kg endotracheal (may be diluted in saline before administration). Anaphylactic shock: 2.5–5 mcg/kg IV; or 50 mcg/kg endotracheal (may be diluted in saline).
Epsiprantel (Cestex)	Anticestodal agent (similar to praziquantel)	See Praziquantel.	See Praziquantel.	Coated tablet.	Dog: 5.5 mg/kg PO. Cat: 2.75 mg/kg PO.
Ergocalciferol (Vitamin D$_2$) (Calciferol, Drisdol)	Vitamin D analogue. Used for vitamin D deficiency and as treatment of hypocalcemia, especially that associated with hypothyroidism. Vitamin D promotes absorption and utilization of calcium.	Overdose may cause hypercalcemia. Avoid use in pregnant animals because it may cause fetal abnormalities. Use cautiously with high doses of calcium-containing preparations.	Should not be used for renal hypoparathyroidism because of inability to convert to active compound. Available as oral solution, tablets, capsules, and injection. Doses for individual patients should be adjusted by monitoring serum calcium concentrations.	400 U tablets (OTC); 50,000 U tablet (1.25 mg); 500,000 U/mL (12.5 mg/mL) injection.	500–2000 U/kg/day PO.
Erythromycin (many brands and generic)	Macrolide antibiotic. Inhibits bacteria by binding to 50S ribosome and inhibiting protein synthesis. Spectrum of activity limited primarily to Gram-positive aerobic bacteria. Used for skin and respiratory infections.	Most common side effect is vomiting (probably caused by cholinergic-like effect or motilin-induced motility). May cause diarrhea in some animals. Do not administer PO to rodents or rabbits.	There are several forms of erythromycin, including the ethylsuccinate and estolate esters, and stearate salt for oral administration. There is no convincing data to suggest that one form is absorbed better than another, and one dose is included for all. Only erythromycin gluceptate and lactate are to be administered IV. Motilin-like effect on GI motility occurs at low dose.	250 mg capsule or tablet.	10–20 mg/kg q8–12h PO. Prokinetic effects at 0.5–1.0 mg/kg.

Drug Name (Trade or Other Names)	Pharmacology and Indications	Adverse Effects and Precautions	Dosing Information and Comments	Formulations	Dosage
Erythropoietin (r-HuEPO) (Epogen, epoetin alfa, [r-HuEPO])	Human recombinant erythropoietin. Hematopoietic growth factor that stimulates erythropoiesis. Used to treat nonregenerative anemia (Compend Cont Education 14: 25–34, 1992; JAVMA 212: 521–528, 1998).	Since this product is a human-recombinant product, it may induce local and systemic allergic reactions in animals. Injection site pain and headache have occurred in people. Seizures also have occurred. Delayed anemia may occur because of cross-reacting antibodies against animal erythropoietin (reversible when drug is withdrawn).	Use has been based on clinical reports in dogs and cats. The only form currently available is a human recombinant product.	2,000 units/mL injection.	Doses range from 35 or 50 U/kg three times/week to 400 U/kg/week SC (adjust dose to hematocrit of 0.30–0.34)
Esmolol (Brevibloc)	β-blocker. Selective for β₁-receptor. The difference between esmolol and other β-blockers is the short duration of action. Indicated for short-term control of heart rate and arrhythimas.	Same as other precautions for β-blockers (see Propranolol).	Indicated for short-term IV therapy only. Doses are based primarily on empiricism or extrapolation of human dose. No clinical studies have been reported in animals.	10 mg/mL injection.	500 mcg/kg, IV, which may be given as 0.05–0.1 mg/kg slowly every 5 min. or 50–200 mcg/kg/min infusion.
Estradiol cypionate (ECP) (ECP, Depo-Estradiol, generic)	Semisynthetic estrogen compound. Used primarily to induce abortion in animals.	High risk of endometrial hyperplasia and pyometra. High doses can produce leukopenia, thrombocytopenia, and fatal aplastic anemia.	Ordinarily, 22 mcg/kg is administered once IM during days 3–5 of estrus, or within 3 days of mating. However, in one study, a dose of 44 mcg/kg was more efficacious than 22 mcg/kg when given during estrus or diestrus.	2 mg/mL injection	Dog: 22–44 mcg/kg IM (total dose not to exceed 1.0 mg). Cat: 250 mcg/cat IM between 40 hrs and 5 days of mating.
Etidronate disodium (Didronel)	Bisphosphonate drug. Used to treat osteoporosis and hypercalcemia. Decreases bone turnover, inhibits osteoclast activity, retards bone resorption and decreases rate of osteoporosis.	Adverse effects not reported for animals. In people, gastrointestinal problems are common.	At high doses may inhibit mineralization of bone. In people, alendronate has replaced etidronate because of side effects.	200, 400 mg tablets; 50 mg/mL injection.	Dog: 5 mg/kg/day PO. Cat: 10 mg/kg/day PO.
Etodolac (Eto-Gesic, veterinary; Lodine, human)	An NSAID of the pyranocarboxylic acid group. Inhibits inflammatory prostaglandins.	NSAIDs may cause gastrointestinal ulceration. Other adverse effects caused by NSAIDs include decreased platelet function and renal injury. In clinical trials with etodolac, some dogs at recommended doses showed weight loss, loose stools, or diarrhea. At high doses, etodolac caused gastrointestinal ulceration in dogs.	Studies in dogs showed etodolac to be more efficacious than placebo for treatment of arthritis.	150 and 300 mg tablets.	Dogs: 10–15 mg/kg, once daily, PO. Cats: Dose not established.
Famotidine (Pepsid)	H-2 receptor antagonist. (See Cimetidine for details.)	See Cimetidine.	See Cimetidine. Clinical studies for famotidine have not been performed, therefore optimal dose for ulcer prevention and healing are not known.	10 mg tablet; 10 mg/mL injection.	0.5 mg/kg q12–24h IM, SC, PO.

Drug Name (Trade or Other Names)	Pharmacology and Indications	Adverse Effects and Precautions	Dosing Information and Comments	Formulations	Dosage
Felbamate (Felbatol)	Anticonvulsant. Usually used when dogs are refractory to other anti-convulsants. Mechanism may be via antagonism at the NMDA receptor and block effects of excitatory amino acids.	Not documented with use in dogs. In people, the most severe reactions have been hepatotoxicity and aplastic anemia. It may increase phenobarbital concentrations.	Dosing has been empirical. See dosage section. Starting doses are 200–400 mg/dog and increased to maximum of 600 mg for small dogs and 1200 mg for large dogs q8h.	120 mg/mL oral liquid, 400 and 600 mg tablets.	Dogs: Start with 15–20 mg/kg q8h PO. Or 200 mg/dog q8h for small dogs and 400 mg/dog q8h for larger dogs. Increase dose gradually by 200 mg increments until seizure control.
Fenbendazole (Panacur, Safe-Guard)	Benzimidazole anti-parasite drugs. (See Albendazole). Effective for treatment of Giardia (AJVR 59:61–63, 1998).	Good safety margin, but vomiting and diarrhea have been reported. No known contraindications.	Dose recommendations based on clinical studies by manufacturer. Granules may be mixed with food. In studies for treatment of Giardia, it was safer than other treatments.	Panacur granules 22.2% (222 mg/gm). 100 mg/mL oral suspension.	50 mg/kg/day × 3 days, PO.
Fentanyl (Sublimaze, generic)	Synthetic opiate analgesic. Approximately 80–100 times more potent than morphine. (See Morphine for more details.)	Adverse effects similar to morphine.	Doses are based on empiricism and experimental studies. No clinical studies have been reported. In addition to fentanyl injection, transdermal fentanyl is available (see below).	250 mg/5 mL injection.	0.02–0.04 mg/kg IV q2h, IM SC or 0.01 mg/kg IV IM SC (with acetylpromazine or diazepam); for analgesia: 0.01 mg/kg, q2h, IV, IM, SC.
Fentanyl transdermal (Duragesic)	Same as for fentanyl. Transdermal fentanyl incorporates fentanyl into adhesive patches applied to skin of dogs and cats. Studies have determined that patches release sustained levels of fentanyl for 72–108 hours in dogs and cats. One 100 mcg/hr patch is equivalent to 10 mg/kg of morphine every 4 hrs, IM.	Adverse effects have not been reported. However, if adverse effects are observed (e.g., respiratory depression, excess sedation, excitement in cats), remove patch and, if necessary, administer naloxone.	Patches available in sizes of 25, 50, 75 and 100 mcg/hr. Patch size is related to release rate of fentanyl. Studies have determined that 25 mcg/hr patches are appropriate for cats; 50 mcg/hr patches are appropriate for dogs 10–20 kg. Follow manufacturer's recommendations carefully when applying patches.	25, 50, 75, and 100 mcg/hr patch.	Cats: 25 mcg patch every 118 hr. Dog: 10–20 kg, 50 mcg/hr patch every 72 hrs.
Ferrous sulfate (many OTC brands)	Iron supplement.	High doses cause stomach ulceration.	Recommendations based on dose needed to increase hematocrit.	Many.	Dog: 100–300 mg/dog q24h PO. Cat: 50–100 mg/cat q24h PO.
Finasteride (Proscar)	Inhibits conversion of testosterone to dihydro-testosterone (DHT). Since DHT stimulates prostate growth, this has been used for benign prostatic hypertrophy.	No adverse effects reported in dogs. Contraindicated in pregnancy.	Doses based on study in dogs (JAVMA 59: 762–764, 1998)	5 mg tablet.	0. 1 mg/kg PO q24 hr (or 5 mg tablet q24h in 10–50 kg dogs).
Florfenicol (Nuflor)	Chloramphenicol derivative with same mechanism of action as chloramphenicol (inhibition of protein synthesis) and broad antibacterial spectrum. It has been used in situations in which chloramphenicol is not available.	Use in dogs and cats has been limited, therefore adverse effects have not been reported. Chloramphenicol has been linked to dose-dependent bone marrow depression, and similar reactions may be possible with florfenicol. However, there does not appear to be a risk of aplastic anemia, as for chloramphenicol.	Dose form is only approved for use in cattle, and these doses have not been thoroughly evaluated in small animals. Doses listed are derived from pharmacokinetic studies. Sustained effect in cattle from IM and SC administration does not appear to be longlasting in dogs. Injectable formulation for cattle has been administered, if necessary, orally to small animals.	300 mg/mL injectable solution.	Dog: 20 mg/kg q6h, PO, IM, q6h. Cat: 22 mg/kg q8h IM, PO.

Drug Name (Trade or Other Names)	Pharmacology and Indications	Adverse Effects and Precautions	Dosing Information and Comments	Formulations	Dosage
Fluconazole (Diflucan)	Azole antifungal drug. Similar mechanism as other azole antifungal agents. Inhibits ergosterol synthesis in fungal cell membrane. Fungistatic. Efficacious against dermatophytes, and variety of systemic fungi.	Adverse effects have not been reported from fluconazole administration. Compared to ketoconazole, has less effect on endocrine function. However, increased liver enzyme plasma concentrations and hepatopathy are possible. Compared to other oral azole antifungals, fluconazole is absorbed more predictably and completely, even on an empty stomach.	Doses for fluconazole are primarily based on studies performed in cats for treatment of cryptococcosis. Efficacy for other infections has not been reported. The primary difference between fluconazole and other azoles is that fluconazole attains higher concentrations in the CNS.	50, 100, 150 or 200 mg tablets; 10 or 40 mg/mL oral suspension; 2 mg/mL IV injection.	Dogs: 10–12 mg/kg/day, PO. Cats: 50 mg/cat q12h PO, or 50 mg/cat per day PO.
Flucytosine (Ancobon)	Antifungal drug. Used in combination with other antifungal drugs for treatment of cryptococcosis. Action is to penetrate fungal cells and is converted to fluorouracil, which acts as antimetabolite.	Adverse effects have not been reported in animals.	Flucytosine is used primarily to treat cryptococcosis in animals. Efficacy is based on flucytosine's ability to attain high concentrations in CSF. Flucytosine may be synergistic with amphotericin B.	250 mg capsule, 75 mg/mL oral suspension.	25–50 mg/kg q6–8h PO (up to a maxiumum dose of 100 mg/kg q12h PO).
Fludrocortisone (Florinef)	Mineralocorticoid. Used as replacement therapy in animals with adrenal atrophy/adrenocortical insufficiency. Has high potency of mineralocorticoid activity compared to glucocorticoid activity.	Adverse effects are primarily related to glucocorticoid effects with high doses. Long-term treatment for hypoadrenocorticism may result in glucocorticoid side effects.	Dose should be adjusted by monitoring patient response (i.e., monitoring electrolyte concentrations.) In some patients, it is administered with a glucocorticoid and sodium supplementation.	100 mcg (0.1 mg) tablets.	Dog: 0.2–0.8 mg per dog or 0.02 mg/kg q24h PO (13–23 mcg/kg). Cat: 0. 1–0.2 mg per cat q24h PO.
Flumazenil (Romazicon)	Benzodiazepine receptor antagonist. Used as reversal agent after benzodiazepine administration in people (not commonly used in veterinary medicine).	No adverse effects reported in animals.	Used primarily to block effects of benzodiazepine drugs. May be used to treat toxicity caused by high doses of benzodiazepines (e.g., diazepam). Although used experimentally for hepatic encephalopathy, it is not recommended for this use.	100 mcg/mL (0.1 mg/mL) injection.	0.2 mg (total dose) as needed IV.
Flumethasone (Flucort)	Potent glucocorticoid anti-inflammatory drug. Potency is approximately 15× that of cortisol. See Dexamethasone for additional details.	See Dexamethasone.	See Dexamethasone. Doses are based on severity of underlying disease (see dose table).	0.5 mg/mL injection.	Dog: 0.0625–0.25 mg/day IV, IM, SC. Cat: 0.03–0.125 mg/day IV, IM, SC. Antiinflammatory: 0.15–0.3 mg/kg q12–24h IV, IM, SC.
Flunixin meglumine (Banamine)	NSAID anti-inflammatory drug. Acts to inhibit cyclooxygenase enzyme (COX), which synthesizes prostaglandins. Other anti-inflammatory effects may occur (such as effects on leukocytes), but have not been well-characterized. Used primarily for short-term treatment of moderate pain and inflammation.	Most severe adverse effects related to gastrointestinal system. Causes gastritis, gastrointestinal ulceration with high doses or prolonged use. Renal ischemia has also been documented. Therapy in dogs should be limited to 4 consecutive days. Avoid use in pregnant animals near term. *Drug interactions:* Ulcerogenic effects are potentiated when administered with corticosteroids.	Not approved for small animals, but has been shown in experimental studies to be an effective prostaglandin synthesis inhibitor. Approved for use in small animals in Europe.	250 mg packet granules; 10, 50 mg/mL injection.	1.1 mg/kg once IV, IM, SC, or 1.1 mg/kg/day 3 day/week PO. Opthalmic: 0.5 mg/kg once IV.

Drug Name (Trade or Other Names)	Pharmacology and Indications	Adverse Effects and Precautions	Dosing Information and Comments	Formulations	Dosage
5-Fluorouracil (Fluorouracil)	Anticancer agent. Antimetabolite. Action is via inhibition with nucleic acid synthesis.	Causes mild leukopenia, thrombocytopenia. CNS toxicity. Do not use in cats.	Used in anticancer protocols. Consult anticancer treatment protocol for precise dosage and regimen.	50 mg/mL vial.	Dog: 150 mg/m^2 once/week IV. Cat: do not use.
Fluoxetine (Prozac)	Antidepressant drug. Used to treat behavioral disorders such as obsessive-compulsive disorders and dominance aggression. Mechanism of action appears to be via selective inhibition of serotonin reuptake and down regulation of 5-HT1 receptors.	Fewer adverse effects (especially antihistamine, antimuscarinic effects) compared to other antidepressant drugs. Serious adverse effects have not been reported in animals, but decreased appetite may be common. In cats, nervousness or increased anxiousness have been observed.	Use of fluoxetine in animals is largely experimental. Doses have been derived empirically and use is based primarily on anecdotal experience. Because of long half-life, acccumulation in plasma may take several days to weeks.	10 and 20 mg capsules; 4 mg/mL oral solution.	Dog: 0.5 mg/kg/day, initially PO, then increase to 1 mg/kg/day, PO (average dose is 10–20 mg/dog). Cat: 0.5–4 mg/cat q24h PO.
Follicle-stimulating hormone (FSH)	See Urofollitropin.				
Fomepizole	See 4-Methylpyrazole.				
Furazolidone (Furoxone)	Oral antiprotozoal drug with activity against Giardia. May have some activity against bacteria in intestine. Not used for systemic therapy.	Adverse effects not reported in animals. In people, mild anemia, hypersensitivity, and disturbance of intestinal flora have been reported.	Clinical studies have not been reported for animals. Doses and recommendations are based on extrapolation from humans. Other drugs, such as fenbendazole, may be preferred for Giardia.	100 mg tablets.	4 mg/kg q12h for 7–10 days PO.
Furosemide (Lasix, generic)	Loop diuretic. Inhibits sodium and water transport in ascending loop of Henle, which produces diuresis. Also may have vasodilating properties, increasing renal perfusion, and decreasing preload.	Adverse effects primarily related to diuretic effect (loss of fluid and electrolytes). Administer conservatively in animals receiving angiotensin-converting enzyme (ACE) inhibitors to decrease risk of azotemia.	Recommendations are based on extensive clinical use of furosemide in animals.	12.5, 20, 50 mg tablets; 10 mg/ml oral solution; 50 mg/mL injection.	Dog: 2–6 mg/kg q8–12h (or as needed) IV, IM, SC, PO. Cat: 1–4 mg/kg q8–24h IV, IM, SC, PO.
Gemfibrozil (Lopid)	Cholesterol lowering agent.	Adverse effects have not been reported in animals.	Used primarily in people to treat hyperlipidemia. Clinical studies have not been performed in animals.	300 mg capsules, 600 mg tablets.	7.5 mg/kg q12h, PO.
Gentamicin (Gentocin)	Aminoglycoside antibiotic. Action is to inhibit bacteria protein synthesis via binding to 30S ribosome. Bactericidal. Broad spectrum of activity except streptococci and anaerobic bacteria.	Nephrotoxicity is the most dose-limiting toxicity. Ensure that patients have adequate fluid and electrolyte balance during therapy. Ototoxicity, vestibulotoxicity also are possible. *Drug interactions:* When used with anesthetic agents, neuromuscular blockade is possible. Do not mix in vial or syringe with other antibiotics.	Dosing regimens are based on sensitivity of organisms. Some studies have suggested that once daily therapy (combining multiple doses into a single daily dose) is as efficacious as multiple treatments. Activity against some bacteria (e.g., *Pseudomonas*) is enhanced when combined with a β-lactam antibiotic. Nephrotoxicity is increased with persistently high trough concentrations.	50 and 100 mg/mL solution for injection.	Dog: 2–4 mg/kg q6–8h, or 6–10 mg/kg q24h IV, IM, SC. Cat: 3 mg/kg q8h, or 9 mg/kg q24h IV, IM, SC.
Glibenclamide	British name for Glyburide				

Drug Name (Trade or Other Names)	Pharmacology and Indications	Adverse Effects and Precautions	Dosing Information and Comments	Formulations	Dosage
Glipizide (Glucotrol)	Sulfonylurea oral hypoglycemic agent. Used as oral treatment in the management of diabetes mellitus, particularly in cats. Response rate is approximately 40%. This drug acts to increase secretion of insulin from pancreas, probably by interacting with sulfonylurea receptors on β-cells. These drugs also may increase sensitivity of existing insulin receptors.	It may cause dose-related vomiting, anorexia, increased bilirubin, and elevated liver enzymes in some cats. Causes hypoglycemia, but less so than insulin. In people, increased cardiac mortality is possible. *Drug Interactions:* Many drug interactions have been reported in people. It is not known if these occur in animals. Use cautiously with β-blockers, antifungal drugs, anticoagulants, fluoroquinolones, sulfonamides, and others (consult package insert).	Oral hypoglycemic agents are successful in people only for non-insulin-dependent diabetes. There has been only limited use in animals. Similar drugs include acetohexamide, chlorpropamide, glyburide, gliclazide, and tolazamide. Since response to oral hypoglycemic agents in cats is unpredictable, it is recommended to use a trial first of at least 4 weeks. If the cat responds, the drug can be continued, otherwise, insulin may be indicated. Feed cats a high-fiber diet when using oral hypoglycemic agents.	5, 10 mg tablets.	2.5–7.5 mg/cat q12h, PO. Usual dose is 2.5 mg/cat initially, then increase to 5 mg/cat, q12h.
Glyburide (Diabeta, Micronase, Glynase)	Sulfonylurea hypoglycemic agent. See Glipizide.	See Glipizide.	See Glipizide.	1.25, 2.5, 5 mg tablet.	0.2 mg/kg daily PO.
Glycerin (generic)	Used to treat acute glaucoma.	No adverse effects reported.		Oral solution.	1–2 mL/kg, up to q8h PO.
Glycopyrrolate (Robinul-V)	Anticholinergic drug (for mechanism, see Atropine.) Glycopyrrolate may have less effect on CNS, compared to atropine, because of lower CSF levels. May have longer duration of action than atropine.	Adverse effects attributed to antimuscarinic (anticholinergic) effects. (see Atropine).	Glycopyrrolate is often used in combination with other agents, particularly anesthetic drugs.	0.2 mg/mL injection.	0.005–0.01 mg/kg IV, IM, SC.
Glucosamine	Combined with chrondroitin sulfate in Cosequin. See Cosequin.				
Gold sodium thiomalate (Myochrysine)	Gold therapy (for mechanism, see Aurothioglucose).	See Aurothioglucose.	Clinical studies have not been performed in animals. Efficacy and safety of this product are not available for animals. Aurothioglucose generally is used more often than Myochrysine.	Injection.	1–5 mg IM on first week, then 2–10 mg IM on second week, then 1 mg/kg once/week IM maintenance.
Gold therapy	See Aurothioglucose, Gold sodium thiomalate, or Auranofin				
Golytely	Oral solution for producing catharsis.	See Polyethylene glycol electrolyte solution.			
Gonadorelin (GnRH, LHRH) (Factrel)	Stimulates synthesis and release of leutinizing hormone (LH) and, to a lesser degree, follicle-stimulating hormone (FSH). Used to induce leutinization.	Adverse effects have not been reported in animals.	Gonadotropin has been used to manage various reproductive disorders. Consult specific reference on reproductive problems in animals to guide therapy.	50 mcg/mL injection.	Dog: 50–100 mcg/dog per day q24–48h IM. Cat: 25 mcg/cat once IM.

Drug Name (Trade or Other Names)	Pharmacology and Indications	Adverse Effects and Precautions	Dosing Information and Comments	Formulations	Dosage
Gonadotropin, chorionic (HCG) (Profasi, Pregnyl, generic, A.P.L.)	Action of hCG is identical to that of leutinizing hormone (LH). Used to induce leutinization in animals.	Adverse effects have not been reported in animals.	Consult specific reference on reproductive problems in animals to guide therapy.	Injection sizes of 5, 10, and 20 thousand units.	Dog: 22 U/kg q24–48h IM, or 44 U once IM. Cat: 250 U/cat once IM.
Gonadotropin-releasing hormone	See Gonadorelin.				
Granisetron (Kytril)	Antiemetic drug that acts by inhibiting serotonin (5-HT) receptors. Used primarily for antiemetic during chemotherapy. '	None reported in dogs or cats.	Doses extrapolated from human uses.	1 mg tablets and 1 mg/mL injection.	0.01 mg/kg IV (in people, dose is 1 mg/person PO).
Griseofulvin (microsize) (Fulvicin U/F)	Antifungal drug. Incorporates into skin layers and inhibits mitosis of fungi. Antifungal activity is limited to dermatophytes.	Adverse effects in animals include: teratogenicity in cats, anemia and leukopenia in cats, anorexia, depression, vomiting, and diarrhea. Do not administer to pregnant cats.	A wide range of doses has been reported. Doses listed here represent the current consensus. Griseofulvin should be administered with food, to enhance absorption.	125, 250, 500 mg tablet, 25 mg/mL oral suspension, 125 mg/mL oral syrup.	50 mg/kg q24h PO (up to a maximum dose of 110–132 mg/kg/day in divided treatments).
Griseofulvin (ultra-microsize) (Fulvicin P/G, GrisPEG)	Same as above.	Same as above.	Same as above. Ultra-microsize is absorbed to a greater extent, and doses should be less than microsize.	100, 125, 165, 250, 330 mg tablets.	30 mg/kg/day in divided treatments PO.
Growth hormone (hGH, Somatrem, Somatropin) (Somatrem and Somatropin. Brand names include Protropin, Humatrope, Nutropin)	Growth hormone, also known as human growth hormone. Used to treat growth hormone deficiencies.	Growth hormone is diabetogenic in all animals. Excess growth hormone causes acromegaly.	There is only limited clinical experience in animals. Dose form must be reconstituted with sterile diluent before use. Prepared solution is stable if refrigerated for 14 days.	5 and 10 mg per vial.	0.1 units/kg three times/week for 4–6 weeks, SC, IM (usual human pediatric dose is 0. 18–0.3 mg/kg/week).
Halothane (Fluothane)	Inhalent anesthetic. Exact mechanism of action unknown.	Adverse effects related to anesthetic effects (e.g., cardiovascular and respiratory depression). Hepatotoxicosis has been reported in people.	Use of inhalent anesthetics require careful monitoring. Dose is determined by depth of anesthesia.	250 mL bottle.	Induction: 3%; maintenance: 0.5–1.5%.
Heparin sodium (Liquaemin ([US]; Hepalean [Canada])	Anticoagulant. Potentiates anticoagulant effects of antithrombin III. Used primarily for prevention of thrombosis.	Adverse effects caused by excessive inhibition of coagulation: bleeding.	Dose adjustments should be performed by monitoring clotting times. For example, dose is adjusted to maintain APTT to 1.5 to 2× normal.	1000 and 10,000 units/mL injection.	100–200 units/kg IV loading dose, then 100–300 units/kg q6–8hr, SC. Low-dose prophylaxis (dog and cat): 70 units/kg q8–12h SC.
Hetastarch	See Hydroxyethyl starch (HES).				
Hycodan	See Hydrocodone bitartrate.				
Hydralazine (Apresoline)	Vasodilator. Antihypertensive. Used to dilate arterioles and decrease afterload. Primarily used for treatment of CHF and other cardiovascular disorders characterized by high peripheral vascular resistance.	Adverse effects attributed to excess vasodilation. Monitor patients for hypotension. May dangerously decrease cardiac output. Allergic reactions (Lupus-like syndrome) have been reported in people and are related to acetylator status, but have not been reported in animals.	Use in heart failure may accompany other drugs, such as digoxin and diuretics. It is advised to monitor patient for hypotension to adjust dosage.	10 mg tablet, 20 mg/mL injection.	Dog: 0.5 mg/kg (initial dose), titrate to 0.5–2 mg/kg q12h PO. Cat: 2.5 mg/cat q12–24h, PO.

Drug Name (Trade or Other Names)	Pharmacology and Indications	Adverse Effects and Precautions	Dosing Information and Comments	Formulations	Dosage
Hydrocodone bitartrate (Hycodan)	Opiate agonist. Used primarily for antitussive action (see Codeine). Hycodan contains homatropine, but other combinations may contain guaifenesin or acetaminophen.	Oral opiate. See Codeine.	Hydrocodone is combined with atropine in the product Hycodan. Atropine can decrease respiratory secretions, but probably does not have significant clinical effects at doses in this preparation (1.5 mg homatropine per 5 mg tablet).	5 mg tablet, and 1 mg/mL syrup.	Dogs: 0.22 mg/kg q4–8 hr PO. Cats: no dose available.
Hydrochlorothiazide (Hydro-Diuril, generic)	Thiazide diuretic. Inhibits sodium reabsorption in distal renal tubules. Used as diuretic and antihypertensive. Since they decrease renal excretion of calcium, they also have been used to treat calcium-containing uroliths.	Do not use in patient with elevated calcium. May cause electrolyte imbalance such as hypokalemia.	Not as potent as loop-diuretics (such as furosemide). Clinical efficacy has not been established in veterinary patients.	10, 100 mg/mL oral solution and 25, 50, and 100 mg tablets.	2–4 mg/kg q12h PO.
Hydrocortisone (Cortef, and generic)	Glucocorticoid anti-inflammatory drug. Hydrocortisone has weaker anti-inflammatory effects and greater mineralocorticoid effects, compared with prednisolone or dexamethasone (see dexamethasone for other details). Also used for replacement therapy.	Adverse effects are attributed to excessive glucocorticoid effects (see Betamethasone).	Dose requirements are related to severity of disease.	5, 10, 20 mg tablet.	Replacement therapy: 1–2 mg/kg q12h PO. Anti-inflammatory: 2.55 mg/kg q12h PO,
Hydrocortisone sodium succinate (Solu-Cortef)	Same as hydrocortisone, except that this is a rapid-acting injectable product.	Same as hydrocortisone.	Same as hydrocortisone. Prepare vials according to manufacturer.	Various size vials for injection.	Shock: 50–150 mg/kg IV. Anti-inflammatory: 5 mg/kg q12h, IV.
Hydroxyethyl starch (HES) (HES, Hetastarch)	Synthetic colloid volume expander (used in same manner as Dextran). Used primarily to treat acute hypovolemia and shock.	Only limited use in veterinary medicine, therefore adverse effects have not been reported. May cause allergic reactions. Coagulopathies rare at usual doses.	Used in critical care situations. Infused via constant rate infusion. HES appears to be more effective and produce fewer side effects than Dextran. Infuse slowly.	Injection.	10–20 mL/kg IV to effect.
Hydroxyurea (Hydrea)	Antineoplastic agent. Used in combination with other anticancer modalities for treatment of certain tumors. Has been used to treat polycythemia vera.	Only limited use in veterinary medicine. No adverse effects have been reported. In people, hydroxyurea causes leukopenia, anemia, thrombocytopenia.	Limited use in veterinary medicine.	500 mg capsule.	Dog: 50 mg/kg PO once daily, 3 days/week. Cat: 25 mg/kg PO once daily, 3 days/week.
Hydroxyzine (Atarax)	Antihistamine, of the piperazine class. Used primarily to treat pruritus in animals.	Side effects of therapy are related primarily to antihistamine effects. Sedation occurs in some animals.	Clinical studies have shown hydroxyzine to be somewhat effective for treatment of pruritus in dogs.	10, 25, 50 mg tablet; 2 mg/mL oral solution.	Dog: 1–2 mg/kg q6–8h IM, PO. Cat: safe dose not established.
Ibuprofen (Motrin, Advil, Nuprin)	Nonsteroidal anti-inflammatory drug (see Flunixin meglumine).	Safe doses have not been established for dogs and cats. Vomiting and severe gastrointestinal ulceration and hemorrhage have been reported in dogs.	Avoid use, especially in dogs.	200, 400, 600, 800 mg tablet.	Safe dose not established.

Drug Name (Trade or Other Names)	Pharmacology and Indications	Adverse Effects and Precautions	Dosing Information and Comments	Formulations	Dosage
Imipenem (Primaxin)	β-lactam antibiotic with broad-spectrum activity. Action is similar to other β-lactam (see Amoxicillin). Imipenem is the most active of all β-lactams. Used primarily for serious, multiple-resistant infections.	Allergic reactions may occur with β-lactam antibiotics. With rapid infusion, or in patients with renal insufficiency, neurotoxicity may occur (seizures). Vomiting and nausea are possible.	Doses and efficacy studies have not been determined in animals. Recommendations are based on studies performed in humans, and extrapolation from humans. Reserve the use of this drug for only resistant, refractory infections. Observe manufacturer's instructions carefully for proper administration. For IV administration, add to IV fluids. For IM administration, add 2 mL lidocaine (1%); suspension is stable for only 1 hour.	250 or 500 mg vials for injection.	3–10 mg/kg, IV, IM q 6–8h.
Imipramine (Tofranil)	Tricyclic antidepressant drug (TCA). Used in people to treat anxiety and depression. Used in animals to treat variety of behavioral disorders, including obsessive-compulsive disorders. Action is via inhibition of uptake of serotonin at presynaptic nerve terminals.	Multiple side effects are associated with TCAs such as antimuscarinic effects (dry mouth, rapid heart rate), and antihistamine effects (sedation). Overdoses can produce life-threatening cardiotoxicity.	Doses are primarily based on empiricism. There are no controlled efficacy trials available for animals. There may be a 2–4 week delay after initiation of therapy before beneficial effects are seen.	10, 25, 50 mg tablets.	2–4 mg/kg, q12–24h, PO.
Indomethacin (Indocin)	NSAID (see Flunixin meglumine).	Causes severe gastrointestinal ulceration and hemorrhage in dogs. Do not use.	Do not use in dogs.		Safe dose has not been established.
Insulin, regular crystalline	Insulin has multiple effects associated with utilization of glucose. Used to treat diabetes mellitus in dogs and cats.	Adverse effects primarily related to overdoses (hypoglycemia).	Doses should be carefully adjusted in each patient, depending on response. Monitor plasma/serum glucose concentrations. For cats with ketoacidosis, alternative dosing regimen has used 0.2 U/kg IM initially, then 0.1 U/kg IM every hour until glucose level is less than 300, then 0.25–0.4 U/kg SC q6h.	100 U/mL injection.	Ketoacidosis: animals < 3 kg, 1 U/animal initially, then 1 U/animal q1h; animals 3–10 kg, 2 U/animal initially then 1 U/animal q1h; animals > 10 kg, 0.25 U/kg initially, then 0.1 U/kg q1h IM (for cats, see dosing information section).
Insulin, NPH isophane	Same as above.	Same as above.	Same as above.	100 U/mL injection.	Dog < 15 kg: 1 units/kg q24h SC (to effect), dog > 25 kg: 0.5 units/kg q24h SC (to effect). Cat: NPH not recommended for cats.
Interferon (interferon α, HuIFN-α) (Roferon)	Human interferon. Used to stimulate the immune system in patients.	Adverse effects have not been reported in animals.	Doses and indications for animals have primarily been based on extrapolation of human recommendations, or limited experimental studies. (JAVMA 199: 1477, 1991). To prepare, add 3,000,000 units to 1 L sterile saline and divide into aliquots and freeze. Thaw as needed for 30 units/mL solution.	3 million U/vial.	Cat: 15–30 U per cat SC or IM once daily for 7 days and repeated every other week.

Drug Name (Trade or Other Names)	Pharmacology and Indications	Adverse Effects and Precautions	Dosing Information and Comments	Formulations	Dosage
Iodide	See Potassium iodide.				
Ipecac Syrup (Ipecac)	Emetic drug. For emergency treatment of poisoning. Active ingredient is thought to be emetine.	No adverse effects with acute therapy for poisoning. Chronic administration can lead to myocardial toxicity.	Available as non-prescription drug. Onset of vomiting may require 20–30 minutes.	Oral solution. 30 mL bottle.	Dog: 3–6 mL per dog PO. Cat: 2–6 mL per cat PO.
Ipodate	Cholecystographic agent. Used as treatment for hyperthyroidism in cats. Used as alternative to methimizole, radiation therapy, or surgery.	No adverse effects reported.	Use of ipodate has been experimental and precise doses have not been evaluated. In one study, 2/3 of treated cats responded.		Cat: 15 mg/kg q12h, PO.
Iron	See Ferrous sulfate.				
Isoflurane (Aerrane)	Inhalent anesthetic. See Halothane.	See Halothane.	See Halothane.	100 mL bottle.	Induction: 5%, maintenance: 1.5–2.5%.
Isoproterenol (Isuprel)	Adrenergic agonist. Stimulates both β_1- and β_2-adrenergic receptors. Used to stimulate heart (inotropic and chronotropic). Also used to relax bronchial smooth muscle for acute treatment of bronchoconstriction.	Adverse effects related to excessive adrenergic stimulation and is seen primarily as tachycardia and tachyarrhythmias.	Short half-life. Must be infused via constant rate infusion or repeated if administered IM, or SC. Recommended for short-term use only.	Ampules for injection, 0.2 mg/mL.	10 mcg/kg q6h IM, SC; or dilute 1 mg in 500 mL of 5% dextrose or Ringer's solution and infuse IV 0.5–1 mL/min (1–2 mcg/min), or to effect.
Isosorbide dinitrate (Isordil, Isorbid, Sorbitrate)	Nitrate vasodilator. Causes vasodilation via generation of nitric oxide. Relaxes vascular smooth muscle, especially venous. Reduces preload in patients with CHF. In people, it is primarily used to treat angina.	Adverse effects are primarily related to overdoses that produce excess vasodilation and hypotension. Tolerance may develop with repeated doses.	Generally, doses are titrated to individual, depending on response.	2.5, 5, 10, 20,30,40 mg tablets; 40 mg capsules.	2.5–5 mg/animal q12h PO (or 0.22–1.1 mg/kg q12h PO).
Isosorbide mononitrate (Monoket)	Same comments as for isosorbide dinitrate, except that this is a biologically active form of isosorbide dinitrate. Compared to isosorbide dinitrate, it does not undergo first-pass metabolism and is completely absorbed orally.	Same as for isosorbide dinitrate and nitroglycerin.	Generally absorbed better than isosorbide dinitrate.	10, 20 mg tablets.	5 mg/dog two doses per day 7 hours apart PO.
Isotretinoin (Accutane)	Keratinization stabilizing drug. Isotretinoin reduces sebaceous gland size and inhibits sebaceous gland activity, and decreases sebum secretion. In people, it is primarily used to treat acne. In animals, has been used to treat sebaceous adenitis.	Absolutely contraindicated in pregnant animals. Adverse effects not reported for animals, although experimental studies have demonstrated that it can cause focal calcification (such as in myocardium and vessels).	Use in veterinary medicine is confined to limited clinical experience and extrapolation from human reports.	10, 20, 40 mg capsules.	1–3 mg/kg/day (up to a maximum recommended dose of 3–4 mg/kg/day PO.
Itraconazole (Sporanox)	Azole (triazole) antifungal drug. See Ketoconazole for mechanism of action. Active against dermatophytes and systemic fungi, such as Blastomyces, Histoplasma and Coccidioides	Itraconazole is better tolerated than ketoconazole. However, vomiting and hepatotoxicosis are possible, especially at high doses. In one study, hepatotoxicosis was more likely at high doses. 10–15% of dogs will develop high liver enzyme levels. High doses in cats caused vomiting and anorexia.	Doses are based on studies in animals in which itraconazole has been used to treat blastomycosis in dogs. In cats, lower doses have been effective for dermatophytes (see dosing section). Other uses or doses are based on empiricism or extrapolation from human literature.	100 mg capsules and 10 mg/mL oral liquid.	Dog: 2.5 mg/kg q12h, or 5 mg/kg q24h PO. Cat: 5 mg/kg q12h PO. For dermatophyte infection in cats: 1.5–3.0 mg/kg (up to 5 mg/kg) q24h, PO for 15 days.

Drug Name (Trade or Other Names)	Pharmacology and Indications	Adverse Effects and Precautions	Dosing Information and Comments	Formulations	Dosage
Ivermectin (Heartguard, Ivomec, Eqvalan liquid)	Antiparasitic drug. Neurotoxic to parasites by potentiating effects of inhibitory neurotransmitter, GABA.	Toxicity may occur at high doses, and in breeds in which ivermectin crosses blood–brain barrier. Sensitive breeds include: collies, Australian shepherds, shelties, and Old English sheepdogs. Toxicity is neurotoxic and signs include: depression, ataxia, difficulty with vision, coma, and death. Ivermectin appears to be safe for pregnant animals. Do not administer to animals under 6 weeks of age. Animals with high microfilaremia may show adverse reactions to high doses.	Doses vary, depending on use. Heartworm prevention is lowest dose, other parasites require higher doses. Heartguard is only form approved for small animals, for other indications, large animal injectable products are often administered orally, IM, or SC to small animals. For demodex therapy. it is advised to start with 100 mcg/kg/day and increase dose by 100 mcg/kg/day to 600 mcg/kg/day (Compendium 20: 459–469, 1998).	1% (10 mg/mL) injectable solution, 10 mg/mL oral solution, 18.7 mg/mL oral paste, 68, 136, and 272 mcg tablets.	Heartworm preventative: 6 mcg/kg q30day PO in dogs and 24 mcg/kg q30d PO in cats. Microfilaricide: 50 mcg/kg PO 2 wks after adulticide therapy. Ectoparasite therapy (dogs and cats): 200–300 mcg/kg IM, SC, PO. Endoparasites (dogs and cats): 200–400 mcg/kg weekly SC, PO. Demodex day for therapy: 600 mcg/kg/60–120 days, PO.
Kanamycin (Kantrim)	Aminoglycoside antibiotic. See Gentamicin, Amikacin for details.	Shares same properties with other aminoglycosides (see Amikacin, Gentamicin).	See Gentamicin.	200,500 mg/mL injection.	10 mg/kg q6–8h IV IM, SC.
Kaopectate (kaolin + pectin) (Kao-Pectate)	Antidiarrheal compound. Kaolin may act as adsorbent for endotoxins and pectin may protect intestinal mucosa.	Side effects are uncommon.	Efficacy has not been established for treatment of diarrhea in animals.	Oral suspension 12 oz.	1–2 mL/kg q2–6h PO
Ketamine (Ketalar, Ketavet, Vetalar)	Anesthetic agent. Exact mechanism of action is not known, but appears to act as dissociative agent. Ketamine has little analgesic activity. Rapidly metabolized and eliminated in most animals.	Causes pain with IM injection. Tremors, spasticity, and convulsive seizures have been reported. Increases cardiac output compared to other anesthetic agents. Do not use in animals with head injury, because it may elevate CSF pressure.	Often used in combination with other anesthetics and anesthetic adjuncts, such as xylazine, acepromazine, or diazepam. IV doses generally less than IM doses.	100 mg/mL injection solution.	Dog:5.5–22 mg/kg, IV, IM (recommend adjunctive sedative or tranquilizer treatment). Cat: 2–25 mg/kg IV, IM (recommend adjunctive sedative or tranquilizer treatment).
Ketoconazole (Nizoral)	Azole (imidazole) antifungal drug. Similar mechanism of action as other azole antifungal agents. Inhibits ergosterol synthesis in fungal cell membrane. Fungistatic. Efficacious against dermatophytes, and variety of systemic fungi, such as Histoplasma, Blastomyces, and Coccidioides.	Adverse effects in animals include: dose-related vomiting, diarrhea, and hepatic injury. Enzyme elevations are common. Do not administer to pregnant animals. Ketoconazole causes endocrine abnormalities, most specifically, inhibition of cortisol synthesis. Drug interactions: Ketoconazole will inhibit metabolism of other drugs (anticonvulsants, cyclosporine, cisapride).	Oral absorption depends on acidity in stomach. Do not administer with antisecretory drugs or antacids. Because of endocrine effects, ketoconazole has been used for short-term treatment of hyperadrenocorticism.	200 mg tablets; 100 mg/mL oral suspension (only available in Canada).	dog: 10–15 mg/kg q8–12h PO. For Malassezia canis infection: 5 mg/kg q24h PO. For hyperadrenocorticism: 15 mg/kg q12h PO. Cat: 5–10 mg/kg q8–12h PO.

Drug Name (Trade or Other Names)	Pharmacology and Indications	Adverse Effects and Precautions	Dosing Information and Comments	Formulations	Dosage
Ketoprofen (Orudis-KT [human OTC tablet]; Ketofen [veterinary injection])	Nonsteroidal anti-inflammatory drug. (See Flunixin meglumine).	All NSAIDs share similar adverse effect of gastrointestinal toxicity. (See Flunixin). Ketoprofen has been administered for 5 consecutive days in dogs, without serious adverse effects. Most common side effect is vomiting. GI ulceration is possible in some animals.	Although not approved in the U.S., ketoprofen is approved for small animals in other countries. Doses listed are based on approved use in those countries. It is available as OTC drug for humans in the U.S.	12.5 mg tablet (OTC), 25, 50, 75 mg Rx ` human form and 100 mg/mL injection for horses.	Dogs and cats: 1 mg/kg q24h PO for up to 5 days. Initial dose can be given via injection at up to 2 mg/kg SC, IM, IV.
Ketorolac trometha-mine (Toradol)	Nonsteroidal anti-inflammatory drug (NSAID). Used for short-term relief of pain and inflammation. Acts by inhibiting cyclooxy-genase enzyme (COX). Use of ketorolac has been evaluated clinic-ally in dogs, but not cats.	NSAIDs may cause gastrointestinal ulcera-tion. Ketorolac may cause gastrointestinal lesions if administered more frequently than every 8 hr. Do not administer more than 2 doses.	Available as 10 mg tablet and injection for IV or IM use. Clinical studies in dogs have shown safety and efficacy. Dosing every 12 hr is recommended to avoid gastrointestinal problems.	10 mg tablets; 15 and 30 mg/mL injection, in 10% alcohol.	Dogs: 0.5 mg/kg, q8–12h PO, IM, IV.
L-Dopa	See Levodopa.				
Lactated Ringer's Solution (many)	Fluid solution for replacement. IV admin-istration.	Administer IV fluids only in carefully monitored patients.	Fluid requirements vary depending on animal's needs (replacement vs maintenance). Consult fluid therapy reference for optimum rate. Rate listed here is for main-tenance and shock.	250, 500, 1000 mL bags.	Maintenance: 40–50 mL/kg/day IV. For shock therapy: dog: 90 mL/kg IV; cat: 60–70 mL/kg IV.
Lactulose (Chronulac, generic)	Laxative. Produces laxative effect by os-motic effect in colon. Lactulose also has been used for treatment of hyper-ammonemia (hepatic encephalopathy), because it decreases blood ammonia con-centrations via lowering pH of colon, thus ammonia in colon is not as readily absorbed.	Excessive use may cause fluid and electro-lyte loss.	In veterinary medicine, clinical studies to establish efficacy are not available. In addition to doses cited, 20–30 mL/kg of 30% solution retention enema has been used in cats.	10 gm/15 mL.	Constipation: 1 mL/4.5 kg q8h (to effect) PO. Hepatic encephalopathy Dog: 0.5 mL/kg q8h PO; hepatic encephalopathy; (cat): 2.5–5 mL/cat q8h PO.
Leucovorin (Folinic acid) (Wellcovorin, and generic)	Leucovorin is a re-duced form of folic acid, which is converted to active folic acid deriva-tives for purine and thymidine synthesis. It is used as antidote for folic acid antagonists.	Allergic reactions have been reported in people.	Used primarily as rescue for overdoses of folic acid antagonists (methotrexate). Clinical studies have not been reported in veterinary medicine. It is not established whether leucovorin will prevent toxicity from trimeth-oprim–sulfonamide administration.	5, 10, 15, 25 mg tablets; 3 or 5 mg/mL injection.	With methotrexate administra-tion: 3 mg/m² IV IM PO. As antidote for pyrimethamine toxicosis: 1 mg/kg q24h PO.
Levamisole (Levasole, Tramisol, Ergamisol)	Antiparasitic drug of the imidazothiazole class. Mechanism of action due to neuromuscular toxicity to parasites. Levamisole has been used for endoparasites in dogs and as micro-filaricide. In people, levamisole is used as immunostimulant to aid in treatment of colo-rectal carcinoma and malignant melanoma.	May produce choliner-gic toxicity. May cause vomiting in some dogs.	In heartworm-positive dogs, it may sterilize female adult heart-worms. Levamisole has also been used as an immunostimulant, how-ever, clinical reports of its efficacy are not available.	0.184 gm bolus; 11.7 gm per 13 gm packet; 50 mg tablet (Ergami-sol).	Dogs (hookworms): 5–8 mg/kg once PO (up to 10 mg/kg PO for 2 days). Microfilaricide: 10 mg/kg PO for 6–10 days. Immunostimulant: 0.5–2 mg/kg 3 times/week PO . Cats:4.4 mg/kg once PO; (for lungworms: 20–40 mg/kg q48h for 5 treatments PO)

Drug Name (Trade or Other Names)	Pharmacology and Indications	Adverse Effects and Precautions	Dosing Information and Comments	Formulations	Dosage
Levodopa (l-dopa) (Larodopa, L-dopa)	Converted to dopamine after crossing blood–brain barrier. Stimulates CNS dopamine receptors. In people, used for treating Parkinson's disease. In animals, has been used for treating hepatic encephalopathy.	Adverse effects in animals have not been reported. In people, dizziness, mental changes, difficult urination, and hypotension are among the reported adverse effects.	Clinical studies have not been reported in veterinary medicine. Titrate dose for each patient.	100, 250, 500 mg tablets or capsules.	Hepatic encephalopathy: 6.8 mg/kg initially, then 1.4 mg/kg q6h.
Levothyroxine sodium (Soloxine, Thyro-Tabs, Synthroid)	Replacement therapy for treating patients with hypothyroidism. Levothyroxine is T-4, which is converted in most patients to the active T-3.	High doses may produce thyrotoxicosis, which is uncommon (compared to people). *Drug interactions:* Patients receiving corticosteroids may have decreased ability to convert T-4 to T-3.	Thyroid supplementation should be guided by testing to confirm diagnosis and post-medication monitoring to adjust dose.	0.1–0.8 mg tablets (in 0.1 mg increments).	Dog: 22 mcg/kg q12h PO (adjust dose via monitoring). Cat: 10–20 mcg/kg/day PO (adjust dose via monitoring).
Lidocaine (Xylocaine, and generic brands)	Local anesthetic. (See Bupivicaine for mechanism of action.) Lidocaine is also used commonly for acute treatment of cardiac arrhythmias. Class-1 antiarrhythmic. Decreases Phase 0 depolarization without affecting conduction. Not useful for supraventricular arrhythmias.	High doses cause CNS effects (tremors, twitches, and seizures). Lidocaine can produce cardiac arrhythmias, but has greater effect on abnormal cardiac tissue than normal tissue. Cats are more susceptible to adverse effects, and lower doses should be used.	When used for local infiltration, many formulations contain epinephrine to prolong activity at injection site. Avoid epinephrine in patients with cardiac arrhythmias. Note that human formulations may contain epinephrine, but no veterinary formulations contain epinephrine. To increase pH, increase onset of action, and decrease pain from injection, one may add 1 mEq sodium bicarbonate to 10 mL lidocaine (use immediately after mixing).	5, 10, 15, 20 mg/mL injection.	Dog (antiarrhythmic): 2–4 mg/kg IV (to a maximum dose of 8 mg/kg over 10 minute period); 25–75 mcg/kg/min IV infusion; 6 mg/kg q1.5h IM. Cat (antiarrhythmic): 0.25–0.75mg/kg IV slowly, or 10–40 mcg/kg/min infusion. For epidural (dog and cat): 4.4 mg/kg of 2% solution.
Lincomycin (Lincocin)	Lincosamide antibiotic, similar in mechanism to clindamycin and erythromycin. Spectrum includes primarily Gram-positive bacteria. Used for pyoderma and other soft-tissue infections.	Adverse effects uncommon. Lincomycin has caused vomiting and diarrhea in animals. Do *not* administer orally to rodents and rabbits.	Action of lincomycin and clindamycin are similar enough that clindamycin can be substituted for lincomycin.	100, 200, 500 mg tablets.	15–25 mg/kg q12h PO. For pyoderma, doses as low as 10 mg/kg q12h have been used.
Liothyronine (Cytomel)	Thyroid supplement. Liothyronine is equivalent to T-3.	Adverse effects have not been reported (see Levothyroxine).	See Levothyroxine. Doses of liothyronine should be adjusted on the basis of monitoring T-3 concentrations in patients.	60 mcg tablet.	4.4 mcg/kg q8h PO. For T-3 suppression test in cats: collect presample for T-4 and T-3, administer 25 mcg q8h for 7 doses, then collect post samples for T-3 and T-4, after last dose.
Lisinopril (Prinivil, Zestril)	ACE-inhibitor. See Captopril for details. Used for treatment of CHF and hypertension.	See Captopril for details. Lisinopril has not been used extensively in animals to document adverse effects. Lisinopril appears to be better tolerated than captopril.	Clinical studies using lisinopril in animals have not been reported. See comments for Captopril and Enalapril. With all ACE-inhibitors, monitor electrolytes and renal function 3–7 days after initiating therapy and periodically thereafter.	2.5, 5, 10, 20, 40 mg tablets.	Dogs: 0.5 mg/kg q24h PO. Cats: no dose established.

Drug Name (Trade or Other Names)	Pharmacology and Indications	Adverse Effects and Precautions	Dosing Information and Comments	Formulations	Dosage
Lithium carbonate (Lithotabs)	Stimulates granulo-poiesis, and elevates neutrophil pool in animals. In people, it is used for treatment of depression. CNS effect is related to decreased concentrations of neurotransmitters.	Adverse effects have not been reported in animals. In people, cardiovascular problems, drowsiness, and diarrhea are among the adverse effects.	Use in animals is not common. It has been used experimentally to increase neutrophils following cancer therapy.	150, 300, 600 mg capsules, 300 mg tablets; 300 mg/5 mL syrup.	Dog: 10 mg/kg q12h PO. Cat: not recommended.
Lomotil	See Diphenoxylate.				
Loperamide (Imodium and generic)	Opiate agonist. Stimulates smooth muscle segmentation in intestine, as well as electrolyte absorption. Used for acute treatment of nonspecific diarrhea.	Diphenoxylate is poorly absorbed systemically and produces few systemic side effects. However, toxicity has been observed in dogs, even at recommended doses. Small dogs and collie-type dogs may be at higher risk. In any animal, excessive use can cause constipation.	Doses are based primarily on empiricism or extrapolation of human dose. Clinical studies have not been performed in animals.	2 mg tablet, 0.2 mg/mL oral liquid.	Dog: 0.1 mg/kg q8–12h PO. Cat: 0.08–0.16 mg/kg q12h PO.
Lufenuron (Program)	Antiparasitic. Used for controlling fleas in animals. Inhibits development in hatching fleas.	Adverse effects have not been reported. Appears to be relatively safe during pregnancy and in young animals.	Lufenuron may control flea development with administration once every 30 days in animals.	45, 90, 135, 204.9, 409.8 mg tablets; 135, and 270 mg suspension per unit pack.	Dogs: 10 mg/kg PO, q30days. Cats: 30 mg/kg PO, q30 days. Cat injection: 10 mg/kg SC every 6 mos.
Lufenuron + milbemycinoxime (Sentinel tablets and Flavor Tabs)	Combination of two antiparasitic drugs. See Lufenuron or Milbemycin. Used to protect against fleas, heartworms, roundworms, hookworms, and whipworms.	See Lufenuron or Milbemycin.	See Lufenuron or Milbemycin.	Milbemycin/lufenuron ratio is as follows: 2.3/46 mg tablets; 5.75/115, 11.5/230, and 23/460 mg Flavor Tabs.	Administer one tablet, q30d. Each tablet formulated for size of dog.
Luteinizing hormone	See Gonadorelin.				
Magnesium citrate (Citroma, Citro-Nesia [Citro-Mag in Canada])	Saline cathartic. Acts to draw water into small intestine vial osmotic effect. Fluid accumulation produces distention, which promotes bowel evacuation. Used for constipation and bowel evacuation prior to certain procedures.	Adverse effects have not been reported in animals. However, fluid and electrolyte loss can occur with overuse. Magnesium accumulation may occur in patients with renal impairment. *Drug interactions:* Magnesium-containing cathartics decrease oral absorption of ciprofloxacin and other fluoroquinolones.	Commonly used to evacuate bowel prior to surgery or diagnostic procedures. Onset of action is rapid.	Oral solution.	2–4 mL/kg PO.
Magnesium hydroxide (Milk of Magnesia)	Same as Magnesium citrate. Magnesium hydroxide also is used as oral antacid to neutralize stomach acid.	Same as Magnesium citrate.	See Magnesium citrate.	Oral liquid.	Antacid: 5–10 mL/kg q4–6h PO. Cathartic (dog): 15–50 mL/kg PO. Cathartic (cat): 2–6 mL/cat q24h PO.
Magnesium sulfate (Epsom salts)	Same as Magnesium citrate.	See Magnesium citrate.	See Magnesium citrate.	Crystals. Many generic preparations.	Dog: 8–25 gm/dog q24h PO. Cat: 2–5 gm/cat q24h PO.
Mannitol (Osmitrol)	Hyperosmotic diuretic. Increases plasma osmolality, which draws fluid from tissues to plasma. Antiglaucoma agent. Used for treatment of edema and reducing intraocular pressure. Mannitol also has been used to promote urinary excretion of certain toxins.	Causes fluid and electrolyte imbalance. Do not use in dehydrated patients. Use cautiously when intracranial bleeding is suspected, because it may increase bleeding. Administration that is too rapid may expand the extracellular volume excessively.	Use only in patients in which fluid and electrolyte balance can be monitored. Once solutions are prepared, discard unused portions.	5–25% solution for injection.	Diuretic: 1 gm/kg of 5–25% solution IV to maintain urine flow. Glaucoma or CNS edema: 0.25–2 gm/kg of 15–25% solution over 30–60 min IV (repeat in 6 hr, if necessary).

Drug Name (Trade or Other Names)	Pharmacology and Indications	Adverse Effects and Precautions	Dosing Information and Comments	Formulations	Dosage
Marbofloxacin (Zeniquin)	Fluoroquinolone antimicrobial. Same mechanism as enrofloxacin and ciprofloxacin. Spectrum includes staphylococci, Gram-negative bacilli, and some Pseudomonas.	Same precautions as enrofloxacin. May cause some nausea and vomiting at high doses. Avoid use in young animals.	Same dosing guidelines as for other fluoroquinolones. Higher doses are needed for organisms with higher MIC values. Safety data not available for cats. Doses published for European use may be lower than U.S. approved dogs.	25, 50, 100 and 200 mg tablets.	Dog: 2.75–5.55 mg/kg, PO.
MCT oil (MCT oil [many sources])	Medium chain triglycerides. Used to treat hepatic encephalopathy.	Adverse effects not reported in veterinary medicine. May cause diarrhea in some patients.	Results of clinical trials using MCT oil have not been reported. Many enteral feeding formulas contain MCT oil (many polymeric formulations).	Oral liquid.	1–2 mL/kg daily in food.
Mebendazole (Telmintic)	Benzimidazole antiparasitic drug. (See Albendazole).	Adverse effects are rare. Occasional vomiting and diarrrhea in dogs. Some reports suggest idiosyncratic hepatic reactions in dogs.	Dose recommendations based upon clinical studies performed by manufacturer.	Each gram of powder contains 40 mg.	22 mg/kg (with food) q24h for 3 days.
Meclizine (Antivert, generic)	Antiemetic and antihistamine. Used for treatment of motion sickness. Action may be caused by central anticholinergic actions. Also may suppress chemoreceptor trigger zone (CRTZ).	Adverse effects have not been reported in animals. Anticholinergic (atropine-like) effects may cause side effects.	Results of clinical studies in animals have not been reported. Use in animals is based on experience in people, or anecdotal experiences in animals.	12.5, 25, 50 mg tablets.	Dog: 25 mg q24h PO (for motion sickness, administer 1 hr prior to travelling). Cat: 12.5 mg q24h PO.
Meclofenamic acid (meclofenamate sodium) (Arquel, Meclofen)	NAID. Used for treatment of arthritis and other inflammatory disorders. (See Flunixin.)	Adverse effects have not been reported in animals, but adverse effects common to other NSAIDs are possible. (See Flunixin).	Results of clinical studies in animals have not been reported. Use in animals is based on experience in people, or anecdotal experiences in animals. Administer with food.	50, 100 mg capsules.	Dog: 1 mg/kg/day for up to 5 days, PO.
Medetomidine (Domitor)	α_2-adrenergic agonist (see Xylazine). Used primarily as sedative, anesthetic adjunct, and analgesia.	α_2-agonists decrease sympathetic output. Cardiovascular depression may occur. Medetomidine will cause an initial bradycardia and hypertension.	May be used for sedation, analgesia, and minor surgical procedures. Should be reversed with equal volume of atipamezole.	1.0 mg/mL injection.	750 mcg/m^2 IV or 1000 mcg/m^2 IM.
Medium chain triglycerides	See MCT oil.				
Medroxyprogesterone acetate (Depo-Provera [injection]; Provera [tablets])	Progestin hormone. Derivative of acetoxyprogesterone. In animals, used as progesterone hormone treatment to control estrous cycle. Also used for management of some behavioral and dermatologic disorders (such as urine spraying in cats and alopecia).	Adverse effects include polyphagia, polydipsia, adrenal suppression (cats), increases risk of diabetes, pyometra, diarrhea, and increases risk of neoplasia.	Clinical studies in animals have studied primarily the reproductive use and effects on behavioral use. Medroxyprogersteone acetate may have fewer side effects than megestrol acetate.	150, 400 mg/mL suspension injection; 2.5, 5, 10 mg tablets.	1.1–2.2 mg/kg q7d IM. For behavioral use 10–20 mg/kg are injected SC. For prostatic disease in dogs, use 3–5 mg/kg IM, SC.

Drug Name (Trade or Other Names)	Pharmacology and Indications	Adverse Effects and Precautions	Dosing Information and Comments	Formulations	Dosage
Megestrol acetate (Ovaban)	See Medroxyprogesterone.	See Medroxyprogesterone.	See Medroxyprogesterone.	5 mg tablets.	Dogs: proestrus: 2 mg/kg q24h PO for 8 days anestrus: 0.5 mg/kg q24h PO for 30 days; behavior: 2–4 mg/kg q24h for 8 days (reduce dose for maintenance). Cats: (dermatologic therapy or urine spraying): 2.5–5 mg/cat q24h PO for one week, then reduce to 5 mg once or twice/week; suppress estrus: 5 mg/cat/day for 3 days, then, 2.5–5 mg once/week for 10 weeks.
Melarsomine (Immiticide)	Organic arsenical compound used for heartworm therapy. Heartworm adulticide. Arsenicals alter glucose uptake and metabolism in heartworms.	Adverse effects: Pulmonary thrombo-embolism (7–20 days after therapy). Anorexia (13% incidence), injection site reaction (myositis) (32% incidence), lethargy or depression (15% incidence). Causes elevations of hepatic enzymes. High doses (3×) can cause pulmonary inflammation and death. If high doses are administered, dimercaprol (3 mg/kg IM) may be used as antidote.	Dose regimens are based on severity of heartworm disease. Consult current reference to determine class of disease (Class 1–4). Class 1 and 2 are least severe. Class 4 is most severe, and should not be treated with adulticide before surgery. Avoid human exposure. (Wash hands after handling, or wear gloves.) Do not freeze solutions after they are prepared.	25 mg/mL injection. After reconstitution, retains potency for 24 hrs.	Administer via deep IM injection. Class 1–2 dogs: 2.5 mg/kg/day for two consecutive days. Class 3 dogs: 2.5 mg/kg once, then, in 1 mo two additional doses 24 hrs apart.
Melphalan (Alkeran)	Anticancer agent. Alkylating agent, similar in action to cyclophosphamide.	Adverse effects related to its action as an anti-cancer agent. Causes myelosuppression.	Used to treat multiple myeloma and certain carcinomas.	2 mg tablets.	1.5 mg/m² (or 0.1–0.2 mg/kg) q24h PO for 7–10 days (repeat every 3 weeks).
Meperidine (Demerol)	Synthetic opioid agonist with activity primarily at the μ-opiate receptor. Similar in action to morphine, except with approximately 1/7 of the potency. 75 mg meperidine (IM) or 300 mg (oral) has similar potency as 10 mg morphine.	Side effects similar to other opiates. See Morphine.	Although comparative clinical studies have not been conducted in animals, meperidine is considered an effective analgesic in dogs and cats, but with short duration.	50, 100 mg tablets; 10 mg/mL syrup; 25, 50, 75, 100 mg/mL injection.	Dog: 5–10 mg/kg IV, IM as often as every 2–3 hrs (or as needed). Cat: 3–5 mg/kg IV, IM every 2–4 hrs (or as needed).
Mepivacaine (Carbocaine-V)	Local anesthetic of the amide class (see Bupivacaine). Medium potency and duration of action, compared to bupivacaine. Compared to lidocaine, longer-acting, but equal potency.	See Bupivacaine. Mepivacaine may cause less irritation to tissues than lidocaine.	See Bupivacaine. For epidural use, do not exceed 8 mg/kg total dose. Duration of epidural is 2.5–3 hrs.	2% (20 mg/mL) injection.	Variable dose for local infiltration. For epidural, 0.5 mL of 2% solution q30sec until reflexes are absent.
6-Mercaptopurine (Purinethol)	Anticancer agent. Anti-metabolite agent that inhibits synthesis of purines in cancer cells.	Many side effects are possible that are common to anticancer therapy (many of which are unavoidable), including bone marrow suppression and anemia.	Used for various forms of cancer, including leukemia and lymphoma. Consult specific anticancer protocol for specific regimen.	50 mg tablets.	50 mg/m² q24h PO.
Meropenem (Merrem)	Carbapenem β-lactam antibiotic similar to imipenem in activity.	Similar risks as other β-lactam antibiotics. Meropenem does not cause seizures as much as imipenem.	Dosing guidelines have been extrapolated from human use, and not tested for efficacy in animals. Meropenem is more soluble than imipenem, and can be injected via bolus.	500 mg in 20 mL vial, or 1 gm vial in 30 mL vial for injection.	20 mg/kg q8h IV; for meningitis 40 mg/kg q8h IV.

Drug Name (Trade or Other Names)	Pharmacology and Indications	Adverse Effects and Precautions	Dosing Information and Comments	Formulations	Dosage
Mesalamine (Asacol, Mesasal, Pentasa)	5-aminosalicylic acid. Used as treatment for colitis. Action is not precisely known, but suppresses inflammation in colon. Component of sulfasalazine.	See Sulfasalazine. Mesalamine alone has not been associated with side effects in animals.	Mesalamine use has not been reported in animals from clinical trials; however, it has been used as a substitute for sulfasalazine in animals that cannot tolerate sulfonamides.	400 mg tablets, 250 mg capsules.	Veterinary dose has not been established. The usual human dose is 400–500 mg q6–8h (also see Sulfasalazine, Olsalazine).
Metamucil	Bulk-forming laxative containing psyllium. See Psyllium for details.				
Metaproterenol (Alupent, Metaprel)	β-adrenergic agonist. β₂-specific. Used primarily for bronchodilation. See Albuterol for further details.	Adverse effects related to excessive β-adrenergic stimulation. See Albuterol.	Results of clinical studies in animals have not been reported. Use in animals (and doses) is based on experience in people, or anecdotal experience in animals. β₂-agonists also have been used in people to delay labor (inhibit uterine contractions).	10, 20 mg tablets; 5 mg/mL syrup; and inhalers.	0.325–0.65 mg/kg q4–6h PO.
Methazolamide (Neptazane)	Carbonic anhydrase inhibitor. Produces less diuresis than others (see Dichlorphenamide and Acetazolamide).	Use cautiously in patients sensitive to sulfonamides. (See Acetazolamide, Dichlorphenamide).	Used to treat glaucoma in patients. May be used with other glaucoma agents. (See Acetazolamide, Dichlorphenamide.)	25, 50 mg tablets.	2–4 mg/kg (to a maximum dose of 4–6 mg/kg) q8–12h PO.
Methenamine hippurate (Hiprex, Urex)	Urinary antiseptic. Converted to formaldehyde in acidic urine to produce antibacterial/antifungal effect. Active against a wide range of bacteria. Resistance does not develop. Less effective against Proteus, which produces an alkaline urine pH. Not effective for systemic infections.	Although formaldehyde formation in bladder may be irritating, in people, high doses were required (>8 gm/day). In animals, no adverse effects have been reported.	Results of clinical studies in animals have not been reported. Use in animals is based on experience in people, or anecdotal experience in animals. Urine must be acidic for methenamine to convert to formaldehyde (monitor pH periodically). pH below 5.5 is optimal. Supplement with ascorbic acid or ammonium chloride to lower pH.	1 gm tablets.	Dog: 500 mg/dog q12h PO. Cat: 250 mg/cat q12h PO.
Methenamine mandelate (Mandelamine, and generic)	Urinary antiseptic. (See Methenamine hippurate.)	See Methenamine hippurate.	See Methenamine hippurate.	1 gm tablets; granules for oral solution; 50 and 100 mg/mL oral suspension.	10–20 mg/kg q8–12h PO.
Methimazole (Tapazole)	Antithyroid drug. Used for treating hyperthyroidism, primarily in cats. Action is to serve as substrate for thyroid peroxidase and decrease incorporation of iodide into throsine molecules.	In people, it has caused agranulocytosis and leukopenia. In cats, lupus-like reactions are possible, such as vasculitis and bone marrow changes. Well-tolerated in dogs.	Use in cats is based on experimental studies in hyperthyroid cats. Methimazole has, for the most part, replaced propylthiouracil for use in cats. Adjust maintenance dose by monitoring T4 levels.	5 and 10 mg tablets.	Cat: 2.5 mg per cat q12h PO × 7–14 days, then 5–10 mg per cat PO q12h, and monitor T4 concentrations.
dl-Methionine	See Racemethionine.				
Methocarbamol (Robaxin-V)	Skeletal muscle relaxant. Depresses polysynaptic reflexes. Used for treatment of skeletal muscle spasms.	Causes some depression and sedation of the CNS.	Results of clinical studies in animals have not been reported. Use in animals (and doses) is based on experience in people, or anecdotal experience in animals.	500, 750 mg tablets; 100 mg/mL injection.	44 mg/kg q8h PO on the first day, then 22–44 mg/kg, q8h PO.
Methohexital (Brevital)	Barbiturate anesthetic. See Thiopental for details. Methohexital is about 2–3 × more potent than pentothal, but with shorter duration.	See Thiopental.	See Thiopental.	0.5-, 2.5-, and 5-gm vials for injection.	3–6 mg/kg IV (give slowly to effect).

Drug Name (Trade or Other Names)	Pharmacology and Indications	Adverse Effects and Precautions	Dosing Information and Comments	Formulations	Dosage
Methotrexate (MTX, Mexate, Folex, Rheumatrex, and generic)	Anticancer agent. Used for various carcinomas, leukemia, and lymphomas. Action is via antimetabolite action. Analogue of folic acid that binds dihydrofolate reductase. Inhibits DNA, RNA, and protein synthesis. In people, methotrexate is also commonly used for autoimmune diseases such as rheumatoid arthritis.	Anticancer drugs cause predictable (and sometimes unavoidable) side effects that include bone marrow suppression, leukopenia, and immunosuppression. Hepatotoxicity has been reported in people from methotrexate therapy. *Drug interactions:* Concurrent use with NSAIDs may cause severe methotrexate toxicity. Do not administer with pyrimethamine, trimethoprim, or sulfonamides.	Use in animals has been based on experimental studies. There is only limited clinical information available. Consult specific anticancer protocols for precise dosage and regimen.	2.5 mg tablets; 2.5 or 25 mg/mL injection.	2.5–5 mg/m² q48h PO (dose depends on specific protocol). Dogs: 0.3–0.5 mg/kg once/week IV. Cats: 0.8 mg/kg IV every 2–3 weeks.
Methoxamine (Vasoxyl)	Adrenergic agonist. Sympathomimetic. α_1-adrenergic agonist. Specific for α_1-receptors.	Adverse effects related to excessive stimulation of α_1-receptor (prolonged peripheral vasoconstriction). Reflex bradycardia may occur.	Used primarily in critical care patients or during anesthesia to increase peripheral resistance and increase blood pressure. Short onset and duration of action.	20 mg/mL injection.	200–250 mcg/kg IM, or 40–80 mcg/kg IV.
Methoxyflurane (Metofane)	Inhalent anesthetic. See Halothane.	See Halothane. Methoxyflurane has been reported to cause hepatic injury in animals. *Drug Interactions:* Labeling recommendations in some countries state that flunixin should not be administered to animals receiving methoxyflurane anesthesia.	See Halothane.	4 oz bottle for inhalation.	Induction: 3%. Maintenance: 0.5–1.5%.
Methylene blue 0.1% (generic, also called New Methylene Blue)	Antidote for intoxication. Used to treat for methemoglobinemia. Methylene blue acts as reducing agent to reduce methemoglobin to hemoglobin.	Methylene blue can cause Heinz body anemia in cats, but is safe when used at therapeutic doses listed here.	Comparison of effects for intoxication has only been performed in experimental studies. One study demonstrated that acetylcysteine produced the best response, methylene blue also was helpful in some cats. (AJVR 56: 1529, 1995)	1% solution (10 mg/mL)	1.5 mg/kg IV, slowly.
Methylprednisolone (Medrol)	Glucocorticoid anti-inflammatory drug. (See Betamethasone). See also Prednisolone. Compared to prednisolone, methylprednisolone is 1.25 × more potent.	Same as for other glucocorticoids (see Betamethasone). Manufacturer suggests that methylprednisolone causes less PU/PD than prednisolone.	Use of methylprednisolone is similar to other corticosteroids. Dose adjustment should be made to account for difference in potency. (See dose section.)	1, 2, 4, 8, 18, 32 mg tablets.	0.22–0.44 mg/kg, q12–24h, PO. Compared to prednisolone, methylprednisolone is 1.25 × more potent.
Methylprednisolone acetate (Depo-Medrol)	Depot form of methylprednisolone. Slowly absorbed from IM injection site, producing glucocorticoid effects for 3–4 weeks in some animals. Used for intralesional therapy, intra-articular therapy, and for inflammatory conditons.	Many adverse effects possible from use of corticosteroids (see Betamethasone).	Use of methylprednisolone acetate should be evaluated carefully because one injection will cause glucocorticoid effects that persist for several days to weeks.	20 or 40 mg/mL suspension for injection.	Dog: 1 mg/kg (or 20–40 mg/dog) IM q1–3weeks. Cat: 10–20 mg/cat IM q1–3 weeks.

Drug Name (Trade or Other Names)	Pharmacology and Indications	Adverse Effects and Precautions	Dosing Information and Comments	Formulations	Dosage
Methylprednisolone sodium succinate (Solu-Medrol)	Same as methyl-prednisolone, except that this is a water-soluble formulation intended for acute therapy when high IV doses are needed for rapid effect. Used for treatment of shock and CNS trauma.	Adverse effects are not expected from single administration; however, with repeated use, other side effects are possible (see Betametha-sone).	Results of clinical studies in animals have not been reported. Use in animals (and doses) is based on experience in people, or anecdotal experience in animals.	1 and 2 gm and 125 and 500 mg vials for injection.	For emergency use: 30 mg/kg IV and repeat at 15 mg/kg in 2–6 hr, IV. For replacement or anti-inflammatory therapy, see Prednisolone.
4-Methylpyrazole (Fomepizole) (Antizol-Vet [Fomepizole])	Antidote for ethylene glycol (antifreeze) intoxication. Inhibits dehydrogenase enzyme that converts ethylene glycol to toxic metabolite. Should be used early for maxi-mum success.	Methylpyrazole was safe and effective in dogs in clinical trials, if used within 8 hours of poisoning.	Used for emergency management of ethyl-ene glycol intoxication. Experimental studies have demonstrated effectiveness in dogs, but, in cats, ethanol is more effective. (JAVMA 209:1880, 1996). Admix 0.9% sodium chloride before administration.	5% solution in a 1.5-mL vial.	20 mg/kg initially, IV, then 15 mg/kg at 12 and 24 hr intervals, then 5 mg at 36 hrs.
Methyltestosterone (Android, generic)	Anabolic androgenic agent. Used for ana-bolic actions or testos-terone hormone replacement therapy (androgenic deficiency). Testosterone has been used to stimulate erythropoiesis.	Adverse effects caused by excessive androgenic action of testosterone. Prostatic hyperplasia is possible in male dogs. Masculinization can occur in female dogs. Hepatopathy is more common with oral methylated testerone formulations.	See also Testosterone cypionate, Testosterone propionate. Use of testosterone androgens has not been evaluated clinical studies in veter-inary medicine. Use is based primarily on experimental evidence or experiences in people.	10, 25 mg tablets.	Dog: 5–25 mg/dog q24–48h PO. Cat: 2.5–5 mg/cat q24–48h PO.
Metoclopramide (Reglan, Maxolon)	Prokinetic drug. Anti-emetic. Stimulates motility of upper gastro-intestinal tract and centrally acting anti-emetic. Action is to inhibit dopamine recep-tors and enhance action of acetylcholine in gastrointestinal tract. Used primarily for gastroparesis and treatment of vomiting. It is not effective for dogs with gastric dilation.	Adverse effects are primarily related to blockade of central dopaminergic receptors. Adverse effects similar to what is reported for phenothiazines (e.g., acepromazine) have been reported, in addi-tion to behavioral changes. Do not use in epileptic patients, or with diseases caused by gastrointestinal obstruction.	Results of clinical studies in animals have not been reported. Use in animals (and doses) is based on experience in people, or anecdotal experience in animals. Most use is for general antiemetic purposes, but doses as high as 2 mg/kg have been used to prevent vomit-ing during cancer chemotherapy.	10, 5 mg tablet; 1 mg/ mL oral solution; 5 mg/ mL injection.	0.2–0.5 mg/kg q6–8h IV IM PO (or 1–2 mg/kg/day via continuous IV infusion, or approximately 0.1–0.2 mg/kg per hr).
Metoprolol tartrate (Lopressor)	Adrenergic blocking agent. β_1-adrenergic blocker. Similar properties to propran-olol, except that meto-prolol is specific for β_1-receptor. Used to control tachyarrhymias and slow heart rate.	Adverse effects are primarily caused by excessive cardiovascu-lar depression (de-creased inotropic effects). May cause heart block. Use cautiously in animals prone to bronchocon-striction.	Results of clinical studies in animals have not been reported. Use in animals (and doses) is based on experience in people, or anecdotal experience in animals.	50, 100 mg tablets; 1 mg/mL injection.	Dog: 5–50 mg/dog (0.5–1.0 mg/kg) q8h PO. Cat: 2–15 mg/cat q8h PO.

Drug Name (Trade or Other Names)	Pharmacology and Indications	Adverse Effects and Precautions	Dosing Information and Comments	Formulations	Dosage
Metronidazole (Flagyl, and generic)	Antibacterial and anti-protozoal drug. Disrupts DNA in organism via reaction with intracellular metabolite. Action is specific for anaerobic bacteria. Resistance is rare. Active against some protozoa, including Giardia; however, other drugs, such as fenbendazole, have been used for Giardia.	Most severe adverse effect is caused by toxicity to CNS. High doses have caused lethargy, CNS depression, ataxia, vomiting, and weakness. Metronidazole may be mutagenic. Fetal abnormalities have not been demonstrated in animals with recommended doses, but use cautiously during pregnancy. Cats may find broken tablets unpalatable.	Metronidazole is one of the most commonly used drugs for anaerobic infections. Although it is effective for giardiasis, other drugs used for giardia include albendazole, fenbendazole, and quinacrine. CNS toxicity is dose-related. Maximum dose that should be administered is 50–65 mg/kg per day in any species. Although tablets have been broken or crushed for oral administration to cats, they find these unpalatable.	250, 500 mg tablet; 50 mg/mL suspension; 5 mg/mL injection.	For anaerobes: dogs: 15 mg/kg q12h, or 12 mg/kg q8h, PO; cats: 10–25 mg/kg q24h, PO. For Giardia: dogs: 12–15 mg/kg q12h for 8 days, PO; cats: 17 mg/kg (1/3 tablet per cat) q24h for 8 days.
Mexiletine (Mexitil)	Antiarrhythmic drug. Used for ventricular arrhythmias. Mechanism of action is to block fast sodium channel. Class IB anti-arrhythmic agent.	May produce arrhythmias. Use cautiously in animals with liver disease.	Results of clinical studies in animals have not been reported. Use in animals (and doses) is based on experience in people, or anecdotal experience in animals.	150, 200, 250 mg capsules.	Dog: 5–8 mg/kg q8–12h PO (use cautiously).
Mibolerone (Cheque-drops)	Androgenic steroid. Used to suppress estrus.	Do not use in Bedlington terriers. Do not use with perianal adenoma or carcinoma. Many bitches show clitoral enlargement or discharge from treatment. Do not use in cats.	Treatment ordinarily is initiated 30 days prior to onset of estrus. It is not recommended to be used for more than 2 years.	55 mcg/mL oral solution.	Dogs: (2.6–5 mcg/kg/day PO) 0.45–11.3 kg, 30 mcg; 11.8–22.7 kg, 60 mcg; 23–45.3 kg, 120 mcg; >45.8 kg, 180 mcg. Cats: safe dose not established.
Midazolam (Versed)	Benzodiazepine. Action is similar to other benzodiazepines (see Diazepam). Used as anesthetic adjunct.	Use very cautiously IV, especially with opiates. IV midazolam has caused serious cardio-respiratory depression.	Routine clinical use is not common. Clinical trials have not been reported. Compared to other benzodiazepines, midazolam can be administered IM.	5 mg/mL injection.	0.1–0.25 mg/kg IV IM (or 0.1–0.3 mg/kg/hr IV infusion).
Milbemycin oxime (Interceptor, Interceptor Flavor Tabs, and Safe Heart)	Antiparasitic drug. Action is similar to ivermectin. Acts as GABA agonist in nervous system of parasite. Used as heartworm preventative, miticide, and micro-filaricide. Used to control infections of hookworm, roundworms, and whipworms. At high doses, it has been used to treat Demodex infections in dogs.	In susceptible dogs (collie breeds), milbemycin may cross the blood–brain barrier and produce CNS toxicicosis (depression, lethargy, coma). At doses used for heartworm prevention, this effect is less likely.	Doses vary, depending on parasite treated. Consult dose column. Treatment of Demodex requires high dose administered daily (JAVMA 207: 1581, 1995). See also Sentinel tablets, which contain milbemycin oxime and lufenuron.	2.3, 5.75, 11.5, and 23 mg tablet.	Dogs: microfilaricide: 0.5 mg/kg: Demodex: 2 mg/kg q24h, PO for 60–120 days; heartworm prevention and control of endoparasites: 0.5 mg/kg q30days PO. Cat: for eartworm and hendoparasite control, 2.0 mg/kg q30d PO.
Milk of Magnesia	See Magnesium hydroxide.				
Mineral oil (generic)	Lubricant laxative. Increases water content of stool. Used to increase passage of feces for treatment of impaction and constipation.	Adverse effects have not been reported. Chronic use may decrease absorption of fat-soluble vitamins.	Use is empirical. No clinical results reported.	Oral liquid.	Dog: 10–50 mL/dog q12h PO. Cat: 10–25 mL/cat q12h PO.

Drug Name (Trade or Other Names)	Pharmacology and Indications	Adverse Effects and Precautions	Dosing Information and Comments	Formulations	Dosage
Minocycline (Minocin)	Tetracycline antibiotic. Similar to doxycycline in pharmacokinetics. (See Docycycline.)	See other tetracycline (Doxycycline). Adverse effects have not been reoported for minocycline. Oral absorption is not affected by calcium products as with other tetracyclines.	Minocycline has received little attention for clinical use in North America. Clinical use has not been reported, but properties are similar to doxycycline.	50, 100 mg tablets; 10 mg/mL oral suspension.	5–12.5 mg/kg q12h PO.
Misoprostol (Cytotec)	Prostaglandin E_2 analogue. Prostaglandins provide a cytoprotective role in the gastrointestinal mucosa. Misoprostol is used to prevent gastritis and ulcers associated with NSAID (aspirin-drugs) therapy.	Adverse effects are caused by effects of prostaglandins. Most common side effect is gastrointestinal discomfort, vomiting and diarrhea. Do *not* administer to pregnant animals; may cause abortion.	Doses and recommendations are based on clinical trials in which misoprostol was administered to prevent gastrointestinal mucosal injury caused by aspirin.	0.1 mg (100 mcg), 0.2 mg (200 mcg) tablets.	Dog: 2–5 mcg/kg q6–8h PO. Cat: dose not established.
Mithramycin	Older name for Plicamycin (Mithracin).				
Mitotane (o,p′-DDD) (Lysodren, op-DDD)	Adrenocortical cytotoxic agent. Causes suppression of adrenal cortex. Used to treat adrenal tumors and pituitary-dependent-hyperadrenocorticism (PDH).	Adverse effects, especially during induction period, include lethargy, anorexia, ataxia, depression, vomiting. Corticosteroid supplementation (e.g., hydrocortisone or prednisolone) may be administered to minimize side effects.	Dose and frequency often is based on patient response. Adverse effects are common during initial therapy. Administration with food increases oral absorption. Maintenance dose should be adjusted on the basis of periodic cortisol measurements and ACTH stimulation tests. (See also Vet Record 122: 486, 1988). Cats usually have not responded to mitotane treatment.	500 mg tablet.	Dogs: For PDH: 50 mg/kg/day (in divided doses) PO for 5–10 days, then 50–70 mg/kg/week PO; for adrenal tumor: 50–75 mg/kg/day for 10 days, then 75–100 mg/kg/week PO.
Mitoxantrone (Novantrone)	Anticancer antibiotic. Similar to doxorubicin in action (see Doxorubicin). Used for leukemia, lymphoma, and carcinomas.	As with all anticancer agents, certain adverse effects are predictable and unavoidable and related to drug's action. Mitoxantrone produces myelosuppression, vomiting, anorexia, and gastrointestinal upset, but may be less cardiotoxic than doxorubicin.	Proper use of mitoxantrone usually follows a specific anticancer protocol. Consult specific protocol for dosing regimen.	2 mg/mL injection.	Dogs: 6 mg/m² IV, every 21 days. Cats: 6.5 mg/m² IV every 21 days.
Morphine (generic)	Opioid agonist, analgesic. Prototype for other opioid agonists. Action of morphine is to bind to μ- and κ-opiate receptors on nerves and inhibit release of neurotransmitters involved with transmission of pain stimuli (such as Substance P). Morphine also may inhibit release of some inflammatory mediatiors. Central edative and seuphoric effects related to μ-receptor effects in brain.	Like all opiates, side effects from morphine are predictable and unavoidable. Side effects from morphine administration include sedation, constipation, and bradycardia. Respiratory depression occurs with high doses. Tolerance and dependence occurs with chronic administration. Cats are more sensitive to excitement than other species.	Effects from morphine administration are dose-dependent. Low doses (0.1–0.25 mg/kg) produce mild analgesia. Higher doses (up to 1 mg/kg) produce greater analgesic effects and sedation. Usually morphine is administered IM, IV, or SC, but delayed-release tablets have been used in dogs experimentally, but dose is higher (1–3 mg/kg q12h). Epidural administration has been used for surgical procedures.	1 and 15 mg/mL injection; 30, 60 mg delayed-release tablets.	Dog: 0.1–1 mg/kg IV IM SC (dose is escalated as needed for pain relief), every 4–6 hrs. Epidural: 0.1 mg/kg. Cat: 0.1 mg/kg IM SC, q3–6h (or as needed).

Drug Name (Trade or Other Names)	Pharmacology and Indications	Adverse Effects and Precautions	Dosing Information and Comments	Formulations	Dosage
Moxidectin (canine form: ProHeart; equine oral gel: Quest; cattle pour-on: Cydectin)	Antiparasitic drug. Neurotoxic to parasites by potentiating effects of inhibitory neurotransmitter, GABA. Used for endo- and ecto-parasites, as well as heartworm prevention.	Toxicity may occur at high doses, and in species in which ivermectin crosses blood–brain barrier (collie-breeds). Toxicity is neurotoxic, and signs include: depression, ataxia, difficulty with vision, coma, and death.	Similar use as ivermectin. Extreme caution is recommended if equine formulation is considered for use in small animals. Toxic overdoses are likely because the equine formulation is highly concentrated.	30, 68, 136 mcg tablets for dogs; 20 mg/mL equine oral gel; and 5 mg/mL cattle pour-on.	Dogs: heartworm prevention 3 mcg/kg q30d PO. 25–300 mcg/kg for endoparasites.
Myochrysine	See Gold sodium thiomalate.				
Naloxone (Narcan)	Opiate antagonist. Used to reverse effects from opiate agonists (such as morphine). Naloxone may be used to reverse sedation, anesthesia, and adverse effects caused from opiates.	Adverse effects are not reported. Tachycardia and hypertension have been reported in people.	Administration may have to be individualized based on response in each patient. Naloxone's duration of action is short in animals (60 min) and may have to be repeated.	20 or 400 mcg/mL injection.	0.01–0.04 mg/kg IV IM SC, as needed, to reverse opiate.
Naltrexone (Trexan)	Opiate antagonist. Similar to naloxone, except that it is longer-acting and administered orally. Used in people for treatment of opiate dependence. In animals, it has been used for treatment of some obsessive-compulsive behavioral disorders.	Adverse effects have not been reported in animals.	Treatment for obsessive-compulsive disorders in animals has been reported with naltrexone. Relapse rates may be high.	50 mg tablets.	For behavior problems: 2.2 mg/kg q12h PO.
Nandrolone deconate (Deca-Durabolin)	Anabolic steroid. Derivative of testosterone. Anabolic agents are designed to maximize anabolic effects, while minimizing androgenic action (see also Methyl testosterone). Anabolic agents have been used for reversing catabolic conditions, increasing weight gain, increasing muscling in animals, and stimulating erythropoiesis.	Adverse effects from anabolic steroids can be attributed to the pharmacologic action of these steroids. Increased masculine effects are common. Increased incidence of some tumors have been reported in people. 17α-methylated oral anabolic steroids (oxymetholone, stanozolol, and oxandrolone) are associated with hepatic toxicity.	Results of clinical studies in animals have not been reported. Use in animals (and doses) is based on experience in people, or anecdotal experience in animals.	Nandrolone decanoate injecton 50, 100, 200 mg/mL.	Dog: 1–1.5 mg/kg/week IM. Cat: 1 mg/kg/week IM.
Naproxen (Naprosyn, Naxen, Aleve [naproxen sodium])	Nonsteroidal anti-inflammatory drug (NSAID). Action is similar to other NSAIDs (see Flunixin).	Naproxen is a potent NSAID. Adverse effects attributed to GI toxicity are common to all NSAID (see Flunixin). Naproxen has produced serious ulceration in dogs, because elimination in dogs is many-fold slower than in people or horses.	Results of clinical studies in animals have not been reported. Use in animals (and doses) is based on pharmacokinetic studies in experimental animals. Caution when using the OTC formulation designed for people, because the tablet size is much larger than safe dose for dogs. 220 mg naproxen sodium is equivalent to 200 mg naproxen.	220 mg tablet (OTC). 25 mg/mL oral suspension; 250, 375, 500 mg tablets (Rx).	5 mg initially, then 2 mg/kg q48h.
Neomycin (Biosol)	Aminoglycoside antibiotic. For mechanism, and other effects, see Gentamicin, Amikacin. Neomycin differs from other aminoglycosides because it is only administered topically or orally. Systemic absorption is minimal from oral absorption.	Although oral absorption is so small that systemic adverse effects are unlikely, some oral absorption has been demonstrated in young animals (calves). Alterations in intestinal bacterial flora from therapy may cause diarrhea.	Neomycin is primarily used for oral treatment of diarrhea. Efficacy for this indication (especially for nonspecific diarrhea) is questionable. Used also for treatment of hepatic encephalopathy.	500 mg bolus; 200 mg/mL oral liquid.	10–20 mg/kg q6–12h PO.

Drug Name (Trade or Other Names)	Pharmacology and Indications	Adverse Effects and Precautions	Dosing Information and Comments	Formulations	Dosage
Neostigmine bromide, and Neostigmine methylsulfate (Prostigmin; Stiglyn)	Anticholinesterase drug. Cholinesterase inhibitor. Inhibits breakdown of acetylcholine at synapse. Antimyasthenic drug. Used primarily for treatment of myasthenia gravis, or as an antidote for neuromuscular blockade caused by nondepolarizing neuromuscular blocking drugs.	Adverse effects are related to drug's pharmacological effects: excessive cholinergic stimulation (muscarinic effects), which include diarrhea, salivation, respiratory problems, vomiting, CNS effects, muscle twitching, or weakness. Atropine is used to treat overdose.	Compared to other drugs in this class (e.g., pyridostigmine) produces more severe muscarinic effects. Neostigmine has been used for diagnostic purposes also (see Edrophonium). When injected for treatment of myasthenia, or diagnosis, it is recommended to use atropine to counteract side effects.	15 mg tablet (neostigmine bromide); 0.25, 0.5 mg/mL injection (neostigmine methylsulfate)	2 mg/kg/day PO (in divided doses, to effect). Injection: antimyasthenic: 10 mcg/kg IM SC, as needed; antidote for neuromuscular block: 40 mcg/kg IM SC; diagnostic aid for myasthenia gravis: 40 mcg/kg IM, or 20 mcg/kg IV.
Nifedipine (Adalat, Procardia)	Calcium-channel blocking drug of the dihydropyridine class. Action is similar to other calcium-channel blocking drugs, except nifedipine is more specific for vascular smooth muscle than cardiac tissue. Used for smooth muscle relaxation, vasodilation.	Adverse effects have not been reported in veterinary medicine. Most common side effect is hypotension.	Use of nifedipine is limited in veterinary medicine. Other calcium-channel blockers, such as diltiazem, are used to control heart rhythm.	10, 20 mg capsules.	Animal dose not established. In people, the dose is 10 mg/per person three times a day and increased in 10 mg increments to effect.
Nitrates	See Nitroglycerin, Isosorbide dinitrate.				
Nitrofurantoin (Macrodantin, Furalan, Furatoin, Furadantin, or generic)	Antibacterial drug. Urinary antiseptic. Action is via reactive metabolites that damage DNA. Therapeutic concentrations are reached only in the urine. Not to be used for systemic infections.	Adverse effects include nausea, vomiting, and diarrhea. Turns urine color rust-yellow brown. Do not administer during pregnancy.	Two dosing forms exist. Microcrystalline is rapidly and completely absorbed. Macrocrystalline (Macrodantin) is more slowly absorbed and causes less gastrointestinal irritation. Urine should be at acidic pH for maximum effect. Administer with food to increase absorption.	Macrodandin and generic 25, 50, 100 mg capsules; Furalan, Furatoin, and generic 50, 100 mg tablets; Furadantin 5 mg/mL oral suspension.	10 mg/kg/day divided into four daily treatments, then, 1 mg/kg at night PO.
Nitroglycerin ointment (Nitrol, Nitrobid, Nitrostat)	Nitrate. Nitrovasodilator. Relaxes vascular smooth muscle (especially venous) via generation of nitric oxide. Used primarily in heart failure to reduce preload, or decrease pulmonary hypertension. In people, used to treat angina pectoris.	Adverse effects from nitrates are related to their pharmacologic action. Most significant adverse effect is hypotension. Methemoglobinemia can occur with accumulation of nitrites, but is a rare problem.	Tolerance can develop with repeated, chronic use. Use should be intermittent for optimum effect. Nitroglycerin has high presystemic metabolism and oral availability is poor. When using ointment, 1 inch of ointment is approximately 15 mg.	0.5, 0.8, 1, 5, 10 mg/mL injection; 2% ointment; transdermal systems (0.2 mg/hr patch).	Dog: 4–12 mg (up to 15 mg) topically q12h. Cat: 2–4 mg topically q12h (or 1/4 inch of ointment per cat).
Nitroprusside (Nitropress)	Nitrate vasodilator. See Nitroglycerin. Nitroprusside is used only as a IV infusion, and patients should be monitored carefully during administration.	Severe hypotension is possible during therapy. Monitor patients carefully during administration. Cyanide is generated via metabolism during nitroprusside treatment, especially at high infusion rates. Cyanide toxicity is possible with nitroprusside therapy. Sodium thiosulfate has been used in people to prevent cyanide toxicity. Methemoglobinemia is possible, and if necessary treated with methylene blue.	Nitroprusside is administered via IV infusion. IV solution should be delivered in 5% dextrose solution (e.g., add 50 mg to 250 mL of 5% dextrose). Protect from light. Discard solutions if color change is observed. Titrate dose carefully in each patient.	50 mg vial for injection.	1–5, up to a maximum of 10 mcg/kg/min IV infusion.

Drug Name (Trade or Other Names)	Pharmacology and Indications	Adverse Effects and Precautions	Dosing Information and Comments	Formulations	Dosage
Nizatidine (Axid)	Histamine H-2 blocking drug. See Cimetidine. Same as cimetidine, except up to 10× more potent.	See Cimetidine and Ranitidine. Side effects from nizatidine have not been reported for animals.	Results of clinical studies in animals have not been reported. Use in animals (and doses) is based on experience in people, or anecdotal experience in animals. Nizatidine and ranitidine have been shown to stimulate gastric emptying and colonic motility via anticholinesterase activity.	150, 300 mg capsules.	Dog: 2.5–5 mg/kg q24h PO.
Norfloxacin (Noroxin)	Fluoroquinolone antibacterial drug. Same action as ciprofloxacin, except spectrum of activity is not as broad as with enrofloxacin or ciprofloxacin.	Adverse effects have not been reported in animals. Some effects are expected to be similar to cipro/enrofloxacin administration.	Use in animals (and doses) is based on pharmacokinetic studies in experimental animals, experience in people, or anecdotal experience in animals.	400 mg tablets.	22 mg/kg q12h PO.
Olsalazine (Dipentum)	Anti-inflammatory drug for treating colitis. Two molecules of aminosalicylic acid joined by an azobond. (See Mesalamine).	See Mesalamine.	See Mesalamine. Olsalazine is used in patients that cannot tolerate sulfasalazine.	500 mg tablets.	Dose not established, but 5–10 mg/kg q8h have been used. (The usual human dose is 500 mg twice daily.)
Omeprazole (Prilosec [formerly Losec]. Equine formulation (a paste) is Gastrogard)	Proton pump inhibitor. Omeprazole inhibits gastric acid secretion by inhibiting the K+/H+ pump. Omeprazole is more potent and longer-acting than most available antisecretory drugs. Used for treatment and prevention of gastrointestinal ulcers.	Side effects have not been reported in animals. However, in people there is concern about hypergastrinemia with chronic use. Drug interactions: Do not administer with drugs that depend on acid stomach for absorption (e.g., ketoconazole).	Due to omeprazole's potency and accumulation in gastric cells, infrequent administration is possible. Lansoprazole is a newer drug of this class, but has not been used in animals.	20 mg capsules and equine paste.	Dog: 20 mg/dog once daily, PO (or 0.7 mg/kg, q24h). Cat: not recommended.
Ondansetron (Zofran)	Antiemetic drug. Ondansetron's action is to inhibit action of serotonin (blocks 5-HT₃ receptors). Used primarily to inhibit vomiting associated with chemotherapy.	Ondansetron adverse effects have not been reported in animals. Some effects may be indistinguishable from concurrent cancer drugs.	Ondansetron has been used infrequently in veterinary medicine due to its expense. Granisetron is a similar drug not yet evaluated in veterinary medicine.	4, 8 mg tablets; 2 mg/mL injection.	0.5 to 1.0 mg/kg, IV or oral 30 min prior to administration of cancer drugs.
o,p'-DDD	See Mitotane (Lysodren).				
Orbifloxacin (Orbax)	Fluoroquinolone antimicrobial. Same mechanism as enrofloxacin and ciprofloxacin. Spectrum includes staphylococci, Gram-negative bacilli, and some Pseudomonas.	Same precautions as enrofloxacin. May cause some nausea and vomiting at high doses. Avoid use in young animals.	Dose range is wide to account for susceptibility of bacteria. Most susceptible bacteria should be treated with low dose, more resistant bacteria, such as Pseudomonas, should be treated with high dose.	5.7, 22.7, and 68 mg tablets.	Dog and cat: 2.5 to 7.5 mg/kg once daily, PO.
Ormetoprim	Trimethoprim-like drug used in combination with sulfadimethoxine. (See Primor.)				
Oxacillin (Prostaphlin, and generic)	β-lactam antibiotic. Inhibits bacterial cell wall synthesis. Spectrum is limited to Gram-positive bacteria, especially staphylococci.	Use cautiously in animals allergic to penicillin-like drugs.	Doses based on empiricism or extrapolation from human studies. No clinical efficacy studies available for dogs or cats. Administer if possible on empty stomach.	250, 500 mg capsules, 50 mg/mL oral solution.	22–40 mg/kg q8h, PO.

Drug Name (Trade or Other Names)	Pharmacology and Indications	Adverse Effects and Precautions	Dosing Information and Comments	Formulations	Dosage
Oxazepam (Serax)	Benzodiazepine. Central-acting CNS depressant. Mechanism of action appears to be via potentiation of GABA-receptor mediated effects in CNS. Used for sedation and to stimulate appetite.	Sedation is most common side effect. Causes polyphagia. In cats, fatal hepatic necrosis has been reported from diazepam.	Doses based on empiricism. There have been no clinical trials in veterinary medicine.	15 mg tablet.	Cats: appetite stimulant: 2.5 mg/cat PO.
Oxtriphylline (Choledyl-SA)	Choline theophyllinate. Methylxanthine bronchodilator, similar in mechanism as theophylline.	See Theophylline.	Adverse effects similar to theophylline (See Theophylline). Some formulations (Theocon) contain oxtriphylline and guaifenesin. When administering slow-release tablet, do not crush tablet.	400, 600 mg tablet. (Oral solutions and syrup available in Canada, but not U.S.).	Dog: 47 mg/kg (equivalent to 30 mg/kg theophylline) q12h PO.
Oxybutynin chloride (Ditropan)	Anticholinergic agent. Inhibits smooth muscle spasms via blocking action of acetylcholine. Used primarily to increase bladder capacity and to decrease spasms of urinary tract.	Adverse effects are related to anticholinergic effects (see Atropine), but are less frequent compared to other anticholinergic drugs. Administer physostigmine for overdose.	Results of clinical studies in animals have not been reported. Use in animals (and doses) is based on experience in people, or anecdotal experience in animals.	5 mg tablets.	Dog: 5 mg/dog q6–8h PO.
Oxyglobin (Oxyglobin)	Hemoglobin glutamer (bovine) used as oxygen-carrying fluid in dogs with varying causes of anemia.	Transient hemoglobinuria. Should not be used in dogs with advanced heart disease. Adverse pulmonary effects can occur from rapid administration. Adverse effects have been skin discoloration, cardiovascular effects, vomiting, diarrhea, and anorexia.	Administer using aseptic technique. Do not administer with other fluids or drugs in the same IV line. Do not mix with other medications. 90% of dose is eliminated in 5–7 days.	13 g/dL polymerized hemoglobin of bovine origin in 125 mL single dose bags.	Dog: One-time dose of 30 mL/kg IV at rate up to 10 mL/kg/hr.
Oxymetholone (Anadrol)	Anabolic steroid. See Nandrolone (there are no differences in efficacy among the anabolic steroids.)	See Nandrolone.	See Nandrolone.	50 mg tablets.	1–5 mg/kg/day PO.
Oxymorphone (Numorphan)	Opioid agonist. Action is similar to morphine, except that oxymorphone is more lipophilic than morphine and 10–15× more potent than morphine.	See Morphine.	See Morphine. There is some evidence that oxymorphone may have fewer cardiovascular effects compared to morphine. Since oxymorphone is more lipophilic, it is readily absorbed from epidural injection.	1.5 and 1 mg/mL injection.	Dogs, cats: analgesia: 0.1–0.2 mg/kg IV, SC, IM (as needed), redose with 0.05–0.1 mg/kg q1–2h. Preanesthetic: 0.025–0.05 mg/kg IM, SC.
Oxytetracycline (Terramycin)	Tetracycine antibiotic. (See Tetracycline). Same mechanism and spectrum as tetracycline. Oxytetracycline may be absorbed to higher extent.	Generally safe. Use cautiously in young animals. See precautions for tetracycline.	Oral dose forms are from large animal use. Use of injectable long-acting forms have not been studied in small animals.	250 mg tablets; 100, 200 mg/mL injection.	7.5–10 mg/kg IV, q12h; 20 mg/kg q12h PO.
Oxytocin (Pitocin and Syntocinon [nasal solution], and generic)	Stimulates uterine muscle contraction via action on specific oxytoxin receptors. Used to induce or maintain normal labor and delivery in pregnant animals. Does not increase milk production, but will stimulate contraction leading to milk ejection.	Adverse effects are uncommon if used carefully. Fetal stress and progression of normal labor should be monitored closely.	Used to induce labor. In people, oxytocin is administered via injection, constant IV infusion, and intranasal solution. Repeat up to 3× every 30–60 min. (maximum dose is 3 units/cat).	10, 20 U/mL injection; and 40 U/mL nasal solution.	Dog: 5–20 units IM, SC, (repeat every 30 min for primary inertia). Cat: 2.5–5 units per cat, IM, IV.

Drug Name (Trade or Other Names)	Pharmacology and Indications	Adverse Effects and Precautions	Dosing Information and Comments	Formulations	Dosage
2-PAM	See Pralidoxime chloride.				
Pancreatic enzym	See Pancrelipase (Viokase).				
Pancrelipase (Viokase)	Pancreatic enzyme. Used to treat pancreatic exocrine insufficiency. Provides lipase, amylase, and protease.	Adverse effects not reported.	Mix with food when administering, approximately 20 minutes prior to feeding.	16,800 U of lipase, 70,000 U of protease, and 70,000 U of amylase per 0.7 gm. Also capsules and tablets.	Dog: Mix 2 tsp powder with food per 20 kg body weight, or 1–3 tsp/0.45 kg of food 20 min prior to feeding. Cat: 1/2 tsp per cat with food.
Pancuronium bromide (Pavulon)	Nondepolarizing neuro-muscular blocker (see Atricurium)	See Atricurium.	See Atricurium.	1, 2 mg/mL injection.	0.1 mg/kg IV, or start with 0.01 mg/kg and additional 0.01 mg/kg doses every 30 min.
Paregoric (Corrective Mixture)	Paregoric (opium tincture) is an outdated product used to treat diarrhea. Paregoric contains 2 mg of morphine in every 5 mL of paregoric.	See opiates (such as Morphine).	Use of paregoric has been replaced by more specific products, such as loperamide or diphenoxylate.	2 mg morphine per 5 mL of paregoric.	0.05–0.06 mg/kg q12h PO.
Paroxetine (Paxil)	Selective serotonin re-uptake inhibitor (SSRI) much like fluoxetine (Prozac) in action. Used for obsessive-compulsive disorders, aggression, and other behavioral problems.	Some effects similar to fluoxetine, but in some animals paroxetine is better tolerated.	Dosing recommendations are empirical.	10, 20, 30, 40 mg tablets.	Cats: 1/8 to 1/4 of a 10 mg tablet daily, PO.
D-penicillamine (Cuprimine, Depen)	Chelating agent for lead, copper, iron, and mercury. Used primarily in animals for treatment of copper toxicity and hepatitis associated with accumulation of copper. It also has been used to treat cystine calculi. Penicillamine has been used in people to treat rheumatoid arthritis.	Do not use in pregnant animals. In people, allergic reactions have been reported, as well as agranulocytosis and anemia.	Administer on an empty stomach (2 hrs before meals).	125, 250 mg capsules and 250 mg tablets.	10–15 mg/kg q12h PO.
Penicillin G, Benzathine (Benza-Pen, and other names)	All benzathine penicillin G is combined with procaine penicillin G in commercial formulation.	See Penicillin G.	Benzathine is not recommended for therapy, because concentrations are too low to be therapeutic.	150,000 U/mL, combined with 150,000 U/mL of procaine penicillin G.	24,000 U/kg q48h IM.
Penicillin G potassium; Penicillin G sodium (many brands)	β-lactam antibiotic. Action is similar to other penicillins (see Amoxicillin). Spectrum of Penicillin G is limited to Gram-positive bacteria and anaerobes.	Same as for other penicillins (see Amoxicillin).	See other penicillins (Amoxicillin).	5–20 million U vials.	20,000–40,000 U/kg q6–8h IV, IM.
Penicillin G, Procaine (generic)	Same as other forms of penicillin G, except procaine penicillin is absorbed slowly, pro-ducing concentrations for 12–24 hrs after injections.	Same as for other penicillins (see Amoxicillin).	Same as other penicillins (amoxicillin). Avoid SC injection with procaine penicillin G.	300,000 U/mL suspension.	20,000–40,000 U/kg q12–24h IM.
Penicillin V (Pen-Vee)	Oral penicillin. Other-wise same as other penicillins. Not highly absorbed, and narrow spectrum in compari-son with other penicillin derivatives.	Same as other penicillin (see Amoxicillin).	Same as other penicil-lins (amoxicillin). Peni-cillin V should be administered on an empty stomach for maximum absorption (250 mg = 400,000 units).	250, 500 mg tablets.	10 mg/kg q8h PO.
Pentazocine (Talwin-V)	Synthetic opiate anal-gesic. Action is as agonist-antagonist (similar to buprenor-phine or butorphanol).	Adverse effects similar to other opiates (see Butorphanol or morphine)	See other opiates.	30 mg/mL injection.	Dog: 1.65–3.3 mg/kg q4h IM. Cat: 2.2–3.3 mg/kg IV, IM, SC.

Drug Name (Trade or Other Names)	Pharmacology and Indications	Adverse Effects and Precautions	Dosing Information and Comments	Formulations	Dosage
Pentobarbital (Nembutal, and generic)	Short-acting barbiturate anesthetic. Action is via nonselective depression CNS. Pentobarbital usually is used as IV anesthetic. Used to control severe seizures in animals. Duration of action may be 3–4 hours.	Adverse effects are related to anesthetic action. (See Thiopental). Cardiac and respiratory depression are common.	Pentobarbital has narrow therapeutic index. When administering IV, inject first half of dose initially, then remainder of calculated dose gradually, until anesthetic effect is achieved.	50 mg/mL.	25–30 mg/kg IV.
Pentoxifylline (Trental)	Methylxanthine. Pentoxifylline is used primarily as a rheological agent in people (increases blood flow through narrow vessels). It may have anti-inflammatory action via inhibition of cytokine synthesis. Used in dogs for some dermatoses (dermatomyositis) and vasculitis.	May cause similar signs as other methylxanthines (see Theophylline). Nausea, vomiting have been reported in people. When broken tablet is administered to cats, the taste is unpleasant.	Results of clinical studies in animals have not been reported. Use in animals (and doses) is based on experience in people, or anecdotal experience in animals.	400 mg tablets.	Dog: dermatologic use: 10 mg/kg q12h PO. For other uses: 10 mg/kg q8–12h PO, or 400 mg/dog for most animals. Cats: 1/4 of a 400 mg tablet (100 mg) q8–12h, PO.
Pepto Bismol	See Bismuth subsalicylate.				
Phenobarbital (Luminal, and generic)	Long-acting barbiturate. See other barbiturates (Thiopental). Phenobarbital's major use is as an anticonvulsant in which it potentiates inhibitory actions of GABA.	Adverse effects are dose-related. Phenobarbital causes polyphagia, sedation, ataxia, and lethargy. Some tolerance develops to side effects after initial therapy. Hepatotoxicity has been reported in some dogs receiving high doses.	Phenobarbital doses should be carefully adjusted via monitoring serum/plasma concentrations. Optimum range for therapeutic effect is 15–40 mcg/mL.	15, 30, 60, 100 mg tablets; 30, 60, 65, and 130 mg/mL injection; 4 mg/mL oral elixir solution.	Dog: 2–8 mg/kg q12h PO. Cat: 2–4 mg/kg q12h PO. Status epilepticus: administer in increments of 10–20 mg/kg IV (to effect).
Phenoxybenzamine (Dibenzyline)	α_1-adrenergic antagonist. Binds α_1-receptor on smooth muscle, causing relaxation. Potent vasodilator. Used primarily to treat peripheral vasoconstriction. In some animals, has been used to relax urethral smooth muscle.	Causes prolonged hypotension in animals. Use carefully in animals with cardiovascular compromise.	Results of clinical studies in animals have not been reported. Use in animals (and doses) is based on experience in people, or limited experimental experience in animals.	10 mg capsules.	Dog: 0.25 mg/kg q8–12h PO, or 0.5 mg/kg q24h. Cat: 2.5 mg/cat q8–12h, or 0.5 mg/kg q12h PO. (In cats, doses as high as 0.5 mg/kg IV have been used to relax urethral smooth muscle.)
Phentolamine (Regitine, [Rogitine in Canada])	Nonselective α-adrenergic blocker. Vasodilator. Blocks stimulation of α-receptors on vascular smooth muscle. Primarily used to treat hypertension.	May cause excess hypotension with high doses or in animals that are dehydrated. May cause tachycardia.	Results of clinical studies in animals have not been reported. Use in animals (and doses) is based on experience in people, or anecdotal experience in animals. Titrate dose for each patient to produce desired vasodilation.	5 mg vials for injection.	0.02–0.1 mg/kg IV.
Phenylbutazone (Butazolidin, and generic)	Nonsteroidal anti-inflammatory drug (NSAID). See Flunixin. Phenylbutazone is used primarily for arthritis and various forms of musculoskeletal pain and inflammation.	Phenylbutazone is generally well-tolerated in dogs, but there is no data for cats. Adverse effects possible are gastrointestinal toxicity (see Flunixin). Do not administer injectable formulation IM. Phenylbutazone causes bone marrow depression in people, which also is possible in dogs.	Doses are based primarily on manufacturer's recommendations and clinical experience. There have been no comparative trials demonstrating efficacy of one NSAID over another. Not approved in U.S. for cats, but has been used in cats in Europe.	100, 200, 400 mg and 1 gm tablets. 200 mg/mL injection.	Dog: 15–22 mg/kg q8–12h (44 mg/kg/day) PO, IV (800 mg/dog maximum). Cat: 6–8 mg/kg q12h IV, PO.

Drug Name (Trade or Other Names)	Pharmacology and Indications	Adverse Effects and Precautions	Dosing Information and Comments	Formulations	Dosage
Phenylephrine (Neosynephrine)	Specific adrenergic agonist; specific for α_1-receptor; same as methoxamine.	Same as methoxamine.	Same as methoxamine. Phenylephrine also is used commonly as topical vasoconstrictor (as in nasal decongestants).	10 mg/mL injection; 1% nasal solution.	0.01 mg/kg q15min IV, 0.1 mg/kg q15min IM, SC.
Phenylpropanolamine (Dexatrim, Propagest and others)	Adrenergic agonist. Used as decongestant, mild bronchodilator, and to increase tone of urinary sphincter. (See Ephedrine, Pseudo-ephedrine).	Adverse effects are attributed to excess stimulation of adrenergic (α and β) receptors. See Ephedrine. Side effects: tachycardia, cardiac effects, CNS excitement, restlessness, and appetite suppression.	Phenylpropanolamine is available in variety of dose forms, usually used for treatment of cough/colds in people. Many preparations contain other ingredients.	15, 25, 30, 50 mg tablets.	1.5–2 mg/kg q12h PO.
Phenytoin (Dilantin)	Anticonvulsant. Depresses nerve conduction via blockade of sodium channels. Also classified as Class-I antiarrhythmic. Commonly used as anticonvulsant in people, but not effective in dogs and not used in cats.	Adverse effects: Sedation, gingival hyperplasia, skin reactions, CNS toxicity. Do not administer to pregnant animals.	Because of short half-life and poor efficacy in dogs, and questionable safety in cats, other anticonvulsants are used as first choice before phenytoin.	30, 125 mg/mL oral suspension; 30, 100 mg capsules; 50 mg/mL injection.	Antiepileptic: dog: 20–35 mg/kg q8h. Antiarrhythmic: 30 mg/kg q8h PO or 10 mg/kg IV over 5 min.
Physostigmine (Antilirium)	Cholinesterase inhibitor. Antidote for anti-cholinergic intoxication, especially intoxication that exhibits CNS signs. Major difference between physostigmine and neostigmine or pyridostigmine is that physostigmine crosses blood–brain barrier and the others do not.	Adverse effects attributed to excessive cholinergic effects (treat overdoses with atropine).	Physostigmine is indicated primarily only for treatment of intoxication. For routine systemic use of anti-cholinesterase drug, neostigmine and pyridostigmine have fewer side effects. When used, frequency of dose may be increased, based on observation of effects.	1 mg/mL injection.	0.02 mg/kg q12h IV.
Phytonadione	See Vitamin K$_1$.				
Phytomenadione	See Vitamin K$_1$.				
Piperacillin (Pipracil)	β-lactam antibiotic of the acylureido-penicillin class. Similar to other penicillins, except with high activity against *Pseudomonas aeruginosa*. Also good activity against streptococci.	Same precautions as for other injectable penicillins (e.g., ampicillin).	Reconstituted solution should be used within 24 hours (or 7 days if refrigerated). Piperacillin is combined with tazobactam (bacta-lactamase inhibitor) in Zosyn.	2-, 3-, 4-, 40-gm vials for injection.	40 mg/kg IV or IM q6h.
Piperazine (many)	Antiparasitic compound. Produces neuromuscular block-ade in parasite through inhibition of neurotransmitter which causes paralysis of worms. Used primarily for treatment of helminth (ascarids) infections.	Remarkably safe in all species.	Used to treat all species for round-worms.	860 mg powder; 140 mg capsules; 170, 340, and 800 mg/mL oral solution.	44–66 mg/kg PO, administered once.
Piroxicam (Feldene, and generic)	Nonsteroidal anti-inflammatory drug (NSAID) of the oxicam class. Clinical effects are similar to other NSAIDs (see Aspirin, Flunixin). Piroxicam has been used for treatment of transitional cell carcinoma in dogs.	Elimination of piroxicam is slow; Use cautiously in dogs. Adverse effects are primarily gastrointestinal toxicity (ulcers); see Flunixin.	Piroxicam is primarily used to treat arthritis and other musculo-skeletal conditions, but there are reports of its activity for treating certain tumors (e.g., transitional cell carcinoma of bladder).	10 mg capsules.	Dog: 0.3 mg/kg q48h PO. Cat: dose not established.

Drug Name (Trade or Other Names)	Pharmacology and Indications	Adverse Effects and Precautions	Dosing Information and Comments	Formulations	Dosage
Pitressin (ADH)	See Vasopressin and Desmopressin.				
Plicamycin (old name is Mithramycin) (Mithracin)	Anticancer agent. Action is to combine with DNA in presence of divalent cations and inhibit DNA and RNA synthesis. Lowers serum calcium. May have direct action on osteoclasts to decrease serum calcium. Used for carcinomas and treatment of hypercalcemia.	Adverse effects have not been reported in animals. In people, hypocalcemia and gastrointestinal toxicity have been reported. May cause bleeding problems. *Drug interactions:* Do not use with drugs that may increase the risk of bleeding (e.g., NSAIDs, heparin, or anticoagulants).	Results of clinical studies in animals have not been reported. Use in animals (and doses) is based on experience in people, or anecdotal experience in animals.	2.5 mg injection.	Dog: antineoplastic: 25–30 mcg/kg/day IV (slow infusion) for 8–10 days; antihypercalcemic: 25 mcg/kg/day IV (slow infusion) over 4 hours.
Polyethylene glycol electrolyte solution (Golytely)	Saline cathartic. (See Magnesium citrate.) Nonabsorbable compounds that increase water secretion into bowel via osmotic effect. Used for bowel evacuation prior to surgical or diagnostic procedure.	Water and electrolyte loss with high doses or prolonged use. (See also Magnesium citrate.)	Used primarily to evacuate bowel as preparation for procedures.	Oral solution.	25 mL/kg, repeat in 2–4 hr PO.
Polysulfated glycosaminoglycan (PSGAG) (Adequan Canine)	Large molecular weight compounds similar to normal constituents of healthy joints. Chondroprotective. Inhibits enzymes that may degrade articular cartilage. Used primarily to treat or prevent degenerative joint disease.	Adverse effects are rare. Allergic reactions are possible. PSGAG has heparin-like effects and may potentiate bleeding problems in some animals.	Doses are derived from empirical evidence, experimental studies, and clinical studies in dogs. (see Compen. Cont. Educat. 16: 501, 1994; or JAVMA 204: 1245, 1994). Although effective for acute arthritis, may not be as effective for chronic arthropathy.	100 mg/mL injection in 5 mL vial (for horses vials are 250 mg/mL).	4.4 mg/kg IM, twice weekly for up to 4 weeks.
Potassium bromide (KBr) (No commercial formulation, but can be formulated by a pharmacist)	Anticonvulsant. Anticonvulsant action is to stabilize neuronal cell membranes. Bromide ordinarily is used in patients refractory to phenobarbital.	Adverse effects are related to high levels of bromide. Signs of toxicosis are CNS depression, weakness, ataxia. Consider using sodium bromide in patients with hypoadrenocorticism.	Bromide usually is administered in combination with phenobarbital. Monitor serum bromide concentrations to adjust dose. Effective plasma concentrations should be 1–2 mg/mL (100–200 mg/dL), but, if used alone (without phenobarbital), higher concentrations of 2–4 mg/mL may be needed. Diets high in chloride will cause shorter half-life and need for higher dose. Sodium bromide can be substituted for potassium bromide.	Usually prepared as oral solution.	Dog and cat: 30–40 mg/kg q24h PO. If administered without phenobarbital, higher doses of up to 40–50 mg/kg may be needed. Adjust doses by monitoring plasma concentrations. Loading doses of 400 mg/kg divided over three days have been administered.
Potassium chloride (generic)	Potassium supplement. Used for treatment of hypokalemia. Usually added to fluid solutions.	Toxicity from high potassium concentrations can be dangerous. Hyperkalemia can lead to cardiovascular toxicity (bradycardia and arrest) and muscular weakness. Oral potassium supplements can cause nausea and stomach irritation.	One gram of potassium chloride provides 13.41 mEq of potassium. When potassium is supplemented in fluids, do not administer at a rate faster than 0.5 mEq/kg/hr.	Various concentrations for injection (usually 2 mEq/mL). Oral suspension and oral solution.	0.5 mEq potassium/kg/day, or supplement 10–40 mEq/500 mL of fluids, depending on serum potassium.
Potassium citrate (generic, Urocit-K)	Alkalinizes urine and may increase urine citric acid. Used for calcium oxalate urolithiasis. Also used for renal tubular acidosis.	Same as potassium chloride.	One gram of potassium citrate provides 9.26 mEq of potassium.	5 mEq tablet. Some forms are in combination with potassium chloride.	2.2 mEq/100 kCal of energy/day PO; or 40–75 mg/kg q12h PO.

Drug Name (Trade or Other Names)	Pharmacology and Indications	Adverse Effects and Precautions	Dosing Information and Comments	Formulations	Dosage
Potassium gluconate (Kaon, Tumil-K, generic)	Same as potassium chloride. Used for renal tubular acidosis.	Same as potassium chloride.	One gram of potassium gluconate provides 4.27 mEq of potassium.	2 mEq tablet; 500 mg tablets; Kaon elixir is 20 mg/15 mL elixir.	Dog: 0.5 mEq/kg q12–24h PO. Cat: 2–8 mEq/day divided twice daily, PO.
Potassium phosphate	Phosphorous supplement. Used for severe hypophosphatemia associated with diabetic ketoacidosis.				0.03–0.12 mmol/kg/hour IV.
Pralidoxime chloride (2-PAM) (2-PAM, Protopam chloride)	Used for treatment of organophosphate toxicosis.	Adverse effects have not been reported.	When treating intoxication, consult poison control center for precise guidelines.	50 mg/mL injection.	20 mg/kg q8–12h (initial dose IV slow); or IM.
Praziquantel (Droncit)	Antiparasitic drug. Action on parasites related to neuromuscular toxicity and paralysis via altered permeability to calcium. Used primarily to treat infections caused by tapeworms.	Vomiting occurs at high doses. Anorexia and transient diarrhea have been reported. Safe in pregnant animals.	Dose recommendations based on label dose supplied by manufacturer.	23, 34 mg tablet. 56.8 mg/mL injection.	Dog: oral dose:<6.8 kg, 7.5 mg/kg PO, once; >6.8 kg, 5 mg/kg PO, once; dog IM SC: ≤ 2.3 kg, 7.5 mg/kg, once; 2.7–4.5 kg, 6.3 mg/kg, once; ≤ 5 kg, 5 mg/kg, once. Cat PO:<1.8 kg, 6.3 mg/kg PO, once; >1.8 kg, 5 mg/kg, once (for Paragonimus, use 25 mg/kg q8h for 2–3 days/cat IM, SC: 5 mg/kg IM SC.
Prazocin (Minipress)	α₁-adrenergic blocker. Relaxes smooth muscle, especially of vasculature. Prazocin is used as vasodilator and to relax smooth muscle (occasionally urethral muscle).	High doses cause vasodilation and hypotension.	Titrate dose to needs of individual patient. Results of clinical studies in animals have not been reported. Use in animals (and doses) is based on experience in people, or anecdotal experience in animals.	1, 2, 5 mg capsule.	0.5–2 mg/animal (1 mg/15 kg) q8–12h PO.
Prednisolone (Delta-cortef, and many others)	Glucocorticoid anti-inflammatory drug. Potency is approximately 4× cortisol. (See Betamethasone for details.)	All glucocorticoids produce expected (and sometimes unavoidable) side effects. See Betamethasone for partial list of side effects.	Doses for prednisolone are based on severity of underlying condition. Doses listed are for dogs. Cats often require 2× the dog dose.	5 and 20 mg tablets.	Dogs (cats often require 2× dogs dose): anti-inflammatory: 0.5–1 mg/kg q12–24h IV, IM, PO initially, then taper to q48h; immunosuppressive: 2.2–6.6 mg/kg/day IV IM PO initially, then taper to 2–4 mg/kg q48h; replacement therapy: 0.2–0.3 mg/kg/day PO. Shock, spinal trauma: see Prednisolone sodium succinate.
Prednisolone sodium succinate (Solu-Delta-Cortef)	Same as prednisolone, except that this is a water-soluble formulation intended for acute therapy when high IV doses are needed for rapid effect. Used for treatment of shock and CNS trauma.	Adverse effects are not expected from single administration; however, with repeated use, other side effects are possible (see Betamethasone).	See Prednisolone.	100, 200 mg vials for injection (10 and 50 mg/mL).	Shock: 15–30 mg/kg IV (repeat in 4–6 hr). CNS trauma: 15–30 mg/kg IV, taper to 1–2 mg/kg q12h.
Prednisone (Deltasone and generic; Meticorten for injection)	Same as prednisolone, except that, after administration, prednisone is converted to prednisolone.	Same as prednisolone.	Same as prednisolone. There are no known contraindications in which prednisolone is preferred over prednisone.	1, 2.5, 5, 10, 20, 25, and 50 mg tablets. 1 mg/mL syrup (Liquid-Pred in 5% alcohol) and 1 mg/mL oral solution (in 5% alcohol); 10, 40 mg/mL prednisone suspension for injection.	Same as prednisolone.
Primidone (Mylepsin, Neurosyn [Mysoline in Canada])	Anticonvulsant. Primidone is converted to phenylethylmalonamide and phenobarbital, both of which have anticonvulsant activity, but most of activity (85%) is probably due to phenobarbital. See Phenobarbital for more details.	Adverse effects are same as for phenobarbital. Primidone has been associated with idiosyncratic hepatotoxicity in dogs. Although some labels caution its use in cats, one study in experimental cats determined that it is safe if used at recommended doses.	See Phenobarbital. When monitoring therapy with primidone, phenobarbital plasma concentrations should be measured to estimate anticonvulsant effect.	50 and 250 mg tablet.	8–10 mg/kg q8–12h as initial dose PO, then is adjusted via monitoring to 10–15 mg/kg q8h.

Drug Name (Trade or Other Names)	Pharmacology and Indications	Adverse Effects and Precautions	Dosing Information and Comments	Formulations	Dosage
Primor (Ormetoprim + Sulfadimethoxine) (Primor)	Antibacterial drug. Ormetoprim inhibits bacterial dihydrofolate reductase, sulfonamide competes with PABA for synthesis of nucleic acids. Bactericidal/bacteriostatic. Broad antibacterial spectrum and active against some coccidia.	Several adverse effects have been reported from sulfonamides (See Trimethoprim/ Sulfonamides). No adverse effects reported from ormetoprim.	Doses listed are based manufacturer's recommendations. Controlled trials have demonstrated efficacy for treatment of pyoderma on once/daily schedule.	Combination tablet (ormetoprim + sulfadimethoxine).	27 mg/kg on first day, followed by 13.5 mg/kg q24h PO.
Procainamide (Pronestyl, Procanamide CR, generic)	Antiarrhythmic drug. Class-I antiarrhythmic used primarily for treatment of ventricular arrhythmias. Action is to inhibit sodium influx into cardiac cell via sodium channel blockade.	Adverse effects include cardiac arrhythmias, cardiac depression, tachycardia, and hypotension. In people, procainamide produces hypersensitivity effects (Lupus-like reactions), but these have not been reported in animals. *Drug interactions:* Cimetidine may increase plasma concentrations.	Since dogs do not produce active metabolite (N-acetyl procainamide), dose may be higher to control some arrhythmias, compared to people. Monitor plasma concentrations during chronic therapy (effective plasma concentrations in experimental dogs are 20 mcg/mL). In animals, there is no evidence that slow-release oral formulations produce longer duration of sustained blood concentraions.	250, 375, 500 mg tablet or capsule; 100, 500 mg/mL injection.	Dog: 10–30 mg/kg q6h PO (q8h for CR-continuous release), (to a maximum dose of 40 mg/kg), 8–20 mg/kg IV, IM; 25–50 mcg/kg/ min IV infusion. Cat: 3–8 mg/kg IM PO q6–8h.
Prochlorperazine (Compazine)	Phenothiazine. Central-acting dopamine (D$_2$) antagonist. Used for sedation, tranquilization, and as antiemetic. Antiemetic action also may be related to α_2- and muscarinic blocking effects.	Causes sedation and other side effects attributed to other phenothiazines (see Acepromazine).	Used primarily as antiemetic in animals. Clinical trials are not available; doses are based primarily on extrapolation and anecdotal experience.	5, 10, 25 mg tablets (prochlorperazine maleate); 5 mg/mL injection (prochlorperazine edisylate).	0.1–0.5 mg/kg q6–8h IM SC.
Progesterone, repositol	See Medroxyprogesterone acetate (Depo-Provera).				
Promethazine (Phenergan)	Phenothiazine with strong antihistamine effects. Used for treatment of allergy and as antiemetic (motion sickness).	Adverse effects include sedation and antimuscarinic (atropine-like) effects. Both phenothiazine effects (see Acepromazine) and anticholinergic (see Atropine) effects are possible in some patients.	Results of clinical studies in animals have not been reported. Use in animals (and doses) is based on experience in people, or anecdotal experience in animals.	6.25 and 25 mg/5 mL syrup; 12.5, 25, 50 mg tablets; 25, 50 mg/mL injection.	0.2–0.4 mg/kg q6–8h IV, IM PO (up to a maximum dose of 1 mg/kg).
Propantheline bromide (Pro-Banthine)	Anticholinergic (antimuscarinic) drug. Blocks acetylcholine receptor to produce parasympatholytic effects (atropine-like effects). (See Atropine). Used to decrease smooth muscle contraction and secretion of gastrointestinal tract. Used to treat vagal-mediated cardiovascular effects.	Side effects are attributed to excess anticholinergic (antimuscarinic) effects (see Atropine). Treat overdoses with physostigmine.	Propantheline has not been evaluated in clinical trials in animals, but propantheline is often the drug of choice for oral therapy in cases in which an anticholinergic effect is desired.	7.5, 15 mg tablet.	0.25–0.5 mg/kg q8–12h PO.
Propiopromazine (Tranvet, Largon)	Phenothiazine sedative. Also has antiemetic, antihistaminic actions.	See other phenothiazines (Acepromazine).	Results of clinical studies in animals have not been reported. Use in animals (and doses) is based on experience in people, or anecdotal experience in animals.	20 mg/mL injection.	1.1–4.4 mg/kg q12–24h.

Drug Name (Trade or Other Names)	Pharmacology and Indications	Adverse Effects and Precautions	Dosing Information and Comments	Formulations	Dosage
Propofol (Rapinovet [veterinary]; Diprivan [human])	Anesthetic. Used for induction or producing short-term general anesthesia. Mechanism of action is not well-defined, but may be barbiturate-like. Propofol may be used as induction agent, followed by inhalation with halothane or isoflurane.	Apnea and respiratory depression is most common adverse effect. Adverse effects attributed to general anesthetic properties.	Propofol is primarily used for general anesthesia, or adjunct for general anesthesia. Propofol's advantage over other agents is smooth, rapid recovery. Use strict aseptic technique for administration. Propofol may be diluted in 5% dextrose, lactated Ringer's solution, and 0.9% saline, but not to less than 2 mg/mL concentration.	1% (10 mg/mL) injection in 20 mL ampules.	6.6 mg/kg IV slowly over 60 sec. Constant rate IV infusions have been used at 2 mg/kg/hr.
Propranolol (Inderal)	β-adrenergic blocker. Nonselective for β_1- and β_2- adrenergic receptors. Class-II antiarrhythmic. Used primarily to decrease heart rate, decrease cardiac conduction, tachyarrhythmias, and decrease blood pressure.	Adverse effects related to β_1-blocking effects on heart. Causes cardiac depression, decreases cardiac output. β_2-blocking effects can cause bronchoconstriction. Decreases insulin secretion.	Usually dose is titrated according to patient's response. Start with low dose and increase gradually to desired effect. Clearance relies on hepatic blood flow; use cautiously in animals with impaired hepatic perfusion.	10, 20, 40, 60 , 80, and 90 mg tablet; 1 mg/mL injection; 4 and 8 mg/mL oral solution.	Dog: 20–60 mcg/kg over 5–10 min IV, 0.2–1 mg/kg PO q8h (titrate dose to effect). Cat: 0.4–1.2 mg/kg (2.5–5 mg/cat) PO q8h.
Propylthiouracil (PTU) (generic, Propyl-Thyracil)	Antithyroid drug. See Methimazole. Compared to methimizole, PTU inhibits conversion of T-4 to T-3.	Adverse effects in cats include hemolytic anemia, thrombocytopenia, and other signs of immune-mediated disease. (JAVMA 184: 806, 1984).	Use of PTU in most cats has been replaced with methimazole.	50 and 100 mg tablets.	11 mg/kg q12h PO.
Prostaglandin F-2α (Dinoprost) (Lutalyse)	Prostaglndin induces leutolysis. Has been used to treat open pyometra in animals. Use for inducing abortion has been questioned.	Side effects include vomiting, diarrhea, and abdominal discomfort.	Use in treating pyometra should be monitored carefully.	5 mg/mL solution for injection.	Pyometra (dog): 0.1–0.2 mg/kg, once daily for 5 days SC; (cat): 0.1–0.25 mg/kg, once daily for 5 days SC. Abortion (dog): 0.025–0.05 mg (25–50 mcg)/kg q12h IM; (cat): 0.5–1 mg/kg IM for 2 injections.
Pseudoephedrine (Sudafed, and many others [some formulations have other ingredients])	Adrenergic agonist. Similar to ephedrine, phenylpropanolamine in action. Used to increase peripheral resistance, as a decongestant, and in animals to treat urinary incontinence.	Side effects attributed to adrenergic effects (excitement, rapid heart rate, arrhythmias) (see Ephedrine, Phenylpropanolamine).	Although clinical trials have not been conducted for comparison, it is believed that pseudoephridine's action and efficacy is similar to ephedrine and phenylpropanolamine.	30, 60 mg tablets; 120 mg capsules; 6 mg/mL syrup.	0.2–0.4 mg/kg (or 15–60 mg/dog) q8–12h PO.
Psyllium (Metamucil, and others)	Bulk-forming laxative. Use for treatment of constipation and bowel evacuation. Action is to absorb water and expand to provide increased bulk and moisture content to the stool, which encourages normal peristalsis and bowel motility.	Adverse effects have not been reported in animals. Intestinal impaction can occur with overuse, or in patients with inadequate fluid intake.	Results of clinical studies in animals have not been reported. Use in animals (and doses) is based on experience in people, or anecdotal experience in animals.	Available as powder.	1 tsp/5–10 kg (added to each meal).
Pyrantel pamoate (Nemex, Strongid)	Antiparasitic drug. Acts to block ganglionic neurotransmission via cholinergic action.	No adverse effects reported.	Dose recommendations based on manufacturer's recommendations.	180 mg/mL paste, and 50 mg/mL suspension.	Dog: 5 mg/kg once PO and repeat in 7–10 days. Cat: 20 mg/kg once PO.

Drug Name (Trade or Other Names)	Pharmacology and Indications	Adverse Effects and Precautions	Dosing Information and Comments	Formulations	Dosage
Pyridostigmine bromide (Mestinon, Regonol)	Anticholinesterase. Same as for neostigmine, except that pyridostigmine has longer duration of action.	Same as for neostigmine, except that adverse effects may persist longer. *Drug interactions:* Since this product contains bromide, use cautiously in patients already receiving bromide (such as potassium bromide for epilepsy.)	Same as for neostigmine.	12 mg/mL oral syrup; 60 mg tablets; 5 mg/mL injection.	Antimyasthenic: 0.02–0.04 mg/kg q2h IV, or 0.5–3 mg/kg q8–12h PO. Antidote for muscle blockade: 0.15–0.3 mg/kg IM, IV.
Pyridoxine	Vitamin B$_6$				
Pyrimethamine (Daraprim)	Antibacterial, antiprotozoal drug. Blocks dihydrofolate reductase enzyme, which inhibits synthesis of reduced folate and nucleic acids. Activity of pyrimethamine is more specific against protozoa than bacteria.	When administered with trimethoprim sulfonamide combinations, anemia has been observed. Folic or folinic acid has been supplemented to prevent anemia, but benefit of this treatment is unclear.	Used either alone or in combination with sulfonamides.	25 mg tablets.	Dog: 1 mg/kg q24h PO for 14–21 days (5 days for *Neosporum caninum*). Cat: 0.5–1 mg/kg q24h PO for 14–28 days.
Quibron	See Theophylline.				
Quinacrine (Atabrine (No longer available in U.S.))	Outdated antimalarial drug. Used occasionally for treatment of protozoa (Giardia). Inhibits nucleic acid synthesis in parasite.	Side effects are common. Vomiting occurs after oral administration.	Doses listed are for treatment of Giardia.	100 mg tablet.	Dog: 6.6 mg/kg q12h PO for 5 days. Cat: 11 mg/kg q24h PO for 5 days.
Quinidine gluconate (Quiniglute, Duraquin)	Antiarrhythmic drug. Class-I antiarrhythmic. Action is to inhibit sodium influx via blockade of sodium channels. Used to treat ventricular arrhythmias and occasionally atrial fibrillation.	Side effects with quinidine are more common than procainamide and include nausea and vomiting. Adverse effects: hypotension, tachycardia (due to antivagal effect). *Drug Interactions:* Co-administration with digoxin may increase digoxin concentrations.	Quinidine is not used as commonly as other Class-I antiarrhytmic drugs. Doses calculated according to amount of quinidine base in each product. 324 mg quinidine gluconate = 202 mg quinidine base.	324 mg tablets; 80 mg/mL injection.	Dog: 6–20 mg/kg q6h IM; 6–20 mg/kg q6–8h PO (of base).
Quinidine polygalacturonate (Cardioquin)	Same as quinidine gluconate.	Same as quinidine gluconate.	Doses calculated according to amount of quinidine base in each product.	275 mg tablets.	Dog: 6–20 mg/kg q6h PO (of base) (275 mg quinidine polygalacturonate = 167 mg quinidine base).
Quinidine sulfate (Cin-Quin, Quinora)	Same as quinidine gluconate.	Same as quinidine gluconate.	Doses calculated according to amount of quinidine base in each product. 300 mg quinidine sulfate = 250 mg quinidine base.	100, 200, 300 mg tablets; 200, 300 mg capsules; 200 mg/mL injection.	Dog: 6–20 mg/kg q6–8h PO (of base); 5–10 mg/kg IV.
Racemethionine (dl methionine) (Uroeze, Methio-Form, and generic. Human forms include Pedameth, Uracid, and generic)	Urinary acidifer. Lowers urinary pH. Also has been used to protect against acetaminophen overdose in people, by restoring hepatic concentrations of glutathione. In people, it also is used to treat dermatitis caused by urinary incontinence (reduces urine ammonia).	Adverse effects have not been reported. Do not use in patients with metabolic acidosis or hepatic function impairment. Do not use in young cats.	Used for urinary acidification. Use for acetaminophen toxicity has been replaced by acetylcysteine.	500 mg tablets, powders added to animal's food; 75 mg/5 mL pediatric oral solution; 200 mg capsules.	Dog: 150–300 mg/kg/day PO. Cat: 1–1.5 gm/cat PO (added to food each day).

Drug Name (Trade or Other Names)	Pharmacology and Indications	Adverse Effects and Precautions	Dosing Information and Comments	Formulations	Dosage
Ranitidine (Zantac)	H-2 antagonist. See Cimetidine for details. Same as cimetidine except 4–10× more potent and longer-acting.	See Cimetidine. Ranitidine may have fewer effects on endocrine function and drug interactions, compared to cimetidine.	See Cimetidine. Pharmacokinetic information in dogs suggests that ranitidine may be administered less often than cimetidine to achieve continuous suppression of stomach acid secretion. Ranitidine may stimulate stomach emptying and colon motility via anticholinesterase action.	75, 150, 300 mg tablets; 150, 300 mg capsules; 25 mg/mL injection.	Dog: 2 mg/kg q8h IV, PO. Cat: 2.5 mg/kg q12h IV, 3.5 mg/kg q12h PO.
Retinoids	See Isotretinoin (Accutane), Retinol (Aquasol-A), or Etretinate (Tegison).				
Retinol	See Vitamin A (Aquasol-A).				
Riboflavin (Vitamin B$_2$)	See Vitamin B$_2$.				
Rifampin (Rifadin)	Antibacterial. Action is to inhibit bacterial RNA synthesis. Spectrum of action includes staphylococci and Mycobacteria. Other susceptible bacteria include streptococci and Mycobacterium. Used in people primarily for treatment of tuberculosis.	Adverse effects not reported in animals. But, in people, hypersensitivity and flu-like symptoms are reported. Drug interactions: Multiple drug interactions are possible. Induces P-450 enzymes. Drugs affected include barbiturates, chloramphenicol, and corticosteroids.	Results of clinical studies in animals have not been reported. Use in animals (and doses) is based on experience in people, or anecdotal experience in animals. Rifampin is highly lipid-soluble and has been used to treat intracellular infections. Administer on an empty stomach.	150, 300 mg capsules;	10–20 mg/kg q24h PO.
Ringer's solution (generic)	IV solution for replacement.	Monitor pulmonary pressure when infusing high doses.	When administering IV fluid solution, monitor rate carefully and electrolyte concentrations.	250, 500, 1000 mL bags for infusion.	40–50 mg/kg day IV, SC, IP.
Salicylate	See Acetylsalicylic acid (Aspirin).				
Selegiline (Deprenyl) (Anipryl [also known as deprenyl, and l-deprenyl], human dose form is Eldepryl)	Action is to inhibit specific monoamine oxidase (MAO type B). Specifically, it appears to inhibit degradation of dopamine in CNS. In people, it is primarily used to treat Parkinson's disease and other neurodegenerative disease (in combination with levodopa). In dogs, it is approved to control clinical signs of pituitary-dependent hyperadrenocorticism (Cushing's Disease) and to treat cognitive dysfunction in geriatric dogs.	Adverse effects have not been reported in dogs. However, amphetamine-like signs can be produced in experimental animals. At high doses in dogs, hyperactivity has been observed (doses > 3 mg/kg).	In dogs, selegiline controlled the clinical signs of >70% of dogs with hyperadrenocorticism. Approximately 20% of dogs failed to respond.	2, 5, 10, 15, and 30 mg tablets.	Dogs: Begin with 1 mg/kg q24h PO. If there is no response within 2 months, increase dose to maximum of 2 mg/kg q24h PO. Cats: dose not established.
Senna (Senokot)	Laxative. Acts via local stimulation or via contact with intestinal mucosa.	Adverse effects not reported for animals.	Doses and indications are not well-established for veterinary medicine. Use is strictly through anecdotal experience.	Granules in concentrate, or syrup.	Cat (syrup): 5 mL/cat q24h; (granules) 1/2 teaspoon per cat q24h (with food).
Septra (sulfmethoxazole + trimethoprim) See Trimethoprim/ sulfonamides (Tribrissen)					

Drug Name (Trade or Other Names)	Pharmacology and Indications	Adverse Effects and Precautions	Dosing Information and Comments	Formulations	Dosage
Sodium bicarbonate (NaHCO₃) (generic, Baking Soda, Soda Mint)	Alkalizing agent. Antacid. Used to treat systemic acidosis or to alkalize urine. Increase plasma and urinary concentrations of bicarbonate.	Adverse effects attributed to alkalizing activity. *Drug interactions:* When administered orally, interaction may occur to decrease absorption of other drugs (partial list includes anticholinergic drugs, ketoconazole, fluoroquinolones, tetracyclines).	When used for systemic acidosis, doses should be adjusted on basis of blood gas measurements or assessment of acidosis. Doses vary depending on underlying condition (see dose section). Note: 8.5% solution = 1 mEq/mL of NaHCO₃.	325, 520, 650 mg tablets; injection of various strengths (4.2% to 8.4%), and 1 mEq/mL.	Acidosis: 0.5–1 mEq/kg IV. Renal failure: 10 mg/kg q8–12h PO. Alkalization of urine: 50 mg/kg q8–12h PO (1 teaspoon is approximately 2 gm).
Sodium chloride (0.9%) (generic)	Sodium chloride is used for IV infusion as replacement fluid.	Not a balanced electrolyte solution. Long-term infusion may cause electrolyte imbalace.	Rate of infusion varies, depending on patient needs.	500, 1000 mL infusion.	40–50 mL/kg/day IV, SC, IP.
Sodium chloride 7.5% (generic)	Concentrated sodium chloride used for acute treatment of hypovolemia.	Not a balanced electrolyte solution. Long-term infusion may cause electrolyte imbalace.	Hypertonic saline is used for short-term infusion for rapid replacement of vascular volume.	Infusion.	2–8 mL/kg IV.
Sodum iodide (20%) (Iodopen, generic)	Used to treat iodine deficiency.	Overuse causes iodism (burning of mouth, gastric irritation, skin lesions).		100 mcg elemental iodide (118 mcg sodium iodide) per mL injection.	20–40 mg/kg q8–12h PO.
Sodium thiomalate	See Gold sodium thiomalate.				
Somatrem Somatropin	See Growth hormone.				
Sotalol (Betapace)	Nonspecific β (β₁ and β₂) adrenergic blocker (Class-II antiarrhythmic). Action is similar to propranolol (1/3 potency); however, its beneficial effect may be caused more by the other antiarrhythmic effects. In addition to being a Class-II antiarrhythmic drug, sotalol may have some Class-III (potassium-channel blocking) activity.	Adverse effects have not been reported for animals, but are expected to be similar to propranolol. Like many antiarrhythmics, it may have some pro-arrhythmic activity. Negative inotropic effects may cause concern in some animals with poor contractility.	There is little reported use in veterinary medicine, but in some animals it has been a beneficial antiarrhythmic, e.g., animals with cardiomyopathy. In people, it may be a more effective maintenance agent for controlling arrhythmias than other drugs.	80, 160, 240 mg.	Dogs: 1–2 mg/kg q12h PO. (Begin with 40 mg/dog q12h, then increase to 80 mg if no response.) Cats: 1–2 mg/kg q12h, PO.
Spironolactone (Aldactone)	Potassium-sparing diuretic. Action is to interfere with sodium reabsorption in distal renal tubule. Spironolactone competitively inhibits the action of aldosterone. Used for treating high blood pressure, and congestion caused by heart failure.	Can produce hyperkalemia in some patients. Do not use in dehydrated patients. *Drug interactions:* NSAIDs may interfere with action. Avoid supplements that are high in potassium.	Spironolactone usually is used with diuretic agent when used for CHF.	25, 50, 100 mg tablets.	2–4 mg/kg/day (or 1–2 mg/kg q12h) PO.
Stanozolol (Winstrol-V)	Anabolic steroid. Stanozolol has been used to decrease negative nitrogen balance in animals with chronic renal failure. There are no documented differences in efficacy among the anabolic steroids. (See Nandrolone.)	See Nandrolone.	See Nandrolone.	50 mg/mL injection; 2 mg tablets.	Dogs: 2 mg/dog (or range of 1–4 mg/dog) q12h PO; 25–50 mg/dog/ week IM. Cats: 1 mg/cat q12h PO; 25 mg/cat/week IM.

Drug Name (Trade or Other Names)	Pharmacology and Indications	Adverse Effects and Precautions	Dosing Information and Comments	Formulations	Dosage
Succimer (Chemet)	Used in treatment of lead toxicosis. Chelates lead and other heavy metals, such as mercury and arsenic.	No known adverse effects.	Doses based studies in dogs. (JAVMA 208: 371, 1996)	100 mg capsule.	10 mg/kg q8h, PO for 5 days, then 10 mg/kg q12h PO for 2 more weeks.
Sucralfate (Carafate, [Sulcrate in Canada])	Gastric mucosa protectant. Antiulcer agent. Action of sucralfate is to bind to ulcerated tissue in gastrointestinal tract to aid healing of ulcers. There is some evidence that sucralfate may act as a cytoprotectant (via prostaglandin synthesis). Used to treat or prevent ulcers.	Adverse effects have not been reported. Not absorbed systemically. Drug interactions: Sucralfate may decrease absorption of other orally administered drugs via chelation with aluminum (such as fluoroquinolones and tetracyclines).	Dosing recommendations are based largely on empiricism. There have not been clinical trials of efficacy in animals with sucralfate. Sucralfate may be administered concurrently with histamine type-2 inhibitors (e.g., cimetidine).	1 gm tablets; 200 mg/mL oral suspension.	Dog: 0.5–1 gm q8–12h PO. Cat: 0.25 gm q8–12h PO.
Sufentanil citrate (Sufenta)	Opiod agonist. Action of fentanyl derivatives is via μ-receptor. See Fentanyl, Morphine. Sufentanil is 5–7× more potent than fentanyl. 13 to 20 mcg of sufentanil produces analgesia equal to 10 mg of morphine.	Adverse effects similar to other opiates (see Morphine).	When used for anesthesia, often animals are premedicated with acepromazine or benzodiazepine.	50 mcg/mL injection.	2 mcg/kg IV, up to a maximum dose of 5 mcg/kg.
Sulfadiazine (generic, combined with trimethoprim in Tribrissen)	Sulfonamides compete with PABA for enzyme that synthesizes dihydrofolic acid in bacteria. Synergistic with trimethoprim. Broad spectrum of activity, including some protozoa. Bacteriostatic.	Adverse effects associated with sulfonamides include: allergic reactions, Type-II and III hypersensitivity, hypothyroidism (with prolonged therapy), keratoconjunctivitis sicca, and skin reactions.	Usually, sulfonamides are combined with trimethoprim or ormetoprim in 5:1 ratio. There is no clinical evidence that one sulfonamide is more or less toxic or efficacious than another sulfonamide.	500 mg tablets.	100 mg/kg IV, PO (loading dose), followed by 50 mg/kg q12h IV, PO (see also Trimethoprim).
Sulfadimethoxine (Albon, Bactrovet, and generic)	See Sulfadiazine.	See Sulfadiazine.	See Sulfadiazine. Sulfadimethoxine has been combined with ormetoprim in Primor.	125, 250, 500 mg tablets; 400 mg/mL injection; 50 mg/mL suspension.	55 mg/kg PO (loading dose), followed by 27.5 mg/kg q12h PO.
Sulfamethazine (many brands [e.g., Sulmet])	See Sulfadiazine.	See Sulfadiazine.	See Sulfadiazine.	30 gm bolus.	100 mg/kg PO (loading dose), followed by 50 mg/kg q12h PO.
Sulfamethoxazole (Gantanol)	See Sulfadiazine.	See Sulfadiazine.	See Sulfadiazine.	500 mg tablets.	100 mg/kg PO (loading dose), followed by 50 mg/kg q12h PO.
Sulfasalazine (Sulfapyridine + Mesalamine) (Azulfidine [Salazopyrin in Canada])	Sulfonamide + anti-inflammatory drug. Used for treatment of colitis. Sulfonamide has little effect, salicylic acid (mesalamine) has anti-inflammatory effects (see Mesalamine).	Adverse effects are all attributed to sulfonamide component. (See Sulfadiazine.) Keratoconjunctivitis sicca has been reported.	Usually used for treatment of idiopathic colitis, often in combination with dietary therapy.	500 mg tablet.	10–30 mg/kg q12h PO (see also Mesalamine, Olsalazine).
Sulfisoxazole (Gantrisin)	See Sulfadiazine. Sulfisoxizole is primarily used only for treating urinary tract infections.	See Sulfadiazine.	See Sulfadiazine.	500 mg tablets; 500 mg/5 mL syrup.	50 mg/kg q8h PO (urinary tract infections).
Tamoxifen (Nolvadex)	Nonsteroid estrogen receptor blocker. Also has weak estrogenic effects. Tamoxifen may also increase release of GNRH. Used as adjunctive treatment for certain tumors.	Adverse effects have not been thoroughly documented in animals. However, in people, tamoxifen causing increased tumor pain has been reported. Do not use in pregnant animals. Drug Interactions: Reacts with antiulcer drugs.	Consult specific anti-cancer protocols for doses and regimens.	10 mg tablets (tamoxifen citrate).	Veterinary dose not established. Human dose is 10 mg q12h PO.

Drug Name (Trade or Other Names)	Pharmacology and Indications	Adverse Effects and Precautions	Dosing Information and Comments	Formulations	Dosage
Taurine (generic)	Nutritional supplement for cats. Used in prevention and treatment of ocular and cardiac disease (cardiomyopathy) caused by taurine deficiency.	Adverse effects have not been reported.	Routine supplementation with taurine may not be necessary in cats that are receiving a balanced diet.	Available in powder.	Dog: 500 mg q12h PO. Cat: 250 mg per cat q12h PO.
Telezol	See Tiletamine.				
Terbutaline (Brethine, Bricanyl)	β-adrenergic agonist. β_2-specific. Used primarily for bronchodilation. See Albuterol for further details.	Adverse effects related to excessive β-adrenergic stimulation. See Albuterol for list of adverse effects.	Used primarily for bronchodilation. May be administered orally, IM, or SC. Terbutaline (and other β_2-agonists) have also been used in people to delay labor (dose in people is 2.5 mg q6h, PO).	2.5, 5 mg tablets, 1 mg/mL injection (equivalent to 0.82 mg/mL).	Dog: 1.25–5 mg/dog q8h PO or 3–5 mcg/kg SC. Cat: 0.1–0.2 mg/kg q12h SC, (or 0.625 mg/cat, (1/4 of 2.5 mg tablet) q12h PO.
Terfenadine	Seldene: No longer available.				
Testosterone cypionate ester (Andro-Cyp, Andronate, Depo-Testosterone, and other forms)	Testosterone ester. Similar effects as methyltestosterone. Testosterone esters are administered IM to avoid first-pass effects. Esters in oil are absorbed more slowly from IM injection. Esters are then hydrolyzed to free testosterone.	See Testosterone, Methyltestosterone.	See Methyltestosterone.	100, 200 mg/mL injection.	1–2 mg/kg q2–4weeks IM (see also Methyltestosterone).
Testosterone propionate ester (Testex, [Malogen in Canada])	Testosterone ester for injection. Similar effects as methyltestosterone. Testosterone esters are administered IM to avoid first-pass effects. Esters in oil are absorbed more slowly from IM injection. Esters are then hydrolyzed to free testosterone.	See Testosterone, Methyltestosterone.	See Methyltestosterone.	100 mg/mL injection.	0.5–1 mg/kg 2–3 times/week IM.
Tetracycline (Panmycin)	Tetracyine antibiotic. Mechanism of action of tetracyclines is to bind to 30S ribosomal subunit and inhibit protein synthesis. Usually bacteriostatic. Broad spectrum of activity including bacteria, some protozoa, Rickettsia, Ehrlichia.	Tetracyclines in general may cause renal tubular necrosis at high doses. Tetracyclines can affect bone and teeth formation in young animals. Tetracyclines have been implicated in drug fever in cats. Hepatotoxicity may occur at high doses in susceptible individuals. *Drug interactions:* Tetracyclines bind to calcium-containing compounds, which decreases oral absorption.	Pharmacokinetic and experimental studies have been conducted in small animals, but no clinical studies. Do not use outdated solutions.	250, 500 mg capsule; 100 mg/mL suspension.	15–20 mg/kg q8h PO; or 4.4–11 mg/kg q8h, IV, IM.
Thenium closylate (Canopar)	Antiparasitic drug. Used to treat hookworms (Ancylostoma and Uncinaria).	Tablet is bitter if coating is broken. May cause occasional vomiting after oral administration.	Doses listed are based on recommendations from manufacturer.	500 mg tablets.	Dogs >4.5 kg: 500 mg PO once, repeat in 2–3 weeks; 2.5–4.5 kg: 250 mg q12h for one day, repeat in 2–3 weeks.

Drug Name (Trade or Other Names)	Pharmacology and Indications	Adverse Effects and Precautions	Dosing Information and Comments	Formulations	Dosage
Theophylline (many brands and generic)	Methylxanthine bronchodilator. Mechanism of action is unknown, but may be related to increased cyclic-AMP, or antagonism of adenosine. There appears to be anti-inflammatory action as well as bronchodilating action.	Adverse effects: nausea, vomiting, diarrhea. With high doses, tachycardia, excitement, tremors, and seizures are possible. Cardiovascular and CNS adverse effects appear to be less frequent in dogs than in people.	Plasma concentrations of theophylline should be monitored in patients receiving chronic therapy to maintain plasma concentrations between 10 and 20 mcg/mL. Doses for slow-release tablets are unique for each product (see Theophylline sustained release and Aminophylline).	100, 125, 200, 250, 300 mg tablets; 27 mg/5 mL oral solution or elixir; injection in 5% dextrose	Dog: 9 mg/kg q6–8h PO. Cat: 4 mg/kg q8–12h PO (see also Aminophylline).
Theophylline sustained-release (Theo-Dur, Slo-bid, Gyrocaps)	Same as theophylline. Sustained-release preparations are used to decrease frequency of administration.	Same as theophylline	Same as theophylline.	100, 200, 300, and 450 mg tablets (Theo-Dur); 50–200 mg capsules (Slo-Bid).	Dog: 20 mg/kg q12h (Theo-Dur); 30 mg/kg q12h (Slo-Bid) PO. Cat: 25 mg/kg q24h (at night) for Theo-Dur and Slo-Bid, PO.
Thiabendazole (Omnizole, Equizole)	Benzimidazole anthelmintic. (See Fenbendazole, Albendazole).	Adverse effects uncommon.	Ordinarily administered to horses and cattle. Experience in small animals is limited.	2 or 4 gm per oz (30 mL) suspension or liquid.	Dog: 50 mg/kg q24h for 3 days, repeat in 1 month; respiratory parasites: 30–70 mg/kg q12h PO. Cat: (Strongyloides): 125 mg/kg q24h for 3 days.
Thiacetarsamide sodium (Caparsolate)	Organic arsenical used for treatment of heartworm infections. Adulticide.	Adverse effects are common, especially anorexia, vomiting, hepatic injury. Pulmonary thromboembolism may occur as consequence of heartworm kill.	Thiacetarsamide is administered via 4 injections over 2 days; however, if severe adverse effects are observed, discontinue regimen. Melarsomine is considered by many experts safer, and has replaced thiacetarsamide for routine treatment.	10 mg/mL.	Dog: 2.2 mg/kg IV twice daily for two days. Cat: Not recommended.
Thiamine (Vitamin B₁) (Bewon and others)	Vitamin B₁ used for treatment of vitamin deficiency.	Adverse effects are rare because water-soluble vitamins are easily excreted. Riboflavin may discolor the urine.	Vitamin B supplements are administered often in combination.	250 mcg/5 mL elixir; tablets of various size from 5 mg to 500 mg; 100 and 500 mg/mL injection.	Dog: 10–100 mg/dog/day PO. Cat: 5–30 mg/cat/day PO (up to a maximum dose of 50 mg/cat/day).
Thiamylal sodium (Surital, Bio-Tal)	No longer available in U.S. Use has been replaced by thiopental.				
Thioguanine (6-TG) (generic)	Anticancer agent. Antimetabolite of purine analog type. Inhibits DNA synthesis in cancer cells.	Adverse effects, as with any anticancer drugs, are expected (see Mercaptopurine). Immunosuppression and leukopenia are common.	Thioguanine is often combined with other agents for treatment of cancer. Consult specific reference on cancer therapy for guidance.	40 mg tablets.	Dog: 40 mg/m² q24h PO. Cat: 25 mg/m², PO q24h, × 1–5 days, then repeat every 30 days.
Thiomalate sodium	See Gold sodium thiomalate.				
Thiopental sodium (Pentothal)	Ultra-short acting barbiturate. Used primarily for induction of anesthesia or for short duration of anesthesia (10–15 min procedures). Anesthesia is produced by CNS depression, without analgesia. Anesthesia is terminated by redistribution in the body.	Adverse effects are related to the anesthetic effects of the drug. Severe adverse effects are caused by respiratory and cardiovascular depression. Overdoses are caused by rapid or repeated injections. Avoid extravasation outside of vein.	Therapeutic index is low. Use only in patients in which it is possible to monitor cardiovascular and respiratory functions. Often administered with other anesthetic adjuncts.	Various size vials from 250 mg to 10 gm. (Mix to desired concentration.)	Dog: 10–25 mg/kg IV (to effect). Cat: 5–10 mg/kg IV (to effect).

Drug Name (Trade or Other Names)	Pharmacology and Indications	Adverse Effects and Precautions	Dosing Information and Comments	Formulations	Dosage
Thiotepa (generic)	Anticancer agent. Alkalylating agent of the nitrogen mustard type (similar to cyclophosphamide). Used for various tumors, especially malignant effusions.	Adverse effects are similar to other anticancer agents and alkylating drugs (many of which are unavoidable). Bone marrow suppression is the most common effect.	One should consult specific cancer chemotherapy protocol for guidance on administration. Thiotepa usually is administered directly in body cavities.	15 mg injection (usually in solution of 10 mg/mL).	$0.2–0.5$ mg/m^2 weekly, or daily for 5–10 days IM, intracavitary, or intratumor.
Thyroid hormone	See Levothyroxine and Liothyronine.				
Thyroid releasing hormone (TRH) (TRH)	Used to detect hyperthyroidism when T4 is not elevated.		Used for diagnostic purposes.	Injection.	Collect baseline T4, followed by 0.1 mg/kg IV. Collect post-TRH T4 sample at 4 hours.
Thyrotropin, Thyroid-stimulating hormone (TSH) (Thytropar)	Thyroid-stimulating hormone is used for diagnostic testing. Stimulates normal secretion of thyroid hormone.	Adverse reactions rare. In people, allergic reactions have occurred.	To prepare solution, add 2 ml NaCL to 10-U vial. Reconstituted solutions retain potency for 2 weeks at 2–8°C. Consult testing laboratory for specific guidelines for thyroid testing.	10-U vial.	Dogs: Collect baseline sample, followed by 0.1 U/kg UIV (maximum dose is 5 U); collect post-TSH sample at 6 h.
Ticarcillin (Ticar, Ticillin)	β-lactam antibiotic. Action similar to ampicillin/amoxicillin. Spectrum similar to carbenicillin. Ticarcillin is primarily used for Gram-negative infections, especially those caused by Pseudomonas.	Adverse effects are uncommon. However allergic reactions are possible. High doses can produce seizures, and decreased platelet function. Drug interactions: Do not combine in same syringe or in vial with aminoglycosides.	Ticarcillin is synergistic with, and often combined with aminoglycosides (e.g., amikacin, gentamicin). 1% lidocaine may be used for reconstitution to decrease pain from IM injection.	6 gm/50 mL vial; vials containing 1, 3, 6, 20, and 30 gm.	33–50 mg/kg q4–6h IV, IM
Ticarcillin + Clavulanate (Timentin)	Same as ticarcillin, except clavulanic acid has been added to inhibit bacterial beta-lactamase and increase spectrum. Clavulanate does not increase activity against Pseudomonas, however.	Same as ticarcillin.	Same as ticarcillin.	3 gm per vial for injection.	Dose according to rate for ticarcillin.
Tiletamine + zolazepam (Telezol, Zoletil)	Anesthetic. Combination of tiletamine (dissociative anesthetic agent similar in action to ketamine) and zolazepam (benzodiazepine similar in action as diazepam). Produces short duration (30 min) of anesthesia.	Wide margin of safety. Side effects include excessive salivation (may be antagonized with atropine), erratic recovery, and muscle twitching.	Administer by deep intramuscular injection. (Consult manufacturer's package insert for dosing information for dogs and cats.)	50 mg of each component per mL.	5–7 mg/kg IM.
Tobramycin (Nebcin)	Aminoglycoside antibacterial drug. Similar mechanism of action and spectrum as amikacin, gentamicin.	Adverse effects similar as amikacin, gentamicin.	Dosing requirements vary depending on bacterial susceptibility. See dose schedules for gentamicin and amikacin.	40 mg/mL injection.	2–4 mg/kg q8h IV, IM, SC.
Tocanide (Tonocard)	Antiarrhythmic drug. Considered an oral analog of lidocaine. Class-I antiarrhythmic.	In dogs, anorexia and gastrointestinal toxicity have been reported. Arrhythmias, vomiting, ataxia also are possible. (In one study, 35% of dogs showed GI effects.)	Limited experience in animals. However, clinical studies demonstrate efficacy. Therapeutic concentrations are 6–10 mcg/mL.	400, 600 mg tablets.	Dog: 15–20 mg/kg q8h PO. Cat: no dose established.

Drug Name (Trade or Other Names)	Pharmacology and Indications	Adverse Effects and Precautions	Dosing Information and Comments	Formulations	Dosage
Trandolapril (Mavik)	Angiotensin-converting enzyme (ACE) inhibitor. Similar in mechanism as captopril and enalapril. Used for management of CHF Converted to active trandolaprilat after administration.	Same adverse effects as for other ACE inhibitors.	Not used extensively in veterinary patients.	1, 2, 4 mg tablets.	Not established for dogs. Dose in people is 1 mg/person/day to start, then increase to 2–4 mg/day.
Triamcinolone (Vetalog, Trimtabs, Aristocort, generic)	Glucocorticoid anti-inflammatory drug. See Betamethasone for details. Triamcinolone has potency that is approximately equal to methylprednisolone (about 5× cortisol and 1.25× prednisolone), although some dermatologists suggest that potency is higher.	Adverse effects are similar to other corticosteroids (see β-methasone).	See Prednisolone. Note that cats may require higher doses than dogs (sometimes 2×).	Veterinary (Vetalog) 0.5 and 1.5 mg tablets. Human form: 1, 2, 4, 8, 16 mg tablets; 10 mg/mL injection.	Anti-inflammatory: 0.5–1 mg/kg q12–24h PO, then taper dose to 0.5–1 mg/kg q48h PO. (However, manufacturer recommends doses of 0.11 to 0.22 mg/kg/day.)
Triamcinolone acetonide (Vetalog)	Same as for triamcinolone, except that injectable suspension is slowly absorbed from IM, or intralesional injection site. Used for intralesional therapy of tumors and similar purposes as methylprednisolone acetate.	See Methylprednisolone acetate. When used for ocular injections, there is some concern that granulomas may occur at injection site.	See Prednisolone.	2 or 6 mg/mL suspension injection. 0.5 and 1.5 mg tablets.	0.1–0.2 mg/kg IM, SC, repeat in 7–10 days. Intralesional: 1.2–1.8 mg, or 1 mg for every cm diameter of tumor q2weeks.
Triamterene (Dyrenium)	Potassium-sparing diuretic. Similar action as spironolactone, except that spironolactone has competitive inhibiting effect of aldosterone, triamterene does not.	See Spironolactone.	Little clinical experience available for triamterene. There is no convincing evidence that triamterene is more effective than spironolactone.	50, 100 mg capsules.	1–2 mg/kg q12h PO.
Tribrissen	See Trimethoprim + sulfonamides.				
Trientine hydrochloride (Syprine)	Chelating agent. Used to chelate copper when penicillamine cannot be tolerated in a patient.	Adverse effects have not been reported in animals.	Used only in patients that cannot tolerate penicillamine. Generally induces less cupriuresis than penicillamine.	250 mg capsules.	10–15 mg/kg q12h PO.
Trifluoperazine (Stelezine)	Phenothiazine. Used for treatment of anxiety, to produce sedation, antiemetic. Action is believed to be via antagonism of dopamine (similar to acepromazine), antiemetic action may be via antimuscarinic action.	Adverse effects not reported in animals, but are expected to be similar to other phenothiazines. See Acepromazine, Prochlorperazine.	Results of clinical studies in animals have not been reported. Use in animals (and doses) is based on experience in people, or anecdotal experience in animals.	10 mg/mL oral solution; 1, 2, 5, 10 mg tablets; 2 mg/mL injection.	0.03 mg/kg IM q12h.
Triflupromazine (Vesprin)	Phenothiazine. Similar action as other phenothiazines, except triflupromazine may have stronger antimuscarinic activity than other phenothiazines. Used for antiemetic action.	Adverse effects have not been reported in animals. Adverse effects possible include anticholinergic effects.	Same as other phenothiazines.	10, 20 mg/mL injection.	0.1–0.3 mg/kg IM PO q8–12h.
Tri-iodothyronine	See Liothyronine.				

Drug Name (Trade or Other Names)	Pharmacology and Indications	Adverse Effects and Precautions	Dosing Information and Comments	Formulations	Dosage
Trimeprazine tartrate (Temaril [Panectyl in Canada])	Phenothiazine with antihistamine activity (similar to promethazine). Used for treating allergies and motion sickness.	Adverse effects similar to promethazine.	There is evidence that trimeprazine is more effective when combined with prednisone for treatment of pruritus. Combination product is Temaril-P.	2.5 mg/5 mL syrup, 2.5 mg tablet.	0.5 mg/kg q12h PO.
Trimethobenzamide (Tigan, and others)	Antiemetic. Mechanism of action is not understood.	Adverse effects not reported in animals.	Efficacy as antiemetic not reported in animals.	100 mg/mL injection; 100, 250 mg capsules.	Dog: 3 mg/kg q8h IM PO. Cat: not recommended.
Trimethoprim + sulfadiazine (Tribrissen, and others)	Combines the antibacterial drug action of trimethoprim and a sulfonamide. Together, the combination is synergistic, with a broad spectrum of activity.	Adverse effects primarily caused by sulfonamide component. (See Sulfadiazine.)	Dosage recommendations vary. There is evidence that 30 mg/kg/day is efficacious for pyoderma; for other infections, 30 mg/kg twice daily has been recommended.	30, 120, 240, 480, 960 mg tablet (all formulations have ratio of 5:1 sulfa:trimethoprim).	15 mg/kg q12h PO, or 30 mg/kg q12–24h PO (for Toxoplasma: 30 mg/kg q12h PO).
Trimethoprim + sulfamethoxazole (Bactrim, Septra, and generic forms)	Combines the antibacterial drug action of trimethoprim and a sulfonamide. Together, the combination is synergistic with a broad spectrum of activity.	Adverse effects primarily caused by sulfonamide component. (See Sulfadiazine.)	Dosage recommendations vary. There is evidence that 30 mg/kg/day is efficacious for pyoderma; for other infections, 30 mg/kg twice daily has been recommended.	480, 960 mg tablet; 240 mg/5 mL oral suspension (all formulations have ratio of 5:1 sulfa:trimethoprim).	15 mg/kg q12h PO, or 30 mg/kg q12–24h PO.
Tripelennamine (Pelamine, PBZ)	Antihistamine (H-1) blocker. Similar in action as other antihistamines (see Chlorpheniramine). Used to treat allergic disease.	Adverse effects similar to other antihistamines. See Chlorpheniramine. Members of this class (ethanolamines) have greater antimuscarinic effects than other antihistamines.	There are no clinical reports of use in veterinary medicine. No evidence that it is more efficacious than other drugs in this class.	25, 50 mg tablets. 20 mg/mL injection.	1 mg/kg q12h PO.
TSH (thyroid-stimulating hormone)	See Thyrotropin.				
Tylosin (Tylocine, Tylan, Tylosin tartrate)	Macrolide antibiotic. (See Erythromycin for mechanisms of action and spectrum of activity.)	May cause diarrhea in some animals. Do not administer orally to rodents or rabbits.	Tylosin is rarely used in small animals. Powdered formulation (tylosin tartrate) has been administered on food for control of signs of colitis in dogs. Tablets are approved for treatment of colitis in Canada.	Available as soluble powder 2.2 gm tylosin per teaspoon (tablets for dogs in Canada).	Dogs and cats: 7–15 mg/kg q12–24h PO. Dogs: (for colitis) 1 mg/kg, 1q8h with food.
Urofollitropin (FSH) (Metrodin)	Stimulates ovulation. Contains FSH. In people, it is used in combination with hCG to stimulate ovulation and induce pregnancy.	Side effects have not been reported in animals. In people, thromboembolism or severe ovarian hyperstimulation syndrome has been reported.	Results of clinical studies in animals have not been reported. Use in animals is based on experience in people.	75 U per vial for injection.	Doses not established.
Ursodiol (Ursodeoxycholate) (Actigall)	Hydrophilic bile acid. Anticholelithic. Used for treatment of liver diseases. Increases bile flow. In dogs, may alter pool of circulating bile acids, displacing the more hydrophobic bile acids. In people, used to prevent or treat gallstones.	Adverse effects not reported in animals. May cause diarrhea.	Results of clinical studies in animals have not been reported. Use in animals (and doses) is based on experience in people, or anecdotal experience in animals. Administer with meals.	300 mg capsules.	10–15 mg/kg q24h PO.

Drug Name (Trade or Other Names)	Pharmacology and Indications	Adverse Effects and Precautions	Dosing Information and Comments	Formulations	Dosage
Valproic acid (Depakene [Valproic acid]; Depakote [Divalproex] [Epival is Canadian brand])	Anticonvulsant. Used, usually in combination with phenobarbital, to treat refractory epilepsy in animals. Action is not known, but may increase GABA concentrations in the CNS.	Adverse effects have not been reported in animals, but hepatic failure has been reported in people. Sedation may be seen in some animals. Do not use in pregnant animals. *Drug interactions:* May cause bleeding if used with drugs that inhibit platelets.	Valproic acid is listed here with divalproex. Divalproex is composed of both valproic acid and sodium valproate. Equivalent oral doses of divalproex sodium and valproic acid deliver equivalent quantities of valproate ion.	125, 250, 500 mg tablets (Depakote); 250 mg capsules; 50 mg/mL syrup (Depakene).	Dog: 60–200 mg/kg q8h PO; or 25–105 mg/kg/day PO, when administered with phenobarbital.
Vancomycin (Vancocin, Vancoled)	Antibacterial drug. Mechanism of action is to inhibit cell wall and cause bacterial cell lysis (via different mechanism as β-lactams). Spectrum includes staphylococci, streptococci, and enterococci (but not Gram-negative bacteria). Used primarily for treatment of resistant staphylococcus and enterococci.	Adverse effects have not been reported in animals. Administer IV; causes severe pain and tissue injury if administered IM or SC. Do not administer rapidly; Use slow infusion, if possible (e.g., over 30 minutes). Adverse effects in people include renal injury (more common with older products that contained impurities), and histamine release.	Vancomycin use is not common in animals, but is valuable for treatment of enterococci or staphylococci that are resistant to other antibiotics. Doses are derived from pharmacokinetic studies in dogs. Monitoring of trough plasma concentrations is recommended to ensure proper dose. Maintain trough concentration above 5 mcg/mL. Infusion solution can be prepared in 0.9% saline or 5% dextrose, but not alkalinizing solutions.	Vials for injection (0.5 to 10 gm).	Dog: 15 mg/kg q6–8h IV infusion. Cat: 12–15 mg/kg, q8h, IV infusion.
Vasopressin (ADH) (Pitressin)	Antidiuretic hormone. Vasopressin is used for treatment of polyuria caused by central diabetes insipidus. Not effective for polyuria caused by renal disease.	Adverse effects have not been reported. Allergic reactions have been reported in people. Increase in blood pressure has been reported in people.	Doses are adjusted on the basis of monitoring of water intake and urine output. See also Desmopressin.	20 U per mL (aqueous).	10 U IV, IM.
Verapamil (Calan, Isoptin)	Calcium-channel blocking drug of the nondihypyridine group. Blocks calcium entry into cells via blockade of slow channel. Produces vasodilation, negative chronotropic effects.	Hypotension, cardiac depression, bradycardia, AV block. May cause anorexia in some patients.	Diltiazem preferred over verapamil in patients with heart failure, because of less cardiac suppression. Oral formulation not absorbed sufficiently (of the active stereoisomer) for adequate effects.	40, 80, 120 mg tablet; 2.5 mg/mL injection.	Dog: 0.05 mg/kg q10–30min IV (maximum cumulative dose is 0.15 mg/kg); oral dose is not established.
Vinblastine (Velban)	Similar to vincristine. Sometimes used as an alternative to vincristine. Do not use to increase platelet numbers (may actually cause thrombocytopenia).	Does not produce neuropathy, as vincristine does, but there may be a higher incidence of myelosuppression. Causes tissue necrosis if injected outside vein.	Vinblastine is used in cancer chemotherapy protocols for various tumors. Consult specific chemotherapy protocol for regimens.	1 mg/mL injection.	2 mg/m² IV (slow infusion) once/week.
Vincristine (Oncovin, Vincasar, generic)	Anticancer agent. Vincristine causes arrest of cancer cell division by binding to microtubules and inhibiting mitosis. Used in combination chemotherapy protocols. Vincristine also increases numbers of functional circulating platelets and is used for thrombocytopenia.	Generally well-tolerated. Less myelosuppressive than other anticancer drugs. Neuropathy has been reported, but is rare. Constipation can occur. Very irritating to tissues. Avoid extravasation outside vein during administration.	Vincristine is used in cancer chemotherapy protocols for various tumors. Consult specific chemotherapy protocol for regimens.	1 mg/mL injection.	Antitumor: 0.5–0.7 mg/m² IV (or 0.025–0.05 mg/kg) once/week. For thrombocytopenia: 0.02 mg/kg IV once/week.
Viokase	See Pancrelipase.				

Drug Name (Trade or Other Names)	Pharmacology and Indications	Adverse Effects and Precautions	Dosing Information and Comments	Formulations	Dosage
Vitamin A (Retinoids) (Aquasol-A)	Vitamin A supplement. See also Isotretinoin (Accutane), or Etretinate (Tegison) for analogues used for other conditions.	Excessive doses can cause bone or joint pain, dermatitis.	Dosing of vitamin is expressed as U or retinol equivalents (RE), or mcg of Retinol. One RE equals 1 mcg of retinol. One RE of vitamin A is equal to 3.33 U of retinol.	Oral solution: 5000 U (1500 RE)/0.1 mL; 10,000-25,000- and 50,000-U tablets.	625–800 U/kg q24h PO. (See dosing information section.)
Vitamin B$_1$	See Thiamine.				
Vitamin B$_2$ (Riboflavin) (Riboflavin)	Vitamin B$_2$ supplement.	Adverse effects are rare, because water-soluble vitamins are easily excreted. Riboflavin may discolor the urine.	Not necessary to supplement in animals with well-balanced diets.	Various size tablets in increments from 10 to 250 mg.	Dog: 10–20 mg/day PO. Cat: 5–10 mg/day PO.
Vitamin B$_{12}$ (Cyanocobalamin) (Cyanocobalamin)	Vitamin B$_{12}$ supplement. Vitamin B$_{12}$ has been used to treat some forms of anemia.	Adverse effects are rare, because water-soluble vitamins are easily excreted.	Not necessary to supplement in animals with well-balanced diets.	Various size tablets in increments from 25 to 1000 mcg, and injections	Dog: 100–200 mcg/day PO, SC. Cat: 50–100 mcg/day PO, SC.
Vitamin C (Ascorbic acid) (see Ascorbic acid)	Used to treat Vitamin C deficiency and occasionally used as urine acidifier. Insufficient data to show that ascorbic acid is effective for preventing cancer or cardiovascular disease.	Adverse effects have not been reported in animals. High doses may increase risk of oxalate stones in bladder.	Not necessary to supplement in animals with well-balanced diets.	Tablets of various sizes and injection.	100–500 mg/day.
Vitamin D	See Dihydrotachysterol or Ergocalciferol.				
Vitamin E (Alpha Tocopherol) (Aquasol E, and generic)	Vitamin considered as antioxidant. Used as supplement and as treatment of some immune-mediated dermatoses.	Side effects have not been reported.	Vitamin E has been proposed as treatment for a wide range of human illnesses, but evidence for efficacy in animals is lacking.	Wide variety of capsules, tablets, oral solution available. (e.g., 1000 U/capsule.)	100–400 U q12h PO, (or 400–600 U q12h PO for immune-mediated skin disease).
Vitamin K$_1$ (Phytonadione, Phytomenadione) (Aqua MEPHYTON [injection], Mephyton [tablets]; Veta-K1 [capsules])	Vitamin K$_1$ used to treat coagulopathies caused by anticoagulant toxicosis (warfarin or other rodenticides). (Anticoagulants deplete Vitamin K in the body, which is essential for synthesis of clotting factors.)	Side effects have not been reported.	Consult poison control center for specific protocol if specific rodenticide is identified. Use Vitamin K$_1$ for acute therapy, because it is more highly bio-available. Administer with food to enhance absorption. Phytonadione and Phytomenadione are synthetic lipid-soluble forms of Vitamin K$_1$. Menadiol is Vitamin K$_4$, which is converted in the body to Vitamin K$_3$ (menadione).	2 or 10 mg/mL injection; Mephyton is 5 mg tablet; Veta-K1 is 25 mg capsule.	Short-acting rodenticides: 1 mg/kg/day IV, IM, SC, PO for 10–14 days. Long-acting rodenticides: 2.5–5 mg/kg/day IV, IM, SC, PO for 3–4 week. Birds: 2.5–5 mg/kg q24h.
Warfarin (Coumadin, generic)	Anticoagulant. Depletes Vitamin K, which is responsible for generation of clotting factors. Used to treat hyper-coagulable disease, prevent thromboembolism.	Adverse effects are attributable to decreased clotting. *Drug interactions:* Other drugs may potentiate warfarin's action (including aspirin, chloramphenicol, phenylbutazone, ketoconazole, cimetidine)	Warfarin response is individualistic. For optimum therapy, adjust dose by monitoring clotting time. For example, in some patients, dose is adjusted to maintain PT to 1.5 to 2 × to 2–2.5 × normal (or INR of 2–3). Consult specific reference for guidance (Current Veterinary Therapy XII, page 868).	1, 2, 2.5, 4, 5, 7.5, 10 mg tablets.	Dogs: 0.1–0.2 mg/kg q24h PO. Cats (thromboembolism): start with 0.5 mg/cat/day, and adjust dose based on clotting time assessment.

Drug Name (Trade or Other Names)	Pharmacology and Indications	Adverse Effects and Precautions	Dosing Information and Comments	Formulations	Dosage
Xylaxine (Rompun, and generic)	α₂-adrenergic agonist. Used primarily for anesthesia and analgesia.	Produces sedation and ataxia. Cardiac depression, heart block, and hypotension are possible with high doses. Produces emesis after IV injection, especially in cats.	Often used in combination with other drugs, e.g., ketamine.	20 and 100 mg/mL injection.	Dog: 1.1 mg/kg IV, 2.2 mg/kg IM. Cat: 1.1 mg/kg im (emetic dose is 0.4–0.5 mg/kg IV).
Yohimbine (Yobine)	α₂-adrenergic antagonist. Used primarily to reverse actions of xylazine or detomidine.	High doses can cause tremors and seizures.	Reverses signs of sedation and anesthesia caused by α₂-agonists.	2 mg/mL injection.	0.11 mg/kg IV, or 0.25–0.5 mg/kg SC, IM.
Zidovudine (AZT) (Retrovir)	Antiviral drug. In people, used to treat AIDS. In animals, has been experimentally used for treatment of FeLV and FIV viral infection in cats. AZT acts to inhibit the viral enzyme, reverse transcriptase, which prevents conversion of viral RNA into DNA.	Anemia and leukopenia are adverse effects. Monitor the PCV in treated cats and perform a CBC periodically.	At this time, experience with using AZT for treating viral disease in animals is largely experimental or anecdotal. Consult a more-detailed reference for guidance (Feline Pract 23: 16, 1995). It may have helped some cats with FIV, and may prevent persistent FeLV.	10 mg/mL syrup; 10 mg/mL injection.	Cats: 15 mg/kg q12h, PO, to 20 mg/kg q8h PO (doses as high as 30 mg/kg/day also have been used).
Zolazepam	See Tiletamine + zolazepam.				

Key to Table Abbreviations:

IM	Intramuscular
IV	Intravenous
OTC	Over the counter (without prescription)
Rx	Prescription only
PO	per os (oral)
SC	Subcutaneous
U	Units
mL	milliliter
mcg	micrograms

DISCLAIMER FOR DOSE TABLES:

Note: Doses listed are for dogs *and* cats, unless otherwise listed. Many of the doses listed are extra-label, or are human drugs not approved for animals administered in an extra-label manner. Doses listed are based on best available information at the time of table editing. The author cannot ensure efficacy or absolute safety of drugs used according to recommendations in this table. Adverse effects may be possible from drugs listed in this table of which authors were not aware at the time of table preparation. Veterinarians using this table are encouraged to consult current literature, product labels and inserts, and the manufacturer's disclosure information for additional information on adverse effects, interactions, and efficacy that were not identified at the time these tables were prepared.

APPENDIX IX

CONVERSION TABLES

Table IX-A.

CONVERSION TABLE OF WEIGHT TO BODY SURFACE AREA (IN SQUARE METERS) FOR DOGS			
kg	m²	kg	m²
0.5	0.06	26.0	0.88
1.0	0.10	27.0	0.90
2.0	0.15	28.0	0.92
3.0	0.20	29.0	0.94
4.0	0.25	30.0	0.96
5.0	0.29	31.0	0.99
6.0	0.33	32.0	1.01
7.0	0.36	33.0	1.03
8.0	0.40	34.0	1.05
9.0	0.43	35.0	1.07
10.0	0.46	36.0	1.09
11.0	0.49	37.0	1.11
12.0	0.52	38.0	1.13
13.0	0.55	39.0	1.15
14.0	0.58	40.0	1.17
15.0	0.60	41.0	1.19
16.0	0.63	42.0	1.21
17.0	0.66	43.0	1.23
18.0	0.69	44.0	1.25
19.0	0.71	45.0	1.26
20.0	0.74	46.0	1.28
21.0	0.76	47.0	1.30
22.0	0.78	48.0	1.32
23.0	0.81	49.0	1.34
24.0	0.83	50.0	1.36
25.0	0.85		

Although the above chart was compiled for dogs, it can also be used for cats. More precise values are represented in the formula BSA in $m^2 = (K \times W^{2/3}) \times 10^{-4}$; where m^2 = square meters, BSA = body surface area, W = weight in g, and K = constant of 10.1 in dogs and 10.0 in cats.

Table IX-B.

	Approximate Equivalents for Degrees Fahrenheit and Celsius*		
°F	°C	°F	°C
0	−17.8	98	36.7
32	0	99	37.2
85	29.4	100	37.8
86	30.0	101	38.3
87	30.6	102	38.9
88	31.1	103	39.4
89	31.7	104	40.0
90	32.2	105	40.6
91	32.7	106	41.1
92	33.3	107	41.7
93	33.9	108	42.2
94	34.4	109	42.8
95	35.0	110	43.3
96	35.5	212	100.0
97	36.1		

*Temperature conversion: °Celsius to °Fahrenheit, (°C)(9/5) + 32°; °Fahrenheit to °Celsius, (°F − 32°)(5/9).

Table IX-C.

	Weight-Unit Conversion Factors	
Units Given	Units Wanted	For Conversion Multiply by
lb	gm	453.6
lb	kg	0.4536
oz	gm	28.35
kg	lb	2.2046
kg	mg	1,000,000.
kg	gm	1000.
gm	mg	1000.
gm	μg	1,000,000.
mg	μg	1000.
mg/gm	mg/lb	453.6
mg/kg	mg/lb	0.4536
μg/kg	μg/lb	0.4536
Mcal	kcal	1000.
kcal/kg	kcal/lb	0.4536
kcal/lb	kcal/kg	2.2046
ppm	μg/gm	1.
ppm	mg/kg	1.
ppm	mg/lb	0.4536
mg/kg	%	0.0001
ppm	%	0.0001
mg/gm	%	0.1
gm/kg	%	0.1

APPENDIX X

HOTLINES EVERY VETERINARIAN SHOULD KNOW

ANIMAL BLOOD BANK HOTLINE—800-243-5759
A 24-hour hotline that focuses on transfusion medicine (particularly blood component therapy), recommending dosages and infusion rates, at no cost to caller

ASPCA NATIONAL ANIMAL POISON CONTROL CENTER (ALLIED AGENCY OF THE UNIVERSITY OF ILLINOIS COLLEGE OF VETERINARY MEDICINE)—888-426-4435
Fee $45 per case; credit cards only; no extra charge for follow-up calls. 900-680-0000—Fee $45 per case. The charge is billed directly to caller's phone. Follow-up calls can be made for no additional charge by dialing 888-426-4435. There is no charge when the call involves a product covered by the Animal Product Safety Service.

DEA TOLL-FREE NUMBER FOR OFFICE OF DIVERSION CONTROL, REGISTRATION SECTION—800-882-9539

EASTERN VETERINARY BLOOD BANK—800-949-EVBB (800-949-3822)
A 24-hour, commercial blood bank that focuses on transfusion medicine; gives recommendations and referrals to distribution centers when it cannot ship the requested product; for complicated cases, offers a paid consultation service.

FOOD ANIMAL RESIDUE AVOIDANCE DATABANK—888-USFARAD (888-873-2723)
E-mail inquiries to FARAD@ncsu.edu or FARAD@ucdavis.edu, or visit the Web site at www.farad.org. Sponsored by the USDA Extension Service; information on animal drugs and chemicals with the potential to cause foodborne residues.

FDA/CVM: DRUGS, DEVICES, ANIMAL FEEDS—888-FDA-VETS (888-332-8387)
Calls to report suspected adverse drug experiences will be forwarded to the CVM's Division of Epidemiology and Surveillance; voice-mail messages can be left during nonbusiness hours.

FDA MEDICAL ADVERTISING LINE—800-AD-US FDA (800-238-7332)
Assists health professionals seeking interpretive information on FDA policy

HEMOPET—949-252-8455
A national, full service, nonprofit blood bank and educational network for animals, in Irvine, CA; accessible 24 hours.

IMPAIRED VETERINARIANS INFORMATION LINE—800-321-1473
Information on, and referrals for assistance with chemical impairment; sponsored by the AVMA.

MIDWEST ANIMAL BLOOD SERVICES—517-851-8244
A 24-hour, commercial all-species blood bank providing blood components, blood-typing services, and transfusion medicine consultation (special emphasis on red blood cell typing and transplantation matching).

NATIONAL PESTICIDE TELECOMMUNICATIONS NETWORK—800-858-7877
Service sponsored by the EPA and Oregon State University provides information about pesticide products and poisonings, toxicology, environmental chemistry, and other pesticide-related issues.

PET LOSS SUPPORT HOTLINES (GRIEF COUNSELING)
530-752-4200—Staffed by University of California Davis veterinary students
630-603-3994—Staffed by Chicago VMA veterinarians and staff
607-253-3932—Staffed by Cornell University veterinary students
352-392-4700; then dial 1 and 4080—Staffed by University of Florida veterinary students
217-244-2273(CARE) or 877-394-2273(CARE)—Staffed by University of Illinois veterinary students
888-ISU-PLSH (888-478-7574)—Staffed by Iowa State University veterinary students and community volunteers
517-432-2696—Staffed by Michigan State University veterinary students
614-292-1823, *e-mail, petloss@osu.edu*—Staffed by The Ohio State University veterinary students
508-839-7966—Staffed by Tufts University veterinary students
540-231-8038—Staffed by Virginia-Maryland Regional College of Veterinary Medicine
509-335-5704—Staffed by Washington State University veterinary students

USDA MEAT AND POULTRY HOTLINE—800-535-4555

USDA VOICE RESPONSE SERVICE—800-545-8732
Up-to-date interstate shipping regulations, emergency notices, and animal care regulations for shipping pets on airlines

USP VETERINARY PRACTITIONERS' REPORTING PROGRAM—800-4-USP-PRN (800-487-7776)
Veterinarians may report any type of problem (adverse reactions, quality concerns, medication errors, etc.) encountered with the use of medical products in animals. Information is shared with manufacturers, regulatory agencies, and the AVMA. Call to make a report or request reporting forms. Reports can also be submitted electronically at *http:/www.usp.org*. Reporting forms are available 24 hours-a-day through our on-demand faxback system. Call our toll-free number, press 1, then enter #9401.

Compiled by the Publications Division, American Veterinary Medical Association. Phone numbers current as of January 1, 2000. From JAVMA 2000; 216: 71 (with permission).

Index

Text in **boldface** denotes chapter discussions

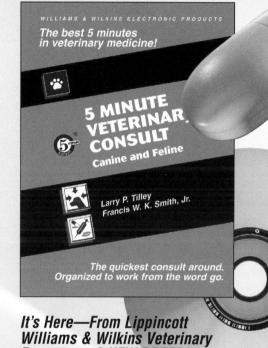
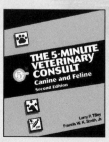
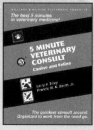
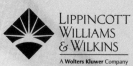
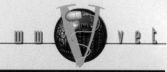